# New This Spring: Online Medical Assisting Simulation

**Clinical Competencies Simulator** introduces students to nonacute medical assisting patient case scenarios, procedure simulators, and quick e-learning exercises based on *ABHES* and *CAAHEP Standards and Guidelines (2003)- CAAHEP Clinical Competence* requirements.

## Six Patient Case Scenarios

A large portion of the core clinical competencies in CAAHEP can be simulated on virtual patients, where the learner can interact with a patient and try out the different tasks that a medical assistant is supposed to be able to perform.

The focus is on vital signs and obtaining patient data, including a chart feature, so that the learner can collect vital signs and make notes about observations that the medical assistant can brief the doctor about.

Virtual patient case scenarios include:

- Blood pressure
- Temperature
- Pulse (including apical pulse)
- Respiratory rate
- Pulse oximeter

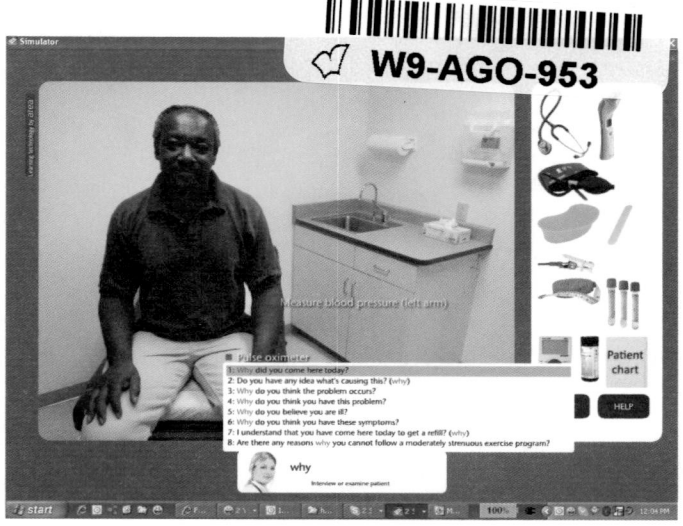

W9-AGO-953

- Patient chart (documentation)
- Body measurements
- Blood glucose
- Pain chart scale
- Brief physician situations

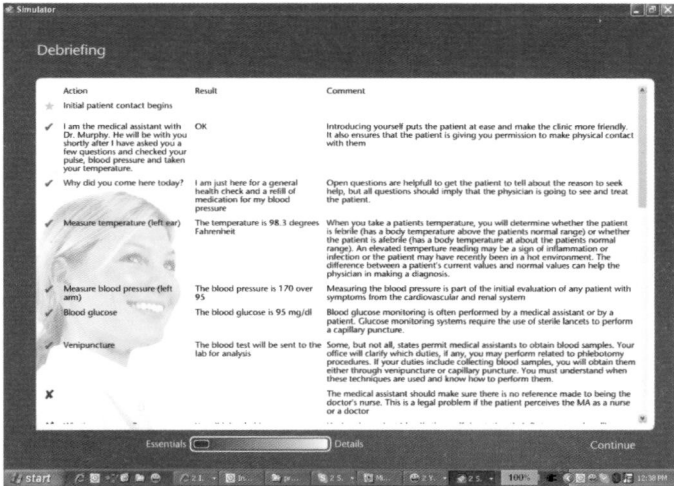

After each simulation, the learner receives elaborate feedback on their performance. The debriefing includes basic patient assessment issues and recommendations for handling patients who have a particular disease.

## Procedure Simulator and Quick E-learning Exercises

A number of procedures are described as part of the necessary clinical competencies that CAAHEP requires a medical assistant to master. Some of these are simple step-by-step procedures, while others are more complex procedures requiring different instruments and devices.

Procedure simulators and quick e-learning exercises can be relevant to emulate these procedures. The difference between full patient simulators (case scenarios) and procedure simulators is that in the latter you focus on the single procedure, e.g., how to check the blood pressure by following a step-by-step procedure or how to run an autoclave.

Procedures include:

- Hand washing
- Practice Standard Precautions
- Blood pressure
- Pulse and respiration
- Temperature
- Wrap items for autoclaving
- Venipuncture
- Capillary puncture
- Specimens for laboratory testing
- ECG
- Spirometry

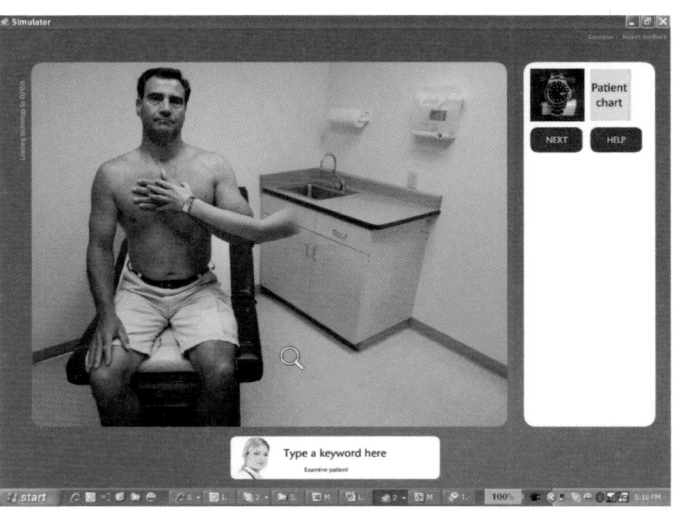

# MEDICAL ASSISTING
## Administrative and Clinical Procedures

**Kathryn A. Booth, RN-BSN, MS, RMA, RPT**
Total Care Programming, Inc.
*Palm Coast, Florida*

**Leesa G. Whicker, BA, CMA (AAMA)**
Central Piedmont Community College
*Charlotte, North Carolina*

**Terri D. Wyman, CMRS**
UMASS Memorial Medical Center
*Worcester, Massachusetts*

**Donna Jeanne Pugh, RN, MSN/ED**
University of Florida College of Nursing
*Jacksonville, Florida*

**Sharion Thompson, BS, RMA**
Bryant and Stratton College, Cleveland Area
*Parma, Ohio*

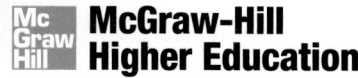
**McGraw-Hill**
**Higher Education**

Boston   Burr Ridge, IL   Dubuque, IA   New York   San Francisco   St. Louis
Bangkok   Bogotá   Caracas   Kuala Lumpur   Lisbon   London   Madrid   Mexico City
Milan   Montreal   New Delhi   Santiago   Seoul   Singapore   Sydney   Taipei   Toronto

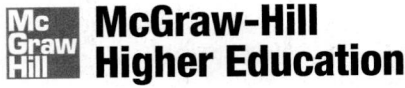

The McGraw-Hill Companies

MEDICAL ASSISTING: ADMINISTRATIVE AND CLINICAL PROCEDURES
Published by McGraw-Hill, a business unit of The McGraw-Hill Companies, Inc., 1221 Avenue of the Americas, New York, NY, 10020.
Copyright © 2009 by The McGraw-Hill Companies, Inc. All rights reserved. Previous editions © 1999 and 2005. No part of this publication may be reproduced or distributed in any form or by any means, or stored in a database or retrieval system, without the prior written consent of The McGraw-Hill Companies, Inc., including, but not limited to, in any network or other electronic storage or transmission, or broadcast for distance learning.

Some ancillaries, including electronic and print components, may not be available to customers outside the United States.

This book is printed on acid-free paper.

1 2 3 4 5 6 7 8 9 0 WCK/WCK 0 9 8

ISBN 978-0-07-337399-7
MHID 0-07-337399-0

Vice President/Editor in Chief: *Elizabeth Haefele*
Vice President/Director of Marketing: *John E. Biernat*
Senior sponsoring editor: *Debbie Fitzgerald*
Managing developmental editor: *Patricia Hesse*
Freelance developmental editor: *Julie Scardiglia*
Executive marketing manager: *Roxan Kinsey*
Lead media producer: *Damian Moshak*
Media producer: *Marc Mattson*
Director, Editing/Design/Production: *Jess Ann Kosic*
Lead project manager: *Susan Trentacosti*
Senior production supervisor: *Janean A. Utley*
Designer: *Srdjan Savanovic*
Senior photo research coordinator: *Carrie K. Burger*
Photo researcher: *Pam Carley*

Media project manager: *Mark A. S. Dierker*
Cover design: *Jenny El-Shamy*
Typeface: *10/12 Slimbach*
Compositor: *ICC Macmillan Inc.*
Printer: *Quebecor World Versailles Inc.*
Cover credits: *Computer, blood draw, applying lead wires: Kathryn Booth, Total Care Programming, Inc.; cover blood pressure: John Lund/Tiffany Schoepp, ©Gettyimages; DAQbilling® Practice Management Software screen shots were provided by Antek HealthWare, LLC. www.antekhealthware.com; background: David Gould, ©Gettyimages*
Credits: The credits section for this book begins on page 1127 and is considered an extension of the copyright page.

### Library of Congress Cataloging-in-Publication Data

Medical assisting : administrative and clinical procedures / Kathryn A. Booth ... [et al.].
    p. ; cm.
    Includes index.
    ISBN-13: 978-0-07-337399-7 (alk. paper)
    ISBN-10: 0-07-337399-0 (alk. paper)
    1. Medical assistants. I. Booth, Kathryn A., 1957-
    [DNLM: 1. Physician Assistants. 2. Interpersonal Relations. 3. Medical Records.
  4. Practice Management, Medical—organization & administration. W 21.5 M48953 2009]
  R728.8.M412 2009
  610.73'7—dc22

2007049727

WARNING NOTICE: The clinical procedures, medicines, dosages, and other matters described in this publication are based upon research of current literature and consultation with knowledgeable persons in the field. The procedures and matters described in this text reflect currently accepted clinical practice. However, this information cannot and should not be relied upon as necessarily applicable to a given individual's case. Accordingly, each person must be separately diagnosed to discern the patient's unique circumstances. Likewise, the manufacturer's package insert for current drug product information should be consulted before administering any drug. Publisher disclaims all liability for any inaccuracies, omissions, misuse, or misunderstanding of the information contained in this publication. Publisher cautions that this publication is not intended as a substitute for the professional judgment of trained medical personnel.

The Internet addresses listed in the text were accurate at the time of publication. The inclusion of a Web site does not indicate an endorsement by the authors or McGraw-Hill, and McGraw-Hill does not guarantee the accuracy of the information presented at these sites.

www.mhhe.com

# Brief Contents

# Contents

## SECTION 3
## Specialty Practices and Medical Emergencies  559

# APPENDIXES

# Procedures

# Preface

*Medical Assisting: Administrative and Clinical Procedures* is a comprehensive textbook for the medical assisting student. It provides the student with information about all aspects of the medical assisting profession, both administrative and clinical, from the general to the specific, it covers the key concepts, skills, and tasks that medical assistants need to know. The book speaks directly to the student, and its chapter introductions, case studies, procedures, and chapter summaries are written to engage the student's attention and build a sense of positive anticipation about joining the profession of medical assisting.

When referring to patients in the third person, we have alternated between passages that describe a male patient and passages that describe a female patient. Thus, the patient will be referred to as "he" half the time and as "she" half the time. The same convention is used to refer to the physician. The medical assistant is consistently addressed as "you."

## New to This Edition

- The *Pocket Guide,* a quick and handy reference to use while working as a medical assistant. It includes Critical Procedure Steps, bulleted lists, and brief information all medical assistants should know. Information is sorted by Administrative, Clinical, and General content.
- Procedures revised to include Procedure Goals and Rationales.
- Each text chapter opener includes a chart indicating Medical Assisting Competencies (CMA and RMA) which are taught in the chapter.
- New "Reflecting On . . ." feature boxes for Legal and Ethical Issues, Communication Issues, Cultural Issues, Professionalism, and HIPAA.
- Virtual Fieldtrips provide simulated activities for each chapter.
- A new chapter—Complementary and Alternative Medicine.
- Updated and expanded information include:
  - Current coding and billing practices, including HIPAA.
  - Use of technology in the medical office—especially more and varied uses of the Internet, including website development, patient education, billing, and coding.

- Clinical diagnostic testing, such as in-office Hemoglobin A1c testing.
- CPR guidelines to comply with the latest American Heart Association guidelines.
- OSHA issues.
- Infection control and antibiotic resistance.
- Expanded Student CD-ROM with applications included in the text. It includes "A Day in the Life of the Medical Assistant" case studies, video clip library, audio glossary, and much more!
- Comprehensive and thoroughly updated Student Workbook. The workbook has been updated to reflect the extensive textbook revisions and there are more questions. The Procedure Competency Checklists have been improved to include more procedure observer comments.

## Patient Education

In this book we focus particularly on patient education and on the role of the medical assistant in encouraging patients to be active participants in their own health care. It is always desirable for patients to be as knowledgeable as possible about their health. Patients who do not understand what is expected of them may become confused, frightened, angry, and uncooperative; educated patients are better able to understand why compliance is important.

Chapter 14 is devoted entirely to patient education. Other chapters cover various aspects of patient interaction—such as Chapter 4, on communicating with the patient, and Chapter 23, on interviewing the patient. Throughout the book, we provide the medical assistant with the information needed to educate patients so that they can participate fully in their health care.

We have also made a consistent effort to discuss patients with special needs. Several chapters in Part 2, Administrative Medical Assisting, and in Part 3, Clinical Medical Assisting, contain special sections of text devoted to the particular concerns of certain patient groups. These groups include the following:

- **Pregnant women.** Pregnancy has profound effects on every aspect of health, all of which must be taken into account when working with pregnant patients. Where appropriate, we have addressed special concerns for pregnant patients, such as positioning them for an examination, recommending changes in diet, and taking care to avoid harming the fetus with drugs or procedures that would ordinarily pose little or no risk to the patient. Chapter 25, on the general physical examination, includes a separate procedure for meeting the needs of the pregnant patient during an examination.

- **Elderly patients.** Special care is often required with elderly patients. The body undergoes many changes with age, and patients may have difficulty adjusting to their changing physical needs. Several chapters deal with the special needs of elderly patients, such as Chapter 14, which discusses instructing patients with hearing impairments.
- **Children.** The special needs of children are complex, because not only their bodies but also their minds and social situations are very different from those of adults. Dealing with children usually means dealing with their parents as well, and medical assistants must hone their communication skills to meet the needs of both patient and parent when working with children. One chapter that focuses on children is Chapter 13, which includes a special text section and a procedure for designing a patient reception area to accommodate children.
- **Patients with disabilities.** Many different diseases and disabilities require extra effort or consideration on the part of the medical assistant. Patients in wheelchairs and patients with diabetes, hemophilia, or visual or hearing impairments all require specific accommodations. For example, Chapter 22 addresses the needs of such patients; it includes a section that discusses the Americans With Disabilities Act and a procedure for making the examination room safe for patients with visual impairments.
- **Patients from other cultures.** Communicating with patients from other cultures, especially when language barriers are involved, poses a special challenge for the medical assistant. In addition, patients from other cultures may have attitudes about medicine or about social interaction that differ sharply from those of the medical assistant's culture. Chapter 4 is one chapter that deals in depth with patients from other cultures. It contains a text section and a Reflecting On . . . Cultural Issues feature about different cultures' attitudes toward medicine.

Because safety is a primary concern for both the patient and the medical assistant, we have emphasized this aspect of medical assisting work. Every clinical procedure includes appropriate icons, discussed in Chapter 20, for safety precautions required by the Occupational Safety and Health Administration (OSHA) guidelines. These icons for the OSHA guidelines appear in order of use within each procedure. If hand washing is necessary more than once, the hand washing icon appears twice. If biohazardous waste is generated during the procedure, the biohazardous waste container icon will appear, and so on.

## Areas of Competence

A key feature of *Medical Assisting* that will enhance its usefulness to both students and instructors is its reference to the areas of competence defined in the 2003 AAMA (American Association of Medical Assistants) Role Delineation Study. The study, which replaces the 1990 DACUM (*Developing A CurriculUM*) analysis, provides a comprehensive list of duties and skills that medical assistants must master at the entry level. The Committee on Accreditation of Allied Health Education Personnel (CAAHEP) requires that all medical assistants be proficient in the 71 entry-level areas of competence when they begin medical assisting work. The opening page of each chapter provides a list of the areas of competence that the chapter covers, and the complete Medical Assistant Role Delineation Chart is provided as an appendix. (A correlation chart also appears in the *Instructor's Resource Binder*.) The chapter-by-chapter listing of areas of competence allows instructors to identify skills that have been covered in the course and helps students find the chapters that cover specific skills and duties.

We have been careful to ensure that the text provides ample coverage of topics used to construct the 2003 American Association of Medical Assistants (AAMA) Role Delineation Study Areas of Competence, the Association of Medical Technologists (AMT) Registered Medical Assistant (RMA) Certified Exam Topics, the National Healthcareer Association (NHA) Medical Assisting Duty/ Task List, the National Occupational Competency Testing Institute (NOCTI) Job Ready Sample Assessment competencies and skills, the Commission on Accreditation of Allied Health Education Programs (CAAHEP) Standards and Guidelines for Medical Assisting Education Programs, and the Secretary's Commission on Achieving Necessary Skills (SCANS) areas of competence. Correlation charts for each of these appears in the *Instructor's Resource Binder*.

## Organization of the Text

*Medical Assisting: Administrative and Clinical Procedures* is divided into three parts.

Part One provides a basic explanation of the role of the medical assistant in a medical practice. It includes an overview of the profession and covers the different types of medical practices, legal and ethical issues—including important information on HIPAA (Health Information Portability and Accountability Act) regulations—and communication with patients, their families, and coworkers.

Part Two explores the administrative duties of the medical assistant, including basic office work, patient interaction, and the financial responsibilities of a medical practice.

Part Three covers the clinical duties of the medical assistant and also provides information on patient assistance; specialty examinations and medical emergencies; and laboratory and other specialized procedures.

Chapter 31, new to this edition, provides essential information on complementary and alternative medicine (CAM). Chapter 41 provides the medical assisting student with information about the externship process and how to prepare to find a position as a medical assistant.

The ordering of chapters within each part allows the student and the instructor to build a knowledge base starting with the fundamentals and working toward an understanding of highly specialized tasks. Part Two introduces the basics of working with office equipment before covering the details of maintaining patient records, scheduling appointments, and processing insurance. Part Three begins with a grounding in principles of asepsis, a concept that is crucial to all clinical procedures. Subsequent chapters lead the student through general and specialized physical examinations, and eventually into the technical details of laboratory testing, drug administration, electrocardiography, and radiology.

Chapters are also grouped into sections when their subjects relate to a broader topic or area of skills. Each section is set apart and the section opener includes the list of chapters within that section.

Each chapter opens with a page of material that includes the CMA and RMA medical assisting competencies covered in the chapter, a list of key terms, the chapter outline, and the learning outcomes the student can expect to achieve after completing the chapter. The main text of each chapter begins with an overview of chapter content and includes a case study for students to consider as they read the chapter. Chapters are organized into topics that move from the general to the specific. Color photographs, anatomic and technical drawings, tables, charts, and text features help educate the student about various aspects of medical assisting. The text features, set off in boxes within the text, include the following:

- **Case Studies** are provided at the beginning of all chapters. They represent situations similar to those that the medical assistant may encounter in daily practice. Students are encouraged to consider the case study as they read each chapter. Case Study Questions in the end-of-chapter review check students' understanding and application of chapter content.

- **Procedures** give step-by-step instructions on how to perform specific administrative or clinical tasks that a medical assistant will be required to perform. A list of the procedures, which follows the Contents, details the procedures found in each chapter.

- **Points on Practice** boxes provide guidelines on keeping the medical office running smoothly and efficiently.

- **Educating the Patient** boxes focus on ways to instruct patients about caring for themselves outside the medical office.

- **Reflecting On . . .** boxes provide specialized information about legal and ethical issues, communication issues, cultural issues, professionalism, and HIPAA.

- **Caution: *Handle With Care*** boxes cover the precautions to be taken in certain situations or when performing certain tasks.

- **Career Opportunities** boxes provide the student with information on various specialized medical professions or duties related to the medical assistant's role within the health-care team.

Each chapter closes with a summary of the chapter material that focuses on the role of the medical assistant. The summary is followed by an end-of-chapter review that consists of the following elements:

- Case Study Questions
- Discussion Questions
- Critical Thinking Questions
- Application Activities
- Virtual Fieldtrip

A list of further readings, including related books and journal articles, will be provided for each chapter within the Instructor's Manual and on McGraw-Hill's medical assisting Online Learning Center. The end-of-chapter questions and activities, as well as the additional online resources, provide supplementary information about the subjects presented in the chapter and allow students to practice specific skills.

The book also includes a glossary and several appendixes for use as reference tools. The glossary lists all the words presented as key terms in each chapter along with a pronunciation guide and the definition of each term. The appendixes include the American Association of Medical Assistants (AAMA) and the Commission on Accreditation of Allied Health Education Programs (CAAHEP) competencies for the medical assistant, the American Medical Technologists (AMT) Registered Medical Assistant (RMA) certified exam topics, the National Healthcareer Association (NHA) medical assisting duty/task list, commonly used prefixes and suffixes, Latin and Greek terms, abbreviations and symbols used in medical terminology, and a comprehensive list of professional organizations and agencies.

# Digital Supplements

**Student CD-ROM.** The Student CD-ROM provides a comprehensive learning program that is correlated to each chapter of the text and reinforces competencies required to become a medical assistant. Short video clips and pictures introduce skills and case studies for application. In addition, numerous interactive exercises and applications are provided for every chapter in the text. The Student CD, included with each student textbook, provides the following menu choices:

- 1 Day in the Life Critical Thinking
- Administrative Practice Activities

# Guided Tour

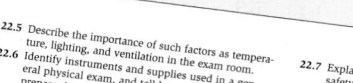

**Case Studies**
represent situations similar to those that the medical assistant may encounter in daily practice.

---

## CHAPTER 22

### Preparing the Exam and Treatment Areas

**KEY TERMS**

accessibility
consumable
fixative
general physical exam
lubricant
occult blood
transcutaneous
    absorption

**MEDICAL ASSISTING COMPETENCIES**

*In preparation for the certification examination, you should know the following areas of competence:*

| COMPETENCY | CMA | RMA |
|---|---|---|
| **Clinical** | | |
| Apply principles of aseptic techniques and infection control, including hand washing | X | X |
| Perform sterilization techniques | X | X |
| Dispose of biohazardous materials | X | X |
| Practice Standard Precautions | X | X |
| Prepare and maintain exam and treatment areas | X | X |
| **General/Legal/Professional** | | |
| Perform risk management procedures | | X |
| Operate and maintain facilities, and perform routine maintenance of administrative and clinical equipment safely | X | X |
| Maintain the physical plant | | X |

**CHAPTER OUTLINE**

- The Medical Assistant's Role in Preparing the Exam Room
- The Exam Room
- Cleanliness in the Exam Room
- Room Temperature, Lighting, and Ventilation
- Medical Instruments and Supplies
- Physical Safety in the Exam Room

**LEARNING OUTCOMES**

After completing Chapter 22, you will be able to:

22.1  Explain the medical assistant's role in preparing the exam room.
22.2  Describe the layout and features of a typical exam room.
22.3  Describe steps to prevent the spread of infection in the exam room.
22.4  Explain how and when to disinfect exam room surfaces.

464

**Chapter Openers**
include the CMA and RMA medical assisting competencies covered in the chapter, a list of key terms, the chapter outline, and the learning outcomes the student can expect to achieve after completing each chapter.

---

22.5  Describe the importance of such factors as temperature, lighting, and ventilation in the exam room.
22.6  Identify instruments and supplies used in a general physical exam, and tell how to arrange and prepare them.
22.7  Explain how to eliminate hazards to physical safety in the exam room.

### Introduction

One of the most important tasks you encounter as a practicing medical assistant is the preparation of the exam room and treatment area. In this chapter you will learn about the common layouts of exam rooms; keeping the rooms clean and stocked with instruments and disposable and consumable supplies; maintaining the comfort of the room; and making the room safe for patients and coworkers. You will also be introduced to the requirements for accessibility established by the Americans With Disabilities Act.

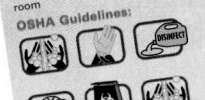

**CASE STUDY**

As a medical assistant, you are reviewing the charts as you prepare for the next day's appointments. You notice that a female patient who is scheduled for her routine gynecological checkup flagged her chart because she has bilateral cataracts.

As you read this chapter, consider the following questions:
1. What are bilateral cataracts, and why were ... on her contact with this patient?
2. What instruments ...
3. What di...

---

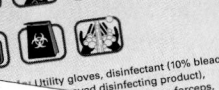

**PROCEDURE 22.1**

### Guidelines for Disinfecting Exam Room Surfaces

**Procedure Goal:** To reduce the risk of exposure to potentially infectious microorganisms in the exam room

**OSHA Guidelines:**

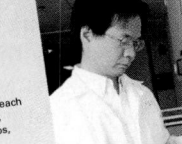

8.  If you keep a container of 10% bleach solution on hand for disinfection purposes, replace the solution daily to ensure its disinfecting potency (Figure 22-4).

Materia... Utility gloves, disinfectant (10% bleach solut... oved disinfecting product), ... sh, tongs, forceps, pap... clea...

M...

**Procedures boxes**
Specific administrative or clinical tasks are illustrated in a step-by-step format.

---

| TABLE 20-1 | Infectious Waste Disposal: Penalties for Not Following Regulations, as Set Forth by OSHA | |
|---|---|---|
| **Type of Violation** | **Characteristics of Violation** | **Penalties for Violation** |
| Other than serious violation | Direct relationship to job safety and health but would probably not result in death or serious physical harm | Fine of up to $7,000 (discretionary) |
| Serious violation | Substantial probability that death or serious physical harm could result; employer knew, or should have known, of the hazard | Fine of up to $7,000 (mandatory) |
| Willful violation | Violation committed intentionally and knowingly | Fine of up to $70,000 with a $5,000 minimum; if violation resulted in death of employee, additional fine and/or up to 6 months' imprisonment |
| Repeated violation | Substantially similar (but not the same) violation found upon reinspection; not applicable if initial citation is under contest | Fine of up to $70,000 |
| Failure to correct prior violation | Initial violation was not corrected | Fine of up to $7,000 for each day the violation continues past the date it was supposed to stop |

### ⚠ CAUTION *Handle With Care*

#### Proper Use of Biohazardous Waste Containers and Handling of Infectious Laundry Waste

Biohazardous waste containers are available in a variety of designs. Frequently, more than one design is used in the clinical setting. These containers are often provided by outside sterilization and waste management companies. Examples of biohazardous waste containers include:

- Bags or containers that are red or have a biohazardous waste label (for any material contaminated with blood or body fluids, such as used dressings or gloves)
- Boxes with biohazardous waste labels (sometimes lined with red bags and used for disposable gowns, examination table covers, and similar items that may be contaminated with blood or body fluids)
- Rigid, leakproof sharps containers that are red or have a biohazardous waste label (for lancets, needles, and other sharp objects)

Every biohazardous waste container has a lid that you must replace immediately after use. In addition, you may not overfill the container, and you must replace it when it is two-thirds full. All biohazardous waste containers must have a fluorescent orange or orange-red label with the biohazard symbol and the word *BIOHAZARD* in a contrasting color (Figure 20-12). Red bags or red containers may be substituted for containers with biohazardous waste labels.

You must follow these guidelines when handling hazardous waste.

- Always wear gloves.
- Place hazardous waste in the appropriate biohazardous waste container immediately or as soon as possible.
- Keep biohazardous waste containers close to the place where the waste material is generated.
- Keep the containers closed when not in use, close them before removing them from the area of use, and keep them upright to avoid any spills.
- If outside contamination of the primary container occurs, place that container in a secondary *continued →*

Infection Control Techniques    425

**CAUTION *Handle With Care* boxes**
cover precautions to be taken when performing certain tasks.

**Points on Practice boxes**
provide guidelines on keeping the medical office running smoothly and efficiently.

**Educating the Patient boxes**
Patient instruction on self-care outside the medical office is the focus

**Reflecting On . . . boxes**
provide specialized information about legal and ethical issues, communication issues, cultural issues, professionalism, and HIPAA.

**Career Opportunities boxes**
provide information on professions and duties related to medical assisting.

**Summary and Review**
A summary of the chapter material and an end-of-chapter review close out each chapter.

## Points on Practice

### Working Efficiently Online

If the medical office where you work is computerized, the system most likely has a modem for sending e-mail and transferring files electronically. The modem may also be used to access various online services and the Internet, a global network of computers. If this access is not currently available in the medical office, it probably will be in the near future. You may be asked to help choose an online servi... vider for the office.

These servi...

that would be useful to the medical office. Other services may not offe... you can. By co...

older than age 65. Although elderly patients can be immunized against influenza each year and influenza-related pneumonia one time, they may have common misconceptions about vaccinations. They may worry about the expense, getting the disease from the vaccine, or the need for a vaccination when they do not feel ill.

Explain to patients who are concerned about the cost of vaccinations that if they are not enrolled in one of the many insurance plans that covers immunization, Medicare Part B covers the cost. For those worried about the potential side effects of immunization, describe the mild symptoms they may encounter, and emphasize that the symptoms are short-lived. You might also mention that compared to the potential dangers of contracting a serious infection, the symptoms are quite mild.

Because older patients are much more likely than younger patients to develop side effects as a result of immunizations, instruct older patients so that they recognize and immediately report any adverse effects. That way, the

physician can treat elderly patients before their illness becomes severe.

**Immunocompromised Patients.** Patients who have an impaired or weakened immune system (are immunocompromised) include those with acquired immunodeficiency syndrome (AIDS) or other immune disorders and those undergoing chemotherapy. Infants may also be considered immunocompromised if they have mothers who are infected with HIV or have AIDS or an unknown immune status.

All immunizations affect the immune system. A patient with a compromised immune system can experience minimal to dangerous effects, depending on the vaccine. Before administration of any immunization, the physician should check the patient's medical history. If the patient is immunocompromised, the dosage may need to be adjusted or administration postponed.

Immunization for immunocompromised patients depends on exactly what disease is present. For example,

## Educating the Patient

### Disease Prevention

As a medical assistant, you can be influential in edu... patients about ways to protect themselves from ... never you have the opportunity for pa... ...uld stress the basic principles ...

- Avoid stress
- Protect against exposure to potentially harmful insects or animals

To provide patients with the knowledge they need, you should educate them in the following subjects:

- Nutrition and diet
- Exercise and weight control
- ...of sexually transmitted diseases

## Reflecting On . . . HIPAA

### Guidelines for HIPAA Privacy Compliance and the Computer

The use of computers is widespread within the typical medical practice. Though the computer is valuable for many administrative functions, it also can be a risk in terms of patient privacy and HIPAA compliance. You must follow special safeguards for computers in order to protect the patient's privacy.

1. Computers are typically placed in or near the patient reception area. Keep the ... screen positioned so that ... unauthorized pers... Screensav...

reenter their password to regain access after an idle period.

3. Always keep your compute... password confide... often, us...

## Career Opportunities

### Registered Health Information Technologist

To gain medical assistant credentials, you must fulfill the requirements of either the American Association of Medical Assistants (for a Certified Medical Assistant) or the American Medical Technologist (for a Registered Health Information Technologist). After obtaining your medical assistant certification or registration, you may wish to acquire additional skills in specialty areas through course work or on-the-job training. Although this course work or training may not lead to an additional certification or degree, it will enable you to expand your role in the medical office and advance your career as the demand for skilled health professionals increases.

#### Skills and Duties

Sometimes called a medical record technician or a medical chart specialist, a Registered Health Information Technologist (RHIT) maintains patient records for a physician or group of physicians. The RHIT is responsible for ensuring that all medical information is accurate and complete. In a hospital, a RHIT deals strictly with health information and has no patient contact. In a small office, however, the RHIT may have additional clerical duties such as answering the telephone.

A patient's medical record includes a medical history and statement of symptoms as well as the results of exams, laboratory tests, and x-rays. The physician's diagnoses and treatment plans are also included. The information in the patient's record may be needed for insurance purposes or to aid in further diagnosis and treatment. In addition, it may be used for research purposes.

The Registered Health Information Technologist checks all patient charts for completeness and accuracy. The RHIT makes sure that all necessary forms related to the patient's care are included, properly filled out, and signed. The RHIT checks to see that all reports and test results are attached to the chart. If necessary, the RHIT speaks with the physician to clarify information about the patient's diagnosis or treatment.

The RHIT must also code the medical record. The RHIT assigns a code to each clinical procedure and diagnosis if this coding has not already been done by another member of the health-care team. In the hospital setting, the RHIT assigns a diagnosis-related group (DRG) to the patient, using a special computer program. The DRG helps determine the reimbursement that the hospital will receive from Medicare or any other insurance provider that uses a DRG system.

The RHIT may also use the coded records to set up a cross-reference index, a type of file that lists the same information under several different headings.

Some medical record technologists specialize in a particular area. Coding is one example. Another is registry, which involves keeping records of all occurrences of certain diseases like bone cancer. The information the registrar collects can be used by individual physicians or as part of a research study.

#### Workplace Settings

The majority of RHITs work in medical record departments of hospitals. Most of the rest work in nursing homes, group practices, and health maintenance organizations (HMOs). A few RHITs work in federal or state government offices, public health departments, health and property insurance companies, or accounting and law firms. Some RHITs are self-employed and work as consultants to nursing homes or physicians' offices.

#### Education

Most Registered Health Information Technologists have completed a two-year associate degree program at a junior or community college. Course work includes biology, anatomy and physiology, medical terminology, data processing, coding, and statistics.

#### Where to Go for More Information

American Health Information Management Association (formerly the American Medical Record Association)
233 N. Michigan Avenue, Suite 2150
Chicago, IL 60601-5800
(312) 233-1100

## REVIEW

### CHAPTER 22

#### CASE STUDY QUESTIONS

Now that you have completed this chapter, review the case study at the beginning of the chapter and answer the following questions:

1. What are bilateral cataracts, and why would this condition be a consideration when you come in contact with this patient?
2. What instruments should be assembled for the physician to use during the exam?
3. What disposable and consumable supplies may reasonably be anticipated for use?
4. What measures can you take to ensure the patient's comfort and safety?

#### Discussion Questions

1. Inadequate hand washing has been identified as a primary cause for transmitting infections. List the circumstances in a medical office when you should wash your hands.
2. Describe each of the four steps in the "PASS" system.
3. Why is it important to keep the exam room neat and clean? What steps will you take to accomplish these tasks?

#### Critical Thinking Questions

1. The Americans With Disabilities Act of 1990 enacted a provision for "reasonable accommodations" for accessibility for the disabled. Identify the accessibility guidelines, and explain why each is important.
2. Risk management is essential in the medical office. What types of problems can occur in the exam room, and what can you do to help prevent them?
3. The Occupational Safety and Health Administration mandates that biohazardous materials must be stored in a separate refrigerator. What is the rationale for this requirement?

#### Application Activities

1. Make a checklist of steps for preparing the exam room. List tasks in the following categories: before/after an exam, daily, weekly, and monthly.
2. Create a fire safety program for a medical office. Present the program to the class. Have the class critique your plan.
3. Draw a floor plan of an exam room. Include the placement of furnishings and any special features the room might need. Be sure to include accommodation... for individuals with disabilities. Present your floor pl... to the class and lead a discussion about the layout of... exam room.

#### Virtual Fieldtrip

*Visit the McGraw-Hill Higher Education Medical Ass... website at www.mhhe.com/medicalassisting3 to com... the following activity:*

Go to the OSHA website and search "Fire Safety." Na... to the first three or four sites listed in the site. Keep ... your search, including:

- The URL of each site visited
- A short synopsis of the information on the sites visited
- Whether the information applies to a medical office
- How the information can be used to develop a fire safety plan for a medical office

Open the CD and complete this chapter's practice activities, play the games, listen to the key terms, and test yourself with the interactive review. E-mail, print, and/or save your results to document your proficiency.

- Clinical Practice Activities
- Anatomy and Physiology Review
- Games: Spin the Wheel, Key Term Concentration, and Challenge
- Interactive Review
- Audio Glossary
- Progress Report
- Online Learning Center

**Online Learning Center.** The Online Learning Center (OLC) is a text-specific website that offers an extensive array of learning and teaching tools, including chapter quizzes with immediate feedback, news-feeds, links to relevant websites, and many more study resources. Log on at www.mhhe.com/medicalassisting3.

**Instructor Productivity CD-ROM.** The Instructor Productivity CD-ROM provides easy-to-use resources for class preparation. The Instructor Productivity CD-ROM includes the following:

- EZTest test generator with over 5000 questions and answer rationales and correlations to AAMA competencies PowerPoint® Presentations
- Correlations to AAMA, AMT, NHA, NOCTI, CAAHEP, and SCANS Standards
- Course syllabi
- Figure browser
- Video clip library
- Lesson plans

# Print Supplements

The *Student Workbook* provides an opportunity for the student to review the material and skills presented in the textbook. On a chapter-by-chapter basis, it provides:

- Vocabulary review exercises, which test knowledge of key terms in the chapter
- Content review exercises, which test the student's knowledge of key concepts in the chapter
- Critical thinking exercises, which test the student's understanding of key concepts in the chapter
- Application exercises, which include figures and practice forms and test mastery of specific skills
- Case studies, which apply the chapter material to real-life situations or problems
- Competency checklists for the procedures in the text

The *Instructor's Resource Binder* provides the instructor with materials to help organize lessons and classroom interactions. It includes:

- A complete lesson plan for each chapter, including an introduction to the lesson, teaching strategies, alternate teaching strategies, case studies, assessment, chapter close, resources, and an answer key to the student textbook

- Procedure competency checklists, reproduced from the *Student Workbook*
- An answer key to the *Student Workbook*
- Charts that show the location in the student textbook, the *Student Workbook,* and the *Instructor's Resource Binder* of material that correlates with the following:
  - The 2003 American Association of Medical Assistants (AAMA) Role Delineation Study Areas of Competence
  - The Association of Medical Technologists (AMT) Registered Medical Assistant (RMA) Certified Exam Topics
  - The National Healthcareer Association (NHA) Medical Assisting Duty/Task List,
  - The National Occupational Competency Testing Institute (NOCTI) Job Ready Sample Assessment competencies and skills
  - The Commission on Accreditation of Allied Health Education Programs (CAAHEP) Standards and Guidelines for Medical Assisting Education Programs competencies
  - The Secretary's Commission on Achieving Necessary Skills (SCANS) areas of competence
- PowerPoint Presentations on the Instructor Productivity CD-ROM
- Computer software for the student and instructor is also available. The Student CD-ROM is packaged with each student textbook.

Together, the Student Edition, the *Student Workbook,* and the *Instructor's Resource Binder* form a complete teaching and learning package. The *Medical Assisting* course will prepare students to enter the medical assisting field with all the knowledge and skills needed to be a useful resource to patients, a valued asset to employers, and a credit to the medical assisting profession.

# Acknowledgments

The publisher and authors would like to thank the reviewers and contributors for their assistance in shaping this revision. We appreciate their suggestions, insights, and commitment to providing information that is relevant and valuable to medical assisting students.

In addition, many people and organizations provided invaluable assistance in the process of illustrating the highly technical and detailed topics covered in the text. Their contributions helped ensure the accuracy, timelines, and authenticity of the illustrations in the book.

We would like to thank the following organizations for providing source materials and technical advice: the American Association of Medical Assistants, Chicago, Illinois; Becton Dickinson Microbiology Systems, Sparks, Maryland; Becton Dickinson VACUTAINER Systems, Franklin Lakes,

New Jersey; Bibbero Systems, Petaluma, California; Burdick, Schaumberg, Illinois; the Corel Corporation, Ottawa, Ontario, Canada; Hamilton Media, Hamilton, New Jersey; Nassau Ear, Nose, and Throat, Princeton, New Jersey; Princeton Allergy and Asthma Associates, Princeton, New Jersey; Richmond International, Boca Raton, Florida; and Winfield Medical, San Diego, California.

We would like to express our appreciation to the following New Jersey physicians and medical facilities for allowing us to photograph a variety of procedures and procedural settings at their facilities: the Eric B. Chandler Medical Center, New Brunswick; Helene Fuld School of Nursing of New Jersey, Trenton; Mercer Medical Center, Trenton; Mercer County Vocational-Technical Health Occupations Center, Trenton; Plainfield Health Center, Plainfield; Princeton Allergy and Asthma Associates, Princeton; the Princeton Medical Group, Princeton; Robert Wood Johnson University Hospital, New Brunswick; Robert Wood Johnson University Hospital at Hamilton, Hamilton; St. Francis Medical Center, Trenton; St. Peter's Medical Center, New Brunswick; Dr. Edward von der Schmidt, neurosurgeon, Princeton; Wound Care Center/Curative Network, New Brunswick.

We would also like to thank the following facilities and educational institutions for graciously allowing us to photograph procedures and other technical aspects related to the profession of medical assisting: Total Care Programming, Henrico, North Carolina; Wildwood Medical Clinic, Henrico, North Carolina; Central Piedmont Community College, Charlotte, North Carolina; Daytona Beach Community College, Daytona Beach, Florida; and Roanoke Rapids Clinic, Roanoke Rapids, Virginia.

# Reviewers

Every area of the text was reviewed by practitioners and educators in the field. Their insights helped shape the direction of the book.

Roxane M. Abbott, MBA
  Sarasota County Technical Institute
  Sarasota, FL

Dr. Linda G. Alford, Ed.D.
  Reid State Technical College
  Evergreen, AL

Suzzanne S. Allen
  Sanford Brown Institute
  Garden City, NY

Ann L. Aron, Ed.D.
  Aims Community College
  Greeley, CO

Emil Asdurian, MD
  Bramson ORT College
  Forest Hills, NY

Rhonda Asher, MT, ASCP, CMA
  Pitt Community College
  Greenville, NC

Adelina H. Azfar, DPM
  Total Technical Institute
  Brooklyn, OH

Joseph H. Balatbat, MD, RMA, RPT, CPT
  Sanford Brown Institute
  New York, NY

Mary Barko, CMA, MA Ed
  Ohio Institute of Health Careers
  Elyria, OH

Katie Barton, LPN, BA
  Savannah River College
  Augusta, GA

Kelli C. Batten, NCMA, LMT
  Medical Assisting Department Chair
  Career Technical College
  Monroe, LA

Nina Beaman, MS, RNC, CMA
  Bryant and Stratton College
  Richmond, VA

Kay E. Biggs, BS, CMA
  Columbus State Community College
  Columbus, OH

Norma Bird, M.Ed., BS, CMA
  Medical Assisting Program Director/Master Instructor
  Pocatello, ID

Kathleen Bode, RN, MS
  Flint Hills Technical College
  Emporia, KS

Natasha Bratton, BSN
  Beta Tech
  North Charleston, SC

Karen Brown, RN, BC, Ed.D.
  Kirtland Community College
  Roscommon, MI

Kimberly D. Brown, BSHS, CHES, CMA
  Swainsboro Technical College
  Swainsboro, GA

Nancy A. Browne, MS, BS
  Washington High School
  Kansas City, KS

Teresa A. Bruno, BA
  EduTek College
  Stow, OH

Marion I. Bucci, BA
  Delaware Technical and Community College
  Wilmington, DE

Michelle Buchman, BSN, RNC
  Springfield College
  Springfield, MO

Michelle L. Carfagna, RMA, ST, BMO, RHE
  Brevard Community College
  Cocoa, FL

Carmen Carpenter, RN, MS, CMA
  South University
  West Palm Beach, FL

Pamela C. Chapman, RN, MSN
Caldwell Community College and Technical Institute
Hickory, NC

Patricia A. Chappell, MA, BS
Director, Clinical Laboratory Science
Camden County College
Blackwood, NJ

Phyllis Cox, MA Ed, BS, MT(ASCP)
Arkansas Tech University
Russellville, AR

Stephanie Cox, BS, LPN
York Technical Institute
Lancaster, PA

Christine Cusano, CMA, CPhT
Clark University–CCI
Framingham, MA

Glynna Day, M.Ed
Dean of Education
Academy of Professional Careers
Boise, ID

Anita Denson, BS
National College of Business and Technology
Danville, KY

Leon Deutsch, RMA, BA, MA Ed
Keiser College
Orlando, FL

Walter R. English, MA, MT(AAB)
Akron Institute
Cuyahoga Falls, OH

Dennis J. Ernst, MT(ASCP)
Center for Phlebotomy Education
Ramsey, IN

C.S. Farabee, MBA, MSISE
High-Tech Institute Inc.
Phoenix, AZ

Deborah Fazio, CMAS, RMA
Sanford Brown Institute–Cleveland
Middleburg Heights, OH

William C. Fiala, BS, MA
University of Akron
Akron, OH

Cathy Flores, BHS
Central Piedmont Community College
Charlotte, NC

Brenda K. Frerichs, MS, MA, BS
Colorado Technical University
Sioux Falls, SD

Michael Gallucci, PT, MS
Assistant Professor of Practice,
Program in Physical Therapy,
School of Public Health,
New York Medical College
Valhalla, NY

Susan C. Gessner, RN, BSN, M Ed
Laurel Business Institute
Uniontown, PA

Bonnie J. Ginman, CMA
Branford Hall Career Institute
Springfield, MA

Robyn Gohsman, RMA, CMAS
Medical Career Institute
Newport News, VA

Cheri Goretti, MA, MT(ASCP), CMA
Quinebaug Valley Community College
Danielson, CT

Marilyn Graham, LPN
Moore Norman Technology Center
Norman, OK

Jodee Gratiot, CCA
Rocky Mountain Business Academy
Caldwell, ID

Donna E. Guisado, AA
North-West College
West Covina, CA

Debra K. Hadfield, BSN, MSN
Baker College of Jackson
Jackson, MI

Carrie A. Hammond, CMA, LPRT
Utah Career College
West Jordan, UT

Kris A. Hardy, CMA, RHE, CDF
Brevard Community College
Cocoa, FL

Toni R. Hartley, BS
Laurel Business Institute
Uniontown, PA

Brenda K. Hartson, MS, MA, BS
Colorado Technical University
Sioux Falls, SD

Marsha Perkins Hemby, BA, RN, CMA
Pitt Community College
Greenville, NC

Linda Henningsen, RN, MS, BSN
Brown Mackie College
Salina, KS

Carol Hinricher, MA
University of Montana College of Technology
Missoula, MT

Elizabeth A. Hoffman, MA Ed., CMA
Baker College of Clinton Township
Clinton Township, MI

Gwen C. Hornsey, BS
Medical Assistant Instructor
Tulsa Technology Center, Lemley Campus
Tulsa, OK

Helen J. Houser, MSHA, RN, RMA
Phoenix College
Phoenix, AZ

Melody S. Irvine, CCS-P, CPC, CMBS
Institute of Business and Medical Careers
Ft. Collins, CO

Kathie Ivester, MPA, CMA(AAMA), CLS(NCA)
North Georgia Technical College
Clarkesville, GA

Josephine Jackyra, CMA
The Technical Institute of Camden County
Sicklerville, NJ

Deborah Jones, BS, MA
High-Tech Institute
Phoenix, AZ

Karl A. Kahley, CHE, BS
Instructor, Medical Assisting
Ogeechee Technical College
Statesboro, GA

Barbara Kalfin Kalish
City College, Palm Beach Community College
Ft. Lauderdale, FL

Cheri D. Keenan, MA Instructor, EMT-B
Remington College
Garland, TX

Barbara E. Kennedy, RN, CPhT
Blair College
Colorado Springs, CO

Tammy C. Killough, RN, BSN
Texas Careers Vocational Nursing Program Director
San Antonio, TX

Jimmy Kinney, AAS
Virginia College at Huntsville
Huntsville, AL

Karen A. Kittle, CMA, CPT, CHUC
Oakland Community College
Waterford, MI

Diane M. Klieger, RN, MBA, CMA
Pinellas Technical Education Centers
St. Petersburg, FL

Mary E. Larsen, CMT, RMA
Academy of Professional Careers
Nampa, ID

Nancy L. Last, RN
Eagle Gate College
Murray, UT

Holly Roth Levine, NCICS, NCRMA, BA, BSN, RN
Keiser College
West Palm Beach, FL

Christine Malone, BS
Everett Community College
Everett, WA

Janice Manning
Baker College
Jackson, MI

Loretta Mattio-Hamilton, AS, CMA, RPT, CCA, NCICS
Herzing College
Kenner, LA

Gayle Mazzocco, BSN, RN, CMA
Oakland Community College
Waterford, MI

Patti McCormick, RN, PHD
President, Institute of Holistic Leadership
Dayton, OH

Stephanie R. McGahee, AATH
Augusta Technical College
Thomson, GA

Heidi M. McLean, CMA, RMA, BS, RPT, CAHI
Anne Arundel Community College
Arnold, MD

Tanya Mercer, BS, RN, RMA
KAPLAN Higher Education Corporation
Roswell, GA

Sandra J. Metzger, RN, BSN, MS. Ed
Red Rocks Community College
Lakewood, CO

Joyce A. Minton, BS, CMA, RMA
Wilkes Community College
Wilkesboro, NC

Grace Moodt, RN, BSN
Wallace Community College
Dothan, AL

Sherry L. Mulhollen, BS, CMA
Elmira Business Institute
Elmira, NY

Deborah M. Mullen, CPC, NCMA
Sanford Brown Institute
Atlanta, GA

Michael Murphy, CMA
Berdan Institute @ The Summit Medical Group
Union, NJ

Lisa S. Nagle, CMA, BS.Ed,
Augusta Technicial College
Augusta, GA

Peggy Newton, BSN, RN
Galen Health Institute
Louisville, KY

Brigitte Niedzwiecki, RN, MSN
Chippewa Valley Technical College
Eau Claire, WI

Thomas E. O'Brien, MBA, BBA, AS, CCT
Central Florida Institute
Palm Harbor, FL

Linda Oliver, MA
Vista Adult School
Vista, CA

Linda L. Oprean, BSN
ACT College
Manassas, VA

Holly J. Paul, MSN, FNP
Baker College of Jackson
Jackson, MI

Shirley Perkins, MD, BSE
Everest College
Dallas, TX

Kristina Perry, BPA
Heritage College
Las Vegas, NV

James H. Phillips, BS, CMA, RMA
Central Florida College
Winter Park, FL

Carol Putkamer, RHIA, MS
Alpena Community College
Alpena, MI

Mary Rahr, MS, RN, CMA-C
Northeast Wisconsin Technical College
Green Bay, WI

David Rice, AA, BA, MA
Career College of Northern Nevada
Reno, NV

Dana M. Roessler, RN, BSN
Southeastern Technical College
Glennville, GA

Cindy Rosburg, MA
Wisconsin Indian Technical College
New Richmond, WI

Deborah D. Rossi, MA, CMA
Community College of Philadelphia
Philadelphia, PA

Donna Rust, BA
American Commercial College
Wichita Falls, TX

Ona Schulz, CMA
Lake Washington Technical College
Kirkland, WA

Amy E. Semenchuk, RN, BSN
Rockford Business College
Rockford, IL

David Lee Sessoms, Jr., M.Ed., CMA
Miller-Motte Technical College
Cary, NC

Susan Shorey, BA, MA
Valley Career College
El Cajon, CA

Lynn G. Slack, BS
ICM School of Business and Medical Careers
Pittsburgh, PA

Patricia L. Slusher, MT(ASCP), CMA
Ivy Tech State College
Kokomo, IN

Deborah H. Smith, RN, CNOR
Southeastern Technical College
Vidalia, GA

Kristi Sopp, AA
MTI College
Sacramento, CA

Nona K. Stinemetz, Practical Nurse
Vatterott College
Des Moines, IA

Patricia Ann Stoddard, MS, RT(R), MT, CMA
Western Business College
Vancouver, WA

Sylvia Taylor, BS, CMA, CPC-A
Cleveland State Community College
Cleveland, TN

Cynthia H. Thompson, RN, MA
Davenport University
Bay City, MI

Geiselle Thompson, M. Div.
The Learning Curve Plus
Cary, NC

Barbara Tietsort, M. Ed.
University of Cincinnati, Raymond Walters
Cincinnati, OH

Karen A. Trompke, RN
Virginia College at Pensacola
Pensacola, FL

Marilyn M. Turner, RN, CMA
Ogeechee Technical College
Statesboro, GA

L. Joleen VanBibber, AS
Davis Applied Technology College
Kaysville, UT

Lynette M. Veach, AAS
Columbus State Community College
Columbus, OH 43215

Antonio C. Wallace, BS
Sanford Brown Institute
Atlanta, GA

Jim Wallace, MHSA
Maric College
Los Angeles, CA

Denise Wallen, CPC
Academy of Professional Careers
Boise, ID

Mary Jo Whitacre, MSN, RN
Lord Fairfax Community College
Middletown, VA

Donna R. Williams, LPN, RMA
Tennessee Technology Center
Knoxville, TN

Marsha Lynn Wilson, BS, MS (ABT)
Clarian Health Sciences Education Center
Indianapolis, IN

Linda V. Wirt, CMA
Cecil Community College
North East, MD

Dr. MaryAnn Woods, PhD, RN
Prof. Emeritus,
Fresno City College
Fresno, CA 93741

Bettie Wright, MBA, CMA
Umpqua Community College
Roseburg, OR

Mark D. Young, DMD, BS
West Kentucky Community and Technical College
Paducah, KY

Cynthia M. Zumbrun, MEd, RHIT, CCS-P
Allegany College of Maryland
Cumberland, MD

# MEDICAL ASSISTING

*Administrative and Clinical Procedures*

# PART *One*

# Introduction to Medical Assisting

"The medical assisting profession is filled with challenges and rewards every day. Everything is important when you are assisting a patient. You should get to know your patient and his family, if possible, in order to understand the patient's specific needs. This is especially true with an elderly patient. Treat your patient like you would want to be treated. Be considerate and concerned, and always maintain a pleasant attitude.

"It is also essential to know your physician well, and how he or she likes to work. Let the physician know all the information the patient has shared with you, to help him or her make a better diagnosis. Keep informed about what the physician has recommended for treatment. The patient will have questions along the way. It's good medicine to be able to give him solid information about his condition and reinforce the doctor's orders when necessary. A skilled physician and an organized, cooperative, receptive medical assistant promote and maintain exceptional patient care."

**Sue Haines**
*Medical Assistant, Princeton, New Jersey*

# SECTION ONE
## Foundations and Principles

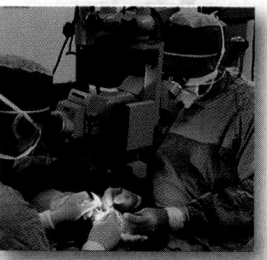
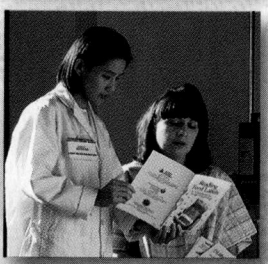
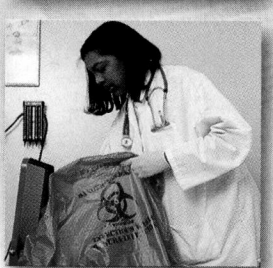
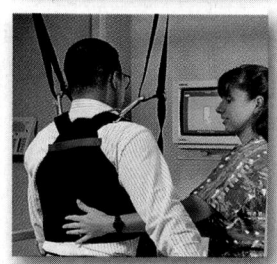
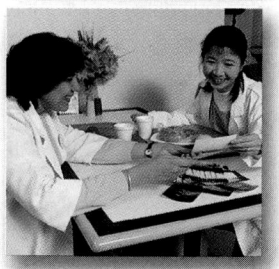
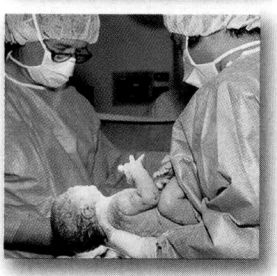

# SECTION 1

# FOUNDATIONS AND PRINCIPLES

# The Profession of Medical Assisting

## MEDICAL ASSISTING COMPETENCIES

*In preparation for the certification examination, you should know the following areas of competence:*

| COMPETENCY | CMA | RMA |
|---|---|---|
| **General/Legal/Professional** | | |
| Be aware of and perform within legal and ethical boundaries | X | X |
| Project a positive attitude | | X |
| Be a "team player" | | X |
| Exhibit initiative | | X |
| Adapt to change | | X |
| Evidence a responsible attitude | | X |
| Be courteous and diplomatic | | X |
| Conduct work within scope of education, training, and ability | | X |
| Be impartial and show empathy when dealing with patients | | X |
| Understand allied health professions and credentialing | | X |

## KEY TERMS

accreditation

American Association of Medical Assistants (AAMA)

Certified Medical Assistant (CMA)

CLIA '88 (Clinical Laboratory Improvement Amendments of 1988)

contaminated

cross-training

externship

HIPAA (Health Insurance Portability and Accountability Act)

managed care organization (MCO)

OSHA (Occupational Safety and Health Act)

practitioner

Registered Medical Assistant (RMA)

résumé

## CHAPTER OUTLINE

- Growth of the Medical Assisting Profession
- Medical Assistant Credentials
- Membership in a Medical Assisting Association
- Training Programs and Other Learning Opportunities
- Accreditation
- Daily Duties of Medical Assistants
- Personal Qualifications of Medical Assistants
- The AAMA Role Delineation Study

## LEARNING OUTCOMES

After completing Chapter 1, you will be able to:

**1.1** Describe the job responsibilities of a medical assistant.

**1.2** Discuss the professional training of a medical assistant.

1.3 Identify the personal characteristics a medical assistant needs.

1.4 Define multiskilled health professional.

1.5 Explain the importance of continuing education for a medical assistant.

1.6 Describe the process and benefits of certification and registration.

1.7 List the benefits of becoming a member of a professional association.

# Introduction

Medical assisting is one of the fastest-growing occupations in allied health care today. Health care is changing at a rapid rate, from advanced technology to implementing cost-effective medicine while maintaining quality patient care. The medical assistant is the perfect complement to this changing industry. Employers are looking for health care professionals who are "generalists." A generalist is someone who is trained in all departments in the facility in which he or she is employed. Medical assistants who graduate from an accredited institution will gain the skills that enable them to multitask. A multitasking professional is someone who is able to work in the administrative areas, the clinical areas, and the financial areas. Employers are seeking credentialed health care professionals who are dedicated to the profession and the patient.

This chapter will introduce the professional standards that are required in medical assisting.

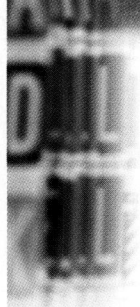

## CASE STUDY

Medical assistants are considered generalists in most medical environments. The following scenarios describe how the medical assistant functions as a generalist or multiskilled professional. As you review the scenarios, make note of the many duties the medical assistant performs.

**Scenario 1** Debbie is 23 years old. She has been working as a medical assistant for 2 years. She is currently working in a family practice office with two doctors, two other medical assistants, and a medical records clerk. Her role is primarily administrative; she is mainly responsible for phone reception and patient check-in and check-out.

A 29-year-old female patient calls complaining of lower back pain. As Debbie listens to the patient describe her condition, she determines the severity of the patient's discomfort and schedules a same-day appointment. When the patient arrives at the office, Debbie greets her at the front desk, verifies her address and insurance information, and escorts her to an exam room. After the physician completes the exam, the patient is instructed to see Debbie on the way out. Debbie reviews the patient's prescriptions and schedules a diagnostic test and laboratory work for the patient at another facility. Debbie then collects the patient co-pay and gives the patient a receipt. After the patient leaves, Debbie prepares the insurance forms for reimbursement and files the patient's chart.

**Scenario 2** Tom is 30 years old. He has been working as a medical assistant for 7 years. He currently works as a clinical medical assistant in an urgent care center that specializes in occupational medicine and basic emergency medicine. He is flexible and works a combination of days, afternoons, and weekends. He normally works with two doctors, two nurses, and four other medical assistants during his shift. The center's patients usually arrive on a walk-in basis.

A 40-year-old man signs in with the receptionist. She helps the patient complete the necessary forms for the medical chart. After the chart is completed, she places the chart at the clinical station. Tom reviews the medical chart and makes note that the patient, a truck driver, is here for an occupational physical. He obtains the protocol from the trucking company file and verifies the testing requested by the company. He then escorts the patient to an exam room and interviews the patient regarding his medical history. He explains all the testing that will be completed and escorts the patient to the laboratory. Tom collects a urine drug screen, following precise directions, and collects a blood specimen. Tom then performs an auditory and visual screening and escorts the patient back to the exam room. The patient is given a gown with instructions on how to put it on. After a few minutes, Tom obtains an EKG on the patient. The patient is now ready for the physical part of the exam, which is performed by the doctor. Tom verifies the information again and gives the chart to the doctor. After the doctor is finished with the exam, Tom returns to the patient, explains how the physical is reported to his employer, and escorts him to the x-ray technician for a chest x-ray. After the patient leaves, Tom completes the paperwork, submits the laboratory work to an outside reference lab, and submits the x-ray to be read by a radiologist.

**Scenario 3** Patty begins her day at 5:00 A.M. Her first stop is the reference laboratory, where she collects all the necessary phlebotomy equipment needed to complete the daily visits. She then drives to the first nursing facility on her route, where she is scheduled to collect blood specimens from 10 patients. She returns to the lab to drop off the specimens and paperwork, and heads out to her second nursing facility to collect blood specimens. She continues to collect specimens throughout the day and returns to the laboratory at 1:30 P.M. She is given her schedule for the following day.

As you read this chapter, consider the following questions:
1. How are the three jobs different?
2. How are the three jobs the same?
3. How do these three medical assistants function as multiskilled health-care professionals?

# Growth of the Medical Assisting Profession

As a medical assistant, you will be an allied health professional trained to work in a variety of health-care settings: medical offices, clinics, and ambulatory care facilities. Your role, with varied and challenging administrative and clinical duties, will be integral to creating a health-care facility that operates smoothly and provides a patient-centered approach to quality health care. Your specific responsibilities will likely depend on the location and size of the facility as well as its medical specialties.

Medical assisting is now one of the fastest-growing occupations. As the health services industry expands, the U.S. Department of Labor projects that medical assisting will be the fastest-growing occupation between 2002 and 2012. The growth in the number of physicians' group practices and other health-care practices that use support personnel will in turn continue to drive up demand for medical assistants.

According to the U.S. Department of Labor Bureau of Statistics, in the year 2002, medical assistants held approximately 365,000 jobs. Of these, 60% were in physicians' offices and approximately 14% were in hospitals, including outpatient and inpatient facilities. Almost 10% were in nursing homes and the offices of other health **practitioners** (those who practice a profession), such as chiropractors, optometrists, and podiatrists. The rest worked mostly in outpatient care centers, public and private educational services, other ambulatory health-care services, state and local government agencies, medical and diagnostic laboratories, nursing care facilities, and employment services. Modern health insurance, Medicare, and Medicaid now make medical care available to more people, and the number of physicians is increasing. Thus, more medical assistants will be needed to run these physicians' offices.

The following factors will also increase job opportunities for medical assistants: growth of outpatient clinics and health maintenance organizations (HMOs), and the population increase. Specifically, greater numbers of older people now require a relatively higher level of medical care. Today, the elderly are the fastest-growing segment of the U.S. population, bringing an increase in demand for health-care services.

## History of the Medical Assisting Profession

With the emergence of formal training programs for medical assistants and the continuous changes in health care today, the role of the medical assistant has become dynamic and wide ranging. These changes have raised the expectations for medical assistants. The knowledge base of the modern medical assistant includes:

- Administrative and clinical skills
- Patient insurance product knowledge (specific to the workers' geographical locations)
- Compliance, especially of OSHA and HIPAA guidelines
- Exceptional customer service
- Practice management
- Current patient treatments and education

The medical assisting profession today requires a commitment to self-directed, lifelong learning. Health care is changing rapidly because of new technology, new health-care delivery systems, and new approaches to facilitating cost-efficient, high-quality health care. A medical assistant who can adapt to change and is continually learning will be in high demand.

## Creating the American Association of Medical Assistants

The seed of the idea for a national association of medical assistants—to be called the **American Association of Medical Assistants (AAMA)**—was planted at the 1955 annual state convention of the Kansas Medical Assistants

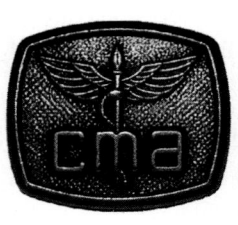 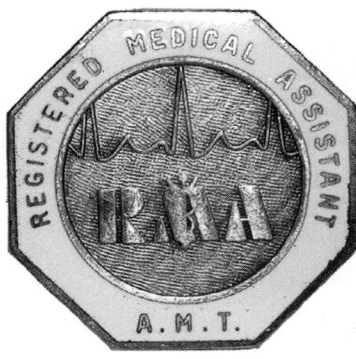

**Figure 1-1.** The pin on the left is worn by members of the American Association of Medical Assistants. The pin on the right is worn by medical assistants registered by the American Medical Technologists.

Society. The next year, at an American Medical Association (AMA) meeting, the AAMA was officially created. In 1978 the U.S. Department of Health, Education, and Welfare declared medical assisting an allied health profession. In the early 1970s the American Medical Technologists (which has been a national certifying body for laboratory personnel since 1939) began a program to register medical assistants at accredited schools. You will read more about the benefits of joining one of these organizations later in the chapter. Figure 1-1 shows the pins worn by medical assistants who are certified by the AAMA and by those registered by the American Medical Technologists.

**The AAMA's Purpose.** The AAMA works to raise standards of medical assisting to a more professional level. It is the only professional association devoted exclusively to the medical assisting profession. Its creator and first president, Maxine Williams, had extensive experience in orchestrating medical assisting projects for the Kansas Medical Assistants Society. She also served as co-chair of the planning committee that formed the AAMA.

**The AAMA Creed.** To maintain the professional standards of the medical assisting profession, the AAMA has developed the following creed, which is reprinted here with the permission of the organization:

> *I believe in the principles and purposes of the profession of medical assisting.*
> *I endeavor to be more effective.*
> *I aspire to render greater service.*
> *I protect the confidence entrusted to me.*
> *I am dedicated to the care and well-being of all people.*
> *I am loyal to my physician-employer.*
> *I am true to the ethics of my profession.*
> *I am strengthened by compassion, courage, and faith.*

**AAMA Code of Ethics.** The AAMA has also established a code of ethics, which is reprinted here with the permission of the organization:

The Code of Ethics of AAMA shall set forth principles of ethical and moral conduct as they relate to the medical profession and the particular practice of Medical Assisting.

Members of AAMA dedicated to the conscientious pursuit of their profession, and thus desiring to merit the high regard of the entire medical profession and the respect of the general public which they serve, do pledge themselves to strive always to:

A. render service with full respect for the dignity of humanity

B. respect confidential information obtained through employment unless legally authorized or required by responsible performance of duty to divulge such information

C. uphold the honor and high principles of the profession and accept its disciplines

D. seek to continually improve the knowledge and skills of medical assistants for the benefit of patients and professional colleagues

E. participate in additional service activities aimed toward improving the health and well-being of the community

# Medical Assistant Credentials

Employers today prefer or even insist that their medical assistants have credentialing within their discipline. Understanding why employers are aggressively recruiting credentialed medical assistants is of utmost importance for medical assisting educators as well as all medical assistants. Listed here are some explanations as to why credentialing is becoming so important for a medical assistant's entry into and advancement within the allied health force.

## Malpractice

The United States continues to be one of the most litigious nations in the civilized world. Disputes that used to be settled by discussion and mediation are now being referred to attorneys and ending up in courts of law. Lawsuit mania is particularly acute in the world of health care. Employers of allied health professionals have correctly concluded that having credentialed personnel or staff will lessen the likelihood of a successful legal challenge to the quality of work of employees.

An accredited medical assisting program is competency based; this means that standards are set by the accrediting body, such as the Accrediting Bureau of Health Education Schools (ABHES) or the Commission on Accreditation of Allied Health Education Programs (CAAHEP), for administrative and clinical competencies. It is the duty of the educational institution to ensure that all medical assisting competencies are learned by medical assisting students and that evidence is clearly documented for each student. Periodic evaluations are performed by the accrediting agencies to ensure the effectiveness of the program. The theory of the competencies as well as the proficiency assessments are components of the CMA examination. For example, administering medications is a competency required of accredited medical assisting programs and is a component of the CMA examination. The CMA credential and the affiliation with a professional organization demonstrate competence and provide evidence of training. They will also lessen the likelihood of a legal challenge to the quality of a medical assistant's work.

## Managed Care Organizations

Managed care is a growing trend in today's health-care industry. The cost limitations imposed by **managed care organizations (MCOs)** are causing mergers and buyouts throughout the nation. Small physician practices are being consolidated or merged into larger providers of health care, such as by hospitals or for-profit organizations, which result in decreased operating expenses. These larger health-care providers can make the delivery of health care more cost-effective. Human resource directors of MCOs place great importance in professional credentials for their employees and therefore are more likely to establish certification or registry as a mandatory professional designation for medical assistants.

## State and Federal Regulations

Certain provisions of the **OSHA (Occupational Safety and Health Act)** and the **CLIA '88 (Clinical Laboratory Improvement Amendments of 1988)** are making mandatory credentialing for medical assistants a logical step in the hiring process. Presently, OSHA and CLIA '88 do not require that medical assistants be credentialed, but there are various components of these statutes and their regulations that can be met by demonstrating that medical assistants in a clinical setting are certified. For example, some physician offices perform moderately complex laboratory testing on site. The medical assistant can perform moderately complex tests if she or he has the appropriate training and skills. The Certified Office Laboratory Technician (COLT) certification offered by the American Medical Technologists is designed to test health-care professionals for the appropriate skills necessary to perform moderately complex laboratory tests under CLIA regulations.

## CMA Certification

The **Certified Medical Assistant (CMA)** credential is awarded by the Certifying Board of the AAMA. The AAMA's certification examination evaluates mastery of medical assisting competencies based on the 2005 Role Delineation Study, discussed later in this chapter. The National Board of Medical Examiners (NBME) also provides technical assistance in developing the tests.

CMAs must recertify the CMA credential every 5 years. This mandate requires you to learn about new medical developments through education courses or participation in an examination. Hundreds of continuing education courses are sponsored by local, state, and national AAMA groups. The AAMA also offers self-study courses through its Continuing Education Department. As described in the AAMA's publication *CMA Today*, the advantages of CMA certification include respect and recognition from peers in the medical assisting profession.

As of June 1998, only applicants of medical assisting programs accredited by the CAAHEP and the ABHES are eligible to take the certification examination. The examination is administered nationwide every January, June, and October at more than 100 test sites. The AAMA offers the *Candidate's Guide to the Certification Examination* to help applicants prepare for the examination. This guide explains the test format and test-taking strategies. It also includes a sample examination with answers and information about study references.

## RMA Registration

The **Registered Medical Assistant (RMA)** credential is given by the American Medical Technologists (AMT), an organization founded in 1939. RMA credentialing by the AMT ensures that you have taken and passed the RMA certification examination for the RMA.

The AMT sets forth certain educational and experiential requirements to earn the RMA credential. These include:

- Graduation from an accredited high school or acceptable equivalent.
- Graduation from a medical assistant program or institution accredited by the ABHES, from a medical assistant program accredited by a regional accrediting commission, or from a formal medical services training program of the U.S. Armed Forces. Alternatively, the applicant can have been employed in the profession of medical assisting for a minimum of 5 years, not more than 2 of which may have been as an instructor in a postsecondary medical assistant program.
- Passing the AMT examination for RMA certification.

## Major Areas of the RMA/CMA Examinations

The RMA and CMA qualifying examinations are rigorous. Participation in an accredited program, however, will help you learn what you need to know. The examinations cover several distinct areas of knowledge. These include:

- General medical knowledge, including terminology, anatomy, physiology, behavioral science, medical law, and ethics

- Administrative knowledge, including medical records management, collections, insurance processing, and the **Health Insurance Portability and Accountability Act (HIPAA)**
- Clinical knowledge, including examination room techniques, medication preparation and administration, pharmacology, and specimen collection

# Membership in a Medical Assisting Association

Professional associations set high standards for quality and performance in a profession. They define the tasks and functions of an occupation. In addition, they provide members with the opportunity to communicate and network with one another. They also present their goals to the profession and to the general public. Becoming a member of a professional association helps you achieve career goals and further the profession of medical assisting.

## Professional Support for CMAs

When you become a member of the AAMA, you will have a large support group of active medical assistants. Membership benefits include:

- Professional publications, such as *CMA Today*
- A large variety of educational opportunities, such as chapter-sponsored seminars and workshops about the latest administrative, clinical, and management topics (Figure 1-2)
- Group insurance

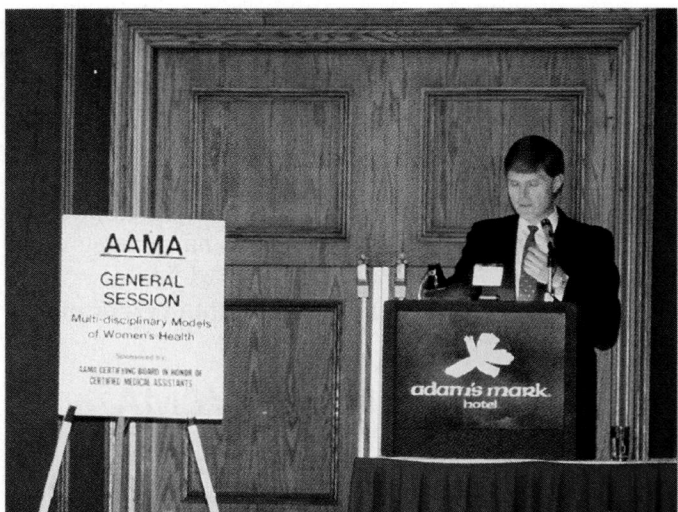

**Figure 1-2.** Local and state chapters of the AAMA and AMT frequently sponsor seminars and workshops on administrative, clinical, or management topics. In this picture, Donald A. Balasa, executive director and staff legal counsel for the AAMA, addresses a group at the annual AAMA national convention.

- Legal information
- Local, state, and national activities that include professional networking and multiple continuing education opportunities
- Legislative monitoring. The AAMA continually works to protect your right to practice as a medical assistant.

## Professional Support for RMAs

The AMT offers many benefits for RMAs. These include:

- Professional publications
- Membership in the AMT Institute for Education
- Group insurance programs—liability, health, and life
- State chapter activities
- Legal representation in health legislative matters
- Annual meetings and educational seminars
- Student membership

# Training Programs and Other Learning Opportunities

Formal programs in medical assisting are offered in a variety of educational settings. They include vocational-technical high schools, postsecondary vocational schools, community and junior colleges, and 4-year colleges and universities. Vocational school programs usually last 1 year and award a certificate or diploma. Community and junior college programs are usually 2-year associate degree programs.

# Accreditation

**Accreditation** is the process by which programs are officially authorized. There are two national entities recognized by the U.S. Department of Education that accredit medical assisting educational programs:

1. The Commission on Accreditation of Allied Health Education Programs (CAAHEP). CAAHEP works directly with the Curriculum Review Board of The American Association of Medical Assistants Endowments to ensure that all accredited schools provide a competency-based education. CAAHEP accredits medical assisting programs in both public and private postsecondary institutions throughout the United States that prepare individuals for entry into the medical assisting profession.
2. Accrediting Bureau of Health Education Schools (ABHES). ABHES accredits private postsecondary institutions and programs that prepare individuals for entry into the medical assisting profession.

Accredited programs must cover the following topics: anatomy and physiology; medical terminology; medical law and ethics; psychology; oral and written communications;

laboratory procedures; and clinical and administrative procedures. High school students may prepare for these courses by studying mathematics, health, biology, keyboarding, office skills, bookkeeping, and information technology. You may obtain current information about accreditation standards for medical assisting programs from the AAMA.

Medical assisting programs must also include an externship. An **externship** is practical work experience for a specified timeframe in an ambulatory care setting, such as physicians' offices, hospitals, or other health-care facilities.

Additionally, the AAMA lists its minimum standards for accredited programs. This list of standards ensures that all personnel—administrators and faculty—are qualified to perform their jobs.

The AAMA requires that administrative personnel exhibit leadership and management skills. They must also be able to fully perform the functions identified in documented job descriptions. Faculty members must develop and evaluate lesson plans, assess student progress toward the program's objectives, and be knowledgeable regarding course content. They must be qualified through work experience and be able to effectively direct and evaluate student learning and laboratory experiences.

The AAMA also has accreditation requirements for financial and physical resources. Each program's financial resources must meet its obligations to students. Schools must also have adequate physical resources—classrooms, laboratories, clinical and administrative facilities, and equipment and supplies.

## The Benefits of Certification/ Registration

Certification or registration is not required to practice as a medical assistant. You may practice with a high school diploma or equivalent. Your career options will be greater, however, if you graduate from an accredited school and you become certified or registered.

Graduation from an accredited program helps your career in three ways. First, it shows that you have completed a program that meets nationally accepted standards. Second, it provides recognition of your education by professional peers. Third, it makes you eligible for registration or certification. Students who graduate from an accredited medical assisting program, such as ABHES or CAAHEP, are eligible to take the CMA or RMA immediately.

## Externships

In an externship you will obtain work experience while completing a medical assisting program. You will practice skills learned in the classroom in an actual medical office environment.

**Externship Requirements.** Externships are mandatory in accredited schools. The length of your externship will vary, depending on your particular program.

Familiarize yourself with the program requirements as soon as possible. You may be able to obtain an externship site of your choice either at a practice already affiliated with the school or at a practice you find on your own.

The externship is offered in cooperative medical offices or hospitals for a predetermined period (several weeks to several months). Another experienced medical assistant, nurse manager, or licensed nurse practitioner in the externship office often becomes your mentor. This mentor advises and supervises you during the externship. Chapter 41 further explains externship.

**Externship Duties.** Your duties will be planned to meet your program's requirements for real-world work experience. Approach the externship with a positive attitude. Accept any guidance, constructive criticism, or praise as a learning experience.

## Other Professional Memberships and Certification

The National Healthcare Association (NHA) was established in 1989 as an information resource and network for today's active health-care professionals. They offer a variety of certification exams and continuing education. Some of the programs and services of the NHA include:

- Certification development and implementation
- Continuing education curriculum development and implementation
- Program development for unions, hospitals, and schools
- Educational, career advancement, and networking services for members
- Registry of certified professionals

Some of the certification examinations offered by the National Healthcare Association include:

- Phlebotomy Technician (CPT)
- EKG/ECG Technician (CET)
- Billing & Coding Specialist
- Medical Transcriptionist (CMT)
- Medical Administrative Assistant (CCMA)
- Medical Laboratory Assistant

The National Healthcare Association certification exams are developed by health-care educators working in their various fields of study. The NHA is a member of The National Organization of Competency Assurance (NOCA).

## Volunteer Programs

Volunteering is a rewarding experience. Before you even begin a medical assisting program, you can gain experience in a health-care profession through volunteer work. As a volunteer, you will get hands-on training and learn what it is like to assist patients who are ill, disabled, or frightened.

You may volunteer as an aide in a hospital, clinic, nursing home, or doctor's office, or as a typist or filing clerk in a medical office or medical record room. Some visiting nurse associations and hospices (homelike medical settings that provide medical care and emotional support to terminally ill patients and their families) also offer volunteer opportunities. These experiences may help you decide if you want to pursue a career as a medical assistant.

The American Red Cross also offers volunteer opportunities for the student medical assistant. The Red Cross needs volunteers for its disaster relief programs locally, statewide, nationally, and abroad.

As part of a disaster relief team at the site of a hurricane, tornado, storm, flood, earthquake, or fire, volunteers learn first-aid and emergency triage skills. Red Cross volunteers gain valuable work experience that may help them obtain a job.

Because volunteers are not paid, it is usually easy to find work opportunities. Just because you are not paid for volunteer work, however, does not mean the experience is not useful for meeting your career goals.

Include information about any volunteer work on your **résumé**—a computer-generated document that summarizes your employment and educational history. Be sure to note specific duties, responsibilities, and skills developed during the volunteer experience. Refer to Chapter 41 for examples of résumés.

## Multiskill Training

Today many hospitals and health-care practices are embracing the idea of a multiskilled health-care professional (MSHP). An MSHP is a cross-trained team member who is able to handle many different duties.

The AAMA includes the word *multiskill* in its definition of the profession of medical assisting:

Medical assisting is a multiskilled allied health profession whose practitioners work primarily in ambulatory settings, such as medical offices and clinics. Medical assistants function as members of the healthcare delivery team and perform administrative and clinical procedures.
An MSHP may be trained to perform certain clinical procedures. She or he is not, however, trained to make judgments or interpretations concerning a patient's diagnosis or treatment, as a physician would.

**Reducing Health-Care Costs.** As a result of health-care reform and downsizing (a reduction in the number of staff members) to control the rising cost of health care, medical practices are eager to reduce personnel costs by hiring multiskilled health professionals. These individuals, who perform the functions of two or more people, are the most cost-efficient employees.

**Expanding Your Career Opportunities.** Career opportunities are vast if you are self-motivated and willing to learn new skills. If you continue to learn about new administrative and clinical techniques and procedures, you will be an important part of the health-care team.

As you read this book, look for a boxed feature titled Career Opportunities. This feature highlights additional skills medical assistants can learn and integrate into their jobs to make themselves more marketable as multiskilled health professionals. Following are several examples of positions for medical assistants with various experience and certifications:

- Office manager
- Certified Office Laboratory Technician (COLT certification)
- ECG technician
- Medical transcriptionist
- Medical biller
- Hospital admissions coordinator
- A professional who performs physical exams for applicants to insurance companies
- An administrative assistant at insurance companies
- Medical Assisting Instructor (with a specified amount of experience and education)

If you are multiskilled, you will have an advantage when job hunting. Employers are eager to hire multiskilled medical assistants and may create positions for them.

You can gain multiskill training by showing initiative and a willingness to learn every aspect of the medical facility in which you are working. When you begin working within a medical facility, establish goals regarding your career path and discuss them with your immediate supervisor. Indicate to your supervisor that you would like to become **cross-trained** in every aspect of the medical facility. Begin your mastery of the department that you are currently working in and branch out to other departments once you master the skills needed for your current position. This will demonstrate a commitment to your profession as well as a strong work ethic. Cross-training is a valuable marketing tool to include on your résumé.

## Daily Duties of Medical Assistants

As a medical assistant, you will be the physician's "right arm." Duties include maintaining an efficient office, preparing and maintaining medical records, assisting the physician during examinations, and keeping examining rooms in order. You may also handle the payroll for the office staff (or supervise a payroll service), obtain equipment and supplies, and serve as the link between the physician and representatives of pharmaceutical and medical supply companies. In small practices you will usually handle all duties. In larger practices you may specialize in a particular duty. As a medical assistant grows in his or her profession, advanced duties may be required, such as Office Practice Management, which may include marketing, and financial and strategic planning.

## Certified Office Laboratory Technician

To gain medical assistant credentials, you must fulfill the requirements of either the American Association of Medical Assistants (obtaining CMA certification) or the American Medical Technologists (obtaining RMA certification). After acquiring your CMA or RMA certification, you may wish to acquire additional skills in specialty areas through course work or on-the-job training. The Certified Office Laboratory Technician certification is awarded by the American Medical Technologists to qualified applicants.

### Nature of the Job

The Certified Office Laboratory Technician is a multi-skilled practitioner qualified by education and experience to perform medical laboratory testing, including CLIA-waived and moderately complex testing. This health-care professional is also trained to perform front and back office tasks, as well as a variety of tasks involving direct patient contact. The position's scope of practice covers many areas and it is necessary to have knowledge of all federal and state regulations applicable to the job.

### Duties and Skills

- Assists others in performing routine administrative and clinical tasks
- Answers telephones
- Processes laboratory specimens
- Assists in the collection and testing of medical specimens
- Depending on state law, performs chemical, biological, hematological, immunologic, microscopic, and bacteriological tests
- Assists with the processing, reading, and reporting of specimens to determine the presence of bacteria, fungi, parasites, or other microorganisms

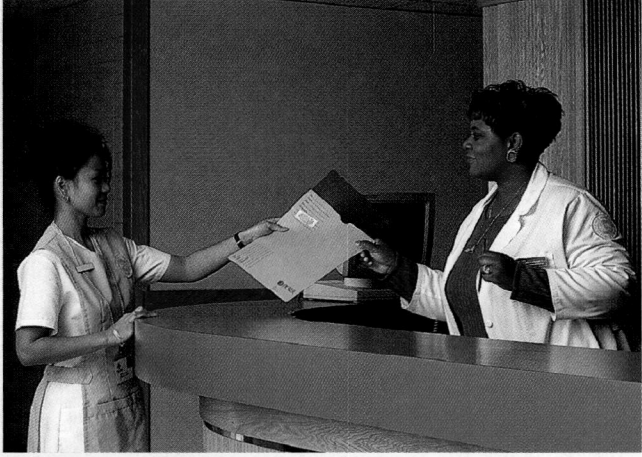

### Educational Requirements

Applicant must have a high school diploma or the equivalent with acceptable training. Often, Certified Office Laboratory Technicians are medical assistants with advanced training.

### Workplace Settings

Most Certified Office Laboratory Technicians work in a physician's office or clinic. She or he may work a flexible schedule that includes evenings and weekends.

### Where to Go for More Information

American Medical Technologists
10700 West Higgins Road, Ste. 150
Rosemont, IL 60018
(847) 823-5169
www.amt1.com

National Healthcare Association
134 Evergreen Place, 9th Floor
East Orange, NJ 07018
(800) 499-9092
infor@nhanow.com

## Entry-Level Administrative Duties

In an entry-level position, your administrative duties may include the following:

- Greeting patients
- Handling correspondence
- Scheduling appointments
- Answering telephones
- Creating and maintaining patient medical records
- Handling billing, bookkeeping, and insurance processing
- Performing medical transcription
- Arranging for hospital admissions

## Advanced Administrative Duties

Your advanced administrative duties may vary according to the practice and may include:

- Developing and conducting public outreach programs to market the physician's professional services
- Negotiating leases of equipment and supply contracts
- Negotiating non-risk and risk managed care contracts
- Managing business and professional insurance
- Developing and maintaining fee schedules
- Participating in practice analysis
- Coordinating plans for practice enhancement, expansion, consolidation, and closure
- Performing as a HIPAA compliance officer
- Providing personnel supervision and employment practices
- Providing information systems management

## Entry-Level Clinical Duties

Your clinical duties may vary according to state law. In an entry-level position, they may include:

- Assisting the doctor during examinations
- Asepsis and infection control
- Performing diagnostic tests, such as spirometry
- Giving injections, where allowed
- Performing electrocardiograms (ECGs)
- Drawing blood for testing
- Disposing of **contaminated** (soiled, or stained) supplies
- Explaining treatment procedures to patients
- Performing first aid and cardiopulmonary resuscitation (CPR)
- Patient education
- Preparing patients for examinations
- Preparing and administering medications as directed by the physician, and following state laws for invasive procedures
- Facilitating treatment for patients from diverse cultural backgrounds and for patients with hearing or vision impairments, or physical or mental disabilities
- Recording vital signs and medical histories
- Removing sutures or changing dressings on wounds
- Sterilizing medical instruments

Other clinical duties may include instructing patients about medication and special diets, authorizing drug refills as directed by the physician, and calling pharmacies to order prescriptions. You may also assist with minor surgery or teach patients about special procedures before laboratory tests, surgery, x-rays, or ECGs.

## Advanced Clinical Duties

As with entry-level clinical duties, your advanced clinical duties may vary according to state law. They may include:

- Initiate an IV and administer IV medications with appropriate training and as permitted by state law

- Report diagnostic study results
- Assist patients in the completion of advanced directives and living wills
- Act as a patient advocate
- Assist with clinical trials

## Entry-Level Laboratory Duties

As an entry-level medical assistant, your laboratory duties may include:

- Performing Clinical Laboratory Improvement Amendments (CLIA)–waived tests, such as a urine pregnancy test, on the premises
- Collecting, preparing, and transmitting laboratory specimens
- Teaching patients to collect specific specimens properly
- Arranging laboratory services
- Meeting safety standards and fire protection mandates

## Advanced Laboratory Duties

As with entry-level laboratory duties, your advanced laboratory duties may vary according to state law. They may include:

- Performing as an Occupational Safety and Health Act (OSHA) compliance officer
- Performing moderately complex laboratory testing with appropriate training and certification

## Specialization

You may also choose to specialize in a specific area of health care. For example, podiatric medical assistants make castings of feet, expose and develop x-rays, and assist podiatrists in surgery. Ophthalmic medical assistants help ophthalmologists (doctors who provide eye care) by administering diagnostic tests, measuring and recording vision, testing the functioning of eyes and eye muscles, and performing other duties. (Chapter 2 fully discusses medical specialties and medical assistant specialties.)

# Personal Qualifications of Medical Assistants

There are several personal qualifications that you must have to be an effective and productive medical assistant. You must enjoy working with all types of people, possess good critical thinking skills, and be able to pay attention to detail. Empathy, willingness to learn, flexibility, self-motivation, professionalism, integrity, and sound judgment are other important traits. Additionally, you must have a neat, professional appearance; possess good communication skills; be able to work in a team environment; and know how to remain calm in a crisis.

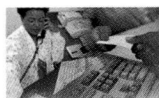
# Recycling in the Medical Office, Hospital, Laboratory, or Clinic

You may easily incorporate recycling procedures into the daily routine of a medical office, hospital, laboratory, or clinic. Medical facilities generate a tremendous amount of recyclable paper material. Recycling may be required by state law. Purchase paper products that can be recycled, or those made of postconsumer recycled materials, and take care in disposing of them. Care should be taken to ensure HIPAA compliance when recycling paper. Shredding is the most effective way to comply with HIPAA regulations.

Some states levy large fines for noncompliance with recycling regulations. It is thus important to have a well-organized office recycling program. There are two essential aspects of recycling: disposal and purchasing. To create a complete recycling program, ensure that materials are disposed of properly and that purchased products have been made from recycled materials.

You may easily call the town's recycling center for guidelines for packaging recycled materials and for a pickup schedule. The recycling center may also provide containers for recyclable materials. You must fulfill all town and state legal recycling requirements.

Most paper products that do not have a glossy coating (like some fax paper) are recyclable. Each recycling center will provide a list of paper materials that can and cannot be recycled.

You must also research disposal techniques for biohazardous materials and follow regulations listed in the office policy manual and OSHA guidelines. These materials cannot be recycled and must be disposed of properly. They must not be mixed with recyclable waste. You will follow the office policy manual and OSHA guidelines for hazardous medical wastes—including blood products, gloves, cotton swabs, body fluids, and sharps (needles or instruments that puncture the skin). These materials must be disposed of following standard guidelines and in a specially designed protective container.

You must keep recycling issues in mind at all times. Always choose products made from recycled materials—including paper (computer paper and letterhead), printer cartridges, pencils, and many other products.

## Critical Thinking Skills

You will develop critical thinking skills over time, as you apply knowledge about and experience with human nature, medicine, and office administration to new situations. Critical thinking skills include quickly evaluating circumstances, solving problems, and taking action.

Critical thinking skills are used every day. One example is prioritizing your work—deciding which are the most important tasks of the day and which are less important. On a day where everything seems to be "top priority," you must use your professional judgment, knowledge of office policies, and experience with physicians and coworkers to determine what should get done first, second, third, and so on.

You must use critical thinking skills to assess how to react to emergency situations. If you see a patient suddenly pass out in the physician's waiting room, you must quickly see that the patient receives first aid, notify a physician, and alert the patient's family.

## Attention to Detail

The profession of medical assisting requires attention to detail. You must check every detail when administering drugs, processing bills and insurance forms, and completing patient charts.

The need for attention to detail is illustrated in the common request to call a patient's pharmacy to order a prescription. You must accurately relay information from the doctor's prescription to the pharmacist. You must ask the pharmacist to read back the information to ensure that he has heard it correctly. Then you must document, in the chart, what has been ordered and when.

## Empathy

Empathy is the ability to "put yourself in someone else's shoes" and to identify with and understand another person's feelings. Patients who are ill, frustrated, or frightened appreciate empathic medical personnel.

Patients require empathy during all medical situations. For example, a patient with the flu may describe how coughing has prevented him from getting a full night's sleep. You may display empathy by saying, "I know how the flu can disrupt sleep. I just got over it last week myself. It's important to rest in bed, though, even if you can't always sleep."

## Willingness to Learn

You must always display a willingness to learn. You will gain new skills more easily and become better acquainted with the administrative and clinical topics and issues related to the practice in which you work if you are willing to learn. Keep an open mind, listen carefully to the professionals with whom you work, observe procedures carefully, listen actively to others, and do your own homework to

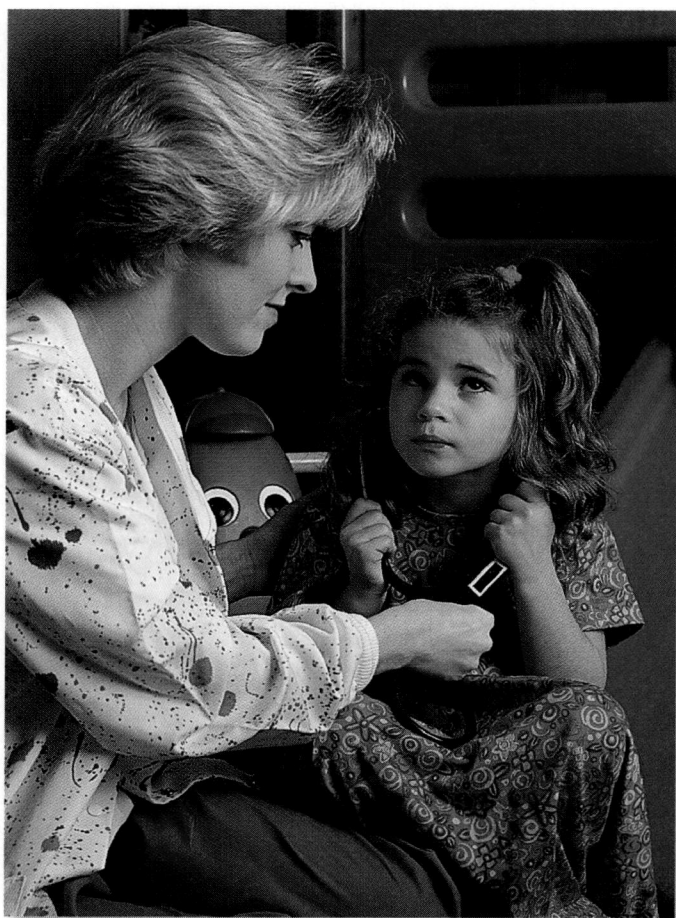

**Figure 1-3.** A medical assistant who works part-time in a pediatric practice might volunteer one day a week at a preschool to learn more about working with children.

learn more about medical topics so you can apply new information to your daily activities. For example, if you work in a pediatric practice, you might take a continuing education class on child development at a local community college, at a YWCA, or in a workshop offered by a professional association such as the AAMA or AMT (Figure 1-3).

## Flexibility

You will encounter new people and situations every day. An attitude of flexibility will allow you to adapt and to handle them with professionalism.

An example of the need for flexibility occurs when a physician's schedule changes to include evening and weekend hours. The staff may also be asked to change schedules. You must make it a priority to be flexible and to meet the employer's needs.

## Self-Motivation

You must be self-motivated and willing to offer assistance with work that needs to be done, even if it is not your assigned job. For example, if you think of a more

efficient way to organize patient check-in, discuss it with your supervisor. She/he may agree and be willing to give your idea a try. If a coworker is on vacation, offer to pitch in and work extra time to keep the office running smoothly.

## Professionalism

You should exhibit courtesy, conscientiousness, and a generally businesslike manner at all times on the job. It is important to act professionally with coworkers, patients, doctors, and others in the work setting. You are an agent of your employer—you represent the doctor or doctors in the practice.

One example of professional behavior includes treating all patients with dignity and kindness. Another is making sure that you have completed and documented all your daily duties before leaving work at the end of each day.

You can start acting like a professional even while you are in the classroom studying to become a medical assistant. Presenting a neat appearance, showing courtesy and respect for peers and instructors, having a good attendance record, and arriving on time to class are all important elements that contribute to professionalism in school and in the workplace.

## Neat Appearance

A medical professional always strives to maintain a neat appearance in the workplace. Personal cleanliness is an important part of maintaining a neat appearance. Your appearance is your first impression to your patients, coworkers, and the physicians you work with. Medical facilities and staff are considered "conservative" work environments. Your appearance should reflect a conservative style. Listed here are a few professional guidelines to follow in the medical environment:

- Your uniforms should be clean, pressed crisply, and in good repair. Your uniform should fit your body type and should not be too large or too small.
- Your shoes should be comfortable, white, clean, and in good condition. Laces should be white and clean. Avoid athletic-looking shoes. Polish your shoes on a daily basis. Only leather shoes that are not open are permitted in a patient treatment area.
- Choose a hairstyle that is flattering and conservative.
- Hair should be clean and pulled back from your face and off your collar if long. Natural colors for hair are the only acceptable color in a medical environment.
- Your nails should be a short working length, no more than one-fourth inch. Nail polish should be pale or clear. A French manicure is acceptable. Acrylic nails should be avoided. Many medical facilities are banning acrylic nails because they pose a risk for infection.
- Avoid heavy perfumes and colognes. Many patients and coworkers could be allergic to perfume and cologne.

- Jewelry should be kept to a minimum and in good taste. No more than one ring should be worn. Rings may tear through latex gloves. Ears can be pierced with one hole, and small earrings are appropriate. Any earrings that dangle can be torn off by a patient, such as pediatric patients. Males should not wear earrings in the medical environment.
- Tattoos should never be in a location where they can be seen by a patient.
- Body piercing and tongue piercing is not acceptable in a medical environment. Patients may view this as a visual threat and question your level of competence. Many physicians will rule you out on the first interview if a body piercing (other than ears) is present.
- Bathe or shower daily and use an antiperspirant.
- Brush your teeth at least twice daily and schedule regular dental visits to maintain oral health and hygiene.
- Schedule regular checkups with your personal physician.
- Get plenty of rest and eat a well-balanced diet.
- If you are not required to wear a uniform, choose clothing that is conservative and business-appropriate. Avoid fad fashions. Wear low-heeled or flat, polished shoes and a lab coat if working with patients.

Some activities may make it difficult to maintain a neat appearance—replacing the toner in the copy machine, for example, or filling the developing solution in the x-ray machine. Always store a spare uniform or business outfit at your workplace.

## Attitude

Your attitude will leave an impression of the type of person you are. In the medical environment, many people depend on you, including coworkers and patients. Your attitude can make or break your career. Professionals always project a positive, caring attitude. They respond to criticism as a learning experience. They take direction from authority without question. They function as a vital member of a medical team. A negative attitude will not be acceptable in a team-oriented medical environment. Many people do not know they have a negative attitude. Ask yourself these questions, and determine if you need to make improvements in your attitude before you begin your new career.

- Do I have repeated conflict with friends or family?
- Have I had a conflict at work that has resulted in voluntary or involuntary termination?
- Do I have conflict with authority figures, such as my instructors?
- Do people make comments about my attitude?

In the workplace environment, professional medical assistants are pleasant, smiling, and conducting themselves in a businesslike and professional manner.

## Integrity and Honesty

People with integrity hold themselves to high standards. Everything they do, every task they complete, is performed with a goal of excellence. Individuals with integrity take extreme pride in everything they do. The characteristics of integrity are honesty, dependability, and reliability. Integrity and honesty are key in providing superior customer service to your patients. You must follow through on everything you say you are going to do. For example, if you tell a patient that you are going to return their call regarding a medication, you must call the patient at the time you indicated. Professionals with integrity are honest with the staff and physicians they work with. If you make an error, be honest about it. In order to have integrity, you must be dependable and reliable. Your office staff and physician must be able to trust you and the decisions you make.

## Diplomacy

Diplomacy is the ability to communicate with patients, coworkers, managers, and physicians in a manner that is not offensive and that both expresses and inspires cooperation. Communicating with diplomacy is communicating with tact. Medical assistants are often exposed to situations that they may not agree with. A professional has the ability to look at both sides of a situation and to handle it with courtesy and professionalism.

## Proper Judgment

You should demonstrate proper judgment in every task. Before making an important decision, you must carefully evaluate each possible outcome.

An example of a situation that requires proper judgment is assessing when an exception should be made in a doctor's schedule of patients. Suppose the next patient on the schedule is in the waiting room. She is having a routine checkup. An unscheduled patient comes in with chest pains. You use proper judgment and allow the patient with chest pains to see the doctor first.

## Communication Skills

Effective communication involves careful listening, observing, speaking, and writing. Communication even involves good manners—being polite, tactful, and respectful. You must use good communication skills during every patient discussion and in every interaction you have with physicians, other staff members, and other professionals with whom your practice does business. (Chapter 4 discusses communication skills.)

## Remaining Calm in a Crisis

There is always the potential for a crisis or emergency in the health-care field. During a crisis you must remain calm and be prepared to handle any situation.

An example of the need for calm and effective action occurs when a patient appears to suffer a stroke while sitting in the waiting room of a busy medical office. You must quickly direct your peers to alert the doctor and remove the other patients from the room while you begin emergency first-aid measures.

## Willingness to Work as a Team Member

Working with and as a member of the health-care team is critical for the overall efficiency of the medical facility. Everyone in the facility has an important job that depends on someone else. It is important to remember that the patient comes first and *everyone* is responsible for the care of that patient. Team dynamics consists of:

- Assisting each other on a daily basis with the duties required
- Avoiding interpersonal conflict with members of the team
- Performing extra responsibilities without questioning or complaining
- Being considerate of all other team members' duties and responsibilities

## Ethical Behavior

Ethics is a system of values that determines right or wrong behavior. Our standard of values is learned by our life experiences. Ethical behavior can have a strong, positive impact on the profession of medical assisting and on the overall reputation of medical assistants in the health-care community. Your professional ethics will involve your relationship with patients and families, your relationship with other allied health professionals, and facilities and your community as a whole. The AAMA Code of Ethics is designed to elevate the profession of medical assisting to a profession of dignity and respect.

## The AAMA Role Delineation Study

In 1996 the AAMA formed a committee whose goal was to revise and update its standards for the accreditation of programs that teach medical assisting. The committee's findings were published in 1997 as the "AAMA Role Delineation Study: Occupational Analysis of the Medical Assisting Profession." The study included a new Role Delineation Chart that outlines the areas of competence you must master as an entry-level medical assistant. The Role Delineation Chart was further updated in 2003 to include additional competencies.

## Areas of Competence

The Medical Assistant Role Delineation Chart, shown in Appendix I, provides the basis for medical assisting education and evaluation. Mastery of the areas of competence listed in this chart is required for all students in accredited medical assisting programs. The chart shows three areas of competence: administrative, clinical, and general. Each of these three areas is divided into two or more narrower areas, for a total of ten specific areas of competence. Within each area, a bulleted list of statements describes the medical assistant's role.

## Uses of the Role Delineation Chart

According to the AAMA, the Role Delineation Chart may be used to:

- Describe the field of medical assisting to other health-care professionals
- Identify entry-level areas of competence for medical assistants
- Help practitioners assess their own current competence in the field
- Aid in the development of continuing education programs
- Prepare appropriate types of materials for home study

## Scope of Practice

Medical assistants are not "licensed" health-care professionals and most often work under another licensed health-care provider, such as a nurse or physician. Licensed health-care professionals may delegate certain duties to a medical assistant, providing she or he has had the appropriate training through an accredited medical assisting program or through on-the-job training provided by the medical facility or physician. Questions often arise regarding the kinds of duties a medical assistant can perform, such as:

- What kinds of clinical duties can a medical assistant lawfully perform?
- Is a medical assistant permitted to start an IV?
- Can a medical assistant run lab tests? If so, which tests are allowed?

There is no universal answer to any of the above questions. There is no single national definition of a medical assistant's scope of practice. Therefore, the medical assistant must research the state in which he or she works to learn about the scope of practice in his or her state. In general, a medical assistant may not perform procedures for which he or she was not educated or trained. The AAMA and AMT are good resources to assist you in your research. The AAMA Role Delineation Chart is also a good reference source that identifies the procedures that medical assistants are educated to perform.

## Summary

There are many kinds of on-the-job training, training programs, and careers for medical assistants. As you make the decision to become a medical assistant, you must evaluate your skills and the type of position you would like to obtain. An important goal will be to obtain a real-life view of the medical assistant's daily administrative, clinical, and laboratory duties. These skills and duties are outlined under the areas of competence listed in the AAMA Role Delineation Chart.

You must also research how to obtain on-the-job training or choose a training program that will adequately teach you those skills, how to conduct a job search, and whether or not to become a certified or registered medical assistant, and take advantage of the benefits of membership in medical assisting organizations such as the AAMA.

Additionally, you must be aware that the medical assisting profession will continue to change. You will need to stay abreast of changes in technology, procedures, and local, state, and federal regulations governing the way you perform daily duties.

# REVIEW

## CASE STUDY QUESTIONS

Now that you have completed this chapter, review the case study at the beginning of the chapter and answer the following questions:

1. How are the three jobs different?
2. How are the three jobs the same?
3. How do these three medical assistants function as multiskilled health-care professionals?

## Discussion Questions

1. Why are more employers recruiting credentialed medical assistants?
2. Explain the importance of continuing education for medical assistants.
3. What is the purpose of the AAMA Role Delineation Chart?
4. Discuss why volunteer work will enhance a medical assistant's career.

## Critical Thinking Questions

1. Describe an effective medical assistant, and explain two ways a new medical assistant may learn to be an efficient and effective employee.
2. How will the "aging boom" affect health care and the profession of medical assisting in the future?
3. What is a self-directed, lifelong learner? How can a medical assistant achieve this goal?
4. Why is it important to stay current on changes in technology and health care?

## Application Activities

1. With a partner, pick one of the following two situations. Without showing your partner, write a description of how you would display the personal attribute stated at the end of the scenario. After you and your partner have written your descriptions, compare them with each other.

Patient Situation

*Patient says: "I have such a horrible headache. I've been feeling tired lately too."*

Attribute You Wish to Display

*Empathy*

Patient Situation

*Doctor: "I'm really backed up on paperwork. Could you come in an hour early tomorrow morning to help me organize it? You will be paid for the overtime."*

Attribute You Wish to Display

*Flexibility*

2. Chose a mentor who displays the personal attributes listed in this chapter and write a few sentences to explain why these attributes apply to her or him.
3. A. Think of all the personal qualifications you possess. List those that will help you as a medical assistant.
   B. List all of the personal qualifications you need to develop or improve in order to work successfully in the career of medical assisting.
   C. Describe the actions you will take to acquire the personal qualifications to become a multiskilled medical assistant.

## Virtual Fieldtrip

*Visit the McGraw-Hill Higher Education Medical Assisting website at www.mhhe.com/medicalassisting3 to complete the following activity:*

Prepare an oral presentation regarding topics such as certification examinations, scope of practice, or accreditation agencies such as ABHES or CAAHEP. Prepare a report using a specified number of references and citations and present your report to the class. Schedule the presentations throughout the course and use available multimedia, such as PowerPoint slides or an overhead projector for the student presentations. Visit the websites of The American Association of Medical Assistants or American Medical Technologists for possible report topics.

Open the CD and complete this chapter's practice activities, play the games, listen to the key terms, and test yourself with the interactive review. E-mail, print, and/or save your results to document your proficiency.

## CHAPTER 2

# Types of Medical Practice

## MEDICAL ASSISTING COMPETENCIES

*In preparation for the certification examination, you should know the following areas of competence:*

| COMPETENCY | CMA | RMA |
|---|---|---|
| **General/Legal/Professional** | | |
| Be aware of and perform within legal and ethical boundaries | X | X |
| Conduct work within scope of education, training, and ability | | X |
| Serve as a liaison between the physician and others | | X |
| Understand allied health professions and credentialing | | X |

## CHAPTER OUTLINE

- Medical Specialties
- Working With Other Allied Health Professionals
- Specialty Career Options
- Professional Associations

## LEARNING OUTCOMES

After completing Chapter 2, you will be able to:

2.1 Describe medical specialties and specialists.
2.2 Explain the purpose of the American Board of Medical Specialties.
2.3 Describe the duties of several types of allied health professionals with whom medical assistants may work.
2.4 Name professional associations that may help advance a medical assistant's career.

## Introduction

Medical assistants are an integral part of a health-care delivery team. It is important to recognize the many different physician specialists and allied health professions. Medical assistants are often asked to call and process insurance referrals to different specialties and diagnostic departments. Therefore, a working knowledge of the different specialties and allied health professionals demonstrates professionalism and competence.

## KEY TERMS

- acupuncturist
- allergist
- anesthetist
- autopsy
- biopsy
- cardiologist
- chiropractor
- dermatologist
- doctor of osteopathy
- endocrinologist
- family practitioner
- gastroenterologist
- gerontologist
- gynecologist
- internist
- massage therapist
- nephrologist
- neurologist
- oncologist
- orthopedist
- osteopathic manipulative medicine (OMM)
- otorhinolaryngologist
- pathologist
- pediatrician
- physiatrist
- physician assistant (PA)
- plastic surgeon
- podiatrist
- primary care physician
- proctologist
- radiologist
- surgeon
- triage
- urologist

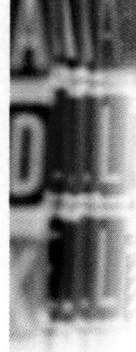

## CASE STUDY

Susan has worked as a medical assistant for 12 years. She is considering furthering her educational background in a different allied health profession. She has a strong interest in nursing and in the laboratory.

As you read this chapter, consider the following questions:

1. What are Susan's career options in nursing? How much further education would she need in order to become a nurse?
2. What are Susan's career options in a laboratory setting? How much further education would she need in order to work in a laboratory?

# Medical Specialties

Since the beginning of the 20th century, some physicians have specialized in particular areas of study. There are now approximately 22 major medical specialties. Within each specialty are several subspecialties. For example, cardiology is a major specialty; pediatric cardiology is a subspecialty. As advances in the diagnosis and treatment of diseases and disorders unfold, the demand for specialized care increases and more medical specialties emerge.

If you graduate from an accredited medical assisting program, you will be well equipped to work with a physician specialist. If you work in the office of a physician specialist, you must continue to learn all the new skills that apply to that specialty. First, however, it is helpful to understand the education and licensing process any medical doctor must undergo to become a board-certified physician.

## Physician Education and Licensure

The educational requirements for physicians are rigorous and take several years to complete. To earn the title MD (doctor of medicine), thereby qualifying as a licensed physician, a student must complete a bachelor's degree with a concentration typically in the sciences. Then she must attend a medical school accredited by the Liaison Committee on Medical Education (LCME). Upon completing medical school, she is awarded the degree of MD, but this is not the end of her required medical training. She must also pass the U.S. Medical Licensing Examination (USMLE). This examination, commonly known as medical boards, has three parts. Part 1 is usually taken after the second year of medical school, part 2 during the fourth year of medical school, and part 3 during the first or second year of postgraduate medical training.

After medical school an MD begins a residency—a period of practical training in a hospital. The first year of residency is known as an internship. Once it is completed an MD can become certified by the National Board of Medical Examiners (NBME). After completing an internship and passing her medical boards, the MD becomes certified as an NBME Diplomate. If she wishes to specialize in a particular branch of medicine, she must complete an additional 2 to 6 years of residency. She also will apply to the American Board of Medical Specialties (ABMS) to take an examination in her specialty area. After passing the examination, she will be board-certified in her area of specialization. For example, a physician who specializes in pediatrics would receive certification from the American Board of Pediatrics.

The ABMS is an organization of many different medical specialty boards. Its primary purpose is to maintain and improve the quality of medical care and to certify doctors in various specialties. This organization helps the member boards develop professional and educational standards for physician specialists.

## Family Practice

**Family practitioners** (sometimes called general practitioners) are MDs or DOs who are generalists and treat all types of illnesses and ages of patients. They do not specialize in a particular branch of medicine. Many patients seek medical care from a family practitioner and may never have visited a medical specialist. Family practitioners are called **primary care physicians** by insurance companies. The term refers to individual doctors who oversee patients' long-term health care. Some people, however, have internists or OB/GYNs as their primary care physician.

A family practitioner sends a patient to a specialist when the patient has a specific condition or disease that requires advanced care. For example, a family practitioner refers a patient with a lump in her breast to an **oncologist,** a specialist who treats tumors, or to a general surgeon. Either of these doctors may order a mammogram or perform a needle biopsy of the lump to determine if it is malignant.

If you work in a general practice, you will encounter patients with many different conditions and illnesses. As in any medical setting, you must become knowledgeable about preventing the transmission of viruses. This important topic is discussed in several parts of this book.

If you work for a general practitioner, you will often be responsible for arranging patient appointments with specialists. It is important, therefore, for you to know about the duties of each medical specialist. One or more of these specialties may interest you, and you may decide to seek a position as a medical assistant for a physician in that specialty.

## Allergy

**Allergists** diagnose and treat physical reactions to substances, including mold, dust, fur, and pollen from plants or flowers. An individual with allergies is hypersensitive to substances such as drugs, chemicals, or elements in nature. An allergic reaction may be minor, such as a rash; serious, such as asthma; or life-threatening, such as swelling of the airways or nasal passages.

## Anesthesiology

**Anesthetists** use medications that cause patients to lose sensation or feeling during surgery. These health-care practitioners administer anesthetics before and during surgery. They also educate patients regarding the anesthetic that will be used and its possible postoperative effects. An anesthesiologist is an MD. A certified registered nurse anesthetist (CRNA) is a registered nurse who has completed an additional program of study recognized by the American Association of Nurse Anesthetists.

## Bariatrics

Bariatrics is the specialty of medicine that deals with the medical and surgical treatment of obesity. Specialists in surgical bariatrics are called bariatric surgeons. Bariatric surgery may be recommended for extremely obese patients who may suffer impaired health as a result of their weight. There are several options available in bariatric surgery, such as gastric banding and gastric bypass.

## Cardiology

**Cardiologists** diagnose and treat cardiovascular diseases (diseases of the heart and blood vessels). Cardiologists also read electrocardiograms (ECGs, which are sometimes referred to as EKGs) for hospital laboratories. They educate patients about the positive role healthy diet and regular exercise play in preventing and controlling heart disease.

## Dermatology

**Dermatologists** diagnose and treat diseases of the skin, hair, and nails. Their patients have conditions ranging from warts and acne to skin cancer. Dermatologists treat boils, skin injuries, and infections. They remove growths—such as moles, cysts, and birthmarks—and they treat scars and perform hair transplants.

## Doctor of Osteopathy

**Doctors of osteopathy,** who hold the title of DO, practice a "whole-person" approach to health care. DOs feel that patients are more than just a sum of their body parts, and they treat the patient as a whole person instead of concentrating on specific symptoms. Osteopathic physicians understand how all the body's systems are interconnected and how each one affects the other. They focus special attention on the musculoskeletal system, which reflects and influences the condition of all other body systems.

One key concept that DOs believe is that structure influences function. If a problem exists in one part of the body, it may affect the function in both that area and other areas. DOs focus on the body's ability to heal itself and they actively engage patients in the healing process. By using **osteopathic manipulative medicine (OMM)** techniques, DOs can help restore motion to these areas of the body, thus improving function and often restoring health.

## Emergency Medicine

Physicians who specialize in emergency medicine work in hospital emergency rooms and outpatient emergency care centers. They diagnose and treat patients with conditions resulting from an unexpected medical crisis or accident. Common emergencies include trauma, such as gunshot wounds or serious injuries from car accidents; other injuries, such as severe cuts; and sudden illness, such as alcohol or food poisoning.

## Endocrinology

**Endocrinologists** diagnose and treat disorders of the endocrine system. This system regulates many body functions by circulating hormones that are secreted by glands throughout the body. An example of a disorder treated by an endocrinologist is hyperthyroidism, an abnormality of the thyroid gland. Symptoms include weight loss, shakiness, and weakness.

## Gastroenterology

**Gastroenterologists** diagnose and treat disorders of the gastrointestinal tract. These disorders include problems related to the functioning of the stomach, intestines, and associated organs.

## Gerontology

**Gerontologists** study the aging process. Geriatrics is the branch of medicine that deals with the diagnosis and treatment of problems and diseases of the older adult. A specialist in geriatrics may also be called a geriatrician. As the population of older adults continues to increase, there will be greater need for physicians who specialize in diagnosing and treating diseases of the elderly.

## Gynecology

Gynecology is the branch of medicine that is concerned with diseases of the female genital tract. **Gynecologists** perform routine physical care and examination of the female reproductive system. Many gynecologists are also obstetricians.

## Internal Medicine

**Internists** specialize in diagnosing and treating problems related to the internal organs. The internal medicine subspecialties include cardiology, critical care medicine, diagnostic laboratory immunology, endocrinology and metabolism, gastroenterology, geriatrics, hematology, infectious diseases, medical oncology, nephrology, pulmonary disease, and rheumatology. Internists must be certified as specialists in these areas.

## Nephrology

**Nephrologists** study, diagnose, and manage diseases of the kidney. They may work in either a clinic or hospital setting. A medical assistant working with a nephrologist may assist in the operation of a dialysis unit for the treatment of patients with kidney disease. In a rural setting a medical assistant might help a doctor operate a mobile dialysis unit that can be taken to the patient's home or to a medical practice that does not have this technology.

## Neurology

Neurology is the branch of medical science that deals with the nervous system. **Neurologists** diagnose and treat disorders and diseases of the nervous system, such as strokes. The nervous system is made up of the brain, spinal cord, and nerves that receive, interpret, and transmit messages throughout the body.

## Nuclear Medicine

Nuclear medicine is a fast-growing specialty related to radiology. Both fields use radiation to diagnose and treat disease, but radiology beams radiation through the body from an outside source, whereas nuclear medicine introduces a small amount of a radioactive substance into the body and forms an image by detecting radiation as it leaves the body. The radiation that patients are exposed to is comparable to that of a diagnostic x-ray. Radiology reveals interior anatomy whereas nuclear medicine reveals organ function and structure. Noninvasive, painless nuclear medicine procedures are used to identify heart disease, assess organ function, and diagnose and treat cancer.

## Obstetrics

Obstetrics involves the study of pregnancy, labor, delivery, and the period following labor called postpartum (Figure 2-1). This field is often combined with gynecology.

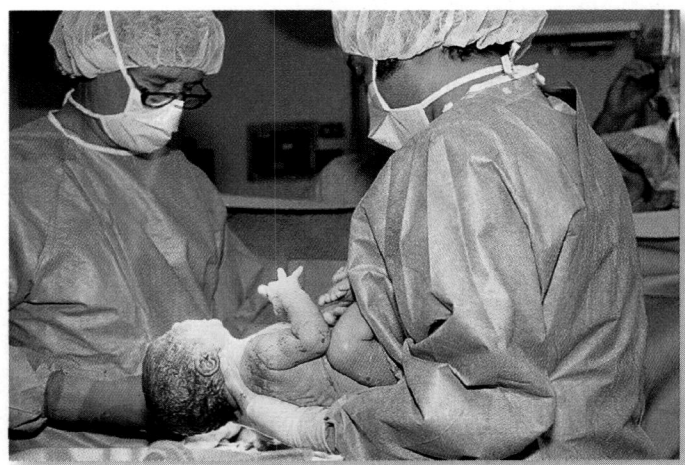

**Figure 2-1.** Obstetricians who are part of a private practice are usually connected with a specific hospital where they help their patients through labor and delivery.

A physician who practices both specialties is referred to as an obstetrician/gynecologist, or OB/GYN.

## Oncology

Oncologists, as stated earlier in the chapter, identify tumors, determine if they are benign or malignant, and treat patients with cancer. Treatment may involve chemotherapy, which is the administration of drugs to destroy cancer cells. Treatment may also involve radiation therapy, which kills cancer cells through the use of x-rays. Oncologists treat both adults and children.

## Ophthalmology

An ophthalmologist is an MD who diagnoses and treats diseases and disorders of the eye. This physician specialist examines patients' eyes for poor vision or disease. Other responsibilities include prescribing corrective lenses or medication, performing surgery, and providing follow-up care after surgery. (Ophthalmologists are sometimes confused with optometrists, but the latter are not MDs; optometrists are doctors of optometry. Optometrists perform eye exams to determine the general health of the eye and to prescribe corrective eyeglasses or contact lenses.)

## Orthopedics

Orthopedics is a branch of surgery that works to maintain function of the musculoskeletal system and its associated structures. An **orthopedist** diagnoses and treats diseases and disorders of the muscles and bones. Some orthopedists concentrate on treating sports-related injuries, either exclusively for professional athletes or for nonprofessionals of all ages. They are called sports medicine specialists.

# Otorhinolaryngology

Otorhinolaryngology involves the study of the ear, nose, and throat. An **otorhinolaryngologist** diagnoses and treats diseases of these body structures. This physician specialist is also referred to as an ear, nose, and throat (ENT) specialist.

# Pathology

Pathology is the study of disease. It provides the scientific foundation for all medical practice. The **pathologist** studies the changes a disease produces in the cells, fluids, and processes of the entire body (sometimes by performing **autopsies,** examinations of the bodies of the deceased) to advance the clinical practice of medicine.

There are two basic types of pathologists. Governments and police departments use forensic pathologists to determine facts about unexplained or violent deaths. Anatomic pathologists often work at hospitals in a research capacity, and they may read **biopsies** (samplings of cells that could be malignant).

# Pediatrics and Adolescent Medicine

Pediatrics is concerned with the development and care of children from birth until 18 years and the diseases of children and adolescents. A **pediatrician** diagnoses and treats childhood diseases and teaches parents skills to keep their children healthy.

# Physical Medicine

Physical medicine specialists **(physiatrists)** are physicians who specialize in physical medicine and rehabilitation. They are certified by the American Board of Physical Medicine and Rehabilitation to diagnose and treat diseases and disorders such as sore shoulders and spinal cord injuries. Physiatrists offer an aggressive, nonsurgical approach to pain and injury. Physical medicine specialists' patients include both adults and children.

# Podiatry

Podiatry is practiced by a licensed doctor of podiatric medicine (D.P.M.). A **podiatrist** is a podiatry professional devoted to the study and treatment of the foot and ankle. A podiatrist's education consists of an undergraduate degree plus a doctoral level 4-year program followed by a 2- or 3-year residency. Podiatrists may independently diagnose, treat, prescribe medication, and perform surgery for disorders of the foot and, in some states, the ankle and leg. There are three board certification possibilities for podiatrists. The Board of Primary Care and Orthopedics is a nonsurgical Board Certification. The Surgical Board of Certification is divided into foot surgery and rear foot and ankle reconstruction surgery. The rear foot and ankle

Board Certification requires at least a 3-year residency to qualify.

# Plastic Surgery

A **plastic surgeon** performs the reconstruction, correction, or improvement of body structures. Patients may be accident victims or disfigured due to disease or abnormal development. Plastic surgery includes facial reconstruction, face-lifts, and skin grafting. Plastic surgery is also used to repair problems like cleft lip and cleft palate.

# Proctology

Proctology is the branch of medicine that diagnoses and treats disorders of the anus, rectum, and intestines. **Proctologists** treat conditions such as colitis, hemorrhoids, fistulas, tumors, and ulcers. Proctologists often work closely with urologists.

# Radiology

Radiology is the branch of medical science that uses x-rays and radioactive substances to diagnose and treat disease. **Radiologists** specialize in taking and reading x-rays.

# Sports Medicine

Sports medicine is an interdisciplinary subspecialty of medicine that deals with the treatment and preventative care of amateur and professional athletes. Sports medicine teams consist of specialty physicians and surgeons, athletic trainers, and physical therapists. Sports medicine is more than treating injuries to the musculoskeletal system. Sports medicine can include an array of treatments, such as prevention and nutritional health. Sports medicine was recognized by the American Board of Medical Specialties in 1989 and continues to grow today.

# Surgery

**Surgeons** use their hands and medical instruments to diagnose and correct deformities and treat external and internal injuries or disease (Figure 2-2). They work with many different specialists to surgically treat a broad range of disorders. General surgeons may, for example, perform operations as diverse as breast lumpectomy and repair of a pacemaker. There are also subspecialties of surgery, such as neurosurgery, vascular surgery, and orthopedic surgery.

# Urology

A **urologist** diagnoses and treats diseases of the kidney, bladder, and urinary system. A urologist's patients include infants, children, and adults of all ages. Urologists also treat male reproductive diseases.

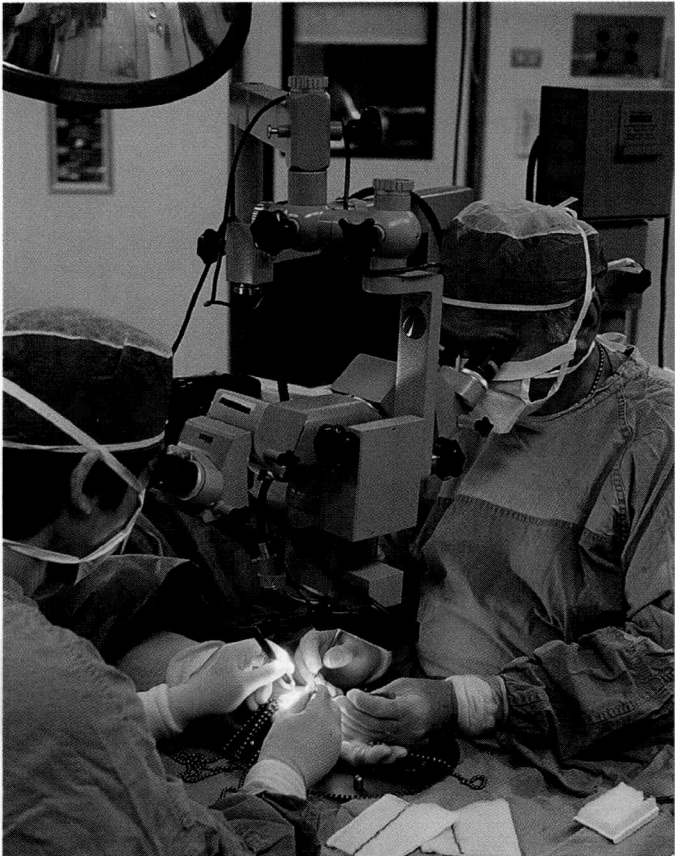

**Figure 2-2.** Most surgeons specialize in a particular type of surgery, such as heart surgery or hand surgery.

# Working With Other Allied Health Professionals

You will always work as a member of a health-care team. That health-care team will include doctors, nurses, specialists, and the patients themselves. You must know the duties of the other allied health professionals in your workplace. Even if you do not work with other allied health professionals in the office, you may contact them through correspondence or by telephone. Understanding the duties of other health-care team members will help make you a more effective medical assistant.

## Acupuncturist

**Acupuncturists** treat people with pain or discomfort by inserting thin, hollow needles under the skin. The points used for insertion are selected to balance the flow of *qi*, or life energy, in the body. The theory of acupuncture relates to Chinese beliefs about how the body works. Qi is composed of two opposite forces called yin and yang. If the flow of qi is unbalanced, insufficient, or interrupted, then emotional, spiritual, mental, and physical problems will result. The acupuncturist works to balance these two

forces in perfect harmony. Although there are variations in types of acupuncture—Chinese, Korean, and Japanese—all practitioners will focus on many pulse points along different meridians, the channels through which qi flows.

## Chiropractor

**Chiropractors** treat people who are ill or in pain without using drugs or surgery. They primarily use manual treatments, although they may also employ physical therapy treatments, exercise programs, nutritional advice, and lifestyle modification to help correct the problem causing the pain. The manual treatments, called adjustments, realign the vertebrae in the spine and restore the function of spinal nerves. Chiropractors use diagnostic testing such as x-rays, muscle testing, and posture analysis to determine the location of spinal misalignments, also called *subluxations.* They then develop a treatment plan based on these findings. The treatment plan generally requires several adjustments per week for several weeks or months. Because the treatment does not involve drugs or surgery, the body needs time for healing and correction to occur.

## Electroencephalographic Technologist

Electroencephalography (EEG) is the study and recording of the electrical activity of the brain. It is used to diagnose diseases and irregularities of the brain. The EEG technologist (sometimes called a technician) attaches electrodes to the patient's scalp and connects them to a recording instrument. The machine then provides a written record of the electrical activity of the patient's brain. EEG technologists work in hospital EEG laboratories, clinics, and physicians' offices.

## Electrocardiograph Technician

The electrocardiograph (ECG/EKG) technician is a trained professional who operates an electrocardiograph machine, as pictured in Figure 2-3. An ECG records the electrical impulses reaching the heart muscles. Physicians and cardiologists use the readings from this machine to detect heart abnormalities and to monitor patients with known cardiac problems. Electrocardiograph technicians work in hospitals.

## Massage Therapist

**Massage therapists** use pressure, kneading, stroking, vibration, and tapping to promote muscle and full-body relaxation as well as to increase circulation and lymph flow. Increasing circulation helps remove blood and waste products from injured tissues and brings fresh blood and nutrients to the areas to speed healing. Massage is one of the oldest methods of promoting healing and is used to treat strains, bruises, muscle soreness or tightness, lower back pain, and dislocations. It can also relieve muscle

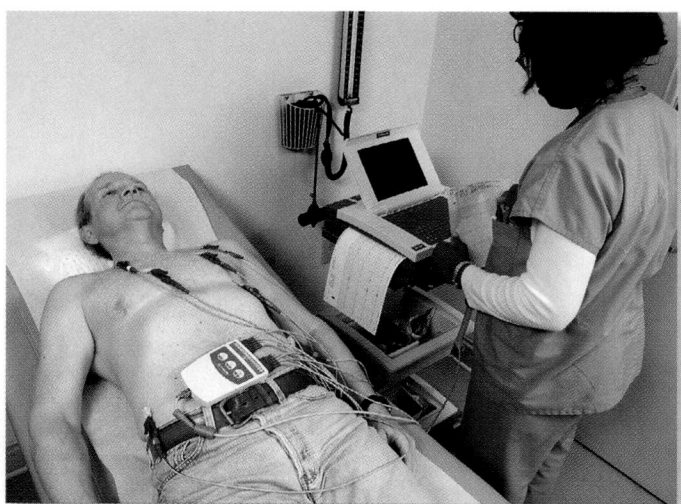

**Figure 2-3.** The electrocardiograph (ECG) technician is responsible for operating an electrocardiograph machine, which detects heart abnormalities and monitors patients with cardiac problems.

spasm, restore motion and function to a body part, and decrease edema.

## Medical Administrative Assistant

A medical administrative assistant assists medical, professional, and technical personnel by providing administrative support. These functions include transcribing dictation and composing correspondence. A medical administrative assistant should also be familiar with application software, such as Microsoft Office. Other functions include maintaining medical and administrative files. A medical administrative specialist may work in a hospital, nursing home, physician's office, or clinic.

## Medical Billing and Coding

Professional medical billers and coders are in very high demand. They perform duties that encompass a wide variety of skills. Medical billers are very knowledgeable in health insurance products offered to patients. They perform a variety of functions, including:

- Reviewing patient insurance coverage
- Educating patients regarding their insurance coverage
- Estimating insurance reimbursement for procedures
- Preparing accurate health-care claims
- Preparing bills and statements
- Working with collection agencies

Medical coders are responsible for abstracting medical information from patient records. They assign a nationally recognized numeric code that correlates to procedures and diagnoses to reimbursement documents such as an HCFA-1500 claim form. A physician will depend on medical codes to accurately code and prepare claim forms. Accu-

rate forms maximize reimbursement and help to ensure ethical standards in medical billing and coding.

## Medical Records Technologist

There are two types of medical records technologists: the Registered Records Administrator (RRA) and the Accredited Records Technician (ART). These technologists are responsible for organizing, analyzing, and evaluating medical records. Other responsibilities include compiling administrative and health statistics, coding symptoms, and inputting and retrieving computerized health data. These positions involve typing medical reports, preparing statistical reports on patient treatments, and supervising clerical personnel in the medical records department. Accredited records technicians and registered records administrators work in hospitals, nursing homes, health maintenance organizations, physicians' offices, and government agencies.

## Medical Technology

*Medical technology* is an umbrella term that refers to the development and design of clinical laboratory tests (such as diagnostic tests), procedures, and equipment. Two types of allied health professionals who work in medical technology are the clinical laboratory technician and the medical technologist.

**Clinical Laboratory Technician.** Clinical laboratory technicians (CLTs) have 1- to 2-year degrees and are responsible for clinical tests performed under the supervision of a physician or medical technologist. They perform tests in the areas of hematology, serology, blood banking, urinalysis, microbiology, and clinical chemistry. Clinical laboratory technicians work in hospital laboratories, commercial laboratories, medical clinics, and physicians' offices.

**Medical Technologist.** Medical technologists perform laboratory tests and procedures with clinical laboratory equipment. They examine specimens of human body tissues and fluids, analyze blood factors, and culture bacteria to identify disease-causing organisms. They also supervise and train technicians and laboratory aides. Medical technologists have 4-year degrees and may specialize in areas such as blood banking, microbiology, and chemistry. These technologists are employed in clinics, hospitals, private practices, colleges, pharmaceutical companies, government, research, and industry.

## Medical Transcriptionist

Medical transcriptionists translate a physician's dictation about patient treatments into comprehensive, typed records. Attorneys, insurance companies, and medical specialists need accurate medical records. Medical transcriptionists work in doctors' offices, hospitals, clinics, laboratories, and radiology departments and for medical transcription services and insurance companies. Medical assistants often have medical transcription duties.

# Medical Office Administrator or Manager

To gain medical assistant credentials, you must fulfill the requirements of either the American Association of Medical Assistants (for a Certified Medical Assistant) or the American Medical Technologists (for a Registered Medical Assistant). After obtaining your medical assistant certification, you may wish to acquire additional skills in specialty areas through course work or on-the-job training. Although this course work or training may not lead to an additional certification or degree, it will enable you to expand your role in the medical office and advance your career as the demand for skilled health professionals increases.

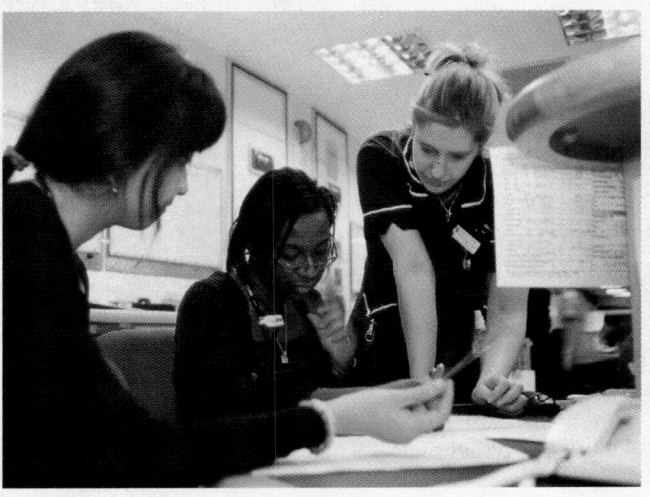

## Skills and Duties

A medical office administrator or manager manages the practice of a single physician (solo practice) or of a group practice. His duties are determined, in part, by the size of the practice. If the practice is large, he may have more managerial duties. If it is small, he may act as the receptionist, secretary, and records clerk. (Occasionally, in a solo practice, the practice nurse performs many or all of these functions.) Large group practices with 10 to 15 physicians may have one medical office administrator or manager, while larger group practices with 40 to 50 physicians (such as managed care organizations) may have a highly trained practice administrator or manager who oversees and coordinates the work of several administrators at multiple practice locations.

The medical office administrator's or manager's reception duties begin with greeting and welcoming new patients. He may provide a medical history form for patients and answer any questions they may have. The administrator must have knowledge of medical terminology in order to answer patients' questions.

This office manager coordinates the practice's records and filing. For example, he ensures that x-rays and test results are attached to the appropriate records and that insurance information is up to date. The medical office administrator or manager may also schedule appointments for patients as well as referrals with other specialists. He may also keep track of the medical and nursing staff schedule. Sometimes the administrator or manager is the person who calls patients ahead of time to confirm their appointments.

In a solo or small practice, the medical office administrator or manager may perform general secretarial tasks, such as handling the mail and answering the telephone. He must have strong computer and application software skills, such as spreadsheet applications and advanced document processing skills, as well as solid accounting skills. In a large practice, the administrator or manager may train and supervise the office staff. It is important that this administrator be knowledgeable in all employment practice laws when in a managerial role. The office administrator may also be responsible for recruiting and hiring medical staff.

## Workplace Settings

Medical office administrators or managers may work in solo practices, group practices, or medical clinics. Specialized health-care facilities, such as nursing homes, may also employ medical office administrators.

## Education

Although medical office administrators or managers may learn the medical terminology they need on the job, they usually acquire their secretarial and clerical background through course work, either in a business/vocational school or in a junior or community college. The educational requirements for a medical office administrator vary with the size of the practice and the extent of the administrator's responsibilities. Upper-level positions require a graduate degree.

*continued* ⟶

## Medical Office Administrator or Manager *(concluded)*

### Where to Go for More Information

American Academy of Medical Administrators
701 Lee Street, Suite 600
Des Plaines, IL 60016
847-759-8601

Medical Group Management Association
104 Inverness Terrace East
Englewood, CO 80112
(303) 799-1111

National Association of Medical Staff Services
2025 Main Street, NW, Suite 800
Washington, DC 20036
202-367-1196

## Mental Health Technician

A mental health technician, sometimes called a psychiatric aide or counselor, works in a variety of health-care settings with emotionally disturbed and mentally retarded patients. This health professional assists the psychiatric team by observing behavior and providing information to help in the planning of therapy. The mental health technician also participates in supervising group therapy and counseling sessions. This technician may work in a psychiatric clinic, specialized nursing home, psychiatric unit of a hospital, or community health center. Other places of employment include crisis centers and shelters. Training varies widely, from on-the-job training to advanced degrees, depending on job responsibilities and medical setting.

## Nuclear Medicine Technologist

A nuclear medicine technologist performs tests to oversee quality control, to prepare and administer radioactive drugs, and to operate radiation detection instruments. This allied health professional is also responsible for correctly positioning the patient, performing imaging procedures, and preparing the information for use by a physician. A nuclear medicine technologist may work in a hospital, public health institution, or physician's office or—with appropriate clinical experience—in a teaching position at a college or university. There are 2- and 4-year training programs. The registration examination is administered by the American Registry of Radiologic Technologists.

## Occupational Therapist

An occupational therapist works with patients who have physical injuries or illnesses, psychologic or developmental problems, or problems associated with the aging process. This health professional helps patients attain maximum physical and mental health by using educational, vocational, and rehabilitation therapies and activities. The occupational therapist may work in a hospital,

clinic, extended care facility, rehabilitation hospital, or government or community agency. To become an occupational therapist, you need a 4-year degree, followed by a 9- to 12-month internship at an accredited hospital. Then you must pass the national board examination in order to earn the title of OTR—registered occupational therapist.

## Pharmacist

Pharmacists are professionals who have studied the science of drugs and who dispense medication and health supplies to the public. Pharmacists know the chemical and physical qualities of drugs and are knowledgeable about the companies that manufacture drugs.

Pharmacists inform the public about the effects of prescription and nonprescription (over-the-counter) medications. Pharmacists are employed in hospitals, clinics, and nursing homes. They may also work for government agencies, pharmaceutical companies, privately owned pharmacies, or chain store pharmacies. Some pharmacists own their own stores. There are three levels of pharmacists, each with different training requirements. A pharmacy technician (CPhT) can typically receive on-the-job training. Formal training, although not required by most states, includes certificate programs and 2-year college programs offering associate degrees in science. Voluntary certification is by examination. A registered pharmacist (RPh) requires 5 years of college training with a bachelor's degree in science. Pharmacists must be registered by the state and must pass a state board examination. A doctor of pharmacy (PharmD) requires 6 to 7 years of college training, which may be followed by a residency in a hospital setting.

## Phlebotomist

Phlebotomists are allied health professionals trained to draw blood for diagnostic laboratory testing. They work in medical clinics, laboratories, and hospitals. Although medical assistants are also trained to draw blood for standard types of tests, phlebotomists are trained at a more advanced level to be able to draw blood under difficult circumstances or in special situations. For example, if a blood sample is needed for a potassium-level test, it must be drawn in a particular manner that only phlebotomists are trained to do. In most states phlebotomists must be certified by the National Phlebotomy Association or registered by the American Society of Clinical Pathologists.

## Physical Therapist

A physical therapist (PT) plans and uses physical therapy programs for medically referred patients. The PT helps these patients to restore function, relieve pain, and prevent disability following disease, injury, or loss of body parts. A physical therapist uses various treatment methods, which include therapy with electricity, heat, cold, ultrasound, massage, and exercise. The physical therapist also helps patients accept their disabilities. A physical therapist may work in a hospital, outpatient clinic, rehabilitation center, home-care agency, nursing home, voluntary health agency, private practice, or sports medicine center. A physical therapist must have a bachelor's degree in physical therapy and must pass a state board examination.

## Physician Assistant

A **physician assistant (PA)** is a health-care provider who practices medicine under the supervision of a physician. Physician assistants are licensed by the state in which they practice. PAs are trained in medicine with a curriculum similar in content but shorter in duration than medical school. Most physician assistants are nationally certified and hold the title PA-C. National certification is maintained through cycles of examinations and continuing medical education.

The scope of the physician assistant's practice corresponds to the supervising physician's practice. Duties may include taking patient histories, performing physical examinations, ordering and interpreting laboratory tests, performing procedures, assisting in surgery, diagnosing medical conditions, and developing and carrying out treatment plans. Physician assistants can prescribe medication in most states. PAs work in a wide variety of health-care settings, including hospitals, clinics, private physician offices, schools, prisons, and governmental agencies. They also serve as faculty in physician assistant programs. Medical assistants may work with physician assistants, particularly in outpatient settings.

## Radiographer

A radiographer (x-ray technician) is one of the most common positions for individuals whose education is in radiologic technology. The radiographer assists a radiologist in taking x-ray films. These films are used to diagnose broken bones, tumors, ulcers, and disease. A radiographer usually works in the radiology department of a hospital. The x-ray technician may, however, use mobile x-ray equipment in a patient's room or in the operating room. A

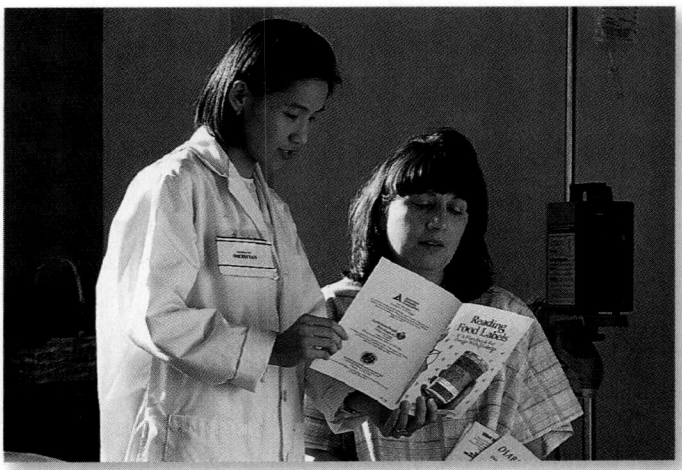

**Figure 2-4.** Registered dietitians work closely with patients who need to modify their food choices for better health.

radiographer may be employed in a hospital, laboratory, clinic, physician's office, government agency, or industry.

## Registered Dietitian

Registered dietitians help patients and their families make healthful food choices that provide balanced, adequate nutrition (Figure 2-4). Dietitians are sometimes called nutritionists. Dietitians may assist food-service directors at health-care facilities and prepare and serve food to groups. They may also participate in food research and teach nutrition classes. Dietitians work in community health agencies, hospitals, clinics, private practices, and managed care settings. They may also teach at colleges and universities, and they serve as consultants to organizations and individuals.

## Radiologic Technologist

A radiologic technologist is a health-care professional who has studied the theory and practice of the technical aspects of the use of x-rays and radioactive materials in the diagnosis and treatment of disease. A radiologic technologist may specialize in radiography, radiation therapy, or nuclear medicine. Radiologic technologists generally work in hospitals; some work in medical laboratories, medical practices, and clinics.

## Respiratory Therapist

A respiratory therapist evaluates, treats, and cares for persons with respiratory problems. The respiratory therapist works under the supervision of a physician and performs therapeutic procedures based on observation of the patient. Using respiratory equipment, the therapist treats patients with asthma, emphysema, pneumonia, and bronchitis. The respiratory therapist plays an active role in newborn, pediatric, and adult intensive care units. The therapist may work in a hospital, nursing home, physician's office, or commercial company that provides emergency oxygen equipment and services to home-care patients.

# Nursing Aide/Assistant

Nursing aides assist in the direct care of patients under the supervision of the nursing staff. Typical functions include making beds, bathing patients, taking vital signs, serving meals, and transporting patients to and from treatment areas. Nursing assistants are often employed in psychiatric and acute care hospitals, nursing homes, and home health agencies. On-the-job training can range from 1 week to 3 months.

# Practical/Vocational Nurse

Licensed practical nurses (LPNs) and licensed vocational nurses (LVNs) provide nursing care to the sick. Both terms refer to the same type of nurse. Duties involve taking and recording patient temperatures, blood pressure, pulse, and respiration rates. They also include administering some medications under supervision, dressing wounds, and applying compresses. LPNs and LVNs are not allowed, however, to perform certain other duties, such as some intravenous (IV) procedures or the administration of certain medications. LPNs/LVNs can obtain additional training to become certified in IV therapy.

Practical/vocational nurses assist registered nurses and physicians by observing patients and reporting changes in their conditions. LPNs/LVNs work in hospitals, nursing homes, clinics, and physicians' offices and in industrial medicine. To meet the needs of the growing aging population in this country, employment opportunities for LPNs and LVNs in long-term care settings have increased.

LPNs/LVNs must graduate from an accredited school of practical (vocational) nursing (usually a 1-year program). They are also required to take a state board examination for licensure as LPNs/LVNs.

# Associate Degree Nurse

Associate degrees in nursing (ADNs) are offered at many junior colleges and community colleges and at some universities. These programs combine liberal arts education and nursing education. The length of the ADN program is typically 2 years. ADNs are also considered RNs if they pass the state boards.

# Diploma Graduate Nurse

Diploma programs are usually 3-year programs designed as cooperative programs between a community college and a participating hospital. The programs combine course work and clinical experience in the hospital.

# Baccalaureate Nurse

A baccalaureate degree refers to a 4-year college or university program. Graduates of a 4-year nursing program are awarded a bachelor of science in nursing (BSN) degree. The curriculum includes courses in liberal arts, general education, and nursing courses. Graduates are prepared to function as nurse generalists and in positions that go beyond the role of hospital staff nurses. BSNs are also considered RNs if they pass the state boards.

# Registered Nurse

A nurse who graduates from a nursing program and passes the state board examination for licensure is considered an RN, indicating formal, legal recognition by the state. The RN is a professional who is responsible for planning, giving, and supervising the bedside nursing care of patients. An RN may work in an administrative capacity, assist in daily operations, oversee programs in hospital or institutional settings, or plan community health services.

Registered nurses work in a variety of settings. These settings include hospitals, nursing homes, public health agencies, industry, physicians' offices, government agencies, and educational settings. Some RNs continue their education to earn master's or doctoral degrees.

# Nurse Practitioner

A nurse practitioner (NP) is an RN who functions in an expanded nursing role. The NP usually works in an ambulatory patient care setting alongside physicians. An NP may work in an independent nurse practitioner practice without physicians. An independent nurse practitioner takes health histories, performs physical exams, conducts screening tests, and educates patients and families about disease prevention.

An NP who works in a physician's practice may perform some duties that a physician would, such as administering physical exams and treating common illnesses and injuries (Figure 2-5). For example, in an OB/GYN practice

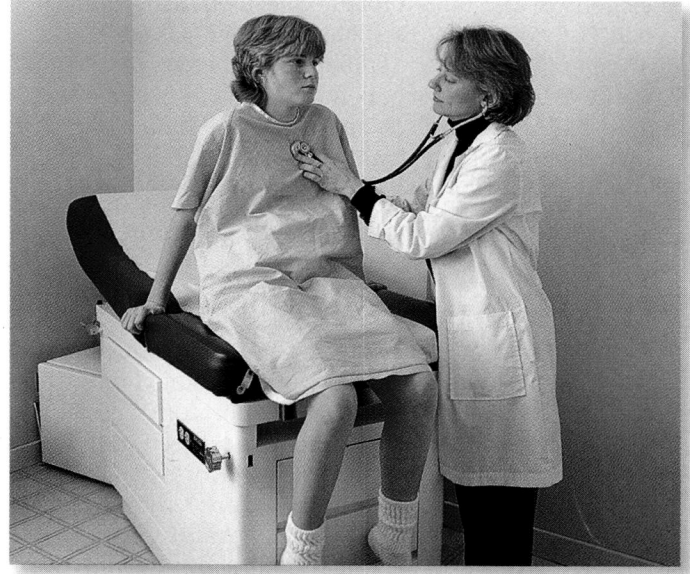

**Figure 2-5.** Many nurse practitioners work in physicians' offices and are trained to perform routine examinations.

the NP can perform a standard annual gynecologic exam, including taking a Pap smear or a culture to test for yeast infection or a bacterial infection. The nurse practitioner usually emphasizes preventive health care.

The NP must be an RN with at least a master's degree in nursing and must complete 4 to 12 months of an apprenticeship or formal training. With specific formal training the student may become a pediatric nurse practitioner, an obstetric nurse practitioner (midwife), or a psychiatric nurse practitioner.

# Specialty Career Options

The various medical specialties can open up many career possibilities for medical assistants. Deciding to specialize may become one of your career goals 5 or more years from now. Remember that you may need additional training or education for some of these positions. Your hard work will be rewarded, however, as you gain additional job responsibilities.

Choosing an area in which to specialize involves research and careful thought. Local and medical college libraries can supply a great deal of information about the areas in which you may specialize. State employment agencies or schools can help you make career choices.

It is also helpful to check the help-wanted section in local newspapers for information about jobs in specialized areas. Many newspapers separate health-care career opportunities into easy-to-find boxed sections. You may also directly contact companies you would like to work for. Ask about job opportunities, and find out what skills and training the employer requires.

## Anesthetist's Assistant

Anesthetist's assistants provide anesthetic care under an anesthetist's direction. Hospitals and high-technology surgical centers frequently employ anesthetist's assistants. These assistants gather patient data and assist in evaluation of patients' physical and mental status. They also record planned surgical procedures, assist with patient monitoring, draw blood samples, perform blood gas analyses, and conduct pulmonary function tests.

## Certified Laboratory Assistant

Certified laboratory assistants perform routine procedures in bacteriology, chemistry, hematology, parasitology, serology, and urinalysis. Laboratory assistants work under the supervision of a medical technologist or hospital anatomic pathologist. They work in laboratories at hospitals, clinics, and physicians' offices and in independent laboratories. One-year training programs are offered by hospitals, vocational schools, and community colleges. Some certified laboratory assistants are medical assistants with advanced training in laboratory testing.

## Dental Assistant

A dental assistant can practice without formal education or training. In this case, on-the-job training is provided. A dental assistant performs many administrative and laboratory functions that are similar to the duties of a medical assistant. For example, a dental assistant may serve as chair-side assistant, provide instruction in oral hygiene, and prepare and sterilize instruments. To perform expanded clinical and chair-side functions such as those of a hygienist, a dental assistant must have at least 1 year of training in theory and clinical application. This formal education also requires work experience in a dental office.

Dental assistants often work in a private practice. They also work in clinics, dental schools, and local health agencies. Insurance companies hire dental assistants to process dental claims.

## Emergency Medical Technician/Paramedic

An emergency medical technician (EMT), sometimes called a paramedic, works under the direction of a physician through a radio communication network. This health professional assesses and manages medical emergencies that occur away from hospitals or other medical settings, such as in private homes, schools, offices, or public areas. An EMT is trained to **triage** patients (to assess the urgency and type of condition presented as well as the immediate medical needs) and to initiate the appropriate treatment for a variety of medical emergencies. While transporting patients to the medical facility, an EMT records, documents, and radios the patient's condition to the physician, describing how the injury occurred. An EMT may work for an ambulance service, fire department, police department, hospital emergency department, private industry, or voluntary care service. Training requirements vary by state but typically require a high school diploma and driver's license, 100 hours of classroom training, and an average of 6 months of practical training on an ambulance squad or in a hospital emergency room.

## Occupational Therapist Assistant

Occupational therapist assistants work under the supervision of an occupational therapist. They help individuals with mental or physical disabilities reach their highest level of functioning through the teaching of fine motor skills, trades (occupations), and the arts. Duties include preparing materials for activities, maintaining tools and equipment, and documenting the patient's progress. Occupational therapist assistants must earn a 2-year degree (OTA).

## Ophthalmic Assistant

An ophthalmic assistant aids ophthalmologists with the routine functions of the practice. This health professional performs simple vision testing, takes medical histories, administers eyedrops, and changes dressings. There are three levels in this category of allied health professional (from most senior to least senior): ophthalmic technologist, ophthalmic technician, and ophthalmic assistant. Duties are determined by the supervising ophthalmologist. Medical assistants can obtain on-the-job training to become an ophthalmic assistant. Although no states currently require certification for these positions, certification examinations are available for each type of category.

## Pathologist's Assistant

Pathologist's assistants work under the supervision of a pathologist. Pathologist's assistants sometimes work with forensic pathologists—professionals who study the human body and diseases for legal purposes, in cooperation with government or police investigations. They may prepare frozen sections of dissected body tissue. Assistants working for anatomic pathologists (professionals who study the human body and diseases in a research capacity) may maintain supplies, instruments, and chemicals for the anatomic pathology laboratory. Pathologist's assistants perform laboratory work about 75% of the workday. Assistants also perform a variety of administrative duties. They work in community hospitals, university medical centers, and private laboratories.

## Pediatric Medical Assistant

A pediatric medical assistant assists the pediatrician in administrative and clinical duties (Figure 2-6). These duties include obtaining medical histories and preparing patients for examination. Other duties include performing routine tests, sterilizing supplies and equipment, typing, filing, and clerical work. This health professional also educates patients and their parents or guardians about follow-up care and maintains patients' records. A pediatric medical assistant should be able to communicate well with children.

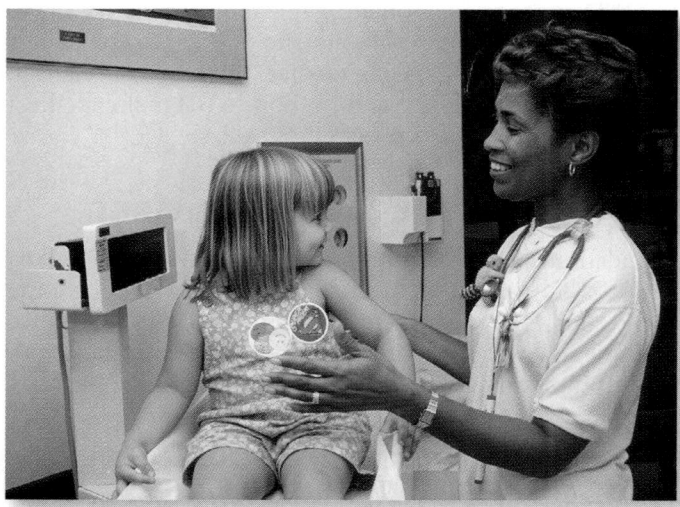

**Figure 2-6.** If you enjoy working with children, you might consider working as a pediatric medical assistant.

Other helpful skills include patience and organizational skills. Pediatric medical assistants work with pediatricians in private practice, hospitals, and clinics.

## Pharmacy Technician

Pharmacy technicians perform specific routine tasks related to record keeping and preparing and dispensing drugs. Duties include preparing medications for administration and making sure patients receive the correct medication. Pharmacy technicians usually work in hospitals or similar facilities under the supervision of a nurse, pharmacist, or other health-care professional. In a commercial pharmacy they work under the pharmacist's supervision. Opportunities are also available with pharmaceutical firms and wholesale pharmaceutical distributors.

Training can be on the job or through certificate programs and 2-year college programs (associate degree). National certification is voluntary by examination and earns the title CPhT (certified pharmacy technician).

## Physical Therapy Assistant

A physical therapy assistant (PTA) works under the direction of a physical therapist to assist with patient treatment. The assistant follows the patient care program created by the physical therapist and physician. This health professional performs tests and treatment procedures, assembles or sets up equipment for therapy sessions, and observes and documents patient behavior and progress (Figure 2-7). A physical therapy assistant may practice in a hospital, nursing home, rehabilitation center, or community or government agency.

## Radiation Therapy Technologist

A radiation therapy technologist assists the radiologist. He may, for example, assist with administering radiation treatment to patients who have cancer. He may also be responsible for maintaining radiation treatment equipment. The technologist shares responsibility with the radiologist for the accuracy of treatment records. A radiation therapy technologist may work in a hospital, laboratory, clinic, physician's office, or government agency. Training requires a high school diploma and graduation from a 2- or 4-year program in radiography.

## Respiratory Therapy Technician

Respiratory therapy technicians work under the supervision of a physician and a respiratory therapist. Respiratory therapists perform procedures such as artificial ventilation. They also clean, sterilize, and maintain the respiratory equipment and document the patient's therapy in the medical record. Respiratory therapy technicians work in hospitals, nursing homes, physicians' offices, and commercial companies that provide emergency oxygen equipment and therapeutic home care.

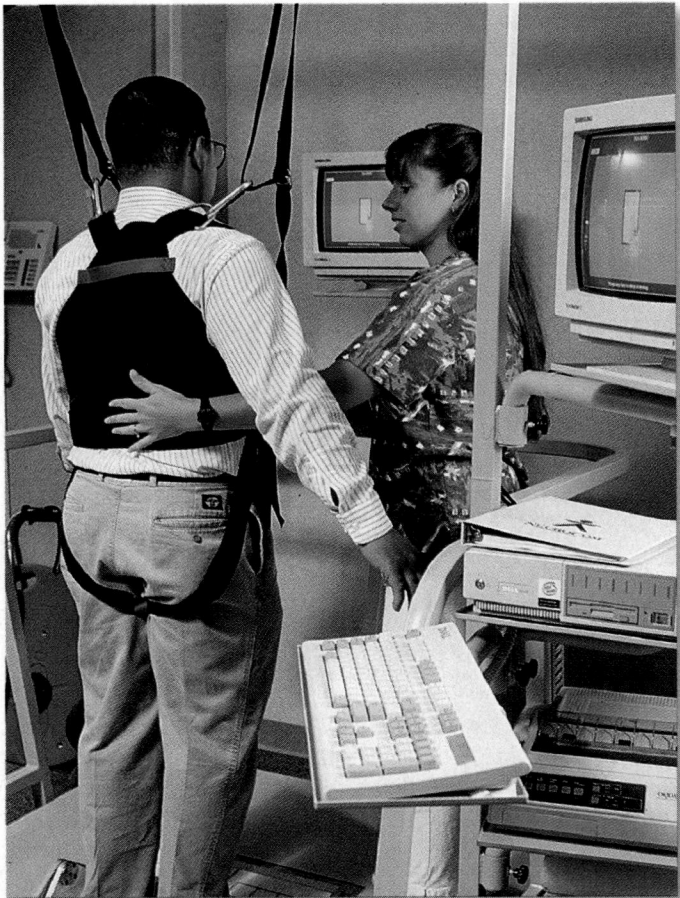

**Figure 2-7.** Physical therapy assistants provide guidance and support to patients who are recovering from a physical injury or from surgery on a limb or joint.

## Speech/Language Pathologist

A speech/language pathologist treats communication disorders, such as stuttering, and associated disorders, such as hearing impairment. This health professional evaluates, diagnoses, and counsels patients who have these problems. A speech/language pathologist may work in a school, hospital, research setting, or private practice or may teach at a college or university.

Speech/language pathologists usually have a master's degree in speech/language pathology or audiology. Certification and licensing requirements vary by state, usually depending on the work setting (public school, private practice, clinic, and so on).

## Surgical Technician

A surgical technician provides patient services under the direction, supervision, and responsibility of a licensed surgeon. This health professional's tasks include obtaining a patient's history and physical data. She then discusses the data with a physician or surgeon to determine what procedures to use to treat the problem. A surgical technician may also assist in performing diagnostic and therapeutic

procedures. She must be calm and have good judgment in the high-pressure environment of the operating room. Surgical technicians work primarily in hospitals and outpatient surgery centers.

Training programs for this position are usually affiliated with 2- and 4-year colleges and with university schools of medicine and allied health. These programs include practical work in the surgery unit of an affiliated hospital.

# Professional Associations

Membership in a professional association enables you to become involved in the issues and activities relevant to your field and presents opportunities for continuing education. It is a good idea to become informed about such associations, even those, such as the American Medical Association, that are open to physicians only. The physician you work for may ask you to obtain information about the group's activities and meetings. Table 2-1 summarizes professional associations related to the field of medicine and medical assisting.

## American Association of Medical Assistants

The American Association of Medical Assistants (AAMA), as described in Chapter 1, was created to serve the interests of medical assistants and to further the medical assisting profession. The AAMA offers self-paced continuing education classes; workshops and seminars at the local, state, and national levels; and job networking opportunities. Other benefits include legal counsel, group health insurance, professional recognition, and member discounts.

## American Association for Medical Transcription

The American Association for Medical Transcription (AAMT) is the professional organization for the advancement of medical transcription. The AAMT also educates medical transcriptionists as medical language specialists. The AAMT offers advice and support to the many medical transcriptionists who are self-employed.

## American College of Physicians

Founded in 1915, the American College of Physicians (ACP) is the largest medical specialty organization in the world. It is the only society of internists dedicated to providing education and information resources to the entire field of internal medicine and its subspecialties.

## American Hospital Association

The American Hospital Association (AHA) is the nation's largest network of institutional health-care providers. These providers represent every type of hospital: rural

## TABLE 2-1 Professional Medical Organizations

| Professional Organization | Membership Requirements | Advantages of Membership |
|---|---|---|
| American Association of Medical Assistants (AAMA) | Interested individuals, including medical assisting students and those who practice medical assisting, may join the AAMA. | Offers flexible continuing education programs; publishes *CMA Today;* offers legal counsel, professional recognition, and various member discounts |
| American Association for Medical Transcription (AAMT) | Interested individuals and those who practice medical transcription may join the AAMT. | Educates and develops medical transcriptionists as medical language specialists; offers advice and support for self-employed medical transcriptionists |
| American College of Physicians (ACP) | Physicians and medical students may join. | Provides education and information resources to the field of internal medicine and its subspecialties |
| American Hospital Association (AHA) | Institutional health-care providers and other individuals may join. | Provides consultant referral service and access to health-care information resources |
| American Medical Association (AMA) | Physicians and medical students may join. | Provides large information source; publishes *Journal of the American Medical Association (JAMA);* offers AMA/Net |
| American Medical Technologists (AMT) | Medical assistants, medical technologists, medical laboratory technicians, dental assistants, and phlebotomy technicians may join. | Offers national certification as Registered Medical Assistant (RMA); offers certification to other health-care professionals, publications, state chapter activities, continuing education programs |
| American Pharmaceutical Association (APhA) | Pharmaceutical professionals and physicians may join. | Helps members improve skills; active in pharmacy policy development, networking, publishing, research, public education |
| American Society of Clinical Pathologists (ASCP) | Any professional involved in laboratory medicine or pathology may join. | Resource for improving the quality of pathology and laboratory medicine; offers educational programs and materials; certifies technologists and technicians |
| American Society of Phlebotomy Technicians (ASPT) | Interested individuals and those who practice phlebotomy may join. | Offers national certification as a phlebotomy technician and continuous education programs |

and city hospitals, specialty and acute care facilities, free-standing hospitals, academic medical centers, and health systems and networks. The AHA works to support and promote the interests of hospitals and health-care organizations across the country. Organizations as well as individual professionals may join the AHA. Membership benefits include use of the AHA consultant referral service, accessed, for example, by hospitals that need experts in areas not addressed by in-house personnel. Members also have access to AHA's health-care information resources, including teleconferencing and AHA database services.

## Joint Commission on Accreditation of Healthcare Organizations (JCAHO)

The Joint Commission on Accreditation of Healthcare Organizations (JCAHO) is a U.S.-based nonprofit organization. It was formed in 1951 with a goal of maintaining and elevating the standards of health-care delivery through the evaluation and accreditation of health-care organizations. JCAHO employs surveyors who are sent to health-care organizations to evaluate their operational practices and facilities. Organizations are given a score from 1 to 100, with 100 being a perfect score. Health-care organizations are highly motivated to do well during a survey because accreditation by JCAHO is a significant factor in gaining reimbursement from Medicare and managed care organizations. In January 2004, JCAHO expanded their focus to include patient safety requirements, such as:

- Improve the accuracy of patient identification
- Improve the safety of high-alert medications, such as electrolyte concentrations
- Eliminate the wrong site, wrong patient, wrong procedure, or wrong surgery
- Improve the safety of using infusion pumps
- Improve the effectiveness of clinical alarm systems
- Reduce the risk of health-care-acquired infections

JCAHO established these requirements to help accredited health-care organizations address issues of patient safety that can lead to adverse events that can result in lawsuits.

## Council of Ethical and Judicial Affairs (CEJA)

The Council of Ethical and Judicial Affairs (CEJA) develops ethics policy for the AMA. It is composed of seven practicing physicians, a resident or fellow, and a medical student. The Council prepares reports that analyze and address timely ethical issues that confront physicians and the medical profession. CEJA maintains and updates the AMA Code of Medical Ethics. This code is widely recognized as the most comprehensive ethics guide for physicians who strive to practice ethically.

## American Medical Association

The American Medical Association (AMA) was founded in 1847. Its members include 300,000 physicians from every medical specialty. The AMA promotes science and the art of medicine and works to improve public health. The AMA is the world's largest publisher of scientific and medical information and publishes ten monthly medical specialty journals. The AMA also accredits medical programs in the United States and Canada.

The AMA provides an online service called AMA/Net for physicians and medical assistants, offering up-to-date information about current medical topics. To use the AMA/Net, the medical office must have a computer, telephone, and modem.

## American Medical Technologists

American Medical Technologists (AMT) was established in 1939 as a not-for-profit organization. The AMT offers national certification as a Registered Medical Assistant (RMA) to medical assisting practitioners. It also offers certification to medical technologists, clinical laboratory technicians, dental assistants, medical administrative specialists, and phlebotomy technicians. Membership benefits include continuing education classes, workshops and seminars, and job networking opportunities.

## American Pharmaceutical Association

The American Pharmaceutical Association (APhA), the national professional society of pharmacists, was founded in 1852. The APhA represents the interests of pharmaceutical professionals, and it strives to help individual members improve their skills. The APhA works to advance the field of pharmacy and the safety of patients. The APhA is active in pharmacy policy development, networking, publishing, research, and public education.

# Summary

There are many medical settings in which you can serve as a medical assistant. Some settings will be in specialized branches of medicine. It is important to gain an understanding of the major areas of medicine, as well as the various subspecialties, in order to choose and plan for the type of setting in which you would like to work.

Learning about various allied health professionals—such as pharmacists, nurse practitioners, and medical transcriptionists—will help you interact with others on the job. Learning about specialty career options—such as physical therapy assistants, certified laboratory assistants, and ophthalmic assistants—can give you ideas about integrating new skills into your job as a multiskilled health professional.

Joining a professional organization will enable you to stay informed about issues and activities in the medical assisting field and the specialty or subspecialty in which you work. Professional organizations also provide other benefits to members, such as group health insurance; job networking opportunities; state or chapter meetings, seminars, workshops, and guest presentations; and member discounts. Membership in a professional organization helps you be recognized as a professional. Therefore, it is an important addition to your résumé.

## CASE STUDY *QUESTIONS*

Now that you have completed this chapter, review the case study at the beginning of the chapter and answer the following questions:

1. What are Susan's career options in nursing? How much further education would she need in order to become a nurse?
2. What are Susan's career options in a laboratory setting? How much further education would she need in order to work in a laboratory?

## Discussion Questions

1. Discuss the different types of physicians, such as podiatrist, chiropractor, MD, and DO. What are the differences in training, education, and board certification?
2. Medical assistants can perform many roles. Discuss the different allied health careers that medical assistants can receive training in, such as phlebotomy assistant, ophthalmic medical assistant, administrative roles, and other positions.
3. How do professional organizations help medical assistants perform their job duties?

## Critical Thinking Questions

1. How might a medical assistant's experience working with a medical specialist differ from her experience working with a general practitioner, in terms of learning about medicine?
2. Why is it important for a medical assistant to be knowledgeable about other allied health-care professionals and their primary duties?
3. How can medical assistants enhance their careers by joining professional organizations such as the AMT or AAMA?

## Application Activities

1. Interview a medical assistant, such as an ophthalmic medical assistant, who has chosen a specialty career option. What additional education or training did she need to obtain the position? What are her administrative and clinical duties? What does she like about her job? What does she find most challenging? How did she come to choose the specialty? Report your findings to the class.
2. Invite a guest speaker to your class who is currently working in an allied health career, such as a pharmacy technician or phlebotomist, to talk about his or her job duties, certifications, and overall involvement in the medical community.
3. Pick three medical specialties and identify the skills required for a medical assistant in each specialty.

## Virtual Fieldtrip

*Visit the McGraw-Hill Higher Education Medical Assisting website at www.mhhe.com/medicalassisting3 to complete the following activity:*

Research a professional organization that interests you the most and research the opportunities that interest you. One opportunity is the professional credentialing offered by the various organizations. Share your research with your classmates.

Open the CD and complete this chapter's practice activities, play the games, listen to the key terms, and test yourself with the interactive review. E-mail, print, and/or save your results to document your proficiency.

# Legal and Ethical Issues in Medical Practice, Including HIPAA

## KEY TERMS

- abandonment
- agent
- arbitration
- assault
- authorization
- battery
- bioethics
- breach of contract
- civil law
- consent
- contract
- corporation
- crime
- criminal law
- defamation
- disclosure
- discrimination
- doctrine of informed consent
- doctrine of professional discretion
- durable power of attorney
- electronic transaction record
- ethics
- expressed contract
- felony
- fraud
- group practice
- implied contract
- informed consent
- law
- law of agency

## MEDICAL ASSISTING COMPETENCIES

**In preparation for the certification examination, you should know the following areas of competence:**

| COMPETENCY | CMA | RMA |
|---|---|---|
| **General/Legal/Professional** | | |
| Identify and respond to issues of confidentiality by maintaining confidentiality at all times and following appropriate guidelines when releasing records or information | X | X |
| Be aware of and perform within legal and ethical boundaries | X | X |
| Determine the needs for documentation and reporting, and document accurately and appropriately | X | X |
| Demonstrate knowledge of and monitor current federal and state health-care legislation and regulations; maintain licenses and accreditation | X | X |
| Follow established policy in initiating or terminating medical treatment | | X |
| Perform risk management procedures | | X |
| Orient and train personnel | | X |
| Maintain liability coverage | | X |
| Conduct work within scope of education, training, and ability | | X |
| Receive, organize, prioritize, and transmit information appropriately | | X |

## KEY TERMS (Concluded)

| | | | |
|---|---|---|---|
| liable | negligence | *qui tam* | *subpoena duces tecum* |
| libel | Notice of Privacy | *res ipsa loquitur* | tort |
| living will | Practices (NPP) | *respondeat superior* | treatment, payments, |
| malpractice claim | partnership | Security Rule | and operations (TPO) |
| minors | Privacy Rule | slander | uniform donor card |
| misdemeanor | protected health | sole proprietorship | use |
| moral values | information (PHI) | subpoena | void |

# CHAPTER OUTLINE

- Medical Law and Ethics
- The Patient-Physician Contract
- Preventing Lawsuits
- Federal Legislation Affecting Health Care
- OSHA Regulations
- Quality Control and Assurance

- HIPAA
- Confidentiality Issues and Mandatory Disclosure
- Code of Ethics
- Labor and Employment Laws
- Legal Medical Practice Models

# LEARNING OUTCOMES

After completing Chapter 3, you will be able to:

**3.1** Define ethics, bioethics, and medical law.

**3.2** Discuss the measures a medical practice must take to avoid malpractice claims.

**3.3** Discuss medical documentation and how it applies to medical law.

**3.4** Discuss the various types of health-care legislation and their impact on medical office practice.

**3.5** Describe Occupational Safety and Health Administration (OSHA) requirements for a medical office.

**3.6** Describe procedures for handling an incident of exposure to hazardous materials.

**3.7** Compare and contrast quality control and quality assurance procedures.

**3.8** Discuss the impact that Health Insurance Portability and Accountability Act (HIPAA) regulations have in the medical office.

**3.9** Explain how to protect patient confidentiality.

**3.10** Describe the different practice management models.

# Introduction

Medical law plays an important role in medical facility procedures and the way we care for patients. We live in a litigious society, where patients, relatives, and others are inclined to sue health-care practitioners, health-care facilities, manufacturers of medical equipment and products, and others when medical outcomes are not acceptable. It is important for a medical professional to understand medical law, ethics, and protected health information as it pertains to Health Insurance Portability and Accountability Act (HIPAA). There are two main reasons for medical professionals to study law and ethics: The first is to help you function at the highest professional level by providing competent, compassionate health care to patients and the second is to help you avoid legal problems that can threaten your ability to earn a living.

A knowledge of medical law and ethics can help you gain perspective in the following three areas:

1. *The rights, responsibilities, and concerns of health-care consumers.* Not only do health-care professionals need to be concerned about how law and ethics impact their respective professions, they must also understand how legal and ethical issues affect patients. As medical technology advances and the use of computers increases, patients want to know more about their options and rights as well as more about the responsibilities of health-care practitioners. Patients want to know who and how their information is used and the options they have regarding health-care treatments. Patients have come to expect favorable outcomes from medical treatment, and when these expectations are not met, lawsuits may result.

2. *The legal and ethical issues facing society, patients, and health-care professionals as the world changes.* Every day new technologies emerge with solutions to biological and medical issues. These solutions often involve social issues, and we are faced with decisions, for example, regarding reproductive rights, fetal stem cell research, and confidentiality with sensitive medical records.

3. *The impact of rising costs on the laws and ethics of health-care delivery.* Rising costs, both of health-care insurance and of medical treatment in general, can lead to questions concerning access to health-care services and the allocation of medical treatment. For example, should everyone, regardless of age or lifestyle, have the same access to scarce medical commodities such as transplant organs or highly expensive drugs.

In today's society, medical treatment and decisions surrounding health care have become complex. It is therefore important to be knowledgeable and aware of the issues and the laws that govern patient care.

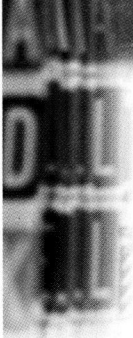
A medical assistant is very busy on a Monday morning. She has drawn blood on a patient that she has known for years and has been very comfortable chatting with this patient. The patient is checking out at the front desk in the reception area, and she notices that he forgot his prescription for Dilantin, a medication for seizure control. She rushes up to the front area and, as he is opening the door, says to him, "Mr. Doe, you forgot your prescription for Dilantin."

As you read this chapter, consider the following questions:
1. Does the medical assistant's comment represent a breach of confidentiality?
2. Has any HIPAA rule been violated? If so, which one?

# Medical Law and Ethics

In order to understand medical law and ethics, it is helpful to understand the differences between laws and ethics. A **law** is defined as a rule of conduct or action prescribed or formally recognized as binding or enforced by a controlling authority, such as local, state, and federal governments. **Ethics** is considered a standard of behavior and a concept of right and wrong beyond what the legal consideration is in any given situation. **Moral values** serve as a basis for ethical conduct. Moral values are formed through the influence of the family, culture, and society.

## Classifications of Law

There are two types of law that pertain to health-care practitioners: criminal law and civil law.

**Criminal Law.** A **crime** is an offense against the state committed or omitted in violation of a public law. **Criminal law** involves crimes against the state. When a state or federal criminal law is violated, the government brings criminal charges against the alleged offender, for example, *Ohio v. John Doe*. State criminal laws prohibit such crimes as murder, arson, rape, and burglary. A criminal act may be classified as a felony or misdemeanor. A **felony** is a crime punishable by death or by imprisonment in a state or federal prison for more than 1 year. Some examples of a felony include abuse (child, elder, or domestic violence), manslaughter, fraud, attempted murder, and practicing medicine without a license.

**Misdemeanors** are less serious crimes than felonies. They are punishable by fines or by imprisonment in a facility other than a prison for 1 year or less. Some examples of misdemeanors are thefts under a certain dollar amount, attempted burglary, and disturbing the peace.

**Civil Law.** **Civil law** involves crimes against the person. Under civil law, a person can sue another person, a business, or the government. Court judgments in civil cases often require the payment of a sum of money to the injured party. Civil law includes a general category of law known as torts. A **tort** is broadly defined as a civil wrong committed against a person or property that causes physical injury or damage to someone's property or that deprives someone of his or her personal liberty and freedom. Torts may be intentional (willful) or unintentional (accidental).

*Intentional Torts.* When one person intentionally harms another, the law allows the injured party to seek a remedy in a civil suit. The injured party can be financially compensated for any harm done by the person guilty of committing the tort. If the conduct is judged to be malicious, punitive damages may also be awarded. Examples of intentional torts include the following:

- Assault. **Assault** is the open threat of bodily harm to another, or acting in such a way as to put another in the "reasonable apprehension of bodily harm."
- Battery. **Battery** is an action that causes bodily harm to another. It is broadly defined as any bodily contact made without permission, In health-care delivery, battery may be charged for any unauthorized touching of a patient, including such actions as suturing a wound, administering an injection, or performing a physical examination.
- Defamation of character. Damaging a person's reputation by making public statements that are both false and malicious is considered **defamation** of character. Defamation of character can take the form of slander and libel. **Slander** is speaking damaging words intended to negatively influence others against an individual in a manner that jeopardizes his or her reputation or means of livelihood. **Libel** is publishing in print damaging words, pictures, or signed statements that will injure the reputation of another.
- False imprisonment. False imprisonment is the intentional, unlawful restraint or confinement of one person by another. Preventing a patient from leaving the facility might be seen as false imprisonment.
- Fraud. **Fraud** consists of deceitful practices in depriving or attempting to deprive another of his or her rights. Health-care practitioners might be accused of fraud

for promising patients "miracle cures" or for accepting fees from patients while using mystical or spiritual powers to heal.

- Invasion of privacy. Invasion of privacy is the interference with a person's right to be left alone. Entering an exam room without knocking can be considered an invasion of privacy. The improper use of or a breach of confidentiality of medical records may be seen as an invasion of privacy.

***Unintentional Torts.*** The most common torts within the health-care delivery system are those committed unintentionally. Unintentional torts are acts that are not intended to cause harm but are committed unreasonably or with a disregard for the consequences. In legal terms, such acts constitute negligence. **Negligence** is charged when a health-care practitioner fails to exercise ordinary care and the patient is injured. The accused may have performed an act or failed to perform an act that a reasonable person would or would not have performed. Under the principles of negligence, civil liability exists only in cases in which the act is judicially determined to be wrongful. Health-care practitioners, for example, are not necessarily liable for a poor-quality outcome in delivering health care. Practitioners become liable only when their conduct is determined to be malpractice, the negligent delivery of professional services.

## Contracts

A **contract** is a voluntary agreement between two parties in which specific promises are made for a consideration. The elements of a contract are important to health-care practitioners because health-care delivery takes place under various types of contracts. To be legally binding, four elements must be present in a contract:

1. Agreement—One party makes an offer and another party accepts it. Certain conditions pertain to the offer:
   - It can relate to the present or the future.
   - It must be communicated.
   - It must be made in good faith and not under duress or as a joke.
   - It must be clear enough to be understood by both parties.
   - It must define what both parties will do if the offer is accepted.

   For example, a physician offers a service to the public by obtaining a license to practice medicine and opening for business. Patients accept the physician's offer by scheduling appointments, submitting to physical examinations, and allowing the physician to prescribe or perform medical treatment. The contract is complete when the physician's fee is paid.
2. Consideration—Something of value is bargained for as part of the agreement. The physician's consideration is providing service; the patient's consideration is payment of the physician's fee.

3. Legal subject matter—Contracts are not valid and enforceable in court unless they are for legal services or purposes. For example, a contract entered into by a patient to pay for services of a physician in private practice would be **void** (not legally enforceable) if the physician was not licensed to practice medicine. **Breach of contract** may be charged if either party fails to comply with the terms of a legally valid contract.
4. Contractual capacity—Parties who enter into the agreement must be capable of fully understanding all its terms and conditions. For example, a mentally incompetent individual or a person under the influence of drugs or alcohol cannot enter into a contract.

**Types of Contracts.** The two main types of contracts are expressed contracts and implied contracts. An **expressed contract** is clearly stated in written or spoken words. A payment contract is an example of an expressed contract. **Implied contracts** are those in which the acceptance or conduct of the parties, rather than expressed words, creates the contract. A patient who rolls up a sleeve and offers an arm for an injection is creating an implied contract.

# The Patient-Physician Contract

A physician has the right, after forming a contract or agreeing to accept a patient under his or her care, to make reasonable limitations on the contractual relationship. The physician is under no legal obligations to treat patients who may wish to exceed those limitations. Under the patient-physician contract, both parties have certain rights and responsibilities.

## Physician Rights and Responsibilities

Physicians have the right to:

- Set up a practice within the boundaries of his or her license to practice medicine
- Set up an office where he or she chooses and to establish office hours
- Specialize
- Decide which services he or she will provide and how those services will be provided

While practicing within the context of an implied contract with the patient, the physician is not bound to:

- Treat every patient with medical care. A physician is free to use his or her discretion to form contracts within his or her practice, with one exception: If a physician is providing care to patients in a hospital emergency room or free clinic, then the physician must treat every patient who comes for treatment.

- Restore the patient to his or her original state of health
- Make a correct diagnosis in every case
- Guarantee the successful result of any treatment or operation. In fact, guarantees of "cures" may constitute fraud on the part of the physician.

Under an implied contract with the patient, the physician has the obligation or responsibility to:

- Use due care, skill, judgment, and diligence in treating patients which peers in the same specialty use
- Stay informed of the best methods of diagnosis and treatment
- Perform to the best of his or her ability, whether or not he or she is to receive a fee
- Furnish complete information and instructions to the patient about diagnoses, options, methods of treatment, and fees for services

**Liability.** All competent adults are liable or legally responsible for their actions, both in their personal lives and their professional careers. It is important as a medical assistant to know and understand your scope of practice within the state you are working. As health-care providers, medical assistants have general liability in the duties they perform, as well as the facility in which they work. By understanding the standard of care and the duty of care, medical assistants can function ethically and legally within their job scope. Medical assistants are held to the "reasonable person standard," which means to carry out your professional and interpersonal relationships without causing harm.

# Patient Rights and Responsibilities

Patients have the right to choose a physician, although some managed care plans may limit choices. Patients also have the right to terminate a physician's services if they wish. Most states have adopted a version of the American Hospital Association's Patient Bill of Rights, which was created in 1973 and revised in 1992. The Patient Bill of Rights is a list of standards that patients can expect in health care. JCAHO requires hospitals to post a copy of the AHA's Patient Bill of Rights and most managed care organizations also require contracted physicians to post a copy of the Patient Bill of Rights.

**Patient Responsibilities.** Patients are also part of the medical team involved in their treatment. Patients have the responsibility under an implied contract to:

- Follow any instructions given by the physician and cooperate as much as possible
- Give all relevant information to the physician in order to reach a correct diagnosis. If a patient fails to inform a physician of any medical conditions he or she may have and an incorrect diagnosis is made, the physician is not liable.

- Follow the physician's orders for treatment
- Pay the fees charged for services provided

**Consent.** **Consent** means that the patient has given permission, either expressed or implied, for the physician to examine him or her, to perform tests that aid in diagnoses, or to treat for a medical condition. When the patient makes an appointment to be examined by a physician, the patient has given implied consent to the examination and any diagnostic testing procedures needed for treatment.

*Informed Consent.* **Informed consent** involves the patient's right to receive all information relative to his or her condition and to make a decision regarding treatment based upon that knowledge. The **doctrine of informed consent** is the legal basis for informed consent and is usually outlined in a state's medical practice acts. Informed consent implies that the patient understands:

- Proposed treatment modes
- Why the treatment was necessary
- The risks involved in the proposed treatment
- Available alternative modes of treatment
- The risks of alternative treatments
- The risks involved if treatment is refused

Adult patients who are of sound mind are usually able to give informed consent. Those patients who cannot give informed consent include the following:

- **Minors** and persons under the age of majority, which excludes emancipated minors, married minors, and mature minors
- The mentally incompetent
- Those who speak a foreign language—interpreters may be necessary

Informed consent is a vital part of the practice of medicine today. Physicians are often sued for negligence because of the failure to adequately inform patients of adverse surgical complications, drug reactions, and alternative treatment modes.

# Preventing Lawsuits

Malpractice litigation not only adds to the cost of health care, it takes a psychological toll on both patients and health-care practitioners. Both sides would probably agree that prevention is preferable to litigation. Health-care practitioners who use reasonable care in preventing professional liability claims are least likely to be faced with defending themselves against malpractice claims.

## Malpractice

**Malpractice claims** are lawsuits by a patient against a physician for errors in diagnosis or treatment. Negligence cases are those in which a person believes that a medical professional did not perform an essential action or performed an improper one, thus harming the patient.

Following are some examples of malpractice:

- Postoperative complications. For example, a patient starts to show signs of internal bleeding in the recovery room. The incision is reopened, and it is discovered that the surgeon did not complete closure (cauterization) of all the severed capillaries at the operation site.

- *Res ipsa loquitur.* This Latin term, which means "the thing speaks for itself," refers to a case in which the doctor's fault is completely obvious. For example, a case in which a surgeon accidentally leaves a surgical instrument inside the patient.

Following are examples of negligence:

- Abandonment. A health-care professional who stops care without providing an equally qualified substitute can be charged with **abandonment.** For example, a labor and delivery nurse is helping a woman in labor. The nurse's shift ends, but all the other nurses are busy and her replacement is late for work. Leaving the woman would constitute abandonment.

- Delayed treatment. A patient shows symptoms of some illness or disorder, but the doctor decides, for whatever reason, to delay treatment. If the patient later learns of the doctor's decision to wait, the patient may believe he has a negligence case.

Negligence cases are sometimes classified using the following three legal terms.

1. *Malfeasance* refers to an unlawful act or misconduct.
2. *Misfeasance* refers to a lawful act that is done incorrectly.
3. *Nonfeasance* refers to failure to perform an act that is one's required duty or that is required by law.

**The Four Ds of Negligence.** The American Medical Association (AMA) lists the following four Ds of negligence:

1. Duty. Patients must show that a physician-patient relationship existed in which the physician owed the patient a duty.
2. Derelict. Patients must show that the physician failed to comply with the standards of the profession. For example, a gynecologist has routinely taken Pap smears of a patient and then, for whatever reason, does not do so. If the patient then shows evidence of cervical cancer, the physician could be said to have been derelict.
3. Direct cause. Patients must show that any damages were a direct cause of a physician's breach of duty. For example, if a patient fell on the sidewalk and damaged her cast, she could not prove that the cast was damaged because it was incorrectly or poorly applied by her physician. It would be clear that the damage to the cast resulted from the fall. If, however, the patient's leg healed incorrectly because of the way the cast had been applied, she might have a case.

4. Damages. Patients must prove that they suffered injury.

To go forward with a malpractice suit, a patient must be prepared to prove all four Ds of negligence.

**Malpractice and Civil Law.** Malpractice lawsuits are part of civil law. Civil law is concerned with individuals' private rights (as opposed to criminal offenses against public law). Under civil law, a breach of some obligation that causes harm or injury to someone is known as a tort. A tort can be intentional or unintentional. Both negligence and breach of contract are considered torts. Breach of contract is the failure to adhere to a contract's terms. The implied physician-patient contract includes requirements such as maintaining patient confidentiality. (Remember that an implied contract is one that is not created by specific, written words, but rather is defined by the conduct of the parties. Usually the parties involved have some special relationship.)

**Settling Malpractice Suits.** Malpractice suits often require a trial in a court of law. Sometimes, however, they are settled through arbitration. **Arbitration** is a process in which the opposing sides choose a person or persons outside the court system, often with special knowledge in the field, to hear and decide the dispute. (Your local or state medical society has information about your state's policy on arbitration.) If injury, failure to provide reasonable care, or abandonment of the patient is proved to have occurred, the doctor must pay damages (a financial award) to the injured party.

If the doctor you work with becomes involved in a lawsuit, you should be familiar with subpoenas. A **subpoena** is a written court order addressed to a specific person, requiring that person's presence in court on a specific date at a specific time. If you were directly involved in the patient case that precipitated the lawsuit, you might be subpoenaed. Another important term to know is *subpoena duces tecum,* which is a court order to produce documents. If you are in charge of patient records at the practice, you may be required to locate, assemble, photocopy, and arrange for delivery of patient records for this purpose.

**Law of Agency.** According to the **law of agency,** an employee is considered to be acting as a doctor's **agent** (on the doctor's behalf) while performing professional tasks. The Latin term *respondeat superior,* or "let the master answer," is sometimes used to refer to this relationship. For example, the employee's word is as binding as if it were the doctor's (so you should never, for example, promise a patient a cure). Therefore, the doctor is responsible, or **liable,** for the negligence of employees. A negligent employee, however, may also be sued directly, because individuals are legally responsible for their own actions. Therefore, a patient can sue both the doctor and the involved employee for negligence. The employer, or the employer's insurance company, can also sue the employee. Most likely, in a case of negligence, the doctor would be sued (because you as an employee are acting on the doctor's behalf), and you are usually covered by the doctor's malpractice insurance.

Some medical assistants choose to obtain malpractice insurance. Obtaining personal malpractice insurance is a professional decision that depends on the type of work or facility in which you are employed. The American Association of Medical Assistants offers medical assisting malpractice insurance through various insurance companies at reduced rates.

**Courtroom Conduct.** Most health-care practitioners will never have to appear in court. If you should be asked to appear, the following suggestions may prove helpful:

- Attend court proceedings as required. Failure to appear in court could result in either charges of contempt of court or the case being forfeited.
- Do not be late for scheduled hearings.
- Bring required documents to court and present them only when requested to do so.
- Before testifying, refresh your memory concerning all the facts observed about the matter in question, such as dates, times, words spoken, and circumstances.
- Speak slowly, clearly, and professionally. Do not use medical terms. Do not lose your temper or attempt to be humorous.
- Answer all questions in a straightforward manner, even if the answers appear to help the opposing side.
- Answer only the question asked, no more and no less.
- Appear well groomed, and dress in clean, conservative clothing.

## Reasons Patients Sue

The following reasons were researched by interviewing families and patients who have sued health-care practitioners:

1. Unrealistic expectations. With the advancements in medical technology today, patients often expect perfection in medical outcomes. They may feel betrayed by the health-care system when a medical outcome is not what was expected.
2. Poor rapport and poor communication. Patients usually do not sue health-care practitioners that they like and trust. Health-care providers who do not return telephone calls or are otherwise unavailable to a patient's family members may be perceived as arrogant, cold, or uncaring. When such perceptions exist, patients and family members are more likely to sue if something goes wrong.
3. Greed and our litigious society. Financial gain is seldom the reason for medical malpractice, but in some cases it may be an influencing factor. Malpractice attorneys sometimes make it very easy for patients to retain their services, such as contingency arrangements.
4. Poor quality of care. Poor quality means that a patient is truly not receiving quality care. Poor quality in "perception" means that the patient believes he or she is not receiving quality care, even if it is not true. Either situation can lead to a malpractice lawsuit.

## Four Cs of Medical Malpractice Prevention

1. Caring. As a health-care professional, caring about your patients and colleagues is your most important asset. Showing patients that you care about them may result in an improvement in their medical condition and, if you are sincere, decreases the likelihood that patients will feel the need to sue if treatment has unsatisfactory results or adverse events occur.
2. Communication. If you communicate in a professional manner and clearly ask for confirmation that you have been understood, you will earn respect and trust with your patients and other members of the allied health team.
3. Competence. Be competent in your skills and job knowledge and maintain and update your knowledge and skills frequently through continuing education.
4. Charting. Documentation is proof of competence. Make sure that all current reports and consultations have been reviewed by the physician and are evident in the chart. Chart every conversation or interaction you have with a patient.

**How Effective Communication Can Help Prevent Lawsuits.** Patients who see the medical office as a friendly place are generally less likely to sue. Physicians, medical assistants, and other medical office staff who have pleasant personalities and are competent in their jobs will have less risk of being sued. Medical assistants can help by:

- Developing good listening skills and nonverbal communication techniques so that patients feel the time spent with them is not rushed
- Setting aside a certain time during the day for returning patients' phone calls
- Checking to be sure that all patients or their authorized representatives sign informed consent forms before they undergo medical or surgical procedures
- Avoiding statements that could be construed as an admission of fault on the part of the physician or other medical staff
- Using tact, good judgment, and professional ability in handling patients
- Making every effort to reach an understanding about fees with the patient before treatment so that billing does not become a point of contention

## Terminating Care of a Patient

A physician may wish to terminate care of a patient. Terminating care is sometimes called withdrawing from a case. Following are some typical reasons a physician may choose to withdraw from a case:

- The patient refuses to follow the physician's instructions.

## LETTER OF WITHDRAWAL FROM CASE

December 12, 2007

Jack Smallwood
Box 3457C
Rogersville, TN 37878

Dear Mr. Smallwood:

This is to inform you of our intent to discontinue medical care to you due to the habitual and continued non-compliance in your medical care. Our records indicate that you have missed several appointments and have not complied with ordered testing. This discontinuance will go into effect 30 days from the date of this letter in order to allow you sufficient time to locate another physician. We will be happy to forward your medical records to the physician of your choice. There is 24-hour medical care available to you at the hospital.

If you need assistance in locating a new physician, please contact your insurance carrier or the Tennessee Medical Society at 1-800-666-9898.

Sincerely,


John Doe, MD

**Figure 3-1.** Physicians are required to inform patients in writing if they wish to withdraw from a case.

- The patient's family members complain incessantly to or about the physician.
- A personality conflict develops between the physician and patient that cannot be reasonably resolved.
- The patient habitually does not pay or fails to make satisfactory arrangements to pay for medical services. A physician may stop treatment of such a patient and end the physician-patient relationship only if adequate notice is given to the patient.
- The patient fails to keep scheduled appointments. To protect the physician from charges of abandonment, all missed appointments should be noted in the patient's chart.

A physician who terminates care of a patient must do so in a formal, legal manner, following these four steps.

1. Write a letter to the patient, expressing the reason for withdrawing from the case and recommending that the patient seek medical care from another physician as soon as possible. Thirty days is the usual norm for finding another physician. Figure 3-1 shows an example of a letter of termination.

2. Send the letter by certified mail with a return receipt requested. This will provide evidence that the patient received the notification by providing a signature on the return receipt.

3. Place a copy of the letter (and the return receipt, when received) in the patient's medical record.

4. Summarize in the patient record the physician's reason for terminating care and the actions taken to inform the patient.

## Standard of Care

You are expected to fulfill the standards of the medical assisting profession for applying legal concepts to practice. According to the AAMA, medical assistants should uphold legal concepts in the following ways:

- Maintain confidentiality
- Practice within the scope of training and capabilities
- Prepare and maintain medical records
- Document accurately
- Use appropriate guidelines when releasing information

- Follow legal guidelines and maintain awareness of health-care legislation and regulations
- Maintain and dispose of regulated substances in compliance with government guidelines
- Follow established risk-management and safety procedures
- Meet the requirements for professional credentialing

Often, state laws dictate what medical assistants may or may not do. For instance, in some states it is illegal for medical assistants to draw blood. No states consider it legal for medical assistants to diagnose a condition, prescribe a treatment, or let a patient believe that a medical assistant is a nurse. In addition to what is stated by law, you and the physician must establish the procedures that are appropriate for you to perform.

## Administrative Duties and the Law

Many of a medical assistant's administrative duties are related to legal requirements. Paperwork for insurance billing, patient consent forms for surgical procedures, and correspondence (such as a physician's letter of withdrawal from a case) must be handled correctly to meet legal standards. Documentation, such as making appropriate and accurate entries in a patient's medical record, is legally important. You may also maintain the physician's appointment book. The appointment book is considered a legal document, especially for tracking missed or canceled appointments.

You may also be responsible for handling certain state reporting requirements. Items that must be reported include births; certain diseases such as acquired immunodeficiency syndrome (AIDS); drug abuse; suspected child abuse or abuse of the elderly; injuries caused by violence, such as knife and gunshot wounds; and deaths. Reports are sent to various state departments, depending on the content of the report. For example, suspected child abuse cases are reported to the state department of social services. Addressing these state requirements is called the physician's public duty.

Phone calls must be handled with an awareness of legal issues. For example, if the physician asks you to contact a patient by phone and you call the patient at work, you should not identify yourself or the physician by name to someone else without the patient's permission. You can say, for example, "Please tell Mrs. Arnot that her doctor's office is calling." If you do not take this precaution, the physician can be sued for invasion of privacy. You must abide by similar guidelines if you are responsible for making follow-up calls to a patient after a procedure or office visit.

## Documentation

Patient records are often used as evidence in professional medical liability cases, and improper documentation can contribute to or cause a case to be lost. Physicians should keep records that clearly show what treatment was performed and when it was done. It is important that physicians be able to demonstrate that nothing was neglected and that the care given fully met the standards demanded by law. One cliché to remember is "If it is not written down, then it was not done." Pay attention to spelling in charts and keep a medical dictionary handy if you are not sure of a spelling. Today's health-care environment requires complete documentation of actions taken and actions not taken. Medical staff members should pay particular attention to the following situations.

**Referrals.** Make sure the patient understands whether the referring physician's staff will make the appointment and notify the patient, or whether the patient must call to set up the appointment. Document in the chart that the patient was referred and the time and date of the appointment, and follow up with the specialist to verify that the appointment was scheduled and kept. Note whether reports of the consultation were received in your office, and document any further care of the patient from the referring physician.

**Missed Appointments.** At the end of the day, a designated person in the medical office should gather all patient charts of those who missed or canceled appointments without rescheduling. Charts should be dated, stamped, and documented "No Call/No Show" or "Canceled/No Reschedule." The appointment book is also considered a legal document; make sure that all missed appointments are documented on the appointment book or in the computer. The treating physician should review these records and note whether follow-up is indicated.

**Dismissals.** To avoid charges of abandonment, the physician must formally withdraw from a case. Be sure that a letter of withdrawal or dismissal has been filed in the patient's records. All mailing confirmations should be filed in the record, such as the return receipt from certified mail.

**All Other Patient Contact.** Patient records should include reports of all tests, procedures, and medications prescribed, including prescription refills. Make sure all necessary informed consent papers have been signed and filed in the chart. Make entries into the chart of all telephone conversations with the patient. Correct documentation requires the initials or signature of the person making the notation on the patient's chart as well as the date and time.

**Medical Record Correction.** Errors made when making an entry in a medical record or errors discovered later can be corrected, but corrections must be made in a certain manner so that if the medical records are ever used in a medical malpractice lawsuit, it will not appear that they were falsified. When deleting information, never black it out, never use correction fluid to cover it up, and never in any other way erase or obliterate the original wording. Draw a line through the original information so that it is still legible. Write or type in the correct information above or below the original line or in the margin. Chapter 9 describes the proper procedure for correcting chart errors.

**Ownership of the Patient Record.** Patients' medical records are considered the property of the owners of the facility where they were created. A physician in a private practice owns his or her charts or records, while records in a hospital or clinic belong to the facility. The facility in which the records were created owns the records, but the patient owns the information they contain. Upon signing a release, patients may usually obtain access to or copies of their medical records depending upon state law. Under HIPAA, patients who ask to see or copy their medical records must be accommodated with few exceptions, such as in mental health records where the physician decides it may be harmful to the patient to see the record. The physician is protected under the **doctrine of professional discretion.**

**Retention and Storage of the Patient Record.** As a protection against legal litigation, records should be kept until the applicable statute of limitations period has elapsed, which is generally two to seven years. In some cases, this involves keeping the medical records for minor patients for a specified length of time after they reach legal age. Some states have enacted statutes for the retention of medical records. Most physicians retain records indefinitely to provide evidence in medical professional liability suits or for tax purposes. The medical record may provide the patient's medical history for future medical treatment.

# Controlled Substances and the Law

You must also follow the correct procedures for the safe-keeping and disposal of controlled substances, such as narcotics, in the medical office. It is important to know the right dosages and potential complications of these drugs, as well as prescription refill rules, in order to understand and interpret the directions of the physician in a legally responsible manner. Prescription pads must be kept secure so that they do not fall into the wrong hands.

# Legal Documents and the Patient

You need to be aware of two legal documents that are typically completed by a patient prior to major surgery or hospitalization: the living will and the uniform donor card. Traditionally, these documents were completed outside the medical office or in the hospital. The current trend, however, is for medical practice personnel, including medical assistants, to assist patients in developing these important documents.

**Living Wills.** A **living will,** sometimes called an advance directive, is a legal document addressed to the patient's family and health-care providers. The living will states what type of treatment the patient wishes or does not wish to receive if she becomes terminally ill, unconscious, or permanently comatose (sometimes referred to as being in a persistent vegetative state). For example, a living will typically states whether a patient wishes to be put on life-sustaining equipment should she become permanently comatose. Some living wills contain DNR (do not resuscitate) orders. These orders mean the patient does not wish medical personnel to try to resuscitate her should the heart stop beating. Living wills are a means of helping families of terminally ill patients deal with the inevitable outcome of the illness and may help limit unnecessary medical costs.

The living will is signed when the patient is mentally and physically competent to do so. It must also be signed by two witnesses. Medical practices can help patients develop a living will, sometimes in conjunction with organizations that make available preprinted living will forms. The Partnership for Caring (based in Washington, D.C.) is one such organization.

Patients who have living wills are asked to name, in a document called a **durable power of attorney,** someone who will make decisions regarding medical care on their behalf if they are unable to do so. Often, a durable power of attorney for health care form is completed in conjunction with a living will.

**The Uniform Donor Card.** In 1968 the Uniform Anatomical Gift Act was passed, setting forth guidelines for all states to follow in complying with a person's wish to make a gift of one or more organs (or the whole body) upon death. An anatomical gift is typically designated for medical research, organ transplants, or placement in a tissue bank. The **uniform donor card** is a legal document that states one's wish to make such a gift. People often carry the uniform donor card in their wallets. Many medical practices offer the service of helping their patients obtain and complete a uniform donor card.

# Confidentiality Issues

The physician is legally obligated to keep patient information confidential. Therefore, you must be sure that all patient information is discussed with the patient privately and shared with the staff only when appropriate. For example, the billing department will have to see patient records to code diagnoses and bill appropriately.

You must avoid discussing cases with anyone outside the office, even if the patient's name is not mentioned. Only the patient can waive this confidentiality right.

# Federal Legislation Affecting Health Care

Congress has passed legislation intended to improve the quality of health care in the United States, to reduce fraud, and to ensure that patients will not be discriminated against by insurance providers. The most significant health-care laws passed in recent years are the Health Care Quality Improvement Act of 1986, the Federal False Claims Act, and the Health Insurance Portability and Accountability

Act (HIPAA) of 1996. HIPAA is discussed in detail in the chapter. The Occupational Safety and Health Administration (OSHA) regulations, which are vitally important to the practice of health care, are also discussed in detail in this chapter.

## Health Care Quality Improvement Act of 1986

The Health Care Quality Improvement Act of 1986 (HCQIA) is a federal statute passed to improve the quality of medical care nationwide. Congress created the Health Care Quality Improvement Act of 1986 because they found that there was an increasing occurrence of medical malpractice and a need to improve the quality of medical care. The act requires professional peer review in certain cases, limits damages professional review, and protects from liability those who provide information to professional review bodies. One of the most important provisions of the HCQIA was the establishment of the National Practitioner Data Bank. The use of the National Practitioner Data Bank was intended to improve the quality of medical care nationwide by encouraging effective professional peer review of physicians. Information that must be reported to the National Practitioner Data Bank includes medical malpractice payments, adverse licensure actions, adverse clinical privilege actions, and adverse professional membership actions. This data bank is a resource to assist state licensing boards, hospitals, and other health-care entities in investigating qualifications of physicians and other health-care practitioners.

## Federal False Claims Act

The Federal False Claims Act is a law that allows individuals to bring civil actions on the behalf of the United States government for false claims made to the federal government, under a provision of the law call *qui tam* (from Latin meaning to bring action for the king and for one's self). The law was enacted because of the rising cost of health care, fraud, and abuse within the health-care industry. As a result, laws have been passed to control three types of illegal conduct:

1. False billing claims. Fraudulently billing for services not performed is prohibited.
2. Kickbacks. Giving financial incentives to a health-care provider for referring patients or for recommending services or products is prohibited under the federal Anti-Kickback Law and by state laws.
3. Self-referrals. Referring patients to any service or facility where the health-care provider has financial interests is prohibited by the Federal Ethics in Patient Referral Act and other federal and state laws.

Violations of laws against health-care fraud and abuse can result in imprisonment and fines, a loss of professional license, a loss of health-care facility staff privileges, and exclusion from participating in federal health-care programs.

# OSHA Regulations

The Occupational Safety and Health Administration (OSHA), a division of the U.S. Department of Labor, has created federal laws to protect health-care workers from health hazards on the job. Medical personnel may accidentally contract a dangerous or even fatal disease by coming into contact with a virus a patient is carrying. Medical assistants may also be exposed to toxic substances in the office. OSHA regulations describe the precautions a medical office must take with clothing, housekeeping, record keeping, and training to minimize the risk of disease or injury. Chapter 20 discusses OSHA in detail.

Some of the most important OSHA regulations are those for controlling workers' exposure to infectious disease. These regulations are set forth in the OSHA Bloodborne Pathogens Protection Standard of 1991. A pathogen is any microorganism that causes disease. Microorganisms are microscopic living bodies such as viruses or bacteria that may be present in a patient's blood or other body fluids (saliva or semen).

Of particular concern to medical workers are the human immunodeficiency virus (HIV), which causes AIDS, and the hepatitis B virus (HBV). AIDS damages the body's immune system and thus its ability to fight disease. AIDS is always fatal. HBV is a highly contagious disease that is potentially fatal. It causes inflammation of the liver and may cause liver failure. Every year, about 8700 health-care workers become HBV-infected at work, and about 200 die from the disease. (Chapter 21 discusses HIV, hepatitis, and other blood-borne pathogens.)

OSHA requires that medical professionals in medical practices follow what are called Standard Precautions. They were developed by the Centers for Disease Control and Prevention (CDC) to prevent medical professionals from exposing themselves and others to blood-borne pathogens. Exposure can occur, for example, through skin that has been broken from a needle puncture or other wound and through mucous membranes, such as those in the nose and throat. If these areas come into contact with a patient's (or coworker's) blood or body fluids, a virus could be transferred from one person to another. Chapter 20 covers standard precautions in more detail.

## Protective Gear

The more exposure that is involved, the more protective clothing you need to wear (Figure 3-2). Procedures that usually involve exposure to blood, other body fluids, or broken skin require gloves. There are several kinds of gloves for different situations.

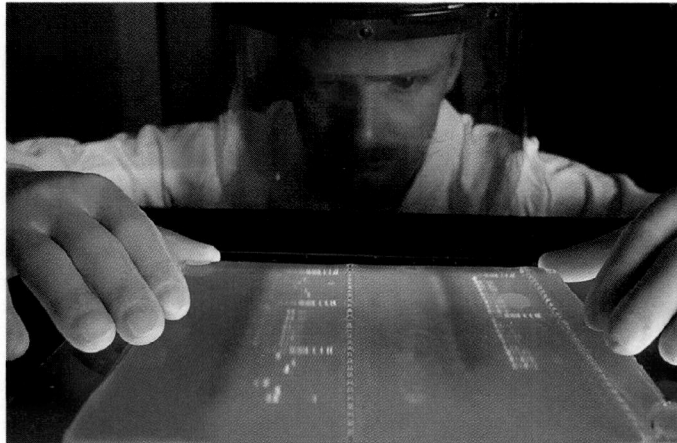

**Figure 3-2.** Researchers must wear full protective gear in a laboratory that studies infectious diseases. Regulations for such gear are set by OSHA.

- Disposable gloves are worn only once and then discarded. Do not use a pair that has been torn or damaged.
- Utility gloves are stronger and may be decontaminated. They are used for housecleaning tasks.
- Examination gloves are used for procedures that do not require a sterile environment.
- Sterile gloves are used for sterile procedures such as minor surgery.

Appropriate masks, goggles, or face shields must be used for procedures in which a worker's eyes, nose, or mouth may be exposed. These are procedures that may involve spraying or splashes—for example, examining blood. If potentially infected substances might get onto a worker's clothing, the worker must wear a protective laboratory coat, gown, or apron. Fluid-resistant material is recommended by OSHA.

The law requires that the physician/employer provide all necessary protective clothing to the employee free of charge. The employer also pays for cleaning, maintaining, and replacing the protective items.

## Decontamination

After a procedure, you must decontaminate all exposed work surfaces with a 10% bleach solution or with a germ-killing solution containing glutoraldohydes approved by the Environmental Protection Agency (EPA). Replace protective coverings on equipment and surfaces if they have been exposed. Regularly decontaminate receptacles such as bins, pails, and cans as part of routine housekeeping procedures. Never pick up broken glass with your hands. Use tongs, even when wearing gloves, so that the sharp glass does not cut the gloves and expose the skin.

Dispose of any potentially infectious waste materials in special "biohazard bags," which are leakproof and labeled with the biohazard symbol (Figure 3-3). Wastes that fall into this category include blood products, body

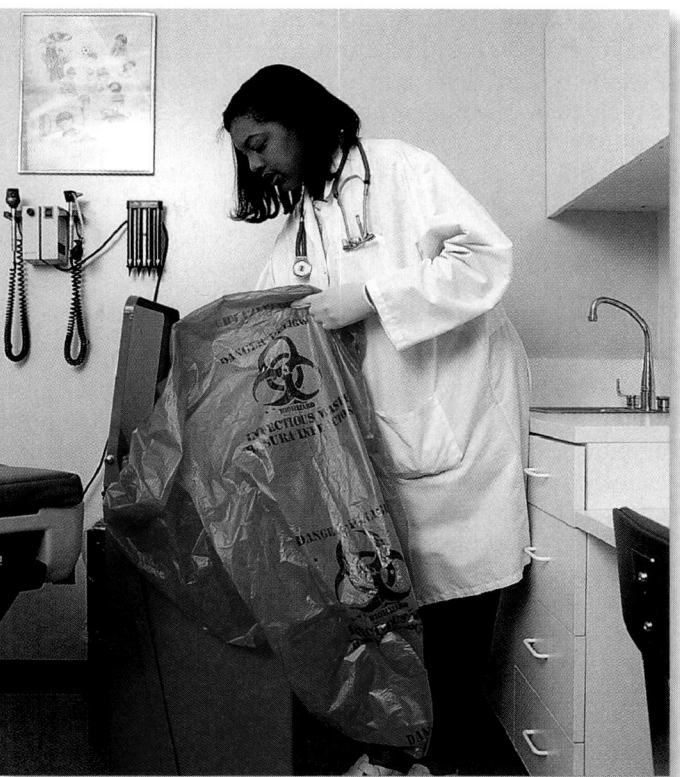

**Figure 3-3.** The medical assistant may be responsible for disposing of wastes such as gloves, table paper, and gauze with body fluids on them in containers that display the biohazard symbol.

fluids, human tissues, and vaccines; table paper, linen, towels, and gauze with body fluids on them; and gloves, diapers, sanitary napkins, and cotton swabs. The next section discusses disposal of sharp instruments ("sharps").

## Sharp Equipment

Disposable sharp equipment that has been used must not be bent, broken, recapped, or otherwise tampered with, so as to prevent possible exposure to medical workers. It should be placed in a leakproof, puncture-resistant, color-coded, and appropriately labeled container. Reusable sharp equipment must be placed as soon as possible into a puncture-resistant container and taken to a reprocessing area.

Both disposable and reusable instruments are sterilized in their appropriate containers. Sterilizing is usually accomplished by means of an autoclave, a machine that uses pressurized steam. Sterilization of disposable instruments is usually handled by an outside waste management company.

## Exposure Incidents

You must give special attention to what to do in case of an exposure incident. This may happen when a medical worker accidentally sticks herself with a used needle. These "puncture exposure incidents" are the most common kind of exposure.

When an exposure incident occurs, the physician/employer must be notified immediately. Quick and proper treatment can help prevent the development of HBV. Timely action can also prevent exposing other people to any infection the worker may have acquired. Reporting the incident to the physician/employer also may encourage him to revise the office's safety procedures in some way to help prevent the same type of incident from happening again.

## Postexposure Procedures

OSHA requires specific postexposure evaluation and follow-up procedures. If an exposure incident occurs, the employer must offer the exposed employee a free medical evaluation by a health-care provider of the employer's choice. The employer must refer the employee to a licensed health-care provider who will counsel the employee about what happened and how to prevent the spread of any potential infection. The health-care provider will also take a blood sample and prescribe the appropriate treatment. The employee has the right to refuse both the medical evaluation and the treatment.

When a medical worker starts a job, the physician/employer is required to offer the worker, at no cost, the opportunity to have an HBV vaccination within 10 days. An employee who refuses vaccination must sign a waiver. The employee can change his mind at any time and decide to have the vaccination. If an employee who declined the HBV vaccination is exposed to a patient who is HBV-positive or who is being tested for HBV, it is recommended that the employee be tested for HBV and receive the vaccination if necessary. (The employee may decline to be tested, however.) If the patient is being tested for HBV, the employee is legally required to be informed of the test results. (This is true for HIV as well, and the employee still has the right to refuse testing.) The employee may agree to give blood but not be tested. The blood sample must be kept on hand for 90 days in case the worker later develops symptoms of HBV or HIV infection and then decides to be tested.

The health-care provider that performs the postexposure evaluation must give the employer a written report stating whether HBV vaccination was recommended and received. The report must also state that the employee, if tested, was informed of the blood test results. Any information beyond this must be kept confidential.

If you plan to do an externship in a medical office, the physician does not have to provide you with the HBV vaccine. She may, however, deny you the opportunity to do the externship if you have not received the vaccination elsewhere. Many accredited medical assisting programs offer the vaccine to their students.

## Laundry

OSHA has regulations for handling potentially infectious laundry. Hospitals have their own laundry facilities because these facilities are cost-effective. Some larger clinics also have their own laundry facilities. Most doctors' offices, however, send laundry out. Laundry must be bagged and labeled. Any wet laundry to be transported should be packed so that it does not leak. The laundry service the medical office uses should abide by all OSHA regulations. Laundry workers must wear gloves and handle contaminated materials as little as possible. Some doctors' offices use only disposable items, such as paper robes, and do not need laundry service.

## Hazardous Materials

You may encounter hazardous equipment and toxic substances in the office. These hazards include vaccines, disinfectants, and laser equipment.

OSHA's Occupational Health and Safety Act of 1970 sets minimum requirements for workplace safety. It also requires employers to keep an inventory of all hazardous materials used in the workplace. Containers of hazardous substances must be labeled in a specific way, listing any potentially harmful ingredients. The employer must post Material Safety Data Sheets (MSDS) about these substances. These sheets specify whether the substance is cancer-causing, list other possible risks, and state OSHA's requirements for controlling exposure. All employees are entitled to be informed about hazardous substances in the workplace and to be trained in how to use them safely.

## Training Requirements

Training requirements are part of OSHA's hazardous substance regulations. Every employee who may be exposed to hazardous or infectious substances on the job must be given free information and training during working hours at least once a year. Training must also be held when a new chemical or piece of medical equipment is introduced into the office or when a procedure changes. Training must cover the following topics:

- How to obtain a copy of the OSHA regulations and an explanation of them
- The causes and symptoms of blood-borne diseases
- How blood-borne pathogens are transmitted
- The facility's Exposure Control Plan and how to obtain a copy
- What tasks might result in exposure
- The use and limitations of all the precautions
- All aspects of personal protective equipment
- All aspects of HBV vaccination
- Emergency procedures
- Postexposure procedures
- Warning labels, signs, and color coding

Beyond this federal law, state training requirements vary. The states of Washington and Florida require medical assistants to take a short course specifically covering HIV laws and precautions. Your instructor will familiarize

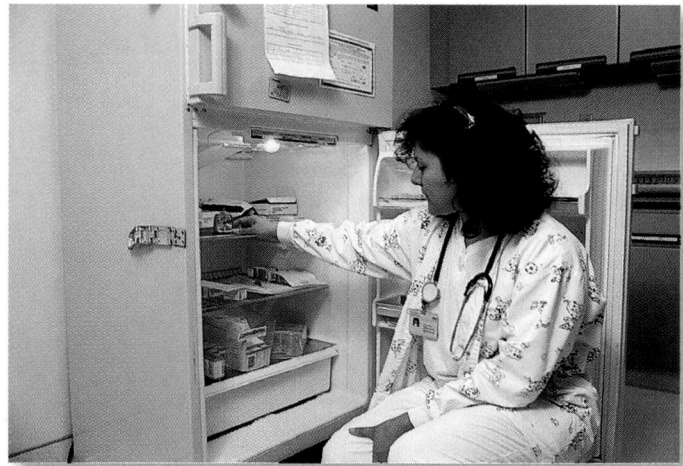

**Figure 3-4.** OSHA laws require blood or other potentially infectious material to be stored separately from food and drinks. Refrigerators storing such material should have working thermometers to ensure proper cooling temperature.

you with your state's policy. OSHA has its own training institute, supports various other training resources, and develops training videotapes and tests for trainees. In some doctors' offices, the laboratory supervisor conducts training for the office staff. Anyone who has gone through a training session can then train others.

## General Regulations

General work area laws restrict eating, drinking, smoking, applying cosmetics or lip balm, and handling contact lenses in the work area. These laws also forbid storing food or drinks in refrigerators that are used to store blood or other potentially infectious material. Refrigerators must have working thermometers to ensure proper cooling temperature (Figure 3-4).

There are also required procedures for various specific on-the-job injuries. For instance, for eye injuries such as burns and chemical splashes, OSHA requires flushing the eye(s) for 15 minutes with a constant water flow.

## Documentation

Lastly, OSHA's record-keeping and documentation requirements are intended to protect the legal rights and safety of everyone in the medical office. The office must have a written Exposure Control Plan describing all precautions against exposure to hazards and blood-borne pathogens and specifying what to do if exposure occurs. Employee medical and exposure records must be kept on file during employment and for 30 years afterward. If an employer retires or closes the practice, the employee records are forwarded to the director of OSHA. Also, a log of occupational injuries and illnesses, OSHA Form 200, must be kept for 5 years. The employer must also keep on

file for 3 years records documenting an employee's training: dates, topics covered, and names and qualifications of the trainers.

## OSHA Inspections

In response to a complaint, or sometimes at random, OSHA may send a compliance officer to inspect a medical office. In 1995 approximately 29,000 inspections were performed. The penalties for not complying with regulations vary according to the severity of the offense. For example, if an inspector finds that the medical assistants have not worn gloves for 2 months because the employer did not make them available, there would be a severe penalty. If four assistants were wearing gloves but one had forgotten to put them on, there would be a lesser penalty. There are reductions for complying on the spot—perhaps no penalty will be charged. In a serious case, the office could be charged up to $10,000 per broken regulation, multiplied by the number of employees. The penalties are paid directly to OSHA, but the money goes into the federal treasury. If a serious violation occurs in a physicians' office laboratory, the laboratory's payments from Medicare may be suspended.

## Quality Control and Assurance

A medical office often has a physicians' office laboratory to perform different types of clinical tests, depending on the physician's specialty and state laws. The Clinical Laboratory Improvement Amendments of 1988 (CLIA '88) lists the regulations for laboratory testing. Physicians must display a certificate from CLIA confirming that their office complies with CLIA regulations. These regulations set standards for the quality of work performed in a laboratory and the accuracy of test results. Congress passed these laws after publicity about deaths caused by errors in the test used to diagnose cancer of the uterus.

According to CLIA '88, there are three categories of laboratory tests: waived tests, moderate-complexity tests, and high-complexity tests. Waived tests, the simplest kind, require the least amount of judgment and pose an insignificant risk to the patient in the event of an error. The laboratory applies for a certificate of waiver from the U.S. Department of Health and Human Services, which grants permission to perform any test on the list of waived tests and to bill it to Medicare or Medicaid. Tests that patients can do at home with kits approved by the department's Food and Drug Administration (FDA), such as the blood glucose test, also fall under this heading.

Most tests are in the moderate-complexity category. Cholesterol testing and checking for the presence or absence of sperm are examples. CLIA lists all waived and moderate-complexity tests and considers all other tests to be of high complexity.

## TABLE 3-1 CLIA '88 Waived Tests

| Urine | Blood | Other Body Fluids and Substances |
|---|---|---|
| • Bilirubin<br>• Glucose<br>• Hemoglobin<br>• Ketones<br>• Leukocytes<br>• Nitrite<br>• pH<br>• Protein<br>• Specific gravity<br>• Urobilinogen<br>• Ovulation<br>• Pregnancy<br>• Drug screen<br>• Nicotine<br>• Microalbumin<br>• Creatinine<br>• Tumor associated antigen (bladder cancer)<br>• Catalase | • Erythrocyte sedimentation rate<br>• Hemoglobin<br>• Microhematocrit<br>• Glucose<br>• Prothrombin time<br>• Ketones<br>• Total cholesterol<br>• HDL cholesterol<br>• LDL cholesterol<br>• Triglycerides<br>• Hemoglobin A1c<br>• Lactate<br>• Lead<br>• Thyroid-stimulating hormone<br>• Mononucleosis<br>• *Helicobacter pylori* antibodies<br>• Lyme disease antibodies<br>• HIV antibodies | • Fecal occult blood<br>• Alcohol in saliva<br>• Influenza A and B<br>• Vaginal Trichomonas<br>• Vaginal pH<br>• Strep A throat swab<br>• Sperm concentration by home screening procedure |

Under CLIA '88, medical assistants are always allowed to perform waived tests. Table 3-1 lists these tests. Medical assistants can also perform moderate-complexity tests as long as the physician can ensure that the assistant is appropriately trained and experienced according to federal guidelines. Some state laws may be stricter than the federal laws, so the medical office should check with the state health department to see if there are any local rules about what kinds of tests medical assistants may perform. As you advance in your career, you will most likely be trained to do more and more types of tests, receiving training either by senior staff members or through outside programs.

## Elements of the Quality Assurance Program

CLIA '88 also requires every medical office to have a quality assurance (QA) program. This program must include a quality control (QC) program specifically for the laboratory. The goal is to track and improve the quality of all aspects of the medical practice—including patient care, laboratory procedures, record keeping, employee evaluations, finances, legal responsibilities, public image, staff morale, insurance issues, and patient education. Documentation is required by QA regulations, to provide evidence that QA procedures are in place in the office. This documentation becomes extremely important if there is an inspection or a legal dispute.

Any QA program must include the following elements:

- Written policies on the standards of patient care and professional behavior
- A QC program

- Training and continuing education programs
- An instrument maintenance program
- Documentation requirements
- Evaluation methods

Software programs are available to help medical offices develop a QA program and procedures manual.

## The Laboratory QC Program

The laboratory QC program must cover testing concerns such as patient preparation procedures, collection of the specimen (blood, urine, or tissue), labeling, preservation and transportation, test methods, inconsistent results, use and maintenance of equipment, personnel training, complaints and investigations, and corrective actions. The accuracy of the tests, and the instruments and chemicals that are used, must be monitored through QC procedures and documented. (Chapter 32 discusses laboratory QC programs in more detail.)

## HIPAA

Today, health care is considered a trillion-dollar industry, growing rapidly with technology and employing millions of health-care workers in numerous fields. The U.S. Department of Labor recognizes 400 different job titles in the health-care industry.

On August 21, 1996, the U.S. Congress passed the Health Insurance Portability and Accountability Act (HIPAA). The primary goals of the act are to improve the portability and continuity of health-care coverage in group and individual markets; to combat waste, fraud, and abuse in health-care insurance and health-care delivery; to promote the use of medical savings accounts; to improve access to long-term care services and coverage; and to simplify the administration of health insurance.

The purposes of the act are to:

- Improve the efficiency and effectiveness of health-care delivery by creating a national framework for health privacy protection that builds on efforts by states, health systems, and individual organizations and individuals
- Protect and enhance the rights of patients by providing them access to their health information and controlling the inappropriate use or disclosure of that information
- Improve the quality of health care by restoring trust in the health-care system among consumers, health-care professionals, and the multitude of organizations and individuals committed to the delivery of care

HIPAA is divided into two main sections of law: Title I, which addresses health-care portability, and Title II, which covers the prevention of health-care fraud and abuse, administrative simplification, and medical liability reform.

## Title I: Health-Care Portability

The issue of portability deals with protecting health-care coverage for employees who change jobs, allowing them to carry their existing plans with them to new jobs. HIPAA provides the following protections for employees and their families:

- Increases workers' ability to get health-care coverage when starting a new job.
- Reduces workers' probability of losing existing health-care coverage.
- Helps workers maintain continuous health-care coverage when changing jobs.
- Helps workers purchase health insurance on their own if they lose coverage under an employer's group plan and have no other health-care coverage available.

The specific protections of this title include the following:

- Limits the use of exclusions for preexisting conditions.
- Prohibits group plans from discriminating by denying coverage or charging extra for coverage based on an individual's or a family member's past or present poor health.
- Guarantees certain small employers, as well as certain individuals who lose job-related coverage, the right to purchase health insurance.
- Guarantees, in most cases, that employers or individuals who purchase health insurance can renew the coverage regardless of any health conditions of individuals covered under the insurance policy.

## Title II: Prevention of Health-Care Fraud and Abuse, Administrative Simplification, and Medical Liability Reform

**HIPAA Privacy Rule.** The HIPAA Standards for Privacy of Individually Identifiable Health Information provide the first comprehensive federal protection for the privacy of health information. The **Privacy Rule** is designed to provide strong privacy protections that do not interfere with patient access to health care or the quality of health-care delivery. This act creates, for the first time, national standards to protect individuals' medical records and other personal health information. The privacy rule is intended to:

- Give patients more control over their health information
- Set boundaries on the use and release of health-care records
- Establish appropriate safeguards that health-care providers and others must achieve to protect the privacy of health information
- Hold violators accountable, with civil and criminal penalties that can be imposed if they violate patients' privacy rights
- Strike a balance when public responsibility supports disclosure of some forms of data—for example, to protect public health

Before the HIPAA Privacy Rule, the personal information that moves across hospitals and doctors' offices, insurers or third-party payers, and state lines fell under a patchwork of federal and state laws. This information could be distributed—without either notice or authorization—for reasons that had nothing to do with a patient's medical treatment or health-care reimbursement. For example, unless otherwise forbidden by state or local law, without the Privacy Rule, patient information held by a health plan could, without the patient's permission, be passed on to a lender who could then deny the patient's application for a home mortgage or a credit card or could be given to an employer who could use it in personnel decisions.

Individually identifiable health information includes:

- Name
- Address
- Phone numbers
- Fax number
- Dates (birth, death, admission, discharge, etc.)
- Social Security number
- E-mail address
- Medical record numbers
- Health plan beneficiary numbers
- Account numbers
- Certificate or license numbers

- Vehicle identifiers and serial numbers, including license plate numbers
- Device identifiers and serial numbers
- Web Universal Resource Locators (URLs)
- Internet Protocol (IP) address numbers

The core of the HIPAA Privacy Rule is the protection, use, and disclosure of **protected health information (PHI).** Protected health information means individually identifiable health information that is transmitted or maintained by electronic or other media, such as computer storage devices. The Privacy Rule protects all PHI held or transmitted by a covered entity, which includes health-care providers, health plans, and health-care clearinghouses. Other covered entities include employers, life insurers, schools or universities, and public health authorities. Protected health information can come in any form or media, such as electronic, paper, or oral, including verbal communications among staff members, patients, and other providers. *Use* and *disclosure* are the two fundamental concepts in the HIPAA Privacy Rule. It is important to understand the differences between these terms.

*Use.* **Use** refers to performing any of the following actions to individually identifiable health information by employees or other members of an organization's workforce:

- Sharing
- Employing
- Applying
- Utilizing
- Examining
- Analyzing

Information is used when it moves within an organization.

*Disclosure.* **Disclosure** occurs when the entity holding the information performs any of the following actions so that the information is outside the entity:

- Releasing
- Transferring
- Providing access to
- Divulging in any manner

Information is disclosed when it is transmitted between or among organizations.

Under HIPAA, *use* limits the sharing of information within a covered entity, whereas *disclosure* restricts the sharing of information outside the entity holding the information.

The Privacy Rule covers the following PHI:

- The past, present, or future physical or mental health or condition of an individual
- Health care that is provided to an individual
- Billing or payments made for health care provided

Information that is not individually identifiable or unable to be tied to the identity of a particular patient is not subject to the Privacy Rule.

*Managing and Storing Patient Information.* Medical facilities have undergone many changes to the way they manage and store patient information. The Privacy Rule compliance was enforced in April of 2003. Many facilities contracted consultants that specialized in HIPAA and became certified in HIPAA compliance. For the health-care provider, the Privacy Rule requires activities such as:

- Notifying patients of their privacy rights and how their information is used
- Adopting and implementing privacy procedures for its practice, hospital, or plan
- Training employees so that they understand the privacy procedures
- Designating an individual to be responsible for seeing that the privacy procedures are adopted and followed
- Securing patient records containing individually identifiable health information so that they are not readily available to those who do not need them

Under HIPAA, patients have an increased awareness of their health information privacy rights, which includes the following:

- The right to access, copy, and inspect their health-care information
- The right to request an amendment to their health-care information
- The right to obtain an accounting of certain disclosures of their health-care information
- The right to alternate means of receiving communications from providers
- The right to complain about alleged violations of the regulations and the provider's own information policies

*Sharing Patient Information.* When sharing patient information, HIPAA will allow the provider to use health-care information for **treatment, payment, and operations (TPO).**

- Treatment. Providers are allowed to share information in order to provide care to patients
- Payment. Providers are allowed to share information in order to receive payment for the treatment provided
- Operations. Providers are allowed to share information to conduct normal business activities, such as quality improvement

If the use of patient information does not fall under TPO, then written authorization must be obtained *before* sharing information with anyone.

Patient information may be disclosed without authorization to the following parties or in the following situations:

- Medical researchers
- Emergencies
- Funeral directors/coroners
- Disaster relief services

- Law enforcement
- Correctional institutions
- Abuse and neglect
- Organ and tissue donation centers
- Work-related conditions that may affect employee health
- Judicial/administrative proceedings at the patient's request or as directed by a subpoena or court order

When using or disclosing PHI, a provider must make reasonable efforts to limit the use or disclosure to the minimum amount of PHI necessary to accomplish the intended purpose. Providing only the minimum necessary information means taking reasonable safeguards to protect an individual's health information from incidental disclosure. State laws may impose more stringent requirements regarding the protection of patient information. Health-care providers and staff should only have access to information they need to fulfill their assigned duties. The minimum necessary standard does not apply to disclosures, including oral disclosures, among health-care providers for treatment purposes. For example, a physician is not required to apply the minimum necessary standard when discussing a patient's medical chart information with a specialist at another hospital.

***Patient Notification.*** Since the effective date of the HIPAA Privacy Rule, medical facilities have made major changes in how they inform patients of their HIPAA compliance. You may have noticed, as a patient yourself, the forms and information packets that are now provided by your health-care providers. The first step in informing patients of HIPAA compliance is the communication of patient rights. These rights are communicated through a document called **Notice of Privacy Practices (NPP).** A notice must:

- Be written in plain, simple language.
- Include a header that reads: "This Notice describes how medical information about you may be used and disclosed and how you can get access to this information. Please review carefully."
- Describe the covered entity's uses and disclosures of PHI.
- Describe an individual's rights under the Privacy Rule.
- Describe the covered entity's duties.
- Describe how to register complaints concerning suspected privacy violations.
- Specify a point of contract.
- Specify an effective date.
- State that the entity reserves to right to change its privacy practices.

The second step in patient notification is to implement a document that explains the policy of the medical facility on obtaining **authorization** for the use and disclosure of patient information for purposes other than TPO. The authorization form must be written in plain language. Some of the core elements of an authorization form include:

- Specific and meaningful descriptions of the authorized information
- Persons authorized to use or disclose protected health information
- Purpose of the requested information
- Statement of the patient's right to revoke the authorization
- Signature and date of the patient

**Security Measures.** Health-care facilities can undertake a number of measures in order to help reduce a breach of confidentiality, including for information that is either stored or delivered electronically (that is, stored in computers or computer networks, or delivered via computer networks or the Internet).

***HIPAA Security Rule.*** In February 2003, the final regulations were issued regarding the administrative, physical, and technical safeguards to protect the confidentiality, integrity, and availability of health information covered by HIPAA. The **Security Rule** specifies how patient information is protected on computer networks, the Internet, disks, and other storage media and extranets. The rapidly increasing use of computers in health care today has created new dangers for breaches of confidentiality. The Security Rule mandates that:

- A security officer must be assigned the responsibility for the medical facility's security
- All staff, including management, receives security awareness training
- Medical facilities must implement audit controls to record and examine staff who have logged into information systems that contain PHI
- Organizations limit physical access to medical facilities that contain electronic PHI
- Organizations must conduct risk analyses to determine information security risks and vulnerabilities
- Organizations must establish policies and procedures that allow access to electronic PHI on a need-to-know basis

Computers are not the only concern regarding security of the workplace. The facility layout can propose a possible violation if not designed correctly. All facilities must take measures to reduce the identity of patient information. Some examples of facility design that can help reduce a breach of confidentiality include the security of patient charts, the reception area, the clinical station, and faxes sent and received.

***Chart Security.*** Patient charts can be kept confidential by following these rules:

- Charts that contain a patient's name or other identifiers cannot be in view at the front reception area or nurse's station. Some offices have placed charts in plain jackets to prevent information from being seen.
- Charts must be stored out of the view of a public area, so that they cannot be seen by unauthorized individuals.

- Charts should be placed on the filing shelves without the patient name showing.
- Charts should be locked when not in use. Many facilities have purchased filing equipment that can be locked and unlocked without limiting the availability of patient information.
- Every staff member who uses patient information must be logged and a confidentiality statement signed. Signatures of staff should be on file with the office.

***Reception Area Security.*** The following steps can be taken to secure the reception area:

- Log off or turn your monitor off when leaving your terminal or computer.
- The computer must be placed in an area where other patients cannot see the screen.
- Many facilities are purchasing flat screen monitors to prevent visibility of the screen.
- The sign-in sheet must be monitored and not left out in patient view. The names of patients must be blacked out so the next patient cannot read the names. It is best to put another system in place and to eliminate the sign-in sheet.
- Many offices are reviewing the reception area with regard to phone conversations. Some offices are creating call centers away from the reception/waiting area.

***Medical Assistant Clinical Station Security.*** Medical assistants should follow these guidelines to protect PHI at the clinical station:

- Log off or turn your monitor off when leaving your terminal or computer.
- When placing charts in exam room racks or in shelves, the name of the patient or other identifiers must be concealed from other patients.
- HIPAA does not have a regulation about calling patients' names in the reception area, but to increase privacy in your facility, you may suggest a numbering system to identify patients.
- When discussing a patient with another staff member or with the physician, make sure your voice is lowered and that all doors to the exam rooms are closed. Avoid discussing patient conditions in heavy traffic areas.
- When discussing a condition with a patient, make sure that you are in a private room or area where no one can hear you.
- Avoid discussing patients in lunchrooms, hallways, or any place in a medical facility where someone can overhear you.

***Fax Security.*** A lot of information is exchanged over the fax machine in a medical office. The fax machine is a vital link among physicians, hospitals, insurance companies, and other medical staff members. Private health information can be exchanged via faxes sent to covered entities.

Here are some recommendations to help safeguard information exchanged via fax machines:

- Fax cover page. State clearly on the fax cover sheet that confidential and protected health information is included. Further state that the information included is to be protected and must not be shared or disclosed without the appropriate authorizations from the patient.
- Location of the fax machine. Keep the fax machine in an area that is not accessible by individuals who are not authorized to view PHI.
- Faxes with protected health information. Faxes that your office receives with PHI must be stored promptly in a protected, secure area.
- Fax number. Always confirm the accuracy of fax numbers to minimize the possibility of faxes being sent to the wrong person. Call people to tell them the fax is being sent.
- Confirmation. Program the fax machine to print a confirmation for all faxes sent, and staple the confirmation sheet to each document sent.
- Training. Train all staff members to understand the importance of safeguarding PHI sent or received via fax.

***Copier Security.*** Medical assistants should follow these guidelines to protect PHI at the copier:

- Do not leave confidential documents anywhere on the copier where others can read the information.
- Do not discard copies in a shared trash container—shred them.
- If a paper jam occurs, be sure to remove from the copier the copy or partial copy that caused the jam.

***Printer Security.*** To maintain the confidentiality of printed materials, medical assistants should follow these guidelines:

- Do not print confidential material on a printer shared by other departments or in an area where others can read the material.
- Do not leave the printer unattended while printing confidential material.
- Before leaving the printing area, make sure all computer disks containing confidential information and all printed material have been collected.
- Be certain that the print job is sent to the right printer location.
- Do not discard printouts in a shared trash container—shred them.

**Violations and Penalties.** Every staff member is responsible for adhering to HIPAA privacy and security regulations to ensure that PHI is secure and confidential. Anyone who uses or shares patient information is ethically obligated to comply with HIPAA. If PHI is abused or confidentiality is breached, the medical facility can incur substantial penalties or even the incarceration of staff. Violations of HIPAA law can result in both civil and criminal penalties.

*Civil Penalties.* Civil penalties for HIPAA privacy violations can be up to $100 for each offense, with an annual cap of $25,000 for repeated violations of the same requirement.

*Criminal Penalties.* Criminal penalties for the knowing, wrongful misuse of individually identifiable health information can result in the following penalties:

- For the knowing misuse of individually identifiable health information: up to $50,000 and/or one year in prison.
- For misuse under false pretenses: up to $100,000 and/or 5 years in prison.
- For offenses to sell for profit or malicious harm: up to $250,000 and/or 10 years in prison.

**Administrative Simplification.** The main key to the set of rules established for HIPAA administrative simplification is standardizing patient information throughout the health-care system with a set of transaction standards and code sets. The codes and formats used for the exchange of medical data are referred to as **electronic transaction records.** Regulated transaction information is given a transaction set identifier. For example, a health-care professional claim would be given an identifier of ASC X12N 837. This is a standard transaction code given to any facility that submits a health-care claim to an insurance company.

Standardized code sets are used for encoding data elements. The following books are used for the standardized code sets for all health-care facilities:

- *ICD-9-CM*, Volumes 1 and 2. This book is used to identify diseases and conditions.
- *CPT 4.* This book is used to identify physician services or procedures.
- *HCPCS.* This book is used to identify health-related services that are not physician or hospital services and procedures, such as radiology or hearing and vision services.

## Frequently Asked Questions About HIPAA

1. May one physician's office send a patient's medical records to another physician's office without the patient's consent?

   *Yes.*

2. Does the HIPAA Privacy Rule prohibit or discourage doctor/patient e-mails?

   *Health-care practitioners can continue to correspond with patients via e-mail, but appropriate electronic safeguards must be in place.*

3. May a patient be listed in a hospital's directory without the patient's consent, and may the directory be shared with the public?

   *The HIPAA Privacy Rule allows hospitals to continue providing directory information to the public unless the patient has specifically chosen not to be included. Hospital directories can include the patient's name, location in the facility, and general condition.*

4. May a patient's family member pick up prescriptions for the patient?

   *The Privacy Rule allows family members to pick up prescriptions, medical supplies, x-rays, or other similar forms of protected health information.*

5. Is a hospital allowed to share patient information with the patient's family without the patient's expressed consent?

   *HIPAA provides that a health-care provider may "disclose to a family member, other relative, or a close personal friend of the individual, or any other person identified by the individual" medical information directly relevant to such a person's involvement with the patient's care or payment related to the patient's care.*

6. Can patients sue health-care providers who do not comply with the HIPAA Privacy Rule?

   *The HIPAA Privacy Rule does not give patients the express right to sue. The patient can file a written complaint with the Secretary of Health and Human Services (HHS) through the office of the Civil Rights. The HHS Secretary then decides whether or not to investigate the complaint.*

7. If a patient refuses to sign an acknowledgement stating that he or she received the health-care provider's notice of privacy practices, must the health-care provider refuse to provide services?

   *The Privacy Rule gives the patient a "right of notice" of privacy practices for protecting identifiable health information. It requires that providers make a "good faith effort" to have patients acknowledge receipt of the notice, but the law does not give health-care practitioners the right to refuse treatment to people who do not sign the acknowledgement.*

# Confidentiality Issues and Mandatory Disclosure

Related to law, ethics, and quality care is the issue of when the medical assistant can disclose information and when it must be kept confidential. The incidents that doctors are legally required to report to the state were outlined earlier in the chapter. A doctor can be charged with criminal action for not following state and federal laws.

Ethics and professional judgment are always important. Consider the question of whether to contact the partners of a patient who has a sexually transmitted disease (STD) and whether to keep the patient's name from those people. The law says that the physician must instruct patients on how to notify possibly affected third parties and give them referrals to get the proper assistance.

If the patient refuses to inform involved outside parties, then the doctor's office may offer to notify current and former partners. The Caution: Handle With Care section addresses this issue.

In general, the patient's ethical right to confidentiality and privacy is protected by law. Only the patient can waive the right to confidentiality. A physician cannot publicize a patient case in journal articles or invite other health professionals to observe a case without the patient's written consent. Most states also prohibit a doctor from testifying in court about a patient without the patient's approval. When a patient sues a physician, however, the patient automatically gives up the right to confidentiality.

Following are six principles for preventing improper release of information from the medical office.

1. When in doubt about whether to release information, it is better not to release it.

2. It is the patient's, not the doctor's, right to keep patient information confidential. If the patient wants to disclose the information, it is unethical for the physician not to do so.

3. All patients should be treated with the same degree of confidentiality, whatever the health-care professional's personal opinion of the patient might be.

4. You should be aware of all applicable laws and of the regulations of agencies such as public health departments.

5. When it is necessary to break confidentiality and when there is a conflict between ethics and confidentiality, discuss it with the patient. If the law does not dictate what to do in the situation, the attending physician should make the judgment based on the urgency of the situation and any danger that might be posed to the patient or others.

6. Get written approval from the patient before releasing information. For common situations, the patient should sign a standard release-of-records form.

## CAUTION *Handle With Care*

# Notifying Those at Risk for Sexually Transmitted Disease

Few things are more difficult for a patient with an STD than telling current and former partners about the diagnosis. In fact, some patients elect not to do so. When patients refuse to alert their partners, the medical office can offer to make those contacts. Often that responsibility lies with the medical assistant.

You are most likely to encounter such a situation if you are a medical assistant working in a family practice, an obstetrics/gynecology practice, or a clinic. Becoming familiar with all facets of the situation—from ensuring patient confidentiality to handling potentially difficult confrontations—will help you best serve the patient.

The first step is to get the appropriate information from the patient who has contracted the STD. Because the patient may be sensitive about revealing former and current partners, help him feel more comfortable. First, spend some time talking about the STD. How much does the patient know about it? Educate him about implications, including the probable short- and long-term effects of the disease. Explain how the STD is transmitted. Alert the patient as to precautions to take so he will not continue to transmit the disease to others. Help the patient understand why it is important for people who may have contracted the disease from him to be told they may have it.

Then, offer to contact the patient's former and current partners. Fully explain each step in the notification process, assuring the patient that his name will not be revealed under any circumstances. Answer any questions and address any concerns about the notification process. If the patient is still reluctant to provide information, give him some time to think about it away from the office, and follow up periodically with a phone call.

Once the patient agrees to reveal names, write down the names and other information, and preferably phone numbers. To make sure you have correct information, read it back to the patient, spelling each person's name in turn and reciting the phone number or address. Write down the phonetic pronunciations of any difficult names. Tell the patient when you will make the notifications.

You now are ready to contact these individuals. Professionals who work with STD patients recommend guidelines for contacting current and former partners to alert them about potential exposure to an STD. Note that these guidelines are applicable only to STDs other than AIDS.

Determine how you will contact each individual: in writing, in person, or by phone.

1. If you use U.S. mail, mark the outside of the addressed envelope "Personal." On a note inside, simply ask the person to call you at the

*continued* ———➤

### Notifying Those at Risk for Sexually Transmitted Disease *(concluded)*

medical office. Do not put the topic of the call in writing.

2. If you make the contact in person, ask where you can talk privately. Even if the person appears to be alone, others may still be able to overhear the conversation.

3. If you use the phone, identify yourself and your office, and ask for the specific individual. Do not reveal the nature of your call to anyone but that person. If pressed, tell the person who answers the phone that you are calling regarding a personal matter.

Once on the phone or alone with the person, confirm that you are talking to the correct person. Mention that you wish to talk about a highly personal matter, and ask if it is a good time to continue the discussion. If not, arrange for a more appropriate time.

Inform the individual that she has come in contact with someone who has an STD. Recommend that the person visit a doctor's office or clinic to be tested for the disease.

Be prepared for a variety of reactions, from surprise to anger. Respond calmly and coolly. Expect to respond to questions and statements such as:

- Who gave you my name?
- Do I have the disease?

- Am I really at risk? I haven't had intercourse recently (or) I've only had intercourse with my spouse.
- I feel fine. I just went to my doctor recently.

Let the person know that you cannot reveal the name of the partner because the information is strictly confidential. Assure the person that you will not reveal her name to anyone either.

Explain that exposure to the disease does not mean a person has contracted it. Encourage the person to get tested to know for sure.

Tell the person that she is still at risk, even if she hasn't had intercourse recently or has had it only with a spouse. Let the person know that someone with whom she came in close contact at some point has contracted the disease.

Even if the person says, "I feel fine," she may still have the disease. Again, stress the importance of getting tested.

Provide your name and phone number for contact about further questions. Recommend local offices and clinics for testing, and provide phone numbers. If the person will come to your office, offer to make the appointment.

Finally, document the results of your call. Log in the original patient's file the date that you completed notification. Include any pertinent details about the notification. Alert the patient when all people on the list have been notified.

---

The AMA has several standard forms for authorization of disclosure and includes disclosure clauses in many other forms. For example, the consent-to-surgery form includes a clause about consenting to picture taking and observation during the surgery. When using a standard form, cross out anything that does not apply in that particular situation. Medical practices often develop their own customized forms.

## Code of Ethics

Medical ethics is a vital part of medical practice and following an ethical code is an important part of your job. Ethics deals with general principles of right and wrong, as opposed to requirements of law. A professional is expected to act in ways that reflect society's ideas of right and

wrong, even if such behavior is not enforced by law. Often, however, the law is based on ethical considerations.

## Bioethics: Social Issues

**Bioethics** deals with issues that arise related to medical advances. Here are three examples of bioethical issues.

1. A treatment for Parkinson disease was developed that uses fetal tissue. Some women, upon learning about this treatment, might get pregnant just to have an abortion and sell the fetal tissue. Is this ethical?

2. If a couple cannot have a baby because of a medical condition of the mother, using a surrogate mother is an option some couples choose. The surrogate mother is artificially inseminated with the sperm of the husband

and carries the baby to term. The couple then raises the child. Ethically speaking, who is the real mother, the woman who bears the child or the woman who raises the child? If the surrogate mother wants to keep the baby after it is born, does she have a right to do so?

3. When a liver transplant is needed by both a famous patient who has had a history of alcohol abuse and a woman who is a recipient of public assistance, what criteria are considered when determining who receives the organ? Who makes the decision? Ethically, treating physicians should not make the decision of allocating limited medical resources. Decisions regarding the allocation of limited medical resources should consider only the likelihood of benefit, the urgency of need, and the amount of resources required for successful treatment. Nonmedical criteria such as ability to pay, age, social worth, perceived obstacles to treatment, patient's contribution to illness, or the past use of resources should not be considered.

Practicing appropriate professional ethics has a positive impact on your reputation and the success of your employer's business. Many medical organizations, therefore, have created guidelines for the acceptable and preferred manners and behaviors, or etiquette, of medical assistants and physicians.

The principles of medical ethics have developed over time. The Hippocratic oath, in which medical students pledge to practice medicine ethically, was developed in ancient Greece. It is still used today and is one of the original bases of modern medical ethics. Hippocrates, the 4th century BC Greek physician commonly called the "father of medicine," is traditionally considered the author of this oath, but its authorship is actually unknown.

Among the promises of the Hippocratic oath are to use the form of treatment believed to be best for the patient, to refrain from harmful actions, and to keep a patient's private information confidential.

The AMA defines ethical behavior for doctors in *Code of Medical Ethics: Current Opinions with Annotations* (Chicago: American Medical Association, 1996). Medical assistants as well as doctors need to be aware of these principles.

A physician shall be dedicated to providing competent medical service with compassion and respect for human dignity.

This concept means that medical professionals will respect all aspects of the patient as a person, including intellect and emotions. The doctor must decide what treatment would result in the best, most dignified quality of life for the patient, and the doctor must respect a patient's choice to forgo treatment.

A physician shall deal honestly with patients and colleagues and strive to expose those physicians deficient in character or competence or who engage in fraud or deception.

Medical professionals, including medical assistants, should respect colleagues, but they must also respect and protect the profession and public welfare enough to report colleagues who are breaking the law, acting unethically, or unable to perform competently. Dilemmas may arise where one suspects, but is not able to prove, for instance, that a coworker has a substance abuse problem or another problem that is affecting performance. Ignoring such a situation in medical practice could cost someone's life as well as lead to lawsuits.

In terms of billing, a doctor should bill only for direct services, not for indirect ones, such as referrals. The doctor also should not bill for services that do not really pertain to the practice of medicine, such as dispensing drugs.

It is also unethical for the doctor to influence the patient about where to fill prescriptions or obtain other medical services when the doctor has a personal financial interest in any of the choices.

A physician shall respect the law and also recognize a responsibility to seek changes in requirements that are contrary to the patient's best interests.

Several legal or employer requirements have come under scrutiny as being contrary to a patient's best interests. Among them are discharging patients from the hospital after a certain time limit for certain procedures, which may be too soon for many patients. Insurance company payment policies have sometimes been criticized as unfair. So have health maintenance organization (HMO) financial policies that may conflict with a doctor's preference in treatment.

A physician shall respect the rights of patients, of colleagues, and of other health professionals and shall safeguard patient confidences within the constraints of law.

A document called the Patient's Bill of Rights, established by the American Hospital Association in 1973 and revised in 1992, lists ethical principles protecting the patient. (The text of the Patient's Bill of Rights appears in Chapter 23.) Some states have even passed this code of ethics into law. Among a patient's rights are the right to information about alternative treatments, the right to refuse to participate in research projects, and the right to privacy.

A physician shall continue to study; apply and advance scientific knowledge; make relevant information available to patients, colleagues, and the public; obtain consultation; and use the talents of other health professionals when indicated.

Keeping up with the latest advancements in medicine is crucial for providing high-quality, ethical care. Most states require doctors to accumulate "continuing education units" to maintain a license to practice. These units are earned by means of educational activities such as courses and scientific meetings. The AAMA requires medical assistants to renew their certification every

## Points on Practice

### AAMA Code of Ethics

The Code of Ethics of the AAMA shall set forth principles of ethical and moral conduct as they relate to the medical profession and the particular practice of medical assisting.

Members of the AAMA dedicated to the conscientious pursuit of their profession, and thus desiring to merit the high regard of the entire medical profession and the respect of the general public which they serve, do pledge themselves to strive always to:

**A.** Render service with full respect for the dignity of humanity

**B.** Respect confidential information obtained through employment unless legally authorized

or required by responsible performance of duty to divulge such information

**C.** Uphold the honor and high principles of the profession and accept its disciplines

**D.** Seek to continually improve the knowledge and skills of medical assistants for the benefit of patients and professional colleagues

**E.** Participate in additional service activities aimed toward improving the health and wellbeing of the community

5 years, by either accumulating continuing education credits through the AAMA or retaking the certification examination.

> A physician shall, in the provision of appropriate patient care, except in emergencies, be free to choose whom to serve, with whom to associate, and the environment in which to provide medical services.

Ethically, doctors can set their hours, decide what kind of medicine to practice and where, decide whom to accept as a patient, and take time off as long as a qualified substitute performs their duties. Doctors may decline to accept new patients because of a full workload. In an emergency, however, a doctor may be ethically obligated to care for a patient, even if the patient is not of the doctor's choosing. The doctor should not abandon that patient until another physician is available.

> A physician shall recognize a responsibility to participate in activities contributing to an improved community. This ethical obligation holds true for the allied health professions as well.

In addition to knowing the physician's codes of ethics, medical assistants should follow the AAMA's Code of Ethics (see the Points on Practice box).

## Labor and Employment Laws

More often than not, medical assistants often find themselves in a supervisory or management role within the medical office. It is not uncommon for a medical assistant to become promoted to an office manager within a medical facility, sometimes in a short period of time after initial employment. It is important to know certain employment

and labor laws in order to perform the managerial tasks within legal and ethical guidelines.

## Title VII of the Civil Rights Act of 1964

This act applies to businesses with 15 or more employees working at least 20 weeks of the year. The law prevents employers from discriminating in hiring or firing or firing on the basis of race, color, religion, sex, or national origin. Some states have laws that also prohibit **discrimination** based on marital status, parenthood, mental health, mental retardation, sexual orientation, personal appearance, or political affiliation. Title VII also addresses and defines sexual harassment.

## Sexual Harassment

Sexual harassment occurs in a variety of circumstances, and anyone may be sexually harassed. A man or a woman may be the victim or harasser, and the victim does not have to be the opposite sex. The victim may be the person being harassed or even a coworker who overhears the harassment. The victim has the responsibility to let the harasser know that the conduct is offensive. The victim should also report any instance of sexual harassment to a supervisor or personnel department. A formal definition of sexual harassment is as follows:

> Unwelcome sexual advances, requests for sexual favors, and other verbal or physical conduct of a sexual nature . . . when submission to such conduct is made either explicitly or implicitly a term or condition of an individual's employment, submission to or rejection of

such conduct by an individual is used as the basis for employment decisions affecting such individual, or such conduct has the purpose or effect of unreasonably interfering with an individual's work performance or creating an intimidating, hostile, or offensive working environment. (Lindgren and Taub, 1993)

## Age Discrimination in Employment Act (ADEA) of 1967

This act applies to businesses with 20 or more employees working at least 20 weeks of the year. It prohibits discrimination in hiring or firing based on age for persons aged 40 or older.

## 1976 Pregnancy Discrimination Act

This is an amendment to Title VII of the Civil Rights Act that makes it illegal to fire an employee based on pregnancy, childbirth, or related medical conditions.

## The Civil Rights Act of 1991

This act provides monetary damages in cases of intentional employment discrimination.

## Titles I and III of the Americans with Disabilities Act of 1990

This act applies to all employers with 15 or more employees working at least 20 weeks during the year. Titles I and III of the act ban discrimination against disabled persons in the workplace, mandate equal access for the disabled to certain public facilities, and require all commercial firms to make existing facilities and grounds more accessible to the disabled.

## 1938 Fair Labor Standards Act

This act prohibits child labor and the firing of employees for exercising their rights under the act's wage and hour standards. It also provides for overtime pay and a minimum wage. New Fair Pay regulations under the act went into effect on August 23, 2004. The new rules guarantee overtime protection to workers earning less that $23,600 annually and continue exemptions of the overtime rule for certain "learned professional employees." Some nurses may receive overtime pay, depending on how they are paid—hourly or salary—and LPNs and other similar health-care employees are guaranteed overtime pay under the new Fair Pay regulations.

## Equal Pay Act of 1963

As an amendment to the Fair Labor Standards Act, this act requires equal pay for men and women doing equal work.

## Family Leave Act of 1991

This act applies to employers with 50 or more employees. It mandates allowing employees to take unpaid leave time for maternity, for adoption, or for caring for ill family members.

# Legal Medical Practice Models

There are four basic types of medical practice:

- Sole proprietorship
- Partnership
- Group practice
- Professional corporation

Laws governing the various types of practice vary, but medical office personnel should be aware of the laws that apply to their employers' practice management models.

## Sole Proprietorship

This type of practice is often referred to as a "solo practice." In this type of practice, a physician practicing alone assumes all the benefits for and liabilities of the business. **Sole proprietorship** practice management is not a popular option as a result of the increased expenses and decreased insurance reimbursements. Therefore, more physicians are joining group practices or professional corporations.

## Partnership

When two or more physicians decide to practice together, they may form a **partnership,** based on a legal contract that specifies the rights, obligations, and responsibilities of each partner. Advantages of partnerships include sharing the workload, expenses, profits, and assets. A disadvantage is that each partner has equal liability for acts of misconduct, losses, and deficits of the practice, unless specified as a contingency in the contract.

## Group Practice

**Group practice** is a medical practice model in which three or more licensed physicians share the collective income, expenses, facilities, equipment, records, and personnel for the practice. Physicians in group practice may be engaged in the same specialty, calling themselves, for example, Associates in Cardiology, or they can be several physicians offering similar specialties, such as ob/gyn and pediatrics.

## Professional Corporations

A **corporation** is a body formed and authorized by state law to act as a single entity. Physicians who form corporations are shareholders and employees of the organization.

There are financial and tax advantages to forming a corporation and the fringe benefits for employees may be greater than in a sole proprietorship or partnership.

In forming a corporation, the incorporators and owners have limited liability in case lawsuits are filed. Sometimes medical practices are "managed" by for-profit corporations that are either formed by outside business interests or subsidiary corporations organized by hospitals. Physicians are hired as salaried employees with bonus options. The management corporation provides the facility, office personnel, employee benefits, human resource services, and operating expenses.

## Summary

You must carefully follow all state, federal, and individual practice rules and laws while performing your daily duties. You must also follow the AAMA Code of Ethics for medical assistants. It is an important part of your duties to help the doctor avoid malpractice claims—lawsuits by the patient against the physician for errors in diagnosis or treatment.

To perform effectively as a medical assistant, you must maintain an office that follows all OSHA regulations for safety, hazardous equipment, and toxic substances. The office also must meet QC and QA guidelines for all tests, specimens, and treatments. It is your responsibility to follow HIPAA guidelines, to ensure patient privacy and confidentiality of patient records, to fully document patient treatment, and to maintain patient records in an orderly and readily accessible fashion.

# REVIEW

## CHAPTER 3

### CASE STUDY QUESTIONS

Now that you have completed this chapter, review the case study at the beginning of the chapter and answer the following questions:

1. Does the medical assistant's comment represent a breach of confidentiality?
2. Has any HIPAA rule been violated? If so, which one?

### Discussion Questions

1. How does the law of agency make it possible for a patient to sue both the medical assistant and the physician for an act of negligence committed by the medical assistant?
2. Under HIPAA, what rights do patients have regarding confidentiality and ownership of their medical records? When does a patient give up the right to confidentiality?
3. How can you prove that the patient gave informed consent?
4. What are two scenarios that would void a contract between physician and patient?
5. Why can't patients schedule appointments at any time of the day?

### Critical Thinking Questions

1. What is an example of a bioethical issue? Give two opposing views of the issue.
2. Explain why a medical record entry that is corrected improperly could damage a malpractice suit against the physician.
3. Describe implied consent and two ways that a patient can accept treatment by implied consent.
4. Discuss the "implied" contract between a physician and a patient.

### Application Activities

1. Research a controversial topic from the following list:
   - Euthanasia
   - Surrogacy
   - Abortion
   - Fetal stem cell research
   - Cloning
   - Emergency contraceptive (morning-after pill)

   Write a three-page report that presents both the pro side and the con side of the issue. Write a closing paragraph that gives your personal opinion and views and how you have been conditioned in that belief, for example, social, cultural, and religious beliefs.
2. Choose teams of four people, and stage debates on the controversial topics listed in question 1. Research your topics thoroughly and present arguments on both sides. Your purpose is to state facts and persuade your audience to your beliefs.

   Rules for the debate:
   - Participants must be courteous and professional
   - Presentations must be factual
   - Opening arguments are four minutes for each side
   - Each side presents, and then for three minutes each side is allowed to counter any fact
   - Closing arguments are five minutes for each side

   Have the class vote on which side was more persuasive.
3. In a medical law textbook or journal, research a malpractice case. Prepare a 10-minute presentation for the class in which you summarize both sides of the case (patient and caregiver). Include when and where the case took place. Explain how the case was settled and whether the settlement took place in a court of law or through arbitration. Close with your opinion about whether the case was settled fairly.
4. Research a piece of legislation on a health-care issue or practice, either a bill passed in the last 5 years or a bill currently being considered in Washington. What impact has this bill had or might this bill have on the medical assisting profession? Summarize your findings in a one- to two-page report.

### Virtual Fieldtrip

*Visit the McGraw-Hill Higher Education Medical Assisting website at www.mhhe.com/medicalassisting3 to complete the following activity:*

As a medical assistant, it is imperative to be knowledgeable about your state regulations regarding medical assisting practice. Research the scope of practice for the state where you will work. The AAMA and American Medical Technologists are good resources for this information. Prepare a one-page summary and share your research with your classmates.

Open the CD and complete this chapter's practice activities, play the games, listen to the key terms, and test yourself with the interactive review. E-mail, print, and/or save your results to document your proficiency.

## CHAPTER 4

# Communication With Patients, Families, and Coworkers

## MEDICAL ASSISTING COMPETENCIES

*In preparation for the certification examination, you should know the following areas of competence:*

| COMPETENCY | CMA | RMA |
|---|:---:|:---:|
| **General/Legal/Professional** | | |
| Recognize and respond to verbal and nonverbal communications by being attentive and adapting communication to the recipient's level of understanding | X | X |
| Be aware of and perform within legal and ethical boundaries | X | X |
| Identify community resources and information for patients and employers | X | X |

## KEY TERMS

active listening
aggressive
assertive
body language
burnout
closed posture
conflict
empathy
feedback
hierarchy
homeostasis
hospice
interpersonal skills
open posture
passive listening
personal space
rapport

## CHAPTER OUTLINE

- Communicating With Patients and Families
- The Communication Circle
- Understanding Human Behavior and How It Relates to the Provider-Patient Relationship
- Types of Communication
- Improving Your Communication Skills
- Communicating in Special Circumstances
- Communicating With Coworkers
- Written Communication Tools and Community Resources
- Managing Stress
- Preventing Burnout

## LEARNING OUTCOMES

After completing Chapter 4, you will be able to:

**4.1** Identify elements of the communication circle.

**4.2** Understand and define the developmental stages of the life cycle.

**4.3** Give examples of positive and negative communication.

**4.4** List ways to improve listening and interpersonal skills.

**4.5** Explain the difference between assertiveness and aggressiveness.

**4.6** Give examples of effective communication strategies with patients in special circumstances.

**4.7** Discuss ways to establish positive communication with coworkers and management.

**4.8** Describe how the office policy and procedures manual is used as a communication tool in the medical office.

**4.9** Describe community resources and how they enhance the services provided by your office.

**4.10** Explain how stress relates to communication and identify strategies to reduce stress.

# Introduction

The ability to recognize human behaviors and the ability to communicate effectively are vital to a medical assistant and the pursuit for success. This chapter has taken a psychological approach to understanding human behavior and the challenges that influence therapeutic communication in a health-care setting. Patients will often have more interaction with the medical assistant than with any other health-care practitioner in the facility. It is important that patients develop a good rapport and feel confident in the care they are receiving from your office. The medical assistant sets the tone for the communication cycle and must be aware of all the obstacles that can affect human communication. As a medical assistant, you are often exposed to all kinds of patients. You will see patients from different cultures, socioeconomic backgrounds, educational levels, ages, and lifestyles. You must be able to communicate with each patient with professionalism and diplomacy.

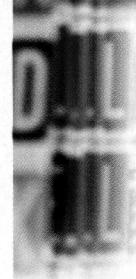

## CASE STUDY

Mary is 23 years old and has been a medical assistant for 6 months. She is currently working in a walk-in clinic in a large urban city. She has interviewed three patients this morning. One patient is a homeless transient male who appears to have some type of mental incapacity; the second is a teenage girl who suspects she might be pregnant; and the third is a well-dressed professional male who complains of a sore throat.

As you read this chapter, consider how you would answer the following questions relative to each of the patients:

1. How will Mary adapt her communication style to communicate with each patient?
2. What types of communication roadblocks will she encounter with each one?
3. What types of communication techniques will she use for each patient?

# Communicating With Patients and Families

Think about the last time you had a doctor's appointment. How well did the staff and physicians communicate with you? Were you greeted cordially and pleasantly invited to take a seat, or did someone thrust a clipboard at you and say "Fill this out"? If you had a long wait in the waiting room or examination room, did someone come in to explain the delay? Did you become frustrated and angry because nobody told you what was happening?

As a medical assistant, you are a key communicator between the office and patients and families. The way you greet patients, explain procedures, ask and answer questions, and attend to the individual needs of patients forms your communication style. Your interaction with the patient sets the tone for the office visit and can significantly influence how comfortable the patient feels in your practice. Developing strong communication skills in the medical office is just as important as mastering administrative and clinical tasks.

Customer service is the most important part of communication to families and patients. Your mastery of clinical and administrative skills is only a portion of your skills; customer service and communication skills are the other 70%.

A definition of customer service includes the following two points:

1. The patient comes first
2. Patient needs are satisfied

In today's health-care environment, patients are consumers and are more educated than ever before. Patients have more options in choosing a physician or a health-care facility. Patients who feel that they were not given exceptional customer service will choose another physician or facility to meet their needs. Another reason a facility must strive for exceptional customer service is that a medical facility grows rapidly from referral business. A medical facility that acquires a reputation for having an "unfriendly" staff will feel the negative impact from that reputation.

Listed here are some examples of customer service in the physician's office:

- Using proper telephone techniques
- Writing or responding to telephone messages
- Explaining procedures to patients
- Expediting insurance referral requests
- Assisting in billing issues
- Answering questions or finding answers to patient questions
- Ensuring that patients are comfortable in your office
- Creating a warm and reassuring environment

From a business perspective, exceptional customer service is vital to a medical facility's success. Any business that does not provide exceptional customer service will not grow and thrive in today's business economy.

# The Communication Circle

As you interact with patients and their families, you will be responsible for giving information and ensuring that the patient understands what you, the doctor, and other members of the staff have communicated. You will also be responsible for receiving information from the patient. For example, patients will describe their symptoms. They may also discuss their feelings or ask questions about a treatment or procedure. The giving and receiving of information forms the communication circle.

## Elements of the Communication Circle

The communication circle involves three elements: a message, a source, and a receiver. Messages are usually verbal or written. (As you will see later in the chapter, some messages are nonverbal.) The source sends the message, and the receiver receives it. The communication circle is formed as the source sends a message to the receiver and the receiver responds (Figure 4-1).

Consider this example, in which Fernando, a medical assistant who works in a physical therapy office, is speaking with Mrs. Riveria, a patient who is having therapy for a back injury. Watch the communication circle at work.

**Fernando:** The physical therapist says you're making great progress and that you can start on some simple back exercises at home. I'd like to go over them with you. Then I'll give you a sheet that illustrates the exercises. How does that sound to you?

**Mrs. Riveria:** I'm a little nervous about doing exercises. I still have some pain when I bend over.

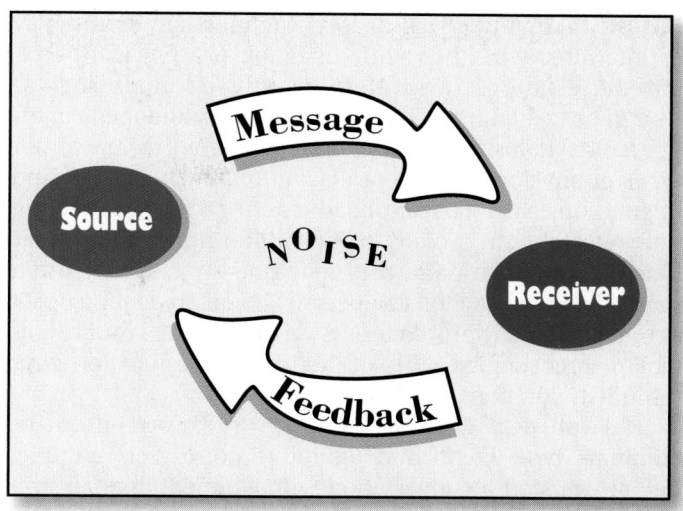

**Figure 4-1.** The process of communication involves an exchange of messages through verbal and nonverbal means.

**Fernando:** I understand. It's important, though, to start using those muscles again. Why don't you show me exactly where it hurts. Then we can go over proper body mechanics, such as bending down to pick something up and getting in and out of chairs, the car, and bed. Then we'll just start with one or two of the exercises and save the rest for next time, when you're feeling more ready.

**Mrs. Riveria:** Yes, I only feel up to doing a little bit today.

The medical assistant (the source) gives a verbal message (about back exercises) to the patient (the receiver). The patient responds by drawing attention to her pain and uneasiness about certain movements. The patient's response is also a message to the medical assistant, who responds in turn. The giving and receiving of information continues within the communication circle until the exchange is finished.

**Feedback.** Another word for response is **feedback,** which is verbal or nonverbal evidence that the receiver got and understood the message. When you communicate information to a patient or ask a patient a question, always look for feedback. For example, if you calculate a pregnant patient's due date and tell her she's 12 weeks pregnant, look for a response. If she responds, "Oh, good, that means I'm out of danger of having a miscarriage," you would respond that whereas most miscarriages occur in the first 12 weeks, some risk of miscarriage remains throughout the pregnancy. If she responds, "I thought I was 14 weeks pregnant," you would need to clarify how you worked out your calculation and compare it with hers, to uncover any discrepancy. Good communication in the medical office requires patient feedback at every step.

**Noise.** Anything that distorts the message in any way or interferes with the communication process can be referred to as noise. Noise refers not only to sounds, such as a siren or jackhammer on the street below the medical office suite. It also refers to room temperature and other types of physical comfort or discomfort, such as pain, and to emotions, such as fear or sadness. If patients are feeling uncomfortable in a chilly or hot room, upset about their illness, or in great pain, they may not pay close attention to what you are saying. Conversely, if you are feeling upset about a personal problem outside work or if you are unwell or preoccupied with all the things you have on your to-do list, you may not communicate well.

As you deal with each patient, try to screen out or eliminate both literal and figurative noise. For example, before you start a conversation with a patient in an examination room, you might ask, "Are you too chilly or too hot? Is the temperature in here comfortable for you?" If there is construction going on outside the building, see if there is a less noisy inner room or office that you might be able to use. If a patient seems nervous or upset, address those feelings before you launch into a factual discussion.

If you are feeling stressed or out of sorts, that feeling constitutes a type of noise. Try to take a "breather" between patients or a break from desk work—walk downstairs, get some fresh air, stretch your legs. Feeling dehydrated or hungry affects your communication efforts too. Limit your caffeine and sugar intake. Drink plenty of water and juice throughout the day. Eat a good lunch and healthful snacks. Leave your personal problems at home.

**Humanizing the Communication Process in the Medical Office.** As highly structured managed care organizations and technological advances rapidly change the face of health care, many patients feel that health care is becoming impersonal. Every time you communicate with patients, you can counteract this perception by playing a humanistic role in the health-care process. Being humanistic means that you work to help patients feel attended to and respected as individuals, not just as descriptions on a chart. Good communication supports this patient-centered approach.

Make a point of developing and using strong communication skills to show patients that you, the doctors, and other staff members care about them and their feelings. Taking care to treat patients as people helps humanize the communication process in the medical office.

# Understanding Human Behavior and How It Relates to the Provider-Patient Relationship

Understanding human behavior is important when you are communicating with patients. Medical assistants are exposed to many different personality types in addition to different illnesses. When you understand why a person is behaving in a certain way, you can adjust your communication style to adapt to that person.

## The Developmental Stages of the Life Cycle

As a professional medical assistant, it is important to understand human growth and development. This understanding will enable you to enhance your communication skills, such as patient education, with patients of all age groups, cultures, and religions. Human growth is not only about the physical development of your patients, but about their psychological growth as well. Many scientists and behaviorists have studied and researched the developmental stages of human life and have developed guidelines to assist us in our patient communication skills. Table 4-1 is an example of a Lifespan Development model created by Erik Erikson (1902–1994). He is best known for his personality development research regarding children.

## Maslow's Hierarchy of Human Needs

Abraham Maslow, a well-known human behaviorist, developed a model of human behavior known as the **hierarchy** (i.e., a classification) of needs. This hierarchy states that human beings are motivated by unsatisfied needs and that certain lower needs have to be satisfied before higher needs, like self-actualization, are met. Maslow felt that people are basically trustworthy, self-protecting, and self-governing and that humans tend toward growth and love. He believed that humans are not violent by nature, but are violent only when their needs are not being met.

**Deficiency Needs.** According to Maslow, there are general types of needs—physiological, safety, love, and esteem—that must be satisfied before a person can act unselfishly. He called these needs *deficiency needs*.

*Physiological Needs.* Physiological needs are humans' very basic needs, such as air, water, food, sleep, and sex. When these needs are not satisfied, we may feel sickness, irritation, pain, and discomfort. These feelings motivate us to alleviate them as soon as possible to establish **homeostasis** (that is, a state of balance or equilibrium). Once those feelings are alleviated, we may think about other things.

*Safety Needs.* People have the need and desire for establishing stability and consistency. These basic needs are security, shelter, and existing in a safe environment.

*Love Needs.* Humans have a desire to belong to groups: clubs, work groups, religious groups, family, and so on. We need to feel loved and accepted by others. Humans are like pack animals—we place great importance in belonging to society.

| TABLE 4-1 | Lifespan Development |
|-----------|---------------------|
| **Life Stage** | **Expected Development** |
| **I. Infant (year 0–1)** | **Trust vs. Mistrust.** The newborn begins to experience a degree of familiarity and begins to trust the world around her. She also begins to trust her own body. |
| **II. Toddler (years 2–3)** | **Autonomy vs. Shame and Doubt.** The child will begin to explore the environment at home and everywhere else. He will begin to gain autonomy (independence) and develop self-control. He can also begin to feel shame and doubt in his abilities. Firm but tolerant parenting is the best practice during this stage. |
| **III. Preschooler (years 3–6)** | **Initiative vs. Guilt.** A child begins to learn new things, and has an active imagination and curiosity about everything. As she grows older, she begins to feel guilt for actions taken, which is a sign that she is developing the capacity for moral judgment. |
| **IV. School Age (years 7–12)** | **Industry vs. Inferiority.** The child becomes exposed to people other than family members, such as teachers and peers, who contribute to his development. He begins to experience feelings of success that can arise from sports, academics, or social acceptance. Failure to experience success at this stage can result in inferiority feelings. |
| **V. Adolescence (years 12–18)** | **Ego Identity vs. Role Confusion.** An adolescent begins to discover who she really is as a preadult human being. She begins to realize how she fits into society (ego identity). When an adolescent is confused about who she is and where she fits in society, role confusion results. Role confusion develops "follower" personality traits, which can lead to inappropriate decision making. |
| **VI. Young Adult (20s)** | **Intimacy vs. Isolation.** A young adult begins to think about marriage, family, and career responsibilities. These issues can come into conflict with the isolation that is an issue in modern society; careers often move people to different cities, and working at home has become more common. |
| **VII. Middle Adult (late 20s to 50s)** | **Generativity vs. Stagnation.** This stage is primarily devoted to raising children. Middle adults have a desire to help future generations and will often teach, write, or become involved in social activism. |
| **VIII. Old Adult (60s and older)** | **Integrity vs. Despair.** Older adults are usually retired and live without children in the house. They tend to question their usefulness at this stage. They begin to notice changes in their physical health and begin to become concerned about these changes. They begin to experience the deaths of relatives, friends, spouses, and, in some cases, their children. |

**Esteem Needs.** Humans like to feel that they are important and have worthiness to society. There are two types of self-esteem. The first results from competence or mastery of a task, such as completing an educational program. The second is the attention and recognition that comes from others.

**Self-Actualization.** The need for self-actualization is "the desire to become more and more what one is, to become everything that one is capable of becoming." To reach this level, a person utilizes many tools to maximize potential, such as education, a fulfilling career, and a balanced personal life.

When working and communicating with patients, remember this hierarchy of human needs and observe what need a patient is deficient in. For example, if an elderly patient has recently lost her husband, she may feel lonely and deficient in the love need. You may see homeless patients who are deficient in their physiological and safety needs. You may have a young girl as a patient who is overweight and has low self-esteem. On the other hand, you may have a high-level executive as a patient who has reached self-actualization. Each of these scenarios would require a communication style adjustment in order for you to effectively communicate with these patients.

# Types of Communication

Communication can be positive or negative. It can also be verbal, nonverbal, or written. To help ensure effective communication with patients, familiarize yourself with these different types of communication. (Chapter 7 discusses written communication.)

## Positive Communication

In the medical office, communication that promotes patients' comfort and well-being is essential. Treating patients brusquely or rudely is unacceptable in the healthcare setting. It is your responsibility—not the patient's—to set the stage for positive communication.

When information—even bad news—is communicated with some positive aspect, patients are more likely to listen attentively and respond positively themselves. For example, you might explain to a patient who is about to get an injection, "This will sting, but only for a couple of seconds. When we're through, you're free to go." You would not just say, "This is going to hurt."

Other examples of positive communication are:

- Being friendly, warm, and attentive ("It's good to see you again, Mrs. Armstrong. I know you're on your lunch hour, so let's get started right away.")
- Verbalizing concern for patients ("Are you comfortable?" "I understand it hurts when I do this; I'll be gentle." "This paperwork won't take long at all.")
- Encouraging patients to ask questions ("I hope I've explained the procedure well. Do you have any questions, or are there any parts you would like to go over again?")
- Asking patients to repeat your instructions to make sure they understand
- Looking directly at patients when you speak to them
- Smiling (naturally, not in a forced way)
- Speaking slowly and clearly
- Listening carefully

## Negative Communication

Most people do not purposely try to communicate negatively. Some people, however, may not realize that their communication style has a negative impact on others. Look for and ask for feedback to help you curb negative communication habits. Ask yourself, "Do the physicians and my other coworkers seem glad to speak with me? Are they open and responsive to me?" "Do patients seem at ease with me, or are they very quiet, turned off, or distant?" (Note that some patients may respond this way because of the way they feel, not because of the way you are communicating with them.) Here are some examples of negative communication:

- Mumbling
- Speaking brusquely or sharply

- Avoiding eye contact
- Interrupting patients as they are speaking
- Rushing through explanations or instructions
- Treating patients impersonally
- Making patients feel they are taking up too much of your time or asking too many questions
- Forgetting common courtesies, such as saying please and thank you
- Showing boredom

A good way to avoid negative communication is to open your eyes and ears to others in service-oriented workplace settings. The next time you buy something at a store, call a company for information over the phone, or eat out at a restaurant, take note of the way the staff treats you. Do they answer your questions courteously? Do they give you the information you ask for? Do they make you feel welcome? What specifically makes their communication style positive or negative? Remember, you can always improve your communication skills.

## Body Language

Verbal communication refers to communication that is spoken. Nonverbal communication is also known as **body language.** Body language includes facial expressions, eye contact, posture, touch, and attention to personal space. In many instances, people's body language conveys their true feelings, even when their words may say otherwise. A patient might say, "I'm OK about that," but if she is sitting with her arms folded tightly across her chest and avoids looking at you, she may not mean what she says.

**Facial Expression.** Your face is the most expressive part of your body. You can often tell whether someone has understood your message simply by his facial expression. For example, when you are explaining a procedure to a patient, look at his expression. Does he seem puzzled? Is his brow wrinkled? Does he look surprised? Facial expressions can give you clues about how to tailor your communication efforts. They also serve as a form of feedback.

**Eye Contact.** Eye contact is an important part of positive communication. Look directly at patients when speaking to them. Looking away or down communicates that you are not interested in the person or that you are avoiding her for some reason.

There may be cultural differences in the ways patients react to eye contact. In some cultures, for example, it is common to avoid eye contact out of respect for someone who is considered a superior. Thus, children may be taught not to look adults in the eye.

**Posture.** The way you hold or move your head, arms, hands, and the rest of your body can project strong nonverbal messages. During communication, posture can usually be described as open or closed.

*Open Posture.* A feeling of receptiveness and friendliness can be conveyed with an **open posture.** In this position, your arms lie comfortably at your sides or in your lap. You face the other person, and you may lean forward in your chair. This demonstrates that you are listening and are interested in what the other person has to say. Open posture is a form of positive communication.

*Closed Posture.* A **closed posture** conveys the opposite, a feeling of not being totally receptive to what is being said. It can also signal that someone is angry or upset. A person in a closed posture may hold his arms rigidly or fold them across his chest. He may lean back in his chair, away from the other person. He may turn away to avoid eye contact. Slouching is a kind of closed posture that can convey fatigue or lack of caring. Watch for patients with closed postures that may indicate tension or pain. Avoid closed postures yourself—they have a negative effect on your communication efforts.

**Touch.** Touch is a powerful form of nonverbal communication. A touch on the arm or a hug can be a means of saying hello, sharing condolences, or expressing congratulations. Family background, culture, age, and gender all influence people's perception of touch. Some people may welcome a touch or think nothing of it. Others may view touching as an invasion of their privacy. In general, in the medical setting, a touch on the shoulder, forearm, or back of the hand to express interest or concern is acceptable.

**Personal Space.** When communicating with others, it is important to be aware of the concept of personal space. **Personal space** is an area that surrounds an individual. By not intruding on patients' personal space, you show respect for their feelings of privacy.

In most social situations, it is common for people to stand 4 to 12 ft away from each other. For personal conversation, you would typically stand between 1½ and 4 ft away from a person. Some patients may feel uncomfortable—and may become anxious—when you stand or sit close to them. Others prefer the reassurance of having people close to them when they speak. Watch patients carefully. If they lean back when you lean forward or if they fold their arms or turn their head away, you may be invading their personal space. If they lean or step toward you, they may be seeking to close up the personal space.

# Improving Your Communication Skills

Sharpening your communication skills should be an ongoing effort and will help you become a more effective communicator. Good communication skills can enhance the quality of your interaction with patients and coworkers alike. Among the skills involved in communication are listening skills, interpersonal skills, therapeutic communication skills, and assertiveness skills.

## Listening Skills

Listening involves both hearing and interpreting a message. Listening requires you to pay close attention not only to what is being said but also to nonverbal cues, such as those communicated through body language.

Listening can be passive or active. **Passive listening** is simply hearing what someone has to say without the need for a reply. An example is listening to a news program on the radio; the communication is mainly one-way. **Active listening** involves two-way communication. You are actively involved in the process, offering feedback or asking questions. Active listening takes place, for example, when you interview a patient for her medical history. Active listening is an essential skill in the medical office.

There are several ways to improve your listening skills:

- Prepare to listen. Position yourself at the same level (sitting, standing) as the person who is speaking and assume an open posture (Figure 4-2).
- Relax and listen attentively. Do not simply pretend to listen to what is being said.
- Maintain eye contact.
- Maintain appropriate personal space.
- Think before you respond.
- Provide feedback. Restate the speaker's message in your own words to show that you understand.
- If you do not understand something that was said, ask the person to repeat it.

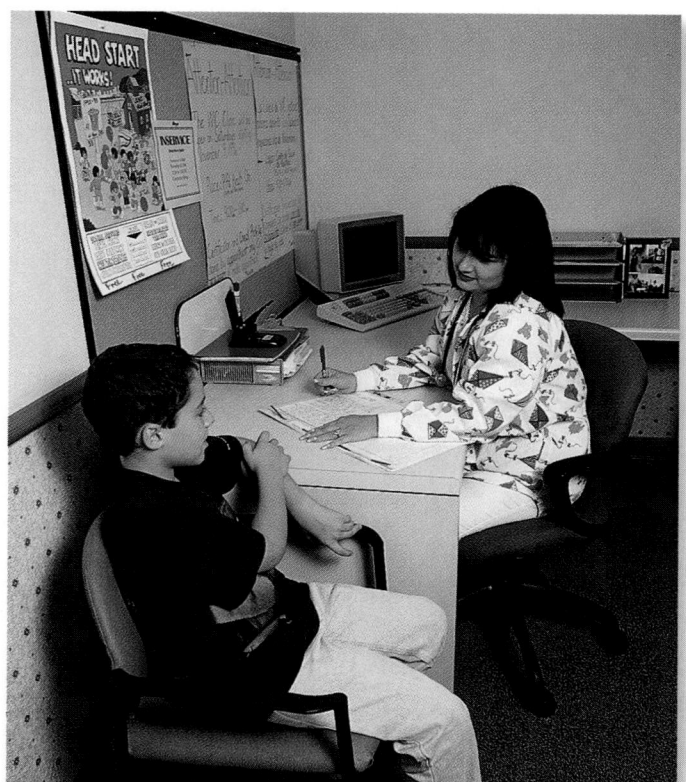

**Figure 4-2.** Active listening requires two-way communication and positive body language.

# Interpersonal Skills

When you interact with people, you use **interpersonal skills.** When you make a patient feel at ease by being warm and friendly, you are demonstrating good interpersonal skills. In addition to warmth and friendliness, valuable interpersonal skills include empathy, respect, genuineness, openness, and consideration and sensitivity.

**Warmth and Friendliness.**  A friendly but professional approach, a pleasant greeting, and a smile get you off to a good start when communicating with patients. When your approach is sincere, patients will be more relaxed and open.

**Empathy.**  The process of identifying with someone else's feelings is **empathy.** When you are empathetic, you are sensitive to the other person's feelings and problems. For example, if a patient is experiencing a migraine headache and you have never had one, you can still let her know you are trying to imagine, or relate to, her situation. In other words, you can acknowledge the severity of her pain and show support and care. You must, however, always remain objective in your interaction with patients.

**Respect.**  Showing respect can mean using a title of courtesy such as "Mr." or "Mrs." when communicating with patients. It can also mean acknowledging a patient's wishes or choices without passing judgment.

**Genuineness.**  Being genuine in your interactions with patients means that you refrain from "putting on an act" or just going through the motions of your job. Patients like to know that their health-care providers are real people. In a medical setting, being genuine means caring for each patient on an individual basis, giving patients the full attention they deserve, and showing respect for them. Being genuine in your communication with patients encourages them to place trust in you and in what you say.

**Openness.**  Openness means being willing to listen to and consider others' viewpoints and concerns and being receptive to their needs. An open individual is accepting of others and not biased for or against them.

**Consideration and Sensitivity.**  You should always try to show consideration toward patients and act in a thoughtful, kind way. You must be sensitive to their individual concerns, fears, and needs.

## Therapeutic Communication Skills

Therapeutic communication is the ability to communicate with patients in terms that they can understand and, at the same time, feel at ease and comfortable in what you are saying. It is also the ability to communicate with other members of the health team in technical terms that are appropriate in a health-care setting. Therapeutic communication techniques are methodologies that can improve communication with patients.

Therapeutic communication involves the following communication skills:

- Being Silent. Silence allows the patient time to think without pressure.
- Accepting. This skill gives the patient an indication of reception. It shows that you have heard the patient and follow the patient's thought pattern. Some indicators of acceptance include nodding; saying "Yes," "I follow what you said," and other such phrases; and body language.
- Giving Recognition. Show patients that you are aware of them by stating their name in a greeting or by noticing positive changes. With this skill, you are recognizing the patient as a person or individual.
- Offering Self. Make yourself available to the needs of the patient.
- Giving a Broad Opening. Allow the patient to take the initiative in introducing the topic. Ask open-ended questions such as "Is there something you'd like to talk about?" or "Where would you like to begin?"
- Offering General Leads. Give the patient encouragement to continue by making comments such as "Go on" or "And then?"
- Making Observations. Make your perceptions known to the patient. Say things like "You appear tense today" or "Are you uncomfortable when you . . . ?" By calling patients' attention to what is happening to them, you encourage them to notice it for themselves so that they can describe it to you.
- Encouraging Communication. Ask patients to verbalize what they perceive. Make statements such as "Tell me when you feel anxious" or "What is happening?" Patients should feel free to describe their perceptions to you, and you must try to see things as they seem to the patients.
- Mirroring. Restate what the patient has said to demonstrate that you understand.
- Reflecting. Encourage patients to think through and answer their own questions. A reflecting dialogue may go like this:
  - Patient: Do you think I should tell the doctor?
  - Medical Assistant: Do you think you should?

  By reflecting patients' questions or statements back to them, you are helping patients feel that their opinions about their health are of value.
- Focusing. Focusing encourages the patient to stay on the topic.
- Exploring. Encourage patients to express themselves in more depth. Try to get as much detail as possible about a patent complaint, but avoid probing and prying if the patient does not wish to discuss it.

- Clarifying. Ask patients to explain themselves more clearly if they provide information that is vague or not meaningful.
- Summarizing. This skill involves organizing and summing up the important points of the discussion and gives the patient an awareness of the progress made toward greater understanding.

**Ineffective Therapeutic Communication.** In the previous section, the focus was on how to communicate effectively in a therapeutic environment. Oftentimes people think they are communicating thoroughly, but they are not. Here are some roadblocks that can interfere with your communication style:

- Reassuring. This type of communication indicates to the patient that there is no need for anxiety or worry. By doing this, you devalue the patient's feelings and give false hope if the outcome is not positive. The communication error here is a lack of understanding and empathy.
- Giving Approval. Giving approval is usually done by overtly approving of a patient's behavior. This may lead the patient to strive for praise rather than progress.
- Disapproving. Being disapproving is done by overtly disapproving of a patient's behavior. This implies that you have the right to pass judgment on the patient's thoughts and actions. Find an alternate attitude when dealing with patients. Adopting a moralistic attitude may take your attention away from the patient's needs and may direct it toward your own feelings.
- Agreeing/Disagreeing. Overtly agreeing or disagreeing with thoughts, perceptions, and ideas of patients is not an effective way to communicate. When you agree with patients, they will have the perception that they are right because you agree with them or because you share the same opinion. Opinions and conclusions should be the patient's, not yours. When disagreeing with patients, you become the opposition to them instead of their caregiver. Never place yourself in an argumentative situation regarding the opinions of a patient.
- Advising. If you tell the patient what you think should be done, you place yourself outside your scope of practice. You cannot advise patients.
- Probing. Probing is discussing a topic that the patient has no desire to discuss.
- Defending. Protecting yourself, the institution, and others from verbal attack is classified as defending. If you become defensive, the patient may feel the need to discontinue communication.
- Requesting an Explanation. This communication pattern involves asking patients to provide reasons for their behavior. Patients may not know why they behave in a certain manner. "Why" questions may have an intimidating effect on some patients.

- Minimizing Feelings. Never judge or make light of a patient's discomfort. It is important for you to perceive what is taking place from the patient's point of view, not your own.
- Making Stereotyped Comments. This type of communication involves using meaningless clichés when communicating with patients. An example of a stereotypical comment is "It's for your own good." These types of comments are given in an automatic, mechanical way as a substitute for a more reasonable and thoughtful explanation.

**Defense Mechanisms.** When working with patients, it is important to observe their communication behaviors. Patients will often develop *defense mechanisms,* which are unconscious, to protect themselves from anxiety, guilt, and shame.

Here are some common defense mechanisms that a patient may display when communicating with the doctor, medical assistant, or other health-care team members:

- Compensation: Overemphasizing a trait to make up for a perceived or actual failing
- Denial: An unconscious attempt to reject unacceptable feelings, needs, thoughts, wishes, or external reality factors
- Displacement: The unconscious transfer of unacceptable thoughts, feelings, or desires from the self to a more acceptable external substitute
- Dissociation: Disconnecting emotional significance from specific ideas or events
- Identification: Mimicking the behavior of another to cope with feelings of inadequacy
- Introjection: Adopting the unacceptable thoughts or feelings of others
- Projection: Projecting onto another person one's own feelings, as if they had originated in the other person
- Rationalization: Justifying unacceptable behavior, thoughts, and feelings into tolerable behaviors
- Regression: Unconsciously returning to more infantile behaviors or thoughts
- Repression: Putting unpleasant thoughts, feelings, or events out of one's mind
- Substitution: Unconsciously replacing an unreachable or unacceptable goal with another, more acceptable one

## Assertiveness Skills

As a professional, you need to be **assertive,** that is, to be firm and to stand by your principles while still showing respect for others. Being assertive means trusting your instincts, feelings, and opinions (not in terms of diagnosing, which only the doctor can do, but in terms of basic communication with patients), and acting on them. For

| TABLE 4-2 | A Comparison of Nonassertive, Assertive, Aggressive, and Nonassertive Aggressive Behavior | | | |
|---|---|---|---|---|
| | **Nonassertive Behavior** | **Assertive Behavior** | **Aggressive Behavior** | **Nonassertive Aggressive Behavior (NAG)** |
| Characteristics of the behavior | Emotionally dishonest, indirect, self-denying; allows others to choose for self; does not achieve desired goal | Emotionally honest, direct, self-enhancing, expressive; chooses for self; may achieve goal | Emotionally honest, direct, self-enhancing at the expense of another, expressive; chooses for others; may achieve goal at expense of others | Emotionally dishonest, indirect, self-denying; chooses for others; may achieve goal at expense of others |
| Your feelings | Hurt, anxious, possibly angry later | Confident, self-respecting | Righteous, superior, derogative at the time and possibly guilty later | Defiance, anger, self-denying; sometimes anxious, possibly guilty later |
| The other person's feelings toward you | Irritated, pity, lack of respect | Generally respected | Angry, resentful | Angry, resentful, irritated, disgusted |
| The other person's feelings about her/himself | Guilty of superior | Valued, respected | Hurt, embarrassed, defensive | Hurt, guilty or superior, humiliated |

Source: Adapted from Alberti, Robert E., and Emmons, Michael, *Your Perfect Right: A Guide to Assertive Behavior,* San Luis Obispo, California: Impact, 1970.

example, when you see that a patient looks uneasy, speak up. You might say, "You look concerned. How can I help you feel more comfortable?" versus asking the patient "What is the matter with you?"

Being assertive is different from being aggressive. When people are **aggressive,** they try to impose their position on others or try to manipulate them. Aggressive people are bossy and can be quarrelsome. They do not appear to take into consideration others' feelings, needs, thoughts, ideas, and opinions before they act or speak.

To be assertive, you must be open, honest, and direct. Be aware of your body position: an open posture conveys the proper message. When you communicate, speak confidently and use "I" statements such as "I feel . . ." or "I think . . ." (Assertiveness is also discussed later in the chapter in the section on communicating with coworkers.)

Developing your assertiveness skills increases your sense of self-worth and your confidence as a professional. Being assertive will also help you prevent or resolve conflicts more peacefully and increase your leadership ability. People look up to and respect professionals who are assertive in the workplace. See Table 4-2 for a comparison of assertive, nonassertive, and aggressive behaviors.

# Communicating in Special Circumstances

If you make an effort to develop good interpersonal skills, most patients will not be difficult to communicate with. You will, however, encounter patients in special circumstances, when they may be anxious or angry. These situations sometimes inhibit communication. Patients from different cultures may pose challenges to communication. Others may have some type of impairment or disability that makes communication difficult. Similarly, young patients, parents with children who are ill or injured, and patients with terminal illnesses may present communication difficulties. Learning about the special needs of these patients and polishing your own communication skills will help you become an effective communicator in any number of situations.

## The Anxious Patient

It is common for patients to be anxious in a doctor's office or other health-care setting. This reaction is commonly known as the "white-coat syndrome." There can be many reasons for anxiety. A patient can become anxious because she is ill and does not know what is wrong with her—she may fear the worst. A patient may have recently been diagnosed with an illness that he knows nothing about, which may necessitate a severe lifestyle change. Fear of bad news or fear that some procedure is going to be painful can create anxiety. Anxiety can interfere with the communication process. For example, because of anxiety a patient may not listen well or pay attention to what you are saying.

Some patients—particularly children—may be unable to verbalize their feelings of fear and anxiety. Watch for signs of anxiety. They may include a tense appearance, increased blood pressure and rates of breathing and pulse, sweaty palms, reported problems with sleep or appetite, irritability, and agitation. Procedure 4-1 will help you communicate with patients who are anxious.

## The Angry Patient

In a medical setting, anger may occur for many reasons. Anger may be a mask for fear about an illness or the outcome of surgery. Anger may come from a patient's feeling of being treated unfairly or without compassion. Anger may stem from a patient's resentment about being ill or injured. Anger may be a reaction to frustration, rejection, disappointment, feelings of loss of control or self-esteem, or an invasion of privacy.

As a medical assistant, you will encounter angry patients and will need to help them express their anger constructively, for the sake of their health. At the same time, you must learn not to take expressions of anger personally; you may just be the unlucky target. A goal with angry patients is to help them refocus emotional energy toward solving the problem. Study the following steps in communicating with an angry patient.

1. Learn to recognize anger and its causes. Anger is easy to recognize in most people, but it can be subtle in others. Patients who speak in a tense tone, are stubborn, or appear to ignore your attempts at communication may be angry.

2. Remain calm and continue to demonstrate genuineness and respect. Communicate that you respect and care about the patient's feelings.

3. Focus on the patient's physical and medical needs.

4. Maintain adequate personal space. Place yourself on the same level as the patient. If the patient is standing, encourage him to sit down. Maintain an open posture to show that you are receptive to listening. Maintain eye contact, but avoid staring at the patient, which can make the person angrier.

5. Avoid the feeling that you need to defend yourself or to give reasons why the patient should not be angry. Instead, listen attentively and with an open mind to what the patient is saying. Most patients' anger will lessen if they know someone is really listening to them and showing an interest in their emotions and needs.

6. Encourage patients to be specific in describing the cause of their anger, their thoughts about it, and their feelings. Be empathic and acknowledge the patient's feelings and perceptions. Follow through with any promises you might make concerning correction of a problem, but avoid totally agreeing or disagreeing with the patient. State what you can and cannot do for the patient.

7. Present your point of view calmly and firmly to help the patient better understand the situation. If patients are receptive to your viewpoint, their perspective may change for the better.

8. Avoid a breakdown in communication. Allow the patient to voice anger. Trying to outtalk the patient or overexplain will only annoy and irritate him. You might also suggest that the patient spend a few moments alone to gather his thoughts or to cool off before continuing any type of communication.

9. If you feel threatened by a patient's anger or if it looks as if the patient's anger may become violent, leave the room and seek assistance from one of the physicians or other members of the office staff. Document any threats in the patient's chart.

## Patients of Other Cultures

Our beliefs, attitudes, values, use of language, and views of the world are unique to us, but they are also shaped by our cultural background. In any health-care setting, you will most likely have contact with patients of diverse cultures and ethnic groups. Each culture and ethnic group has its own behaviors, traditions, and values. Rather than viewing these differences as barriers to communication, strive to understand and be tolerant of them.

As a medical professional, it is important to understand the cultural differences of the patients who come to your medical office for care. Many medical facilities are located in heavily populated ethnic locations, and it is important that the medical staff understand the differences among patient cultures. A medical assistant who is employed in a medical facility in which the majority of its patients are Latino should learn as much as possible about the specific Latin culture in her area in order to provide good customer service. It is also important to understand the difference between stereotyping and generalizing. *Stereotyping* is a negative statement about the specific traits of a group that is applied unfairly to an entire population. A *generalization* is a statement about common trends within a group, but it is understood that further investigation is needed to determine if the trend applies to an individual. Listed in the next sections are common ethnic cultures and some generalizations that will enhance your communication.

Remember that the beliefs of other cultures are neither superior nor inferior to your own. They are simply different. Never allow yourself to make value judgments or to stereotype a patient, a culture, or an ethnic group. Each patient is an individual in her own right.

# PROCEDURE 4.1

## Communicating With the Anxious Patient

**Procedure Goal:** To use communication and interpersonal skills to calm an anxious patient

**Materials:** None

**Method:**

1. Identify signs of anxiety in the patient.
2. Acknowledge the patient's anxiety. (Ignoring a patient's anxiety often makes it worse.)

   *Rationale*

   Good therapeutic communication techniques can help reduce patient anxiety.

3. Identify possible sources of anxiety, such as fear of a procedure or test result, along with supportive resources available to the patient, such as family members and friends. Understanding the source of anxiety in a patient and identifying the supportive resources available can help you communicate with the patient more effectively.
4. Do what you can to alleviate the patient's physical discomfort. For example, find a calm, quiet place for the patient to wait, a comfortable chair, a drink of water, or access to the bathroom (Figure 4-3).
5. Allow ample personal space for conversation. Note: You would normally allow a 1½- to 4-ft distance between yourself and the patient. Adjust this space as necessary.
6. Create a climate of warmth, acceptance, and trust.
   a. Recognize and control your own anxiety. Your air of calm can decrease the patient's anxiety.
   b. Provide reassurance by demonstrating genuine care, respect, and empathy.
   c. Act confidently and dependably, maintaining truthfulness and confidentiality at all times.
7. Using the appropriate communication skills, have the patient describe the experience that is causing anxiety, her thoughts about it, and her feelings. Proceeding in this order allows the patient to describe what is causing the anxiety and to clarify her thoughts and feelings about it.

   *Rationale*

   The use of open-ended questioning will result in more information about the patient's feelings of anxiety.

   a. Maintain an open posture.
   b. Maintain eye contact, if culturally appropriate.
   c. Use active listening skills.
   d. Listen without interrupting.
8. Do not belittle the patient's thoughts and feelings. This can cause a breakdown in communication, increase anxiety, and make the patient feel isolated.
9. Be empathic to the patient's concerns.
10. Help the patient recognize and cope with the anxiety.
    a. Provide information to the patient. Patients are often fearful of the unknown. Helping them understand their disease or the procedure they are about to undergo will help decrease their anxiety.
    b. Suggest coping behaviors, such as deep breathing or other relaxation exercises.
11. Notify the doctor of the patient's concerns.

    *Rationale*

    The physician must be aware of all aspects of the patient's health, including anxiety, to allow for optimal patient care. Part of your job as a medical assistant is to act as a liaison between the patient and the physician.

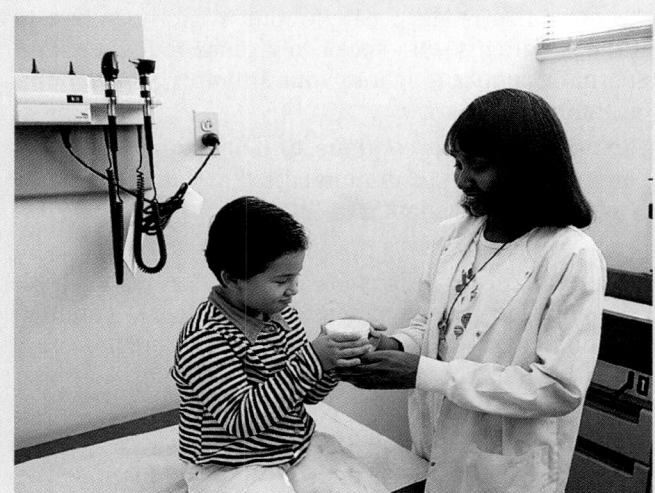

**Figure 4-3.** You can calm children's anxiety by spending time talking with them, playing a game, reading a story, or just offering a glass of water.

# Reflecting On . . . Cultural Issues

## Multicultural Attitudes About Modern Medicine

Patients' cultural backgrounds have a great effect on their attitudes toward health and illness. Patients from different cultural backgrounds often have beliefs about the causes of illness, what symptoms mean, and what to expect from health-care professionals that are different from those of modern medicine. Understanding some of these perceptions, behaviors, and expectations will help you communicate effectively with patients of different cultures.

### Beliefs About Causes of Illness

Some cultures have beliefs about the causes of illness that differ sharply from accepted notions in the mainstream culture. As an example, many cultures believe that some illnesses are caused by hot or cold forces in the body. Some believe that winds and drafts cause illness or that illness can be caused by blood that is too thick or too thin. Others believe that having bad feelings toward others can create ill health.

Because of such beliefs, it may be hard to obtain information from patients about possible reasons for their medical problems. It may also be hard for some patients to realize the importance of taking medication to treat certain illnesses. In this case, you may have to be very persuasive and firm when giving the patient instructions for medication usage. It may be helpful or necessary to involve other family members in persuading the patient.

### How Symptoms Are Presented and What They Mean

People from different cultures may differ in the way they perceive and report symptoms. Some may express pain very emotionally because their culture may feel that suppressing pain is harmful. In contrast, people from other cultures may not admit that they are in pain, thinking that acknowledging pain is a sign of weakness. People of all cultures may be more likely to report physical symptoms of illness than they are to report psychologic symptoms. Be aware of nonverbal indications of pain or other symptoms.

### Treatment Expectations

Patients from other cultures may be totally unaccustomed to some of the practices of modern medicine. Patients of certain ethnic or cultural groups often consult other types of healers before seeing a doctor. They are likely to have different expectations of treatment from each.

Patients from other cultures may be wary of certain treatments because these treatments are so different from what they are accustomed to. This is especially true of some of the medical procedures and interventions considered to be state-of-the-art, such as laser surgery or diabetes management.

When dealing with patients of other cultures, keep in mind their perspectives on health care. Try to avoid generalizations and cultural stereotyping, however, because there can be a variation of attitudes within ethnic groups. Treat each patient as an individual, and you will be providing the best care possible.

---

The Reflecting On . . . Cultural Issues box on this page discusses different cultural views of health care.

**Asian Patients.** Out of respect to the health-care provider, Asian patients may agree to any directives provided without any intention of following through. Make sure the reasons for compliance are explained and emphasized. Avoid hand gestures, such as beckoning with the index finger, as it is insulting to Filipinos and Koreans. Wives may defer to their husbands in decision making. Involve family members in decision making.

**Middle Eastern Patients.** Within Middle Eastern culture, family members may be demanding because they may see it as their duty to ensure that the patient receives the best care possible. They may repeat their demands and speak loudly to emphasis their expectations. Sexual segregation is usually extremely important. Maintain a woman's modesty at all times. The patient may insist on a same-sex physician and medical staff. Women may defer to their husbands for decision making regarding their own and their children's health.

**Hispanic Patients.** In Hispanic cultures, personal relationships are important. Ask about the patient's family and interests before focusing on health issues. Among more traditional women, being fat is seen as being healthy. Because many Hispanic foods are high in fat and sodium, nutritional counseling may be necessary for diabetics and patients with high blood pressure.

**The Language Barrier.** Patients who cannot speak or understand English may have difficulty expressing their needs or feelings effectively. You may need to speak through an interpreter to gather and convey information or to discuss sensitive issues with a patient. Instead of using medical terms, which can be difficult to translate, try to say the same thing using basic, familiar words and simple phrases.

If the patient comes to the office often, take the time to learn some basic phrases in the patient's native language, such as "How are you feeling today?" and "Is there anything I can get you?" Even if the rest of your conversation must take place in English, your small efforts will be much appreciated.

## The Patient With a Visual Impairment

When communicating with a patient who has a visual impairment, be aware of what you say and how you say it. Since people with visual impairments cannot usually rely on nonverbal clues, your tone of voice, inflection, and speech volume take on greater importance.

Following are some suggestions for communicating with a patient who has a visual impairment.

- Use large-print materials whenever possible.
- Make sure there is adequate lighting in all patient areas.
- Use a normal speaking voice.
- Talk directly and honestly. Explain instructions thoroughly.
- Don't talk down to the patient; preserve the patient's dignity.

## The Patient With a Hearing Impairment

Hearing loss can range from mild to severe. How you communicate depends on the degree of impairment and on whether the patient has effective use of a hearing aid.

Following are some tips to help you communicate effectively with a hearing-impaired patient.

- Find a quiet area to talk, and try to minimize background noise.
- Position yourself close to and facing the patient. The patient will rely on visual clues such as the movement of your lips and mouth, your facial expression, and your body language (Figure 4-4).
- Speak slowly, so the patient can follow what you are saying.
- Remember that elderly patients lose the ability to hear high-pitched sounds first. Try speaking in lower tones.
- Speak in a clear, firm voice, but do not shout, especially if the patient wears a hearing aid.

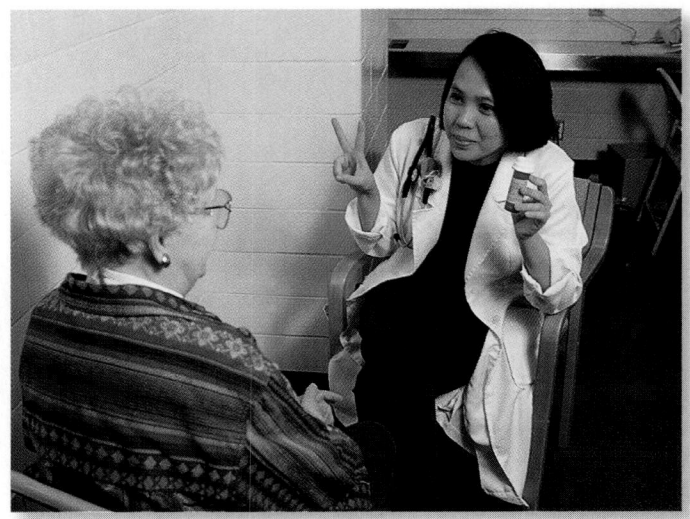

**Figure 4-4.** When communicating with a patient who has a hearing impairment, position yourself close to the patient and use gestures and effective body language.

- To verify understanding, ask questions that will encourage the patient to repeat what you said.
- Whenever possible, use written materials to reinforce verbal information.

## The Patient Who Is Mentally or Emotionally Disturbed

There may be times when you will need to communicate with patients who are mentally or emotionally disturbed. When dealing with this type of patient, you need to determine what level of communication the patient can understand. Keep these suggestions in mind to improve communication.

- It is important to remain calm if the patient becomes agitated or confused.
- Avoid raising your voice or appearing impatient.
- If you do not understand, ask the patient to repeat what he said.

## The Elderly Patient

Medical assistants now spend at least 50% of their time caring for older patients. Be aware of the vast differences in the capabilities of people of this age group. Do not stereotype all elderly patients as frail or confused. Most are not, and each patient deserves to be treated according to her own individual abilities.

Always treat elderly patients with respect. Regardless of their physical or mental state, elderly patients are adults. Do not talk down to them. Use the title "Mrs." or "Mr." to address older people unless they ask you to call them by their first name.

**Denial or Confusion.** Some elderly patients deny that they are ill. For example, in a survey of elderly people, the majority of whom had at least one chronic condition, 85% reported that they were in good or excellent health (Bradley and Edinberg, 1990). Patients' perception of how they feel may be quite different from their actual state of health.

The reverse situation can also occur. Elderly patients may overreact to a problem and consider themselves sicker than they really are. They may become dependent, passive, or anxious. Elderly patients may also over- or underestimate their ability to perform certain tasks or to deal with certain limitations.

Elderly patients may be confused if they have some impairment in memory, judgment, or other mental abilities. Signs of confusion can occur with Alzheimer disease, senility, depression, head injury, or misuse of medications or alcohol. Elderly patients may or may not be aware of their condition. They may have difficulty understanding instructions.

The following tips can help you communicate with elderly patients.

- Act as if you expect the patient to understand.
- Respond calmly to any confusion on the patient's part.
- Tell the truth. Use facts. Do not go along with misconceptions or make up explanations.
- Use simple questions and terms, but avoid using baby talk or speaking to the patient as if he were a child.
- Explain points slowly and clearly, using concrete terms rather than abstract expressions. Say, for example, "You may feel a pinprick and a sting when I put the needle in" instead of "You may feel some discomfort in your arm."
- Ask the patient to relax and speak slowly.
- If you do not understand the patient, simply say that you cannot understand her well and ask her to repeat what she said. Do not say you understand when in fact you do not. It is important not to belittle the patient. It is equally important to inform yourself about what could be very important information.

**The Importance of Touch.** Because they often live alone, many elderly patients experience a lack of physical touch. Using touch—offering to hold a patient's hand or placing an arm around his shoulder—communicates that you care about the patient's well-being.

## Terminally Ill Patients

Terminally ill patients are often under extreme stress and can be a challenge to treat. It is important that health-care professionals respect the rights of terminal patients and treat them with dignity. It is also important that you communicate with the family and offer support and empathy as their loved one accepts her condition. You should also provide information on **hospice,** which is an area of medicine that works with terminally ill patients and their families. Hospice workers often go to the home of the terminally ill patient or work with patients in facilities. Hospice care is usually staffed with RNs who have specialized training in issues related to death and dying. They work with the family and patient in the beginning, assisting with medications, and they end by making arrangements with the funeral home and coroner.

Elisabeth Kübler-Ross, a world-renowned authority in the areas of death and dying, developed a model of behavior that patients will experience on learning their condition. This is called the Stages of Dying or Stages of Grief. This model is widely used today in work with terminally ill patients.

Kübler-Ross's Stages of Dying include five stages, which usually—but not always—progress in the following order:

1. Denial. Patients are in direct denial or periods of disbelief. This defense is generally temporary.
2. Anger. Patients may suddenly realize what is really happening and respond with anger. They can become difficult patients in this stage and display temper tantrums and fits of rage.
3. Bargaining. Patients attempt to make deals with physicians, clergy, and family members. Patients at this stage may become more cooperative and congenial.
4. Depression. The patient will begin to show signs of depression, such as withdrawal, lethargy, and sobbing. The patient's body is beginning to deteriorate, and the patient may experience more pain and realize that relationships with family and friends will soon be gone.
5. Acceptance. Patients accept the fact that they are dying. They will begin arrangements for when they expire, making funeral or burial requests. The patient's family needs the most support at this stage.

Even though these stages have been generalized to dying, many experts have applied them to the grieving process as well.

## The Young Patient

A doctor's office can be a frightening place for children. They often associate the doctor's office with getting a shot or being sick. Sometimes parents have misled their children about what to expect from a visit to the doctor. When dealing with children, it is better to recognize and accept their fear and anxiety than to dismiss these emotions. When children realize that you take their feelings seriously, they are more apt to be receptive to your requests and suggestions.

Explain any procedure, no matter how basic (such as testing a reflex with a reflex hammer), in very simple terms. Let the child examine the instrument.

Other suggestions include using praise ("You were very brave") and always being truthful. Do not tell children that a procedure will not hurt if it will, or you will lose their trust.

As children get older, you can use more detailed descriptions when explaining procedures. Remember that after the age of 7 or 8, children can tell if they are being talked down to or treated like babies. Encourage them to participate actively in their care, and direct any questions or instructions to them, when appropriate. You should also respect the adolescent's request not to have a parent present during private conversations.

## Parents

Parents are naturally concerned about their children and are likely to be worried or anxious when a child is ill. Children often react to a situation based on how they see their parents react. Reassuring parents and keeping them calm can also help children relax.

## The Patient With AIDS and the Patient Who Is HIV-Positive

Patients with acquired immunodeficiency syndrome (AIDS) and patients who have the human immunodeficiency virus (HIV), the virus that causes AIDS, have a grave illness to deal with. They also face a society that often stigmatizes them, saying they have only themselves to blame. These patients often feel guilty, angry, and depressed.

To communicate effectively with these patients, you need accurate information about the disease and the risks involved. Take the initiative to educate yourself about AIDS and HIV. Patients will have many questions. Part of your role as a good communicator will be to answer as many questions as you can. If a patient asks a question you cannot answer, tell the physician so he can respond quickly.

Above all, remember that HIV is not transmitted through casual or common physical contact, such as brushing by a person in a crowded hall or shaking hands. It is transferred only through bodily fluids. Patients with AIDS and those who are HIV-positive need to know you are not afraid to be near them, to touch them, or to talk to them. Like any patient whose body is being ravaged by a serious illness, these patients need human contact (verbal and physical) and they need to be treated with dignity.

## Patients' Families and Friends

Family members or friends sometimes accompany a patient to the office. These individuals can provide important emotional support to the patient. Always ask patients if they want a family member or friend to accompany them to the examination room, however. Do not just assume their preference. Acknowledge family members and friends, and communicate with them as you do with patients. They should be kept informed of the patient's progress, whenever possible, to avoid unnecessary anxiety on their part. You must always protect patient confidentiality, however. Too often, health-care workers think that it is acceptable to discuss patient cases in detail with family members, even without the consent of the patient.

# Communicating With Coworkers

The quality of the communication you have with coworkers greatly influences the development of a positive or negative work climate and a team approach to patient care. In turn, the workplace atmosphere ultimately affects your communication with patients.

## Positive Communication With Coworkers

In your interactions with coworkers, use the same skills and qualities that you use to communicate with patients. Have respect and empathy; be caring, thoughtful, and genuine; and use active listening skills. These skills will help you develop **rapport,** which is a harmonious, positive relationship, with your coworkers (Figure 4-5).

Following are some rules for communication in the medical office.

- Use proper channels of communication. For example, if you are having problems getting along with a coworker, try first to work it out with her. Do not go over her head and complain to her supervisor. Your coworker may not have realized the effect of her behavior and may wish to correct it without involving her supervisor. If you go to the supervisor right away, working relationships can become even more strained.

- Have the proper attitude. You can avoid conflict and resolve most problems if you maintain a positive attitude. A friendly approach is much more effective than a hostile approach. Remember that many problems are simply the result of misinformation or lack of communication.

- Plan an appropriate time for communication. If you have something important to discuss, schedule a time

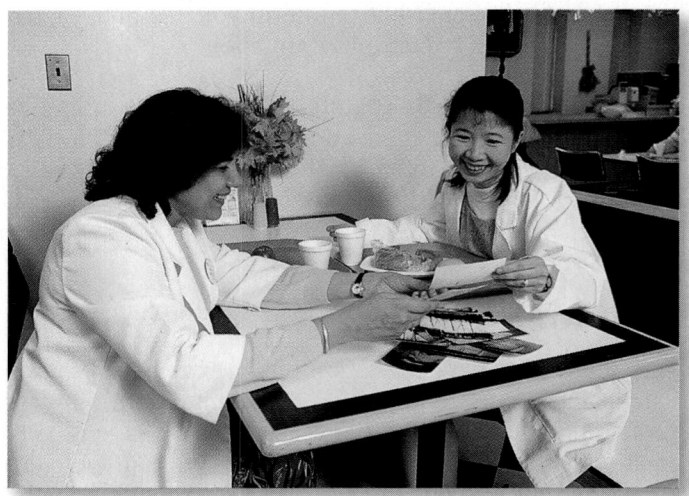

**Figure 4-5.** Rapport with coworkers is easy to build when you are open, friendly, and thoughtful.

to do so. For example, if you want to talk with the office manager about renewing the lease of a piece of office equipment, tell him you would like to discuss that topic and ask him to let you know a time that is convenient.

As an example of good communication with coworkers, consider this exchange between Mai Lee, a medical assistant, and Margot, a coworker in a pediatric practice. Note the way Mai Lee demonstrates assertiveness.

**Mai Lee:** I know you spent a lot of time choosing the new toys for the reception area. I love the wooden safari animal puzzles.

**Margot:** Thanks. I think the children really enjoy themselves now.

**Mai Lee:** I wanted to mention to you, though, that I'm concerned about the toy tea set with miniature cupcakes and sandwiches. Anything that's smaller than a golf ball is a choking hazard to infants and toddlers.

**Margot:** I don't think the little ones pay much attention to the tea set. It's mostly for older kids.

**Mai Lee:** Yes, but I'm still afraid that a baby could put one of those pieces in his mouth. What if we put up a little shelf in the play area that is low enough for kids 4 years old or more to reach but high enough to be out of reach of the babies. We could put the tea set on it in a clear plastic box and any other toys with small parts.

**Margot:** I see your point. Sounds like a good idea to me.

Mai Lee started with a statement that acknowledged the coworker's situation and feelings. Then she stated her own opinion. When her coworker disagreed, she repeated her concern, describing what might happen if the situation remained unchanged. Then she made a constructive suggestion for solving the problem without hurting the coworker's feelings. As you interact with coworkers, be sensitive to the timing of your conversations, the manner in which you present your ideas and thoughts, and your coworkers' feelings.

# Communicating With Management

Positive or negative communication can affect the quality of your relationships with your supervisor or manager. For example, problems arise when communication about job responsibilities is unclear or when you feel that your supervisor does not trust or respect you, or vice versa.

Consider these suggestions when communicating with your direct supervisor:

- Keep your supervisor informed. If the office copier is not working properly, talk to your supervisor about it before a breakdown occurs that will hold everyone up. If several patients express the same types of complaint about the examination rooms, make sure

the right people are told. If the doctor asks you to call a patient and you reach the patient, tell the doctor.

- Ask questions. If you are unsure about an administrative task or the meaning of a medical term, for example, do not hesitate to ask your supervisor. It is better to ask a question before acting than to make a mistake. It is also better to ask than to risk annoying someone because you carried out a task or wrote a term incorrectly. Asking your supervisor or manager a question means that you respect him or her professionally.

- Minimize interruptions. For example, before launching into a discussion, make sure your supervisor has time to talk. Opening with "Can I interrupt you for a moment, or should I come back?" or "Do you have a minute to talk?" goes a long way toward establishing good communication. It is also better to go to your supervisor when you have several questions to ask rather than to interrupt her repeatedly.

- Show initiative. Any manager or supervisor will greatly appreciate this quality. For example, if you think you can come up with a more efficient way to get the office newsletter written and distributed, write out a plan and show it to your supervisor. He or she is likely to welcome any ideas that improve office efficiency or patient satisfaction.

# Dealing With Conflict

**Conflict,** or friction, in the workplace can result from opposition of opinions or ideas or even from a difference in personalities. Conflict can arise when the lines of communication break down or when a misunderstanding occurs. Conflict can also result from prejudices or preconceived notions about people or from lack of mutual respect or trust between a staff member and management. Whatever the cause, conflict is counterproductive to the efficiency of an office.

Following these suggestions can help prevent conflict in the office and improve communication among coworkers.

- Do not "feed into" other people's negative attitudes.

- For example, if a coworker is criticizing one of the doctors, change the subject or walk away.

- Try your best at all times to be personable and supportive of coworkers. For example, everyone has bad days. If a coworker is having a bad day, offer to pitch in and help or to run out and get her lunch if she is too busy to go out.

- Refrain from passing judgment on others or stereotyping them (women are bad at math, men don't know how to communicate, and so on). Coworkers should show respect for one another and try to be tolerant and nonjudgmental.

- Do not gossip. You are there to work. Act professionally at all times.
- Do not jump to conclusions. For example, if you get a memo about a change in your schedule that disturbs you, bring your concern to your supervisor. She may be able to be flexible on certain points. You do not know until you ask.

# Written Communication Tools and Community Resources

Communication is not effective if it is communicated incorrectly. It is important to be knowledgeable in the policies and procedures in your medical facility and the community resources that you have implemented into your facility. Many offices provide written documentation regarding the policies and procedures in their unique setting.

## The Policy and Procedures Manual

The policy and procedures manual is a key written communication tool in the medical office. No discussion of communication in the medical office would be complete without a description of this important document. The manual is used by permanent employees as well as by temporary employees who may be hired when others are ill or on vacation, or when there is an unusually heavy workload. The manual covers all office policies and clinical procedures. It is usually developed as a joint effort by the physician (or physicians) and the staff (often the medical assistant).

**Policies.** Policies are rules or guidelines that dictate the day-to-day workings of an office. Although individual policies vary from office to office, most medical office manuals describe the following policy areas:

- Office purposes, objectives, and goals as set down by the physician(s)
- Rules and regulations
- Job descriptions and duties of staff personnel
- Office hours
- Dress code
- Insurance and other benefits
- Vacation, sick leave, and other time away from the office
- Salary and performance evaluations
- Maintenance of equipment and supplies
- Mailings
- Bookkeeping
- Scheduling of appointments and maintenance of patient records
- OSHA guidelines

The policy section of the manual also typically describes the chain of command for the office, or the person to whom each employee reports. This information is sometimes presented in chart form and called an organizational chart. For example, the receptionist, secretary, medical assistant, and billing person might report to the office manager. The office manager, in turn, might report directly to the physician or physicians. This chain of command varies from office to office, depending on the size and needs of the practice.

**Procedures.** Detailed instructions for specific procedures are covered in the procedures section of the manual. The areas discussed include clinical procedures and quality assurance programs.

Each clinical procedure should include instructions about the following:

- Purpose of the test, clinical application, and usefulness
- Specimen required and collection method; special patient preparation or restrictions
- Reagents, standards, controls, and media used; special supplies
- Instrumentation, including calibration and schedules
- Step-by-step directions

## Community Resources

There are many community resources available in your local area that provide needed services to patients. The medical facility often works with outside resources such as laboratories, home health-care agencies, and social service agencies. It is beneficial to the patient if the medical assistant is familiar with services that could assist with his or her care. Good customer service is founded on providing or researching services that can assist in the goal of patient health and well-being. Some community resources include:

- Alcoholics Anonymous
- Shelters for abused individuals
- Hospice care
- Mental health services
- Meals on Wheels
- PASSPORT
- Easter Seals
- Various state agencies, such as health insurance for the indigent; Women, Infants, and Children (WIC); etc.
- Support groups for grief, obesity, and various diseases

If a medical assistant discovers that an external community resource is needed for a patient, the medical assistant should first discuss with the physician the needs of the patient. If the physician is in agreement, then the medical assistant can arrange for services. The first step in developing a community resource library is to gather a listing of local agencies. You will need the correct name,

# PROCEDURE 4.2

## Identifying Community Resources

**Procedure Goal:** To create a list of useful community resources for patient referrals

**Materials:** Computer with Internet access, phone directory, printer

**Method:**

1. Determine the needs of your medical office and formulate a list of community resources.

   ### Rationale

   It is important to understand the specific needs of your patients and be able to assist them with finding outside assistance when necessary.

2. Use the Internet to research the names, addresses, and phone numbers of local resources such as Meals on Wheels, state and federal agencies, home health-care agencies, long-term nursing facilities, mental health agencies, and local charities. Use the phone directory to assist in local agencies as well.

3. Contact each resource and request information such as business cards and brochures. Some agencies may send a representative to meet with you regarding their services.

   ### Rationale

   If patients can access information easily, they are more likely to avail themselves of the services available to them.

4. Compile a list of community resources with the proper name, address, phone number, e-mail address, and contact name. Include any information that may be helpful to the office.

5. Update and add to the information often because outdated information will only frustrate you and your patients, creating even more anxiety.

6. Post the information in a location where it is readily available.

---

address, phone number, contact person, and directions for submitting a referral for each resource listed. It may take some research on your part to locate and organize this information. The Internet and phone directory can be useful tools. Contact the community resource and request information, such as brochures, newsletters, and referral applications. Type up an inventory sheet of your resources and make sure that all appropriate departments have a copy. A filing drawer can be used to organize and maintain the informational material regarding each resource. See Procedure 4-2 about Identifying Community Resources.

## Other Communication Resources

Often a medical office will work with an external business or facility to assist with the care of a patient. Such facilities can include reference laboratories, insurance companies, office equipment suppliers, and maintenance companies. It is efficient if you follow the protocol of each organization in order to maximize the level of service that you receive from them. For example, many reference laboratories, such as Lab Corp, have reference manuals available to medical facilities. These manuals can provide answers to questions about obtaining the correct amount of a specimen for testing. Insurance manuals such as the annual Medicare changes and coding reference books can provide you with updated information. Insurance company manuals provide information regarding precertifying procedures

or referrals. Even the office equipment can be repaired and maintained with little disruption to the daily office flow if protocol is followed. Make sure that you familiarize yourself with these important resources to assist in your daily communication interactions.

## Managing Stress

Stress can be a barrier to communication. For example, if you are feeling very pressured at work, you might snap at a coworker or patient, or you might forget to give the physician an important message.

Professionals in the health-care field may experience high levels of stress in their daily work environment. Stress can result from a feeling of being under pressure, or it can be a reaction to anger, frustration, or a change in your routine. Stress can increase your blood pressure, speed up your breathing and heart rate, and cause muscle tension. To minimize stress—for the sake of your health as well as for good communication in the office—it is helpful to understand some basic information about stress.

### Stress—Good or Bad?

A certain amount of stress is normal. A little bit of stress—the kind that makes you feel excited or challenged by the task at hand—can motivate you to get things done and push you toward a higher level of productivity. Ongoing stress, however, can be overwhelming and affect you physically. For example, it can lower your resistance to colds and increase your risk for developing heart disease, diabetes, high blood pressure, ulcers, allergies, asthma, colitis, and cancer. It can also increase your risk for certain autoimmune diseases, which cause the body's immune system to attack normal tissue. The Points on Practice boxes list the potential causes of stress and ways to reduce stress.

## Reducing Stress

Some stress at work is inevitable. An important goal is to learn how to manage or reduce stress. Take into account your strengths and limitations, and be realistic about how much you can handle at work and in your life outside work. Pushing yourself a certain amount can be motivating.

Pushing yourself too much is dangerous. The Points on Practice box lists tips for reducing stress.

## Points on Practice

### Potential Causes of Stress

- Death of a spouse or family member
- Divorce or separation
- Hospitalization (yours or a family member's) due to injury or illness
- Marriage or reconciliation from a separation
- Loss of a job or retirement
- Sexual problems
- Having a new baby
- Significant change in your financial status (for better or worse)
- Job change
- Children leaving or returning home
- Significant personal success, such as a promotion at work
- Moving or remodeling your home
- Problems at work, such as your boss's retiring, that may put your job at risk
- Substantial debt, such as a mortgage or overspending on credit cards

## Points on Practice

### Tips for Reducing Stress

- Maintain a healthy balance in your life among work, family, and leisure activities.
- Exercise regularly.
- Eat balanced, nutritious meals and healthful snacks.
- Avoid foods high in caffeine, salt, sugar, and fat.
- Get enough sleep.
- Allow time for yourself, and plan time to relax.
- Rely on the support that family, friends, and coworkers have to offer. Don't be afraid to share your feelings.
- Try to be realistic about what you can and cannot do. Do not be afraid to admit that you cannot take on another responsibility.
- Try to set realistic goals for yourself. Remember that there are always choices, even when there appear to be none.
- Be organized. Good planning can help you manage your workload.
- Redirect excess energy constructively—clean your closet, work in the garden, do volunteer work, have friends over for dinner, exercise.
- Change some of the things you have control over. Keep yourself focused. Focus your full energy on one thing at a time, and finish one project before starting another.
- Identify sources of conflict, and try to resolve them.
- Learn and use relaxation techniques, such as deep breathing, meditation, or imagining yourself in a quiet, peaceful place. Choose what works for you.
- Maintain a healthy sense of humor. Laughter can help relieve stress. Joke with friends after work. Go see a funny movie.
- Try not to overreact. Ask yourself if a situation is really worth getting upset or worried about.
- Seek help from social or professional support groups, if necessary.

# Preventing Burnout

**Burnout** is the end result of prolonged periods of stress without relief. Burnout is an energy-depleting condition that will affect your health and career. Certain personality types are more prone to burnout than others. If you are a highly driven, perfectionist-type person, you will be more susceptible to burnout. Experts often refer to such a person as a characteristic Type A personality. A more relaxed, calm, laid-back individual is considered a Type B person. Type B personalities are less prone to burnout but have the potential to suffer from it, especially if they work in health care.

According to some experts on stress, there are five stages that lead to burnout (Miller and Smith). The road to burnout follows this path:

1. The Honeymoon Phase. During the honeymoon phase, your job is wonderful. You have boundless energy and enthusiasm, and all things seem possible. You love the job and the job loves you. You believe it will satisfy all your needs and desires and solve all your problems. You are delighted with your job, your coworkers, and the organization.

2. The Awakening Phase. The honeymoon wanes and the awakening stage starts with the realization that your initial expectations were unrealistic. The job isn't working out the way you thought it would. It doesn't satisfy all your needs, your coworkers and the organization are less than perfect, and rewards and recognition are scarce.

   As disillusionment and disappointment grow, you become confused. Something is wrong, but you can't quite put your finger on it. Typically, you work harder to make your dreams come true. But working harder doesn't change anything and you become increasingly tired, bored, and frustrated. You question your competence and ability, and start losing your self-confidence.

3. The Brownout Phase. As brownout begins, your early enthusiasm and energy give way to chronic fatigue and irritability. Your eating and sleeping patterns change, and you indulge in escapist behaviors such as partying, overeating, recreational drugs, alcoholism, and binge shopping. You become indecisive and your productivity drops. Your work deteriorates. Coworkers and managers may comment on it.

   Unless interrupted, brownout slides into later stages. You become increasingly frustrated and angry and project the blame for your difficulties onto others. You are cynical, detached, and openly critical of the organization, superiors, and coworkers. You are beset with depression, anxiety, and physical illness.

4. The Full-Scale Burnout Phase. Unless you wake up and interrupt the process or someone intervenes, brownout drifts remorselessly into full-scale burnout. Despair is the dominant feature of this final stage. It may take several months to get to this phase, but in most cases it takes three to four years. You experience an overwhelming sense of failure and a devastating loss of self-esteem and self-confidence. You become depressed and feel lonely and empty.

   Life seems pointless, and there is a paralyzing, "what's the use" pessimism about the future. You talk about "just quitting and getting away." You are exhausted physically and mentally. Physical and mental breakdowns are likely. Suicide, stroke, or heart attack is not unusual as you complete the final stage of what all started with such high hopes, energy, optimism, and enthusiasm.

5. The Phoenix Phenomenon. You can arise from the ashes of burnout (like a phoenix), but it takes time.

   First, you need to rest and relax. Don't take work home. If you're like many people, the work won't get done and you'll only feel guilty for being "lazy."

   Second, be realistic in your job expectations as well as your aspirations and goals. Whoever you're talking to about your feelings can help you, but be careful. Your readjusted aspirations and goals must be yours and not those of someone else. Trying to be and do what someone else wants you to be or do is a sure-fire recipe for continued frustration and burnout.

## Reflecting On . . . Communication Issues

### Scope of Practice

A medical assistant is a representative of the physician. Patients often will view you as a health-care practitioner with medical decision-making ability. The physician will diagnose and prescribe treatment to a patient based on his or her examination and diagnostic test results. A medical assistant is not allowed to give his or her opinions on the decisions that are made by the physician. By doing so, a medical assistant will find him- or herself in an "advising" position, which could cause legal complications for the practice or physician. "Advising" is out of the scope of practice for a medical assistant and could be considered practicing medicine, which is illegal in most states.

Third, create balance in your life. Invest more of yourself in family and other personal relationships, social activities, and hobbies. Spread yourself out so that your job doesn't have such an overpowering influence on your self-esteem and self-confidence.

# Summary

As a medical assistant, you are a key communicator between the office and patients and families. The way you greet patients, the way you explain procedures, the manner in which you ask and answer questions, and your attentiveness to patients' individual needs combine to form your communication style. Effective communication skills—which include listening, interpersonal, and assertiveness skills—will help you improve your communication style. These skills will also enable you to develop good communication with patients under special circumstances. Patients with special needs include those who are anxious or angry, elderly, and from other cultures and who have hearing or visual impairments.

Good communication skills also enable you to develop satisfying and professional working relationships with co-workers and managers. Effective communication helps the office function smoothly, helps reduce conflicts and stress, and helps motivate individuals to achieve personal and professional goals.

## CASE STUDY QUESTIONS

Now that you have completed this chapter, review the case study at the beginning of the chapter and answer the following questions:

1. How will Mary adapt her communication style to communicate with each patient?
2. What types of communication roadblocks will she encounter with each one?
3. What types of communication techniques will she use for each patient?

## Discussion Questions

1. Discuss the difference between verbal and nonverbal communication. Give examples of each.
2. Suggest some of the communication problems that can arise with patients from other cultures. How might you deal with these problems?
3. Discuss defense mechanisms and apply them to everyday communication with friends, family, and classmates.

## Critical Thinking Questions

1. You notice that you have not been feeling well lately, and you suspect that it is job-related stress. What kinds of activities can you take part in to help reduce stress and prevent job burnout?
2. How does learning about the cultural differences related to ethnic groups enhance a medical assistant's professional development?
3. An established patient has just recently lost her husband of 56 years and is very depressed. Which stage of the Kübler-Ross model best describes this patient?

## Application Activities

1. With a partner or group, take turns using body language to indicate a variety of emotions and see if the others can correctly guess what message you are sending.
2. With a group of classmates, create an outline for an office policy and procedures manual. Identify sections that might need updating on an ongoing basis and why the updating might be necessary.
3. With a partner, take turns being blindfolded and communicate a list of activities each of you wants the other person to do. For example:
   - Walk to the bathroom
   - Purchase a candy bar out of the vending machine
   - Find the light switch
   - Turn on a computer

   This activity will teach you how to communicate with someone who depends on you and allows the partner to feel what it is like to depend on someone.

## Virtual Fieldtrip

*Visit the McGraw-Hill Higher Education Medical Assisting website at www.mhhe.com/medicalassisting3 to complete the following activity:*

Research the predominant ethnic group in your location and write a one-page report on the perspectives members of various cultures may have on their attitudes about health care.

Open the CD and complete this chapter's practice activities, play the games, listen to the key terms, and test yourself with the interactive review. E-mail, print, and/or save your results to document your proficiency.

# PART
## *Two*

# Administrative Medical Assisting

"In my 15 years as a medical assistant and transcriptionist in a large cardiology practice, I have gained invaluable experience that enhances the care of our patients. Cardiology patients require complex care. State-of-the-art equipment, pleasant office surroundings, and a well-educated, warm, and caring staff are key elements in helping patients feel at ease. As I work with patients, I do everything I can to help them feel comfortable in the office. Using reassuring words and good listening skills helps them overcome the anxieties they may have about their illness or a test they are about to have performed.

"Administrative duties are as important as clinical duties. For example, make sure the medical transcription work space is quiet and comfortable. Transcription requires intense concentration to ensure accuracy. Accuracy in all administrative tasks contributes to the success of each patient's treatment plan."

**Kaye H. Listug**
*Medical Assistant, La Mesa, California*

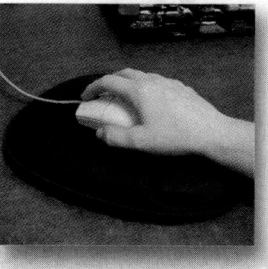

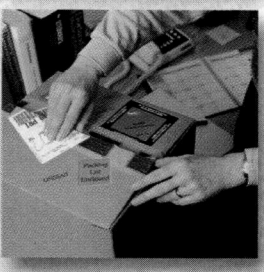

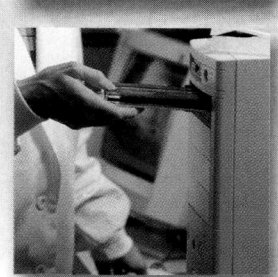

## SECTION ONE
### Office Work

## SECTION TWO
### Interacting With Patients

## SECTION THREE
### Financial Responsibilities

# SECTION 1

## OFFICE WORK

# Using and Maintaining Office Equipment

## MEDICAL ASSISTING COMPETENCIES

*In preparation for the certification examination, you should know the following areas of competence:*

| COMPETENCY | CMA | RMA |
|---|---|---|
| **Administrative** | | |
| Perform basic clerical skills | X | X |
| **General/Legal/Professional** | | |
| Respond to and initiate written communications by using correct grammar, spelling, and formatting techniques | X | X |
| Explain general office policies and procedures | X | X |
| Identify community resources and information for patients and employers | X | X |
| Perform an inventory of supplies and equipment | X | X |
| Operate and maintain facilities, and perform routine maintenance of administrative and clinical equipment safely | X | X |
| Perform quality control procedures | X | X |
| Maintain the physical plant | | X |
| Evaluate and recommend equipment and supplies for practice | | X |
| Project a positive attitude | | X |
| Exhibit initiative | | X |
| Evidence a responsible attitude | | X |
| Conduct work within scope of education, training, and ability | | X |
| Receive, organize, prioritize, and transmit information appropriately | | X |

## KEY TERMS

- abuse
- cover sheet
- covered entity
- disclaimer
- electronic media
- interactive pager
- lease
- maintenance contract
- microfiche
- microfilm
- service contract
- troubleshooting
- voice mail
- warranty

## CHAPTER OUTLINE

- Office Communication Equipment
- Office Automation Equipment
- Purchasing Decisions
- Maintaining Office Equipment

# LEARNING OUTCOMES

After completing Chapter 5, you will be able to:

5.1 Describe the types of office equipment used in a medical practice.

5.2 Explain how each piece of office equipment is used.

5.3 List the steps in making purchasing decisions for office equipment.

5.4 Compare and contrast leasing and buying.

5.5 Describe a warranty, a maintenance contract, and a service contract, and discuss the importance of each.

5.6 Identify when troubleshooting is appropriate and what actions may be taken.

5.7 List the information included in an equipment inventory.

5.8 Explain how HIPAA law applies to faxing confidential patient information.

5.9 Explain how HIPAA law applies to telephone conversations and conversations with patients.

# Introduction

Today's medical office requires many different types of clerical equipment in order to function effectively and smoothly. The role of the medical assistant includes learning how to evaluate, purchase or lease, operate, and maintain this essential equipment.

Think how difficult it would be to communicate with others outside the office without the use of a communication system, which could include telephones, e-mail, beepers or pagers, interactive pagers, text messaging, answering machines, and fax machines. How limited would a medical practice become if the recording of the care given to a patient had to done *without* the use of a computer? What if all patient billing, bank deposits, and payroll management had to be done *without* the use of a calculator or business accounting software? Without a paper shredder, each piece of confidential paper would have to be torn many times before discarding. Possibly the most difficult of all tasks would be the duplication of endless documents by hand instead of using a copy machine!

In this chapter you will be learning about the use and maintenance of many important pieces of administrative medical office equipment. Additionally, you just might come away with a new appreciation of the importance they play in the function of the efficient medical practice.

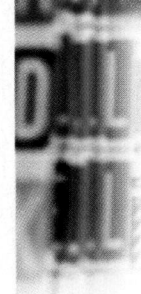

## CASE STUDY

Meg is a CMA and is the first to arrive each morning at the busy medical practice where she works. As she unlocks the back door, she is thinking about the entry process. She knows she will set off an alarm as she enters and that she must go immediately to the security alarm box on the nearby wall and type in her security code number to turn off the system.

Meg walks through the office to the administrative section of the practice. As she walks, she notices the fire extinguisher hanging on the wall. She makes a note to herself to call the maintenance company today to notify them that the expiration date on the extinguisher is this month. They will replace the old one with a new extinguisher.

Meg next turns on all the lights in the administrative and clinical areas. As she walks through the quiet office, she sees three messages in the fax machine that have come in overnight. She picks them up and scans them quickly before she places them in the center of her desk. She notices that the late-night pick-up specimen boxes are empty. She now knows that all items placed there last evening at the close of the day were picked up by the lab.

She switches on the copy machines. On the top display is a four-digit number that indicates the number of copies each machine has made this month. Because it is the first of the month, she will call the leasing company today to report that number. Her office is billed based on how many copies are made each month.

Sitting at her desk, Meg turns off the telephone answering machine, which has been in operation throughout the night. There are four messages. As she listens, she makes careful notes before she discards each message and turns off the system. She knows that the phone will start ringing soon.

Meg turns on her computer and reviews all the tasks ahead of her today as a CMA in a busy medical practice. She has received e-mail from another doctor's office asking her to call about a new referral. Another e-mail is requesting medical records. Meg prints out two computer lists of appointments scheduled for the day, placing one in the front office and one in the back office for easy reference.

Next, she moves to the patient medical charts already pulled from the medical chart area the night before. She makes sure they are in chronological order. Comparing the charts against the computer list of appointments, she makes sure she has a chart for every name on the list.

A quick look around the administrative office helps her to identify items that need to be restocked. She checks and restocks the supply of pens and forms, and makes sure the copier tray is filled with paper. Making her way into the patient reception area, she turns on the soft lighting and music, tidies the magazines, feeds the fish in the fish tank, picks up the physician's morning newspaper at the front door, and unlocks the front door.

There is one more thing Meg must check before she settles in to her day's work. She makes her way to the break room and makes a big pot of coffee for all the staff. With a steaming coffee mug in hand, Meg walks back to her desk. Let the day begin!

As you read this chapter, consider the following questions:

1. What factors might go into the choice of an answering machine over the use of an answering service?
2. What backups for system failure might be important for the equipment in a medical office?
3. How could a misdialed phone number on the fax machine impact the life of a patient?
4. Why is routine maintenance of all office equipment important?

# Office Communication Equipment

When you think of equipment for a medical office, you probably imagine x-ray machines, blood pressure monitors, and stethoscopes. You will, however, find many other kinds of equipment in a medical practice. Medical offices also use business communication equipment, including telephones, facsimile machines, computers, and photocopiers. Part of your responsibilities as a medical assistant is maintaining and operating the medical office's communication equipment.

Just as medical equipment has evolved over the years, so has office equipment. The office communication equipment available not so many years ago handled only the most basic tasks. Today's technology allows almost instantaneous communication of information throughout the world. This instant communication can be critical for the fast-paced medical profession, where information often translates to the need for immediate treatment, sometimes in life-threatening situations. Communicating effectively within a medical office can be as vital as providing the correct treatment to patients—and often ensures that they receive such treatment (Figure 5-1).

## Telephone Systems and Call Handling

The telephone is one of the most important pieces of communication equipment in a medical practice. Not only is it the primary instrument patients use to communicate with the office, but it is also the primary means of communication with other doctors, hospitals, laboratories, and other businesses important to the practice.

**Multiple Lines.** Few practices can function with just one or two telephone lines because if those lines are in use, no other calls can be placed or received. Most medical

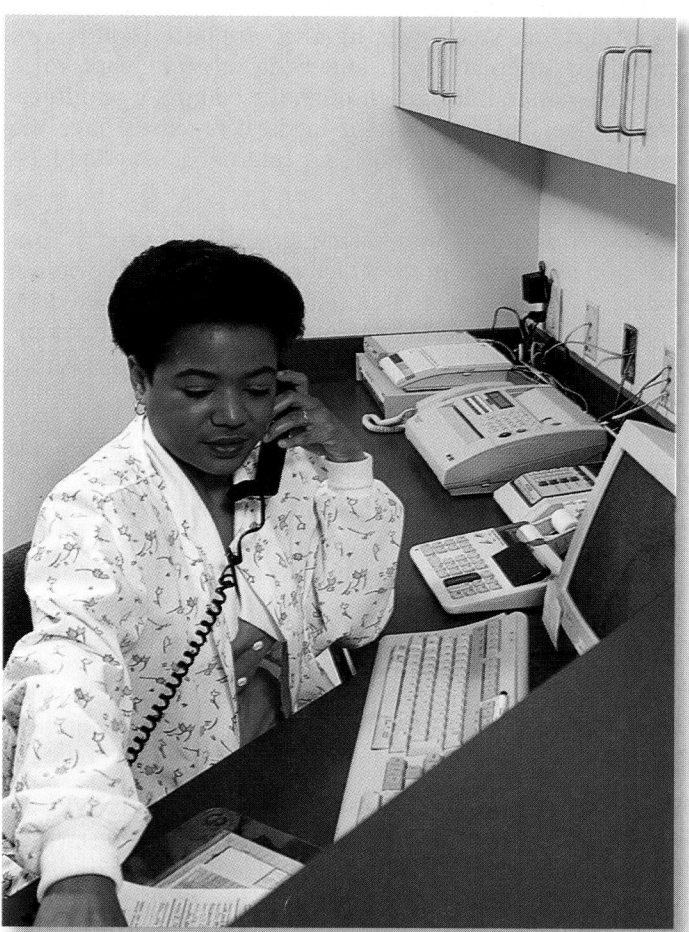

**Figure 5-1.** Most medical offices today rely on many up-to-date pieces of communication equipment.

offices have a telephone system that includes several telephones and telephone lines. The key telephone system with multiple buttons is a traditional choice in medical practices. This system has multiple lines for incoming or outgoing calls, an intercom line, and a button for putting a call on hold. The larger a practice becomes, the greater will be the demand on the phone system. Larger practices may need complex communications systems to handle all their needs.

A telephone system can be set up so that all incoming calls ring on all the telephones in the office. A more common setup in busy practices is to use a switchboard, a device that receives all calls. The receptionist then routes calls to the appropriate telephone extensions.

An alternative to the use of a switchboard and receptionist is an automated voice response unit. This unit will automatically answer all calls. A recorded voice offers the caller various options for routing of the call. Once the caller selects an option, the system automatically routes the call to another detailed menu or to the designated department. The use of automated voice response units can provide greater flexibility for the medical staff, as well as enhanced service to the patient. However, the use of more than three menu levels may be frustrating to callers.

Advances in technology and the advent of the Internet is dramatically changing voice communications. Technologies such as Voice over Internet Protocol (VoIP), also known as Internet Voice, allow the integration of voice and data communication through the computer and Internet service. This means that medical practices have the option of using the computer for Internet access and telephone conversations.

**Voice Mail.**  An automated menu is often used in conjunction with **voice mail,** which is a form of an answering machine. If the office is closed, the call is answered by voice mail, and the caller can leave a message. The advantage of a voice-mail system is that the caller never receives a busy signal.

**Patient Courtesy Phone.**  Some offices have a patient courtesy phone, which provides an outside local phone line strictly for the use of patients. Long-distance calls can be blocked from this phone. The addition of such a line leaves office lines free for business calls. The patient courtesy phone is usually located in the reception area. A patient courtesy phone provides a line of communication for patients to call for transportation or to contact work or family as needed. It is helpful to post a sign near the phone to indicate guidelines for its use. Calls are usually limited to three minutes.

**Cellular (Cell) Phones—Personal and Business Use.**  The use of cell phones has become widespread. Today, physicians, medical practice employees, and patients may all be carrying their own personal cell phones into the medical office. With all that technology available at the touch of a button, it is important to address cell phone etiquette. Generally, it is appropriate to turn off all personal cell phones inside a physician's office. The patient should be shown this consideration by the physician and staff, and the physician and staff deserve the same consideration from the patient. Many medical facilities post signs near their doors to ask the public to turn off all cell phones before entering. Cell phone calls from outside the practice are usually an interruption to the communication among the physician, the staff, and the patient. More importantly, the use of personal cell phones can interfere with other electronic equipment that may be functioning inside the medical practice.

However, cell phones do play an important part in the business functioning of the medical office. Physicians may use a cell phone to respond quickly to a message from staff or a hospital. Office staff may use personal cell phones in the case of emergency, when traditional phone systems fail. Some medical practices will even issue a cell phone to key employees who conduct business for the practice outside the office. In addition, patients may use their cell phones to call for a taxi after a doctor's appointment. If your medical office allows staff and patients to use cell phones, make sure that it is clearly noted in which areas cell phone use is permitted.

**Leaving a Message on an Answering Machine or Fax Machine.**  On occasion, it is also important to leave a message on a patient's answering machine or to send a message to a patient's fax machine. It is now required by HIPAA law that you use these pieces of equipment correctly and confidentially. The goal in calling a patient's home is to speak directly to the patient or to leave a message with enough information to get the patient to call back. It is unlawful to disclose confidential patient information to anyone but the patient. The law requires that you guard the patient's private medical information. HIPAA requires that you *never* leave any information if unsure of the phone number dialed. As a medical assistant, you cannot ensure that only the intended patient will receive any message left on an answering machine or sent to a fax machine. To guard the patient's privacy, *state only the following information:*

- The name of the individual for whom the message is intended
- The date and time of the call
- The name of your office or practice
- Your name as the contact person in the office
- The phone number of your office or practice
- The hours the office is open for a return call
- A request for a return call

Be especially careful of the hasty and indiscriminate use of fax machines. HIPAA law states that the best format for the use of fax machines involves the use of a locked mailbox at the receiver's end of the transmission. Most in-home users, however, will not have this feature. It is always best to simply fax a request containing only the same information that was recommended for answering machines.

# Reflecting On . . . HIPAA

## Avoiding Abuse of Patient Confidentiality

HIPAA law describes **abuse** as a practice or behavior that is not indicative of sound medical or fiscal activity. Improper or careless use of a patient's answering system or fax machine can be viewed as abusive behavior in the eyes of the law. It is imperative that the patient's right to privacy be carefully guarded at all times. If in doubt that the patient's privacy might be violated by leaving a verbal or written message on a machine, it is best to leave no message at all.

**Answering Machine.** Many offices use a telephone answering machine to answer calls after office hours, on weekends and holidays, and when the office is closed for any reason. A typical recorded message announces that the office is closed and states when it will reopen. The message must always indicate how the caller can reach the doctor or the answering service in an emergency.

An answering machine may be programmed simply to play a taped message from the office, or it may also record messages from callers. If callers can leave messages, you have a responsibility to check the answering machine to retrieve them at the start of each day and after the lunch break.

**Answering Service.** Instead of, or in addition to, an answering machine, many medical offices use an answering service. Unlike answering machines, answering services provide people to answer the telephone. They take messages and communicate them to the physician on call. The doctor on call is responsible for handling emergencies that may occur when the office is closed, such as at night or on weekends or holidays. Upon receiving a message from the answering service, the doctor calls the patient.

Answering services can be used in a number of ways. The doctor's office may use an answering machine to record calls of a routine nature and give the number of the answering service to call in emergencies. Alternatively, the answering service may have a direct connection to the doctor's office, picking up calls after a certain number of rings day or night or during specific hours.

Although most answering services provide satisfactory, sometimes even outstanding, service, it is good practice to check up on the service every so often by calling it during its coverage hours. This quality check ensures that the service meets office standards and expectations.

Some answering services specialize in medical practices. These medical specialty services will ask the medical practice to give specific directives for the triage of calls. Always ask any service for references before signing a contract for service.

## Pagers (Beepers)

Physicians often need to be reached when they are out of the office, so many carry pagers. Pagers or beepers are small electronic devices that give a signal to indicate that someone is trying to reach the physician. Today, this is considered an outdated technology, but it is still used in some areas.

**Technology of Paging.** Each paging device is assigned a telephone number. When someone calls that number, the pager picks up the signal and beeps, buzzes, or vibrates to indicate that a call has been made. Most pagers have a window that displays the caller's telephone number so that the person who has been paged can return the call promptly. Certain models display a short message. Some pagers store telephone numbers so that the receiver can return several calls without having to write down the numbers.

**Paging a Physician.** Many telephone messages can wait until the physician returns to the office or calls in for messages. When a message needs to be delivered immediately, however, paging is an efficient response. The paging process is as simple as making a telephone call.

1. A list of pager numbers for each physician in the practice should be kept in a prominent place in the office, such as by the main switchboard. Make sure you know where these numbers are kept. Look up the telephone number for the pager of the physician you need to contact.

2. Dial the telephone number for the pager.

3. You will hear the telephone ringing and the call picked up. Listen for a high-pitched tone, which signals the connection between the telephone and the pager.

4. To operate most pagers, you need to dial the telephone number you wish the physician to call, followed by the pound sign (#), located below the number 9 on a push-button telephone. (Some pager services have an operator and work much like an answering service. Give the operator a message, and the operator will contact the physician.)

5. Listen for a beep or a series of beeps signaling that the page has been transmitted. Then hang up the phone. The physician will call the number at his earliest convenience.

## Interactive Pagers (I-Pagers)

**Interactive pagers** (I-pagers) are designed for two-way communication. The individual carrying the pager is paged in much the same way as the traditional pager. The

# Points on Practice

## Routing Calls Through an Automated Menu

An automated menu system answers calls for you and separates requests into categories so that you can deal with them efficiently. You may already be familiar with automated menus, which are widely used by many large businesses. Someone who calls an automated system hears a recorded message identifying the business. The message gives the caller a list of options from which to choose to identify the purpose of the call. The caller selects an option by pressing the corresponding button on her push-button telephone. If she does not have a push-button telephone, her call is automatically routed so that she can talk to a person or leave a voice-mail message. For example, the voice response may say, "Press or say 1 for appointments. Press or say 2 for prescription renewals. Press or say 3 for referrals."

How does an automated menu system save time and effort in a medical office? You don't have to answer calls as they come in but can instead reserve a block of time in which to listen and respond to messages. This system allows you to complete other work without interruption. Though this practice is efficient, this is a policy that needs to be approved by the office manager and physicians within the practice before it is implemented. Some medical offices maintain a philosophy that places the importance of a patient's call above all other office tasks. Always ask the supervisor

in charge of the office how you should use the automated system.

To set up an automated system, you need to plan specific categories from which patients can choose. Categories may include but are not limited to (1) making and changing appointments, (2) asking billing questions, (3) asking medical questions of the doctors or nurses, (4) reporting patient emergencies, and (5) receiving calls from another doctor's office.

When the caller presses the code for a patient emergency, the call rings in the office because it needs to be answered immediately. You or other staff members can respond to calls in the other categories in a timely fashion. Questions for doctors or nurses can be routed immediately to the appropriate voice mail, bypassing the front office lines.

Automated menu systems can be set up by telephone vendors listed in the Yellow Pages. When choosing an automated telephone system, be careful that callers do not become lost in the process. It is a good idea to set up a system that allows callers to return easily to the main menu. Be sure to build in an option for rotary dial telephones as well. Following up on messages promptly will also help callers feel comfortable with your voice-mail system, so you should check for messages at least once every hour.

pager can be set on "Audio" or "Vibrate" to alert the carrier that a message is coming in. However, the interactive pager screen displays a printed message and allows the physician to respond by way of a mini keyboard.

The physician can respond to the printed page by typing a return message (done by typing with the thumbs). The physician can respond back in real time to the office. The office computer and the physician enter into a conversation much like e-mail or an Internet chat room. Many problems can be handled quickly and efficiently in this manner. Additionally, because the I-pager can function silently, the physician can communicate with her office while in a meeting without disturbing others.

Each interactive pager has its own wireless Internet address. The user types in the receiving party's e-mail address and creates a message on a monitor screen. The interactive pager will give the sender the status of his message by indicating on the screen when the message has been sent, received, or read.

I-pagers can communicate with other I-pagers as well. I-pagers also have broadcast capability, meaning the sender can send to more than one receiver at a time. For

this reason, practices with multiple physicians may find them very helpful.

Interactive pagers can also send messages to traditional telephones. The message is typed into the pager, and the system "calls" the telephone number. When answered, an electronic-type voice reads the message to the individual who has answered.

## Facsimile Machines

Critical documents, such as laboratory reports or patient records, often need to be sent immediately to locations outside the office. Documents can be sent by means of a facsimile machine, or fax machine. A fax machine scans each page, translates it into electronic impulses, and transmits those impulses over the telephone line. When they are received by another fax machine, they are converted into an exact copy of the original document.

A fax machine in a medical office should have its own telephone line. A separate line ensures that transmission of incoming and outgoing faxes will not be interrupted and that the machine will not tie up a needed telephone line when sending or receiving information.

**Benefits of Faxing.** A fax machine can send an exact copy of a document within minutes. The cost for sending a fax is the same as for making a telephone call to that location. For a short document, this is usually less expensive than an overnight mail service.

Many fax machines have a copier function and can be used as an extra copy machine. This function may only be useful, however, if the machine uses plain paper. The telephone for the fax may also be used as an extra extension for outgoing calls, if needed. Procedure 5-1 details the correct steps for using a facsimile (fax) machine.

# PROCEDURE 5.1

## Using a Facsimile (Fax) Machine

**Procedure Goal:** To correctly prepare and send a fax document, while following all HIPAA guidelines to guard patient confidentiality

**Materials:** Fax machine, fax line, cover sheet with statement of disclaimer, area code and phone number of fax recipient, document to be faxed, telephone line, and telephone

### Method:

1. Prepare a **cover sheet,** which provides information about the transmission. Cover sheets can vary in appearance but usually include the name, telephone number, and fax number of the sender and the receiver; the number of pages being transmitted; and the date of the transmission. Preprinted cover sheets can be used.

    *Rationale*

    The fax should clearly identify where it originated and to whom it is being sent. If another recipient receives the fax in error, they will know who to notify regarding the error.

2. All cover sheets must carry a statement of disclaimer to guard the privacy of the patient. A **disclaimer** is a statement of denial of legal liability. (A sample cover sheet is shown in Figure 5-2.) A disclaimer should be included on the cover sheet and may read something like the following:

    *This fax contains confidential or proprietary information that may be legally privileged. It is intended only for the named recipient(s). If an addressing or transmission error has misdirected the fax, please notify the author by replying to this message. If you are not the named recipient, you are not authorized to use, disclose, distribute, copy, print, or rely on this fax and should immediately shred it.*

    *Rationale*

    This step helps guard the privacy of the patient.

3. Place all pages of the document, including the cover sheet, either facedown or face up in the fax machine's sending tray, depending on the directions stamped on the sending tray.

4. If the documents are placed facedown, write the area code and fax number on the back of the last page.

5. Dial the telephone number of the receiving fax machine, using either the telephone attached to the fax machine or the numbers on the fax keyboard. Include the area code for long-distance calls.

6. When using a fax telephone, listen for a high-pitched tone. Then press the "Send" or "Start" button, and hang up the telephone. This step completes the call circuit in older-model fax machines. Your fax is now being sent. Newer fax machines do not require this step.

    *Rationale*

    This step completes the call circuit in older-model fax machines.

7. If you use the fax keyboard, press the "Send" or "Start" button after dialing the telephone number. This button will start the call.

8. Watch for the fax machine to make a connection. Often a green light appears as the document feeds through the machine.

9. If the fax machine is not able to make a connection, as when the receiving fax line is busy, it may have a feature that automatically redials the number every few minutes for a specified number of attempts.

10. When a fax has been successfully sent, most fax machines print a confirmation message. When a fax has not been sent, the machine either prints an error message or indicates on the screen that the transmission was unsuccessful.

*continued* ⟶

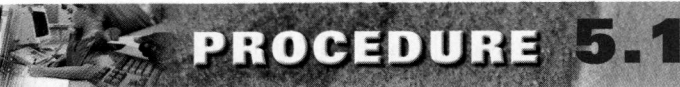

# PROCEDURE 5.1

## Using a Facsimile (Fax) Machine *(concluded)*

### Rationale
This message confirms to the sender that the fax has been sent or indicates that the fax needs to be sent again.

11. Attach the confirmation or error message to the documents faxed. File appropriately.

### Rationale
This step ensures thorough documentation related to the fax.

12. If required by office policy, the sender should call the recipient to confirm the fax was received.

---

## City Medical Associates
555 London Street  Strathspey, PA  19919

---

Janet Michaels, MD              INTERNAL MEDICINE              Scott J. Michaels, MD

---

### FACSIMILE COVER SHEET

Date: _____

To: _____    From: _____

Fax #: _____    Fax #: _____

# of pages (including this cover sheet): _____

Message: _____
_____
_____
_____
_____

The information contained in this transmission is privileged and confidential, intended only for the use of the individual or entity named above. If the reader of this message is not the intended recipient, you are hereby notified that any dissemination, distribution, or copying of this communication is strictly prohibited. If you have received this transmission in error, do not read. Please immediately respond to the sender that you have received this communication in error and then destroy or delete it. Thank you.

**Figure 5-2.** Every document that is sent by fax transmission should include a cover sheet, which provides details about the transmission. A disclaimer should be included on the cover sheet.

**Thermal Paper Versus Plain Paper.** Older fax machines print on rolls of specially treated paper called electrothermal, or thermal, paper, which reacts to heat and electricity. Thermal paper tends to fade over time, so documents received on this type of paper may need to be photocopied. Most models of fax machines use plain copy paper instead of thermal paper, avoiding the need for making copies. Information is transferred to the plain paper by either a carbon ribbon or a laser beam.

**Receiving a Fax.** Faxes can be received 24 hours a day if the fax machine is turned on and has an adequate supply of paper (Figure 5-3). Newer-model fax machines have memories and can store and receive documents. If the fax machine is not already sending or receiving a fax, the fax telephone rings, or the machine buzzes briefly, signaling the start of a transmission. The transmission begins shortly thereafter, with the machine printing out the document as it is sent. When completed, the machine may print a transmission report that includes the number of pages, the date and time, and the originating fax number. Chapter 6 discusses sending and receiving faxes via computers, scanners, servers, and the Internet.

## Typewriters

Typewriters are used very little in a medical practice. They may still be used to complete medical forms brought in by patients or sent from an insurance company. These forms can be completed more clearly when the information is typed instead of handwritten.

**Models and Features.** Although typewriter models differ in features, all use a standard keyboard. Most typewriters have replaceable cartridge ribbons for printing and a second correction ribbon for corrections.

A wide variety of electric and electronic typewriter models are available. Although both are powered by electricity, they differ in their ability to perform certain functions. Electronic typewriters can store limited amounts of information for further use, but electric typewriters cannot. Both electric and electronic typewriters provide a selection of features, including, but not limited to, automatic carriage return, automatic centering, self-correction, and changeable typefaces or fonts. Today,

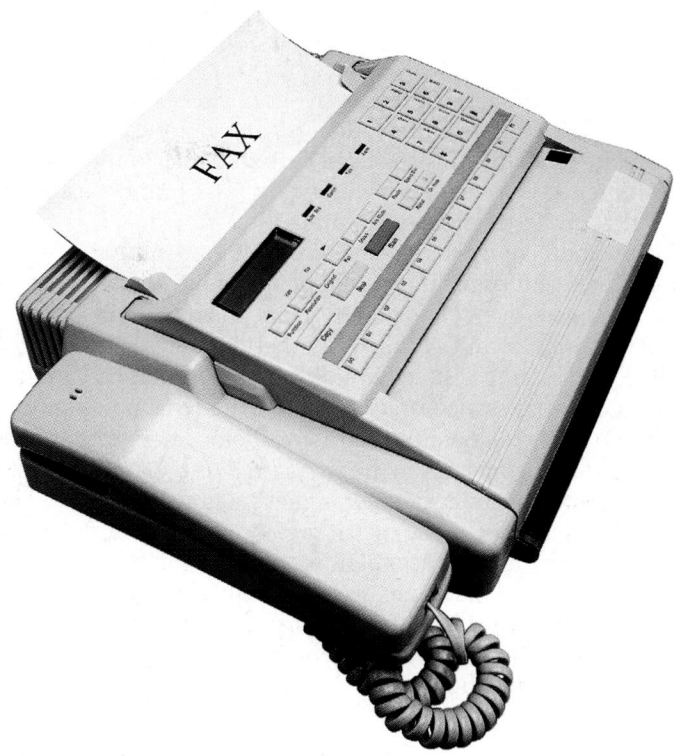

**Figure 5-3.** A fax machine scans a document, translates it into electronic impulses, and then transmits those impulses over the telephone line.

most medical practices use computers with word processing software and scanners to create and manipulate word documents.

## Office Automation Equipment

Using automated equipment enables you to perform a task more easily and quickly than doing it manually. For example, adding numbers on a calculator is a much faster process than doing it on paper. Many of the administrative tasks in a medical practice can be accomplished with the assistance of automated equipment, allowing you more time to perform other tasks.

## Reflecting On . . . HIPAA

### HIPAA and Faxing

Faxed material may include protected health information. For this reason, fax machines should never be placed in patient examination rooms or reception areas where unauthorized persons may be able to view incoming or outgoing documents. Only staff members with a "need to know" should have access to faxed and other confidential information.

# Photocopiers

A photocopier, also called a copier or copy machine, instantly reproduces office correspondence, forms, bills, patient records, and other documents. Before photocopiers were available, offices used carbon paper to reproduce documents as they were being typed. The number of copies that could be made was limited.

A photocopier takes a picture of the document it is to reproduce and prints it on plain paper using a heat process. Photocopiers use either liquid or dry toner, a form of ink. They can make an unlimited number of copies. Photocopiers do not require treated or otherwise special paper. Various kinds of paper can be used in the machine, including office stationery and colored paper. Many photocopiers accept different sizes of paper, from the standard 8½- by 11-inch paper to 8½- by 14-inch legal paper and even larger.

Photocopiers come in many models, from desktop machines for limited use to industrial models for continual heavy use. The machines vary in features and speed. All styles of machines are available through purchase or lease. Procedure 5-2 describes the correct method for using a photocopier machine.

**Special Features.** Copiers offer a wide range of special features. They may collate (assemble sets of multiple pages in order) and staple pages, punch holes, enlarge or reduce images, and produce double-sided copies (print on both sides of the page). Some can also adjust contrast and even track the cost of a job via a specific code input into the machine. Photocopiers produce black-and-white copies as well as color copies. Some copiers can make transparencies (text and images printed on clear acetate), which physicians often use for presentations. Copiers can even be configured to electronically scan documents for electronic communications, and to send and receive facsimiles.

One of the more useful features of photocopiers is the help function. Selecting this function displays directions in plain English that explain how to fix a paper jam or deal with other routine copier problems. Some copiers are even programmed to indicate that service is needed.

## Adding Machines and Calculators

For handling tasks such as patient billing, bank deposits, and payroll, many medical practices depend on adding machines and calculators. The difference between the

# PROCEDURE 5.2

## Using a Photocopier Machine

**Procedure Goal:** To produce copies of documents

**Materials:** Copier machine, copy paper, documents to be copied

**Method:**

1. Make sure the machine is turned on and warmed up. It will display a signal when it is ready for copying.

2. Assemble and prepare your materials, removing paper clips, staples, and self-adhesive flags.

   *Rationale*

   This step helps avoid loose items getting caught in the copier and provides for optimum efficiency.

3. Place the document to be copied in the automatic feeder tray as directed, or upside down directly on the glass. The feeder tray can accommodate many pages; you may place only one page at a time on the glass. Automatic feeding is a faster process, and you should use it when you wish to collate or staple packets. Page-by-page copying is best if you need to copy a single sheet or to enlarge or reduce the image. To use any special features, such as making double-sided copies or stapling

the copies, press a designated button on the machine.

4. Set the machine for the desired paper size.

   *Rationale*

   The copier will select the paper size automatically if the size is not selected. This could result in a waste of paper.

5. Key in the number of copies you want to make, and press the "Start" button. The copies are made automatically.

6. Press the "Clear" or "Reset" button when your job is finished.

   *Rationale*

   The machine is now ready for the next user and will not perform unwanted functions on the next document.

7. If the copier becomes jammed, follow the directions on the machine to locate the problem (for example, there may be multiple pieces of paper stuck inside the printer), and dislodge the jammed paper. Most copy machines will show a diagram of the printer and the location of the problem.

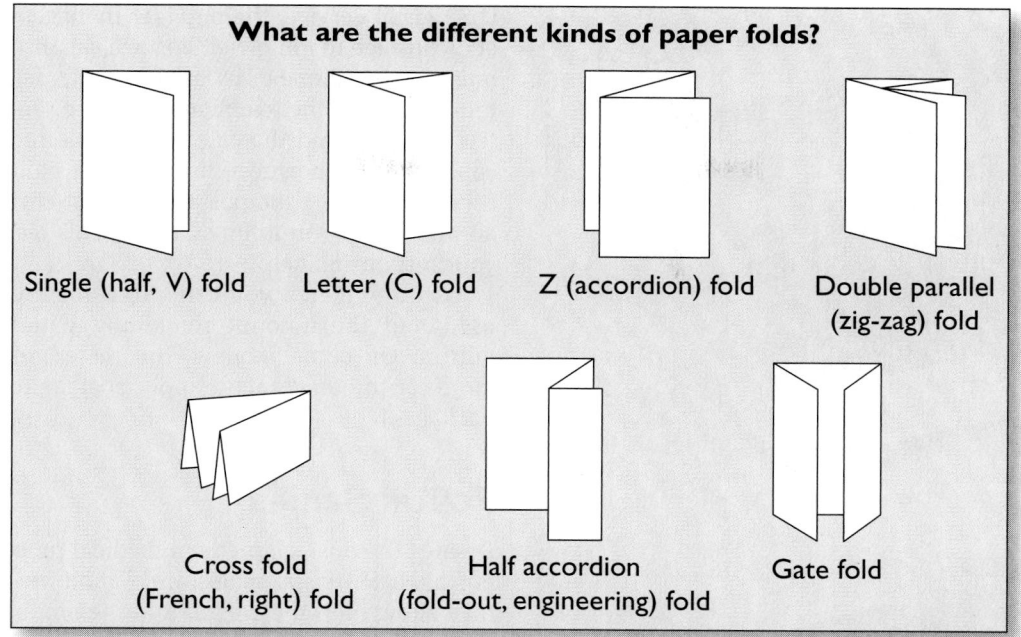

**Figure 5-4.** Folding machines can make many different kinds of paper folds.

two types of machines is minimal. Adding machines typically plug into an outlet and produce a paper tape on which calculations are printed. Calculators are more often battery or solar powered, with memory to store figures. Calculators are portable and usually do not produce a paper tape.

**Routine Calculations.** Both adding machines and calculators are sufficient for most routine office calculations. These machines perform basic arithmetic functions, such as addition, subtraction, multiplication, and division. Many of today's models perform such specialized functions as computing percentages and storing data. Some are even computerized.

**Checking Your Work.** It is easy to hit an incorrect key or to key in a number twice when using an adding machine or a calculator. Therefore, check all mathematical computations.

If the machine produces a paper tape, check the numbers on the tape against the numbers you are adding. The paper tape is especially useful when adding a long series of numbers. Without a printed record, you must perform the same calculations again to make sure the total is correct.

## Folding and Inserting Machines

Letter-folding equipment can help minimize the amount of time staff spends preparing large volumes of outgoing mail. Letter folders are also used for creating folded brochures. A medical practice may use folding and inserting machines for a variety of items, including invoices, newsletters, checks, statements, letters, and flyers.

Lower-end folding equipment requires letters to be fed manually. The speed of this machine is limited to the speed an individual can feed in letters, which is typically about 200 pieces per hour. An automatic feeder is required for faster folding. Letter-folding machines can make many different types of folds, including standard business letter folds (c-fold), accordion folds (z-fold), single folds, right-angle folds, and brochure folds (Figure 5-4). Most machines can fold more than one sheet of paper together, but do not allow stapled pages to be fed and folded.

Many special features are available that may help the processing of mail and brochures. Batch counters and stackers help to prevent a letter folding machine from folding more sheets than desired. A jogger helps align stacks of paper and dissipates static electricity. Some machines are better designed for certain types of paper, such as glossy or carbonless paper. Inserters are used to insert a folded document into an envelope.

## Postage Meters

Every medical office uses the U.S. Postal Service. Patient bills, routine correspondence, purchase orders, and payments are just some of the items typically sent by mail. (See Chapter 7 for additional information on mailing correspondence.)

Although some medical offices use stamps, most use a postage meter. A postage meter is a machine that applies postage to an envelope or package, eliminating the need for postage stamps (Figure 5-5). There are often two parts to a postage meter: the meter, which belongs to the post office, and the mailing machine, which the practice can own. The meter actually applies the postage, and the mailing machine does the rest, such as sealing the envelope.

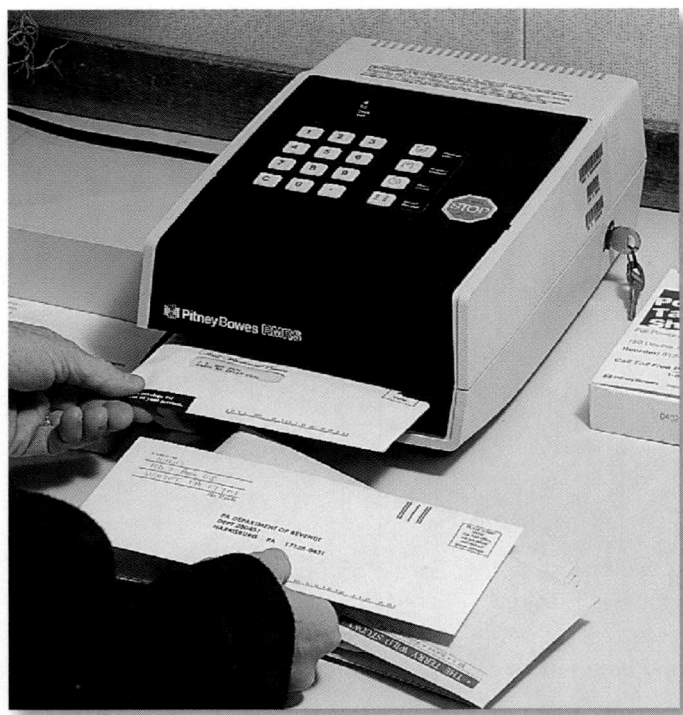

**Figure 5-5.** The postage meter is a convenient and cost-effective way to apply postage to office correspondence and packages.

**Benefits of Using a Postage Meter.** There are several advantages to using a postage meter instead of purchasing stamps. It saves frequent trips to the post office. It also saves money for the office by providing the exact amount of postage needed for each item. When you have to use a combination of stamps, you may exceed the minimum required postage. It is unlikely as well as impractical for a practice to keep every denomination of stamps on hand.

Some postage meters can imprint envelopes with the name of your medical practice or with a message at the same time postage is applied. The message appears immediately to the left of the postal mark, at the top of the envelope.

Many types of postage meters are available, from basic models for a small office to advanced models for large businesses. The latest machines include automatic date setting, memory to program a large mailing, and display alerts for low postage or the need for ribbon replacement. Some models can apply postage to parcels without the use of labels or tape. Procedure 5-3 describes how to use a postage meter.

**Prepaying for Postage.** To use a postage meter, you must prepay the postage. You can take your meter to the post office to add postage, or you can use a postage meter service. A service maintains the postal account for you. Although the money in each account is the property of the

U.S. Postal Service, the provider manages the account and adds postage to the meter. Postage can also be added to the meter by telephone or by modem, with data sent directly to the meter over the telephone line. The process takes only a few minutes, and the call is often toll-free. Before postage can be added, however, money must be deposited into an account. Keeping the postage account current ensures that all mail is sent on a timely basis. This task may be one of your responsibilities.

On any meter, you can check the amount of postage used and the amount remaining with the touch of a button. On some models, the meter must have $10 or more for the machine to apply postage to an envelope or package.

## Postal Scales

Besides the postage meter, a medical practice also needs a postal scale. Postal scales are a good investment because they show both the weight and the amount of postage required. Some postage meters include an electronic scale. If you need a postal scale but one is not available, you can use any scale that weighs in ounces. When using a simple scale, you can then translate the weight into the correct postage by using a current postal rate chart, available from the U.S. Postal Service.

## Posting Mail

Before you begin posting mail, make sure the envelope or package is complete, with all materials included. After applying the proper postage, place the postmarked envelope or package in the area of your office designated for mail pickup.

## Dictation-Transcription Equipment

Physicians usually do not type their own correspondence, patient records, or other documents. Medical assistants, although not professional medical transcriptionists, may be asked to transcribe recorded words into written text. Using dictation-transcription equipment is the most efficient way to complete this task. *Dictation* is another word for speaking; *transcription* is another word for writing. Together they mean to transform spoken words into written form.

**Dictation-Transcription Equipment with Standard Options.** Medical assistants performing transcription will generally use a desktop dictation-transcription machine, a unit similar in size and appearance to a telephone. A small attachment resembles a handheld tape recorder. The machine includes special controls to record and play magnetic tapes, a cassette, or a disk. Standard features usually include controls for starting, stopping,

# PROCEDURE 5.3

## Using a Postage Meter

**Procedure Goal:** To correctly apply postage to an envelope or package for mailing, according to U.S. Postal Service guidelines

**Materials:** Postage meter, addressed envelope or package, postal scale

**Method:**

1. Check that there is postage available in the postage meter.

   *Rationale*

   For the postage meter to function, there must be money in your postal account. Contact the company that is managing your account or your local post office for more information.

2. Verify the day's date.

   *Rationale*

   U.S. Postal Service guidelines prohibit mailing envelopes and packages that are postmarked with an incorrect date.

3. Check that the postage meter is plugged in and switched on before you proceed

4. Locate the area where the meter registers the date. Many machines have a lid that can be flipped up, with rows of numbers underneath. Months are represented numerically, with the number "1" indicating the month of January, "2" indicating February, and so on. Check that the date is correct. If it is incorrect, change the numbers to the correct date.

5. Make sure that all materials have been included in the envelope or package. Weigh the envelope or package on a postal scale. Standard business envelopes weighing up to 1 oz require the minimum postage (the equivalent of one first-class stamp). Oversize envelopes and packages require additional postage. A postal scale will indicate the amount of postage required.

6. Key in the postage amount on the meter, and press the button that enters the amount. For amounts over $1, press the "$" sign or the "Enter" button twice.

   *Rationale*

   This feature verifies large amounts, catching errors in case you mistakenly press too many keys.

7. Check that the amount you typed is the correct amount. Envelopes and packages with too little postage will be returned by the U.S. Postal Service. Sending an envelope or package with too much postage is wasteful to the practice.

8. While applying postage to an envelope, hold it flat and right side up (so that you can read the address). Seal the envelope (unless the meter seals it for you). Locate the plate or area where the envelope slides through. This feature is usually near the bottom of the meter. Place the envelope on the left side, and give it a gentle push toward the right. Some models hold the envelope in a stationary position. (If the meter seals the envelope for you, it is especially important that you insert it correctly to allow for sealing.) The meter will grab the envelope and pull it through quickly.

9. For packages, create a postage label to affix to the package. Follow the same procedure for a label as for an envelope. Affix the postmarked label on the package in the upper-right corner.

10. Check that the printed postmark has the correct date and amount and that everything written or stamped on the envelope or package is legible.

---

backing up and fast forwarding, volume and tone control, speed control, headphones, and a counter (Figure 5-6).

**Dictation-Transcription Equipment with Special Controls.** More specialized controls include scanning, which allows reviewing a tape's contents quickly, and indicator strips, which mark important material. Some machines are also equipped with an automatic backspace control, which rewinds the tape slightly each time it is stopped so that no words are missed. For the recording process, the machine may be equipped with an insert control, to allow placement of additional dictation in the middle of existing dictation. The machine may also include a voice-activated sensor for hands-free recording. After a transcribed document has been approved, the erase function cleans the tape, preparing it for the next dictation.

**Dictating.** Before a tape can be transcribed, it must be recorded. The physician information can take several

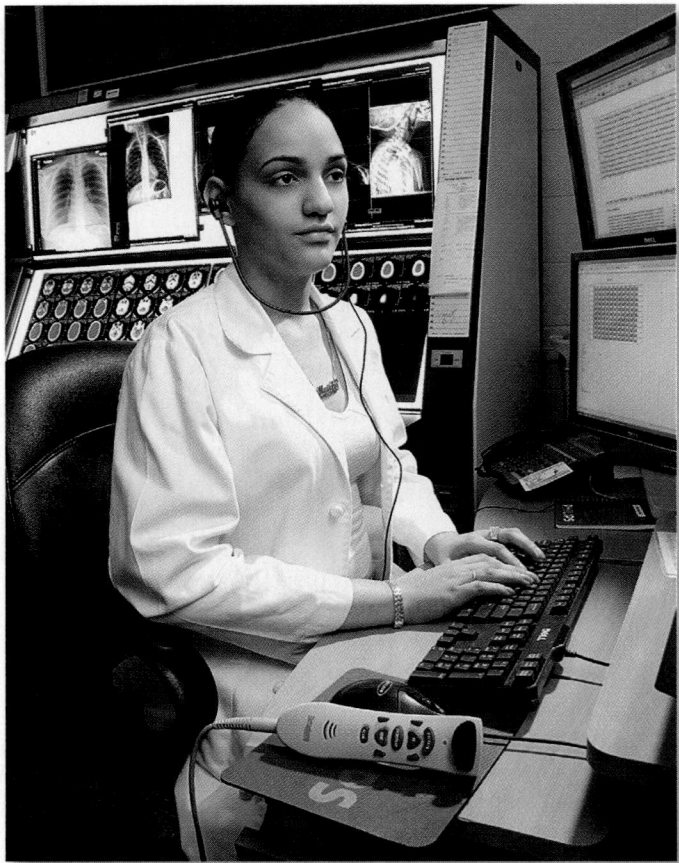

**Figure 5-6.** One of the responsibilities of a medical assistant may be to use dictation-transcription equipment.

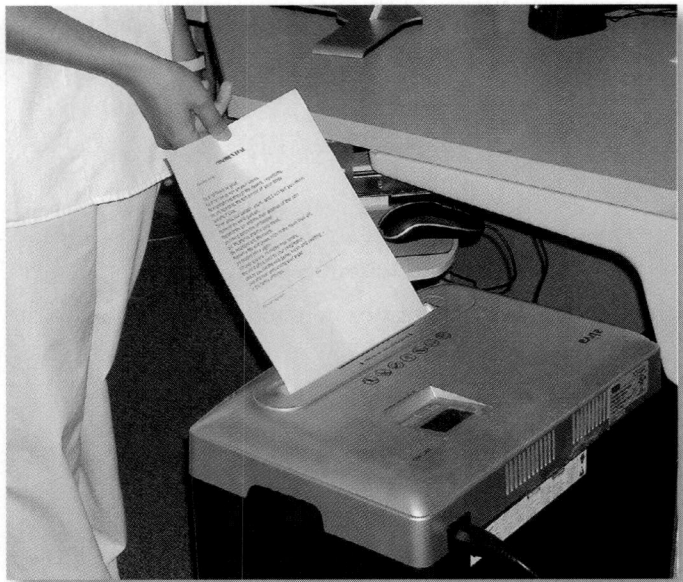

**Figure 5-7.** As a medical assistant, you may be asked to use a paper shredder to destroy confidential documents that are no longer needed by the practice.

steps, which can make the transcription process faster, easier, and more accurate:

1. Indicate the date and the type of document being dictated and provide explicit instructions about the document. For example, it is helpful to indicate that the document is a letter and that it is to be produced on office stationery and mailed to a patient.
2. Spell out all names and addresses as well as any unfamiliar terms.
3. Indicate punctuation by saying, for example, "comma" or "begin new paragraph."
4. Speak clearly and slowly. Neither eat while dictating nor record in a noisy environment, if at all possible.

Procedure 5-4 shows you how to operate a dictation-transcription machine. Chapter 9 describes the medical transcription process in greater detail.

## Check Writers

Medical practice personnel need to write checks to pay for equipment, supplies, and payroll. This common office procedure can be automated by using a check writer, which is a machine that imprints checks. Procedure 5-5

details the correct steps for operating a check-writing machine. The safety advantage of using such a machine is that the name of the payee (the person receiving the check) and the amount of the check, once imprinted, cannot be altered.

**Voiding a Check.** If the information on an imprinted check is incorrect, it cannot be changed. Therefore, you must issue a new check and void the previous one. To void the check, write "VOID" in clear letters across it, or use a VOID stamp with red ink. Then file the check with the office bank records so that the practice's money manager is aware that it has been voided.

## Paper Shredders

Paper shredders are quite common in medical practices. A paper shredder, such as the one shown in Figure 5-7, is often used when confidential documents, such as patient records, need to be destroyed. Paper shredders cut documents into tiny pieces to make them unreadable.

The most common type of shredder cuts paper into ribbonlike strips, which differ in width, depending on the model. Other shredders cut the paper in two directions, forming small pieces. Some paper shredders offer additional options, such as an electronic eye that automatically starts the machine when paper is inserted and stops when it is done. Other features available are paper jam detection, automatic reverse, and automatic shutdown when the machine gets too hot.

**How to Shred Materials.** A paper shredder is ready to use when it is turned on. To shred a document, insert it into the feed tray at the top of the shredder. The machine feeds the paper through hundreds of knifelike cutters,

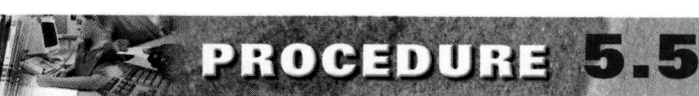

# PROCEDURE 5.4

## Using a Dictation-Transcription Machine

**Procedure Goal:** To correctly use a dictation-transcription machine to convert verbal communication into the written word

**Materials:** Dictation-transcription machine, audiocassette or magnetic tape or disk with the recorded dictation, word processor or computer, and printer

**Method:**

1. Assemble all the necessary equipment.
2. Select a transcription tape, cassette, or disk for dictation. Select any transcriptions marked "Urgent" first. If there are none, select the oldest dated transcription first.

   *Rationale*

   The items marked "urgent" are needed as soon as possible. The other items need to be completed in the order in which they were received for the smoothest flow of work within the office.
3. Turn on all equipment and adjust it according to personal preference.

   *Rationale*

   Making adjustments for comfort and proper body alignment will help you avoid injury and strain.
4. Prepare the format and style for the selected letter or form.
5. Insert the tape or cassette and rewind.

   *Rationale*

   The tape or cassette will be positioned at the end of the transcription.
6. While listening to the transcription tape, cassette, or disk, key in the text.
7. Adjust the speed and volume controls as needed.
8. Proofread and spell check final document, making any corrections.

   *Rationale*

   This step ensures a professional and accurate document.
9. Print the document for approval and signature.
10. Turn off all equipment. Place the transcription tape, cassette, or disk in the proper storage area.

# PROCEDURE 5.5

## Using a Check-Writing Machine

**Procedure Goal:** To produce a check using a check-writing machine

**Materials:** Check-writing machine, blank checks, office checkbook or accounting system

**Method:**

1. Assemble all equipment.
2. Turn on the check-writing machine.
3. Place a blank check or a sheet of blank checks into the machine.
4. Key in the date, the payee's name, and the payment amount. The check-writing machine imprints the check with this information, perforating it with the payee's name. The perforations are actual little holes in the paper, which prevent anyone from changing the name on the check.
5. Turn off the check-writing machine.
6. A doctor or another authorized person then signs the check.

   *Rationale*

   The check is not valid without the proper signature.
7. To complete the process, record the check in the office checkbook or accounting system.

   *Rationale*

   To maintain accurate records, all financial transactions must be promptly and accurately recorded.

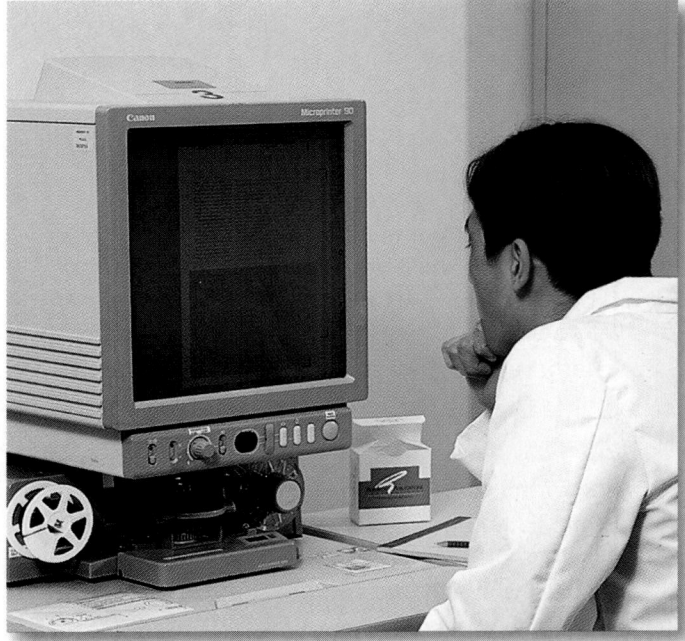

**Figure 5-8.** Storing information on microfilm helps reduce the amount of storage space needed by the practice.

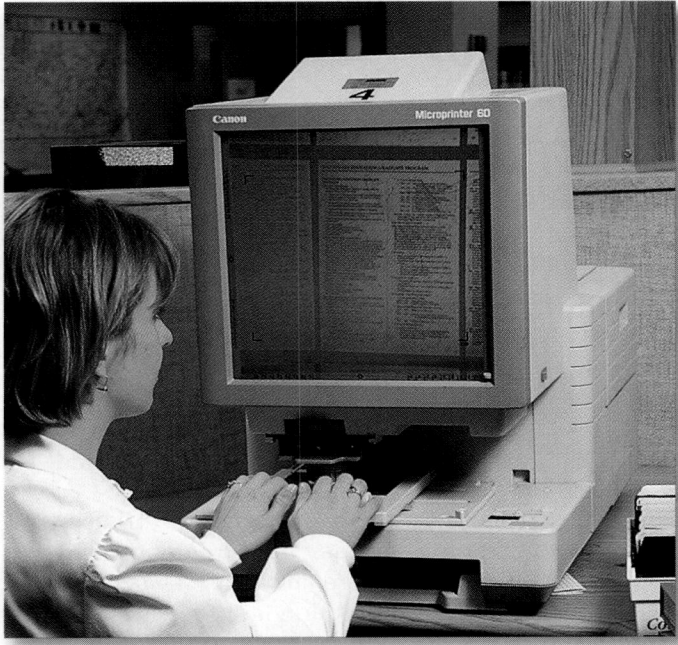

**Figure 5-9.** Special equipment must be used to read text that has been converted to microfiche.

instantaneously shredding the paper. A basket attached beneath the shredder catches the bits of paper. Different models can accommodate different amounts of paper through the cutters. Shredder baskets must be emptied periodically to allow room for additional shredded paper. Some shredders signal when the basket is full. It is very important not to wear loose-fitting clothing while operating a shredder to avoid accident and personal injury.

**When to Shred Materials.** Medical practices need to eliminate old patient records or other sensitive materials. These items cannot simply be thrown into the trash because of confidentiality problems. The shredder is an effective disposal solution. If records have incorrect information that has been corrected on subsequent documents, the old records are shredded so that the incorrect information is not mistakenly placed in the patient's folder. A document that has been shredded cannot be put back together. Therefore, do not decide on your own to shred a document. The physician or office manager will set guide-

lines regarding when a document should be shredded. If you are not sure whether to shred a document, check with a senior staff member before beginning the process.

## Microfilm and Microfiche Readers

If all information were stored on paper in file folders, medical offices would need additional rooms to hold it all. Therefore, some medical offices store information on microfilm or microfiche. **Microfilm** is a roll of film imprinted with information and stored on a reel. Film can also be stored in cartridges, to protect the film from being touched. **Microfiche** is film imprinted with information and stored in rectangular sheets.

Information stored on microfilm and microfiche is dramatically reduced in size. Because each roll or sheet can hold a large amount of material, less storage space is required than for comparable paper files. Because the information is so tiny, however, reading it requires special machines, such as those shown in Figures 5-8 and 5-9.

## Reflecting On . . . HIPAA

### HIPAA and Shredding

Shredding is an important way to responsibly handle confidential information that is no longer needed. Many medical practices contract with a shredding company to come into the practice, remove, and shred designated materials. Using another company for this task does not relieve the medical practice of the responsibility for the confidential materials. The healthcare provider is still considered the **covered entity** and must comply with HIPAA law. It is important to contract only with companies that also abide by HIPAA law.

Although considered to be old technology, the use of microfilm and microfiche is still in use in many medical practices today. Even if your office does not store records on microfilm or microfiche, you may still need to have a reader because back issues of medical journals and other publications are often available only in these formats.

**Models and Features.** Microfilm and microfiche machines come in many different sizes. Most medical offices use a desktop model to conserve space. The main difference between a desktop model and other models is size. The features and controls are similar.

Basic controls on microfilm and microfiche readers allow adjustment of the image—zooming into an area, focusing, and rotating it—and fast-forwarding to other parts of the film. Advanced controls include image editing, an odometer that measures the amount of film scanned, and search functions that can be connected to a computer to locate specific items.

**Reading and Printing.** For ease of use, you should label and date each roll of microfilm or each microfiche sheet with the information it contains. Then you will be able to locate information easily when you need it.

Because the film is stored in different formats, microfilm and microfiche require different mechanisms to read them. For example, microfilm requires a roller attachment; microfiche requires a flat surface. Newer models can accommodate different formats with the use of detachable, interchangeable reading mechanisms.

Microfilm is inserted onto a rod and threaded onto the microfilm reader. Microfiche is placed directly on the glass tray of a microfiche reader. If you are unsure, check the directions in the manual for your reader.

The reading process is similar for all machines, with information displayed on a large screen. The screen displays only a small portion of the information stored on the film. You can fast-forward through the film to read additional information. Most machines allow you to print out the image on the screen.

# Purchasing Decisions

As a medical assistant, you may be involved in making purchasing decisions for office equipment. For example, the physician or office manager may ask you to investigate whether the practice needs a certain piece of equipment, such as a new photocopier or microfiche reader. To make a sound decision about whether the office will benefit from such a purchase, you will need to conduct thorough research.

## Evaluating Office Needs

The first step in evaluating the equipment needs of a health-care office is the research process. Make note of the equipment that is already available and consider the different tasks the equipment can perform. To obtain a complete list of office needs, consult other staff members for their ideas.

When considering replacing an old piece of equipment, ask what advantages the new piece of equipment offers over the current one. Create a list of equipment on hand, and a list of any new products the office staff recommends. Compare the benefits offered by the new product to the capability of the currently used equipment. Many medical magazines review medical office equipment periodically and are good resources to consult in making your purchasing decisions. Go online to shop and compare products, features, and prices. Discuss with the office manager the budget for the equipment under consideration. Consider calling a supplier for more detailed information.

**Contacting Suppliers.** Put together a list of the features you would like in your machine. Then contact suppliers who sell models that offer those features. You can call or e-mail the manufacturer directly to find out the name of a local vendor. Many manufacturers prepare brochures giving information about their products. Request that this information be sent to you.

Go online or look in the Yellow Pages for office supply stores and other companies that sell office equipment. Obtain product and pricing information on each model. For certain equipment, such as photocopiers, a sales representative will come to your office to demonstrate and discuss the product.

**Evaluating Warranty Options.** Most products come with a warranty. A **warranty** is a contract that guarantees free service and replacement of parts for a certain period, usually 1 year. Warranties are valid only for

## Reflecting On . . . HIPAA

### HIPAA and Electronic Media

According to HIPAA law, transmissions that are physically moved from one location to another using magnetic tape, disk, or compact disk media are considered **electronic media**. This form of patient information must be handled in the same confidential manner as patient records. All patient information, regardless of the form, is required by HIPAA law to be guarded by the health-care provider.

specified service and repairs. They usually do not cover accidents, vandalism, acts of God (such as damage caused by floods or earthquakes), or mistreatment of the machine. In most cases, warranty repairs must be made at an authorized service center.

If you want more coverage than the warranty allows, consider buying an extended warranty. Extended warranties increase the amount of time that equipment is covered. For expensive pieces of equipment or parts, the additional cost of an extended warranty may be justified.

After you purchase a product, you must fill out the warranty card and mail it to the manufacturer. File the receipt in a safe place in the office where it can easily be retrieved.

**Preparing a Recommendation.** After you have obtained all the information, you are ready to evaluate it. To compare and contrast the different models, construct a chart. Place the product model names in columns across the top. Down the left side, list factors that will influence the purchase decision: cost, warranty options (including the length of the warranty and the price of an extended warranty), special features, and delivery time. Then fill in the information. This chart will provide an easy-to-use summary of your research.

Finally, analyze the list, and choose the product that will best meet the needs of the office. Meet with the physician or office manager to discuss your recommendation.

## Leasing Versus Buying Equipment

Once the product has been selected, there is one more decision to make: whether to lease or to buy the item. When buying a product, the purchaser becomes the owner of the product. Owners are free to do with the product anything they choose, which may include selling it to someone else.

For most large pieces of office equipment, such as photocopiers, there is also an option to **lease** the equipment. Leasing, or renting, usually involves an initial charge and a monthly fee. On average, the initial charge is equal to about two monthly payments. The ownership of a leased piece of equipment is retained by the leasing company.

**Lease Agreement.** A lease is for a specified time, after which time the equipment is returned to the seller (Figure 5-10). Some leases allow purchase of the equipment at the end of the rental period for an additional payment. The details of the purchase option are covered in the lease agreement.

Metropolitan Office Systems

Lease Agreement

Customer (Location)

*Standard Education Corporation*
Full Legal Name (Please Print)

*119 Washington Blvd.*
Address

*Spokane,* *WA* *98548*
City County State Zip

Billing Contact

Dealer:

Customer (Billing address, if different)

Full Legal Name (Please Print)

Address

City County State Zip

Phone

| Quantity | Description: Make, Model, and Serial Number | Quantity | Description: Make, Model, and Serial Number |
|---|---|---|---|
| *1* | *FT 6655 Copier AA3365430358* | | |
| *1* | *Sorter A337502010902* | | |
| *1* | *Document Feeder A338506* | | |
| *1* | *RT314 Large-capacity Tray* | | |

Minimum Lease Term: *60* Months

Payment Due: *X* Monthly; ___ Quarterly; ___ Annually; ___ Other: *$455.46*

Amount of Monthly Payment With Sales, Use, and Property Tax: *$482.78*

Advance Payment of *$965.56* (Tax Included) by Check #___
___ First Month's Rent
*X* First and Last
___ Security Deposit (Without Tax)
___ Other

Documentation Fee $ *-0-*

**Figure 5-10.** Read lease agreements carefully.

**Advantages of Leasing.** When you lease a product, your office does not own it, but you have several advantages.

1. Leasing allows purchasers to keep more of their money. The initial cost of obtaining the machine is a fraction of the full cost of purchasing it. Therefore, the remainder of the money can earn interest in the bank or be used for other expenses. Leasing is advantageous when you do not have enough money to buy the equipment but need the services it provides. In addition, leasing allows businesses to update equipment every few years at the end of each lease period. Updating may not be as affordable if you buy equipment.

2. Often the company that leases the product is also responsible for servicing it.

3. In most cases, businesses are able to take lease payments as a tax deduction each year.

Leasing is not always the best solution. It is important to weigh the advantages of leasing against the advantages of buying equipment for your medical practice.

**Negotiating.** Whether you decide to lease or buy equipment, always ask whether the price is firm or if there is room for negotiation. Many discounted rates are never extended to the customer simply because the customer did not ask. Although some equipment prices are non-negotiable, terms can sometimes be negotiated on more expensive pieces of equipment. Companies that lease office equipment are often flexible in determining the monthly payment. Equipment companies may accept smaller payments in the beginning of the rental or purchase agreement period, and require larger payments near the end.

In a competitive market, some suppliers may match their competitors' prices. When purchasing several pieces of equipment at the same time, a supplier may be able to offer some savings on the total cost of the purchase or provide some service, such as delivery, free of charge.

# Maintaining Office Equipment

Office equipment must be regularly maintained to provide high-quality service. Daily or weekly maintenance, such as cleaning the glass on the photocopier or replacing toner, can be performed by the office staff. However, more extensive maintenance should be done by the equipment supplier. Consult the equipment manual for details about the care of each piece of equipment.

## Equipment Manuals

The best source of information about maintaining a piece of equipment is the manual that comes with it. This booklet gives basic information about the equipment, including how to set it up, how it works, special features, and problems you may encounter. The information in an equipment manual is extremely valuable. If the manual is lost, call the manufacturer to obtain another one. Equipment manuals should be stored where they can be retrieved easily. Some large pieces of office equipment provide racks or slots on the side of the equipment for storage of the manual.

## Maintenance and Service Contracts

Equipment suppliers provide standard maintenance contracts when office equipment is purchased. A **maintenance contract** specifies when the equipment will be cleaned, checked for worn parts, and repaired. A standard maintenance contract may include regular checkups as well as emergency repairs.

In addition, some suppliers offer a **service contract,** which covers services that are not included under the standard maintenance agreement. A service contract may cover emergency repairs not covered under standard maintenance. In some cases, service contracts are combined with maintenance contracts in one document.

It is important to keep track of all maintenance performed on your equipment. Many offices keep a maintenance log, where staff members record the date and purpose of each service call. This log is helpful in identifying whether equipment should be replaced because of the need for frequent servicing.

## Troubleshooting

When a piece of equipment stops functioning properly, what is the correct course of action? One option is to call a service supplier. However, you can also take steps to

## Points on Practice

### Equipment Manual Tips

It is helpful to write the following information on the inside front cover of the equipment manual upon initial setup. If there is a problem with the equipment that requires a maintenance call, this valuable information will be quick and easy to retrieve.

1. The date of purchase or lease
2. The serial number of the equipment
3. The phone number of the company contracted to repair the equipment

determine and correct the problem yourself. This process is called **troubleshooting.** Resolving the problem can save you the cost of a service call that may not be covered by the standard agreement.

The first step in troubleshooting is to eliminate possible simple causes of a problem. For example, if the equipment is powered by electricity, make sure that it is plugged into a functioning outlet and that it is turned on. Are all doors and other openings in their correct positions? Are all machine connections firmly in place?

If you cannot discover a simple cause for the problem, it is time to test the machine to determine what it is failing to do. In the case of a malfunctioning photocopier, for example, try making a copy and note the response. Write down any error messages the machine provides.

Next, consult the equipment manual. Many manuals devote a section to troubleshooting. If you cannot find the solution after reading the manual, call the manufacturer or the place of purchase for additional assistance. Be prepared to explain the steps you have already taken toward resolving the problem.

## Backup Systems

Occasionally, more than one piece of equipment can be affected by a single problem. For example, if the electricity goes off, all electrical equipment will go out at once. To avoid losing important information and records, it is important to have backup systems in place.

**Computers.** Computers should be placed on a backup system. The company that services the computer system usually sets this up. Computer backup may occur either automatically off-site over the phone lines or on-site, which may require that a staff member manually plug in a backup tape every night before going home. Computer backup usually occurs at midnight, when the office is not using the system. Computer backup ensures that all information will be retrievable even if the computers suffer a catastrophic failure.

**Telephones.** The use of cell phones in addition to traditional phones offers a backup to communication in the event that phone service is interrupted. Cell phones are also helpful during emergency weather conditions.

**Electricity.** An emergency generator may supply emergency power for lighting in key hallways and exam rooms. Interior rooms and halls can quickly become very dark and hazardous when the electricity is unexpectedly cut off.

**Battery Power.** Battery power backup is a key component of security and warning system backups. Audio warning signals sound when it is time to replace the batteries in smoke and security detectors. All batteries should routinely be replaced every six months.

**Fire Extinguishers.** Fire extinguishers need to be serviced or replaced once a year to ensure maximum performance. The office may choose to contract with a local company to provide this annual maintenance evaluation.

## Equipment Inventory

Each piece of equipment is an asset of a business. It is part of the business's net worth and should be listed on the medical practice's balance sheet. Therefore, taking inventory of office equipment provides relevant information for the practice's money manager. It may also indicate whether old equipment is due for replacement.

There are many different ways to take an office equipment inventory. Figure 5-11 shows one example. Many offices use a master inventory sheet to survey all equipment at a glance. The master sheet usually includes such general information as equipment name and purchase price, and the quantity of each type of equipment.

### EQUIPMENT INVENTORY

| ITEM | PURCHASE DATE | PURCHASE PRICE |
|------|---------------|----------------|
| 1. TotalOffice oak desk | 07/25/06 | $295.00 |
| 2. TotalOffice rolling desk chair | 02/19/06 | $119.00 |
| 3. TotalOffice 4-drawer file cabinet | 12/21/07 | $150.00 |
| 4. TotalOffice 2-drawer file cabinet | 08/05/07 | $100.00 |
| 5. HYtech Pentium 100 computer | 03/10/08 | $1150.00 |
| 6. HYtech 14-inch monitor | 03/10/08 | $200.00 |

**Figure 5-11.** An equipment inventory sheet includes equipment names and the quantity of each type of equipment.

Many offices also keep more detailed information about each individual piece of equipment in files or on a single sheet of paper. Detailed information may include the following:

- Name of the equipment, including the brand name
- Brief description of the equipment
- Model number and registration number
- Date of purchase
- Place of purchase, including contact information
- Estimated life of the product
- Product warranty
- Maintenance and service contracts

All equipment inventories should be updated periodically.

## Summary

In many ways, state-of-the-art office equipment is as important for a medical office as its medical equipment. Although every office does not have the same equipment, common equipment may include telephones, electronic typewriters, computers, pagers, fax machines, dictation-transcription equipment, folding equipment, photocopiers, adding machines and calculators, postage meters, check writers, paper shredders, and microfilm or microfiche readers.

As a medical assistant, you may be expected not only to operate this equipment but also to help make purchasing decisions by researching various purchasing options. This research includes obtaining information about product features, warranties, and maintenance. You may also be involved in researching information regarding the advantages and disadvantages of leasing and buying equipment.

Equipment is an asset for a medical office. The office staff needs to maintain a comprehensive inventory of the products leased and purchased. It is important to keep up-to-date with new technologies that will help the administrative office function smoothly and efficiently.

# REVIEW

## CHAPTER 5

### CASE STUDY QUESTIONS

Now that you have completed this chapter, review the case study at the beginning of the chapter and answer the following questions:

1. What factors might go into the choice of an answering machine over the use of an answering service?
2. What backups for system failure might be important for the equipment in a medical office?
3. How could a misdialed phone number on the fax machine impact the life of a patient?
4. Why is routine maintenance of all office equipment important?

### Discussion Questions

1. Why is office equipment important to the medical office? Give at least three examples of pieces of typical office equipment, and describe their use in the medical office.
2. Compare and contrast the advantages and disadvantages of buying and leasing equipment.
3. What are some features of a standard product warranty?
4. Describe a scenario in which an interactive pager might be helpful in a medical office.

### Critical Thinking Questions

1. Imagine that you are responsible for the maintenance of the office equipment in a busy medical practice. What weekly, monthly, and yearly checks might you perform? How would you document these checks?
2. You think that your office needs a new photocopier. Explain how you would justify this need to the office manager.
3. You have been asked to fax confidential patient information to another medical office. What precautions will you take to protect this information?
4. The fax machine in your office is malfunctioning. Explain the steps you might take to troubleshoot the problem.
5. Typewriters and microfiche machines are not commonly used in medical offices today. What technology has replaced them?

### Application Activities

1. Your office frequently uses temporary employees to help with copying. The office manager asks you to write directions for the use of the photocopier, to be posted near the machine. Using the computer, create a sign suitable for posting.
2. Your office is moving soon, and you have been asked to assist in the design of a new communication system for the practice. What features would you include in the new system?
3. You have been asked to design a cover sheet for the fax machine for your office. Using the computer, design a cover sheet with a disclaimer.
4. Go online and research three different types of photocopiers. Write a report describing each. Be sure to include the equipment name, manufacturer, warranty options, price, advantages to buying or leasing, features, and recommendations for use.

### Virtual Fieldtrip

*Visit the McGraw-Hill Higher Education Medical Assisting website at www.mhhe.com/medicalassisting3 to complete the following activity:*

Use the American Association of Medical Assistants and the U.S. Department of Health and Human Services websites. Prepare an oral presentation about one of the following topics:

- HIPAA law and the use of fax machines
- HIPAA law and the use of answering machines
- The advantages and disadvantages of an automated phone system
- The appropriate use of a cell phone while on the job

Ask your instructor how many references and citations you should minimally include in your research. Present your report to the class, using all available multimedia, including PowerPoint slides or an overhead projector if possible.

Open the CD and complete this chapter's practice activities, play the games, listen to the key terms, and test yourself with the interactive review. E-mail, print, and/or save your results to document your proficiency.

## CHAPTER 6

# Using Computers in the Office

## MEDICAL ASSISTING COMPETENCIES

*In preparation for the certification examination, you should know the following areas of competence:*

| COMPETENCY | CMA | RMA |
|---|---|---|
| **Administrative** | | |
| Perform basic clerical skills | X | X |
| **General/Legal/Professional** | | |
| Respond to and initiate written communications by using correct grammar, spelling, and formatting techniques | X | X |
| Identify and respond to issues of confidentiality by maintaining confidentiality at all times and following appropriate guidelines when releasing records or information | X | X |
| Be aware of and perform within legal and ethical boundaries | X | X |
| Utilize computer software and electronic technology to maintain office systems | X | X |
| Maintain the physical plant | | X |
| Evaluate and recommend equipment and supplies for practice | | X |
| Adapt to change | | X |
| Evidence a responsible attitude | | X |
| Receive, organize, prioritize, and transmit information appropriately | | X |

## KEY TERMS

bandwidth

CD-ROM

central processing unit (CPU)

clock speed

cursor

database

dot matrix printer

DSL (digital subscriber line)

electronic mail (e-mail)

hard copy

hardware

icon

ink-jet printer

instruction set

Internet

LAN

laser printer

modem

motherboard

mouse

multimedia

multitasking

network

optical character recognition (OCR)

random-access memory (RAM)

read-only memory (ROM)

scanner

screen saver

## KEY TERMS *(Concluded)*

| | | |
|---|---|---|
| software | tower case | VPN |
| touch pad | trackball | WAN |
| touch screen | tutorial | zip drive |

# CHAPTER OUTLINE

- The Computer Revolution
- Types of Computers
- Components of the Computer
- Using Computer Software
- Selecting Computer Equipment
- Security in the Computerized Office
- Computer System Care and Maintenance
- Computers of the Future

# LEARNING OUTCOMES

After completing Chapter 6, you will be able to:

**6.1** List and describe common types of computers.

**6.2** Identify computer hardware and software components and explain the functions of each.

**6.3** Describe the types of computer software commonly used in the medical office.

**6.4** Discuss how to select computer equipment for the medical office.

**6.5** Explain the importance of security measures for computerized medical records, including HIPAA compliance.

**6.6** Describe the basic care and maintenance of computer equipment.

**6.7** Identify advances in computer technology and explain their importance to the medical office.

# Introduction

The practice of medicine has grown to be increasingly complex:

- Never before has so much medical information been available for the physician.
- Never before has the practice of billing and collecting for medical services rendered and also the scheduling and coordinating of services among multiple providers been so complicated.
- Never before has a "super computer" been more needed to assist with all aspects of a busy practice. We live in the age of information. The need for a device to organize and correlate all this information has never been greater.

The computer has become an integral tool of the medical office. It is used to organize and categorize thousands of bits of information required to accurately record patient care, transmit information to others at distant points, and maintain an orderly record of all the activities of the business.

In this chapter you will learn about the many aspects of using a computer in a medical practice. Regardless of your past experience with computers, after you complete this chapter, you will have a growing awareness and respect for the marvelous technology it represents. You may even become enthusiastic about the possibilities of its many uses.

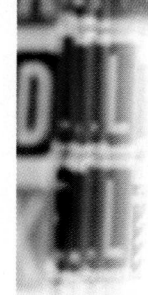 **CASE STUDY**

The big day has come at last! Today the new computer system will be installed. Everyone on staff will be involved in learning the new system and using it every day. For a while, everyone will be expected to learn the new system while continuing to maintain the old way of doing things. That will be no small effort for this busy medical office. Some of the office staff are nervous and edgy, whereas others are excited and looking forward to a new experience. Everyone agrees it is going to be a big change.

Chris is a medical assistant and is excited and eager to get started. She has been waiting for this day ever since she studied the use of computers in medical assisting school. She knows the next few weeks are going to be full of training and building data sets. She knows she is going to be an integral part of the creation of a new way of getting things done. Chris is excited.

Alicia, a medical assistant who works with Chris, thinks that life would be much easier if the administration had just chosen to leave things the way they were. Alicia is not alone in thinking that computers are just an unnecessary inconvenience. The truth is, Alicia is a little afraid that she will not be able to learn the new system. She has tried to ask questions and express her concerns about the new computer system. But each time she tried to talk to one of the computer specialists, she felt stupid and clumsy. They spoke in a language she didn't understand, and she was too intimidated to tell them she didn't understand what they were talking about. Alicia will go along with this new system just to keep her job. But she has decided that she is definitely not going to waste her time learning anything more than she absolutely has to.

As you read this chapter, consider the following questions:

1. Are you more like Chris or Alicia? What background do you bring to the study of computers that makes you feel the way you do?
2. Why is it important for an office to continue to use the manual system at the same time that it converts to a computerized system?
3. Who should be trained in the use of a new computer system in a medical practice? Why?
4. Which group do you think would be the most difficult to train in an average medical practice?
    a. Those who think like Chris?
    b. Those who think like Alicia?
    c. The physicians?
5. What would be the best way to approach the group you just identified?

# The Computer Revolution

Over the past decade computers have revolutionized the way we live and work. Computers make many tasks easier because they process information with great speed and accuracy. They are also capable of storing vast amounts of information in a small space.

In today's world, computer skills are essential for most career choices, and medical assisting is no exception. As a medical assistant, you need to understand the fundamentals of computers and their uses. This knowledge will enable you to perform many office tasks with ease.

In addition, the more you know about computers, the more easily you will be able to solve or avoid computer problems.

# Types of Computers

Four basic types of computers are used today: supercomputers, mainframe computers, minicomputers, and personal computers. Each type of computer is suitable for a certain type of work in a particular kind of workplace.

## Supercomputers

Supercomputers are the biggest, fastest, and most complex computers in use. They are primarily used in research in medicine and are considered to be the hope of the medicine of tomorrow. They are used for genetic coding and for DNA and cancer research.

## Mainframe Computers

Often used by government facilities and large institutions, including universities and hospitals, mainframes can process and store huge quantities of information. Mainframe computers are used for large governmental service programs such as Medicare and Medicaid.

## Minicomputers

Minicomputers are smaller than mainframes but larger than personal computers. Minicomputers have traditionally been used in network settings. A **network** is a system that links several computers together. In this environment a minicomputer typically functions as a server, which is a computer used as a centralized storage location for shared information. However, personal computers are becoming as powerful as minicomputers and may eventually replace them.

## Personal Computers

Also called microcomputers, personal computers can be found in homes, offices, and schools. They are ideal for these settings because they are small, self-contained units. Because users have different needs, personal computers are available in three different types: desktop, notebook, and subnotebook.

**Desktop.** The most common type of personal computer, a desktop model fits easily on a desk or other flat surface. The system unit of many newer desktop models is housed in a **tower case,** which extends vertically instead of horizontally. A tower case—often placed on the floor next to the desk—allows more surface area at the workstation (Figure 6-1). Both large and small medical offices commonly use desktop computers. Information is displayed on a monitor screen. Monitors may be flat, resembling a framed picture. In many health-care facilities, these flat-screen monitors are commonly LCD (liquid crystal diode) monitors. Monitors may also resemble a standard television screen. LCD screens provide for better privacy because they can't be seen from the side. They also generate less heat.

**Laptop and Notebook.** A laptop computer is small—about the size of a thick magazine—and weighs

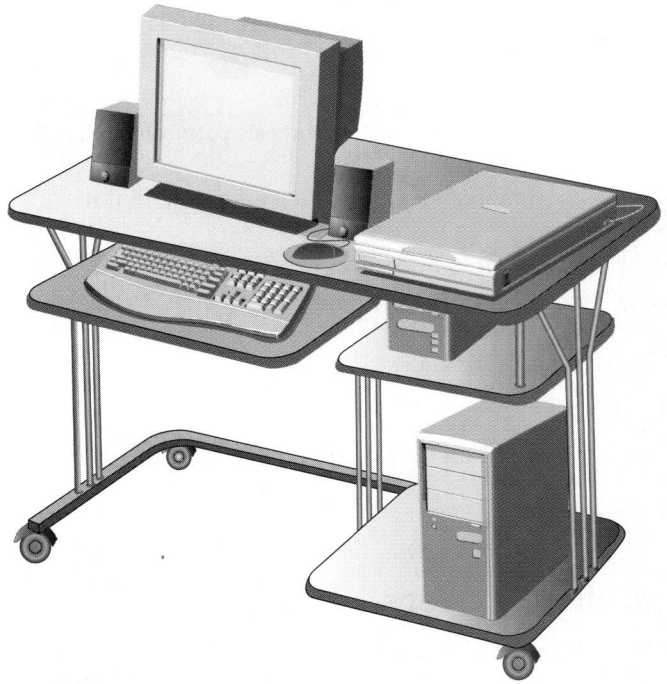

**Figure 6-1.** Offices can free up much-needed desktop space by using computers in tower cases, which can be kept on the floor.

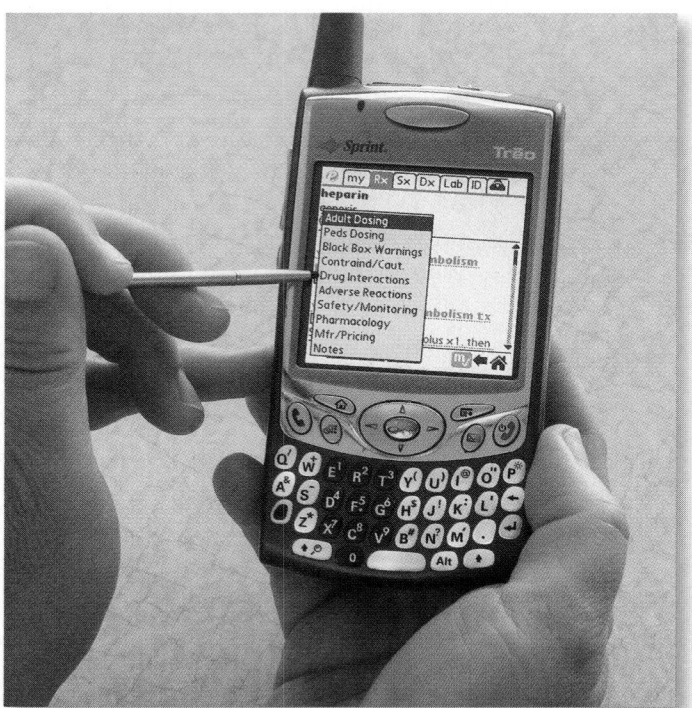

**Figure 6-2.** A handheld computer or PDA like this one can be used as a handy reference to look up medications or perform calculations in the medical office. Handheld computers are also used as part of a sophisticated computer network for the physician to enter and receive patient data.

only a few pounds. Laptops operate either on battery power or on an AC adapter. As advances in technology make laptops smaller, more powerful, and less expensive, they are becoming increasingly popular. Their portability makes them especially convenient for students, for those who travel, and for anyone who desires fast and easy access to the Internet. Using laptops and their smaller counterparts, notebook computers, physicians and other health-care professionals can instantly communicate with the medical office computer, accessing data and information from other locations.

**Subnotebook.** A subnotebook computer (sometimes called a palmtop) is about the size of your palm and is extremely light. Because they are so small, subnotebooks generally do not perform all the functions of desktop or laptop computers. The keyboard of a subnotebook does not contain all the extra function keys found on a standard keyboard, and the keys themselves are quite small. For these reasons, subnotebooks are not used for large keying tasks such as word processing. They may, however, be useful for health-care professionals who need to receive and enter small amounts of patient data from locations outside the medical office.

**Personal Digital Assistant (PDA).** PDAs are common in medical offices and other health-care facilities. Doctors often look up medications and other reference information (Figure 6-2). They may also enter data that is transferred into a patient's chart.

## Components of the Computer

Computer components are divided into hardware and software. **Hardware** comprises the physical components of a computer system, including the monitor, keyboard, and printer. **Software** is a set of instructions, or a program, that tells the computer what to do. Software includes both the operating system and applications that run on the operating system.

### Hardware

The computer's hardware serves four main functions: inputting data, processing data, storing data, and outputting data. Various hardware components are needed to perform each of these functions (Figure 6-3). In order to work, hardware devices must be connected by a cable, such as a USB or serial cable.

**Input Devices.** For a computer to handle information, such as patient records, the data must first be entered, or input. Several types of input devices may be used to enter data into the computer. Keyboards, pointing devices, modems, and scanners are input devices. After information is entered into the computer, it can be displayed on the monitor, processed, or stored.

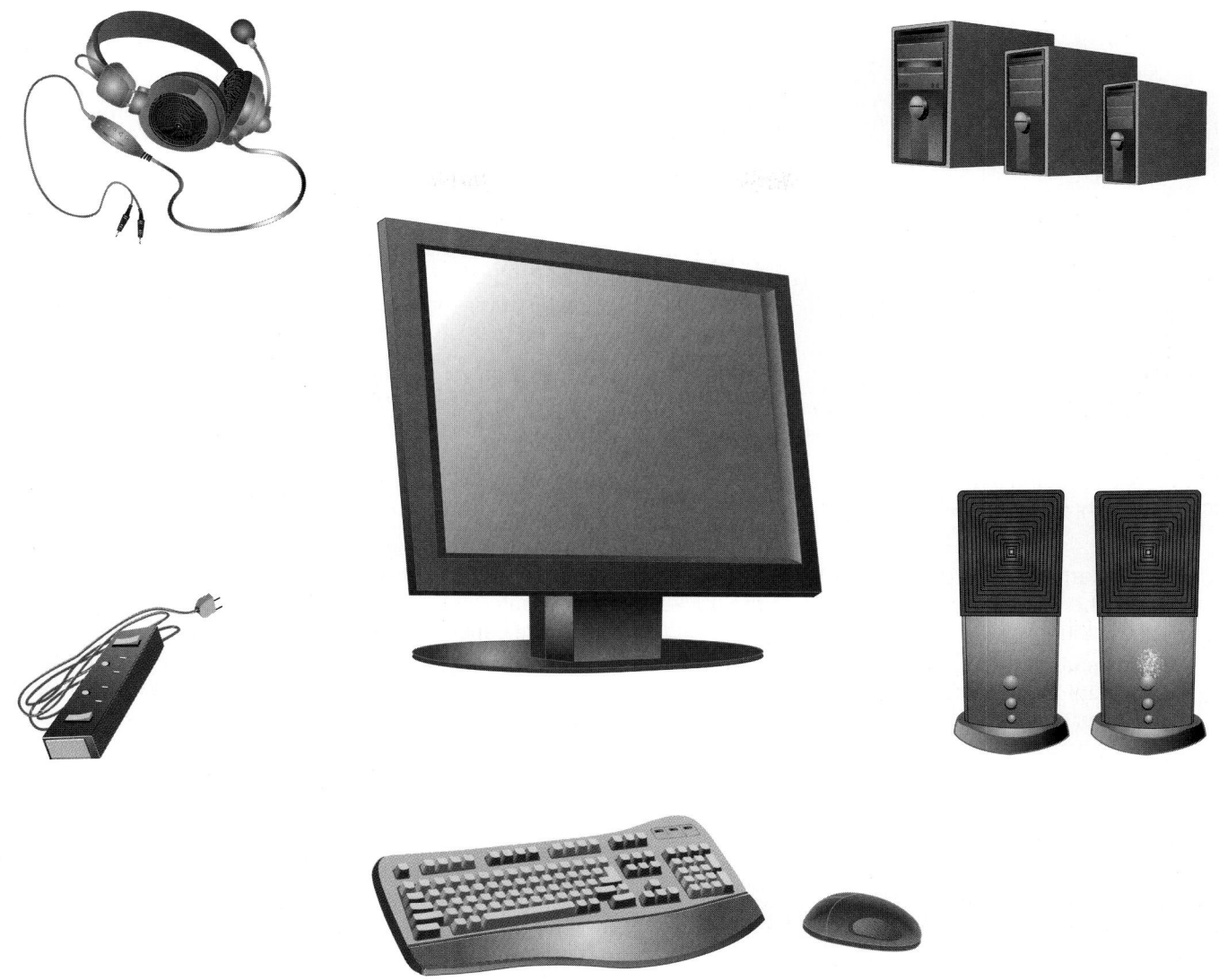

**Figure 6-3.** Some components of a computer system.

*Keyboard.* The keyboard is the most common input device. The main part of a keyboard resembles a typewriter. Most keyboards have several additional keys, however. A typical keyboard contains the following:

- Standard typewriter keys to enter letters, numbers, symbols, and punctuation marks
- Separate numerical keypad for entering numbers faster and more easily
- Arrow keys to move the **cursor,** a blinking line or cube on the computer screen showing where the next character that is keyed will appear
- Function keys to perform such tasks as saving and printing files

When you use the keyboard, it is important to position your hands properly to avoid injury. The Caution: Handle With Care section provides tips for preventing and coping with carpal tunnel syndrome, a condition resulting from repetitive motion.

*Pointing Device.* Many sophisticated software programs need not only a keyboard but also a pointing device to enter information into the computer. When you move the pointing device, an arrow appears. You can point and click the arrow on various buttons that appear on the screen. The four common types of pointing devices are the mouse, the trackball, the touch pad, and the touch screen.

1. A **mouse,** the most common pointing device, has two or three buttons on top and a rolling ball on the bottom. As you move the mouse across a flat surface or mouse pad, you cause a light-sensing device on the bottom to move. This controls an arrow on the screen that points at the desired button or object on the screen. Then, as shown in Figure 6-4, you push one of the buttons on the mouse to access a function, such as opening a file. A laser mouse detects movement through a laser and does not have a ball.

2. A **trackball** is similar to a mouse except that the rolling ball is on the top of the device instead of on the

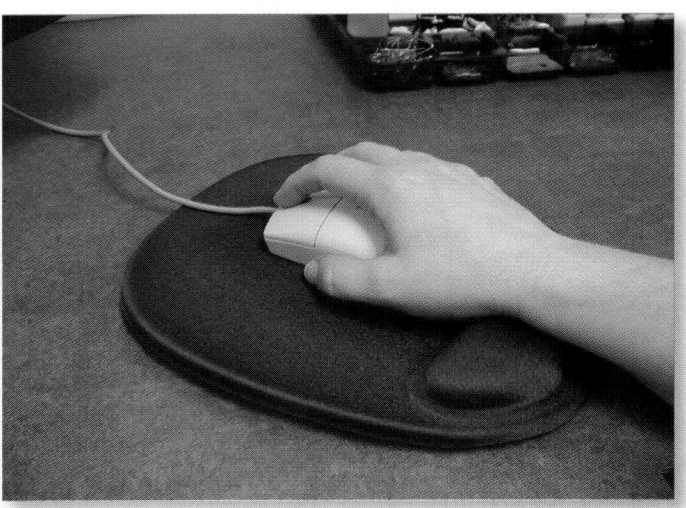

**Figure 6-4.** Using a mouse, you can point and click to access a variety of functions.

bottom. Rather than pushing a trackball across a pad, you roll the ball with your fingers while the trackball remains stationary.

3. A **touch pad** is a form of pointing device and is common on laptop and notebook computers. It is a small, flat device that is highly sensitive to the touch. To move the arrow on the screen, you simply slide your finger across the touch pad. To click on an item, you push a button similar to that on a mouse or trackball, or you tap your finger on the touch pad.

4. A **touch screen** is a monitor screen that is illuminated at the touch of a pen, wand, or finger. When an object is touched on the screen, the touch itself acts as a pointing device and conveys information to the computer. Touch screens are increasingly being used in clinical and hospital settings.

*Modem.* This term **modem** is a shortened form of the words *modulator-demodulator*. A modem is used to transfer information from one computer to another over telephone lines. Because modems allow information to be transferred both to and from a computer, they are considered input/output devices. The speed at which a modem transfers data is called the bit rate. Modem speeds are continually being improved. Modems are essential for any medical office that needs to transfer files electronically, as when submitting insurance claim forms.

A cable modem is a modem that operates over cable television lines to provide fast Internet access. **DSL (digital subscriber line)** modems operate over telephone lines but use a different frequency than a telephone frequency. This type of modem allows computer Internet access and telephone use at the same time.

An advanced type of modem is a fax modem. This device allows the computer to send and receive files much as a fax machine does. A fax modem is not quite as versatile as a regular fax machine, however. The information being sent must first be input into the computer. In addition, without the use of a scanner, you cannot use a fax modem to send a patient record with handwritten notes on it.

*Scanner.* A **scanner** is a device used to input printed matter and convert it into a format that can be read by the computer. Scanners are useful in the medical office because patient reports from another doctor, a hospital, or another outside source can be easily entered into the computer. Scanners are also making it possible to move into a paperless medical system. Using a scanner is much faster than keyboarding, or inputting the information with a keyboard. Three types of scanners are available:

1. Handheld scanners are generally the least expensive but are more difficult to use and produce lower-quality results than the other two types.

2. A single-sheet scanner feeds one sheet of paper through at a time and looks similar to a single-sheet printer.

3. A flatbed scanner is the most expensive type of scanner but is the easiest to use and produces the highest-quality input. It works much like a small photocopier: the paper lies flat and still on a glass surface while the machine scans it. Photocopiers can be configured with a scanning capability and can transmit the images of scanned documents to computers.

**Processing Devices.** There are two major processing components inside the system unit, or computer cabinet. The **motherboard** is the main circuit board that controls the other components in the system. The **central processing unit (CPU),** or microprocessor, is the primary computer chip responsible for interpreting and executing programs. The CPU is considered the most important piece of hardware in a computer system. It interprets instructions from software programs.

CPUs have three central elements that define their function: bandwidth, clock speed, and instruction set. **Bandwidth** is a measurement of how much information can be sent or processed with one single instruction, and is calculated in bits or bytes. **Clock speed** is a measurement of how many instructions per second the CPU can process. Clock speed is measured in megahertz (MHz) or gigahertz (GHz). An **instruction set** includes the groups of instructions from installed programming that a CPU can employ. The greater the bandwidth and clock speed, the faster and more powerfully the CPU can execute programs. The more programs are installed, the more versatile the CPU is.

**Storage Devices.** One of the main tasks of a computer is to store information for later retrieval. The computer uses memory to store information either temporarily or permanently. Several types of drives are used for permanent information storage.

*Memory.* Computers use two types of memory to store data: **random-access memory (RAM)** and read-only memory (ROM). RAM is temporary, or programmable,

## CAUTION *Handle With Care*

# Carpal Tunnel Syndrome

As the number of computers used in the home and workplace has escalated in recent years, the number of cases of carpal tunnel syndrome has also risen dramatically. Carpal tunnel syndrome is a hand disorder that is often associated with computer use. The term for this condition comes from the name for a canal (the carpal tunnel) located in the wrist. Several tendons pass through this tunnel, allowing the hand to open and close.

Carpal tunnel syndrome results from repetitive motion, such as keyboarding, for hours at a time. This motion may cause swelling to develop around the tendons and carpal tunnel. The swelling compresses the nerve. The people most likely to develop carpal tunnel syndrome are workers whose jobs require them to perform repetitive hand and finger motions.

## Symptoms

The symptoms associated with carpal tunnel syndrome include the following:

- Tingling or burning in the hands or fingers
- Weakness or numbness in the hands or fingers
- Hands that go to sleep frequently
- Difficulty opening or closing the hands
- Pain that stems from the wrist and travels up the arm

## Tips for Prevention

If you use a keyboard for extended periods, you should practice proper techniques to prevent carpal tunnel syndrome (Figure 6-5).

- While seated, hold your arms relaxed at your sides, and check to make sure that your keyboard is positioned slightly higher than your elbows. As you input, keep your elbows at your sides, and relax your shoulders (see Figure 6-5).
- Use only your fingers to press keys, and do not use more pressure than necessary. Use a wrist rest, and keep your wrists relaxed and straight.

- When you need to strike difficult-to-reach keys, move your whole hand rather than stretching your fingers. When you need to press two keys at the same time, such as "Control" and "F1," use two hands.
- Try to break up long periods of keyboard work with other tasks that do not require computer use.

## Tips for Relieving Symptoms

If you have symptoms of carpal tunnel syndrome, try these suggestions for relief.

- Elevate your arms.
- Wear a splint on the hand and forearm.
- Discuss your symptoms with a physician, who may prescribe medication.

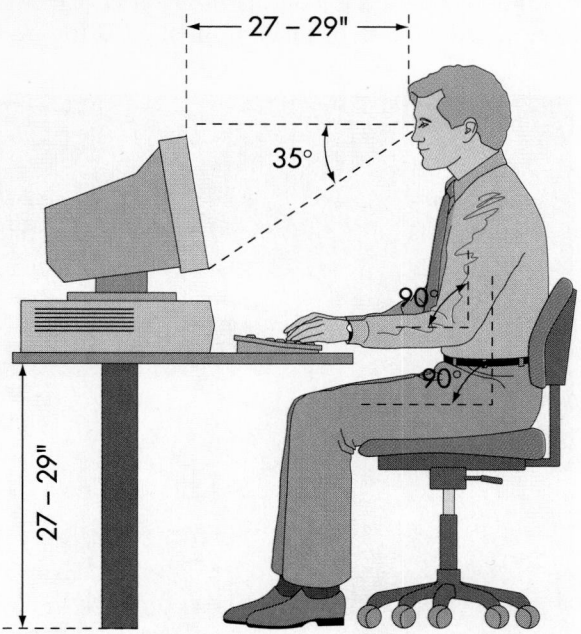

**Figure 6-5.** Maintaining proper posture and hand positions helps to avoid strain or injury of the back, eyes, neck, or wrist when keyboarding.

memory. While you are working on a software program, the computer is accessing RAM. In general, the more RAM that is available, the faster the computer will perform. As software programs become more sophisticated, they require more RAM.

**Read-only memory (ROM)** is permanent memory. The computer can read it, but you cannot make changes

to it. The purpose of ROM is to provide the basic operating instructions the computer needs to function.

***Hard Disk Drive.*** The hard disk drive is where information is stored permanently for later retrieval. Software programs and important data are usually stored on the hard disk for quick and easy access. The amount of hard disk space needed to store software programs is increasing rapidly. The more software programs you want to store, the larger the hard disk you will need.

***Diskette Drive.*** A diskette drive can read from and write to diskettes (also called disks). Rigid 3.5-inch disks were once commonly used but they are now considered outdated technology. The use of CDs has quickly taken the place of disks because they have a much greater storage capacity.

***CD-ROM Drive.*** CD-ROMs look just like audio compact discs, but they contain software programs. The term **CD-ROM** stands for "compact disc—read-only memory." The main advantage of a CD-ROM over a diskette is its ability to store large amounts of data. CD-ROMs can be used to back up information from the hard drive.

CD-ROM drives have become standard equipment on most personal computers. Although many software packages are available on both CD-ROM and diskettes, some large programs are available only on CD-ROM. These programs include multimedia applications such as medical encyclopedias. **Multimedia** refers to software that uses more than one medium—such as graphics, sound, and text—to convey information (Figure 6-6).

Some computers have a CD burner or recorder (CD-R), which allows information to be taken from one CD (or any other source) and "burned" to a CD. CD-Rs work when software to operate the burner is installed in the computer. This software provides instruction for the burner operation.

***Tape Drive.*** This storage device is used to back up (make a copy of) the files on the hard disk. The information is copied onto magnetic tapes that resemble audiotapes. If the hard drive malfunctions, you will have a copy of the information on these tapes.

It is possible to back up information onto diskettes. Most hard disks, however, contain so much information that a large number of diskettes would be required to back up all the data. With most tape drives, the entire contents of the hard disk can be stored on one or two tapes. Store these tapes at night in a fireproof container.

***Jump Drive.*** A jump drive is an externally attached drive that is small enough to be carried on a key chain, yet holds 16 gigabytes or more of data. (Gigabytes are a measurement of memory space.) It also may be called a flash drive, a pen drive, a key drive, a memory key, a flash key, or simply a USB drive. It provides easy portability for large bodies of data. It may be used for backup operations in a medical practice when stored off-premise.

***Zip Drive.*** A **zip drive** is a high-capacity floppy disk drive developed by Iomega®. Zip drives are slightly larger and about twice as thick as a conventional floppy disk.

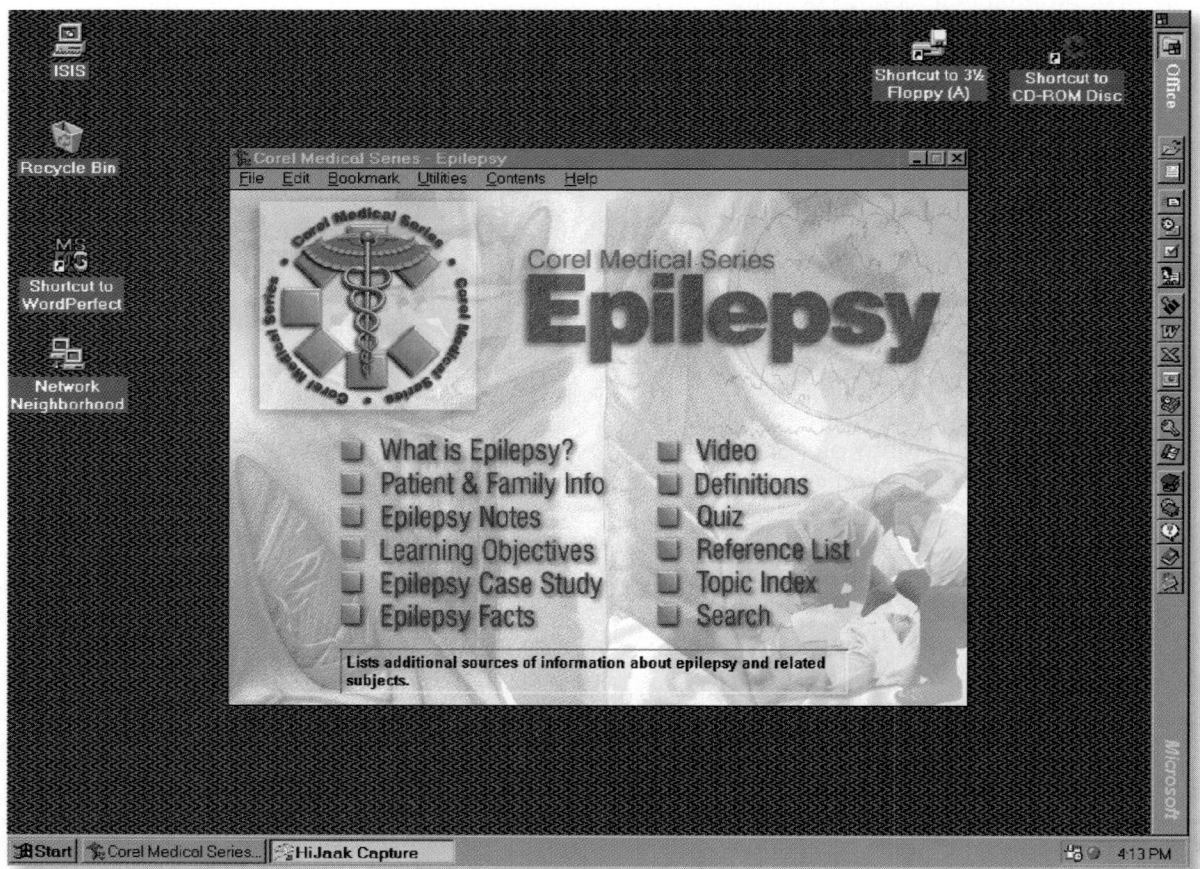

**Figure 6-6.** A CD-ROM provides features, such as video and sound, that are not possible in a standard printed book.

Zip drives can hold up to 750 MB of data. They are durable and relatively inexpensive. They may be used for backing up hard disks and transporting large files.

***DVD.*** DVD (digital video disc) is optical disc storage technology. It is similar to CD technology except it is bigger and faster. It can hold movie-like video, including audio, photos, and computer data. One double-sided, dual-layer disk can store about eight hours of high-quality video.

**Output Devices.** Output devices are used to display information after it has been processed. A monitor and a printer are two output devices needed in the medical office.

***Monitor.*** A standard computer monitor looks like a television screen or may be an LCD flat screen. It displays the information that is currently active, such as a word processing document, an Internet link, or e-mail. Monitors are available in color and a variety of sizes. They also come in a flat-screen model that conserves desk space. All of the software programs that are used today, including multimedia applications, require a color monitor to run.

Color monitors vary in the number of colors they can display and in the resolution of the images. *Resolution* refers to the crispness of the images and is measured in dot pitch. The lower the dot pitch, the higher the resolution. For example, a monitor with a 0.26 dot pitch displays sharper images than a monitor with a 0.39 dot pitch. Using a high-resolution monitor can help you avoid eye strain.

***Printer.*** A printer is required to produce a **hard copy,** which is a readable paper copy or printout of information (Figure 6-7). You will need a printer to print out correspondence, patient reports, bills, insurance claims, and other documents. Printer resolution is noted in terms of dots per inch (dpi). The higher the dpi, the better the print quality. Printer output varies, depending on the type of printer and the model. The three most commonly used printers are dot matrix, ink-jet, and laser.

1. **Laser printers** are high-resolution printers that use a technology similar to that of photocopiers. Laser printers are the fastest and produce the highest-quality output. Laser printers are more expensive than dot matrix or ink-jet printers.

2. **Ink-jet printers** also form characters using a series of dots, but they are nonimpact printers in which the dots are created by tiny drops of ink. Many ink-jet printers are capable of printing in both black and color. Because of their high-quality output and affordable prices, ink-jet printers are popular for home and small-office use.

3. **Dot matrix printers** create characters by placing a series of tiny dots next to one another. The dot matrix printer is the only type that is an impact printer, which means that it makes an impression on the paper as it prints. It is the least expensive of the three types. It is also slower and noisier, and produces a lower-quality output than the other types. It represents older technology in printing and is the least popular type of printer. Because it is an impact printer, however, it is the only type that is capable of producing multiple copies with carbon paper or other multicopy forms.

Because each type of printer has advantages and disadvantages, some medical offices may purchase more than one type. For example, a medical office may have a dot matrix printer for creating internal memos and multipage insurance forms and a laser printer for creating documents whose quality resembles that of typeset documents.

A current trend in printers is the "all-in-one" model (Figure 6-8), which functions not only as an ink-jet printer

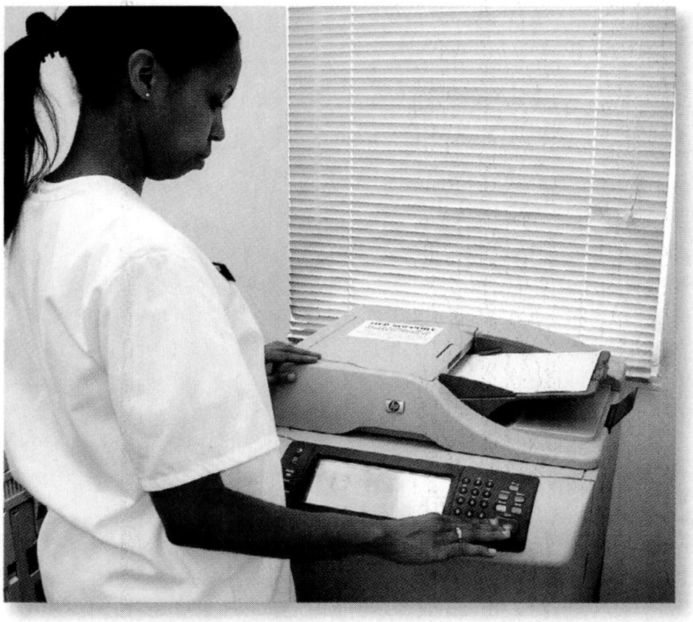

**Figure 6-7.** You may need to print out hard copies of documents to send to patients, vendors, insurance companies, or other doctors' offices.

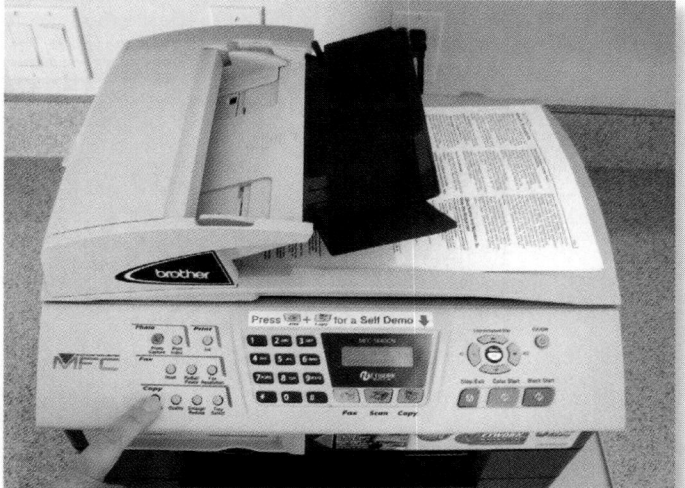

**Figure 6-8.** An "all-in-one" printer can send and receive faxes, print, and copy. Some models like this one can be networked to more than one computer in the medical office.

but also as a fax machine, scanner, and photocopier. This type of machine may be convenient for a small medical office that requires each of these functions but does not have space for four separate devices. In addition, purchasing an all-in-one unit is usually more economical than purchasing the machines separately.

# Software

Computer software is generally divided into two categories: operating system and application software. The operating system controls the computer's operation. Application software allows you to perform specific tasks, such as scheduling appointments.

**Operating System.**  When you turn on a computer, the operating system starts working, providing instructions that the computer needs to function. Examples of operating system software include Microsoft Windows XP and Vista, Linux, and DOS. Most computers come pre-installed with Windows XP or Vista.

Operating system software is sometimes referred to as the platform for the system. Most medical practices use IBM-compatible personal computers, which are most suitable for businesses that use computers primarily to manipulate words. Apple computers are used by businesses,

such as advertising agencies or design firms that are extensively involved in graphics, visual images, or desktop publishing.

***DOS.***  DOS and OS/2 are the original operating systems created for IBM and IBM-compatible computers. They are considered to be old and very limiting computer technology. A pointing device, such as a mouse, is not interfaced with the operation. Instead, "F" or "function" keys are used to indicate the functions to be performed.

***Windows.***  This operating system employs a graphical user interface (GUI) instead of a command line interface. With a GUI, menu choices are identified by **icons,** or graphic symbols (Figure 6-9). For example, the "Print" command is usually identified by a button with a tiny illustration of a printer on it. To print a document, you move the pointing device until the arrow is on the printer icon and then click the button.

An important advantage of the Windows operating system over DOS is that it is easier to learn because you do not have to remember commands. Another benefit of Windows is that it is a **multitasking** system—users can run two or more software programs simultaneously. You could, for example, enter patient information into a **database,** a collection of records created and stored on the computer, while a word processing program is running in

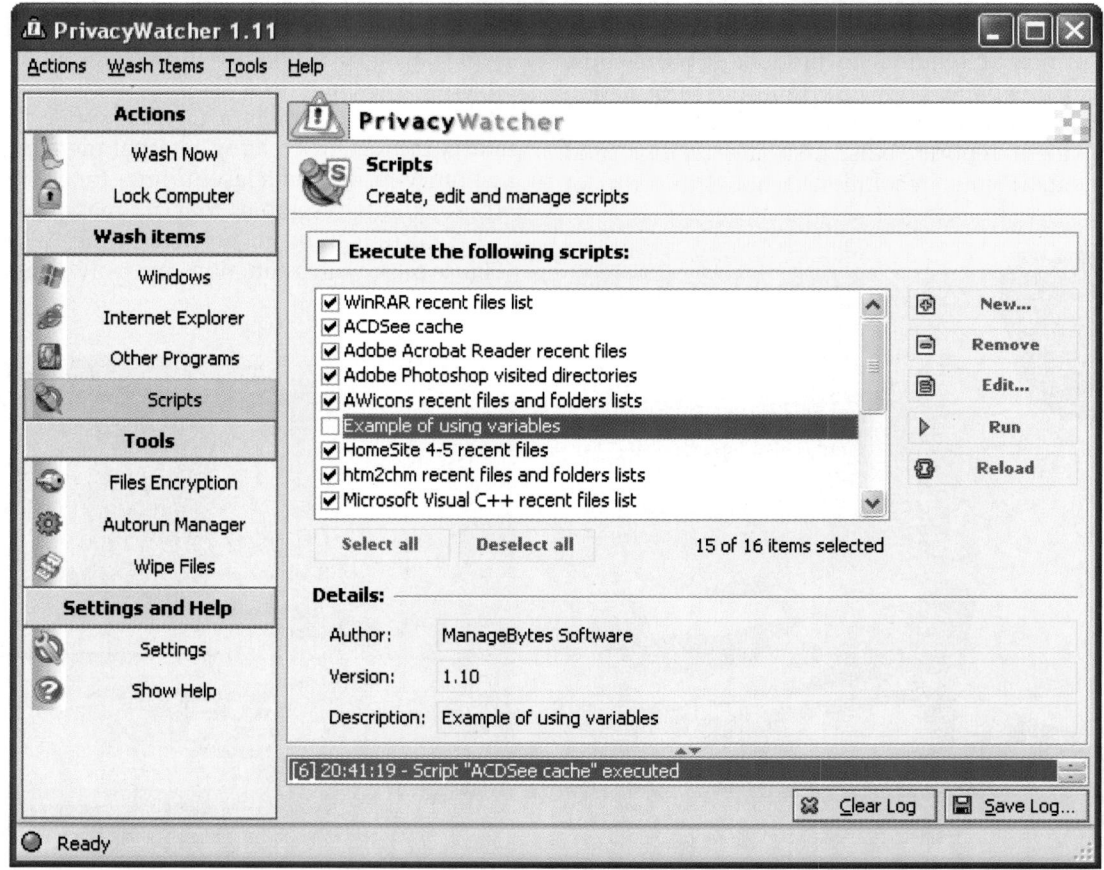

**Figure 6-9.**  An online help system allows you to access helpful information when you are using a software program, while protecting the privacy of the patient.

the background. DOS is not a multitasking system; you can run only one application at a time.

***Windows XP.*** Windows XP is a Windows operating system that is reliable and versatile. In most businesses, Windows XP has become the standard operating system for IBM and IBM-compatible computers. Most new computers are shipped with Windows XP preinstalled, and many software programs are being written to run exclusively under this operating system.

With the release of Windows Vista in 2007, medical offices may replace their XP systems with Vista.

**Applications.** Most of the software sold in stores is application software. An example of application software is Microsoft® Office. Microsoft® Office includes word processing (Word), presentation software (PowerPoint), spreadsheets (Excel), database management (Access), and desktop publishing (Publisher). Medical Manager®, Medware®, Medasis, and MediSoft™ are practice management applications. These software packages are specifically designed to meet the needs of a medical practice. Standard computer practice management software packages can be purchased. In addition, custom-made computer practice management software can be designed to meet the needs of a particular practice. Word processing, database, and accounting software are just a few examples of the wide variety of applications available.

**Optical Character Recognition.** **Optical character recognition** or **OCR** software enables the conversion of images to text so they can be treated like any other type of Word document. An OCR system includes an optical scanner for reading text and state-of-the-art software for analyzing images. An OCR system enables an article or patient file to be fed into an optical scanner, where it is transferred into an electronic computer file. It is then possible to manipulate and edit the file using a word processor.

# Using Computer Software

Computer software has been developed for nearly every office function imaginable. Using software, you can complete tasks with greater speed, accuracy, and ease than with a manual system. Learning how to use the software correctly, however, is the key to getting the most out of your computer system.

## Word Processing

In the medical office, as in any office, word processing is a common computer application. It has replaced the typewriter for writing correspondence and reports, transcribing physicians' notes, and performing many other functions. Correcting errors is easy on a word processor, and you can save documents for later retrieval and modification. With word processing, a form letter can be merged with a patient mailing list to create letters that are personalized with patients' names.

## Database Management

A database is a collection of records created and stored on a computer. In a medical office, databases are used to store patient records such as billing information, medical chart data, and insurance company facts. These records can be sorted and retrieved in many ways and for a variety of purposes. You may be asked to find, add to, or modify information in a database. For example, you might use a database to determine all the patients covered by a particular insurance company.

## Accounting and Billing

Accounting and billing software is extremely useful in an office environment. It enables you to perform many tasks, including keeping track of patients' accounts, creating billing statements, preparing financial reports, and maintaining tax records. (You will learn more about billing and accounting functions in Chapters 17 and 18.)

## Appointment Scheduling

Instead of writing in an appointment book, you can use software to schedule appointments. Some scheduling packages allow you to enter patient preferences, such as day of the week and time, and then to list available appointments based on that information. If the office system is on a network, scheduling software is particularly valuable, because more than one user can access the appointment schedule at a time.

## Electronic Transactions

Using a computer equipped with a modem and communications software, you can perform several types of electronic transactions. This technology enables you to send and receive information instantaneously rather than waiting the days or weeks required for regular mail. Common electronic transactions include sending insurance claims and communicating with other computer users. Electronic medical records can easily be sent anywhere in seconds.

**Sending Insurance Claims.** Insurance claims can be submitted electronically directly from the medical office to an insurance company. This procedure enables claims to be processed quickly and efficiently. (Chapter 15 discusses health insurance billing procedures.)

**Communicating.** The ability to communicate and share information with other computer users and systems is important in many medical offices. This communication may take place through electronic mail, online services, and the Internet. The Points on Practice section gives valuable ideas for saving time online.

***Electronic Mail.*** Commonly known as e-mail, **electronic mail** is a method of sending and receiving messages almost instantly through a network. Through e-mail, it is possible to communicate with computer users in your own office,

## Creating a Form Letter

**Procedure Goal:** To use a word processing program to create a form letter

**Materials:** Computer equipped with a word processing program, printer, form letter to be created, 8½-by-11-inch paper.

**Method:**

1. Turn on the computer. Select the word processing program.

2. Use the keyboard to begin entering text into a new document.

3. To edit text, press the arrow keys to move the cursor to the position at which you want to insert or delete characters, and enter the text. Either type directly or use the "Insert" mode to type over and replace existing text.

4. To delete text, position the cursor to the left of the characters to be deleted and press the "Delete" key. Alternatively, place the cursor to the right of the characters to be deleted and press the "Backspace" key (the left-pointing arrow usually found at the top right corner of the keyboard).

5. If you need to move an entire block of text, you must begin by highlighting it. In most Windows-based programs, you first click the mouse at the beginning of the text to be highlighted. Then you hold down the left mouse button, drag the mouse to the end of the block of text, and release your finger from the mouse. The text should now be highlighted. Choose the button or command for cutting text. Then move the cursor to the place where you want to insert the text, and select the button or command for retrieving or pasting text.

6. As you input the letter, it is important to save your work every 15 minutes or so. Some programs do this automatically. If yours does not, use the "Save" command or button to save the file. Be sure to save the file again when you have completed the letter.

### Rationale

The document must be saved periodically so that if power is lost or if part of the document is accidentally deleted, at least part of the document is still retrievable.

7. Carefully proofread the document and use the spell checker, correcting any errors in spelling or formatting.

### Rationale

Your documents should contain no spelling or grammatical errors and should be professional in appearance.

8. Print the letter using the "Print" command or button.

# Reflecting On . . . HIPAA

## HIPAA and E-mail

HIPAA law requires that all transactions containing patient health information be protected. Consider the following guidelines when sending e-mail within a medical practice:

1. Do not send email containing protected health information without specific written authorization from the patient.

2. Always check the patient's medical record and the computer system for any special instructions for contacting the patient through e-mail. Follow all patient requests. When in doubt, do not send an e-mail. Check with the office manager or supervisor.

3. Maintain virus protection to guard your computer system against viruses, which commonly infect a computer system through e-mail.

across town, or on the other side of the world. Unlike regular mail, e-mail operates in real time.

As the use of e-mail has increased, e-mail etiquette rules designed especially for Internet use have become important. By requiring employees to use appropriate, professional language in all electronic communications, employers limit their liability risk and maintain their professional image. E-mail etiquette is established when a practice creates a written e-mail policy spelling out the "dos" and "don'ts" concerning the use of the company's e-mail system. The implementation of e-mail etiquette rules can be monitored by using e-mail management software and response tools.

**Online Services.** These services, known as *servers*, provide a means for health-care professionals to communicate with one another. Most online services contain forums that offer information and discussion groups focusing on a wide range of medical topics. Health-care workers can learn about the latest medical research and technology or exchange ideas with others in their field. In addition, some online services provide access to medical databases such as MEDLINE®, created by the National Library of Medicine. Users can search MEDLINE® for records and abstracts from thousands of medical journals from around the world.

**Internet.** The **Internet** is a global network of computers. Through the Internet, you can communicate with millions of computer users around the world. E-health or medical information and products are easy to access worldwide through the use of the Internet. Many large medical facilities, universities, and other organizations—such as the National Institutes of Health (NIH) and the Centers for Disease Control and Prevention (CDC)—provide medical resources, databases, and other information on the Internet. Users can visit Internet sites to find multimedia textbooks, presentations, and links to other related sites on the Internet. Table 6-1 describes some popular medical resources available on the Internet.

Search engines are specialized websites that search other websites for information. The user connects with the search engine and indicates a topic of interest. Typically, a box is provided for the topic and then the user selects a box marked "Go." The search engine electronically searches for the information requested and lists many different website

| TABLE 6-1 Medical Resources on the Internet | | |
|---|---|---|
| **Organization** | **Web Address** | **Description** |
| American Medical Association | www.ama-assn.org | News announcements and press releases; articles from *JAMA* and other AMA journals; links to other medicine-related Internet sites |
| eMedicineHealth | www.emedicinehealth.com | Health resource center where you can learn about health issues and the latest treatments available |
| MedlinePlus® | http://medlineplus.gov | A service of the U.S. National Library of Medicine and NIH; site includes current health news, medical encyclopedia, and directories for doctors, dentists, and hospitals |
| National Institutes of Health | www.nih.gov | Medical news and current events; press releases; biomedical information about health issues; scientific resources; links to Internet sites of related government agencies |
| National Library of Medicine | www.nlm.nih.gov | Internet site for world's largest biomedical library; research and development activities; connections to online medical information services |
| *New England Journal of Medicine* | http://content.nejm.org | Articles and abstracts; archives of past issues |
| Virtual Hospital | http://radiology.uiowa.edu | Information on a variety of health issues, medical resources, tutorials, and multimedia textbooks |
| WebMD Health® | www.webmd.com | Trustworthy, credible, and timely health information written by experts in medicine, journalism, and health communications |

# Working Efficiently Online

If the medical office where you work is computerized, the system most likely has a modem for sending e-mail and transferring files electronically. The modem may also be used to access various online services and the Internet, a global network of computers. If this access is not currently available in the medical office, it probably will be in the near future. You may even be asked to help choose an online service or Internet provider for the office.

These services, known as *Internet Service Providers (ISPs)*, allow access to a network of servers that provides a means for health-care professionals to communicate with one another.

## Choosing an Online Service

Compare several services for the following features:

- The speed and accessibility of services. A cable modem or DSL through the phone line has faster speeds for communicating information than a regular phone line service. Plus these services are always on and do not interfere with the telephone service at the facility.
- Free trial membership. Many services offer a free 1-month membership to try out the service. The trial periods enable office staff members to test several services to determine which one best suits their needs.
- Local access telephone number. Make sure the service provides an access number within the local dialing area of the office. If it does not, the office will be charged long-distance telephone rates each time someone goes online. These fees are separate from the online service's rates and can add up quickly.
- Extra fees. Although access to most of the information found in online services is included in the membership fee, some providers charge extra for premium or extended services. If you want to read or print out the full text of an article in a medical journal, for example, some providers charge an additional fee. Make sure you consider these extra fees when comparing costs of online services.
- Availability of health-care information. Some online services provide discussion groups (commonly known as chat rooms) and resources that would be useful to the medical office. Other services may not offer as much relevant information. By comparing several services, you can determine which service best meets the needs of the practice.

## Sending and Receiving E-Mail

When using e-mail, follow these guidelines to manage your online time efficiently.

- Use computerized address books. As part of the e-mail system, most services provide an online address book in which you can store frequently used e-mail addresses. Instead of wasting time searching for an e-mail address in a standard card file, you simply click on the person's name in the address book and the mail is automatically sent to that person. You can also use the address book to send the same e-mail message to several people at once.
- After sending an e-mail, watch for any alert that the message did not go through. If an alert appears, check the address again and resend the e-mail.

## Doing Research

Although a great deal of valuable information can be found through online services and the Internet, searching for this information can be time-consuming. The following tips are provided to make the most of your online time.

- Use the favorite places feature. Keep a list of favorite places, or sites that you visit frequently.
- Refine your searches. Searching for *arthritis*, for example, might produce hundreds of references that you would have to read through to determine their relevance. Narrowing your search to *juvenile rheumatoid arthritis*, on the other hand, would produce fewer references but would provide more exact matches.
- Download files. *Download* means to transfer a file to the hard disk. Instead of reading through information while you are online, download the files and later retrieve them or print them to read later.

link options for the user. Examples of popular search engines include "Google™" and "Yahoo!®."

## Research

The advent of CD-ROM technology has revolutionized the world of research and education. Not only can an immense amount of information be contained on one compact disc, but the CD-ROM usually provides additional information in the form of videos and sound (see Figure 6-6). A CD-ROM encyclopedia, for example, might also provide spoken pronunciations of medical terms. This type of software may help patients—especially children—understand the human body as well as various medical conditions.

## Software Training

Software programs may seem quite complex. Most people need a period of training before they feel comfortable using the application. Several methods of training— some from outside sources and some provided by the software manufacturer—are available.

**Classes.** Many computer vendors offer training classes for the software packages they sell. In addition, community colleges and high schools sometimes offer adult education classes for a variety of applications, including word processing and communications. These classes may be at the beginner, intermediate, or advanced level.

**Tutorials.** Many software packages come with a **tutorial,** which is a small program designed to give users an overall picture of the product and its functions. The tutorial usually provides a step-by-step walk-through and exercises in which you can try out your newly acquired knowledge.

**Documentation.** Nearly all software manufacturers provide some type of documentation with their programs. Documentation is usually in the form of written instruction manuals or online help that is accessed from within the program.

*Manuals.* Some manuals provide detailed information on software operation and may include an index and sections on troubleshooting and commonly asked questions. Other manuals may simply give installation instructions and brief information on program basics. This type of manual may refer users to the software's online help.

*Online Help.* In most software applications, users access the online help screen by clicking on a "Help" button or by pressing a certain function key, such as "F1." The online help usually provides a "Contents" section (see Figure 6-9), in which you can browse for topics. An index, in which you can search for key words, is also provided.

**Technical Support.** A software company's technical support service is designed to assist you with problems that go beyond the scope of the user's guide or manual. A call to technical support is important when you encounter a problem that cannot be solved by simple problem-solving techniques. By calling a toll-free number, you can access a knowledgeable team who will listen to the description of the problem and suggest solutions over the phone.

Before calling technical support:

- Check the system for errors to the best of your ability.
- Check your manual for answers. Ask your supervisor for assistance.
- Have the software registration number available.
- Be prepared to follow the instructions of the technical support personnel.
- Allow uninterrupted time to spend on the phone with the technical support person.
- Plan to call from a location that gives ready access to the computer with the problem.

Technical support is also helpful when you are upgrading software. Some software companies automatically notify their customers of available upgrades. The technical support service is always a good source of information regarding the latest products and their applications.

## Selecting Computer Equipment

Most medical offices are computerized. If the decision is made to upgrade the system, you may be a part of the decision-making process in selecting equipment. As a medical assistant who will be using the system, you may be asked for your input in selecting software, adding a network, or choosing a vendor.

The first step for helping in the selection process is to learn as much as you can about hardware and software. You can get information by taking an introductory computer class at an adult school or community college; by reading computer magazines or books; or by talking to friends, relatives, or coworkers who use computers.

## Upgrading the Office System

Computer hardware is changing and improving at such a rapid pace that a system seems to become outdated almost as soon as it is purchased. In addition, more advanced software is introduced every day, and this software requires more advanced hardware to run. Consequently, an office system purchased only a year or two ago may need to be upgraded. Sometimes an upgrade simply requires replacement or addition of certain components. For instance, a laser printer can take the place of a dot matrix printer, or a CD-ROM drive can be added. In other cases, such a solution is not possible or cost-effective, so an entirely new system must be purchased.

## Selecting Software

After a decision is made regarding the type of software needed, such as an accounting program, a specific product must be chosen. To make an informed decision, you can read software reviews in computer magazines or trade publications. Check with other medical offices to get opinions on software packages. A crucial step in selecting software is to make sure the office computer system meets the minimum system requirements listed on the software box.

## Adding a Network

There are several advantages to adding a network to the computer system in a medical office. A computer network enables users to share software programs and files and allows more than one person to work on the same patient's information at one time. While you are working on a patient's insurance claim, for example, another medical assistant might be inputting billing information. Some medical offices are virtually paperless. They use a highly sophisticated network with a notebook or desktop computer in every examination room. Doctors input information into patients' computerized charts. If a doctor is in her office and a patient is waiting, a staff member at the front desk sends an e-mail message to the doctor's desktop computer, and a beep sounds as an alert. Networks also allow large medical facilities to communicate with employees via e-mail. For instance, an internal memo about changes in office policies may be sent by e-mail to all employees. For networks to operate, the computer must have either a network interface card or wireless connection to the network. Networks can be run with Windows®, Novell®, or Unix® network operating systems.

## Virtual Private Networks

When a group of two or more computer systems are linked together, it is known as a network system. Local-area networks are called **LAN**s. The computers in this system are geographically close together (for example, in the same building). Wide-area networks are known as **WAN**s. The computers in this network are farther apart and are connected by telephone lines. Virtual private networks, known as **VPN**s, are used to connect two or more computer systems. They are also constructed using public telephone lines. They use the Internet as the medium for transporting data. VPNs use encryption and other security methods to ensure that only authorized users can access the network. This type of network makes it possible for physicians to access patient records in a secure manner from a variety of locations.

## Choosing a Vendor

When purchasing computer equipment, you should look for a reputable vendor who not only offers a reasonable price but also provides training, service, and technical support. A first step might be to check with personnel in other medical offices that use a computer system. Find out which dealer they use and if they are satisfied with the system, salespeople, and support. You can also ask dealers for names of references—medical offices that have purchased systems from them. It is a good idea to get cost estimates from at least three vendors, and it is preferable to buy all hardware components from the same vendor.

# Security in the Computerized Office

Although security measures are important in any office, they are especially important in a computerized medical office. Great care must be taken to safeguard confidential files, make backup copies on a regular basis, and prevent system contamination. HIPAA law requires that privacy and security procedures are in place to prevent the misuse of health information. These procedures must also ensure confidentiality.

## Safeguarding Confidential Files

Much of the information collected in a medical office is confidential. Just as with paper records, confidential information stored on the computer should be accessible only to authorized personnel. Two common ways to provide security in a computerized office are to employ passwords and to install an activity-monitoring system.

**Passwords.** In many hospitals and physicians' offices, each employee who is allowed access to computerized patient files is given a password. The employee must enter the password into the computer when using the files. Access codes or passwords only allow the user into approved areas according to the individual's job description. If you are given a password, do not divulge it to anyone else unless your office manager asks you to do so. If an employee leaves or is fired, the user account should be deleted.

**Activity-Monitoring Systems.** In conjunction with passwords, some health-care facilities use a computer system that monitors user activity. Whenever someone accesses computer records, the system automatically keeps track of the user's name and the files that have been viewed or modified. In this way, problems or security breaches can be traced back to specific employees.

## Making and Storing Backup Files

For securing important computer files, it is essential to routinely make diskette or tape backups of them (Figure 6-10). How often backups are made varies among medical offices; your supervisor will tell you the policy for your office. Just as important as making the backups is storing them properly. Backup files should not be stored near the original

# Reflecting On . . . HIPAA

## Guidelines for HIPAA Privacy Compliance and the Computer

The use of computers is widespread within the typical medical practice. Though the computer is valuable for many administrative functions, it also can be a risk in terms of patient privacy and HIPAA compliance. You must follow special safeguards for computers in order to protect the patient's privacy.

1. Computers are typically placed in or near the patient reception area. Keep the computer screen positioned so that it is not visible to unauthorized personnel or patients. Screensavers can be used to minimize the amount of time any information is visible on the screen.

2. All computers should automatically log the user off after a period of no activity. The computer should require that all users must reenter their password to regain access after an idle period.

3. Always keep your computer username and password confidential. Change your password often, using a variety of numbers, symbols, and both lower- and uppercase letters.

4. Consider the use of practice management software, which can track users and follow their activity within a computer system.

5. Formal policies should be developed for every practice regarding the transfer and acceptance of outside protected health information. When using any computer system, always follow practice policy to assure that protected health information is being transferred in a secure and compliant manner.

files. Ideally, they should be kept outside the medical office—perhaps at the physician's home—so that they will be secure in case of fire, burglary, or other catastrophe at the office.

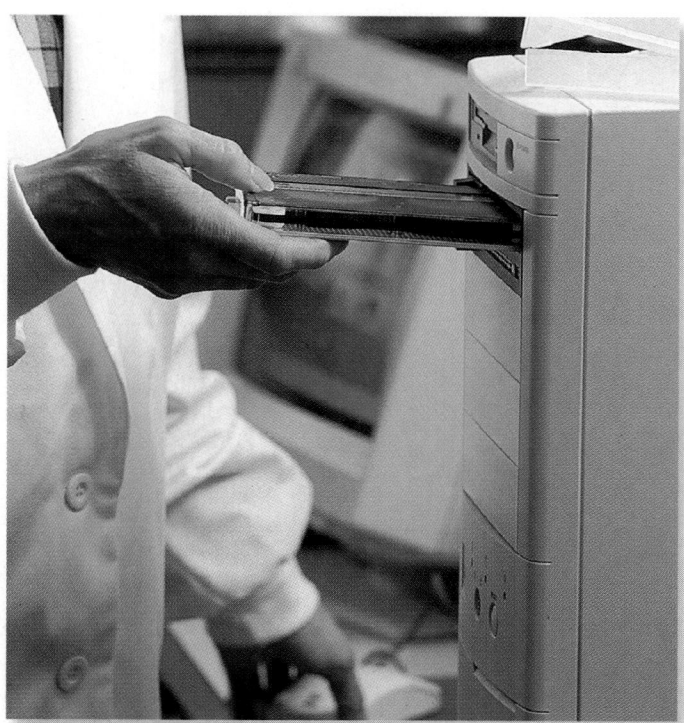

**Figure 6-10.** It is important to back up computer files and store them properly.

## Preventing System Contamination

Another important security issue in the computerized medical office is computer viruses. Computer viruses are programs written specifically to contaminate the hard disk by damaging or destroying data.

Viruses can be passed from computer to computer through shared diskettes that have been infected. Computer viruses can also be spread through infected files retrieved from online services, the Internet, e-mails, and electronic bulletin boards. Several software programs are available to detect and correct computer viruses. Most are fairly inexpensive but provide an invaluable service.

## Computer System Care and Maintenance

Like a car, a computer needs routine care and maintenance to stay in sound condition. The computer user's manual outlines the steps required. Also, a good general rule is not to eat or drink near the computer. Crumbs and spilled liquids can damage the system components and storage devices.

### System Unit

The system unit should be placed in a well-ventilated location, with nothing blocking the fan in the back of the cabinet. To keep the system's delicate circuitry from being damaged by an electrical power surge, you should use a power strip with a surge protector. You plug the computer into the power strip and then plug the power strip into the electrical outlet (see Figure 6-3).

## Monitor

A **screen saver** automatically changes the monitor display at short intervals or constantly shows moving images on the computer monitor or screen. All Windows® operating systems come equipped with screen savers. A wide variety of screen savers are also available as separate software packages. Adding a screen cover to a monitor will protect the monitor.

To protect their screens, many monitors "power down" after a certain period of inactivity. If no one uses the computer for 30 minutes, for example, the monitor screen goes blank. To resume using the computer after the screen saver has been activated or the monitor has powered down, simply touch any key or move the mouse.

In addition, the computer monitor power settings can be set to meet the needs of the health-care facility. Powering down can also be adjusted to suit the facility's needs.

## Printer

Maintenance of a printer generally consists of replacing the ink cartridge, or toner cartridge. When the cartridge needs to be changed, the ink on your printouts becomes very light and colors become faded. Some integrated computer and printer systems automatically provide a "Low Ink" message on the screen when printer cartridges need replacing. The message appears when the "Print" command is given. A graph indicates the amount of ink left in the cartridge. Ink can be ordered online through a link provided with the printer program. Replacement is usually a simple process, described in the printer manual.

## Information Storage Devices

Jump drives, CD-ROMs, diskettes, and magnetic tapes are highly sensitive devices. Even a small scratch may cause permanent damage or make it impossible to retrieve data. To avoid problems, handle and store disks and tapes properly.

**Jump Drives.**   Jump drives are connected to the computer through a USB port (Figure 6-11). This port should be protected when the drive is not attached to the computer, so be certain to put the cap back on the drive when you are transporting the drive to another location.

**CD-ROMs.**   Figure 6-12 shows the proper way to handle a CD-ROM. When you pick it up, touch only the edges or the edge and the hole in the center. CD-ROMs should be stored in the clear plastic case in which they are packaged, sometimes called a jewel case. If a CD-ROM becomes dusty or smudged with fingerprints, clean it by rubbing it gently with a soft cloth. Always rub from the center to the outside. *Never* rub in a circular motion.

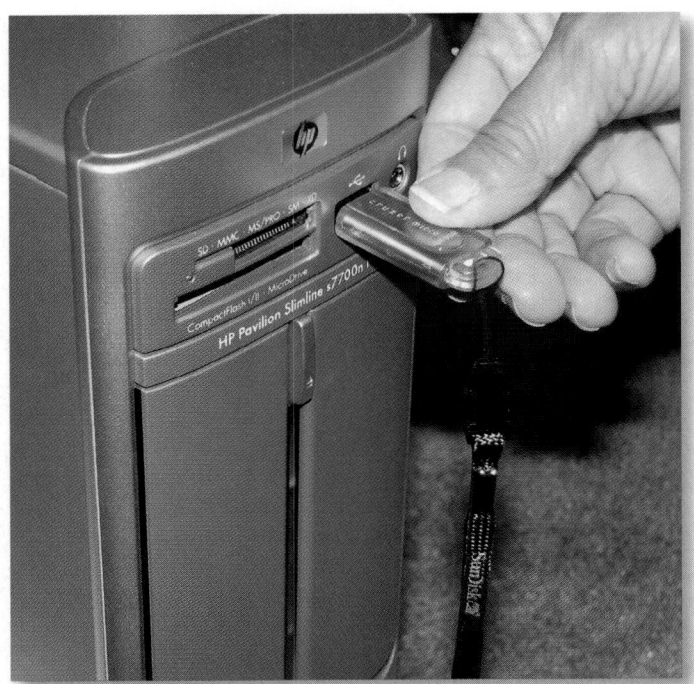

**Figure 6-11.**   A jump drive is a small portable storage device that attaches to the USB port and can store and move up to 16 gigabytes of electronic data.

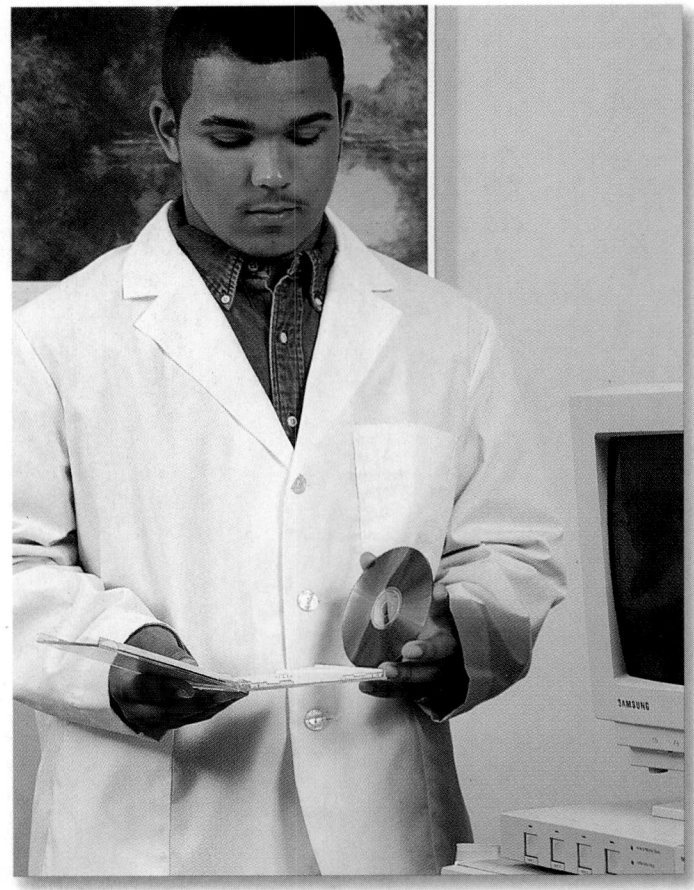

**Figure 6-12.**   When handling a CD-ROM, be careful not to touch the flat surface of the disc.

**Diskettes.** Diskettes should be kept away from magnetic fields, such as a paper clip holder that has a magnet in it. They should also be kept out of direct sunlight and away from extreme temperatures. Although 3.5-inch disks are sturdy, they should be handled with care. They should be labeled appropriately and stored in a durable storage case.

**Magnetic Tapes.** Magnetic tapes should be treated much the same as you would treat audiotapes. They should be stored in a relatively cool, dry place, away from magnetic fields.

## Computer Disaster Recovery Plan

When any business is dependent on computer technology for daily functioning, a computer disaster recovery plan for the business must be in place. A recovery plan offers a possible solution if the primary computer system should fail or "crash," making all information on the hard drive unavailable.

In a medical practice, it is important to discuss the computer disaster recovery plan with the staff so that everyone knows the part they will play if the computer system fails. As devices, systems, and networks become more complex, there are simply more things that can go wrong. As a result, computer disaster recovery plans have become more important and more sophisticated.

A computer disaster recovery plan will vary from practice to practice. However, all plans should include these elements:

1. Minimizing damage to equipment. Automatic warnings are built into computer systems to indicate when a fatal error has occurred. Warnings also provide direction to help prevent loss of information and minimize damage to the computer equipment.

2. Retrieving information. A backup computer system should copy all of the information in the primary computer system every day. If the main system fails, this backup system will allow all the information to be retrieved and not permanently lost.

   This backup system can either be automated or manual. An example of an automated system is a second computer, networked to the first, to which information is regularly backed up in the event the primary computer system fails. With this type of backup, the operation of the office can continue while the primary system is repaired or replaced. An example of a manual backup system, which is less useful, is a handwritten list of patients and the procedures performed each day.

3. Protecting protected health information. Even during an office emergency, such as a computer failure, health-care professionals are still required to carefully guard the privacy of the patient records. If an electronic or manual backup system is implemented, safeguards to protect patient information must still be observed.

Disaster recovery planning can be purchased as a software application or a service, or it can be developed within an organization.

## Computers of the Future

Computers are evolving at such a rapid pace that it is virtually impossible to predict the changes that will take place even in the next few years. Some important new technologies, however, have already been introduced in the medical office and will be improved in the near future. Telemedicine, CD-R technology, and speech recognition technology are only three examples of new computer technologies. Undoubtedly, more will be explored and developed every year.

### Telemedicine

*Telemedicine* refers to the use of telecommunications to transmit video images of patient information. These images are already used to provide medical support to physicians caring for patients in rural areas. The use of telemedicine and advancements in computer technology allow medical practices to quickly access vast amounts of current medical information.

### CD-R and DVD-R Technology

While CD-ROMs and DVDs can only be *read* by the computer, CD-R (compact disc–recordable) media and DVD-Rs can be read *and* written to. CD-R and DVD-R technology allows you to use compact discs like diskettes—to store data and information. Recordable CDs and DVDs, however, can store much more information than diskettes can.

### Speech Recognition Technology

Speech recognition technology enables the computer to comprehend and interpret spoken words. The user simply speaks into a microphone instead of inputting information with a keyboard or a scanner. Because every human voice is different, however, and the English language is vast and complex, this technology is difficult to perfect. As speech recognition technology becomes more advanced, more accurate, and less expensive, it will most likely gain widespread acceptance. It has a great deal of potential, including the ability to virtually eliminate the need for medical assistants to transcribe physicians' notes.

## Summary

As a medical assistant, you should familiarize yourself with the types of computers available and the hardware and software components that make up a computer system. A variety of software programs are used in the medical office, including word processing, database management, accounting and billing, appointment scheduling, and electronic transactions, such as submitting insurance claims. Other computer technology you need to know about includes modems, scanners, and CD-ROM and DVD software.

Whether you are converting to a computerized office or simply upgrading an existing system, learn the guidelines for selecting computer hardware and software. In a computerized office it is also important to know how to secure computerized files and to care for and maintain computer equipment.

Computer technology is advancing so quickly that it is not possible to predict what tools might soon be available for the medical office. Regardless of what the future holds, the need for good equipment management will continue to be an important part of the role of the medical assistant.

## CASE STUDY QUESTIONS

Now that you have completed this chapter, review the case study at the beginning of the chapter and answer the following questions:

1. Are you more like Chris or Alicia? What background do you bring to the study of computers that makes you feel the way you do?
2. Why is it important for an office to continue to use the manual system at the same time that it converts to a computerized system?
3. Who should be trained in the use of a new computer system in a medical practice? Why?
4. Which group do you think would be the most difficult to train in an average medical practice?
   a. Those who think like Chris?
   b. Those who think like Alicia?
   c. The physicians?
5. What would be the best way to approach the group you just identified?

## Discussion Questions

1. Compare and contrast the three kinds of printers. What are the advantages of each?
2. What do you think is in the future in the development of computers? Describe your vision of the typical medical office and its use of computers 25 years from now.
3. A new computer system has just been installed at your office. How would you encourage and assist a fellow employee in learning the new system?
4. Compare and contrast bandwidth, clock speed, and instruction set.
5. Though the computer is valuable for many administrative functions, it also can be a risk in terms of patient privacy and HIPAA compliance. Describe some special computer safeguards that protect the patient's privacy.
6. Describe optical character recognition (OCR) software and how it is useful.

## Critical Thinking Questions

1. A technical problem is detected on the computer at your desk. What would you do? Explain in detail.
2. A fellow employee asks to use your password to the computer because she has forgotten hers. How do you respond and why?
3. Summarize the proper care and maintenance of computer diskettes and CDs. How does proper care reduce problems?

4. Which do you think is a better choice for a medical practice: a LAN, WAN, or VPN system?
5. Think about the future. What do you think the future holds for computers in the medical office?

## Application Activities

1. Go online and research the purchase of a new software package for a medical encyclopedia. Which would you recommend for purchase by your office and why?
2. Look through computer magazines or trade journals for descriptions or reviews of the latest software upgrades for your computer system. Describe what new benefits the upgrades offer and how each feature would benefit a medical practice.
3. Research one of the technological advances mentioned in this chapter—telemedicine, CD-R technology, or speech recognition technology—to learn more about it. Find out how the technology benefits the medical office. Write and present a full report on your topic.
4. Review Table 6-1. Research medical resources on the Internet and find three additional organizations, giving their websites and a brief description of each site.

## Virtual Fieldtrip

*Visit the McGraw-Hill Higher Education Medical Assisting website at www.mhhe.com/medicalassisting3 to complete the following activity:*

Use the American Association of Medical Assistants and the U.S. Department of Health and Human Services websites as well as websites about wireless technology. Prepare a one-page report about one of the following topics:

- The future use of laptop, notebook, and palmtop computers in a medical practice
- The increasing use of wireless configuration for computer access and what it could mean to a medical practice
- An overview of pointer devices used today and what might be used in the future
- HIPAA laws and their application to electronic mail

Ask your instructor how many references and citations you should minimally include in your paper.

Open the CD and complete this chapter's practice activities, play the games, listen to the key terms, and test yourself with the interactive review. E-mail, print, and/or save your results to document your proficiency.

# Managing Correspondence and Mail

## KEY TERMS

annotate

body

clarity

complimentary closing

concise

courtesy title

dateline

editing

enclosure

full-block letter style

identification line

inside address

key

letterhead

margin

modified-block letter style

notations

optical character reader (OCR)

proofreading

salutation

signature block

simplified letter style

subject line

template

## MEDICAL ASSISTING COMPETENCIES

### In preparation for the certification examination, you should know the following areas of competence:

| COMPETENCY | CMA | RMA |
|---|---|---|
| **Administrative** | | |
| Perform basic clerical skills | X | X |
| **General/Legal/Professional** | | |
| Respond to and initiate written communications by using correct grammar, spelling, and formatting techniques | X | X |
| Identify and respond to issues of confidentiality by maintaining confidentiality at all times and following appropriate guidelines when releasing records or information | X | X |
| Be aware of and perform within legal and ethical boundaries | X | X |
| Utilize computer software and electronic technology to maintain office systems | X | X |
| Use appropriate medical terminology | | X |
| Receive, organize, prioritize, and transmit information appropriately | | X |
| Understand allied health professions and credentialing | | X |

## CHAPTER OUTLINE

- Correspondence and Professionalism
- Choosing Correspondence Supplies
- Written Correspondence
- Effective Writing
- Editing and Proofreading
- Preparing Outgoing Mail
- Mailing Equipment and Supplies
- U.S. Postal Service Delivery
- Other Delivery Services
- Processing Incoming Mail

# LEARNING OUTCOMES

After completing Chapter 7, you will be able to:

**7.1** List the supplies necessary for creating and mailing professional-looking correspondence.

**7.2** Identify the types of correspondence used in medical office communications.

**7.3** Describe the parts of a letter and the different letter and punctuation styles.

**7.4** Compose a business letter.

**7.5** Explain the tasks involved in editing and proofreading.

**7.6** Describe the process of handling incoming and outgoing mail.

**7.7** Compare and contrast the services provided by the U.S. Postal Service and other delivery services.

# Introduction

Communication skills are important in every profession. Written materials are tangible demonstrations of an office staff's ability to communicate and conduct business.

Others often evaluate the entire medical practice by the work of one employee. When a letter, form, or document is carelessly prepared and sent into the community, the physician may be judged as "careless." However, when a letter or general business correspondence is constructed in a neat, concise, and well-organized fashion, the physician is often judged to be organized and competent. The skill demonstrated in the creation of a simple business letter reflects on the medical skills of the physician and the

practice. Professional image is conveyed in written correspondence.

Because written documents also serve as legal records, all documents must be prepared with great care and attention to detail. The administrative role of the medical assistant includes the creation of documents that are consistently accurate and clear.

In this chapter you will learn how to write effectively. You will develop skills in composing a business letter. You will learn different styles and formats of writing and will learn how to professionally manage all forms of correspondence commonly used in an ambulatory care setting.

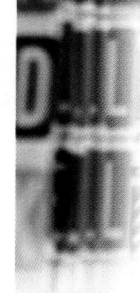

## CASE STUDY

Paula and Tom are medical assistants whose duties include making sure the daily correspondence is created and on the physician's desk before they go home at the end of the day. Today, they are working together to complete these tasks.

Paula will key into the computer letters of referral to other physicians. She is using a template saved within the computer to easily and quickly turn out many different letters. She is simply keying in different fields of information with the specifics for each patient referral. She then prints out a draft copy for proofreading and review by the physician or office manager. Once reviewed, corrected, and approved, she will print out the final letters onto the more expensive letterhead of the office. She will also copy the address from the letters and complete a mailing envelope for each letter.

Tom is assisting as he takes each completed letter and attaches all materials noted as enclosures to each letter. He then folds each letter and its enclosures carefully and inserts them into the properly addressed envelope. Next, he determines the weight of each envelope and the best choice for mailing it. He sorts the mailing into separate piles for different mail handling. The routine mailing is run through the stamp machine. The appropriate forms for the specialty mailing are created and attached. Tom makes sure copies of all mailings are carefully placed in the patient's chart. Both Paula and Tom know the importance of careful and accurate handling of all patient correspondence.

As you read this chapter, consider the following questions:

1. Why is it important to accurately and carefully prepare correspondence for an ambulatory setting? What could the poor management of documents and correspondence mean to a medical practice?

2. What are the differences between the language used in an informal or casual letter and that used in a formal or professional business letter?

3. What are some appropriate shortcuts that can assist in the daily management of correspondence and mailing?

4. What are some factors to consider in choosing the best mode of delivery for letters and parcels?

# Correspondence and Professionalism

As in any business, correspondence from health-care professionals to patients and colleagues must be handled carefully, with appropriate attention to content and presentation. By learning how to create, send, and receive correspondence and other types of mail, you can ensure positive, effective communication between your office and others. Well-written, neatly prepared correspondence is one of the most important means of communicating a professional image for the medical office (Figure 7-1).

# Choosing Correspondence Supplies

The first step in preparing professional-looking correspondence is choosing the right supplies. Many offices already have most of these supplies on hand. However, you may be responsible for choosing and ordering such supplies. You may need to make decisions about letterhead paper, envelopes, labels, invoices, and statements.

## Letterhead Paper

**Letterhead** refers to formal business stationery on which the doctor's (or office's) name and address are printed at the top. In most cases, the office phone number is listed, along with the names of all the associates in the practice. Letterhead is used for correspondence with patients, colleagues, and vendors. Letterhead is used only for the first page of a letter. If a letter is more than one page, all additional pages of the letter are printed on standard bond paper or a plain paper.

Letterhead paper can be cotton fiber bond (sometimes called rag bond) or sulfite bond. Cotton fiber bond is usually more expensive than other types of paper. Cotton bond contains a watermark, which is an impression or pattern that can be seen when the paper is held up to the light. A watermark indicates that the paper is of high quality. The most popular cotton bond used for letterhead is 25% cotton because it is economical, but all higher grades can be used.

The two most common sizes of letterhead paper are standard and legal. Standard or letter-size paper is 8½ × 11 inches. Legal size is 8½ × 14 inches. Most general business correspondence is done on standard size. Legal size paper, as the name indicates, is used for legal documents, especially very lengthy documents.

A formal invitation or announcement may be engraved or embossed. Embossing involves a process where the letters are pressed into the paper. The letters are often set in gold or silver.

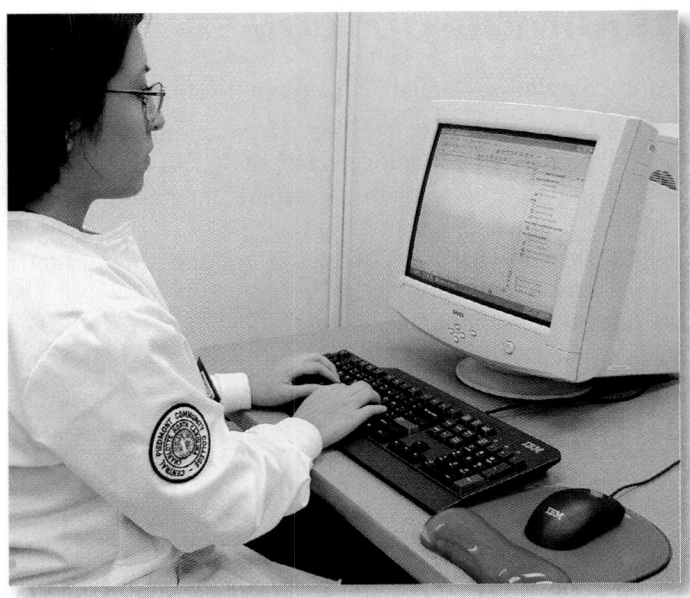

**Figure 7-1.** The correspondence that goes out of and comes into a medical office is vital to a well-run practice.

## Envelopes

Envelopes are used for correspondence, invoices, and statements. Typically, business letterhead, matching envelopes, and sometimes invoice and statement letterhead are printed together.

Familiarize yourself with the several types of envelopes used in the medical office.

- The most common envelope size used for correspondence is the No. 10 envelope (also called business size). It measures 4⅛ by 9½ inches.

- Envelopes used for invoices and statements can range from No. 6 (3⅝ by 6½ inches) to No. 10. These envelopes commonly have a transparent window that allows the address on the invoice or statement to show through, saving time and reducing the potential for errors involved in retyping the address.

- Smaller payment-return envelopes—preaddressed to the doctor's office—are often included along with a bill, for the patient's convenience.

- Tan Kraft envelopes, also called clasp envelopes, are available in many sizes and are used to send large or bulky documents.

- Padded envelopes are used to send documents or materials, such as slides, that may be damaged in the normal course of mail handling.

- The stock and quality of the envelope should always match the stationery. An office typically has two grades of envelopes with a return address. One is a less expensive stock and quality of paper with a block format return address printed in black. The second is a more expensive stock and quality of paper with a block format return address printed in black or a dark color.

## Labels

Address labels, printed from a computerized mailing list, can greatly speed the process of addressing envelopes for bulk mailings. For example, you may have to send a notice of a change in office hours or a quarterly office newsletter to a large number of patients in a practice.

You may choose to set up a system for frequently used labels. Many practices write referrals and other business letters to the same addresses again and again. For fast and easy access, it is helpful to print out labels a full page at a time of the same address. Pages of labels can then be stored in alphabetized folders near the transcription desk. Excel databases can also be set up to print labels and to insert names and addresses in standardized **templates.**

## Invoices and Statements

There are several different types of invoices and statements in use today. They include:

- Preprinted invoices (used to send an original bill)
- Preprinted statements (used to send a reminder when an account is 30 or more days past due)
- Computer-generated invoices and statements
- Superbills (discussed in Chapter 17)
- Data mailers (used to send information)

# Written Correspondence

A letter is a form of communication—much like holding a conversation in person. The recipient will form an impression of the physician or the office based on the letter. Therefore, letters must be clear and well written and must politely convey the appropriate information.

Commonly used paragraphs and even entire letter formats, or templates, are used repeatedly in some practices. It is handy to save these bodies of text in the computer for quick and easy repeated access. With very few keystrokes, the material can be selected and displayed quickly. Then minor changes specific to the letter or document can be added.

It is also helpful to use the cut, paste, and copy features in word processing software to quickly piece together a correspondence that uses sentences or paragraphs from other documents. Large and small bodies of text can easily be moved from document to document, saving time for the medical assistant.

## Types of Correspondence in the Medical Office

As a medical assistant, you will be responsible for preparing routine letters at the doctor's request. You may transcribe some letters from the doctor's dictation and compose others from notes.

The purpose of most letters is to explain, clarify, or give instructions or other information. Correspondence includes letters of referral; letters about scheduling, canceling, or rescheduling appointments; patient reports for insurance companies; instructions for examinations or laboratory tests; answers to insurance or billing questions; and cover letters or form letters to order supplies, equipment, or magazine subscriptions.

## Parts of a Business Letter

Figure 7-2 illustrates the parts of a typical business letter. Details about format may vary from office to office.

**Margin.** The **margin** is the space around the edges of a form or letter that is left blank. The standard setting for margin in business correspondence is one inch.

**Letterhead.** The letterhead is the preprinted portion of formal business stationary.

**Dateline.** The **dateline** consists of the month, day, and year. It should begin about three lines below the preprinted letterhead text on approximately line 15. The month should always be spelled out, and there should be a comma after the day.

**Inside Address.** The **inside address** contains all the necessary information for correct delivery of the letter. The inside address spells out the name and address of the person to whom the letter is being sent. In general, you should:

- **Key,** or type, the inside address on the left margin, two to four spaces down from the date. It should be two, three, or four lines in length.
- Include a **courtesy title** (Dr., Mr., Mrs., and so on) and the intended receiver's full name. Note: If Dr. is used, it is not followed by MD after the name. For example, either of these forms is acceptable: Dr. John Smith; John Smith, MD. This form is not acceptable: Dr. John Smith, MD.
- Include the intended receiver's title on the same line with the name, separated by a comma, or on the line below it.
- Include the company name, if applicable.
- Use numerals for the street address, except the single numbers one through nine, which should be spelled out—for example, Two Markham Place.
- Spell out numerical names of streets if they are numbers less than ten.
- Spell out the words *Street, Drive,* and so on.
- Include the full city name; do not abbreviate.
- Use the two-letter state abbreviation recommended by the U.S. Postal Service (USPS) (Table 7-1).
- Leave one space between the state and the zip code; include the zip + 4 code, if known.

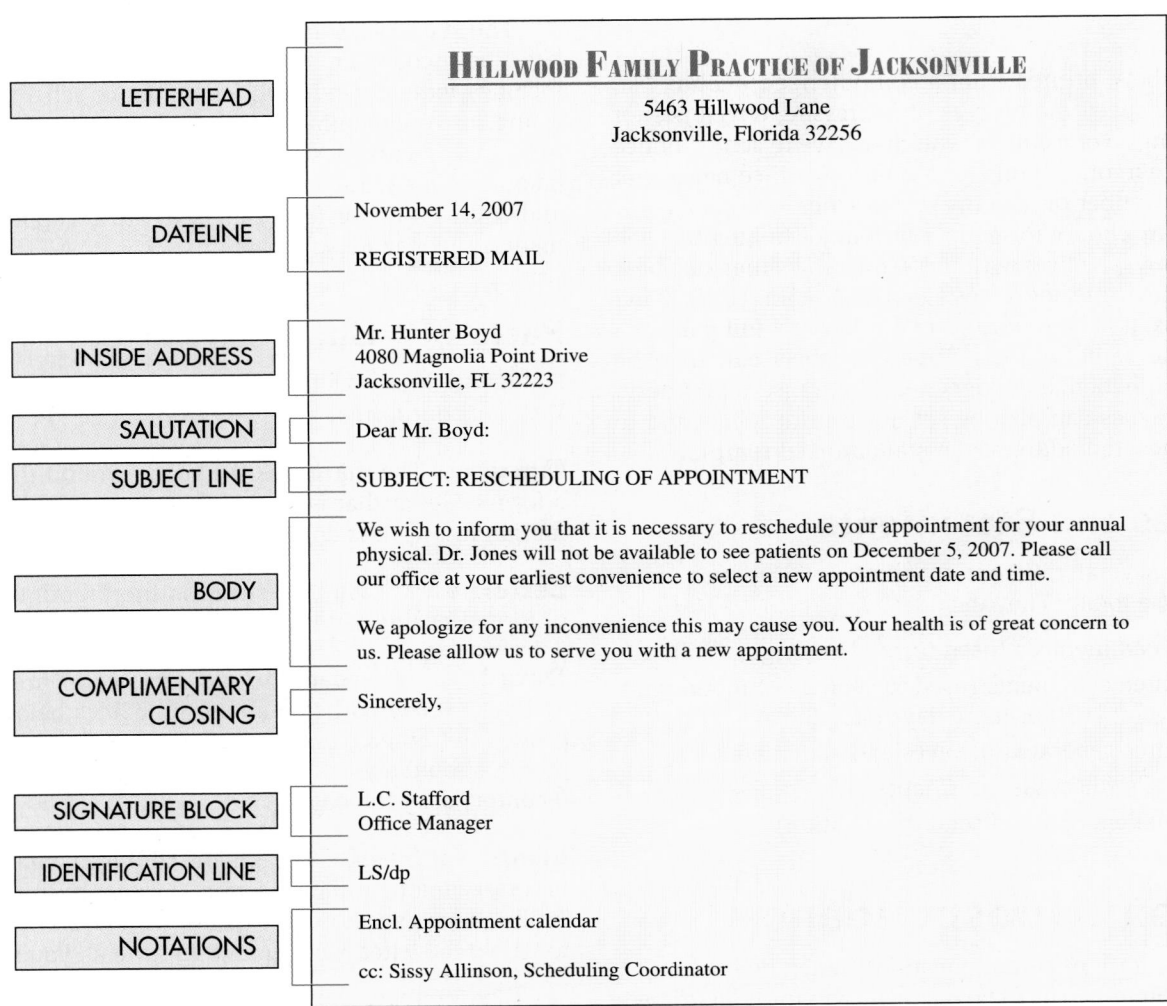

**Figure 7-2.** Knowing the parts of a typical business letter enables medical assistants to create written communications that reflect well on the office.

| TABLE 7-1 | USPS State Abbreviations | | |
|-----------|--------------|--------|--------------|
| **State** | **Abbreviation** | **State** | **Abbreviation** |
| Alabama | AL | Idaho | ID |
| Alaska | AK | Illinois | IL |
| Arizona | AZ | Indiana | IN |
| Arkansas | AR | Iowa | IA |
| California | CA | Kansas | KS |
| Colorado | CO | Kentucky | KY |
| Connecticut | CT | Louisiana | LA |
| Delaware | DE | Maine | ME |
| District of Columbia | DC | Maryland | MD |
| Florida | FL | Massachusetts | MA |
| Georgia | GA | Michigan | MI |

## TABLE 7-1    USPS State Abbreviations (concluded)

| State | Abbreviation | State | Abbreviation |
|---|---|---|---|
| Hawaii | HI | Minnesota | MN |
| Mississippi | MS | Pennsylvania | PA |
| Missouri | MO | Puerto Rico | PR |
| Montana | MT | Rhode Island | RI |
| Nebraska | NE | South Carolina | SC |
| Nevada | NV | South Dakota | SD |
| New Hampshire | NH | Tennessee | TN |
| New Jersey | NJ | Texas | TX |
| New Mexico | NM | Utah | UT |
| New York | NY | Vermont | VT |
| North Carolina | NC | Virginia | VA |
| North Dakota | ND | Washington | WA |
| Ohio | OH | West Virginia | WV |
| Oklahoma | OK | Wisconsin | WI |
| Oregon | OR | Wyoming | WY |

**Attention Line.**   An attention line is used when a letter is addressed to a company but sent to the attention of a particular individual. If you do not know the name of the individual, call the company directly to inquire the name of the appropriate contact person. A colon between the word *Attention* and the person's name is optional.

**Salutation.**   When addressing a person by name, use a **salutation,** a written greeting such as "Dear," followed by Mr., Mrs., or Ms., and the person's last name. The salutation should be keyed at the left margin on the second line below the inside address. A colon should follow. When you do not know the name, it is becoming common practice to use the business title or department in the salutation, as in "Dear Sir," "Dear Laboratory Director," or "Dear Claims Department." This also avoids confusion if you do not know the gender of a person with a name such as Pat or Chris.

**Subject Line.**   A **subject line** is sometimes used to bring the subject of the letter to the reader's attention. The subject line is not required. However, if it is used, it should be keyed on the second line below the salutation. The subject line may be flush with the left margin, indented five spaces, or centered to the page. The subject line should be limited to two to three words and should be keyed in all capital letters to capture the attention of the reader.

**Body.**   The **body** of the letter begins two lines below the salutation or subject line. The text is single-spaced with double-spacing between paragraphs.

If the body contains a list, set the list apart from the rest of the text. Leave an extra line of space above and

below the list. For each item in the list, indent five to ten spaces from each margin. Single-space within items, but leave an extra line between items. A bulleted list has a small, solid, round circle before each item.

**Complimentary Closing.**   The **complimentary closing** is placed two lines below the last line of the body. Capitalize only the first word of the closing. "Sincerely" is a common closing. "Very truly yours" and "Best regards" are also acceptable closings in business correspondence.

**Signature Block.**   The **signature block** contains the writer's name on the first line and the writer's business title on the second line. The block is aligned with the complimentary closing and typed three to four lines below it, to allow space for the signature.

**Identification Line.**   The letter writer's initials followed by a colon or slash and the typist's initials are sometimes included in the letter. These initials are called the **identification line.** This line is typed flush left, two lines below the signature block.

**Notations.**   **Notations** include information such as the number of **enclosures** that are included with the letter and the names of other people who will be receiving copies of the letter (sometimes referred to as cc's, or carbon copies). If there are enclosures, a notation should appear flush left, one or two lines below the identification line (or one or two lines below the signature block, if no identification line is present). You may abbreviate the word *Enclosure* by typing "Enc," "Encl," or "Encs" (with or without punctuation, depending on the style of the letter you are writing). The copy notation, "cc," appears after the enclosure notation and includes one or more names or initials.

## Punctuation Styles

Two different styles of punctuation are used in correspondence: open punctuation and mixed punctuation. A writer should use one punctuation style consistently throughout a letter.

**Open Punctuation.**   This style uses no punctuation after the following items when they appear in a letter:

- The word *Attention* in the attention line
- The salutation
- The complimentary closing
- The signature block
- The enclosure and copy notations

**Mixed Punctuation.**   This style includes the following punctuation marks used in specific instances:

- A colon after *Attention* in the attention line
- A colon after the salutation
- A comma after the complimentary closing
- A colon or period after the enclosure notation
- A colon after the copy notation

## Letter Format

Follow these general formatting guidelines for all letters.

- With paper 8½ inches wide, it is common to use 1-inch margins on the left and right.
- Roughly center the letter on the page according to the length of the letter. For shorter letters, you can use wider margins and start the address farther down the page. For longer letters, use standard margins but start higher up on the page.
- Single-space the body of the letter. Double-space between paragraphs or parts of the letter.
- Use short sentences (no more than 20 words on average).
- Include at least two sentences in each paragraph.
- Divide long paragraphs—more than 10 lines of type— into shorter ones.

For multipage letters, use letterhead for the first page and blank paper for the subsequent pages. (When you order letterhead, be sure to order blank paper of the same type as the letterhead for subsequent sheets.) Using a 1-inch margin at the top, include a heading with the addressee, date, and page number on all pages following the first one. Resume typing or printing the text about three lines below the heading.

## Letter Styles

Different letter styles are used for different purposes. Your office is likely to have a preferred style in place. The four most common letter styles are full-block, modified-block, modified-block with indented paragraphs, and simplified.

**Full-Block Style.**   The **full-block letter style,** also called block style, is typed with all lines flush left. Figure 7-3 shows an example of the block letter style. This style may include a subject line two lines below the salutation. Block-style letters are quick and easy to write because there are no indented paragraphs to slow the typist. Block style is one of the most common formats used in the medical office.

**Modified-Block Style.**   The **modified-block letter style** is similar to full block but differs in that the dateline, complimentary closing, signature block, and notations are aligned and begin at the center of the page or slightly to the right. This type of letter has a traditional, balanced appearance.

**Modified-Block Style with Indented Paragraphs.**   This style is identical to the modified-block style except that the paragraphs are indented one-half inch.

**Simplified Style.**   The **simplified letter style** is a modification of the full-block style. Figure 7-4 shows an example of the simplified letter style. The salutation is omitted, eliminating the need for a courtesy title. A subject line in all-capital letters is placed between the address and the body of the letter. The subject line summarizes the main point of the letter but does not actually use the word *subject*. All text is typed flush left. The complimentary closing is omitted, and the sender's name and title are typed in capital letters in a single line at the end of the letter. Note that this letter style always uses open punctuation, so it is both easy to read and quick to type. In most situations in a medical office, however, the simplified letter style may be too informal.

## Effective Writing

To create effective, professional correspondence that reflects well on the practice, be sure that you use an appropriate style, clear and **concise** language, and the active voice. Though there are many forms of written communication other than a business letter, all of them must be written in such as way as to convey information clearly. Most medical practices make use of internal memos and external forms of communication, including all types of business letters. Following are some general tips to help you write more effectively.

- Before you write, know the type of person to whom you are writing. Is the letter to a physician, a patient, a vendor, or fellow staff members? Decide if the tone should be formal or more relaxed.

**ABC PUBLISHERS, INC.**

July 10, 2007

Ms. Lara Erickson
2594 Hughes Boulevard
Hamilton City, NJ 08999

Dear Ms. Erickson:

SUBJECT: SHIPMENT DELAY

Thank you for contacting us regarding your order for *Smith and Doe's New Medical Dictionary*. Due to an unexpectedly heavy demand for the book, we are experiencing delays in processing and shipping orders.

We expect to ship your book in four weeks, around August 15. Because of this delay, we offer you the option of canceling your order with a full refund. If you would like to cancel at this point, please fill out and return the enclosed postcard. If we do not hear from you, your order will be shipped when ready.

We are sorry for any inconvenience this delay may cause you. Please be assured that ABC Publishers values its customers and always endeavors to fulfill orders in a timely fashion.

Sincerely yours,

*Andrew Williams*

Andrew Williams
Customer Service Manager

AW/cjc
Enclosure

*117 New Avenue New York, NY 10000*

**Figure 7-3.** The full-block letter style is quicker and easier to type than other styles.

**ABC PUBLISHERS, INC.**

July 10, 2007

Ms. Lara Erickson
2594 Hughes Boulevard
Hamilton City, NJ 08999

SHIPMENT DELAY

Thank you for contacting us regarding your order for *Smith and Doe's New Medical Dictionary*. Due to an unexpectedly heavy demand for the book, we are experiencing delays in processing and shipping orders.

We expect to ship your book in four weeks, around August 15. Because of this delay, we offer you the option of canceling your order with a full refund. If you would like to cancel at this point, please fill out and return the enclosed postcard. If we do not hear from you, your order will be shipped when ready.

We are sorry for any inconvenience this delay may cause you. Please be assured that ABC Publishers values its customers and always endeavors to fulfill orders in a timely fashion.

*Andrew Williams*

ANDREW WILLIAMS, CUSTOMER SERVICE MANAGER

AW/cjc
Enclosure

*117New Avenue  New York, NY  10000*

**Figure 7-4.** The simplified letter style is considered by some executives to be the most readable style for correspondence.

- Know the purpose of the letter before you begin, and make sure your letter accurately conveys that purpose.
- Be concise. Use short sentences. Be brief. Be specific.
- Do not use unnecessary words. Use the simplest way to say what you mean.
- Show **clarity** in your writing; state your message so that it can be understood easily.
- Use the active voice whenever possible. Voice shows whether the subject of a sentence is acting or is being acted upon. Here is an example of the active voice:

    "Dr. Huang is seeing 18 patients today."

    Here is an example of the same sentence, written in the passive voice:

    "Eighteen patients will be seen by Dr. Huang today."

    Note that the active voice is more direct and livelier to read.
- Use the passive voice, however, to soften the impact of negative news:

    "Your account will be turned over to a collection agency if we do not receive payment promptly."

    It would sound harsher to say:

    "We will turn over your account to a collection agency if we do not receive payment promptly."
- Always be polite and courteous.
- Always check spelling and the accuracy of dates and monetary figures.
- Always check your grammar. Do not use slang.
- Avoid leaving "widows and orphans" or dangling words and phrases. These are words and short phrases at the end or beginning of paragraphs that are left to sit alone at the top or bottom of a page or column or separated from the rest of the thought. Do not start a paragraph at the bottom of a page if the rest of the sentence must be continued on the next page.

# Editing and Proofreading

Editing and proofreading take place after you create the first draft of a letter. **Editing** involves checking a document for factual accuracy, logical flow, conciseness, clarity, and tone. **Proofreading** involves checking a document for grammatical, spelling, and format errors. When possible, ask another person to proofread your work as well. *Never* skip over the very important steps of editing and proofreading!

## Tools for Editing and Proofreading

Reference books can help you prepare letters that appear professional. Keep the following tools available.

**Dictionary.**  An up-to-date dictionary gives you more than definitions of words. A dictionary tells you how to spell, divide, and pronounce a word and what part of speech it is, such as a noun or adjective. A dictionary can be accessed on the Internet or in book form.

**Medical Dictionary.**  It is nearly impossible for even the most experienced health-care professional to be familiar with every medical term and its correct spelling. A medical dictionary will serve as a handy reference for terms with which you are unfamiliar or about which you would like more information. Like a regular dictionary, a medical dictionary can also be accessed on the Internet or in book form. However, a medical dictionary in book form may not have the most updated terms. Like other medical books, a medical dictionary usually needs to be replaced frequently.

Becoming familiar with some of the prefixes and suffixes commonly used in medical terms can help you understand the meanings of many words. Appendix IV at the back of the book lists some common medical prefixes and suffixes.

**Thesaurus.**  A thesaurus provides synonyms or similar words to a word you are using. It helps you avoid repetition in your writing and helps you find a word for an idea you have in mind. A thesaurus can be found in word processing programs, in print, and online.

***Physicians' Desk Reference (PDR).***  The *PDR* is a dictionary of medications. Published yearly, it provides up-to-date information on both prescription and nonprescription drugs. Consult the *PDR* for the correct spelling of a particular drug or for other information about its usage, side effects, contraindications, and so on.

**English Grammar and Usage Manuals.**  These manuals answer questions concerning grammar and word usage. They usually contain sections on punctuation, capitalization, and other details of written communication.

**Word Processing Spelling Checkers.**  Most word processing programs used in medical offices have built-in spelling checkers. There are also programs designed specifically to check spelling in medical documents. These spelling checkers include most common medical terms that would not be found in a regular software program.

Spelling checkers pick up many spelling errors and often give suggestions for correct spellings. If you indicate the choice you meant to input, the program automatically replaces the misspelled word. These programs may not detect all spelling errors, however. They should not be relied on as the only means of checking a document. For example, spelling checkers cannot tell you that you used the wrong word if you type the word *form* instead of *from*, because *form* is also a correctly spelled word.

You may be able to add words that are not currently recognized by the spelling checker in your computer. Use this feature to add medical terms. A word of caution is important here! Before you add the word to the computer's dictionary, be sure to look up the exact spelling in a medical dictionary. The computer will recognize only the spelling you add. If you place the *wrong* spelling in the computer, your spelling checker will not correct it.

When you type e-mails, take special care to use correct grammar and punctuation. Spelling checkers are available in most e-mail programs and should be used at the completion of the e-mail. The e-mail spelling checker does not automatically point out mistakes as you type.

Some software packages offer grammar-checking and style-checking features. These programs can identify certain problems, but the person using them still needs to know basic rules of grammar and style to correct errors.

## Editing

The editing process ensures that a document is accurate, clear, and complete; free of grammatical errors; organized logically; and written in an appropriate style. It is a good idea to leave some time between the writing and editing stages so that you can look at the document in a fresh light. As you edit, you must examine language usage, content, and style.

**Language Usage.** Learn basic grammar rules. When in doubt, refer to a grammar handbook or reference manual. Make sure all sentences are complete. Continually ask yourself, Is this the best way to convey what I want to say? Do my word choices reflect the overall tone of the document? For example, in a business letter, you would avoid choosing phrases that are too casual such as, "Thanks a million" or "Take it easy." These expressions are inappropriate for a business letter.

**Content.** A business letter should contain all the necessary information the writer intends to convey. If you are editing someone else's letter and something appears to be missing, check with the writer. She or he may have omitted information by mistake.

The content of a letter should follow a logical thought pattern. Create a clean, concise letter by:

- Stating the purpose of the letter in the first sentence
- Discussing one topic at a time
- Changing paragraphs when you change topics

- Listing events in chronological order
- Sticking to the subject
- Selecting words carefully
- Reading over what you have written before printing

**Style.** Use a writing style that is appropriate to the reader. A letter written to a patient is likely to require a different style than one written to a physician.

## Proofreading

Proofreading means thoroughly checking a document for errors. After editing a document, put it aside for a short time before proofreading it. Ideally, have a coworker proofread your work. Someone else will often notice errors that you may miss. There are three types of errors that can occur when preparing a document: formatting, data, and mechanical.

**Formatting Errors.** These errors involve the positioning of the various parts of a letter. They may include errors in indenting, line length, or line spacing. To avoid these errors, take the following two steps:

1. Scan the letter to make sure that the indentions are consistent, that the spacing is correct, and that the text is centered from left to right and top to bottom.
2. Follow the office style.

**Data Errors.** Data errors involve mistyping monetary figures, such as a balance on a patient statement. Verify the accuracy of all figures by checking them twice or by having another coworker check them.

**Mechanical Errors.** Mechanical errors are errors in spelling, punctuation, spacing between words, and division of words. Mechanical errors also include reversing words or characters, typing them twice, or omitting them altogether. Here are some tips to help you avoid mechanical errors.

- Learn basic spelling, punctuation, and word division rules. When in doubt, be sure to check a manual on English usage. Table 7-2 presents some basic rules

| TABLE 7-2 | Basic Rules of Writing |
|---|---|
| **Word Division** | Divide:<br>• According to pronunciation<br>• Compound words between the two words from which they derive<br>• Hyphenated compound words at the hyphen<br>• After a prefix<br>• Before a suffix<br>• Between two consonants that appear between vowels<br>• Before *-ing* unless the last consonant is doubled; in that case, divide before the second consonant |

| TABLE 7-2 | Basic Rules of Writing *(concluded)* |
|---|---|
| | Do not divide:<br>• Such suffixes as *-sion, -tial,* and *-gion*<br>• A word so that only one letter is left on a line |
| **Capitalization** | Capitalize:<br>• All proper names<br>• All titles, positions, or indications of family relation when preceding a proper name or in place of a proper noun (not when used alone or with possessive pronouns or articles)<br>• Days of the week, months, and holidays<br>• Names of organizations and membership designations<br>• Racial, religious, and political designations<br>• Adjectives, nouns, and verbs that are derived from proper nouns (including currently copyrighted trade names)<br>• Specific addresses and geographic locations<br>• Sums of money written in legal or business documents<br>• Titles, headings of books, magazines, and newspapers |
| **Plurals** | • Add *s* or *es* to most singular nouns (Plural forms of most medical terms do not follow this rule.)<br>• With medical terms ending in *is,* drop the *is* and add *es:*<br>    metastasis/metastases<br>    epiphysis/epiphyses<br>• With terms ending in *um,* drop the *um* and add *a:*<br>    diverticulum/diverticula<br>    atrium/atria<br>• With terms ending in *us,* drop the *us* and add *i:*<br>    calculus/calculi<br>    bronchus/bronchi<br>(Two exceptions to this are virus/viruses and sinus/sinuses.)<br>• With terms ending in *a,* keep the *a* and add *e:*<br>    vertebra/vertebrae |
| **Possessives** | To show ownership or relation to another noun:<br>• For singular nouns, add an apostrophe and an *s*<br>• For plural nouns that do not end in an *s,* add an apostrophe and an *s*<br>• For plural nouns that end in an *s,* just add an apostrophe |
| **Numbers** | Use numerals:<br>• In general writing, when the number is 11 or greater<br>• With abbreviations and symbols<br>• When discussing laboratory results or statistics<br>• When referring to specific sums of money<br>• When using a series of numbers in a sentence<br><br>Tips:<br>• Use commas when numerals have more than three digits<br>• Do not use commas when referring to account numbers, page numbers, or policy numbers<br>• Use a hyphen with numerals to indicate a range |

concerning the mechanics of writing. Table 7-3 lists some of the most commonly misspelled medical terms and other words.

- Check carefully for transposed characters or words.
- Avoid dividing words at the end of a line. Most word processing programs automatically wrap words to the next line, so if you are writing on a computer, word division should not present a problem.

Creating a business letter involves many steps. Procedure 7-1 organizes these steps for you.

# Preparing Outgoing Mail

After you have created, edited, and proofread a letter, you need to prepare it for mailing. This preparation includes having the letter signed, preparing the envelope, and folding and inserting the letter into the envelope (Figure 7-5). It will then be ready for postage to be calculated and affixed.

## Signing Letters

After the letter is complete—it has been proofread and the envelope and enclosures have been prepared—it is ready for signing. Some doctors authorize other staff members to sign for them. If you have been authorized to sign letters, you should sign the doctor's name and place your initials after the doctor's signature.

If the doctor prefers to sign all letters, you should place the letter on the doctor's desk in a file folder marked "For Your Signature." If the letter is of an urgent nature, give it to the doctor as soon as possible. Otherwise, you can collect several letters in the folder and present the entire group for signing at one time. However, all prepared work should be given to the physician at the end of the day.

## Preparing the Envelope

To ensure the quickest delivery of mail, the USPS has issued several guidelines for preparing envelopes. The USPS uses electronic **optical character readers (OCRs)** to help speed mail processing. OCRs read the last two lines of an address and sort the mail accordingly. To take advantage of this technology, envelopes must be no smaller than $3\frac{1}{2}$ by 5 inches and no larger than $6\frac{1}{8}$ by $11\frac{1}{2}$ inches. They must be addressed in a specific format that can be read by the OCR. Use USPS guidelines for addressing envelopes.

| TABLE 7-3 Commonly Misspelled Medical Terms and Other Words | | | |
|---|---|---|---|
| **Medical Terms** | | | |
| abscess | dissect | leukocyte | prescription |
| aerobic | eosinophil | malaise | prophylaxis |
| anergic | epididymis | menstruation | prostate |
| anesthetic | epistaxis | metastasis | prosthesis |
| aneurysm | erythema | muscle | pruritus |
| anteflexion | eustachian | neuron | psoriasis |
| arrhythmia | fissure | nosocomial | psychiatrist |
| asepsis | flexure | occlusion | pyrexia |
| asthma | fomites | ophthalmology | respiration |
| auricle | glaucoma | oscilloscope | rheumatism |
| benign | glomerular | osseous | roentgenology |
| bilirubin | gonorrhea | palliative | scirrhous |
| bronchial | hemocytometer | parasite | serous |
| calcaneus | hemorrhage | parenteral | specimen |
| capillary | hemorrhoids | parietal | sphincter |
| cervical | homeostasis | paroxysm | sphygmomanometer |
| chancre | humerus | pericardium | squamous |
| choroid | ileum | perineum | staphylococcus |
| chromosome | ilium | peristalsis | surgeon |
| cirrhosis | infarction | peritoneum | vaccine |
| clavicle | inoculate | pharynx | vein |
| curettage | intussusception | pituitary | venous |
| cyanosis | ischemia | plantar | wheal |
| defibrillator | ischium | pleurisy | |
| desiccation | larynx | pneumonia | |
| diluent | leukemia | polyp | |

**Other Words**

| | | | |
|---|---|---|---|
| absence | defendant | its | pronunciation |
| accept | definite | it's | psychiatry |
| accessible | dependent | labeled | psychology |
| accommodate | description | laboratory | pursue |
| accumulate | desirable | led | questionnaire |
| achieve | development | leisure | rearrange |
| acquire | dilemma | liable | recede |
| adequate | disappear | liaison | receive |
| advantageous | disappoint | license | recommend |
| affect | disapprove | liquefy | referral |
| aggravate | disastrous | maintenance | relieve |
| all right | discreet | maneuver | repetition |
| a lot | discrete | miscellaneous | rescind |
| already | discrimination | misspelled | résumé |
| altogether | dissatisfied | necessary | rhythm |
| analysis | dissipate | noticeable | ridiculous |
| analyze | earnest | occasion | schedule |
| apparatus | ecstasy | occurrence | secretary |
| apparent | effect | offense | seize |
| appearance | eligible | oscillate | separate |
| appropriate | embarrass | paid | similar |
| approximate | emphasis | pamphlet | sizable |
| argument | entrepreneur | panicky | stationary |
| assistance | envelope | paradigm | stationery |
| associate | environment | parallel | stomach |
| auxiliary | exceed | paralyze | subpoena |
| balloon | except | pastime | succeed |
| bankruptcy | exercise | persevere | suddenness |
| believe | exhibit | persistent | supersede |
| benefited | exhilaration | personal | surprise |
| brochure | existence | personnel | tariff |
| bulletin | fantasy | persuade | technique |
| business | fascinate | phenomenon | temperament |
| category | February | plagiarism | temperature |
| changeable | fluorescent | pleasant | thorough |
| characteristic | forty | possession | transferred |
| cigarette | grammar | precede | truly |
| circumstance | grievance | precedent | tyrannize |
| clientele | guarantee | predictable | unnecessary |
| committee | handkerchief | predominant | until |
| comparative | height | prejudice | vacillate |
| complement | humorous | preparation | vacuum |
| compliment | hygiene | prerogative | vegetable |
| concede | incidentally | prevalent | vicious |
| conscientious | indispensable | principal | warrant |
| conscious | inimitable | principle | Wednesday |
| controversy | insistent | privilege | weird |
| corroborate | irrelevant | procedure | |
| counsel | irresistible | proceed | |
| courtesy | irritable | professor | |

# Creating a Letter

**Procedure Goal:** To follow standard procedure for constructing a business letter

**Materials:** Word processor or personal computer, letterhead paper, dictionaries or other sources

**Method:**

1. Format the letter according to the office's standard procedure. Use the same punctuation and style throughout.

   *Rationale*

   Consistency in format creates a professional-looking document.

2. Start the dateline three lines below the last line of the printed letterhead. (Note: Depending on the length of the letter, it is acceptable to start between two and six lines below the letterhead.)

   *Rationale*

   The letter should be centered both vertically and horizontally on the page for visual appeal.

3. Two lines below the dateline, type in any special mailing instructions (such as REGISTERED MAIL, CERTIFIED MAIL, and so on).

4. Three lines below any special instructions, begin the inside address.

   Type the addressee's courtesy title (Mr., Mrs., Ms.) and full name on the first line. If a professional title is given (M.D., RN, Ph.D.), type this title after the addressee's name instead of using a courtesy title.

   *Rationale*

   A professional title is used when available in professional correspondence. Never use both a courtesy title and professional title at the same time.

5. Type the addressee's business title, if applicable, on the second line.

   Type the company name on the third line. Type the street address on the fourth line, including the apartment or suite number.

   Type the city, state, and zip code on the fifth line. Use the standard two-letter abbreviation for the state, followed by one space and the zip code.

6. Two lines below the inside address, type the salutation, using the appropriate courtesy title (Mr., Mrs., Ms., Dr.) prior to typing the addressee's last name.

   *Rationale*

   The salutation uses a courtesy title. Do not include the professional title or the addressee's first name in the salutation.

7. Two lines below the salutation, type the subject line, if applicable.

8. Two lines below the subject line, begin the body of the letter. Single-space between lines. Double-space between paragraphs.

9. Two lines below the body of the letter, type the complimentary closing.

10. Leave three blank lines (return four times), and begin the signature block. (Enough space must be left to allow for the signature.) Type the sender's name on the first line. Type the sender's title on the second line.

    *Rationale*

    Adequate space must be left for the signature. If the signer has a long signature, more than three blank lines may be left. Typing the name allows the addressee to understand who sent the letter if the sender's signature is not legible.

11. Two lines below the sender's title, type the identification line. Type the sender's initials in all capitals and your initials in lowercase letters, separating the two sets of initials with a colon or a forward slash.

12. One or two lines below the identification line, type the enclosure notation, if applicable.

13. Two lines below the enclosure notation, type the copy notation, if applicable.

14. Edit the letter.

    *Rationale*

    Make appropriate changes to clarify the meaning of the letter.

15. Proofread and spell check the letter.

    *Rationale*

    Every letter must be read again to assure there are no errors.

## How to Fold a Standard Letter

A business letter is folded twice into horizontal thirds and placed into an envelope. This insures a little privacy in the letter. The letter is also easy to unfold after opening the envelope. The following diagram shows how a letter is normally folded. This type of fold is used regardless of letter style.

If the letter needs to have the address face out an envelope window, make the second fold in the same location but opposite direction. The letter will then be folded in a Z shape and the address can be positioned to face out the window of the envelope.

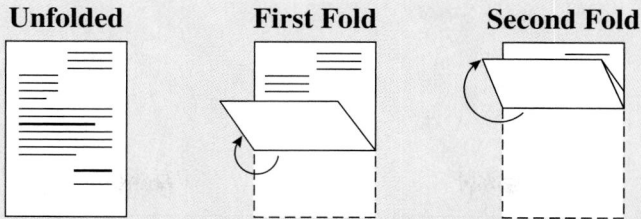

| Unfolded | First Fold | Second Fold |

Make a second horizontal crease one third from the top of the letter where the bottom of the letter had been folded to. Tuck the bottom into this crease and fold the top over it. The letter will be folded into thirds. It will fit any standard envelope.

If you are folding the letter so the address faces out the envelope window, fold the letter toward the back instead of the front. The letter address will appear through the envelope window, but it will still be folded in thirds.

**Figure 7-5.** It is important to fold a business letter correctly.

**Address Placement.** The address must be placed in a certain location on the envelope for reading by the OCR (Figure 7-6). The area the OCR can read has the following characteristics:

- It is bordered by a 1-inch margin on both the left and right sides of the envelope.
- It has a ⅝-inch margin on the bottom. The top of the city/state/zip code line (the last line in the address block) must be no higher than 2¼ inches from the bottom edge of the envelope.
- An area 4½ inches wide in the bottom right corner of the envelope should be left clear. The OCR reads the address and prints a bar code that corresponds to the zip code in this area.

**Address Format.** When you type an address, follow these format guidelines:

- Type or machine-print (for example, by computer) the address. (The OCR cannot read handwriting.) Using all CAPS for the address is suggested. The OCR cannot read fancy script fonts.
- Single-space the lines and use the block format. Use only one or two spaces between numbers and words in the address.

- Use only USPS-approved abbreviations for location designations, as presented in Table 7-4.
- Put the addressee's name on the first line of the address block, the department (if any) on the second line, and the company name on the third line. If the letter is to go to someone's attention at a company, put the company name on the first line and "Attention: [Name]" on the second line.
- The line above the city, state, and zip code should contain the street address or post office box number. Include suite or apartment numbers on the same line as the street address.
- The last line of the address must include the city, state, and zip code. Use the zip + 4 code whenever possible.
- Include the hyphen in the zip + 4 code, for example, 08520-6142. Obtain current zip codes by logging on to the USPS Web page at http://zip4.usps.com.
- Type any special notations (such as SPECIAL DELIVERY, CERTIFIED, or REGISTERED) two lines below the postage in all-capital letters. This information should appear outside the area the OCR can read.
- Type any handling instructions (such as PERSONAL or CONFIDENTIAL) three lines below the return address. This information should also be outside the area the OCR can read.

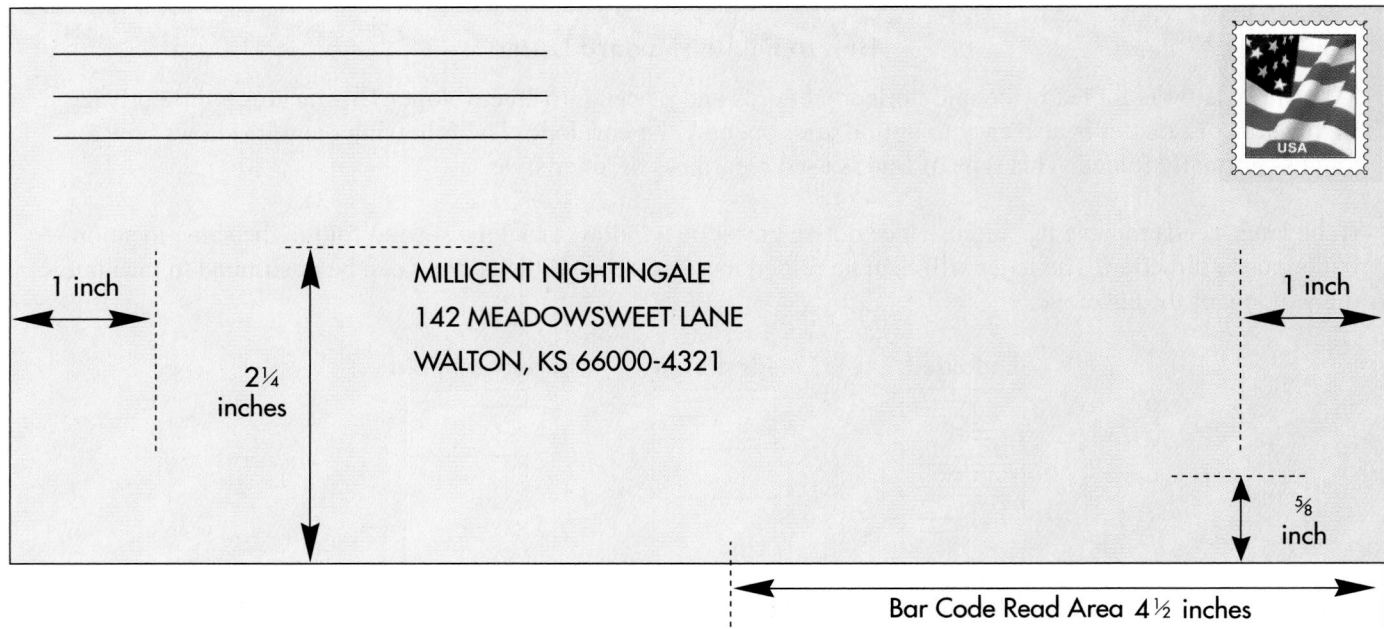

MILLICENT NIGHTINGALE
142 MEADOWSWEET LANE
WALTON, KS 66000-4321

1 inch

1 inch

2¼ inches

⅝ inch

Bar Code Read Area 4½ inches

**Figure 7-6.** Following this format for typing an envelope ensures that it can be processed by USPS electronic equipment.

| TABLE 7-4 | USPS Abbreviations | | |
|---|---|---|---|
| **Word** | **Abbreviation** | **Word** | **Abbreviation** |
| Avenue | AVE | Highway | HWY |
| Boulevard | BLVD | Junction | JCT |
| Center | CTR | Lane | LN |
| Circle | CIR | North | N |
| Corner | COR | Parkway | PKY |
| Court | CT | Place | PL |
| Drive | DR | Plaza | PLZ |
| East | E | South | S |
| Expressway | EXPY | West | W |

- Letters going to foreign countries should have the name of the country on the last line of the address block in all-capital letters.
- Some letters may be appropriate for interoffice or company mail systems. These letters are usually placed in a large envelope with multiple address lines. The enveloped can be reused many times by crossing out the previous name and address and using the next line. Place interoffice mail in a specially designated area or basket for pickup. Be sure not to mix it with outgoing mail.

## Folding and Inserting Mail

Letters and invoices must be folded neatly before they are inserted into the envelopes. The proper way to fold a letter depends on the type of envelope into which the letter will fit.

- With a small envelope, fold the enclosure in half lengthwise, and insert it.
- With a regular business-size envelope, fold the letter in thirds. Fold the bottom third up first, then the top third down, and insert the letter.

- With a window envelope, use an accordion fold. Fold the bottom third up. Then, fold the top third back so that the address appears in the window and insert the enclosure.

Before folding the letter, double-check that it has been signed, that all enclosures are included, and that the address on the letter matches the one on the envelope. Any enclosures that are not attached to the letter should be placed inside the folds so that they will be removed from the envelope along with the letter. (See Chapter 5 for information about folding and inserting machines.)

# Mailing Equipment and Supplies

The proper equipment and supplies will help you handle the mail efficiently and cost-effectively. In addition to letterhead, blank stationery for multipage letters, and envelopes, you will need some standard supplies. The USPS provides forms, labels, and packaging for items that need special attention, such as airmail, Priority Mail, Express Mail, certified mail, or registered mail. Private delivery companies, such as United Parcel Service (UPS) and Federal Express (FedEx), also provide shipping supplies to their customers.

## Airmail Supplies

In the past, any piece of mail that was transported by air was designated as airmail. Today nearly all first-class mail outside a local area is routinely sent by air. However, airmail services are still available for some packages and for most mail going to foreign countries.

If you are sending an item by airmail, attach special airmail stickers, available from the post office, on all sides. (The word *AIRMAIL* can also be neatly written on all sides.) Special airmail envelopes for letters can be purchased from the USPS.

## Envelopes for Overnight Delivery Services

For correspondence or packages that must be delivered by the next day, a number of overnight delivery services are available through the USPS and private companies. Most companies require the use of their own envelopes and mailing materials. Make sure you keep adequate supplies on hand.

## Postal Rates, Scales, and Meters

Postal rates and regulations change periodically, and every medical office should have a copy of the latest guidelines. These guidelines are available from the USPS. Chapter 5 describes postal scales and meters.

# U.S. Postal Service Delivery

The USPS offers a variety of domestic and international delivery services for letters and packages. As a result of a comprehensive USPS Transformation Plan in 2002, many new services were added to the post office. As a result, the post office became much better able to compete with other mail and package delivery services. Following are some of the services you will be most likely to use in a medical office setting.

## Regular Mail Service

Regular mail delivery includes several classes of mail as well as other designations such as Priority Mail and Express Mail. The class or designation determines how quickly a piece of mail is delivered.

**First-Class Mail.** Most correspondence generated in a medical office—letters, postcards, and invoices—is sent by first-class mail. Items must weigh 11 ounces or less to be considered first-class. (An item over 11 ounces that requires quick delivery must be sent by Priority Mail, which is discussed later in the chapter.) The cost of mailing a first-class item is based on its weight. The standard rate is for items 1 ounce or less that are not larger than 6⅛ inches high, 11½ inches wide, and ¼ inch thick. Additional postage is required for items that are heavier or larger. Postage for postcards is less than the letter rate. First-class mail is forwarded at no additional cost.

**Second-Class Mail.** Second-class mail is not used by most medical offices. This class of mail is designed for the delivery of newspapers and periodicals only.

**Third-Class Mail.** Third-class mail is also known as bulk mail. It is not often used in medical offices. Bulk mail is used for the mailing of books, catalogs, and other printed material that weighs less than 16 ounces. This class of mailing is available only to authorized mailers.

**Fourth-Class Mail.** Fourth-class mail is also called parcel post. It is used for items that weigh at least 1 pound but not more than 70 pounds and that do not require speedy delivery. Rates are based on weight and distance. There is a special fourth-class rate for mailing books, manuscripts, and some types of medical information.

**Priority Mail.** Priority class is useful for heavier items that require quicker delivery than is available for fourth-class mail. Any first-class item that weighs between 11 ounces and 70 pounds requires Priority Mail service. Although the rate for Priority Mail varies with the weight of the item and the distance it must travel, the USPS offers a flat rate for all material that can fit into its special Priority Mail envelope. The USPS guarantees delivery of Priority Mail items in 2 to 3 days.

**Express Mail.** Express Mail is the quickest USPS service. Different types are available, including next-day and second-day delivery. Express Mail deliveries are made

365 days a year. Rates vary, depending on the weight and the specific service. A special flat-rate envelope is also available. Items sent by Express Mail are automatically insured against loss or damage. You can drop off packages at the post office or arrange for pickup service.

## Special Postal Services

The USPS offers a variety of special mail delivery services in addition to the regular classes of mail. These services may require an additional fee above and beyond the cost of postage.

**Special Delivery.** Use special delivery if you want an item delivered as soon as it reaches the recipient's post office. Delivery of the item is typically made before the regularly scheduled mail delivery. Special delivery service is available within certain distance limits and during certain hours.

**Certified Mail.** Certified mail offers a guarantee that the item has been received. The item is marked as certified mail and requires the postal carrier to obtain a signature on delivery (Figure 7-7). The signature card is then returned to the sender. The card should be added to the patient's file. This documentation is evidence that the document was not only mailed but also received. The receiver's name is clearly printed along with the signature. The certified mail signature card becomes a legal document, which may be important in court.

**Return Receipt Requested.** You may request a return receipt to obtain proof that an item was delivered. The receipt indicates who received the item and when. You can obtain a return receipt for various types of mail. This type of mail service is very important when a medical practice requires proof that a letter was received. The receipt should be carefully added to the patient record. It may become an important legal document and may be required at a later date in a court of law.

**Registered Mail.** Use registered mail to send items that are valuable, irreplaceable, or otherwise important. Registered mail provides the sender with evidence of mailing and delivery. It also provides the security that an item is being tracked as it is transported through the postal system. Because of this tracking process, delivery may be slightly delayed.

To register a piece of mail, take it to the post office and indicate the full value of the item. Both first-class mail and Priority Mail can be registered.

## International Mail

The USPS offers both surface (via ship) and airmail service to most foreign countries. Information on rates and fees is available from the post office.

There are various types of international mail, which are similar to the domestic classes. The USPS also provides international Express Mail and Priority Mail services, along with special mail delivery services such as registered mail, certified mail, and special delivery.

## Tracing Mail

If a piece of registered or certified mail does not reach its destination by the expected time, you can ask the post office to trace it (Figure 7-8). You will need to present your original receipt for the item. You can also trace mail on the Internet through a UPC symbol that is scanned at the post office.

# Other Delivery Services

In addition to the USPS, other companies provide mail and package delivery services across the world. UPS, FedEx, and DHL are three of the largest and most popular of these companies. DHL is one of the newest companies. The costs and types of services vary.

## United Parcel Service

United Parcel Service (UPS) delivers packages and provides overnight letter and express services. You can either drop off packages at a UPS location or have them picked up at your office. Fees vary with the services provided, such as ground or air. Packages are automatically insured against theft or damage.

## Express Delivery Services

Companies such as Federal Express and DHL provide several types of quick delivery services for letters and packages. Rates vary according to weight, time of delivery, and, in some cases, whether you have the package picked up at your office or drop it off at one of the company's local branches.

## Messengers or Couriers

When items must be delivered within the local area on the same day, local messenger services are an option. Many messenger companies are listed in the Yellow Pages of the telephone book.

# Processing Incoming Mail

Mail is an important connection between the office and other professionals and patients. Often an office has an established procedure for handling the mail. It is best to set aside a specific time of the day to process all the incoming mail at once rather than trying to do a little bit at a time.

Although it sounds simple, processing mail involves more than merely opening envelopes. In general, it

**Back side of signature card**

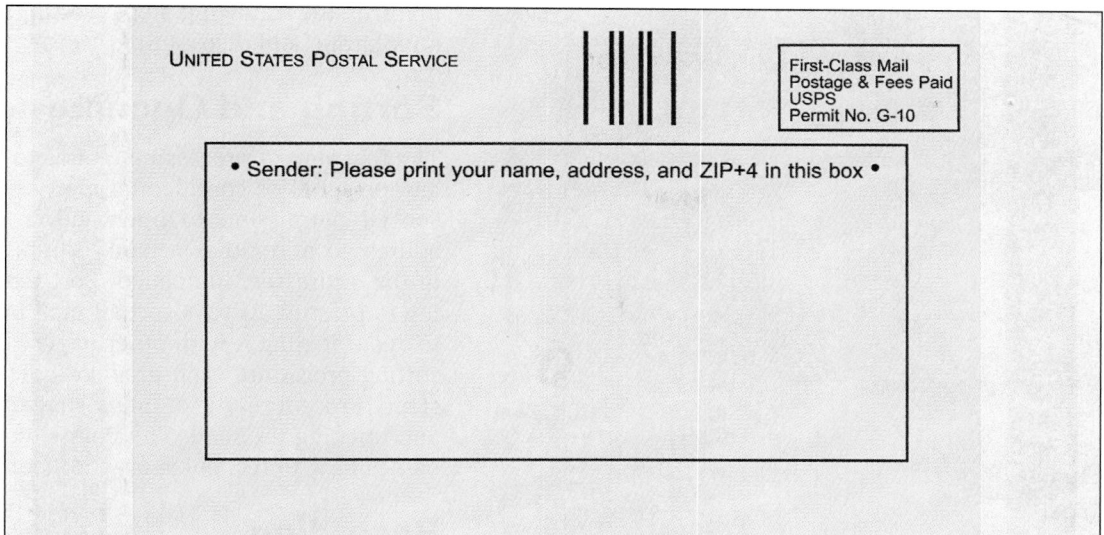

**Front side of signature card**

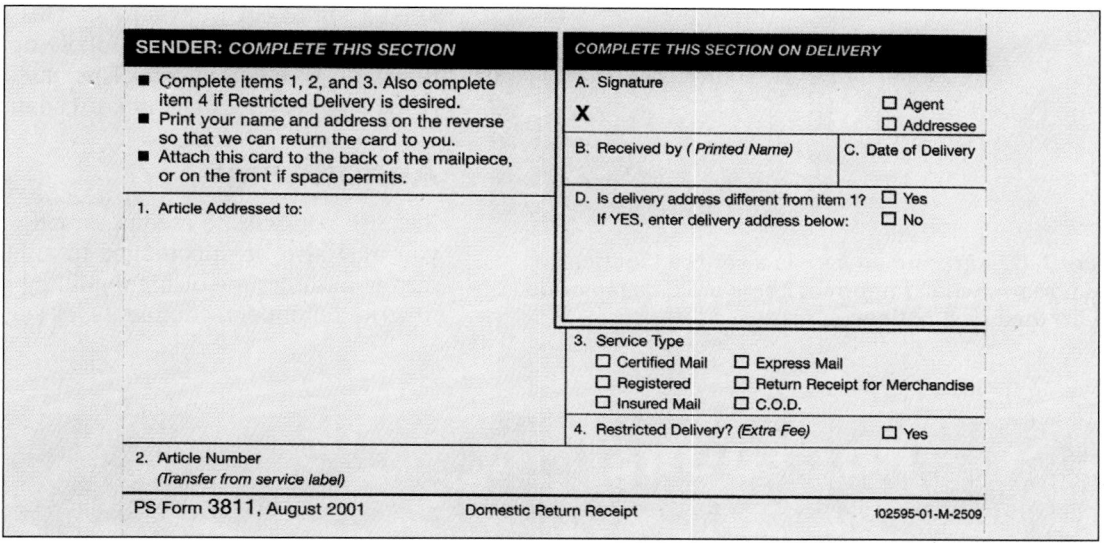

**Certified mail receipt**

**Figure 7-7.** Certified mail offers a guarantee that the item has been received. The item is marked as certified mail and requires the postal carrier to obtain a signature on delivery. Registered mail provides the sender with evidence of mailing and delivery.

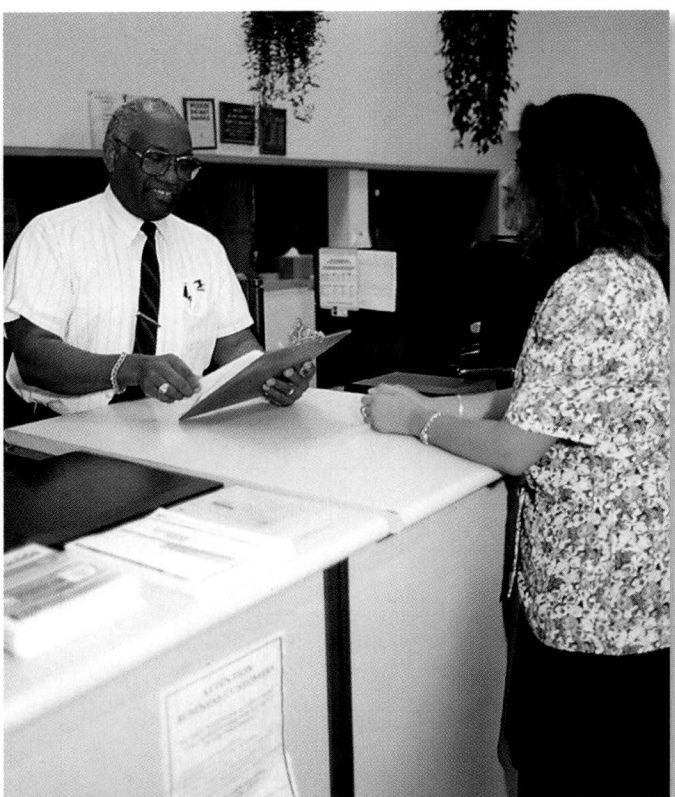

**Figure 7-8.** Tracing an item is a service that post offices perform when important items are delayed or do not reach their destinations.

involves the following steps: sorting, opening, recording, annotating, and distributing.

## Sorting and Opening

The first step in processing mail is to sort it. Always place any personal or confidential mail aside. Unless you have special permission to open, never open personal mail addressed to another person. Carefully lay it on the desk of the addressee, unopened. Sort remaining mail according to priority. Always sort all mail in an uncluttered area to avoid mixing it with other paperwork. Follow a regular sorting procedure each time so that you do not miss any steps. Procedure 7-2 outlines suggested steps for sorting and opening the mail. The Points on Practice section discusses how to recognize urgent incoming mail.

## Recording

Keep a log of each day's mail. This daily record lists the mail received and indicates follow-up correspondence and the date it is completed. This method helps in tracing items and keeping track of correspondence.

## Annotating

Because you will be reading much of the incoming mail, you may also be encouraged to annotate it. To **annotate** means to underline or highlight key points of the letter or to write reminders, comments, or suggested actions in the

## PROCEDURE 7.2

### Sorting and Opening Mail

**Procedure Goal:** To follow a standard procedure for sorting, opening, and processing incoming office mail

**Materials:** Letter opener, date and time stamp (manual or automatic), stapler, paper clips, adhesive notes

**Method:**

1. Check the address on each letter or package to be sure that it has been delivered to the correct location.

2. Sort the mail into piles according to priority and type of mail. Your system may include the following:

   - Top priority. This pile will contain any items that were sent by overnight mail delivery in addition to items sent by registered mail,

   certified mail, or special delivery. (Faxes and e-mail messages are also top priority.)

   - Second priority. This pile will include personal or confidential mail.

   - Third priority. This pile will contain all first-class mail, airmail, and Priority Mail items. These items should be divided into payments received, insurance forms, reports, and other correspondence.

   - Fourth priority. This pile will consist of packages.

   - Fifth priority. This pile will contain magazines and newspapers.

   - Sixth priority. This last pile will include advertisements and catalogs.

3. Set aside all letters labeled "Personal" or "Confidential." Unless you have permission to

*continued* ⟶

# Sorting and Opening Mail (concluded)

open these letters, only the addressee should open them.

4. Arrange all the envelopes with the flaps facing up and away from you.

5. Tap the lower edge of the envelope to shift the contents to the bottom. This step helps to prevent cutting any of the contents when you open the envelope.

6. Open all the envelopes.

### Rationale

It is more efficient to open all the envelopes first and then remove the contents.

7. Remove and unfold the contents, making sure that nothing remains in the envelope.

8. Review each document, and check the sender's name and address.

   • If the letter has no return address, save the envelope, or cut the address off the envelope, and tape it to the letter.

   • Check to see if the address matches the one on the envelope. If there is a difference, staple the envelope to the letter, and make a note to verify the correct address with the sender.

9. Compare the enclosure notation on the letter with the actual enclosures to make sure that all items are included. Make a note to contact the sender if anything is missing.

10. Clip together each letter and its enclosures.

11. Check the date of the letter. If there is a significant delay between the date of the letter and the postmark, keep the envelope.

### Rationale

It may be necessary to refer to the postmark in legal matters or cases of collection.

12. If all contents appear to be in order, you can discard the envelope.

13. Review all bills and statements.

   • Make sure the amount enclosed is the same as the amount listed on the statement.

   • Make a note of any discrepancies.

14. Stamp each piece of correspondence with the date (and sometimes the time) to record its receipt. If possible, stamp each item in the same location—such as the upper-right corner.

### Rationale

It may be necessary to refer to the date in legal matters or in cases of collection.

---

margins or on self-adhesive notes. Annotating may involve pulling a patient's chart or any previous related correspondence from a file and attaching it to the letter.

## Distributing

Sort letters into separate batches for distribution. These batches might include correspondence that requires the physician's attention, payments to be directed to the person in charge of billing, and correspondence that requires your attention. Each batch should be presented to the appropriate person in a file folder or arranged with the highest-priority items on top. You may be given specific instructions on how to distribute magazines, newspapers, and advertising circulars.

## Handling Drug and Product Samples

Many physicians receive a number of drug and product samples in the mail. Handling procedures vary from office to office. Samples of nonprescription products, such as hand creams or cough drops, may be placed in the patient treatment area for patient distribution as directed by the physician.

The physician may ask that you put samples of any new prescription drugs in the consultation room for him to evaluate. Store all other drug samples in a locked cabinet reserved solely for such samples. Sort and label the samples by category, such as antibiotics, sedatives, painkillers, and so on. Never give samples to patients or use them yourself unless directed by the physician. If the doctor directs you to give samples to a patient, make sure to write this information in the patient's chart and date the entry.

When a box of samples is outdated, you should properly dispose of them, following all state and DEA regulations. You will most likely use the disposal company that handles your biomedical waste to dispose of unused, outdated sample medications. Flushing samples down the sink or toilet is no longer allowed because of the possibility of polluting the environment. Samples should not be placed in the trash where unauthorized individuals could take the medications. Your local pharmacy may also have a program for disposing of outdated medications.

### How to Spot Urgent Incoming Mail

How can you tell if a piece of incoming mail is urgent? First-class mail marked "Urgent" tells you that it requires immediate attention. Here are some other signals to look for (Figure 7-9).

#### Overnight Mail

Any package that has been sent by an overnight carrier or by USPS Express Mail should be considered urgent and should be opened immediately.

#### Certified Mail

Certified mail requires your signature on delivery. The sender used certified mail to be sure that the item would be sent to the proper person.

#### Registered Mail

Items sent by registered mail typically are valuable, irreplaceable, or otherwise important. Registered mail provides the sender with evidence of mailing and delivery.

#### Special Delivery

An item sent by special delivery is likely to be delivered sometime before the normal mail delivery—possibly even on a Sunday or holiday. The sender requested special delivery to ensure that the item would be delivered promptly after it was received at the addressee's post office.

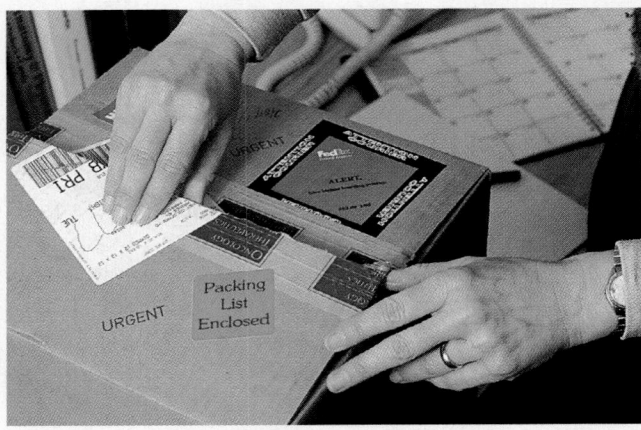

**Figure 7-9.** Urgent materials receive top priority upon arrival at an office.

## Summary

As a medical assistant, you are responsible for many of the tasks involved in writing correspondence and processing outgoing and incoming mail in the medical office. Proper and efficient management of correspondence and mail is essential to promoting a positive, professional office image.

Choosing the proper letterhead and envelope helps to ensure professional-looking correspondence. Knowing the parts of a letter and the various letter styles and formats used in the business environment today helps you create effective correspondence. Knowing how to edit and proofread and how to use writing reference materials helps ensure that your letters are clear, concise, and well-written.

Familiarity with the types of mail and delivery services available enables you to choose the proper services to meet the office's mailing needs. Following proper procedures and recommended USPS guidelines ensures that office mail will be received in the most timely manner. Handling incoming mail is an important responsibility. Following an established procedure allows you to process and route the mail efficiently.

## CASE STUDY QUESTIONS

Now that you have completed this chapter, review the case study at the beginning of the chapter and answer the following questions:

1. Why is it important to accurately and carefully prepare correspondence for an ambulatory setting? What could the poor management of documents and correspondence mean to a medical practice?
2. What are the differences between the language used in an informal or casual letter and that used in a formal or professional business letter?
3. What are some appropriate shortcuts that can assist in the daily management of correspondence and mailing?
4. What are some factors to consider in choosing the best mode of delivery for letters and parcels?

## Discussion Questions

1. Why is it important to closely follow the basic rules of writing when creating a business letter?
2. Name and describe the five steps involved in processing incoming mail.
3. You have been asked to create a basic business letter format for use within a medical practice. Summarize the format, describing the placement of each part of the letter.
4. Name and describe the different types of invoices and statements and their use in a medical practice.

## Critical Thinking Questions

1. You have been asked to mail a letter to a patient, withdrawing the services of the practice. What type of mail service would you use and why?
2. The physician tells you to make sure that all patient letters that address withdrawing the services of the practice are "well documented." What does the physician mean? What would you do?
3. Imagine that your coworker is out sick. You must make sure all the work is handled. Which is more important—typing referral letters or sorting the mail? Why? How might you proceed if you are responsible for both but don't have the time to complete both?

4. You need a quick and easy way to remember the parts of a business letter and how they are placed. How are you going to remember them?

## Application Activities

1. You are employed in Dr. Angelo Carillo's office. A young patient of yours, Rodney Sills, has broken his wrist, and Dr. Carillo says that Rodney will be unable to participate in gym class for 10 weeks. Create a letter notifying his gym instructor of the situation.
2. Prepare a No. 10 business envelope using the USPS guidelines for addressing envelopes. Include the following information.

   Return address:
   Dr. Angelo Carillo, 123 Winding Way, Suite 2, Rockland, NJ 09876

   Mailing address:
   ABC Insurance, 987 Hill Street, Marrakesh, CA 01234

   Attention:
   Susan Jones, Claims Department

   Special Instructions:
   Certified Mail

3. Using proper letter formatting technique and the basic rules of writing reviewed in this chapter, correct the following letter:

   September 18th, 2007

   Mountainside Hospital
   Samuel Adams, Educational Coordinator
   1 Mountainside Lane
   San Francisco, California, 94112

   Dear mr. Adams:
   I am writing in response to your letter of the 10th. I am very interested in presenting a talk at your Health Fare in February. I am aviaable to speak on either the 20th or the 21st.

   If there is any flexibility in scheduling, I would prefer to present my talk in the afternoon. Also, please let me know how long I should prepare to speak. I am including a copy of an article I recently wrote on the same subject for the local paper.

   I am looking forward to hearing from you.
   Sincerely,
   Enclosure
   Dr. Angelo Carillo AC/SCB

# REVIEW

## CHAPTER 7

4. Create flashcards for use in class and for individual study. Use all the key terms and definitions in this chapter, 20 commonly misspelled words from Table 7-3, and 10 common USPS abbreviations from Table 7-4.

### Virtual Fieldtrip

*Visit the McGraw-Hill Higher Education Medical Assisting website at www.mhhe.com/medicalassisting3 to complete the following activity:*

Use the American Association of Medical Assistants and other websites related to effective writing. Prepare an oral presentation about one of the following topics:

- The parts of a business letter and why each part is important

- Styles of business letters and the circumstances for using each type
- Techniques for becoming an effective writer
- Tools for editing and proofreading
- The process of preparing an envelope and mailing

Ask your instructor how many references and citations you should minimally include in your research. Present your report to the class, using all available multimedia, including PowerPoint slides or an overhead projector if possible.

Open the CD and complete this chapter's practice activities, play the games, listen to the key terms, and test yourself with the interactive review. E-mail, print, and/or save your results to document your proficiency.

## CHAPTER 8

# Managing Office Supplies

## MEDICAL ASSISTING COMPETENCIES

*In preparation for the certification examination, you should know the following areas of competence:*

| COMPETENCY | CMA | RMA |
|---|:---:|:---:|
| **Administrative** | | |
| Perform basic clerical skills | X | X |
| **General/Legal/Professional** | | |
| Respond to and initiate written communications by using correct grammar, spelling, and formatting techniques | X | X |
| Recognize and respond to verbal and nonverbal communications by being attentive and adapting communication to the recipient's level of understanding | X | X |
| Be aware of and perform within legal and ethical boundaries | X | X |
| Identify community resources and information for patients and employers | X | X |
| Perform an inventory of supplies and equipment | X | X |
| Operate and maintain facilities, and perform routine maintenance of administrative and clinical equipment safely | X | X |
| Perform quality control procedures | X | X |
| Maintain the physical plant | | X |
| Exercise efficient time management | | X |
| Exhibit initiative | | X |
| Adapt to change | | X |
| Evidence a responsible attitude | | X |
| Use appropriate medical terminology | | X |
| Receive, organize, prioritize, and transmit information appropriately | | X |

## KEY TERMS

- disbursement
- durable item
- efficiency
- expendable item
- inventory
- invoice
- Material Safety Data Sheet (MSDS)
- purchase order
- purchasing groups
- reputable
- requisition
- unit price

## CHAPTER OUTLINE

- Organizing Medical Office Supplies
- Taking Inventory of Medical Office Supplies
- Ordering Supplies

## LEARNING OUTCOMES

After completing Chapter 8, you will be able to:

**8.1** Give examples of vital, incidental, and periodic supplies used in a typical medical office.

**8.2** Describe how to store administrative and clinical supplies.

**8.3** Implement a system for tracking the inventory of supplies.

**8.4** Schedule inventories and ordering times to maximize office efficiency.

**8.5** Locate and evaluate supply sources.

**8.6** Use strategies to obtain the best-quality supplies while controlling cost.

**8.7** Follow procedures for ordering supplies.

**8.8** Check a supply order and pay for the supplies.

## Introduction

The purpose of a medical office or clinic is to deliver appropriate care to those in need. However, no medical office can function without adequate supplies. It is therefore essential that the medical assistant routinely evaluate and replenish the office's supplies before a shortage is noted.

In this chapter, you will focus on the importance of adequate administrative and clinical supplies in the daily operation of a typical medical practice. You will learn to evaluate, replace, organize, and pay for expendable items used routinely in a practice.

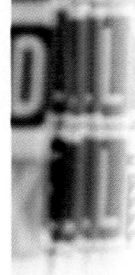

## CASE STUDY

The administration of the hospital where you are employed has made the decision to open a series of clinics across the city to provide ambulatory care to patients in their neighborhoods. As an experienced medical assistant, you have been asked to plan for the purchase of expendable items for stocking in the new clinics. What a task! How will you determine what items to provide for each clinic and the amount to order? Do you know where to go to get the best price for the best products? Who is the best vendor in each area? What about discounts for volume buying? Where do you start? You need a plan or a system to help organize your thoughts and then your actions.

As you read this chapter, consider the following questions:

1. What is an *expendable* item? What items would you list on the expendable administrative supply list? The clinical supply list? The general supply list?

2. What factors would you consider about each office as you determine the appropriate supplies?

3. How would you recommend that the supplies be stored with inventory management in mind?

## Organizing Medical Office Supplies

Purchasing and maintaining administrative and medical supplies are essential skills that you will use in managing the office. You will be responsible for taking inventory of equipment and supplies, evaluating and recommending equipment and supplies, and negotiating prices with suppliers. When managing office supplies, your goal is to achieve **efficiency,** which is the ability to produce the desired result with the least effort, expense, and waste.

The word *supply* refers to an **expendable item,** or an item that is used and then must be restocked, such as prescription pads (Figure 8-1). Ideally, office supplies are stored on labeled shelves. More **durable items,** or pieces of equipment that are used indefinitely—such as telephones, computers, and examination tables—are not

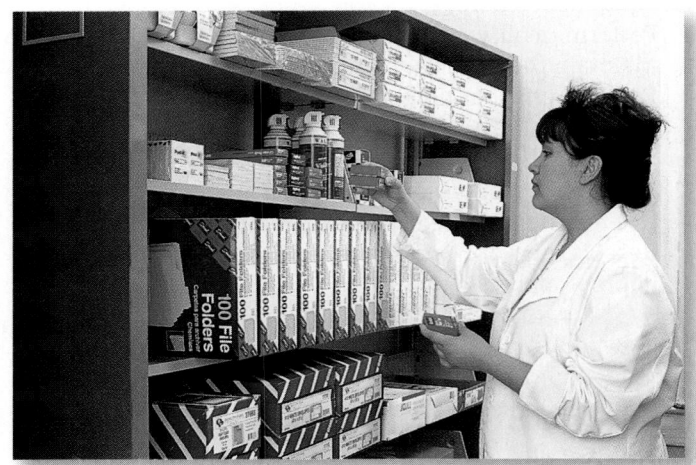

**Figure 8-1.** Making sure that supplies are in order is a continuous process that ensures an efficient, well-prepared office.

considered supplies. Also included in the category of durable items is medical equipment, such as stethoscopes and reflex hammers. Chapter 5 discusses ordering durable administrative items.

## Determining Responsibility for Organizing Supplies

It is recommended that the responsibility for organizing office supplies lie with one to two individuals. Often this responsibility is given to the medical assistant. In a small practice, one medical assistant may be able to handle this responsibility. A practice with several physicians may require more help to manage supplies. When two medical assistants handle this responsibility, one is often assigned to handle administrative items and the other to handle clinical (medical) supplies. In a very large practice, a third assistant might handle computer, copier, and fax supplies.

## Categorizing Supplies

Most supplies in the medical office fall into two main categories: administrative and clinical. Examples of administrative supplies include items that are used in the office portion of the practice, such as stationery, insurance forms, pens, pencils, and clipboards. Clinical supplies are medically related and include alcohol swabs, tongue depressors, disposable tips for otoscopes, and disposable sheaths for thermometers.

General supplies are used by both patients and staff. Examples of general supplies include paper towels, liquid hypoallergenic soap, and facial and toilet tissue.

**The Supply List.**  You will need to determine what items in your office are used routinely and reordered systematically. Keep a list of these items, and update it as needed. This master supply list is usually kept in the office procedures manual. Appropriate sections of this list may be posted on the cabinets where the items are stored.

One good way to help keep track of supplies is to categorize them according to their importance within the practice. Although all supplies in your office are necessary, some supplies are more important than others. You may find it helpful to identify an item in one of three categories: vital, incidental, and periodic use. Table 8-1 will help you determine vital, incidental, and periodic supplies for your office.

**Vital Supplies.**  These items are absolutely essential for the functioning of the practice. They include paper examination table covers and prescription pads. Without these items, the physician would be unable to work in a clean examination environment or to readily prescribe medication for patients during office visits. Another type of vital supply is an item that requires a special order, such as a printed form. Special orders take time to obtain, so they must be ordered well before supplies run low.

**Incidental Supplies.**  These supplies are needed in the office but do not threaten the efficiency of the office if the supply runs low. Incidental supplies include staples and rubber bands, which can be purchased quickly and easily at a local stationery store.

**Periodic Supplies.**  These supplies require ordering only occasionally. For example, if your office uses appointment books, you will order them only once or twice a year, probably in small numbers. The urgency of ordering some periodic items can depend on the size of the office. A multi-physician office, for example, would require more appointment books than a single-physician office. Another example of a periodic item might be holiday cards to send to the physician's colleagues and patients.

## Storing Office Supplies

Storing office supplies requires good organizational skills and attention to detail. Many people in an office use these supplies, so the items should be stored neatly and in an orderly way. In addition, it is important to store supplies safely to prevent loss or theft, damage, or deterioration.

**Location.**  In a small medical office, supplies are generally kept near the areas of the office where they are used. Administrative supplies are usually stored behind or adjacent to the reception area, with clinical supplies stored near the examination rooms. If the practice has a laboratory, pertinent supplies are stored in or near the laboratory. Offices that have separate supply rooms offer more storage space.

Small medical offices may not have ample space for storage. It may be tempting to store boxes on the floor behind the air conditioning unit, stacked up close to the ceiling, or in potentially hazardous locations, such as near a source of heat. It is essential that supplies be stored according to the guidelines described by JCAHO (Joint Commission for Accreditation of Health Organizations).

Items may not be stored on the floor; instead, they must be raised off the floor, as on a crate or shelf, to avoid contamination by water. Items stored close to the ceiling are considered a fire hazard. JCAHO standards require that supplies stored on the top shelf of a closet or storage area be at least 18 inches below the ceiling.

Avoid storing any boxes or supplies near a water heater, air conditioning unit, heater, or stove. Many expendable items and their packaging are combustible and can quickly become a fire hazard. Air conditioning units may drip water on the floor. If boxes of expensive forms are stored nearby, they can quickly become ruined as water seeps unnoticed into the packaging.

**Storage Cabinets.**  Each storage cabinet should be labeled with a list of its contents. Keep all stock of one item together.

Finding supplies is easier if you keep small items at eye level. Put large, bulky goods, such as reams of

## TABLE 8-1 Typical Supplies in a Medical Office

### Administrative Supplies

Appointment books, daybooks (still used in noncomputerized offices)
Back-to-school/back-to-work slips
Clipboards
Computer supplies
Copy and facsimile (fax) machine paper
File folders, coding tabs
HIPAA forms (Notice of Privacy Practices, authorization forms, disclosure logs, request to inspect/copy medical record forms, request for amendment forms, acknowledgment of request for amendment forms)
History and physical examination sheets/cards
Insurance forms: disability, HMO and other third-party payers, life insurance examinations, Veterans Administration, workers' compensation

Insurance manuals
Local welfare department forms
Patient education materials
Pens, pencils, erasers
Rubber bands, paper clips
Registration forms
Social Security forms
Stamps
Stationery: appointment cards, bookkeeping supplies (ledgers, statements, billing forms), letterhead, second sheets, envelopes, business cards, prescription pads, notebooks, notepads, telephone memo pads

### Clinical Supplies

Alcohol swabs
Applicators
Bandaging materials: adhesive tape, gauze pads, gauze sponges, elastic bandages, adhesive bandages, roller bandages (gauze and elastic)
Cloth or paper gowns
Cotton, cotton swabs
Culture tubes
50% dextrose solution
Disposable sheaths for thermometers
Disposable tips for otoscopes
Gloves: sterile, examination
Hemoccult test kits
Iodine or Betadine pads
Lancets
Lubricating jelly
Microscopic slides and fixative
Needles, syringes
Nitroglycerin tablets

Safety pins
Silver nitrate sticks
Suture removal kits
Sutures
Thermometer covers
Tongue depressors
Topical skin freeze
Urinalysis test sticks
Urine containers
Injectable medications: diazepam (Valium), diphenhydramine hydrochloride (Benadryl), epinephrine (Adrenalin), furosemide (Lasix), isoproterenol (Isuprel), lidocaine (Xylocaine: 1%, 2%, and plain), meperidine hydrochloride (Demerol), morphine, phenobarbital, sodium bicarbonate, sterile saline, sterile water
Other medicines, chemicals, solutions, ointments, lotions, and disinfectants, as needed

### General Supplies

Liquid hypoallergenic soap
Paper cups
Paper towels

Tampons
Tissues: facial, toilet

stationery, on lower shelves. Label boxes and containers clearly so that all employees can readily find what they need and so that the inventory process is easier.

As you initially arrange items on storage shelves, label the shelves. Reserve enough space to completely stock each item. Do not put anything but the appropriate item in each designated space. This easy system allows for a quick review when you reorder supplies.

To reduce the risk of errors on reorders, keep each item's original label attached to it. Cover the label with clear tape, if necessary. If you must replace a worn label, do it immediately when needed, making sure the new label has the same detailed information as the old one. Bottles with pouring spouts should be labeled on the side opposite the spout to prevent the liquid from dripping onto the label. Use a laundry marking pen to label linens with the name of your office. Linen services usually premark linens with the name of the company or the practice.

Many items have a shelf life after which they are no longer usable. By not over-ordering and by rotating supplies—using older ones first—your office will be able to use items during their shelf life. This is true not only for perishable items such as medications, but also for linens and paper, which can deteriorate. Keep in mind when stocking medications or chemicals that a more recent shipment may have an earlier expiration date than a previous shipment. Always check expiration dates when storing supplies.

Store all items based on the expiration date for the items. The oldest items should be stored in the front and the newer items stored in the rear of the cabinet. Be sure to rotate the inventory every time you add new stock, placing the newly received stock at the back of each shelf. Sometimes items expire before they are used. Check every item for the expiration date before use. Discard all expired items carefully and appropriately according to JCAHO and OSHA standards.

**Administrative Supplies.** In addition to such expendable items as pens, pencils, and paper clips, paper products are important to a medical office. In general, paper products should be stored flat in their original boxes or wrappings to prevent pages from bending or curling. Information booklets may be stored upright to save space. Envelopes and other paper goods with gummed surfaces must be kept dry to prevent them from sticking together.

**Clinical Supplies.** The rules of good housekeeping and asepsis (see Chapter 19) apply to storage areas for clinical supplies. These areas must be kept clean and protected from damage and exposure to the elements.

All dressings and most bandaging materials must be kept sterile. For example, gauze that may be used to bandage an open wound must be sterile. Elastic rolled bandages, which do not touch open wounds, must be clean but not necessarily sterile.

Chemicals, drugs, and solutions should be kept in a cool, dark place because light and heat cause some substances to deteriorate. Store all liquids in their original containers. Line cabinets with plastic-coated shelf paper, and wipe it frequently with a damp cloth.

Store all poisons and narcotics separately from all other products. Narcotics must be stored securely out of sight in a locked cabinet. Never store strong acids near alkaline solutions or flammable items near sources of heat. Solutions that will be stored for a considerable length of time should have a small amount of space at the top of the bottle to allow for heat expansion.

Some liquids should be stored in the refrigerator. Check each item for specific storage instructions. If storage space is limited, consider eliminating some items—especially bulky ones that are rarely used or items that a patient can purchase at surgical supply stores.

Clinical refrigerators may be needed to store certain clinical supplies that require refrigeration. Never store food items and clinical items in the same refrigerator. A clinical refrigerator must be kept at a constant temperature to properly maintain the chemical integrity of lab supplies. Monitoring and recording the date and temperature of the clinical refrigerator should be completed once a week or per office protocol.

# Taking Inventory of Medical Office Supplies

The list of supplies your office uses regularly and the quantities you have in storage constitute the office **inventory.** Keeping track of the office's inventory is a job that requires careful planning, attention to detail, and basic math skills. Accurate inventory activity ensures that the office never runs out of much-needed supplies.

## Understanding Your Responsibilities

It is important to have an understanding with the doctor or doctors in the practice about the extent of your responsibilities for maintaining supplies. Some doctors are more involved with the details of running an office than others. Your responsibilities may grow as you become more experienced. The doctor, however, usually takes care of certain duties, such as meeting with drug company representatives or authorizing large purchases.

Generally you will be responsible for overseeing the flow of supplies bought and used, calculating the budget for supplies, selecting supplies and vendors, following correct purchasing and payment procedures, and storing the goods properly.

All efficient offices will have a process for everyone within the practice to record their supply needs. The process may be as simple as a notebook stored at the front desk or a supply list positioned in a key location. As a supply need in the office is noted, it can be recorded by anyone on the supply list for the next order. It is then important that the medical assistant who is compiling the order check all the inventory cards, reorder reminder cards, and supply lists before ordering.

**The Inventory Filing System.** To oversee the flow of inventory efficiently, you will need a filing system (see Procedure 8-1). This system consists of several elements:

- The list of supplies (discussed earlier in the chapter)
- An itemized inventory
- An inventory card or record page for each item
- A list of the names and addresses of current vendors
- A file of current catalogs from vendors (including some vendors not currently used, for comparison shopping)
- A want list of brands or items that the office does not currently use but may want to try in the future
- Files for **invoices,** or bills from vendors, and completed order forms

# Step-by-Step Overview of Inventory Procedures

**Procedure Goal:** To set up an effective inventory program for a medical office

**Materials:** Pen, paper, file folders, vendor catalogs, index cards or loose-leaf binder and blank pages, reorder reminder cards, vendor order forms

**Method:**

1. Define with your physician/employer the extent of your responsibility in managing supplies. Know whether the physician's approval or supervision is required for certain procedures, whether any systems have already been established, and if the physician has any preference for a particular vendor or trade-name item. If your medical practice is large, determine which medical assistant is responsible for each aspect of supply management.

2. Know what administrative and clinical supplies should be stocked in your office. Create a formal supply list of vital, incidental, and periodic items, and keep a copy in the office's procedures manual.

3. Start a file containing a list of current vendors with copies of their catalogs.

4. Create a wish list of brands or products the office does not currently use but might like to try. Inform other staff members of the list so that they can make entries.

5. Make a file for supply invoices and completed order forms. (Keep these documents on file for at least 3 years.)

   ## Rationale
   Keep completed documents for future reference as well as for legal protection, if needed.

6. Devise an inventory system of index cards, loose-leaf pages, or a computer spreadsheet for each item. List the following data for each item on its card:
   - Date and quantity of each order
   - Name and contact information for the vendor and sales representative
   - Date each shipment was received
   - Total cost and unit cost, or price per piece for the item
   - Payment method used
   - Results of periodic counts of the item

   - Quantity expected to cover the office for a given period of time
   - Reorder quantity (the quantity remaining on the shelf that indicates when reorder should be made)

7. Have a system for flagging items that need to be ordered and those that are already on order. For example, mark their cards or pages with a self-adhesive tab or note. Make or buy reorder reminder cards to put into the stock of each item at the reorder quantity level.

   ## Rationale
   Having a system in place makes your job easier and will also make it easier for anyone else taking over the task at a later date.

8. Establish with the physician a regular schedule for taking inventory. Every 1 to 2 weeks is usually sufficient. As a backup system for remembering to check stock and reorder, estimate the times for these activities. Mark them on your calendar, or create a tickler file on your computer.

   ## Rationale
   A regular schedule means inventory and ordering will not be forgotten.

9. Order at the same times each week or month, after inventory is taken. However, if there is an unexpected shortage of an item, and more than a week or so remains before the regular ordering time, place the order immediately.

10. Fill in the vendor's order form (or type a letter of request). Order by telephone, fax, e-mail, or online. Online ordering will expedite the order. Follow procedures that have been approved by the physician or office manager. When placing an order, have all the necessary information at hand, including the correct name of the item and the order and account numbers. Record the order information in the inventory file for that item. Be sure to obtain from the vendor an estimated arrival time for the order, and mark that date and order number on your calendar.

11. When ordering online, save the website to "Favorites" for easy, one-click future access. Select the website and establish an account with the company. To establish an account, you will need to give information about your office practice, including the name of the practice,

*continued* ⟶

## Step-by-Step Overview of Inventory Procedures (concluded)

contact name, the address, the phone number, an e-mail address, and a payment source. Ask about adding the practice to any special contact lists for promotional materials and discounts.

12. When you receive the shipment, record the date and the amount received on the item's inventory card or record page. Check the shipment against the original order and the packing slip inside the package to ensure that the right items, sizes, styles, packaging, and amounts have arrived. If there is any error, immediately call or e-mail the vendor, with the catalog page and the inventory card or record page at hand.

### Rationale

Items should be unpacked and checked immediately so that if a problem is discovered, it will be relatively easy to prove that the error or problem is with the shipment and not caused by office personnel.

13. Check the invoice carefully against the original order and the packing slip, making sure that the bill has not already been paid. Sign or stamp the invoice to show that the order was received.

14. Write a check to the vendor to be signed by the physician. (Check writing procedures are described in Chapter 18.) Be sure to show the physician the original order, packing slip, and invoice. Record the check number, date, and amount of payment on the invoice, and initial it or have the physician do so. Write the invoice number on the front of the check.

### Rationale

Writing the invoice number on the check will ensure that the payment is posted to the correct account. Writing the check number and date on the invoice will be useful for future reference if there is a payment dispute.

15. Mail the check and the vendor's copy of the invoice to the vendor within 30 days, and file the office copy of the invoice with the original order and packing slip.

---

- Reorder reminder cards to indicate when an in-stock item should be reordered
- Color-coded, removable self-adhesive flags to indicate "Need to Order" or "On Order"
- An inventory and ordering schedule
- Order forms for each vendor (may be multicopy forms, fax forms, electronic forms, or e-mail forms)

**The Inventory Card or Record Page.** The inventory card or record page for each item or category of items may be a 4-by-6-inch index card, a page in a loose leaf binder, or a spreadsheet stored in the computer system (Figure 8-2). These methods make it easy to group together the items that need to be ordered at any given time. Records help you monitor how quickly items are used and how much should be ordered each time.

Some information may change. As you become more proficient at monitoring inventory or as the practice grows or diminishes in size, you may find that quantities, vendors, or reorder quantities need to be adjusted. With the help of the doctor or office manager, you will be able to determine the ideal quantity of each item to have on hand, depending on the size of the practice, the available storage space, and the ordering schedule.

It is important to check the storage areas regularly, preferably at specific times, and to count the items on hand. When the supply of an item begins to run low, you (or another staff member) should flag the inventory card or record page to indicate the need to reorder it at the next regular ordering time.

Color-coded, removable self-adhesive flags on the inventory card or record page are an efficient way to track inventory. A red flag, for example, might indicate that a supply needs to be ordered. A yellow flag might be substituted when the item has been ordered.

**Reorder Reminder Cards.** Reorder reminder cards (Figure 8-3) are usually brightly colored cards inserted directly into stock on the supply shelf to indicate when it is time to reorder an item. For example, if you have determined that four boxes of staples is a sufficient quantity to keep on hand and your office supply orders are filled in 2 business days, you might place the reorder reminder card between the third and fourth boxes of staples. The reorder quantity on the inventory card or record page for staples would indicate "four boxes."

The reorder reminder cards also remind other staff members to tell you when an item is in short supply. In some offices, the medical assistant labels the reminder card with the name and bar code number of the supply item, such as "staples 002345." This method allows any staff member to pull the card when the last box of staples before the reminder card is taken from the supply shelf. The staff

## (ITEM NAME)  *Exam Table Paper 21"*

**ORDER QUANTITY** _____ 12 _____  **REORDER POINT** _____ 4 _____

| ORDER | QTY | REC'D | UNIT COST | PRICE | PREPAID | ON ACCT. | ORDER | QTY | REC'D | UNIT COST | PRICE | PREPAID | ON ACCT. |
|---|---|---|---|---|---|---|---|---|---|---|---|---|---|
| 1/4 | 12 | 1/8 | $12.25 | $147.00 | Check 1214 | X | | | | | | | |
| 2/5 | 12 | 2/9 | $12.25 | $147.00 | Check 2110 | X | | | | | | | |
| | | | | | | | | | | | | | |
| | | | | | | | | | | | | | |

**INVENTORY COUNT**

| | JAN. | FEB. | MAR. | APR. | MAY | JUNE | JULY | AUG. | SEPT. | OCT. | NOV. | DEC. |
|---|---|---|---|---|---|---|---|---|---|---|---|---|
| DATE _____ | 7 | 10 | | | | | | | | | | |
| DATE _____ | | | | | | | | | | | | |

**ORDER SOURCE**

Smith Physician's Supply Co.

493 Carlton Avenue

South Union, NJ 07422

908-899-6123   Contact: Martin Kohn

**UNIT PRICE**

12 – $147.00

36 – $441.00

**Figure 8-2.** The inventory card, record page, or computer spreadsheet is the primary inventory-tracking tool in managing medical office supplies.

member can then place the card in a "To Be Ordered" envelope. Some offices can reorder simply by scanning the bar code. Staff members in some offices request supplies by writing them in an order book or on an order list.

**Inventory Reminder Kits.** Some mail-order supply vendors sell inventory kits, complete with cards and tabs or flags. Computerized inventory systems are also available. Shelves still need to be checked and counts logged on to the computer, however. Therefore, smaller offices generally do not benefit as much as larger ones from a computerized inventory system.

## Scheduling Inventory and Ordering

Establish a regular schedule for counting the supplies in the office. Taking inventory every 1 or 2 weeks is usually sufficient. Estimating when you will probably need to reorder a particular item—and putting that date on your calendar or in your appointment book—is also helpful. You and the physician can determine how often storage areas should be checked.

**Established Ordering Times.** You should have established ordering times, such as the same day each week or month, after inventory is taken. For example, you

might take inventory the first Tuesday of every month and order supplies the first Thursday of every month.

A regular schedule for taking inventory and ordering helps all staff members remember when they must give their requests to you. Although you may need to adjust the ordering time occasionally, try to adhere to the schedule to avoid the expense and inconvenience of rush orders.

## When to Order Ahead of Schedule

When you take inventory, and the spare supply of an item has not been reached but is close to the placement of the reorder reminder card, you must decide whether you should reorder then or wait until the next regular ordering time. You will probably find it is more efficient to go ahead and order rather than wait. Ordering early assures you that the supply will not be depleted before the next regular ordering time.

Ordering ahead of schedule can be especially important if there is a large demand for a particular product and manufacturers' production levels have not caught up with that demand. This situation can occur if there has been an outbreak of a particular flu or virus, or if the Food and Drug Administration has determined that a certain product is harmful, resulting in higher demand for an alternative product.

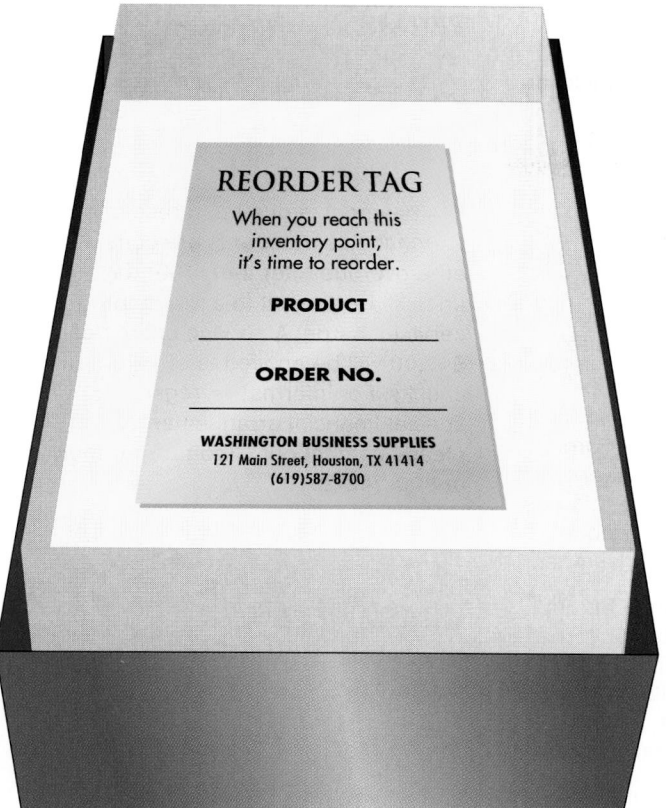

**Figure 8-3.** Reorder reminder cards are usually brightly colored cards inserted directly into the spare stock of an item on the supply shelf to indicate when it is time to reorder the item.

**Unanticipated Shortage of a Supply Item.** If the supply of an item reaches the reorder reminder card, and there is still a long time before the next regular ordering time, place the order immediately so that you do not risk running out of the item.

To help you oversee inventory effectively, finish one container before opening a new one. Keep all stock of the same item in one place. The need to count inventory of an item in more than one location or container increases the likelihood of errors. If an item is kept in more than one location, as in the case of multiple exam rooms, inventory is best maintained per room.

As a medical assistant, you want to be sure that there are always sufficient quantities of supplies to keep the office running efficiently. It is unwise to stock spare supplies in too great a quantity, however, because the administrative budget is not likely to support such expenditures. In addition, spare quantities of supplies can be a storage problem.

# Ordering Supplies

Ordering supplies requires a procedure to deal with vendors and to order and check supplies. You can avoid common purchasing mistakes by understanding the most efficient way to order supplies for your office.

## Locating and Evaluating Supply Vendors

A vendor will most likely already be in place when you join a practice. You should, however, be aware of competitors' prices, services, and other incentives intended to attract your office as a customer. Sometimes the incentives—such as bonus supplies with certain purchases—can represent sizable savings. Remember also that your time has a dollar value to the practice, and services that save you time are worth comparing when evaluating vendors.

Obtaining recommendations from other medical offices is a good way to locate office-supply dealers who sell items at reasonable prices and are also reputable. **Reputable** vendors fulfill orders accurately with quality items, deliver products in good condition, and charge fair prices. Keep in mind when evaluating vendors that the physician may have preferences for certain trade names or vendors.

**Gathering Competitive Prices.** The costs of maintaining a medical practice are continually rising. Saving money on supplies through careful purchasing strategies is one way to help your physician/employer reduce spending. The medical assistant is often largely responsible for comparison pricing, ordering, and establishing and maintaining relationships with vendors. Your awareness of the most up-to-date information about vendors and supplies is valuable to your physician/employer. Discuss prices with the physician, who in turn may want to discuss them with an accountant.

**Setting Up a Supply Budget.** The average medical practice spends 4% to 6% of its annual gross income on administrative, clinical, and general supplies. If an office is spending more than 6%, it may be time to reevaluate the office's spending practices. Remember, though, that any budget is only a guide. A budget is meant to serve your office, not the reverse. You and your physician/employer may need to adjust the supply budget based on prices and discounts available from vendors.

**Comparing Vendors.** To collect competitive data from vendors, contact them by telephone or in writing to request catalogs and other forms of product information. If you are not in charge of routing mail, make sure that supply-related mail, such as product catalogs and sale notices, is routed to you. Catalogs usually include basic information, such as the dealer's name, address, and telephone number, order numbers for items, and vendor policy (Figure 8-4). When investigating a vendor, obtain the following information:

- Prices—costs for supplies, delivery, and any other services; special discounts; minimum quantities applicable; bonus supplies with purchases
- Quality—product descriptions, illustrations, trade names, recommendations for use, durability, guarantees

## BY PHONE

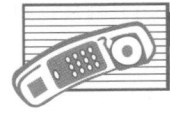

Call our toll-free number:
(800) BIBBERO
(800-242-2376)
Monday thru Friday,
6:00 A.M. – 5:00 P.M. (PST)

## BY MAIL

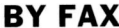

Complete order form and mail to:
Bibbero Systems, Inc.
1300 N. McDowell Blvd.
Petaluma, CA 94954-1180

## BY FAX

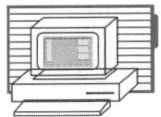

Complete order form and transmit via
FAX to : 800-242-9330
Our FAX line is open 24 hours daily.

## BY ONLINE ORDER

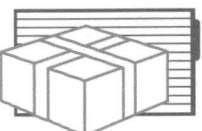

Log on to our convenient website at www.bibbero.com, 24 hours a day.

## SHIPPING POLICY

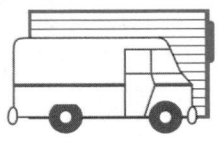

Stock items are normally shipped the same day.

## FREE DELIVERY

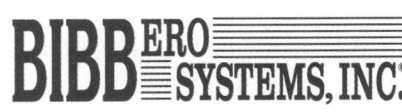

Free delivery on pre-paid orders totaling $300.00 or more.

Fill out the enclosed order form located in the center of this catalog, and return in the enclosed postage-paid envelope to:

**Bibbero Systems, Inc.**
**1300 N. McDowell Blvd.**
**Petaluma, CA 94954-1180**

If you are in a hurry, call us toll free at: 800-242-2376 or FAX us at 800-242-9330. Our Customer Service Department will be happy to assist you.

For items requiring custom imprinting, please enclose with your order the following information, either typed or printed: Name, Specialty, Address, City/State & Zip Code, Telephone Number and State License Number.

Send us your specifications for any type of special form—Patient Registration, History Forms, Dividers, Charts, etc. – and we will furnish quotes at no charge. We can print single page or multiple part forms.

**Please Note:** All custom printed orders are subject to an overrun or underrun variance of 10%.

Stock orders received by 11:00 A.M. are normally shipped the same day. Out-of-stock items are automatically back ordered. Custom printed orders normally leave our plant within 10-15 working days after proof approval.

Combined stock and custom printed orders are shipped together, if requested. All orders are shipped via the best method available to your location. Common carriers are used for large volume orders. Overnight air and 2nd day delivery services are available on request.

All orders prepaid by check, Visa, MasterCard or American Express totaling $300.00 or more will be shipped freight free within the continental U.S. This offer excludes furniture, cabinets, and special order items. We regret that the high cost of shipping outside the 48 contiguous states prohibits us from extending this service; we will use the most economical shipping method available to your location.

## TERMS

Full payment is due upon receipt of merchandise. Accounts are considered overdue after thirty (30) days and will be subject to a 1% monthly service charge. A service charge of $10.00 will be applied to all returned checks. For information regarding special financial arrangements, please contact our Credit Department at 800-242-2376.

## GUARANTEE!

Your Satisfactio n Guaranteed!

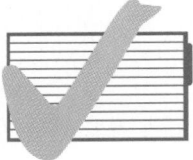

We guarantee our stock products. Return any of our stock products within 60 days of purchase for full credit, exchange or refund of your purchase price. After 60 days, your return will be subject to prior approval and a 15% restocking charge. All returns must have an authorization number. Call our Customer Service Department at 800-242-2376 for your authorization number and enclose it with your return. Opened and/or partially used packages cannot be returned. Personalized items, made to order, special orders and unlocked or opened software cannot be returned.

*We accept Visa, MasterCard,*
*& American Express*
*for all your purchases.*

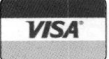 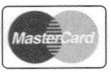 

**BIBB**ERO **SYSTEMS, INC.**

**Figure 8-4.** Examine supply catalogs and websites carefully to find out vendors' company policies.

- Service—availability of products, delivery time and procedures, sales representative availability, damaged-goods policy
- Payment policies

# Competitive Pricing and Quality

Part of your responsibility in managing office supplies is to stay informed about the pricing and quality of competitors to your vendors. Savings can add up quickly, and ongoing comparison pricing can save the practice hundreds of dollars a year.

**Unit Pricing.** Because many medical items come in a variety of package sizes, you need to be aware of how much the office is actually paying per item. To calculate an item's **unit price,** divide the total price of the package by the quantity, or number of items. For example, if a package of 12 pens costs $12, the unit price, or price per pen, is $1 ($12 divided by 12 pens). If another vendor provides the same type of pen in a package of 18 for $17.10, the unit price is 95 cents ($17.10 divided by 18 pens). The second set of pens is the better buy.

Unit prices are generally lower at larger quantities. Therefore, it makes sense to place one large order for a nonperishable item to cover the office until the next ordering time. Generally, however, you should not order more than a year's supply of any one item, particularly if the item is custom-printed. Addresses, insurance codes, or additions to medical staff can change. When placing quantity discount orders, always consider the following factors: whether the supply can be used within a reasonable time, the possibility of spoilage or deterioration, the amount of storage space in the office, and whether the doctor will continue to use the item. Avoid overspending by not ordering more of an item than is reasonable or necessary.

**Rush Orders.** Unexpected rush orders usually cost the office more money than regularly scheduled orders. (In some cases, a vendor may not charge extra to a steady customer, but these cases would be exceptions.) To avoid rush orders, be aware of approximately how long the vendor takes to deliver an order. You can obtain this information from the vendor policy and by keeping accurate records of your own experience with deliveries.

**Mail-Order Companies.** Using large, established mail-order companies often saves money for the medical office, but there may be less control over orders and a greater potential for hidden costs. The neighborhood pharmacy may also offer discounts, but ordering from wholesalers or directly from the manufacturer is usually more economical. The Points on Practice section provides helpful information about cost-efficient ordering by telephone or fax or through an online service.

**Purchasing Groups.** **Purchasing groups** are groups of physicians that order supplies together to obtain a quantity discount. For example, several medical offices associated with a nearby hospital may order through the hospital. In return for this convenience, the physicians pay dues and guarantee the vendors a certain amount of business. Some programs require members to spend a certain percentage of their supply budget through the group. Groups may also require that members not disclose the group's prices to other physicians. Large medical practices that participate in these groups usually save an average of 20% on supplies. The savings are not usually significant for small offices.

**Group Buying Pools.** If a medical office wants to use local vendors instead of, or in addition to, a purchasing group or if it is too small to benefit from a purchasing group, it can still pool resources with other area offices to qualify for quantity discounts. Even if the offices are ordering different items, discounts are based on the total order and savings can range from 10% to 20%. Under this arrangement the offices must usually take responsibility for distributing the items among themselves. A buying pool is convenient for medical practices that are in the same building or office complex (Figure 8-5).

**Cost Controls.** Medical practices are increasingly interested in saving money and controlling costs in general. Physician reimbursement is constantly being reevaluated. As a result, more than ever, physicians are interested in controlling the operating costs of their practices. Managing expenses within the practice is a very important responsibility for the medical assistant. What may seem to be just a small reduction in cost to the practice can actually result in a substantial reduction to office expenses over the course of a year. As a medical assistant, it is your job to constantly look for ways to reduce costs within the practice without sacrificing quality.

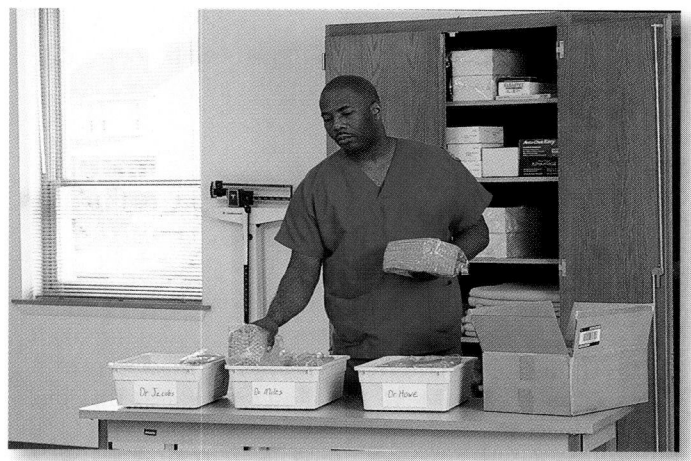

**Figure 8-5.** Ordering jointly with other offices can cut expenses for everyone.

## Benefits of Using Local Vendors

There are many potential vendors, including local dealers, mail-order companies, and nearby pharmacies. Try to establish good credit and business relationships with reputable local vendors. These companies often charge a little more than mail-order companies. Still, spending most of the office's supply budget through one favored local dealer often results in discounts, special service in the event of an emergency, and information about upcoming

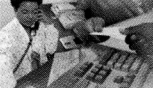

# Points on Practice

## Ordering by Telephone or Fax or Online

You may occasionally purchase office supplies at a local office supply store, but most often you will order them without leaving your office. Three common ways to do so are by telephone, by facsimile (or fax) machine, and through an online service. Here are tips to help make sure every order—no matter which option you choose—is successfully placed.

### Ordering by Telephone

1. Clear communication is a must when ordering by telephone. Speak slowly, and enunciate your words carefully to make sure you are understood. It is also a good idea to spell each word of the practice's name and the address to ensure proper delivery. Use expressions like "S as in Sam, P as in people" to clarify your spelling.

2. Ask the representative taking your order to repeat the order. Check that every item is included with the appropriate price, quantity, style, and color.

3. Confirm the expected delivery date so that you will know if something is late. Also confirm how payment will be made, to prevent unexpected delays.

4. Record the name and telephone number of the person who takes the order in case there is a problem with the order. Get an order number (sometimes called a confirmation number) in case you have to call back with a question or a change in your order.

5. If possible, avoid placing telephone orders on Mondays and Fridays, when call volume is typically high.

### Ordering by Fax

1. When ordering by fax, use the form provided by the vendor if one is available. This form uses the format to which the supply company is accustomed and will speed the processing of your order.

2. Type your order, or write it neatly and legibly, to prevent miscommunication. Fill out the form completely. Make sure you indicate quantities, descriptions, and prices (including shipping) for each item you order.

3. Proofread your order before you send it. Checking the accuracy of the order now will save time later.

4. Follow up by telephone to make sure your order was received and understood and to confirm the delivery date and payment requirements.

### Ordering Online

1. Ordering online requires a computer and a modem connection to the Internet or to an online service. Before ordering online, make sure you are fully familiar with the equipment and the process, or have your supervisor or the supply company's sales representative oversee your initial orders.

2. Type your name and address accurately.

3. If pictures of supplies are not available online, consult the company's printed catalog or CD-ROM catalog. If you do not have access to a catalog, read the online text descriptions carefully, checking trade names and specifications, to select the appropriate merchandise (Figure 8-6). If you have questions, consult the supply company by telephone.

4. When you have completed the selections, the online service will display your order so that you can confirm it. Check that all the information is accurate, including your name, address, and telephone number.

5. If you have an account with the company, you may type in your account number to place the order. Otherwise, you may wish to arrange to make payment on delivery. If you prefer to pay by credit card, first make sure that the company is reputable and that it uses a security system that prevents your number from being read by anyone unauthorized to do so.

If, despite your best efforts, your order is processed incorrectly, take appropriate action immediately. Although ordering by telephone or fax or online is convenient, it still requires additional time to package items that must be returned.

*continued* ⟶

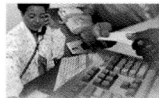

# Points on Practice

## Ordering by Telephone or Fax or Online *(concluded)*

By law, orders that you place must be fulfilled within a reasonable time. The Federal Trade Commission (FTC) monitors purchases by telephone, fax, and online services to protect consumers. The FTC requires supply companies to provide merchandise within 30 days or to give you the option of canceling the order and receiving a full refund.

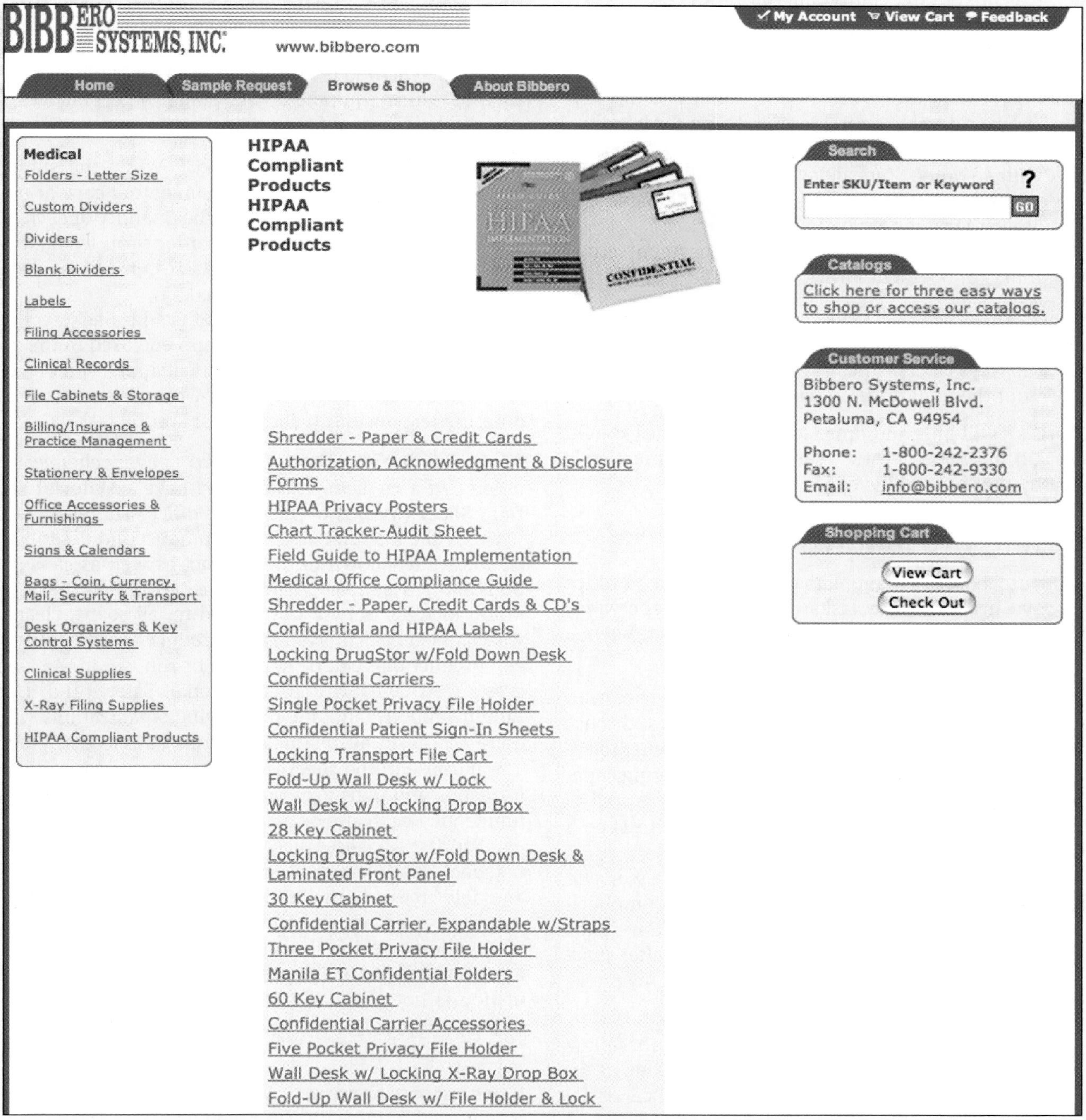

---

**BIBBERO SYSTEMS, INC.**    www.bibbero.com

✓ My Account   ▽ View Cart   ☞ Feedback

| Home | Sample Request | Browse & Shop | About Bibbero |

**Medical**
Folders - Letter Size
Custom Dividers
Dividers
Blank Dividers
Labels
Filing Accessories
Clinical Records
File Cabinets & Storage
Billing/Insurance & Practice Management
Stationery & Envelopes
Office Accessories & Furnishings
Signs & Calendars
Bags - Coin, Currency, Mail, Security & Transport
Desk Organizers & Key Control Systems
Clinical Supplies
X-Ray Filing Supplies
HIPAA Compliant Products

**HIPAA Compliant Products**
**HIPAA Compliant Products**

Shredder - Paper & Credit Cards
Authorization, Acknowledgment & Disclosure Forms
HIPAA Privacy Posters
Chart Tracker-Audit Sheet
Field Guide to HIPAA Implementation
Medical Office Compliance Guide
Shredder - Paper, Credit Cards & CD's
Confidential and HIPAA Labels
Locking DrugStor w/Fold Down Desk
Confidential Carriers
Single Pocket Privacy File Holder
Confidential Patient Sign-In Sheets
Locking Transport File Cart
Fold-Up Wall Desk w/ Lock
Wall Desk w/ Locking Drop Box
28 Key Cabinet
Locking DrugStor w/Fold Down Desk & Laminated Front Panel
30 Key Cabinet
Confidential Carrier, Expandable w/Straps
Three Pocket Privacy File Holder
Manila ET Confidential Folders
60 Key Cabinet
Confidential Carrier Accessories
Five Pocket Privacy File Holder
Wall Desk w/ Locking X-Ray Drop Box
Fold-Up Wall Desk w/ File Holder & Lock

**Search**
Enter SKU/Item or Keyword  **?**
[          ] GO

**Catalogs**
Click here for three easy ways to shop or access our catalogs.

**Customer Service**
Bibbero Systems, Inc.
1300 N. McDowell Blvd.
Petaluma, CA 94954

Phone:   1-800-242-2376
Fax:     1-800-242-9330
Email:   info@bibbero.com

**Shopping Cart**
( View Cart )
( Check Out )

---

**Figure 8-6.**   Ordering online is easy and convenient. Be certain to read the details of your order before sending the order.

sales and specials. Local dealers may also offer more personal assistance, perhaps even a salesperson's help with taking inventory, to compete with larger vendors whose business is based primarily on catalog sales. The extra service may be worth the higher cost.

Buying from local vendors can also provide a public relations benefit for physicians; it means keeping business in the community. However, specialty items may need to be ordered from other vendors. For example, letterhead should be ordered from a reliable printer, whether that printer is located in the community or out of state.

## Payment Schedules

Another factor that affects the cost of supplies is the payment schedule. Many vendors do not charge for handling if an order is prepaid. Others offer a discount for enclosing a check with an order. Some delay billing for 30 to 90 days, allowing the physician to keep the money in the bank, collecting interest for a longer period.

The vendor's invoice usually describes payment terms. Two examples of payment terms are:

1. If the invoice says "Net 30," you have 30 days in which to pay the total amount.
2. "1% 10 Days Net 30" means that you will get a savings of 1% of the total price by paying within 10 days.

Copies of all bills and order forms for supplies should be kept on file for at least 7 years in case the practice is audited by the Internal Revenue Service (IRS).

## Ordering Procedures

Ordering procedures for supplies vary from office to office but always involve these tasks: completing paperwork, checking orders received, correcting errors in shipments, and making payment.

**Order Forms.** Before ordering merchandise, you should inquire about a vendor's ordering options, discuss them with the physician, and determine which method is best for the office. Many vendors now have ordering capability through telephone, fax, e-mail, and online as well as traditional written order forms. Always be sure to keep a copy of each order you submit.

Before you place an order, gather all the necessary information, such as correct names of items, item numbers, and order and account numbers. This information helps ensure the accuracy of the order. Immediately after placing the order, note all order information on the inventory card or record page for that item.

**Purchase Requisitions.** You will need to follow any special ordering procedures established in your medical office. The specific procedures and the medical assistant's level of authority vary from one office to another. Sometimes placing an order requires a **requisition** (a formal request from a staff member or doctor), which is given to the medical assistant who does the actual ordering. The

doctor's approval may be necessary for large purchases—for example, for orders that total more than $300. Recurring orders may not require the doctor's approval, but you may need to get approval before ordering a new brand or quantities of a particular item over a certain amount.

In a group practice where doctors order different items and several staffers are in charge of ordering, procedures for ordering can be complicated. One common way to simplify matters is to use **purchase orders,** forms that authorize a purchase for the practice. Figure 8-7 shows a sample purchase order. Purchase orders are usually preprinted with consecutive numbers. The medical assistant submits approved purchase orders to the vendor for fulfillment. This method is most often used for expensive items, such as office equipment, but some large practices also use purchase orders for supplies.

**Checking Orders Received.** When the shipment of supplies arrives, record on the inventory card or record page the date received as well as the quantity of each item. Check the shipment against the order form to make sure the correct items—in the correct sizes, styles, packaging, and quantity—have been delivered.

Then check the contents against the packing slip (a description of the package contents) enclosed in the package. This checking takes time, but catching even one error is worth the time taken. If several people on a staff have ordering responsibility, they can share the task.

**Material Safety Data Sheets.** Every chemical item ordered in a medical practice must have a **Material Safety Data Sheet (MSDS)** on file in the office. This sheet is provided by the manufacturer of the product and describes the chemical breakdown of the product as well as safety cautions and procedures to follow in using it. Items that require MSDS include, but are not limited to, all soaps, cleansers, waxes, reagents, clinical testing products, inks, toners, and any product that can be splashed or rubbed on the skin or eyes. JCAHO, OSHA (Occupational Safety and Health Administration), and other surveying organizations will require MSDS on all products used in the medical practice. The purpose of the sheet is to provide important safety information about the item that may be critical in the event of unintended exposure or potentially dangerous reactions.

For fast and easy access, organize these sheets in a notebook in alphabetical order. As new items are ordered and delivered, add the MSDS into the master notebook. As a medical assistant, you must always check the MSDS notebook when stocking the supply shelves to ensure that all items stocked are included in the notebook. If MSDS information is not included with the item, either immediately request the information from the vendor or go online to print information directly from the product manufacturer.

**Correcting Errors.** All errors in a shipment should be reported immediately to the vendor so that the records can be corrected and missing supplies can be delivered. When you call to report errors, be sure you have all the paperwork in front of you. You will need the invoice

## PURCHASE ORDER

Submitted by: _____

Order Number: _____

Date Ordered: _____

Date Required: _____

SHIP TO:   Dr. Carlotta Montoni
201 Oak Walk, Suite 32
Gilead, PA 19034

PHONE:   215-610-4120

| | ITEM | DESCRIPTION/MODEL | COLOR | SIZE | QUANTITY | PRICE EACH | TOTAL |
|---|---|---|---|---|---|---|---|
| 1. | | | | | | | |
| 2. | | | | | | | |
| 3. | | | | | | | |
| 4. | | | | | | | |
| 5. | | | | | | | |
| 6. | | | | | | | |
| 7. | | | | | | | |
| 8. | | | | | | | |
| | | | | | | TOTAL | |

Approved: _____   Date: _____

**Figure 8-7.** A purchase order, when approved by the physician or office manager, is an authorization from the practice for a purchase.

number, order date, name of the person who placed the order, name of the person who took the order, and a list of questions or a description of the complaint. If a catalog was used in ordering, have it open to the appropriate page. Always record the name and title of the person you speak with when reporting the error.

**Invoices.** Typically the vendor sends an invoice to the medical office, either accompanying the merchandise or separately. This invoice also should be checked carefully against the original order and the packing slip. Be sure to check the arithmetic as well. Then sign or stamp the invoice to confirm that the order was received. If an item you order is temporarily out of stock, the vendor usually sends an invoice stamped "Back Ordered." Later, when the item is back in stock, the vendor will ship it to your office.

Make sure the invoice has not already been paid. It is a good habit to record the check number, date, and amount of payment on the invoice. You may initial it or have the doctor initial it.

**Disbursements.** An invoice is paid with a **disbursement** (payment of funds) to a vendor. Disbursements may be made in cash or by check or money order. Usually you will write a check to the vendor and have the physician sign it. Be sure to show the physician the original order,

packing slip, and invoice. On the front of the check, record the invoice number. Finally, mail the check to the vendor with the vendor's copy of the invoice. File the office copy of the invoice, along with the original order and the packing slip, according to your inventory filing system (Figure 8-8).

If you make a cash disbursement, obtain a receipt to keep on file. If you are the one responsible for maintaining the practice's financial records and presenting them to the accountant, you may also be responsible for recording the payment information in the office's accounting books.

## Avoiding Common Purchasing Mistakes

Even the most watchful professional can make purchasing mistakes. The best you can do is to educate yourself about common mistakes and try to avoid them. For example, be aware of the possibility of dishonest telephone solicitations. A caller may claim to be a sales representative for the manufacturer of the office photocopier, offering bargains on paper or toner. The caller may require advance payment to be sent to a post office box. The bargains may never arrive.

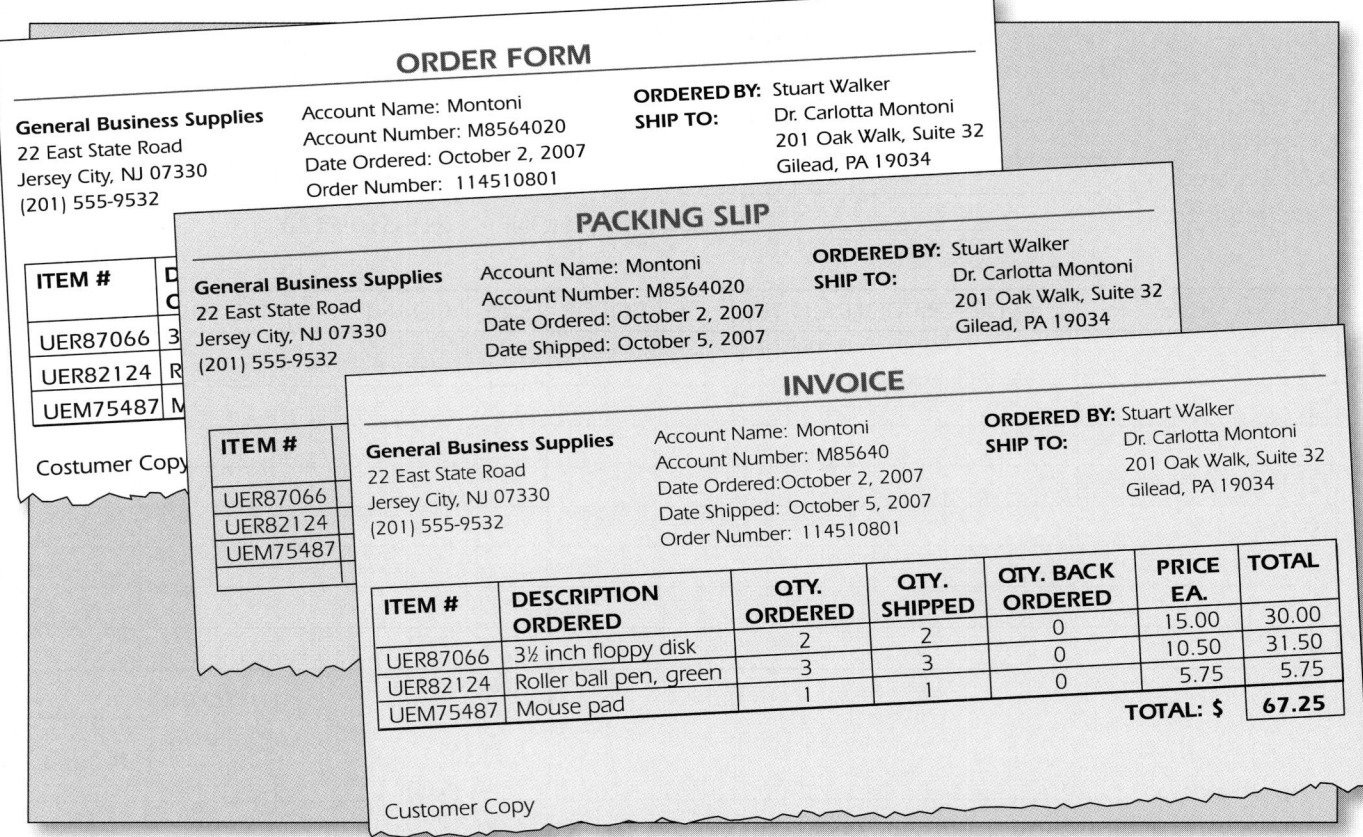

**Figure 8-8.** Check the information on the vendor invoice against the original order and the packing slip to make sure there are no errors.

The best way to deal with these solicitations is to tell the caller that your office does not purchase supplies by telephone. If a telephone offer appears to be legitimate and to offer substantial savings, ask for the name and telephone number of the firm so that you can return the call at a more convenient time. Then you can verify the number with the telephone company and check the firm's name with the Better Business Bureau.

Another disreputable tactic some vendors use is bait and switch: The price of one item is lowered to attract the customer, but that item is always "sold out" and the customer is encouraged to buy a more expensive one. A vendor may also mislead you by raising the price of an item you have been ordering without informing you. Always confirm the current price, check invoices as they come in, and record everything in the item's file. Having your inventory card or record page open while ordering will prompt you to notice and question price changes. If there is an honest error, a reputable firm will readily and courteously correct it.

Problems can also be avoided by carefully supervising a new vendor's sales representative until a comfortable, professional rapport has been established. Discuss your inventory system with representatives, and ask them questions about their procedures.

# Summary

A typical medical practice uses both administrative and clinical office supplies. Supplies can be categorized as vital, incidental, and periodic.

Keeping track of supplies involves creating supply lists and taking inventory. You must know the storage requirements for various kinds of supplies. An inventory filing system can help you organize office supply tasks. Maintaining adequate supplies and well-organized storage space contributes to the smooth running of the office.

You will also locate, evaluate, and establish and maintain working relationships with vendors. It is important to be adept at comparison pricing and to stay abreast of competitors' product quality, pricing policies, and services.

Just as cost-effectiveness is stressed in medical care, it is important to look for ways to control costs when ordering supplies. Checking orders carefully and avoiding dishonest telephone solicitations are two examples of ways to control costs.

## CASE STUDY *QUESTIONS*

Now that you have completed this chapter, review the case study at the beginning of the chapter and answer the following questions:

1. What is an *expendable* item? What items would you list on the expendable administrative supply list? The clinical supply list? The general supply list?
2. What factors would you consider about each office as you determine the appropriate supplies?
3. How would you recommend that the supplies be stored with inventory management in mind?

## Discussion Questions

1. As a new employee, what questions would you want to ask about the process of ordering supplies within the office?
2. Describe some ways you can avoid common purchasing mistakes.

## Critical Thinking Questions

1. During a routine inventory inspection, you notice that the supply of prescription pads is extremely low for typical office use. Could there be a problem within the office other than just the need to order more pads from the printer? What would you do?
2. You share the responsibility of ordering supplies with another medical assistant in the office. You are checking supplies and ordering regularly, but the other employee is allowing items to become completely depleted. What would you do?
3. You discover that an error has been made in a shipment from a vendor. What should you do?

## Application Activities

1. Using vendor catalogs, make a list of ten typical office supply items for a medical practice. Create a fictional office supply list and ordering schedule (including quantities and prices) for the practice.
2. Select a supply company catalog, and become familiar with it. Imagine that you are a sales representative for that company, and make a presentation to your class as if it were a typical medical practice. Your goal is to have the medical office choose your company as its vendor. Be prepared to answer questions about how your company handles various customer concerns.
3. Make a diagram of an office supply cabinet, indicating how you would label and store items for maximum efficiency. Try to use several of the inventory elements discussed in the chapter.

## Virtual Fieldtrip

*Visit the McGraw-Hill Higher Education Medical Assisting website at www.mhhe.com/medicalassisting3 to complete the following activity:*

Use the Sterling Medical Products website and the Lights and Sirens website to research and comparatively price any five items commonly used in a medical practice. Based on your research, which company would you recommend to the office manager and why?

Open the CD and complete this chapter's practice activities, play the games, listen to the key terms, and test yourself with the interactive review. E-mail, print, and/or save your results to document your proficiency.

# CHAPTER 9

# Maintaining Patient Records

## KEY TERMS

documentation

electronic health records (EHR)

electronic medical records (EMR)

individual identifiable health information (IIHI)

informed consent form

noncompliant

objective

patient record/chart

POMR

sign

SOAP

subjective

symptom

transcription

transfer

## MEDICAL ASSISTING COMPETENCIES

*In preparation for the certification examination, you should know the following areas of competence:*

| COMPETENCY | CMA | RMA |
|---|---|---|
| **Administrative** | | |
| Perform basic clerical skills | X | X |
| Prepare, organize, and maintain medical records | X | X |
| File medical records | X | X |
| Maintain medication and immunization records | X | X |
| Screen and follow up on patient test results | X | X |
| **General/Legal/Professional** | | |
| Respond to and initiate written communications by using correct grammar, spelling, and formatting techniques | X | X |
| Identify and respond to issues of confidentiality by maintaining confidentiality at all times and following appropriate guidelines when releasing records or information | X | X |
| Be aware of and perform within legal and ethical boundaries | X | X |
| Determine the needs for documentation and reporting, and document accurately and appropriately | X | X |
| Project a positive attitude | | X |
| Evidence a responsible attitude | | X |
| Be courteous and diplomatic | | X |
| Conduct work within scope of education, training, and ability | | X |
| Use appropriate medical terminology | | X |
| Receive, organize, prioritize, and transmit information appropriately | | X |
| Understand allied health professions and credentialing | | X |

# CHAPTER OUTLINE

- Importance of Patient Records
- Contents of Patient Charts
- Initiating and Maintaining Patient Records
- The Six Cs of Charting
- Types of Medical Records

- Appearance, Timeliness, and Accuracy of Records
- Computer Records
- Medical Transcription
- Correcting and Updating Patient Records
- Release of Records

# LEARNING OUTCOMES

After completing Chapter 9, you will be able to:

**9.1** Explain the purpose of compiling patient medical records.

**9.2** Describe the contents of patient record forms.

**9.3** Describe how to create and maintain a patient record.

**9.4** Identify and describe common approaches to documenting information in medical records.

**9.5** Discuss the need for neatness, timeliness, accuracy, and professional tone in patient records.

**9.6** Discuss tips for performing accurate transcription.

**9.7** Explain how to correct a medical record.

**9.8** Explain how to update a medical record.

**9.9** Identify when and how a medical record may be released.

# Introduction

The medical assistant plays a major role in writing and maintaining patient records. These records document the evaluation and treatment given to the patient. Patient records are critical to the care of the patient. Without accurate and complete patient records, medical care could easily be compromised.

Patient records have many parts or sections that describe these facets of every patient:

- Personal information or data
- Physical and mental condition

- Medical history
- Medical care
- Medical future if the patient is referred to other physicians

In this chapter you will learn how to carefully manage the records of the patient. You will understand that if the medical care is not documented, in a legal sense, the medical care did not occur at all.

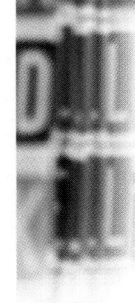

## CASE STUDY

A man is waiting at the busy family practice door on Monday morning as Paul, the medical assistant, arrives to open the office. He instantly recognizes the man as Christopher Hansen, a patient of Dr. Jones's and the first scheduled patient of the day. Mr. Hansen states that he is very ill and needs to see a doctor as soon as possible. Paul assists Mr. Hansen to an examination room and picks up the patient chart from the rack that holds the charts for the day's patients.

As Paul begins to check the patient's vital signs, he asks Mr. Hansen what brings him to the doctor today. The patient grips his lower right side as he responds that his stomach hurts a lot. The patient also reports running a temperature between 100.5°F and 101.3°F for a full day and that he has not been able to eat in the last day because of his stomach pains. Paul knows that this information is important to chart in the permanent record as *subjective* information that has been stated by the patient.

Paul carefully writes down the vital signs for inclusion in the patient chart. He continues his evaluation with an abdominal exam to identify the exact area of tenderness. Paul knows that this information is important to chart in the permanent record as *objective* information that has been observed by the medical professional.

Paul is charting information in the patient record using the SOAP charting method:

- S for subjective
- O for objective
- A for assessment
- P for plan

Paul notifies the physician that the patient is ready for his exam. Dr. Jones completes the record after he evaluates the patient and makes entries to the chart for assessment and the plan for care. The medical record reflects the good clinical management that the patient receives.

As you read this chapter, consider the following questions:

1. Why is an accurate medical record important to the care of a patient?
2. Why is interviewing the patient important to the medical evaluation?
3. What are the six Cs of charting and what do they mean to you as a medical assistant?
4. What are the differences between the conventional and the POMR systems of keeping charts?
5. What are some helpful tips you might use as you perform transcription?

# Importance of Patient Records

One of your most important duties as a medical assistant will be filling out and maintaining accurate and thorough patient records. **Patient records,** also known as **charts,** contain important information about a patient's medical history and present condition. Patient records serve as communication tools as well as legal documents. They also play a role in patient and staff education and may be used for quality control and research. Patient records may either be paper or electronic.

Regardless of the type of record, the patient chart provides physicians with all the important information, observations, and opinions that have been recorded about a patient. The health-care professional can read the complete patient medical history and information about treatment and outcomes. The information in the records can also be sent to other physicians or health-care specialists if the patient needs further treatment, changes physicians, or moves to a new location. The information recorded provides a "map" or plan to follow for the continuity of patient care. The medical chart also serves as supporting documentation for billing and coding purposes, and as a legal document that is admissible in a court of law. Medical records include the following general information about the patient:

- Address and phone number
- Insurance coverage
- Name of the person responsible for payment
- Occupation
- Medical history
- Current complaint or condition
- Health-care needs
- Medical treatment plan or services received

- Radiology and laboratory reports (sometimes)
- Response to care

Standard patient records are usually assembled for new patients well before their actual use. It is the medical assistant's responsibility to make sure there are adequate patient records prepared to meet the needs of the practice.

## Legal Guidelines for Patient Records

Patient records are important for legal reasons. As a general rule, if information is not documented, no one can prove that an event or procedure took place. Medical records are used in lawsuits and malpractice cases to support a patient's claim of malpractice against a doctor and to support the doctor in defense against a claim. Medical records must be retained for 7 years; for pediatric records, the guideline is 7 years from the age of majority. Many legal experts suggest that medical records be kept for 10 years instead of the legally required 7 years.

All medical care, evaluation, and instruction given to the patient by the physician must be documented. Every chart entry must be clear, accurate, legible, dated, and per HIPAA guidelines, written in blue ink. The patient chart is a legal document. Always consider how the patient record would present if it was called into a court of law for review.

Additionally, it is very important to document when a patient is **noncompliant.** *Noncompliant* is a medical term used to describe a patient who does not follow the medical advice he or she is given. After a clear record has been made of the directions given to a patient for optimum health, it is essential to record the level of patient compliance. For example, after you have instructed a patient, you may write in her chart that "Patient stated she understood all direction. Written instruction given to patient." If it is determined that a patient did *not* follow the medical advice, it is then essential to chart this as well. The physician may wish to withdraw from the care of a patient because of the patient's noncompliance. Without a proper and accurate documentation of the patient's noncompliance, the physician may not be able to withdraw care without becoming legally liable. Additionally, documented noncompliance can be used in the physician's defense in a malpractice suit if it can be proven that, due to patient noncompliance, the physician was not solely responsible for inadequate medical care or result.

## Standards for Records

Records that are complete, accurate, and well documented can be convincing evidence that a doctor provided appropriate care. On the other hand, altered, incomplete, inaccurate, or illegible records may imply that a doctor's entire medical practice is below standard.

It is important to understand that the physicians in a practice are not the only people who chart medical records within that practice. However, if an employee of the practice charts inappropriately or inaccurately in a patient's chart, in a court of law, the physician is held responsible for that action. All records, both medical and financial, are the responsibility of the physician. As a medical assistant, you are responsible to the patient and the physician for both the medical and administrative procedures you perform and the accurate recording of those procedures.

## Additional Uses of Patient Records

Patient records serve as ongoing references about individual patients' medical care. They are also valuable for patient education, quality of treatment, and research.

**Patient Education.** Patient records can be used to educate patients about their own conditions and treatment plans. The physician can point out how test results have changed or how the patient's general health has improved or lessened. The physician can also emphasize the importance of following treatment instructions. The medical assistant in turn may use some of this information in educating the patient about his condition or its management. Records can also be used to educate the health-care staff about unusual medical conditions, patient progress, or results of treatment plans.

**Quality of Treatment.** Patient records may be used to evaluate the quality of treatment a facility or doctor's office provides. Auditing groups, such as peer review organizations or the Joint Commission on Accreditation of Healthcare Organizations (JCAHO), may review the charts to monitor whether the care provided and the fees charged meet accepted standards. Records also provide statistics for health-care analysis and future health-care plans and policy decisions.

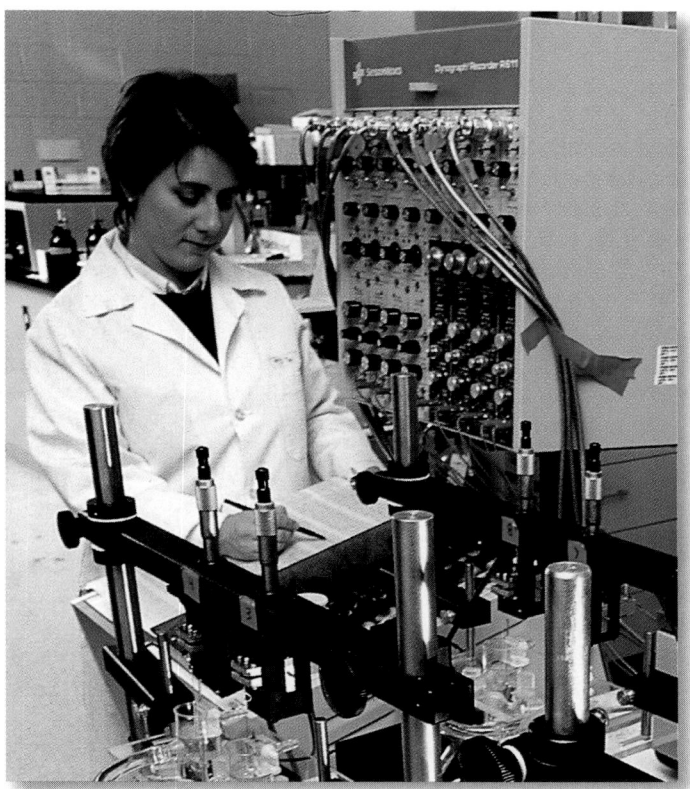

**Figure 9-1.** Medical researchers may rely on data gathered from patient records.

**Research.** Patient records also play an important role in medical research. For example, a medical research team may be testing a new hypertension drug with volunteers who fit a certain medical category—perhaps men between the ages of 45 and 54 who have high blood pressure. Carefully kept records are valuable sources of data about patient responses, behavior, symptoms, side effects, and outcomes (Figure 9-1).

Information in charts may spur researchers to begin a study. For example, the records may show that 80% of all patients taking a particular heart medication experience dizziness. Researchers can investigate why this reaction might be happening.

## Contents of Patient Charts

You will fill out a record for each new patient who comes to the office. Although each physician's office has its own forms and medical charts, in general, all records must contain certain standard information.

### Standard Chart Information

Standard chart information covers a spectrum of different, carefully detailed notes and facts about a patient, from his medical history to the doctor's diagnosis and comments on follow-up care. You must have an understanding of what each part means.

**Patient Registration Form.** Initial registration information is collected at the beginning of the first patient visit. All legal, financial, and demographic information is usually placed on the left side of the patient chart. The patient registration part of the record should list the date of the patient's current visit, the patient's age, address, Social Security number, DOB (date of birth), medical insurance, occupation, marital status, number of children, and the name of the person to contact in an emergency.

Some patient registration forms include family medical history and a list of medical problems. This information is usually placed at the front or top half of the chart for easy reference. Figure 9-2 is an example of a patient registration form.

**Patient Medical History.** The medical history section includes the patient's past medical history (including illnesses, surgeries, known allergies, or current medications), family medical history, and social and occupational history (including diet, exercise, smoking, and use of alcohol or drugs). Usually, the history form ends with a section for the patient to describe the condition or complaint that is the reason for her visit. Medicare and managed care insurance now require that the patient's complaint be entered into the medical record. Known as the chief complaint, this information should be recorded in the patient's own words.

**Physical Examination Results.** Sometimes a form is used to record the results of a general physical examination. Figure 9-3 shows a combination medical history and physical examination form.

**Results of Laboratory and Other Tests.** Test results include findings from tests performed in the office and those received from other doctors, hospitals, or independent laboratories or other outside sources. Some offices use a laboratory summary sheet to help the doctor detect significant changes more easily.

Test results received from sources outside the practice are best organized in sections within this part of the medical chart. Each section is determined by the source of the information. For example, all reports from a particular hospital may be grouped together in one section. Each section from outside sources should be arranged in chronological order, with the latest report on the top.

**Records From Other Physicians or Hospitals.** Incoming records from other sources must be entered into the patient's chart. A copy of the patient's written request authorizing release of the records from the other sources must also be included.

**Doctor's Diagnosis and Treatment Plan.** The doctor's diagnosis must be recorded, along with the treatment plan, which may consist of treatment options, the final treatment list, instructions to the patient, and any medications prescribed. The doctor may also put specific comments or impressions on record. All of this information is recorded with every patient visit.

**Operative Reports, Follow-Up Visits, and Telephone Calls.** Continuation of the record lasts as long as the patient is under the doctor's care. You should record and date all procedures, surgeries, follow-up care, and additional notes the doctor makes regarding the patient's case. You can use continuation forms to add more pages. In addition, you may keep a separate log of telephone calls to and from the patient.

**Informed Consent Forms.** Informed consent forms, such as the one shown in Figure 9-4, verify that a patient understands the treatment offered and the possible outcomes or side effects of the treatment. Consent forms may specify what the outcome might be if the patient receives no treatment. They may also describe alternative treatments and possible risks. The patient signs the consent form but may withdraw consent at any time.

**Hospital Discharge Summary Forms.** The discharge summary form generally includes information that summarizes the reason the patient entered the hospital; tests, procedures, or operations performed in the hospital; medications administered in the hospital; and the disposition, or outcome, of the case. Elements of the form may include the following:

- Date of admission
- Brief history
- Date of discharge
- Admitting diagnosis
- Operations and procedures or hospital course (course of action taken in the hospital)
- Complications
- Instructions to the patient for follow-up care after discharge from the hospital
- Physician's signature

**Correspondence With or About the Patient.** All written correspondence from the patient or from other doctors, laboratories, or independent health-care agencies must be kept in the patient's chart. Each piece of correspondence should be marked or stamped with the date the doctor's office received the document.

# Information Received by Fax

Some information—such as laboratory results, physician comments, or correspondence—may be received by fax transmission. Always request that the original be mailed if possible.

# Dating and Initialing

You must be careful not only to date everything you put into the patient chart but also to initial the entry. This system makes it easy to tell which items the assistant enters into the chart and which items others enter. In many practices the physician initials reports before they are filed to prove that he saw them.

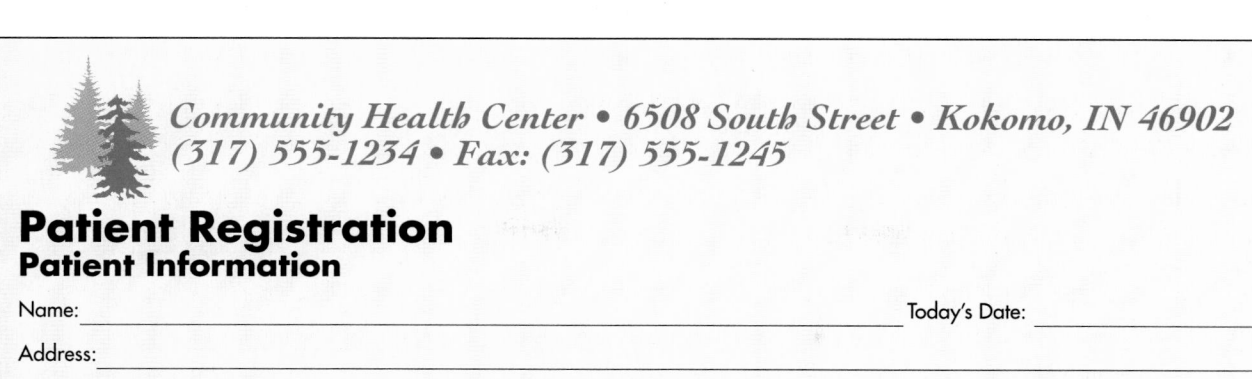

*Community Health Center • 6508 South Street • Kokomo, IN 46902*
*(317) 555-1234 • Fax: (317) 555-1245*

# Patient Registration
## Patient Information

Name: _____ Today's Date: _____

Address: _____

City: _____ State: _____ Zip Code: _____

Telephone (Home): _____ (Work): _____ (Cell): _____

Birthdate: _____ Age: _____ Sex: M  F   No. of Children _____ Marital Status: M  S  W  D

Social Security Number: _____ Employer: _____ Occupation: _____

Primary Physician: _____

Referred by: _____

Person to Contact in Emergency: _____

Emergency Telephone: _____

Special Needs: _____

## Responsible Party

Party Responsible for Payment:          Self          Spouse          Parent          Other

Name (If Other Than Self): _____

Address: _____

City: _____ State: _____ Zip Code: _____

## Primary Insurance

Primary Medical Insurance: _____

Insured party:     Self     Spouse     Parent     Other

ID#/Social Security No.: _____ Group/Plan No.: _____

Name (If Other Than Self): _____

Address: _____

City: _____ State: _____ Zip Code: _____

## Secondary Insurance

Secondary Medical Insurance: _____

Insured party:     Self     Spouse     Parent     Other

ID#/Social Security No.: _____ Group/Plan No.: _____

Name (If Other Than Self): _____

Address: _____

City: _____ State: _____ Zip Code: _____

**Figure 9-2.**   The patient registration form is often the first document used in initiating a patient record.

# The Medical Center at Springfield
## Medical History

Name _____ Age _____ Sex _____ S  M  W  D
Address _____ Phone _____ Date _____

Occupation _____ Ref. by _____
Chief Complaint _____

Present Illness _____
_____
_____
_____
_____

History —Military _____
    —Social _____
    —Family _____
    —Marital _____
    —Menstrual _____ Menarche _____ Para. _____ LMP _____
    —Illness  Measles  Pert.  Var.  Pneu.  Pleur.  Typh.  Mal.  Rh. Fev.  Sc. Fev.  Diphth.  Other
    —Surgery _____
    —Allergies _____
    —Current Medications _____

## Physical Examination

Temp. _____ Pulse _____ Resp. _____ BP _____ Ht. _____ Wt. _____
General Appearance _____ Skin _____ Mucous Membrane _____
Eyes: _____ Vision _____ Pupil _____ Fundus _____
Ears: _____
Nose: _____
Throat: _____ Pharynx _____ Tonsils _____
Chest: _____ Breasts _____
Heart: _____
Lungs: _____
Abdomen: _____
Genitalia: _____
Rectum: _____
Pelvic: _____
Extremities: _____ Pulses: _____
Lymph Nodes: _____ Neck _____ Axilla _____ Inguinal _____ Abdominal _____
Neurological: _____
Diagnosis: _____
_____
_____

Treatment: _____
_____
_____

Laboratory Findings: _____
Date _____ Blood _____
_____
_____

Date _____ Urine _____
_____
_____
_____
_____
_____

**Figure 9-3.** In some doctors' offices, the medical history form and the physical examination form are combined.

## THE OAK HILLS MEDICAL CENTER
### Oak Hills, MA

CONSENT TO OPERATION, ADMINISTRATION OF ANESTHETICS,
AND RENDERING OF OTHER MEDICAL SERVICE

Patient: _____ Age: _____
Date: _____ Time: _____

1. I AUTHORIZE AND DIRECT _____ , with the associates
   and assistants of his/her choice, to perform upon myself the following operation
   _____
   _____
   _____

   If any unforeseen conditions arise in the course of the operation or in the postoperative period, calling in their judgment for other operations or procedures, I further request and authorize them to do whatever is deemed advisable for my health and well-being.

2. The positive and negative aspects of autologous blood transfusions (receiving my own blood donated prior to surgery), designated blood transfusions (donated in advance by family/friends for my use), or homologous blood transfusions (from general donor population) have been explained to me. I understand autologous and designated transfusions can be accommodated only for nonemergency surgery.

6. I certify that I understand the above consent to operation and that the explanations referred to have been made.

_____          _____
Witness (of signature only)          Signature

**Figure 9-4.** Patients are asked to sign informed consent forms to confirm that they understand the treatment offered.

# Initiating and Maintaining Patient Records

Besides the receptionist, you will often be the first health-care professional that new patients talk with when they visit a doctor's office. During your first contact with a patient, you will initiate a patient record. Recording information in the medical record is called **documentation.** Complete, thorough documentation ensures that the doctor will have detailed notes about each contact with the patient and about the treatment plan, patient responses and progress, and treatment outcomes.

## Initial Interview

You usually perform the following tasks on your own, depending on the doctor's practice and your experience and background. Familiarize yourself with each task.

**Completing Medical History Forms.** You will help new patients fill out medical history forms or questionnaires. You may retrieve current patients' records from the files to update them. Type the patient's name and other identifying information on the first page and on all subsequent pages of the form.

You may interview patients to fill in some of the remaining blanks about medical history. Some doctors prefer to ask patients questions themselves. Others believe that people sometimes talk more freely with an assistant than they do with the doctor.

**Documenting Patient Statements.** You will record any signs, symptoms, or other information the patient wishes to share. Document this information in the patient's own words, not your interpretation of the words. Record this data in specific detail. For example, if the patient drinks alcohol, you should record the number of drinks per week, the type of liquor consumed, and whether

# Reflecting On . . . HIPAA

## Guidelines for Handling Protected Health Information Within the Medical Record

HIPAA (the Health Insurance Portability and Accountability Act) became law on August 21, 1996. This new law required that all health-care providers be in compliance by April 2003. HIPAA law states that all patients have rights regarding their health information, which is known as Protected Health Information (PHI). A patient's PHI is stored in the patient's record chart. Federal law protects the individual's rights to know about how her or his PHI is used and disclosed.

The term *use* means the employment, application, utilization, sharing, examination or analysis of **individual identifiable health information (IIHI)**. For example, when a medical assistant keys in a patient's health insurance number to determine the status of payment from the insurance company, the patient's PHI is being used. The term *disclosure* means the release or transfer in any way of patient IIHI beyond the confines of the health-care practice to which the information was given. For example, when a medical assistant gives patient information to another medical office to which the patient is being referred, PHI is being disclosed.

Patients have the following rights under HIPAA law:

1. *The right to notice of privacy practices.* Because it is unlikely that your patients will be reading federal laws, the law states it is your responsibility to give them a copy of the laws that protect them concerning their PHI. Patients must receive a written notice of privacy practices on their first visit to a health-care provider. They should sign a form stating they have received this information. This signed form must be carefully filed in the patients' medical record.

2. *The right to limit or request restriction on their PHI and its use and disclosure.* This means that patients can limit how your office uses their medical information, and how much of that information is shared. For example, a patient with a history of sexually transmitted disease may not wish to have that information released to the orthopedic physician who is setting his broken arm. It is not necessary. In general, only the minimal amount of patient information should be released to meet the current needs of the patient. This is called the "Need to Know" general rule.

3. *The right to confidential communications.* This means that patients can request to receive PHI in a manner other than during a medical appointment. For example, your patients may request that you call them at a variety of different numbers, including home, work, or cell phone number. The patient does not have to explain the request. The law says you must make a reasonable effort to communicate with the patient in a confidential manner as the patient requests.

4. *The right to inspect and obtain a copy of their PHI.* This means that patients have a right to request and receive a copy of their own medical records. There are a few exceptions to this rule; however, in general, the medical assistant receives and processes all patient requests for medical records. It is important to always follow the protocols established in your office for medical record copying. It is considered an acceptable practice to act on a request within 30 days of the request, and to charge a reasonable fee to cover the expense for copying supplies and labor.

5. *The right to request an amendment to their PHI.* Health-care providers have the right to require that a request to amend a record be made in writing. The request may be denied if the health-care provider receiving the request is not the original recorder of the PHI, or if the PHI is believed to be accurate and complete. All requests for amendment and response must be carefully documented and filed in the medical chart.

6. *The right to know if their PHI has been disclosed and why.* Providers are required to keep a written record of every disclosure made of a patient's PHI. You must also keep a written record of any request by the patient for this information and the response of the health-care provider. This information is usually filed in the patient's medical record. When making a disclosure of information, always record the date of the disclosure, the name and address of the person receiving the PHI, a brief summary of the information released, and the purpose of the disclosure.

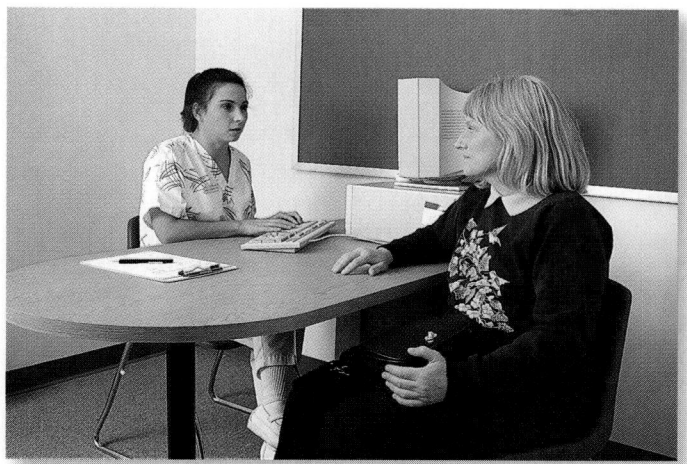

**Figure 9-5.** Conduct interviews with patients in a private or semiprivate room to make them feel more comfortable.

the drinking has affected the patient's behavior and health. Chart this information by writing "Patient states that . . ." and then, whenever possible, complete the sentence with the exact words the patient used.

Conduct the interview in a private room or in a semi-private office away from the reception area, as shown in Figure 9-5. Patients usually do not like to discuss their medical or personal problems in front of others. Your opinion of the patient, such as "the patient seems mentally unstable," is your own and should not be discussed or documented. The Points on Practice section will help you take information from elderly patients.

**Documenting Test Results.** Put a copy in the chart of any test results, x-ray reports, or other diagnostic results that the patient has brought with him. You may also record this information on a separate test summary sheet in the chart.

**Examination Preparation and Vital Signs.** In many instances, you will prepare patients for examination. You will record vital signs, medication the patient is currently taking, and any responses to treatment. Before you leave a patient, ask, "Is there anything else you would like the doctor to know?" The patient may be more comfortable sharing further information with you than with the doctor.

## Follow-Up

After you record the initial interview and background information, the doctor decides what entries will be made regarding examinations, diagnosis, treatment options and plans, and comments or observations about each case. You will then maintain the patient record by performing some or all of the following duties:

- Transcribing notes the doctor dictates about the patient's progress, follow-up visits, procedures, current status, and other necessary information

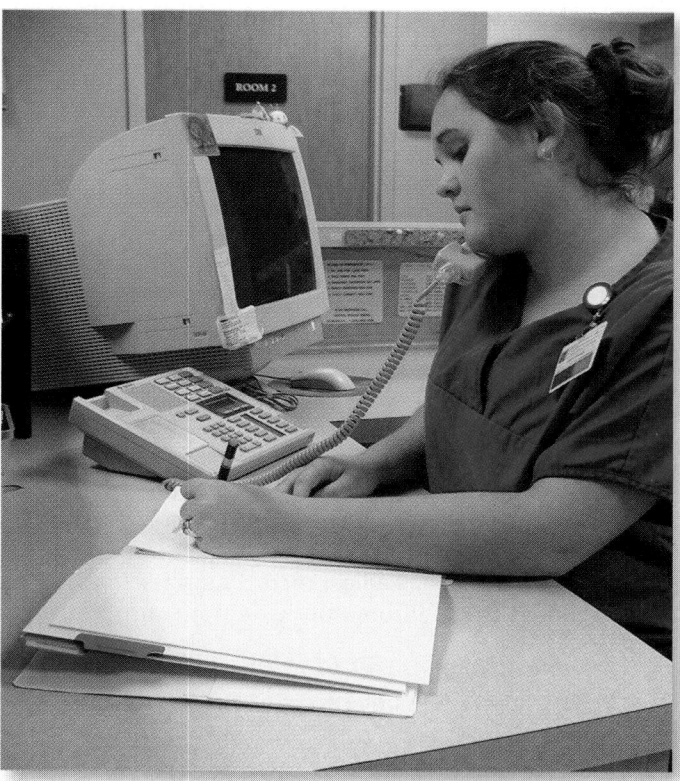

**Figure 9-6.** All telephone conversations to and from the patient must be logged in the patient record.

- Note that transcription by the medical assistant does not occur in all practices.
- Posting laboratory test results or results of examinations in the medical record or on the summary sheet
- Recording telephone calls from the patient and calls that the doctor or other office staff members make to the patient (Figure 9-6)
  - Telephone calls can be an important part of good follow-up care. Calls must be dated, and the content of the conversations must be documented. You must initial the entry. Even if the doctor did not reach the patient, the call should be recorded and dated. State whether the doctor got an answer, left a message on an answering machine or with a person, and so on. Legally, if an item is not in the record, it did not happen.
- Recording medical instructions or discharge instructions the doctor gives
  - At the doctor's request, you may counsel or educate the patient regarding the treatment regimen or home-care procedures the patient must follow. This information must be entered into the record, dated, and initialed. Some offices make carbon copies or photocopies of patient instructions.

Procedure 9-1 provides information about how to prepare a patient medical record/chart.

# PROCEDURE 9.1

## Preparing a Patient Medical Record/Chart

**Procedure Goal:** To assemble new patient record/charts

**Materials:** File folder, labels as appropriate (alphabet, numbers, dates, insurance, allergies, etc.), forms (patient information, advance directives, physician progress notes, referrals, laboratory forms), hole punch

**Method:**

1. Carefully create a chart label according to practice policy. This label may include the patient's last name followed by the first name, or it may be a medical record number for those offices that utilize numeric or alphanumeric filing

   ### Rationale
   The label must be correct to help avoid filing errors.

2. Place the chart label on the right edge of the folder, extending the label the length of the tab on the folder.

3. Place the date label on the top edge of the folder, updating the date according to the practice's policy. (The date is usually updated annually, provided the patient has come into the office within the last year.)

   ### Rationale
   It makes it easy to identify current patient records for retrieval as well as identify records for purging if the patient has not been seen for a specified amount of time (often, three years).

4. If alpha or numeric filing labels are utilized, place a patient name label on the chart according to the practice's policy.

5. Punch holes in the appropriate forms for placement within the patient's medical record/chart.

6. Place all the forms in appropriate sections of the patient's medical record/chart.

## The Six Cs of Charting

To maintain accurate patient records, always keep these six Cs in mind when filling out and maintaining charts: *C*lient's (patient's) words, *C*larity, *C*ompleteness, *C*onciseness, *C*hronological order, and *C*onfidentiality.

1. Client's words. Be careful to record the patient's exact words rather than your interpretation of them. For instance, if a client says, "My right knee feels like it's thick or full of fluid," write that down. Do not rephrase the sentence to say, "Client says he's got fluid on the knee." Often the patient's exact words, no matter how odd they may sound, provide important clues for the physician in making a diagnosis.

2. Clarity. Use precise descriptions and accepted medical terminology when describing a patient's condition. For instance, "Patient got out of bed and walked 20 feet without shortness of breath" is much clearer than "Patient got out of bed and felt fine."

3. Completeness. Fill out completely all the forms used in the patient record. Provide complete information that is readily understandable to others whenever you make any notation in the patient chart.

4. Conciseness. While striving for clarity, also be concise, or brief and to the point. Abbreviations and

specific medical terminology can often save time and space when recording information. For instance, you can write "Patient got OOB and walked 20 ft w/o SOB." OOB and SOB are standard abbreviations for "out of bed" and "shortness of breath," respectively. Every member of the office staff should use the same abbreviations to avoid misunderstandings. Table 9-1 lists some common medical abbreviations.

5. Chronological order. All entries in patient records must be dated to show the order in which they are made. This factor is critical, not only for documenting patient care but also in case there is a legal question about the type and date of medical services.

6. Confidentiality. All the information in patient records and forms is confidential, to protect the patient's privacy. Only the patient, attending physicians, and the medical assistant (who needs the record to tend to the patient and/or to make entries into the record) are allowed to see the charts without the patient's written consent. Never discuss a patient's records, forward them to another office, fax them, or show them to anyone but the physician unless you have the patient's written permission to do so. (Review the section, Reflecting On . . . HIPAA: Guidelines for Handling Protected Health Information Within the Medical Record.)

## TABLE 9-1    Common Medical Abbreviations

| Abbreviation | Meaning | Abbreviation | Meaning |
|---|---|---|---|
| AIDS | acquired immunodeficiency syndrome | inj. | injection |
| a.m.a. | against medical advice | IV | intravenous |
| b.i.d./BID | twice a day | MI | myocardial infarction |
| BP | blood pressure | MM | mucous membrane |
| bpm | beats per minute | NPO | nothing by mouth |
| CBC | complete blood count | NYD | not yet diagnosed |
| C.C. | chief complaint | OOB | out of bed |
| CNS | central nervous system | OPD | outpatient department |
| CPE | complete physical examination | OR | operating room |
| CV | cardiovascular | PH | past history |
| D & C | dilation and curettage | PT | physical therapy |
| Dx | diagnosis | Pt | patient |
| ECG/EKG | electrocardiogram | q.i.d./QID | four times a day |
| ER | emergency room | ROS/SR | review of systems/systems review |
| FH | family history | s.c./subq. | subcutaneously |
| Fl/fl | fluid | SOB | shortness of breath |
| GBS | gallbladder series | S/R | suture removal |
| GI | gastrointestinal | stat | immediately |
| GU | genitourinary | t.i.d./TID | three times a day |
| GYN | gynecology | TPR | temperature, pulse, respirations |
| HEENT | head, ears, eyes, nose, throat | UCHD | usual childhood diseases |
| HIV | human immunodeficiency virus | VS | vital signs |
| I & D | incision and drainage | WNL | within normal limits |
| ICU | intensive care unit | | |

# Types of Medical Records

You should be familiar with the different approaches to documenting patient information. The most common methods are conventional/source-oriented and problem-oriented medical records.

## Conventional, or Source-Oriented, Records

In the conventional, or source-oriented, approach, patient information is arranged according to who supplied the data—the patient, doctor, specialist, or someone else. The medical form may have a space for patient remarks, followed by a section for the doctor's comments.

These records describe all problems and treatments on the same form in simple chronological order. For example, a patient's broken wrist would be recorded on the same form as her stomach ulcer. Although easy to initiate and maintain, this system presents some difficulty in tracking the progress of a specific ailment, such as the patient's ulcer. The doctor has to search the entire record to find information on that one problem.

## Problem-Oriented Medical Records

One way to overcome the disadvantages of the conventional approach is to use the problem-oriented medical record (POMR) system of keeping charts. This approach,

## Talking With the Older Patient

If you work in a practice that specializes in geriatrics or in any practice with older patients, certain communication skills will help you in your job. You may find yourself in various situations in which knowing how to talk with the older patient will be a necessary skill. Taking a medical history and helping a patient describe her symptoms are two such situations. The following tips will help you and the patient communicate with each other more effectively.

1. Make sure you select a private setting for the patient interview.

2. Many older patients are hard of hearing, but *not deaf.* Speak slightly more slowly than you normally would. Speak clearly and loudly (but do not shout—shouting will insult and anger an older patient who does hear well). Enunciate well, and use a lower tone of voice (elderly people lose the ability to hear high-frequency sounds first). If the patient asks you to repeat a question, rephrase it instead of repeating it verbatim.

3. Look at the patient directly so that she knows you care about what she has to say and so that you can make sure she understands what you tell or ask her.

4. You can show respect for the patient's age by addressing the patient with Mr., Mrs., Ms., or Miss, unless the patient asks to be called by his or her first name.

5. Be patient. Some older patients live alone or in relative isolation and may be out of practice with the two-way communication skills that make a conversation or interview go smoothly. The simple act of being interviewed, even for what may seem to you a straightforward medical history, may unsettle the older patient. For example, he may need to stop and think of a word here and there. Do not supply the word. Wait and let the patient think of it on his own. Also, do not rush through your questions. Rushing will only make the patient feel anxious and incompetent if she feels she cannot keep up with you.

6. Practice active listening skills. Pay attention to the patient's verbal and nonverbal cues. Do not interrupt the patient. After the patient finishes giving each answer, repeat it, to give him a chance to correct you if you misheard or misunderstood.

7. If you are interviewing the patient to obtain a medical history, explain before you begin the type of questions you will ask and how the information will be used.

8. If you need to use medical terminology, try also to express the same information in lay terms. For example, you might ask, "Do you use a diuretic or pill to help you eliminate fluids?"

9. Be cheerful and friendly but not sugary-sweet. Do not talk down to older patients; they are not stupid.

10. Avoid sounding surprised or excited by any answer to a question or to any information the patient gives.

11. Under no circumstances use endearments such as dear, honey, or sweetie.

12. Look for ways to make a connection so that the patient feels relaxed and comfortable. For example, in the course of taking a patient's history, you might find out that he enjoys swimming. Ask him to tell you about it.

13. Show an interest in the patient as a person. Ask about something she is interested in. For example, a patient might be wearing a piece of handmade jewelry. Ask where it came from. She might have a wonderful story to tell.

---

developed by Lawrence L. Weed, MD, makes it easier for the physician to keep track of a patient's progress. The information in a POMR includes the database; problem list; educational, diagnostic, and treatment plan; and progress notes.

**Database.** The database includes a record of the patient's history; information from the initial interview with the patient (for example, "Patient unemployed—second time in past 12 months"); all findings and results from physical examinations (such as "Pulse 105 bpm, BP 210/80"); and any tests, x-rays, and other procedures.

**Problem List.** Each problem a patient has is listed separately, given its own number, and dated. You then identify a problem by its number throughout the record.

You can also list work-related, social, or family problems that may be affecting the patient's health. For instance, the problem list for the example patient who is unemployed might include, "Severe stomach pain, worse at night and after eating."

You can alert the doctor to the fact that the patient has lost two jobs within 1 year. Such radical life changes can often provoke strong physical reactions. In this patient's case the elevated blood pressure may be related to the job losses, and stress may be causing the stomach pain.

When you document problems, be careful to distinguish between patient signs and symptoms. **Signs** are objective, or external, factors—such as blood pressure, rashes, or swelling—that can be seen or felt by the doctor or measured by an instrument. **Symptoms** are subjective, or internal, conditions felt by the patient, such as pain, headache, or nausea. Together, signs and symptoms help clarify a patient's problem.

**Educational, Diagnostic, and Treatment Plan.** Each problem should have a detailed educational, diagnostic, and treatment summary in the record. The summary contains diagnostic workups, treatment plans, and instructions for the patient. Here is an example.

*Problem 2, Stomach Pain, 2/2/XX [date]*
- *Upper GI exam negative, CBC normal.*
- *Prescribed over-the-counter antacid, 2 tablets by mouth t.i.d. after each meal.*
- *Set up appointment for patient with Dr. R. Neil at stress-management clinic (Broughten Professional Center) for Monday, February 4, at 4:30 p.m.*
- *Patient's anxiety is high. Recheck in 1 week.*

**Progress Notes.** Progress notes are entered for each problem listed in the initial record. The documentation always includes—in chronological order—the patient's condition, complaints, problems, treatment, and responses to care. Here is an example.

*Problem 2, Stomach Pain, 2/9/XX. Patient enrolled in stress-reduction class. Reports stomach pain has diminished—"I can eat without pain; only a little discomfort at night." Vital signs improved: pulse 85 bpm, BP 115/70, respiration 20. Reduced antacid to one tablet by mouth two times daily after meals. Anxiety much reduced. Recheck anxiety level in 2 weeks.*

## SOAP Documentation

Many medical records, such as the POMR format, emphasize the **SOAP** approach to documentation, which provides an orderly series of steps for dealing with any medical case. SOAP documentation lists the patient's symptoms, the diagnosis, and the suggested treatment.

Information is documented in the record in the following order.

1. S: **Subjective** data come from the patient; they describe his or her signs and symptoms and supply any other opinions or comments.
2. O: **Objective** data come from the physician and from examinations and test results.
3. A: *Assessment* is the diagnosis or impression of a patient's problem.
4. P: *Plan* of action includes treatment options, chosen treatment, medications, tests, consultations, patient education, and follow-up.

Whether you keep conventional or POMR charts, you can include all these steps for each problem. Figure 9-7 shows an example of SOAP notes. If you abbreviate any term when entering data into the records, use only approved medical abbreviations. For example, use "5 g" instead of "5 grams." Several resources, including those published by JCAHO and the American Medical Association, list approved medical abbreviations for measurements, instructions for taking medication, and other topics. Keep these references readily available in the office.

# Appearance, Timeliness, and Accuracy of Records

You must ensure that the medical records are complete. They must also be written neatly and legibly, contain up-to-date information, and present an accurate, professional record of a patient's case.

## Neatness and Legibility

A medical record is useless if the doctor or others have difficulty reading it. You should make sure that every word and number in the record is clear and legible. Follow these tips to keep charts neat and easy to read.

- Use a good-quality pen that will not smudge or smear.
- HIPAA requires that all original documents be maintained in the patient's medical record. Blue ink is considered the best choice for charting. It is easy to confuse an original written in black ink with a copy. Blue ink will copy as black, making the original and copy look different, which can reduce the possibility of error. Blue ink is also more difficult to match, making any additions to the medical record easy to spot, which can cut down on fraudulent entries. For these reasons, blue ink is the best choice for documentation.
- Use highlighting pens to call attention to specific items such as allergies. Be aware, however, that unless the office has a color copier, most colored ink will photocopy black or gray. Highlighting-pen marks may not be visible on a photocopy.

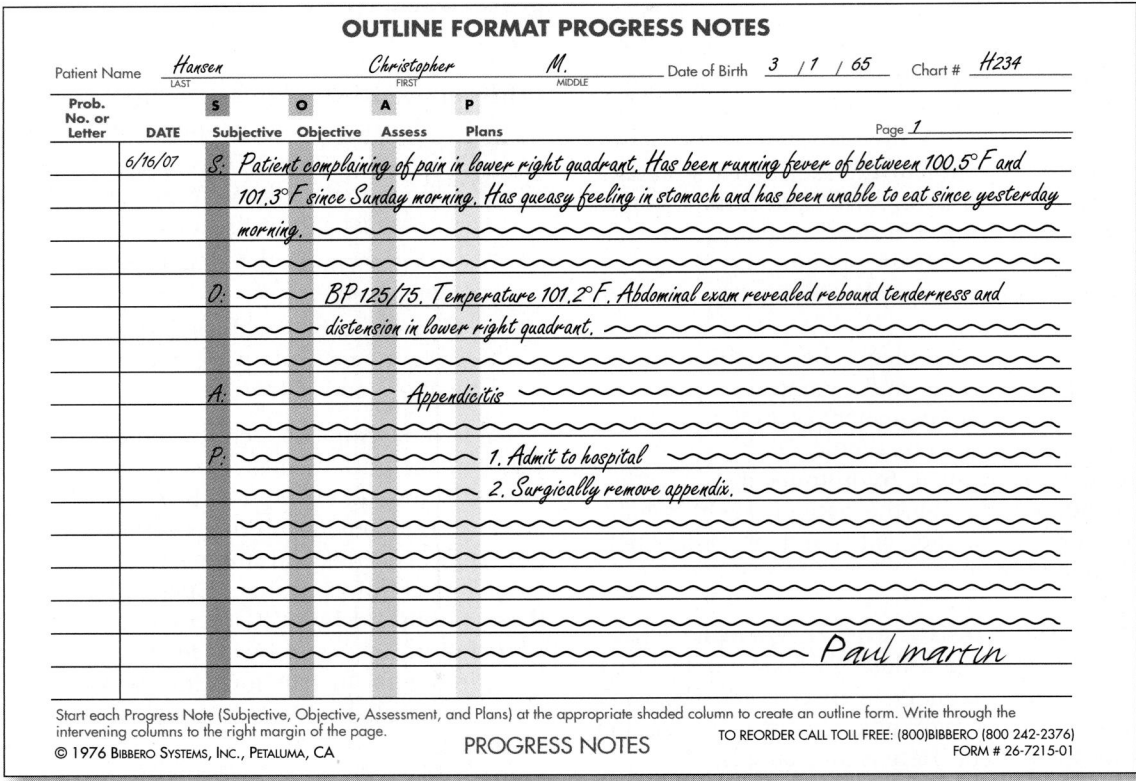

**OUTLINE FORMAT PROGRESS NOTES**

Patient Name _Hansen_ (LAST) _Christopher_ (FIRST) _M._ (MIDDLE) Date of Birth _3_ / _1_ / _65_ Chart # _H234_

| Prob. No. or Letter | DATE | S Subjective | O Objective | A Assess | P Plans | Page _1_ |

6/16/07

S: Patient complaining of pain in lower right quadrant. Has been running fever of between 100.5°F and 101.3°F since Sunday morning. Has queasy feeling in stomach and has been unable to eat since yesterday morning.

O: BP 125/75. Temperature 101.2°F. Abdominal exam revealed rebound tenderness and distension in lower right quadrant.

A: Appendicitis

P: 1. Admit to hospital
2. Surgically remove appendix.

_Paul Martin_

Start each Progress Note (Subjective, Objective, Assessment, and Plans) at the appropriate shaded column to create an outline form. Write through the intervening columns to the right margin of the page.

**PROGRESS NOTES**

TO REORDER CALL TOLL FREE: (800)BIBBERO (800 242-2376)
FORM # 26-7215-01

© 1976 BIBBERO SYSTEMS, INC., PETALUMA, CA

**Figure 9-7.** The SOAP approach to documentation is one way to organize information in a patient record.

- Make sure all handwriting is legible. Take time to write names, numbers, and abbreviations clearly.
- Make any corrections to the chart by following Procedure 9-2, Correcting Medical Records.

## Timeliness

Medical records should be kept up to date and should be readily available when a doctor or another health-care professional needs to see them. Follow these guidelines to ensure that a doctor can find the most recent information on a patient when it is needed.

- Record all findings from exams and tests as soon as they are available.
- If you forget to enter a finding into the record when it is received, record both the original date of receipt and the date the finding was entered into the record.
- To document telephone calls, record the date and time of the call, who initiated it, the information discussed, and any conclusions or results. You can either enter the telephone call directly into the record or make a note referring the doctor to a separate telephone log kept in the record.
- Establish a procedure for retrieving a file quickly in case of emergency. Should the patient be in a serious

accident, for example, the emergency doctor will need the patient's medical history immediately.

## Accuracy

The physician must be able to trust the accuracy of the information in the medical records. You must make it a priority always to check the accuracy of all data you will enter in a chart. To ensure accurate data, follow these guidelines.

- Never guess at or assume knowledge of names, procedures, medications, findings, or any other information about which there is some question. Always check all the information carefully. Make the extra effort to ask questions of the physician or senior staff member and to verify information.
- Double-check the accuracy of findings and instructions recorded in the chart. Have all numbers been copied accurately? Are instructions for taking medication clear and complete?
- Make sure the latest information has been entered into the chart so that the physician has an accurate picture of the patient's current condition.

Procedure 9-2 explains how to correct a medical chart.

## Professional Attitude and Tone

Part of creating timely, accurate records is maintaining a professional tone in your writing when recording information. Record information from the patient using his own words. Also record the doctor's observations and comments as well as any laboratory or test results. Do not record your personal, subjective comments, judgments, opinions, or speculations about a patient's words, problems, or test results. You may call attention to a particular problem or observation, for example, by attaching a note to the chart. Do not, however, make such comments part of the patient's record.

## Computer Records

In some offices the computer is used for more than just storing financial, billing, and insurance information. Some hospitals, clinics, and even individual physicians use computer software and hardware to create and store patient records. These **electronic health records (EHR)** or **electronic medical records (EMR)** are created and recorded on a desktop or even some type of portable computer. When medical records are kept electronically it is essential that the facility have policies in place to ensure security and confidentiality of records. In addition, electronic files must be backed-up on a regular basis to avoid accidental loss of data. Whether you are documenting by hand or electronically, accuracy is always important. Careful key entry is essential to maintain accurate electronic files.

### Advantages of Computerizing Records

In a setting in which several terminals in a network are connected to a main computer, computerizing medical records presents several advantages. A physician can call up the record on her own or another computer monitor whenever the record is needed, review or update the file, and save it to the central computer again (see Figure 9-8).

Computerized records can also be used in teleconferences, where people in different locations can look at the same record on their individual computer screens at the same time. Records can also be sent by modem to the physician's home computer so that the physician will have a patient's records on hand for calls after hours. Computer access to patient records is also helpful for health-care providers with satellite offices in different cities or different parts of a city. Review the Points on Practice box for information about electronic health records.

Computers are useful for tickler files (files that need periodic attention). For example, they can alert staff members about patients who are due for yearly checkups and patients who require follow-up care. Some hospitals have begun to use electronically scanned images of patients'

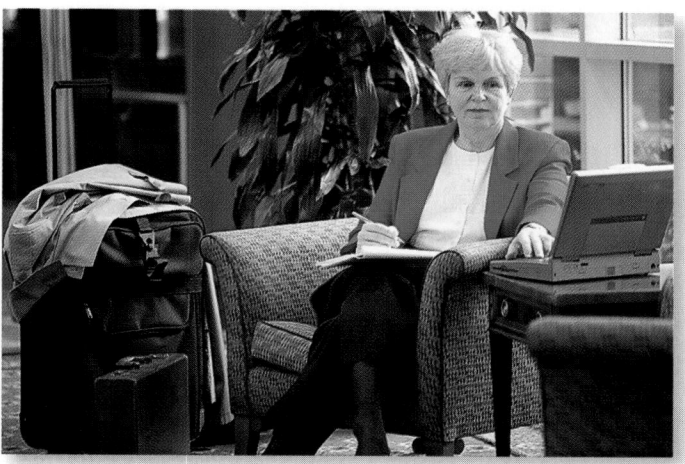

**Figure 9-8.** Computerized medical records, laptop computers, and the Internet provide physicians with easy access no matter where they are.

thumbprints to keep track of records. This system saves time and helps maintain the security of patient records. (Review Chapter 6 for more information on the use of computers in the medical practice.)

### Security Concerns

Protecting the confidentiality of patient records in computer files is the greatest concern of electronic health records. Just as paper health care records are kept secure, so should the electronic health care records be secure. Review Chapter 6 for more information about maintaining computer confidentiality.

## Medical Transcription

Your knowledge of abbreviations, medical terminology, and medical coding will be invaluable when transcribing a doctor's notes or dictation (either recorded or direct). **Transcription** means transforming spoken notes into accurate written form. These written notes are then entered into the patient record. As is the case with information in medical charts, all dictated materials are confidential and should be regarded as potential legal documents. They are part of the patient's continuing case history. They often include findings, treatment stages, prognoses, and final outcomes. Always date and initial all transcription pages.

Strive to make transcribed material accurate and complete. Good grammar, spelling, and an accurate use of medical abbreviations and terminology are important in maintaining patient records. Use the medical dictionary and the medical computer spelling check to verify the spelling or meaning of words. Ask the physician only if you cannot find something in a reference source. Above-average typing or word processing accuracy and speed are also important. (See Chapter 5, Procedure 5-4, Using a Dictation-Transcription Machine.)

# Working With Electronic Health Records

Electronic health records (EHRs) are essentially a computer-based or a digital recording of patient information. They are also called computer records, electronic medical records (EMR), electronic charts, and computer health records. Paper records can be lost and information is not consistent. In addition, handwriting is often illegible. EHRs provide a multitude of advantages, including the following:

- Access. Electronic records can be accessed by health-care providers at various locations, including the laboratory, pharmacy, and even the medical records department.
- Availability. Information is immediately available, so health-care providers do not have to wait for the paper document to get written and sent. The data is entered and then immediately viewed at any electronic record location.
- Security. Electronic records provide security through special passwords for each individual entering the records. Passwords can be set to open access to only the parts necessary for the type of health-care provider.
- Safety. Sophisticated programs help prevent patient identification errors by including a picture of each patient as part of the patient record.
- Extra Features. Electronic software programs can alert the health-care provider to abnormal results to tests or the need for routine tests to be performed. More sophisticated programs can document health trends, provide voice recognition, and convert notes to complete sentences.

As a medical assistant working with electronic records, you should keep the following in mind:

- Become familiar with the software and hardware used at your facility. Make sure you are not focused on the computer when you are with the patient. Becoming comfortable with the system you are using will help you to focus on the patient. If necessary, take notes and enter them in the computer when the patient is not present until you become comfortable.
- Retrieve the patient record carefully just as you would a paper record. Make sure you have identified the patient with at least two identifiers such as the name, date of birth, and/or medical record number.
- Keep your password information secure. Change the password on a regular basis or as directed by the health-care facility.
- Secure the computer that maintains the electronic records and keep a backup of electronic files.
- Check your entries carefully before hitting the enter button. An EHR is a legal document just like a paper chart.

# Transcribing Direct Dictation

At times the physician may wish to dictate material directly to you. He may want to get observations, comments, or treatment options into the record immediately rather than waiting until a more convenient time to dictate the material into a recorder. Follow these guidelines.

- Use a writing pad with a stiff backing or place the pad on a clipboard to make it easier to write quickly. Use a good ballpoint pen that will not smear or drag on the paper.
- Use incomplete sentences and phrases to keep up with the physician's pace. For example, say "Patient home Friday, re-check 2 wks" instead of "The patient is going home on Friday. We should see him again in 2 weeks."

- Use abbreviations for common phrases (*w/o* for "without," *s/b* for "should be," and so on); for medical terms (*q.d.* for "every day," *mg* for "milligrams," and so on); and for medications or chemicals.
- If a term, phrase, prescription, or name is unclear, ask for clarification right away (say "Excuse me, could you repeat that phrase, please?").
- If the physician speaks with a pronounced accent, ask her to speak more slowly than normal.
- Read the dictation back to the physician to verify all terms, names, figures, and other information for accuracy.
- Enter the notes into the patient record, and date and initial the notes.

# Medical Transcriptionist

*To gain medical assistant credentials, you must fulfill the requirements of either the American Association of Medical Assistants (for a Certified Medical Assistant) or the American Medical Technologists (for a Registered Medical Assistant). After obtaining your medical assistant certification or registration, you may wish to acquire additional skills in specialty areas through course work or on-the-job training. Although this course work or training may not lead to an additional certification or degree, it will enable you to expand your role in the medical office and advance your career as the demand for skilled health professionals increases.*

## Skills and Duties

A medical transcriptionist creates written health records for patients based on the physician's dictation or notes. The records may be typewritten or input on a computer. Some transcriptionists work for a single physician; others work for a small or large group.

To create a patient record, the transcriptionist listens to an audiocassette containing information dictated by the physician. Typical information on the tape includes the physician's diagnosis and treatment of the patient. Using dictation equipment, the transcriptionist can slow down or stop and start the cassette tape as she types.

The medical transcriptionist must have excellent typing skills and a good command of medical terminology to make sure that medical terms are used accurately and spelled correctly. She will often need to edit the physician's notes to make sure that the language follows standard English grammar and usage. Sometimes she must also reorganize the physician's comments to create an understandable and easy-to-follow medical record. After she finishes transcribing the record, the medical transcriptionist checks it for correct spelling and punctuation. This last step is called proofreading.

## Workplace Settings

Medical transcriptionists may work in the medical records department of a hospital or in a nursing home, clinic, laboratory, physician's practice, insurance company, or emergency or immediate health-care center. Some transcriptionists work for medical transcribing firms; others are self-employed and work out of their homes.

## Education

Medical transcriptionists usually complete a training program at a 4-year college or university, junior or community college, vocational institute, or adult education center. They receive instruction in medical terminology, anatomy and physiology, pharmaceuticals, laboratory procedures, and medical treatments. Some transcriptionists concentrate on a particular specialty area, such as pathology, and acquire specialized training in that area. Medical transcriptionists can become certified if they meet the qualifying standards of the American Association for Medical Transcription.

## Where to Go for More Information

American Association for Medical Transcription
P.O. Box 576187
Modesto, CA 95355

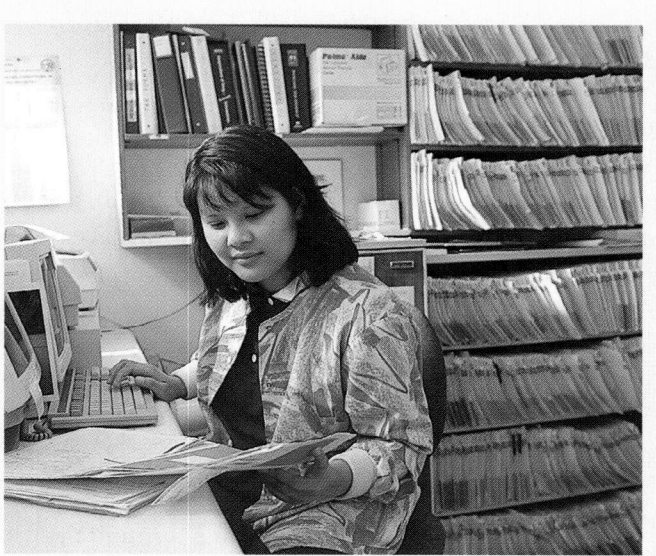

# Transcription Aids

Keep a library of medical, secretarial, and transcription reference books and medical terminology texts near the transcription workstation. Abbreviations can save time, but you should use only those that are accepted as standard. Reference books will help you find the correct word quickly and easily and help you apply proper grammar, style, and usage to the copy.

# Correcting and Updating Patient Records

In legal terms, medical records are regarded as having been created in "due course." All information in the record should be entered at the time of a patient's visit and not days, weeks, or months later. Information corrected or added some time after a patient's visit can be regarded as "convenient" and may damage a doctor's position in a lawsuit.

## Using Care With Corrections

If changes to the medical record are not done correctly, the record can become a legal problem for the physician. A physician may be able to more easily explain poor or incomplete documentation than to explain a chart that appears to have been altered after something was originally documented. You must be extremely careful to follow the appropriate procedures for correcting patient records.

Mistakes in medical records are not uncommon. The best defense is to correct the mistake immediately or as soon as possible after the original entry was made. Procedure 9-2 shows you how to correct the patient record.

## Updating Patient Records

All additions to a patient's record—test results, observations, diagnoses, procedures—should be done in a way that no one could interpret as deception on the physician's part. In a note accompanying the material, the physician should explain why the information is being added to the record. In some cases the material may simply be a physician's recollections or observations on a patient visit that occurred in the past. Each item added to a record must be dated and initialed. Sometimes a third party may be asked to witness the addition. Procedure 9-3 shows you how to maintain medical records properly.

Most hospitals and clinics have detailed guidelines for late entries to a patient's chart. You must follow these guidelines carefully to avoid potential legal problems (see Procedure 9-2).

## PROCEDURE 9.2

### Correcting Medical Records

**Procedure Goal:** To follow standard procedures for correcting a medical record

**Materials:** Patient file, other pertinent documents that contain the information to be used in making corrections (for example, transcribed notes, telephone notes, physician's comments, correspondence), good ballpoint pen

**Method:**

1. Always make the correction in a way that does not suggest any intention to deceive, cover up, alter, or add information to conceal a lack of proper medical care.

2. When deleting information, never black it out, never use correction fluid to cover it up, and never in any other way erase or obliterate the original wording. Draw a line through the original information so that it is still legible.

   *Rationale*

   All entries to a medical chart, even errors, must be legible according to law.

3. Write or type in the correct information above or below the original line or in the margin. The location on the chart for the new information should be clear. You may need to attach another sheet of paper or another document with the correction on it. Note in the record "See attached document A" or similar wording to indicate where the corrected information can be found.

4. Place a note near the correction stating why it was made (for example, "error, wrong date; error, interrupted by phone call.") This indication can be a brief note in the margin or an attachment to the record. As a general rule of thumb, do not make any changes without noting the reason for them.

   *Rationale*

   By noting the reason as well as the correction, you clearly indicate that the correction is intentional and necessary.

5. Enter the date and time, and initial the correction.

   *Rationale*

   No correction to a medical chart is complete or acceptable without these elements.

6. If possible, have another staff member or the physician witness and initial the correction to the record when you make it.

# PROCEDURE 9.3

## Maintaining Medical Records

**Procedure Goal:** To document continuity of care by creating a complete, accurate, timely record of the medical care provided at your facility

**Materials:** Patient file, other pertinent documents (test results, x-rays, telephone notes, correspondence), blue ballpoint pen, notebook, keyboard, transcribing equipment

**Method:**

1. Verify that you have the correct chart for the records to be filed.

   *Rationale*

   You do not want to record information in the wrong patient chart.

2. Transcribe dictated doctor's notes as soon as possible, and enter them into the patient record.

   *Rationale*

   Delays increase the chance of making errors in transcribing and recording the information. Also, for legal reasons, medical information should be entered into the record in a timely fashion.

3. Spell out the names of disorders, diseases, medications, and other terms the first time you enter them into the patient record, followed by the appropriate abbreviation (for example: "congestive heart failure [CHF]"). Thereafter, you may use the abbreviation alone.

   *Rationale*

   Using only abbreviations could cause confusion.

4. Enter only what the doctor has dictated. Do *not* add your own comments, observations, or evaluations. Use self-adhesive flags or other means to call the doctor's attention to something you have noticed that may be helpful to the patient's case. Date and initial each entry.

   *Rationale*

   Should the file be examined later in a legal proceeding, your notes and comments will be taken as part of the official record.

5. Follow office procedure to record routine or special laboratory test results. They may be posted in a particular section of the file or on a separate test summary form. If you use the summary form, make a note in the file that the results were received and recorded. Place the original laboratory report in the patient's file if required to do so by office policy. Date and initial each entry. Always note in the chart the date of the test and the results, whether or not test result printouts are filed in the record.

6. Make a note in the record of all telephone calls to and from the patient. Date and initial the entries. These entries may also include the doctor's comments, observations, changes in the patient's medication, new instructions to the patient, and so on. If calls are recorded in a separate telephone log, note in the patient's record the time and date of the call and refer to the log. It is particularly important to record such calls when the patient resists or refuses treatment, skips appointments, or has not made follow-up appointments.

   *Rationale*

   These entries can demonstrate that a doctor made every effort to provide quality care and that the patient is demonstrating noncompliant behavior.

7. Read over the entries for omissions or mistakes. Ask the doctor to answer any questions you have.

   *Rationale*

   If it is not written down, from a legal perspective, it did not happen.

8. Make sure that you have dated and initialed each entry.

9. Be sure that all documents are included in the file.

10. Replace the patient's file in the filing system as soon as possible.

# Release of Records

All physical medical records, including x-rays, test results, and physician notes created by the doctor, are considered the property of that doctor. However, the information contained within the physical record belongs to the patient and is regarded as confidential. Even though the doctor owns the records, no one can see them or obtain information from them without the patient's written consent. However, the law may require the doctor to release them, as in the case of a patient with a contagious disease or when the records are subpoenaed by a court.

## Procedures for Releasing Records

Physicians often receive requests from lawyers, other physicians, insurance companies, government agencies, and the patient himself for copies of a patient's records. Follow these steps for releasing medical information.

1. Obtain a signed and newly dated release from the patient authorizing the **transfer** of specific information—that is, giving information to another party outside the physician's office. *Verbal consent in person or over the telephone is not considered a valid release.* The release form should be filed in the patient's record.

2. Make photocopies of the original material. Copy and send only those portions of the record covered by the release and usually only records originating from your facility. Unless the patient specifically requests that you do so, you should not release records that were obtained from other sources, such as consultations or tests done in a hospital. Do not send original documents. (If a record will be used in a court case, however, you must submit the original unless the judge specifies that a photocopy is acceptable.) If you cannot make copies, as in the case of x-rays, send the originals, and tell the recipient that they must be returned (Figure 9-9). Follow up with the recipient until the originals have been returned and are placed in the patient's files. Often, the recipient is asked to sign a statement of responsibility for the original records until they are returned to the office. Document in the chart who has possession of the original document, the date the recipient received the originals, and the date they are returned.

3. Call the recipient to confirm that all materials were received. Avoid faxing confidential records. There is no way to tell who will see documents sent by fax.

## Special Cases

It may not always be immediately clear who has the right to sign a release-of-records form. When a couple divorces, for example, both parents are still considered legal guardians of their children, and either one can sign a release form authorizing transfer of medical records. If a patient dies, the patient's next of kin or legally authorized representative, such as the executor of the estate, may see the records or authorize their release to a third party. When you are in doubt regarding who is authorized to sign, *always* ask your supervisor before releasing confidential medical records.

## Confidentiality

When children reach age 18, most states consider them adults with the right to privacy. No one, not even their parents, may see their medical records without the children's written consent. Some states extend this right to privacy to emancipated minors who are under the age of 18 and living on their own or are married, a parent, or in the armed services. This is particularly the case with minors seeking care for STDs, birth control, and drug or alcohol counseling. In these instances, the minor is considered a "mature minor" and her treatment cannot be discussed with her parents without her permission, even though the parents may still be held responsible for payment of such treatment through insurance or self-payment unless the patient pays for treatment at the time of service.

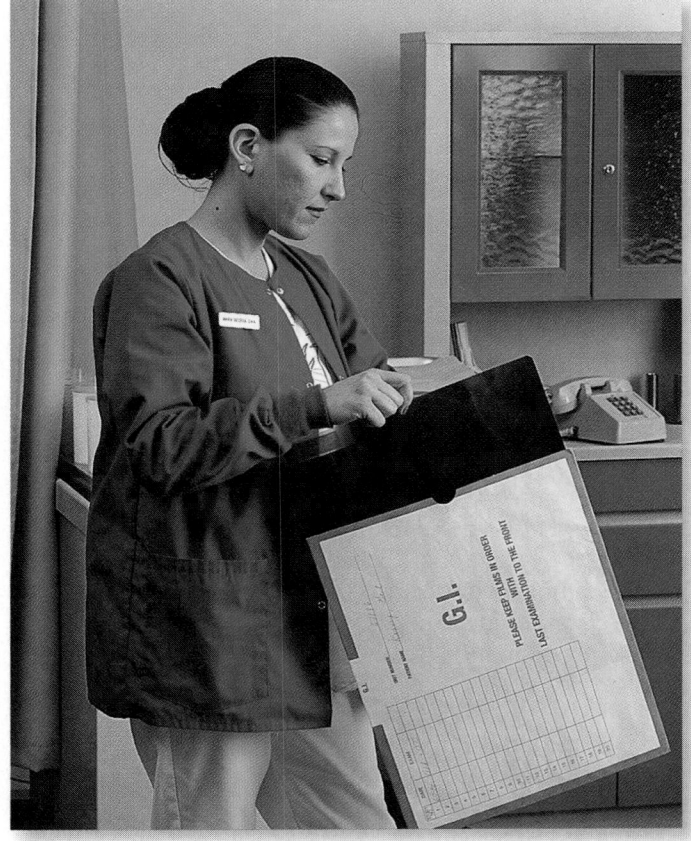

**Figure 9-9.** When you are preparing a patient record to be transferred, never send original material. One exception to this rule is x-rays, which should be sent with a request that the recipient return them as soon as possible.

The main legal and ethical principle to keep in mind is that you must protect each patient's right to privacy at all times.

## Summary

The medical assistant must properly prepare and maintain patient records. Patient records, also known as charts, contain important information about a patient's medical history and present condition. Patient records serve as communication tools as well as legal documents. They also play a role in patient and staff education and may be used for quality control and research. The six Cs of charting are the client's words, clarity, completeness, conciseness, chronological order, and confidentiality.

You should be familiar with the most common methods for documenting patient information, which include the conventional, or source-oriented, and the problem-oriented medical record approaches. You must ensure not only that the medical records are complete but also that they are neat, legible, contain up-to-date information, and present an accurate and professional record of a patient's care.

Part of maintaining patient records includes transcribing physician's notes—that is, transforming spoken notes into accurate written form. In addition, you must know the guidelines for how to correct and update a patient record and how to legally release it to a third party by obtaining written consent from the patient.

# REVIEW

## CHAPTER 9

## CASE STUDY QUESTIONS

Now that you have completed this chapter, review the case study at the beginning of the chapter and answer the following questions:

1. Why is an accurate medical record important to the care of a patient?
2. Why is interviewing the patient important to the medical evaluation?
3. What are the six Cs of charting and what do they mean to you as a medical assistant?
4. What are the differences between the conventional and the POMR systems of keeping charts?
5. What are some helpful tips you might use as you perform transcription?

## Discussion Questions

1. Select one of the six Cs of charting and discuss why it is important to maintain accurate patient records.
2. Why is confidentiality regarding medical charting so difficult to maintain? Name three areas of concern in daily chart management that could lead to a loss of confidentiality, and discuss.
3. Discuss the procedures for releasing medical records.

## Critical Thinking Questions

1. A patient wants to take his medical records and x-rays to another physician's office. He insists that the records belong to him. How would you handle this situation?
2. Identify the elements of SOAP charting for the following scenario: A patient has come to see the doctor complaining of asthma. She says she has been wheezing and coughing for two days. The patient's vital signs are P–102, B/P–146/100, R–28, T–98.6. Following examination, the physician determines the patient is having an asthma attack. She gives you an order to give the patient a breathing treatment using the nebulizer and 2.5 mg of albuteral sulfate. Then you are to take her vital signs again.

## Application Activities

1. After reading the following description of a patient's condition, list the patient's signs and symptoms.

   A 72-year-old man with no history of gastrointestinal problems was complaining of fatigue, back pain, appetite loss, and nausea. The patient had a hemoglobin of about 7 g, indicating marked anemia. His blood pressure was low (95/70), his heartbeat erratic—from 55 to 85 bpm—and his white blood cell count elevated.

   While in the office he experienced a headache and ringing in his right ear. A CT scan taken the next day revealed an abdominal aortic aneurysm containing a large clot. The scan also revealed a small lesion in the lining of the stomach.

2. Role-play in groups of three students. One student should play the patient, one the medical assistant, and one the observer. Role-play a scenario in which the patient requests to have her medical records released to another physician. The medical assistant should explain to the patient the process for the release of her medical records.

   The observer should not speak but should observe and take notes on the scenario as acted out by the other two students. The observer should compare the scenario to the steps provided in the text for the release of records. Note what is done well and what needs improvement.

   Each student should rotate through all three roles.

3. Photocopy the blank combination medical history and physical examination form shown in Figure 9-3. Fill out the form by using the following patient information:

   For medical history section: Date: 2/14/07; the patient is Heather R. MacEntee, age 35, living at 344 Westwind Lane, Apartment 28, Round Tree, IL 60012; telephone (708) 333-5555. She is a real estate broker, married, with a 6-year-old child. Her father died at age 55; her mother is 62 and has congestive heart disease. She has no siblings. The family has a history of heart disease and diabetes. The patient had chickenpox and mumps at age 7 and surgery for an ovarian cyst at 22. She has an allergy to ragweed but is not taking any medications at present.

   For physical examination section: Ms. MacEntee weighs 142 lb, is 5 ft 10 in tall, and her temperature and respiration are normal. Her pulse is 74, her blood pressure is 110/75, and her chest sounds are normal. Her chief complaint is discomfort in the area of the gallbladder. She has intense pain after eating. Blood tests are normal. The doctor's initial impression is suspected gallstones, and an ultrasound scan of the gallbladder is ordered. Treatment plan depends on the scan results.

4. Working in small groups, discuss which part of a medical record you consider to be the most important and why.

5. Go on the Internet and look up the *Medical Transcriptionists Bill of Rights* for discussion in your class.

### Virtual Fieldtrip

*Visit the McGraw-Hill Higher Education Medical Assisting website at www.mhhe.com/medicalassisting3 to complete the following activity:*

The practice manager has asked you to research and make recommendation for improvement in maintaining patient records within the office. The goal is to save time and cost.

- Describe how you would evaluate the current system, and the needs of the office.
- What website might you visit to get tips for smoother management and maintenance of patient records?
- Who might you invite to your office to assist you?

Open the CD and complete this chapter's practice activities, play the games, listen to the key terms, and test yourself with the interactive review. E-mail, print, and/or save your results to document your proficiency.

# Managing the Office Medical Records

## KEY TERMS

- active file
- alphabetic filing system
- closed file
- compactible file
- cross-referenced
- file guide
- inactive file
- indexing
- indexing rules
- lateral file
- middle digit
- numeric filing system
- out guide
- records management system
- retention schedule
- sequential order
- tab
- terminal digit
- tickler file
- unit
- vertical file

## MEDICAL ASSISTING COMPETENCIES

*In preparation for the certification examination, you should know the following areas of competence:*

| COMPETENCY | CMA | RMA |
|---|---|---|
| **Administrative** | | |
| Perform basic clerical skills | X | X |
| Prepare, organize, and maintain medical records | X | X |
| File medical records | X | X |
| **General/Legal/Professional** | | |
| Respond to and initiate written communications by using correct grammar, spelling, and formatting techniques | X | X |
| Identify and respond to issues of confidentiality by maintaining confidentiality at all times and following appropriate guidelines when releasing records or information | X | X |
| Be aware of and perform within legal and ethical boundaries | X | X |
| Determine the needs for documentation and reporting, and document accurately and appropriately | X | X |
| Demonstrate knowledge of and monitor current federal and state health-care legislation and regulations; maintain licenses and accreditation | X | X |
| Explain general office policies and procedures | X | X |
| Identify community resources and information for patients and employers | X | X |
| Evaluate and recommend equipment and supplies for practice | | X |
| Evidence a responsible attitude | | X |
| Conduct work within scope of education, training, and ability | | X |
| Receive, organize, prioritize, and transmit information appropriately | | X |

## CHAPTER OUTLINE

- The Importance of Records Management
- Filing Equipment
- Filing Supplies

- Filing Systems
- The Filing Process
- Inactive and Closed File Storage

## LEARNING OUTCOMES

After completing Chapter 10, you will be able to:

**10.1** Describe the equipment and supplies needed for the filing of medical records.

**10.2** List and describe the various types of filing systems.

**10.3** Discuss the benefits of each type of system.

**10.4** Discuss the advantages of color coding the files.

**10.5** Explain how to set up and use a tickler file.

**10.6** Describe each of the five steps in the filing process.

**10.7** Explain the steps to take in trying to locate a misplaced file.

**10.8** List and describe the basic file storage options and the advantages of each.

**10.9** Identify criteria for determining whether files should be retained, stored, or discarded.

# Introduction

The role of the medical assistant is both clerical and clinical in nature. The most important clerical function is the careful management of the patient chart, or record. The management of these individual files is vital to the care of each patient and to the smooth operation of the medical office.

In this chapter you will learn about various options for handling large volumes of patient records. As you work through this chapter, you will begin to have an appreciation for the very important task of records management, and you will develop an organized approach to maintaining these critical files. As you read, watch for helpful tips that teach you how to locate and access patient records quickly and efficiently.

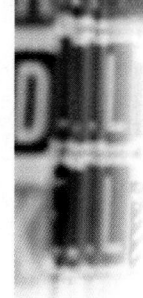

## CASE STUDY

It is the new calendar year and time to update the patient files. The office manager explains that the law in this state requires that all medical offices maintain patient records, or charts, for *seven years* from the last medical treatment or consult. The charts of current patients, of patients who have contacted the office within the last year, or of patients who have an unpaid balance are kept in the front of the office for easy access. Added to the front of each current chart will be a new sticker that indicates the new calendar year; the new sticker is placed directly on top of the previous year's sticker.

All other charts will be moved to a separate chart storage room, organized alphabetically, and grouped according to the last year in which there was contact with the patient. These older charts must remain readily available in case:

- The patient returns to the practice
- Records are subpoenaed by a court of law
- Records are requested for a medical history

The office manager reminds the staff that all original charts belong to the physician who owns the practice. Copies can be made *only* when the patient signs a release authorizing the distribution to another party. When copies are made, a notation must be added to the chart that copying occurred and the date. In this state, even with a subpoena, physicians must have patient permission to release records to the court. Originals are *never* taken out of the medical office.

At this same time, the staff will purge the chart room and shred the oldest charts. All charts that have had no activity in the last eight years will be either pulled apart and shredded in a shredding machine in the office or picked up by a local company that will shred the documents for the physician. It is essential, the office manager points out, that all documents be shredded, not just thrown away, in order to guard the confidential content of the documents.

As you read this chapter, consider the following questions:
1. What are advantages and disadvantages of different file systems?
2. What security measures might be used to protect patient files?
3. What is a tickler system and how is it set up?
4. Identify several storage options for closed charts. Which is the most secure? The easiest? The most cost-efficient?

# The Importance of Records Management

The information contained in the patient medical records is the most valuable information in a medical office. For a practice to operate smoothly and efficiently, it is critical that these records be organized in a way that makes them easily retrievable. Maintaining a well-organized, easy-to-use records management system is essential to providing good patient care. The **records management system** refers to the way patient records are created, filed, and maintained. When such a system is not in place, valuable time is wasted searching for important information. In addition, vital medical data can be lost.

# Filing Equipment

Filing equipment generally refers to the place where records, or files, are housed. Although there are various types of equipment, two of the most common options are shelves and cabinets. The choice of whether to use filing shelves or filing cabinets is often made according to space considerations and personal preference.

## Filing Shelves

Files can be kept on shelves, which resemble traditional shelves, as shown in Figure 10-1. Files are stacked upright on the shelves in filing containers such as boxes or large heavy-duty envelopes. Some shelf systems have doors that slide from side to side or above or below the files. These doors can be locked for security. Other shelf systems have no front covers. Some rolling file units are on wheels for ease of transporting a shelf system easily. Filing shelves are often long, sometimes extending the full length and height of an office wall or room. An advantage of keeping files on shelves is that it allows several people to retrieve and return files at the same time.

## Filing Cabinets

Filing cabinets are sturdy pieces of office furniture, usually made of metal or wood. They contain a series of pullout drawers in which files are hung. Filing cabinets, unlike shelves, are best used by one person at a time because the drawer setup provides limited maneuvering room. In addition, cabinets require more floor space than filing shelves. About twice the depth of the file drawer is needed to allow it to fully open.

Although shelves are horizontal by design, filing cabinets can stand vertically or horizontally. A **vertical file** features pullout drawers that usually contain a metal frame or bar equipped to handle letter-size or legal-size documents. Hanging file folders are hung on this frame, with identifying names facing out. Vertical files may have two, three, four, or six drawers.

Horizontal filing cabinets, called **lateral files,** often feature doors that flip up and pullout drawers. Files are arranged with sides facing out. Lateral files require more wall space but do not extend as far into the room as vertical file drawers.

## Compactible Files

Some offices have limited space in which to house filing cabinets or shelves. These offices may choose to use a variation of shelf filing, called compactible files. **Compactible files** are kept on rolling shelves that slide along permanent tracks in the floor.

When not in use, these files can be stored close together—even one on top of another—to conserve space. When needed, they can be rolled out into an open area so that the staff can easily use them. Compactible files can be moved manually or automatically with the touch of a button.

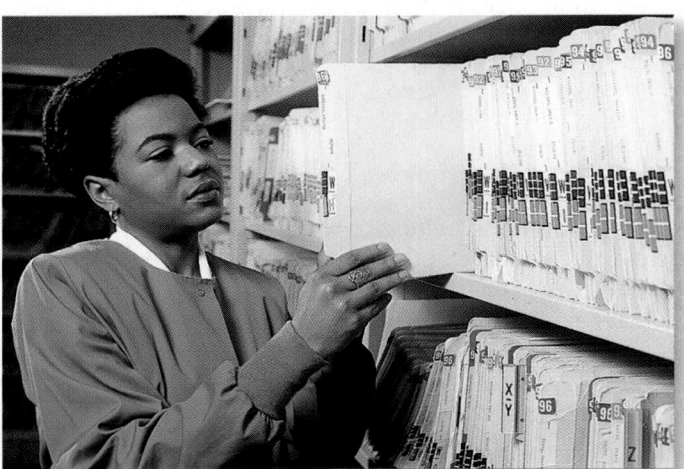

**Figure 10-1.** Files kept on shelves are easily accessible.

## Rotary Circular Files

Rotary circular files are another option to consider when space is limited. These files are stored in a circular fashion, similar to a revolving door, and are accessed by rotating the files. They also can be operated either manually or electronically.

## Plastic or Cardboard Tubs or Boxes

Files may be suspended in hanging files in plastic or cardboard file boxes. While this system may be adequate for a small number of files, the system is less efficient for larger numbers of files because it would require numerous boxes.

Tubs or boxes resemble open drawers. They may have a lid or be open. When not in use, all tubs or boxes must be locked in a secure storage area to protect patient confidentiality. Additionally, open tubs or boxes collect dust and are inappropriate for storage in a dirty warehouse storage area. All tubs or boxes must be stored off the floor, either on shelves or on platforms, to avoid water damage. This is a JCAHO requirement and is routinely checked during a survey.

Tubs or boxes are often stacked to save space, which can make it very difficult to locate files. JCAHO also requires that nothing be stacked within 18 inches of the ceiling. Tubs and boxes appear portable, but are usually very heavy once filled. Care should be taken to avoid injury when moving these files.

## Labeling Filing Equipment

Regardless of which type of filing equipment your office uses, files should be clearly labeled on the outside of the drawer so that you do not have to open doors or drawers to know the contents. Labeling allows you to go directly to the appropriate place when retrieving a file. The label lists the range of files the drawer or shelf contains. For example, if the drawer includes all the files of patients whose last names begin with the letters A, B, C, and D, the drawer should be labeled "A–D."

## Security Measures

All filing equipment must be secured to protect the confidentiality of medical records. *Never* place patient records in an unsecured filing system.

Most filing cabinets come with a lock and key. To protect filing shelves in a separate room, you can lock the file room. Security of the keys to that room then becomes an important issue. The number of staff members who have keys to that room should be limited—perhaps just the head doctor and the office manager. Every staff member does not need a key to the filing equipment. When the office manager comes into the office each morning, she can unlock the files. Because the files remain open during the day, it is important to make sure they are not placed in areas where unauthorized people can obtain access to them. Posting a sign on the file room door stating "Authorized Personnel Only" helps ensure that files remain secure. To ensure office security after hours, some practices install alarm systems.

Keys and locks bring a measure of security only when they are *used*. Many office staffs become lazy and routinely overlook locking file rooms and cabinets. Security survey teams will always ask to see the keys to any locked door or cabinet and ask the staff to demonstrate that they work. Within a medical office, conducting regular security drills at the same time that fire drills are held will aid staff in staying sharp and aware of security risks.

## Equipment Safety

Safety is an important consideration for filing systems. For example, opening more than one drawer in a vertical file cabinet at the same time may cause it to fall forward. If the bottom drawer in a vertical file is left open, someone can easily trip over it. Shelves can be dangerous if staff members need to climb a ladder to retrieve files from the highest level.

Safety guidelines for each piece of equipment should be posted prominently in the office. Make sure that every staff member knows where the rules are posted. Then,

## Reflecting On . . . HIPAA

### Safeguarding Protected Health Information

HIPAA law requires that every covered entity have appropriate safeguards to ensure the protection of the patient's confidential health information. Safeguards include administrative, technical, and physical measures of protection. These measures must provide a "reasonable safeguard" for protected health information from any disclosure that violates HIPAA law, whether intentional or unintentional. The use of locked, fireproof filing cabinets to store patient paper records is an important element of providing a physical safeguard for records. Computer equipment that stores electronic patient records should also be kept secure through these physical measures.

make sure that everyone follows the rules to prevent possible injury.

## Purchasing Filing Equipment

You may never be involved in the purchase of filing equipment because most medical offices already have filing systems in place. Occasionally, however, you may be responsible for setting up an office's filing system—for example, if your practice opens a new office. You may also need to buy equipment as the number of patients in the practice grows.

In either case, you will need to determine where to position the files. When purchasing filing cabinets or shelves, you need to determine how much office space is available for files. This information, along with the number of file folders to be included, will help you figure out how many cabinets or shelves to purchase. An office supply store or office supply catalog can provide you with a list of available products.

# Filing Supplies

Once you have chosen your filing equipment, the next step is selecting filing supplies. Figure 10-2 features an assortment of filing supplies commonly used by medical practices.

## File Folders

The most basic filing supply is the file folder, often referred to as a manila folder. This folder is made of heavy paper folded in half to form a pocket that can hold papers.

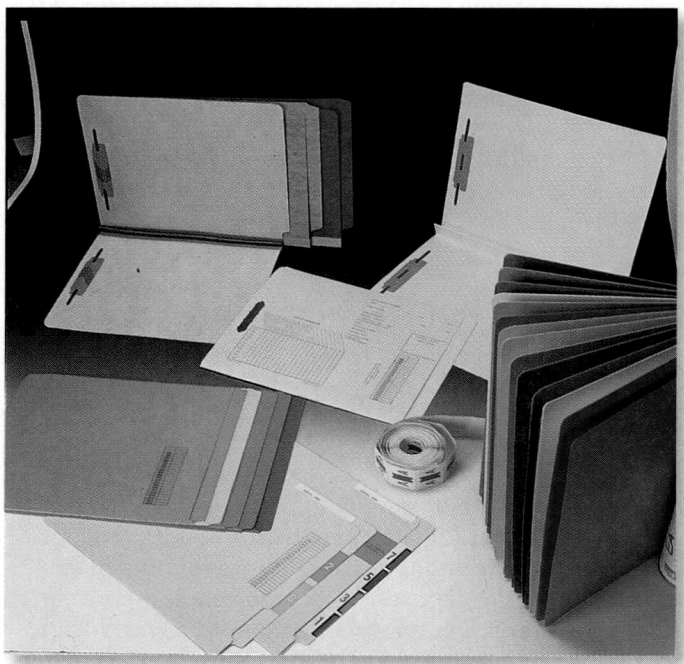

**Figure 10-2.** Medical offices use a wide variety of filing supplies.

File folders come in two sizes: letter size, which is 8½ by 11 inches, and legal size, which is 8½ by 14 inches.

**Tabs.** An important feature of file folders is the **tab,** the tapered rectangular or rounded extension at the top of the folder. Tabs may extend the full length of the folder, as with straight-cut folders, but they are usually cut to extend partway across a folder.

Using folders with a variety of tab cuts makes it easier to read the names on the tabs. One common type of folder is the third-cut folder. Tabs are one-third the width of the folder and appear at the left, center, or right side. Fourth-cut tabs are smaller. Tabs extend one-fourth the width of the folder and occupy one of four positions—left, left-center, right-center, or right.

**Labels.** The tabs on file folders are used to identify the contents of the individual folder. You can write directly on the tab area in pen or pencil. When creating a label manually, it is critical that each label be printed very clearly. A more desirable option is typing or printing a label and affixing it to the tab. This method is consistently easier to read and lends a more professional appearance. Printing labels can be easier from label templates that are available at any office supply store. These templates allow you to use a word processing program, such as Microsoft Office, to create several neatly printed labels at once or one at a time. Tabs should be covered with transparent tape to prevent smudging.

No matter what filing system your office uses, it is important to be consistent in preparing file labels. If all the files are labeled with the patient's last name, followed by the patient's first name and middle initial (for example, Brown, Emma L.), you should not prepare a label for a new folder giving the patient's name in a different order (for example, James P. Regan). Each member of a family must have a separate file.

## File Jackets

File folders cannot be suspended inside filing cabinet drawers. File folders must be placed inside file jackets, or hanging file folders. These jackets resemble file folders, but feature metal or plastic hooks on both sides at the top, which hook onto the metal bars inside the drawers. Like file folders, jackets come in letter and legal size.

Plastic tabs, either colored or clear, and blank inserts are supplied to identify the contents of hanging file folders. The information is typed or printed on the insert and placed in the plastic tab, which is inserted into the hanging file folder. All inserts should be prepared in a consistent and legible style.

## File Guides

To identify a group of file folders in a file drawer, you may use **file guides,** which are heavy cardboard or plastic inserts. For example, if a drawer contains the files for patients whose last names begin with the letters A through C, the guides might separate A from B and B from C.

## Out Guides

Another filing supply is an **out guide.** An out guide is a marker made of stiff material. It is used as a placeholder when a file has been removed from the filing system. Some out guides include pockets that can hold the name of the file that belongs in that place or the name of the individual who took the file, and its due date for return. On another type of out guide, you can write the information on the out guide and cross it out when the file is returned. Out guides can be used for both shelf and cabinet filing.

Although out guides are not essential, they are extremely helpful in ensuring that files are returned to their proper places. Out guides also save the time and effort necessary to go through files to determine where a particular file belongs. Out guides work well when the entire staff, including the physicians, makes a dedicated effort to use the system.

## File Sorters

File sorters are large envelope-style folders with tabs in which files can be stored temporarily. File sorters are used to hold patient records that will be returned to the files during the day or at the end of the day. The sorters help keep files in order and prevent them from being lost.

## Binders

Some offices keep patient records in three-ring binders rather than in file folders. The binders are labeled on the outside spine. Documents are three-hole-punched and then placed inside the binder. Tab sheets are used to separate individual records. A binder can conveniently hold many records.

Binders are stronger than a file folder but require more storage space. Inactive patient records can be transferred to a file folder for off-premise storage. The binder can then be used again. Binders are especially effective in the management of active patient records.

## Purchasing Filing Supplies

Although you may never have to buy filing equipment, buying filing supplies may be one of your regular responsibilities as a medical assistant. (See Chapter 8 for a discussion of how to manage office supplies.)

# Filing Systems

A filing system is a method by which files are organized. Any of a variety of filing systems may be used, but every system places patient records in some sort of **sequential order**—one after another in a pattern, or sequence, that can be predicted. It is important to find out which filing system your office is using and to follow it exactly. Any deviation can result in lost or misplaced records. Never make any changes in the filing system without first consulting the doctors and other staff members in the practice.

The most common filing system for maintaining patient files in sequential order is the alphabetic system. It is simple and easy to use.

## Alphabetic

In the **alphabetic filing system,** files are arranged in alphabetic order, as shown in Figure 10-3. Files are labeled with the patient's last name first, followed by the first, or given, name and the middle initial.

There are specific rules to follow when filing personal names alphabetically. These rules are called **indexing rules** (Table 10-1). Indexing rules are rules used as guidelines for the sequencing of files based on current business practice. They define a consistent method for the ordering of filed materials. The Association of Records, Managers, and Administrators monitors and updates these suggested methods periodically. In this way, the best, most efficient management of paper records is continually being re-evaluated for maximum outcomes. From time to time, individual medical practices may choose to deviate from some of these accepted

**Figure 10-3.** Most medical practices file patient records according to the alphabetic filing system.

## TABLE 10-1 Rules for Alphabetic Filing of Personal Names

In alphabetizing, treat each part of a patient's name as a separate unit, and look at the units in this order: last name, first name, middle initial, and any subsequent names or initials. Disregard punctuation.

| Name | Unit 1 | Unit 2 | Unit 3 | Unit 4 |
|------|--------|--------|--------|--------|
| Stephen Jacobson | JACOBSON | STEPHEN | | |
| Stephen Brent Jacobson | JACOBSON | STEPHEN | BRENT | |
| B.T. Jacoby | JACOBY | B | T | |
| C. Bruce Hay Jacoby | JACOBY | C | BRUCE | HAY |
| D. Jones | JONES | D | | |
| David Jones | JONES | DAVID | | |
| Kwong Kow Ng | NG | KWONG | KOW | |
| Philip K. Ng | NG | PHILIP | K | |

Treat a prefix, such as the O' in O'Hara, as part of the name, not as a separate unit. Ignore variations in spacing, punctuation, and capitalization. Treat prefixes—such as De La, Mac, Saint, and St.—exactly as they are spelled.

| Name | Unit 1 | Unit 2 | Unit 3 | Unit 4 |
|------|--------|--------|--------|--------|
| A. Serafino Delacruz | DELACRUZ | A | SERAFINO | |
| Victor P. De La Cruz | DELACRUZ | VICTOR | P | |
| Irene J. MacKay | MACKAY | IRENE | J | |
| Walter G. Mac Kay | MACKAY | WALTER | G | |
| Kyle N. Saint Clair | SAINTCLAIR | KYLE | N | |
| Peter St. Clair | STCLAIR | PETER | | |

Treat hyphenated names as a single unit. Disregard the hyphen.

| Name | Unit 1 | Unit 2 | Unit 3 | Unit 4 |
|------|--------|--------|--------|--------|
| Victor Puentes-Ruiz | PUENTESRUIZ | VICTOR | | |
| Jean-Marie Vigneau | VIGNEAU | JEANMARIE | | |

A title, such as Dr. or Major, or a seniority term, such as Jr. or 3d, should be treated as the last filing unit, to distinguish names that are otherwise identical.

| Name | Unit 1 | Unit 2 | Unit 3 | Unit 4 |
|------|--------|--------|--------|--------|
| Dr. George B. Diaz | DIAZ | GEORGE | B | DR |
| Major George B. Diaz | DIAZ | GEORGE | B | MAJOR |
| James R. Foster, Jr. | FOSTER | JAMES | R | JR |
| James R. Foster, Sr. | FOSTER | JAMES | R | SR |
| Sister Theresa | SISTER | THERESA | | |

*Source:* Adapted from William A. Sabin, *The Gregg Reference Manual*, 8th ed. (Columbus, OH: Glencoe/McGraw-Hill, 1996), 288–295.

practices. However, indexing rules are generally the norm for most medical practice filing systems.

Indexing rules define each separate part of a person's name or title as a **unit.** Indexing rules then describe the order to display and manage each unit in an alphabetized system. Proper indexing begins with listing the patient's last name first, followed by the patient's first name and then middle name. This is considered the correct order for the units of a patient's name. The correct order for the full name is determined by the order of the alphabet. If an initial is used instead of a name, the single initial is viewed as the entire unit. For example, if a patient's name of record is Jones, D., his or her name will precede Jones, David, in an alphabetized system.

Many names have additional parts beyond three basic units. Indexing rules give direction, as much as is possible, to combine these additional parts to maintain the three-part basic unit model for indexing. For example, all hyphenated names are always considered to be one name. If a patient's last name is Terry-Jones, it is properly alphabetized as Terryjones. In the same manner, prefixes to names are treated as part of the name. For example, von Trapp would be properly indexed as Vontrapp. An abbreviated name is combined with the unit. For example, St. Mary would be combined to form Stmary. The abbreviation for a first name, such as Wm. for William, is filed as Wm without the use of a period. It is not spelled out.

Last names beginning with Mc or Mac can be properly filed in alphabetic order as spelled. Not as frequently, the office manager may choose to treat the letters Mc and Mac as completely separate categories for filing purposes. Check with your office manager to determine which system is used in your office. Either system works well and is considered acceptable practice.

Always remember that each individual must have her own separate file and must be identified by her own name. Even though patients may share a family name, always use each individual's first and second name as much as possible. For example, do not refer to a married woman named Mary Anne Smith as Mrs. John Smith. Instead, her file should read Smith, Mary Anne. It is also important to use the legal name of the patient for all filing, even though the individual may commonly use another name. For example, a minor may commonly use the family name of a stepfather, even when the child has not been legally adopted. Always request and use legal names for all medical records.

Titles are considered to be the fourth indexing unit only when followed by a complete name. This is especially important when the title is needed to distinguish patients with the same name. For example, military titles may be helpful in determining the difference between the files of Jones, Harry W Commander, and Jones, Harry W Ensign. If the title is not followed by a complete name, the title then becomes the first indexing unit. For example, it is proper to index Sister Theresa as written. The title "Sister" is the first index.

Terms of seniority, such as Jr. or Sr., or an academic degree, such as PhD and M.D., are appropriate to use only to distinguish one identical name from another. In these cases, the seniority or academic degree is listed as unit four. Identical names are then alphabetized by this fourth unit.

Indexing rules apply to all alphabetizing done within a medical practice. The business side of the practice can use indexing rules to set up files for vendors, hospitals, clinics, and insurance companies. The first unit when listing any company name is the first word exactly as it is listed and spelled by the company. The words "The," "A," and "An" are articles and are used as the last indexing unit to distinguish otherwise identically named companies from one another. For example, The Stevenson's Homecare Supplies company would properly be listed as Stevenson's (unit 1), Homecare (unit 2), Supplies (unit 3), and The (unit 4).

Indexing rules are designed to keep alphabetizing simple. Although the alphabetic system is simple, you must know the exact spelling of a patient's name to retrieve a file. You must also know the rules of indexing.

## Numeric

A **numeric filing system** organizes files by numbers instead of by names. In this system each patient name is assigned a number. New patients are assigned the next unused number in sequence. Then, instead of being filed by name, the files are arranged in numeric order—1, 2, 3, 4, and so on. The resulting files are sequential by the order in which patients have come to the practice.

Only the numbers are indicated on the files. Patient names are recorded elsewhere. Such a system is often used when patient information is highly confidential—as in the case of HIV-positive patients—and patients' identities need to be protected, as well as in large offices where alphabetic filing systems become too cumbersome.

The numeric system can be expanded to indicate the location of files. For example, if the last three numbers represent the patient's number, the number 113306 may represent the file of the 306th patient, which can be found in the eleventh filing cabinet in the third drawer.

A numeric system must include a master list of patients' names and corresponding numbers. To ensure confidentiality, the office manager should keep the list in a secure place. The physician should hold a duplicate copy, which must also be kept under lock and key. Since folders are filed in numeric order, it should not be necessary for other staff members to have this list.

To find a patient's file number using a computer system, a staff member might input a password or access code, and then type in the first three letters of the patient's last name. If the patient's last name were Mulligan, for example, the staff member would type in Mul. The computer would then show all patients whose last names begin with Mul. The staff member would scroll the names, find the patient, highlight the patient name, and hit the "Enter" key. The computer would then give the number of the patient's chart.

**Terminal digit** filing is often used in conjunction with a general numerical system. Numbers are assigned in small groups of two or three numbers, similar to a social security number, and are read from right to left. Filing is done numerically, starting with the lowest number and moving to the highest, according to the last group of numbers. For example, all files ending in 00 are filed first. They are then followed by files ending in 01, etc.

**Middle digit** filing is similar to terminal digit filing. Middle digit filing uses the middle group of numbers as the primary index.

Numeric, terminal digit, and middle digit filing can all be used in combination with color coding to add even more information to the filing system.

## Color Coding

Color coding is used when there is a need to distinguish files within a filing system. For example, you may wish to find at a glance all the office's new patients, all patients on Medicare, or all patients whose last names begin with the letters WI. Coding by color can help you do so quickly and easily.

Patient records can be color-coded in a variety of ways. File folders are available in a range of colors, as are filing labels, plastic tabs, and stickers.

**Using Classifications.** To make the best use of color, you must first identify the classifications that are important to your office. For example, is it important to be able to identify all new patients easily? (A new patient is a patient who has never been seen in the practice or has not been seen at the practice in 3 years.) Once you select the classifications, choose a different color for each.

Then file the information by color, within the filing system. For example, all new patients may be kept in red folders, or you can attach a red sticker or red filing label to the folders.

An example of a typical color-coding system might be based on a combination of patient factors. The records of patients under the age of 18 might be color-coded blue. The records of patients over the age of 65 might be color-coded red. The records of patients who are insulin-dependent might be color-coded green. The records of patients who are hemophiliacs might be coded with a half-red/half-white sticker. In an emergency situation, as when a patient with diabetes passes out while in the office, the color coding could give staff quick and vital information at a glance.

After a color-coding system is finalized, the codes should be prominently posted on a chart in the file room so that all staff members are aware of them. This chart will help to ensure that records are filed correctly. Remember to update color-coded files consistently, coding new ones and revising older ones as a patient's status changes.

**Using Color in an Alphabetic Filing System.** One way to use color-coded filing is in conjunction with an alphabetic filing system. After files are organized alphabetically, each letter of the alphabet is assigned a color. Then the first two letters of each patient's last name are color-coded, usually with colored tabs.

The colored tabs are attached to the top of straight-edged or tabbed file folders. For example, if the letter S is coded as light blue and the letter M is coded as light green, all names starting with SM—like Smith—would have light-blue and

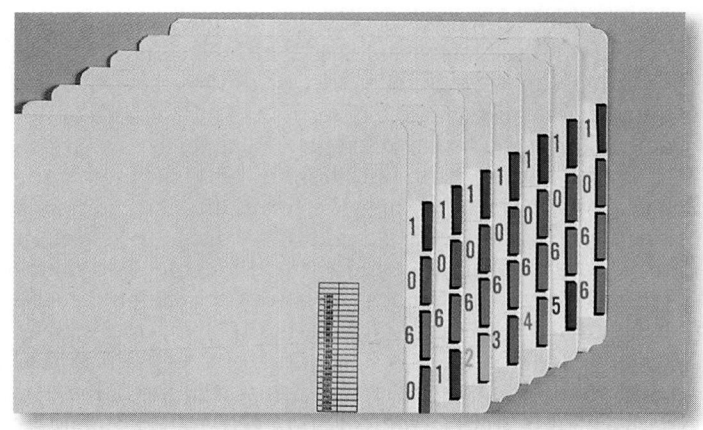

**Figure 10-4.** Color coding can make it easy to find a misfiled record.

light-green colored tabs at the top of the folders. The name Snyder would be filed under a different color combination, such as light blue (for S) and peach (for N). Because the colors will be the same in each segment of the file drawer, a color-coded system makes it easy to tell at a glance if files are filed correctly.

**Using Color in a Numeric Filing System.** Color can be used in a similar way with numeric systems. The numerals 1 to 9 may each be assigned a distinct color, as shown in Figure 10-4. Then, numerals 1, 21, 31, 41, and 51, for example, would share the same color in the ones place of their numeric designation.

As with the alphabetic system, color coding helps identify numeric files that are out of place. There are exceptions, however. For example, if a numeric system uses white stickers for the numeral 2 and red stickers for the numeral 3, the number 134 filed in place of 124 would be spotted immediately as a red sticker in a row of white, but the number 128 misfiled in the same spot could go unnoticed. Procedure 10-1 explains how to use your knowledge of alphabetic and numeric filing and color coding to set up a patient records system.

## Tickler Files

To avoid losing track of important dates, many medical practices use tickler files. A **tickler file** is a date-ordered reminder file. Think of your home calendar; many of us write important activities on our home calendar, creating an informal tickler file for our personal activities. Any office activity that needs to be scheduled ahead of time can be noted and a reminder placed in the file. For example, reminders to order supplies or send patient checkup cards can be entered. When the task has been completed, the note can be crossed off the list or removed from the file and thrown away. Someone in the office should be assigned the responsibility of regularly checking the tickler files. Tickler files can be checked daily or, at a

# PROCEDURE 10.1

## Creating a Filing System for Patient Records

**Procedure Goal:** To create a filing system that keeps related materials together in a logical order and enables office staff to store and retrieve files efficiently

**Materials:** Vertical or horizontal filing cabinets with locks, file jackets, tabbed file folders, labels, file guides, out guides, filing sorters

**Method:**

1. Evaluate which filing system is best for your office—alphabetic or numeric. Make sure the doctor approves the system you choose.

### Rationale

The purpose of a filing system is to provide accessibility of all medical records for the entire staff.

2. Establish a style for labeling files, and make sure that all file labels are prepared in this manner. Place records for different family members in separate files.

3. Avoid writing labels by hand. Use a keyboard, a label maker, or preprinted adhesive labels.

4. Set up a color-coding system to distinguish the files (for example, use blue for the letters A–C, red for D–F, and so on). Create a chart, suitable to be hung in a professional file room, that indicates the color-coding system.

5. Use file guides to divide files into sections.

6. Use out-guides as placeholders to indicate which files have been taken out of the system. Include a charge-out form to be signed and dated by the person who is taking the file.

### Rationale

To quickly and easily identify a missing file and its location.

7. To keep files in order and to prevent them from being misplaced, use a file sorter to hold those patient records that will be returned to the files during the day or at the end of the day.

8. Develop a manual explaining the filing system to new staff members. Include guidelines on how to keep the system in good order.

---

minimum, once a week. It is important to check tickler files frequently because they work only if they are used regularly.

You can organize tickler files in a variety of ways. The most common method, discussed in Procedure 10-2, is to allot one file folder to each month of the year. Tickler files can also be organized by day of the week or week of the month. This method is most useful if there are responsibilities that occur regularly on a certain day of the week or in a certain week within the month. If there are so many notes in a monthly folder that it becomes cumbersome to deal with, it may be best to organize weekly files.

Some offices keep their tickler files in three-ring binders, with tabs separating the months. Notes can be written on three-hole-punched sheets of paper, with pages added as needed. Binders offer essentially unlimited space.

Computers systems also offer tickler files in the form of a calendar. When the computer is turned on, it lists, for example, "Things to Do Today" with the tickler information posted for that date. Reminders can be set for tasks that must be done on a regular basis, such as daily, weekly, or monthly, or on a one-time basis.

## Supplemental Files

Occasionally you may need to set up additional files to supplement the medical records filing system. For example, you may wish to keep some information separate from the primary file, such as older patient records or insurance information. You may also be asked to create temporary files, such as copies of patient records in the primary files. In these cases you set up supplemental files. Supplemental files allow you to keep this additional information about each patient without cluttering up the primary filing cabinets and without making it difficult to find information.

Supplemental files are usually created using the same system as the primary files, but they are kept in a different location. Depending on frequency of use, they may be stored in a less accessible, but equally secure area of the office. If you are keeping supplemental files, it is important to distinguish their content from that of the primary files. For example, you may decide that all information pertaining to certain subjects—such as patient diagnosis and treatment—will be kept in the primary files and that all other information—such as insurance company payments

## Setting Up an Office Tickler File

**Procedure Goal:** To create a comprehensive office tickler file designed for year-round use

**Materials:** 12 manila file folders, 12 file labels, pen or typewriter, paper

**Method:**

1. Write or type 12 file labels, 1 for each month of the year. Abbreviations are acceptable. Do *not* include the current calendar year, just the month.

2. Affix one label to the tab of each file folder.

3. Arrange the folders so that the current month is on the top of the pile. Months should follow in chronological order.

4. Write or type a list of upcoming responsibilities and activities. Next to each activity, indicate the date by which the activity should be completed. Leave a column after this date to indicate when the activity has been completed. Use a separate sheet of paper for each month.

### Rationale

Each sheet should clearly indicate when the activity has been completed and by whom. Each sheet should be filed within the appropriate month's folder.

5. File the notes by month in the appropriate folders.

### Rationale

This will create a neat and orderly way to collect tickler notes for each month.

6. Place the folders, with the current month on top, in order, in a prominent place in the office, such as in a plastic box mounted on the wall near the receptionist's desk.

7. Check the tickler file at least once a week on a specific day, such as every Monday. Assign a backup person to check it in case you happen to be out of the office.

8. Complete the tickler activities on the designated days, if possible. Keep notes concerning activities in progress. Be sure to note when activities are completed and by whom.

### Rationale

Keep a record of responsibilities and completed activities in case a question concerning the activity or responsibility comes up at a later date.

9. At the end of the month, place that month's file folder at the bottom of the tickler file. If there are notes remaining in that month's folder, move them to the new month's folder.

### Rationale

Incomplete activities must be moved to the new month to be sure they are not overlooked.

10. Continue to add new notes to the appropriate tickler files.

### Rationale

To provide for continual update to the tickler system.

for each patient—will be kept in the supplemental files. This designation will help you and other office staff members know exactly where to go to retrieve specific information.

# The Filing Process

Pulling and filing patient records and filing individual documents may be among your responsibilities as a medical assistant. Some practices require that records be returned to the files as soon as they are no longer in use. In other practices the timing is up to you. Still other offices schedule a specific time at the end of each day to file the current day's records and pull those for the next day.

Records waiting to be filed should be placed temporarily in a file return area, as shown in Figure 10-5. To protect

patient privacy, this place should be in a secure area of the office. Clear rules should designate who may handle these files and under what conditions.

# How to File

Essentially, you will be filing three types of items: new patient record folders, individual documents that belong in existing patient record folders, and patient record folders that have previously been filed. There are five steps involved in filing: inspecting, indexing, coding, sorting, and storing.

**Inspecting.** The first step in the filing process is to make sure the item is ready to be filed. Inspect the document or patient record folder for a mark, notation, or

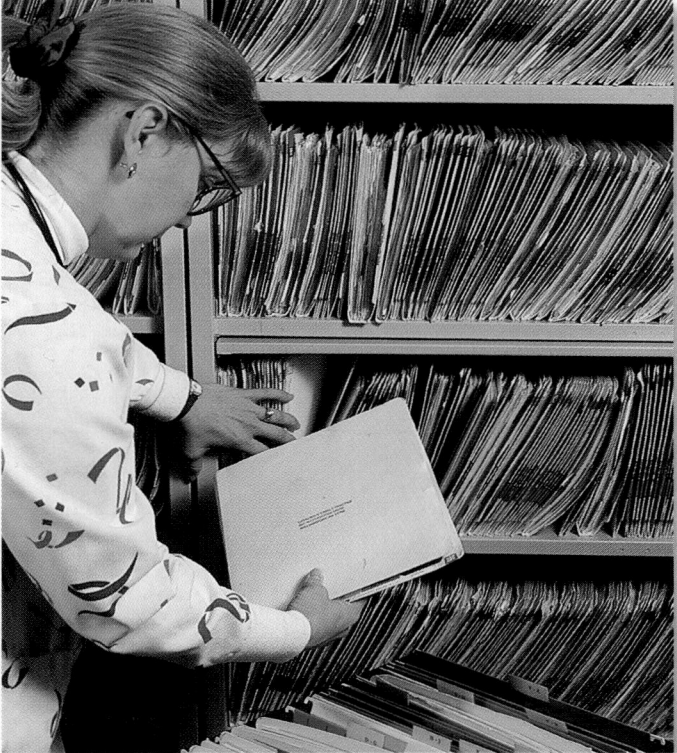

**Figure 10-5.** In some practices, patient records are filed once at the end of the day. Throughout the day, records are placed in a file sorter in a secure area of the office.

stamp indicating that it is ready to be filed. For example, it may be initialed by the physician or stamped with the word *File* on a self-adhesive flag attached to the upper right corner. Some offices have staff members simply place folders ready for filing in a specially designated box or bin.

Remove paper clips, rubber bands, and any extraneous material that does not need to be filed. Staple loose papers to keep them together, per your specific office's protocol. Documents are less bulky when stapled than when held together by clips or rubber bands.

If the document to be filed is much smaller than standard size, it may become lost in the file or even fall out. You may want to use tape or rubber cement to attach it to a standard-size piece of paper before filing it within the folder. When small documents have wording on both sides of the paper, they can be placed in standard-size clear plastic envelopes and then filed.

**Indexing.** **Indexing** is another term for naming a file. Names should be chosen carefully because that is how the file will be known, retrieved, and replaced. Patient names are traditionally used as the file names for patient records.

If you are using a numeric system, you can assign a number instead of a name. Most offices that use a numeric system use computer software to create new patient charts

and assign numbers. As part of the indexing process, color-code the file (if you use color coding in your system).

Note that some files can logically be placed in more than one location. Such files should be **cross-referenced** or filed in two or more places, with each place noted in each file. When cross-referencing a file, you may create a cross-reference form that gives the correct location to look for the file. For instance, an elderly woman might refer to herself as Mrs. John Smith. If you cannot remember her legal name, in the area where *Smith, John, Mrs.* would be located, you would place a mock folder that reads "Smith, John, Mrs., SEE Smith, Christine." You would then place the form under any heading where it is possible to look for that file. You may wish to attach it to a blank file, cutting the file folder in half so that no other documents are mistakenly filed in it.

Indexing can also be used as a step to ensure that folders are filed properly. You can take the opportunity to decide whether the name and color of the file folder are accurate or should be changed in any way.

**Coding.** This step can be skipped when filing patient record folders that have previously been filed. Coding means to put an identifying mark or phrase on a document to ensure that it is placed in the correct file. To code a record, simply mark the patient's name, the number, or the subject title of the file folder. If appropriate, you can underline or highlight key words on the document itself.

It is important to use a phrase or identifying code that anyone who will review the file can easily understand. Avoid medical jargon whenever possible because some terms may not be familiar to everybody. If you are unsure whether a code will be understood, attach a brief explanation to the front of the file folder for reference.

**Sorting.** If you have more than one folder to be filed, you must sort the files that have accumulated. Sort them in the order in which they are kept—such as alphabetically or numerically. Sorting saves you time later when you return the files to their proper places. If you will not be filing the folders immediately, store them in a temporary location, such as a file sorter. The final step in the filing process is to store the files in the appropriate filing equipment.

**Storing.** Documents should be stored neatly within their file folders in the proper sequence.

Careful attention to file storage will make your job easier. Make sure the folders are in good condition. Change them whenever they appear damaged or torn to prevent file contents from spilling out during the retrieval and filing process. If a file contains too many documents, divide it into two or more folders, and label each one (for example, Glass, Ann M.—Folder 1 of 2; Glass, Ann M.—Folder 2 of 2). Also be sure when labeling records that consist of more than one chart that the content of each chart is clear (Folder 1 of 2, records prior to 2002; Folder 2 of 2, records from 2002 forward). Make sure to replace labels that are no longer legible.

## Limiting Access to Files

Some offices restrict the number of people who can retrieve and return files. Limiting the number of people with access to the file room adds an extra measure of security to the practice. To obtain a file, staff members must fill out a requisition slip with their name and the name of the patient, as shown in Figure 10-6.

A record of who has the file is kept either in a notebook or on index cards in special boxes. The record includes the name of the file, the name of the borrower, the date the file was borrowed, and the date it is due back.

Under *no* circumstances should original patient medical records ever leave the practice. Photocopies can be made, if necessary. (Chapter 9 provides specific guidelines on releasing medical records to individuals and organizations outside your medical office.)

## Filing Guidelines

There are specific rules for each filing system as well as general guidelines, or helpful hints, applicable to any system. Following these guidelines will help you file more efficiently.

- Each time you pull or file a patient record, glance at its contents. You should be familiar with the typical contents and the order of a patient record folder to help avoid filing errors.
- Keep files neat. Make sure that documents fit neatly into the file folders. Papers should not extend beyond the edge of the folder. Do not place too many papers in each file folder. Folders should be able to stay closed when laid on a flat surface.
- When inserting documents into folders already in place in the drawer, lift the folders up and out of the drawer. Attempting to force documents into a folder inside the drawer can damage the documents.
- Do not crowd the file drawer. Leave extra space to allow for leafing through the files and for retrieving and replacing files easily. Where possible, use a combination of uppercase and lowercase letters to label folders. This format is easier to read than labels written completely in capital letters.
- Choose file guides with a different tab position than your folders to help them stand out. Do not place guides so close together that they hide one another. A good rule of thumb is to position guides at least 5 inches apart.
- If you are unsure whether to cross-reference a file, do it. It is better to err on the side of providing too many cross-references than too few.
- File regularly so that you are not overwhelmed with too many folders to file.
- Store only files in filing cabinets or on filing shelves.
- Do not store office equipment or supplies where files belong.

## Springfield Medical Associates
### Patient File Requisition Slip

Patient: _____

File Given to: _____

Date: _____

Time: _____

Due Back: _____

**Figure 10-6.** Some offices limit the personnel who have access to the file room. Staff members must fill out a requisition slip with their name and the name of the patient to obtain a patient record.

- Train all staff members who will retrieve and replace files to make sure they have a thorough understanding of the system. Update them on any changes.
- Periodically evaluate your office's filing system. The Points on Practice section will help you with this task.

## Locating Misplaced Files

Even in the best filing systems, there is a chance of temporarily misplacing or even losing patient medical records. No matter how good a system is, people still make errors. If a file is misplaced, here are steps you can take to try to locate it.

1. Determine the last time you or anyone else in the practice knew the file's location.
2. Go to that location, and retrace the steps of the last person who handled the file. Look for the file along the way.
3. Look in the filing cabinet where the file belongs. Check neighboring files. Possibly the file was simply put in the wrong place. Look inside other thicker files to determine if the missing file was accidentally placed inside another file.
4. Check underneath the files in the drawer or shelf to see if the file slipped out.
5. Check the pile of items to be filed or the file sorter envelope.
6. Consider possible cross-references or similar indexes (for example, similar patient names) for the file. Check those headings to see if the file was accidentally placed there.

7. Check with other staff members to determine if they have seen the file.

8. Check to make sure the missing file was not filed under the patient's *first* name instead of the last.

9. Stand back from the file cabinet and view the *top* of the folders looking at only the first three letters of the last names. A misfiled file will stand out.

10. If using a color-coded system, look for the color of the misfiled chart.

11. Even though files should always be kept in a secure area, occasionally individuals who are not part of the office staff, such as visiting physicians, may be in the area and may inadvertently pick up a file with their own materials. If you think someone could have taken the file, call the person immediately.

12. Ask another staff person to complete steps 1 through 7 to double-check your search.

13. Straighten the office, taking care to check through all piles of information where a file could be lodged.

If the misplaced file is not found within a reasonable time—24 to 48 hours—it may be considered lost. Losing a file has potentially devastating consequences. It may not be possible to duplicate the information within the file, but you can try to re-create it in a new file.

To do so, meet with the physician and office staff members to review the information needed. Record their recollections of information in the file. Note on the file document that it is a duplicate, and that the information is not official.

Then consult other office records that may include information related to the file. Contact insurance companies, laboratories, and other information providers for copies of original documents previously included in the lost file. Place copies of those records in the new file, or excerpt information. If the physician considers it appropriate, tell the patient whose file has been misplaced about its status and the steps you have taken to re-create it.

## Points on Practice

## Evaluating Your Office Filing System

In a typical medical office, you retrieve and file documents daily using a filing system that may have been set up when the practice first opened. Now it is time to take a critical look at that system and determine how well it meets your needs.

The filing system you have probably does an adequate or better-than-average job of fulfilling the needs of the practice. Otherwise, retrieving and filing patient records would have become annoyingly inefficient. It is always beneficial to see where improvements can be made, however. Even a good filing system can be enhanced to increase office efficiency and save staff members valuable time.

Here are some simple guidelines for evaluating your filing system.

1. How well do you think your filing system meets your needs? Rate it on a scale of 1 to 10, with 10 representing the best. Survey staff members to determine their ratings, and calculate a composite number. *Based on this feedback, does your filing system seem to do a poor, adequate, or exceptional job?*

2. Note the type of system you use—for example, alphabetic or numeric. Then list the various reasons why files are retrieved from the system. *Would another system, a combination of systems (such as alphanumeric), or the addition of color coding save time or offer other benefits?*

3. Survey the office staff to determine whether there have been difficulties in retrieving or filing or problems with lost or misplaced files. Solicit suggestions for improvement. *If there have been problems, what steps could you take to avoid future difficulties?* (You might even ask your local office-supply representative for ideas.)

4. Consult personnel at other, similar medical practices to determine which filing system works for them. Compare and contrast their systems with yours. *How would their systems work in your office?*

Before making any major changes to your filing system, evaluate each idea in terms of the time and effort it will require and the benefits it will deliver. For example, changing from an alphabetic to a numeric system may provide a relatively small benefit to your office but require a great deal of time to prepare new files and re-file current documents. In that case implementing a numeric system is probably not worthwhile.

If you do make changes to your system, make sure that all staff members are retrained on how to file documents. It is well worth the extra time required at the start to prevent having to locate misplaced files in the future.

## Active Versus Inactive Files

At any given time, there are files that you use frequently and files that you use infrequently or not at all. Files that you use frequently are called **active files.** Files that you use infrequently are called **inactive files.** What constitutes an active, as opposed to an inactive, file? It depends on your individual practice. In a heart specialist's office, a patient who has not been seen for a year may be considered inactive, while in a dentist's office, a year may simply indicate one missed appointment.

There is a third category of files, called closed files. **Closed files** are files of patients who have died, have moved away, or for some other reason no longer consult the office. Although closed files could be moved immediately to storage, they are usually treated in the same manner as inactive files. That is, they are kept in the office for a certain length of time to make sure that there are no requests for the information in the file.

Medical records must be retained for 7 years; however, the Federal False Claims Act requires financial records be kept for 10 years. Because financial records and insurance claims must be backed up by the medical record, the American Health Information Management Association (AHIMA) and many legal experts are suggesting that medical records also be kept for 10 years instead of the legally required 7 years.

The physician must determine when a patient file is deemed inactive or closed. You and the physician can meet regularly, perhaps once a month or once a quarter, to review these files.

## Inactive and Closed File Storage

No office has unlimited space. Therefore, you may regularly need to transfer inactive and closed files from the office's filing area to a storage area.

## Basic Storage Options

Before you can transfer files, you need to determine how and where they will be stored. The design and layout of file storage should make even older stored files easily accessible so that they can be periodically evaluated for retention or elimination.

There are many ways to store inactive files. For example, they can be stored in their original paper state or transferred into another format, such as onto a computer disk or tape or into microfilm or microfiche. Files can even be electronically coded with bar codes for immediate retrieval with a computer system. Regardless of the medium chosen for storing and preserving documents, keeping related material together and retrieving it should be made as easy as possible. Inactive files also must be kept secure, just as active ones are.

**Paper Storage.** If you choose to store files in their original form, you will be storing them as paper files. Paper files are often stored in boxes labeled with their contents. Choose boxes that are uniform in size so that they will stack well. Lift-off lids enable easy access to the contents of the box.

Paper files are bulky to store. They require roughly the same amount of space as they occupied in the office's primary files. Paper files preserve the original documents, however, and these documents can be important when providing evidence of medical treatment in legal proceedings. If paper files start to become brittle, they should be transferred to another storage medium.

**Computer Storage.** If storage space is limited, there are a number of paperless options for storing files. Options include storing files on computer tapes, recordable CDs or DVDs, jump or flash drives, and external hard drives. To store records or information electronically, the office needs a computer system that can transfer documents to some type of electronic or digital format, and then read them when they are retrieved from storage. (See Chapter 6 for more information about using computers in the medical office.)

The easiest way to transfer documents directly into the computer is to use a scanner. This device copies a document onto the computer's hard drive. This process saves countless hours of re-keying (re-entering) documents into the computer. Many scanners also have the capability of copying graphics and handwritten notes.

The document is then labeled and saved. When documents were originally created electronically on the computer, they can be similarly transferred to CD, DVD or tape, or external hard drive and then deleted from the computer's internal hard drive. CDs, DVDs, external hard drives, and tapes are dated and stored in file boxes or other containers.

Electronic documents are usually on the hard drive of the computer. However, the information should also be stored in a backup system in case the hard drive crashes and information is lost.

If documents are stored directly on the hard drive of the computer system, a variety of computer software programs will help in managing these records. This software checks files automatically using different criteria, such as the date the file was established or last updated. This software will help you make decisions about how long documents should be stored. When considering computer record management programs, look for user friendliness, speed and response time, and whether the features of the program meet your needs.

**Microfilm, Microfiche, and Cartridges.** Other paperless storage options include microfilm, microfiche, and film cartridges. (Chapter 5 discusses these storage options.)

When considering transferring files to these formats, explore microfilm services, which index and transfer files for a fee. Using a service helps ensure that files are correctly indexed and thus easily found later on. Always have the microfilm service sign a confidentiality agreement.

# Storage Facilities

You may wish to store files in a remote area of your office building, such as an unused closet or office. Check to make sure that the area is secure, accessible, and safe for storing files (for example, do not store files where hazardous materials are stored). The practice may have to pay additional rent if the space is not within the confines of its office suite.

If there is no space in the building, consider a neighboring building, perhaps one in the same office complex.

Many buildings rent space that can be used to store records. If you pursue this option, you will be responsible for managing the storage of records, including transporting them to the space, positioning them, and retrieving them as needed.

Certain storage facilities, called commercial records centers, will do some of the work for you (Figure 10-7). For a monthly fee, these centers typically house and manage stored documents. When evaluating commercial records centers, inquire about whether they will retrieve and/or deliver boxes or files and whether there is an on-site work area if someone needs to review the files at the storage location.

Beware of general storage facilities that are not specially equipped for document management. These facilities may not address safety concerns by taking precautions for fire or floods, for example.

Maintain a separate list of files stored off-site. This list can save a wasted trip to the storage site if a needed file is not housed there. The list also provides a valuable record if files are damaged or destroyed. Remember to update the list as new files are moved into storage and old files are taken out of storage and destroyed.

# Storage Safety

No matter where you store files, you must consider the issue of safety as well as security. Paper, computer, and film files are easily damaged and destroyed by fire, water, and extreme temperatures. Old, brittle paper files are particularly susceptible. Therefore, it is wise to evaluate the storage site and to take some basic precautions.

- Choose a site with moderate temperatures year-round and adequate ventilation.
- Select storage containers that can withstand intense heat and are waterproof. When possible, use metal or plastic boxes that are designated as fireproof and waterproof. Cardboard boxes, although often used for storage, are not as strong or durable. If cardboard storage boxes are used, they need to be placed on shelving well off the floor to avoid water damage.
- Choose a site equipped with a smoke alarm, sprinkler system, and fire extinguishers.
- Select a site that is above ground and away from flood hazards. One way to find out if a site is susceptible to

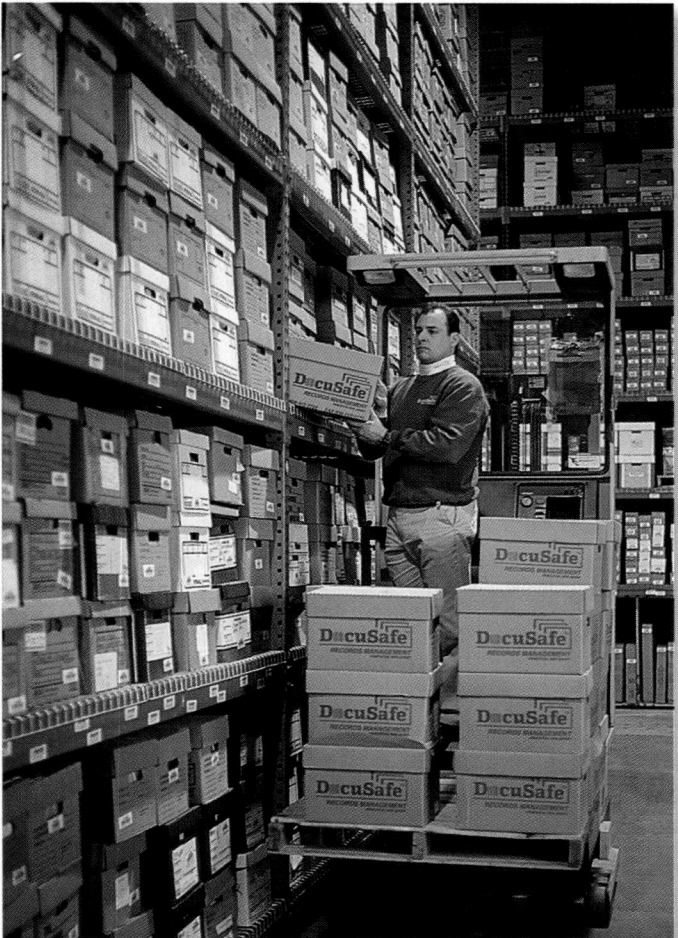

**Figure 10-7.** Commercial records centers manage stored documents for medical practices. Look for a center with personnel who retrieve and deliver boxes or files directly to your office.

flooding is to inquire whether the facility has flood insurance, a requirement for sites at risk.

- Choose a site that is kept locked, is regularly patrolled, or has an alarm system, to prevent theft or vandalism.
- Remove old, brittle files as soon as possible, or transfer them into another format. They can then be placed in file storage again.
- Ask for references from people at other offices who have stored files at the site. Talk to these people about what they like and dislike about the storage facility and any problems they have had in storing or retrieving documents.
- If you are storing files in another form—on computer disk or microfiche—inquire about any special precautions the site owner takes to ensure safety.

Taking the time to thoroughly research storage options ultimately saves time and effort as you manage stored files.

# Retaining Files in the Office

Every office will develop a length of time appropriate for the long-term storage of files. Most practices develop a records retention program.

Typically the doctor decides—based on the potential need for the information—how long to keep inactive or closed patient files in the office before sending them to storage. Working with the doctor, you should prepare a retention schedule. A **retention schedule** specifies how long to keep different types of patient records in the office after files have become inactive or closed. The schedule also details when files should be moved to a storage area and how long they should be kept in storage before being destroyed. The retention schedule should be posted in the file room to make certain that all staff members are aware of it.

Although the doctor decides how long to keep inactive or closed patient records in the office, there are legal requirements for retaining certain types of information, which determine how long these documents must be stored.

- According to the National Childhood Vaccine Injury Act of 1986, doctors must keep all immunization records on file in the office permanently. These records should not be put in storage.
- The Labor Standards Act states that doctors must keep employee health records for 3 years.
- The statute of limitations—the law stating the time period during which lawsuits may be filed—varies by state for civil suits. The most common length of time is 2 years. If a case involves a child or someone mentally incompetent, the statute of limitations extends the deadline. Regardless of the statute of limitations, it is always advisable for doctors to seek legal advice before destroying any records.
- Many legal consultants advise that doctors maintain patient records for at least 7 years to protect themselves against malpractice suits.

- The Internal Revenue Service usually requires doctors to keep financial records for up to 10 years. Doctors are required to keep medical records of minors previously under their care for 2 to 7 years after the child reaches legal age, depending on the state. Some doctors keep these records indefinitely.
- The American Medical Association, the American Hospital Association, and other groups generally suggest that doctors keep patient records for up to 10 years after a patient's final visit or contact.

For the most updated and complete list of required record retention periods according to HIPAA law, go to the HIPAA advisory website. At this website you will also find a number of other federal recordkeeping laws required that have specific record-keeping requirements.

This guide is updated annually. State and local retention requirements can be obtained from offices with which you regularly conduct business, such as insurance companies, state and local agencies, and medical associations. If you do business in more than one state, follow the schedule that requires the longest retention time for materials. Also, if your state's retention requirements are more stringent than HIPAA laws, follow your state's requirements.

When counting years in a retention schedule, remember not to count the year in which the document was produced but to begin counting with the following year. This way, documents produced near the end of a calendar year will be tracked more efficiently. Procedure 10-3 summarizes the steps for setting up a records retention program.

When records can finally be eliminated, they cannot simply be thrown away. Even old records hold confidential information about patients. Therefore, they must be completely destroyed by shredding. Be careful not to destroy records prematurely, because they often cannot be re-created. It is vital that you retain a list of documents that have been destroyed.

## PROCEDURE 10.3

## Developing a Records Retention Program

**Procedure Goal:** To establish a records retention program for patient medical records that meets office needs as well as legal and government guidelines

**Materials:** Updated guide for record retention as described by federal and state law (Go to the HIPAA Advisory website), file folders, index cards, index box, paper, pen or typewriter

**Method:**

1. List the types of information contained in a typical patient medical record in your office. For example, a file for an adult patient may include the patient's case history, records of hospital stays, and insurance information.

2. Research the state and federal requirements for keeping documents. Contact your appropriate state office (such as the office of the insurance commissioner) for specific state requirements, such as rules for keeping records of insurance payments and the statute of limitations for initiating lawsuits. If your office does business in more than one state, be sure to research all applicable regulations. Consult with the attorney who represents your practice.

*continued ⟶*

# Developing a Records Retention Program *(concluded)*

3. Compile the results of your research in a chart. At the top of the chart, list the different kinds of information your office keeps in patient records. Down the left side of the chart, list the headings "Federal," "State," and "Other." Then, in each box, record the corresponding information.

4. Compare all the legal and government requirements. Indicate which one is for the longest period of time.

### Rationale
Retaining all records for the longest period of time required by the laws governing your organization will assure that you are in compliance with all laws.

5. Meet with the doctor to review the information. Working together with the physician, prepare a retention schedule. Determine how long different types of patient records should be kept in the office after a patient leaves the practice and how long records should be kept in storage. Although retention periods can vary based on the type of information kept in a file, it is often easiest to choose a retention period that covers all records. For example, all records could be kept in the office for 1 year after a patient leaves the practice and then kept in storage for another 9 years, for a total of 10 years. Determine how files will be destroyed when they have exceeded the retention requirements. Usually, records are destroyed by paper shredding. Purchase the appropriate equipment, or contract with a shredding company as necessary.

### Rationale
Shredding complies with HIPAA privacy rules regarding protected health information (PHI).

6. Put the retention schedule in writing, and post it prominently near the files. In addition, keep a copy of the schedule in a safe place in the office. Review it with the office staff.

7. Develop a system for identifying files easily under the retention system. For example, for each file deemed inactive or closed, prepare an index card or create a master list containing the following information:
   - Patient's name and Social Security number
   - Contents of the file
   - Date the file was deemed inactive or closed and by whom

- Date the file should be sent to inactive or closed file storage (the actual date will be filled in later; if more than one storage location is used, indicate the exact location to which the file was sent)
- Date the file should be destroyed (the actual date will be filled in later)

   Have the card signed by the doctor and by the person responsible for the files. Keep the card in an index box or another safe place. This is your authorization to destroy the file at the appropriate time.

8. Use color coding to help identify inactive and closed files. For example, all records that become inactive in 2008 could be placed in green file folders or have a green sticker with 08 placed on them and moved to a supplemental file. Then, in January 2010, all of these files could be pulled and sent to storage.

9. One person should be responsible for checking the index cards once a month to determine which stored files should be destroyed. Before retrieving these files from storage, circulate a notice to the office staff stating which records will be destroyed. Indicate that the staff must let you know by a specific date if any of the files should be saved. You may want to keep a separate file with these notices.

10. After the deadline has passed, retrieve the files from storage. Review each file before it is destroyed. Make sure the staff members who will destroy the files are trained to use the equipment properly. Develop a sheet of instructions for destroying files. Post it prominently with the retention schedule, near the machinery used to destroy the files.

### Rationale
To guard patient confidentiality and follow all HIPAA laws governing the protection of patient information.

11. Update the index card, giving the date the file was destroyed and by whom.

12. Periodically review the retention schedule. Update it with the most current legal and governmental requirements. With the staff, evaluate whether the current schedule is meeting the needs of your office or whether files are being kept too long or destroyed prematurely. With the doctor's approval, change the schedule as necessary.

## Registered Health Information Technologist

*To gain medical assistant credentials, you must fulfill the requirements of either the American Association of Medical Assistants (for a Certified Medical Assistant) or the American Medical Technologists (for a Registered Health Information Technologist). After obtaining your medical assistant certification or registration, you may wish to acquire additional skills in specialty areas through course work or on-the-job training. Although this course work or training may not lead to an additional certification or degree, it will enable you to expand your role in the medical office and advance your career as the demand for skilled health professionals increases.*

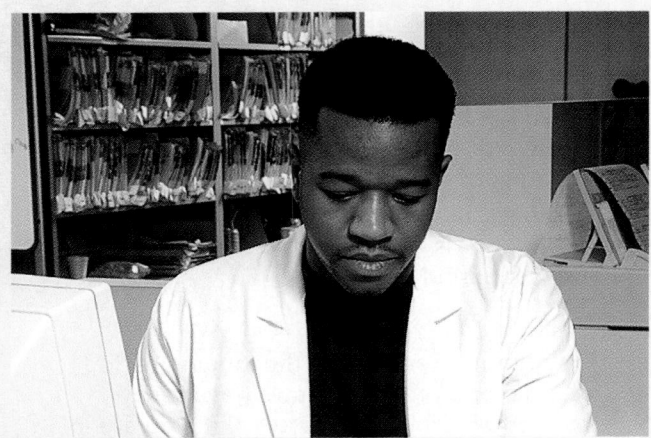

### Skills and Duties

Sometimes called a medical record technician or a medical chart specialist, a Registered Health Information Technologist (RHIT) maintains patient records for a physician or group of physicians. The RHIT is responsible for ensuring that all medical information is accurate and complete. In a hospital, a RHIT deals strictly with health information and has no patient contact. In a small office, however, the RHIT may have additional clerical duties such as answering the telephone.

A patient's medical record includes a medical history and statement of symptoms as well as the results of exams, laboratory tests, and x-rays. The physician's diagnoses and treatment plans are also included. The information in the patient's record may be needed for insurance purposes or to aid in further diagnosis and treatment. In addition, it may be used for research purposes.

The Registered Health Information Technologist checks all patient charts for completeness and accuracy. The RHIT makes sure that all necessary forms related to the patient's care are included, properly filled out, and signed. The RHIT checks to see that all reports and test results are attached to the chart. If necessary, the RHIT speaks with the physician to clarify information about the patient's diagnosis or treatment.

The RHIT must also code the medical record. The RHIT assigns a code to each clinical procedure and diagnosis if this coding has not already been done by another member of the health-care team. In the hospital setting, the RHIT assigns a diagnosis-related group (DRG) to the patient, using a special computer program. The DRG helps determine the reimbursement that the hospital will receive from Medicare or any other insurance provider that uses a DRG system.

The RHIT may also use the coded records to set up a cross-reference index, a type of file that lists the same information under several different headings.

Some medical record technologists specialize in a particular area. Coding is one example. Another is registry, which involves keeping records of all occurrences of certain diseases like bone cancer. The information the registrar collects can be used by individual physicians or as part of a research study.

### Workplace Settings

The majority of RHITs work in medical record departments of hospitals. Most of the rest work in nursing homes, group practices, and health maintenance organizations (HMOs). A few RHITs work in federal or state government offices, public health departments, health and property insurance companies, or accounting and law firms. Some RHITs are self-employed and work as consultants to nursing homes or physicians' offices.

### Education

Most Registered Health Information Technologists have completed a two-year associate degree program at a junior or community college. Course work includes biology, anatomy and physiology, medical terminology, data processing, coding, and statistics.

### Where to Go for More Information

American Health Information Management Association (formerly the American Medical Record Association)
233 N. Michigan Avenue, Suite 2150
Chicago, IL 60601-5800
(312) 233-1100

# Summary

The organization of a practice's filing system depends on how files need to be retrieved. Alphabetic systems are the most common. Numeric systems are sometimes used in practices with patients who require a high level of confidentiality, such as those who are HIV-positive.

Color coding may be used to further identify files. In addition, special types of files, such as tickler files or supplemental files, are sometimes used.

The five steps in the filing process are inspecting, indexing, coding, sorting, and storing. Failure to follow each of the steps in order can result in misplaced or lost files.

Typically, only active files are kept in the practice's main file area. When patient records are determined to be inactive or closed, they are transferred to storage—either elsewhere in the office or outside the practice in a special storage facility. Files may be stored in a variety of formats: paper, microfilm or microfiche, recordable CDs, jump drives, or on the computer. Regardless of where files are stored and in what format, they must be kept safe and secure.

The amount of time that stored files are retained depends on legal, state, and federal guidelines. Offices manage the storage and destruction of files by developing a records retention program. Because even old files contain confidential information, they must be destroyed in an approved manner, not simply thrown away.

# REVIEW

## CHAPTER 10

### CASE STUDY *QUESTIONS*

Now that you have completed this chapter, review the case study at the beginning of the chapter and answer the following questions:

1. What are advantages and disadvantages of different file systems?
2. What security measures might be used to protect patient files?
3. What is a tickler system and how is it set up?
4. Identify several storage options for closed charts. Which is the most secure? The easiest? The most cost-efficient?

### Discussion Questions

1. Why is it important to use a filing system to keep medical records? What could happen if a filing system is not instituted or not followed consistently in a medical practice?
2. What is the importance of HIPAA law in the development of a medical record filing system?
3. What important behaviors should an efficient medical record technologist demonstrate?
4. What do you think is the best way to organize a filing system for a medical practice and why?

### Critical Thinking Questions

1. One of the other medical assistants tells you that you really don't have to keep medical charts once the patient is no longer with the practice. What would be your response?
2. What special concerns might arise when storing records on the computer rather than in traditional (hard copy) paper files? Why do you think major clinics such as the Mayo Clinic use a completely electronic or computerized file storage system?
3. What filing system would you choose for a series of numbered insurance claim forms for patients? Why?

### Application Activities

1. Arrange these ten patient names in order as they would appear in an alphabetic filing system.
   Jordan, Larry W.
   Everett James
   Angie Jones
   John B. James
   Florence Glenn Jones
   Stafford, Samantha L.
   A. James Ingersol
   Stafford, G. E.
   Sarah Coats
   Curtis W. Weaver
2. Using your class list, develop a numeric filing system and a master list that matches each number to a specific person. Then set up an alphabetic filing system based on students' last names. Discuss with your classmates which system is most useful in an educational setting and why.
3. Set up a personal tickler file for yourself, containing personal responsibilities—such as errands, appointments, and social engagements—for the coming week. Keep your notes in a file folder or on a calendar until all activities have been completed. At the end of the week, write a brief paragraph explaining the format of your tickler system and if you found the process helpful. Give several examples to support your answer.
4. Obtain an office-supply catalog that features filing supplies. Put together a product order to set up a patient records filing system for a midsized medical office serving approximately 100 patients. Assume that the practice has already purchased the appropriate equipment, such as filing cabinets or shelves.

### Virtual Fieldtrip

*Visit the McGraw-Hill Higher Education Medical Assisting website at www.mhhe.com/medicalassisting3 to complete the following activity:*

Research the laws in your state regarding the retention of medical records. Compare your state laws to the two states nearest your state. Determine which state has the better laws, explaining your response. What guidelines for record retention would you recommend for a medical practice in your state?

Open the CD and complete this chapter's practice activities, play the games, listen to the key terms, and test yourself with the interactive review. E-mail, print, and/or save your results to document your proficiency.

# SECTION 2

# INTERACTING WITH PATIENTS

# CHAPTER 11

# Telephone Techniques

## KEY TERMS

enunciation
etiquette
facsimile machine
pitch
pronunciation
telephone triage

## MEDICAL ASSISTING COMPETENCIES

*In preparation for the certification examination, you should know the following areas of competence:*

| COMPETENCY | CMA | RMA |
|---|---|---|
| **Administrative** | | |
| Perform basic clerical skills | X | X |
| Recognize emergencies; perform first aid and CPR | | X |
| Recognize and respond to verbal and nonverbal communications by being attentive and adapting communication to the recipient's level of understanding | X | X |
| Demonstrate proper telephone techniques | X | X |
| Identify and respond to issues of confidentiality by maintaining confidentiality at all times and following appropriate guidelines when releasing records or information | X | X |
| Be aware of and perform within legal and ethical boundaries | X | X |
| Determine the needs for documentation and reporting, and document accurately and appropriately | X | X |
| Instruct individuals according to their needs | X | X |
| Project a positive attitude | | X |
| Exhibit initiative | | X |
| Adapt to change | | X |
| Evidence a responsible attitude | | X |
| Be courteous and diplomatic | | X |
| Be impartial and show empathy when dealing with patients | | X |
| Serve as a liaison between the physician and others | | X |
| Receive, organize, prioritize, and transmit information appropriately | | X |
| Understand allied health professions and credentialing | | X |

## CHAPTER OUTLINE

- Using the Telephone Effectively
- Communication Skills
- Managing Incoming Calls
- Types of Incoming Calls
- Using Proper Telephone Etiquette
- Taking Messages
- Telephone Answering Systems
- Placing Outgoing Calls
- Telephone Triage
- Telecommunications
- Facsimile (Fax) Machines

# LEARNING OUTCOMES

After completing Chapter 11, you will be able to:

**11.1** Explain the importance of communication skills.

**11.2** Explain how to manage incoming telephone calls.

**11.3** Describe how the Health Insurance Portability and Accountability Act (HIPAA) applies to telephone communications.

**11.4** Describe the procedure for calling a prescription renewal into a pharmacy.

**11.5** Compare the types of calls the medical assistant handles with those the physician or other staff members handle.

**11.6** Describe how to handle various types of incoming calls from patients and from others.

**11.7** Discuss the importance of proper telephone etiquette.

**11.8** Describe the procedures for taking telephone messages.

**11.9** Explain how to retrieve calls from an answering service.

**11.10** Describe the procedures for placing outgoing calls.

**11.11** Explain the function of telephone triage in the medical office.

**11.12** Explain the uses of a facsimile machine in a medical office.

# Introduction

In this chapter, you will learn key terms associated with telephone techniques. You will be able to utilize a telephone professionally and effectively while handing various types of calls that are either received or initiated by a medical office. These types of calls will vary and can include calls about patient illness and injury, filling prescriptions, or requests for test results; calls from other medical offices; or calls from sales representatives. After completing this chapter, you will understand which calls may be handled by the medical assistant and which require the physician's attention.

Most medical offices have policies and procedures on handling or routing incoming calls, especially emergency calls. This chapter helps you identify which calls are considered emergencies and how to properly route these calls.

In addition, after reading this chapter, you will be able to demonstrate proper telephone etiquette by using common courtesy, proper pronunciation, tone, and enunciation while speaking. You will learn how to effectively handle difficult telephone situations or complaints and how to properly document messages taken.

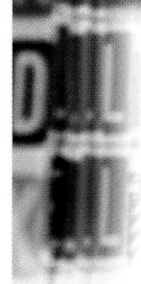

## CASE STUDY

A 54-year-old male patient calls in to the office and, as the medical assistant, you answer the phone. The patient obviously has shortness of breath and states rapidly, "I need to see the doctor right away."

After you establish the patient's name, you learn that the patient complains of pain in his jaw area that lasts for about 5 minutes and then goes away. He also states that he was mowing the lawn when he started sweating heavily and having difficulty breathing. Once he was inside the house, he did have some nausea and vomited once.

As you read this chapter, consider the following questions:

1. What would your first response to the patient be?
2. Explain how you would handle this situation.
3. What type of incoming call was this?
4. What type of condition did this patient's symptoms indicate?
5. What are some other symptoms of this condition?

# Using the Telephone Effectively

The telephone is an important tool for promoting the positive, professional image of a medical practice. When you answer the telephone, you may be the first contact a person has with the practice. The impression you leave can be either positive or negative. Your job is to ensure that it is positive.

Good telephone management leaves callers with a positive impression of you, the physician, and the practice. Poor telephone management can result in bad feelings, misunderstandings, and an unfavorable impression. The telephone image you present should convey the message that the staff is caring, attentive, and helpful. Showing concern for a patient's welfare is a quality that patients rate highly when evaluating health-care professionals. In addition, you must sound professional and knowledgeable when handling telephone calls. Learning and using proper telephone management skills will help keep patients informed and ensure their satisfaction with the medical practice.

# Communication Skills

The telephone is a communication and public relations tool that is essential to the operation of the medical office. Good communication skills are important in telephone management—they help to project a positive image and to satisfy the needs and expectations of the patient. Individuals who engage in good and effective communication employ the following communications skills:

- Using tact and sensitivity
- Showing empathy
- Giving respect
- Being genuine
- Displaying openness and friendliness
- Refraining from passing judgment or stereotyping others
- Being supportive
- Asking for clarification and feedback
- Paraphrasing to ensure an understanding of what others are saying
- Being receptive to patients' needs
- Knowing when to speak and when to listen
- Exhibiting a willingness to consider other viewpoints and concerns

As a medical assistant, you can also apply the five Cs of communication to use the telephone effectively:

- Completeness—The message must contain all necessary information
- Clarity—The message must be legible and free from ambiguity
- Conciseness—The message must be brief and direct
- Courtesy—The message must be respectful and considerate of others
- Cohesiveness—The message must be organized and logical

# Managing Incoming Calls

Telephone calls must always be answered promptly. The procedures for answering calls may vary. Guidelines are usually presented in the office policy and procedures manual. In general, you should greet callers with your name and the office name. Some people may feel awkward using their own name when answering the telephone. Introducing yourself to callers, however, lets them know that they are speaking to a real person, not simply an anonymous voice.

No matter how hurried you are, you should be courteous, calm, and pleasant on the telephone, devoting your full attention to the caller. If the caller does not give a name, ask for it. Many calls result in pulling the patient's file, so it is important to obtain the correct name and date of birth of the patient.

## Guidelines for Managing Incoming Calls

The following guidelines will help you manage incoming calls:

- Answer the telephone promptly by the second or third ring. Hold the telephone to your ear, or use a headset to hold the ear piece securely against your ear. Do not cradle the telephone with your shoulder; doing so can cause muscle strain.
- Hold the mouthpiece about an inch away from your mouth and leave one hand free to write with.
- Greet the caller first with the name of the medical office and then with your name.
- Identify the caller. Demonstrate your willingness to assist the caller by asking, "Mrs. Hernandez, how may I help you?"
- Be courteous, calm, and pleasant no matter how hurried you are.
- Identify the nature of the call and devote your full attention to the caller.
- At the end of the call, say goodbye and use the caller's name.

## Following HIPAA Guidelines

As you learned in Chapter 3, the Health Insurance Portability and Accountability Act (HIPAA) was originally created in 1996 and has additions as recent as April 2006. This act is concerned with the privacy and confidentiality of patient information, including information communicated via the telephone.

In compliance with HIPAA guidelines, all medical providers have standards or written policies that require the following to be in a secure area where no one can see or overhear:

- Medical records
- Clerical forms
- Financial forms and reports
- Computer monitors
- Conversations
- Verbal reports

All employees must comply with the guidelines to safeguard patient information, including when talking on the telephone with a patient.

Health-care providers are allowed to disclose patient information for the purpose of treatment, payment, and health-care operations (known as TPO). Any use of this information outside of these reasons would require a written authorization from the patient. Exceptions include emergency situations or information that is required by governmental agencies for compliance. Follow the medical provider's policy and procedures for disclosing patient information.

## Screening Calls

Part of the responsibility of answering the telephone involves screening calls before you transfer them. Each office has its own policy about calls that should be put through right away, those that should be returned later, and those that should be handled by other staff members. The Points on Practice section describes some guidelines for screening calls.

## Routing Calls

In general, there are three types of incoming calls to a doctor's office: calls dealing mainly with administrative issues, emergency calls that require immediate action by the doctor, and calls relating to clinical issues that require the attention of the doctor, nurse, nurse practitioner, or physician assistant.

**Calls Handled by the Medical Assistant.** The most common calls to a medical office involve administrative and clinical issues. As a medical assistant, you will be able to handle most of these calls yourself. They will concern the following matters:

- Appointments (scheduling, rescheduling, canceling)
- Questions concerning office policies, fees, and hours
- Billing inquiries
- Insurance questions
- Other administrative questions
- X-ray and laboratory reports
- Reports from hospitals regarding a patient's progress
- Reports from patients concerning their progress
- Requests for referrals to other doctors

- Requests for prescription renewals, which must be approved by the doctor unless approval is indicated on the patient's chart. Prior to the renewal, you should take the phone call, discuss it with the physician, chart it, and have the physician sign off on the chart.
- Complaints from patients about administrative matters

Depending on the practice, the office manager or someone in the billing department may handle some administrative calls. The calls you handle may include scheduling appointments, receiving or requesting reports or information, insurance and billing questions, and general inquiries, such as those concerning office hours.

**Calls Requiring the Doctor's Attention.** Certain calls will require the doctor's personal attention. These include the following:

- Emergency calls
- Calls from other doctors
- Patient requests to discuss test results, particularly abnormal results
- Reports from patients concerning unsatisfactory progress
- Requests for prescription renewals (unless previously authorized on the patient's chart)
- Personal calls

Occasionally the patient may prefer to discuss symptoms only with the doctor. These requests should be honored. Depending on the doctor's preference and availability, you may call the doctor to the telephone to handle calls of this nature as they are received. Otherwise, the calls will be returned when the doctor has time available. Do not state a specific time the doctor will return the call. (Most doctors have a set time, such as a half hour in the late morning or at the end of the day, for returning nonemergency patient calls.)

In certain practices some of these calls may be handled by others on the staff, such as a nurse practitioner or physician assistant. For example, a nurse practitioner may be able to order a renewal of a regular prescription, provide advice for the care of a sprain, or answer well-baby questions or questions about the side effects of a drug.

**The Routing List.** Each medical office has a standard policy that documents how incoming telephone calls are to be routed and handled. A routing list, such as the one shown in Figure 11-1, specifies who is responsible for the various types of calls in the office and how the calls are to be handled. For example, the routing list indicates which calls should be put through to the doctor immediately and which ones can be returned later.

The routing procedure may simply identify the general title of the person responsible for handling a call. When more than one person in the office has the same title, however, the name of the individual who has that particular responsibility should be specified.

## HANDLING INCOMING TELEPHONE CALLS

| | Route to doctor immediately | Take message for doctor | Route to nurse or assistant |
|---|---|---|---|
| Emergencies: bleeding, drug/allergic reaction, difficulty breathing, injury, pain, poisoning, shock, unconsciousness, incoherence or hysteria | X | | |
| Calls from other physicians | if possible | | |
| Patient progress report | | X | |
| Patient request for laboratory report | | X (if abnormal) | Melissa (if normal) |
| Patient questions re medication | | X | |
| Patient questions re billing or insurance | | | Jerry |
| Patient complaints | | | Melissa |
| Appointments | | | Melissa |
| Prescription renewals or refills | | X | |
| Office business | | | Jerry |
| Personal business | | X | |
| Salespeople | | | Jerry |

**Figure 11-1.**   A routing list identifies which office staff member is responsible for each type of incoming call.

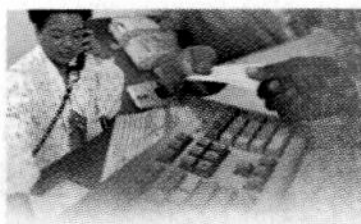

## Points on Practice

### Screening Incoming Calls

Each medical office has its own policy about how to screen incoming calls before transferring them to the appropriate person. Calls come not only from patients but also from other physicians, hospital personnel, pharmacists, insurance company personnel, sales representatives, and family members and friends of patients. Here are some general tips for screening calls.

*Find out who is calling.* A polite way to do this is to say, "May I ask who is calling?" Another option is, "May I tell Dr. who is calling?"

*Ask what the call is in reference to.* When a caller asks to speak with the physician, you should ask the purpose of the call. Depending on the answer, you may determine that you or someone else in the office can handle the situation without disturbing the physician. The response may be as simple as solving a billing problem or clarifying instructions. Remember, however, that emergency calls should be transferred to the physician right away.

*Decide whether the call should be put through.* Although most calls are routed to the appropriate person, any callers who refuse to identify themselves should not be put through. In such a case suggest that the caller write a letter to the physician and mark it "Personal."

*Determine what to do if the matter is personal.* The physician may ask you to take a message in these instances. Inform the caller that the physician will return the call as soon as possible.

# Types of Incoming Calls

In dealing with incoming telephone calls, you will encounter a variety of questions and requests from numerous people. Many incoming calls are from patients. You will also receive calls from other people, including attorneys, other physicians, pharmaceutical sales representatives, and other salespeople.

## Calls from Patients

Patients call the medical office for a variety of reasons, including rescheduling appointments and requesting prescription renewals. If you will be discussing clinical matters over the telephone, it is a good idea to pull the patient's chart. The information in the chart may enable you to address any problems quickly. Having the chart handy also allows you to document the conversation immediately.

Always keep in mind that the physician is legally responsible for your actions, including relaying information to patients over the telephone. The office policy manual typically specifies what you may and may not discuss with patients. If you are uncertain about giving particular information to a patient, it is best to have the physician return the patient's call.

**Appointment Scheduling.** Follow office procedures for making or changing appointment times over the telephone. Ask the patient to provide his name, a telephone number during the day where he can be reached, and the reason for the visit. The medical assistant should repeat the information back to the patient to verify all information before ending the call. (Scheduling appointments is discussed in Chapter 12.)

**Billing Inquiries.** If a patient calls about a billing problem, you will need to pull the patient's chart and billing information. With this information, you can compare the charges with the actual services performed.

If a patient claims to have been overcharged, check to see if the correct fee was charged. If you find that an error was made, apologize and tell the patient the office will send a corrected statement. Ask the patient to wait for the new statement before sending payment. If in fact the proper fee was charged, it may be helpful to speak to the physician before responding to the patient. The physician may be able to tell you if there were special circumstances regarding the visit or charge in question. Allowing the patient to pay the bill in installments is usually an acceptable option.

If a patient is dissatisfied, document all appropriate comments and relay the information to the physician. If a bill has not been paid, ask if there are special circumstances affecting the patient's ability to pay. Always give this information to the physician or office manager.

**Requests for Laboratory or Radiology Reports.** If a patient calls the office requesting the results of tests, pull the patient's chart to see if the report has been received.

If it has not, suggest that the patient call back in a day or two. Some offices will call the laboratory or radiology office for the results.

In some offices you may be authorized to give laboratory results by telephone if they are normal, or negative, so the patient does not have to wait for results to be mailed. Make a note on the patient's chart if you provide any information about test results. If a test result is abnormal, the physician will need to speak with the patient. In such a case tell the patient that the office has received the results and that the physician will call as soon as possible. Then place the patient's chart and the telephone message on the physician's desk.

**Questions About Medications.** One of the most common types of calls from patients involves questions about medication. A patient may ask about using a current prescription or may want to renew an existing prescription.

*Prescription Renewals.* Calls for prescription renewals occur frequently and may come from the patient's pharmacy or from the patient. A pharmacist usually calls to check before dispensing refills if more than a year has passed since the original prescription was written. If the physician has indicated on the patient's chart that renewals are approved, you may authorize the pharmacy to renew a prescription. In any other case, only the physician may authorize renewals. If the physician authorizes a renewal, you may be asked to telephone it in to the patient's pharmacy. See Procedure 11-1. All renewals must be documented in the patient's medical record, with the date and the medical assistant's initials.

*Old Prescriptions.* Patients may call to ask if they can use a medication that was prescribed for a previous condition. In these instances, recommend that the patient come in for an appointment. Explain why the medication should not be used: it may be old and no longer effective, the current problem may not be the same as the previous one, the medication may not be helpful, and using the medication may mask the current condition's symptoms and make a diagnosis difficult.

If the patient does not want to make an appointment, relay the information to the physician. The physician will probably want to speak with the patient.

**Reports on Symptoms.** Sometimes patients call the office about symptoms they wish to discuss with the physician. Here are tips for handling such calls.

- Listen attentively to the patient.
- If the patient is in real distress, try to schedule an appointment that day or as soon as possible.
- Write down all the patient's symptoms completely, accurately, and immediately. In many instances the physician may be able to suggest simple emergency relief measures that you can relay to the patient. These measures may make the patient comfortable until the time of the appointment.

## Calling a Prescription Refill into a Pharmacy

**Procedure Goal:** To accurately and efficiently place a telephone call to a pharmacy to refill a patient's prescription

**Materials:** Patient chart with written order or prescription with the following information: the name of the drug, the drug dosage, the frequency and mode of administration, the number of refills authorized, and the name and phone number of the pharmacy

**Method:**

1. Gather all materials and information necessary, checking for the doctor's written order (or prescription) in the chart. Seek clarification as needed. Schedule II and III drugs cannot be filled by a telephone order (refer to Chapter 37 for more information).

    *Rationale*

    You must have complete and accurate information before placing the call.

2. Follow your office policy regarding refills. Typically, refills are called in the day they are received. An example policy may be posted at the facility and may state: "Nonemergency prescription refill requests must be made during regular business hours. Please allow 24 hours for processing."

3. Communicate the policy to the patient. You should know the policy and the time when the refills will be reviewed. For example, you might state, "Dr. Alexander will review the prescription between patients and it will be telephoned within one hour to the pharmacy. I will call you back if there is a problem."

    *Rationale*

    Letting the patient know the policy demonstrates good communication skills and will result in less misunderstandings as to when the prescription will be available for pickup.

4. Obtain the patient's chart or reference the electronic chart to verify you have the correct patient and that the patient is currently taking the medication. Check the patient's list of medications, which are usually part of the chart.

5. Telephone the pharmacy. Identify yourself by name, the practice name, and the doctor's name.

    *Rationale*

    Only an identified representative from a medical practice can authorize a prescription refill.

6. State the purpose of the call. (Example: "I am calling to request a prescription refill for a patient.")

7. Identify the patient. Include the patient's name, date of birth, address, and phone number.

    *Rationale*

    It is essential that the correct drug be prescribed for the correct patient according to doctor's order.

8. Identify the drug (spelling the name when necessary), the dosage, the frequency and mode of administration, and any other special instructions or changes for administration (such as "take at bedtime").

    *Rationale*

    Accuracy and complete information is essential for medication administration.

9. State the number of refills authorized.

10. If leaving a message on a pharmacy voicemail system set up for physicians, state your name, the name of the doctor you represent, and your phone number before you hang up.

    *Rationale*

    If the pharmacist has any questions, he must be able to reach the physician.

11. Document the entire process in the patient's medical chart. Sign and date the entry per office policy.

12. File the chart appropriately.

**Progress Reports.** Physicians often ask patients to call the office to let them know how a prescribed treatment is working. If a patient has a satisfactory progress report to make to the doctor, it is not necessary that the patient speak to the physician. It is important that the medical assistant relay the information to the doctor and log the call in the patient's medical record immediately. You may also be responsible for making routine follow-up calls to patients to verify that they are following treatment instructions.

**Requests for Advice.** Although a patient may ask you for your medical opinion, do not give medical advice of any kind. Explain that you are not trained to make a diagnosis or licensed to prescribe medication. Stress that the patient must see the physician. If the patient cannot come into the office, assure her that the physician will return the call or that you will call back after discussing the problem with the physician. Occasionally a patient wants to speak only with the physician, not other staff members. You must honor this request.

In some cases the physician may feel that a patient's symptoms warrant immediate attention and will insist on seeing the patient before prescribing any treatment. If the patient refuses to come to the office, note the reason on the chart, and suggest a visit to the emergency room or to a nearby physician. For legal reasons, it is important to document such conversations completely in the patient's chart, including the refusal of treatment. It is always appropriate and professional to offer to take a message to have the physician return the call.

**Complaints.** Even when an office provides the highest-quality care, complaints still occur. When a patient calls with a complaint, such as a billing error, it is important to listen carefully, without interrupting. Take careful notes of all the details, and read them back to the caller to ensure that you have written them down correctly. Let the caller know the person to whose attention you will bring the complaint and, if possible, when to expect a response.

Always apologize to the caller for any inconvenience the problem may have caused, even if the problem occurred through no fault of the office. Make sure the proper person receives the information about the complaint.

Sometimes a patient who calls with a complaint is angry. Responding to this type of call can be difficult and uncomfortable. Your first priority is to stay calm and try to pacify the caller. Follow these guidelines when dealing with an angry caller.

- Listen carefully, and acknowledge the patient's anger. By understanding the problem, you will be better able to work toward a solution.
- Remain calm, and speak gently and kindly. Do not act superior or talk down to the patient. Do not interrupt the patient. Do not return the anger or blame.
- Let the patient know that you will do your best to correct the problem. This message will convey that you care.
- Take careful notes, and be sure to document the call.
- Do not become defensive.
- Never make promises you cannot keep.
- Follow up promptly on the problem.
- Any time a staff member has a difficult time with a patient, it is important to inform the physician, even when the situation is resolved. Always inform the physician immediately if an angry patient threatens legal action against the office.

**Emergencies.** Emergency calls must be immediately routed to the physician. Emergency situations include serious or life-threatening medical conditions, such as severe bleeding, a reaction to a drug, injuries, poisoning, suicide attempts, loss of consciousness, or severe burns. Table 11-1 lists symptoms and conditions that require immediate help.

| TABLE 11-1 | Symptoms and Conditions That Require Immediate Medical Help |
|---|---|

- Unconsciousness
- Lack of breathing or trouble breathing
- Severe bleeding
- Pressure or pain in the abdomen that will not go away
- Severe vomiting or bloody stools
- Poisoning
- Injuries to the head, neck, or back
- Choking
- Drowning
- Electrical shock
- Snakebites
- Vehicle collisions
- Allergic reactions to foods or insect stings
- Chemicals or foreign objects in the eye
- Fires, severe burns, or injuries from explosions
- Human bites or any deep animal bites
- Heart attack. Symptoms include chest pain or pressure; pain radiating from the chest to the arm, shoulder, neck, jaw, back, or stomach; nausea or vomiting; sweating; weakness; shortness of breath; pale or gray skin color.
- Stroke. Symptoms include seizures, severe headache, slurred speech, and sudden inability or difficulty in moving a body part or one side of the body.
- Broken bones. Symptoms include being unable to move or put weight on the injured body part. The injured part is very painful or looks misshapen.
- Shock. Symptoms include paleness; feeling faint and sweaty; weak, rapid pulse; cold, moist skin; confusion or drowsiness.
- Heatstroke (sunstroke). Symptoms include confusion or loss of consciousness; flushed skin that is hot and may be moist or dry; strong, rapid pulse.
- Hypothermia (a drop in body temperature during prolonged exposure to cold). Symptoms include becoming increasingly clumsy, unreasonable, irritable, confused, and sleepy; slurred speech; slipping into a coma with slow, weak breathing and heartbeat.

# Handling Emergency Calls

**Procedure Goal:** To determine whether a telephone call involves a medical emergency and to learn the steps to take if it is an emergency call

**Materials:** Office guidelines for handling emergency calls; list of symptoms and conditions requiring immediate medical attention; telephone numbers of area emergency rooms, poison control centers, and ambulance transport services; telephone message forms or telephone message log

**Method:**

1. When someone calls the office regarding a potential emergency, remain calm.

   ### Rationale

   This attitude will help calm the caller and enable you to gather necessary information in the most efficient manner.

2. Obtain the following information, taking accurate notes:

   a. The caller's name

   b. The caller's telephone number and the address from which the call is being made

   ### Rationale

   It may be necessary for you to put the call on hold or to hang up so that you can call for medical assistance. Before you do so, however, be sure to read the information back to the caller to ensure that you have written it down correctly.

   c. The caller's relationship to the patient (if it is not the patient who is calling)

   d. The patient's name (if the patient is not the caller)

   e. The patient's age

   f. A complete description of the patient's symptoms

   g. If the call is about an accident, a description of how the accident or injury occurred and any other pertinent information

   h. A description of how the patient is reacting to the situation

   i. Treatment that has been administered

3. Read back the details of the medical problem to verify them.

### Rationale

Details are necessary to determine whether or not an emergency exists and the steps you next need to take.

4. If necessary, refer to the list of symptoms and conditions that require immediate medical attention to determine if the situation is indeed a medical emergency.

## If the Situation Is a Medical Emergency:

1. Put the call through to the doctor immediately, or handle the situation according to the established office procedures.

   ### Rationale

   Medical emergencies take precedence over all other matters.

2. If the doctor is not in the office, follow established office procedures. They may involve one or more of the following:

   a. Transferring the call to the nurse practitioner or other medical personnel, as appropriate

   b. Instructing the caller to hang up and dial 911 to request an ambulance for the patient

   c. Instructing the patient to be driven to the nearest emergency room

   d. Instructing the caller to telephone the nearest poison control center for advice and supplying the caller with its telephone number

   e. Paging the doctor

## If the Situation Is Not a Medical Emergency:

1. Handle the call according to established office procedures.

2. If you are in doubt about whether the situation is a medical emergency, treat it like an emergency. You must always alert the doctor immediately about an emergency call, even if the patient declines to speak with the doctor.

   ### Rationale

   It is better to be overly cautious than to let an emergency go untreated. The doctor should be the one to decide how to handle these situations.

If someone calls the office on behalf of a patient who is experiencing any of these symptoms or conditions, you may instruct the caller to dial 911 to request an ambulance. Procedure 11-2 describes the steps for handling emergency calls. The physician should be called to the telephone immediately to offer assistance.

## Other Calls

Besides calls from patients, a medical office receives many other types of calls. For example, family members and friends of patients may call the physician at the office. The use of the office telephone is never appropriate for personal calls. The physician will let you know how to handle these calls. In addition, personal cell phone use should also be limited to essential calls only.

Remember that a patient's information is confidential. HIPAA requires medical providers to obtain authorization from the patient before any information can be disclosed. This is usually in the form of a written authorization, signed by the patient, and indicates what type of information may be given out and to whom. The following are guidelines for managing calls from attorneys, other physicians, and salespeople.

**Attorneys.** Refer to the procedures listed in your practice's office policy manual regarding how to handle calls from attorneys. Follow the office guidelines closely, and ask the physician how to proceed if you receive a call that does not fall within the guidelines. Remember, never release any patient information to an outside caller unless the physician has asked you to do so.

**Other Physicians.** Patients at your practice may be referred to surgeons, specialists, and other physicians for consultations. Consequently, you may receive calls from those physicians' offices. Route those calls to the physician if the caller requests that you do so. Always remember to ask if the call is about a medical emergency. Also keep in mind that you may not give out any patient information—even to another physician—unless you have a written, signed release from the patient.

**Salespeople.** As a medical assistant, you will probably be the contact for salespeople, unless the office policy manual states that another staff member should handle this duty. On the telephone, ask the salesperson to send you information about any new products or equipment. Pharmaceutical sales representatives may want to meet with the physician. Forward such messages to the physician with a request to let you know when to schedule the appointment. Many physicians see pharmaceutical sales representatives on certain days at certain times. Sometimes they limit the number of representatives they will see in one day. Make sure you know your office policy.

# Using Proper Telephone Etiquette

Handle all telephone calls politely and professionally. Use proper telephone **etiquette,** or good manners, so you feel confident in your role of providing quality care and assistance. Adhering to the guidelines that follow will help ensure that your telephone conversations are pleasant and constructive.

## Your Telephone Voice

Customer service is critical when using the telephone. When you speak on the telephone, your voice represents the medical office. It must present your message effectively and professionally. Because you cannot rely on body language or facial expressions to help you communicate over the telephone, it is important to make the most of your telephone voice. Use the following tips to make your voice pleasant and effective.

- Speak directly into the receiver. Otherwise, your voice will be difficult to understand.
- Smile. The smile in your voice will convey your friendliness and willingness to help.
- Visualize the caller, and speak directly to that person.
- Convey a friendly and respectful interest in the caller.
- You should sound helpful and alert.
- Use language that is nontechnical and easy to understand. Never use slang.
- Speak at a natural pace, not too quickly or too slowly.
- Use a normal conversational tone.
- Try to vary your pitch while you are talking. **Pitch** is the high or low level of your speech. Varying the pitch of your voice allows you to emphasize words and makes your voice more pleasant to listen to.
- Make the caller feel important.

**Pronunciation.** Proper **pronunciation** (saying words correctly) is one of the most important telephone skills. Sometimes last names are difficult to pronounce. Ask patients, "How do you pronounce your name?" to make them feel welcome and important. When clarifying the spelling of a word or name, it is common practice to state the letter and then a word that begins with the letter. Examples include D as in dog, V as in Victor, M as in Mary, N as in Nancy, and B as in balloon.

**Enunciation.** **Enunciation** (clear and distinct speaking) is the opposite of mumbling. Good enunciation helps the person you are speaking to understand you, which is especially important when you are trying to convey medical information.

Speaking clearly over the telephone is very important because the speaker cannot be seen. Correct interpretation of the message is determined by hearing the words precisely. Activities such as chewing gum, eating, or propping the phone between the ear and shoulder hinder proper enunciation.

**Tone.**  Because you are not face-to-face with the caller, the most important measurements of good telephone communication are voice quality and tone. Always speak with a positive and respectful tone.

## Making a Good Impression

In a sense your telephone duties include public relations skills. How you handle telephone calls will have an impact on the public image of the medical practice.

**Exhibiting Courtesy.**  Using common courtesy is a characteristic of professional office personnel. Courtesy is expressed by projecting an attitude of helpfulness. Always use the person's name during the conversation, and apologize for any errors or delays. When ending the conversation, be sure to thank the caller before hanging up.

**Giving Undivided Attention.**  Do not try to answer the telephone while continuing to carry out another task. This practice may lead to errors in message taking and may give the caller the impression that you are uncaring or uninterested. Give the caller the same undivided attention you would if the person were in the office. Listen carefully to get the correct information.

**Putting a Call on Hold.**  Although you should try not to put a caller on hold, there will be times when it is unavoidable. You may receive a call on another line, or a situation in the office may prevent you from devoting your full attention to the caller. Sometimes you may have to check a file or ask someone else in the office a question on behalf of the caller. Before putting a call on hold, however, always let the caller state the reason for the call. This step is essential so that you do not inadvertently put an emergency call on hold.

The medical office may have a standard procedure for placing a call on hold. Typically, you will ask the caller the purpose of the call, state why you need to place the call on hold, explain how long you expect the wait to be, and ask the caller if this wait is acceptable. If you think the wait will be long, offer to call back rather than asking the caller to hold. Being kept on hold too long or too often makes people think the staff is inattentive to their needs. You should return to the caller on hold at no more than two-minute intervals and inquire whether or not the caller wants to remain on hold.

If you know you can return to the line shortly, you can put the caller on hold, then attend to the problem. If you need to answer a second call, get the second caller's name and telephone number, and put that call on hold until you have completed the first call. You can then return to the second call.

**Handling Difficult Situations.**  At times it will be impossible to give your undivided attention to a caller because of a pressing issue or emergency in the office. If the call itself is not an emergency one, it is best to ask if you can call back. Explain that you are currently handling an urgent matter, and offer to return the call in a few minutes. Most people will appreciate your honesty. Return the call in a reasonable amount of time, and be sure to apologize for the inconvenience.

**Remembering Patients' Names.**  When patients are recognized by name, they are more likely to have positive feelings about the practice. Using a caller's name during a conversation makes the caller feel important. If you do not recognize a patient's name, it is better to ask "Has it been some time since you've seen the doctor?" rather than to ask if the patient has been to the practice before.

**Checking for Understanding.**  When communicating by telephone, you do not have visual signals to convey the caller's feelings and level of understanding of the information you are discussing. Consequently, you must ask certain questions in the right way. If a call is long or complicated, summarize what was said to be sure that both you and the caller understand the information. Ask if the caller has any questions about what you have discussed. If a situation requires a lengthy conversation, it might be best to have the patient come into the office.

**Communicating Feelings.**  Whenever information is conveyed over the telephone, feelings are also communicated. When dealing with a caller who is nervous, upset, or angry, try to show empathy (an understanding of the other person's feelings). Communicating with empathy helps the caller feel more positive about the conversation and the medical office.

**Ending the Conversation.**  It is not useful to let a conversation run on if you can effectively complete the call sooner. Before hanging up, however, take a few seconds to complete the call so that the caller feels properly cared for and satisfied. You can complete the call by summarizing the important points of the conversation and thanking the caller. Then let the caller hang up first. When you put the receiver down, never slam it—even if the caller has already hung up. Remember that all your actions reflect the professional image of the medical practice. Patients in the waiting room may see you when you are talking on the telephone.

## Taking Messages

Always have paper and a pen or pencil near the telephone so that you are prepared to write down messages (Figure 11-2). Proper documentation protects the physician

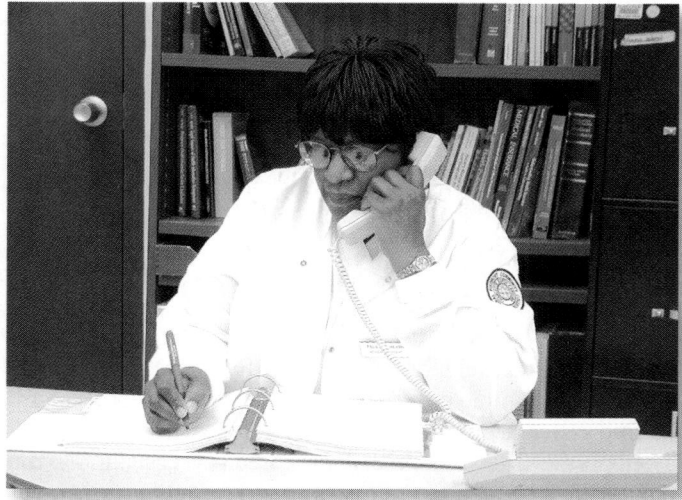

**Figure 11-2.** Use one hand or a telephone rest to hold the telephone so that the hand you write with is free to take messages.

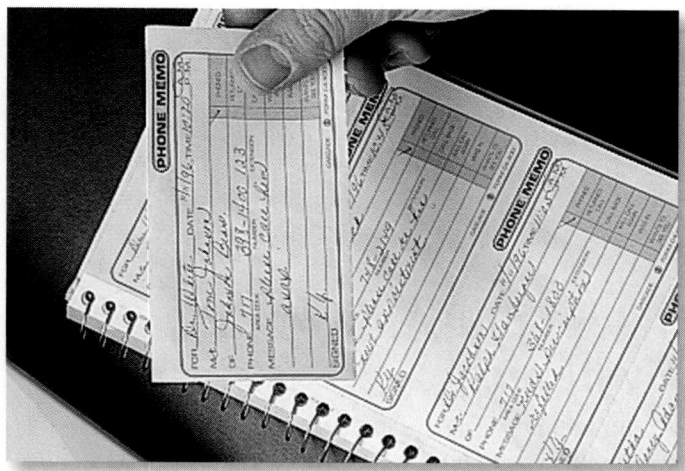

**Figure 11-3.** When using a telephone message pad or telephone log, be sure to fill out the form completely and accurately.

if the caller takes legal action. A record of telephone calls should also be included in a patient's file or electronic health record as part of a complete medical history.

## Documenting Calls

Documenting telephone calls is essential in a medical office. You can use telephone message pads, a manual telephone log book, or an electronic (computerized) telephone log (Figure 11-3). Again, remember that many calls (for example, those concerning clinical problems or referrals) and the actions or decisions they lead to need to be documented in patients' charts. Every entry into a patient's chart is considered a legal document; therefore, the information must be accurate and legible. Accurate documentation helps guard against lawsuits.

**Telephone Message Pads.** You can use telephone message pads, which often come in brightly colored paper, to record the following information:

- Date and time of the call
- Name of the person for whom you took the message
- Caller's name
- Caller's telephone number (including area code and extension, if any)
- A description or an action to be taken, including comments such as "Urgent," "Please call back," "Wants to see you," "Will call back," or "Returned your call"
- The complete message, such as "Dr. Stephenson wants to reschedule the committee meeting."
- Name or initials of the person taking the call

**The Manual Telephone Log.** Some medical offices use spiral-bound, perforated message books with carbon-less forms to record messages. The top copy, or original, of

each message is given to the appropriate person, and a copy is kept in the book for future reference.

**The Electronic Telephone Log.** Some medical offices use an electronic or computer-based system to record messages. The message is keyed in as it is received. A copy of the message can be stored in an electronic record, printed out, or e-mailed as needed.

**Tips for Taking Messages.** The following suggestions will help you provide accurate documentation for incoming messages:

- Always have a pen or pencil and paper on hand.
- Jot down notes as the information is given.
- Verify information, especially the spelling of patient or caller names and the correct spelling of medications.
- Verify the correct callback number.
- When taking a phone message for the physician, never make a commitment on behalf of the physician by saying, "I'll have the physician call you." An appropriate response would be, "I will give your message to the physician."

## Ensuring Correct Information

When you are taking a message, be sure to get the proper spelling of the caller's name. Repeat the spelling to the caller to make sure it is correct. If it is necessary to pull the patient's chart, ask for the patient's date of birth, in case there are two patient's with the same name. When you have taken down all the necessary information, repeat the key points to the caller for verification.

## Maintaining Patient Confidentiality

Do not repeat information over the telephone when the information is confidential. This point is especially important if patients or others in the office may overhear the conversation. You must also maintain patient confidentiality when handling written telephone messages. If a confidential message must be brought to the doctor's attention, do not leave it on the doctor's desk where it can be seen by someone else. Instead, put the message in a file folder marked "Confidential" and place the folder on the desk. Follow the same procedure when handling confidential faxes.

# Telephone Answering Systems

An office telephone system can range from a single telephone line to a complex multiline system. Most medical offices use one or more of the following pieces of equipment and services to provide efficient management of telephone calls: an automated voice mail system, an answering machine, and an answering service. Chapter 5 describes these systems. One of your telephone responsibilities may be to retrieve messages from the practice's answering service. Procedure 11-3 describes how to do so.

# Placing Outgoing Calls

You will often be required to place outgoing calls on behalf of the medical office. You may need to return calls, obtain information, provide patient education, or arrange patient consultations with other physicians. Occasionally, you may be asked to assist with long-distance calls. Seek assistance as needed for these calls. It is important to determine the time zone and the time of day in the location you are calling before you place a call. Time zones can be determined by checking the front of the phone book, going online, or speaking with a telephone operator.

# Locating Telephone Numbers

Before you can place an outgoing call, of course, you must have the correct telephone number. If you are calling a patient, the telephone number should be in the patient's chart. To find other telephone numbers, you may need to consult a telephone directory or call for directory assistance. You may also go to the Internet to find a phone directory.

The medical office should have at least one telephone directory, or telephone book, for the local calling area and perhaps additional directories for surrounding areas. Use these books to locate telephone numbers for outside calls. The office may also have a card file, a list, or an electronic record of commonly used telephone numbers, or these numbers may be listed in the office policy manual.

If you need to find a long-distance telephone number, many offices use the directory assistance service. You can reach this service by dialing 1-[area code]-555-1212. Use directory assistance only when you have exhausted other options, however, because most long-distance carriers

## PROCEDURE 11.3

## Retrieving Messages from an Answering Service

**Procedure Goal:** To follow standard procedures for retrieving messages from an answering service

**Materials:** Telephone message pad, manual telephone log, or electronic telephone log

**Method:**

1. Set a regular schedule for calling the answering service to retrieve messages.

   *Rationale*

   Having a regular schedule ensures that you do not miss any messages.

2. Call at the regularly scheduled time(s) to see if there are any messages.

3. Identify yourself, and state that you are calling to obtain messages for the practice.

   *Rationale*

   The service will only give information to approved personnel from the practice.

4. For each message, write down all pertinent information on the telephone message pad or telephone log, or key it into the electronic telephone log. Be sure to include the caller's name and telephone number, time of call, message or description of the problem, and action taken, if any.

5. Repeat the information, confirming that you have the correct spelling of all names.

   *Rationale*

   Many names sound alike on the phone. It is easy to make a mistake. Accurate information is important to assure that the correct medical chart is pulled and reviewed.

6. When you have retrieved all messages, route them according to the office policy.

charge a fee each time you use the service. If you are required to call out of the country, you will need to use an international dialing code. These codes, as well as area codes and long distance numbers, can be located through the Internet as well as through directory assistance.

## Applying Your Telephone Skills

You can apply the telephone skills you use for answering incoming calls when placing outgoing calls. Here are additional tips for handling outgoing calls.

- Plan before you call. Have all the information you need in front of you before you dial the telephone number. Plan what you will say, and decide what questions to ask so that you will not have to call back for additional information.
- Double-check the telephone number. Before placing a call, always confirm the number. If in doubt, look it up in the telephone directory. If you do dial a wrong number, be sure to apologize for the mistake.
- Allow enough time, at least a minute or about eight rings, for someone to answer the telephone. When calling patients who are elderly or physically disabled, allow additional time.
- Identify yourself. After reaching the person to whom you placed the call, give your name and state that you are calling on behalf of the doctor or practice.
- Ask if you have called at a convenient time and whether the person has time to talk with you. If it is not a good time, ask when you should call back.
- Be ready to speak as soon as the person you called answers the telephone. Do not waste the person's time while you collect your thoughts.
- If you are calling to give information, ask if the person has a pencil and piece of paper available. Do not begin with dates, times, or instructions until the person is ready to write down the information.

## Arranging Conference Calls

It may be necessary for you to schedule conference calls with patients, hospitals, or other doctors to discuss tests or surgical results. When dealing with several people, suggest several time slots in case someone is not available at a particular time. Also keep in mind the various time zones in the country. Make sure that all the conference-call participants are given the proper time in their time zone to expect the call.

# Telephone Triage

Some physicians delegate to other staff members some of the clinical decision making that is done over the telephone. In these instances, **telephone triage** is used as a process of deciding what necessary action to take. The word *triage* refers to the screening and sorting of emergency incidents. Performing triage correctly is an important skill. You should learn as much as possible about triage techniques.

## Learning the Triage Process

Proper training of office staff is vital in providing safe, sound, and cost-effective medical care over the telephone. An increasing number of medical practices are preparing guidelines for the telephone staff to follow when patients call the office with specific medical problems or questions.

Guidelines are often written for common questions, such as how to deal with sniffles and fevers during cold and flu season or how to make a child with chickenpox more comfortable. Members of the telephone staff must realize, however, that their responsibility is to determine whether a caller needs additional medical care. They cannot diagnose or treat the patient's problem.

Office guidelines outline the specific information the telephone staff must obtain from the patient. In general, this information is the same type as that obtained during an office visit. It should include the patient's age, symptoms, when the problem began, and the patient's level of anxiety about the problem.

## Categorizing Patient Problems and Providing Patient Education

After the patient information is obtained, the guidelines help the staff categorize the problem according to severity. The telephone staff then decides if the problem can be handled safely with advice over the telephone, whether the patient needs to come into the office, or whether the problem requires immediate attention at an emergency room.

If a problem is deemed appropriate for telephone management, the guidelines may include recommendations for nonprescription treatment that may relieve symptoms and anxiety. This information falls under the category of patient education. Advise the caller that recommendations are based on the symptoms and are not a diagnosis. Remember that only the doctor is authorized to make a diagnosis and prescribe medication. Ask the caller to repeat any instructions you give, and tell the patient to call back within a specified time if symptoms worsen. Be sure to document the critical elements of the conversation that relate to the patient's health status.

## Taking Action

Clinical triage involves determining the extent of medical emergencies and deciding on the appropriate action. If a caller is having chest pains, you would be performing a type of triage by instructing him to go to the emergency room as soon as possible. Telephone triage is also used in handling common minor medical problems and questions. Whatever the nature of the problem, the situation must be dealt with appropriately to protect the health and safety of the patient.

# Telecommunications

An automated telephone system is used in many hospitals and larger ambulatory care settings. When a call is answered, a recorded voice identifies departments or services the caller can reach by pressing a specified number on the telephone keypad. This telephone system and menu provide a convenient way for patients or callers to reach the direct service or department needed.

# Facsimile (Fax) Machines

**Facsimile machines,** more commonly referred to as fax machines, are commonly used in physicians' offices. A fax is sent over telephone lines from one fax modem to another. Fax machines may be used to send referrals, reports, insurance approvals, or medication refill approvals. Per HIPAA guidelines, a patient's confidentiality must be protected by placing the fax machine in a secure location that only authorized personnel can access. Federal and state laws also must be followed in maintaining or faxing medical records. The physician's office should develop guidelines to follow when faxing information about patients.

See Chapter 5 for more information regarding using a fax machine.

# Summary

The telephone is an important communication tool in the medical office. Your telephone manner will reflect the professionalism of the office. Medical offices commonly receive several types of calls, and there are varying ways to handle these calls.

Special attention should be given to documenting incoming telephone calls and ensuring accuracy. HIPAA guidelines must be followed to maintain patient confidentiality. This applies to telephone conversations and computer monitors as well as medical records. Telephone etiquette involves practicing proper pronunciation and enunciation, using common courtesy and a respectful tone of voice, giving undivided attention to callers, and accommodating patients' requests and needs. Placing outgoing calls requires the same careful attention as taking incoming calls. Telephone triage is the art of determining the level of urgency of each call and how it should be handled or routed.

## CASE STUDY *QUESTIONS*

Now that you have completed this chapter, review the case study at the beginning of the chapter and answer the following questions:

1. What would your first response to the patient be?
2. Explain how you would handle this situation.
3. What type of incoming call was this?
4. What type of condition did this patient's symptoms indicate?
5. What are some other symptoms of this condition?

## Discussion Questions

1. What is the purpose of screening calls that come into the medical office?
2. List five communication skills that are used in effective communication.
3. Name five of the most common types of calls received in the medical office that can be handled by the medical assistant.
4. Describe the procedure for calling a prescription renewal into a pharmacy.
5. Name five symptoms or conditions that require immediate medical help.
6. List five examples of calls received by a medical office that require a doctor's attention.
7. What act does HIPAA stand for, and what is the purpose of the act?

## Critical Thinking Questions

1. As a medical assistant, how would you make a positive impression over the phone?
2. Describe how you would handle a situation in which an angry patient calls to complain that he was overcharged for a recent office visit.
3. How would you handle a call from a patient who discusses symptoms he or she is experiencing?
4. A 12-year-old female patient had lab tests performed. The patient's mother calls and requests to know her daughter's lab results. What is HIPAA policy regarding this information? What should you do?

5. List the five Cs of communication and define what each means.
6. How does the way you handle telephone calls impact the public image of the medical practice?

## Application Activities

1. With a partner, role-play a scenario in which a patient calls the medical office to report that he or she is experiencing chest pain. You can review Procedure 11-2 in order to demonstrate how to handle this emergency situation. If possible, ask a third student to observe and comment.
2. When speaking with patients on the telephone, how might you demonstrate the following qualities? Give several examples for each quality.
   a. concern
   b. attentiveness
   c. friendliness
   d. respect
   e. empathy
3. Your doctor's schedule is full for the day, and you have been told not to schedule any other patients. Demonstrate how you would handle the following caller: The patient states she is sick with a cough and congestion. She insists that she needs to be seen today.
4. Define telephone triage. Give examples of three different patient calls and how you would triage each call.
5. Write a paragraph about how to make a good impression in your telephone duties.

## Virtual Fieldtrip

*Visit the McGraw-Hill Higher Education Medical Assisting website at www.mhhe.com/medicalassisting3 to complete the following activity:*

Using the Internet, research telephone etiquette and ways to handle difficult callers. Then write a brief summary of one of the most helpful articles you read, describing what you learned. Print the articles to share with the class.

Open the CD and complete this chapter's practice activities, play the games, listen to the key terms, and test yourself with the interactive review. E-mail, print, and/or save your results to document your proficiency.

# CHAPTER 12

# Scheduling Appointments and Maintaining the Physician's Schedule

## KEY TERMS

- advance scheduling
- agenda
- cluster scheduling
- double-booking system
- itinerary
- locum tenens
- matrix
- minutes
- modified-wave scheduling
- no-show
- open-hours scheduling
- overbooking
- time-specified scheduling
- underbooking
- walk-in
- wave scheduling

## MEDICAL ASSISTING COMPETENCIES

*In preparation for the certification examination, you should know the following areas of competence:*

| COMPETENCY | CMA | RMA |
|---|---|---|
| **Administrative** | | |
| Perform basic clerical skills | X | X |
| Schedule and oversee appointments | X | X |
| Schedule inpatient and outpatient admissions and procedures | X | X |
| Manage the physician's professional schedule and travel | | X |
| Recognize and respond to verbal and nonverbal communications by being attentive and adapting communication to the recipient's level of understanding | X | X |
| Identify and respond to issues of confidentiality by maintaining confidentiality at all times and following appropriate guidelines when releasing records or information | X | X |
| Explain general office policies and procedures | X | X |
| Instruct individuals according to their needs | X | X |
| Utilize computer software and electronic technology to maintain office systems | X | X |
| Project a positive attitude | | X |
| Adapt to change | | X |
| Evidence a responsible attitude | | X |
| Be courteous and diplomatic | | X |
| Be impartial and show empathy when dealing with patients | | X |
| Serve as a liaison between the physician and others | | X |
| Receive, organize, prioritize, and transmit information appropriately | | X |

# CHAPTER OUTLINE

- The Appointment Book
- Appointment Scheduling Systems
- Arranging Appointments

- Special Scheduling Situations
- Scheduling Outside Appointments
- Maintaining the Physician's Schedule

# LEARNING OUTCOMES

After completing Chapter 12, you will be able to:

**12.1** Explain the importance of the appointment book in maintaining the schedule in the medical office.

**12.2** Identify common scheduling abbreviations.

**12.3** Identify different types of appointment scheduling systems.

**12.4** Discuss ways to arrange appointments for patients.

**12.5** Explain how to handle special scheduling situations.

**12.6** Explain how to properly document no-shows and late patients.

**12.7** Describe how to schedule appointments that are outside the medical office.

**12.8** Discuss ways to keep an accurate and efficient physician schedule.

# Introduction

As a medical assistant, you need to know all aspects of how to create and utilize an appointment book. In this chapter you will learn to identify the different types of scheduling systems, how each is used, and which type of practice each system would work best in. You will also learn how to handle many types of scheduling situations within the office, including patient appointments, emergencies, pharmaceutical representatives, and the scheduling of outside appointments with other medical facilities. Legal aspects of the appointment book are discussed, and proper documentation is stressed. Additional topics include appointment cards, reminder mailings, reminder calls, and recall notices for patients.

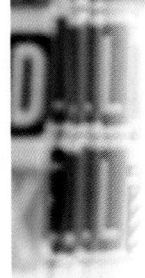

## CASE STUDY

A 71-year-old female patient has a routine follow-up appointment with the physician regarding her medications. Her appointment is at 9:00 A.M. and lasts about 15 minutes. As the patient is checking out at the reception desk, she trips and falls, hitting her head on the corner of the reception desk. There is a bleeding wound on her forehead, and she complains of a headache. The physician and another medical assistant obtain a stretcher and move the patient to an exam room to assess her injuries. It is expected that this emergency will take at least 45 minutes to handle. You are managing the schedule for the day. The physician has a full schedule for this morning and has already worked in a couple of additional appointment times for patients who need to be seen this morning for acute problems.

The next scheduled appointment is for a 24-year-old male who needs an employment physical for a new job he is to start next week. He must have the physical performed prior to his first day. His appointment is scheduled for 9:15 A.M. and is expected to last 30 minutes. At 9:45 A.M., two patients are scheduled for the same 15-minute appointment. One has a sore throat, and the other is scheduled for a wound check. The afternoon schedule has two appointment openings: the first at 2:00 P.M., which is for 15 minutes, and the second at 4:15 P.M., also for 15 minutes.

As you read this chapter, consider the following questions:
1. How would you adjust the schedule to allow for the emergency?
2. If it is necessary to reschedule patients, who should be rescheduled and when?
3. Would you explain anything to the patients in the waiting room about the emergency? If so, what would you say?

# The Appointment Book

Time is a treasured commodity for both patients and physicians. Scheduling appointments in an organized fashion shows respect for everyone's time and creates an efficient patient flow. A well-managed appointment book is the key to establishing this efficiency.

Scheduling is dependent upon the physician's preferences and habits, the facilities available, and the patient's need. Although most patients understand that they may have to wait in the reception area before they are seen by the physician, few patients are willing to wait more than 20 minutes. Offices that routinely have long waiting times can end up with dissatisfied patients and other problems. Some patients, in an attempt to avoid a long wait, may deliberately arrive after their scheduled appointment times. Accommodating these latecomers can throw the office schedule off track. Other patients may become resentful and decide to seek medical care with a competing practice.

Even in a well-run office, however, unexpected events can disrupt the schedule. Some patients arrive early, some arrive late, and others do not arrive at all. Some appointments take longer than expected, for example, if the physician needs to spend extra time with a patient. In addition, emergency appointments sometimes need to be squeezed into the schedule. For these reasons, making an office schedule flow smoothly can be a challenge. Through good planning and scheduling, a medical practice can run smoothly despite these obstacles.

## Preparing the Appointment Book

Before you can begin scheduling appointments, you need to prepare the appointment book. The first step is to establish the **matrix,** or basic format, of the appointment book. In order to create the matrix, you need to block off times on the schedule during which the doctor is not available to see patients. Time would be blocked off the schedule, for example, when the doctor is away for the following reasons:

- Hospital rounds
- Surgery
- Lunch
- Vacation days
- Holidays
- Scheduled meetings (for example, pharmaceutical, medical supply company, or in-service meetings)

The day's schedule is then built around this matrix. See Figure 12-1 for an example of a matrix.

## Obtaining Patient Information

When the matrix has been established, you can begin scheduling appointments. You must obtain and enter certain patient information for each appointment. At some practices personnel enter the information into both traditional paper appointment books and computerized systems. Then, if the computer fails to work for some reason, the office has the book for reference. Some doctors who have been in practice for many years are used to the appointment book method and do not want to give it up for a computer system. Other offices are completely computerized. Using either the book or computer method, obtain the necessary patient information:

- Patient's full name. Obtain the correct spelling of the patient's name.
- Home and work telephone numbers. Repeat phone numbers to ensure accuracy.
- Purpose of the visit. Use a brief description and utilize approved abbreviations when possible. Do not create your own abbreviations.

## Commonly Used Abbreviations

If you are the person who maintains the appointment book, you will find that certain procedures and conditions occur frequently. To save space and time when entering information, use these abbreviations:

| | |
|---|---|
| BP | blood pressure check |
| can | cancellation |
| c/o | complains of |
| cons | consultation |
| CP | chest pain |
| CPE | complete physical examination |
| ECG | electrocardiogram |
| FU | follow-up appointment |
| GI | gastrointestinal |
| I & D | incision and drainage |
| inj | injection |
| lab | laboratory studies |
| N & V | nausea and vomiting |
| NP | new patient |
| NS | no-show patient |
| P & P | Pap smear (Papanicolaou smear) and pelvic examination |
| Pap | Pap smear |
| PMS | premenstrual syndrome |
| pt | patient |
| PT | physical therapy |
| re | recheck |
| ref | referral |
| RS | reschedule |
| Rx | prescription |
| sig | sigmoidoscopy |
| SOB | shortness of breath |
| S/R | suture removal |
| STD | sexually transmitted disease |
| surg | surgery |
| URI | upper respiratory infection |
| US | ultrasound |
| UTI | urinary tract infection |

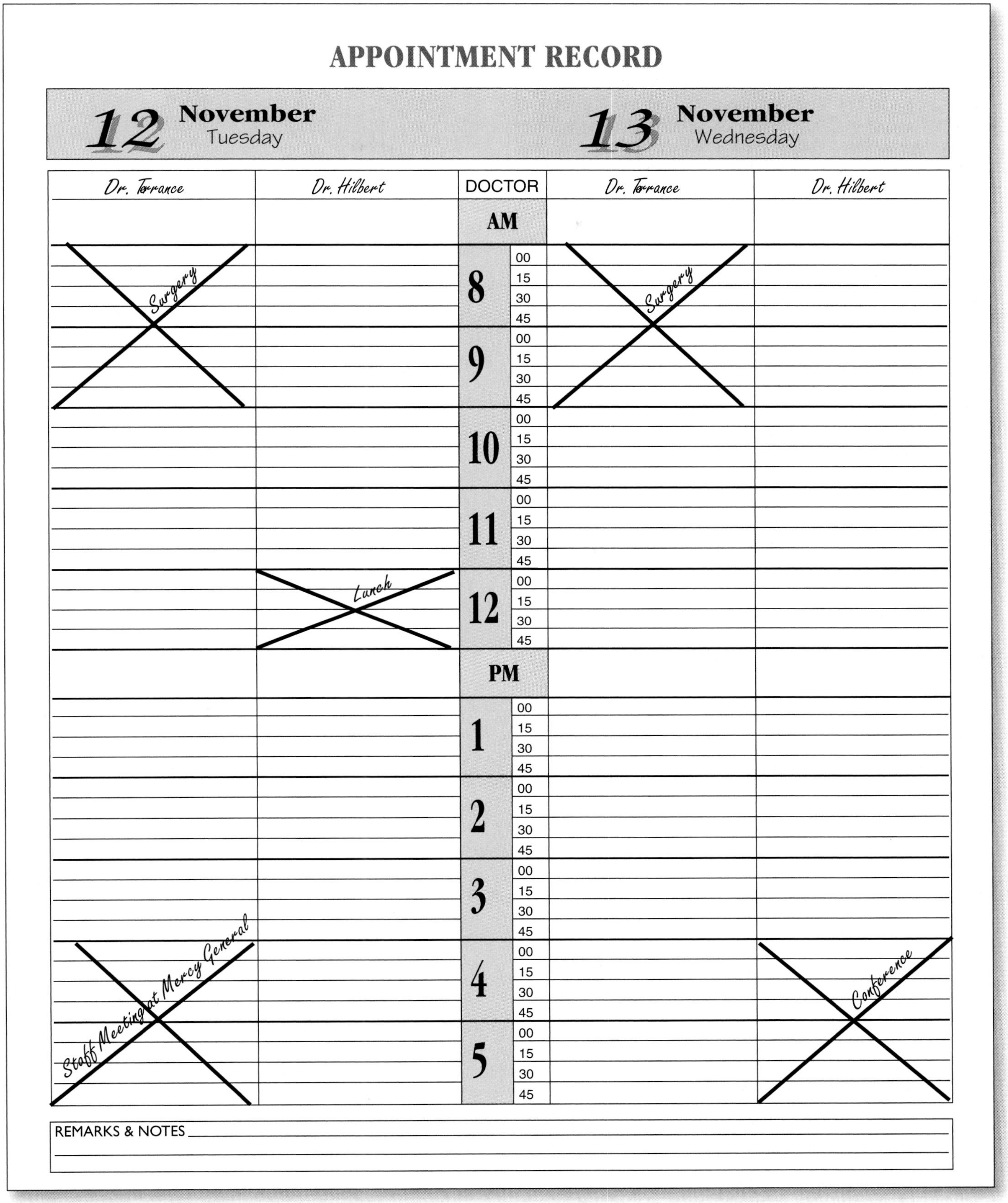

# APPOINTMENT RECORD

| | | DOCTOR | | |
|---|---|---|---|---|
| **12** November Tuesday | | | **13** November Wednesday | |

| Dr. Torrance | Dr. Hilbert | DOCTOR | Dr. Torrance | Dr. Hilbert |
|---|---|---|---|---|
| | | **AM** | | |
| Surgery | | **8** 00 15 30 45 | Surgery | |
| | | **9** 00 15 30 45 | | |
| | | **10** 00 15 30 45 | | |
| | | **11** 00 15 30 45 | | |
| | Lunch | **12** 00 15 30 45 | | |
| | | **PM** | | |
| | | **1** 00 15 30 45 | | |
| | | **2** 00 15 30 45 | | |
| | | **3** 00 15 30 45 | | |
| Staff Meeting at Mercy General | | **4** 00 15 30 45 | | Conference |
| | | **5** 00 15 30 45 | | |

REMARKS & NOTES _____

**Figure 12-1.** It is important to establish a matrix in the appointment book so that appointments are not scheduled for times when the doctor will be out of the office.

## Determining Standard Procedure Times

If you are to schedule appointments efficiently, you must have an estimate of how long visits will take. Working with the physician or physicians in your practice, create a list of standard procedure times. Also indicate on the list how much time to allow for tests that are commonly performed in the practice. This list, kept beside the appointment book, helps you identify which openings are appropriate for the procedure or test involved. This list is intended as a guide only, as each patient visit is unique. The lengths and types of tests and procedures will depend on the practice. Following are typical lengths of common procedures:

| | |
|---|---|
| Complete physical examination | 30–60 minutes |
| New patient visit | 30 minutes or more |
| Follow-up office visit | 5–10 minutes |
| Emergency office visit | 15–20 minutes |
| Prenatal examination | 15 minutes |
| Pap smear and pelvic examination | 15–30 minutes |
| Minor in-office surgery, such as a mole removal | 30 minutes |
| Suture removal | 10–20 minutes |

## A Legal Record

The appointment book is considered a legal record. Some experts advise holding on to old appointment books for at least 3 years. Because the appointment book could be used as evidence in legal proceedings, entries must be clear and easy to read. Management consultants suggest that because the appointment book is a legal medical document, the schedule should be written in blue ink and never with a pencil. Never erase a name or use correction fluid to blot the name out. Instead, draw a single line through the name and beside it write "can" for canceled or "NS" for a no-show patient. Also write the date, time, and reason (if known) why the appointment was missed or canceled, then initial the entry. This information should also be documented in the patient's chart.

Some offices permit the use of pencil to allow for changes or corrections if necessary. If pencil is used, at the end of each day you or another designated staff member should write directly over the penciled entries in ink to create a permanent document.

# Appointment Scheduling Systems

There are several possible appointment scheduling systems. The method chosen usually depends on the type of practice and the physician's preferences. No matter which method your office uses, it should be regularly reviewed to see whether it is meeting its goals: a smooth flow of patients and minimal waiting time.

## Open-Hours Scheduling

In the **open-hours scheduling** system, patients arrive at their own convenience with the understanding that they will be seen on a first-come, first-served basis, unless there is an extreme emergency. Depending on how many other patients are ahead of them, they may have a considerable wait. The open-hours system eliminates the problems caused by broken appointments (because there are no appointments), but it increases the possibility of inefficient downtime for the doctor. In addition, with this system the medical assistant cannot pull patients' charts before they arrive.

Most private practices have replaced the open-hours system with scheduled appointments. Open-hours systems are sometimes still used by rural practices and by practices specializing in urgent care, such as emergency centers. An open-hours system still requires the use of an appointment book, to record patients as they come into the office. You must also still establish a matrix so that you will know when a doctor is out of the office.

## Time-Specified Scheduling

**Time-specified scheduling** (also called stream scheduling) assumes a steady stream of patients all day long at regular, specified intervals. Most minor medical problems, such as sore throats, earaches, or blood pressure follow-ups, usually require only 10- to 15-minute appointment slots. More time may be required for appointments such as physical exams, which usually require 60 minutes, or new patient visits, which usually require 30 minutes (Figure 12-2). When a visit requires more time, you simply assign the patient additional back-to-back slots.

## Wave Scheduling

**Wave scheduling** works effectively in larger medical facilities that have enough departments and personnel to provide services to several patients at the same time. This method of scheduling is based on the reality that some patients will arrive late and that others will require more or less time than expected with the physician. Wave scheduling has the flexibility to allow for appointments that require more time than anticipated or for patients who miss appointments. The goal of wave scheduling is to begin and end each hour with the overall office schedule on track. You determine the number of patients to be seen each hour by dividing the hour by the length of the average visit. If the average is 15 minutes, for example, you schedule four patients for each hour. An example of wave scheduling would be:

| | | | |
|---|---|---|---|
| 10:00 A.M. | Patient A | 555-5683 | Sore throat |
| 10:00 A.M. | Patient B | 555-7322 | Low back pain |
| 10:00 A.M. | Patient C | 555-4673 | FU B/P |
| 10:00 A.M. | Patient D | 555-2854 | B12 inj |

You ask all four to arrive at the beginning of the hour and have the physician see them in the order of their

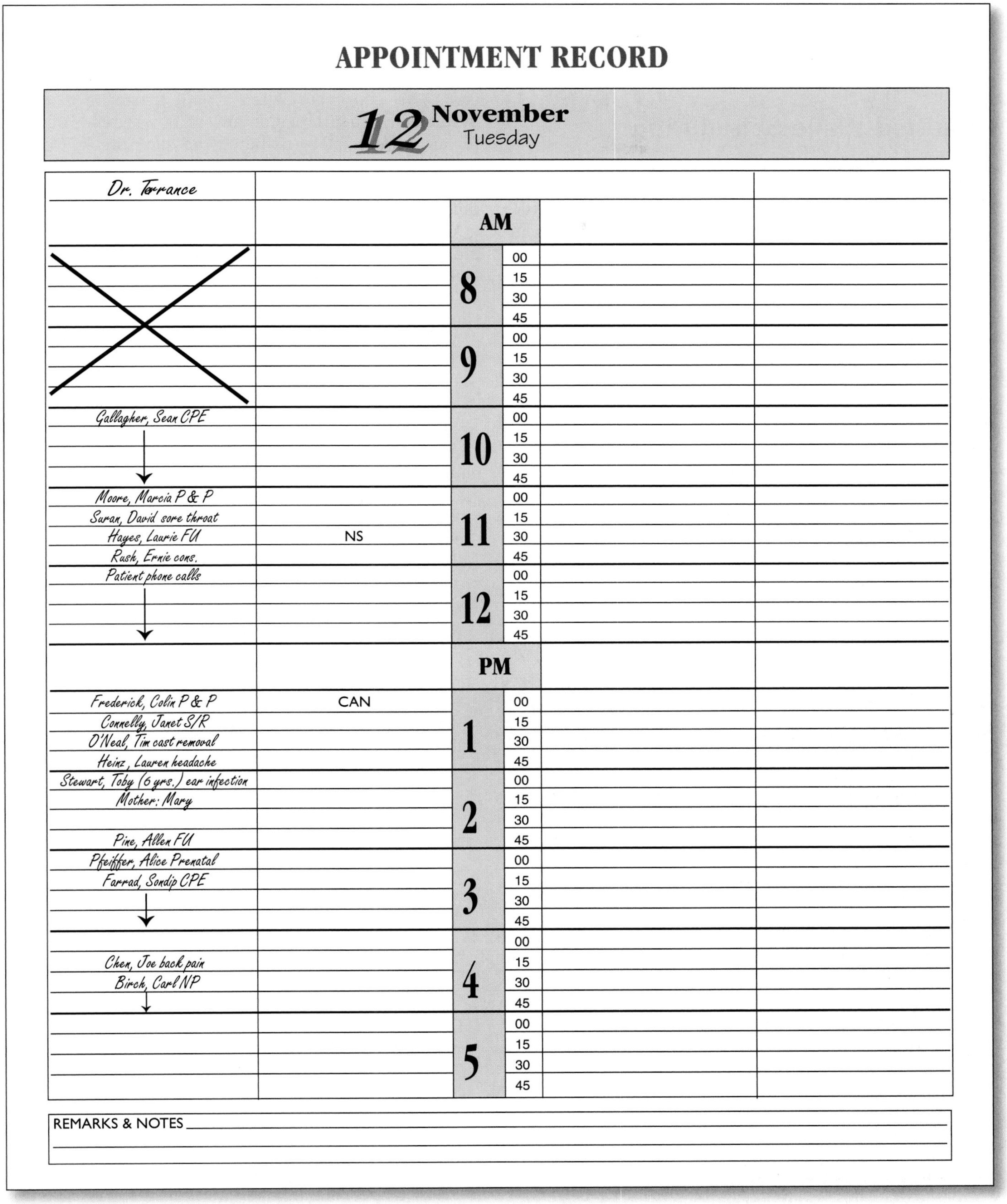

# APPOINTMENT RECORD

## 12 November Tuesday

**Dr. Terrance**

| | | AM | | |
|---|---|---|---|---|
| | | **8** | 00 | |
| | | | 15 | |
| | | | 30 | |
| | | | 45 | |
| | | **9** | 00 | |
| | | | 15 | |
| | | | 30 | |
| | | | 45 | |
| Gallagher, Sean CPE | | **10** | 00 | |
| ↓ | | | 15 | |
| | | | 30 | |
| | | | 45 | |
| Moore, Marcia P & P | | **11** | 00 | |
| Suran, David sore throat | | | 15 | |
| Hayes, Laurie FU | NS | | 30 | |
| Rush, Ernie cons. | | | 45 | |
| Patient phone calls | | **12** | 00 | |
| | | | 15 | |
| ↓ | | | 30 | |
| | | | 45 | |
| | | PM | | |
| Frederick, Colin P & P | CAN | **1** | 00 | |
| Connelly, Janet S/R | | | 15 | |
| O'Neal, Tim cast removal | | | 30 | |
| Heinz, Lauren headache | | | 45 | |
| Stewart, Toby (6 yrs.) ear infection | | **2** | 00 | |
| Mother: Mary | | | 15 | |
| | | | 30 | |
| Pine, Allen FU | | | 45 | |
| Pfeiffer, Alice Prenatal | | **3** | 00 | |
| Farrad, Sondip CPE | | | 15 | |
| ↓ | | | 30 | |
| | | | 45 | |
| | | **4** | 00 | |
| Chen, Joe back pain | | | 15 | |
| Birch, Carl NP | | | 30 | |
| ↓ | | | 45 | |
| | | **5** | 00 | |
| | | | 15 | |
| | | | 30 | |
| | | | 45 | |

REMARKS & NOTES _____
_____

**Figure 12-2.** Time-specified appointment scheduling is commonly used in the medical office.

actual arrival. The main problem with wave scheduling is that patients may realize they have appointments at the same time as other patients. The result may be confusion and possibly annoyance or anger.

## Modified-Wave Scheduling

The wave system can be modified in several ways. With **modified-wave scheduling,** as shown in Figure 12-3, patients might be scheduled in 15-minute increments. Another option is to schedule four patients to arrive at planned intervals during the first half hour, leaving the second half hour unscheduled. Appointments that are anticipated to require more time should be scheduled at the beginning of the hour. Appointments that are expected to be less time-consuming should be scheduled in 10- to 20-minute time slots. This method allows time for catching up before the next hour begins.

## Double Booking

With a **double-booking system,** two or more patients are scheduled for the same appointment slot. Unlike the wave or modified-wave system, however, the double-booking system assumes that both patients will actually be seen within the scheduled period. If the types of visits are usually short (5 minutes, for example), it is reasonable to book two patients for one 15-minute opening. If

both patients require the entire 15 minutes, however, the office falls behind schedule.

Double-booking scheduling is especially useful when one patient does not necessarily need to see the physician. This can occur when a patient can be managed by a nurse practitioner or physician assistant, such as for an immunization or blood pressure check. Double-booking scheduling works most effectively in practices in which more than one patient can be attended to at a time.

Double-booking can be helpful if a patient calls with a problem and needs to be seen that day but no appointments are available. You could double-book this patient with an already scheduled patient. In such cases you should explain that the caller might have to wait a bit before being seen by the doctor.

## Cluster Scheduling

As the name suggests, **cluster scheduling** groups similar appointments together during the day or week. (This system is also called categorization scheduling.) For example, you might cluster all physical examinations between 9:00 A.M. and 11:00 A.M. on Tuesdays and Thursdays. Cluster scheduling is also helpful in offices where specialized equipment or services (such as physical therapy or ultrasound) are available only at certain times. Procedure 12-1 explains how to create a cluster schedule.

## PROCEDURE 12.1

### Creating a Cluster Schedule

**Procedure Goal:** To set up a cluster schedule

**Materials:** Calendar, tickler file, appointment book, colored pencils or markers (optional)

**Method:**

1. Learn which categories of cases the physician would like to cluster and on what days and/or times of day.
2. Determine the length of the average visit in each category.
3. In the appointment book, cross out the hours in the week that the physician is typically not available.

   *Rationale*

   This creates the matrix of physician availability around which appointments can be booked.

4. Block out one period in midmorning and one in mid-afternoon for use as buffer, or reserve, times for unexpected needs.
5. Reserve additional slots for acutely ill patients. The number of slots depends on the type of practice.

   *Rationale*

   There needs to be room in the schedule for emergency appointments that cannot wait.

6. Mark the appointment times for clustered procedures. If desired, color-code the blocks of time. For example, make immunization clusters pink, blood pressure checks green, and so forth.

   *Rationale*

   Blocking the time or color coding it indicates that a specific type of appointment should be booked in this location.

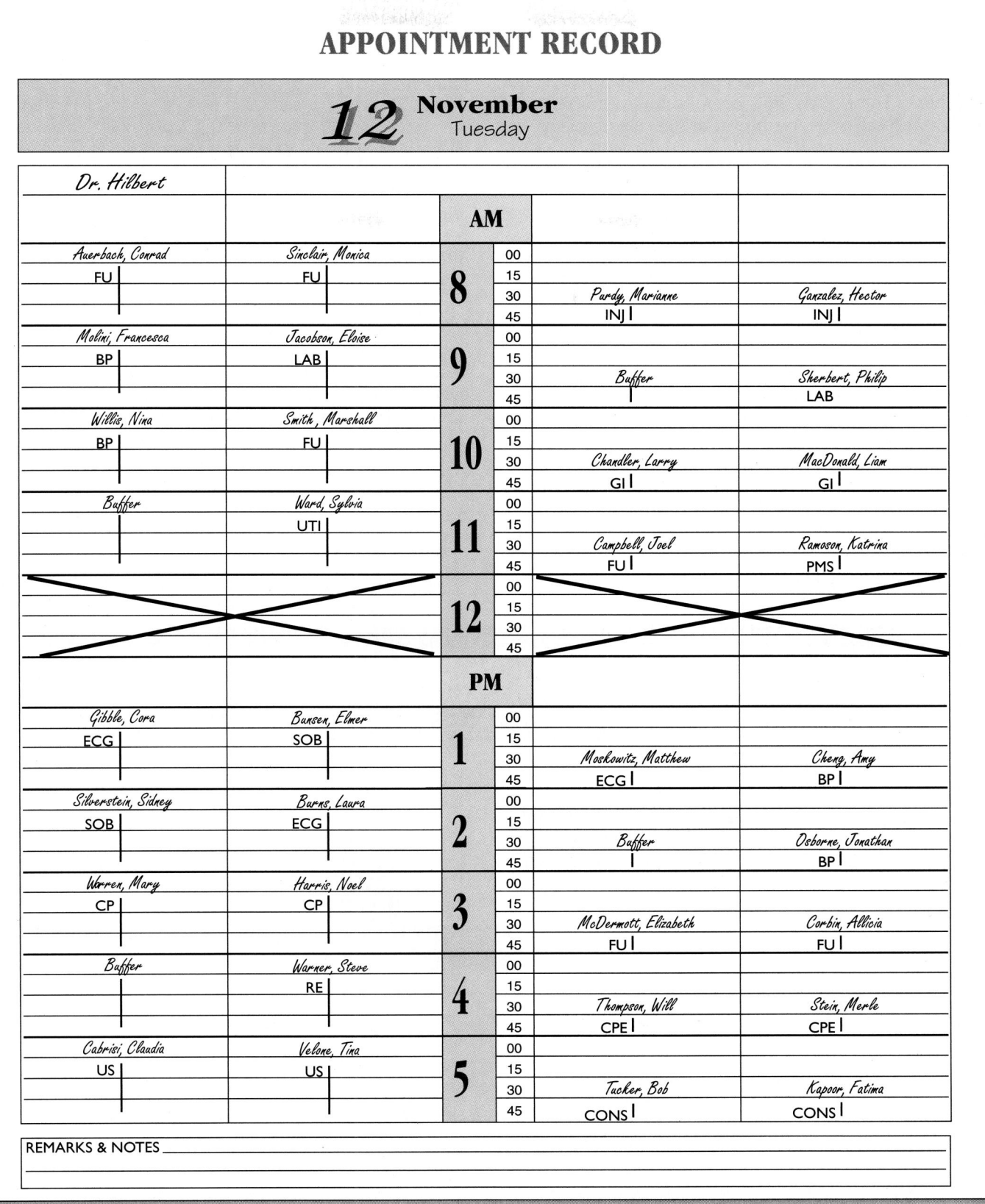

**Figure 12-3.** Modified-wave scheduling allows more flexibility than wave scheduling.

## Advance Scheduling

In some specialties patients might be booked weeks or months in advance, as for annual gynecologic examinations. In such practices **advance scheduling** is used. It is still advisable to leave a few slots open each day, however, for patients who call with unexpected or unusual problems.

## Combination Scheduling

Some practices combine two or more scheduling methods. For example, they might use cluster scheduling for new patients and double-booking for quick follow-ups.

## Computerized Scheduling

Computerized scheduling systems are becoming more common in medical offices because they have several advantages over handwritten systems (Figure 12-4). For example, they can be programmed to "lock out" selected appointment slots so that those slots will always be available for emergencies. Another advantage of using a computerized system is that the scheduling information can be accessed from all terminals located within the practice. Computerized systems can also help staff members identify patients who often are late, forget their appointments altogether, or cancel. In addition, the computer can identify patients who may require additional time with the physician because of special needs. Computerized scheduling also provides the doctor with a variety of reports about the scheduling practices of the office, which can help improve efficiency.

## Arranging Appointments

Whether you are arranging appointments in person or by telephone, be polite and courteous. In scheduling an appointment, try to offer the patient a choice between two different dates, with either a morning or afternoon time slot. Once the patient decides on the date and time, always confirm the appointment by repeating it to the person before printing it in the schedule. If you are scheduling the appointment in person, write the appointment date and time on an appointment card to give to the patient. Whenever possible, try to accommodate the patient's needs while still maintaining a smoothly flowing schedule.

### New Patients

A patient who has not been established at a medical practice is considered a new patient. Patients who have not been seen by the practice in three or more years are also considered to be new patients. Appointments for new

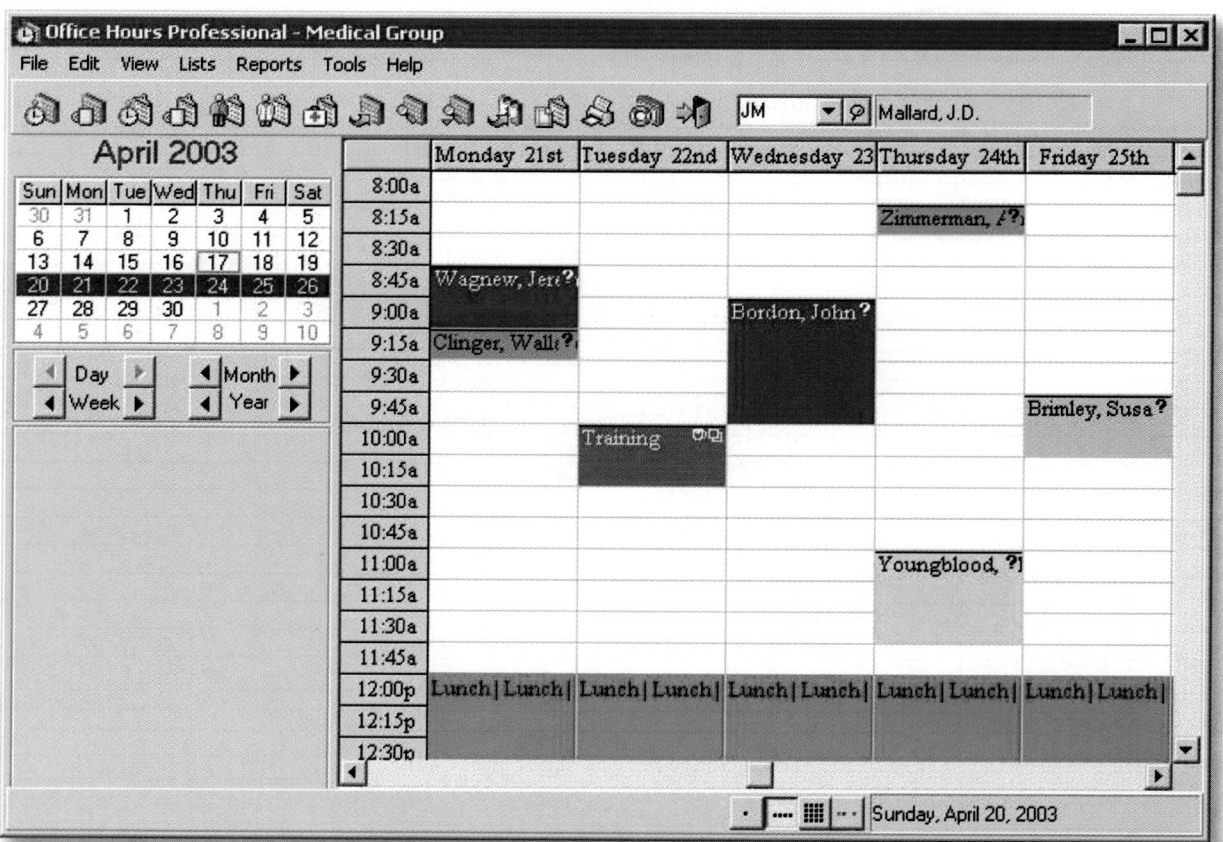

**Figure 12-4.** Many medical offices use computerized scheduling instead of or in addition to a traditional appointment book.

patients are most often arranged over the telephone. Be sure to obtain all the necessary information, including the correct spelling and pronunciation of the person's name, home address, daytime telephone number, and date of birth. It is helpful to obtain insurance information at the time of new patient scheduling so that insurance verification can be made before the patient comes into the office.

When arranging the appointment, keep in mind that some physicians prefer to schedule new patients at certain times of the day, such as first thing in the morning. When scheduling an appointment for a new patient, make sure to allow enough time for filling out forms. Have the new patient arrive 15 to 30 minutes early to do this. Information about the office may be mailed out prior to the first appointment, including a patient information brochure, medical history forms, and a patient registration form. The patient should be instructed to complete the forms and bring the completed forms with him for the first appointment.

## Return Appointments

It is always good practice to ask patients returning to the reception area if they need to schedule another appointment. It may be helpful to routinely schedule return appointments at the same time and/or day that the patient has had previously. Getting them to make the appointment then will save you from having to do so by telephone later on. When patients call to arrange appointments, use the telephone techniques outlined in Chapter 11.

## Appointment Reminders

Some patients may have trouble remembering their next appointment, especially if they arrange it far in advance. To help patients keep track of their appointments, you can use several types of appointment reminders.

**Appointment Cards.** In many offices the medical assistant fills out and hands the patient an appointment reminder card, like the one shown in Figure 12-5. To reduce

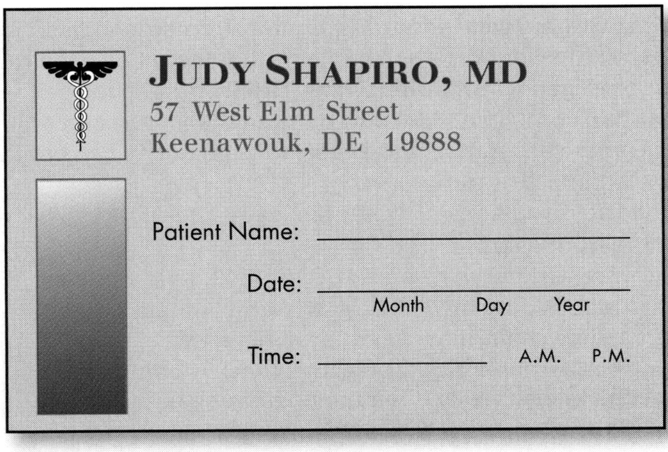

JUDY SHAPIRO, MD
57 West Elm Street
Keenawouk, DE 19888

Patient Name: _____

Date: _____
　　　　　Month　　Day　　Year

Time: _____ A.M. P.M.

**Figure 12-5.** Before patients leave the office, be sure to give them an appointment card if they are scheduled to return to the office.

the chance of error, enter the appointment in the appointment book first, then fill out the card. Otherwise, when the patient takes the appointment card, you have to rely on your memory when entering the appointment in the book.

**Reminder Mailings.** When making a follow-up appointment in person, you can ask the patient to address to himself a postcard on which you have written the next appointment's date and time. This postcard serves as a backup in case the patient loses the original appointment reminder card. Place the postcard in the tickler file under the day when it should be sent (usually a week before the appointment). Reminder mailings can also be sent to patients who make appointments over the telephone. In this case, of course, you must address the postcard for the tickler file yourself. Reminder mailings are useful when appointments are made many months in advance or are for geriatric patients.

**Reminder Calls.** Depending on office policy and available time, you might also call patients 1 or 2 days before their appointments to confirm the scheduled time. This technique can be especially helpful for patients with a history of late arrivals or for **no-shows** (patients who do not call to cancel and do not come to the appointment). Writing patients' phone numbers next to their names in the appointment book makes it convenient for you to make appointment reminder calls.

**Recall Notices.** Some offices book appointments no more than a few weeks in advance, or may not have the next year's schedule available when a patient is to book a return appointment. In either case, if your office has such a policy, you need a way to make sure patients do not forget to call for appointments that are 6 months—or even a year—away from their last appointments.

Suppose, for example, that the physician tells a patient she should have an annual breast examination. How can you help her remember to call to schedule one at the appropriate time? One way is to use a system of recall notices. In a tickler file enter the patient's name under the month when she should call the office. When the time arrives, send a form letter reminding her that she will soon be due for a breast examination and asking her to call for an appointment.

# Special Scheduling Situations

Although a great deal of scheduling is routine, creativity and flexibility are necessary for scheduling some special cases. These special situations often involve patients, but they may also involve physicians.

## Patient Scheduling Situations

On some days all patients will keep their appointments and arrive on time. On many other days, however, patients may walk in without appointments, arrive late for scheduled appointments, or miss appointments entirely. Being prepared for these possibilities allows you to handle them better and to keep the office schedule running as smoothly as possible.

**Emergencies.** Your training as a medical assistant will help you recognize the signs of an emergency. In some instances you will refer the caller to the nearest hospital emergency room or instruct the caller to call Emergency Medical Services (EMS) for an ambulance. In other instances you will ask the caller to come to the office right away. It is vital that doctors see emergency patients before patients who are already in the waiting area or on the schedule. It is best to explain to waiting patients that there has been an emergency (without giving details). This announcement helps them understand and accept the delay and also gives them an opportunity to reschedule their appointments. The Points on Practice section provides guidelines for scheduling emergency appointments. Procedure 11-1 in Chapter 11 details how to handle emergency calls.

**Referrals.** Sometimes other doctors refer patients to the practice for second opinions or special consultations. Patients seeking second opinions before deciding on surgery, often at the request of his or her insurance carrier,

should be fit into the schedule as soon as possible. Other referred patients should also be seen quickly, as a matter of professional courtesy to the referring doctor as well as good business practice.

Many office manuals contain a listing of referral physicians and facilities, including the names of facilities or specialty physicians, their addresses, and their phone numbers. When arranging a referral, try to give the patient two referral names to choose from, along with the referral phone numbers and addresses. When choosing the referral names of either physicians or facilities, be sure that the facility accepts the patient's insurance. All referrals should be documented in the patient's medical record.

**Fasting Patients.** Some procedures and tests require patients to fast (refrain from eating or drinking anything beginning the night before). Scheduling these patients as early in the day as possible shows consideration for their needs. When scheduling appointments that require the patient to fast, be sure to inform the patient of the need to fast and when fasting should start.

**Patients With Diabetes.** Like fasting patients, patients with diabetes can use extra consideration when you schedule their appointments. In general, patients who take

## Points on Practice

## Scheduling Emergency Appointments

As a multiskilled medical assistant, you will be well prepared to tell the difference between acute conditions that are emergencies and those that are not. Guidelines on types of emergencies to be seen in the office and types to be referred elsewhere will vary. If you have any doubt, interrupt the physician to ask for instructions.

Even with buffer times built into the daily schedule, emergencies are still disruptive to most practices. Your ability to stay calm, respond quickly, and remain flexible will be of great comfort to the emergency patient and to others in the waiting area. Read the following story to see how an emergency situation can be handled skillfully.

### The Situation

It is 4:15 P.M. in a busy family practice. The telephone rings. The caller is the father of a 10-year-old boy. Maria, the medical assistant, can hear the panic in his voice. His son Kyle has injured his knee while playing football with friends. Kyle cannot straighten the knee, and it is quite swollen.

Maria consults the physician, who suspects torn cartilage. The physician tells Maria to have the father wrap ice in a towel, apply it to Kyle's knee, and bring him in immediately. Maria relays this advice to the father and asks him how soon he can get to the office.

"It will take about 25 minutes," he replies.

The office schedule includes a buffer time opening at 4:30, but based on the father's estimate, Kyle cannot possibly arrive until 4:40. Maria notes that Mrs. Griffin, a good-natured retiree, is scheduled to come in for her weekly blood pressure check at 4:45 P.M. Hers is the last scheduled appointment of the day.

### The Solution

Mrs. Griffin lives about 5 minutes from the office. Maria calls her home and explains that there has been an emergency. She offers Mrs. Griffin three choices: she can come in at 4:30 and be seen then; she can arrive at the usual time and expect to wait; or she can be rescheduled for tomorrow.

"No problem," Mrs. Griffin says cheerfully. "I'll come right over."

Mrs. Griffin arrives at 4:35. At 4:40, Kyle hobbles in, supported by his father. Maria greets them and offers Kyle a chair on which to prop his foot.

Mrs. Griffin's blood pressure check is complete at 4:45. Kyle waits only 5 minutes before he is seen.

Thanks to Maria's quick thinking, the office stays on schedule—essentially by switching one appointment for another.

insulin must eat meals and snacks at regular times. This routine keeps their blood sugar from dropping too low—a condition that can result in confused thinking or even loss of consciousness. Therefore, you might want to avoid scheduling patients with diabetes for slots in late morning, close to lunchtime. If the schedule is running late by the time these patients arrive, they will be waiting in your reception area at a time when they really need to eat.

If the physician sees several patients with diabetes, you might also ask him about keeping appropriate snacks on hand to offer these patients in emergencies. Most patients with diabetes, however, carry their own emergency snacks with them to treat low blood sugar.

**Repeat Visits.** Some patients need regular appointments, such as for prenatal checkups or physical therapy. If possible, schedule these appointments for the same day and time each week. Establishing a routine helps patients remember their appointments and simplifies the office schedule.

**Late Arrivals.** If the practice has patients who are routinely late and gentle reminders to be on time have not helped, you might try booking them toward the end of the day. Even if a patient arrives late for a late-afternoon appointment, the doctor has already seen most of the day's patients and the late patient will not disrupt the schedule. Document late arrivals or missed appointments in the patient's chart. With documentation, patients who are habitually late can be called to discuss the reasons for their lateness. The goal of the discussion should be to find a solution so that patients can make their appointments on time and the schedule will run smoothly.

**Walk-Ins.** From time to time, a patient (or a person who has not visited the practice before) may arrive without an appointment and still expect to see the doctor. These people are called **walk-ins.** Office policies on how to handle walk-ins vary. If the person is experiencing an emergency, handle the situation as you would handle any emergency. Otherwise, you might politely explain that the doctor is fully booked for the day and offer to schedule an appointment in the usual manner. If, by chance, the doctor is available and willing to see the walk-in, you should still ask the person to call to schedule appointments in the future. If your physician's office has a policy of no walk-ins, post a sign in the lobby or waiting area stating that patients are seen by appointment only.

**Cancellations.** When patients call to cancel appointments, thank them for calling, and try to reschedule the appointment while they are on the telephone. If patients say they will call later to reschedule, note this information in the appointment book.

You should also write "canceled" in the appointment book and draw a single line through the patient's name. To avoid confusion, cancel the first appointment *before* entering the patient's rescheduled appointment. Remember that the appointment book is a legal record. If you forget to cross out the name at the time of the first appointment, it may later seem that the doctor saw the patient twice. It is also important to note the cancellation in the patient's medical record. This notation can protect the practice from possible legal action. For example, a patient whose incision became infected could not blame the doctor if the patient canceled an appointment for a dressing change.

You may be able to fill slots created by cancellations by calling patients who have appointments scheduled for later in the day or week. Some patients may be willing to come in earlier than planned. When you make appointments, you can ask patients if they would be interested in coming in earlier if openings occur. Placing the names of interested patients in a tickler file can save time later.

**Missed and Wrong-Day Appointments.** It is important for legal reasons to document a no-show in the appointment book and patient record. Always inform the physician of any missed appointments in case the patient's condition requires a follow-up. The physician may want you to call the patient with a polite reminder that the patient has missed an appointment and needs to reschedule. There may have been a misunderstanding about the time, or the patient may simply have forgotten the appointment. Some offices, especially ones that use computerized scheduling systems, send out form letters when patients miss appointments. If failure to keep the appointment could endanger the patient's health, mention this possibility to the patient, or ask the physician to tell the patient over the telephone.

Sometimes a patient may show up on the wrong day for his or her appointment. If the patient lives in the local area, rescheduling makes sense. But if the patient made special transportation arrangements or traveled from a long distance, it may be best to try to work the patient into the schedule for the day. When in doubt about the best course of action, consult with the doctor or office manager.

## Physician Scheduling Situations

Not all scheduling problems result from patients. Sometimes physicians disrupt the office schedule. They may be called away on an emergency, may be delayed at the hospital, or may simply arrive late. In any event, the appointment schedule may get off track.

Physicians are only human and may occasionally be late for appointments. Some physicians are frequently late, however, either when arriving in the morning or when returning from lunch or from regular meetings. If this situation occurs in your office, you might approach it in several ways.

At a staff meeting you could mention that the morning or afternoon schedule often seems to get off to a late start. Then you might ask if anyone has suggestions for improving this situation. The physician may recognize that she is the cause of the problem and decide to resolve it.

If the physician does not take responsibility for the problem, however, you may need to adjust the office schedule to handle the situation. Suppose, for example, that the first patient appointment slot is at 8:30 A.M., but the physician usually does not arrive until 8:35 A.M. You could simply avoid scheduling patients between 8:30 and 8:45 A.M. If a physician is often 15 minutes late returning from lunch or from meetings, you might leave open the first appointment slot after the normal arrival time. In effect, you build buffer time into the schedule.

# Scheduling Outside Appointments

You may be responsible for arranging patient appointments outside the medical office. These appointments may include:

- Consultations with other physicians
- Laboratory work
- X-rays
- Other diagnostic tests
- Hospital stays
- Surgeries

Before scheduling these appointments, ask the doctor for an order that identifies the exact procedures to be performed and specifies when the results will be needed. Always verify the patient's type of insurance before choosing which facility or physician the referral will be sent to. Insurance companies that are HMOs (health maintenance organizations) often will arrange the referral themselves. The medical assistant or secretary sending the referral completes the necessary forms and faxes them to the insurance company. The insurance company will authorize the referral and notify the office when approved. Sometimes referrals, if not urgent, can take 30 days or longer to approve.

Once authorization has been obtained, then talk with the patient to find convenient appointment times. This habit is not only courteous but also gives patients a sense of control over situations they may find a bit frightening. Some doctors' offices may have you call the outside laboratory or hospital with all information concerning the patient and then give the patient the number to call to set up the appointment. This approach is often easier for patients. They then have the telephone number in case they need to reschedule.

If you are calling to make the appointment for the patient, tell the medical assistant, scheduling secretary, or admissions clerk what consultation, test, or procedure is required. Then find out what your office or the patient must do to prepare for the appointment. For example, the admitting doctor may need to complete a preadmission evaluation for a patient who is to be hospitalized.

When arrangements have been made, inform the patient, and note on the chart that you have done so. You may also provide the patient with a completed referral slip or, in the case of laboratory work, a laboratory request slip. Procedure 12-2 explains how to schedule

## PROCEDURE 12.2

### Scheduling and Confirming Surgery at a Hospital

**Procedure Goal:** To follow the proper procedure for scheduling and confirming surgery

**Materials:** Calendar, telephone, notepad, pen

**Method:**

1. Elective surgery is usually performed on certain days when the doctor is scheduled to be in the operating room and a room and an anesthetist are available. The patient may be given only one or two choices of days and times. (For emergency surgery the first step is to reserve the operating room.)

2. Call the operating room secretary. Give the procedure required, the name of the surgeon, the time involved, and the preferred date and hour.

3. Provide the patient's name (including birth name, if appropriate), address, telephone number, age, gender, Social Security number, and insurance information.

*Rationale*

This ensures that the hospital has the correct patient information for the admission.

4. Call the admissions office (or day-stay surgery office). Arrange for the patient to be admitted on the day of surgery or the day before (depending on the surgery to be performed). Ask for a copy of the admissions form for the patient record.

5. Some hospitals want patients to complete preadmission forms. In such cases, request a blank form for the patient. Depending on hospital policy, tell the patient to arrive for the appointment a few minutes early to complete the appropriate paperwork.

6. Confirm the surgery and the patient's arrival time 1 business day before surgery.

*Rationale*

This helps to ensure that the patient will not forget about the appointment date and time.

and confirm appointments for surgery. (You will find additional information on preparing patients for surgery in Chapter 14.)

# Maintaining the Physician's Schedule

The schedules of busy physicians are not limited to office visits with patients and hospital rounds. Physicians also need to attend professional meetings, travel to conferences, present speeches to colleagues, complete paperwork, and perform other duties. Your job is to help physicians make the most efficient use of their time.

One way is to avoid overbooking appointments with patients. **Overbooking** (scheduling more patients than can reasonably be seen in the time allowed) creates stress for the physician and the staff, and eventually causes the office schedule to fall behind.

The opposite problem, **underbooking**—leaving large, unused gaps in the schedule—does not make the best use of the physician's time. Of course, you have no control over patients who cancel appointments. If you cannot reschedule another patient for the empty slot, the physician can use the time to catch up on telephone calls to patients or to attend to other matters.

At times you will have to cancel appointments because the physician has been delayed or called away by an emergency. Apologize to waiting patients on behalf of the physician, and offer them a choice. Explain that they can wait in the office (give an estimated waiting time), leave to run errands and return later, or reschedule their appointments for another day. Documentation should be noted in the patient's chart that because of an emergency in the office, the appointment had to be rescheduled. Be sure to write the date of the rescheduled appointment in the chart. Always make sure patients who need immediate attention are seen by another physician.

## Reserving Operating Rooms

If the doctor in your office plans to perform surgery at a hospital, you will need to call the operating room secretary to reserve the facility. Give the preferred days and times, the type of surgery, and the length of time the doctor will need the operating room. After the day and time are set, provide the secretary with all relevant patient information. Relay any requests from the doctor, such as the blood type and units of blood that may be needed. It may also be your responsibility to make arrangements for surgical assistants, an anesthetist, and a hospital bed for the patient following surgery.

## Stocking the Medical Bag

Some physicians see patients at skilled nursing facilities and elsewhere outside the office. You must enter these visits on the appointment schedule, taking into account the

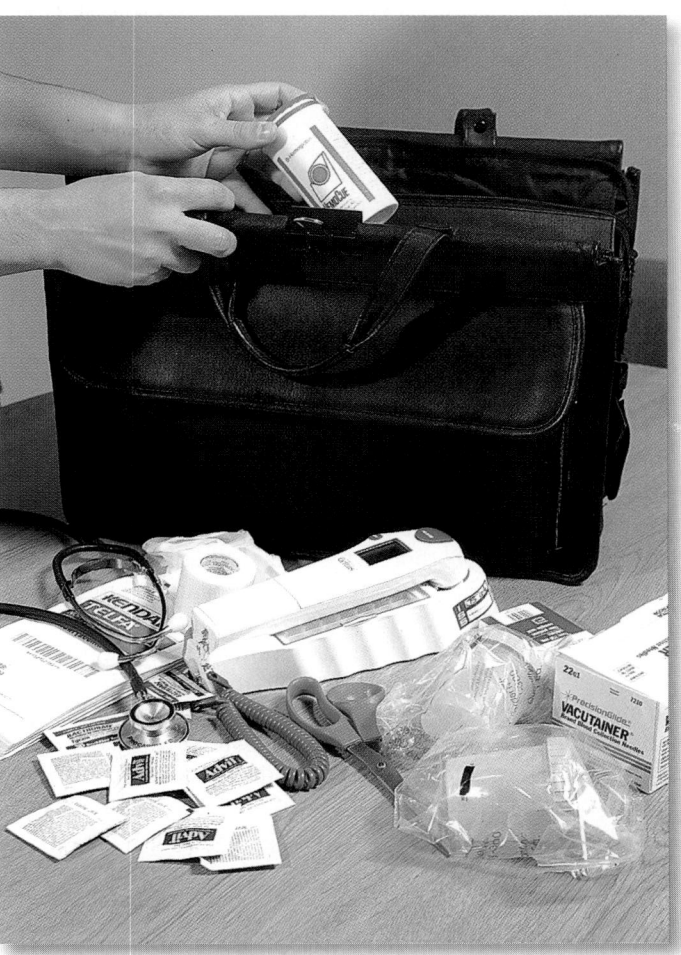

**Figure 12-6.** You may be responsible for keeping the physician's medical bag stocked with supplies.

necessary travel time. For these visits, you may be responsible for stocking the physician's medical bag, as shown in Figure 12-6. The supplies vary depending on the practice, but the following items are commonly included:

- Adhesive tape, bandages, dressings
- Biohazard container
- Sphygmomanometer and blood pressure cuff
- Containers for specimens
- Medications—antibiotics, epinephrine, digitalis
- Microscope slides and fixative
- Ophthalmoscope
- Otoscope
- Penlight
- Personal protective equipment (for example, sterile latex gloves, protective face shield, and protective gown)
- Prescription pads and pens
- Scissors
- Sterile dressing forceps
- Sterile swabs

- Sterile syringes and needles
- Stethoscope
- Thermometers

Post a list of all the necessary items in the area where you check, clean, and restock the medical bag. The expiration dates on the medications and supplies should be checked routinely. It is important that no one borrow any supplies from the medical bag. In the event of an emergency, the bag must always be fully stocked.

## Scheduling Pharmaceutical Sales Representatives

Drug manufacturers often send pharmaceutical sales representatives into medical offices with printed information about new drugs as well as free samples that can be given to patients. These representatives are sometimes called detail persons. Some doctors do not want to meet with pharmaceutical representatives. Other doctors are willing to spend a few minutes if time permits and if the products are likely to be useful to the practice. Some doctors set aside a certain time 1 or 2 days a week to see detail persons. When a pharmaceutical representative who is unknown to you comes into the office, ask for a business card and check with the doctor before scheduling an appointment (Figure 12-7). (Storing drug samples is discussed in Chapter 8.)

## Making Travel Arrangements

You may be responsible for arranging transportation and lodging when physicians attend meetings, speaking engagements, and other events out of town. You may contact the airline, car rental agency, hotel, or other services yourself, or you may work through a travel agent. In either case request confirmation of travel and room reservations. You may also be responsible for picking up tickets or

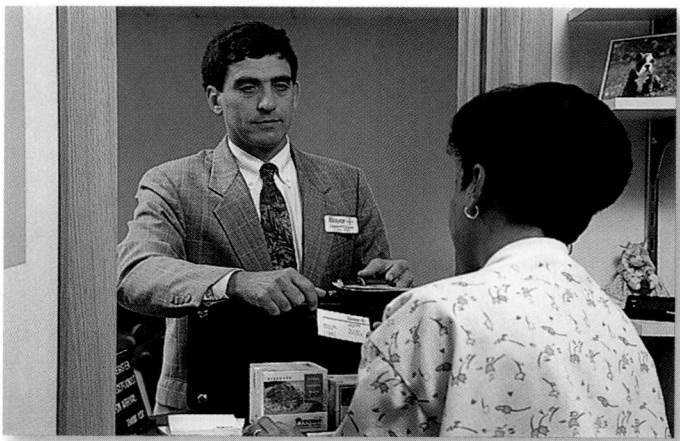

**Figure 12-7.** If pharmaceutical representatives come into the office without an appointment, you can ask them to leave a business card.

seeing that they are mailed to the office if time permits before the trip.

Before the day of departure, obtain an itinerary from the travel agent, or create one yourself. An **itinerary** is a detailed travel plan, listing dates and times of flights and events, locations of meetings and lodgings, and telephone numbers. Give several copies to the physician, and keep one for the office.

You must schedule and confirm professional coverage of the practice during the physician's absence. This coverage may be important for legal reasons. A **locum tenens,** or substitute physician, may be hired to see patients while the regular physician is away. (*Locum tenens* is Latin for "one occupying the place of another.") You may have more than one locum tenens on call, depending on the practice. In some areas special firms provide a locum tenens and other temporary medical and nursing help.

## Planning Meetings

You may help the doctor set up meetings of professional societies or committees. To do so, you will need to know how many people are expected to attend, how long the meeting will last, and the purpose of the meeting. In addition, ask the doctor if a meal is to be served.

Some groups always meet at the same location. If there is no established meeting place, you must choose and reserve one. Select a location with an adequately sized meeting room, sufficient parking, and, if needed, food services. Be sure also to arrange for necessary equipment, such as a microphone, podium, or overhead projector. Many conference centers and hotels have an on-site catering manager or conference manager to assist you with these arrangements. When the facility has been booked, mail a notice to all those expected to attend the meeting. On the notice provide the topic, names of the speakers, date, time, place, and admission costs or fees associated with attending.

With direction from the physician, you may also be responsible for creating the meeting's agenda. An **agenda** is a list of topics to be discussed or presented at a meeting in order of presentation. You may be asked to prepare the **minutes,** or the report of what was discussed and decided at the meeting.

## Scheduling Time With the Physician

You and the physician should meet regularly to go through the tickler file and make sure necessary paperwork is prepared on time. Examples of recurring deadlines include those for state medical license renewal, Drug Enforcement Agency registrations, and documentation of the physician's continuing medical education (CME) requirements. Table 12-1 lists items that are often part of a physician's schedule.

## TABLE 12-1  Common Items on a Physician's Schedule

### Payments, Dues, and Fees

- Association dues
- Health insurance premium
- Payment for laundry service
- Liability insurance premium
- Life insurance premium
- Office rent
- Property insurance premium
- Paychecks for staff
- Payment for janitorial services
- Payment for leased equipment
- Taxes
  - Quarterly federal tax payments
  - Quarterly state tax payments
  - Annual federal and state tax filing deadline

### Time Commitments

- Committee meetings
- Conventions

### Renewals and Accreditations

- Facility accreditation
  - State requirements
  - Certificate of necessity
  - Laboratory registration
  - Federal requirements
  - Ambulatory surgical centers
  - Physician office laboratory
- Medical license renewal
- Narcotics licenses renewal
- Drug Enforcement Agency registrations
- CME accreditations

# Summary

Properly scheduling appointments in the medical office ensures a steady, efficient flow of patients. Setting up a matrix in the appointment book is the first step in scheduling appointments.

There are various appointment scheduling systems, including open-hours scheduling, wave scheduling, and cluster scheduling. Arranging appointments involves scheduling new and return patients and includes appointment reminder techniques. Special scheduling situations may occur, such as emergencies, referrals, and missed appointments. These situations may involve either patients or physicians. You may also be responsible for scheduling outside appointments for patients, as for testing or surgery.

Maintaining the physician's schedule includes such responsibilities as making travel arrangements and planning meetings. Meeting regularly with the physician helps ensure the smooth running of the office.

# REVIEW

## CHAPTER 12

### CASE STUDY QUESTIONS

Now that you have completed this chapter, review the case study at the beginning of the chapter and answer the following questions:

1. How would you adjust the schedule to allow for the emergency without falling behind schedule?
2. If it is necessary to reschedule patients, who should be rescheduled and when?
3. Would you explain anything to the patients in the waiting room about the emergency? If so, what would you say?

### Discussion Questions

1. Describe situations that could cause the office to run behind schedule.
2. List the different types of appointment scheduling systems and briefly describe each.
3. Why is it important to note missed appointments and cancellations in the patient record and in the appointment book?
4. What is a matrix and why is it necessary?
5. List how long each of the following appointments should be scheduled for:
   a. earache
   b. CPE
   c. wound check
   d. Pap
   e. suture removal
   f. establish NP w/Rx prn
6. List the information that should be documented in the appointment book when scheduling.
7. Discuss how you would feel in a situation in which you had an extended wait in a physician's office. What could the medical assistant or office personnel do to ease your frustration?

### Critical Thinking Questions

1. A persistent pharmaceutical representative continues to come into the office without an appointment. How would you handle this situation?

2. The physician is running about an hour and a half behind schedule and the schedule is completely filled. Describe how you would handle this problem.
3. What do you say to a patient who wishes to schedule an appointment, but is reluctant to tell you the reason for the appointment? Would you make the appointment?
4. Right after lunch, a patient walks into the office and requests to see the physician. The patient does not have an appointment and is complaining of pain in her stomach that will not go away. She has vomited a few times and looks very pale. How should you handle this situation?
5. Describe the best scheduling system for the following types of physician offices:
   a. A large practice with four physicians and with x-ray and lab facilities that are available anytime
   b. A small practice with two physicians and with lab facilities that are available only between 8:00 A.M. and 10:00 A.M.

### Application Activities

1. A patient arrives at 10:00 A.M. for an appointment. When you check the schedule, the patient is not listed for an appointment for today. The patient produces an appointment card that clearly states that he has an appointment on this date at 10:00 A.M. You check tomorrow's schedule and realize that the patient is scheduled for the next day at 10:00 A.M. The medical office staff member who filled out the appointment card had made a mistake. The schedule for today is completely full and is already running behind. The patient is leaving the country for two months tomorrow morning and must see the physician today. What should you do?
2. A patient is a no-show for an appointment today. List where this should be documented. Discuss why it is important to document a no-show appointment.
3. Dr. Thompson, the only physician in your office, is out of town at a medical meeting. She is due back tomorrow morning. At 4:00 P.M., Dr. Thompson calls to say that a blizzard has closed the airport and she will be forced to stay away for another day. You look at tomorrow's schedule. She has a full patient load. What should you do?

## Virtual Fieldtrip

*Visit the McGraw-Hill Higher Education Medical Assisting website at www.mhhe.com/medicalassisting3 to complete the following activity:*

Visit The American Association of Medical Assistants website and other websites about medical practice scheduling. Prepare an oral presentation regarding topics such as electronic scheduling, different methods of medical appointment scheduling, scheduling for patients with special needs, and methods to help avoid underbooking and overbooking appointments. Present your report to the class, using all available multimedia, including PowerPoint slides or an overhead projector.

Open the CD and complete this chapter's practice activities, play the games, listen to the key terms, and test yourself with the interactive review. E-mail, print, and/or save your results to document your proficiency.

# Patient Reception

## KEY TERMS

access

Americans With
　Disabilities Act

color family

contagious

differently abled

infectious waste

interim room

Older Americans Act
　of 1965

teletype (TTY) device

## MEDICAL ASSISTING COMPETENCIES

*In preparation for the certification examination, you should know the following areas of competence:*

| COMPETENCY | CMA | RMA |
|---|---|---|
| **Administrative** | | |
| Perform basic clerical skills | X | X |
| Provide patients with methods of health promotion and disease prevention | X | X |
| Identify community resources and information for patients and employers | X | X |
| Perform an inventory of supplies and equipment | X | X |
| Operate and maintain facilities, and perform routine maintenance of administrative and clinical equipment safely | X | X |
| Maintain the physical plant | | X |
| Evaluate and recommend equipment and supplies for practice | | X |
| Project a positive attitude | | X |
| Adapt to change | | X |
| Evidence a responsible attitude | | X |
| Be courteous and diplomatic | | X |

## CHAPTER OUTLINE

- First Impressions
- The Importance of Cleanliness
- The Physical Components
- Keeping Patients Occupied and Informed
- Patients With Special Needs

## LEARNING OUTCOMES

After completing Chapter 13, you will be able to:

**13.1** Identify the elements that are important in a patient reception area.

**13.2** Discuss ways to determine what furniture is necessary for a patient reception area and how it should be arranged.

**13.3** List the housekeeping tasks and equipment needed for this area of the office.

**13.4** Summarize the Occupational Safety and Health Administration (OSHA) regulations that pertain to a patient reception area.

**13.5** List the physical components associated with a comfortable and accessible patient reception area.

**13.6** List the physical components associated with a safe and secure patient reception area.

**13.7** List the types of reading material appropriate to a patient reception area.

**13.8** Describe how modifications to a reception area can accommodate patients with special needs.

**13.9** Identify special situations that can affect the arrangement of a reception area.

# Introduction

Going to the doctor's office can be an emotional and sometimes even a frightening event for many people. The office staff can do much to make the entry into the medical environment easier and less intimidating.

This chapter describes the patient reception area. As you look at the reception area and patient bathrooms through the eyes of patient needs, you begin to see ways to make the rooms both inviting and functional. Additionally, you will learn about the special needs of disabled patients. Well-planned and pleasant surroundings can do much to set the stage for a successful interaction between the patient and the doctor and other medical staff.

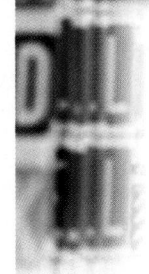

## CASE STUDY

A 70-year-old patient has just arrived for his first appointment with his new primary care physician. He recently moved to Florida to be near his grown children, and today he meets his new doctor. He is apprehensive and concerned that he won't like this new doctor. He takes a deep breath and opens the door into the medical office reception room.

The first thing he notices is the cool air, which is in stark contrast to the hot humid air outside. As he enters the area, he sees a comfortable, spacious room decorated in soft color tones. The chairs and sofas are arranged in small conversational groupings. Neatly stacked on the tables is a colorful array of many different types of magazines. Playing softly in the corner of the room is a television tuned to a health channel. At the end of the room are a sliding glass window and a countertop with a sign-in clipboard. Crossing the room, he notices a family with small children playing with blocks in an adjoining room marked "Children's Reception Area." He sees a courtesy phone for patient use located in a nearby alcove. He adds his name to the list on the clipboard, noticing that all the patient names above his own have been blacked out. The glass window immediately opens and a neatly dressed medical assistant with a pleasant smile speaks to him, calling him by name. He is beginning to think this doctor might be all right after all.

As you read this chapter, consider the following questions:

1. What basic elements are *required* in every patient reception area? What other nonessential elements are nice to include as well?
2. Why is it important to think of the front patient area as the "patient reception area" and not the "waiting room"?
3. What special accommodations in the reception area are important to patients with disabilities?

# First Impressions

The reception area plays a significant role in a patient's experience at the doctor's office. It is the first area patients see when entering the office. It is also a place where they have to spend time waiting for their appointments.

The appearance of the reception area creates an impression of the practice. Is the office bright and cheerful, cool and modern, or warm and cozy? The impression created by the reception area reflects on the quality of care patients can expect to receive. For example, old, tattered, or dirty furniture in the reception area will give patients the impression that the medical practice is unsuccessful and outdated. A carefully designed and well-maintained patient reception area, on the other hand, can attract and keep patients in the practice. It also ensures a pleasant and comfortable experience while they wait to receive medical care.

## Reception Area

The reception area includes a reception window or desk, as shown in Figure 13-1, where patients check in for their appointments. Windows are not soundproof. Care should

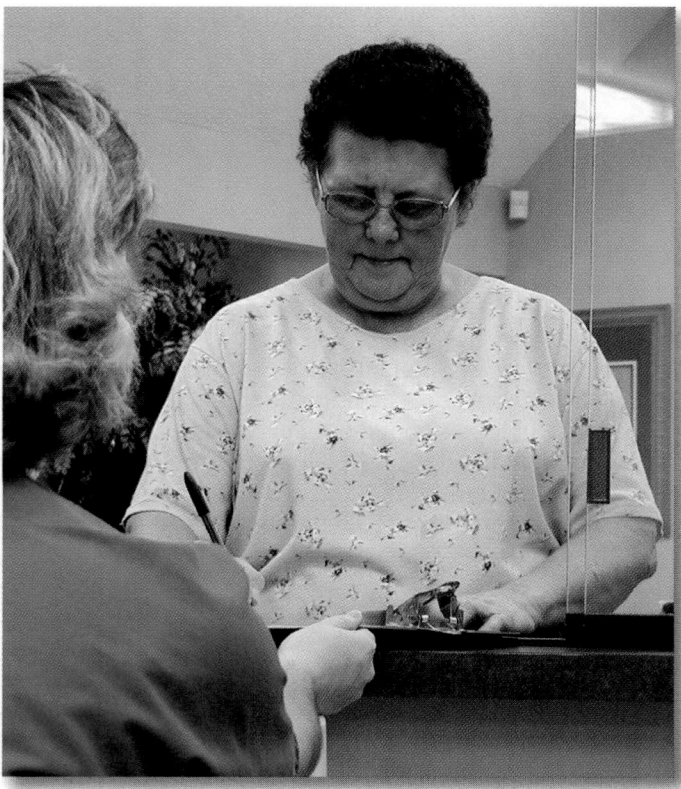

**Figure 13-1.** A receptionist's desk or window, where patients can check in, is part of every patient reception area.

be taken by employees to minimize noise and conversation behind the window.

The reception area also includes chairs and couches for patients to sit on while waiting. Most patient reception areas are arranged using the same basic organizational concepts. The impressions they create can vary widely, however, depending on the elements chosen to enhance this part of the office.

Do not refer to the patient reception area as the "waiting room." The term has a negative connotation and implies that the patient and family members should expect a long wait. A more positive descriptive term to use is the "reception area."

**Medical Office Information.** As a convenience to patients, the business cards of all the physicians practicing at the location should be available. These cards are best placed at the reception window or desk, where patients can access them easily.

Other information about the practice is usually posted near the reception desk, including insurance information, workers' compensation information, and a reminder to turn off all cell phones.

**Lighting.** Most medical offices use fairly bright lighting in the reception area, allowing patients to see their surroundings easily. Subdued lighting, like that sometimes used in restaurants, could be hazardous because it could cause patients to trip over or bump into hard-to-see objects.

In addition, bright lighting is essential for reading, which is a common activity in the patient reception area. Bright lighting also conveys an impression of cleanliness.

Lighting should not be so bright that it becomes bothersome, however. Extremely bright light can be harsh on the eyes and create an annoying glare. A specialist, such as an electrician or lighting showroom salesperson, can help determine the appropriate level of lighting for the patient reception area.

**Room Temperature.** Patients will be uncomfortable if the reception area is too hot or too cold. In an uncomfortable setting, waiting time can seem much longer than it really is. Therefore, maintaining an average, comfortable temperature is important.

The thermostat should be kept at a temperature that feels comfortable to you and to the office staff. You might periodically survey patients to see if they are comfortable and adjust the setting accordingly. Many elderly people feel cold because of lowered metabolisms. You may want to increase the temperature setting for a geriatric practice or if the office sees a large number of elderly patients. The room temperature in the reception area may be a bit cooler than in the examination rooms, where patients may be required to disrobe.

**Music.** Many medical offices pipe music through speakers to the reception area as well as elsewhere in the office. The music provides a soothing background sound. Because the music is meant to calm patients, it should be chosen accordingly. Classical music, light jazz, and soft rock are appropriate choices, whereas heavy metal and rap music are not. Some offices use prepared tapes or compact discs. Others tune in to a local radio station.

The music should reflect the interests of the patients. If the office serves an older population, you might choose oldies or classical music. Try soft rock for an obstetrics/gynecology practice or children's folk music for a pediatric practice.

## Decor

The patient reception area gets its distinctive look from the way it is decorated. With the appropriate elements, the decor can create whatever impression is desired—warm and friendly, modern and elegant, and so on. Some suggestions follow. It is wise to consult a professional decorator, if possible.

**Colors and Fabrics.** Colors and fabrics are the primary elements that make up a room's decor. Colors can be used throughout the room—on walls, furniture, carpeting, and other items. Fabrics are used primarily on furniture and draperies.

When using several colors, it is important to decorate in color families to avoid a jarring, unprofessional look. A **color family** is a group of colors that work well together. Colors fall within two basic areas, cool and warm. Using all cool colors—like white, blue, and mauve—creates a more harmonious impression in the reception area than mixing cool colors with warm ones like red, orange, and hot pink. When

## Medical Receptionist

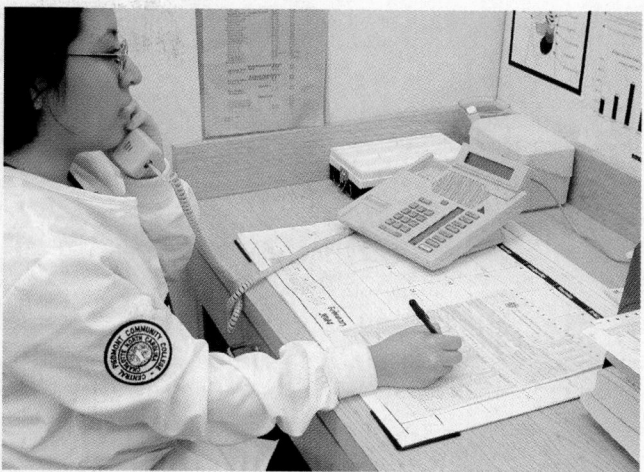

*To gain medical assistant credentials, you must fulfill the requirements of either the American Association of Medical Assistants (for a Certified Medical Assistant) or the American Medical Technologists (for a Registered Medical Assistant). After obtaining your medical assistant certification, you may wish to acquire additional skills in specialty areas through course work or on-the-job training. Although this course work or training may not lead to an additional certification or degree, it will enable you to expand your role in the medical office and advance your career as the demand for skilled health professionals increases.*

### Skills and Duties

A medical receptionist answers telephone calls; performs triage on calls, contacting the physician or nurse with urgent needs; directs calls; assists patients with completing forms; receives patients and initiates the necessary paperwork; receives payments from patients and posts payments to patient accounts; covers all duties at the patient reception desk; schedules patient appointments; schedules surgeries; arranges referrals to other practices; calls patients as necessary; notifies patients of changes or cancellations and prioritizes appointments for rescheduling; updates patient information; maintains office bulletin boards; schedules and coordinates appointments and meetings for the physician; uses the computer to both input and retrieve data; operates the fax machine, the letter folding machine, the postage machine, and other administrative office equipment as needed; orders postage; compiles the daily mail; distributes mail to staff; maintains the patient reception area; creates patient handouts as necessary; establishes and maintains the filing system; inventories and orders office supplies as needed; and performs other administrative duties as needed.

### Workplace Settings

Medical receptionists work in medical practices, including all medical specialties, as well as in outpatient clinics, hospital clinics, and all medical facilities.

### Education

Medical receptionists must be a high school graduate and must complete medical receptionist training as required by state law.

### Where to Go for More Information

The American Association of Medical Assistants
20 N. Wacker Drive, Suite 1575
Chicago, IL 60606
(312) 899-1500

choosing the color family, consider the mood you want to create. Bright colors produce a lively atmosphere, whereas softer, muted colors create a relaxing one.

Fabrics, too, add to the atmosphere in the room. Heavy fabrics like velvet or brocade are more formal, whereas lightweight or sheer fabrics create a soft, delicate appearance. Patterns on fabrics or wallpaper can immediately change the mood of the room. No matter what the design, fabrics should be easy to clean and maintain.

Many medical offices are carpeted, and carpets come in a variety of colors and patterns. Carpeting is attractive, and helps reduce noise. Carpeting also provides a comfortable cushion when people walk through the office.

Carpeting should be easy to clean and durable enough to handle a large volume of patient traffic. Wall-to-wall carpeting is preferable to scatter rugs, which can cause injuries if someone slips on or trips over them and falls.

Professional services can be contracted to deliver a clean, fresh entry carpet on a regular basis. These rubber-backed carpets lie directly on any floor surface and are commonly used at entranceways and hallways or areas of heavy traffic to catch soil from being "walked" into the rest of the office. Unlike scatter rugs, these heavyweight professional carpets lay flat and are not a hazard for tripping or falling. The service brings a fresh carpet and removes the soiled carpeting as scheduled.

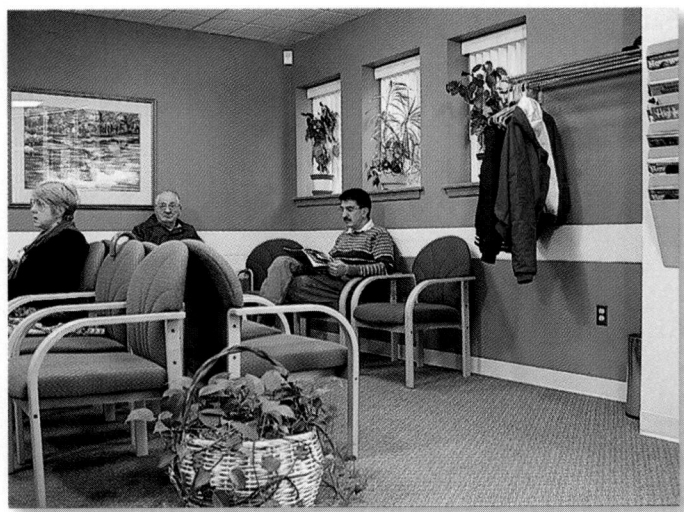

**Figure 13-2.** Specialty items—such as plants, paintings, and coat racks—enhance the patient reception area.

**Specialty Items.** Some offices include specialty items, or accessories, as part of the decor (Figure 13-2). Examples of such items include coat racks, aquariums, plants, paintings, sculptures, mobiles, and children's toys. Some items are meant to add a finishing touch, completing the desired atmosphere. Others may help to interest waiting patients by providing an activity, such as watching the fish in an aquarium.

*Choosing Accessories.* Although specialty items enhance the office decor, keep the number of accessories to a minimum. Too many pieces can give the room a cluttered look. Try to select specialty items that will be pleasing or helpful to patients. A clock is one example. Another useful item is a coat rack, which helps prevent clutter by providing a place for coats, umbrellas, and briefcases. Avoid accessories such as scented candles or potpourri that may be offensive to some people or cause allergic reactions.

*Keeping Safety in Mind.* When selecting specialty items for the medical office, be sure to consider the issue of safety. Follow these guidelines to avoid potential hazards in the patient reception area.

- Do not include any item smaller than a golf ball. Small items present a choking hazard for young children.
- Avoid objects that can be easily pulled apart and then swallowed.
- Avoid easily breakable items, such as glass vases, that might cause cuts or other injuries to patients.
- Choose furniture with rounded, not sharp, corners.
- Coffee tables or other low tables with sharp corners can be a hazard especially to the elderly and to small children.
- Secure heavy wall hangings, shelves, and coat racks to the wall so that there is no risk of their falling.
- It is preferable to display artificial plants rather than living ones. Living plants may irritate patients who

have allergies or present a poisoning hazard if parts of the plants are eaten by toddlers.

- If possible, build large, heavy items (such as fish tanks) into the wall to avoid climbing children and the danger of the items falling.
- Make sure all items in the reception area get a careful daily dusting before patients arrive. Artificial flowers and plants will need to be washed upside-down in soap and water occasionally to remove any potential allergens such as dust.

## Furniture

Buying furniture for a patient reception room requires thoughtful planning. Although the office in which you work will no doubt be furnished already, it is a good idea to learn the steps and decisions involved in choosing furniture. You may be included in future purchasing decisions if the office expands or moves to a new location or if the doctor wants to redecorate.

Furniture styles vary to suit the office decor. Most important, seating furniture should be firm, comfortable, safe, and easy to get in and out of. In addition, washable and fireproof fabric on the furniture minimizes care and maximizes safety. Close color coordination of the seating, floors, and walls may be difficult for an elderly person with failing eyesight. When possible, it is best to have chairs that contrast the carpet color to help prevent accidental falls.

The reception area should have enough furniture so that all patients and family members or friends who accompany them can sit, no matter how busy the office schedule. Forcing people to stand while they wait for an appointment makes the wait seem much longer. The American Medical Association (AMA) suggests that seating be sufficient to accommodate the number of patients, family members, and friends who may be in the office during a 2-hour time period. When calculating this number, be generous in allowing for family members. In some types of practices, such as pediatrics, all patients are accompanied by at least one parent or guardian and sometimes siblings as well.

**Arranging Furniture.** The furniture arrangement can make the office seem comfortable or uncomfortable. If furniture is too close together, patients do not have sufficient space to move around easily or to stretch their legs. They may feel cramped. To ensure that patients have adequate room, a good rule of thumb is to allow 12 square feet of space per person. By this measurement, a 120-square-foot room (10 feet by 12 feet) can accommodate ten people comfortably.

The furniture arrangement should allow maximum floor space. Patients should be able to stretch out their legs when seated and to walk around the reception area if they wish (Figure 13-3). Placing chairs against the wall usually produces the greatest amount of floor area. Additional seating in the middle of the room can be placed

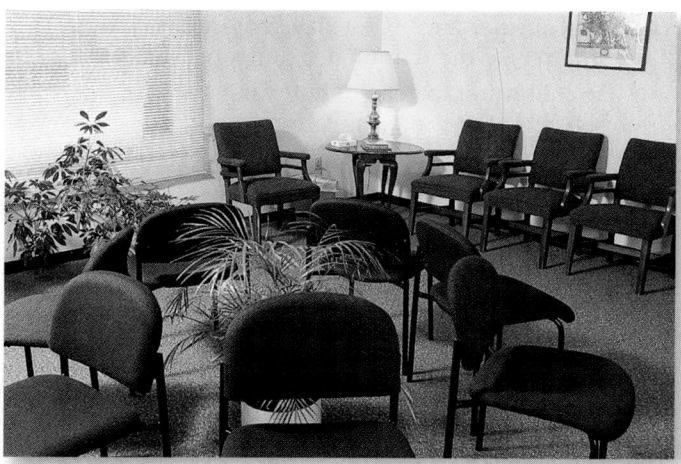

**Figure 13-3.** The furniture in a patient reception area can be arranged in a variety of ways.

back-to-back to conserve space. Seats should be grouped so that families or friends can sit together. Remember to reserve room for patients in wheelchairs. This area should be carefully marked. Always allow enough space for wheelchairs with extended leg supports.

**Ensuring Privacy.** Some patients come to the office alone and value their privacy. Placing single chairs or small groups of chairs in corners of the room offers patients some measure of privacy.

Some medical offices offer more complete privacy in the form of an **interim room,** a room in which people can talk or meet without being seen or heard from the patient reception area. This interim room provides an ideal location for medical staff to confer privately with patients about appointments or bills. It also allows patients to make private telephone calls and allows people to feed or diaper babies in privacy. Not every office has the luxury of space for such a room, but it provides a valuable service to patients when it is possible.

**Accommodating Children.** A pediatric reception area caters to a unique age group of patients. Reception areas for children usually have the same basic setup as those for adults, but special accommodations for children are also made.

In addition to regular chairs, for example, child-size chairs may be available. Some reception areas include playhouses or play furniture, such as small tables. The decor may also be made appealing to young children by the use of bright colors and storybook characters. It is important to make the setting feel familiar and comfortable. The reception desk may stock rolls of stickers or other inexpensive prizes to give to young patients after they have seen the doctor. Later in the chapter, you will learn how to set up a pediatric reception area.

Some pediatricians' offices have a well reception area and a sick reception area to separate children who are contagious from well children. **Contagious** means having a disease or condition that can easily be transmitted to others.

# The Importance of Cleanliness

No matter how tastefully it is decorated, the reception area will be unappealing if it is not clean. Patients expect a physician's office to maintain a high standard of cleanliness. The perception is that a messy or dirty reception area or patient bathroom reflects a practice that does not meet minimum standards for cleanliness. A practice with a spotless, attractive reception area reassures patients that they have chosen a practice with high standards of cleanliness.

## Housekeeping

Keeping the patient reception area clean usually falls within the duties of the medical assistant. In most cases you will be responsible for supervising the work of a professional cleaning service. In a small medical office you may be required to clean the area yourself, using appropriate antibacterial agents and a vacuum. Cleaning should occur daily, with emergency cleanups as needed.

Because professional services generally clean in the evening after business hours, you will probably not be present while the housekeeping staff is working. You may be asked to provide feedback to the cleaning company, however. It may also be your responsibility to outline the tasks you expect workers to complete, including any special requests.

One way of communicating with the cleaning staff is to create a Cleaning Communications Notebook. Arrange with the cleaning staff to leave the notebook open every evening in the same place. Date all entries. Write short, concise directions about any special requests for cleaning. Describe the nature of any stain so the service can best treat it. Sign each entry. Be sure to comment when something is done especially well. Like all of us, your cleaning staff likes to hear when they have done a particularly nice job!

**Tasks.** Although housekeeping tasks vary from office to office, basic routines are applicable to areas such as the patient reception room. The Caution: Handle With Care section gives more information about maintaining a clean reception area.

Whether or not the office employs a professional cleaning service, you or another staff member will need to check for cleanliness throughout the day. As patients spend time in the office, items may become dirty or be moved out of place. Taking time between patient appointments or at midday to spot-clean small areas that have become dirty and straighten items will help keep the patient reception area in good condition.

**Equipment.** If you, and not a professional service, are responsible for cleaning, the person in charge of the office budget will approve the purchase of cleaning equipment and supplies. Examples of cleaning equipment include handheld and upright vacuums, mops, and brooms. Supplies include trash bags, cleaning solutions, rags, and buckets. It is a good idea to have some basic cleaning materials on hand in case an emergency cleanup job is needed during office hours. Always wear gloves when doing cleaning of any kind.

## Cleaning Stains

If furniture, carpet, or other items in the reception area become stained, it is important to remove the stains quickly. Follow these tips for stain removal.

- Try to remove the stain right away. The longer a stain remains, the more difficult it is to remove.
- Blot as much of the stain as possible before rubbing it with a cleaning solution.
- Take special precautions in handling stains involving blood, feces, and urine. Put on latex gloves before blotting or scraping up the stain.
- Wipe the area with a cleaning solution and water.

- Blood, urine, and feces may require special cleaners with an enzyme that breaks down organic waste.
- Use cold water instead of hot water because hot water often sets stains into the fabric.
- Keep all cleaning materials within easy reach for quick action when a stain occurs.

## Removing Odors

Odors are particularly offensive in a doctor's office because people expect a high level of cleanliness and cannot readily leave to escape the odor. Some odors that may occasionally be present in a medical practice include those of urine, feces, vomit, body odors, and laboratory chemicals. A good ventilating system with charcoal filters can help minimize odors. If the system has temporary high-speed blowers, they can be activated as well. Disinfectant sprays and deodorant scents may also help.

## CAUTION *Handle With Care*

### Maintaining Cleanliness Standards in the Reception Area

Cleanliness is one of the hallmarks of a medical office. Not only is cleanliness required in the examination and testing rooms, it is also expected in the patient reception area. A messy patient reception area reflects poorly on the physician and on the practice. Maintaining standards of cleanliness helps ensure that the reception area is presentable at all times.

As a medical assistant, you may be involved—along with the physician, office manager, and other staff members—in setting cleanliness standards for the office. Standards are general guidelines. In addition to setting standards, you will need to specify the tasks required to meet each standard. A checklist of the tasks required to meet all standards is a helpful document to create as well.

The following list outlines standards you may want to consider. Specific housekeeping tasks for meeting those standards are included in parentheses.

1. Keep everything in its place. (Complete a daily visual check for items that are out of place. Return all magazines to racks. Push chairs back into place.)
2. Dispose of all trash. (Empty trash cans. Pick up trash on the floor or on furniture.)
3. Prevent dust and dirt from accumulating on surfaces. (Wipe or dust furniture, lamps, and artificial plants. Polish doorknobs. Clean mirrors, wall hangings, and pictures.)

4. Spot-clean areas that become dirty. (Remove scuff marks. Clean upholstery stains.)
5. Disinfect areas of the reception area if they have been exposed to body fluids. (Immediately clean and disinfect all soiled areas.)
6. Handle items with care. (Take precautions when carrying potentially messy or breakable items. Do not carry too much at once.)

After the standards have been established, type and post them in a prominent place for the office staff to see. The checklist of cleaning activities may be posted, but the person responsible for cleaning the office should also keep a copy.

You should also produce a schedule of specific daily and weekly cleaning activities. Less frequent housekeeping duties, such as laundering drapes, shampooing the carpet, and cleaning windows and blinds, can be noted in a tickler file so that they will be performed on a regular basis.

It is always a good idea to have a second staff member responsible for periodically working with the medical assistant on housekeeping responsibilities. That person may also be responsible for handling cleaning duties when the medical assistant is away from the office.

One odor that can be prevented is smoke. Display "Thank You for Not Smoking" signs prominently in the patient reception area. Do not provide ashtrays, and ask smokers to leave the office if they insist on smoking. Not only does smoking produce an offensive odor, it also may affect the health of other patients in the reception area. People who have asthma or other breathing disorders, or who are feeling unwell for any reason, are particularly sensitive to smoke and strong odors.

## Infectious Waste

There may be times when you will need to clean up infectious waste. **Infectious waste** is waste that can be dangerous to those who handle it or to the environment. Infectious waste includes human waste, human tissue, and body fluids such as blood and urine. It also includes any potentially hazardous waste generated in the treatment of patients, such as needles, scalpels, cultures of human cells, and dressings.

Although infectious waste is not commonly generated in the patient reception area, it can be—as when a patient vomits or bleeds on the rug or on furniture. If that situation should occur, you must clean up the waste promptly.

Infectious waste must be handled in accordance with federal law. Your office may choose to purchase commercially prepared hazardous waste kits for use in cleaning up spills. After cleaning infectious waste from the patient reception area, deposit it in a biohazard container. Disinfect the site to eliminate possible contamination of other patients.

## OSHA Regulations

Federal safety precautions for the workplace are mandated by the Occupational Safety and Health Administration (OSHA), a government agency. OSHA has developed general guidelines for most businesses as well as special rules for health-care practices. To determine whether the requirements are being met, OSHA periodically inspects medical offices. If the rules are not followed, medical offices may be required to pay penalties in addition to correcting the problem. All employees in a medical office must be thoroughly trained in following OSHA guidelines.

Among the OSHA requirements is regular cleaning of walls, floors, and other surfaces. OSHA requires the use of disinfectants to combat bacteria as part of a routine cleaning schedule. In addition, OSHA mandates that broken glass, which may be contaminated, be picked up using a dustpan and brush or tongs. It should not be picked up by hand, even if one wears gloves.

## The Physical Components

No one arrangement of a reception area is necessarily better than another. As long as the arrangement provides clear pathways and comfortable places to sit, the reception area will be functional.

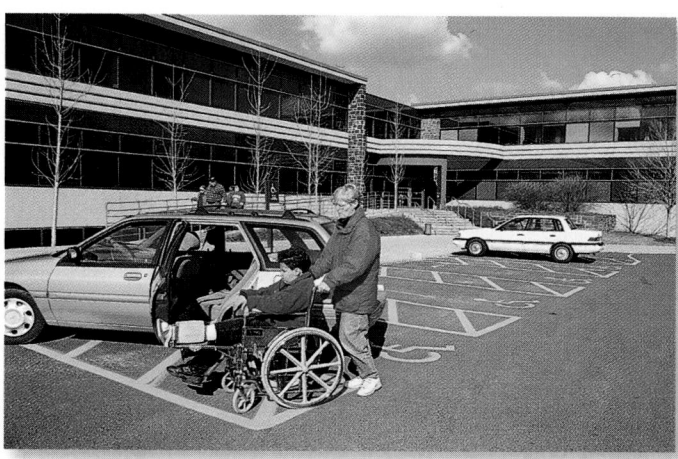

**Figure 13-4.** Patients should have easy, clear access from the parking lot to the medical office door.

## Office Access

The path patients must take to get from the parking area or street to the office and then back out again is called the office **access.** Some offices have easy access and some do not (Figure 13-4).

**Parking Arrangements.** Although some patients walk to the medical office or take public transportation, the majority of patients probably travel by car. Patients who drive to the office need a place to park.

The office can offer either on-street parking or a parking lot. On-street parking requires patients to fend for themselves. They may have to put money into parking meters, and parking spaces may be difficult to find. Both the money required and the potential problems in finding parking spots limit the ease with which patients can gain access to the office.

A free parking lot improves office access. Parking lots should be well lit for safety. To determine the number of parking spaces the office needs, calculate the average length of time a patient spends in the office from arrival to departure and the number of appointments scheduled during that time period. Allow one parking spot per appointment if most patients drive to the office and fewer if many use public transportation. In your count be sure to include parking spaces for office staff. Periodically reevaluate the office's parking needs because they may change over time. All offices must also provide handicapped parking space for patients.

**Entrances.** The entrance to the office should be clearly marked so that patients can find the office easily. The name of the practice and of the doctor or doctors should be on the door or beside the door. Just outside the doorway should be a doormat to help control the amount of dirt tracked into the office. If the office door opens directly to the outside, people inside will feel a sudden change in temperature each time the door is opened in hot or cold weather. A foyer or double-door arrangement helps minimize the effects of the weather and helps keep the office at a consistent, comfortable temperature.

Doorways must be wide enough to accommodate patients using wheelchairs and walkers. Hallways should be extra wide to allow patients in wheelchairs to turn around or to allow two wheelchairs to pass one another. The Americans With Disabilities Act, discussed later in this chapter, requires that doorways have a minimum width of 32 inches and that hallways have a minimum width of 5 feet. Well-lit hallways, without obstructions, are required.

## Safety and Security

Safety and security are important concerns in any public building, and they are especially important in a doctor's office. To ensure safety of the patients and staff, such as protection from hazardous wiring or poorly lit hallways, there are guidelines for businesses, some of which pertain to the patient reception area. In addition, the medical office must be secure from burglary.

**Building Exits.** Make sure you and the office staff are familiar with all building exits. It may be necessary to leave the office quickly, as during a fire, flood, or other emergency. You and other staff members must be prepared to assist and direct patients toward the exits in such a situation.

Ideally, the office should have at least two doorways that lead directly to the outside or to a hallway that leads to stairs. This arrangement affords patients and staff members the speediest, most direct route outside in case of an emergency. All exits must be clearly labeled with illuminated red "Exit" signs. These signs normally have a backup power system, such as a battery, so that they will remain lit even during a power outage.

Having two or more exits also allows staff members to enter and leave the office during nonemergency situations without disrupting people in the patient reception area. Deliveries can be made at the second entrance, further minimizing interruptions.

**Smoke Detectors.** By law, a medical office is required to install smoke detectors that sound an alarm when triggered by heat or smoke. The office staff should be trained in the proper procedure if the smoke alarm sounds—including how to evacuate patients from the building efficiently. Smoke detectors must be checked regularly to ensure that they are operating properly.

**Security Systems.** No matter where the medical office is located, a security alarm system is a wise investment, even if the office building is patrolled by security personnel. A security alarm system offers valuable protection for the confidential patient information housed in a medical office. After the alarm system is installed, all office staff members should thoroughly familiarize themselves with it. They should be able to arm and disarm it easily and know what to do if it is accidentally activated. Each member of the staff should have her or his own individually assigned security access number. This number is required to authorize locking or unlocking the system. Like a credit card, bank, or other security PIN (personal identification number), it should never be shared.

# Keeping Patients Occupied and Informed

Many patients who come into a medical office are ill, anxious, and concerned about their health. While they wait in the reception area, they need a way to stay occupied so that the time seems to pass quickly. In addition, patients may want to be informed about a particular medical condition or about general health issues. To meet these patient needs, most medical offices provide reading materials in the patient reception area. They may also offer television or educational videotapes.

## Reading Materials

The most common activity in a patient reception area is probably reading. Although some patients bring their own books or magazines, most patients expect to find reading materials at the medical office (Figure 13-5). Magazines and books are probably the most popular types of reading materials, but a variety of others may also be available.

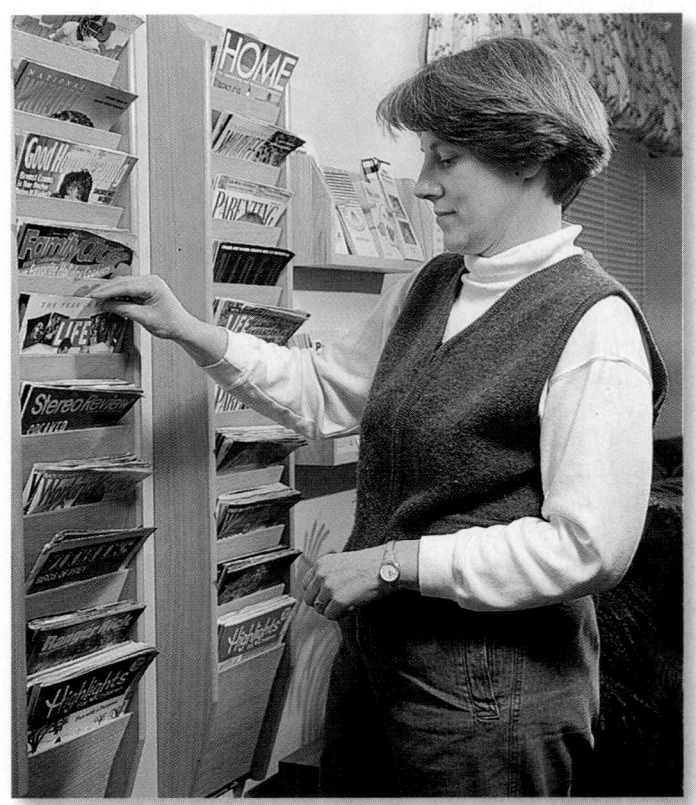

**Figure 13-5.** Reading materials can be organized on tables or in a wall rack.

**Magazines and Books.** Choosing the right mix of reading material to interest all patients is a challenge. You may know doctors' offices that have a wonderful selection of magazines and books and others that have a poor selection. Your judgment of the selection, however, is based on how those publications match your interests. The Points on Practice section gives guidelines on selecting magazines for the medical office. In addition to reading materials for adults, most offices also have children's books and magazines for younger patients and family members.

You or someone on the office staff should be sure to screen publications for medical content. You can then alert the doctors to articles that might stimulate patients' questions.

**Patient Information Packet.** One type of reading material other than magazines is a patient information packet. This document is an easy way to inform patients about the practice. The packet can be designed in many ways, from a simple flyer to a formal folder with pockets to hold individual sheets of information. Topics covered in the packet can range from billing and insurance processing policies to biographical information on each physician in a group practice. Read Chapter 14 to learn more about how to develop the contents of a patient information packet.

**Medical Information.** Another type of reading material commonly found in reception areas is medical brochures. Patients may be interested in information that pertains to their general health or to a specific condition. Brochures on a variety of topics are available to medical offices either free of charge or for a nominal fee. These brochures are usually produced by nonprofit associations that specialize in a disease or condition, such as the American Cancer Society, and by pharmaceutical companies.

Before displaying pamphlets and brochures in the reception area, be sure to read them thoroughly. Make sure they provide accurate information. You may also want to review them to prepare for questions patients may ask. The physician may also want to review them for medical accuracy.

**Bulletin Board.** Most patient reception areas feature a bulletin board. Bulletin boards often highlight area meetings, such as those of support groups, and offer other current information. To encourage patients to look at the bulletin board, change the format and content frequently. An interesting design with bright colors and bold headlines attracts

## Points on Practice

# Tailoring Office Magazines to Patient Interests

It is a common sight: Patients waiting their turn for an appointment pick up one of the many magazines in the reception area. Sometimes it is hard to choose — because every magazine is interesting or because none of them are.

As a medical assistant, you may be responsible for selecting magazines for the office's reception area. The right selection can make the difference between a pleasant wait and a tedious one. Follow these guidelines to compile a suitable mix of magazines that will be of interest to a majority of patients.

1. Patients in some practices immediately share a common ground. They fall within the category of the practice's specialty — for example, geriatrics or pediatrics. Some magazines may be a natural fit for this category. A geriatric practice, for example, may provide publications geared toward senior citizens. A pediatric practice may offer parenting and children's magazines.

2. People waiting in a doctor's office usually have an interest in their health. Therefore, health magazines geared toward the general public are good choices. Of course, the reception area is not the place for the highly technical medical journals, with graphic pictures, that the doctor may receive or for religious materials of any kind.

3. Make sure the magazines cover a variety of interests. The more topics available, the greater the chance that someone will be interested in one of them. Instead of subscribing to several magazines on one topic, try to limit subscriptions to one magazine per topic, unless the topic is of special interest to most patients.

4. Choose magazines that cover topics in a general way — travel, news, sports, fashion, or entertainment. Delving into these areas too specifically — as in a tennis magazine rather than one on a variety of sports — may not interest many patients.

5. Remove torn or out-of-date magazines from the patient reception area. Replenish them with a fresh supply as soon as possible.

6. The best way to determine patients' interests is to ask for feedback. Develop a form on which patients can indicate their hobbies, interests, and favorite types of magazines. Periodically display the form in the reception area, and encourage patients to make suggestions.

readers. Depending on your time and inclination, you might change the bulletin board every week, month, or season.

Items on a reception area bulletin board should be tailored to patient interests. For example, an obstetrics/gynecology practice specializing in infertility might display recent birth announcements from its patients. The bulletin board might also feature support groups for parents trying to conceive, information on the latest medical studies of fertility drugs, and magazine clippings on parenting issues.

Other, more general items for display on any physician's bulletin board might include the following:

- Government reports on food and drugs
- Nutrition information
- Requests from the American Red Cross or the local blood bank for blood donors
- Pamphlets or flyers distributed by nonprofit health-care organizations, such as the American Heart Association
- Flyers on upcoming health fairs
- Blood pressure or other health screening notices
- Newspaper or magazine articles on interesting medical issues
- Community notices for food drives or similar charity events

The bulletin board might also feature information about staff members in the practice. Do not allow the bulletin board to become cluttered with advertising or business cards.

Finally, the bulletin board is an ideal place to display the office brochure. Put some extra copies of the brochure in an open envelope tacked to the bulletin board to encourage patients to take one home. To keep the bulletin board up to date, all time-sensitive materials, such as notices about a class or seminar, should be removed as soon as the date of the scheduled event has passed (Figure 13-6).

## Television and Videotapes

Although reading remains the primary pastime in patient reception areas, watching television and videotapes is becoming a more common activity in physicians' offices across the country. Many patient reception areas now include a television, which can be tuned to regular stations or can play preselected videos. Physicians may provide informative health-care videos of general interest to their patients or videos that meet the more specific interests of the practice.

## Items for Children

Many patient reception areas include items to occupy children while they wait. Because children—even sick ones—do not usually like to sit still for long periods, these items may include toys, games, videos, and books (Figure 13-7). If the pediatric reception area separates sick children from well children, the "well" side may include more active entertainment, such as an indoor slide or playhouse. The "sick" side may provide quieter games and activities, such as books and puzzles.

Choose toys carefully. You do not want children—even well ones—to be too active in the reception area because they might disrupt other patients and their families. Avoid balls, jump ropes, and other toys meant for outside use. Puzzles and blocks are good choices because they encourage quieter play. All toys should be easy to clean and, for safety and health reasons, should not include stuffed animals. Stuffed animals are not appropriate because they are not easily kept clean. They can be a source of infection or the small parts on them can be a choking hazard. You might informally ask parents and children if they like the play items or if they would prefer other types of toys. Procedure 13-1 explains how to set up a pediatric playroom.

**Figure 13-6.** Check the office bulletin board frequently for outdated information.

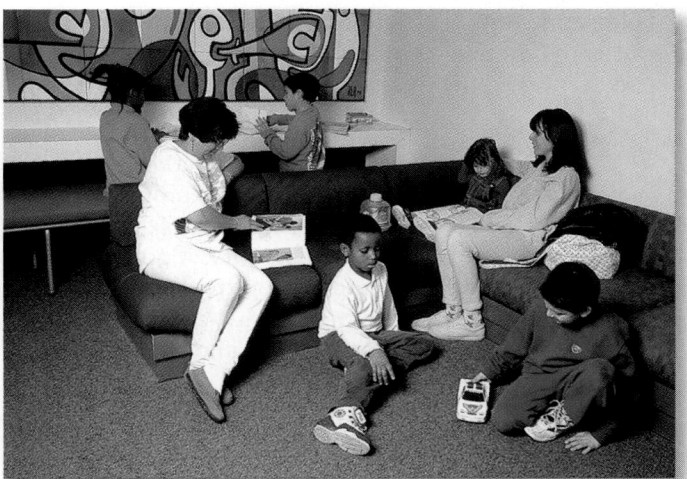

**Figure 13-7.** Toys and games that encourage quiet play are well suited to a reception area in a pediatric practice.

## PROCEDURE 13.1

## Creating a Pediatric Playroom

**Procedure Goal:** To create a play environment for children in the patient reception area of a pediatric practice

**Materials:** Children's books and magazines, games, toys, nontoxic crayons and coloring books, television and videocassette recorder (VCR), children's videotapes, child- and adult-size chairs, child-size table, bookshelf, boxes or shelves, decorative wall hangings or educational posters (optional)

**Method:**

1. Place all adult-size chairs against the wall. Position some of the child-size chairs along the wall with the adult chairs.

2. Place the remainder of the child-size chairs in small groupings throughout the room. In addition, put several chairs with the child-size table.

3. Put the books, magazines, crayons, and coloring books on the bookshelf in one corner of the room near a grouping of chairs.

4. Choose toys and games carefully. Avoid toys that encourage active play, such as balls, or toys that require a large area. Make sure that all toys meet safety guidelines. Watch for loose parts

or parts that are smaller than a golf ball. Toys should also be easy to clean.

### Rationale
Helps ensure safety in the patient reception area

5. Place the activities for older children near one grouping of chairs and the games and toys for younger children near another grouping. Keep the toys and games in a toy box or on shelves designated for them. Consider labeling or color-coding boxes and shelves and the games and toys that belong there to encourage children to return the games and toys to the appropriate storage area.

6. Place the television and VCR on a high shelf, if possible, or attach it to the wall near the ceiling. Keep children's videos behind the reception desk, and periodically change the video in the VCR.

### Rationale
Doing so helps ensure safety in the patient reception area. Videos and video equipment are easily damaged or destroyed by young patients.

7. To make the room more cheerful, decorate it with wall hangings or posters.

## Patients With Special Needs

Some patients who come into the medical office will be disabled—that is, they were born with or have acquired a condition that limits or changes their abilities. A more positive way of referring to these patients is **differently abled.** For example, people who are paralyzed from the waist down are differently abled; so are people who are visually impaired. This does not mean that these people cannot perform the same tasks that other people can. They may simply need special accommodations to do so.

## Americans With Disabilities Act

Differently abled individuals are often singled out for their differences and are sometimes discriminated against. For example, if a company building does not have access ramps for wheelchairs, workers in wheelchairs cannot qualify for jobs there. This would violate the American With Disabilities Act, which prevents discrimination based solely on a person's physical disability.

**Preventing Discrimination.** In 1990 a law was enacted to prevent certain types of discrimination. The **Americans With Disabilities Act** is a federal civil rights act forbidding discrimination on the basis of physical or mental handicap. This act maintains the rights of differently abled (disabled) people in many areas, including jobs, transportation, and access to public buildings. The act relates to medical practices (and reception areas) in that an office must be able to accommodate any patient who wants to see the physician.

**Differently Abled Patients.** Differently abled patients may have special needs. With some forethought and planning, the office can accommodate these needs. Ensuring wheelchair access through doors and hallways, as mentioned earlier, is just one way. Using ramps instead of steps, as shown in Figure 13-8, allows easier access not only for wheelchair users but also for others who have limited mobility. Allowing additional space in the reception area for wheelchairs, walkers, crutches, and guide dogs accommodates several types of differently abled

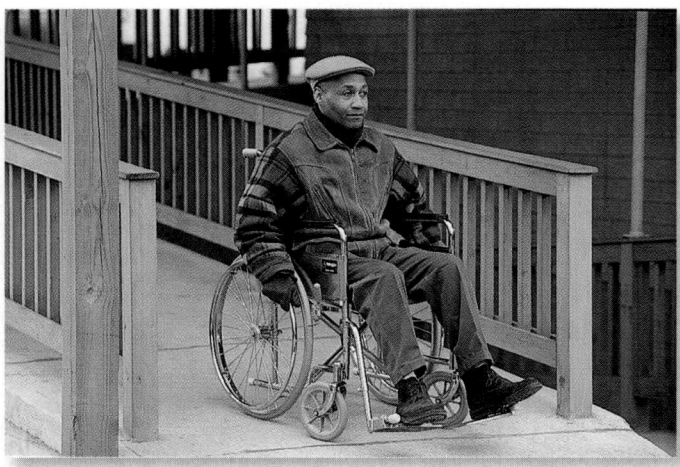

**Figure 13-8.** Ramps allow patients who use wheelchairs access to the medical office.

patients. Procedure 13-2 explains how to organize the patient reception area to meet the special needs of patients who are physically challenged.

Many offices do not make special accommodations for patients with vision or hearing impairments. Post prominent signs in the reception area with information that patients need to know. A staff member should offer to assist patients with hearing or vision impairments as needed from the reception area to the examination room when it is their turn to see the doctor.

Patients who are hearing impaired may request that a certified sign language interpreter be present to assist in communicating with the medical staff. If requested, it is required by federal law that the physician provide and pay for this interpreter.

It is also helpful, but not required by law, to provide a **teletype (TTY) device** for hearing-impaired patients. This specially designed telephone looks very much like a laptop computer with a cradle for the receiver of a traditional telephone. The receiver is placed in the cradle, and the hearing-impaired patient can then type the communication on the keyboard. The message can be received by another TTY or relayed through a specialty relay service.

Some states offer a relay service for patients with hearing impairments or those with speech disabilities. When an individual accesses this service through the TTY, the service then places the call using voice. It is important to understand that a relay service could call a medical office to make an appointment for a patient. The medical assistant needs to be careful to respond appropriately and not mistake the call as an unwanted marketing call.

## Older Americans Act of 1965

A growing proportion of the American population is elderly. Like those who are disabled, many elderly people face discrimination. One reason for the discrimination may be that with age come medical conditions and disorders that create physical limitations.

The **Older Americans Act of 1965** was passed by Congress to eliminate discrimination against the elderly. Among other benefits, the act guarantees elderly citizens the best possible health care regardless of ability to pay, an adequate retirement income, and protection against abuse, neglect, and exploitation.

What does the Older Americans Act mean for the medical office reception area? If the practice serves elderly patients, the office staff must be sensitive to their special needs. The patient reception area should be as comfortable as possible for patients with arthritis, failing eyesight, and other common ailments of the elderly. Make sure there are a few straight-backed chairs, which are easier to get into and out of than soft sofas. Arms on chairs provide support when sitting and standing for patients who are unsteady. In addition, straight-backed chairs offer greater back support than low chairs or couches with sinking cushions. These chairs should be located near the front door and near the examination rooms.

Place reading materials within easy reach of the chairs so that elderly patients do not have to get up from their chairs for them. Have large-print books and magazines available, if possible, for patients with poor eyesight. You might also offer magnifying glasses for patients who like to use them. In addition, make sure that the print on all office signs is large and easy to read. The patient reception area and restrooms should be well lit to help everyone, including elderly patients, see more clearly.

## Special Situations

Patients in a medical practice are usually a diverse group of people. Their interests, needs, and medical conditions can have an impact on the design of the reception area.

**Patients from Diverse Cultural Backgrounds.** The United States has long been called a melting pot because of its mixture of people and cultures. Each culture lends its own special qualities, and together the cultures combine to create a unique blend of people called Americans.

You may work in a neighborhood that has a distinct culture or one in which many cultures are represented. To help patients feel comfortable, make the reception area reflect aspects of their cultural backgrounds whenever possible. This effort will help patients feel more welcome.

Suppose, for example, that the medical office where you work serves many Latino patients. Posting signs in Spanish and English acknowledges the fact that both languages are spoken in that neighborhood. Providing reading materials, such as newspapers and magazines, in a second language—for both adults and children—is another way to show respect and interest. Decorating the office for Spanish holidays in addition to American ones demonstrates that you care about what is important to patients. Displaying artwork created by local artists and artisans is another idea.

# PROCEDURE 13.2

## Creating a Reception Area Accessible to Differently Abled Patients

**Procedure Goal:** To arrange elements in the reception area to accommodate patients who are differently abled

**Materials:** Ramps (if needed), doorway floor coverings, chairs, bars or rails, adjustable-height tables, magazine rack, television/VCR or DVD player, large-type and Braille magazines

**Method:**

1. Arrange chairs, leaving gaps so that substantial space is available for wheelchairs along walls and near other groups of chairs. Keep the arrangement flexible so that chairs can be removed to allow room for additional wheelchairs if needed.

### Rationale
To meet all the requirements of the Americans With Disabilities Act

2. Remove any obstacles that may interfere with the space needed for a wheelchair to swivel around completely. Also remove scatter rugs or any carpeting that is not attached to the floor. Such carpeting can cause patients to trip and create difficulties for wheelchair traffic.

### Rationale
Helps ensure safety in the patient reception area

3. Position coffee tables at a height that is accessible to people in wheelchairs.

4. Place office reading materials, such as magazines, at a height that is accessible to people in wheelchairs (for example, on tables or in racks attached midway up the wall).

5. Locate the television and VCR within full view of patients sitting on chairs and in wheelchairs so that they do not have to strain their necks to watch.

6. For patients who have a vision impairment, include reading materials with large type and in Braille.

7. For patients who have difficulty walking, make sure bars or rails are attached securely to walls 34 to 38 inches above the floor, to accommodate requirements set forth in the Americans With Disabilities Act. Make sure the bars are sturdy enough to provide balance for patients who may need it. Bars are most important in entrances and hallways, as well as in the bathroom. Consider placing a bar near the receptionist's window for added support as patients check in.

### Rationale
To meet all the requirements of the Americans With Disabilities Act

8. Eliminate sills of metal or wood along the floor in doorways. Otherwise, create a smoother travel surface for wheelchairs and pedestrians with a thin rubber covering to provide a graduated slope. Be sure that the covering is attached properly and meets safety standards.

### Rationale
Helps ensure safety in the patient reception area

9. Make sure the office has ramp access.

### Rationale
To meet all the requirements of the Americans With Disabilities Act

10. Solicit feedback from patients with physical disabilities about the accessibility of the patient reception area. Encourage ideas for improvements. Address any additional needs.

### Rationale
Doing so lets patients know that their comfort and well being are important to you.

---

**Patients Who Are Highly Contagious.** Patients may have to come into the physician's office when they are highly contagious. This fact is a concern for all patients, but it is especially critical for patients who are immunocompromised. Immunocompromised patients have an immune system—which protects against disease—that is not functioning at a normal level. Because these pa-tients do not have the normal ability to fight off disease, they are at greater risk than the average person for becoming sick. Patients undergoing chemotherapy and patients with AIDS, for example, have compromised immune systems.

To protect patients who are immunocompromised, as well as other patients and staff members, you may need to separate a highly contagious patient from them. Instead of having contagious patients wait in the reception area, for example, you might bring them directly into an examination room to wait. By screening patients for highly contagious conditions and taking precautions, you can minimize the chances of exposing other people unnecessarily.

## Summary

The patient reception area is where patients are received before they are seen by the physician. The area's appearance creates an immediate and lasting impression on patients. Patients may notice elements such as temperature, lighting, decor, and cleanliness, all of which influence their perception of the practice.

Offices with well-planned, pleasant reception areas provide a comfortable experience for waiting patients. Important elements include easy access from the outside, safety measures that meet federal requirements, and appropriate furnishings, reading material, and other entertainment to make the wait as enjoyable as possible. Special accommodations for patients who are young, elderly, differently abled, and from diverse cultural backgrounds help create a welcoming environment.

## CASE STUDY QUESTIONS

Now that you have completed this chapter, review the case study at the beginning of the chapter and answer the following questions:

1. What basic elements are *required* in every patient reception area? What other nonessential elements are nice to include as well?
2. Why is it important to think of the front patient area as the "patient reception area" and not the "waiting room"?
3. What special accommodations in the reception area are important to patients with disabilities?

## Discussion Questions

1. What is the Americans With Disabilities Act, and what impact does it have on the patient reception area and patient bathrooms?
2. What is the Older Americans Act, and what impact does it have on the patient reception area and patient bathrooms?
3. What psychological effect does a cheerful, inviting reception room have on the patient?
4. Why do you think it is important to think of disabled patients as "differently abled"?
5. Do you think it projects a negative image to place magazines in the reception area when we do not want the patients to consider the space to be a "waiting room"? Explain your answer.

## Critical Thinking Questions

1. What special difficulties might patients in wheelchairs have in a small, overcrowded reception area?
2. Who is responsible if a patient or family member or friend is hurt in the reception area or bathroom? What could be the possible consequences?
3. What would be the best design for a pediatric reception area and bathroom? Describe it.
4. What is the responsibility of the medical practice in the unlikely event of a fire?
5. Which arrangement is best for a reception area? Why?
6. Why is OSHA involved in the management of the reception area?

## Application Activities

1. Design a reception area bulletin board for a family practitioner's office. List at least six items to include, and draw a rough sketch for placing these items on a rectangular bulletin board.
2. Develop a daily checklist for closing down a patient reception area at the end of the day. Be sure to include any housekeeping chores.
3. Visit a patient reception area at a clinic or a doctor's or dentist's office. Notice the decor, furniture arrangement, specialty items, and reading materials. Note what you like and dislike about the area. Then write down suggestions for improvement. Compare your results with those of your classmates.
4. Create a design for a desirable layout for a medical practice using cutouts of cardboard that represent chairs, tables, and other elements within a patient reception area. Design the entire layout to scale. In a one-page summary, explain how your plan meets safety requirements for a physician practice.
5. Develop a one-page questionnaire for patients to determine if the reception area meets their needs. Be sure to include questions that relate to the needs of differently abled patients.

## Virtual Fieldtrip

*Visit the McGraw-Hill Higher Education Medical Assisting website at www.mhhe.com/medicalassisting3 to complete the following activity:*

- Explore the occupation of a medical receptionist and compare and contrast the duties, responsibilities, education, and pay with that of a medical assistant.
- Write a one-page summary of your research, including websites accessed, for presentation to the class. You may wish to go online and visit websites in addition to the site suggested for this exercise.

Open the CD and complete this chapter's practice activities, play the games, listen to the key terms, and test yourself with the interactive review. E-mail, print, and/or save your results to document your proficiency.

# Patient Education

## KEY TERMS

consumer education
dementia
modeling
philosophy
return demonstration
screening

## MEDICAL ASSISTING COMPETENCIES

*In preparation for the certification examination, you should know the following areas of competence:*

| COMPETENCY | CMA | RMA |
|---|---|---|
| Recognize and respond to verbal and nonverbal communications by being attentive and adapting communication to the recipient's level of understanding | X | X |
| Explain general office policies and procedures | X | X |
| Instruct individuals according to their needs | X | X |
| Provide patients with methods of health promotion and disease prevention | X | X |
| Identify community resources and information for patients and employers | X | X |
| Project a positive attitude | | X |
| Be courteous and diplomatic | | X |
| Conduct work within scope of education, training, and ability | | X |
| Be impartial and show empathy when dealing with patients | | X |
| Serve as a liaison between the physician and others | | X |
| Use appropriate medical terminology | | X |

## CHAPTER OUTLINE

- The Educated Patient
- Types of Patient Education
- Promoting Good Health Through Education
- The Patient Information Packet
- Educating Patients With Special Needs
- Patient Education Prior to Surgery
- Additional Educational Resources

## LEARNING OUTCOMES

After completing Chapter 14, you will be able to:

**14.1** Identify the benefits of patient education.

**14.2** Explain the role of the medical assistant in patient education.

**14.3** Discuss factors that affect teaching and learning.

**14.4** Describe patient education materials used in the medical office.

**14.5** Explain how patient education can be used to promote good health habits.

**14.6** Identify the types of information that should be included in the patient information packet.

**14.7** Discuss techniques for educating patients with special needs.

**14.8** Explain the benefits of patient education prior to surgery, and identify types of preoperative teaching.

**14.9** List educational resources that are available outside the medical office.

# Introduction

Health education should be a lifelong pursuit for all of us. The ultimate goal of all medical professionals is to encourage and teach healthy habits and behaviors to all patients. People first have to understand what is good for them, and then they have to make a decision to follow that advice. In patient education, the medical assistant both shares information and encourages patients to make good health decisions.

In this chapter you will learn about the medical assistant's role in patient education. You will sharpen your skills in recognizing and overcoming road blocks to education. You will become more comfortable with teaching and demonstrating procedures to others. Most importantly, you will begin to recognize the incredible responsibility of the medical assistant to correctly lead others to their highest level of health.

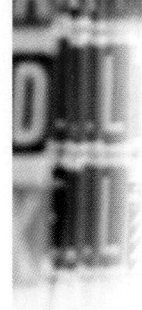

## CASE STUDY

Laura is a 26-year-old pregnant patient with hypertension (high blood pressure). She is taking blood pressure medication, but her pressure is becoming increasingly difficult to manage as she progresses with her pregnancy. The doctor has ordered a 24-hour urine collection test to help determine if Laura is in a dangerous state of preeclampsia. It is your task as medical assistant to explain to Laura the process of urine collection that she must follow. You know that she is not going to want to carry a large jug of urine to work with her and keep it on ice all day. You know that she is not likely to accurately follow the procedures of the test. But you also know it is imperative that the doctor accurately gather this test information for the health of this woman and the infant she carries.

After first reading the 24-hour urine collection procedure yourself and ensuring that you understand it thoroughly, you sit with Laura in a quiet place and explain the test and the need for accuracy. You then listen to her and evaluate her level of understanding. You listen for any cues she gives that indicate difficulties in completing the test as ordered. Thinking creatively, you suggest that Laura conduct the test on a Sunday when she can stay at home during the day and bring the specimen directly to the doctor's office early on Monday morning. You give her all the test lab items she will need, explaining each item. Additionally, you give her written instructions that she can take with her and a phone number to call with any questions she may have over the weekend. You encourage her as she leaves. By doing everything you can to ensure this patient's compliance, you contribute to the chances that both she and her baby will be strong and healthy throughout her pregnancy and delivery.

As you read this chapter, consider the following questions:
1. What might be important to consider when creating an educational plan for a patient? How might the plan vary according to the individual?
2. What factors could block effective patient education?
3. What specific behaviors do you associate with talking down to a patient?
4. Why are good listening skills an important part of teaching?

# The Educated Patient

Patient education is an essential process in the medical office. It encourages patients to take an active role in their medical care. It results in better compliance with treatment programs. When patients are suffering from illness, disease, or injury, education can often help them regain their health and independence more quickly. Simply put, patient education helps patients stay healthy. Educated patients are more likely to comply with instructions if they understand the why behind the instructions. Also, educated patients are more likely to be satisfied clients of the practice.

Patients benefit from education and the medical office benefits as well. Preoperative instruction to surgical patients, for example, lessens the chance that procedures will have to be rescheduled because surgical guidelines were not followed. Educated patients will also be less likely to call the office with questions. Thus, the office staff will have to spend less time on the telephone.

Patient education takes many forms and includes a variety of techniques. It can be as simple as answering a question that comes up during a routine visit. Patient education can involve printed materials. It can also be participatory, as with a demonstration of the procedure for changing a bandage or for giving oneself an insulin injection. No matter what type of patient education is used, the goal is the same—to help patients help themselves attain better health. Procedure 14-1 will help you create a patient education plan.

As a medical assistant, you play a vital role in the process of patient education, primarily because of your constant interaction with patients in the office. Although the initial visit is a good time to assess the need for patient education, the educational process can and should be ongoing. Continue to assess patients' needs at every visit, and be aware of situations in which you can share meaningful and helpful information.

## Types of Patient Education

Patient education can take many forms. Any instructions—verbal, written, or demonstrative—that you give to patients are a type of patient education. Most formal types of

---

## PROCEDURE 14.1

### Developing a Patient Education Plan

**Procedure Goal:** To create and implement a patient teaching plan

**Materials:** Pen, paper, various educational aids (such as instructional pamphlets and brochures), and/or visual aids (such as posters, videotapes, or DVDs)

**Method:**

1. Identify the patient's educational needs. Consider the following:
   a. The patient's current knowledge
   b. Any misconceptions the patient may have
   c. Any obstacles to learning (loss of hearing or vision, limitations of mobility, language barriers, and so on)
   d. The patient's willingness and readiness to learn (motivation)
   e. How the patient will use the information

   *Rationale*

   All instruction must begin at the patient's point of need.

2. Develop and outline a plan using the various educational aids available. Include the following areas in the outline:
   a. What you want to accomplish (your goal)
   b. How you plan to accomplish it
   c. How you will determine if the teaching was successful

   *Rationale*

   Developing an educational plan ensures that all patient needs will be addressed.

3. Write the plan. Try to make the information interesting for the patient.

4. Before carrying out the plan, share it with the physician to get approval and suggestions for improvement.

5. Perform the instruction. Be sure to use more than one teaching method. For instance, if written material is being given, be sure to explain or demonstrate the material instead of simply telling the patient to read the educational materials.

6. Document the teaching in the patient's chart.

   *Rationale*

   All patient education must be documented in the patient's medical chart for continuity of care and as a legal record.

7. Evaluate the effectiveness of your teaching session. Ask yourself:
   a. Did you cover all the topics in your plan?
   b. Was the information well received by the patient?
   c. Did the patient appear to learn?
   d. How would you rate your performance?

8. Revise your plan as necessary to make it even more effective.

   *Rationale*

   Being an effective teacher means continually evaluating the methods that you use.

patient education involve some printed information. They may also include visual materials, such as videotapes and DVDs. Patient educational materials inform patients and enable them to become involved in their own medical care.

## Printed Materials

Printed educational materials come in a variety of formats. They can be as simple as a single sheet of paper, or they can be several sheets that are folded or stapled together to form a booklet.

**Brochures, Booklets, and Fact Sheets.** Many medical offices have materials available that explain procedures performed in the medical office or give information about specific diseases and medical conditions. For example, women who have had a cesarean section delivery may be given a fact sheet describing simple exercises they can do in bed to help regain strength in the abdominal muscles. Some printed materials provide information to help patients stay healthy, such as tips for eating low-fat foods. Many educational aids are prepared by pharmaceutical companies and are provided free of charge to medical offices. Others may be written by the physician or members of the office staff. You may be asked to help prepare some of these materials.

Anytime written materials of any kind are given to a patient, it must be noted in the patient's chart. Be sure to document exactly which brochure or leaflet was distributed.

**Educational Newsletters.** A popular patient education tool is the medical office newsletter. Newsletters contain timely, practical health-care tips. Regular newsletters can also offer updates on office policies, information about new diagnostic tests or equipment, and news about the office staff. Newsletters are often written by the doctor or office staff. Some publishing companies and medical groups also offer newsletters that can be customized to a particular practice.

**Community-Assistance Directory.** Patients often require the assistance of health-related organizations within the community. For example, an elderly patient may need the services of a visiting nurse or a meals-on-wheels food program. Other patients may need the services of a day-care center, speech therapist, or weight clinic. A written community resource directory prepared by the office is a valuable aid for referring patients to appropriate agencies.

## Visual Materials

Many patients are better able to comprehend complicated medical information when it is presented in a visual format. When using visual educational materials, it is usually best to provide corresponding written materials that patients can keep for reference.

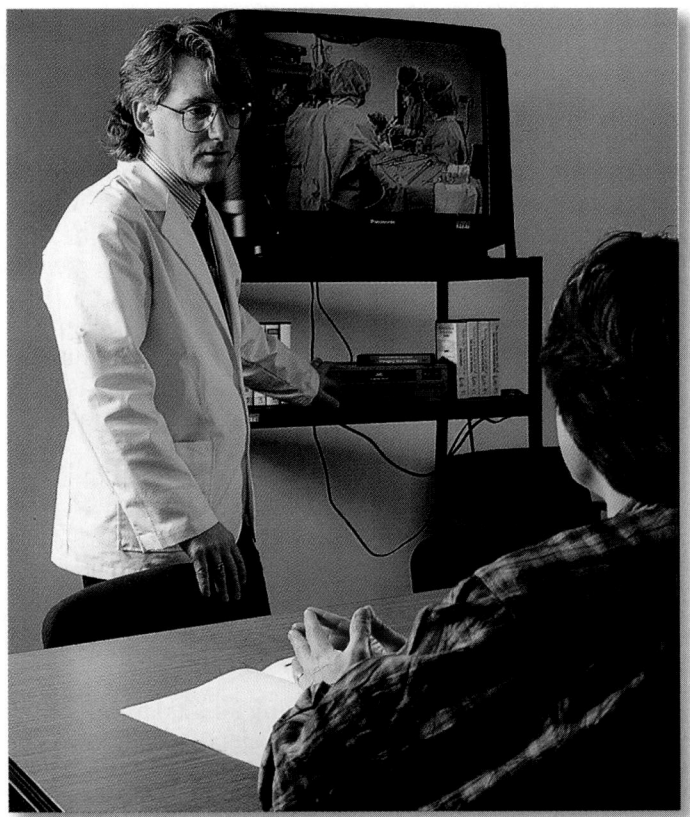

**Figure 14-1.** Videotapes and DVDs are an excellent educational aid for the medical office because of their visual format.

**Videotapes and DVDs.** Videotapes and DVDs are often used to educate patients about a variety of topics and to instruct them in self-care techniques (Figure 14-1). The use of videotapes is especially effective when teaching about complex subjects and procedures. Examples of helpful videotapes used in patient education include videos on self-breast examination, dressing change, and infant care.

**Seminars and Classes.** Many physicians conduct or arrange educational seminars or classes for their patients. For example, an obstetrician might offer classes in childbirth preparation for patients and their partners.

**Online Health Information.** There are many wonderful online health information websites. Ask the doctor which websites to recommend to patients for general consumer health information. Be sure to recommend only sites that have been visited by a member of the office medical staff.

# Promoting Good Health Through Education

One of the most important goals of patient education is to promote good health. Health is not just the absence of illness. It is a complex concept that involves the body, mind, emotions, and environment. Health involves physical, mental, emotional, spiritual, and social influences working together as a whole.

Maintaining or improving your health is the best way to protect yourself against disease and illness. **Consumer education**—education that is geared, both in content and language, toward the average person—has helped Americans become more aware of the importance of good health. As a result, many people are beginning to take greater responsibility for their own health and well-being.

There are many ways to achieve good health. You can develop healthful habits, take steps to protect yourself from injury, and take preventive measures to decrease the risk of disease or illness. Patient education in the medical office should help patients achieve these goals.

## Healthful Habits

When educating patients about good health, you can recommend several specific guidelines. Patient education can be used to promote good health habits by teaching patients the importance of

- Good nutrition, including limiting fat intake and eating an adequate amount of fruits, vegetables, and fiber
- Regular exercise

- Adequate rest (7 to 8 hours of sleep a night)
- The dangers of smoking and drug use
- The limiting of alcohol consumption
- Safe-sex practices
- The benefits of a balanced lifestyle of work and leisure activities (moderation)
- The benefits of safety practices

Whenever possible, these guidelines should be recommended to patients of all ages. Good health should be a top priority in life. Although it is best to incorporate healthful behavior before illness develops, remind patients that it is never too late to work toward improving their health. It is also important for medical assistants to act as models of good health practices for their patients.

## Protection from Injury

Many accidents happen because people fail to see potential risks and do not develop plans of action. Following safety measures at home, at work, at play, and while traveling can help prevent injury. A discussion of ways to avoid accidents and injury should be part of the educational process. Table 14-1 lists tips for preventing injury at home and at work.

## TABLE 14-1 Tips for Preventing Injury

**At Home**

- Install smoke detectors, carbon monoxide detectors, and fire extinguishers.
- Keep all medicines, chemicals, and household cleaning solutions out of reach of children. Purchase products in childproof containers. Lock or attach childproof latches to all cabinets, medicine chests, and drawers that contain poisonous items.
- Keep chemicals in their original containers, and store them out of children's reach.
- Install adequate lighting in rooms and hallways.
- Install railings on stairs.
- Use nonskid backing on rugs to help prevent falls, or remove rugs altogether.
- In the bathroom use nonskid mats or strips that stick to the tub floor.
- Stay with young children when they are in the bathroom.
- Don't rely on bath seats or rings as a safety device for babies and children.
- Set the water temperature on the water heater at 120°F.
- Practice good kitchen safety: Store knives and kitchen tools properly. Unplug small appliances when not in use. Wipe up spills immediately.
- Shorten long electrical cords and speaker wires, or secure them with electrical tape. Avoid plugging too many electrical appliances into the same outlet.

- Never use appliances in the bathtub or near a sink filled with water.
- Exercise caution when using electrical appliances. Use outlet covers when outlets are not in use.
- To reach high places, use proper equipment, such as stepladders, not chairs.
- Use child gates.
- When cooking, take care to turn all handles of pots and pans inward, toward the cooking surface, to avoid spills and burns.

**At Work**

- Use appropriate safety equipment and protective gear, as required.
- Lift heavy objects properly: Bend at the knees, not at the waist. As you straighten your legs, bring the object close to your body quickly. That way, strong leg muscles do the lifting, not weaker back muscles.
- Never attempt to move furniture on your own. Request that a member of the office building maintenance staff be engaged to do so.
- Use surge protectors on computer and other electronic equipment to prevent overloading outlets.
- Make sure hallways, entrance areas, work areas, offices, and parking lots are well lit.
- If your job involves desk work, practice proper posture when sitting. Do not sit for long periods of time. Get up and stretch, or walk down the hall and back.

Facts from the latest National Safety Council data (2003) provide information on in-home deaths of people of all ages. These facts indicate that the home is not as safe as people think. According to this data, people are most likely to die in the home in the following ways:

- Falls (33%)
- Poisoning by solids (29%)
- Fires and burns (10%)
- Suffocation by ingestion (5%)
- Drowning (3%)
- Mechanical suffocation (2%)
- Poisoning by gases or vapors (1%)
- All other (15%)

Another essential aspect of educating patients about injury prevention is teaching them about the proper use of medications. A prescription includes specific instructions for taking the medication. Emphasize to the patient that these instructions must be followed exactly. In addition, the patient must not change the dosage or mix medications of any kind without first checking with the physician. Patients who do not adhere to these rules run the risk of potentially dangerous side effects. Tell patients to report to the physician any unusual reactions experienced when taking medications.

When providing a patient with a new prescription, always ask the patient if he has told the doctor about all the medications he is already taking, including herbs, vitamins, and over-the-counter (OTC) medications. If the patient tells you that he has not, immediately inform the physician before the patient leaves the office. Medications taken together can change the desired drug response. The physician needs to know about *all* drugs as well as herbal preparations and OTC medications that the patient is taking.

## Preventive Measures

Preventive health care is an area in which patient education plays a vital role. Patients need to know that they can decrease their chances of getting certain illnesses and diseases by taking preventive measures and avoiding certain behaviors. Preventive techniques can be described on three levels: health-promoting behaviors, screening, and rehabilitation.

**Health-Promoting Behaviors.** The first level of disease and illness prevention involves adopting the health-promoting behaviors described in the section titled Healthful Habits. This primary level of prevention also includes educating patients about the symptoms and warning signs of disease. One example is informing patients about the warning signs of cancer. The first letters of these warning signs spell the word *caution.* They are as follows:

- **C**hange in bowel or bladder habits
- **A** sore that does not heal

- **U**nusual bleeding or discharge
- **T**hickening or lump in a breast or elsewhere
- **I**ndigestion or difficulty in swallowing
- **O**bvious change in a wart or mole
- **N**agging cough or hoarseness

**Screening.** The second level of disease prevention is screening. **Screening** involves the diagnostic testing of a patient who is typically free of symptoms. Screening allows early diagnosis and treatment of certain diseases. Examples of screening tests include mammography and Pap smears for women and prostate examinations for men.

Annual screening is important to health maintenance. Although the requirements may differ according to the age and condition of the patient, most annual screenings usually include:

- Routine blood work
- Urinalysis
- Chest x-ray
- EKG or ECG (electrocardiogram)
- Physical examination (PE)

**Rehabilitation.** The third level of disease prevention involves the rehabilitation and management of an existing illness. At this level the disease process remains stable, but the body will probably not heal any further. The objective is to maintain functionality and avoid further disability. Examples of this level of prevention include stroke rehabilitation programs, cardiac rehabilitation, and pain management for a condition such as arthritis.

# The Patient Information Packet

When patients come to the medical practice, they need to learn not only about health and medical issues but also about the medical office itself. The patient information packet explains the medical practice and its policies. Unlike most other patient education materials, the patient information packet deals mainly with administrative matters rather than with medical issues.

The patient information packet may be as simple as a one-page brochure or pamphlet. It may be a multi-page brochure or a folder with multiple-page inserts.

## Benefits of the Information Packet

The patient information packet is a simple, effective, and inexpensive way to improve the relationship between the office and the patients. It provides important information about the practice and the office staff. This information helps patients feel more comfortable with the qualifications of the health-care professionals involved in their care. The packet may help clarify the roles that each office staff member has in patient care.

The information packet also informs patients of office policies and procedures. Patients will learn the doctor's office hours, how to schedule appointments, the office's payment policies, and other administrative details. This information helps limit misunderstandings about these procedures.

The patient information packet also benefits the office staff. It is both an excellent marketing tool and an aid to running the office more smoothly. Providing patients with a prepared information packet saves staff time by answering a number of potential patient inquiries. The information packet is also a good way to acquaint new office staff members with office policies.

## Contents of the Information Packet

Regardless of what material the information packet contains, it must be written in clear language so that patients are able to read and understand it. All materials should be written at a sixth-grade level for reading ease of all patients. Information should not be presented in a technical medical style. Because you may be responsible for preparing portions of the policy packet, you should be familiar with the contents of a typical packet.

**Introduction to the Office.** A brief introduction serves to welcome the patient to the office. It may be helpful to summarize the office's philosophy of patient care. The office's **philosophy** means the system of values and principles the office has adopted in its everyday practices.

**Physician's Qualifications.** The packet commonly contains information about the physician's professional qualifications and training. It includes details about education, internship, and residency. It may list credentials such as board certification or board eligibility in a certain medical specialty. It may also list the physician's membership in professional societies. The information packet for a group practice may contain a paragraph or a page for each physician.

**Description of the Practice.** It is helpful to include a brief description of the practice, particularly if it is a specialty practice. Explaining the types of examinations or procedures that are commonly performed in the office may be useful. It may also be helpful to list any special services the office provides, such as physical examinations for employment, workers' compensation cases, or other occupational services. Be sure to make medical terms and specialties clear by avoiding the use of initials. Spell out everything the first time the reference is made and place the appropriate initials in parentheses.

**Introduction to the Office Staff.** Many patients are not familiar with the qualifications and duties of the various members of the office staff. It is a good idea, therefore, to identify the staff positions according to their responsibilities and duties. Patients need to understand that some duties commonly thought to be a nurse's responsibilities may also be performed by a medical assistant. It

may be helpful to include the professional credentials and licenses of key staff members.

**Office Hours.** This section should list the exact days and hours the office is open, including holidays. In addition, patients need to know what to do if an emergency occurs outside regular office hours. Tell the patient what number to call first (for example, the answering service, 911, or the hospital emergency room) and what to do next. Include the telephone number and address of the emergency room at the hospital with which the doctor is affiliated. Assure patients that the doctor or a physician partner can be reached at all times through the answering service. Some practices have multiple offices, and the physicians rotate from office to office on a regular schedule. List all office addresses and phone numbers along with directions to all office sites.

**Appointment Scheduling.** This section of the packet should explain the procedure for scheduling and canceling appointments. You might suggest that patients can benefit by scheduling routine checkups and visits as far in advance as possible. Also note if certain times of the day are reserved for sudden or unexpected office visits.

In this section encourage patients to be on time for appointments. Explain the problems that result from late or broken appointments. If the office charges a fee for breaking an appointment without advance notice, mention it here. Be careful to address these sensitive areas with a positive, nonthreatening tone. The office's written material should simply state the office policies and the problems that can result when functioning outside the policies.

**Telephone Policy.** Providing the office's telephone policies in the information packet can help reduce the number of unnecessary calls to the office and thus save time for the office staff. Explain which procedures can be handled over the telephone and which cannot. Explain procedures such as calling in for prescription renewals or laboratory test results. If the physician returns patients' calls at a certain time of day, mention that policy in this section. Some practices bill patients for telephone calls in which medical advice is given but not for follow-up calls. For example, if a parent of a child who was vomiting uncontrollably called the physician to get immediate medical advice, the call might be billed. If the physician called to inform a patient of test results, however, the call would not be billed. It is important that patients know about these policies, particularly because many insurance plans do not cover charges for medical advice given over the phone, so the patient will be responsible for these charges.

Some offices (particularly pediatric offices) schedule a certain time of the day for patients (or parents and guardians) to call the physician for answers to their questions. This type of policy benefits both the office and the patients. The patients (or parents) have the assurance that they can speak with the physician about their concerns, and the office is spared interruptions during other times of the day.

**Payment Policies.**    Inform patients of the office's policies regarding payment and billing. State whether payment is expected at the time of a visit or whether the patient can be billed. List accepted forms of payment (for example, cash, personal checks, and credit cards). It is not common practice to mention specific fees in an information packet.

**Insurance Policies.**    Advise patients to bring proof of insurance coverage and the proper claim forms (if standard claim forms are not accepted by their insurance carrier) when they visit the office. State whether the office submits claim forms directly to the insurance company or whether the patient has this responsibility. If the office or a billing service bills the insurance carrier, also include information regarding whether claims are submitted manually, using paper claims, or electronically. Outline the practice's policy for handling Medicare coverage, including whether or not the office accepts assignment on Medicare claims. If the office does not submit insurance claims directly, explain that the staff will help patients fill out insurance forms when necessary. Advise the patient of the office's policy for form completion. Include the amount of time that the patient should allow for completion and any fees that the office charges. Generally, there is no charge for the first insurance claim form; however, some offices charge for secondary insurance forms.

**Patient Confidentiality Statement.**    The information packet must include a copy of the office privacy policy. Complete information regarding the privacy policy and HIPAA regulations can be found in Chapter 3 in the section titled HIPAA Privacy Rules. It is important to remember that the first step in informing patients of HIPAA compliance is the communication of patient rights. These rights are communicated through the Notice of Privacy Practices (NPP), which must adhere to the following specifications:

- Be written in plain, simple language.
- Include a header that reads "This notice describes how medical information about you may be used and disclosed and how you can get access to this information. Please review carefully."
- Describe the medical office's uses and disclosures of personal health information.
- Describe an individual's rights under the Privacy Rule.
- Describe the medical office's duties regarding patient privacy.
- Describe how patients can register complaints concerning suspected privacy violations.
- Specify a point of contact.
- Specify an effective date.
- State that the medical office reserves to right to change its privacy practices.

The information packet must also state that no information from patient files will be released without a signed authorization from the patient. Each patient who receives a copy of the privacy notice should sign a document stating that he received the privacy notice and had the opportunity to have his questions about the notice answered. This document should remain in the patient's medical file.

**Other Information.**    The patient information packet may include the practice's policy on referrals. It may provide information about access to available community health resources or agencies. It may also include special instructions for common office procedures (for example, whether the patient needs to fast before a procedure or to avoid certain foods).

## Distributing the Information Packet

For the information packet to be effective, you must make sure that new patients receive and read it. One way is to hand the packet to new patients at the time of their first office visit and briefly review the contents with them (Figure 14-2). Explain that they can find answers to many questions in the packet. Encourage patients to take the packet home, read the information, and keep it handy for future reference.

When new patients make an appointment, many offices send them a copy of the information packet if there is enough time before the appointment to get it to them by regular mail. (It is a nice gesture to include a detailed map or written directions to the office for new patients who are not familiar with the area.) Patients can review the packet and the Consent for Treatment form before coming to the

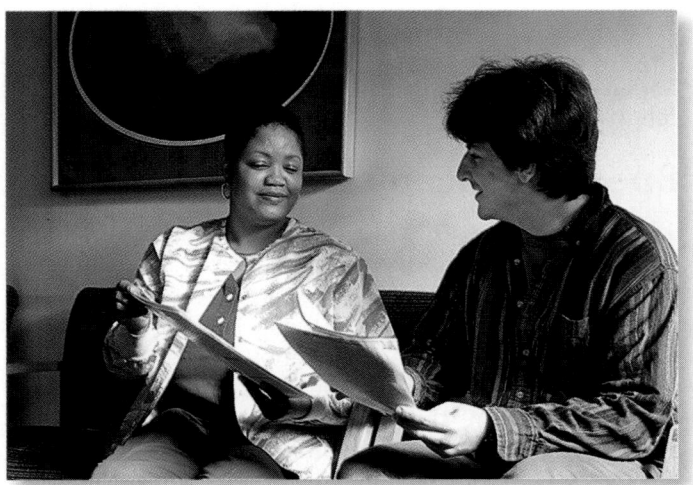

**Figure 14-2.**    Give patients the patient information packet on their first visit to the office, or mail it prior to their first appointment.

## Consent for Treatment
### Dr. Harry W. Jones Jr. and Associates

I voluntarily give my permission to the health-care providers of Dr. Harry W. Jones Jr. and such assistants and other health-care providers as they may deem necessary to provide medical services to me. I understand by signing this form, I am authorizing them to treat me for as long as I seek care from Dr. Harry W. Jones Jr., or until I withdraw my consent in writing.

_____

**Signature of Patient or Guardian**                                                       **Date**

_____

**Printed Name of Patient or Guardian**                                        **Relationship to Patient**


## Statement of Financial Responsibility/Assignment of Benefits
### Dr. Harry W. Jones Jr. and Associates

I acknowledge that I am legally responsible for all charges in connection with the medical care and treatment provided by Dr. Harry W. Jones Jr. and Associates. I assign and authorize payments to Dr. Harry W. Jones Jr. I understand my insurance carrier may not approve or reimburse my medical services in full due to usual and customary rates, benefit exclusions, coverage limits, lack of authorization, or medical necessity. I understand I am responsible for fees not paid in full, co-payments, and policy deductibles and co-insurance except where my liability is limited by contract or State or Federal law.

_____

**Signature of Patient or Guardian**                                                       **Date**

_____

**Printed Name of Patient or Guardian**                                        **Relationship to Patient**


A duplicate or faxed copy of this form is considered the same as the original document.

**Figure 14-3.** Sample patient Consent for Treatment form.

office (Figure 14-3). Additional copies of the packet should be placed in an accessible area in the office so that patients can take them home.

## Special Concerns

Some practices serve patients who cannot read well or who do not speak or understand English. It may be necessary to create a second information packet that is written in very simple terms and that presents information through pictures and charts. The information packet can also be translated into one or more languages.

It is important that patients understand the office's policies and procedures. Additional one-on-one explanations may be required. Patients should still receive the printed materials to take home, however. Family members or friends may be able to read the materials for them, reinforcing what they learned in the office.

It is important to match the learning materials to the patient's needs and to their level of understanding. When possible, consider the patient's cultural background, age, medical condition, emotional state, learning style, educational background, disabilities, religious background, and readiness to learn when providing new materials. Even if a patient understands new materials, she still has the right to refuse treatment and information. If this occurs, notify the doctor and document the event in the patient's chart.

## Educating Patients With Special Needs

During your career as a medical assistant, you will probably encounter many patients with special needs. Each patient's individual circumstances will affect your approach to patient education. In all cases try to see situations from the point of view of the patient. In many instances you can enlist the support of family or friends to aid in the educational process.

## Elderly Patients

You will probably be called on to provide care for more and more elderly patients as the number of older people continues to grow. Patient education for elderly patients is especially valuable because it can help them prevent or manage health problems and remain independent. You may need to educate some older people about the importance of taking measures to protect their health.

You may work with elderly patients who have hearing or vision problems or physical limitations that restrict their ability to perform certain tasks. Keep the following suggestions in mind when working with elderly patients.

- Treat each patient as an individual. This point is perhaps the most important to remember when dealing with elderly patients. Some older people have trouble understanding directions. Try to communicate with them at the highest level they can understand. Never talk down to patients.
- Put instructions in writing. Because some elderly patients have problems with memory, detailed written instructions are an essential aspect of patient care. Patients can refer to the instructions as necessary or can ask a relative to do so.
- Adjust procedures as needed. When demonstrating a procedure to elderly patients, keep in mind any physical limitations they may have and adjust the procedure accordingly. Make sure patients understand the instructions by asking them to perform the procedure for you.

## Patients With Mental Impairments

Patients with impaired mental functions include those with **dementia,** Alzheimer's disease, mental retardation, drug addictions, and emotional problems. These patients can be challenging to deal with because communication may be difficult. Tact and empathy are important. A key to dealing with these patients is to speak at their level of understanding. Again, you must try to meet patients' needs without talking down to them.

## Patients With Hearing Impairments

Patients with hearing impairments may have conditions ranging from mild impairment to total hearing loss. It is a common mistake to treat these patients as though they have mental impairments. Although you may have difficulty communicating with these patients, remember that their inability to hear has nothing to do with their level of intelligence. The Educating the Patient section provides techniques for educating patients who have hearing impairments.

## Patients With Visual Impairments

As with hearing impairment, the level of visual impairment can vary significantly from patient to patient. Determining the severity of a patient's condition allows you to tailor your instruction to the patient's needs.

For those with mildly impaired vision, the approach may be as simple as providing instructional materials printed in large type. In addition, you can demonstrate

## Reflecting On . . . Cultural Issues

### Respecting Patients' Cultural Beliefs

Patients come from many diverse cultures and often have different beliefs about the causes and treatments of illness. These differences may affect their treatment expectations, as well as their willingness to follow medical directions. When talking with patients, it is important to understand and respect their cultural beliefs. Patients may not be willing to accept instructions or consent to treatment based on their cultural background. Consider these simple steps when giving instructions to patients of diverse cultures:

1. Speak slowly and clearly.
2. Request a translator as needed.

3. Ask for and look for feedback from the patient, indicating that she understands and intends to follow the patient instructions.
4. Ask the patient if there is any reason that she will not be able to follow the instructions.
5. Address any concerns addressed by the patient, notifying the doctor if the concerns will mean that patient is not likely to follow instructions.
6. Provide educational resources in the patient's primary language, if available.

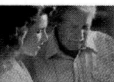

# Educating the Patient

## Instructing Patients With Hearing Impairments

Educating patients who have hearing impairments need not be difficult if you pay a little extra attention in the following areas.

- Try to eliminate all background noise. Talk in a quiet room, if possible.
- Make sure the room is well lit.
- Face the patient, and make sure the patient can see your mouth. Having the patient watch your mouth movements can help him understand what you are saying.
- Speak loudly and clearly, but do not shout. Use visual aids as necessary.
- Tell patients to let you know right away if they cannot hear you or do not catch something you have said. Even patients who do not have hearing impairments often appear to understand what a medical professional is saying rather than admit they are confused. It is a good idea to ask patients to repeat information to you to check

their understanding. Also, periodically ask if they would like you to go over any particular part of the explanation or instructions again.

Loss of hearing can cause people to withdraw and feel isolated. Being empathic and patient greatly enhances the educational process.

### Elderly Patients With Hearing Loss

Most people experience a gradual loss of hearing as they get older. In addition to the preceding suggestions, try to talk in a lower pitch whenever possible. As people get older, they often lose the ability to hear higher tones first.

### Patients Who Wear Hearing Aids

When talking to a patient who wears a hearing aid, it is best to speak at a normal level. Many hearing aids make a normal voice louder but filter out loud noises. If you raise your voice, the hearing aid may filter it out. Consequently, the patient may hear only broken speech.

---

procedures in a well-lit area and close to the patients. For more severe visual impairment, adjust the level of instruction appropriately. For example, to demonstrate how to use a particular knob on a wheelchair, you might actually place the patient's hand on the knob and discuss its function.

When speaking to someone who has a visual impairment, remember to use a normal tone of voice. A patient with a visual impairment does not necessarily also have a hearing impairment. Although you should never talk down to patients, you need to verify that they understand all verbal instructions. Have the patient repeat all instructions to you.

Giving procedural instructions may be a challenge, depending on the patient's ability to perform certain tasks. Suggest that patients ask a family member or friend to help them with procedures they have trouble doing on their own.

# Patient Education Prior to Surgery

One instance in which patient education is vital to a successful outcome is the instruction given before a patient undergoes a surgical procedure. Although exact instructions vary according to the procedure, their purpose is to prepare the patient for the procedure and to aid the patient during the recovery period. Instructions may include verbal, written, and demonstrative techniques (Figure 14-4).

## The Role of the Medical Assistant

Patients generally receive information about the need for surgery and its nature from the physician. Educating and preparing patients for surgery will probably be your responsibility, however. You may provide support and explanations to patients. You must verify that they understand any information they may have been given by other members of the health-care team. Preoperative instruction may include discussion of postoperative care issues, such as temporary dietary restrictions.

You may also be responsible for determining whether patients have all the information they need before surgery, from both an educational and a legal standpoint. All patients who are undergoing a surgical procedure must first sign an informed consent form. As stated in Chapter 9, this legal document provides specific information about the surgical procedure, including its purpose, the possible risks, and the expected outcome. The informed consent form, along with documentation of all preoperative instruction, must be put in the patient's chart.

## Benefits of Preoperative Education

Preoperative education has many benefits. It increases patients' overall satisfaction with their care. It helps reduce patient anxiety and fear, use of pain medication, complications

Revised: 2003.06.12 Non-Hospital Medical/Surgical Facility: Schedule S-04

## Patient Surgical Consent Form

Your surgeon for this procedure is: ______________________________

I hereby authorize and request the surgeon, along with any assistants he/she feels are necessary, to perform upon me the following operation(s):

______________________________________________________________

I understand that the nature and purpose of the above mentioned procedure(s) is/are to:

______________________________________________________________

______________________________________________________________

I also authorize the surgeon to do any therapeutic procedure or investigation that in his/her judgment may be advisable for my well-being.

The nature of the planned operation has been thoroughly explained to me by my surgeon and I have decided to proceed with this form of therapy over other alternative methods. The risks, benefits, and alternatives, including doing nothing, have been explained to me. I understand that the practice of medicine and surgery is not an exact science and I acknowledge that no guarantees have been made about the results of the operation or procedure planned. Furthermore, the risks and complications inherent in the operation have been explained to me and I accept these.

I further give permission to have such anesthetics administered to me as the surgeon or the anesthetist deems necessary or advisable.

Pictures may be taken of the treatment site for record purposes. I understand that these photographs/videos will be the property of the attending physician.

☐ I DO agree to allow these pictures to be used for publication or teaching purposes.

☐ I DO NOT agree to allow these pictures to be used for publication or teaching purposes.

If I agree, I understand that my name and identity will be kept confidential and protected.

I agree to keep the office of the surgeon informed of my post-operative progress and I agree to cooperate with instructions given for my post-operative care.

Patient or Legal Guardian (Signature) ______________________________

Patient or Legal Guardian (Please Print) ______________________________

Surgeon as Witness (Signature) ______________________________

Surgeon as Witness (Please Print) ______________________________

Date ________ (Year) ________ (Month) ________ (Day)

______________________________________________________________

I hereby acknowledge receiving a copy of the post-operative instructions which have been reviewed with me. I understand the advice and restrictions given and agree to abide by them. I will notify my doctor immediately if any unusual bleeding, respiratory problems, or acute pain occurs after my discharge from this surgical facility.

Patient (Signature) ____________________ Witness (Signature) ____________________

Patient (Please Print) ____________________ Witness (Please Print) ____________________

Date ________ (Year) ________ (Month) ________ (Day)

**Figure 14-4.** Sample patient Surgical Consent form.

following surgery, and recovery time. Letting the patient know what to expect during the surgery and afterward allows the patient to emotionally and educationally prepare for all aspects of the surgical procedure.

## Types of Preoperative Teaching

Three types of teaching should occur during the preoperative period: factual, sensory, and participatory. The combination of these teaching methods gives the patient an overall understanding of the surgical procedure.

**Factual.** Factual teaching informs the patient of details about the procedure. You should tell the patient what will happen during the surgery, when it will happen, and why the procedure is necessary. Factual information also includes restrictions on diet or activity that may be necessary both before and after surgery. Procedure 14-2 describes how to inform patients of guidelines for surgery.

**Sensory.** Give patients a description of the physical sensations they may have during the procedure. All five

# PROCEDURE 14.2

## Informing the Patient of Guidelines for Surgery

**Procedure Goal:** To inform a preoperative patient of the necessary guidelines to follow prior to surgery

**Materials:** Patient chart, surgical guidelines

**Method:**

1. Review the patient's chart to determine the type of surgery to be performed and then ask the patient what procedure is being performed.

### Rationale

Doing so confirms that the patient knows what surgery is being performed.

2. Tell the patient that you will be providing both verbal and written instructions that should be followed prior to surgery.

3. Inform the patient about policies regarding makeup, jewelry, contact lenses, wigs, dentures, and so on.

4. Tell the patient to leave money and valuables at home.

5. If applicable, suggest appropriate clothing for the patient to wear for postoperative ease and comfort.

6. Explain the need for someone to drive the patient home following an outpatient surgical procedure.

### Rationale

Driving after even simple surgery can be very dangerous. Surgery can be cancelled if a patient does not identify a responsible driver before surgery occurs.

7. Tell the patient the correct time to arrive in the office or at the hospital for the procedure.

8. Inform the patient of dietary restrictions. Be sure to use specific, clear instructions about what may or may not be ingested and at what time

the patient must abstain from eating or drinking. Also explain these points:

a. The reasons for the dietary restrictions

b. The possible consequences of not following the dietary restrictions.

### Rationale

Surgery can be cancelled if the patient has not followed dietary instructions.

9. Ask patients who smoke to refrain from or reduce cigarette smoking during at least the 8 hours prior to the procedure. Explain to the patient that reducing smoking improves the level of oxygen in the blood during surgery.

10. Suggest that the patient shower or bathe the morning of the procedure or the evening before.

11. Instruct the patient about medications to take or avoid before surgery.

### Rationale

Surgery can be cancelled if the patient has not followed medication instructions.

12. If necessary, clarify any information about which the patient is unclear.

13. Provide written surgical guidelines, and suggest that the patient call the office if additional questions arise.

### Rationale

Patients may not understand or remember verbal instructions. Written instructions can be taken home and reviewed again

14. Document the instruction in the patient's chart.

### Rationale

All patient education must be documented in the patient's medical chart for continuity of care and as a legal record.

senses may be involved: feeling, seeing, hearing, tasting, and smelling.

**Participatory.** Participatory teaching includes demonstrations of techniques that may be necessary or helpful during the postoperative period. Aspects of postoperative care include cleaning the wound, changing the dressing, and applying ice packs.

During this phase of teaching, you need to first describe the technique to the patient and then demonstrate it. The patient should repeat the demonstration for you. This practice is called **return demonstration.** If any aspects of the technique are unclear to the patient, you should demonstrate the technique again. The patient should be capable of performing the procedure properly. This process of teaching a new skill by having the patient observe and imitate is called **modeling.**

## Using Anatomical Models

An anatomical model is a useful tool in preoperative education. As shown in Figure 14-5, looking at a lifelike model—and being able to see the actual body structures—helps patients better understand their condition. A model also allows patients to see how the surgical procedure will help correct their problem.

It may be difficult for a patient to visualize exactly what will take place in some surgical procedures. For example, think of arthroscopy of the knee. When told that the doctor will insert a viewing instrument into the knee, patients probably have no idea of the size of this scope. As a result, they may be particularly fearful of the procedure. Using a model to show exactly what will happen can ease patients' fears.

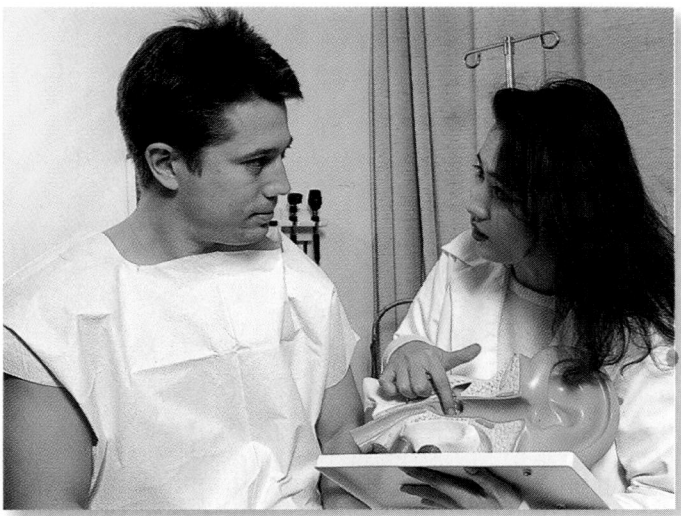

**Figure 14-5.** An anatomical model can help patients visualize what will happen during surgery.

## Helping Relieve Patient Anxiety

When you provide preoperative education, be aware that the fear and anxiety of patients who are about to undergo a surgical procedure can adversely affect the learning process. Consequently, allow extra time for repetition and reinforcement of material.

Always consider your choice of words carefully, stressing the positive rather than the negative whenever possible. Involving family members in the educational process is often beneficial, particularly if the patient is especially apprehensive about the surgery. Remember to present your instructions and explanations in straightforward language that they can understand. Family members can often help relieve the patient's anxiety.

## Verifying Patient Understanding

The key to the success of any educational process is verifying that patients have actually understood the information. A good way to check for understanding is to have patients explain in their own words what they have learned. In addition, have them engage in return demonstrations.

## Additional Educational Resources

Besides the resources available in the medical office, a vast number of outside resources are available for patient education. You can use these resources to obtain information for your own use in patient education, or you can mention them to patients who are looking for additional information. Following are several sources of patient education materials:

- Libraries and patient resource rooms. Most public libraries have an assortment of books, magazines, and electronic databases pertaining to health and medical topics. Many hospitals provide patient resource rooms, which include a variety of educational materials—such as books, brochures, and videotapes—for public use.

- Computer resources. A great deal of up-to-date medical information can be accessed through online services and CD-ROMs. The Internet is another widely used source of medical information. It will be helpful to suggest specific, reputable websites for patient research to ensure that the information obtained is valid.

- Community resources. Many local social service agencies provide specialized health information related to such topics as nursing home care, visiting nurses' care, counseling, and rehabilitation. Most of these agencies are listed in the telephone book. Area hospitals, the library, and the local chamber of commerce are other good sources for these services.

## TABLE 14-2 Patient Resource Organizations

Alzheimer's Disease Education and Referral Center
P.O. Box 8250
Silver Spring, Maryland, 20907-8250
(800) 438-4380
Fax: (301) 495–3334

American Academy of Pediatrics
141 Northwest Point Boulevard
Elk Grove Village, IL, 60007-1098
(847) 434-4000

American Cancer Society
19 West 56th Street
New York, New York 10019
(212) 586-8700

American Diabetes Association
ATTN: National Call Center
1701 North Beauregard Street
Alexandria, VA 22311
(800)-DIABETES [(800) 342-2383]

American Dietetic Association
120 South Riverside Plaza
Suite 2000
Chicago, IL 60606-6995
(800) 877-1600, ext. 4793

American Heart Association
National Center
7272 Greenville Avenue
Dallas, TX 75231
(800) 242-8721

Arthritis Foundation
P.O. Box 7669
Atlanta, GA 30357-0669
(404) 872-7100
(404) 965-7888
(800) 568-4045

Asthma and Allergy Foundation of America
1233 20th Street, NW
Suite 402
Washington, DC 20036
(800) 7ASTHMA [(800) 727-8462]

Centers for Disease Control and Prevention
Department of Health and Human Services
1600 Clifton Road
Atlanta, GA 30333
(404) 639-3311

National AIDS Hotline
995 Market Street #200
San Francisco, California 94103
(800) 342-2437
(800) 344-SIDA (Español)
(800) AIDS-TTY (hearing-impaired)

National Cancer Institute
NCI Public Inquiries Office
6116 Executive Boulevard
Room 3036A
Bethesda, MD 20892-8322
(800) 4-CANCER

National Clearinghouse for Alcohol and Drug Information
P.O. Box 2345
Rockville, MD 20847-2345
(800) 729-6686
TDD: (800) 487-4889
(877) 767-8432 (Español)

National Health Information Center
P.O. Box 1133
Washington, DC 20013-1133
(800) 336-4797
(The information specialists at this agency can provide telephone numbers for associations that deal with specific diseases or problems.)

National Kidney Foundation
30 East 33rd Street
New York, NY 10016
(800) 622-9010

National Organization for Rare Disorders
55 Kenosia Avenue
P.O. Box 1968
Danbury, CT 06813-1968
(203) 744-0100
(800) 999-6673 (voicemail only)
TDD Number: (203) 797-9590
Fax: (203) 798-2291

President's Council on Physical Fitness and Sports
Department W, 200 Independence Avenue, SW
Room 738-H
Washington, D.C. 20201-0004
(202) 690-9000
Fax: (202) 690-5211

- Associations. Thousands of health organizations and associations can be contacted for information about preventive health care and virtually every known disease or disorder. The names, addresses, telephone numbers, and websites of these organizations are provided in several directories, which are available at most libraries or online. Table 14-2 provides a sample list of patient resource organizations.

# Occupational Therapy Assistant

*To gain medical assistant credentials, you must fulfill the requirements of either the American Association of Medical Assistants (for a Certified Medical Assistant) or the American Medical Technologists (for a Registered Medical Assistant). After obtaining your medical assistant certification or registration, you may wish to acquire additional skills in specialty areas through course work or on-the-job training. Although this course work or training may not lead to an additional certification or degree, it will enable you to expand your role in the medical office and advance your career as the demand for skilled health professionals increases.*

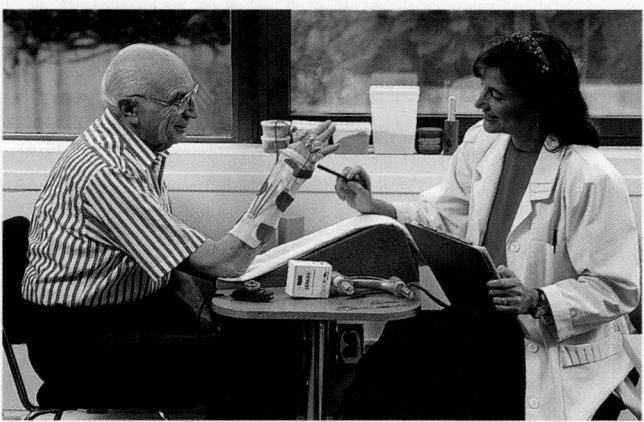

## Skills and Duties

An occupational therapy assistant helps patients learn, or relearn, basic and special skills they need to function in their daily lives. Patient interaction is the focus of the occupational therapy assistant's job. An occupational therapy assistant works under the supervision of an occupational therapist.

Occupational therapists teach many different types of skills to many different types of patients. These skills include the following:

- Basic life skills, such as dressing and feeding oneself or moving about at home. For example, patients with partial paralysis or nerve damage resulting from a stroke may need this type of help.

- Vocational skills, such as typing. These skills will help patients with disabilities get jobs to support themselves.

- Designing and supervising arts and crafts activities. These activities serve as recreation and help patients develop fine motor skills in a nonthreatening, pleasant atmosphere.

- Helping accident victims who have an injured limb or a prosthetic device learn new ways to perform simple tasks. A patient with a prosthetic hand, for example, may need help learning to open jar lids.

- Working with patients who have behavioral or emotional disturbances. Occupational therapy may help these patients express their feelings in constructive ways, by building an interest in music, drama, or art.

The occupational therapy assistant also performs a number of clerical and administrative tasks. He checks inventories, orders supplies, and helps maintain the equipment in his workplace. He may also be responsible for paperwork, including writing reports on therapy sessions with patients.

## Workplace Settings

Occupational therapy assistants often work in hospitals. They may also find work in clinics or long-term care facilities, such as retirement communities with assisted-care services, nursing homes, or rehabilitation centers. Some occupational therapists are employed in educational settings, including occupational workshops and schools for children with special needs.

## Education

Community colleges and vocational schools offer 2-year programs for an associate degree in occupational therapy assisting. By completing a program approved by the American Occupational Therapy Association and passing a qualifying test, you can become a Certified Occupational Therapy Assistant (COTA).

## Where to Go for More Information

The American Occupational Therapy Association
4720 Montgomery Lane
P.O. Box 31220
Bethesda, MD 20824-1220
(301) 652-2682
TDD: (800) 377-8555
Fax: (301) 652-7711

American Society of Hand Therapists
401 North Michigan Avenue
Chicago, IL 60611
(312) 321-6866

# Summary

Patient education plays a key role in many aspects of patient care. Knowledgeable patients are able to take an active approach to their own medical care. They are also likely to be aware of the benefits of activities that promote and protect their health.

There are many reasons for patient education in the medical office. Patients need to understand their medical conditions and to be prepared for necessary procedures. Many opportunities exist to educate patients about the benefits of good health. In addition, patients need to be informed of the policies of the medical office.

Many educational resources are available to both medical assistants and patients. The key for medical assistants is to take advantage of all opportunities to educate patients and to match this teaching to the needs of individual patients.

## CASE STUDY QUESTIONS

Now that you have completed this chapter, review the case study at the beginning of the chapter and answer the following questions:

1. What might be important to consider when creating an educational plan for a patient? How might the plan vary according to the individual?
2. What factors could block effective patient education?
3. What specific behaviors do you associate with talking down to a patient?
4. Why are good listening skills an important part of teaching?

## Discussion Questions

1. Why is it important to educate patients about how to take care of themselves?
2. Patients spend less time in the hospital than ever before. How does this change the role of private medical offices and the role of medical assistants in those practices?
3. What are some good ways to get patients to read printed materials?
4. How would you educate patients with diverse cultural backgrounds?

## Critical Thinking Questions

1. In this chapter, you have learned that patient education is an essential process in the medical office. In your own words, describe why.
2. You are measuring the vital signs of an overweight woman. She becomes visibly upset when you ask her to step on the scale. The office has many brochures with tips on promoting good health and exercise. How might you bring up the subject of proper diet and exercise?

## Application Activities

1. Practice your patient education skills by role-playing giving health-care instructions to a person who comes from a culture other than your own. Ask another student to watch and evaluate your teaching method.
2. Write the section of a patient information brochure that describes the general roles of the medical office staff. Exchange your writing sample with that of another student, and critique each other's work.
3. With a partner, role-play a medical assistant giving procedural instructions to a patient with a hearing impairment. Then switch roles, and offer suggestions for improving each other's teaching techniques.

## Virtual Fieldtrip

*Visit the McGraw-Hill Higher Education Medical Assisting website at www.mhhe.com/medicalassisting3 to complete the following activity:*

Search the Internet for ideas on patient pamphlets that might be helpful to patients with diabetes and heart disease. What samples can you provide that you have either downloaded or created yourself?

Open the CD and complete this chapter's practice activities, play the games, listen to the key terms, and test yourself with the interactive review. E-mail, print, and/or save your results to document your proficiency.

# SECTION 3

# FINANCIAL RESPONSIBILITIES

## CHAPTER 15

# Health Insurance Billing Procedures

## MEDICAL ASSISTING COMPETENCIES

*In preparation for the certification examination, you should know the following areas of competence:*

| COMPETENCY | CMA | RMA |
|---|---|---|
| **Administrative** | | |
| Use manual and computerized bookkeeping systems | | X |
| Maintain records for accounting and banking purposes | | X |
| Apply managed care policies and procedures | X | X |
| Analyze and apply third-party guidelines | X | X |
| Complete insurance claim forms | X | X |
| Use the physician fee schedule | | X |
| Identify and respond to issues of confidentiality by maintaining confidentiality at all times and following appropriate guidelines when releasing records or information | X | X |
| Be aware of and perform within legal and ethical boundaries | X | X |
| Determine the needs for documentation and reporting, and document accurately and appropriately | X | X |
| Utilize computer software and electronic technology to maintain office systems | X | X |
| Evidence a responsible attitude | | X |
| Conduct work within scope of education, training, and ability | | X |
| Use appropriate medical terminology | | X |
| Receive, organize, prioritize, and transmit information appropriately | | X |

## KEY TERMS *(Concluded)*

| | | |
|---|---|---|
| participating physicians | premium | third-party payer |
| pre-authorization | referral | TRICARE |
| pre-certification | remittance advice (RA) | X12 837 Health Care Claim |
| preferred provider organization (PPO) | resource-based relative value scale (RBRVS) | |

## KEY TERMS

allowed charge

assignment of benefits

balance billing

benefits

birthday rule

capitation

Centers for Medicare and Medicaid Services (CMS)

CHAMPVA

clearinghouse

coinsurance

coordination of benefits

copayment

deductible

disability insurance

elective procedure

electronic data interchange (EDI)

exclusion

explanation of benefits (EOB)

fee-for-service

fee schedule

formulary

health maintenance organization (HMO)

liability insurance

lifetime maximum benefit

Medicaid

Medicare

Medicare + Choice Plan

Medigap

Original Medicare Plan

# CHAPTER OUTLINE

- Basic Insurance Terminology
- Types of Health Plans
- The Claims Process: An Overview
- Fee Schedules and Charges
- Preparing and Transmitting Health-Care Claims

# LEARNING OUTCOMES

After completing Chapter 15, you will be able to:

**15.1** Define Medicare and Medicaid.

**15.2** Discuss TRICARE and CHAMPVA health-care benefits programs.

**15.3** Distinguish between HMOs and PPOs.

**15.4** Explain how to manage a workers' compensation case.

**15.5** List the basic steps of the health insurance claim process.

**15.6** Describe your role in insurance claims processing.

**15.7** Apply rules related to the coordination of benefits.

**15.8** Describe the health-care claim preparation process.

**15.9** Explain how payers set fees.

**15.10** Complete a Centers for Medicare and Medicaid Service (CMS-1500) claim form.

**15.11** Identify three ways to transmit electronic claims.

# Introduction

Health-care claims are a critical part of the reimbursement process. Accurate claims sent to payers mean that physicians receive the maximum appropriate payment for the services they provide. Patients are also concerned with their health-care plans, asking "How much will my insurance pay?" "How much will I owe?" "Why are this doctor's fees different from my previous doctor's fees?"

You will handle questions such as these every day. Not only must you correctly prepare health-care claims, but you will also review patients' insurance coverage, explain the physician's fees, estimate what charges payers will cover, and prepare claims for patients. This chapter prepares you for these tasks by explaining the types of health-care insurance patients have, how payers set the charges they pay for providers' services, and how to transmit complete and accurate claims. This chapter also gives you the information you need about patients' financial responsibilities for services so that you can figure out how much patients should pay and how much will be billed to their health-care plans.

## CASE STUDY

A patient has a $100 deductible that he has not met this year. He has 80% insurance coverage (of allowed charges) once the deductible is met. The charges for the initial visit today are $150 and the insurance carrier approves the entire amount ($150).

As you read this chapter, consider the following questions:

1. How much should this patient pay?
2. How much will he owe for his next visit this year, which is expected to have a charge of $200?
3. Assuming that the patient in the case study has a managed care policy, what type of policy does he probably have?
4. What term would you use to describe the part of the payment that is based on 20% of the charges?
5. If you did not know whether the deductible had been met, what procedure would you follow?

# Basic Insurance Terminology

The first step in understanding insurance is to learn some basic terminology. Medical insurance, which is also known as health insurance, is a written contract in the form of a policy between a policyholder and a health plan (insurance carrier). The policyholder may also be called the insured, the member, or the subscriber.

Under the insurance policy, the policyholder pays a **premium,** which is the charge for keeping the insurance policy in effect. In exchange, the health plan provides **benefits**—payments for medical services—for a specified time period. The policy may cover dependents of the policyholder, such as a spouse or children. The contract may specify a **lifetime maximum benefit,** which is a total sum that the health plan will pay out over the patient's life.

There are actually three participants under insurance contracts. The patient (policyholder) is the *first party,* and the physician who provides medical services is the *second party.* A patient-physician contract is created when a physician agrees to treat a patient who seeks medical services. Through this unwritten contract, the patient is legally responsible for paying for services. The patient may have a policy with a health plan, the *third party,* which agrees to carry the risk of paying for those services and therefore is called a **third-party payer.**

Depending on the type of health plan, the policyholder may pay a **deductible**—a fixed dollar amount that must be paid or "met" once a year, in addition to the premium, before the third-party payer begins to cover medical expenses. The patient may also have to pay **coinsurance,** a fixed percentage of covered charges after the deductible is met. The coinsurance rate presents the health plan's percentage of the charge followed by the insured's percentage, such as 80-20, which means the insurance carrier would pay 80% of allowed charges and the patient would be responsible for the remaining 20%. If the patient belongs to a managed care health plan, such as a health maintenance organization (HMO), the patient often must pay a **copayment,** a small fixed fee that is collected at the time of the visit. The health plan then pays the covered amount of the charges.

Some expenses, such as routine eye examinations or dental care, may not be covered under the insured's contract. Uncovered expenses are **exclusions.** Many plans offer a prescription drug benefit. Such benefits usually require the use of drugs that are listed on the plan's **formulary,** a list of approved brands.

An **elective procedure** describes a medical procedure that is medically necessary but is not required to sustain life and that is requested for payment to the third-party payer by the patient or the physician. Some elective procedures are paid for by third-party payers while others are not. **Pre-authorization** is authorization or approval for payment from a third-party payer requested in advance of a specific procedure. **Pre-certification** is a determination of the amount of money that will be paid by a third-party payer for a specific procedure before the procedure is performed.

Two special types of insurance are liability insurance and disability insurance. **Liability insurance** covers injuries that are caused by the insured or that occurred on the insured's property. If an individual (or company) has home, business, automobile, or health liability insurance, the injured person can claim benefits under the insured's policy. To obtain details about coverage, contact the liability insurance company.

**Disability insurance** is a type of insurance that may be provided by an employer for its employees or purchased privately by self-employed individuals. Disability insurance is activated when the insured is injured or disabled. When the insured cannot work, the insurance company pays the insured a prearranged monthly amount that covers the insured's normal expenses.

# Types of Health Plans

All insurance companies have their own rules about benefits and procedures. Many companies also have their own manuals, printed or online, which you must keep handy in the office for reference. Representatives of the insurance companies are available to work with you, however, to answer questions and help ensure that claims are correctly filed. Their business depends on it. Never hesitate to contact an insurance company. Many have toll-free numbers and websites for just this purpose.

There are many sources of health plans in the United States. The majority of individuals with insurance are covered by group policies, usually through their employers. Some people have individual plans. Many are covered under a government plan. Still others—over 40 million Americans—have no health-care insurance.

Traditionally, each insurance plan issued each of their providers an identification number, similar to the policy number given to each subscriber. Since the advent of HIPAA, individual insurers can no longer issue identifying numbers. Every physician and provider who submits a claim to any insurance carrier must obtain a specific provider number, known as a National Provider Identifier (NPI).

During the transition period, while providers obtain their NPIs, CMS is allowing previous provider numbers to be used on the CMS-1500 claim form. However, qualifiers to identify the type of provider number being used must also appear on the claim form. Table 15-1 lists the approved non-NPI numbers and the qualifiers that identify them.

## Fee-for-Service and Managed Care Plans

There are two major types of health plans: fee-for-service plans and managed care plans. **Fee-for-service** plans, the oldest and most expensive type, repay policyholders for costs of health care due to illnesses and accidents. The policy lists the medical services that are covered. The amount charged for services is controlled by the physician who provides them. The benefit may be for all or part of the charges (as with the 80/20 plans discussed previously).

## TABLE 15-1 National Uniform Claim Committee (NUCC) Non-NPI Qualifiers

These qualifiers are for use in CMS-1500 (and X12 837) if the provider does not have an NPI. These identifiers may be used in the following fields: 17a, 19, 24I, 32a, and 32b.

| Qualifier | Description |
| --- | --- |
| 0B | State License Number |
| 1B | Blue Shield Provider Number |
| 1C | Medicare Provider Number |
| 1D | Medicaid Provider Number |
| 1G | Provider UPIN Number |
| 1H | CHAMPA Identification Number |
| E1 | Employer's Identification Number |
| G2 | Provider Commercial Number |
| LU | Location Number |
| N5 | Provider Plan Network Identification Number |
| SY | Social Security Number (this may not be used for Medicare) |
| X5 | State Industrial Accident Provider Number |
| ZZ | Provider Taxonomy |

Managed care plans, in contrast, control both the financing and the delivery of health care to policyholders. They enroll policyholders, and they also enroll physicians and other providers, controlling the delivery of health care. The managed care organizations (MCOs) that set up managed care health plans reach agreements with physicians and other health-care providers that control fees. Many people who are insured through their employers are covered by some form of a managed care plan.

Physicians who enroll with managed care plans are called **participating physicians.** They have contracts with the MCOs that stipulate physician fees, the credentials they must have, and their responsibilities and that also explain the MCO's duties. For example, the MCO must usually publish the participating physicians' names in booklets and on a website so that policyholders can choose a provider from the list.

Managed care plans pay their participating physicians in one of two ways—either by contracted fees or a fixed prepayment called **capitation.** In a capitated managed care plan, providers are paid a fixed amount per month to provide necessary, contracted services to patients who are plan members. The rate the provider is paid is based on several factors, including the number of plan members in the insured pool and their ages. The capitated rate per enrollee is paid to the provider even if the provider does not provide any medical services to the patient during the time period covered by the payment. Similarly, the provider receives the same capitated rate if a patient is treated more than once during the time period. In other plans, negotiated per-service fees are paid. These fees are less than the regular rate for a service that the provider normally charges.

As shown in Figure 15-1, more than half of all health plans are **preferred provider organizations (PPO).** A PPO is a managed care plan that establishes a network of providers to perform services for plan members. In exchange for the PPO sending them patients, the physicians agree to

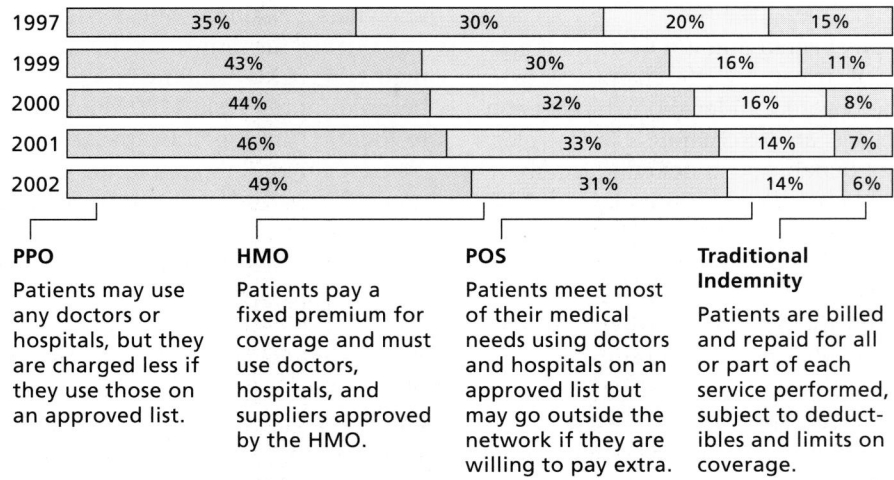

**Figure 15-1.** Types of health plans.
*Source:* Mercer's National Survey of Employer Sponsored Health Plans, 2003.
Copyright 2003, The Managed Care Information Center.

charge discounted fees. Plan members may usually choose to receive care from other doctors or providers outside the network, but they are responsible for paying a higher percentage of the charges for these visits.

Another common type of managed care system is a **health maintenance organization (HMO).** Physicians with HMO contracts are often paid a capitated rate, or they may be employees of the organization who are paid salaries. Patients who enroll in an HMO pay premiums and usually also pay a copayment, often $10 to $20, at the time of the office visit. No other fees are required for any covered service that a member needs. In HMOs, patients must usually choose from a specific group of health-care providers for care. If they seek services from a provider who is not in the health plan, the HMO does not pay for the care. Patients also pay for excluded services.

# Medicare

Several federal programs provide health care. The largest is **Medicare,** which provides health insurance for citizens aged 65 and older. Certain patients under the age of 65 may also be entitled to Medicare. Such patients include those who are blind or widowed or who have serious long-term disabilities, such as chronic joint pain or kidney failure. The Medicare program is managed by the **Centers for Medicare and Medicaid Services (CMS).**

**Part A.**    Medicare has two parts. Part A is hospital insurance, which is billed by hospitals (or other health-care facilities). It pays most of the benefits for the following individuals:

- A patient who has been hospitalized (as an inpatient) up to 90 days for each benefit period. A benefit period begins the day a patient goes into the hospital and ends when that patient has not been hospitalized for 60 days.

    The 90-day benefit period is divided into two parts. The Medicare benefit period is 60 days, after which the patient enters into a 30-day period called coinsurance days. During this 30-day period, the patient must pay an additional per-day payment. If the hospital stay extends beyond the 30 coinsurance days, the patient may use up to 60 lifetime reserve days, which also include a per-day charge.

- A patient who has been an inpatient in a skilled nursing facility (SNF) for no more than 100 days in each benefit period. A benefit period is usually 1 calendar year.

- A patient who is receiving medical care at home.

- A patient who has been diagnosed as terminally ill and needs hospice care. Medicare defines *terminally ill* as having a prognosis (prediction of the probable course of a disease in an individual and the chances of recovery) of 6 months or less to live. A hospice is a medical organization that provides pain relief and other end-of-life care to terminally ill patients and emotional support for these patients and their families.

- A patient who requires psychiatric treatment. Currently Medicare covers only 190 days of psychiatric hospitalization in a patient's lifetime.

- A patient who requires respite care. In certain circumstances, Medicare provides for a respite, or short break, for the person who cares for a terminally ill patient at home. The terminally ill patient is moved to a care facility for the respite.

Anyone who receives Social Security benefits is automatically enrolled in Part A and does not have to pay a premium. Individuals aged 65 or older who are not eligible for Social Security benefits may enroll in Part A, but they must pay premiums for the coverage.

**Part B.**    Part B helps pay for a wide range of outpatient procedures and supplies. For example, it covers physician services, outpatient hospital services, diagnostic tests, clinical laboratory services, and outpatient physical and speech therapy as long as these services are considered medically necessary. Individuals entitled to Part A benefits automatically qualify for Part B benefits. In addition, U.S. citizens and permanent residents over the age of 65 are also eligible. Part B is a voluntary program; eligible persons may or may not take part in it. However, those desiring Part B must enroll, because coverage is not automatic. The Medicare beneficiary has a six-month timeframe to apply, beginning three months prior to his 65th birthday until three months after it. If the deadline is missed, the beneficiary must wait until open enrollment, which is from January 1–March 31 of each year. Unlike Part A, Part B coverage is not premium-free. In 2006, Part B coverage cost $88.50 per month, and the premium usually increases annually.

Each Medicare enrollee receives a health insurance card. This card lists the beneficiary's name, sex, effective dates for Part A and Part B coverage, and Medicare number. The Medicare number is assigned by CMS and usually consists of the Social Security number followed by an alpha or alphanumeric suffix.

**Types of Medicare Plans.**    Medicare beneficiaries can choose from among a number of insurance plans, including traditional fee-for-service and Medicare + Choice, which consists of a group of different managed care plans.

*Fee-for-Service: The Original Medicare Plan.*    The Medicare fee-for-service plan, referred to by Medicare as the **Original Medicare Plan,** allows the beneficiary to choose any licensed physician certified by Medicare. Each time the beneficiary receives services, a fee is billable. Part of this fee is generally paid by Medicare and part is due from the beneficiary. An annual deductible of $100 is the patient's responsibility. If the patient sees a participating provider, Medicare pays 80% of approved charges directly to the provider and the patient is responsible for the remaining 20% as well as any disallowed charges. A Medicare beneficiary may choose a provider who does not participate in the Medicare program and who does not accept Medicare's allowable as payment in full (known as accepting assignment). In that case, the patient pays the provider's charges and is reimbursed by Medicare at 80% of the allowed charge. This arrangement usually results in an increased out-of-pocket expense for the patient.

To pay these bills, individuals enrolled in Medicare Part B Original Medicare Plan often buy additional insurance called a **Medigap** plan. These plans frequently reimburse the patient's Part B deductible and pick up the 20% of the Medicare allowed charge. If Medicare does not pay a claim, Medigap is not required to pay the claim either. Although private insurance carriers offer Medigap plans, coverage and standards are regulated by federal and state law. In exchange for Medigap coverage, the policyholder pays a monthly premium. A number of different options are available. These choices are labeled A through J. Monthly premiums vary widely across the different plan levels as well as within a single plan level, depending on the insurance company selected. While coverage varies from policy to policy, a set of core benefits is common to all Medigap plans, including the Part B coinsurance amount (usually 20% of approved charges) after the deductible ($100).

### *Medicare + Choice Plans.*

Medicare also offers a group of plans called the **Medicare + Choice Plans.** Beneficiaries can choose to enroll in one of three major types of plans instead of the Original Medicare Plan:

1. Medicare Managed Care Plans
2. Medicare Preferred Provider Organization Plans (PPO)
3. Medicare Private Fee-for-Service Plans

*Medicare Managed Care Plans* charge a monthly premium and a small copayment for each office visit, but not a deductible. Like private payer managed care plans, Medicare managed care plans often require patients to use a specific network of physicians, hospitals, and facilities. Some plans offer the option of receiving services from providers outside the network for a higher fee. However, they offer coverage for services not reimbursed in the Original Medicare Plan, such as physical examinations and inoculations. Participants are generally required to select a primary care provider (PCP) from within the network. The PCP provides treatment and manages the patient's medical care through **referrals.**

In the *Medicare Preferred Provider Organization Plan (PPO)*, patients pay less to use doctors within a network, but they may choose to go outside the network for additional costs, such as a higher copayment or higher coinsurance. Patients do not need a PCP, and referrals are not required.

Under a *Medicare Private Fee-for-Service Plan*, patients receive services from the provider they choose, as long as Medicare has approved the provider or facility. The plan is operated by a private insurance company that contracts with Medicare to provide services to beneficiaries. The plan sets its own rates for services, and physicians are allowed to bill patients the amount of the charge not covered by the plan. A copayment may or may not be required.

## Medicaid

**Medicaid,** also run by CMS, is a health-benefit program designed for low-income, blind, or disabled patients; needy families; foster children; and children born with birth defects. Medicaid is a health cost assistance program, not an insurance program. The federal government provides funds to all 50 states to administer Medicaid (covering specified mandated services), and states add their own funds (for optional services in addition to the federally funded services). Every state has a program to assist with medical expenses for citizens who meet its qualifications. Such programs may have different names and slightly different rules, but they provide basically the same assistance. This assistance includes:

- Physician services
- Emergency services
- Laboratory services and x-rays
- SNF care
- Early diagnostic screening and treatment for minors (those aged 21 and younger)
- Vaccines for children

**Accepting Assignment.** A physician who agrees to treat Medicaid patients also agrees to accept the established Medicaid payment for covered services. This agreement is called accepting assignment. It means that the physician will accept the amount of money that Medicaid will pay as payment in full for the Medicaid-covered service. If the physician's fee is higher than the Medicaid payment, the patient cannot be billed for the difference. The physician can bill the patient for services that Medicaid does not cover, however. It is important to note that, as a federally funded assistance program, Medicaid is known as the *payer of last resort*. This means that if a patient is covered by both a private insurance plan and Medicaid, the private plan must be billed before Medicaid. It is considered fraud to knowingly bill Medicaid if another insurance company provides medical coverage for a patient.

**Medi/Medi.** Older or disabled patients who have Medicare and who cannot pay the difference between the bill and the Medicare payment may qualify for Medicare and Medicaid. This type of coverage is known as Medi/Medi. In such cases, Medicare is the primary payer, and Medicaid is the secondary payer. The patient with Medi/Medi is never billed for a balance unless the service provided is a noncovered service, or Medicare/Medicaid states that the patient may be billed.

**State Guidelines.** Medicaid benefits can vary greatly from state to state. Eligibility for Medicaid is based on how much income the patient reported for the previous month. It is important to understand the Medicaid guidelines in your state so that your office's Medicaid reimbursement is prompt and trouble-free. Here are some suggestions:

- Do not submit a claim to Medicaid without verification of Medicaid membership and benefit eligibility.

Doing so may constitute fraud. You should always contact Medicaid to verify eligibility.

- Ensure that the physician signs all claims, unless claims are submitted electronically, in which case the physician's signature is kept on file. Then send them to the state's Medicaid-approved contractor (which pays on behalf of the state) or to the state department that administers Medicaid (for example, the state department of social services or public health). Check the regulations with the state Medicaid office if you are unsure where to send the claim.
- Unless the patient has a medical emergency, Medicaid often requires authorization before services are performed. Authorization must be obtained from the state Medicaid office in advance.
- Check the time limit on claim submissions. It can be as short as 2 months or as long as 1 year. Verify deadlines with your local Medicaid office.
- Meet the deadlines. If a Medicaid claim is submitted after the time limit, the claim may be rejected.
- Treat Medicaid patients with the same professionalism and courtesy that you extend to other patients. Simply because a patient qualifies for Medicaid assistance does not mean that the patient is in any way inferior to those with private insurance.

## TRICARE and CHAMPVA

The U.S. government provides health-care benefits to families of current military personnel, retired military personnel, and veterans through the TRICARE and CHAMPVA programs. Unless you work in a military-related facility, you will probably see TRICARE and CHAMPVA patients only for emergency services or for nonemergency care that a military base cannot provide.

**TRICARE.** Run by the Defense Department, **TRICARE** is not a health insurance plan. Rather, it is a health-care benefit for families of uniformed personnel and retirees from the uniformed services, including the Army, Navy, Marines, Air Force, Coast Guard, Public Health Service, and National Oceanic and Atmospheric Administration (Figure 15-2). TRICARE offers families three choices of health-care benefits:

1. TRICARE Prime, a health maintenance organization
2. TRICARE Extra, a managed care network of health-care providers that families can use on a case-by-case basis without a required enrollment
3. TRICARE Standard, a fee-for-service plan

Another program, TRICARE for Life, is aimed at Medicare-eligible military retirees and Medicare-eligible family members. TRICARE for Life offers the opportunity to receive health care at a military treatment facility to individuals aged 65 and older who are eligible for both Medicare and TRICARE.

In the past, individuals became ineligible for TRICARE once they reached age 65, and they were required to enroll

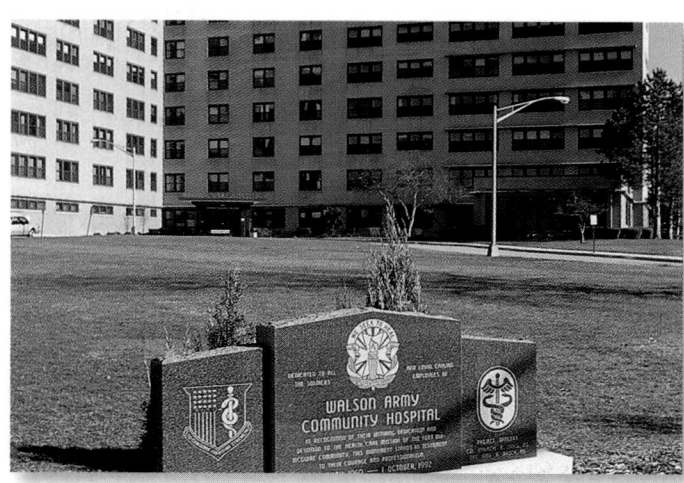

**Figure 15-2.** TRICARE covers health-care services for family members of military personnel and military retirees at facilities such as the military base hospital pictured here.

in Medicare to obtain any health-care coverage. Beneficiaries could still seek treatment at military treatment facilities, but only if space was available. Under TRICARE for Life, enrollees in TRICARE who are aged 65 and older can continue to obtain medical services at military hospitals and clinics as they did before they turned 65. TRICARE for Life acts as a secondary payer to Medicare; Medicare pays first, and the remaining out-of-pocket expenses are paid by TRICARE.

**CHAMPVA.** **CHAMPVA** (Civilian Health and Medical Program of the Veterans Administration) covers the expenses of the families (dependent spouses and children) of veterans with total, permanent, service-connected disabilities. It also covers surviving spouses and dependent children of veterans who died in the line of duty or as a result of service-connected disabilities.

**TRICARE and CHAMPVA Eligibility.** You must verify TRICARE eligibility. All TRICARE patients should have a valid identification card. To receive TRICARE benefits, eligible individuals must be enrolled in the Defense Enrollment Eligibility Reporting System (DEERS), a computer database.

Eligibility for CHAMPVA is determined by the nearest Veterans Affairs medical center. Contact this center if any questions arise. Patients can choose the doctor they wish after CHAMPVA eligibility is confirmed.

Under TRICARE and CHAMPVA, participating doctors have the option of deciding whether to accept patients on a case-by-case basis. Make sure you know the policy of the doctor or doctors in your office on this issue.

## Blue Cross and Blue Shield

Many people think that Blue Cross and Blue Shield (BCBS) is one large corporation. Rather, it is a nationwide federation of nonprofit and for-profit service organizations that provide prepaid health-care services to BCBS subscribers. Each local organization operates under its own state laws, and specific plans for BCBS can vary greatly.

## Workers' Compensation

Workers' compensation insurance covers employment-related accidents or diseases. Federal law requires employers to purchase and maintain a certain minimum amount of workers' compensation insurance for their employees. Workers' compensation laws vary from state to state. In most states, workers' compensation includes these benefits:

- Basic medical treatment.
- A weekly amount paid to the patient for a temporary disability. This amount compensates workers for loss of job income until they can return to work.
- A weekly or monthly sum paid to the patient for a permanent disability.
- Death benefits.

- Rehabilitation costs to restore an employee's ability to work again.

Not all medical practices accept workers' compensation cases. Make sure you know your office's policy. Records management of workers' compensation varies by state. If you see a patient privately and then she comes to you for a work-related illness or injury, be sure to keep the medical and financial records of the private care and the care related to the workers' compensation case separate. Because the employer and the insurer have contracted with the physician to provide care, they have the right to see any and all treatment and applicable financial records related to the workers' compensation claim without patient consent. It is up to the office to maintain the patient's confidentiality related to any care provided to her that is not related to the workers' compensation claim and keeping separate files makes it easier to do so.

Procedure 15-1 outlines the steps for verifying a patient's workers' compensation coverage.

## PROCEDURE 15.1

### Verifying Workers' Compensation Coverage

**Procedure Goal:** To verify workers' compensation coverage before accepting a patient

**Materials:** Telephone, paper, pencil

**Method:**

1. Call the patient's employer and verify that the accident or illness occurred on the employer's premises or at an employment-related work site.

2. Obtain the employer's approval to provide treatment. Be sure to write down the name and title of the person giving approval, as well as his phone number.

   *Rationale*

   Without approval, treatment costs may not be covered.

3. Ask the employer for the name of its workers' compensation insurance company. (Employers are required by law to carry such insurance. It is a good policy to notify your state labor department about any employer you encounter that does not have workers' compensation insurance, although you are not required to do so.)

   You may wish to remind the employer to report any workplace accidents or injuries that result in a workers' compensation claim to the state labor department within 24 hours of the incident.

*Rationale*

Without this form on file, the claims may not be approved.

4. Contact the insurance company and verify that the employer does indeed have a policy with the company and that the policy is in good standing.

   *Rationale*

   The insurance company will not pay for services without a valid policy.

5. Obtain a claim number for the case from the insurance company. This claim number is used on all bills and paperwork.

   *Rationale*

   All invoices must include the claim number in order for the practice to receive payment.

6. At the time the patient starts treatment, create a patient record. If the patient is already one of the practice's regular patients, create separate medical and financial records for the workers' compensation case.

   *Rationale*

   This is the legal procedure to protect the patient confidentiality with regard to private medical care. Confidentiality does not exist with regard to care related workers' compensation cases.

# The Claims Process: An Overview

From the time the patient enters a doctor's office until the time the insurer pays the practice for that office visit and associated services, several steps are carried out. In brief, the doctor's office performs the following services:

- Obtains patient information
- Delivers services to the patient and determines the diagnosis and fee (Table 15-2)
- Records charges and codes, records payment from the patient, and prepares health-care claims
- Reviews the insurer's processing of the claim, remittance advice, and payment

Most medical assistants use a medical billing program to support administrative tasks such as:

- Gathering and recording patient information
- Verifying patients' insurance coverage
- Recording procedures and services performed
- Filing insurance claims and billing patients
- Reviewing and recording payments

Billing programs streamline the important process of creating and following up on health-care claims sent to payers and bills sent to patients. For example, a large medical practice with a group of providers and thousands of patients may receive a phone call from a patient who wants to know the amount owed on an account. With a billing program, the medical assistant can key the first

## TABLE 15-2 Common Abbreviations Used in Claims Form Processing

| Abbreviations Related to Diagnosis | | Abbreviations Related to Procedures | |
|---|---|---|---|
| AHF | Acute heart failure | AKA | Above-knee amputation |
| Ca | Cancer | BKA | Below-knee amputation |
| CC | Chief complaint | Bx | Biopsy |
| CHF | Congestive heart failure | CABG | Coronary artery bypass graft |
| CO | Complains of | CT | Computed tomography |
| COPD | Chronic obstructive pulmonary disease | CXR | Chest x-ray |
| CVA | Cerebrovascular accident | D & C | Dilation and curettage |
| DJD | Degenerative joint disease | ERCP | Endoscopic retrograde cholangiopancretography |
| DVT | Deep vein thrombosis | I & D | Incision and drainage |
| Dx | Diagnosis | IF | Internal fixation |
| ESRD | End-stage renal disease | IVP | Intravenous pyelogram |
| ESRF | End-stage renal failure | MRI | Magnetic resonance imaging |
| FAS | Fetal alcohol syndrome | PE | Physical examination |
| FBD | Fibrocystic breast disease | PET | Positron emission tomography |
| FM | Fibromyalgia | PFT | Pulmonary function test |
| FUO | Fever of unknown origin | PTCA | Percutaneous transluminal coronary angioplasty |
| Fx | Fracture | T & A | Tonsillectomy and adenoidectomy |
| GI | Gastrointestinal | | |
| HA | Headache | TKA | Total knee arthroplasty |
| HPV | Human papillomavirus | Tx | Treatment |
| Hx | History | | |
| JRA | Juvenile rheumatoid arthritis | | |
| RO | Rule out | | |
| SOM | Serous otitis media | | |

few letters of the patient's last name and the patient's account data will appear on the screen. The outstanding balance can then be communicated to the patient. Billing programs are also used to exchange health information about the practice's patients with health plans. Using **electronic data interchange (EDI)**, similar to the technology behind ATMs, information is sent quickly and securely.

# Obtaining Patient Information

You will need certain information to be able to complete insurance claims and bill correctly for the patients of the medical practice where you work. This information is usually completed on a patient registration form, as shown in Chapter 9.

**Basic Facts.**   When the patient first arrives, obtain or verify the following personal information:

- Name of patient (be sure to get the correct spelling of the patient's legal name)
- Current home address
- Current home telephone number
- Date of birth (month, day, and the four digits of the year)
- Social Security number
- Next of kin or person to contact in case of an emergency

Obtain the following insurance information:

- Current employer (may be more than one)
- Employer address and telephone number
- Insurance carrier and effective date of coverage
- Insurance group plan number
- Insurance identification number
- Name of subscriber or insured

Depending on state law, obtain the following release signatures:

- Patient's signature on a form authorizing release of information to the insurance carrier
- Patient's signature on a form for assignment of benefits

**Eligibility for Services.**   After you obtain personal and insurance information and release signatures from the patient, scan or copy the patient's insurance card, front and back, to include in the patient's record. Also verify the effective date of insurance coverage because services performed before this date may be excluded from claims. To reduce possible payment problems, remind the patient before a service is performed if it might not be covered. Many offices now have a patient sign a waiver of liability form, giving the reason it is believed that a procedure will not be covered. By signing the form, the patient agrees to accept responsibility for payment should the insurer not pay for the service.

**Coordination of Benefits.**   **Coordination of benefits** clauses are legal clauses in insurance policies that prevent duplication of payment. These clauses restrict payment by insurance companies to no more than 100% of the cost of covered benefits. In many families, husband and wife are both wage earners. They and their children are frequently eligible for health insurance benefits through both employers' plans. In such cases the two insurance companies coordinate their payments to pay up to 100% of a procedure's cost. A payment of 100% includes the policyholder's deductible and copayment. The *primary,* or main, plan is the policy that pays benefits first. Then the *secondary,* or supplemental, plan pays the deductible and copayment. A policyholder's primary plan is always his employer group health plan. If both a husband and wife have insurance through their employers, the husband's plan is his primary plan and the wife's insurance plan is her primary plan. To determine which plan is the primary for dependents, in many states, the **birthday rule** is followed. It states that the insurance policy of the policyholder whose birthday comes first in the calendar year is the primary payer for all dependents.

For example, if a husband's birthday is July 14 and his wife's birthday is June 11, following the birthday rule, the wife's insurance plan is the primary payer for their children and the husband's is the secondary payer. If a husband and wife were born on the same day, the policy that has been in effect the longest is the primary payer.

The birthday rule is applied in most states in which dependents are covered by two or more medical plans. Not all states are covered by the birthday rule, so be sure to check with your state's insurance commission whenever you are in doubt. Table 15-3 describes widely used coverage guidelines.

# Delivering Services to the Patient

To ensure accuracy in claims processing, any services delivered to the patient in the office by the physician or other members of the health-care team must be entered into the patient record. Referrals to outside physicians or specialists must be entered into the record.

**Physician's Services.**   The physician who examines the patient notes the patient's symptoms in the medical record. The physician also notes a diagnosis and treatment plan (including prescribed medications) and specifies if and when the patient should return for a follow-up visit. After completing the visit with the patient, the physician writes the diagnosis, treatment, and sometimes the fee on a charge slip and instructs the patient to give you the charge slip before leaving.

**Medical Coding.**   The next step is to translate the medical terminology on the charge slip from precise descriptions of medical services into procedural and diagnostic codes on the health-care claim. This step, which is critical to the provider and to reimbursement, is the topic of Chapter 16.

## TABLE 15-3 Guidelines for Determining Primary Coverage

- If the patient has only one policy, it is primary.

- If the patient has coverage under two plans, the plan that has been in effect for the patient for the longest period of time is primary. However, if an active employee has a plan with the present employer and is still covered by a former employer's plan as a retiree or a laid-off employee, the current employer's plan is primary.

- If the patient is also covered as a dependent under another insurance policy, the patient's plan is primary.

- If an employed patient has coverage under the employer's plan and additional coverage under a government-sponsored plan, the employer's plan is primary. An example of this is a patient enrolled in a PPO through employment who is also on Medicare.

- If a retired patient is covered by the plan of the spouse's employer and the spouse is still employed, the spouse's plan is primary, even if the retired person has Medicare.

- If the patient is a dependent child covered by both parents' plans and the parents are not separated or divorced (or have joint custody of the child), the primary plan is determined by which parent has the first birth date in the calendar year (the birthday rule).

- If two or more plans cover the dependent children of separated or divorced parents who do not have joint custody of their children, the children's primary plan is determined in this order:

  1. The plan of the custodial parent
  2. The plan of the spouse of the custodial parent (if the parent has remarried)
  3. The plan of the parent without custody

**Referrals to Other Services.** You may be asked to secure authorization from the insurance company for additional procedures. If so, contact the insurance company to explain the procedures and obtain approval and an authorization number. Enter this referral number in the billing program.

Frequently you will be asked to arrange an appointment for the referred services, particularly if the physician believes they are urgently needed. For example, a physician may send a patient for a specialist's evaluation or x-ray on the same day the patient visits your office.

## Preparing the Health-Care Claim

Everyone who receives services from a doctor in the practice where you work is responsible for paying the practice for those services. When the patient brings you the charge slip from the doctor, you may perform one or more of the following procedures, depending on the policy of your practice:

- Prepare and transmit a health-care claim on behalf of the patient directly to the insurance company.
- Accept payment from the patient for the full amount. The patient will submit a claim to the insurance carrier for reimbursement.
- Accept an insurance copayment.

**Filing the Insurance Claim.** If you are going to transmit the claim directly to the payer, you will prepare

an insurance claim, often electronically. After the physician reviews the claim, you will transmit the claim to the insurance carrier for payment. The billing program will create a log of transmitted claims, or a register such as the one shown in Figure 15-3 may be maintained.

**Time Limits.** Claims must be filed in a timely manner. Time limits for filing claims vary from company to company. For example, some insurers will not pay a claim unless it is filed within 6 months of the date of service. The limits for commercial payers such as Blue Cross and Blue Shield vary from state to state.

Medicare states that for services rendered from January 1 to September 30, claims must be filed by December 31 of the following year; for services rendered from October 1 through December 31, claims must be filed no later than December 31 of the second year following the service.

Medicaid states that claims must be filed no later than 1 year from the date of service. The time frame for refiling rejected claims varies by state. In Indiana, for example, if you filed a claim for a service performed on January 2, 2008, and the claim was rejected on May 31, 2008, you would have until May 31, 2009, to refile the claim.

Although Medicare and Medicaid allow quite a long time for claims to be filed, it is poor business practice to wait so long. In the typical medical practice, claims are transmitted within a few business days after the date of service. Many large practices file claims every day or twice a week.

| Patient's Name | Insurance Company | Claim Filed | | Payment Received | | Difference (owed by patient) |
|---|---|---|---|---|---|---|
| | | Date | Amount | Date | Amount | |
| | | | | | | |
| | | | | | | |
| | | | | | | |
| | | | | | | |
| | | | | | | |
| | | | | | | |
| | | | | | | |
| | | | | | | |
| | | | | | | |
| | | | | | | |
| | | | | | | |

**Figure 15-3.** After submitting a claim to an insurer, track each claim in an insurance claim register, such as the one pictured here.

## Insurer's Processing and Payment

Your transmitted claim for payment will undergo a number of reviews by the insurer. Currently, much of the review process occurs electronically.

**Review for Medical Necessity.** The insurance carrier reviews each claim to determine whether the diagnosis and accompanying treatment are compatible and whether the treatment is medically necessary, as explained in Chapter 16.

**Review for Allowable Benefits.** The claims department also compares the fees the doctor charges with the benefits provided by the patient's health insurance policy. This review determines the amount of deductible or coinsurance the patient owes. This amount—that is, what the patient owes—is called subscriber liability.

**Payment and Remittance Advice.** After reviewing the claim, the insurer pays a benefit, either to the subscriber (patient) or to the practice, depending on what recipient the claim requested. With the payment, the insurer sends a **remittance advice (RA),** also called an **explanation of benefits (EOB).** A patient who receives the payment gets the original RA, and the practice receives a copy (and vice versa). The RA or the EOB explains the medical claim. For each service submitted to an insurer, the RA or EOB form gives the following information:

- Name of the insured and identification number
- Name of the beneficiary
- Claim number
- Date, place, and type of service (coded)
- Amount billed by the practice
- Amount allowed (according to the subscriber's policy)

- Amount of subscriber liability (coinsurance, copayment, deductible, or noncovered services)
- Amount paid and included in the current payment
- A notation of any services not covered and an explanation of why they were not covered (for example, many insurance plans do not cover a woman's annual gynecologic examination and only a certain dollar amount of well-baby visits for infants)

## Reviewing the Insurer's RA and Payment

Verify all information on the RA, line by line, using your records for each patient represented on the RA. In a large practice, you will frequently receive payment and an RA for multiple patients at one time. An example of a Medicare RA, which is called a Medicare Remittance Notice, is shown in Figure 15-4.

If all numbers on the RA agree with your records, you can make the appropriate entries in the insurance follow-up log for claims paid. In a small practice, the insurance follow-up log is used to track filed claims, using such information as patient name, date the claim was filed, services the claim reflects, notations about the results of the claim, and any balance due from the patient. Larger practices tend to track claims on computer in a file called, for example, "Unpaid Claims." If all the numbers do not agree, you will need to trace the claim with the insurance company.

When a claim is rejected, the RA states the reason. You will need to review the claim, examining all procedural and diagnosis codes for accuracy and comparing the claim with the patient's insurance information. You will probably need to contact the insurance company by telephone to find out how to resolve the claim problem.

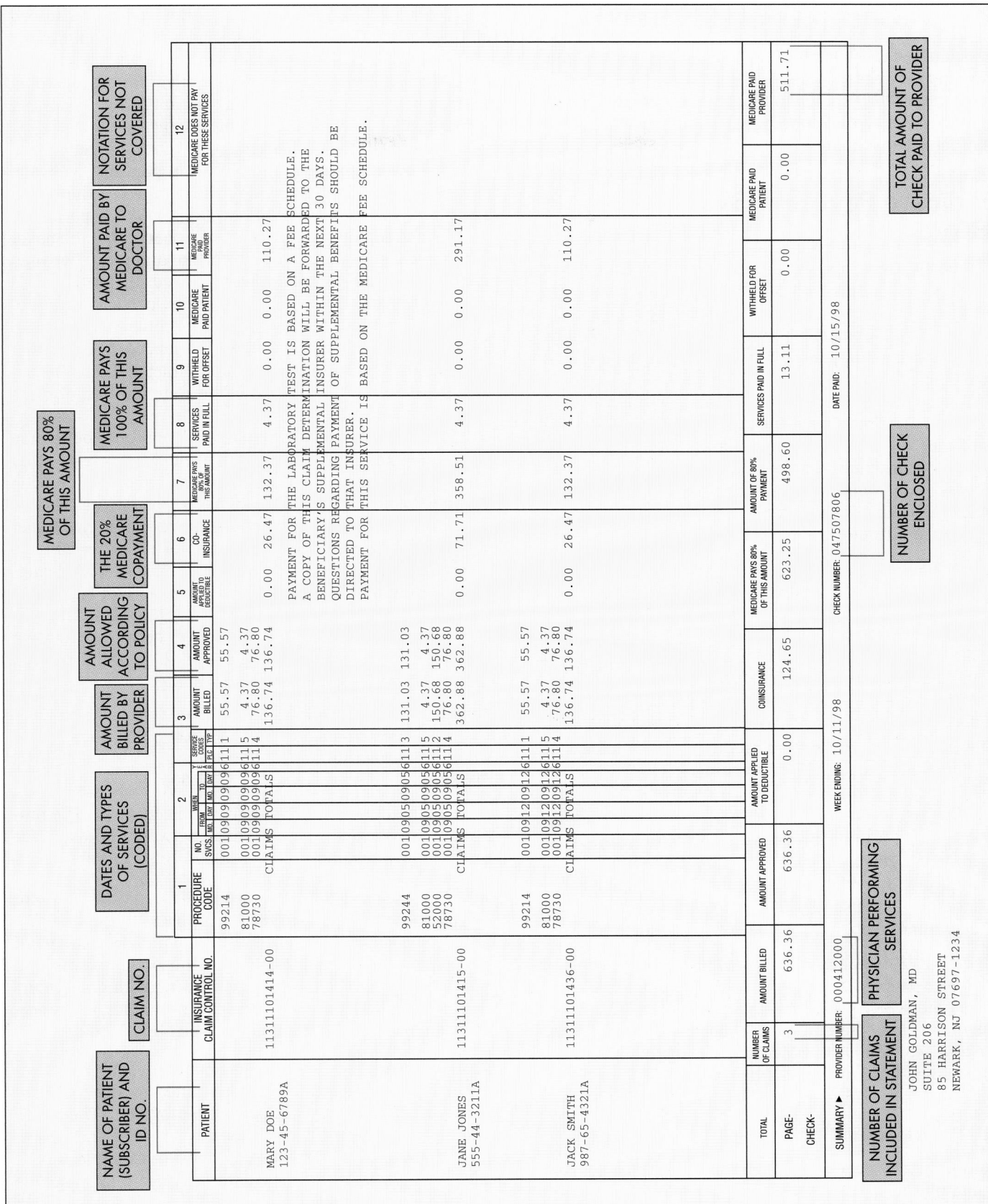

**Figure 15-4.** The insurer sends the remittance advice form to the medical practice.

# Fee Schedules and Charges

Physicians establish a list of their usual fees for the procedures and services they frequently perform. The usual fees are those that they charge to most of their patients most of the time under typical conditions. These fees are listed on the office's **fee schedule.**

## Medicare Payment System: RBRVS

Third-party payers also set the fees they are willing to pay providers, and often these fees are less than the physician's fee schedule. Most payers base their fees on the amounts that Medicare allows because the Medicare method of fee setting takes into account important factors other than only the usual fees.

The payment system used by Medicare is called the **resource-based relative value scale (RBRVS).** The RBRVS establishes the relative value units for services, replacing providers' consensus on fees (the "usual" or historical charges) with amounts based on resources (what each service really costs to provide).

There are three parts to an RBRVS fee:

1. The nationally uniform relative value unit (RVU). The relative value of a procedure is based on three cost elements: the physician's work, the practice cost (overhead), and the cost of malpractice insurance. For example, the relative value unit for a simple office visit, such as to administer a flu shot, is much lower than the relative value for a complicated encounter such as planning the treatment of uncontrolled diabetes in a patient.

2. A geographic adjustment factor (GAF). A geographic adjustment factor is used to adjust each relative value to reflect a geographical area's relative costs, such as office rents.

3. A nationally uniform conversion factor (CF). A uniform conversion factor is a dollar amount used to multiply the relative values to produce a payment amount. It is used by Medicare to make adjustments according to changes in the cost-of-living index.

When RBRVS fees are used, providers receive considerably lower payments than when usual fees are used. Each part of the RBRVS—the relative values, the geographic adjustment, and the conversion factor—is updated each year by CMS. The year's Medicare fee schedule (MFS) is published by CMS in the *Federal Register.*

## Payment Methods

Most third-party payers use one of three methods for reimbursing physicians:

1. Allowed charges
2. Contracted fee schedule
3. Capitation

**Allowed Charges.** Many payers set an **allowed charge** for each procedure or service. This amount is the most the payer will pay any provider for that work. The term *allowed charge* has many equivalent terms, including *maximum allowable fee, maximum charge, allowed amount, allowed fee,* or *allowable charge.*

The physician's usual charge is often greater than a plan's allowed charge. If the physician participates in the plan, only the allowed charge can be billed to the payer. The plan's rules govern whether the provider is permitted to bill a patient for the part of a usual charge that the payer does not cover. Billing a patient for the difference between a higher usual fee and a lower allowed charge is called **balance billing.** Under most contracts, participating providers may not bill the patient for the difference. Instead, the provider must write off the difference, meaning that the amount of the difference is subtracted from the patient's bill and never collected. The common term for this write-off is *adjustment.*

For example, Medicare-participating providers may not receive an amount greater than the Medicare-allowed charge that is based on the Medicare fee schedule. The Original Medicare Plan is responsible for paying 80% of this allowed charge (after patients have met their annual deductible). Patients are responsible for the other 20%.

Here is an example of a Medicare billing. A Medicare-participating provider reports a usual charge of $200 for a service, and the Medicare-allowed charge is $84. The provider must write off the difference between the two charges. The patient is responsible for 20% of the allowed charge, not of the provider's usual charge:

| | |
|---|---|
| Provider's usual fee: | $200.00 |
| Medicare-allowed charge: | $84.00 |
| Medicare pays 80% | $67.20 |
| Patient pays 20% | $16.80 |

The total that the provider can collect is $84. The provider must write off the difference between the usual fee and the allowed charge, or $116.00 in this example.

**Contracted Fee Schedule.** Some payers, particularly PPOs, establish fixed fee schedules with their participating physicians. The terms of the plan determine what percentage of the charges, if any, the patient owes and what percentage the payer covers. Participating providers can typically bill patients their usual charges for procedures and services that are not covered by the plan.

**Capitation.** The fixed prepayment for each plan member in capitation contracts is determined by the managed care plan that initiates contracts with providers. The plan's contract with the provider lists the services and procedures that are covered by the cap rate. For example, a typical contract with a primary care provider might include the following services:

- Preventive care, including well-child care, adult physical exams, gynecological exams, eye exams, and hearing exams

- Counseling and telephone calls
- Office visits
- Medical care, including medical care services such as therapeutic injections and immunizations, allergy immunotherapy, electrocardiograms, and pulmonary function tests
- The local treatment of first-degree burns, the application of dressings, suture removal, the excision of small skin lesions, the removal of foreign bodies or cerumen from the external ear

These services are covered in the per-member charge for each plan member who selects the PCP. Noncovered services can be billed to patients using the physician's usual rate. Plans often require the provider to notify the patient in advance that a service is not covered and to state the fee for which the patient will be responsible.

## Calculating Patient Charges

The patients of medical practices have a variety of health plans, so they have different financial responsibilities. In addition to premiums, patients may be obligated to pay deductibles, copayments, coinsurance, excluded and over-limit services, and balance billing.

All payers require patients to pay for excluded (non-covered) services. Physicians generally can charge their usual fees for these services. Likewise, in managed care plans that set limits on the annual usage (or other period) of covered services, patients are responsible for usage beyond the allowed number. For example, if one preventive physical examination is permitted annually, additional preventive examinations are paid for by the patient.

## Communications With Patients About Charges

When patients have office visits with a physician who participates in the plan under which they have coverage, such as a Medicare-participating (PAR) provider, they generally sign an **assignment of benefits** statement. When this occurs, the provider agrees to prepare health-care claims for patients, to receive payments directly from the payers, and to accept a payer's allowed charge. Patients are billed for charges that payers deny or do not pay. When patients have encounters with nonparticipating (nonPAR) providers, the procedure is usually different. To avoid the difficulty of collecting payments at a later date from a patient, practices may require that the patient either (1) assigns benefits or (2) pays in full at the time of services.

Many times patients want to know what their bills will be. For example, suppose a patient receives a bill for $100 from your practice. She calls to say that she has paid her deductible for the year, so her insurance company should have paid 80% of the bill. You call the patient's insurance company and learn that she still has to pay $100 to meet her deductible. If she pays the $100 bill in full, her deductible will then be met. You would have to explain these facts to the patient.

To estimate patients' bills, you should check with the payer to find out:

- The patient's deductible amount and whether it has been paid in full, the covered benefits, and coinsurance or other patient financial obligations
- The payer's allowed charges for the services that the provider anticipates providing

If the patient's request comes after the appointment, the encounter form can be used to tell the payer what procedures are going to be reported on the patient's claim to determine the likely payer reimbursement.

Patients should always be reminded of their financial obligations under their plans, including claim denials, according to practice procedures. The practice's financial policy regarding payment for services is usually either displayed on the wall of the reception area or included in a new patient information packet. The policy should explain what is required of the patient and when payment is due. For example, the policy may state the following:

- For unassigned claims: Payment for the physician's services is expected at the end of your appointment, unless you have made other arrangements with our practice manager.
- For assigned claims: After your insurance claim is processed by your insurance company, you will be billed for any amount you owe. You are responsible for any part of the charges that are denied or not paid by the carrier. All patient accounts are due within 30 days of the date of the invoice you receive.
- For managed care members: Copayments must be paid before patients leave the office.

It is also a good practice to notify patients in advance of the probable cost of procedures that are not going to be covered by their plan. For example, many private plans as well as Medicare do not pay for most preventive services, such as annual physical examinations. Many patients, however, consider preventive services a good idea and are willing to pay for them. Patients should be asked to agree in writing to pay for any noncovered services. A letter of agreement, also known as a waiver of liability, should also specify why the service will not be covered and the cost of the procedure. In the case of Medicare, a form called the Advance Beneficiary Notice (ABN) (Figure 15-5) is given to the patient to sign. It explains the charges that the patient is likely to have to pay.

## Preparing and Transmitting Health-Care Claims

Health-care claims are a critical communication between medical offices and payers on behalf of patients. Processing claims is a major task in most offices, and the numbers

Patient's Name: _____                    Medicare # (HICN): _____

### ADVANCE BENEFICIARY NOTICE (ABN)

NOTE: You need to make a choice about receiving these health care items or services.

We expect that Medicare will not pay for the item(s) or service(s) that are described below. Medicare does not pay for all of your health care costs. Medicare only pays for covered items and services when Medicare rules are met. The fact that Medicare may not pay for a particular item or service does not mean that you should not receive it. There may be a good reason your doctor recommended it. Right now, in your case, **Medicare probably will not pay for –**

| **Items or Services:** |
| --- |
| |
| **Because:** |
| |

The purpose of this form is to help you make an informed choice about whether or not you want to receive these items or services, knowing that you might have to pay for them yourself. Before you make a decision about your options, you should **read this entire notice carefully.**

- Ask us to explain, if you don't understand why Medicare probably won't pay.
- Ask us how much these items or services will cost you (**Estimated Cost: $_____**), in case you have to pay for them yourself or through other insurance.

PLEASE CHOOSE **ONE** OPTION.  CHECK **ONE** BOX.  **SIGN & DATE** YOUR CHOICE.

☐ **Option 1. YES.   I want to receive these items or services.**

I understand that Medicare will not decide whether to pay unless I receive these items or services. Please submit my claim to Medicare. I understand that you may bill me for items or services and that I may have to pay the bill while Medicare is making its decision. If Medicare does pay, you will refund to me any payments I made to you that are due to me. If Medicare denies payment, I agree to be personally and fully responsible for payment. That is, I will pay personally, either out of pocket or through any other insurance that I have. I understand I can appeal Medicare's decision.

☐ **Option 2. NO.   I have decided not to receive these items or services.**

I will not receive these items or services. I understand that you will not be able to submit a claim to Medicare and that I will not be able to appeal your opinion that Medicare won't pay.

_____                    _____
   **Date**                          **Signature of patient or person acting on patient's behalf**

**NOTE: Your health information will be kept confidential.** Any information that we collect about you on this form will be kept confidential in our offices. If a claim is submitted to Medicare, your health information on this form may be shared with Medicare. Your health information which Medicare sees will be kept confidential by Medicare.

OMB Approval No. 0938-0566      Form No. CMS-R-131-G    (June 2002)

**Figure 15-5.**   Advance Beneficiary Notice.
*Source:* Centers for Medicare and Medicaid Services.

can be huge. For example, a 40-physician group practice with 55,000 patients served annually typically processes 1000 claims daily!

## HIPAA Claims and Paper Claims

Two types of claims are in use: (1) the predominant HIPAA electronic claim transaction and (2) the older CMS-1500 paper form. The electronic claim transaction is the HIPAA Health-Care Claim or Equivalent Encounter Information; it is commonly referred to as the "HIPAA claim." Its official name is **X12 837 Health Care Claim.** The paper format is the "universal claim" known as the CMS-1500 claim form (formerly, the HCFA-1500).

As of October 2003, Medicare mandates the X12 837 transaction for all Medicare claims except those from very small practices. Third-party payers may continue to accept paper transactions. But practices that elect to use paper claims must have two versions of their medical billing software: one to capture the necessary data elements for HIPAA-compliant electronic Medicare claims and another version to generate CMS-1500 claims. Also, under HIPAA regulations, only medical offices that do not handle any other HIPAA-related transactions can still use paper claims. It is anticipated that eventually, for cost reasons, all payers will require electronic submissions and add this provision to their contracts with providers.

**Preparing HIPAA Claims.** The information entered on claims is called data elements. Many elements, such as the patient's personal and insurance information, are entered in the billing program before patients' appointments, based on forms patients fill out and on communications with payers. After patients' office visits, their claims are completed when the medical assistant enters the billing transactions—the services, charges, and payments—as detailed on the superbill (encounter form). The medical assistant then instructs the software to prepare claims for editing and transmission.

Follow these tips when entering data in medical billing programs:

- Enter data in all capital letters
- Do not use prefixes for people's names, such as Mr., Ms., or Dr.
- Unless required by a particular insurance carrier, do not use special characters such as hyphens, commas, or apostrophes
- Use only valid data in all fields; avoid words such as "same"

The X12 837 transaction requires many data elements, and all must be correct. Most billing programs or claim transmission programs automatically reformat data such as dates into the correct formats. These data elements are reported in five major sections:

1. Provider
2. Subscriber (the insured or policyholder)
3. Patient (who may be the subscriber or another person) and payer
4. Claim details
5. Services

Not all data elements are required. Some are considered situational and are required only when a certain condition applies. When it does apply, then that data element also becomes required. For example, if a claim involves pregnancy, the date of the last menstrual period is required. If the claim does not involve pregnancy, that date should not be reported.

Before the HIPAA mandate for standard transactions, some payers required additional records, such as their own information sheet, when providers billed them. Some payers also used their own coding systems. The HIPAA Electronic Health Care Transactions and Code Sets (TCS) mandate means that health plans are required to accept the standard claim submitted electronically.

Other standard transactions also support the claim process, such as advising the office of claim status, payment, and other key information. These transactions standards apply to the treatment, payment, and operations information that is exchanged between medical offices and health plans. Each electronic transaction has both a title and a number. Each number begins with X12, which is the number of the EDI format, followed by a unique number that stands for the transaction. Here are some examples of titles and numbers that medical assistants may encounter while processing X12 837 health-care claims:

| Number | Title |
|---|---|
| X12 276/277 | Claim status inquiry and response |
| X12 270/271 | Eligibility inquiry and response |
| X12 278 | Referral authorization inquiry and response |
| X12 835 | Payment and remittance advice |
| X12 820 | Health plan premium payments |
| X12 834 | Enrollment in and withdrawal from a health plan |

**Preparing Paper Claims.** The process for preparing paper claims is similar to the X12 837 claim. Usually, the medical billing program is updated with information about the patient's office visit. Then the program is instructed to print the data on a CMS-1500 paper form, shown in Figure 15-6. This claim may be mailed or faxed to a third-party payer.

Because of the HIPAA mandate, the paper claim is not widely in use; however, the information it contains is essentially very similar to the X12 837. For this reason, you should study Procedure 15-2, Completing the CMS-1500 Claim Form. This exercise will give you a good understanding of the data elements needed on all claims.

The CMS-1500 contains 33 form locators, which are numbered items. Form locators 1–13 refer to the patient and the patient's insurance coverage. Form locators 14–33 contain information about the provider and the transaction information, including the patient's diagnoses, procedures, and charges.

CARRIER

**NUCC**
National Uniform Claim Committee

# HEALTH INSURANCE CLAIM FORM

APPROVED BY NATIONAL UNIFORM CLAIM COMMITTEE XX/XX

☐☐ PICA | PICA ☐☐

1. MEDICARE ☐ (Medicare #)   MEDICAID ☐ (Medicaid #)   CHAMPUS ☐ (Sponsor's SSN)   CHAMPVA ☐ (VA File #)   GROUP HEALTH PLAN ☐ (SSN or ID)   FECA BLK LUNG ☐ (SSN)   OTHER ☐ (ID) | 1a. INSURED'S I.D. NUMBER   (FOR PROGRAM IN ITEM 1)

2. PATIENT'S NAME (Last Name, First Name, Middle Initial) | 3. PATIENT'S BIRTH DATE MM ┊ DD ┊ YY   SEX M ☐ F ☐ | 4. INSURED'S NAME (Last Name, First Name, Middle Initial)

5. PATIENT'S ADDRESS (No., Street) | 6. PATIENT RELATIONSHIP TO INSURED   Self ☐ Spouse ☐ Child ☐ Other ☐ | 7. INSURED'S ADDRESS (No., Street)

CITY | STATE | 8. PATIENT STATUS   Single ☐ Married ☐ Other ☐ | CITY | STATE

ZIP CODE | TELEPHONE (Include Area Code) ( ) | Employed ☐ Full-Time Student ☐ Part-Time Student ☐ | ZIP CODE | TELEPHONE (INCLUDE AREA CODE) ( )

9. OTHER INSURED'S NAME (Last Name, First Name, Middle Initial) | 10. IS PATIENT'S CONDITION RELATED TO: | 11. INSURED'S POLICY GROUP OR FECA NUMBER

a. OTHER INSURED'S POLICY OR GROUP NUMBER | a. EMPLOYMENT? (CURRENT OR PREVIOUS) ☐ YES ☐ NO | a. INSURED'S DATE OF BIRTH MM ┊ DD ┊ YY   SEX M ☐ F ☐

b. OTHER INSURED'S DATE OF BIRTH MM ┊ DD ┊ YY   SEX M ☐ F ☐ | b. AUTO ACCIDENT?   PLACE (State) ☐ YES ☐ NO | b. EMPLOYER'S NAME OR SCHOOL NAME

c. EMPLOYER'S NAME OR SCHOOL NAME | c. OTHER ACCIDENT? ☐ YES ☐ NO | c. INSURANCE PLAN NAME OR PROGRAM NAME

d. INSURANCE PLAN NAME OR PROGRAM NAME | 10d. RESERVED FOR LOCAL USE | d. IS THERE ANOTHER HEALTH BENEFIT PLAN? ☐ YES ☐ NO   *If yes*, return to and complete item 9 a-d.

**READ BACK OF FORM BEFORE COMPLETING & SIGNING THIS FORM.**

12. PATIENT'S OR AUTHORIZED PERSON'S SIGNATURE I authorize the release of any medical or other information necessary to process this claim. I also request payment of government benefits either to myself or to the party who accepts assignment below.

SIGNED _____ DATE _____

13. INSURED'S OR AUTHORIZED PERSON'S SIGNATURE I authorize payment of medical benefits to the undersigned physician or supplier for services described below.

SIGNED _____

PATIENT AND INSURED INFORMATION

14. DATE OF CURRENT: MM ┊ DD ┊ YY ◄ ILLNESS (First symptom) OR INJURY (Accident) OR PREGNANCY(LMP) | 15. IF PATIENT HAS HAD SAME OR SIMILAR ILLNESS. GIVE FIRST DATE MM ┊ DD ┊ YY | 16. DATES PATIENT UNABLE TO WORK IN CURRENT OCCUPATION FROM MM ┊ DD ┊ YY TO MM ┊ DD ┊ YY

17. NAME OF REFERRING PROVIDER OR OTHER SOURCE | 17a.   17b. NPI# | 18. HOSPITALIZATION DATES RELATED TO CURRENT SERVICES FROM MM ┊ DD ┊ YY TO MM ┊ DD ┊ YY

19. RESERVED FOR LOCAL USE | 20. OUTSIDE LAB? ☐ YES ☐ NO   $ CHARGES

21. DIAGNOSIS OR NATURE OF ILLNESS OR INJURY. (RELATE ITEMS 1,2,3 OR 4 TO ITEM 24E BY LINE)
1. ⌊___ . __   3. ⌊___ . __
2. ⌊___ . __   4. ⌊___ . __
| 22. MEDICAID RESUBMISSION CODE   ORIGINAL REF. NO.
23. PRIOR AUTHORIZATION NUMBER

24.
| A. DATE(S) OF SERVICE | | B. Place of Service | C. EMG | D. PROCEDURES, SERVICES, OR SUPPLIES (Explain Unusual Circumstances) | | E. DIAGNOSIS POINTER | F. $ CHARGES | G. DAYS OR UNITS | H. EPSDT Family Plan | I. ID. QUAL. | J. RENDERING PROVIDER ID. # |
|---|---|---|---|---|---|---|---|---|---|---|---|
| From MM DD YY | To MM DD YY | | | CPT/HCPCS | MODIFIER | | | | | | |
| 1 | | | | | | | | | | NPI # | |
| 2 | | | | | | | | | | NPI # | |
| 3 | | | | | | | | | | NPI # | |
| 4 | | | | | | | | | | NPI # | |
| 5 | | | | | | | | | | NPI # | |
| 6 | | | | | | | | | | NPI # | |

25. FEDERAL TAX I.D. NUMBER   SSN ☐ EIN ☐ | 26. PATIENT'S ACCOUNT NO. | 27. ACCEPT ASSIGNMENT? (For govt. claims, see back) ☐ YES ☐ NO | 28. TOTAL CHARGE $ | 29. AMOUNT PAID $ | 30. BALANCE DUE $

31. SIGNATURE OF PHYSICIAN OR SUPPLIER INCLUDING DEGREES OR CREDENTIALS (I certify that the statements on the reverse apply to this bill and are made a part thereof.)

SIGNED _____ DATE _____
| 32. SERVICE FACILITY LOCATION INFORMATION   a.   b. | 33. BILLING PROVIDER INFORMATION & PHONE #   a.   b.

PHYSICIAN OR SUPPLIER INFORMATION

www.nucc.org

FOLD HERE / USE ENVELOPE NO. 1500E

**Figure 15-6.** The CMS-1500 is a paper health insurance claim form.

# PROCEDURE 15.2

## Completing the CMS-1500 Claim Form

**Procedure Goal:** To complete the CMS-1500 claim form correctly

**Materials:** Patient record, CMS-1500 form, typewriter or computer, patient ledger card or charge slip

**Method:**

*Note:* The numbers below correspond to the numbered fields on the CMS-1500.

### Patient Information Section

1. Place an *X* in the appropriate insurance box.

    *Rationale*

    Check marks are not recognized by computer programs.

    1a. Enter the insured's insurance identification number as it appears on the insurance card.

    *Rationale*

    If the insurance identification number is incorrect, payment will be denied.

2. Enter the patient's name in this order: last name, first name, middle initial (if any).

3. Enter the patient's birth date using two digits each for the month and day. For example, for a patient born on February 9, 1954, enter 02-09-1954. Indicate the sex of the patient: male or female.

4. If the insured and the patient are the same person, enter SAME. If not, enter the policyholder's name. For TRICARE claims, enter the sponsor's (service person's) full name. For Medicare, leave blank.

5. Enter the patient's mailing address, city, state, and zip code.

6. Enter the patient's relationship to the insured. If they are the same, mark SELF. For TRICARE, enter the patient's relationship to the sponsor. For Medicare, leave blank.

7. Enter the insured's mailing address, city, state, zip code, and telephone number. If this address is the same as the patient's, enter SAME. For Medicare, leave blank.

8. Indicate the patient's marital, employment, and student status by placing an *X* in the boxes.

9. Enter the last name, first name, and middle initial of any other insured person whose policy might cover the patient. If the claim is for Medicare and the patient has a Medigap policy, enter the patient's name again. Keep in mind that block 9 is for secondary insurance coverage; block 11 is for the patient's primary insurance plan.

    9a. Enter the policy or group number for the other insured person. If this is a Medigap policy, enter MEDIGAP before the policy number. If Medicare, leave blank.

    9b. Enter the date of birth and sex of the other insured person (field 9).

    9c. Enter the other insured's employer or school name. (Note: If this is a Medicare claim, enter the claims-processing address for the Medigap insurer from field 9. If this is a Medicaid claim and other insurance is available, note it in field 1a and in field 2, and enter the requested policy information.

    9d. Enter the other insured's insurance plan or program name. If the plan is Medigap and CMS has assigned it a nine-digit number called PAYERID, enter that number here. On an attached sheet, give the complete mailing address for all other insurance information, and enter the word ATTACHMENT in 10d.

10. Place *X*s in the appropriate YES or NO boxes in a, b, and c to indicate whether the patient's place of employment, an auto accident, or other type of accident precipitated the patient's condition. If an auto accident is responsible, for PLACE, enter the two-letter state postal abbreviation for the location of the accident.

    For Medicaid claims, enter MCD and the Medicaid number at line 10d. For all other claims, enter ATTACHMENT here if there is other insurance information. Be sure the full names and addresses of the other insurers appear on the attached sheet. Also, code the insurer as follows: MSP Medicare Secondary Payer, MG Medigap, SP Supplemental Employer, MCD Medicaid.

    *Rationale*

    If any of these questions are answered *yes*, a workers' compensation plan, automobile insurer, or other liability insurer may be responsible for charges.

11. Enter the insured's policy or group number. For Medicare claims, fill out this section only if

*continued* ⟶

# Completing the CMS-1500 Claim Form *(continued)*

there is other insurance primary to Medicare; otherwise, enter NONE and leave fields 11a–d blank.

### Rationale

The word NONE lets Medicare know that there is no payer primary to Medicare. Without this notation, Medicare will assume another payer is primary.

**11a.** Enter the insured's date of birth and sex as in field 3, if the insured is not the patient.

**11b.** Enter the employer's name or school name here. This information will determine if Medicare is the primary payer.

**11c.** Enter the insurance plan or program name.

**11d.** Place an *X* to indicate YES or NO related to another health benefit plan. If YES, you must complete 9a through 9d. Failure to do so will cause the claim to be denied.

  *Note:* It is important to remember that section 11 is for the primary insurer and section 9 is for any secondary insurance coverage.

**12.** Have the patient or an authorized representative sign and date the form here. If a representative signs, have the representative indicate the relationship to the patient.

### Rationale

The signature indicates that the patient has given permission to release medical information to the insurance company and is required for payment. If a signature is kept on file in the office, indicate by inserting "Signature on file."

**13.** Have the insured (the patient or another individual) sign here.

### Rationale

Required for payment to be sent directly to the provider. Otherwise, payment will be sent to the patient.

## Physician Information Section

**14.** Enter the date of the current illness, injury, or pregnancy, using eight digits.

**15.** Enter date patient was first seen for illness or injury. Leave it blank for Medicare.

**16.** Enter the dates the patient is or was unable to work. This information could signal a workers' compensation claim.

**17.** Enter the name of the referring physician, clinical laboratory, or other referring source.

**17a.** If the provider does not have an NPI, enter the appropriate two-digit qualifier in the small space immediately to the right of 17a. Next to this, enter the appropriate provider identifier (refer to Table 15-1 for these qualifiers).

**17b.** If the provider has an NPI number, enter it here.

### Rationale

This number identifies the referring physician. NPI numbers are replacing all other provider identifiers.

**18.** Enter the dates the patient was hospitalized, if at all, with the current condition.

**19.** Use your payer's current instructions for this field. Some payers require you to enter the date the patient was last seen by the referring physician or other medical professional. Other payers ask for certain identifiers. If an NPI is not available, be sure to use the appropriate non-NPI qualifier to identify the identifier used.

**20.** Place an *X* in the YES box if a laboratory test was performed outside the physician's office, and enter the test price if you are billing for these tests. Ensure that field 32 carries the laboratory's exact name and address and the insurance carrier's nine-digit provider identification number (PIN). Place an *X* in the NO box if the test was done in the office of the physician who is billing the insurance company.

**21.** Enter the multidigit *International Classification of Diseases, 9th edition, Clinical Modification* (ICD-9-CM) code number diagnosis or nature of injury (see Chapter 16). Enter up to four codes in order of importance. *Note:* Some insurers are allowing up 6 or 8 diagnoses, particularly on electronic claims. Be sure to check with each carrier for its regulations.

### Rationale

The first code should relate to the primary reason the patient was seen.

*continued* ⟶

# PROCEDURE 15.2

## Completing the CMS-1500 Claim Form *(continued)*

**22.** Enter the Medicaid resubmission code and original reference number if applicable.

**23.** Enter the prior authorization number if required by the payer.

### Rationale

If prior authorization was required and not obtained, the claim will be denied.

**24.** The six service lines in block 24 are divided horizontally to accommodate NPI and other proprietary identifiers. The upper shaded area may also be used to provide supplemental information regarding services provided, but you must verify requirements for the use of this area with each payer prior to use. Otherwise, use the nonshaded areas.

**24A.** Enter the date of each service, procedure, or supply provided. Add the number of days for each, and enter them, in chronological order, in field 24G.

**24B.** Enter the two-digit place-of-service code. For example, 11 is for office, 12 is for home, and 25 is for birthing center. Your office should have a list for reference.

**24C.** EMG stands for *emergency care*. Check with provider to see if this information is needed. If it is required and emergency care was provided, enter *Y*; if it is not required or care was not on an emergency basis, leave this field blank. For Medicare, leave blank.

**24D.** Enter the CPT/HCPCS codes with modifiers for the procedures, services, or supplies provided (see Chapter 16).

**24E.** Enter the diagnosis code (or its reference number—1, 2, 3, or 4—depending on carrier regulations) that applies to that procedure, as listed in field 21.

### Rationale

Identifies the medical necessity for each procedure or service performed

**24F.** Enter the dollar amount of fee charged.

**24G.** Enter the days or units on which the service was performed. If a service took 3 days or was performed 3 times, as listed in 24A, enter 3.

**24H.** This field is Medicaid-specific for early periodic screening diagnosis and treatment programs.

**24I.** If the provider does not have an NPI, enter the appropriate qualifier, indicating the identification number being used in the shaded area. If an NPI is being used, leave this area blank.

**24J.** If a non-NPI number is being used, enter the insurance-company-assigned nine-digit physician PIN in the shaded area. If an NPI is available, use the NPI number, placing it in the nonshaded area next to the premarked NPI in field 24I.

**25.** Enter the physician's or care provider's federal tax identification number or Social Security number.

**26.** Enter the patient's account number assigned by your office, if applicable.

**27.** Place an *X* in the YES box to indicate that the physician will accept Medicare or TRICARE assignment of benefits. The check will be sent directly to the physician.

**28.** Enter the total charge for the service.

**29.** Enter the amount already paid by any primary insurance company or the patient, if it pertains to his deductible. Do not enter payments by the patient if it pertains to the coinsurance amount. For primary Medicare claims, leave blank.

### Rationale

Bill the insurance carrier for the full charge owed to the office. The physician's allowed amounts are based on this and must be consistent each time a claim is filed. If the coinsurance is deducted prior to billing the insurer, it may be assumed that the provider has decreased his charges and the payment from the insurer will be decreased.

**30.** Enter the balance due your office (subtract field 29 from field 28 to obtain this figure). For primary Medicare claims, leave blank.

**31.** Have the physician or service supplier sign and date the form here.

### Rationale

The provider is verifying that the services were provided, which is required for payment.

**32.** Enter the name and address of the organization or individual who performed the services. If performed in the patient's home, leave this field blank.

**a.** In field 32a, enter the NPI for the service facility.

*continued* ⟶

### Completing the CMS-1500 Claim Form (concluded)

b. Use field 32b if the service facility does not yet have an NPI. In this case, enter the appropriate two-digit qualifier immediately followed by the identification number being used. Do not place any spaces or punctuation between the qualifier and the identification number.

33. List the billing physician's or supplier's name, address, zip code, and phone number.

a. In field 33a, enter the NPI of the billing provider.

b. If the billing provider does not yet have an NPI, enter the non-NPI qualifier in field 33b, immediately followed by the identification number being used. Do not place any spaces or punctuation between the qualifier and the identification number.

## Transmission of Electronic Claims

Practices handle the transmission of electronic claims—which may be called electronic media claims, or EMC—in a variety of ways. Some practices transmit claims themselves; others hire outside vendors to handle this task for them.

Claims are prepared for transmission after all required data elements have been posted to the medical billing software program. The data elements that are transmitted are not seen physically, as they would be on a paper form. Instead, these elements are in a computer file.

Three major methods are used to transmit claims electronically: direct transmission to the payer, clearinghouse use, and direct data entry.

**Transmitting Claims Directly.** In the direct transmission approach, medical offices and payers exchange transactions directly. To do this, providers and payers need the necessary information systems, including a translator and communications technology, to conduct electronic data interchange (EDI).

**Using a Clearinghouse.** Many offices whose medical billing software vendors do not have translation software must use a **clearinghouse** in order to send and receive data in the correct EDI format. Clearinghouses can take in nonstandard formats and translate them into the standard format. To ensure that the standard format is compliant, the clearinghouse must receive all the required data elements from the physician. Clearinghouses are prohibited from creating or modifying data content.

Medical offices may use a clearinghouse to transmit all their claims, or they may use a combination of direct transmission and a clearinghouse. For example, they may send claims directly to Medicare, Medicaid, and a few other major commercial payers, and use a clearinghouse to send claims to other payers.

**Using Direct Data Entry.** Online direct data entry (DDE) is offered by some payers. It uses an Internet-based service into which employees key the standard data elements. Although the data elements must meet the HIPAA standards requirements regarding content, they do not have to be formatted for EDI. Instead, they are loaded directly in the health plans' computer.

## Generating Clean Claims

Although health-care claims require many data elements and are complex, often simple errors prevent you from generating "clean" claims—that is, those accepted for processing by the payer. Claims should be carefully checked before transmission or printing (Figure 15-7). Be alert for these common errors:

- Missing or incomplete service facility name, address, and identification for services rendered outside the office or home. This includes invalid ZIP codes or state abbreviations.
- Missing Medicare assignment indicator or benefits assignment indicator.
- Missing part of the name or the identifier of the referring provider.
- Missing or invalid subscriber's birth date.
- Missing information about secondary insurance plans, such as a spouse's payer.

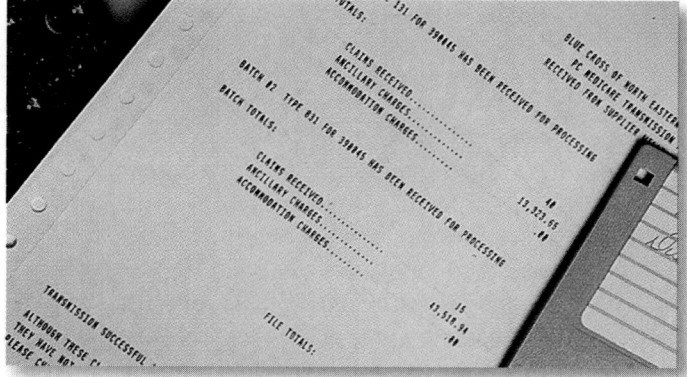

**Figure 15-7.** Print out the claims report to check for any errors that might make the payer reject a claim.

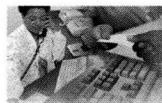

## Points on Practice

# Data Elements for HIPAA Electronic Claims

The X12 837 health-care claim has many of the same data elements as are required to correctly complete a paper claim, but some elements require understanding new terms. Here are tips for locating these types of information.

## Reporting Provider Information

The *billing provider* is the entity that is transmitting the claim to the payer. Medical offices often use a billing service or a clearinghouse to serve as the billing provider and transmit their claims. When this is done, the outside organization is the billing provider, and the practice is the *pay-to provider* that receives the payment from the insurance carrier. If an office sends claims directly to the payer, it is the billing provider and there is no additional pay-to provider to report.

Another term associated with claim preparation is *rendering provider.* It is common to have a billing provider (such as a clearinghouse), a pay-to provider (the office), and a rendering provider, the physician who, as a member of the practice, treats the patient.

## Reporting Taxonomy Information

A *taxonomy code* is a 10-digit number that stands for a physician's medical specialty. Physicians select the taxonomy code that most closely matches their education, license, or certification. The code is reported on claims because payment for some services is impacted by the particular specialty of the doctor performing them and by payers' contracts. For example, nuclear medicine is usually a higher-paid specialty than internal medicine. An internist who also has a specialty in nuclear medicine would report the nuclear medicine taxonomy code when billing for that service and use the internal medicine taxonomy code when reporting internal medicine claims. Many medical billing programs store the necessary taxonomy codes. The user selects the correct specialty, and the code is correctly selected for reporting on the claim.

## Reporting HIPAA National Identifiers

HIPAA *national identifiers* must be established for the following:

- Employers
- Health-care providers
- Health plans
- Patients

*Identifiers* are numbers of predetermined length and structure, such as a person's Social Security number. As the HIPAA rules establishing these identifiers are passed, the correct data elements must be reported on the claim. For example, the employer identifier has been adopted; it is the Employer Identification Number (EIN) issued by the Internal Revenue Service.

Until the identifiers for the three other entities are adopted, these rules are in effect:

- For health care providers, report the tax identification number or Social Security number
- For health plans, report the appropriate code; here are some common codes

| Code | Definition |
|------|------------|
| 09 | Self-pay |
| 12 | Preferred provider organization (PPO) |
| 15 | Indemnity insurance |
| BL | Blue Cross/Blue Shield |
| CH | TRICARE |
| CI | Commercial insurance company |
| HM | Health maintenance organization |
| MB | Medicare Part B |
| MC | Medicaid |
| WC | Workers' compensation health claim |

- For patients, report the policyholder's health plan identification number

---

- Missing payer name and/or payer identifier, required for both primary and secondary payers.

Many offices use a specialized software program called a "claim scrubber" to check claims before they are released and to allow errors to be fixed. Clearinghouses also apply software checks to claims they receive and transmit back reports of errors or missing information to the sender.

## Claims Security

Electronic data about patients are stored on a computer system. Most medical offices use computer networks in which personal computers are connected to a local area network (LAN), so users can exchange and share information and hardware. The LAN is linked to remote networks such as the Internet by a router that determines the best route for data to travel across the network. Packets of data traveling between the LAN and the Internet—such as electronic claims—must usually pass through a firewall, a security device that examines information (for example, e-mails) that enter and leave a network, determining whether to forward them to their destination.

The HIPAA rules set standards for protecting individually identifiable health information when it is maintained or transmitted electronically. Medical offices must protect the confidentiality, integrity, and availability of this information. A number of security measures are used:

- Access control, passwords, and log files to keep intruders out
- Backups (saved copies of files) to replace items after damage to the computer
- Security policies to handle violations that do occur

Medical assistants participate in the protection of patients' health information. One way is to select a good password for your computer. Never give out your password, nor allow anyone to use a computer terminal where you are logged in. Before you walk away from a computer, be sure you log out. Doing so will require that anyone else needing to use the computer logs in, using her or his own password. Here are tips for selecting a good password:

- Always use a combination of letters and numbers that are not real words and also not an obvious number string such as 123456 or a birth date.

- Do not use a user ID (log-on or sign-on) as a password.
- Even if it has both numbers and letters, it is not secret.
- Select a mixture of both uppercase and lowercase letters if the system can distinguish between them, and, if possible, include special characters such as @, $, or &.
- Use a minimum of six or seven alphanumeric characters. The optimal minimum number varies by system, but most security experts recommend a length of at least six or seven characters.
- Change passwords periodically, but not too often.

Forcing frequent changes can actually make security worse because users are more likely to keep passwords written down.

## Summary

Part of your responsibilities as a medical assistant will be to make sure that health-care claims are processed accurately. When accurate claims are sent to payers, physicians receive the maximum appropriate payment for the services they provide.

As a medical assistant, you will handle patients' questions about their health-care plans and claims. You will review patients' insurance coverage, explain the physician's fees, estimate what charges payers will cover, estimate how much patients should pay, and prepare complete and accurate health-care claims for patients.

## CASE STUDY *QUESTIONS*

Now that you have completed this chapter, review the case study at the beginning of the chapter and answer the following questions:

1. How much should this patient pay?
2. How much will he owe for his next visit this year, which is expected to have a charge of $200?
3. Assuming that the patient in the case study has a managed care policy, what type of policy does he probably have?
4. What term would you use to describe the part of the payment that is based on 20% of the charges?
5. If you did not know whether the deductible had been met, what procedure would you follow?

## Discussion Questions

1. How do HMOs and PPOs compare?
2. How would you explain the purpose of the assignment of benefits form to a patient?
3. Why do insurers coordinate benefits?
4. How would you explain to a patient what an allowable charge is?

## Critical Thinking Questions

1. How is the increasing cost of medical procedures affecting the insurance industry?
2. Why is it important to remind patients of their financial obligations?
3. What are the advantages of electronic claims?

## Application Activities

1. Apply the birthday rule in this situation: Both parents of the patient have health-care coverage through their employers. The father's birthday is December 5 and the mother's is June 4. Which plan is primary for the child?
2. A patient's insurance policy states: Annual deductible: $300; Coinsurance: 70-30. This year, the patient has made payments totaling $533 to all providers. Today, the patient has an office visit (fee: $80). The patient presents a credit card for payment of today's bill. What is the amount that the patient should pay?
3. A patient is a member of an HMO with a capitation plan and a $10 copayment. The usual charges for the day's services would be $480. What does the patient pay?
4. You need to calculate how much a patient needs to pay. He is a member of a preferred provider organization (PPO) that has a contract that allows all members a 25% discount. The patient's total bill for services rendered today is $300.00. The patient has a copayment of 20%. The patient states that he can only pay $50.00 today. Does the patient have enough to cover the amount due today?

## Virtual Fieldtrip

*Visit the McGraw-Hill Higher Education Medical Assisting website at www.mhhe.com/medicalassisting3 to complete the following activity:*

Visit a Medicaid website and determine the requirements to qualify for Medicaid services in your state. Write a one-page summary for submission to your instructor.

Open the CD and complete this chapter's practice activities, play the games, listen to the key terms, and test yourself with the interactive review. E-mail, print, and/or save your results to document your proficiency.

# Medical Coding

## KEY TERMS

- add-on code
- Alphabetic Index
- code linkage
- compliance plan
- conventions
- cross-reference
- *Current Procedural Terminology* (CPT)
- diagnosis (Dx)
- diagnosis code
- E code
- E/M code
- established patient
- global period
- HCPCS Level II codes
- Health Care Common Procedure Coding System (HCPCS)
- *International Classification of Diseases, Ninth Revision, Clinical Modification* (ICD-9-CM)
- modifier
- new patient
- panel
- procedure code
- Tabular List
- V code

## MEDICAL ASSISTING COMPETENCIES

*In preparation for the certification examination, you should know the following areas of competence:*

| COMPETENCY | CMA | RMA |
|---|:---:|:---:|
| **Administrative** | | |
| Apply managed care policies and procedures | X | X |
| Analyze and apply third-party guidelines | X | X |
| Perform procedural and diagnostic coding | X | X |
| Complete insurance claim forms | X | X |
| Use the physician fee schedule | | X |
| Identify and respond to issues of confidentiality by maintaining confidentiality at all times and following appropriate guidelines when releasing records or information | X | X |
| Be aware of and perform within legal and ethical boundaries | X | X |
| Determine the needs for documentation and reporting, and document accurately and appropriately | X | X |
| Demonstrate knowledge of and monitor current federal and state health-care legislation and regulations; maintain licenses and accreditation | X | X |
| Utilize computer software and electronic technology to maintain office systems | X | X |
| Evidence a responsible attitude | | X |
| Conduct work within scope of education, training, and ability | | X |
| Use appropriate medical terminology | | X |
| Receive, organize, prioritize, and transmit information appropriately | | X |

## CHAPTER OUTLINE

- Diagnosis Codes: The ICD-9-CM
- Procedure Codes: The CPT
- HCPCS
- Avoiding Fraud: Coding Compliance

# LEARNING OUTCOMES

After completing Chapter 16, you will be able to:

**16.1** Explain the purpose and format of the ICD-9-CM volumes that are used by medical offices.

**16.2** Describe how to analyze diagnoses and locate correct codes using the ICD-9-CM.

**16.3** Identify the purpose and format of the CPT.

**16.4** Name three key factors that determine the level of Evaluation and Management codes that are selected.

**16.5** Identify the two types of codes in the Health Care Common Procedure Coding System (HCPCS).

**16.6** Describe the process used to locate correct procedure codes using CPT.

**16.7** Explain how medical coding affects the payment process.

**16.8** Define fraud and provide examples of fraudulent billing and coding.

# Introduction

Welcome to an introduction to the world of coding! In order to correctly report on health-care claims the conditions that patients have and the services they receive during office visits, medical assistants need to understand the basics of medical coding. Medical coding is the translation of medical terms for diagnoses and procedures into code numbers selected from standardized code sets. Codes on health-care claims explain to payers that the services patients received were medically necessary and complied with the payer's rules. Finding the correct codes can require detective work! The reward is accurate claims that bring the maximum appropriate reimbursement to the physicians in your medical office.

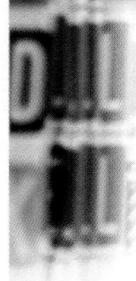

## CASE STUDY

A patient who has asthma has an office visit for her chest pain and shortness of breath. The physician performs a cardiovascular stress test using submaximal treadmill (with continuous electrocardiographic monitoring, physician supervision, and interpretation/report) to assess the patient's heart function. While the patient is in the office, the physician also evaluates her asthma and increases her prescription for asthma medication.

As you read this chapter, consider the following questions:

1. How would you select the ICD-9 and CPT codes for a health-care claim for this visit?
2. What diagnosis and procedure codes will result in the correct payment for these services?
3. How should the claim show the medical necessity of the procedures?
4. Locate the ICD-9 code for the patient's asthma. How many digits are required? What code did you assign?
5. Locate the CPT code for the cardiovascular stress test. What information did you use to select it from the list of related codes?

# Diagnosis Codes: The ICD-9-CM

Patients present to physicians with a description of their medical problems, called their chief complaints (CC) in the documentation of their visits. To diagnose a patient's condition, the physician follows a complex process of decision making based on the patient's statements, an examination, and the physician's evaluation of this information. The physician establishes a **diagnosis (Dx)** that describes the primary condition for which a patient is receiving care. Additional conditions or symptoms that affect the patient's management are called coexisting conditions. These conditions may be related or totally unrelated to the primary condition, but if they currently affect the patient's condition or treatment, they must also be noted in the chart, coded, and reported to the insurance carrier. The diagnoses listed on a health-care claim form should prove medical necessity for the treatment provided.

The diagnosis is communicated to the third-party payer through a **diagnosis code** on the health care claim.

The diagnosis codes used in the United States are found in the ***International Classification of Diseases, Ninth Revision, Clinical Modification,*** commonly referred to as the **ICD-9-CM** or simply ICD-9. Also available on CD-ROM, this code set is based on a system maintained by the World Health Organization (WHO) of the United Nations.

The use of the ICD-9 codes in the health-care industry is mandated by Health Insurance Portability and Accountability Act (HIPAA) for reporting patients' diseases, conditions, or their signs and symptoms if no actual diagnosis has been assigned. The codes are updated every year and new ICD-9 manuals are available every October. Medical offices should have the current year's reference book and should update office forms and computer programs that contain diagnosis codes; using outdated codes can result in denied claims.

## Using the ICD-9

To find the correct diagnosis codes, you follow a five-step process, working with the diagnostic information provided by the physician and the ICD-9 manual. Coding becomes easier with practice, but do not be tempted to take shortcuts. Every case is different, and additional terms or digits may be necessary to make a diagnosis code as specific as possible. If a step is skipped, important information may be missed. If more than one diagnosis is described in a patient's chart, work on only one diagnosis at a time to avoid coding errors, which may result in decreased or denied payment of a patient's claim.

The ICD-9-CM used in medical offices has two parts, the Tabular List, known as Volume 1, and the Alphabetic Index, known as Volume 2, which is actually found at the beginning of the manual.

**Diseases and Injuries: Tabular List, Volume 1.** The **Tabular List** has 17 chapters of disease descriptions and codes, with two additional types of codes and five appendixes.

**Diseases and Injuries: Alphabetic Index, Volume 2.** The **Alphabetic Index** provides the following:

- An index of the disease descriptions in the Tabular List
- An index in table format of drugs and chemicals that cause poisoning
- An index of external causes of injury, such as accidents and poisonings

Diagnoses are listed two ways in the ICD-9, as illustrated in Figure 16-1. In the Alphabetic Index, diagnoses

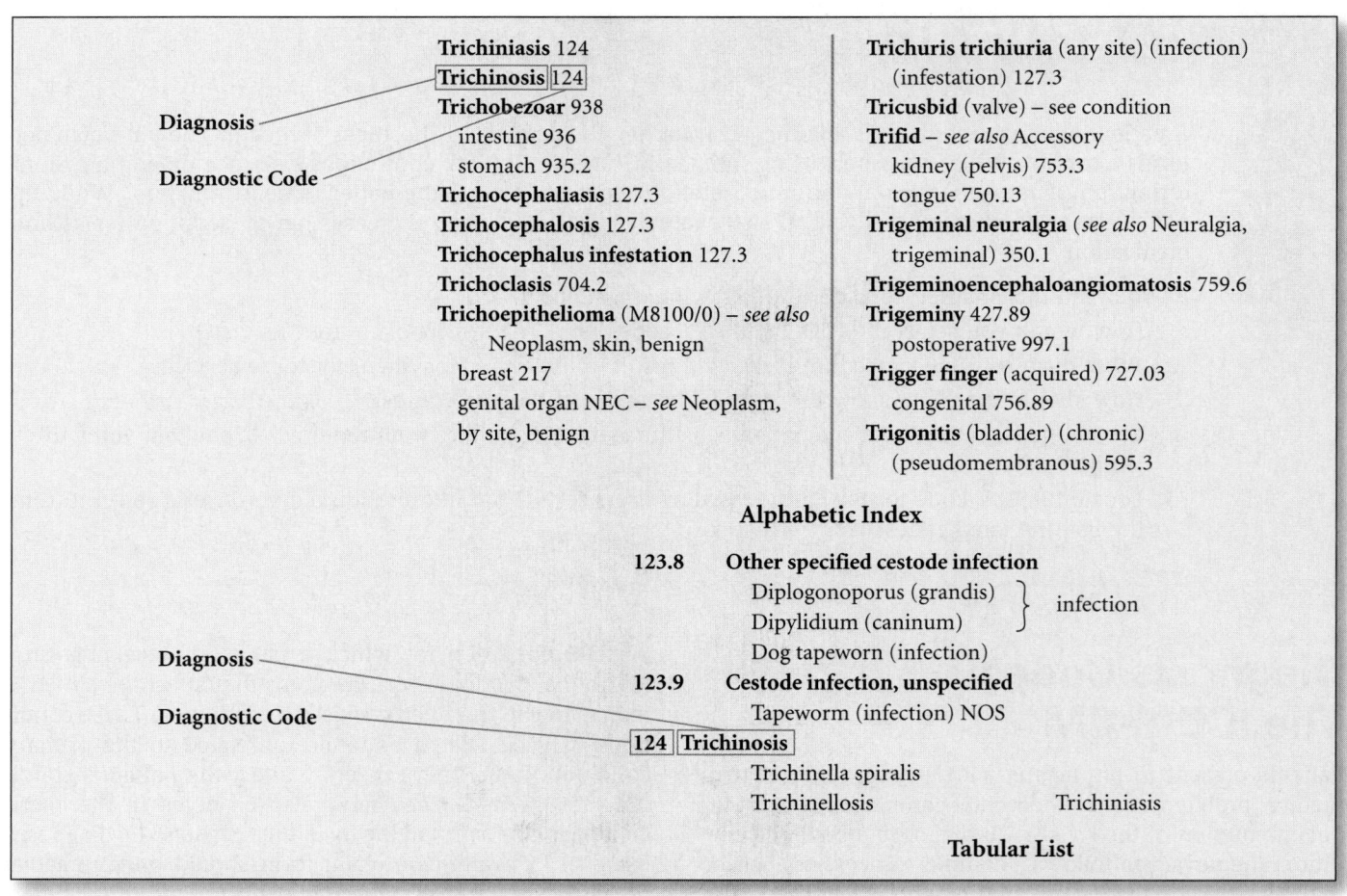

**Figure 16-1.** ICD Alphabetic Index and Tabular List.
*Source:* International Classification of Diseases, Ninth Revision, Clinical Modification, 2006, Volumes 1 and 2.

appear in alphabetic order with at least the main portion of their corresponding diagnosis codes. In the Tabular List, the diagnosis codes are listed in numerical order with additional instructions that are necessary to choose the final diagnosis code. Both the Alphabetic Index and the Tabular List are used to find the right code. The Alphabetic Index is *never* used alone because it does not contain all the necessary information. After you locate a code in the index, look it up in the Tabular List. Notes in this list may suggest or require the use of additional codes, or indicate that conditions should be coded differently because of exclusion from a category.

Although the official order of the volumes puts the Tabular List before the Alphabetic Index, the correct use is to examine the Alphabetic Index when you are researching a term and then to verify your selection in the Tabular List. For this reason, commercial printers usually reverse the order, printing the Alphabetic Index at the front and the Tabular List behind it.

## The Alphabetic Index

The Alphabetic Index contains all the medical terms in the Tabular List. For some conditions, it also has common terms that are not found in the Tabular List. The index is organized by the condition, not by the body part in which it occurs. To use the Alphabetic Index, think about what is wrong (the problem) and not where the problem occurred. For example, you would find the term *wrist fracture* by looking under *fracture* (the condition) and then, below it, *wrist* (the location), rather than by looking under *wrist* to find *fracture*. In fact, if you look up the word *wrist*, you will be told "See also condition," telling you to look up the problem with the wrist.

The assignment of the correct code begins with looking up the medical term that describes the patient's condition in the Alphabetic Index. The following example illustrates the index's format. Each main term is printed in boldface type and is followed by its code number. For example, if the diagnostic statement is "the patient presents with blindness," the main term *blindness* is located in the Alphabetic Index.

**Blindness** (acquired) (congenital) (both eyes) 369.00
    blast 921.3
       with nerve injury—see Injury, nerve, optic
    Bright's—see Uremia
    color (congenital) 368.59
      acquired 368.55
      blue 368.53
      green 368.52
      red 368.51
      total 368.54
    concussion 950.9
    cortical 377.75

Any other terms that are needed to select correct codes are printed and indented after the main term. These terms, called *subterms*, may show the cause or source of the disease, or describe a particular type or body site for the main

term. In this shortened example, the main term *blindness* is followed by five additional terms, each indicating a different type—such as color blindness—for this medical condition. Additionally, when coding color blindness, note that each of its subterms, which denote the actual type of color blindness, has its own code. When cross-referencing with the tabular index, you will note that the main code of 368 represents a visual disturbance. The fourth digit (after the decimal point) of 5 represents color vision deficiencies, and the fifth digit changes to indicate the type of color blindness.

Other helpful terms, in parentheses, known as *nonessential terms*, may also be shown. Nonessential terms are those that assist you in choosing the correct code, but it is not mandatory that they be present within the code description. In the example, any of the terms *acquired, congenital,* and/or *both eyes* may be in the diagnostic statement, such as "the patient presents with blindness acquired in childhood."

Some entries use **cross-references.** If the cross-reference *see* appears after a main term, you *must* look up the term that follows the word *see* in the index. The *see* reference means that the main term where you first looked is not correct; another category must be used. In the previous example, to code *Bright's,* the term *Uremia* must be located.

## The Tabular List

The diseases, conditions, and injuries in the Tabular List are organized into chapters according to the source or body system. The Tabular List also includes two kinds of supplementary codes, V codes and E codes, which will be discussed later in the chapter. The organization of the Tabular List and the ranges of codes each chapter covers are shown in Table 16-1.

**Code Structure.** ICD-9-CM diagnosis codes are made up of three, four, or five digits, and a description. The system uses three-digit categories for diseases, injuries, and symptoms. Many of these categories are divided into four-digit codes. Some codes are further subdivided into five-digit codes. For example:

415 Acute pulmonary heart disease *[three digits]*
    415.1 Pulmonary embolism and infarction *[four digits; more specific]*
        415.11 Iatrogenic pulmonary embolism and infarction *[five digits; most specific]*

When listed in the ICD-9, four- and five-digit diagnosis codes should be reported on claims because they represent the most specific diagnosis documented in the patient medical record. If available, the use of fourth and fifth digits is not optional; payers require them. For example, Centers for Medicare and Medicaid Services (CMS) rules state that a Medicare claim will be rejected when the most specific code available is not used. In the above example, it would be incorrect to use code 415 or 415.1, because code 415.11 is available and it is required that the

## TABLE 16-1  Tabular List Organization

### Classification of Diseases and Injuries

| Chapter | Categories |
|---|---|
| 1 Infectious and Parasitic Diseases | 001–139 |
| 2 Neoplasms | 140–239 |
| 3 Endocrine, Nutritional, and Metabolic Diseases, and Immunity Disorders | 240–279 |
| 4 Diseases of the Blood and Blood-Forming Organs | 280–289 |
| 5 Mental Disorders | 290–319 |
| 6 Diseases of the Central Nervous System and Sense Organs | 320–389 |
| 7 Diseases of the Circulatory System | 390–459 |
| 8 Diseases of the Respiratory System | 460–519 |
| 9 Diseases of the Digestive System | 520–579 |
| 10 Diseases of the Genitourinary System | 580–629 |
| 11 Complications of Pregnancy, Childbirth, and the Puerperium | 630–679 |
| 12 Diseases of the Skin and Subcutaneous Tissue | 680–709 |
| 13 Diseases of the Musculoskeletal System and Connective Tissue | 710–739 |
| 14 Congenital Anomalies | 740–759 |
| 15 Certain Conditions Originating in the Perinatal Period | 760–779 |
| 16 Symptoms, Signs, and Ill-Defined Conditions | 780–799 |
| 17 Injury and Poisoning | 800–999 |
| **Supplementary Classifications** | |
| V Codes—Supplementary Classification of Factors Influencing Health Status and Contact with Health Services | V01–V83 |
| E Codes—Supplementary Classification of External Causes of Injury and Poisoning | E800–E999 |

most specific code be used. Always keep in mind that the minimum code contains 3 digits, but if a 4th digit is available, it must be used, and if a 5th digit is available, it also must be used. The fourth and fifth digits are preceded by a decimal point.

**V Codes and E Codes.** Two additional types of codes follow the chapters of the Tabular List:

1. **V codes** identify encounters for reasons other than illness or injury, such as annual checkups, immunizations, and normal childbirth. The descriptions for V codes are found throughout the main portion of the Alphabetic Index. A V code can be used either as a primary code for an encounter or as an additional code. You should be aware that some insurance carriers, such as Medicare, do not cover V codes, so the charges associated with them may become the patient's responsibility.

2. **E codes** identify the external causes of injuries and poisoning. E (for external) codes are used for injuries resulting from various environmental events, such as transportation accidents, accidental poisoning by drugs or other substances, falls, and fires. An E code is never used alone as a diagnosis code. It always supplements a code that identifies the injury or condition itself. E codes are often used in collecting public health information. The alphabetic descriptions for E codes are found at the end of the Alphabetic Index in two sections. Section 2 is the alphabetic Table of Drugs and Chemicals, which is used to identify drugs and chemicals responsible for poisonings. Immediately following this, in Section 3, is the alphabetic index for all E codes.

Both V and E codes are alphanumeric; they contain letters followed by numbers. For example, the code for a complete physical examination of an adult is V70.0. The code for a fall from a ladder is E881.0. The same rule for specificity applies to E and V codes regarding 4th and 5th digits; that is, if a 4th or 5th digit is available, it must be utilized or the code will be rejected by the insurance carrier.

# ICD-9-CM Conventions

A list of abbreviations, punctuation, symbols, typefaces, and instructional notes appears at the beginning of the ICD-9. These items, called **conventions,** provide guidelines for using the code set. Here are some important conventions:

- NOS. This abbreviation means "not otherwise specified," or "unspecified." It is used when a condition cannot be described more specifically. In general, codes with *NOS* should be avoided unless no other option is available. The physician should be asked for more specific information to help select a more specific code, if possible. Most of the NOS codes end with the number 9.
- NEC. This abbreviation means "not elsewhere classified." It is used when the ICD-9 does not provide a code specific enough for the patient's condition. Only use these codes when you are sure a more specific code does not exist. In general, the NEC codes end with the number 8.
- [ ] Brackets. These are used around synonyms, alternative wordings, or explanations.
- ( ) Parentheses. These are used around descriptions that do not affect the code, that is, nonessential or supplementary terms.
- : Colon. This is used in the Tabular List after an incomplete term that needs one of the terms that follow to make it assignable to a given category.
- } Brace. This encloses a series of terms, each of which is modified by the statement that appears to the right of the brace.
- § Section mark symbol. This symbol, preceding a code, denotes the placement of a footnote at the bottom of the page that is applicable to all subdivisions in that code. Not all editions of ICD-9 utilize the section mark symbol.
- *Includes.* This note indicates that the entries following it refine the content of a preceding entry. For example, after the three-digit diagnosis code for acute sinusitis, the word *includes* is followed by the types of conditions that the code covers.
- *Excludes.* These notes, which are boxed and italicized, indicate that an entry is not classified as part of the preceding code. The note may also give the correct location of the excluded condition.
- *Use additional code.* This note indicates that an additional code should be used, if available. The additional code is always listed after the primary code. For instance, when looking up a urinary tract infection NOS (599.0), you are asked to also code the causative

organism (if given), such as *E. coli* (041.4). The complete coding sequence would be 599.0, 041.4.

- *Code first underlying disease.* This instruction appears when the category is not to be used as the primary diagnosis. These codes may not be used as the first code; they must always be preceded by another code for the primary diagnosis. An example of this would be any diabetic complication, such as diabetic retinopathy for a noninsulin-dependent diabetic. Under diabetic retinopathy (362.01), you are instructed to *Code first diabetes* (250.5). The correct coding order would be 250.50, 362.01. The fifth digit with the diabetes code indicates *noninsulin-dependent diabetes not stated as uncontrolled.* You will note when coding diabetes that the instructions state that all diabetes codes require fifth digits.

**Locating the Diagnosis in the Patient Chart.** If the physician uses a SOAP note format (Chapter 9), you can locate the diagnosis in the assessment area. If a more "free-hand" approach is used, a little detective work may be needed.

Example #1, from a Patient Medical Record:
CC: *Chest and epigastric pain; feels like a burning inside. Occasional reflux.*
Exam: *Abdomen soft, flat without tenderness. No bowel masses or organomegaly.*
Dx: *Peptic ulcer.*

The diagnosis is peptic ulcer.

Now, decide what the main term is for the condition or the diagnosis. For the diagnosis in the above scenario, the main term is *ulcer.* The word *peptic* (meaning stomach) describes the type of ulcer and is considered a subterm. Because there is an exact diagnosis, the pain and reflux will not be coded.

Example #2:
The diagnosis is sebaceous cyst. Look under *cyst,* the condition, and not *sebaceous,* the descriptive subterm. Many entries in the Alphabetic Index are cross-referenced, so if you look up a descriptive word, the ICD-9 will lead you to alternate words to assist you in finding the correct description. For example, *sebaceous* is followed by instructions in parentheses that say "(*see also* Cyst, sebaceous)." Be sure to follow all cross-reference instructions.

Once you find the description, locate the code given for that description; it is usually to the right of the description or just below it. Now go to Volume 1, the Tabular Index, to verify the code. Be sure to read all instructions in this section because there are often more specific instructions in the Tabular Index that will help you find the right code or affirm that you have the correct code.

Examples:

1. For the first diagnosis of peptic ulcer, the main 3-digit code for peptic ulcer is 533. The 4th digit, 9, indicates

that the ulcer is not specified as acute or chronic and there is no mention of hemorrhage or perforation. The 5th digit, 0, is chosen as there is no mention of obstruction. The final code for the peptic ulcer is 533.90.

2. In the second scenario, the sebaceous cyst, the main code is 706, which denotes diseases of the sebaceous glands. The 4th digit, 2, indicates that the "disease" is a sebaceous cyst. In this example, there is no 5th digit, so the final code for a sebaceous cyst is 706.2.

In both of these cases, the level of specificity of each diagnosis was greatly increased by the addition of the 4th and 5th digits, underlining the importance of these "optional" additions to the main codes; they truly are not optional at all.

Lastly, don't forget to look for instructions for additional codes that may be needed to completely code the diagnosis. These instructions may include *Code also* and *Code first underlying condition*, as well as *includes* and *excludes* notes that assist you in deciding on the correct code or codes.

Procedure 16-1 outlines the steps for locating an ICD-9-CM code.

## A New Revision: The ICD-10-CM

The tenth edition of the ICD was published by the World Health Organization (WHO) in the mid-1990s. In the United States, the new *Clinical Modification* (ICD-10-CM) is being reviewed by health-care professionals. It is

## PROCEDURE 16.1

## Locating an ICD-9-CM Code

**Procedure Goal:** To analyze diagnoses and locate the correct ICD code.

**Materials:** Patient record, charge slip or superbill, ICD-9-CM manual

**Method:**

1. Locate the patient's diagnosis.
   a. This information may be located on the superbill (encounter form) or elsewhere in the patient's chart. If it is on the superbill, verify documentation in the medical chart.

   *Rationale*
   All diagnosis codes must be referenced in the patient's medical record for legal purposes.

2. Find the diagnosis in the ICD's Alphabetic Index. Look for the condition first, then locate the indented subterms that make the condition more specific. Read all cross-references to check all the possibilities for a term, including its synonyms and any eponyms.

   *Rationale*
   The goal is to attain the highest level of specificity possible to avoid denial of the claim.

3. Locate the code from the Alphabetic Index in the ICD's Tabular List.

   *Rationale*
   *Never* code directly from the Alphabetic Index. Important coding instructions are found only in the Tabular Index.

4. Read all information to find the code that corresponds to the patient's specific disease or condition.
   a. Study the list of codes and descriptions. Be sure to pick the most specific code available. Check for the symbol that shows that a four- or five-digit code is required.

   *Rationale*
   When available, 4th and 5th digits are mandatory for accurate coding. Claims will be denied if these "optional" digits are available and not used when submitting a claim.

5. Carefully record the diagnosis code(s) on the insurance claim and proofread the numbers.
   a. Be sure that all necessary codes are given to completely describe each diagnosis. Check for instructions stating an additional code is needed. If more than one code is needed, be sure instructions are followed and the codes are listed in the correct order.

   *Rationale*
   Coding order is important for claims to be considered "clean" and paid in a timely fashion.

expected to be adopted as the Health Insurance Portability and Accessibility Act (HIPAA)-required diagnosis code set before 2010. Major changes include the following:

- The ICD-10 contains more than 2000 categories of diseases, many more than the ICD-9. This creates more codes to permit more specific reporting of diseases and newly recognized conditions, such as SARS.

- Codes are alphanumeric, containing a letter followed by up to five numbers. The sixth digit is added to capture clinical details. For example, all codes that relate to pregnancy, labor, and childbirth include a digit that indicates the patient's trimester.

- Codes will often combine diagnoses and symptoms, which will reduce the number of codes needed to fully describe many conditions.

- Codes are added to show which side of the body is affected when a disease or condition can be involved with the right side, the left side, or bilaterally.

- E codes and V codes are incorporated throughout ICD-10 and will no longer be found in supplemental classifications. Additionally, the E code section on injuries is greatly expanded to allow for greater specificity.

- Unlike ICD-9, which also includes a Volume 3 specifically for hospital procedures, ICD-10 will not include procedures. A separate volume called ICD-10-PCS (Procedure Coding System) is also being developed.

Because the ICD-10 codes are much more specific, providers will have to give detailed diagnosis information so that the most accurate code can be assigned, but it is generally acknowledged that experienced ICD-9 coders will require only brief training to work effectively and efficiently with ICD-10.

# Procedure Codes: The CPT

After an office visit, each procedure and service performed for a patient is reported on health-care claims using a **procedure code.** These codes represent medical procedures, such as surgery and diagnostic tests, and medical services, such as a physical examination to evaluate a patient's condition. Medical assistants often choose procedure codes based on the information given to them by the physician on the charge slip and use them to report physicians' services.

The most commonly used system of procedure codes is found in the *Current Procedural Terminology,* a book published by the American Medical Association (AMA) that is commonly known as **CPT.** CPT is the HIPAA-required code set that translates descriptions for physicians' procedures into 5-digit codes.

An updated edition of the CPT is published every January to reflect changes in medical practice. Newly developed procedures are added and old ones are revised or, if they have become obsolete, are deleted. These changes are also available in a computer file because some medical offices use a computer-based version of the CPT.

Medical offices should have the current year's CPT available for reference and keep forms up to date. Like ICD-9 codes, if current codes are not used, medical claims are often denied. Previous years' books should also be kept in case there is a question about health-care claims that were previously submitted.

## Organization of the CPT Manual

CPT codes are organized into six main sections:

| Section | Range of Codes |
|---|---|
| Evaluation and Management | 99201–99499 |
| Anesthesiology | 00100–01999, 99100-99140 |
| Surgery | 10021–69990 |
| Radiology | 70010–79999 |
| Pathology and Laboratory | 80048–89356 |
| Medicine (except for anesthesia) | 90281–99199, 99500–99602 |

Except for the first section, the CPT reference book is arranged in numerical order. Codes for evaluation and management, which describe care given by the physician, are listed first, out of numerical order, because they are used most often.

Each section opens with important guidelines that apply to its procedures. This material should be checked carefully before a procedure code is chosen. The sections of the CPT are divided into categories. These in turn are further divided into headings according to the type of test, service, or body system. Code number ranges included on a particular page are found in the upper-right corner. This helps to locate a code quickly after using the index. An example is shown in Figure 16-2.

Locate correct procedure codes by first looking up the term in the CPT's index, which is found at the back of the manual. Boldfaced main terms may be followed by descriptions and groups of indented subterms. The correct code is selected by reviewing each description and indented term under the main term.

Although it may seem tempting to record the procedure code directly from the index, resist the shortcut. Explanations and notes in the guidelines and main sections more accurately lead to finding main numbers and modifiers that reflect the services performed. That is the only way to ensure reimbursement at the highest allowed level.

**Add-On Codes.** A plus sign (+) is used for **add-on codes,** indicating procedures that are usually carried out in addition to another procedure. For example, code 90471 covers one immunization administration and code 90472 covers administering an additional shot. Add-on codes are never reported alone. They are used together with the primary code.

**Modifiers.** One or more two-digit **modifiers** (up to three per procedure) may be assigned to the five-digit main number. Modifiers are written in a separate column on the CMS-1500 Claim Form (Centers for Medicare and Medicaid Services Claim Form; see Figure 15-6). The use of a modifier

# Surgery

## General

(10000-10020 have been deleted. To report see 10060, 10061)

**10021** Fine needle aspiration; without imaging guidance
🔁 *CPT Assistant* Aug 02:10; *CPT Changes: An Insider's View* 2002

**10022** with imaging guidance
🔁 *CPT Changes: An Insider's View* 2002

(For radiological supervision and interpretation, see 76003, 76360, 76393, 76942)

(For percutaneous needle biopsy other than fine needle aspiration, see 20206 for muscle, 32400 for pleura, 32405 for lung or mediastinum, 42400 for salivary gland, 47000, 47001 for liver, 48102 for pancreas, 49180 for abdominal or retroperitoneal mass, 60100 for thyroid, 62269 for spinal cord)

(For evaluation of fine needle aspirate, see 88172, 88173)

## Integumentary System

### Skin, Subcutaneous and Accessory Structures

#### Incision and Drainage

(For excision, see 11400, et seq)

**10040** Acne surgery (eg, marsupialization, opening or removal of multiple milia, comedones, cysts, pustules)

**10060** Incision and drainage of abscess (eg, carbuncle, suppurative hidradenitis, cutaneous or subcutaneous abscess, cyst, furuncle, or paronychia); simple or single

**10061** complicated or multiple

**10080** Incision and drainage of pilonidal cyst; simple

**10081** complicated

(For excision of pilonidal cyst, see 11770-11772)

**10120** Incision and removal of foreign body, subcutaneous tissues; simple

**10121** complicated

(To report wound exploration due to penetrating trauma without laparotomy or thoracotomy, see 20100-20103, as appropriate)

(To report debridement associated with open fracture(s) and/or dislocation(s), use 11010-11012, as appropriate)

**10140** Incision and drainage of hematoma, seroma or fluid collection
🔁 *CPT Changes: An Insider's View* 2002

(If imaging guidance is performed, see 76360, 76393, 76942)

**10160** Puncture aspiration of abscess, hematoma, bulla, or cyst
🔁 *CPT Changes: An Insider's View* 2002

(If imaging guidance is performed, see 76360, 76393, 76942)

**10180** Incision and drainage, complex, postoperative wound infection

(For secondary closure of surgical wound, see 12020, 12021, 13160)

## Excision—Debridement

(For dermabrasions, see 15780-15783)

(For nail debridement, see 11720-11721)

(For burn(s), see 16000-16035)

**11000** Debridement of extensive eczematous or infected skin; up to 10% of body surface

**+ 11001** each additional 10% of the body surface (List separately in addition to code for primary procedure)

(Use 11001 in conjunction with code 11000)

**11010** Debridement including removal of foreign material associated with open fracture(s) and/or dislocation(s); skin and subcutaneous tissues
🔁 *CPT Assistant* Mar 97:1, Apr 97:10, Aug 97:6

**11011** skin, subcutaneous tissue, muscle fascia, and muscle
🔁 *CPT Assistant* Mar 97:1, Apr 97:10, Aug 97:6

**11012** skin, subcutaneous tissue, muscle fascia, muscle, and bone
🔁 *CPT Assistant* Mar 97:1, Apr 97:10, Aug 97:6

**11040** Debridement; skin, partial thickness
🔁 *CPT Assistant* Fall 93:21, May 96:6, Feb 97:7, Aug 97:6

**11041** skin, full thickness
🔁 *CPT Assistant* Fall 93:21, May 96:6, Feb 97:7, Aug 97:6

**11042** skin, and subcutaneous tissue
🔁 *CPT Assistant* Winter 92:10, May 96:6, Feb 97:7, Aug 97:6

**11043** skin, subcutaneous tissue, and muscle
🔁 *CPT Assistant* May 96:6, Feb 97:7, Apr 97:11, Aug 97:6

**11044** skin, subcutaneous tissue, muscle, and bone
🔁 *CPT Assistant* Fall 93:21, Mar 96:10, May 96:6, Feb 97:7, Apr 97:11, Aug 97:6

(Do not report 11040-11044 in addition to 97601, 97602)

**Figure 16-2.** Examples of CPT codes, surgical section.
*Source*: American Medical Association, *Current Procedural Terminlolgy*, copyright 2006.

shows that some special circumstance applies to the service or procedure the physician performed. For example, in the surgery section, the modifier -62 indicates that two surgeons worked together, each performing part of a surgical procedure during an operation. Each physician will be paid part of the amount normally reimbursed for that procedure code. Appendix A of the CPT explains the proper use of each modifier. Some section guidelines also discuss the use of modifiers with the section's codes.

### Category II Codes, Category III Codes, and Unlisted Procedure Codes.
Category II codes are optional, supplemental tracking codes used to track healthcare performance measures, such as programs and counseling to avoid tobacco use. Category III codes are temporary CPT codes for emerging technology, services, and procedures. If available, these codes should be used instead of the *unlisted codes* found throughout the CPT manual.

When no code is available to completely describe a procedure, a code for an unlisted procedure is selected. Unlisted procedure codes are used for new services or procedures that have not yet been assigned codes in CPT. When these codes are used, which is rare, a written explanation of the procedure or service is needed.

## Evaluation and Management Services

To diagnose conditions and plan treatments, physicians use a wide range of time, effort, and skill for different patients and circumstances. Evaluation and management codes (**E/M codes**) are often considered the most important of all CPT codes because they can be used by all physicians in any medical specialty.

The E/M section guidelines explain how to code different levels of these services. Three key factors documented in the patient's medical record help determine the level of service:

1. The extent of the patient history taken
2. The extent of the examination conducted
3. The complexity of the medical decision making

Payers also want to know whether the physician treated a **new patient** or an **established patient.** Physicians often spend more time during new patients' visits than during visits from established patients, so the E/M codes for the two types of patients are separate. For reporting purposes, the CPT considers a patient "new" if that person has not received professional services from the physician within the past three years. An established patient is one who has seen the physician within the past three years. (Note that the current visit need not be for a problem treated previously.) Most insurers also consider a patient to be an established patient if, within the past 3 years, she had seen a different physician in the same practice with the same specialty as the "new" physician she is seeing. Emergency patients are not classified as either new or established patients.

The CPT has a range of five codes each for new-patient or established-patient encounters. The lowest-level code is often called a Level I code; the highest-level code is a Level V code. For example, code 99213 is the Level III code for an established patient's office visit. The higher the level, the more labor-intensive the service.

The location of the service is also important because different E/M codes apply to services performed in a physician's office or other outpatient location, a hospital inpatient room, a hospital emergency department, a nursing facility, an extended-care facility, or a patient's home.

## Surgical Procedures

Figure 16-2 illustrated a series of codes from the integumentary part of the surgical section. Codes listed in the surgery section represent all the procedures that are normally a part of that operation, including preoperative testing, local anesthesia, the surgery itself, and routine follow-up care. This combination of services is called a *surgical package.* Payers assign a fee to each of these codes that pays for all the services provided under them. If other than local anesthesia is used, an anesthesia code would be used by the anesthesiologist billing for his services.

The period of time that is covered for follow-up care is called the **global period.** For example, the global period for repairing a tendon might be set at 15 days. A global period for major surgery such as an appendectomy might be set at 100 days. During the global period, any care provided related to the surgical procedure is included in the surgical fee and cannot be billed separately; any attempt to do so is called *unbundling* and is considered fraud. If a patient is seen for an unrelated problem, the procedure may be billed separately using a modifier (24 for E/M services, 79 for a surgical procedure), identifying the procedure as being unrelated. After the global period ends, additional services related to the initial surgery can be reported separately for payment.

To make the coding process more efficient, medical offices often list frequently used procedures and their applicable CPT codes on superbills. After seeing the patient, the physician checks off the appropriate procedures or services. An example of a dermatology practice's superbill is shown in Figure 16-3. This sample superbill lists the E/M codes for new and established patient office visits as well as common procedures for the office. If superbills are used in the office, it is important to remember to update both the ICD-9 and CPT codes on the superbills and in any computer programs when the new manuals are available each year.

## Laboratory Procedures

Organ or disease-oriented **panels** listed in the pathology and laboratory section of the CPT include tests frequently ordered together. An electrolyte panel, for example, includes tests for carbon dioxide, chloride, potassium, and sodium. Each element of the panel has its own procedure code. However, when the tests are performed together, the code for the panel must be used rather than the separate procedure codes. To

## VALLEY ASSOCIATES, P.C.
### David Rosenberg, M.D. - Dermatology
555-321-0987
FED I.D. #06-2345678

| PATIENT NAME | | | | APPT. DATE/TIME | | | |
|---|---|---|---|---|---|---|---|
| Scott Yeager | | | | 10/14/2007 | | 11:00am | |

| PATIENT NO. | | | | DX | | | |
|---|---|---|---|---|---|---|---|
| YEAGESCO | | | | 1. 919.7 superficial foreign body without | | | |
| | | | | 2. major open wound. Infected | | | |
| | | | | 3. | | | |
| | | | | 4. | | | |

| DESCRIPTION | ✓ | CPT | FEE | DESCRIPTION | ✓ | CPT | FEE |
|---|---|---|---|---|---|---|---|
| **EXAMINATION** | | | | **PROCEDURES** | | | |
| **New Patient** | | | | Acne Surgery | | 10040 | |
| Problem Focused | | 99201 | | I&D Cyst/Abscess | | 10060 | |
| Expanded Problem Focused | ✓ | 99202 | 50 | I&D Multiple | | 10061 | |
| Detailed | | 99203 | | I&D Remove Foreign Body | ✓ | 10120 | 60 |
| Comprehensive | | 99204 | | Debridement | | 11000 | |
| Comprehensive/Complex | | 99205 | | Paring/Curett. (Benign) | | 11055 | |
| **Established Patient** | | | | Paring/Curett. (2-4) | | 11056 | |
| Minimum | | 99211 | | Paring/Curett. (Over 4) | | 11057 | |
| Problem Focused | | 99212 | | Excision Skin Tags (1-15) | | 11200 | |
| Expanded Problem Focused | | 99213 | | Cyrosurgery | | 17340 | |
| Detailed | | 99214 | | Skin Biopsy | | 11100 | |
| Comprehensive/Complex | | 99215 | | Skin Biopsy (EA additional) | | +11101 | |

**Figure 16-3.** Superbill with procedure codes.

code a panel correctly, the physician must order each test listed within the panel and there must be a need for each of them. If a panel is appropriate but one or two laboratory tests are ordered that are not included in the panel, code the panel and then the additional tests separately.

If each test in a panel or procedure in a surgical package is listed separately, it will unbundle the panel or package. The review performed by the insurance carrier's claims department will rebundle the services under the appropriate code, which could delay payment. Remember that when unbundling is done intentionally or repeatedly to receive more payment than is correct, the claim is likely to be considered fraudulent.

## Immunizations

Injections and infusions of immune globulins, vaccines, toxoids, and other substances require two codes, one for giving the injection and one for the particular vaccine or toxoid that is given. An E/M code is not used along with the codes for immunization unless a significant evaluation and management service is also performed and documented appropriately by the doctor.

## HCPCS

The **Health Care Common Procedure Coding System,** commonly referred to as **HCPCS,** was developed by the Centers for Medicare and Medicaid Services (CMS) for use in coding services for Medicare patients. The HCPCS (pronounced "hic-picks") coding system has two levels:

1. HCPCS Level I codes are more commonly known as CPT codes.
2. **HCPCS Level II codes,** issued by CMS, are called national codes and cover many supplies, such as sterile trays, drugs, injections, and DME (durable medical

equipment). If both CPT and HCPCS have an appropriate code, the HCPCS Level II code should be used, especially for Medicare claims, because they are generally more specific then the CPT codes. Level II codes also cover services and procedures not included in the CPT.

The HCPCS codes for Level II have five characters, either numbers, letters, or a combination of both. At times there are also two-character modifiers, either two letters or a letter with a number. These modifiers are different from the CPT modifiers, but may be used with CPT codes as well as with Level II codes. For example, HCPCS modifiers may indicate social worker services or equipment rentals.

Examples of Level II codes are:

| Code Number | Description |
| --- | --- |
| A0225-QN | Ambulance service, neonatal transport, base rate, emergency transport, one way, furnished directly by the provider of services |
| E0781 | Ambulatory infusion pump |
| G0001 | Routine venipuncture |
| G0104 | Colorectal cancer screening; flexible sigmoidoscopy |
| Q0091 | Screening Papanicolaou (Pap) smear; obtaining, preparing, and conveyance of cervical or vaginal smear to laboratory |
| V5299 | Hearing service, miscellaneous |

In medical offices where the HCPCS system is used, regulations issued by CMS are reviewed to determine the correct code and modifier for claims.

## Using the CPT

Before you can use the CPT manual, you must first become familiar with the format and guidelines regarding the use of CPT. To begin with, read the introduction and main section guidelines and notes for each section. For example, look at the guidelines for the evaluation and management section. They include definitions of key terms, such as *new* and *established patient, chief complaint, concurrent care,* and *counseling.* They also explain the method for selecting E/M codes. You may find it helpful to actually highlight important information within the guidelines and section notes.

The next step is to find the procedures and services provided by the office. As with diagnosis codes, these may be found on the superbill, but remember to check the patient's chart to verify that documentation on the procedures and services exists within the medical chart (if it is not written down, it did not happen). When coding E/M codes, remember that you must keep in mind *where* the service took place, as well as whether the patient is a new client or an established patient. You may find it easiest to go directly to the E/M section in the front of the CPT

manual to choose the correct code. For all other procedures, you will need to use the alphabetic listing of procedures found in the back of the CPT manual.

The number or number range in the index to the right of the description represents the coding possibilities for the description. If a hyphen is between 2 codes, this indicates a code range and each code in the range will need to be checked in the numeric index to choose the correct code. Code numbers with commas between them indicate that there is more than one location possibility. Again, all codes will have to be checked. In some cases, the patient's medical record may show an abbreviation, an *eponym* (a person or place for which a procedure is named), or a synonym. For example, the record might state "treated for bone infection." In CPT's index, the entry for "Infection, Bone," is followed by the instruction "See Osteomyelitis." The greater your knowledge of anatomy and physiology and terminology, the easier it will be for you to code.

Example 1: To find the code for "dressing change," first look alphabetically in the index for that procedure. Then find the procedure code in the body of the CPT to be sure the code accurately reflects the service performed. The procedure code 15852 explains the dressing change is for "other than burns" and "under anesthesia (other than local)." (A dressing change without anesthesia would be included in an E/M code.) Per the notes in CPT, a dressing for a burn is found in procedure codes 16010–16030.

Example 2: To code the excision of a vaginal cyst, you would first look under "Excision" (the main term). There is a listing for the subterm "Cyst" beneath "Excision," followed by a list of organs, regions, or structures involved. Note that each subterm is indented under the main term. Additionally, the subterms relating to cyst locations are indented even further under that subterm. This is a common occurrence in the CPT manual. Look for "Vagina" to find the code (57135). Another way to find the code is to look under "Vagina" as the main term and then find the listing for "Cyst Excision" as a subterm beneath it.

Once you decide on the appropriate CPT code(s), the next step is to check for any applicable modifiers. The use of modifiers can greatly enhance your reimbursement and can cut down on claim inquiries from the insurance carrier, but the ability to use modifiers correctly and proficiently will require practice. Appendix A contains all CPT modifiers and many times the section guidelines also contain information regarding the use of modifiers within that section.

Example: A bilateral breast reconstruction requires the modifier -50. Find the code for "breast reconstruction with free flap": 19364. To show the insurance carrier that the procedure was performed on both breasts, attach the -50: 19364-50. (Some insurers will require that you list the code once and then a second time

# PROCEDURE 16.2

## Locating a CPT Code

**Procedure Goal:** To locate correct CPT codes

**Materials:** Patient record, superbill or charge slip, CPT manual

**Method:**

1. Find the services listed on the superbill (if used) and in the patient's record.

   a. Check the patient's record to see which services were documented. For E/M procedures, look for clues as to the location of the service, extent of history, examination, and medical decision making that were involved.

   ### Rationale

   Every billed procedure or service must be backed up by the medical record.

2. Look up the procedure code(s) in the alphabetic index of the CPT manual.

   a. Verify the code number in the numeric index, reading all notes and guidelines for that section.

   b. If a code range is noted, look up the range and choose the correct code from the range given. If the correct description is not found, start the process again. Use the same process if multiple codes are given.

   ### Rationale

   CPT codes must accurately reflect the services or procedures provided to the patient. Payment is based on the codes chosen and must be backed up by the medical record.

3. Determine appropriate modifiers.

   a. Check section guidelines and Appendix A to choose a modifier if needed to explain a situation involving the procedure being coded, such as bilateral procedure, surgical team, or a discontinued procedure.

   ### Rationale

   The goal of coding is specificity. Modifiers, when available for the circumstance, provide specificity to CPT codes.

4. Carefully record the procedure code(s) on the health-care claim. Usually the primary procedure, the one which is the primary reason for the encounter or visit, is listed first.

   ### Rationale

   Transposed figures will represent procedures other than those performed, affecting claim status and reimbursement.

5. Match each procedure with its corresponding diagnosis. The primary procedure is often (but not always) matched with the primary diagnosis.

   ### Rationale

   Matching each procedure to the correct diagnosis gives the insurance carrier the reason the procedure was done, which verifies medical necessity.

---

with the modifier: 19364, 19364-50.) The insurance company will often pay the full charge for the first procedure and then pay the second procedure at 50%.

Once all procedures and services have been assigned a CPT code and modifier as needed, carefully enter the 5-digit code(s) and modifiers in the appropriate area of the CMS-1500 form. After the procedure code is verified, it is posted to the health-care claim. The primary procedure, often the one that is most labor intensive or is the principal reason for the patient's encounter, is listed first and is often matched with the primary diagnosis.

Be sure to match up each procedure with its applicable diagnosis. This step verifies medical necessity for the insurance carrier.

Procedure 16-2 outlines the correct steps for locating a CPT code.

# Avoiding Fraud: Coding Compliance

Physicians have the ultimate responsibility for proper documentation and correct coding as well as for compliance with regulations. Medical assistants help ensure maximum appropriate reimbursement for reported services by submitting correct health-care claims. These claims, as well as the process used to create them, must comply with the rules imposed by federal and state law and with payer requirements.

# Code Linkage

On correct claims, each reported service is connected to a diagnosis that supports the procedure as necessary to investigate or treat the patient's condition. Insurance company representatives analyze this connection between the diagnostic and the procedural information, called **code linkage,** to evaluate the medical necessity of the reported charges. Correct claims also comply with many other regulations from government agencies.

The possible consequences of inaccurate coding and incorrect billing include:

- Denied claims
- Delays in processing claims and receiving payments
- Reduced payments
- Fines and other sanctions
- Loss of hospital privileges
- Exclusion from payers' programs
- Prison sentences
- Loss of the physician's license to practice medicine

To avoid errors, the codes on health-care claims are checked against the medical documentation. A code review, also known as a coding audit, checks these key points:

- Are the codes appropriate to the patient's profile (age, gender, condition; new or established), and is each coded service billable?
- Is there a clear and correct link between each diagnosis and procedure?
- Have the payer's rules about the diagnosis and the procedure been followed?
- Does the documentation in the patient's medical record support the reported services?
- Do the reported services comply with all regulations?

# Insurance Fraud

Almost everyone involved in the delivery of health care is a trustworthy person devoted to patients' welfare. However, some people are not. For example, according to the Department of Health and Human Services (DHHS), in 1 year alone, the federal government recovered more than $1.3 billion in judgments, settlements, and other fees in health-care fraud cases. Fraud is an act of deception used to take advantage of another person or entity. For example, it is fraudulent for people to misrepresent their credentials or to forge another person's signature on a check.

Claims fraud occurs when physicians or others falsely represent their services or charges to payers. For example, a provider may bill for services that were not performed (phantom billing), overcharge for services, or fail to provide complete services under a contract. A patient may exaggerate an injury to get a settlement from an insurance company or ask a medical assistant to change a date on a chart so that a service is covered by a health plan.

A number of coding and billing practices are fraudulent. Investigators reviewing physicians' billings look for patterns like these:

- Reporting services that were not performed.
  Example: A lab bills Medicare for a general health panel (CPT 80050), but fails to perform one of the tests in the panel.
- Reporting services at a higher level than was carried out.
  Example: After a visit for a flu shot, the provider bills the encounter as an evaluation and management service plus a vaccination.
- Performing and billing for procedures that are not related to the patient's condition and therefore not medically necessary.
  Example: After reading an article about Lyme disease, a patient is worried about having worked in her garden over the summer and requests a Lyme disease diagnostic test. Although no symptoms or signs have been reported, the physician orders and bills for the Lyme disease test.
- Billing separately for services that are bundled in a single procedure code.
  Example: When a physician orders a comprehensive metabolic panel (CPT 80053), the provider bills for the panel as well as for a quantitative glucose test, which is in the panel.
- Reporting the same service twice.

Note that HIPAA calls for penalties for giving remuneration to anyone eligible for benefits under federal health-care programs. The forgiveness or waiver of copayments may violate the policies of some payers; others may permit forgiveness or waiver if they are aware of the reasons for the forgiveness or waiver, such as the patient's inability to pay (be sure to have documentation of such inability to avoid charges of discrimination). Routine forgiveness or waiver of copayments or deductibles constitutes fraud when billing federal programs such as Medicare or TRICARE. The physician practice should ensure that its policies on copayments are consistent with applicable law and with the requirements of their agreements with payers.

# Compliance Plans

To avoid the risk of fraud, medical offices have a **compliance plan** to uncover compliance problems and correct them. A compliance plan is a process for finding, correcting, and preventing illegal medical office practices. Its goals are to:

- Prevent fraud and abuse through a formal process to identify, investigate, fix, and prevent repeat violations relating to reimbursement for health-care services provided

## Medical Coder, Physician Practice

Medical coding specialists work in a number of health-care settings, including medical practices, hospitals, government agencies, and insurance companies. Coders who work in physician practices review patients' medical records and assign diagnosis and procedure codes. They are knowledgeable about the coding rules and procedures for physicians' work, which are different than those for coding hospital services. The position of medical coding specialist is growing in importance in physician practices. Accurate coding is a critical part of ensuring that claims follow the legal and ethical requirements of Medicare and other third-party payers as well as HIPAA regulations. Accurate coding also ensures optimum reimbursement for submitted claims.

Medical office employees may gain required health-care work experience and then attain coding positions through coding education from seminars or college classes. Certification as a professional coder offers an excellent route to success as a medical coder in the medical practice setting. Some employers require certification for employment; others state that certification must be earned after a certain amount of time in the position, such as 6 months. Coding classes followed by examinations are used to obtain certification. Three physician-office coding certifications are available. All require a high school diploma or equivalent.

- The American Health Information Management Association offers the Certified Coding Associate (CCA) credential and the Certified Coding Specialist—Physician-based (CCS-P) credential. The CCA is an entry-level title; completion of either a training program or 6 months' job experience is recommended. The CCS-P requires at least 3 years of coding experience.

- The American Academy of Professional Coders offers the Certified Professional Coder (CPC) credential, also requiring coursework and on-the-job experience. AAPC also offers an entry-level certification, the CPC-A (apprentice). Once documentation for two years of work experience as a coder is received and if the CPC-A maintains the required number of CEUs (continuing education units), the credential will be converted to a CPC.

Medical assistants who hold these credentials and have coding experience may advance to coding management and coding compliance auditor positions. Becoming expert in a specialty such as surgical coding also offers advancement opportunities.

---

- Ensure compliance with applicable federal, state, and local laws, including employment laws and environmental laws as well as antifraud laws
- Help defend physicians if they are investigated or prosecuted for fraud by showing the desire to behave compliantly and thus reduce any fines or criminal prosecution

When a compliance plan is in place, it demonstrates to payers such as Medicare that honest, ongoing attempts have been made to find and fix weak areas of compliance with regulations. The development of this written plan is led by a compliance officer and committee with the intention to (1) audit and monitor compliance with government regulations, especially in the area of coding and billing, (2) develop written policies and procedures that are consistent, (3) provide for ongoing staff training and communication, and (4) respond to and correct errors.

Although coding and billing compliance are the plan's major focus, it covers all areas of government regulation of medical practices, such as equal employment opportunity (EEO) regulations (for example, hiring and promotion policies) and OSHA regulations (for example, fire safety

and handling of hazardous materials such as blood-borne pathogens).

# Summary

The ICD-9-CM is used for diagnostic coding in the United States. ICD-9 codes are required for reporting patients' conditions on health-care claims. Codes are made up of three, four, or five numbers and a description. New codes are issued annually, and current codes should be used because they can affect billing and reimbursement.

The ICD-9 has two volumes that are used in outpatient medical practices: the Tabular List (Volume 1) and the Alphabetic Index (Volume 2). To find a code, use the Alphabetic Index first. Its main terms may be followed by related subterms. The codes themselves are organized into 17 chapters and are listed in numerical order in the Tabular List. Code categories consist of three-digit groupings of a single disease or a related condition. Further clinical detail is shown by 4th or 5th digit code modifiers that give further specificity to the diagnosis code. When available, these 4th and 5th digits must be used. The conventions, notes, and guidelines within the ICD-9 manual must be observed to correctly select codes.

Diagnosis codes, known as V codes, identify encounters for reasons other than illness or injury and are used for healthy patients receiving routine services (physical exams), for therapeutic encounters such as chemotherapy, for a problem that is not currently affecting the patient's condition (such as a family history of cancer), and for preoperative evaluations. Diagnostic E codes, which are never used as primary codes, classify the illnesses and injuries resulting from various environmental events.

CPT provides a standardized list of five-digit procedure codes for medical, surgical, and diagnostic services. Add-on codes and modifiers may also be selected.

CPT is divided into six sections: (1) evaluation and management, (2) anesthesiology, (3) surgery, (4) radiology, (5) pathology and laboratory, and (6) medicine. The three main factors that influence the level of service for coding purposes are the type and extent of (1) history, (2) examination, and (3) medical decision making. Surgical packages and laboratory panels should be coded as single procedures rather than broken into component parts (unbundling).

The Health Care Common Procedure Coding System (HCPCS), used to code Medicare services and that more recently has been adopted by some private payers, has codes from CPT (Level I) as well as Level II national codes.

Diagnoses and procedures must be correctly linked when services are reported for reimbursement because payers analyze this connection to determine the medical necessity of the charges. Correct claims also comply with all applicable governmental regulations and requirements. Codes should be appropriate and well documented within the patient's medical record, as well as compliant with each payer's rules.

A medical practice compliance plan addresses compliance concerns of governmental regulations (for example, HIPAA), as well as government and private payers. Furthermore, having a formal process in place is a sign that the practice has made a good-faith effort to achieve compliance in coding.

# REVIEW

## CHAPTER 16

## CASE STUDY QUESTIONS

Now that you have completed this chapter, review the case study at the beginning of the chapter and answer the following questions:

1. How would you select the ICD-9 and CPT codes for a health-care claim for this visit?
2. What diagnosis and procedure codes will result in the correct payment for these services?
3. How should the claim show the medical necessity of the procedures?
4. Locate the ICD-9 code for the patient's asthma. How many digits are required? What code did you assign?
5. Locate the CPT code for the cardiovascular stress test. What information did you use to select it from the list of related codes?

## Discussion Questions

1. What are the differences among the three code sets discussed in the chapter?
2. Are *see* cross-references in the Alphabetic Index of the ICD-9 followed by codes? Why?
3. Would you expect to locate codes for the following services or procedures in CPT? What range or series of codes would you investigate?
   a. Routine obstetric care including antepartum care, cesarean delivery, and postpartum care
   b. Echocardiography (cardiac)
   c. Radiologic examination, nasal bones, complete
   d. Home visit for evaluation and management of an established patient
   e. Drug test for amphetamines
   f. Anesthesia for cardiac catheterization
4. Why are both the ICD-9 and CPT codes updated each year?
5. What three main changes in coding will be included in the ICD-10-CM revision?
6. What is the value of modifiers in coding?

## Critical Thinking Questions

1. What is the proper order in which to select a diagnosis code?
2. What are some of the possible consequences of inaccurate coding and incorrect billing?
3. Why is accurate coding important to the financial management of a medical practice?
4. How can improving physicians' documentation of diagnoses and procedures help ensure compliance?
5. A patient asked a medical assistant to help her out of a tough financial spot. Her medical insurance authorized her to receive four radiation treatments for her condition, one every 35 days. Because she was out of town, she did not schedule her appointment for the last treatment until today, which is 1 week beyond the approved period. The health plan will not reimburse her for this procedure. The patient asks the MA to change the date on the record to last Wednesday so that it will be covered, explaining that no one will be hurt by this change, and anyway, she pays the insurance company plenty.

   What type of action is the patient asking the MA to do? How should the request be handled?
6. What does the existence of a compliance plan in the workplace indicate about the medical practice?

## Application Activities

1. A. A female patient is taking a medication that is known to affect the lining of the endometrium. She received an endometrial biopsy and pelvic ultrasound to monitor changes. What type of ICD-9 code is used to describe the medical need for these services?

   B. A patient fell off a ladder while on the job, spraining his left ankle and fracturing the right femur. In addition to the main code, what type of ICD-9 code is used to report his diagnosis?
2. Review Figure 16-2. What is the correct code for nail debridement?
3. Underline the main term in each of the following diagnoses and then determine the correct ICD-9 codes.
   a. Cerebral atherosclerosis
   b. Spasmodic asthma with status asthmaticus
   c. Congenital night blindness
   d. Recurrent inguinal hernia with obstruction
   e. Incomplete bundle branch heart block

4. Find the following codes in the index of CPT. Underline the key term you used to find the code.
   a. Intracapsular lens extraction
   b. Coombs test
   c. X-ray of duodenum
   d. Unlisted procedure, maxillofacial prosthetics
   e. DTAP immunization
5. Review Table 16-1, Tabular List Organization. What is the category number range for congenital abnormalities?
6. According to Figure 16-1, the ICD Alphabetic Index and Tabular List, what is the diagnosis code for Trichocephalus infestation?
7. According to Figure 16-3, the superbill with procedure codes, what is the correct code for a detailed evaluation of a new patient?

## Virtual Fieldtrip

*Visit the McGraw-Hill Higher Education Medical Assisting website at www.mhhe.com/medicalassisting3 to complete the following activity:*

Use the American Association of Medical Assistants and other websites related to medical practice coding.

Prepare an oral presentation about one of the following topics:

- Code structuring
- The Alphabetic Index and its use
- The Tabular List and its use
- Special codes such as V codes and E codes
- A career in medical billing

Ask your instructor how many references and citations you should minimally include in your research. Present your report to the class, using all available multimedia including PowerPoint slides or an overhead projector if possible.

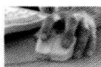 Open the CD and complete this chapter's practice activities, play the games, listen to the key terms, and test yourself with the interactive review. E-mail, print, and/or save your results to document your proficiency.

# Patient Billing and Collections

## KEY TERMS

accounts payable (A/P)
accounts receivable (A/R)
age analysis
charge slip
class action lawsuit
credit
credit bureau
cycle billing
damages
disclosure statement
encounter form
legal custody
open-book account
punitive damages
single-entry account
statement
statute of limitations
superbill
written-contract account

## MEDICAL ASSISTING COMPETENCIES

*In preparation for the certification examination, you should know the following areas of competence:*

| COMPETENCY | CMA | RMA |
|---|:---:|:---:|
| **Administrative** | | |
| Perform basic clerical skills | X | X |
| Prepare, organize, and maintain medical records | X | X |
| Maintain accounts payable and receivable | X | X |
| Perform billing and collection procedures | X | X |
| Post adjustments | X | X |
| Process a credit balance | X | X |
| Process refunds | X | X |
| Post collection agency payments | X | X |
| Be aware of and perform within legal and ethical boundaries | X | X |
| Determine the needs for documentation and reporting, and document accurately and appropriately | X | X |
| Utilize computer software and electronic technology to maintain office systems | X | X |

## CHAPTER OUTLINE

- Basic Accounting
- Standard Payment Procedures
- Standard Billing Procedures
- Standard Collection Procedures
- Credit Arrangements
- Common Collection Problems

## LEARNING OUTCOMES

After completing Chapter 17, you will be able to:

17.1 Discuss the importance of accounts receivable to a medical practice.
17.2 Explain how to accept and account for payment from patients.
17.3 Prepare an invoice.
17.4 Manage a billing cycle efficiently.
17.5 Describe standard collection techniques.
17.6 Explain how to perform a credit check.
17.7 Identify credit arrangements.
17.8 Recognize common collection problems.

# Introduction

Medical assisting is a multifaceted career. As such, a person in that career may be required to take on many duties in the medical office that are administrative in nature. The medical office has customers who have various payment arrangements, such as third-party payers (usually insurance carriers) and payment plans, and who may also have large outstanding balances. A proper understanding and administration of billing—for both third-party payers and patients—as well as payment collection methods is therefore required.

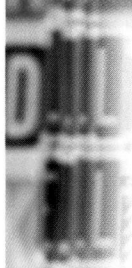

## CASE STUDY

One of the patients in your medical office has an insurance plan that covers 95% of his charges. He has already paid his yearly deductible of $200 for this year. He came into the physician's office to receive physical therapy three times a week for one week. Each visit is charged at $42.

As you read this chapter, consider the following questions:

1. What is the total owed for this patient's visits?
2. How much of the total, if any, is not covered by insurance and should be billed to the patient?

# Basic Accounting

In any business, basic accounting involves managing accounts receivable and accounts payable. **Accounts receivable (A/R)** is the term for income, or money, owed to the business. **Accounts payable (A/P)** is the term for money owed by the business. In a medical practice, accounts receivable represents the money patients owe in return for medical services. Accounts payable describes the money the medical practice must pay out to run the practice.

Billing and collections are vitally important tasks because they convert the practice's accounts receivable into readily available income, or cash flow, from which the accounts payable can be paid. Unless billing and collections are carried out effectively, a practice might have plenty of money due in accounts receivable without having enough cash flow for accounts payable.

There are methods of improving billing and collection procedures to increase income for the practice. You will need to know about standard payment, billing, and collection procedures as well as about credit arrangements and common problems in collecting payment.

# Standard Payment Procedures

Most physicians prefer to collect payment from patients at each office visit. Immediate payment not only brings income into the practice faster, but it saves the cost of preparing and mailing bills and collecting on past-due accounts. For these reasons, many physicians' offices post a small sign at the reception desk that states, for example, "Payment is requested when services are rendered unless other arrangements are made in advance."

As a medical assistant, you are responsible for collecting these payments. If the patient cannot pay at the time of the visit, it is your responsibility to bill for the physician's services. A bill, the paperwork sent to patients to inform them of payment or balance due, is referred to as an invoice.

# Determining Appropriate Fees

A fee schedule is a price list for the medical practice. Figure 17-1 shows an example. The fee schedule lists the services the doctor offers and the corresponding charges for those services. Fees are not randomly assigned. They reflect the cost of services, the doctor's experience, charges of other doctors in the area, and other factors. Sometimes the fee allowed by insurance policies is a determining factor. The practice may use a particular system to determine how much to charge for each service. Following are descriptions of these systems.

**Usual and Customary Fees.**  A usual fee is the fee a doctor charges for a service or procedure. A customary fee is either the average fee charged for a service or procedure by all comparable doctors in the same region or the 90th percentile of all fees charged by comparable doctors in the same region for the same procedure. There is a growing tendency, however, to determine fees by national rather than regional trends.

**Relative Value Unit.**  Section 121 of the Social Security Act Amendments of 1994 required CMS to develop a methodology for a resource-based system. This system was created to determine practice expense relative value units (RVUs) for all Medicare physician fee schedule services. Effective January 1, 1999, Phase 1 of resource-based practice expense was put into effect.

## John Q. Davis, MD

### Adult and Pediatric Urology-Infertility

| SERVICE RENDERED | CPT | FEE | SERVICE RENDERED | CPT | FEE |
|---|---|---|---|---|---|
| Initial OV | 99204 | $100.00 | Condyloma Treatment | 54050 | $40.00 |
| Follow-up Visit | 99214 | $65.00 | Cystoscopy | 52000 | $300.00 |
| Fertility Consultation | 99243 | $140.00 | Catheterization | 93975 | $45.00 |
| Office Consultation | 99244 | $140.00 | Vasectomy | 55250 | $775.00 |
| Hospital Admission | 99223 | $150.00 | Ultrasonic Guide Needle Biopsy | 76942 | $395.00 |
| Hospital Consultation | 99254 | $150.00 | | | |
| ER Visit | 99284 | $75.00–$150.00 | Prostate Biopsy | 55700 | $325.00 |
| | | | Biopsy Gun | A9270 | $45.00 |
| Hospital Visit | 99232 | $55.00 | Uroflowmeter | 51741 | $80.00 |
| Urinalysis w/ Micro | 81000 | $14.00 | Renal Ultrasound | 76775 | $295.00 |
| Culture | 87086 | $45.00 | Scrotal Ultrasound | 76870 | $295.00 |
| Stone Analysis | 32360 | $60.00 | Acidic Acid | 99070 | $20.00 |
| Venipuncture | 36415 | $10.00 | Foley Catheter Starter Set | A4329 | $35.00 |

**Figure 17-1.** The fee schedule shows the charges for services provided by the practice.

For each medical service, an RVU is assigned that reflects the following factors:

- The doctor's skill and time required
- The professional liability expenses related to that service, such as malpractice insurance
- The overhead costs associated with that service

The RVUs are converted to dollar amounts. These dollar amounts form the basis of the RVU fee schedule. This schedule creates uniform payments that are adjusted for geographic differences.

This methodology has reduced the growth rate of spending for doctors' professional services, related services and supplies, and other Medicare Part B services.

## Processing Charge Slips

Fees must be determined in order to create a **charge slip,** the original record of the doctor's services and the charges for those services. Figure 17-2 shows an example of a charge slip. Charge slips are also called fee slips or transaction slips. They are usually numbered consecutively. They may be preprinted with common services and charges for the practice. Charge slips are used in several ways.

Some doctors keep a pad of charge slips on their desk. After seeing a patient, they fill in the services and charges on the charge slip. They give the charge slip to the patient and ask the patient to give it to you on the way out of the office.

In other offices, you may write the patient's name on the charge slip and give the slip to the doctor along with the patient's medical record. The doctor then fills in the services performed and asks you to fill in the charges according to the fee schedule. If questions arise about the fee for a particular service, you can refer to the fee schedule and tell the patient how much that service will cost.

## Accepting Payment

When the patient comes to you with the charge slip, you complete the charge slip and ask for payment. There are several effective yet diplomatic ways to request payment. Two examples are, "For today's visit, the total charge is $50. How would you like to pay?" and "The charge for your laboratory work today is $80. Would you like to pay for that now?" The first example is the preferred method because in the second example, asking the patient if he would like to pay for the service now leaves him open to say, "No, bill me," which will slow your cash flow and cost the practice the expense of sending an invoice. Most practices accept several forms of

| DATE | DESCRIPTION–CODE | CHARGE | PAYMENT | CURRENT BALANCE |
|------|------------------|--------|---------|-----------------|

(918) 555-9680                                          Tax ID No. 11-0004004

*Patricia Belden, MD*
111 Roosevelt Boulevard
Lawrence, OK 77527

| 99205 | Office Visit, New Patient | 36425 | Venipuncture | 59025 | NST |
| 99215 | Office Visit, Established Patient | 57454 | Colposcopy with Biopsy | 54150 | Circumcision |
| 99213 | Office Visit, Established, Brief | 57511 | Cryosurgery | 58300 | IUD Insertion |
| 88155 | Pap | 58100 | Endometrial Biopsy | 57170 | Diaphragm Fitting |
| 84703 | Urine Pregnancy Test | 56600 | Vulva Biopsy | | |

NAME _____ DX _____      No. 0005807

**Figure 17-2.** A charge slip shows the services performed for a patient and the charges for those services.

payment, including cash, check, debit card, credit card, and insurance. Insurance payment is discussed in detail in Chapter 15.

**Cash.** If the patient chooses to pay in cash, count the money carefully to be sure you have received the proper amount. Next, record the payment on the patient's ledger card and give the patient a receipt. (Patient ledger cards are explained in Chapter 18.)

Some practices use a combination charge slip/receipt, known as a superbill, which is discussed later in the chapter. If your practice does not, prepare a cash receipt manually, as shown in Figure 17-3. Then place the money in the cash drawer or cash box.

**Check.** If the patient pays by check, be sure the check is written properly, including the current date. The amount of the check should match the total amount listed on the charge slip, unless the patient has made prior arrangements to pay only part of the amount. The name of the doctor or practice should appear in the "Pay to the Order of" section and should be properly spelled. The check should be signed by the person whose name is printed on the check. After accepting the check, endorse it immediately, and deposit it in the practice bank account. If a check is returned for insufficient funds, notify the patient immediately, asking for payment in full by another payment method. It is acceptable to also charge the patient an additional fee for the inconvenience and expense of processing the bad check. Most offices then see that patient on a *cash only* basis unless the patient can provide a current credit card.

**Debit Card.** Some patients may pay through the use of a debit card. A debit card looks like a credit card but is used differently. When the patient presents a debit card for payment, he is allowing the immediate removal of funds from his checking or savings account to the account of the practice. If there are insufficient funds in the patient's account to cover the payment, it is known immediately and other arrangements can be made with the patient. A debit card is processed much like a credit card. It is read by swiping it through an electronic reader that transmits the information to the patient's bank or credit union. The patient must input his PIN (personal identification number), which is a four-digit number, to release the funds for transfer.

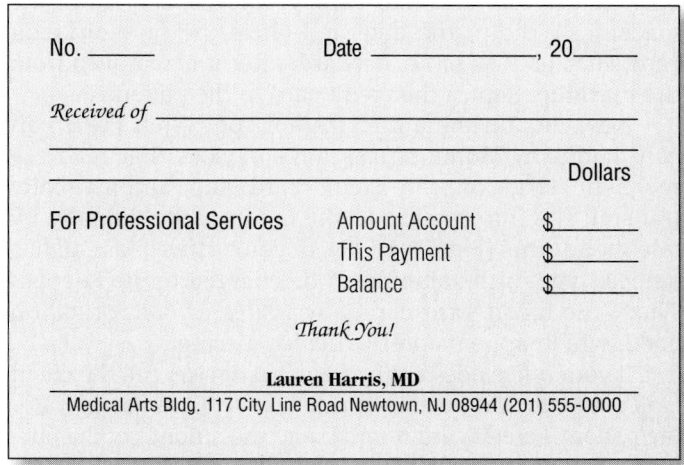

**Figure 17-3.** After writing a receipt for cash, record the payment on the patient's ledger card.

**Credit Card.** Many doctors' offices accept credit cards, such as Visa or MasterCard. This payment method offers advantages for both the practice and the patient. For the practice, it provides prompt payment from the credit card company, thus increasing cash flow. It also reduces the amount of time and money spent on preparing and mailing invoices, thus decreasing expenses. For the patient, it is convenient and allows a large bill to be paid in several smaller amounts, usually once a month.

Credit cards have one major disadvantage for the practice—cost. The credit card company deducts a percentage of each charge for its collection service, usually between 1% and 5%. If a patient charges $100 in services on a credit card, for example, the practice receives only $95 to $99. The credit card company keeps the difference. A disadvantage for patients is the accrued interest charges on unpaid balances.

If the practice accepts credit card payments, the American Medical Association (AMA) suggests several guidelines.

- Do not set higher fees for patients who pay by credit card.
- Do not encourage patients to use credit cards for payment.
- Do not advertise outside the office that the practice accepts credit cards.

If a patient chooses to pay by credit card, process the transaction carefully to ensure that the credit card company charges the patient correctly. To begin, inform the patient of the amount due and ask for the credit card.

Check the expiration date on the front of the credit card. If the card has expired, it cannot be used for payment. If the card has not expired, it may be swiped through an electronic reader or recorded through the use of a credit card machine that mechanically records the information on the card. To operate a credit card machine, place the credit card in the machine and place a credit card voucher on top of it. Slide the imprint arm firmly to the right and back across the machine. Remove the voucher from the machine. Write in the date and circle the type of credit card, such as Visa or MasterCard, after it is removed from the machine. Return the credit card to the patient.

Next, obtain the authorization code from the credit card company. Some offices have devices that read the magnetic strip on the credit card and automatically transmit the information to the credit card company by telephone line (Figure 17-4). If your office has such a device, type in the amount to be charged on its keypad. Then, the credit card company issues an authorization code, which appears on the device's screen.

If your office does not have such a device, call the credit card company for the authorization code. Give the operator the patient's credit card number and the amount of the payment. The operator then gives you the authorization code.

Write the authorization code in the box marked "Authorization" on the credit card voucher. Initial the

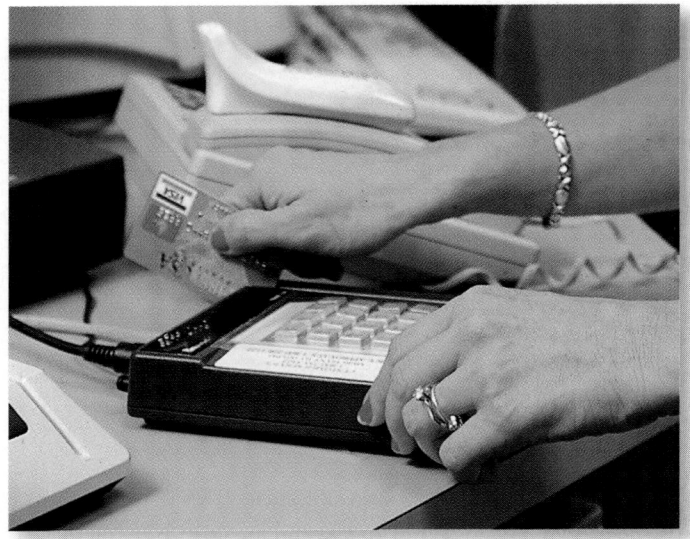

**Figure 17-4.** Using a device like this one, you can swipe the patient's card through the machine and obtain instant authorization from the credit card company.

voucher in the appropriate box. Then, fill in the services provided and the amount of the charges. Enter the total charges in the box marked "Total."

Give the voucher to the patient to sign. Compare the patient's signature on the voucher with the signature on the back of the credit card (they should, of course, be identical). Keep one copy of the voucher for the office. Give the other copy and the credit card to the patient.

## Using the Pegboard System for Posting Payments

While not often used, some physicians' offices still use the pegboard system to post payments and generate receipts for patients. If your office uses the pegboard system, you may use the pegboard to record the payment on the ledger card and receipt simultaneously. You handle this task in basically the same way, whether the patient pays immediately or later, in response to a bill. (See Chapter 18 for more information about pegboard systems.)

## Determining Payment Responsibility

Generally the patient is responsible for payments for medical services. To help promote timely payments, however, you need to know exactly who is responsible for them.

**Third-Party Liability.** Third-party liability refers to the responsibility of the patient's insurance company to pay for certain medical expenses, which may include doctors' services. Each practice decides how to handle its patients' health insurance claims.

Some practices do not accept any insurance, although these practices are rare. The patient must pay the doctor directly and file an insurance claim for reimbursement. If you work in such a practice, you must give the patient the necessary medical information to fill out the insurance claim. A completed superbill or encounter form (discussed later in this chapter) provides the information.

Practices increasingly handle all their patients' insurance paperwork to ensure accuracy, timely submission, and prompt payment. Some practices charge a fee for handling patients' insurance claims, although for some insurance plans such as Medicare, participating providers are required to submit claim forms except under very specific circumstances. Some practices handle paperwork only for patients who find it particularly difficult, such as those who are frail or disabled.

If you work in an office that handles insurance paperwork, you can submit insurance claims manually or electronically. Regardless of which method you use, be sure to use the proper forms, complete them correctly, and submit them within the time limits set by insurers to ensure timely and accurate reimbursement. (Procedures for completing insurance forms and filing claims are discussed in Chapter 15.)

TRICARE, which provides health insurance for dependents of active-duty and retired military personnel, operates differently from other insurers. TRICARE pays the doctor through a local fiscal agent. Patients pay any copayments and deductible amounts. You must adjust for the difference between the billed fees and the amounts received from TRICARE and the patient (known as the allowed or approved amount). If a TRICARE patient fails to pay the patient's portion, you may take steps to obtain payment just as you would with any other patient.

**Responsibility for Minors.**　When a child's parents are married, either parent may consent (agree) to treatment for the minor child (child younger than age 18). Both parents are responsible for payment for the minor's treatment. If you must send them a bill, you should address it to both parents to ensure payment. There is one exception to this process. Anyone younger than the age of 18 who is no longer living at home and is self-supporting is considered an emancipated minor and is responsible for payment. For example, a 16-year-old girl who is pregnant and leaves her parents' home to set up a household with her boyfriend is considered an emancipated minor. In addition to this example, emancipation may also occur if a minor is in the military, is married, or obtains a court order.

Divorce or separation can create confusion about which parent can consent to the child's treatment and which of the two is responsible for payment. The parent who has **legal custody,** or the court-decreed right to make decisions about a child's upbringing, is the parent who has consent ability and payment responsibility. A divorced couple's legal and financial arrangements are considered private information, however. Therefore, you should assume that the parent who brings the child for treatment has consent ability and payment responsibility. The physician should inform the responsible parent of this assumption before providing treatment. Occasionally, a custodial parent brings in a minor for care and states that the other parent is responsible for medical bills. Any time someone states that someone else is responsible for his or her bill, it is important to have documentation to support the claim. Otherwise, if the office policy is that payment is due at the time of service, whoever brings the child in for treatment should expect to pay for the service at the time of the visit. Some practices have a policy of asking for a copy of the divorce agreement so that proof of responsibility for payment can be filed in the patient record. It is important to know the policy of your medical practice.

**Responsibility for Elderly Patients and Patients With Disabilities.**　Sometimes elderly patients or patients with disabilities are brought in for medical care. The medical assistant may be asked to send the bill to another party. In general, it is considered good practice to request proof of legal guardianship before sending the bill to another person. Always check your medical practice's policies to learn how to handle these situations correctly and confidentially.

**Overpayments.**　Occasionally an overpayment is discovered. If this occurs, check the remittance advice carefully in the insurance and patient responsibility areas. If funds are owed to the patient, make an adjustment to her account noting the overpayment and issue a check to the patient. If the insurance carrier made the overpayment, contact them. Often the carrier will simply decrease the next payment made to the physician in the amount of the overpayment. The account with the overpayment is then debited by that amount and the appropriate patient's account is credited for the amount of the overpayment.

**Professional Courtesy.**　As a matter of professional courtesy, a doctor may treat some patients free of charge or for just the amount covered by the patient's insurance. These patients often include other doctors and their families, the practice's staff members (including medical assistants) and their families, other health-care professionals (including pharmacists and dentists), clergy members, and hospital employees. If the patient is part of a managed care organization or has Medicare, the provider must collect any copayment or deductible as part of the contracted agreement with the insurance carrier. It is considered fraud to consistently not collect copayments or deductibles if the collection of such payments is stipulated in the provider-insurer contract.

Be sure you know the doctor's policy so that you do not bill these patients in error. If, for example, the doctor agrees to accept only the amount paid by the patient's insurance, note this professional courtesy on the patient's ledger card and do not request payment from the patient.

# Standard Billing Procedures

If the physician extends credit to patients, you need to know how to prepare invoices. You also have to manage related billing responsibilities, such as establishing and maintaining billing cycles.

## Preparing Invoices

As a medical assistant, part of your job may be to prepare an invoice to mail to the patient who does not pay when services are rendered or who makes only a partial payment. Figure 17-5 shows an invoice with an itemized list of services. You can obtain most of the information for the invoice from the patient ledger card. The invoice should include the following information:

- Physician's name, address, and telephone number
- Patient's name and address
- Balance (if any) from the previous month(s)
- Itemized list of services and charges, by date, for the current month
- Payments from the patient or insurer during the month
- Total balance due

Whatever invoicing procedure you use, enclose a self-addressed envelope with the invoice to encourage prompt payment. Some offices have found that using a lightly colored return envelope, such as pale yellow, actually encourages faster payment because the color stands out against the usual white envelopes, jogging the patient's memory to "pay that one."

**Using Codes on the Invoice.** Write the name of each procedure on the itemized list, or use abbreviations for common procedures, such as OV for office visit. If you use abbreviations, be sure that an explanation of the abbreviations appears with the invoice. (Many practices use invoices with a key to the abbreviations printed at the bottom.) Using an itemized list on invoices is standard procedure in most physicians' offices and is required by all health insurance plans. After completing the invoice, fold it in thirds, and mail it in a typewritten or window business envelope.

**Using the Patient's Ledger Card as an Invoice.** A common alternative to writing or typing the invoice, you may photocopy the patient's ledger card and fold the photocopy so that the patient's address shows through the window in a window envelope. If you prepare invoices this way, be sure there are no stray marks or comments written on the card. Also, be sure the photocopy is clean and easy to read.

**Generating the Invoice by Computer.** In computerized offices, you may print out an invoice for each patient account that has a balance due. Follow the instructions in the software manufacturer's manual. You can then fold the printouts and mail them in window envelopes.

**Using an Independent Billing Service.** Large practices may have invoices handled by an independent billing service. The billing service may rapidly copy ledger cards or produce computer-generated invoices from the office computer for patients with balances due. Then it mails the invoices to patients, usually with an envelope for sending payment directly to the physician's office.

**Sending Claims Electronically to Insurance Companies.** Claims to insurance companies may be prepared by hand using paper claims or physicians' offices that have a computer and modem may bill insurance companies electronically, as discussed in Chapter 15.

## Using the Superbill

Some doctors' offices use a **superbill,** which includes the charges and procedure codes (CPT) for services rendered on that day, including appropriate diagnoses and codes (ICD-9), an invoice for payment or insurance copayment, and all the information for submitting an insurance claim. In many facilities, the superbill is also known an **encounter form.** Figure 17-6 shows an example of a superbill. Having all this information on one form saves time and paperwork. These forms are often printed on NCR (no-carbon-required) paper with copies for the practice, patient, and insurance company. Encounter forms can also be generated and transmitted electronically as part of electronic health records.

Complete as much of the superbill as possible at the beginning of the patient's visit. (See Procedure 17-1 for specific instructions.) Some practices use a computerized version of the superbill, printing it out instead of completing the initial information by hand. Attach the superbill to the patient's medical record, and give them both to the doctor before he sees the patient. The doctor circles or checks the appropriate procedures and diagnoses after seeing the patient and it is returned to the front desk to begin the billing cycle.

## Managing Billing Cycles

Many practices send out their bills just after the end of each month. You can send out bills at any regular time, however, such as once a week or twice a month. You may also send bills at a particular time of the month at the patient's request.

**Cycle billing** is a common billing system that bills each patient only once a month but spreads the work of billing over the month. Using this system, you send invoices to groups of patients every few days.

For example, you may bill on the fifth of the month for patients whose last names begin with A through D. Then, on the tenth of the month, you may bill patients whose names begin with E through H, and so on. In a larger office with more patients, you may prefer to bill more frequently but to smaller groups of patients.

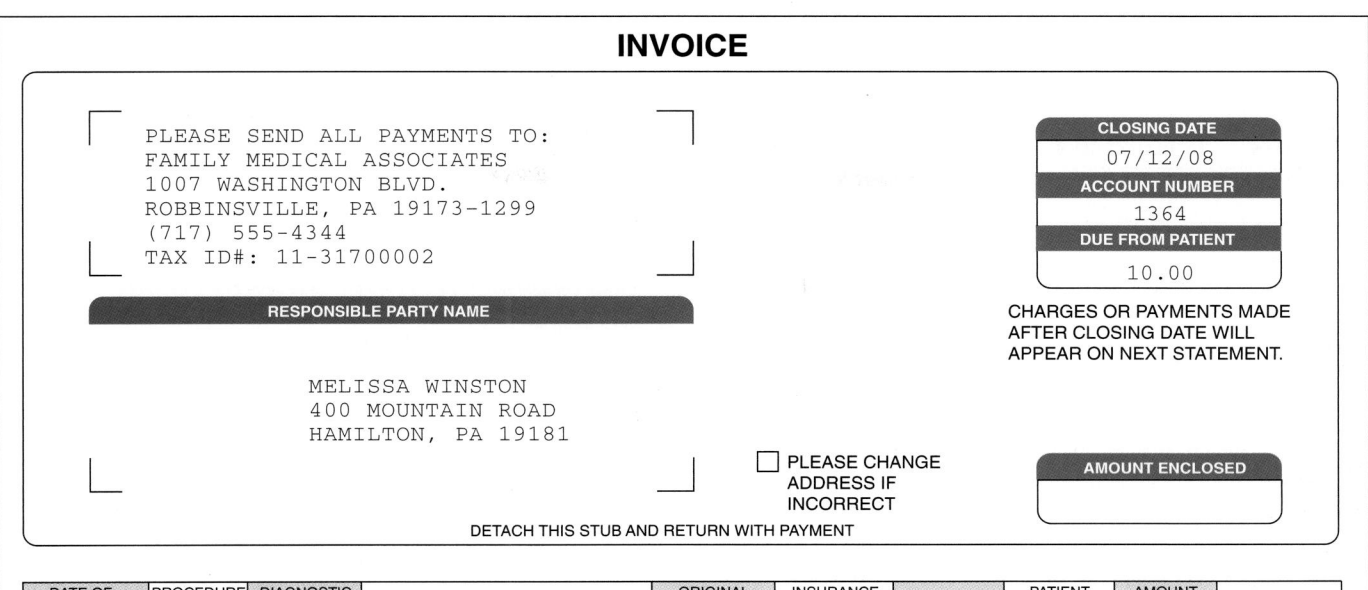

# INVOICE

PLEASE SEND ALL PAYMENTS TO:
FAMILY MEDICAL ASSOCIATES
1007 WASHINGTON BLVD.
ROBBINSVILLE, PA 19173-1299
(717) 555-4344
TAX ID#: 11-31700002

| CLOSING DATE |
| --- |
| 07/12/08 |
| **ACCOUNT NUMBER** |
| 1364 |
| **DUE FROM PATIENT** |
| 10.00 |

CHARGES OR PAYMENTS MADE
AFTER CLOSING DATE WILL
APPEAR ON NEXT STATEMENT.

**RESPONSIBLE PARTY NAME**

MELISSA WINSTON
400 MOUNTAIN ROAD
HAMILTON, PA 19181

☐ PLEASE CHANGE
ADDRESS IF
INCORRECT

**AMOUNT ENCLOSED**

DETACH THIS STUB AND RETURN WITH PAYMENT

| DATE OF SERVICE | PROCEDURE CODE | DIAGNOSTIC CODE | SERVICE DESCRIPTION | ORIGINAL CHARGE | INSURANCE PAID | ADJ. | PATIENT PAID | AMOUNT DUE | DUE FROM |
| --- | --- | --- | --- | --- | --- | --- | --- | --- | --- |
| 5/13/08 | 99213 | 473.9 | EXT PAT-INTER | 50.00 | 40.00 | .00 | .00 | 10.00 | PAT |
| 5/13/08 | 92567 | 473.9 | TYMPANOGRAM | 35.00 | 35.00 | .00 | .00 | .00 | INS |
| 5/02/08 | 99203 | 706.2 | NEW PAT-INTER | 80.00 | 70.00 | .00 | 10.00 | .00 | INS |

PLEASE NOTE: ANY BALANCE NOW DUE BY THE PATIENT HAS BEEN SUBMITTED TO
THE PATIENT'S INSURANCE (IF ANY) AND PROCESSED AND IS NOW THE
RESPONSIBILITY OF THE PATIENT.

| ACCOUNT NO. | SOCIAL SECURITY # | CURRENT | OVER 30 DAYS | OVER 60 DAYS | OVER 90 DAYS | OVER 120 DAYS | INSURANCE PENDING | DUE FROM PATIENT |
| --- | --- | --- | --- | --- | --- | --- | --- | --- |
| 1364 | 140-62-0000 | 10.00 | .00 | .00 | .00 | .00 | .00 | 10.00 |

**Figure 17-5.** The invoice shows an itemized list of services and charges, organized by date, for the current month.

# Lakeridge Medical Group
## 262 East Pine Street, Suite 100
## Santa Cruz, CA 95062

☐ **PRIVATE**  ☐ **BLUECROSS**  ☐ **IND.**  ☐ **MEDICARE**  ☐ **MEDI-CAL**  ☐ **HMO**  ☐ **PPO**

| PATIENT'S LAST NAME | FIRST | ACCOUNT # | BIRTHDATE / / | SEX ☐ MALE ☐ FEMALE | TODAY'S DATE / / |
|---|---|---|---|---|---|
| INSURANCE COMPANY | SUBSCRIBER | | PLAN # | SUB. # | GROUP |

| ASSIGNMENT: I hereby assign my insurance benefits to be paid directly to the undersigned physician. I am financially responsible for non-covered services. SIGNED: (Patient, or Parent, if Minor)   DATE: / / | RELEASE: I hereby authorize the physician to release to my insurance carrers any information required to process this claim. SIGNED: (Patient, or Parent, if Minor)   DATE: / / |
|---|---|

| ✔ | DESCRIPTION | M/Care | CPT/Mod | DxRe | FEE | ✔ | DESCRIPTION | M/Care | CPT/Mod | DxRe | FEE | ✔ | DESCRIPTION | M/Care | CPT/Mod | DxRe | FEE |
|---|---|---|---|---|---|---|---|---|---|---|---|---|---|---|---|---|---|
| | OFFICE CARE | | | | | | PROCEDURES | | | | | | INJECTIONS/IMMUNIZATIONS | | | | |
| | NEW PATIENT | | | | | | Tread Mill (In Office) | | 93015 | | | | Tetanus | | 90718 | | |
| | Brief | | 99201 | | | | 24 Hour Holter | | 93224 | | | | Hypertet | J1670 | 90782 | | |
| | Limited | | 99202 | | | | If Medicare (Set up Fec) | | 93225 | | | | Pneumococcal | | 90732 | | |
| | Intermediate | | 99203 | | | | Physician Interpret | | 93227 | | | | Influenza | | 90724 | | |
| | Extended | | 99204 | | | | EKG w/Interpretation | | 93000 | | | | TB Skin Test (PPD) | | 86585 | | |
| | Comprehensive | | 99205 | | | | EKG (Medicare) | | 93005 | | | | Antigen Injection-Single | | 95115 | | |
| | | | | | | | Sigmoidoscopy | | 45300 | | | | Multiple | | 95117 | | |
| | ESTABLISHED PATIENT | | | | | | Sigmoidoscopy, Flexible | | 45330 | | | | B12 Injection | J3420 | 90782 | | |
| | Minimal | | 99211 | | | | Sigmoidos., Flex. w/Bx. | | 45331 | | | | Injection, IM | | 90782 | | |
| | Brief | | 99212 | | | | Spirometry, FEV/FVC | | 94010 | | | | Compazine | J0780 | 90782 | | |
| | Limited | | 99213 | | | | Spirometry, Post-Dilator | | 94060 | | | | Demerol | J2175 | 90782 | | |
| | Intermediate | | 99214 | | | | | | | | | | Vistaril | J3410 | 90782 | | |
| | Extended | | 99215 | | | | | | | | | | Susphrine | J0170 | 90782 | | |
| | Comprehensive | | 99215 | | | | LABORATORY | | | | | | Decadron | J0890 | 90782 | | |
| | | | | | | | Blood Draw Fee | | 36415 | | | | Estradiol | J1000 | 90782 | | |
| | CONSULTATION-OFFICE | | | | | | Urinalysis, Chemical | | 81005 | | | | Testosterone | J1080 | 90782 | | |
| | Focused | | 99241 | | | | Throat Culture | | 87081 | | | | Lidocaine | J2000 | 90782 | | |
| | Expanded | | 99242 | | | | Occult Blood | | 82270 | | | | Solumedrol | J2920 | 90782 | | |
| | Detailed | | 99243 | | | | Pap Handling Charge | | 99000 | | | | Solucortef | J1720 | 90782 | | |
| | Comprehensive 1 | | 99244 | | | | Pap Life Guard | | 88150-90 | | | | Hydeltra | J1690 | 90782 | | |
| | Comprehensive 2 | | 99245 | | | | Gram Stain | | 87205 | | | | Pen Procaine | J2510 | 90788 | | |
| | Dr. | | | | | | Hanging Drop | | 87210 | | | | | | | | |
| | Case Management | | 98900 | | | | Urine Drug Screen | | 99000 | | | | INJECTIONS - JOINT/BURSA | | | | |
| | | | | | | | | | | | | | Small Joints | | 20600 | | |
| | Post-op Exam | | 99024 | | | | SUPPLIES | | | | | | Intermediate | | 20605 | | |
| | | | | | | | | | | | | | Large Joints | | 20610 | | |
| | | | | | | | | | | | | | Trigger Point | | 20550 | | |
| | | | | | | | | | | | | | MISCELLANEOUS | | | | |

| DIAGNOSIS: | ICD-9 | | | | | | | | |
|---|---|---|---|---|---|---|---|---|---|
| __ Abdominal Pain | 789.0 | __ Gout | 274.0 | __ C.V.A. - Acute | 436. | __ Electrolyte Dis. | 276.9 | __ Herpes Simplex | 054.9 |
| __ Abscess (Site) | 682.9 | __ Asthma | 493.90 | __ Cere. Vas. Accid. (Old) | 438 | __ Fatigue | 780.7 | __ Herpes Zoster | 053.9 |
| __ Adverse Drug Rx | 995.2 | __ Asthmatic Bronchitis | 493.90 | __ Cerumen | 380.4 | __ Fibrocys. Br. Dis | 610.1 | __ Hydrocele | 603.9 |
| __ Alcohol Detox | 291.8 | __ Atrial Fib. | 427.31 | __ Chestwall Pain | 786.59 | __ Fracture (Site) | 829.0 | __ Hyperlipidemia | 272.4 |
| __ Alcoholism | 303.90 | __ Atrial Tachi. | 427.0 | __ Cholecystitis | 575.0 | __ Open/Close | | __ Hypertension | 401.9 |
| __ Allergic Rhinitis | 477 | __ Bowel Obstruct. | 560.9 | __ Cholelithiasis | 574.00 | __ Fungal Infect. (Site) | 110.8 | __ Hyperthyroidism | 242.9 |
| __ Allergy | 995.3 | __ Breast Mass | 611.72 | __ COPD | 492.8 | __ Gastric Ulcer | 531.90 | __ Hypothyroidism | 244.9 |
| __ Alzheimer's Dis. | 290.1 | __ Bronchitis | 490 | __ Cirrhosis | 571.5 | __ Gastritis | 535.0 | __ Labyrinthitis | 386.30 |
| __ Anemia | 285.9 | __ Bursitis | 727.3 | __ Cong. Heart Fail. | 428.9 | __ Gastroenteritis | 558.9 | __ Lipoma (Site) | 214.9 |
| __ Anemia - Pernicious | 281.0 | __ Cancer, Breast (Site) | 174.9 | __ Conjunctivitis | 372.30 | __ G.I. Bleeding | 578.9 | __ Lymphoma | 202.8 |
| __ Angina | 413.9 | __ Metastatic (Site) | 199.1 | __ Contusion (Site) | 924.9 | __ Glomerulonephritis | 583.9 | __ Mit. Valve Prolapse | 424.0 |
| __ Anxiety Synd. | 300.00 | __ Colon | 153.9 | __ Costochondritis | 733.99 | __ Headache | 784.0 | __ Myocard. Infarction (Area) | 410.9 |
| __ Appendicitis | 541 | __ Cancer, Rectal | 154.1 | __ Depression | 311. | __ Headache, Tension | 307.81 | __ M.I., Old | 412 |
| __ Arterioscl. H.D. | 414.0 | __ Lung (Site) | 162.9 | __ Dermatitis | 692.9 | __ Migraine (Type) | 346.9 | __ Myositis | 729.1 |
| __ Arthritis, Osteo. | 715.90 | __ Skin (Site) | 173.9 | __ Diabetes Mellitus | 250.00 | __ Hemorrhoids | 455.6 | __ Nausea/Vomiting | 787.0 |
| __ Rheumatoid | 714.0 | __ Card. Arrhythmia (Type) | 427.9 | __ Diabetic Ketosis | 250.1 | __ Hernia, Hiatal | 553.3 | __ Neuralgia | 729.2 |
| __ Lupus | 710.0 | __ Cardiomyopathy | 425.4 | __ Diverticulitis | 562.11 | __ Inguinal | 550.9 | __ Nevus (Site) | 216.9 |
| | | __ Cellulitis (Site) | 682.9 | __ Diverticulosis | 562.10 | __ Hepatitis | 573.3 | __ Obesity | 278.0 |

**DIAGNOSIS: (IF NOT CHECKED ABOVE)**

| SERVICES PERFORMED AT: ☐ Office ☐ E.R.  ☐ ☐  ☐ CLAIM CONTAINS NO ORDERED REFERRING SERVICE | REFERRING PHYSICIAN & I.D. NUMBER |
|---|---|

| RETURN APPOINTMENT INFORMATION: 5 - 10 - 15 - 20 - 30 - 40 - 60  [ DAYS] [ WKS.] [ MOS.] [ PRN] | NEXT APPOINTMENT M - T - W - TH - F - S  DATE / / TIME:  AM PM | ACCEPT ASSIGNMENT? ☐ YES ☐ NO | DOCTOR'S SIGNATURE |
|---|---|---|---|

| INSTRUCTIONS TO PATIENT FOR FILING INSURANCE CLAIMS: | ☐ CASH | TOTAL TODAY'S FEE | |
|---|---|---|---|
| 1. Complete upper portion of this form, sign and date. 2. Attach this form to your own insurance company's form for direct reimbursement. **MEDICARE PATIENTS - DO NOT SEND THIS TO MEDICARE. WE WILL SUBMIT THE CLAIM FOR YOU.** | ☐ CHECK #  ☐ VISA  ☐ MC  ☐ CO-PAY | OLD BALANCE  TOTAL DUE  AMOUNT REC'D. TODAY | |

INSUR-A-BILL ® BIBBERO SYSTEMS, INC. • PETALUMA, CA • UP. SUPER. © 6/94 (BIBB/STOCK)

**Figure 17-6.** A superbill is a form that can also be used as a charge slip and invoice, and can be submitted with insurance claims.

## How to Bill With the Superbill

**Procedure Goal:** To complete a superbill accurately

**Materials:** Superbill, patient ledger card, patient information sheet, fee schedule, insurance code list, pen

**Method:**

1. Make sure the doctor's name and address appear on the form.

   *Rationale*

   The doctor must have the superbill to add the charges and diagnoses for the visit.

2. From the patient ledger card and information sheet, fill in the patient data, such as name, sex, date of birth, and insurance information.

3. Fill in the place and date of service.

4. Attach the superbill to the patient's medical record, and give them both to the doctor.

   *Rationale*

   The doctor must have the superbill to add the charges for the day.

5. Accept the completed superbill from the patient after the patient sees the doctor. Make sure that the doctor has indicated the diagnosis and the procedures performed. Also make sure that an appropriate diagnosis is listed for each procedure.

   *Rationale*

   Ensures medical necessity for payment by the insurance carrier.

6. If the doctor has not already recorded the charges, refer to the fee schedule for procedures that are marked. Then fill in the charges next to those procedures.

   *Rationale*

   Each procedure must have a charge to ensure accurate billing.

7. In the appropriate blanks, list the total charges for the visit and the previous balance (if any).

8. Calculate the subtotal.

9. Fill in the amount and type of payment (cash, check, money order, or credit card) made by the patient during this visit.

   *Rationale*

   This helps to ensure accurate posting to the patient's account.

10. Calculate and enter the new balance.

11. Have the patient sign the authorization-and-release section of the superbill.

    *Rationale*

    Without this signature (or one on file), there is no permission to release information to the insurance carrier, nor is there agreement for the carrier to pay the provider directly.

12. Keep a copy of the superbill for the practice records. Give the original to the patient along with one copy to file with the insurer.

# Standard Collection Procedures

Although most patients pay invoices within the standard 30-day period, some do not. When a patient does not pay an invoice during the standard period, you need to take steps to collect the payment. For example, you may need to call or write the patient to determine the reason for non-payment or to set up a payment arrangement.

Whether you use telephone calls, notes, or letters, there are laws, such as statutes of limitations, and professional standards to guide your efforts to collect overdue payments from patients.

# State Statute of Limitations

A **statute of limitations** is a state law that sets a time limit on when a collection suit on a past-due account can legally be filed. The time limit varies with the type of account.

**Open-Book Account.** An **open-book account** is one that is open to charges made occasionally as needed. Most of a physician's long-standing patients have this type of account. An open-book account uses the last date of payment or charge for each illness as the starting date for determining the time limit on that specific debt.

**Written-Contract Account.** A **written-contract account** is one in which the physician and patient sign an agreement stating that the patient will pay the bill in more than four installments. Some states allow longer time limits for these accounts than for open-book accounts. Written-contract accounts are regulated by the Truth in Lending Act, discussed later in this chapter.

**Single-Entry Account.** A **single-entry account** is an account with only one charge, usually for a small amount. For example, someone vacationing in your area might come in for treatment of a cold. This person's account would list only one office visit. If the vacationer did not become a regular patient, the account would be considered a single-entry account. Some states impose shorter time limits on single-entry accounts than on open-book accounts.

## Using Collection Techniques

Individual practices have their own ways of approaching the task of collection. Most begin the process with telephone calls, letters, or statements.

**Initial Telephone Calls or Letters.** When calling a patient (or sending a letter) about collections, be friendly and sympathetic. (Do not call a patient at work and leave a message. That type of phone call is an invasion of privacy. Call the patient at home unless you have permission to call the patient at work and you have been unable to reach the patient at home.) The first phone call to the patient should occur if payment has not been received after 30–45 days (remember the patient received his first bill at the time of the visit, so the invoice received in the mail is essentially a second notice of payment due). Assume that the patient forgot to pay or was temporarily unable to pay. You should ask the patient for the full amount due. If the patient states that he cannot afford full payment, ask him what amount he feels could be sent (you should have a minimum amount in mind), and obtain a date you can expect to receive the payment. If you do not receive the payment within 24 hours of the stated date, an initial collection letter may be sent. This letter may need to be more urgent in tone because the patient did not respond to your phone call and the tone of any subsequent letters will be still more urgent. Standard collection letters, such as the one shown in Figure 17-7, are available for you to fill in the details, or you can create a letter to reflect the style of the practice.

**Preparing Statements.** You might send the patient a statement for an account that is 30 days past due. A **statement** is similar to an invoice except that it contains a courteous reminder that payment is due. This reminder can be a typewritten note on the statement, a brightly colored sticker, or a separate handwritten note attached to the statement.

If an account is 60 days past due, you could send a collection letter that says, for example, "If you are unable to pay your account in full this month, please telephone our office at (number) to make payment arrangements."

If an account is 90 days past due, your collection letter can contain stronger wording. For example, it might say, "Please let us know when you plan to pay the $250 past-due balance. We have sent you three monthly reminders. If you cannot pay in full now, please contact us at (number) to make payment arrangements. We want to be understanding but need your cooperation."

If an account is 120 days or more past due, you can send a final letter. It might state, "Every courtesy has been extended to you in arranging for payment of your long overdue account. Unless we hear from you by (date), the account will be given to (name of collection agency) for collection." Be sure to note the cutoff date on the patient's ledger card. By law, you cannot threaten to send an account to a collection agency unless it will actually be sent on that cutoff date. Therefore, you must be sure you are ready to do so before you send such a letter. This collection letter should be mailed by certified mail with return receipt so you have proof that the letter was sent and that the intended recipient received the letter.

If you still cannot collect payment, the physician may indeed choose to hire an outside collection agency. Once an agency has taken over the account, there should not be any more correspondence on this matter between the physician's office and the patient. If the patient contacts you or sends a payment after the account has been sent to collection, you are to refer the patient to the collection agency.

## Preparing an Age Analysis

**Age analysis** is the process of classifying and reviewing past-due accounts by age from the first date of billing. A monthly age analysis, such as that shown in Figure 17-8, helps you keep on top of past-due accounts and determine which ones need follow-up.

You can do an age analysis by computer (most computer programs generate one automatically) or by hand. An age analysis should list all patient account balances, when the charges originated, the most recent payment date, and any special notes concerning the account.

In a single doctor's office or a small group practice, information for the age analysis may come from the patient ledger cards. You may place color-coded tags on the patient ledger cards to indicate the number of days past due. For example, a yellow tag might be placed on the ledger card of an account that is 60 days past due. An orange tag might be used for an account that is 90 days past due. A red tag might be used for an account that is 120 days or more past due. In a large practice, however, age analysis is typically done on the computer. The use of patient ledger cards has been phased out as more practices have become computerized.

# City Medical Group

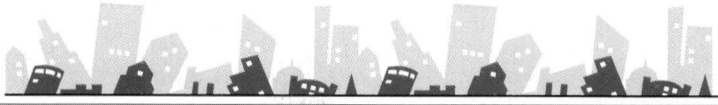

1234 Wayne Street
Smithtown, OR 93689
(503) 555-1217

**Internal Medicine**
Marianne Harris, MD
Karen Payne-Johnson, MD

May 5, 2008

Mr. J. J. Andrews
1414 First Avenue
Smithtown, OR 93668

Dear Mr. Andrews:

It has been brought to my attention that your account in the amount of <u>$240.00</u> is past due.

Normally at this time the account would be placed with a collection agency. However, we would prefer to hear from you regarding your preference in this matter.

(    )    Payment in full is enclosed.

(    )    Payment will be made in _____ days.

(    )    I would like to make regular weekly/monthly payments of $ _____ until this account is paid in full. My first payment is enclosed.

(    )    I would prefer that you assign this account to a collection agency for enforcement of collection. (Failure to return this letter within 30 days will result in this action.)

(    )    I don't believe I owe this amount for the following reason(s):

Signed: _____

Please indicate your preference and return this letter within 30 days. Please do not hesitate to call if you have any questions regarding this matter.

Sincerely,

Diana Sanchez
Office Manager

**Figure 17-7.** Standard collection letters are available for you to fill in the details.

# ACCOUNTS RECEIVABLE–AGE ANALYSIS

**Date:** October 1, 2008

| Patient | Balance | Date of Charges | Most Recent Payment | 30 days | 60 days | 90 days | 120 days | Remarks |
|---|---|---|---|---|---|---|---|---|
| Black, K. | 120.00 | 5/24 | 5/24 | | | 75.00 | 45.00 | 3rd Notice |
| Brown, R. | 65.00 | 8/30 | 8/30 | 65.00 | | | | |
| Green, C. | 340.00 | 8/25 | | | | | | Medicare filed |
| Jones, T. | 500.00 | 6/1 | 6/30 | | 125.00 | 125.00 | 250.00 | 3rd Notice |
| Perry, S. | 150.00 | 7/28 | 7/28 | 75.00 | 75.00 | | | 1st Notice |
| Smith, J. | 375.00 | 6/15 | 7/1 | | | 375.00 | | 2nd Notice |
| White, L. | 200.00 | 6/24 | 7/5 | 20.00 | 30.00 | 150.00 | | 2nd Notice |

**Figure 17-8.** An age analysis organizes past-due accounts by age.

## Following Laws That Govern Debt Collection

Federal and state laws govern debt collection. Table 17-1 outlines the penalties for violating laws that regulate credit and debt.

**Fair Debt Collection Practices Act of 1977.** This act (also called Public Law 95-109) governs the methods that can be used to collect unpaid debts. It prevents you from threatening to take an action either that is illegal or that you do not actually intend to take. The aim of this law is to eliminate abusive, deceptive, or unfair debt collection practices. For example, the law requires that after you have said you are going to give an account to a collection agency if it is not paid within 1 month, you must actually do so. Not doing what you threaten to do can be construed as harassment, and your practice can be liable for a harassment charge. Following are guidelines for sending letters and making calls requesting payment from patients.

- Do not call the patient before 8 A.M. or after 9 P.M. Calling outside those hours can be considered harassment.
- Do not make threats or use profane language. For example, do not state that an account will be given to a collection agency in 7 days if it will not be.
- Do not discuss the patient's debt with anyone except the person responsible for payment. If the patient is represented by a lawyer, discuss the problem only with the lawyer, unless the lawyer gives you permission to talk to the patient.
- Do not use any form of deception or violence to collect a debt. For example, do not pose as a government employee or other authority figure to try to force a debtor to pay.

## TABLE 17-1 Laws That Govern Credit and Collections

| Law | Requirements | Penalties for Breaking Law |
|-----|-------------|---------------------------|
| Equal Credit Opportunity Act (ECOA) | • Creditors may not discriminate against applicants on the basis of sex, marital status, race, national origin, religion, or age.<br>• Creditors may not discriminate because an applicant receives public assistance income or has exercised rights under the Consumer Credit Protection Act. | • If an applicant sues the practice for violating the ECOA, the practice may have to pay **damages** (money paid as compensation), penalties, lawyers' fees, and court costs.<br>• If an applicant joins a class action lawsuit against the practice, the practice may have to pay damages of up to $500,000 or 1% of the practice's net worth, whichever is less. (A **class action lawsuit** is a lawsuit in which one or more people sue a company that wronged all of them the same way.)<br>• If the Federal Trade Commission (FTC) receives many complaints from applicants stating that the practice violated the ECOA, the FTC may investigate and take action against the practice. |
| Fair Credit Reporting Act (FCRA) | • This act requires credit bureaus to supply correct and complete information to businesses to use in evaluating a person's application for credit, insurance, or a job. | • If one applicant sues the practice in federal court for violating the FCRA, the practice may have to pay damages, **punitive damages** (money paid as punishment for intentionally breaking the law), court costs, and lawyers' fees.<br>• If the FTC receives many complaints from applicants stating that the practice violated the FCRA, the FTC may investigate and take action against the practice. |
| Fair Debt Collection Practices Act (FDCPA) | • This act requires debt collectors to treat debtors fairly. It also prohibits certain collection tactics, such as harassment, false statements, threats, and unfair practices. | • If one debtor sues the practice in a state or federal court for violation of the FDCPA, the practice may have to pay damages, court costs, and lawyers' fees.<br>• If the debtor joins a class action suit against the practice, the practice may have to pay damages of up to $500,000 or 1% of the practice's net worth, whichever is less.<br>• If the FTC receives many complaints from debtors stating that the practice violated the FDCPA, the FTC may investigate and take action against the practice. |
| Truth in Lending Act (TLA) | • This act requires creditors to provide applicants with accurate and complete credit costs and terms, clearly and obviously. | • If one applicant sues the practice in a federal court for violation of the TLA, the practice may have to pay damages, court costs, and lawyers' fees.<br>• If the FTC receives many complaints from applicants stating that the practice violated the TLA, the FTC may investigate and take action against the practice. |

**Telephone Consumer Protection Act (TCPA) of 1991.** This act protects telephone subscribers from unwanted telephone solicitations, commonly known as telemarketing. The act prohibits autodialed calls to emergency service providers, cellular and paging numbers, and patients' hospital rooms. It prohibits prerecorded calls to homes without prior permission of the resident, and it prohibits unsolicited advertising via fax machine.

These regulations do not apply to people who have an established business relationship with the telemarketing firm or people who have previously given the telemarketing firm permission to call. The law also does not apply to

## Points on Practice

### Choosing a Collection Agency

If a patient does not respond to your final collection letter or has twice broken a promise to pay, the doctor may choose to seek the help of a collection agency. This step should be taken carefully, however. Some collection agencies use illegal and unethical tactics to obtain payment. For example, some collectors have made repeated, profane phone calls to frighten debtors. Others have threatened debtors with prison for nonpayment. A good collection agency reflects the humanitarian and ethical standards of the medical profession.

To help select an effective—and ethical—collection agency, ask for a referral from the doctor's colleagues, fellow specialists, or hospital associates. You may also contact one of the following organizations:

American Collectors Association International
ACA International
P.O. Box 390106
Minneapolis, MN 55439
(952) 926–6547

Medical Collection Agency
517 S. Livingston Ave.
Livingston, NJ 07039
Toll Free: 1-877-77-Collect
Phone: 1-973-740-0044
Fax: 1-973-740-1119

After obtaining a referral, contact the agency and request samples of its letters, reminder notices, and other print material for debtors. Be sure this material is courteous and reflects the way you would handle the collection. Also, be sure the agency uses a persuasive approach rather than simply suing debtors. Ask if the agency reports cases that deserve special consideration to the doctor's office.

Determine what methods the agency uses for out-of-town accounts. For example, it may use out-of-town services to help with those collections. Ask the agency about its collection percentage and fees for large, small, and out-of-town accounts. Be sure the percentages and fees are appropriate for the collection amounts.

After selecting a collection agency, supply all pertinent data to the agency, such as the patient's name, address, and full amount of the debt. Mark the patient's ledger card so that you do not call or write to the patient about the debt. If the patient contacts the office about the account, refer the patient to the collection agency.

If you receive any payments from the debtor, alert the collection agency immediately. (The agency takes a portion of any payments it collects.) Also, contact the agency if you learn anything new about the patient's address or employer.

telemarketing calls placed by tax-exempt nonprofit organizations, such as charities.

Although most provisions of this federal law do not apply to medical practices, you should be aware of the law. One way to avoid an unknowing violation of this law is to limit your calls to patients to the hours between 8 A.M. and 9 P.M. (some states, however, have exceptions for the TCPA provisions). Also, place your calls yourself. Do not use an automated dialing device for calls to patients.

## Observing Professional Guidelines for Finance Charges and Late Charges

According to the AMA, it is appropriate to assess finance charges or late charges on past-due accounts if the patient is notified in advance. Advance notice may be given by posting a sign at the reception desk, giving the patient a pamphlet describing the practice's billing practices, or including a note on the invoice.

The physician must adhere to federal and state guidelines that govern these charges. The physician should also use compassion and discretion when assigning charges, especially in hardship cases.

## Using Outside Collection Agencies

If your collection efforts do not result in payment, the doctor may wish to select a collection agency to manage the account. Because collection agencies keep a percentage of any funds they collect for their clients (usually between 40% and 60% of the collected amount), the office staff should use all reasonable methods to collect unpaid balances prior to sending an account to collection. Because doctors adhere to the humanitarian and ethical standards of the medical profession, they must be careful to avoid collection agencies that use harsh or harassing collection practices. The Points on Practice section gives information about selecting an outside collection agency.

When giving a patient's account to an agency, supply the following information about the patient:

- Full name and last known address
- Occupation and business address
- Name of spouse, if any
- Total debt
- Date of last payment or charge on the account
- Description of actions you took to collect the debt
- Responses to collection attempts

Color-coded tabs on the patient ledger cards make this information easy to gather. Note on the patient ledger card that the account has been given to a collection agency. When the agency reports progress toward a settlement, record that information on the card too.

After the account is given to the agency, do not send bills to or contact the patient in any way. If the patient wants to discuss payment, refer the patient to the agency. If the patient sends a payment, forward it to the agency; or, if the agency and the practice agree, keep the payment for the practice and forward the collection fee to the agency.

The arrangement with the agency should give the doctor the final word on the uncollected account. In other words, the doctor should decide whether to write off the debt or take the matter to court.

## Insuring Accounts Receivable

To protect the practice from lost income because of non-payment, the practice may buy accounts receivable insurance. One type of accounts receivable policy pays when a large number of patients do not pay and the physician must absorb the lost income. It protects the practice's cash flow and helps ensure that the practice will have sufficient income to cover expected expenses.

# Credit Arrangements

Sometimes a doctor agrees to extend credit to a patient who is unable to pay immediately. This situation is not uncommon when a patient's medical bills are high. By extending **credit,** the doctor gives the patient time to pay for services, which are provided on trust. If the doctor knows the patient well, she may offer credit without checking the patient's credit history. However, to avoid charges of discrimination under the Equal Credit Opportunity Act (ECOA), you will normally perform a credit check prior to extending credit. The ECOA is discussed in further detail later in the chapter.

## Performing a Credit Check

To perform a credit check, be sure you have the most current information. You will need the patient's address, telephone number, and Social Security number and the patient's employer's name, address, and telephone number. With this information you can verify employment and generate a credit bureau report.

**Employment Verification.** Explain to the patient that you will be calling his employer to verify employment. Many employers have someone designated to handle such calls. The patient may be able to give you that name before you call the place of employment.

After calling, record the updated information on the patient's registration card, along with any credit references you obtain from the patient.

**Credit Bureau Report.** A **credit bureau** is a company that provides information about the creditworthiness of a person seeking credit. If a patient's credit history is in question, you may request a report from a credit bureau. A sample credit report is shown in Figure 17-9. A credit bureau collects information about an individual's payment history on credit cards, student loans, and similar accounts. Three leading national credit bureaus are TRW Inc., Equifax Inc., and Trans Union Credit Information Company.

The physician may decide not to extend credit, based on the credit report. If so, the Fair Credit Reporting Act states that you must inform the patient in writing that credit was denied based on the credit report. You must also provide the name and address of the credit bureau; however, you do not need to discuss the information obtained from the report. The patient may contest the credit report and may correct any incorrect information the credit bureau may have. Once the information has been corrected, the provider may then decide to extend the patient credit.

## Following Laws Governing Extension of Credit

When you help the doctor decide whether to grant credit to a patient, you must comply with certain laws governing extension of credit.

**Equal Credit Opportunity Act.** This act states that credit arrangements may not be denied based on a patient's sex, race, religion, national origin, marital status, or age. Also, credit cannot be denied because the patient receives public assistance or has exercised rights under the Consumer Credit Protection Act, such as disputing a credit card bill or a credit bureau report.

Under the Equal Credit Opportunity Act, the patient has a right to know the specific reason that credit was denied. Some reasons might include having too little income or not being employed for a certain period of time. Vague reasons about not meeting minimum standards or not receiving enough points on a credit-scoring system are not acceptable.

**Truth in Lending Act.** This act is Regulation Z of the Consumer Credit Protection Act. The Truth in Lending Act covers credit agreements that involve more than four

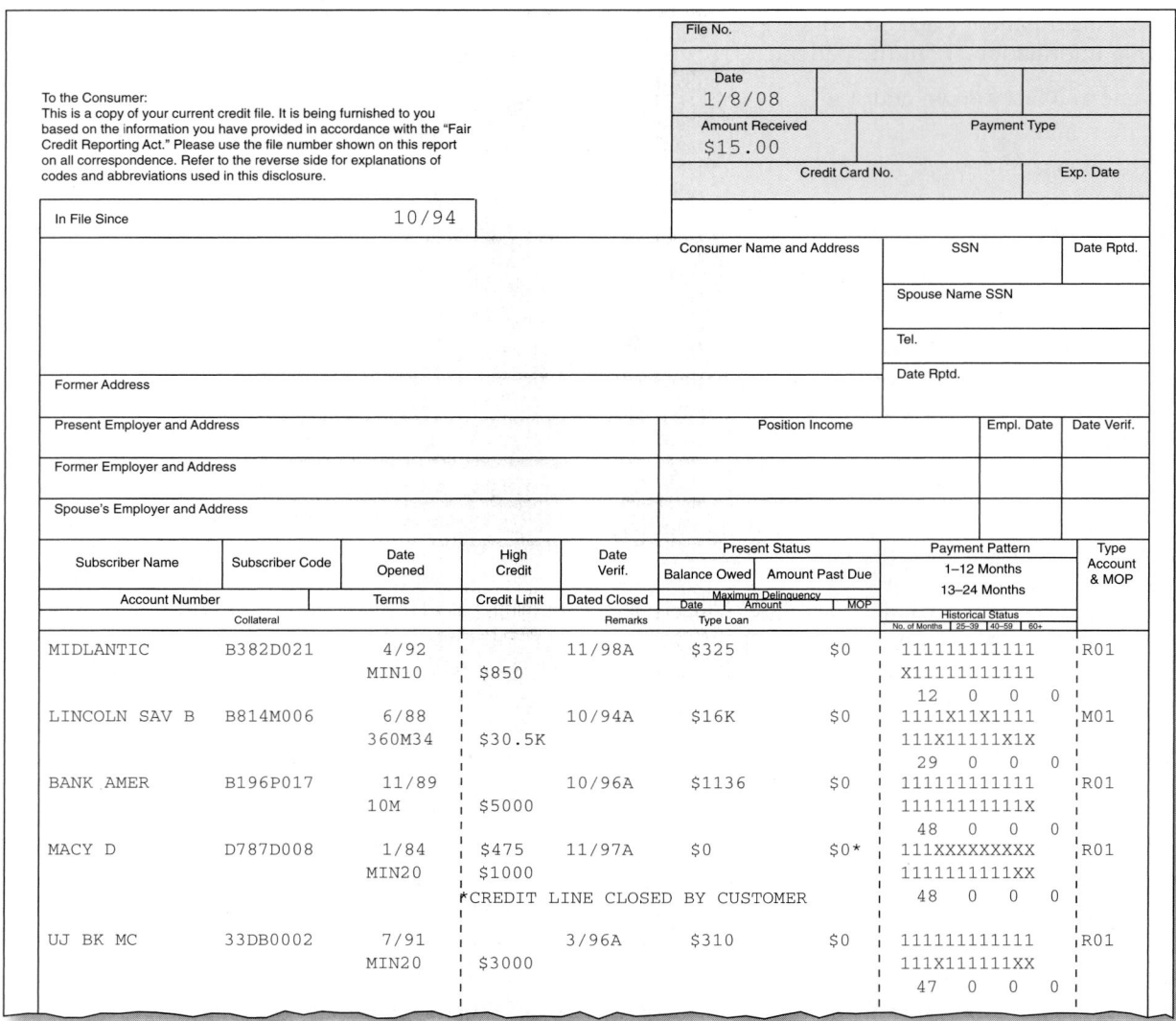

To the Consumer:
This is a copy of your current credit file. It is being furnished to you based on the information you have provided in accordance with the "Fair Credit Reporting Act." Please use the file number shown on this report on all correspondence. Refer to the reverse side for explanations of codes and abbreviations used in this disclosure.

File No.

Date
1/8/08

Amount Received
$15.00

Payment Type

Credit Card No.

Exp. Date

In File Since          10/94

Consumer Name and Address

SSN

Date Rptd.

Spouse Name SSN

Tel.

Date Rptd.

Former Address

Present Employer and Address

Position Income

Empl. Date   Date Verif.

Former Employer and Address

Spouse's Employer and Address

| Subscriber Name | Subscriber Code | Date Opened | High Credit | Date Verif. | Present Status | | Payment Pattern | Type Account & MOP |
|---|---|---|---|---|---|---|---|---|
| | | | | | Balance Owed | Amount Past Due | 1–12 Months 13–24 Months | |
| Account Number | | Terms | Credit Limit | Dated Closed | Maximum Delinquency Date \| Amount \| MOP | | Historical Status No. of Months \| 25–39 \| 40–59 \| 60+ | |
| Collateral | | | | | Remarks | Type Loan | | |
| MIDLANTIC | B382D021 | 4/92 MIN10 | $850 | 11/98A | $325 | $0 | 111111111111 X11111111111 12   0   0   0 | R01 |
| LINCOLN SAV B | B814M006 | 6/88 360M34 | $30.5K | 10/94A | $16K | $0 | 1111X11X1111 111X11111X1X 29   0   0   0 | M01 |
| BANK AMER | B196P017 | 11/89 10M | $5000 | 10/96A | $1136 | $0 | 111111111111 11111111111X 48   0   0   0 | R01 |
| MACY D | D787D008 | 1/84 MIN20 | $475 $1000 | 11/97A | $0 | $0* | 111XXXXXXXXX 111111111XX 48   0   0   0 | R01 |
| | | | *CREDIT LINE CLOSED BY CUSTOMER | | | | | |
| UJ BK MC | 33DB0002 | 7/91 MIN20 | $3000 | 3/96A | $310 | $0 | 111111111111 111X111111XX 47   0   0   0 | R01 |

**Figure 17-9.** Credit reports are generated by credit bureaus.

payments. It requires the physician and patient to discuss, sign, and retain copies of a **disclosure statement** (frequently called a federal Truth in Lending statement), which is a written description of the agreed terms of payment (Figure 17-10).

According to the Truth in Lending Act, a disclosure statement must meet the following two requirements.

1. The agreement must be discussed with the patient when the terms are first determined. The physician and the patient must agree on the payment terms.
2. Both the physician and the patient must sign the document to indicate mutual agreement on the written terms.

Further, a disclosure statement must include the following six pieces of information:

1. The amount of total debt (the amount for which the patient is receiving credit).

2. The amount of the down payment (which is sometimes greater than the weekly or monthly payments that follow).
3. The amount of each payment (which may be weekly or monthly or for another period) and the date it is due. (Frequently the total number of payments to be made after the down payment is also included.)
4. The due date for the final payment.
5. The interest rate, if interest is to be paid, expressed as an annual percentage.
6. The total finance charges, if any. (If interest is charged, the total amount of interest accrued during the course of the debt will be entered here.)

The practice and the patient should each keep a copy of the signed disclosure agreement.

Under the Truth in Lending Act, you must send the patient a statement of account at the end of each billing cycle.

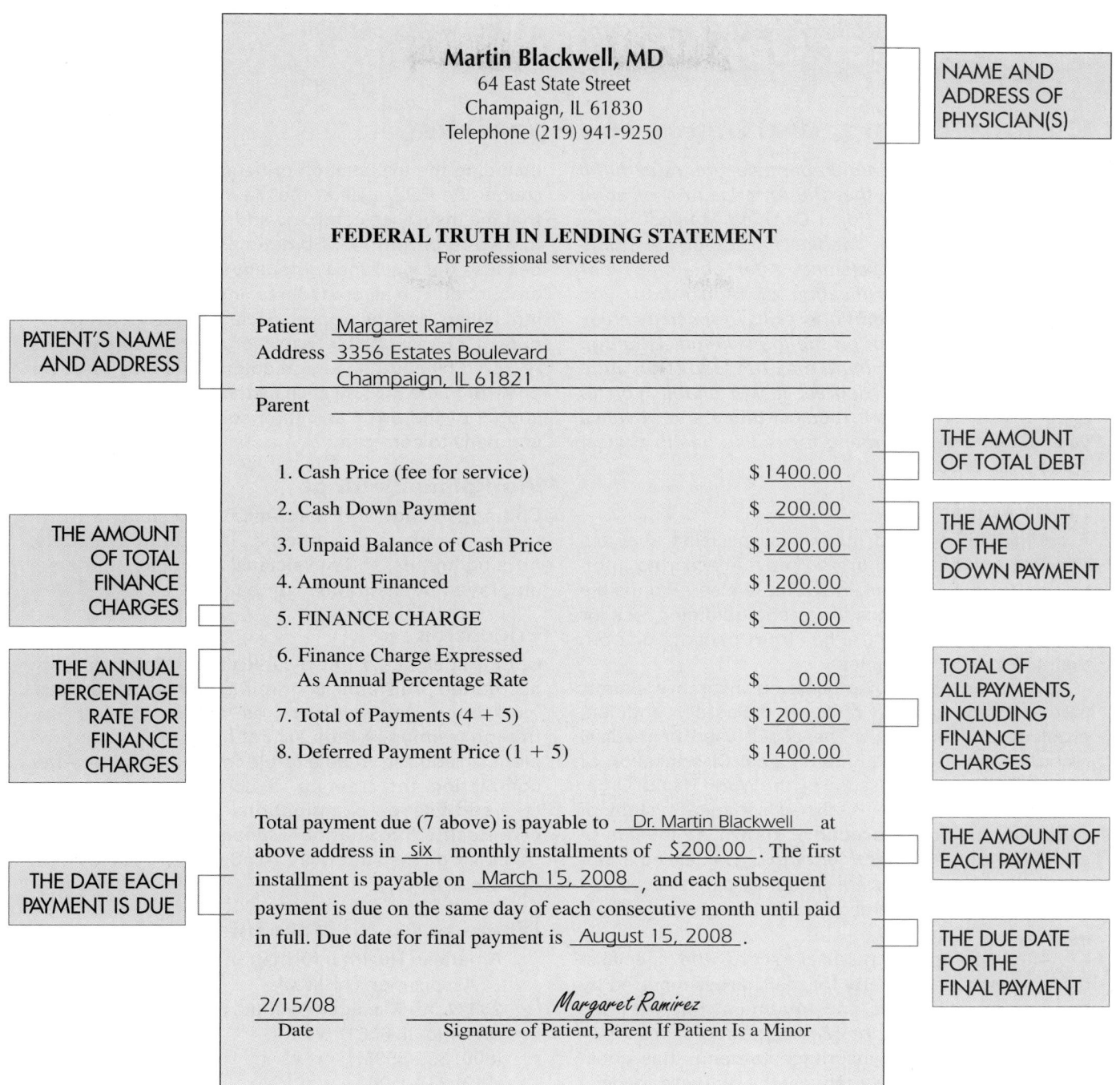

**Figure 17-10.** The federal Truth in Lending Act mandates that a written disclosure statement be completed and signed by the physician and patient.

This statement must include the previous balance, any payments or charges, the periodic and annual interest rates, finance charges (if any) for the billing cycle, the new balance, and a description of how the new balance was obtained.

## Extending Credit

If the doctor decides to extend credit, several possible arrangements can be made. Two common arrangements are the unilateral decision and the mutual agreement.

**Unilateral Decision.** The doctor may decide that the patient will be billed every month for the full amount owed and should make whatever payment is possible each month. This type of arrangement is considered a unilateral decision of the doctor and is not regulated by the Truth in Lending Act.

**Mutual Agreement.** Another option is a mutual, or bilateral, agreement between physician and patient. They might agree that the patient will be billed for the full

## Coding, Billing, and Insurance Specialist

*To gain medical assistant credentials, you must fulfill the requirements of either the American Association of Medical Assistants (for a Certified Medical Assistant) or the American Medical Technologists (for a Registered Medical Assistant). After obtaining your medical assistant certification or registration, you may wish to acquire additional skills in specialty areas through course work or on-the-job training. Although this course work or training may not lead to an additional certification or degree, it will enable you to expand your role in the medical office and advance your career as the demand for skilled health professionals increases.*

### Skills and Duties

A coding, billing, and insurance specialist analyzes the data in patients' charts to provide accurate information for insurance claims. She is also responsible for processing insurance forms and obtaining fees for procedures performed, either from patients or from their insurance companies.

For the purpose of processing insurance claims, there is a code for every recognized disease, condition, problem, and diagnosis. The codes used in medical records come from the International Classification of Disease (ICD) system, issued by the World Health Organization (WHO). There is also a separate system of codes for medical procedures, known as the *Physicians' Current Procedural Terminology,* released annually by the AMA. Coders are encouraged to take courses each year to stay informed about coding changes and updates.

After coding the medical record, the specialist bills the responsible party for the charges incurred by the patient's diagnosis and treatment. She may bill the patient, Medicare or Medicaid, and/or an insurance company. If the insurance company has questions about a bill, it may request the patient's medical records to verify that a particular procedure was medically necessary.

The coding, billing, and insurance specialist may also assist patients with the claims process. She can explain what information the patient must provide to streamline the process. When patients are responsible for submitting claims to their insurance companies, the coding, billing, and insurance specialist may tell the patient what forms to use and assist the patient with the forms completion.

The coding, billing, and insurance specialist also processes responses from the insurance companies, including the explanation of benefits (EOB) form. She checks the EOB against the claim form to make sure that the insurance company addressed all procedures that were performed. Sometimes a balance remains because the insurance company did not pay the total amount due on all procedures. In those cases the coding, billing, and insurance specialist sends a bill to the patient or responsible party, or adjusts balances as required by contracted agreement. She may discover an error in the EOB. In such instances she looks for the source of the error and then contacts the insurance company to correct it.

### Workplace Settings

Coding, billing, and insurance specialists work in many health-care settings, including hospitals, nursing homes, and physicians' practices. Some are employed by insurance companies.

### Education

Coding specialists may receive their training through accredited programs, continuing education courses, workshops, and seminars, as well as through on-the-job training. A high school diploma or its equivalent is required to be eligible for this training. After completing the training, a coding specialist may take certification examinations through the American Health Information Management Association (AHIMA) or the American Academy of Professional Coders (AAPC).

### Where to Go for More Information

American Health Information Management
   Association (AHIMA)
233 North Michigan Avenue, Suite 2150
Chicago, IL 60611-5800
(800) 335-5535
(312) 233-1100
Fax: (312) 233-1090

American Academy of Professional
   Coders (AAPC)
2480 South 3850 West, Suite B
Salt Lake City, UT 84120
(800) 626-CODE (2633)
Fax: (801)-236-2258

amount owed each month and will pay a minimum amount each month. If the physician does not assess finance charges, and if the total number of payments is four or fewer, this type of agreement is also not covered by the Truth in Lending Act. If the physician and patient make a bilateral agreement that includes more than four payments, or if the physician assesses finance charges, the agreement is subject to the requirements of the Truth in Lending Act.

# Common Collection Problems

There are two common collection problems that medical practices encounter. The first is patients who cannot pay—also called hardship cases—and the second is patients who have moved and have not received an invoice.

## Hardship Cases

A physician may decide to treat some patients without charge—or at a deep discount—simply because they cannot pay. These patients may be poor, uninsured or underinsured, or elderly and on a limited income. They may be patients who have suffered a severe financial loss or family tragedy. Medical ethics require physicians to provide care to individuals who need it, regardless of their ability to pay. Nevertheless, free treatment for hardship cases is at the physician's discretion.

Keep in mind that under ECOA, if a patient is given free or reduced-fee treatment based on her inability to pay and another patient under similar circumstances is treated, she must also be extended the same financial consideration or a charge of discrimination may be levied against the physician. Some providers treat such patients for urgent problems and then refer the patients to federally funded clinics that are allowed to provide free or reduced-fee services related to their government funding.

## Patient Relocation and Address Change

Sometimes an invoice remains unpaid because the patient has moved without leaving a forwarding address and has not received the invoice. Obviously, you will have a problem if you are trying to call such a patient about an invoice.

Remember not to discuss a debt with anyone except the person responsible for the charges. When you make a telephone call for collection, however, you may ask a third party for the patient's new address. If the third party claims not to know the new address, do not call again unless there is reason to believe that the third party has learned of the person's address since the first inquiry. You may ask the post office for a forwarding address, but if the patient cannot be located, the patient may be labeled a "skip." It is acceptable to refer the patient to the office collection agency. Be sure to keep the returned invoice stamped by the post office as "addressee unknown" or "no forwarding address" to prove a reasonable attempt to collect the debt.

# Summary

Most doctors prefer to obtain payment by cash, check, or credit card at the time medical services are provided. As a medical assistant, you may assign the fee for these services and collect payment. For various reasons, however, some patients cannot pay immediately. To accommodate these patients, the doctor may want to extend credit. If so, you may be asked to check credit references or to obtain a credit report.

When patients have made credit arrangements with the doctor, you must regularly prepare invoices from information on the patient ledger cards. To simplify this task, you may use a multipurpose superbill and send out invoices in billing cycles.

If patients do not pay their bills within 30 days, you may be asked to act as the doctor's collection agent. Through telephone calls and collection letters, you can try tactfully to collect payments. Federal and state laws govern collections and carry harsh penalties for infractions, so it is important to be knowledgeable of these laws and regulations.

If your efforts to collect a payment are not effective, the doctor may ask you to help find an outside collection agency. A good collection agency should reflect the humanitarian standards of the medical profession. You will need to supply the agency with the pertinent account information.

# REVIEW

## CHAPTER 17

## CASE STUDY QUESTIONS

Now that you have completed this chapter, review the case study at the beginning of the chapter and answer the following questions:

1. What is the total owed for this patient's visits?
2. How much of the total is not covered by insurance and should be billed to the patient?

## Discussion Questions

1. Discuss the procedure for handling a parent who brings in a child for care and asks you to bill the other parent.
2. What information is required to prepare invoices?
3. What are some of the techniques used in the task of collections?
4. Discuss the difference between a unilateral and a bilateral or mutual agreement.

## Critical Thinking Questions

1. What are the most common collection problems? Give examples of how you would handle these problem cases. Who has the final decision on who receives discounted rates for services?
2. How is the use of a debit card a more reliable payment method than accepting a check from a patient?

## Application Activities

1. With a partner, role-play a scenario in which you, as a medical assistant, are making an initial request for payment over the phone to a patient who is late in paying a bill but has not yet been sent any collection letters. Your partner should act as the patient, offering any information or explanation she wants.

2. Explain to another student the difference between accounts receivable and accounts payable. Use an example of each in your explanation.
3. Using the guidelines described in this chapter, write a collection letter to a fictional patient. The patient owes the doctor $125, and the account is 60 days past due. Share your letter with a classmate to analyze how well you complied with federal collection guidelines.

## Virtual Fieldtrip

*Visit the McGraw-Hill Higher Education Medical Assisting website at www.mhhe.com/medicalassisting3 to complete the following activity:*

Go online and visit a website that offers "free" credit reports. Some examples are:

- Free Credit Report Instantly
- Free3BureauCreditReport
- Credit Smart

Write one to two paragraphs answering these questions. Is the credit report really "free"? Do you have to join first? Specifically state the disclaimer. What do the warnings on the website say?

Open the CD and complete this chapter's practice activities, play the games, listen to the key terms, and test yourself with the interactive review. E-mail, print, and/or save your results to document your proficiency.

## CHAPTER 18

# Accounting for the Medical Office

## MEDICAL ASSISTING COMPETENCIES

*In preparation for the certification examination, you should know the following areas of competence:*

| COMPETENCY | CMA | RMA |
|---|:---:|:---:|
| **Administrative** | | |
| Prepare a bank deposit record | X | X |
| Post NSF checks | X | X |
| Reconcile a bank statement | | X |
| Establish and maintain a petty cash fund | | X |
| Use manual and computerized bookkeeping systems | | X |
| Maintain records for accounting and banking purposes | | X |
| Process employee payroll | | X |
| Analyze and apply third-party guidelines | X | X |
| Be aware of and perform within legal and ethical boundaries | X | X |
| Determine the needs for documentation and reporting, and document accurately and appropriately | X | X |
| Evidence a responsible attitude | | X |
| Receive, organize, prioritize, and transmit information appropriately | | X |

## KEY TERMS

ABA number
asset
bookkeeping
cash flow statement
cashier's check
certified check
check
counter check
dependent
employment contract
endorse
Federal Unemployment Tax Act (FUTA)
gross earnings
journalizing
limited check
money order
negotiable
net earnings
patient ledger card
pay schedule
payee
payer
pegboard system
petty cash fund
power of attorney
quarterly return
reconciliation
State Unemployment Tax Act (SUTA)
tax liability
third-party check
tracking
traveler's check
voucher check

## CHAPTER OUTLINE

- The Business Side of a Medical Practice
- Bookkeeping Methods
- Banking for the Medical Office
- Managing Accounts Payable
- Managing Disbursements
- Handling Payroll
- Calculating and Filing Taxes
- Managing Contracts

## LEARNING OUTCOMES

After completing Chapter 18, you will be able to:

18.1 Describe traditional bookkeeping systems, including single-entry and double-entry.

18.2 Explain the benefits of performing bookkeeping tasks on the computer.

18.3 List banking tasks in a medical office.

18.4 Describe the logistics of accepting, endorsing, and depositing checks from patients and insurance companies.

**18.5** Reconcile the office's bank statements.

**18.6** Give several examples of disbursements.

**18.7** Record disbursements in a disbursement journal.

**18.8** Set up and maintain a petty cash fund.

**18.9** Create employee payroll information sheets.

**18.10** Compute an employee's gross earnings, total deductions, and net earnings.

**18.11** Prepare an employee earnings record and payroll register.

**18.12** Set up the practice's tax liability accounts.

**18.13** Complete federal, state, and local tax forms.

**18.14** Submit employment taxes to government agencies.

**18.15** Describe the basic parts of an employment contract.

# Introduction

Accounting is another of the administrative competencies in the medical assisting career. A person in this career may be required to take on many duties in the medical office that would typically be done by an office manager. This chapter describes the key areas of accounting and bookkeeping that may be encountered.

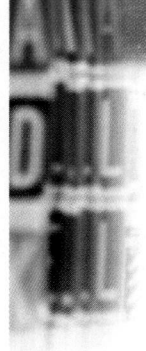

## CASE STUDY

Ben is a medical assistant at a family practice clinic. A patient gave him a check for $85 for payment on her account.

As you read this chapter, consider the following question:

1. What should Ben do to properly record the payment?

# The Business Side of a Medical Practice

A medical practice is a business. If it is to prosper, its income must exceed its expenses. In other words, it must produce a profit. To determine whether the business is making a profit, you may be asked to do **bookkeeping,** or systematic recording of business transactions. Your records will later be analyzed by an accountant or by a more experienced medical assistant.

Bookkeeping and banking are two key responsibilities of medical assistants. To fulfill these responsibilities, you need an understanding of basic accounting systems and certain financial management skills.

## Importance of Accuracy

Whenever you do bookkeeping or banking, strive for 100% accuracy. Because bookkeeping records form a chain of information, an undetected error at the first link will be carried through all other links in the chain. Undetected errors can result in billing a patient twice for the same visit, omitting bank deposits, or making improper payments to suppliers. These actions can result in lost money—and patients—for the practice.

# Establishing Procedures

A set procedure not only helps you remember important aspects of bookkeeping and banking but also helps ensure that your books are accurate. Here are some general suggestions for maintaining accuracy in bookkeeping and banking procedures for a medical practice.

- Maintain the practice's bookkeeping and banking procedures in a logical and organized way.
- Be consistent. Always handle the same kinds of transactions in exactly the same way. For example, endorse all checks with the same information, regardless of who wrote them or when you will be depositing them.
- Use check marks as you work to avoid losing your place if you are interrupted. For example, place a red check mark on each check stub as you reconcile the bank statement.
- Write clearly, and always use the same type of pen. If more than one person performs bookkeeping and banking tasks, each person might use a different color ink to identify her work. It is recommended that as few people as possible perform these tasks, however. You may use pencil for trial balances and worksheets, but you should use pen for bookkeeping entries.

- Double-check your work frequently to detect—and correct—any errors. To correct errors, draw a straight line through the incorrect figure, and write the correct figure above it. Do not erase errors or delete them with correction fluid or tape.
- Keep all columns of figures straight, so that decimal points align correctly.

Using set procedures will help you organize your work, help ensure accuracy, and make you a more valuable member of the practice staff.

# Bookkeeping Methods

Bookkeeping methods within a medical practice may be computerized or manual. Computerized bookkeeping is the most commonly used type of bookkeeping system. Three types of manual accounting systems may be used by medical practices that are not computerized: single-entry, double-entry, and pegboard. All bookkeeping systems record income, charges (money owed to the practice), disbursements (money paid out by the practice), and other financial information. The choice of system is based on the size and complexity of the practice.

## Bookkeeping on the Computer

Physicians or office managers who choose to set up the practice's bookkeeping system on the computer enjoy several important benefits over traditional bookkeeping methods. Computerized bookkeeping saves time; many repetitive tasks are done by the computer. The computer also performs mathematic calculations. Most bookkeeping software programs include built-in tax tables, which can calculate tax liabilities and so on.

As discussed in Chapter 6, many bookkeeping software programs or practice management software programs are available on the market. Any bookkeeping software package performs the same tasks as manual bookkeeping methods, so knowing these tasks is essential to performing computerized bookkeeping. Understanding these tasks is an essential part of managing books on a computer. The practice in which you work may already have a computerized bookkeeping program in place, which you should learn. It is also a good idea to stay current by reading computer software magazines. You may learn about a new software program you might recommend to the physician or office manager, or you may read about a new or more efficient way to use the practice's current software program.

## Single-Entry System

As the name implies, the single-entry system requires only one entry for each transaction. Therefore, it is the easiest system to learn and use. Unlike the double-entry system, however, the single-entry system is not self-balancing. In addition, it does not detect errors as readily and has fewer accuracy checkpoints. This system is also more likely to

produce errors because information must be posted (copied) separately to each of the bookkeeping forms.

The single-entry system uses several basic records, as well as auxiliary records:

- A daily log (also called a general ledger, day sheet, or daily journal) to record charges, payments, and adjustments (or write-offs)
- Patient ledger cards or an accounts receivable ledger, which shows how much each patient owes
- A checkbook register or cash payment journal, which shows the practice expenses
- Payroll records, which show salaries, wages, and payroll deductions
- Petty cash records, which show disbursements for minor office expenses

The double-entry and pegboard systems, discussed later in this chapter, also use these records.

**Daily Log.** The daily log is a chronological list of the charges to patients and the payments received from patients each day, as shown in Figure 18-1. In the daily log, you write the name of each patient seen that day. Across from the name, you record the service provided, the fee charged, and the payment received (if any). This process is called **journalizing.** You then post (copy) the charges and payments from the daily log to patient ledger cards (described in the next section). Using a daily or monthly cash control sheet, you record checks and cash received as well as deposits made each day.

Some physicians keep a daily log at their desks for entering information after they see each patient. In such cases, it may be helpful to write the name of each scheduled patient in the log to provide an appointment list. You may be responsible for this task.

In other offices, the medical assistants maintain the daily log. You can obtain the information for the log from charge slips and from checks received from patients or insurance companies. (Note: A charge slip is the original record of the doctor's services and the charge for those services. Some practices use a combination charge slip/receipt, which automatically creates a receipt to tear off for the patient. Typically, a charge slip/receipt includes a duplicate copy underneath to use for bookkeeping purposes. Remember, you need to track charges *and* receipts for payment, regardless of whether the practice uses separate charge slips and receipts or a combination.) There may also be records of outside visits, such as to nursing homes or hospital emergency rooms.

Be sure to record any night calls or other unscheduled visits in the daily log. Simply check with the physician each morning. If the physician has not noted the charge amount on a charge slip/receipt or record of outside visits, remember to apply the correct fee.

Record in the daily log all payments that come in the mail. If a check from an insurance company includes payment for more than one patient (which frequently is the

| Hour | Patient | Service Provided | Charge | Paid |
|------|---------|------------------|--------|------|
| 1 | | | | |
| 2 | | | | |
| 3 | | | | |
| 4 | | | | |
| 5 | | | | |
| 6 | | | | |
| 7 | | | | |
| 8 | | | | |
| 9 | | | | |
| 10 | | | | |
| 11 | | | | |
| 12 | | | | |
| 13 | | | | |
| 14 | | | | |
| 15 | | | | |
| 16 | | | | |
| | | Totals | | |

Dr. _____    Date _____

**Figure 18-1.** A daily log is used to record charges and payments.

case), post the appropriate amount to each patient ledger card. The information will be found on the EOB (explanation of benefits) attached to the check.

If extra columns are available, you can record additional financial information in the daily log. For example, in addition to showing the total amount charged to the patient, you can show a breakdown of that total into the amounts generated by different physicians in a group practice or by different functions of the office, such as laboratory or x-ray.

At the end of each day, total the charges and receipts in the daily log, and post these totals to the monthly summary of charges and receipts. To double-check your totals, perform the following procedures:

- Ensure that the day's total cash and check receipts are the same as the day's total bank deposit.
- Ensure that the sum of the day's charges for each type of service is the same as the total of the day's charges.

**Patient Ledger Cards.** Another bookkeeping task is preparing a patient ledger card for each patient. The **patient ledger card** includes the patient's name, address, home and work telephone numbers, and the name of the person who is responsible for the charges (if different from the patient). The ledger card also lists the patient's insurance information, Social Security number, employer's name,

and any special billing instructions. Figure 18-2 shows an example of a patient ledger card.

You use the patient ledger card to record charges incurred by the patient, payments received, adjustments made, and the resulting balance owed to the doctor. Because these cards document the financial transactions of the patient account, they are sometimes called account cards. In some practices, they are photocopied for use as monthly statements.

The information for the patient ledger cards comes from the daily log or from charge slips. It is best to complete all the cards at the end of the day. If this is not possible, you may complete them as time permits during the day. To prevent double or omitted postings, put a small check mark next to each entry in the daily log after you post it to the proper ledger card.

Take great care when posting, because errors on ledger cards will be reflected on invoices. To ensure accuracy, add up the total charges and receipts from the ledger cards, and make sure the information matches the total charges and receipts in that day's daily log.

**Accounts Receivable.** Every day, you must also update the accounts receivable record, which shows the total owed to the practice (the amount able to be received but not yet received). Total up the items on the accounts receivable record, and then total up the outstanding balances on

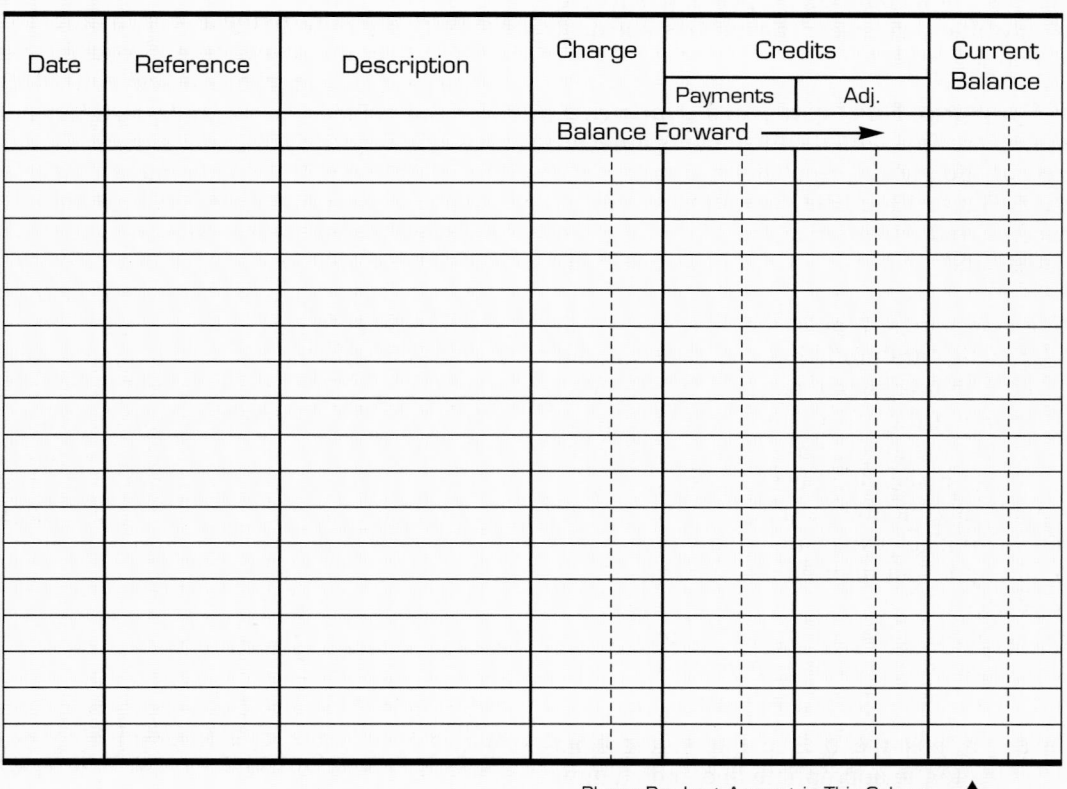

Patient's Name    Jonathan Jackson

Home Phone    (612) 555-9921    **Work Phone**   (612) 555-1000

Social Security No.   111-21-4114

Employer    Ashton School District

Insurance    National Insurance Co.

Policy #    123-4-56-788

**Person Responsible for Charges (if Different from Patient)** _____

**JONATHAN JACKSON**
123 Fourth Avenue
Ashton, MN 70809-1222

| Date | Reference | Description | Charge | Credits | | Current Balance |
|------|-----------|-------------|--------|---------|---|-----------------|
| | | | | Payments | Adj. | |
| | | Balance Forward ⟶ | | | | |
| | | | | | | |
| | | | | | | |
| | | | | | | |
| | | | | | | |
| | | | | | | |
| | | | | | | |
| | | | | | | |
| | | | | | | |
| | | | | | | |
| | | | | | | |
| | | | | | | |
| | | | | | | |
| | | | | | | |
| | | | | | | |
| | | | | | | |
| | | | | | | |
| | | | | | | |

Please Pay Last Amount in This Column ▲

OV—Office Visit      C—Consultation      EX—Examination
X—X-ray      NC—No Charge      INS—Insurance
ROA—Received on Account      MA—Missed Appointment

**Figure 18-2.** Patient ledger cards are used to show how much each patient owes.

the patient ledger cards. The two numbers should match. If they do not, recheck your work to find the cause of the discrepancy.

**Accounts Payable.** Accounts payable are the amounts the practice owes to vendors (the amount able to be paid but not yet paid). If your responsibilities include accounts payable, keep careful records of equipment and supplies ordered, and compare orders received against the invoices. In the checkbook register, keep detailed and accurate records of accounts paid.

**Record of Office Disbursements.** The record of office disbursements is a list of the amounts paid for such items as medical supplies, office rent, office utilities, employee wages, postage, and equipment over a certain period of time. It shows the **payee** (the person who will receive the payment), the date, the check number, the amount paid, and the type of expense. Figure 18-3 is an example of a disbursement record.

A checkbook register may be used to record office disbursements. As an alternative, a disbursement journal or the bottom section of the daily log may be used to record office disbursements. For income tax purposes, this record should include only office expenses. The doctor's personal expenses should not be listed here.

**Summary of Charges, Receipts, and Disbursements.** Charges, receipts, and disbursements are usually summarized at the end of each month, quarter, or year, as shown in Figure 18-4. The summary is used to compare the income and expenses of the current period with the income and expenses from any previous period.

By analyzing summaries, a physician can see which functions of the practice are profitable, the total amount charged for services, the payments received for services, the total cost of running the office, and a breakdown of expenses into various categories. Based on this information, the physician can make vital business decisions. For example, after analyzing monthly summaries, the physician may decide to budget expenses differently, collect payments more promptly, cut unprofitable services, or expand profitable services.

Although an accountant may prepare these reports, an experienced medical assistant can prepare them. If you are asked to prepare them, follow these guidelines.

- Every business day, post the total charges and receipts from the daily log to the appropriate line and column of the monthly summary.
- Every business day, also post the disbursements from the record of office disbursements to the appropriate lines and columns of the monthly summary.
- At the end of the month, total the columns on the monthly summary.
- At the end of each quarter, post the charges, receipts, and disbursements for each of the previous 3 months to the quarterly summary. Then, total each column.

- At the end of the year, post the charges, receipts, and disbursements for each of the previous 12 months (or 4 quarters) to the annual summary. Then, total each column.

Remember that the total charges and total receipts in any summary should be almost the same. They may not be identical, because some bills may not have been fully collected. Procedure 18-1 offers a plan for setting up a medical practice bookkeeping system.

## Double-Entry System

The double-entry accounting system is based on an accounting equation:

$$\text{Assets} = \text{Liabilities} + \text{Owner's Equity}$$

**Assets** are goods or properties that have a dollar value, such as the medical practice building, bank accounts, office equipment, and accounts receivable. Owner's equity (also called capital, net worth, or proprietorship) is the owner's right to the value of the assets. Liabilities are amounts owed by the practice to creditors, such as a mortgage on the building and accounts payable. Liabilities decrease the value of the assets. In other words, in a medical practice, the owner (the physician) has the rights to the value of the practice's assets, once the liabilities have been subtracted. An example of this would be the purchase of an office computer system for which a loan has been taken out. If the equipment cost is $45,000 with a $20,000 deposit and a $25,000 loan still owed, the equation would look like this: $45,000 = $25,000 + $20,000.

Because both sides of the accounting equation must always balance (agree), every transaction is recorded as an entry on each side of the equation. Thus, there are two entries, or a double entry. The double-entry system is accurate, detects errors easily, and provides the most complete information about the practice and its contribution to the physician's net worth. It is complex, however, and requires a great deal of time and skill to master. If it is used in a medical practice, an accountant usually establishes and maintains the system, and the medical assistant simply keeps a daily log.

## Pegboard System

The **pegboard system** lets you write each transaction once while recording it on four different bookkeeping forms. The pegboard system is called the one-write system and used to be the most widely used bookkeeping system in medical practices. With the advancement of computerized medical billing and records, this system is seldom used in actual practice. However, understanding the principles of this system will be an essential part of your training as a medical assistant and will help you understand the concepts behind the computerized accounting system.

A pegboard system usually includes a lightweight board with pegs on the left or right edges. The pegs match holes that are punched in daily log sheets, patient ledger

**Record of Office Disbursements**

April 2008

| DATE | PAYEE | CK. NO. | TOTAL AMOUNT | TYPES OF EXPENSES | | | | | | | | | | |
|---|---|---|---|---|---|---|---|---|---|---|---|---|---|---|
| | | | | RENT | UTILITIES | POSTAGE | LAB./X-RAY | MEDICAL SUPPLIES | OFFICE SUPPLIES | WAGES | INSURANCE | TAXES | TRAVEL | MISC. |
| 01 | Philips' Med. Suppl. | 1778 | 125.00 | | | | | 125.00 | | | | | | |
| 01 | Postage | 1779 | 16.85 | | | 16.85 | | | | | | | | |
| 02 | Medi Path | 1780 | 32.50 | | | | 32.50 | | | | | | | |
| 02 | Quik Service Co. | 1781 | 82.40 | | | | | | 82.40 | | | | | |
| 02 | Philips' Med. Suppl. | 1782 | 92.00 | | | | | 92.00 | | | | | | |
| 02 | Jean Medina | 1783 | 77.06 | | | | | | | 77.06 | | | | |
| 05 | State Dept. of Rev. | 1784 | 189.16 | | | | | | | | | 189.16 | | |
| 06 | General Insurance | 1785 | 165.92 | | | | | | | | 165.92 | | | |
| 07 | Postage | (Cash) | 5.19 | | | 5.19 | | | | | | | | |
| 07 | Micah Smith | (Cash) | 15.00 | | | | | | | | | | 15.00 | |
| 08 | IRS | 1786 | 419.41 | | | | | | | | | 419.41 | | |
| 12 | Quik Service Co. | 1787 | 124.00 | | | | | | 124.00 | | | | | |
| 13 | City Laundry | 1788 | 75.00 | | | | | | | | | | | 75.00 |
| 13 | National Insurance | 1789 | 189.00 | | | | | | | | 189.00 | | | |
| 14 | Broyer Assoc. | 1790 | 1 500.00 | 1 500.00 | | | | | | | | | | |
| 14 | Postage | (Cash) | 12.11 | | | 12.11 | | | | | | | | |
| 15 | City Gas Co. | 1791 | 125.00 | | 125.00 | | | | | | | | | |
| 19 | Jean Medina | 1792 | 85.92 | | | | | | | 85.92 | | | | |
| 19 | Postage | (Cash) | 8.95 | | | 8.95 | | | | | | | | |
| 21 | Philips' Med. Suppl. | 1793 | 85.00 | | | | | 85.00 | | | | | | |
| 25 | Medi Path | 1794 | 67.90 | | | | 67.90 | | | | | | | |
| 24 | Micah Smith | (Cash) | 10.00 | | | | | | | | | | 10.00 | |
| 24 | Elena Paxson | 1795 | 126.00 | | | | | | | 126.00 | | | | |
| 27 | Postage | 1796 | 17.32 | | | 17.32 | | | | | | | | |
| 28 | Johnson Assoc. | 1797 | 123.45 | | | | 123.45 | | | | | | | |
| | Total | | 3770.14 | 1500.00 | 125.00 | 60.42 | 223.85 | 302.00 | 206.40 | 288.98 | 354.92 | 608.57 | 25.00 | 75.00 |

**Figure 18-3.** A record of office disbursements lists the amounts paid over a certain period of time.

## Quarterly Summary of Charges, Receipts, and Disbursements, 2008

| | MONTH | 1 CHARGES | 2 RECEIPTS | 3 DISBURSE-MENTS | Types of Disbursements: 4 WAGES | 5 RENT & UTILITIES | 6 OFFICE EXPENSES | 7 GENERAL MEDICAL | 8 X-RAY/ LAB. | 9 TAXES | 10 PERSONAL | 11 MISC. |
|---|---|---|---|---|---|---|---|---|---|---|---|---|
| 1 | Jan. | 15400.00 | 14800.00 | 6218.14 | 3349.50 | 1625.00 | 129.86 | 93.45 | 241.86 | 589.02 | 100.00 | 89.45 |
| 2 | Feb. | 18255.00 | 18950.00 | 7050.40 | 3872.80 | 1683.08 | 235.00 | 118.72 | 266.00 | 611.20 | 186.60 | 77.00 |
| 3 | Mar. | 13850.00 | 13250.00 | 6530.14 | 3666.10 | 1702.85 | 43.85 | 243.11 | 187.02 | 577.00 | 88.11 | 22.10 |
| 4 | | | | | | | | | | | | |
| 5 | Subtotal | 47505.00 | 47000.00 | 19798.68 | 10888.40 | 5010.93 | 408.71 | 455.28 | 694.88 | 1777.22 | 374.71 | 188.55 |
| 6 | | | | | | | | | | | | |
| 7 | Apr. | | | | | | | | | | | |
| 8 | May | | | | | | | | | | | |
| 9 | June | | | | | | | | | | | |
| 10 | | | | | | | | | | | | |
| 11 | Subtotal | | | | | | | | | | | |
| 12 | | | | | | | | | | | | |
| 13 | July | | | | | | | | | | | |
| 14 | Aug. | | | | | | | | | | | |
| 15 | Sept. | | | | | | | | | | | |
| 16 | | | | | | | | | | | | |
| 17 | Subtotal | | | | | | | | | | | |
| 18 | | | | | | | | | | | | |
| 19 | Oct. | | | | | | | | | | | |
| 20 | Nov. | | | | | | | | | | | |
| 21 | Dec. | | | | | | | | | | | |
| 22 | | | | | | | | | | | | |
| 23 | Subtotal | | | | | | | | | | | |
| 24 | | | | | | | | | | | | |
| 25 | Grand Total | | | | | | | | | | | |
| 26 | | | | | | | | | | | | |
| 27 | | | | | | | | | | | | |
| 28 | | | | | | | | | | | | |
| 29 | | | | | | | | | | | | |
| 30 | | | | | | | | | | | | |
| 31 | | | | | | | | | | | | |
| 32 | | | | | | | | | | | | |
| 33 | | | | | | | | | | | | |
| 34 | | | | | | | | | | | | |
| 35 | | | | | | | | | | | | |
| 36 | | | | | | | | | | | | |

**Figure 18-4.** Creating a summary of charges, receipts, and disbursements is a regular bookkeeping task, performed monthly, quarterly, or yearly.

# PROCEDURE 18.1

## Organizing the Practice's Bookkeeping System

**Procedure Goal:** To maintain a bookkeeping system that promotes accurate record keeping for the practice

**Materials:** Daily log sheets, patient ledger cards, and check register, or computerized bookkeeping system; summaries of charges, receipts, and disbursements

**Method:**

1. Use a new daily log sheet each day. For each patient seen that day, record the patient name, the relevant charges, and any payments received, calculating any necessary adjustments and new balances. If you're using a computerized system, enter the patient's name, the relevant charges, and any payments received and adjustments made in the appropriate areas. The computer will calculate the new balances.

### Rationale

Each day's transactions must be accurately and promptly recorded.

2. Create a ledger card for each new patient, and maintain a ledger card for all existing patients. The ledger card should include the patient's name, address, home and work telephone numbers, and insurance company. It should also contain the name of the person responsible for the charges (if different from the patient). Update the ledger card every time the patient incurs a charge or makes a payment. Be sure to adjust the account balance after every transaction. In a computerized system, a patient

record is the same as a ledger card. This record must also be maintained and updated.

### Rationale

The information on each patient's ledger card must match that of the daily log.

3. Record all deposits accurately in the check register. File the deposit receipt—with a detailed listing of checks and money orders deposited—for later use in reconciling the bank statement. The deposit amount should match the amount of money collected by the practice for that day.

4. When paying bills for the practice, enter each check in the check register accurately, including the check number, date, payee, and amount before writing the check.

### Rationale

Record payments first so the step will not be skipped once the check is written.

5. Prepare and/or print a summary of charges, receipts, and disbursements every month, quarter, or year, as directed. Be sure to double-check all entries and calculations from the monthly summary before posting them to the quarterly summary. Also, double-check the entries and calculations from the quarterly summary before posting them to the yearly summary.

### Rationale

Double-checking all entries ensures mistakes are found and corrected as soon as possible.

---

cards, charge slips/receipts, and deposit slips. The holes allow the forms to be aligned while stacked on top of each other. Information, entered on only one form, is simultaneously transferred to the form(s) below. Generally these forms are printed on NCR (no-carbon-required) paper. If not, you must place carbon paper between the forms.

**Starting the Business Day.** Place a daily log sheet on the pegboard at the beginning of each day. Then, place the stack of charge slips/receipts on the pegs, aligning the top line of the first charge slip/receipt with the daily log top line. Because the charge slips/receipts are shingled, or layered one over the other from top to bottom, alignment of the first aligns all the others. The charge slips/receipts

are prenumbered. This numbering promotes good cash control and theoretically prevents embezzlement.

**Upon Patient Arrival.** As each patient comes into the office, place the patient's ledger card under the next available charge slip/receipt. Be sure to align the card's first blank line with the carbon strip on the charge slip/receipt. Write the date, the patient's name, and the patient's previous balance on the charge slip section. The information will automatically be recorded in the daily log and on the patient ledger card.

**Attaching the Charge Slip/Receipt to the Patient Chart.** Next, remove the charge slip/receipt and attach it to the patient chart so that the doctor will see it. After examining the patient, the doctor fills in the appropriate charges on the charge slip/receipt, indicates when the next appointment is needed, and gives the charge slip/receipt to the patient.

**Before the Patient Leaves.** The patient comes to you with the completed charge slip/receipt, and you again place the ledger card between the charge slip/receipt and the daily log. Check to be sure you align it properly. On the charge slip/receipt, write the charge slip/receipt number, date, procedure (or code), charges, payments, new balance, and the date and time of the next appointment (if any). As you write this information, it should be automatically transferred onto the ledger card and daily log. Finally, tear off the receipt, and give it to the patient. You can now return the patient ledger card to the file.

**Payments After the Patient Visit.** If you receive payments sometime after the patient visit, either by mail or in person, record them on the patient ledger card and daily log as you normally would. Record charges for doctor visits to hospitalized patients or other out-of-office visits in the same way. If required, you can use the pegboard system to record bank deposits and petty cash disbursements in the daily log, but you will need the appropriate overlapping forms.

**Returned Checks.** If a patient's check does not clear due to nonsufficient funds, you must adjust the account accordingly. NSF payments are first deducted from the office checking account. The patient's account is then updated with a negative payment (noted in parentheses in the payment column) for the amount of the check, adding that amount back to the patient balance. An office fee may also be charged for the inconvenience of dealing with the NSF check. Depending on office policy, the patient may now be seen on a *cash only* basis by the practice.

**End of the Day.** At the end of each day, total and check the arithmetic (addition and subtraction) in all columns. If you find an error, correct it immediately by drawing a line through it and making a new entry on the next available writing line. Remember to make the correction on the patient ledger card also and to issue a new receipt to the patient. To balance a pegboard, after adding the figures in each column, use the following formula for the column totals:

Previous balance + Today's charges − (Payments + adjustments) = New accounts receivable total

# Banking for the Medical Office

Besides bookkeeping, you may be responsible for handling the banking for the practice. Because a practice may use traditional (manual) or electronic (computerized) banking methods, you should be familiar with both. Regardless of which method you use, remember to keep all banking materials secure because they represent the finances of the practice. For example, to prevent theft of checks, always put the checkbook in a securely locked place when it is not in use. Also, file deposit receipts promptly. If they are lost, you have no proof that a deposit was made. Lack of proof could cost the practice thousands of dollars. If you ever suspect checks are stolen from your office, contact the bank and police department as soon as possible.

## Banking Tasks

Banking tasks for the medical practice include:

- Writing checks
- Accepting checks
- Endorsing checks
- Making deposits
- Reconciling bank statements

To perform these tasks properly, you must be familiar with several terms and concepts related to banking.

**Checks.** A **check** is a bank draft or order for payment. The person who writes the check is called the **payer.** By writing a check, the payer directs the bank to pay a sum of money on demand to the payee. In order to be considered **negotiable** (legally transferable from one person to another), a check must:

- Be written and signed by the payer or maker
- Include the amount of money to be paid, considered a promise to pay a specified sum
- Be made payable to the payee or bearer
- Be made payable on demand or on a specific date
- Include the name of the bank that is directed to make payment

**Other Negotiable Papers.** You may receive other negotiable paper in addition to standard personal and business checks.

- A **cashier's check** is a check issued on bank paper signed by a bank representative. It is usually purchased by individuals who do not have checking accounts.
- A **certified check** is a payer's check written and signed by the payer and stamped "Certified" by the bank. This certification means that the bank has already drawn money from the payer's account to guarantee that the check will be paid when submitted. (The money is set aside to cover this specific check.) Few banks offer certified checks anymore.
- A **money order** is another kind of certificate of guaranteed payment. Money orders may be purchased from banks (bank money orders) or post offices (postal money orders) or from some convenience stores.

**Check Codes.** The face (front) of every check contains two important items: the American Banking Association (ABA) number and the magnetic ink character recognition

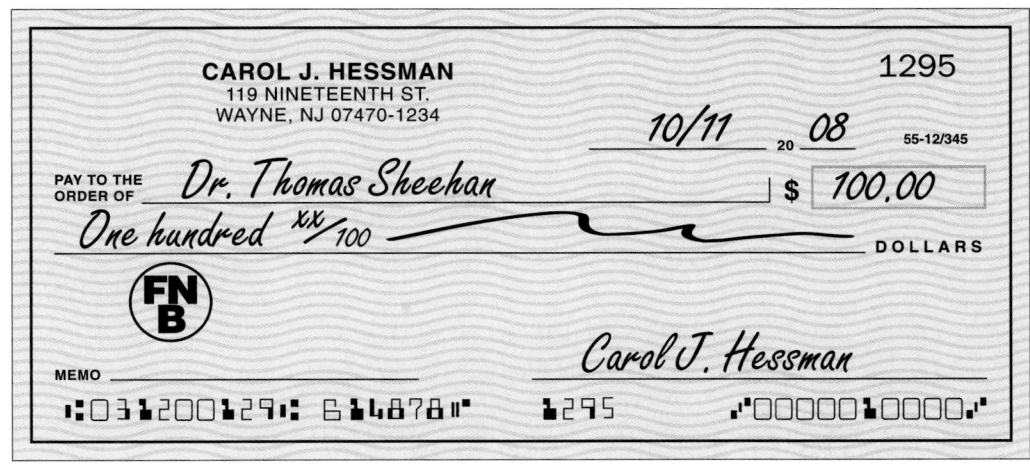

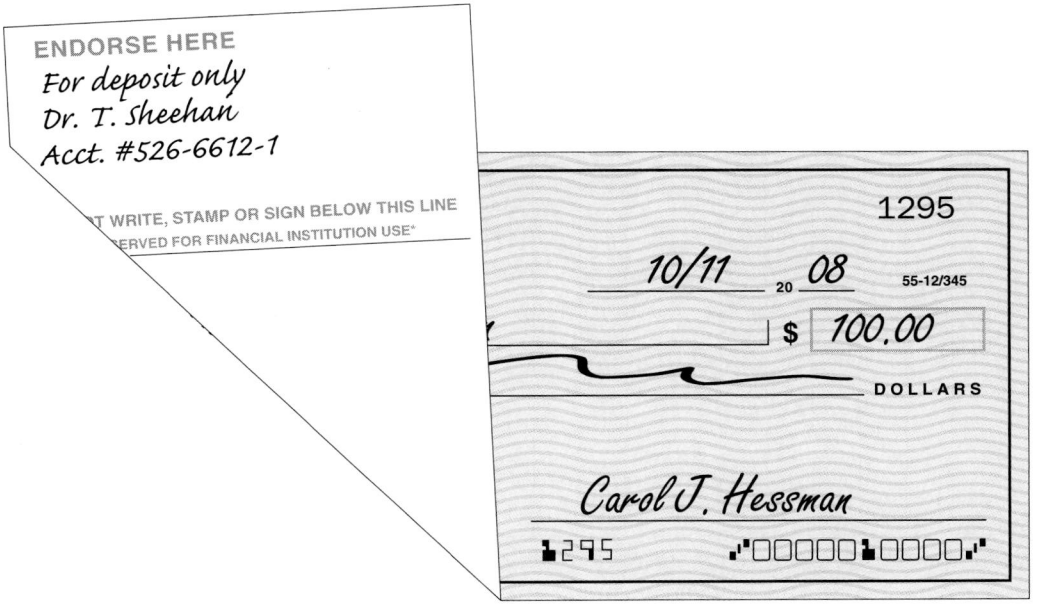

ENDORSE HERE
For deposit only
Dr. T. Sheehan
Acct. #526-6612-1

T WRITE, STAMP OR SIGN BELOW THIS LINE
ERVED FOR FINANCIAL INSTITUTION USE*

**Figure 18-5.** After verifying that a patient's check is correct, immediately endorse it with "For Deposit Only," the name of the practice, and the account number.

(MICR) code. The **ABA number** appears as a fraction, such as 60–117/310, on the upper edge of all printed checks. It identifies the geographic area and specific bank on which the check is drawn.

Found at the bottom of a check, the MICR code consists of numbers and characters printed in magnetic ink, which can be read by MICR equipment at the bank. This code enables checks to be read, sorted, and recorded by computer.

**Types of Checking Accounts.** A physician is likely to have three different types of checking accounts: a personal account, a business account for office expenses, and an interest-earning account. The interest-earning account will be used for paying special expenses, such as property taxes and insurance premiums. Most of your work will be with the business checking account. You may sometimes, however, make payments from, or transfer money to, the interest-earning account, as directed.

**Accepting Checks.** Before accepting any check, review it carefully. First be sure the check has the correct date, amount, and signature and that no corrections have been made. Figure 18-5 shows a correctly written and endorsed check. Do not accept a **third-party check** (one made out to the patient rather than to the practice) unless it is from a health insurance company. Also, do not accept a check marked "Payment in Full" unless it actually does pay the complete outstanding balance. You may accept a check signed by someone other than the payer if the person who signed the check has power of attorney. **Power of attorney** gives a person the legal right to handle financial matters for another person who is unable to do so. Frequently power of attorney is granted to a patient's spouse, son, or daughter.

Be sure to follow the policy of your practice when accepting a check. For example, if a patient is new or unfamiliar, office policy may require you to request patient identification and to compare the signature on the

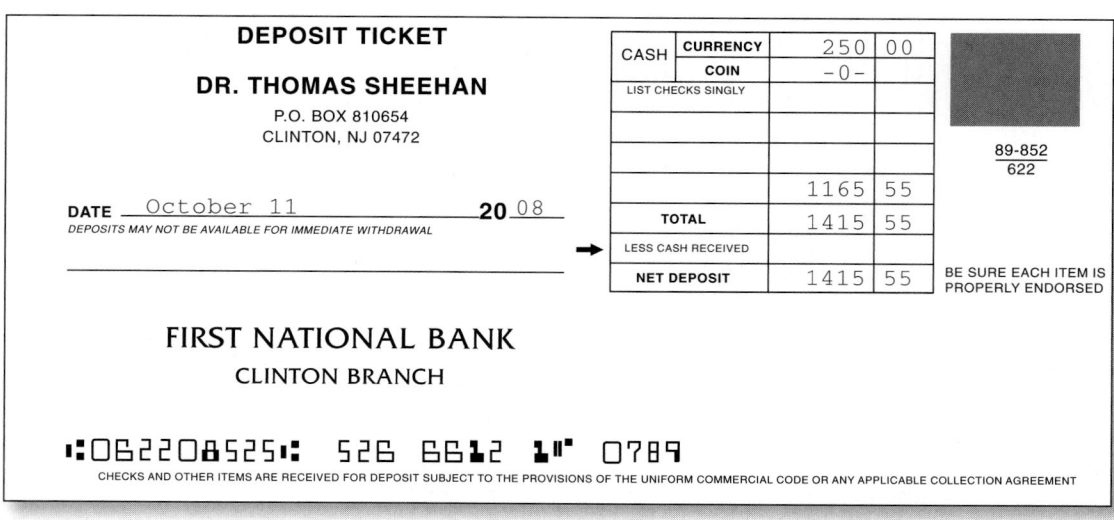

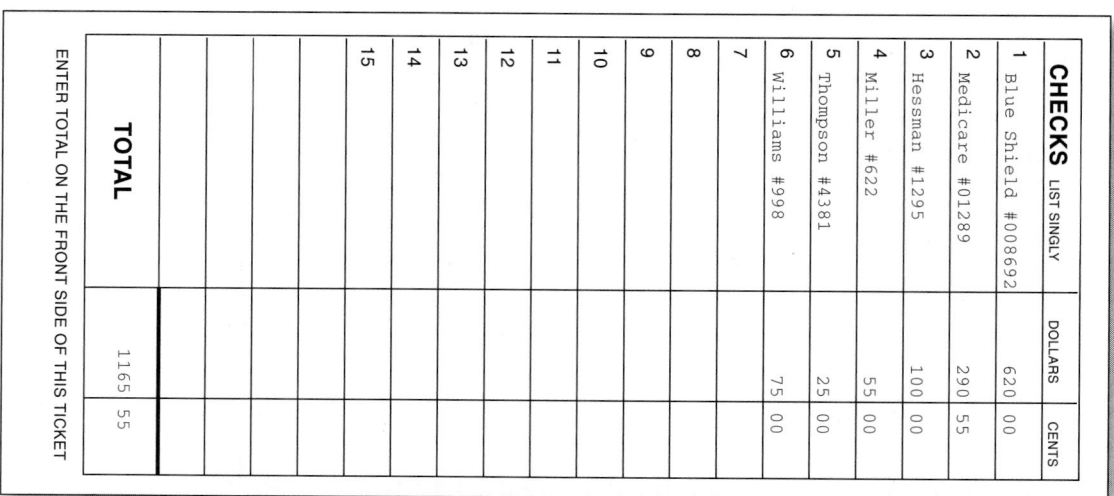

**Figure 18-6.** List each check on the deposit slip, including the check number and amount.

identification with the signature on the check. Policy may also require that you not accept a check for more than the amount due.

**Endorsing Checks.** After accepting a check, immediately **endorse** it by writing the name of the doctor or the practice on the back. Include the words "For Deposit Only" and the account number. (For convenience, this statement may be made into a rubber stamp.) This type of endorsement, known as a restrictive endorsement, prevents the check from being cashed if it is lost or stolen because the only way the check can be redeemed is by deposit into the specified account.

Be sure to endorse the check in ink, using a pen or rubber stamp. Place the endorsement in the 1.5-inch area indicated on the back of the check. Most personal and business checks have a number of lines or a shaded area preprinted on the checks for this purpose. Leave the rest of the back of the check blank for the use of the bank.

**Completing the Deposit Slip.** After endorsing the check, post the payment to the patient ledger card, and put the check with others to be deposited. Then, fill out a deposit slip, as shown in Figure 18-6. The account number is printed on deposit slips in MICR numbers that match those on the checks. As mentioned, these numbers enable checks and deposit slips to be read, sorted, and recorded by computer.

Banks will accept a list of deposited items on something other than the bank-provided deposit slip if the bank's deposit slip is attached. For example, if you are depositing 50 checks, you may create a computer printout listing the payers' names, check numbers, amount of each check, and total. You can then attach the printout to a deposit slip with the total written on the deposit slip. Another method is to attach a calculator or adding machine tape listing the individual check amounts and a total.

**Making the Deposit.** Plan to deposit checks and cash into the practice's bank account in person at the bank, as described in Procedure 18-2. Avoid sending cash through the mail, but if it is absolutely necessary to do so, use registered mail. Always obtain a deposit receipt from the bank.

# PROCEDURE 18.2

## Making a Bank Deposit

**Procedure Goal:** To prepare cash and checks for deposit and to deposit them properly into a bank account

**Materials:** Bank deposit slip and items to be deposited, such as checks, cash, and money orders

**Method:**

1. Divide the bills, coins, checks, and money orders into separate piles.

2. Sort the bills by denomination, from largest to smallest. Then, stack them, portrait side up, in the same direction. Total the amount of the bills, and write this amount on the deposit slip on the line marked "Currency."

   ### Rationale

   This is the order necessary for the teller to easily verify your totals. The deposit slip separates bill totals from coin totals.

3. If you have enough coins to fill coin wrappers, put them in wrappers of the proper denomination. If not, count the coins, and put them in the deposit bag. Total the amount of coins, and write this amount on the deposit slip on the line marked "Coin."

4. Review all checks and money orders to be sure they are properly endorsed with a restrictive endorsement. List each check on the deposit slip, including the check number and amount. If you do not keep a list of the check writers' names in the office, record this information on the deposit slip also.

5. List each money order on the deposit slip. Include the notation "money order" or "MO" and the name of the writer.

6. Calculate the total deposit (total of amounts for currency, coin, checks, and money orders). Write this amount on the deposit slip on the line marked "Total." Photocopy the deposit slip for your office records.

   ### Rationale

   Doing so provides a legal record for your office.

7. Record the total amount of the deposit in the office checkbook register.

   ### Rationale

   So that an accurate balance is recorded

8. If you plan to make the deposit in person, place the currency, coins, checks, and money orders in a deposit bag. If you cannot make the deposit in person, put the checks and money orders in a special bank-by-mail envelope, or put all deposit items in an envelope and send it by registered mail.

9. Make the deposit in person or by mail.

10. Obtain a deposit receipt from the bank. File it with the copy of the deposit slip in the office for later use when reconciling the bank statement.

    ### Rationale

    For accurate recordkeeping

---

In a busy physician's office, you may need to make deposits every day. If the physician has a limited practice, you may make deposits less frequently. Keep in mind, however, that making deposits more frequently increases cash flow and reduces the risk of lost or bounced checks.

**Reconciling Bank Statements.** Another banking task is reconciling the bank statement. **Reconciliation** involves comparing the office's financial records with the bank records to ensure that they are consistent (all numbers agree) and accurate. In most practices this task is performed once a month when the practice receives the monthly checking account statement from the bank. An example of a bank statement is shown in

Figure 18-7. The process of reconciliation is explained in Procedure 18-3.

## Electronic Banking

Compared with traditional banking methods, electronic banking has several advantages. Electronic banking can improve productivity, cash flow, and accuracy. The use of electronic banking can also speed up many banking tasks.

If your medical office uses electronic banking, your basic tasks will be the same as in an office that uses traditional banking methods. How these tasks are performed, however, may be quite different. When you use electronic banking, you are still responsible for recording

# 1st First State Bank of Englewood

CN 1
Englewood WI 54534-0001

PAGE 1

ACCOUNT NO.      518-833-3

STATEMENT PERIOD
07/19/08 TO 08/20/08

||I₁₁₁|₁|₁|₁|₁||₁|₁||₁||₁₁₁₁₁|₁|₁|₁|₁|₁|₁|₁₁₁₁₁||₁₁|₁₁₁|₁||
CAROL J CHARLESTON
APT 49
1013 HUGHES DR
LAWRENCE SQUARE WI 54690-1226

## YOUR ACCOUNT SUMMARY

| DEPOSIT ACCOUNTS | BALANCE |
|---|---|
| CHECKING ACCOUNT | 2,088.08 |
| SAVINGS ACCOUNT | 6.54 |
| TOTAL | 2,094.62 |

## CHECKING ACCOUNT

CAROL J CHARLESTON

SUMMARY OF ACCOUNT    518-833-3

| | |
|---|---|
| BEGINNING BALANCE ON 07/18/08 | 3,055.24 |
| DEPOSITS AND CREDITS | +3,819.02 |
| CHECKS & WITHDRAWALS | −4,786.18 |
| ENDING BALANCE ON 08/20/08 | 2,088.08 |

CHECKS PAID: 38

| CHECK | AMOUNT | DATE PAID | REFERENCE# | CHECK | AMOUNT | DATE PAID | REFERENCE# |
|---|---|---|---|---|---|---|---|
| CHECK | 450.00 | 07/19/08 | 81569110 | 2226 | 181.00 | 08/12/08 | 05105878 |
| 2202 | 146.23 | 07/31/08 | 29521570 | 2227 | 24.74 | 08/19/08 | 06120827 |
| 2203 | 122.03 | 07/29/08 | 29141271 | 2228 | 140.00 | 08/12/08 | 05022086 |
| 2210* | 43.00 | 07/29/08 | 07046380 | 2229 | 148.71 | 08/16/08 | 27248941 |
| 2211 | 60.09 | 08/01/08 | 04597911 | 2230 | 53.16 | 08/13/08 | 27852752 |
| 2214* | 123.59 | 07/24/08 | 29470425 | 2231 | 50.00 | 08/14/08 | 01018325 |
| 2215 | 47.70 | 07/19/08 | 12357289 | 2232 | 50.00 | 08/13/08 | 05080148 |
| 2216 | 9.00 | 07/22/08 | 05479786 | 2233 | 15.00 | 08/16/08 | 04709533 |
| 2217 | 30.00 | 07/26/08 | 29841864 | 2234 | 13.95 | 08/19/08 | 06008593 |
| 2218 | 19.00 | 07/30/08 | 04330539 | 2235 | 123.59 | 08/14/08 | 27050650 |
| 2219 | 12.00 | 07/24/08 | 04037820 | 2236 | 50.00 | 08/13/08 | 05099115 |
| 2220 | 35.93 | 07/24/08 | 04068844 | 2237 | 50.00 | 08/15/08 | 03014667 |
| 2221 | 10.00 | 08/12/08 | 05091269 | 2238 | 20.00 | 08/16/08 | 04675854 |
| 2222 | 23.48 | 07/24/08 | 29465653 | 2239 | 47.70 | 08/14/08 | 06172997 |
| 2223 | 242.43 | 07/26/08 | 29804419 | 2240 | 24.74 | 08/19/08 | 06120925 |
| 2224 | 150.00 | 07/30/08 | 29405827 | 2243* | 400.00 | 08/14/08 | 29652307 |
| 2225 | 830.00 | 08/07/08 | 02242873 | 2344 | 400.00 | 08/14/08 | 29652306 |

**Figure 18-7.** Each month you will receive a current bank statement, which you should reconcile with the previous statement and your checkbook register.

and depositing checks, just as if you were using traditional methods, but you will see these differences.

- Rather than your recording each check in a paper checkbook and determining the new balance, the computer software calculates the new balance for you.
- Rather than your reconciling the office bank statement on paper, the computer software does it automatically.
- Rather than putting the checkbook and banking forms in a securely locked place at the end of the day, you use a computer password for security.

Many medical office software programs are available today. Each one has a different interface, uses different menus, and prompts you for information in different ways. Certain general concepts apply to all. For specific information, consult the user's manual that comes with your practice's computer software. All software will allow you to perform the following tasks:

- Record deposits
- Pay bills
- Display the checkbook
- Balance the checkbook

**Record Deposits.** If you select "Record Deposits," a message on the computer screen prompts you to enter information about each check to be deposited that day. This information usually includes the check writer's name and the amount of the check. The check's ABA number may also be requested. After you enter this information, the computer gives you a chance to double-check it. If all the information is correct, you continue entering and checking the other deposits, one at a time. You can then select a command to print a deposit slip that contains the information you have just entered. To make the deposit, place the cash and checks in a deposit bag along with the computerized deposit slip and the bank's deposit slip.

**Pay Bills.** The bill-paying function allows you to log checks that you write into a computerized checkbook register. For each check you want to write, a message on the computer screen should prompt you for information, such as the payee and the amount of the check. The computer should also give you a chance to verify and correct this information before moving on to the next check or printing the actual checks.

Some software programs automatically assign the next available check number to each new check you enter. To double-check that the computer-assigned check numbers match those on the actual checks, print a list of the checks you have entered and compare it with the checks before mailing them.

**Display the Checkbook.** The checkbook display function allows you to review the electronic checkbook register. Although you cannot change information that appears in the register, you can print it out. Thus, you can be sure the checks have been recorded properly, and you can check your latest balance.

If you select "Display Checkbook" from the "Banking" menu, the computer displays a list of all checks that have been entered into the register. Information includes check number, date, payee, and amount. Scrolling up and down reveals all the checks in the register. (Some banks also allow you to access this information by telephone. The Points on Practice section gives more information about telephone banking.)

**Balance Checkbook.** The "Balance Checkbook" option electronically reconciles the monthly bank statement. After you enter the appropriate date or dates, the computer screen displays all the checks and deposits that were logged into the register in the order they were posted. Figure 18-8 shows an example of this function.

The next screen highlights each check or deposit that has not been seen on a previous bank statement. You are prompted to indicate whether that item appears on the current statement, usually using Y for yes and N for no. After the computer queries these items, it may ask you to enter any items that appear on the current bank statement but are not in the checkbook, such as service charges.

Finally, a message on the screen prompts you to enter the current account balance from the bank statement. Then, the computer reconciles the bank statement. It will alert you if the system balance does not agree with the balance on the bank statement. If the balance does not agree, recheck the information you entered for possible error. If your work is correct, and the balances still do not agree, call the bank to determine if a bank error has been made.

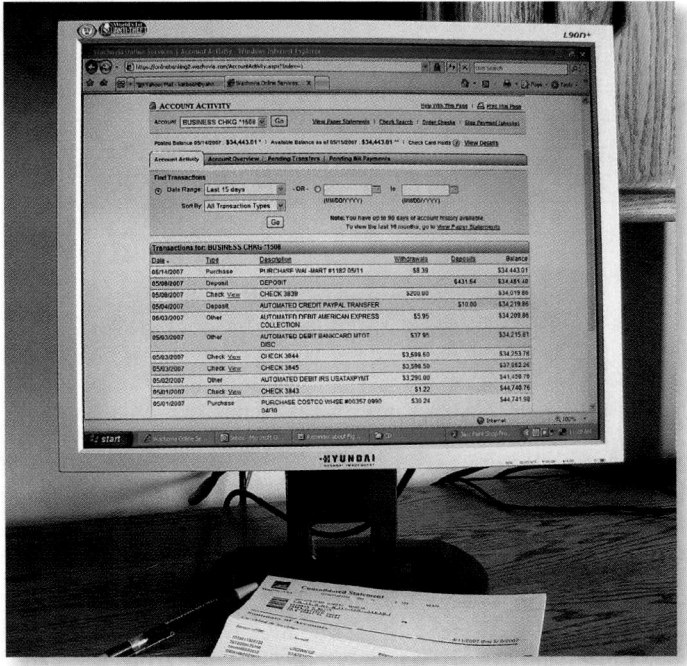

**Figure 18-8.** Electronic banking will allow you to see the "Balanced Checkbook" on the screen.

# PROCEDURE 18.3

## Reconciling a Bank Statement

**Procedure Goal:** To ensure that the bank record of deposits, payments, and withdrawals agrees with the practice's record of deposits, payments, and withdrawals

**Materials:** Previous bank statement, current bank statement, reconciliation worksheet (if not part of current bank statement), deposit receipts, red pencil, check stubs or checkbook register, returned checks

### Method:

1. Check the closing balance on the previous statement against the opening balance on the new statement. The balances should match. If they do not, call the bank.

2. Record the closing balance from the new statement on the reconciliation worksheet (Figure 18-9). This worksheet usually appears on the back of the bank statement.

3. Check each deposit receipt against the bank statement. Place a red check mark in the upper right corner of each receipt that is recorded on the statement. Total the amount of deposits that do *not* appear on the statement. Add this amount to the closing balance on the reconciliation worksheet.

### Rationale

Deposits not appearing on the statement have not been recorded by the bank at the time the statement was created.

4. Put the returned checks in numerical order. (Your bank may send you several sheets consisting of photocopies of checks instead of the actual checks.)

5. Compare each returned check with the bank statement, making sure that the amount on the check agrees with the amount on the statement. Place a red check mark in the upper-right corner

---

## HOW TO BALANCE YOUR CHECKING ACCOUNT

1. Subtract any service charges that appear on this statement from your checkbook balance.
2. Add any interest paid on your checking account to your checkbook balance.
3. Check off (✔) in your checkbook register all checks and pre-authorized transactions listed on your statement.
4. Use the worksheet to list checks you have written, ATM withdrawals, and Point of Sale transactions which are not listed on your statement.

| | | |
|---|---|---|
| 5. Enter the closing balance on the statement. | $ | . |
| 6. Add any deposits not shown on the statement. | + | . |
| 7. Subtotal | $ | . |
| 8. Subtract total transactions outstanding (from worksheet on right). | − | . |
| 9. Account balance (should match balance in your checkbook register). | $ | . |

### IF YOUR ACCOUNT DOES NOT BALANCE

a. Check your addition and subtraction first on this form and then in your checkbook.
b. Be sure the deposit amounts on your statement are the same as those in your checkbook.
c. Be sure all the check amounts on your statement agree with the amounts entered in your checkbook register.
d. Be sure all checks written prior to this reconcilement period but not listed on the statement are listed on the worksheet.
e. Verify that all MAC® ATM, Point of Sale, and other pre-authorized transactions have been recorded in your checkbook register.
f. Review last month's statement to be certain any corrections were entered into your checkbook.

### WORKSHEET
#### Transactions Outstanding

| Number or Date | Amount |
|---|---|
| | |
| | |
| | |
| | |
| | |
| | |
| | |
| | |
| | |
| | |
| | |
| | |
| | |
| | |
| | |
| TOTAL | |

**Figure 18-9.** Use the reconciliation worksheet on the back of the bank statement to reconcile the statement with your checkbook register.

*continued* ⟶

## Reconciling a Bank Statement (concluded)

of each returned check that is recorded on the statement. Also, place a check mark on the check stub or check register entry. Any checks that were written but that do not appear on the statement and were not returned are considered "outstanding" checks. You can find these easily on the check stubs or checkbook register because they have no red check mark.

6. List each outstanding check separately on the worksheet, including its check number and amount. Total the outstanding checks, and subtract this total from the bank statement balance.

### Rationale

These checks have not cleared yet. The total of these checks will still appear in the medical practice balance.

7. If the statement shows that the checking account earned interest, add this amount to the checkbook balance.

### Rationale

You did not know about accrued interest until receiving the statement.

8. If the statement lists such items as a service charge, check printing charge, or automatic

payment, subtract them from the checkbook balance.

### Rationale

You did not know about these charges until receiving the statement.

9. Compare the new checkbook balance with the new bank statement balance. They should match. If they do not, repeat the process, rechecking all calculations. Double-check the addition and subtraction in the checkbook register. Review the checkbook register to make sure you did not omit any items. Ensure that you carried the correct balance forward from one register page to the next. Double-check that you made the correct additions or subtractions for all interest earned and charges.

10. If your work is correct, and the balances still do not agree, call the bank to determine if a bank error has been made. Contact the bank promptly because the bank may have a time limit for corrections. The bank may consider the bank statement correct if you do not point out an error within 2 weeks (or other period, according to bank policy).

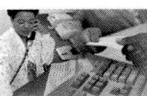

## Points on Practice

## Telephone Banking

Telephone banking is a form of electronic banking that enables you to access your bank's computer system by phone to obtain account information and perform simple banking tasks. To use telephone banking, you should have a push-button telephone, the telephone personal identification number (TPIN) assigned to your practice by the bank, and the telephone number that accesses the telephone banking system.

The telephone banking system prompts you for information. You use the push-button pad on the telephone to provide the information. For example, an automated voice may ask you to press 1 to inquire about deposits or 2 to inquire about withdrawals. Telephone banking is especially useful for the following banking tasks:

- Checking the current balance of an account
- Determining whether deposited funds are available

- Obtaining the date and amount of the last few deposits and the last few checks paid (usually the last three)
- Finding out if a specific check has been paid
- Transferring funds between accounts (if the practice has more than one account)
- Stopping payment on checks

Although this form of electronic banking is especially useful for some services, you cannot use it to manage all banking tasks. For example, you cannot use it to make deposits or reconcile a bank statement. However, it can be quite convenient for the day-to-day banking tasks just listed. If you have a hearing impairment and have a telecommunications device for the deaf (TDD) installed on the telephone, you can bank by phone.

# PROCEDURE 18.4

## Setting Up the Accounts Payable System

**Procedure Goal:** To set up an accounts payable system

**Materials:** Disbursements journal, petty cash record, payroll register, pen

**Method:**

### Setting Up the Disbursements Journal

1. Write in column headings for the basic information about each check: date, payee's name, check number, and check amount.
2. Write in column headings for each type of business expense, such as rent and utilities.
3. Write in column headings (if space is available) for deposits and the account balance.
4. Record the data from completed checks under the appropriate column headings.

### Setting Up the Petty Cash Record

1. Write in column headings for the date, transaction number, payee, brief description, amount of transaction, and type of expense.
2. Write in a column heading (if space is available) for the petty cash fund balance.

3. Record the data from petty cash vouchers under the appropriate column headings.

### Setting Up the Payroll Register

1. Write in column headings for check number, employee name, earnings to date, hourly rate, hours worked, regular earnings, overtime hours worked, and overtime earnings.
2. Write in column headings for total gross earnings for the pay period and gross taxable earnings.
3. Write in column headings for each deduction. These may include federal income tax, Federal Insurance Contributions Act (FICA) tax, state income tax, local income tax, and various voluntary deductions.
4. Write in a column heading for net earnings.
5. Each time you write payroll checks, record earning and deduction data under the appropriate column headings on the payroll register.

# Managing Accounts Payable

As you learned in Chapter 17, accounts payable are the practice's expenses (money leaving the business), and accounts receivable reflect a practice's income (money coming into the business). This section focuses on accounts payable, including payroll. A basic accounting principle to bear in mind is that when a practice's income exceeds its expenses, it has a profit. When a practice's expenses exceed its income, it has a loss.

Because of this relationship between income and expenses, most practices try to reduce expenses by controlling accounts payable. As a medical assistant, you play an important role in helping control accounts payable and maximize profits.

Accounts payable fall into three main groups:

1. Payments for supplies, equipment, and practice-related products and services
2. Payroll, which may be the largest of the accounts payable
3. Taxes owed to federal, state, and local agencies

A practice's accounting system usually consists of several elements. These elements include the daily log,

patient ledger cards, the checkbook, the disbursements journal, the petty cash record, and the payroll register.

The daily log and patient ledger cards are used primarily for accounts receivable. The disbursements journal, petty cash record, and payroll register are used primarily in accounts payable. Procedure 18-4 tells you how to set up and use these accounting tools effectively.

# Managing Disbursements

A disbursement is any payment the physician's office makes for goods or services. One of the most common disbursements is payment for office supplies. Other disbursements include payments for equipment, dues, rent, taxes, salary, and utilities. No matter what type of disbursement you make on behalf of the practice, you must keep accurate records of the purchase and the payment.

## Managing Supplies

In most practices, the physician authorizes one person to handle the purchasing of supplies and other products. This person is usually the office manager or medical assistant.

Guidelines for purchasing supplies are discussed in detail in Chapter 8. When buying clinical or office supplies, keep these six principles in mind to control expenses.

1. Order only the necessary supplies, and order them only in the proper amounts. Buying too much reduces cash flow. Buying too little may cause you to run out of needed items and you may have to reorder too often.

2. Combine orders when possible. You may save money and time by placing a larger order for several items at once rather than placing a smaller order each time an item is needed.

3. Follow your practice's purchasing guidelines, if any. For example, you may have to get the physician's approval for purchases over a specific dollar amount. Employees may have to submit purchase orders (formal requests for goods or services).

4. Buy from reputable suppliers. They are more likely to provide on-time delivery and satisfactory handling of your order. If your office does not already have a list of reliable suppliers, ask for recommendations from other practices.

5. Get the best-quality supplies for the best price.

6. For clinical supplies, consider the amount for which insurance companies will reimburse the practice. For example, if your office does only a few throat cultures a year, it might make more sense to send those patients elsewhere for the test than to stock the supplies required. The small reimbursement amount for a few throat cultures may not justify purchasing the supplies. Also consider shelf life. Do not buy large amounts of clinical supplies that will expire before use.

## Writing Checks

Virtually all disbursements are made by check. Paying by check gives the practice complete, accurate records of all financial transactions.

Before writing a check, make sure the checking account balance is up-to-date and large enough to cover the check you want to write. Enter the date, check number, payee information, and reason for the payment on the check stub, and then subtract the amount of each check from the previous balance, enter the new balance, and carry that balance forward to the next stub. Do this step before writing the check so the payment entry is not accidentally omitted from the disbursement journal.

If you use a pegboard system, you will automatically record the date, check number, payee, and check amount on the check register as you write out the check. You must note the reason for payment and the new balance manually, however. Record that information in the appropriate spaces on the register.

If you make an error when completing a check, write VOID in ink across the front of the check in large letters so that it cannot be used again. Then file the voided check in numerical order with the returned checks.

After filling out the check properly, detach it from the checkbook and give it to the doctor to sign, along with the invoice to be paid. (With experience, you may be trusted to sign checks under a certain amount.) Mark the date, check number, and amount paid on the invoice. Make a copy of the invoice for your records. Keep these copies with supporting documents, such as order forms or packing slips, in a paid-invoice file. Then, mail the check and the original invoice to the payee in a neatly hand-addressed or typewritten envelope. If you use a window envelope, be sure the payee's address shows through the window.

**Commonly Used Checks.** Most practices use checks from a standard checkbook, or they use **voucher checks,** business checks with stubs attached. Voucher checks come in several styles. A common style is a large, ring-bound checkbook, with three checks to a page. A perforation divides each check from its matching stub, which the practice retains.

Limited checks are sometimes used for payroll. A **limited check** states that it is void after a certain time limit. Many practices use checks that are void after 90 days. Some limited check accounts may also limit the amount for which a limited check may be written.

**Other Types of Checks.** You or the physician may sometimes need to use other types of checks. The physician may use a cashier's check to pay certain types of taxes. A cashier's check is purchased from a bank, written on the bank's own checking account, and signed by a bank official.

The physician may use a certified check to pay certain taxes or to buy property. A certified check is a standard check that the bank verifies and certifies before it is used. This certification means that funds have been set aside to guarantee payment of the check.

A **counter check** is a special bank check that allows the depositor to withdraw funds from her account only. It states, "Pay to the Order of Myself Only." The physician may use a counter check when she wants to withdraw money but has forgotten her checkbook.

A physician may use **traveler's checks** when attending an out-of-town conference or whenever using a personal check or carrying a lot of cash is not appropriate. Printed in $10, $20, $50, and $100 denominations, these checks must be signed at the location where they are purchased (usually a bank). To use traveler's checks, the physician fills in the payee's name and signs it in a second place. She must sign it in the payee's presence so the payee can ensure that the signatures match.

## Recording Disbursements

You may record disbursements in a check register, in a disbursements journal, or on the bottom section of the daily log.

If you use a disbursements journal, follow these steps to record disbursements.

1. When beginning a new journal page, give each column a heading to reflect the type of expense, such as utilities or rent.
2. For each check, fill in the date, payee's name, check number, and check amount in the appropriate columns.
3. Determine the expense category of the check.
4. Record the check amount in the column for that type of business expense.
5. If you must divide a check between two or more expense columns, record the total in the check amount column. Then record the amount that applies to each type of expense in the appropriate column. The total amount must equal the sum of the amounts listed between the columns.

Recording disbursements in columns for each type of expense allows you to total and track expenses by category. **Tracking** (watching for changes) is important because it helps control expenses. Before tracking, check your calculations by performing a trial balance.

1. Total the check amount column.
2. Find the total for each expense column.
3. Add together all the expense column totals. The combined expense column total should match the total in the check amount column.
4. If the amounts do not match, recheck every entry until you find the error. When you find it, draw a line through it, and record the correct information neatly above it or to the side.
5. When the two amounts match (or balance), carry forward all column totals to the disbursements journal for the next month. Remember to prepare summaries and perform balances at the end of every month, quarter, and year.

## Managing Petty Cash

Occasionally, you may need to make small (petty) cash disbursements for minor expenses such as postage-due fees or holiday decorations (Figure 18-10). To avoid writing checks for such small amounts, you may pay for them from the **petty cash fund** (also known as the revolving fund), cash kept on hand in the office for small purchases. The doctor should determine the amount of the petty cash account (usually $50) and the minimum amount of cash to be kept on hand (such as $15).

**Starting and Maintaining a Petty Cash Fund.** To start the fund with $50, write a check to "Petty Cash" or "Cash" for that amount. Enter the check in the miscellaneous column of the monthly disbursement record. Then, cash the check. Because this money will be used for small disbursements, be sure to get some of it in pennies,

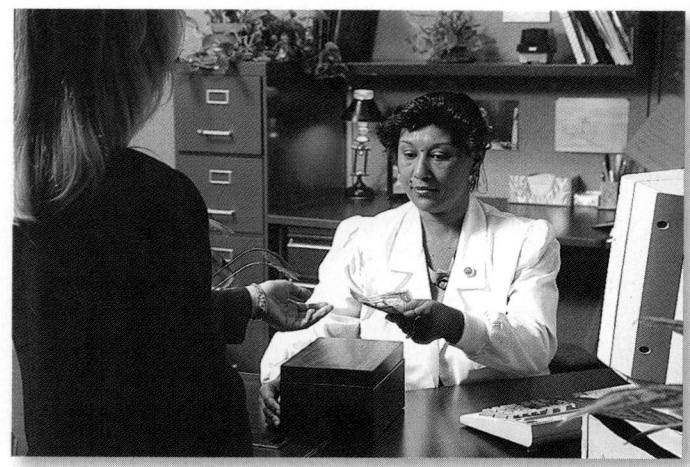

**Figure 18-10.** You may be in charge of maintaining the practice's petty cash fund. Count cash carefully, and keep accurate records about purchases made.

nickels, dimes, quarters, and dollar bills. Put this money in a special petty cash box, along with a stack of petty cash vouchers.

For each payment from the petty cash fund, obtain a receipt or create a petty cash voucher. The voucher should record the transaction number, date, amount paid, purpose of the expense, your signature (as the person issuing the money), and the signature of the person receiving it. Keep the receipt for any item purchased, along with the completed voucher, in the petty cash box to verify expenses later.

Also, document each petty cash withdrawal on a petty cash record form. Include the transaction number, date, payee, a brief description, amount, and type of expense (such as office expense, auto expense, or miscellaneous expense). If a space is provided, calculate and record the new balance in the petty cash fund.

**Replenishing the Petty Cash Fund.** At the end of the month (or whenever the fund is low), compare the latest petty cash balance to the money in the petty cash box. If you have not kept a running balance, total the receipts and vouchers, then count the cash on hand. Subtract the total amount on the receipts and vouchers (for example, $35) from the original balance (for example, $50). The difference ($15) should equal the cash on hand in the petty cash box ($15).

To replenish the account, write a check to "Cash" or "Petty Cash" for the amount spent ($35). Cash the check and add the money to the box, bringing the total back up to the original amount of $50. Record the check for $35 on the disbursement record. Also, total the receipts and vouchers by expense category. Record those totals in the appropriate columns on the disbursement record.

## Understanding Financial Summaries

The physician may periodically analyze the income and expenses of the practice. Financial summaries provide an easy-to-read report on the business transactions for a given period, such as a month or a year.

An accountant usually prepares financial summaries. Although you will probably not have to create these summaries, you should understand how they are prepared.

**Statement of Income and Expense.** Also called a profit-and-loss statement, a statement of income and expense highlights the practice's profitability. It shows the physician the practice's total income and then lists and subtracts all expenses.

**Cash Flow Statement.** A **cash flow statement** shows how much cash is available to cover expenses, to invest, or to take as profits. The cash flow statement begins with the cash on hand at the beginning of the period and shows the income and disbursements made during that period. It concludes with the new amount of cash on hand at the end of the period.

**Trial Balance.** The doctor may review trial balances periodically to ensure that the books balance. The combined expense column total should match the total in the check amount column. If the amounts do not match, recheck every entry until you find the error.

# Handling Payroll

You may be responsible for handling the office payroll (Table 18-1). If so, your duties may include:

- Obtaining tax identification numbers
- Creating employee payroll information sheets
- Calculating employees' earnings
- Subtracting taxes and other deductions
- Writing paychecks
- Creating employee earnings records
- Preparing a payroll register
- Submitting payroll taxes

| TABLE 18-1 Payroll Duties | |
|---|---|
| **Frequency** | **Duties** |
| Upon assuming payroll responsibilities | Apply for an employer identification number (EIN) with Form SS-4 if the physician does not already have an EIN. |
| Whenever a new employee is hired | Have the employee complete an Employee's Withholding Allowance Certificate (Form W-4) and Employment Eligibility Verification (Form I-9). Record the employee's name and Social Security number from the employee's Social Security card. |
| Every payday | Withhold federal income tax as well as state and local income taxes (if any). Withhold the employee's share of FICA taxes (for Social Security and Medicare). Record a matching amount for the employer's share. Calculate how much the practice must pay for each employee's federal and state unemployment tax. |
| Monthly or biweekly (depending on your deposit schedule) | Deposit withheld income taxes, withheld and employer Social Security taxes, and withheld and employer Medicare taxes. |
| Quarterly (by April 30, July 31, October 31, and January 31) | File Employer's Quarterly Federal Tax Return (Form 941). With the return, pay any taxes that were not deposited earlier. Deposit federal unemployment tax, if over $100. |
| At least once a year | Have all employees update their W-4 forms. |
| On or before January 31 | Give employees their Wage and Tax Statements (Form W-2), which show total wages and various withheld taxes. File Employer's Annual Federal Unemployment (FUTA) Tax Return (Form 940) with tax amount due. |
| On or before February 28 | File Transmittal of Wage and Tax Statements (Form W-3) along with the government's copies of the W-2 forms. |

## Applying for Tax Identification Numbers

Every employer—whether a single physician or a corporate practice—must have an employer identification number (EIN). An EIN is required by law for federal tax accounting purposes. An EIN is obtained by completing Form SS-4 (Application for Employer Identification Number) and submitting it to the Internal Revenue Service (IRS). Some states also require employer tax reports, for which the practice must have a state identification number, obtained from the proper state agency.

## Creating Employee Payroll Information Sheets

The practice must maintain up-to-date, accurate payroll information about each employee. You should prepare a payroll information sheet for each employee. Each sheet should have the following information:

- The employee's name, address, Social Security number, and marital status
- An indication that the employee has completed an Employment Eligibility Verification (Form I-9), verifying that the employee is a U.S. citizen, a legally admitted alien, or an alien authorized to work in the United States
- The employee's pay schedule, number of dependents, payroll type, and voluntary deductions

**Pay Schedule.** On the payroll information sheet, list the employee's **pay schedule,** showing how often the employee is paid. Common pay schedules are weekly, biweekly, and monthly.

**Number of Dependents.** Record the number of **dependents** (people who depend on the employee for financial support). Dependents may include a spouse, children, and other family members.

You can find the number of dependents on the Employee's Withholding Allowance Certificate (Form W-4), which should have been completed when the employee was hired (Figure 18-11). Remember to keep the completed W-4 forms in the physician's personnel file, and update them at least annually.

**Payroll Type.** List the employee's payroll type—hourly wage, salary, or commission—on the payroll information sheet. An hourly wage is a set amount of money per hour of work. A salary is a set amount of money per pay period, regardless of the number of hours worked. A commission is a percentage of the amount an employee earns for the employer. Salespeople, for example, are often paid by commission.

**Voluntary Deductions.** Finally, document the voluntary deductions to be taken from the employee's check. These may include additional federal withholding taxes, contributions to a 401(k) retirement plan, or payments to a company health insurance plan. Employees who want additional federal taxes taken out of their paycheck will indicate this deduction on their W-4 form.

## Gross Earnings

**Gross earnings** refers to the total amount of income earned before deductions. Gross earnings must be calculated for each employee as a first step in the payroll process.

**Calculating Gross Earnings.** For every payroll period, use data from the payroll information sheet to compute each employee's gross earnings. For an hourly employee, use this equation:

Hourly Wage × Hours Worked = Gross Earnings

An employee who earns $10 per hour and works 35 hours, for example, has gross earnings of $350 ($10 × 35 hours) per week.

For a salaried employee, use the salary amount as the gross earnings for the pay period, no matter how many hours the employee worked. An employee who earns a weekly salary of $400, for example, receives that amount whether she worked 30, 40, or 50 hours during that week.

**Fair Labor Standards Act.** The Fair Labor Standards Act primarily affects employees who earn hourly wages. It limits the number of hours they may work, sets their minimum wage, and regulates their overtime pay. It also requires the employer to record the number of hours they work, usually on a time card or in a time book.

For hourly employees, this act mandates payment of:

- Time and a half (1½ times the normal hourly wage) for all hours worked beyond the normal 8 in a regular workday.
- Time and a half for all hours worked on the sixth consecutive day of the work week.
- Twice the normal wage (double time) for all hours worked on the seventh consecutive workday.
- Double time, plus normal holiday pay, for all hours worked on a company-approved holiday.

The Fair Labor Standards Act also requires overtime payments for part-time hourly employees for every hour worked beyond the normal 8 in a day or 40 in a week.

## Making Deductions

The law requires all employers to withhold money from employees' gross earnings to pay federal, state, and local (if any) income taxes and certain other taxes. In addition, employees may wish you to make certain voluntary deductions. For example, you might be asked to deduct an amount for child care, if the practice or hospital provides on-site child care. You might also deduct employee contributions to health insurance premiums.

# Form W-4 (2007)

**Purpose.** Complete Form W-4 so that your employer can withhold the correct federal income tax from your pay. Because your tax situation may change, you may want to refigure your withholding each year.

**Exemption from withholding.** If you are exempt, complete **only** lines 1, 2, 3, 4, and 7 and sign the form to validate it. Your exemption for 2007 expires February 16, 2008. See Pub. 505, Tax Withholding and Estimated Tax.

**Note.** You cannot claim exemption from withholding if (a) your income exceeds $850 and includes more than $300 of unearned income (for example, interest and dividends) and (b) another person can claim you as a dependent on their tax return.

**Basic instructions.** If you are not exempt, complete the **Personal Allowances Worksheet** below. The worksheets on page 2 adjust your withholding allowances based on itemized deductions, certain credits, adjustments to income, or two-earner/multiple job situations. Complete all worksheets that apply. However, you may claim fewer (or zero) allowances.

**Head of household.** Generally, you may claim head of household filing status on your tax return only if you are unmarried and pay more than 50% of the costs of keeping up a home for yourself and your dependent(s) or other qualifying individuals.

**Tax credits.** You can take projected tax credits into account in figuring your allowable number of withholding allowances. Credits for child or dependent care expenses and the child tax credit may be claimed using the **Personal Allowances Worksheet** below. See Pub. 919, How Do I Adjust My Tax Withholding, for information on converting your other credits into withholding allowances.

**Nonwage income.** If you have a large amount of nonwage income, such as interest or dividends, consider making estimated tax payments using Form 1040-ES, Estimated Tax for Individuals. Otherwise, you may owe additional tax. If you have pension or annuity income, see Pub. 919 to find out if you should adjust your withholding on Form W-4 or W-4P.

**Two earners/Multiple jobs.** If you have a working spouse or more than one job, figure the total number of allowances you are entitled to claim on all jobs using worksheets from only one Form W-4. Your withholding usually will be most accurate when all allowances are claimed on the Form W-4 for the highest paying job and zero allowances are claimed on the others.

**Nonresident alien.** If you are a nonresident alien, see the Instructions for Form 8233 before completing this Form W-4.

**Check your withholding.** After your Form W-4 takes effect, use Pub. 919 to see how the dollar amount you are having withheld compares to your projected total tax for 2007. See Pub. 919, especially if your earnings exceed $130,000 (Single) or $180,000 (Married).

---

## Personal Allowances Worksheet (Keep for your records.)

**A** Enter "1" for **yourself** if no one else can claim you as a dependent . . . . . . . . . . . **A** _____

**B** Enter "1" if:
- You are single and have only one job; or
- You are married, have only one job, and your spouse does not work; or
- Your wages from a second job or your spouse's wages (or the total of both) are $1,000 or less.

. . . **B** _____

**C** Enter "1" for your **spouse**. But, you may choose to enter "-0-" if you are married and have either a working spouse or more than one job. (Entering "-0-" may help you avoid having too little tax withheld.) . . . . **C** _____

**D** Enter number of **dependents** (other than your spouse or yourself) you will claim on your tax return . . . . . . . . **D** _____

**E** Enter "1" if you will file as **head of household** on your tax return (see conditions under **Head of household** above) . . . **E** _____

**F** Enter "1" if you have at least $1,500 of **child or dependent care expenses** for which you plan to claim a credit . . . **F** _____
(**Note.** Do **not** include child support payments. See Pub. 503, Child and Dependent Care Expenses, for details.)

**G** **Child Tax Credit** (including additional child tax credit). See Pub 972, Child Tax Credit, for more information.
- If your total income will be less than $57,000 ($85,000 if married), enter "2" for each eligible child.
- If your total income will be between $57,000 and $84,000 ($85,000 and $119,000 if married), enter "1" for each eligible child plus "1" **additional** if you have 4 or more eligible children. **G** _____

**H** Add lines A through G and enter total here. (**Note.** This may be different from the number of exemptions you claim on your tax return.) ▶ **H** _____

For accuracy, complete all worksheets that apply.
- If you plan to **itemize or claim adjustments to income** and want to reduce your withholding, see the **Deductions and Adjustments Worksheet** on page 2.
- If you have **more than one job** or are **married and you and your spouse both work** and the combined earnings from all jobs exceed $40,000 ($25,000 if married) see the **Two-Earners/Multiple Jobs Worksheet** on page 2 to avoid having too little tax withheld.
- If **neither** of the above situations applies, **stop here** and enter the number from line H on line 5 of Form W-4 below.

------------------------ Cut here and give Form W-4 to your employer. Keep the top part for your records. ------------------------

| Form **W-4** | **Employee's Withholding Allowance Certificate** | OMB No. 1545-0074 |
|---|---|---|
| Department of the Treasury Internal Revenue Service | ▶ Whether you are entitled to claim a certain number of allowances or exemption from withholding is subject to review by the IRS. Your employer may be required to send a copy of this form to the IRS. | 20**07** |

| **1** Type or print your first name and middle initial. | Last name | **2** Your social security number |
|---|---|---|

| Home address (number and street or rural route) | **3** ☐ Single ☐ Married ☐ Married, but withhold at higher Single rate. **Note.** If married, but legally separated, or spouse is a nonresident alien, check the "Single" box. |
|---|---|
| City or town, state, and ZIP code | **4** If your last name differs from that shown on your social security card, check here. You must call 1-800-772-1213 for a replacement card. ▶ ☐ |

**5** Total number of allowances you are claiming (from line **H** above **or** from the applicable worksheet on page 2) — **5** _____

**6** Additional amount, if any, you want withheld from each paycheck. . . . . . . . . . . . . . . **6** $ _____

**7** I claim exemption from withholding for 2007, and I certify that I meet **both** of the following conditions for exemption.
- Last year I had a right to a refund of **all** federal income tax withheld because I had **no** tax liability **and**
- This year I expect a refund of **all** federal income tax withheld because I expect to have **no** tax liability.

If you meet both conditions, write "Exempt" here . . . . . . . . . . . . . . ▶ **7** _____

Under penalties of perjury, I declare that I have examined this certificate and to the best of my knowledge and belief, it is true, correct, and complete.

**Employee's signature**
(Form is not valid unless you sign it.) ▶ _____ **Date** ▶ _____

**8** Employer's name and address (Employer: Complete lines 8 and 10 only if sending to the IRS.) | **9** Office code (optional) | **10** Employer identification number (EIN)

**For Privacy Act and Paperwork Reduction Act Notice, see page 2.** | Cat. No. 10220Q | Form **W-4** (2007)

---

**Figure 18-11.** Update all Employee's Withholding Allowance Certificates (W-4 forms) at least once a year.

You must deposit all employee deductions and employer payments into separate accounts. Monies from these **tax liability** accounts are used to pay taxes to appropriate government agencies.

**Income Taxes.** You must withhold enough money to cover the employee's federal income tax for the pay period. You can determine this amount by finding the employee's number of exemptions (from Form W-4) and referring to the tax tables in *Circular E, Employer's Tax Guide,* published by the IRS.

Consult the state and local tax tables for other income taxes. These taxes may be simpler to calculate. For example, they may be 4% and 1% of the employee's gross earnings, respectively.

**FICA Taxes.** For FICA tax, withhold from the employee's check half of the tax owed for the pay period. Pay the other half from the practice's accounts. The amount of FICA tax that funds Social Security differs from the amount that funds Medicare. Report these two amounts separately. Check IRS *Circular E* for the latest FICA tax percentages and level of taxable earnings.

**Unemployment Taxes.** Federal unemployment tax is not a deduction from employees' paychecks, but it is based on their earnings. It is paid by the practice. The **Federal Unemployment Tax Act (FUTA)** requires employers to pay a percentage of each employee's income, up to a certain dollar amount. The percentage may be reduced if the employer also pays state unemployment taxes.

States calculate unemployment taxes differently. Some states tax employers and employees; others tax only employers. State unemployment tax usually varies with the employer's past employment record. Employers with few layoffs, such as physicians, have lower tax rates than those with many layoffs. To compute state unemployment tax, apply the assigned tax rate to each employee's earnings, up to a maximum for the calendar year. For details, consult your state unemployment insurance department.

**Workers' Compensation.** Some states require employers to insure their employees against possible loss of income resulting from work-related injury, disability, or disease. Although state laws vary, they typically require doctors to carry this insurance with a state insurance fund or state-authorized private insurer. Usually, a medical practice's insurance agent will audit the payroll books annually and then issue a bill for the workers' compensation premium due.

## Calculating Net Earnings

Add each employee's required and voluntary deductions together to determine the total deductions. Then, subtract the total deductions from the gross earnings to get the employee's **net earnings,** or take-home pay. Use the following equation:

Gross Earnings − Total Deductions = Net Earnings

The exception to this rule may be contributions the employee makes to the employer retirement plan, if available. When sponsored by an employer, as with a 401(k) account, these deductions are often taken before taxes are calculated, reducing the employee's taxable income, which encourages the employee to take part in these plans.

## Preparing Paychecks

The way you prepare the practice's payroll will depend on the system the practice uses. In a small practice, you may write paychecks manually. In this case, write the check amount for the employee's net earnings, and deduct the check amount from the office checkbook. Payroll may also

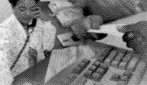 **Points on Practice**

### Handling Payroll Through Electronic Banking

An electronic funds transfer system (EFTS) enables you to handle the practice's payroll without writing payroll checks manually. The physician must sign up for EFTS with the bank, and employees must supply their bank account numbers to the employer. Then, the bank electronically deposits employees' paychecks into their bank accounts, as directed.

Most employees like to have their paychecks deposited automatically. The money is available on the day of deposit, and no one has to worry about losing a paycheck, getting to the bank before it closes, or carrying a paycheck around. Also, employees still receive a check stub along with a notification of deposit, so they can track their earnings and deductions.

Contact your bank for more information and specific procedures for setting up EFTS and electronic payroll.

# PROCEDURE 18.5

## Generating Payroll

**Procedure Goal:** To handle the practice's payroll as efficiently and accurately as possible for each pay period

**Materials:** Employees' time cards, employees' earnings records, payroll register, IRS tax tables, check register

**Method:**

1. Calculate the total regular and overtime hours worked, based on the employee's time card. Enter those totals under the appropriate headings on the payroll register.

   ### Rationale
   Time calculations and the separation of regular and overtime hours must be accurate in order for the paycheck to be correct.

2. Check the pay rate on the employee earnings record. Then multiply the hours worked (including any paid vacation or paid holidays, if applicable) by the rates for regular time and overtime (time and a half or double time). This yields gross earnings.

   ### Rationale
   An accurate gross earnings calculation is the basis for taxes and deductions.

3. Enter the gross earnings under the appropriate heading on the payroll register. Subtract any nontaxable benefits, such as health-care or retirement programs.

4. Using IRS tax tables and data on the employee earnings record, determine the amount of federal income tax to withhold based on the employee's marital status and number of exemptions. Also compute the amount of FICA tax to withhold for Social Security (6.2%) and Medicare (1.45%).

   ### Rationale
   This is required by law.

5. Following state and local procedures, determine the amount of state and local income taxes (if any) to withhold based on the employee's marital status and number of exemptions.

   ### Rationale
   This is required by law.

6. Calculate the employer's contributions to FUTA and to the state unemployment fund, if any. Post these amounts to the employer's account.

7. Enter any other required or voluntary deductions, such as health insurance or contributions to a 401(k) fund.

8. Subtract all deductions from the gross earnings to get the employee's net earnings.

9. Enter the total amount withheld from all employees for FICA under the headings for Social Security and Medicare. Remember that the employer must match these amounts. Enter other employer contributions, such as for federal and state unemployment taxes, under the appropriate headings.

   ### Rationale
   These deductions are required by law.

10. Fill out the check stub, including the employee's name, date, pay period, gross earnings, all deductions, and net earnings. Make out the paycheck for the net earnings.

11. Deposit each deduction in a tax liability account.

---

be handled through electronic banking; see the Points on Practice section.

If the practice uses a payroll service, you may supply time cards or payroll data to the service by mail or electronically. The service calculates all the deductions, prepares paychecks, and mails them to the practice for distribution.

No matter how paychecks are prepared, they should include information about how the check amount was determined. This information usually appears on the check stub. It should match the information on the em-

ployee earnings records and payroll register. Procedure 18-5 explains the process for generating payroll.

## Maintaining Employee Earnings Records

You need to keep an employee earnings record for each employee (Figure 18-12). When you create the record, list the employee's name, address, phone number, Social Security number, birth date, spouse's name, number of

| Name | | Soc. Sec. No. | | Dependents | | Year | |
|------|--|---------------|--|------------|--|------|--|

Name_____ Soc. Sec. No. _____ Dependents _____ Year _____

Address_____ Birth Date _____ Deductions _____

_____ Job Title _____

Employed on _____ Pay Rate

| | Date | Rate |
|--|------|------|
| | | |
| | | |

Spouse_____ Terminated on _____ Record of Changes

Phone Reason

| Check Number | Period Number | Earnings | | | Deductions | | | | | Net Pay | Cumulative FICA |
|--------------|---------------|----------|----|-------|------|----------|-------|-----|-----|---------|-----------------|
| | | Regular | OT | Total | FICA | Fed. Tax | State | SUI | SDI | | |
| | | | | | | | | | | | |
| | | | | | | | | | | | |
| | | | | | | | | | | | |
| | | | | | | | | | | | |
| | | | | | | | | | | | |
| | | | | | | | | | | | |
| | | | | | | | | | | | |
| | | | | | | | | | | | |
| 1st Quarter Total | | | | | | | | | | | |
| | | | | | | | | | | | |
| | | | | | | | | | | | |
| | | | | | | | | | | | |
| | | | | | | | | | | | |
| | | | | | | | | | | | |
| | | | | | | | | | | | |
| | | | | | | | | | | | |
| | | | | | | | | | | | |
| 2d Quarter Total | | | | | | | | | | | |
| | | | | | | | | | | | |
| | | | | | | | | | | | |
| | | | | | | | | | | | |
| | | | | | | | | | | | |
| | | | | | | | | | | | |
| | | | | | | | | | | | |
| | | | | | | | | | | | |
| | | | | | | | | | | | |
| 3d Quarter Total | | | | | | | | | | | |
| | | | | | | | | | | | |
| | | | | | | | | | | | |
| | | | | | | | | | | | |
| | | | | | | | | | | | |
| | | | | | | | | | | | |
| | | | | | | | | | | | |
| | | | | | | | | | | | |
| | | | | | | | | | | | |
| 4th Quarter Total | | | | | | | | | | | |

**Figure 18-12.** Earnings records show the earning history of each employee at your practice.

| Emp. No. | Name | Earnings to date | Hrly. Rate | Reg. Hrs. | OT Hrs. | OT Earnings | TOTAL GROSS | Earnings Subject to Unemp. | Earnings Subject to FICA | Social Security (FICA) | Medicare | Federal W/H | State W/H | Health Ins. | Net Pay | Check No. |
|---|---|---|---|---|---|---|---|---|---|---|---|---|---|---|---|---|
| 0010 | Scott, B. | 9,823.14 | 14.00 | 70.00 | | | 980.00 | 980.00 | 980.00 | 60.50 | 14.10 | 147.92 | 15.10 | 25.00 | 717.38 | 11747 |
| 0020 | Wilson, J. | 14,290.38 | 17.00 | 70.00 | 6.50 | 153.00 | 1343.00 | 1343.00 | 1343.00 | 83.26 | 19.47 | 160.45 | 15.85 | 67.50 | 996.47 | 11748 |
| 0030 | Diaz, J. | 2,750.26 | 5.50 | 46.25 | | | 254.37 | 254.37 | 254.37 | 15.77 | 3.68 | 38.20 | 3.75 | | 192.97 | 11749 |
| 0040 | Ling, W. | 2,240.57 | 6.80 | 30.00 | | | 204.00 | 204.00 | 204.00 | 12.66 | 2.96 | 26.02 | 3.12 | | 159.54 | 11750 |
| 0050 | Harris, E. | 2,600.98 | 10.00 | 23.50 | | | 235.00 | 235.00 | 235.00 | 14.57 | 3.41 | 33.52 | 3.36 | | 180.14 | 11751 |
| | | | | | | | | | | | | | | | | |
| | | | | | | | | | | | | | | | | |

Pay Period 6/1–6/14

**Figure 18-13.** A payroll register is designed to summarize information about all employees and their earnings.

dependents, job title, employment starting date, pay rate, and voluntary deductions.

Then, for each pay period, record the employee's gross earnings, individual deductions, net earnings, and related information. Properly completed earnings records show each employee's earning history.

## Maintaining a Payroll Register

A payroll register summarizes vital information about all employees and their earnings (Figure 18-13). At the end of each pay period, record each employee's earnings to date, hourly rate, hours worked, overtime hours, overtime earnings, and total gross earnings. Also, list the gross earnings subject to unemployment taxes and FICA, all required and voluntary deductions, net earnings, and the paycheck number.

## Handling Payroll Electronically

Manual payroll preparation and related tasks may take an hour per week for each employee. To save time and to provide the convenience for employees of having their paychecks automatically deposited, some practices handle payroll tasks electronically.

If you work in a relatively small practice, you may handle all payroll tasks in the office, using accounting or payroll software. If you work in a large practice, you may prepare payroll information on the computer and transmit it by modem to an outside payroll service for processing. Depending on which system and software the practice has, you may use the computer to:

- Create, update, and delete employee payroll information files
- Prepare employee paychecks, stubs, and W-2 forms
- Update and print employee earnings records

- Update all appropriate bookkeeping records, such as the payroll ledger and general ledger, with payroll data

To perform these payroll functions electronically, follow the specific instructions in the software manual or get instructions from the payroll service. Generally, you would follow these steps.

Select an option from the "Payroll" menu. Wait for the prompt, then select the appropriate employee from a list of employees.

To create an employee payroll information file for a new employee, input the same information that you would record manually on an employee payroll information sheet: name, address, Social Security number, marital status, pay schedule, number of dependents, payroll type, and voluntary deductions. Print two copies of the employee payroll information file—one for the employee and one for the physician's personnel file.

To update an employee payroll information file when an employee moves, marries, has a child, or wants to change deductions, select "Update Employee File." After making the changes, print out two copies of the file. Show one to the employee to confirm that the information is correct. Then have the employee sign and date it. Keep the signed copy for the physician's personnel file, and give the other to the employee. To ensure that payroll information is always correct and current, you should update it once a year for every employee.

To delete an employee payroll information file when an employee leaves the practice, select "Terminate Employee." Remember to print out and file a copy of this information before deleting it, because the physician is required to keep employees' payroll records for 4 years.

To generate paychecks and stubs, select the employee from the list of employees and choose the "Print Paycheck" option. Then, answer each prompt displayed by the computer (for example, hours worked). The computer has the employee's pay rate, payroll type, and deductions on file and automatically calculates the employee's net earnings, generates a paycheck, and prints a pay stub with the appropriate information.

To create an employee earnings record, select this option and follow the prompts for the needed information. Depending on the software used, each employee's earnings record may be updated automatically every time you generate a paycheck or make changes to other payroll files.

# Calculating and Filing Taxes

In many practices, medical assistants set up tax liability accounts for money withheld from paychecks. These accounts are used to submit this money to appropriate agencies.

## Setting Up Tax Liability Accounts

It is important to hold the money deducted from paychecks until it can be sent to the appropriate government agencies. Deductions from employees' paychecks for federal, state, and local income taxes and FICA taxes, as well as employer payments based on payroll, such as federal and state unemployment taxes, must be deposited until payment is due. For these accounts, choose a bank that is authorized by the IRS to accept federal tax deposits. If the practice makes other paycheck deductions, as for workers' compensation or a 401(k) plan, maintain accurate records for this money as well.

Each time you prepare paychecks, deposit the withheld money into the proper account as dictated by your particular practice. Record the deposited amounts as debits in the practice's checking account.

## Understanding Federal Tax Deposit Schedules

You will probably deposit federal income taxes and FICA taxes (which together are known as employment taxes) on a quarterly, monthly, or biweekly (every-other-week) schedule. Every November IRS personnel decide which deposit schedule your office should use for the next year.

If the IRS does not notify you about this matter, determine your deposit schedule based on the total employment taxes your office reported on the previous year's Employer's Quarterly Federal Tax Returns (Form 941). For example, if your office reported $50,000 or less in employment taxes during the past year, you would make monthly employment tax deposits the present year. If your office reported more than $50,000 during the past year, you would make semimonthly tax deposits.

There are exceptions to the monthly or semimonthly tax deposit schedules: the $500 rule and the $100,000 rule. The $500 rule applies to employers who owe less than $500 in employment taxes during a tax period (such as a quarter). These employers do not have to make a deposit for that period. The $100,000 rule applies to employers who owe $100,000 or more in employment taxes on any one day during a tax period. These employers must deposit the tax by the next banking day after the day that ceiling is reached.

## Submitting Federal Income Taxes and FICA Taxes

Some businesses must submit federal income taxes and FICA taxes to the IRS by electronic funds transfer (EFT). The EFT program, known as TAXLINK, began in 1995. Since then, more taxpayers have been required to use it each year. If your practice is not required to use EFT but wishes to do so voluntarily, contact the IRS, Cash Management Site Office, to enroll.

If your practice does not use EFT, you must submit these employment taxes with a Federal Tax Deposit (FTD) Coupon (Form 8109) (see Figure 18-14). FTD Coupons are supplied by the IRS. They are printed with the physician's name, address, and EIN. They have boxes for filling in the type of tax and the tax period for which the deposit is being made.

To make the deposit, write a single check or money order for the total amount of federal income taxes and FICA taxes withheld during the tax period. Make the check payable to the bank where you make the deposit. This must be a Federal Reserve Bank or another bank authorized to make payments to the IRS. Also, complete the FTD Coupon. Then, mail or deliver the check and FTD Coupon to the bank. The bank will give you a deposit receipt.

If you work in a practice with a large payroll, you may need to make deposits every few days. In most practices, however, you will probably make deposits once a month. Then, every 3 months, a more complete accounting is required on a **quarterly return,** called the Employer's Quarterly Federal Tax Return (Form 941).

## Submitting FUTA and SUTA Taxes

FUTA taxes provide money to workers who are unemployed. If the practice owes more than $100 in federal unemployment tax at the end of the quarter, deposit the tax amount with an FTD Coupon (Form 8109). At the end of

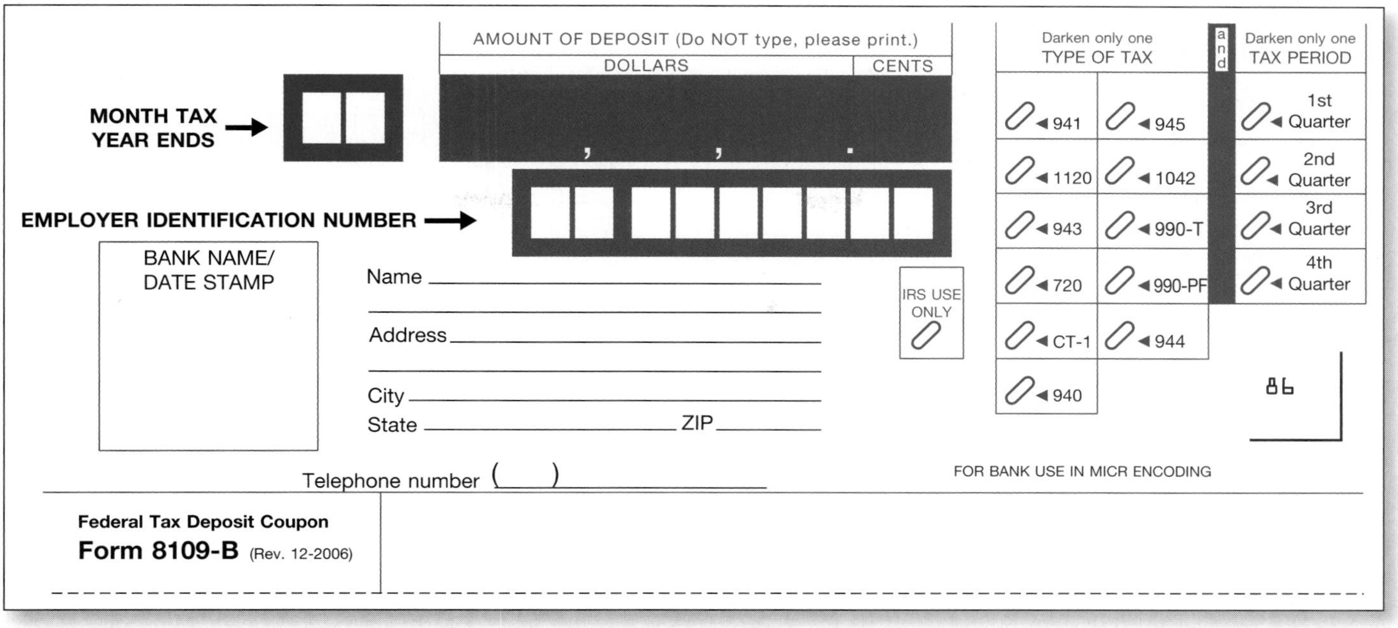

AMOUNT OF DEPOSIT (Do NOT type, please print.)

DOLLARS | CENTS

MONTH TAX YEAR ENDS

EMPLOYER IDENTIFICATION NUMBER

BANK NAME/ DATE STAMP

Name

Address

City

State ZIP

Telephone number ( )

IRS USE ONLY

Darken only one TYPE OF TAX

941 | 945
1120 | 1042
943 | 990-T
720 | 990-PF
CT-1 | 944
940

and

Darken only one TAX PERIOD

1st Quarter
2nd Quarter
3rd Quarter
4th Quarter

86

FOR BANK USE IN MICR ENCODING

Federal Tax Deposit Coupon

Form 8109-B (Rev. 12-2006)

**Figure 18-14.** Practices that do not use TAXLINK to submit taxes electronically must submit federal income and FICA taxes with a Federal Tax Deposit (FTD) Coupon (Form 8109).

the year, file an Employer's Annual Federal Unemployment (FUTA) Tax Return (Form 940) with any final taxes owed (Figure 18-15).

Generally, an employer must pay FUTA taxes if employees' wages total more than $1500 in any quarter (3-month period) and if those employees are not seasonal or household workers. The FUTA tax, which is 6.2%, is applied to the first $7000 of income for a year.

Some states are also governed by a **State Unemployment Tax Act (SUTA)**. These taxes are filed along with FUTA taxes. Make sure you know the laws governing unemployment taxes in your state.

## Filing an Employer's Quarterly Federal Tax Return

Each quarter, file an Employer's Quarterly Federal Tax Return (Form 941) with the IRS (Figure 18-16). This tax return summarizes the federal income and FICA taxes (employment taxes) withheld from employees' paychecks.

As a general rule, you should file Form 941 at the nearest IRS office by the last day of the first month after the quarter ends. If the practice has deposited all taxes on time, you have an additional 10 days after the due date to file.

## Handling State and Local Income Taxes

Send withheld state and local income taxes to the proper agencies, using their forms, procedures, and schedules. If required, prepare quarterly or other tax forms for the state and local governments.

## Filing Wage and Tax Statements

After the end of each year, file a Wage and Tax Statement (Form W-2) with the appropriate federal, state, and local government agencies for each employee who had federal income and FICA taxes withheld during the previous year (Figure 18-17). Also, supply copies of Form W-2 to each employee.

Form W-2 shows the employee's total taxable income for the previous year. It also shows the exact amount of federal income taxes and FICA taxes (for Social Security and Medicare) withheld, along with the amounts of state and local taxes withheld (if any).

Along with the W-2 forms, submit Form W-3, a Transmittal of Wage and Tax Statements (Figure 18-18). This form lists the employer's name, address, and EIN and summarizes the amount of all employees' earnings and the federal income taxes and FICA taxes withheld.

# Managing Contracts

An **employment contract**—a written agreement of employment terms between employer and employee—may be considered a benefit because it increases employee job security. It also allows the employer to attract and keep the best employees. Although contracts are rarely offered to medical assistants, you should be aware of them because they may be used for doctors and executive management of a practice and because they may be used for medical assistants in the future.

Form **940 for 2006:** Employer's Annual Federal Unemployment (FUTA) Tax Return

850106

Department of the Treasury — Internal Revenue Service

OMB No. 1545-0028

**(EIN)**
**Employer identification number** ☐ ☐ — ☐ ☐ ☐ ☐ ☐ ☐ ☐

**Name** (not your trade name)

**Trade name** (if any)

**Address**

Number     Street     Suite or room number

City     State     ZIP code

**Type of Return**
(Check all that apply.)

☐ a. Amended

☐ b. Successor employer

☐ c. No payments to employees in 2006

☐ d. Final: Business closed or stopped paying wages

Read the separate instructions before you fill out this form. Please type or print within the boxes.

**Part 1: Tell us about your return. If any line does NOT apply, leave it blank.**

1   If you were required to pay your state unemployment tax in ...

   **1a One state only,** write the state abbreviation . . .   **1a** ☐ ☐

   - OR -

   **1b More than one state** (You are a multi-state employer) . . . . . . . . . . . . . . .   **1b** ☐ Check here. Fill out Schedule A.

2

**Part 2: Determine your FUTA tax before adjustments for 2006. If any line does NOT apply, leave it blank.**

3   Total payments to all employees . . . . . . . . . .   **3** ☐ .

4   Payments exempt from FUTA tax . . . . . . . .   **4** ☐ .

   Check all that apply:   **4a** ☐ Fringe benefits   **4c** ☐ Retirement/Pension   **4e** ☐ Other

   **4b** ☐ Group term life insurance   **4d** ☐ Dependent care

5   Total of payments made to each employee in excess of $7,000 . . . . . . . . . . . . . . . . . .   **5** ☐ .

6   **Subtotal** (line 4 + line 5 = line 6) . . . . . . . . .   **6** ☐ .

7   **Total taxable FUTA wages** (line 3 – line 6 = line 7) . . .   **7** ☐ .

8   FUTA tax before adjustments (line 7 × .008 = line 8) . . . . . . . . . .   **8** ☐ .

**Part 3: Determine your adjustments. If any line does NOT apply, leave it blank.**

9   If ALL of the taxable FUTA wages you paid were excluded from state unemployment tax, multiply line 7 by .054 (line 7 × .054 = line 9). Then go to line 12 . . . . . .   **9** ☐ .

10   If SOME of the taxable FUTA wages you paid were excluded from state unemployment tax, OR you paid ANY state unemployment tax late (after the due date for filing Form 940), fill out the worksheet in the instructions. Enter the amount from line 7 of the worksheet onto line 10   **10** ☐ .

Form **940-V**

Department of the Treasury
Internal Revenue Service

**Payment Voucher**

OMB No. 1545-0028

2006

► **Do not staple or attach this voucher to your payment.**

1 Enter your employer identification number (EIN).

2
**Enter the amount of your payment.** ►

Dollars     Cents

3 Enter your business name (individual name if sole proprietor).

Enter your address.

Enter your city, state, and ZIP code.

**Figure 18-15.**   Tax dollars filed with FUTA tax returns (Form 940) provide money to workers who are unemployed.

Form **941 for 2007:** **Employer's QUARTERLY Federal Tax Return**

Form (Rev. January 2007)

Department of the Treasury — Internal Revenue Service

990107

OMB No. 1545-0029

**(EIN)**
**Employer identification number** ☐☐ — ☐☐☐☐☐☐☐

**Name** *(not your trade name)*

**Trade name** *(if any)*

**Address**
Number        Street                    Suite or room number

City                    State        ZIP code

**Report for this Quarter of 2007**
**(Check one.)**

☐ **1:** January, February, March

☐ **2:** April, May, June

☐ **3:** July, August, September

☐ **4:** October, November, December

Read the separate instructions before you fill out this form. Please type or print within the boxes.

**Part 1: Answer these questions for this quarter.**

1 Number of employees who received wages, tips, or other compensation for the pay period including: *Mar. 12* (Quarter 1), *June 12* (Quarter 2), *Sept. 12* (Quarter 3), *Dec. 12* (Quarter 4)   **1**

2 Wages, tips, and other compensation . . . . . . . . . .   **2**

3 Total income tax withheld from wages, tips, and other compensation . . . . . .   **3**

4 If no wages, tips, and other compensation are subject to social security or Medicare tax .   ☐ Check and go to line 6.

5 Taxable social security and Medicare wages and tips:

| | Column 1 | | Column 2 |
|---|---|---|---|

**5a** Taxable social security wages        × .124 =

**5b** Taxable social security tips        × .124 =

**5c** Taxable Medicare wages & tips        × .029 =

**5d** Total social security and Medicare taxes (*Column 2*, lines 5a + 5b + 5c = line 5d) .   **5d**

6 Total taxes before adjustments (lines 3 + 5d = line 6) . . . . . . . . . . .   **6**

7 **TAX ADJUSTMENTS** (Read the instructions for line 7 before completing lines 7a through 7h.):

**7a** Current quarter's fractions of cents . . . . . . . . . . .

**7b** Current quarter's sick pay . . . . . . . . . . .

**7c** Current quarter's adjustments for tips and group-term life insurance

**7d** Current year's income tax withholding (attach Form 941c) . .

**7e** Prior quarters' social security and Medicare taxes (attach Form 941c)

Under penalties of perjury, I declare that I have examined this return, including accompanying schedules and statements, and to the best of my knowledge and belief, it is true, correct, and complete.

X **Sign your name here**

Date        /        /

Print your name here

Print your title here

Best daytime phone ( ) —

**Part 6: For paid preparers only** *(optional)*

Paid Preparer's Signature

Firm's name

Address                                    EIN

ZIP code

Date   /   /   Phone ( ) —     SSN/PTIN

☐ Check if you are self-employed.

**Figure 18-16.** Most practices make tax deposits monthly and then make a more complete accounting once every 3 months on the Employer's Quarterly Federal Tax Return (Form 941), the first page of which is shown here.

| 22222 | Void ☐ | **a** Employee's social security number | **For Official Use Only ▶**<br>OMB No. 1545-0008 | | |
|---|---|---|---|---|---|
| **b** Employer identification number (EIN) | | | **1** Wages, tips, other compensation | **2** Federal income tax withheld | |
| **c** Employer's name, address, and ZIP code | | | **3** Social security wages | **4** Social security tax withheld | |
| | | | **5** Medicare wages and tips | **6** Medicare tax withheld | |
| | | | **7** Social security tips | **8** Allocated tips | |
| **d** Control number | | | **9** Advance EIC payment | **10** Dependent care benefits | |
| **e** Employee's first name and initial / Last name / Suff. | | | **11** Nonqualified plans | **12a** See instructions for box 12 | |
| | | | **13** Statutory employee / Retirement plan / Third-party sick pay | **12b** | |
| | | | **14** Other | **12c** | |
| | | | | **12d** | |
| **f** Employee's address and ZIP code | | | | | |

| **15** State | Employer's state ID number | **16** State wages, tips, etc. | **17** State income tax | **18** Local wages, tips, etc. | **19** Local income tax | **20** Locality name |
|---|---|---|---|---|---|---|
| | | | | | | |

Form **W-2** Wage and Tax Statement **2007** Department of the Treasury—Internal Revenue Service

Copy A For Social Security Administration — Send this entire page with Form W-3 to the Social Security Administration; photocopies are **not** acceptable.

Cat. No. 10134D

For Privacy Act and Paperwork Reduction Act Notice, see back of Copy D.

**Do Not Cut, Fold, or Staple Forms on This Page — Do Not Cut, Fold, or Staple Forms on This Page**

**Figure 18-17.** A Wage and Tax Statement (Form W-2) records the total amount of taxes withheld during the previous year for each employee.

## Legal Elements of a Contract

An employment contract is a legal agreement between two or more people to perform an act in exchange for payment. To be binding, the contract must include these main elements:

- An agreement between two or more competent people to do something legal
- Names and addresses of the people involved
- Consideration (whatever is given in exchange, such as money, work, or property)
- Starting and ending dates, as well as date(s) the contract was signed
- Signatures of the employer and employee

## A Medical Assistant Contract

Some medical practices use employment contracts for medical assistants. This type of contract would include these elements:

- A description of your duties and your employer's duties
- Plans for handling major changes in job responsibilities
- Salary, bonuses, and other forms of compensation
- Benefits, such as vacation time, sick days, life insurance, and participation in pension plans
- Grievance procedures
- Exceptional situations under which the contract may be terminated by either you or your employer
- Termination procedures and compensation
- Special provisions, such as job sharing, medical examinations, or liability coverage

If you are offered an employment contract, study it closely. Consider any local laws that may apply, and have a lawyer or business adviser review the contract.

## Summary

The administrative and accounting duties of the medical assistant may involve several aspects of financial control through the proper understanding and management of

## DO NOT STAPLE

| 33333 | **a** Control number | For Official Use Only ▶ OMB No. 1545-0008 | | |
|---|---|---|---|---|

| **b** Kind of Payer ▶ | 941 ☐  CT-1 ☐ | Military ☐  Hshld. emp. ☐ | 943 ☐  Medicare govt. emp. ☐ | 944 ☐  **Third-party sick pay** ☐ |
|---|---|---|---|---|

| **1** Wages, tips, other compensation | **2** Federal income tax withheld |
|---|---|
| **3** Social security wages | **4** Social security tax withheld |

| **c** Total number of Forms W-2 | **d** Establishment number |
|---|---|

| **5** Medicare wages and tips | **6** Medicare tax withheld |
|---|---|

| **e** Employer identification number (EIN) |
|---|

| **7** Social security tips | **8** Allocated tips |
|---|---|

| **f** Employer's name |
|---|

| **9** Advance EIC payments | **10** Dependent care benefits |
|---|---|
| **11** Nonqualified plans | **12** Deferred compensation |
| **13** For third-party sick pay use only | |
| **14** Income tax withheld by payer of third-party sick pay | |

| **g** Employer's address and ZIP code |
|---|
| **h** Other EIN used this year |

| **15** State    Employer's state ID number | **16** State wages, tips, etc. | **17** State income tax |
|---|---|---|
| | **18** Local wages, tips, etc. | **19** Local income tax |

| Contact person | Telephone number ( ) | For Official Use Only |
|---|---|---|
| Email address | Fax number ( ) | |

Under penalties of perjury, I declare that I have examined this return and accompanying documents, and, to the best of my knowledge and belief, they are true, correct, and complete.

Signature ▶                Title ▶                Date ▶

Form **W-3** Transmittal of Wage and Tax Statements  **2007**    Department of the Treasury
Internal Revenue Service

**Send this entire page with the entire Copy A page of Form(s) W-2 to the Social Security Administration. Photocopies are not acceptable.**

**Do not** send any payment (cash, checks, money orders, etc.) with Forms W-2 and W-3.

## What's New

**Relocation of form ID on Form W-3.** For consistency with the revisions to Form W-2, we relocated the form ID number ("33333") to the top left corner of Form W-3.

## Reminder

**Separate instructions.** See the 2007 Instructions for Forms W-2 and W-3 for information on completing this form.

## Purpose of Form

Use Form W-3 to transmit Copy A of Form(s) W-2, Wage and Tax Statement. Make a copy of Form W-3 and keep it with Copy D (For Employer) of Form(s) W-2 for your records. Use Form W-3 for the correct year. **File Form W-3 even if only one Form W-2 is being filed.** If you are filing Form(s) W-2 electronically, **do not** file Form W-3.

## When To File

File Form W-3 with Copy A of Form(s) W-2 by February 29, 2008.

## Where To File

Send this entire page with the entire Copy A page of Form(s) W-2 to:

**Social Security Administration
Data Operations Center
Wilkes-Barre, PA 18769-0001**

**Note.** If you use "Certified Mail" to file, change the ZIP code to "18769-0002." If you use an IRS-approved private delivery service, add "ATTN: W-2 Process, 1150 E. Mountain Dr." to the address and change the ZIP code to "18702-7997." See Publication 15 (Circular E), Employer's Tax Guide, for a list of IRS-approved private delivery services.

**For Privacy Act and Paperwork Reduction Act Notice, see the back of Copy D of Form W-2.**

**Figure 18-18.**    Submit a Transmittal of Wages and Tax Statements (Form W-3) with the W-2 forms.

accounts receivable and accounts payable. The use of standard bookkeeping and banking procedures is necessary in order to maintain the business of the office in proper form. The tasks involved may include the following:

- Using daily logs of charges and receipts for patient accounts

- Depositing cash and checks in bank accounts
- Summarizing patient charges and receipts
- Reconciling bank accounts to the practice records
- Disbursing funds for petty cash and office purchases
- Managing payroll for employees
- Preparing tax forms for payroll processing
- Assisting with contracts of the practice

## CASE STUDY QUESTIONS

Now that you have completed this chapter, review the case study at the beginning of the chapter and answer the following question:

1. What should Ben do to properly record the payment?

## Discussion Questions

1. Name three things that are required in a single-entry accounting system.
2. Discuss the meaning of a payroll deduction.
3. Why is the reconciliation of the bank statement so important?
4. Discuss the advantages and disadvantages of electronic banking.
5. When creating a payroll information sheet, name what it should contain.

## Critical Thinking Questions

1. Why is it important for an employer to have an Employer Identification Number?
2. From an employer's perspective, when might a medical assistant contract be advisable?
3. Name some of the banking tasks of the medical practice.
4. Generating payroll is a very important part of a medical assistant's job. What could be the result if the payroll is inaccurate?

## Application Activities

1. Record the following disbursements made on September 9, 2007, in a disbursements journal: Check no. 1234, payee—Tom Jones (electrician), check amount—$125; Check no. 1235, payee—Postmaster (postage), check amount—$32; Check no. 1236, payee—Gateway Property Management (rent), check amount—$900
2. A medical assistant in a medical practice is hired to work 8 hours a day, 4 days a week at an hourly rate of $10.00/hour. Checks are issued every 2 weeks. Her total deductions each week equal 10% of her gross earnings. What are her gross earnings per week? What is her "take home" pay in each check?
3. Prepare your personal federal income tax return, using information from the Wage and Tax Statement (Form W-2) and the Employee's Withholding Allowance Certificate (Form W-4) provided by your employer.

## Virtual Fieldtrip

*Visit the McGraw-Hill Higher Education Medical Assisting website at www.mhhe.com/medicalassisting3 to complete the following activity:*

Imagine that you are a medical assistant in a busy medical practice. You are assisting a new employee with the completion of the W-4 form. Go online and visit the U.S. government website and any other sites that offer information about how to complete the W-4 form. Then answer the following questions for submission to your instructor.

1. What general instruction would you give the employee?
2. Is claiming "exempt" the same thing as claiming "0"?
3. Under what conditions will the employee be exempt from any income tax withholding?

Open the CD and complete this chapter's practice activities, play the games, listen to the key terms, and test yourself with the interactive review. E-mail, print, and/or save your results to document your proficiency.

# PART Three

## Clinical Medical Assisting

"One of the most important things you must remember when assisting with patients is to put yourself in the patient's place. How would you feel if you were told to do something you didn't know how to do? Wouldn't you want to know ahead of time what will be expected of you?

"As a medical assistant, it is your job to anticipate the physician's every need during a physical exam. Compare the process with that of surgery, where the doctor is handed an instrument even before he asks for it. You should try to make as smooth a transition as possible from one step to the next; everyone benefits."

**Diane Morlock**
*Medical Assisting Instructor,*
*Stautzenberger College,*
*Toledo, Ohio*

# SECTION ONE
## The Medical Office Environment

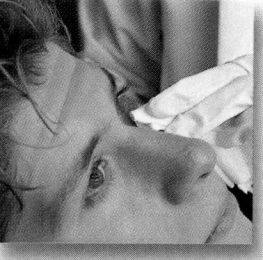

# SECTION TWO
## Assisting With Patients

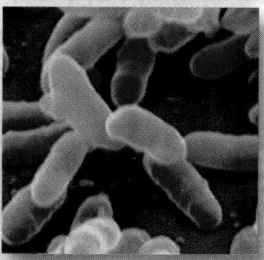

# SECTION THREE
## Specialty Practices and Medical Emergencies

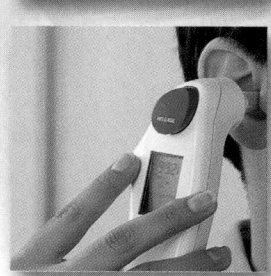

# SECTION FOUR
## Physician's Office Laboratory Procedures

# SECTION FIVE
## Nutrition, Pharmacology, and Diagnostic Equipment

# SECTION SIX
## Externship

# SECTION 1

## THE MEDICAL OFFICE ENVIRONMENT

# Principles of Asepsis

## MEDICAL ASSISTING COMPETENCIES

*In preparation for the certification examination, you should know the following areas of competence:*

| COMPETENCY | CMA | RMA |
|---|:---:|:---:|
| **Clinical** | | |
| Apply principles of aseptic techniques and infection control, including hand washing | X | X |
| **General/Legal/Professional** | | |
| Provide patients with methods of health promotion and disease prevention | X | X |

## CHAPTER OUTLINE

- History of Infectious Disease Prevention
- Microorganisms and Disease
- Infectious Diseases
- Drug-Resistant Microorganisms

- The Disease Process
- The Body's Defenses
- The Cycle of Infection
- Breaking the Cycle

## KEY TERMS

antibodies
antigen
asepsis
carrier
endogenous infection
exogenous infection
fomite
immunity
induration
macrophage
microorganism
monocyte
opportunistic infection
pathogen
phagocyte
reservoir host
resident normal flora
subclinical case
susceptible host
vector
virulence

## LEARNING OUTCOMES

After completing Chapter 19, you will be able to:

**19.1** Explain the historical background of infectious disease prevention.
**19.2** Identify the types of microorganisms that cause disease.
**19.3** List some infectious diseases, and identify their signs and symptoms.
**19.4** Discuss the importance of preventing antibiotic resistance in a health-care setting.
**19.5** Describe ways you can help prevent antibiotic resistance in health-care settings.
**19.6** Explain the disease process.
**19.7** Explain how the body's defenses protect against infection.
**19.8** Describe the cycle of infection.
**19.9** Identify and describe the various methods of disease transmission.
**19.10** Explain how you can help break the cycle of infection.

# Introduction

Our bodies are amazing structures that defend us against infections under normal circumstances. As you read this chapter, you will learn about disease-causing microorganisms, how the body defends itself against infections, and ways that infections might occur. You will also learn about antibiotic-resistant organisms and the importance of educating patients regarding the proper use of antibiotics. The chapter focuses on the history of disease prevention, disease processes, the body's defenses, and the cycle of infection.

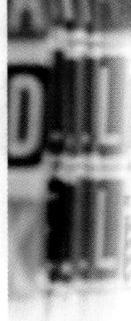

## CASE STUDY

A 14-year-old girl comes to your office with symptoms of diarrhea, flatulence, greasy stools, stomach cramps, and nausea. In the past 2 weeks, the patient has lost 10 pounds. During the patient interview, you find out from her mother that the family went camping about 3 weeks earlier. You also discover that the patient drank from a stream while on a hike. The patient shares with you that she saw beavers in the stream during the hike. No other family members are exhibiting any symptoms. After several laboratory tests, the patient is diagnosed with giardiasis, a parasitic infection often carried by beavers. The incubation period for Giardia is 1 to 2 weeks; however, adults do not always show signs of the infection. Risk factors for infection with Giardia include children in child care settings, people in close contact with infected persons, people who drink or swim in contaminated water, and people who have contact with infected animals. The patient is placed on antimicrobial therapy.

As you read this chapter, consider the following questions:

1. What part of the cycle of infection caused the problem for the patient?
2. How could the patient have avoided this infection?
3. Why are the other family members not showing symptoms of the infection?
4. Should the patient's family members be tested for the infection?

# History of Infectious Disease Prevention

Throughout history, doctors have tried to solve the problem of infection: what causes it, how it spreads, how to prevent it, and how to treat it. Some infections, such as the plague in the Middle Ages, have changed the course of history. Table 19-1 briefly describes some of the scientists who made early contributions in the prevention of infectious disease.

During the past century, remarkable advances have taken place in knowledge regarding the causes, prevention, and treatment of infectious disease. The threat of

| TABLE 19-1 | A Brief History of Infectious Disease Prevention |
|---|---|
| **Scientist** | **Contribution** |
| Edward Jenner (1749–1823) | Developed first effective vaccine<br>Used cowpox to vaccinate against smallpox |
| Ignaz Semmelweis (1818–1865) and Oliver Wendell Holmes (1809–1894) | Promoted hand washing as a means of reducing the spread of puerperal fever to women in childbirth |
| Louis Pasteur (1822–1895) | Helped develop the germ theory of infectious disease, stating that disease is caused by microorganisms |
| Joseph Lister (1827–1912) | Helped develop the germ theory<br>Introduced aseptic techniques in medicine through the use of antiseptics on wounds, surgical sites, and surgical instruments |
| Robert Koch (1843–1910) | Developed a set of proofs, known as Koch's Postulates, that microbes caused disease |
| Sir Alexander Fleming (1881–1955) | Discovered penicillin |

## TABLE 19-2 Microbial Pathogens and Their Characteristics

| Classification | Characteristics | Example | Disease |
|---|---|---|---|
| **Prions\*** | • Infectious particle made of protein<br>• Very small<br>• No nucleic acid<br>• Reproduction unknown | Pr P | Creutzfeldt-Jakob disease (CJD)<br>Bovine spongiform encephalopathy (BSE) (Mad Cow Disease) |
| **Viruses** | • DNA or RNA surrounded by protein coat<br>• Reproduced in living cells only<br>• Very small<br>• Acellular | varicella-zoster virus | Chickenpox |
| **Bacteria** | • Single celled<br>• Reproduce quickly<br>• Mostly asexual reproduction | Vibrio cholerae | Cholera |
| **Protozoans** | • Single celled<br>• Reproduction mostly asexual | Entamoeba hystolytica | Amebic dysentery |
| **Fungi** | • Multicellular<br>• Reproduction is sexual & asexual | Candida albicans | Candidiasis |
| **Helminths** | • Multicellular<br>• Parasitic<br>• Contain specialized organs<br>• Reproduction is sexual | Enterobius vermicularis | Pinworms |

*\*Although there is evidence that prions are directly responsible for several diseases that cause progressive brain degeneration, such as spongiform encephalopathies, there are scientists who believe that prions merely aid another unknown infectious agent in causing disease. Prion research is ongoing.*

infection, however, is as great as it has ever been. Medical science still wrestles with relatively new infectious diseases, such as acquired immunodeficiency syndrome (AIDS) and Ebola virus disease. In addition, some established diseases continue to challenge researchers because they have become resistant to antibiotics used to treat them. Some examples of established diseases that have become resistant to antibiotics are methicillin-resistant *Staphylococcus aureus* (MRSA), vancomycin-resistant *Staphylococcus aureus* (VRSA), and multidrug-resistant tuberculosis. As a medical assistant, you need to understand how to perform specific tasks to control infection and prevent disease transmission. Prior to this, you need to understand the disease process and spread of infection.

## Microorganisms and Disease

**Microorganisms** live all around us. They are found in and on our bodies, in the air we breathe, in the water we drink, and on almost every surface we touch. There is great variety in the types of pathogenic microorganisms. Successful **pathogens** (microorganisms capable of causing disease) have developed ways to evade the host defenses. There are pathogens in each classification of microorganism. Some examples of these are given in Table 19-2. Additional discussion about microorganisms and disease will be covered later in this chapter and in Chapter 33.

Although everyone is surrounded by microorganisms, people are able to avoid infection most of the time for the following three reasons:

1. The majority of microorganisms are either beneficial or harmless. Pathogens, microorganisms capable of causing disease, comprise only a small portion of the total number of microorganisms that exist in a given environment.
2. The human body has a wide variety of defenses that allow people to resist infection.
3. Conditions must be favorable for a pathogen to grow and to be transmitted to a person who is susceptible (sensitive) to infection.

## Infectious Diseases

Identifying the signs and symptoms of some infectious diseases can help protect health-care workers and patients from exposure to pathogens. It is important that you become familiar with some of the more common infectious diseases, including common signs and symptoms.

### Chickenpox (Varicella)

Chickenpox, or varicella, is a contagious viral infection with an incubation period of 7 to 21 days. Patients with chickenpox experience an itchy rash that begins as tiny, red bumps and eventually becomes fluid-filled blisters. The blisters break and dry into scabs, usually within a few days. The rash may cover most of the body. Patients may also run a slight fever, have a headache, and experience general malaise. The infection is spread through direct or indirect transmission as well as by droplets, or airborne secretions. Patients should be isolated for about a week following the initial eruption of the rash, until all the blisters have scabbed over. In 1996 the Food and Drug Administration (FDA) approved a live vaccine for chickenpox, and it was recently added to the immunization schedule for children. Many states require reporting chickenpox cases to the state or county department of health, although there are no national requirements for reporting them.

## Common Cold

Common colds are viral infections of the upper respiratory tract. They are transmitted from person to person through direct or indirect contact. The patient does not have to be isolated. It is important, however, that commonsense precautions be taken to avoid spreading the infection to others. For example, advise the patient to use tissues when coughing or sneezing, and have the patient and family wash their hands frequently and, if possible, use disposable dishware while the patient is ill. Incubation normally lasts for 2 to 3 days.

## Croup

Croup is a condition characterized by a harsh, barking cough, difficulty breathing, hoarseness, and low-grade fever. The leading cause of croup is Human parainfluenza virus I, but it may also be caused by an allergy, a foreign body, or a new growth obstructing the upper airway. Croup is most common in infants and young children. Symptoms of croup may be lessened by humidifying the air in the child's room, encouraging rest, and giving clear, warm fluids. If croup accompanies a bacterial respiratory infection, the doctor may prescribe antibiotics. As with the common cold, have the patient and family take commonsense precautions to prevent spreading the respiratory infection to others.

## Diphtheria

Diphtheria is a bacterial infection, primarily of the nose, throat, and larynx. The patient may experience pain, fever, and respiratory obstruction. Untreated, diphtheria is generally fatal. The incubation period is between 2 and 5 days. The patient must be isolated from others and undergo antibiotic therapy until tissue cells taken from the nose and the throat show negative results. Once a leading cause of death among young children, diphtheria is now rare in the United States because of widespread immunization. Cases of diphtheria must be reported to the state or county health department.

## Epstein-Barr Virus

Epstein-Barr virus is a common human virus. The CDC estimates that nearly 95% of adults in the United States have, at some time, been infected with the virus. Thirty-five percent to 50% of adolescents who become infected develop infectious mononucleosis. The symptoms of infectious mononucleosis are fever, sore throat, swollen lymph nodes, and, occasionally, spleen and liver involvement. Recovery from the symptoms of infectious mononucleosis usually occurs within two months. However, the virus remains dormant in the person's throat for life. Occasionally, the virus reactivates and is associated two types of tumors: Burkitt's lymphoma and carcinoma of the nasopharynx.

## Haemophilus Influenzae Type B

Haemophilus influenzae type B (Hib) is a frequent cause of bacterial infections—including blood infections, epiglottitis, and pneumonia—in infants and young children in the United States. It is spread through direct, indirect, and droplet transmission. The incubation period is approximately 3 days. The patient may experience upper respiratory symptoms, fever, drowsiness, body aches, and diminished appetite. The infection can also cause bacterial meningitis (a swelling or inflammation of the tissue covering the spinal cord and brain) and should be carefully monitored.

## Hepatitis

Hepatitis is a viral infection of the liver. There are several different viruses that cause hepatitis. Depending on the virus, transmission can be spread either through the blood or through the fecal-oral route. Hepatitis will be covered in greater detail in Chapter 21.

## HIV/AIDS

Human immunodeficiency virus (HIV) is the virus implicated as the cause of acquired immune deficiency syndrome (AIDS). HIV/AIDS will be covered in greater detail in Chapter 21.

## Influenza (Flu)

Nearly everyone has experienced symptoms of influenza, or the flu: fever, chills, headaches, body aches, and upper respiratory congestion. Isolation and other commonsense precautions can greatly reduce transmission of this viral infection. In addition, two types of vaccines are available to help prevent the flu. A live, attenuated (weakened) virus is given as a nasal spray and is approved for healthy individuals aged 5 through 49. This type of vaccine is not recommended for pregnant women. An inactivated (dead) virus is given as an intramuscular injection. This type of vaccine is approved for healthy individuals older than 6 months of age and people with chronic medical conditions.

The CDC recommends that the following people receive a yearly flu vaccination:

- People with an increased risk of flu complications
- Individuals older than age 50
- Anyone in close contact with people at risk for complications

# Measles (Rubeola)

Measles, also called rubeola, is an infectious viral disease spread through droplets or direct transmission. Normally, the disease requires 8 to 13 days for the initial symptom of fever to appear. The characteristic itchy rash appears 14 days after exposure. Patients should follow isolation procedures for 7 days after the rash first appears. Children younger than the age of 3 are especially at risk for contagion and should be kept apart from family members who have contracted the disease. The CDC requires reporting measles to the state or county health department.

# Meningitis

Meningitis is an inflammation and infection of the protective coverings of the brain and spinal cord, and the fluid that surrounds these tissues. Meningitis is caused by an infection with a virus or bacteria. Viral meningitis is usually milder than bacterial meningitis. It clears up in a week or two without specific treatment. Viral meningitis is also called aseptic meningitis.

Bacterial meningitis is a serious, life-threatening condition that requires immediate medical treatment. Severe bacterial meningitis can result in brain damage and even death. It affects more men than women. At highest risk are the elderly, children younger than 5, and people with chronic illnesses. Risk groups include children in daycare or schools, military recruits, anyone with a damaged spleen, and college students living in dorms or other close environments. The Centers for Disease Control and Prevention (CDC) recommend everyone in these risk groups receive meningococcal vaccination.

Between 5% and 20% of the population normally carry the bacteria that cause meningitis. These bacteria are commonly found in the nose and throat. Occasionally, a person who carries these bacteria develops meningitis. A person with an ear or sinus infection is at greater risk for meningitis. In addition, persons who have certain types of skull fractures also have a higher risk for developing meningitis.

For patients older than age 2, symptoms may include the following:

- A red, blotchy rash
- Confusion and delirium (delusions or hallucinations)
- Coma (in severe cases)
- Discomfort looking into bright lights
- Headache
- High fever and chills
- Nausea and vomiting
- Pain in the arms, legs, and abdomen
- Sleepiness
- A stiff neck and back

The classic symptoms of fever, headache, and neck stiffness may be absent or difficult to detect in newborns and small infants. The infant may only appear slow or inactive, be irritable, have vomiting, or be feeding poorly.

Some forms of bacterial meningitis are contagious. The bacteria are spread through the exchange of respiratory and throat secretions (for example, coughing, kissing, laughing, or sneezing). It can also be spread to individuals who have had close or prolonged contact with an infectious patient who has meningitis caused by *Neisseria meningitidis* (also called meningococcal meningitis) or Hib. Any health-care worker who has had direct contact with an infectious patient's oral secretions would be considered at increased risk of acquiring the infection. The CDC requires reporting meningitis to the state or county health department.

# Mumps

Mumps is a viral infection that primarily affects the salivary glands. The incubation period lasts from 2 to 3 weeks. The patient may experience pain, especially related to parotitis (inflammation of the parotid gland near the ear), and fever. Isolation procedures should be followed until glandular swelling stops. You must report all cases of mumps to the state or county health department.

# Pertussis (Whooping Cough)

Pertussis, or whooping cough, is an acute, highly contagious bacterial infection of the respiratory tract. Symptoms include slight fever, sneezing, runny nose, and quick, short coughs. The characteristic "whoop" occurs during the inhaled breath that follows a severe coughing fit. The patient should be isolated for 3 weeks after the onset of the spasmodic coughs. Whooping cough cases must be reported to the state or county health department.

# Poliomyelitis (Polio)

Poliomyelitis, more commonly called polio, is an acute viral disease involving the gray matter of the spinal cord. It is caused by any of three related viruses, and it occurs in three different forms:

1. Inapparent, in which a patient may experience fever, sore throat, headache, and vomiting
2. Nonparalytic, in which a patient experiences the same symptoms as the inapparent type but in a more severe form, and in which pain and stiffness occur in the neck, back, and legs
3. Paralytic, in which a patient has the same symptoms as the nonparalytic form, followed by recovery and then signs of central nervous system paralysis

Although polio outbreaks occur worldwide, polio's current incidence in the United States is rare. Since the 1950s, the incidence of polio has decreased as a result of the routine immunization of most children. In the United States, vaccinations are generally administered by injection to protect against all three types of polio viruses. There is no drug treatment once the disease begins. Report all cases of polio to the state or county health department.

## Roseola

Roseola is a rose-colored rash thought to be caused by a human herpes virus. The disease affects infants and young children. Its incubation period lasts between 5 and 15 days. Symptoms include sudden, high fever; sore throat; swollen lymph nodes; and after several days, a rash. Although seizures may sometimes accompany cases involving a very high fever, the disease is usually not serious.

## Rubella (German Measles)

Rubella, or German measles, is a highly contagious viral disease. It is transmitted through direct or droplet transmission, and incubation normally occurs in 16 to 18 days, although periods as long as 23 days have been recorded. Symptoms are mild and include fever and an itchy rash. Because of effective vaccination programs, the occurrence of rubella is diminishing. Fetuses of pregnant women who are not immune to rubella are at the greatest risk because the disease can cause birth defects in a fetus during the first trimester of pregnancy. Report rubella to the state or county department of health.

## Streptococcal Pharyngitis

Streptococcal pharyngitis (strep throat) is a bacterial infection of the throat. It is a common infection among children and adolescents. Patients experience severe throat pain with redness and swelling of the pharyngeal mucosa. They may also have fever, headache, nausea, and abdominal pain. Streptococcal pharyngitis is treated with antibiotics. Occasionally, complications occur due to strep infection. These include scarlet fever (scarlatina), rheumatic fever, and acute post-streptococcal glomerulonephritis.

**Scarlet Fever (Scarlatina).** Scarlet fever, also known as scarlatina, commonly accompanies strep throat. It occurs when the bacteria causing strep throat become systemic. In addition to the symptoms of strep throat (fever, sore throat, and swollen glands), the patient experiences the characteristic "strawberry rash" (tiny, bright red spots) that progresses from the trunk and neck to the face and extremities, along with nausea and vomiting. Incubation occurs in 1 to 3 days, and the patient may be kept isolated for 7 days. A shorter isolation period may be allowed if symptoms indicate the infection is not severe.

**Rheumatic Fever.** Rheumatic fever can occur several weeks after the patient's apparent recovery from strep throat. It is thought to be an autoimmune disorder. Research suggests that **antibodies** made by the body against Streptococci cross react with heart tissues. Antibodies are highly specific proteins that attach themselves to foreign substances. The heart valves are especially prone to damage by these antibodies, resulting in the need for valve replacement later in life. The signs and symptoms of rheumatic fever are carditis (inflammation of the heart), electrocardiogram changes, joint pain and inflammation, and fever.

**Acute Post-Streptococcal Glomerulonephritis.** Acute post-streptococcal glomerulonephritis, a complication of strep throat, is an inflammation of part of the filtering unit of the kidney (glomerulus). Damage to the glomerulus causes inadequate filtering of the blood. Signs of acute glomerulonephritis include swelling in the hands and feet, decreased urine output, hypertension, and increased protein in the urine.

## Tetanus

Tetanus is an acute, often fatal infectious bacterial disease. The infection follows the introduction of pathogenic spores, which enter the body through a contaminated puncture wound. If the disease process is not halted, the patient can experience lockjaw (a motor disturbance resulting in difficulty opening the mouth) and, eventually, paralysis. Incubation of the disease is normally 3 to 21 days. Patients with tetanus do not need to be isolated, but you must report cases to the state or county health department.

## Tuberculosis

Tuberculosis, also called TB, is an infectious bacterial disease that mainly affects the lungs but can also involve other organs. TB is the leading infectious killer of adults worldwide. A patient infected with tuberculosis may not have any symptoms. The body's immune system often destroys the bacteria, leaving only a scar or spot on the lungs. Sometimes, however, the infection spreads, and the patient exhibits these symptoms:

- Night sweats
- Productive and prolonged cough
- Fever
- Chills
- Fatigue
- Unexplained weight loss
- Diminished appetite
- Bloody sputum

**Incidence of Tuberculosis.** Since 1992, the incidence in the United States has been declining. Incidence remains high or on the increase in many states, however, particularly in some urban centers. You may encounter patients with tuberculosis, and you can never relax your vigilance when working in environments where there is any risk of infection.

Many factors contribute to the continued high incidence of tuberculosis. You may work with patients who are affected by some or all of these factors:

- Infection with HIV increases the risk for developing tuberculosis after exposure to the pathogen
- The population of the United States is shifting to include a larger percentage of people from countries where there is a higher incidence of tuberculosis

- The number of people living in environments known to pose increased risk, such as long-term institutional settings, homeless centers, and medically underserved neighborhoods, has increased
- The public health-care system is unable to meet the needs of its constituents, resulting in patients who remain untreated
- New drug-resistant strains of the tuberculosis pathogen are appearing, requiring longer and more potent therapy regimens, which are harder to enforce and with which many patients do not comply

Understanding how tuberculosis is transmitted and managed will help you apply the principles of infection control.

**Transmission of Tuberculosis.** *Mycobacterium tuberculosis,* the microorganism responsible for tuberculosis infection, is spread through droplet transmission. The bacteria can spread through the air near an infected person when the person breathes, coughs, sneezes, or talks.

When another person inhales the bacteria, they travel through that person's respiratory system to lodge in the alveoli. From there, the bacteria can eventually spread throughout the body.

The most effective way to break the growth cycle of the tuberculosis pathogen is to contain the bacteria at the source. Containing the pathogen at this point prevents its entrance into another host. Containment measures are discussed in the Points on Practice box.

**Increasing Resistance to Tuberculosis.** Another way to break the pathogenic growth cycle is to decrease the susceptibility of the host. Early diagnosis, prompt treatment, and compliance with the treatment regimen have a positive impact on the outcome of tuberculosis. Risk factors for infection include the following:

- HIV infection or any disease state that weakens the immune system
- Intravenous drug use
- Previous tuberculosis infection
- Diabetes mellitus, a disorder characterized by a deficiency of the hormone insulin
- End-stage renal disease, a type of kidney disease
- Low body weight

**Preventing Tuberculosis.** A vaccine is available for the prevention of TB. Bacille Calmette-Guérin (BCG) is used in countries with a high rate of tuberculosis. BCG is not commonly used in the United States because it is not especially effective in adults. It also interferes with the tuberculin skin test by causing a false-positive result.

The CDC recommends vaccinating children who are continually exposed to TB and cannot be removed from the source of the exposure. They also recommend vaccinating certain health-care workers who work with patients with a high percentage of TB infection.

## Points on Practice

## Preventing the Spread of Tuberculosis

Containing the tuberculosis bacteria is the single best means of preventing the spread of the disease. There are specific measures that should be taken by the patient and the office personnel. Containment measures include the following:

### Patient Measures

- Instruct patients in the correct procedure for covering the mouth when sneezing, coughing, laughing, or yawning. Explain that patients should properly dispose of tissues or other materials that have been used to block a sneeze or a cough and should thoroughly wash their hands afterward.
- Instruct patients that they should always take their tuberculosis medication as directed. If they miss a dose or are having problems taking the medicine, they should call the office.
- Have patients avoid close contact with other people. They should avoid going to school, work,

or any public place until instructed to do so by the doctor.
- Patients should air out their room as often as possible, even in the winter. Moving air to the outside reduces the number of tuberculosis bacteria in the room.

### Office Measures

- When you must perform a procedure that induces coughing, conduct the procedure in an area with negative air pressure, such as inside a protective booth. Negative air pressure acts to draw contaminated air out of the immediate area and into a filtration system.
- When you work with a patient who is infectious, wear a personal respirator to prevent inhalation of the bacteria. Be sure also to apply standard sanitization, disinfection, and sterilization techniques to instruments and equipment.

**Treating Tuberculosis.** Tuberculosis infection must be confirmed by a Mantoux tuberculin skin test, in which you administer tuberculin intradermally with a needle and syringe. If the test results are positive, the skin area turns red and becomes raised and hard, which is termed **induration.** A positive test result reveals that a patient has had previous exposure to tuberculosis, either from immunization (common outside the United States) or from coming in contact with the tuberculosis bacteria. If a patient tests positive for tuberculin sensitivity, further tests, including chest x-rays and sputum examination, are performed.

The specific treatment of a patient with active tuberculosis depends on the part of the body affected and the type of tuberculosis involved. In all cases, however, drug therapy must be begun immediately. Emphasize to patients the importance of completing the entire course of treatment (12 to 18 months on medication). As a medical assistant, you can help patients comply with the treatment by providing education about the following:

- The disease
- The expected course of treatment
- The anticipated outcome
- Measures patients can take to prevent the spread of the disease

Patients with active pulmonary tuberculosis should be hospitalized in a facility approved for treating the disease. They should also be placed in an isolation room with negative air pressure. Visitors should be kept to a minimum. Patients may be discharged to their homes after starting TB therapy, even though they may still be infectious. Transmission is less likely to occur after treatment has begun.

# Drug-Resistant Microorganisms

Resistance to antimicrobial agents is a severe problem. Drug-resistant pathogens are the cause of many infections. It is the responsibility of physicians, medical staff, and patients to use antibiotics wisely. Bacteria and other microorganisms that have developed resistance to antimicrobial drugs include the following:

- MRSA—methicillin/oxacillin-resistant *S. aureus*
- VRE—vancomycin-resistant enterococci
- VISA—vancomycin-intermediate *S. aureus*
- VRSA—vancomycin-resistant *S. aureus*
- ESBLs—extended-spectrum beta-lactamases, which are resistant to cephalosporins and monobactams
- PRSP—penicillin-resistant *Streptococcus pneumoniae*

MRSA and VRE are the most common multidrug-resistant organisms in patients who reside in nonhospital health-care facilities (for example, nursing homes and other long-term-care facilities). Persons outside of health-care facilities are increasingly at risk for becoming colonized with MRSA.

Community-associated MRSA, an infection found in otherwise healthy individuals, is on the rise in the United States. PRSP are more common in patients seeking care in physicians' offices and clinics, especially in pediatric settings.

## Risk Factors

There are a number of risk factors for both the development of and infection with drug-resistant organisms. These risk factors include the following:

- Advanced age
- Invasive procedures, which include dialysis, the presence of invasive devices, and urinary catheterization
- Previous use of antimicrobial agents
- Repeated contact with the health-care system
- Severity of the illness
- Underlying diseases or conditions, especially chronic renal disease, insulin-dependent diabetes mellitus, peripheral vascular disease, and dermatitis or skin lesions.

## Preventing Antibiotic Resistance in Health-Care Settings

In response to a growing concern over the emergence of antibiotic-resistant infections, the CDC began the Campaign to Prevent Antimicrobial Resistance in Healthcare Settings. This campaign has four strategies to reduce the incidence of antibiotic-resistant microorganisms:

1. Prevent infection
2. Diagnose and treat infection appropriately
3. Use antibiotics carefully
4. Prevent transmission of infections

# The Disease Process

Many types of diseases affect humans. An infectious disease is one that is caused by the action of a microorganism. An infection begins when the microorganism finds a human host, that is, a body in which it can survive, multiply, and thrive. To grow, a microorganism requires specific conditions, which include three things: (1) the proper temperature, (2) pH (a measure of the body's acid-base balance), and (3) moisture level. The temperature within the human body (98.6°F, or 37°C), the body's neutral pH, and the body's dark, moist environment are prime conditions for the growth of microorganisms.

Some pathogens nearly always cause disease, whereas others cause disease less often or only under certain circumstances. A microorganism's disease-producing power is called **virulence.** When microorganisms damage the body, they do so in many ways:

- By depleting nutrients or other materials needed by the cells and tissues they invade
- By reproducing themselves within body cells

- By making body cells the targets of the body's own defenses
- By producing toxins, or poisons, that damage cells and tissues

Once exposed to a pathogenic organism, the body goes through 4 stages of illness:

1. Incubation period. This period begins at the first exposure and ends when the first symptoms appear.
2. Prodromal stage. This stage begins with the first onset of symptoms. This stage is generally short, lasting only from one to two days.
3. Invasion period. During this stage, the numbers of organisms are greatest and symptoms are most pronounced.
4. Convalescent period. During this time, the patient regains his or her normal health status.

Patients can be contagious during any of these stages, though patients are generally most contagious during the invasion period.

## The Body's Defenses

People are constantly exposed to multitudes of pathogens, but the bodies of healthy individuals have built-in defenses against them. The condition of being resistant to pathogens and the diseases they cause is called **immunity.**

The body has several first lines of defense. These serve as nonspecific physical or chemical barriers to any invader. They include:

- Skin—a strong mechanical barrier that resists penetration

- Sweat glands—structures that mechanically flush microbes from skin surfaces
- Mucous membranes—mechanical barriers that prevent microbe adherence
- Cilia—structures that line the respiratory tract; they act as "brooms" to remove substances trapped in mucus (Figure 19-1)
- Lacrimal glands—structures that produce tears to mechanically flush the eyes
- Saliva—a substance that mechanically pushes microorganisms to the stomach
- Hydrochloric acid—an acid found in the stomach that acts as a chemical barrier to ingested microbes
- Lysozyme—an enzyme found in tears and saliva that acts as a chemical barrier for the eyes and mouth

In addition to the first lines of defense, other factors help to protect the body. **Resident normal flora** are microorganisms found in the body. They consist of bacteria, fungi, and protozoa that have taken up residence either in or on the human body. Some of these organisms neither help nor harm the host and some are beneficial, creating a barrier against pathogens. Resident normal flora produce substances that can harm invaders or simply starve them by using up the resources pathogens need to live. The skin, nose, mouth, vagina, rectum, and intestines are all colonized by resident normal flora. Table 19-3 summarizes the anatomic sites colonized and gives examples of organisms found at those sites. These organisms live in balance most of the time, dependent on the health of the host. They can become pathogenic when they enter tissues normally not populated by them or when the host's defenses are compromised.

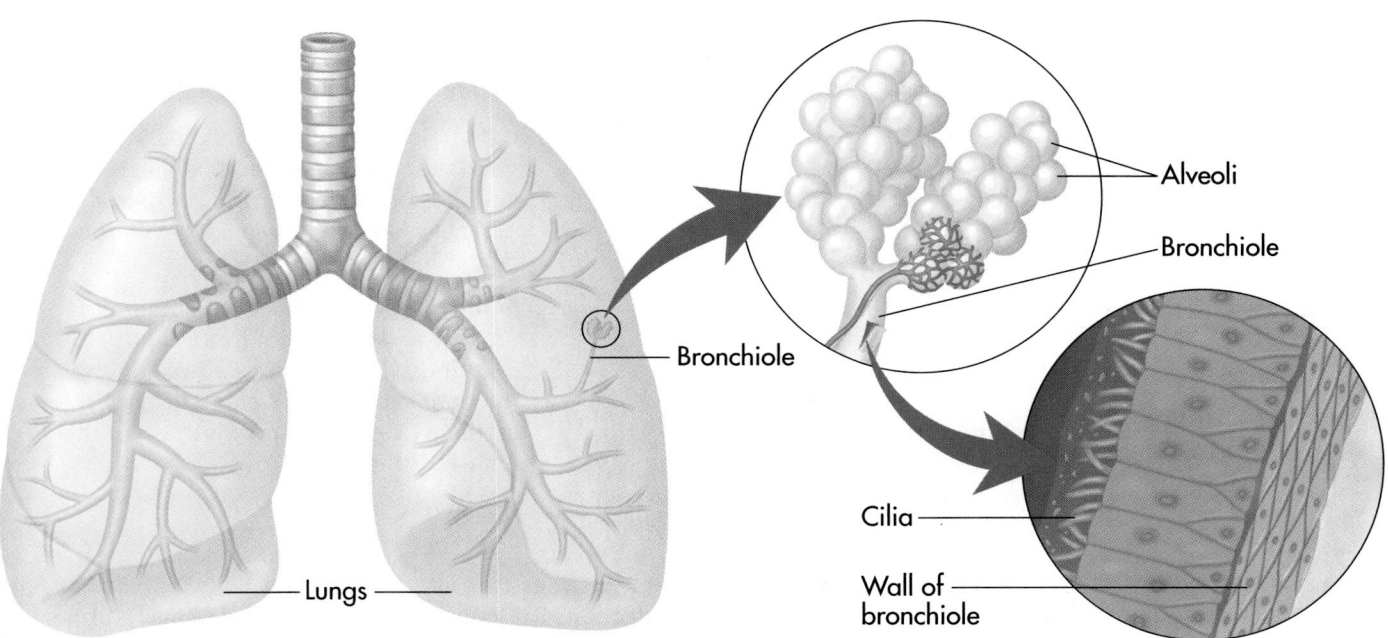

**Figure 19-1.** The sweeping motion of cilia that line the respiratory tract helps rid the body of foreign particles and some microorganisms.

## TABLE 19-3  Sites Containing Well-Established Flora and Representative Examples

| Anatomic Sites | Common Organisms | Characteristics |
|---|---|---|
| **Skin** | Bacteria: *Staphlococcus, Micrococcus, Corynebacterium,* | Microbes live only in upper dead layers of epidermis, glands, and follicles; dermis and layers below are sterile |
| | Fungi: *Malassezia yeast* | Dependent on skin lipids for growth |
| | Arthropods: *Demodix mite* | Present in sebaceous glands and hair follicles |
| **Gastrointestinal tract** Oral cavity | Bacteria: *Streptococcus, Neisseria, Staphylococcus, Lactobacillus,* | |
| | Fungi: *Candida* species | Can cause thrush |
| | Protozoa: *Trichomonas tenax, Entamoeba gingivalis* Colononize the epidermal layer of cheeks, gingiva, pharynx; surface of teeth; found in saliva in huge numbers | Frequent the gingiva of persons with poor oral hygiene |
| Large intestine and rectum | Bacteria: *Bacteroides, Clostridium, fecal streptococci, Lactobacillus, coliforms (Esherichia, Enterobacter)* | Sites of lower gastrointestinal tract other than large intestine and rectum have sparse or nonexistent flora Flora consists predominantly of strict anaerobes; other microbes are aerotolerant or facultative |
| | Fungi: *Candida* | |
| | Protozoa: *Entamoeba coli, Trichomonas hominis* | Feed on waste materials in the large intestine |
| **Upper respiratory tract** | Microbial population exists in the nasal passages, throat, and pharynx; owing to proximity, flora is similar to that of oral cavity | Trachea and bronchi have a sparse population; smaller breathing tubes and alveoli have no normal flora and are essentially sterile |
| **Genital tract** | Bacteria: *Lactobacillus, Streptococcus, Corynebacterium, Escherichia,* | In females, flora occupies the external genitalia and vaginal and cervical surfaces; internal reproductive structures normally remain sterile. Flora responds to hormonal changes during life. |
| **Urinary tract** | Bacteria: *Staphlylococcus, Streptococcus, coliforms* | In females, flora exists only in the first portion of the urethral mucosa; the remainder of the tract is sterile. In males, the entire reproductive and urinary tract is sterile except for a short portion of the anterior urethra. |
| | Fungi: *Candida* | Cause of yeast infections |

A person's defenses may be compromised by poor health, inadequate nutrition, or poor hygiene. A break in the skin caused by injury can leave a person especially vulnerable to microorganisms. This type of opening in the body provides the organisms with an unprotected point of entry. Drugs can also weaken the body's ability to fight infection. For example, anticancer drugs may kill healthy cells along with cancer cells. Disorders of the immune system, such as AIDS, interfere with the body's natural ability to fight infection. Because people are constantly surrounded by pathogens, the body's natural defenses against pathogens are crucial to survival. If people do not have these defenses, they are potentially vulnerable to infection by every microorganism they encounter, including the body's resident normal flora.

Infections by microorganisms that can cause disease only when a host's resistance is low are called **opportunistic infections.** Examples of opportunistic infections are pneumonia caused by *Pneumocystis carinii* (a protozoan) and oral candidiasis, which is caused by *Candida* (a fungus found commonly in the mouth, intestinal tract, and vagina). Both of these infections are common in AIDS patients.

In most cases, when microorganisms successfully evade the body's first lines of defense and invade body tissues, the immune system begins to neutralize and destroy them. The immune system includes nonspecific defenses, humoral defenses (fluid mechanisms), and cell-mediated defenses. The immune system also involves the spleen, lymph nodes, tonsils, thymus, lungs, liver, and kidneys, all of which contain lymphatic tissue. Lymphatic tissue is a filtering network of connective tissue containing large numbers of lymphocytes. Lymphocytes are specialized white blood cells that combat infectious agents.

## Nonspecific Defense

A microorganism that invades the human body is subjected to a variety of host defenses. Initially, the defense mechanisms are nonspecific. These nonspecific defenses include inflammation and phagocytosis.

**Inflammation.** Following an injury or invasion by a pathogen, the body begins a response known as inflammation. Signs of inflammation include redness, localized heat, swelling, and pain. The purposes of inflammation are to

1. Summon immunologic agents to the site
2. Begin tissue repair
3. Destroy invading microorganisms

This "call to action" by the body includes the following steps:

1. Initial constriction of blood vessels followed very shortly by dilation of blood vessels, causing redness and heat
2. Fluid leakage from local vessels, resulting in local swelling
3. Scar tissue formation, at which point the inflammatory response decreases

Inflammation is a useful initial tool for fighting foreign invaders. However, when inflammation becomes chronic, it can create new problems in the body. Chronic inflammation can damage tissues, resulting in a permanent loss of function. An example of the damage chronic inflammation can do is seen in rheumatoid arthritis.

**Phagocytosis.** Another type of nonspecific defense is the process known as phagocytosis. This process occurs

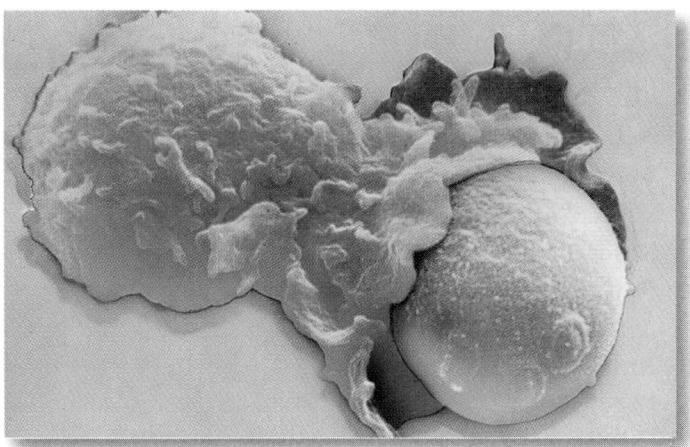

**Figure 19-2.** Phagocytes protect the body from infection by finding, surrounding, and digesting intruding microorganisms.

when special white blood cells called **phagocytes** engulf and digest pathogens. (Figure 19-2 shows how a phagocyte "swallows" a pathogen.) A pouch forms around the pathogen as it is engulfed. The phagocyte secretes enzymes and metabolites into the pouch, destroying the trapped material.

Phagocytes constantly search for and destroy foreign invaders. There are three main types of phagocytes: neutrophils, **monocytes,** and **macrophages.** Neutrophils are important in the inflammatory response. When tissues are injured, neutrophils travel to the site of injury and begin engulfing bacteria. Pus contains large numbers of neutrophils. Monocytes are phagocytes that are formed in bone marrow and circulate throughout the blood for a very short period of time. They then migrate to specific tissues and are called macrophages. Macrophages are slightly larger and more specialized than monocytes. Macrophages are found in the lymph nodes, liver, spleen, lungs, bone marrow, and connective tissue. Macrophages play several roles in humoral and cell-mediated immunity, including delivering **antigens** (foreign substances) to the lymphocytes involved in these defenses.

## Humoral Immunity

One type of humoral protection is provided by antibodies. This defense involves two types of lymphocytes: B cells (also called B lymphocytes) and T cells (also known as T lymphocytes). When the body is invaded by antigens, helper T cells activate B cells to produce antibodies, which combine with the antigens to neutralize them. Although the initial response to a major invasion by an antigen may not be a highly effective defense, memory B cells are produced for the appropriate antibody. A later invasion by the same antigen will be quickly and effectively countered. Specific antibodies are produced in response to specific antigens. These antibodies

## TABLE 19-4  Types of Immunity

Immunity to a disease can be acquired in a variety of ways: naturally, artificially, actively, and passively.

| Active Immunity | Passive Immunity |
|---|---|
| Body produces its own antibodies; provides long-term immunity | Antibodies produced outside of the body are introduced into the body; provides only temporary immunity |
| **Natural Active Immunity** | **Natural Passive Immunity** |
| Results from exposure to disease-causing organism | Results when antibodies from the mother cross the placenta to the fetus |
| **Artificial Active Immunity** | **Artificial Passive Immunity** |
| Results from administration of a vaccine with killed or weakened organisms | Results from immunization with antibodies to a disease-causing organism |

act as a homing device to attract phagocytes, which then engulf and destroy the antigen.

The formation of antibodies gives the body immunity from a particular disease. Immunity can be active or passive, natural or artificial (Table 19-4).

- Active immunity is a long-term immunity in which the body produces its own antibodies. Active immunity can be natural or artificial.

- Passive immunity results when antibodies produced outside the body enter the body. Passive immunity can be natural or artificial.

- Natural active immunity results from exposure to organisms that cause a disease, such as mumps. Although the person becomes sick with the disease, the body produces antibodies that prevent the individual from having the disease again if re-exposed. A fetus acquires natural passive immunity when the mother's antibodies move across the placenta. Natural passive immunity lasts only a short time, usually a few weeks after birth.

- Artificial active immunity results from the administration of an immunization or a vaccine. There are several types of vaccines available. Some vaccines are made from whole organisms that have been either killed or altered in a way that makes them unable to cause disease. Examples of vaccines produced from whole organisms are the influenza vaccines. Both live and dead virus influenza vaccines are available. Vaccines can also be made from purified substances found on or in a pathogen. More recently, vaccine research is studying the use of DNA techniques to produce vaccines. New DNA vaccines for West Nile Virus and HIV are on the horizon. All of these methods of immunization induce the formation of antibodies without causing disease.

- Natural passive immunity occurs when the mother transfers immunity to her unborn fetus through the placenta or to the newborn through breast milk. This type of immunity is temporary.

- Artificial passive immunity occurs as a result of injecting premade antibodies that provide temporary protection for people who have been exposed to serious disease, such as hepatitis and tetanus. Artificial passive immunity lasts only a short time, usually a few weeks.

The other type of humoral defense is called complement. Complement is a group of proteins that circulates in the blood and body fluids. It is always present in low amounts. When activated by antibodies, however, complement can multiply rapidly and destroy pathogens. It helps the white blood cells ingest microorganisms, sometimes making a hole in the microorganisms' cells that causes the cells to rupture and be destroyed. The main reason that most bacteria do not cause disease is that complement proteins destroy many species of bacteria.

## Cell-Mediated Immunity

In addition to their role in humoral immunity, T cells are instrumental in cell-mediated immunity. Cell-mediated immunity differs from humoral immunity in that T cells do not form antibodies to combat antigens. Instead, they directly attack the invader. Several different types of T cells are involved in the attack process. Helper T cells activate the killer T cells, which bind with the antigen and kill it. Suppressor T cells slow down or stop the attack after the antigen is destroyed. Memory T cells are formed and will respond quickly to another attack by the same antigen.

Cell-mediated defenses against infection often result in inflammation of the affected area. Inflammation occurs when phagocytes enter the area, stick to the lining of the blood vessels, and come out of the vessels to attack the infecting agent. Small blood vessels then dilate and leak fluid, resulting in swelling, redness, and warmth. This process often causes fever, which is a common response to many infections and may play a part in fighting infection. The fever results when endogenous pyrogen, a product of phagocytic cells, acts on the area of the brain that controls the body's temperature.

# The Cycle of Infection

Five elements make up the cycle of infection (Figure 19-3). These five parts must all be present for infection to occur:

1. Reservoir host
2. Means of exit
3. Means of transmission
4. Means of entrance
5. Susceptible host

## Reservoir Host

The infection cycle begins when the pathogen invades the reservoir host. The **reservoir host** is an animal, insect, or human whose body is capable of sustaining growth of a pathogen. Many pathogens require a reservoir host to provide nutrition and a place to multiply.

The presence of the pathogen in the reservoir host may cause an infection in the host. At times, however, the host avoids full infection. A human **carrier** is a reservoir host who is unaware of the presence of the pathogen and so spreads the disease. The carrier exhibits no symptoms of infection. A human host also may have a **subclinical case,** which is a manifestation of the infection that is so slight that it is unnoticeable. The host experiences only some of the symptoms of the infection or milder symptoms than in a full case. A wide range of diseases can be manifested subclinically.

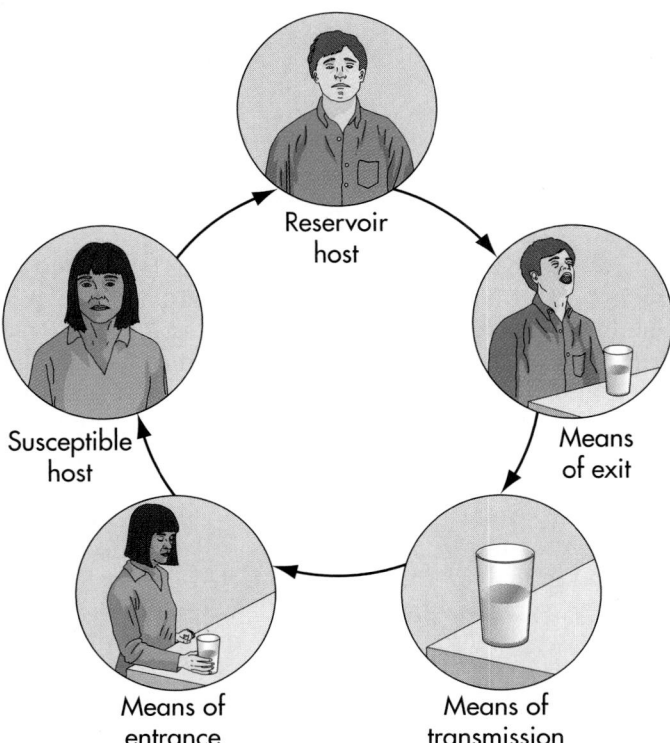

**Figure 19-3.** The cycle of infection must be broken at some point to prevent the spread of disease.

An infection in the reservoir host may be either endogenous or exogenous. An **endogenous infection** is one in which an abnormality or malfunction in routine body processes has caused normally beneficial or harmless microorganisms to become pathogenic. An **exogenous infection** is one that is caused by the introduction of a pathogen from outside the body.

## Means of Exit

The next step in the cycle of infection is the pathogen's exiting from the reservoir host. Common routes of exit include the following:

- Through the nose, mouth, eyes, or ears
- In feces or urine
- In semen, vaginal fluid, or other discharge through the reproductive tract
- In blood or blood products from open wounds

## Means of Transmission

To reproduce after it has exited from the reservoir host, the pathogen must spread to another host by some means of transmission. The means may be direct or indirect. Direct transmission occurs when the pathogen moves immediately from one host to another. This type of transmission may happen through contact with the infected person or with the discharges of the infected person, such as saliva or blood.

Indirect transmission is possible only if the pathogen is capable of existing independently of the reservoir host. In this case, the pathogen survives until a new host encounters it and the pathogen takes up residence in that new host.

**Airborne Transmission.** Pathogens can be transmitted to a new host through the air. For example, microorganisms may enter the respiratory tract of a new host by inhalation. Respiratory diseases such as influenza, or flu, are often transmitted this way.

Pathogens may be inhaled from a variety of sources, such as soil particles or secretion droplets. When people inhale contaminated soil particles, fungal diseases may be contracted. If contaminated droplets are inhaled, diseases including influenza, chickenpox, and tuberculosis may be contracted. Because pathogens can spread relatively rapidly through airborne transmission, they may cause large epidemics among susceptible people.

**Blood-Borne Transmission.** Pathogens can also enter a new host through contact with blood or blood products. Blood-borne pathogens (discussed in greater detail in Chapter 21) may be transmitted in a variety of ways:

- Indirectly, as when pathogens are transferred through blood transfusions, needlesticks, or improperly sterilized dental equipment
- Directly, as when the contaminated blood of one person comes into contact with another person's broken skin or mucous membrane, or when a pregnant woman transmits a disease to her fetus across the placenta

**Transmission During Pregnancy or Birth.** If a mother becomes infected during her pregnancy, she can pass on pathogens to the fetus. An infection may be transmitted while the fetus is in the mother's uterus, which may result in damage to the fetus. This transmission is a form of blood-borne transmission.

Some blood-borne infections that produce only mild symptoms in the mother may be devastating to the fetus (for example, rubella). Other infections, such as herpes, gonorrhea, syphilis, or streptococcal infections, may infect the baby during passage through the birth canal. An infection that is present in a child at the time of birth is said to be congenital.

**Foodborne Transmission.** A new host may be exposed to pathogens by ingesting contaminated food or liquids. Food can become contaminated when it is handled by an infected person who has poor hygiene habits, such as a customer at a self-service salad bar who did not wash his hands. The amount of contamination needed in a food to make someone ill varies. People who produce less stomach acid may become infected with a smaller dose of pathogens than those with higher acid production because stomach acid kills many microorganisms. An example of a pathogen transmitted by ingestion is a strain of *Escherichia coli* bacteria, commonly known as E. coli, which can cause severe food poisoning.

**Vector-Borne Transmission.** A living organism that carries microorganisms from an infected person to another person is known as a **vector.** The most common carriers are insects such fleas, flies, mosquitoes, and ticks.

- Fleas carry the organism responsible for plague. Though the number of cases in the United States is very low, plague has been identified as a possible bioterrorism agent.
- Common houseflies carry pathogens from garbage and feces on their bodies and feet. When they land on food, they mechanically transfer these microorganisms to the food.
- Mosquitoes are carriers of several diseases of importance in the United States. They carry the organisms responsible for West Nile Virus and malaria.
- Ticks carry the microorganisms responsible for Lyme disease and Rocky Mountain spotted fever.

**Transmission by Touching.** Direct or indirect contact through touch is another method of transmitting infection. Direct transmission occurs through contact with an infected person's mucous membranes. Sexually transmitted diseases are spread through the direct contact of one mucous membrane with another (in the penis, vagina, urethra, mouth, or anus) during sexual activity.

Indirect transmission occurs through contact with **fomites.** A fomite is any inanimate reservoir of pathogenic microorganisms. Any object that can be contaminated

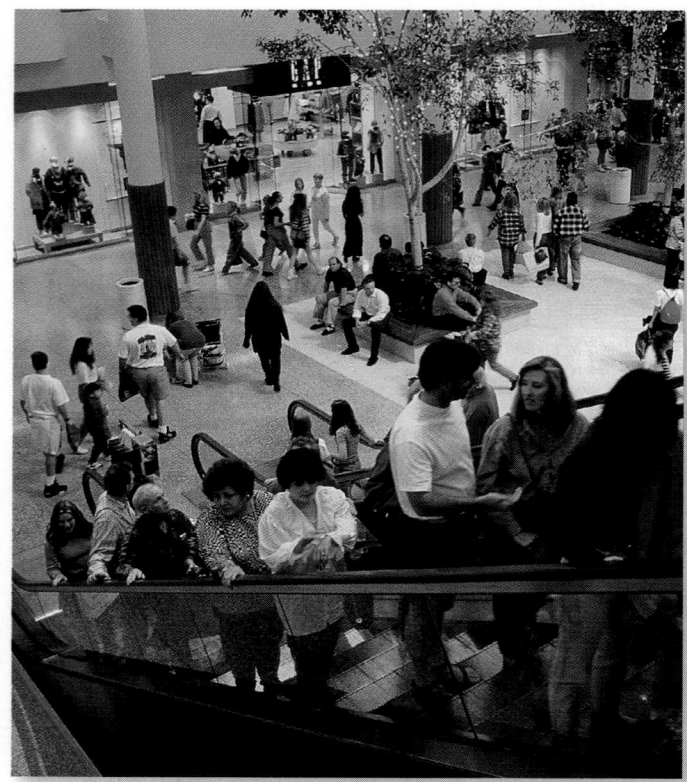

**Figure 19-4.** Because many people touch stair railings, they are common fomites for disease transmission.

by an infected person and then can transmit the infective agent to a susceptible host is considered a fomite. These objects can include drinking glasses, door knobs, shopping cart handles, pencils, and almost any surface or object that can temporarily hold microorganisms (Figure 19-4).

## Means of Entrance

Just as the pathogen needs a means of exit from the reservoir host, it also needs a means of entrance into the new host. Pathogens can enter a new host through any cavity lined with mucous membrane, such as the mouth, nose, throat, vagina, or rectum. They can also enter through the ears, eyes, intestinal tract, urinary tract, reproductive tract, or breaks in the skin. Most pathogens can take advantage of any means of exit and entry. For example, the droplets from an infected child's sneeze can land on a toy in a common play area. The next child to pick up the toy can transfer the infected droplets to his own nose, spreading the infection.

## Susceptible Host

A final requirement must be met for the infection cycle to remain intact. The person into whom the pathogen has been transmitted must be an individual who has little or no immunity to infection by that organism. This individual is called a **susceptible host.**

Susceptibility is determined by a variety of factors. Some of these factors are related to the host, some to the pathogen, and some to the environment. Factors related to the host include the following:

- Age
- Genetic predisposition to certain illnesses
- Nutritional status
- Other disease processes
- Stress levels
- Hygiene habits
- General health

Factors related to the pathogen include the number and concentration of pathogens, the strength (virulence) of the pathogen, and the point of entry. Environmental factors, such as the living conditions of the host and the host's exposure to hazardous substances, also affect susceptibility.

Once a new host has been infected, the cycle can continue. This host becomes the reservoir host and eventually transmits the pathogen to yet another host.

## Environmental Factors in Disease Transmission

The climate, food, water, animals, insects, and people in a community may greatly influence the types and courses of infection there. In a highly dense population, the infection rate may be higher than in a low-density population because pathogens spread more quickly from person to person when people are in closer proximity. Proximity is one reason for the increase in respiratory disease during seasons when people are indoors for long periods.

Animals can play a role in infection. Infections related to pathogens are found in domestic and wild animals. Unpasteurized milk from an infected cow may cause disease. Some pathogens can infect animals and people. Butchers, hunters, and people in occupations dealing with animals may be at greater risk than other individuals for infection by those pathogens.

The environment affects the incidence of diseases carried by insects. Whether a potentially disease-carrying insect is in a certain area depends on whether that area has the appropriate climate and environment the insect needs to live. For instance, in tropical regions, malaria is spread by the female *Anopheles* mosquito (Figure 19-5). In other areas, ticks may carry Rocky Mountain spotted fever or Lyme disease.

Economic and political factors influence the pattern of infection transmission. They help determine the cleanliness of an area, the availability of medical care, and people's knowledge about preventing infection. Other factors that influence infection transmission include the availability

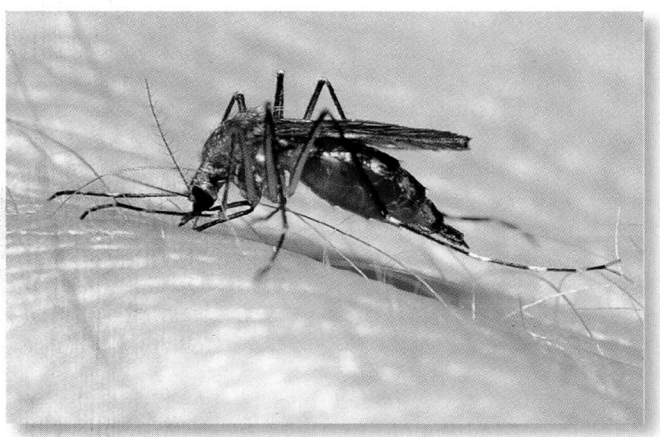

**Figure 19-5.** The female *Anopheles* mosquito carries malaria-causing parasites, transmitting them to humans when it bites.

of transportation, urbanization, population growth rates, and sexual behavior.

## Breaking the Cycle

The principles of **asepsis** must be applied to break the cycle of infection and its spread. Asepsis is the condition in which pathogens are absent or controlled. In medical settings, where many people are hosts to pathogens and many others are susceptible, asepsis can break the cycle by preventing the transmission of pathogens.

Specific measures to help break the cycle of infection include:

- Maintaining strict housekeeping standards to reduce the number of pathogens present
- Adhering to government guidelines to protect against diseases caused by pathogens
- Educating patients in hygiene, health promotion, and disease prevention

You will learn more about specific ways of promoting asepsis in Chapter 20.

## Summary

As doctors and scientists have learned more about the causes of infection, they have developed principles and practices of asepsis.

To protect patients and yourself, you need to know how pathogens cause disease, how disease is transmitted, and how to prevent the spread of infection. You will also use this knowledge to help your employer educate patients about ways they can remain healthy and reduce their risk of contracting diseases.

# REVIEW

## CHAPTER 19

### CASE STUDY *QUESTIONS*

Now that you have completed this chapter, review the case study at the beginning of the chapter and answer the following questions:

1. What part of the cycle of infection caused the problem for the patient?
2. How could the patient have avoided this infection?
3. Why are the other family members not showing symptoms of the infection?
4. Should the patient's family members be tested for the infection?

### Discussion Questions

1. Why would patients who reside in long-term care facilities be at greater risk for infection with a multi-drug resistant microorganism?
2. Differentiate active, passive, and natural active immunities.
3. Discuss ways in which vector-borne disease transmission can be controlled.

### Critical Thinking Questions

1. Why are people, as a rule, able to avoid infections?
2. Why is the previous use of antibiotics a risk factor for the development of antibiotic-resistant microorganisms?
3. In order for a disease to be transmitted to a person, that person must be susceptible. Which susceptibility factors does a person have control over and how can he or she control these factors?

### Application Activities

1. With another student, role-play a scenario involving a medical assistant and a patient with newly diagnosed tuberculosis. Include information about containing the spread of infection. Document this teaching in the patient's medical record.
2. Create a poster for your office describing the cycle of infection. You might choose a specific disease to illustrate the cycle.
3. With another student, role-play a scenario involving a medical assistant and a patient. The medical assistant should use various media to explain and teach the patient about a specific infectious disease.

### Virtual Fieldtrip

*Visit the McGraw-Hill Higher Education Medical Assisting website at www.mhhe.com/medicalassisting3 to complete the following activity:*

Use the National Institutes of Health's website and search the term *influenza*. Keep a journal of your trip. Include the following information:

- Trail map (describe where your search led you)—this should include the URL of each link you found useful and a short synopsis of the information found at the link
- List of information useful to patients
- List of information useful to staff

Plan how you will use this information in a medical practice.

Open the CD and complete this chapter's practice activities, play the games, listen to the key terms, and test yourself with the interactive review. E-mail, print, and/or save your results to document your proficiency.

## CHAPTER 20

# Infection Control Techniques

## MEDICAL ASSISTING COMPETENCIES

*In preparation for the certification examination, you should know the following:*

| COMPETENCY | CMA | RMA |
|---|---|---|
| **Clinical** | | |
| Apply principles of aseptic techniques and infection control, including hand washing | X | X |
| Wrap items for autoclaving | X | X |
| Perform sterilization techniques | X | X |
| Dispose of biohazardous materials | X | X |
| Practice Standard Precautions | X | X |
| **General/Legal/Professional** | | |
| Determine the needs for documentation and reporting, and document accurately and appropriately | X | X |
| Demonstrate knowledge of and monitor current federal and state health-care legislation and regulations; maintain licenses and accreditation | X | X |
| Perform risk management procedures | | X |
| Instruct individuals according to their needs | X | X |
| Provide patients with methods of health promotion and disease prevention | X | X |
| Perform quality control procedures | X | X |

## KEY TERMS

antiseptic

autoclave

bacterial spore

biohazardous materials

biohazardous waste container

contraindication

disinfectant

immunization

nosocomial infection

Occupational Safety and Health Administration (OSHA)

personal protective equipment (PPE)

sanitization

Standard Precautions

sterilization

sterilization indicator

ultrasonic cleaning

Universal Precautions

vaccine

## CHAPTER OUTLINE

- The Medical Assistant's Role in Infection Control
- Infection Control Methods
- Medical Asepsis
- Sanitization
- Disinfection
- Surgical Asepsis
- Sterilization
- OSHA Blood-Borne Pathogens Standard and Universal Precautions
- Reporting Guidelines
- Guideline for Isolation Precautions in Hospitals
- Immunizations: Another Way to Control Infection
- Educating Patients About Preventing Disease Transmission

# LEARNING OUTCOMES

After completing Chapter 20, you will be able to:

**20.1** Describe the medical assistant's role in infection control.

**20.2** Describe methods of infection control.

**20.3** Compare and contrast medical and surgical asepsis.

**20.4** Describe how to perform aseptic hand washing.

**20.5** Compare and contrast the procedures for sanitization, disinfection, and sterilization.

**20.6** Describe measures used in sanitization.

**20.7** List various methods used in disinfection and the advantages and disadvantages of each.

**20.8** Discuss the goal of surgical asepsis.

**20.9** Explain what an autoclave is and how it operates.

**20.10** List the steps in the general autoclave procedures.

**20.11** Explain how to wrap and label items for sterilization in an autoclave.

**20.12** Describe how to complete the sterilization procedure using an autoclave.

**20.13** Define the Blood-Borne Pathogens Standard and Universal Precautions as described in the rules and regulations of the Occupational Safety and Health Administration (OSHA).

**20.14** Explain the role of Universal Precautions in the duties of a medical assistant.

**20.15** List the procedures and legal requirements for disposing of hazardous waste.

**20.16** Describe Centers for Disease Control and Prevention (CDC) requirements for reporting cases of infectious disease.

**20.17** Discuss the need for specific guidelines for isolating patients in health-care settings.

**20.18** Describe the appropriate use of personal protective equipment in various situations.

**20.19** Explain the purpose of immunization.

**20.20** Describe your role in educating patients about immunizations.

**20.21** Explain how to educate patients in preventing disease transmission.

# Introduction

Although our bodies ordinarily are quite capable in their defense against pathogens, patients coming into an office for treatment may be more susceptible to infections. In this chapter you will learn methods of infection control and their respective processes. You will also be introduced to OSHA Guidelines, the Blood-Borne Pathogens Standard, reporting guidelines established by the CDC (Centers for Disease Control and Prevention), and the procedures for isolating patients. The importance of immunizations and patient education regarding immunizations will be stressed as a method of infection control.

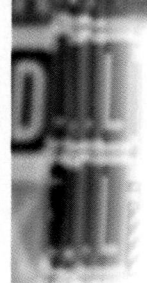

# CASE STUDY

The medical assistant employed at the doctor's office was scratched on the hand last week by her kitten, and the scratch subsequently became infected. The office was very busy this week with patients, and the medical assistant assisted with ten Category I minor surgical procedures. Three days later, six of the ten surgical patients returned to the office with infected surgical sites.

While reading this chapter, consider the following questions:

1. How might the patients have been infected?
2. What steps should the medical assistant have taken to prevent these infections?
3. How does the Blood-Borne Pathogens Standard apply to the medical assistant?
4. If the medical assistant did not observe the regulation, what penalties, if any, could be imposed by OSHA?

# The Medical Assistant's Role in Infection Control

As you learned in Chapter 19, the cycle of infection is one in which pathogens grow and are transmitted from one host to another. To control infectious diseases, this cycle must be broken. You can help break the cycle by applying the principles of infection control to specific tasks in the office setting. These tasks include:

- Following correct sanitization, disinfection, and sterilization procedures
- Helping patients understand basic disease prevention techniques and recognize infectious diseases
- Administering immunizations and educating patients about the importance of immunizations and schedules for obtaining them

# Infection Control Methods

As a medical assistant, you will take measures to eliminate the elements that must be present for disease to occur. To do so, you must have a thorough knowledge of the two types of asepsis:

- Medical asepsis, or clean technique, which is based on maintaining cleanliness to prevent the spread of microorganisms and to ensure that there are as few microorganisms in the medical environment as possible
- Surgical asepsis, or sterile technique, which depends on a completely sterile environment that eliminates all microorganisms

Medical asepsis and surgical asepsis are required by law. Each individual who works in a medical setting must recognize the importance of asepsis and strictly adhere to aseptic procedures in daily routines.

# Medical Asepsis

The medical office can be the host to many pathogens. Therefore, strict, controlled asepsis is crucial. All employees in the medical office must observe and practice the principles of asepsis to ensure a safe environment for patients and staff.

You can promote asepsis through vigilant cleanliness. Every day before patients arrive, you must inspect the office for any surfaces or objects that may be dirty or contaminated. Keeping the office clean reduces the number of microorganisms on surfaces.

## Office Procedures

Other physical aspects of the medical office also contribute to asepsis (Figure 20-1).
They include:

- A reception room that has designated waiting areas for well and sick people. If there is not enough space, sick

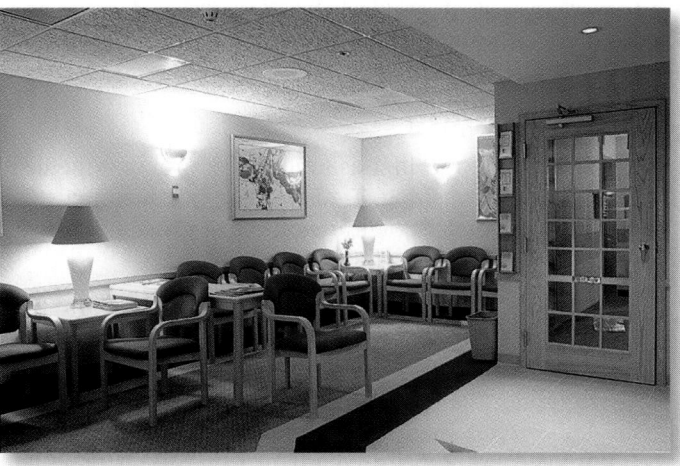

**Figure 20-1.** Asepsis begins in the reception area and waiting room of a medical office. These areas should be kept well lit, well ventilated, and free from dust and dirt. A rest room should be accessible to patients from the waiting area.

patients should be led immediately to an examination room. You may need to explain this policy to well people who have been waiting so that no one thinks other patients are getting preferential treatment.

- An office that is cleaned daily.
- An office that is well lit and ventilated, has no drafts, and has a temperature of approximately 72°F.
- Furniture that is kept in good repair and is replaced when necessary.
- A strict "no eating or drinking" policy.
- Trash that is emptied as necessary, at least once daily.
- An insect-free environment.
- A sign stating that any safety or health hazard be reported to the receptionist.
- A sign asking that patients use tissues for coughs or sneezes, put all waste in the trash can, and tell the receptionist if they are nauseated or have to use the restroom. (Ideally, the reception area should be equipped with a restroom for emergencies.)

## Asepsis During Medical Assistant Procedures

Many of the procedures you perform require aseptic techniques to prevent cross contamination from one place to another. For instance, when opening a sterile container, you should rest its lid face-up instead of facedown. Placing it facedown contaminates the inside of the lid, making it unsuitable to be put back on the sterile container. When administering tablets or capsules, you should pour them into the bottle cap or a cup rather than into your hand to prevent the transfer of microorganisms from your hand onto the medication. To prevent cross contamination, you must also follow guidelines about the types of protective gear to wear during a procedure. (Personal protective equipment is discussed later in this chapter.)

## Hand Washing

The single most important aseptic procedure for a medical assistant is hand washing. Transmission by touching is the most common means of transmitting pathogens. Hands should be washed at the following times:

- At the beginning of the day, after breaks, before and after using the restroom, before and after lunch, and before leaving for the day
- Before and after using gloves, handling specimens or waste, seeing each patient, handling clean or sterile supplies, and performing any procedure
- After blowing your nose or coughing

Aseptic hand washing removes accumulated dirt and microorganisms that could cause infection under the right conditions. Procedure 20-1 describes how to perform aseptic hand washing.

## Other Aseptic Precautions

You need to make certain precautions part of your daily routine. For example, take these safeguards:

- Avoid leaning against sinks, supplies, or equipment.
- Avoid touching your face or mouth.
- Use tissues when you cough or sneeze, and always wash your hands afterward.
- Whenever possible, avoid working directly with patients when you have a cold.
- Wear gloves and a mask if you have a cold and must work with patients.
- Stay home if you have a fever, and remain there until you have maintained a normal temperature for 24 hours.

## Sanitization

**Sanitization** is the scrubbing of instruments and equipment with special brushes and detergent to remove blood, mucus, and other contaminants or media where pathogens can grow. Sanitization is used to clean items that touch only healthy, intact skin. For other equipment, sanitization is the first step before disinfection and sterilization. Instruments and equipment that you can sanitize and reuse without further disinfection or sterilization include the following:

- Blood pressure cuff
- Ophthalmoscope (an instrument containing a mirror and lenses used to examine the interior of the eye)
- Otoscope (an instrument used for inspecting the ear)
- Penlight
- Reflex hammer

- Stethoscope
- Tape measure
- Tuning fork

## Collecting Instruments for Sanitization

Sanitize instruments as soon as possible after use. If you cannot sanitize them immediately, place them in a sink or container filled with water and a neutral-pH detergent solution so that blood and tissue will not dry on the instrument. In a surgical setting, use a special receptacle of disinfectant solution for collecting contaminated instruments. In an examination setting, place instruments in a sink or a container that can be transported to a sink. Take care when placing instruments in sinks or basins. You can damage pieces of equipment if you drop them carelessly into a receptacle. Nicks or scratches can affect their function and can provide opportunities for bacterial contamination.

When you are ready to begin the sanitization procedure, put on properly fitting, intact utility gloves. They are the barrier between your skin and any infectious material on the instruments and equipment to be cleaned. When you work with instruments that may be contaminated with blood, body fluids, or tissue, you may want the additional protection of a mask, eye protection, or protective clothing.

Separate the sharp instruments from all other equipment (Figure 20-4). Separating them reduces the risk of blunting sharp edges or points, damaging other equipment, and injuring yourself.

## Scrubbing Instruments and Equipment

Begin by draining the disinfectant or detergent solution in which the equipment was soaking. Rinse each piece of equipment in hot running water, and handle only one item at a time (by its handles where applicable). Scrub each item using hot, soapy water and a small plastic scrub brush. Never use metal brushes or steel wool, which can scratch and damage instruments. Pay careful attention to hinges, ratchets, and other nooks and crannies where it is possible for contaminated material to collect (Figure 20-5). Use brushes of different sizes to clean all areas of each item.

Use a detergent specially formulated for medical instruments and equipment. This type of detergent is low-sudsing, has a neutral pH, and is formulated to dissolve blood and blood products. Equipment and instrument manufacturers provide guidelines for sanitizing various types of products. For example, stainless steel items must be sanitized differently from chrome-plated instruments. Follow manufacturers' guidelines when you are working with their products.

After scrubbing all surfaces and removing all visible stains and residue, rinse instruments individually, and

# Aseptic Hand Washing

**Procedure Goal:** To remove dirt and microorganisms from under the fingernails and from the surface of the skin, hair follicles, and oil glands of the hands

**OSHA Guidelines:** This procedure does not involve exposure to blood, body fluids, or tissues.

**Materials:** Liquid soap, nailbrush or orange stick, paper towels

**Method:**

1. Remove all jewelry (plain wedding bands may be left on and scrubbed).
2. Turn on the faucets using a paper towel, and adjust the water temperature to moderately warm. (Sinks with knee-operated faucet controls prevent contact of the surface with the hands.)
3. Wet your hands and apply liquid soap. Use a clean, dry, paper towel to activate soap pump. Liquid soap, especially when dispensed with a foot pump, is preferable to bar soap.

*Rationale*

There is less available area for dirt to accumulate on a liquid soap dispenser than on bar soap, and there is a smaller chance of dropping the soap dispenser into the sink or onto the floor.

4. Work the soap into a lather, making sure that all of both hands are lathered. Rub vigorously in a circular motion for 2 minutes. Keep your hands lower than your forearms so that dirty water flows into the sink instead of back onto your arms. Your fingertips should be pointing down. Interlace your fingers to clean between them, and use the palm of one hand to clean the back of the other (Figure 20-2). It is important that you wash every surface of your hands.

*Rationale*

Microorganisms are found on every surface of the hand and if not washed away can be transferred to the patient.

5. Use a nailbrush or orange stick to dislodge dirt around your nails and cuticles (Figure 20-3).

*Rationale*

Microorganisms under the nails are not directly subjected to the running water and must be dislodged so that they can be washed away.

6. Rinse your hands well, keeping the hands lower than your forearms and not touching the sink or faucets.

7. With the water still running, dry your hands thoroughly with clean, dry paper towels and then turn off the faucets using a clean, dry paper towel. Discard the towels.

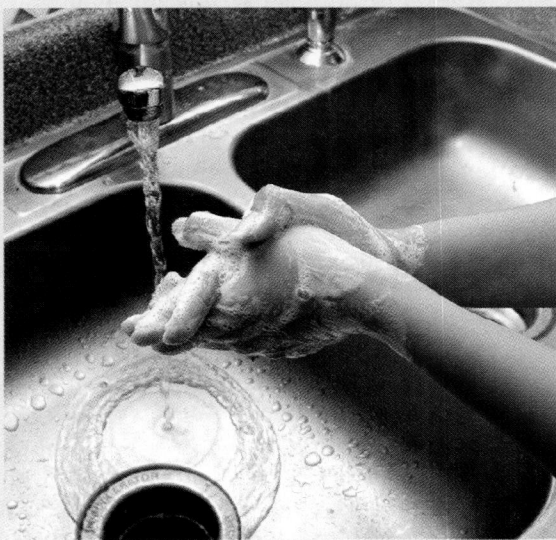

**Figure 20-2.** When you wash your hands, be sure to clean all surfaces, including the palms, between the fingers, and under the fingernails.

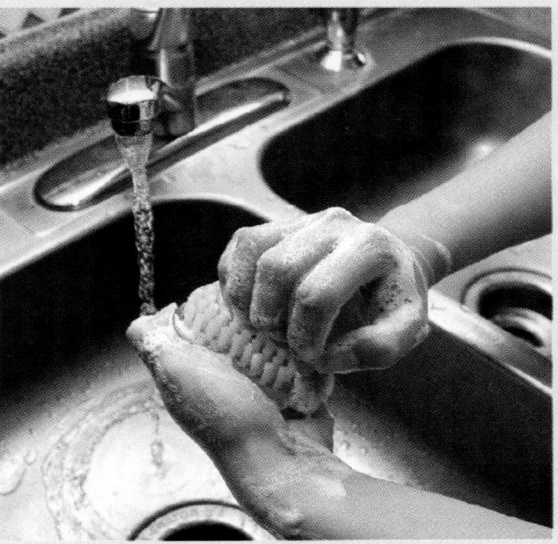

**Figure 20-3.** The nails and cuticles require additional attention to ensure that all dirt is removed.

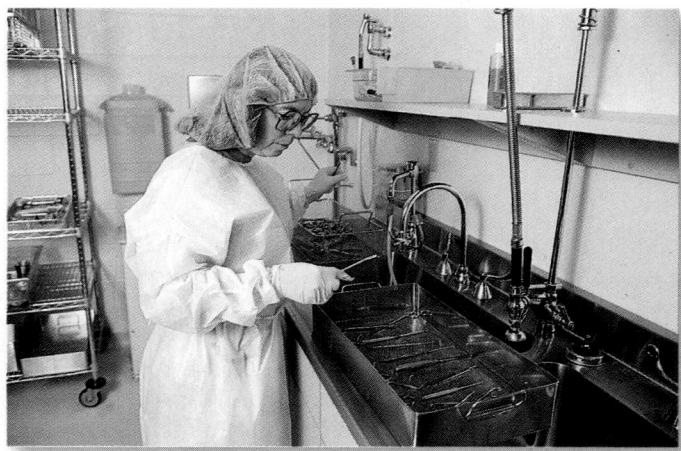

**Figure 20-4.** When working with instruments and equipment, separate pointed or sharp-edged instruments from all others.

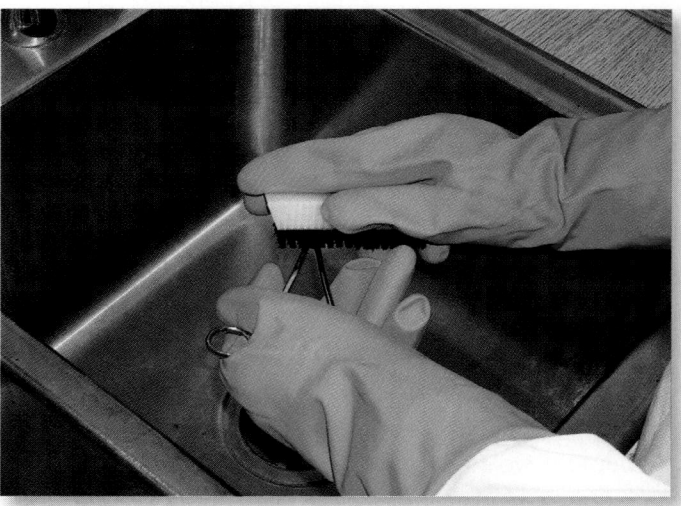

**Figure 20-5.** Clean all areas of an instrument, using a brush for hard-to-reach surfaces.

place each one on a clean towel. Roll the instrument in the towel to remove most of the moisture. Then dry the instrument thoroughly, and examine it closely to be sure that it is operating correctly. Be sure that all moving parts operate smoothly and that surfaces are free from nicks, scratches, and other imperfections. Instruments that need only to be sanitized can be returned to trays or bins for storage. Wrap items that require disinfection and **sterilization** (complete destruction of all living organisms) in a clean covering, and set them aside for those processes.

## Rubber and Plastic Products

To sanitize rubber and plastic products, you may need to soak them only for a short period or not at all. Some rubber and plastic products fade or discolor if left in a detergent solution. When you sanitize these products, be sure to follow manufacturers' guidelines.

## Syringes and Needles

Disposable syringes and needles have replaced reusable ones in medical offices. Using disposable instruments helps reduce the risk of infection to both patients and health-care personnel.

## Ultrasonic Cleaning

Delicate instruments or those with moving parts should be sanitized by using ultrasonic cleaners. **Ultrasonic cleaning** involves placing instruments in a special bath. The cleaner generates sound waves through a cleaning solution, loosening contaminants. Ultrasonic cleaning is safe for even very fragile instruments. If your medical office sanitizes instruments with an ultrasonic cleaner, follow the manufacturer's guidelines for operating the device.

Instruments with points or sharp edges and instruments made of different types of metal should be separated

from other equipment. The ultrasonic cleaning process can cause one metal to disintegrate and fuse with another metal, rendering all instruments useless. Place all instruments with hinges or ratchets in the ultrasonic cleaner in the open position. If such an instrument is placed in the cleaner in the closed position, contaminated material can become trapped between the two surfaces.

After the instruments have been in the ultrasonic cleaner for the recommended cleaning time, remove them and rinse them under cool running water. Be sure to remove all the ultrasonic cleaning fluid. Then dry the instruments, and wrap them for storage or for disinfection and sterilization.

You can reuse ultrasonic cleaning solution for several cleaning baths. Replace it according to the care and maintenance procedures outlined by the manufacturer of the cleaning device.

## Disinfection

Sanitization is often only the beginning of the process of eliminating microorganisms. After sanitization, some instruments and equipment require only disinfection before being used again. Disinfection of other items, however, is merely the second step in infection control, performed before the process of sterilization. You must wear gloves when handling instruments during disinfection procedures because instruments requiring disinfection are considered to be contaminated.

To destroy microorganisms, a disinfectant solution must reach every surface of an instrument; however, disinfection cannot kill all microorganisms. **Bacterial spores** (thick-walled, reproductive bodies capable of resisting harsh conditions) and certain viruses have been known to survive disinfection with strong chemicals and boiling water. It is essential to understand this limitation of disinfection when you work with instruments and equipment.

Disinfection is usually sufficient for instruments that do not penetrate a patient's skin or that come in contact only with a patient's mucous membranes or other surfaces not considered sterile. Instruments and equipment that you can disinfect and reuse without sterilization include the following:

- Enamelware
- Endotracheal tubes (tubes used to establish an artificial airway through the nose, mouth, or direct tracheal route)
- Glassware
- Laryngoscopes (tubes equipped with lighting and used to examine the interior of the larynx through the mouth)
- Nasal specula (instruments used to enlarge the opening of the nose to permit viewing)

Note that you must sterilize any instrument or piece of equipment, including those just listed, if there is visible contamination with blood or blood products before another use, even if disinfection is commonly considered sufficient. Sterilization is the only reliable measure you can take to eliminate blood-borne pathogens.

## Using Disinfectants

**Disinfectants** are cleaning products applied particularly to instruments and equipment to reduce or eliminate infectious organisms. They are used primarily on inanimate materials. In contrast, cleaning products that are used on human tissues as anti-infection agents are called **antiseptics.**

There are no clear indications that an item has been properly and completely disinfected. To ensure the optimum effectiveness of disinfectants, follow the manufacturers' guidelines carefully when using them.

Other factors may also have an impact on the effectiveness of a disinfectant. For example, if the disinfectant solution has been used many times, it may not be as powerful as a fresh solution. When wet items are put in the disinfectant bath, the surface moisture may dilute the solution. Traces of the soap used in the sanitization process can alter the chemical makeup of the disinfectant, making it nonlethal to pathogens. Evaporation can also alter the chemical makeup of the solution.

## Choosing the Correct Disinfectant

Manufacturers' guidelines are the most accurate and up-to-date sources of information about the type of disinfectant to use on a given product. Generally, disinfect instruments and equipment by using one or more of the following agents:

- Germicidal soap products
- Alcohol
- Acid products
- Formaldehyde

- Glutaraldehyde
- Household bleach
- Iodine and iodine compounds

Each of these disinfectants has advantages and disadvantages. Before using any disinfectant product or procedure, it is important to understand some general guidelines about disinfectant use as well as specific concerns with each approach.

**Germicidal Soap Products.** Research has shown that the use of soap in the process of disinfection is less important than the scrubbing and rinsing steps. Germ-killing additives may increase the effectiveness of soap products, however, and a soap-and-water disinfection may be sufficient for items that do not come in contact with a patient's mucous membranes.

**Alcohol.** Alcohol (70% isopropyl) is commonly used to clean instruments and equipment that would be damaged by immersion in soap and water or other disinfectant solutions. It is a corrosive product, however, and can cause damage to the skin if it is used excessively.

**Acid Products.** The killing power of concentrated acid products such as phenol (carbolic acid) is quite high. In a concentrated form, acid products are also extremely corrosive and toxic to tissue and should be used with care.

**Formaldehyde.** Formaldehyde is a corrosive and an irritant to body tissue. It is commonly used as a preservative in a 10% solution. In a 5% solution, it can be used as a germicidal agent and a sporicidal agent. Formaldehyde must be used at room temperature because its effectiveness is reduced in cooler environments. After disinfecting items with formaldehyde, rinse them thoroughly with distilled or sterile water before using them on patients.

**Glutaraldehyde.** Glutaraldehyde (known more commonly by the trade names Cidex, Cidexplus, and Glutarex) is used in chemical sterilization processes, but you can also use it as a disinfectant. Immersing instruments or equipment in a bath of glutaraldehyde for 10 to 30 minutes is sufficient for disinfection. Any chemical used in this "cold disinfection" method must be rated as a sterilant and registered with the EPA.

**Household Bleach.** Bleach (sodium hypochlorite) is commonly used in laboratory settings to provide a measure of protection against transmission of the human immunodeficiency virus (HIV). It is an effective disinfectant when used in a 10% solution. Bleach is used to disinfect surfaces and to soak rubber equipment before sanitization. Ventilation may be necessary when you use bleach because the fumes should not be inhaled for a prolonged period.

**Iodine and Iodine Compounds.** Iodine products are used as both disinfectants (solutions stronger than 2%) and antiseptics (solutions weaker than 2%). They are somewhat corrosive, however, and their effectiveness is limited by the presence of blood products, mucus, or soap.

## Handling Disinfected Supplies

After disinfecting equipment, handle it with care to prevent contaminating any surface that may later come in contact with a patient. Use sterile transfer forceps, or sterilizing forceps, to remove items from whatever disinfection unit is used. Always wear gloves to handle disinfected items, and make sure you store disinfected equipment in a clean, moisture-free environment.

# Surgical Asepsis

Surgical asepsis takes medical asepsis to a higher level. The aim of surgical asepsis is to keep the surgical environment completely free of all microorganisms. To accomplish this, you will be responsible for sterilizing surgical instruments prior to their use during sterile procedures. You may also be asked to assist with various surgical procedures, such as closing a wound or removing a cyst. The sterile technique of surgical asepsis must be maintained for even simple, minor operations and injections (Figure 20-6). Keep in mind, however, that the more extensive the procedure, the greater the risk of infection.

# Sterilization

Sterilization is required for all instruments or supplies that will penetrate a patient's skin or come in contact with any other normally sterile areas of the body. Sterilization is also required for all instruments that will be used in a sterile field, even if they will not actually be used on a patient. An item is considered either sterile or unsterile. If you doubt the status of an item, consider it unsterile.

Before sterilizing an item, you must first sanitize it and, sometimes, disinfect it. Instruments and equipment that need to be sterilized include the following:

- Curettes (spoon-shaped instruments for removing material from the wall of a cavity or other surface)
- Instruments used during surgical procedures
- Suture removal instruments
- Vaginal specula (instruments used to enlarge the opening of the vagina and allow examination of the vagina and cervix)

Sterilize instruments and equipment by one of the following methods:

- Autoclaving
- Chemical (cold) processes

## The Autoclave

The primary method for sterilizing instruments and equipment is the use of pressurized steam in an **autoclave** (Figure 20-7). This device forces the temperature of steam above the boiling point of water (212°F, or 100°C). There are two reasons why sterilization by autoclave is such a widely accepted method of sterilization:

1. Steam autoclaves can operate at a lower temperature than is required for dry heat sterilization. The moist heat from steam more quickly permeates the clean, porous wrappings in which all instruments are placed prior to loading them into the unit.
2. The moisture causes coagulation of proteins within microorganisms at a much lower temperature than is possible with dry heat. When cells containing coagulated protein cool, their cell walls burst, resulting in the death of the microorganisms.

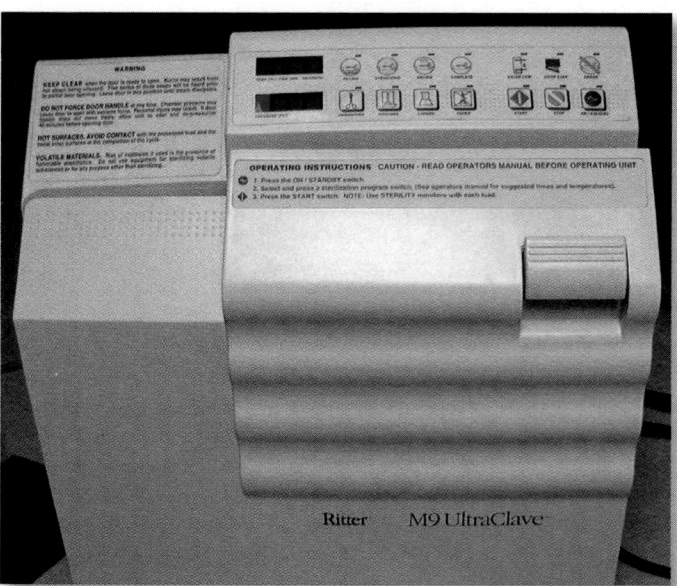

**Figure 20-7.** Steam autoclaving is the most common method of sterilizing instruments and equipment. Understanding the gauges and timer is essential to proper operation of an autoclave.

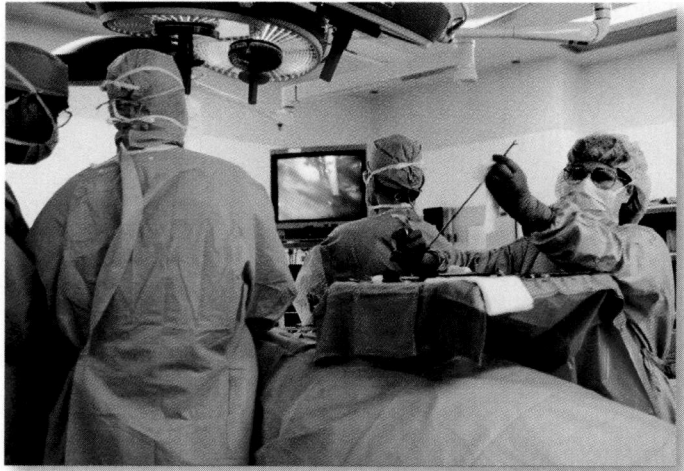

**Figure 20-6.** Surgical asepsis must be strictly adhered to even for minor procedures.

**General Autoclave Procedures.** In general, the autoclave process involves your taking the following steps:

1. Prepare sanitized and disinfected instruments and equipment for loading into the autoclave by wrapping them in muslin or special porous paper or plastic bags or envelopes and labeling each pack. (Include sterilization indicators.)

2. Check the water level in the autoclave and add distilled water if necessary.

3. Preheat the autoclave according to the manufacturer's guidelines. (Some models require putting instruments in before preheating.)

4. Perform any required quality control procedures (besides including sterilization indicators in instrument packs).

5. Load the instruments and equipment into the autoclave. Allow adequate space around the items to ensure that steam reaches all areas.

6. Choose the correct setting based on the type of load (unwrapped items, pouches, packs, liquids, etc.). If the autoclave is not automatic, set the autoclave for the correct time after the correct temperature and pressure have been reached.

7. Run the autoclave through the sterilization cycle, including drying time.

8. Remove the instruments and equipment from the autoclave.

9. Store the instruments and equipment properly for the next use. Rotate stored items so that packages with the oldest date are used first.

10. Clean the autoclave and the surrounding work area.

During each step of the process, assume that the instruments and equipment are contaminated, and follow **Universal Precautions:**

- Wear gloves to avoid contamination by blood, body fluids, or tissues.
- Take measures to protect against needlesticks or cuts—for example, by using forceps to handle sharps.
- Wash your hands thoroughly after all cleaning procedures.

Universal Precautions will be discussed in greater detail later in this chapter.

***Wrapping and Labeling All Items.*** Wrap items in porous fabric, paper, or plastic when placing them in the autoclave. This material helps surround the items with the correct levels of moisture and heat. Instruments and equipment that are to be used immediately after autoclaving can be placed on trays with material above and below the items. Items that are to be stored or that must be sterile when used must be wrapped and sealed before autoclaving. Refer to Procedure 20-2 for wrapping and labeling instructions.

A number of products are available for wrapping items for sterilization. Muslin (140 count) is the most commonly

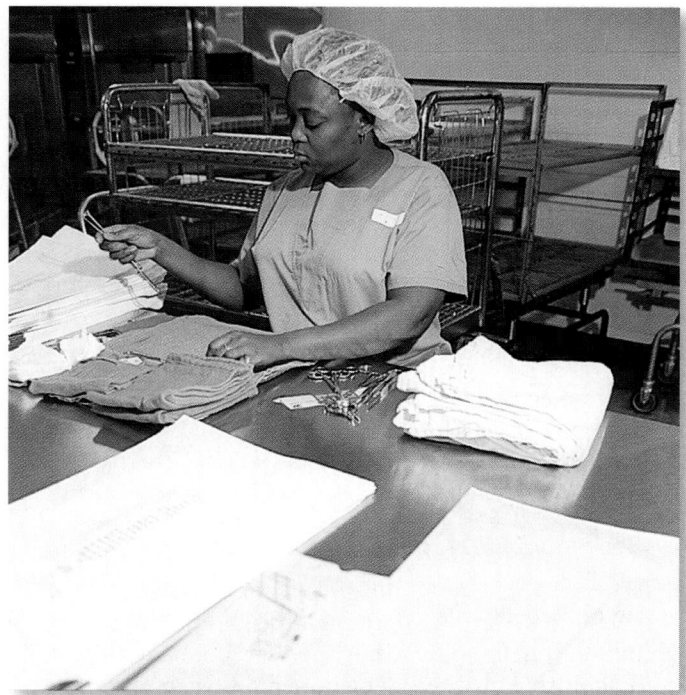

**Figure 20-8.** Many wrapping products are available for use when instruments or equipment are autoclaved.

used wrapping fabric. Other products include permeable paper, disposable nonwoven fabric, and clear plastic envelopes with one side made of permeable material. Figure 20-8 shows several common wrapping products.

Instruments that will be used together must be wrapped together to form a sterile pack. Take care to wrap the pack loosely so that the steam can reach the instruments inside. Position the instruments so they do not touch each other inside the pack. After using a pack, consider all items (even those not used) unsterile and return them for sanitization, disinfection, and sterilization.

Clearly label each pack to identify the item or items inside the wrapping and the person who completed the procedure. The label must also include the date so that packs are not used after their expiration dates. A 30-day period is generally considered the maximum shelf life for a sterile pack wrapped in cloth (6 months for airtight pouches).

***Preheating the Autoclave.*** Be careful to check for solution that may have boiled over and for deposits that may have formed on any of the inner surfaces. Make sure the water reservoir is filled to the proper level with distilled water. Also check the discharge lines and valves to make sure there are no obstructions. If lines or valves are blocked, air may remain trapped inside the chamber, rendering the load unsterile.

Following this inspection, preheat the unit according to the manufacturer's guidelines. Loading cold instruments into an overheated chamber can cause excess condensation, so be sure to understand and follow the preheating instructions.

# Wrapping and Labeling Instruments for Sterilization in the Autoclave

**Procedure Goal:** To enclose instruments and equipment to be sterilized in appropriate wrapping materials to ensure sterilization and to protect supplies from contamination after sterilization

**OSHA Guidelines:**

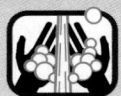 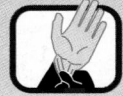 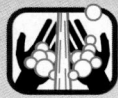

(See Figure 20-14, p. 427.)

**Materials:** Dry, sanitized, and disinfected instruments and equipment; wrapping material (paper, muslin, gauze, bags, envelopes); sterilization indicators; autoclave tape; labels (if wrapping does not include space for labeling); pen

**Method:**

For wrapping instruments or equipment in pieces of paper or fabric:

1. Wash your hands and put on gloves before beginning to wrap the items to be sterilized.

2. Place a square of paper or muslin on the table with one point toward you. With muslin, use a double thickness. The paper or fabric must be large enough to allow all four points to cover the instruments or equipment you will be wrapping. It must also be large enough to provide an overlap, which will be used as a handling flap.

3. Place each item to be included in the pack in the center area of the paper or fabric "diamond" (Figure 20-9A). Items that will be used together should be wrapped together. Take care, however, that surfaces of the items do not touch each other inside the pack. Inspect each item to make sure it is operating correctly. Place hinged instruments in the pack in the open position. Wrap a small piece of paper, muslin, or gauze around delicate edges or points to protect against damage to other instruments or to the pack wrapping.

*Rationale*

Overcrowding instruments may prohibit sterilization by interfering with steam penetration.

4. Place a sterilization indicator inside the pack with the instruments. Position the indicator correctly, following the manufacturer's guidelines.

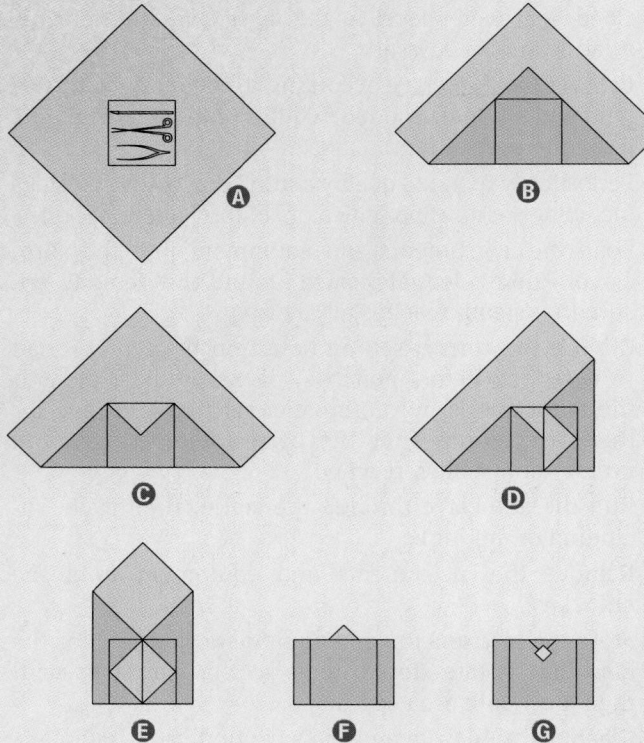

**Figure 20-9.** Follow this sequence when you wrap instruments in a paper or fabric pack for sterilization in an autoclave.

*Rationale*

A sterilization indicator must always be placed inside the pack so that you can be sure the contents have been sterilized properly.

5. Fold the bottom point of the diamond up and over the instruments in to the center (Figure 20-9B). Fold back a small portion of the point (Figure 20-9C).

*Rationale*

This "handle" will be used later, when the sterile pack is opened.

6. Fold the right point of the diamond in to the center. Again, fold back a small portion of the point to be used as a handle (Figure 20-9D).

7. Fold the left point of the diamond in to the center, folding back a small portion to form a

*continued* →

# PROCEDURE 20.2

## Wrapping and Labeling Instruments for Sterilization in the Autoclave *(concluded)*

handle. The pack should now resemble an open envelope (Figure 20-9E).

8. Grasp the covered instruments (the bottom of the envelope) and fold this portion up, toward the top point (Figure 20-9F). Fold the top point down over the pack, making sure the pack is snug but not too tight.

9. Secure the pack with autoclave tape (Figure 20-9G). A "quick-opening tab" can be created by folding a small portion of the tape back onto itself. The pack must be snug enough to prevent instruments from slipping out of the wrapping or damaging each other inside the pack but loose enough to allow adequate circulation of steam through the pack.

10. Label the pack with your initials and the date. List the contents of the pack as well. If the pack contains syringes, be sure to identify the syringe size(s).

### Rationale
Dating helps you keep up with the date the pack expires. Items should be easily identified without opening the pack.

11. Place the pack aside for loading into the autoclave.

12. Remove gloves, dispose of them in the appropriate waste container, and wash your hands.

For wrapping instruments and equipment in bags or envelopes:

1. Wash your hands and put on gloves before beginning to wrap the items to be sterilized.

2. Insert the items into the bag or envelope as indicated by the manufacturer's directions. Hinged instruments should be opened before insertion into the package.

### Rationale
This allows steam to penetrate inside the hinge.

3. Close and seal the pack. Make sure the sterilization indicator is not damaged or already exposed.

### Rationale
If the sterilization indicator is damaged or already exposed, you have no way of knowing if the sterilization cycle was completed.

4. Label the pack with your initials and the date. List the contents of the pack as well. The pens or pencils used to label the pack must be waterproof; otherwise, the contents of the pack and date of sterilization will be obliterated.

### Rationale
Dating helps you keep up with the date the pack expires. Items should be easily identified without opening the pack.

5. Place the pack aside for loading into the autoclave.

6. Remove gloves, dispose of them in the appropriate waste container, and wash your hands.

---

**Understanding Autoclave Settings.** Modern autoclaves are designed to operate as automatically as possible; however, manual autoclaves are still used. Because you are responsible for the sterility of the items processed by the autoclave, you must be able to identify the various gauges and interpret their readings correctly.

Manual autoclaves have three gauges and a timer. The jacket pressure gauge shows the outer chamber's steam pressure. The chamber pressure gauge shows the inner chamber's steam pressure. The temperature gauge shows the temperature inside the inner, or sterilization, chamber. The timer allows you to control the number of minutes that the load is exposed to the high-temperature, pressurized steam.

Exact temperature and pressure requirements vary with the model and type of autoclave as well as with the instruments and packaging in the load. In general, the temperature must reach 250°F to 270°F (121°F to 132°C), and the chamber pressure gauge must show 15 to 30 pounds of pressure. Follow the manufacturer's instructions precisely for each autoclave load. Procedure 20-3 describes the general steps to follow for running a load through the preheated autoclave.

**Storing Sterilized Supplies.** After packs and instruments are sterilized in the autoclave, you must store them in a clean, dry location. The method you use to wrap an item for sterilization determines the item's sterile shelf life. As a general rule, double-layer fabric- or paper-wrapped packages are considered sterile for 30 days. The manufacturers of other wrapping products provide their own guidelines for sterile shelf life.

Return items for sanitization, disinfection, and sterilization after the sterile shelf life period has elapsed. Do not reuse any wrapping or labeling products. Instead, process each item as if it had never been cleaned.

***Cleaning the Autoclave and Work Area.*** Clean the autoclave after each use to prevent accumulation of deposits that might affect the unit's operation. You may use an all-purpose cleaner, although specific cleaning products are available for use with autoclaves.

You are responsible for ensuring that routine cleaning is done correctly and thoroughly. When you clean the unit, also check for signs of cracking or wear in gaskets, drain valves, and tubing. Check the level of distilled water in the reservoir. Service representatives who specialize in the maintenance of your unit should periodically clean and check all seals and gauges.

The work area around the autoclave unit should be divided into two areas: one for nonsterile, not-yet-autoclaved items and one for sterile equipment as it is removed from the unit. Each area should be clearly marked. Do not use supplies from one area in the other. Be sure to move any sterile packs or equipment to the correct storage areas when cleaning the counters and other work surfaces. If anything is spilled on a sterile pack or instrument, return the item for sanitization, disinfection, and sterilization.

***Sterilization Indicators and Quality Control.*** It is important to monitor all sterilization procedures. This is

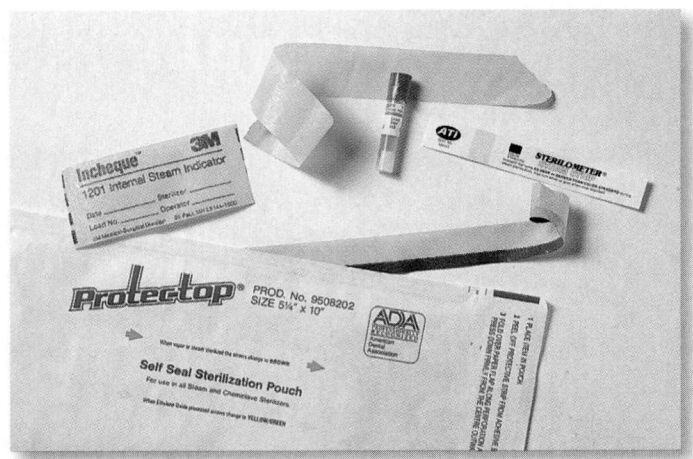

**Figure 20-10.** Sterilization indicators are manufactured in many sizes and shapes.

accomplished through the use of various types of indicators and quality control measures.

**Sterilization indicators** are tags, inserts, tapes, tubes, or strips that confirm that the items in the autoclave have been exposed to the correct volume of steam at the correct temperature for the correct length of time. Several types of indicators are available (Figure 20-10).

You place tags or inserts within the load, whereas you affix tapes to the outside of wrapped instrument packs. These types of indicators have designated areas or words

# PROCEDURE 20.3

## Running a Load Through the Autoclave

**Procedure Goal:** To run a load of instruments and equipment through an autoclave, ensuring sterilization of items by properly loading, drying, and unloading them

**OSHA Guidelines:**

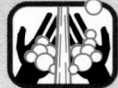 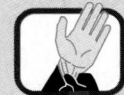 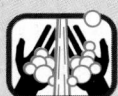

(See Figure 20-14, p. 427.)

**Materials:** Dry, sanitized, and disinfected instruments and equipment, both individual pieces and wrapped packs; oven mitts; sterile transfer forceps; storage containers for individual items

**Method:**

1. Wash your hands and put on gloves before beginning to load items into the autoclave.

2. Rest packs on their edges, and place jars and containers on their sides.

3. Place lids for jars and containers with their sterile sides down.

4. If the load includes plastic items, make sure no other item leans against them.

*Rationale*

Pressure that results from the high temperatures can cause plastic items to bend or warp.

5. If your load is mixed—containing both wrapped packs and individual instruments—place the tray containing the instruments below the tray containing the wrapped packs (Figure 20-11).

*Rationale*

This arrangement prevents any condensation that forms on the instruments from dripping onto the wrapped packs, saturating the wrapping.

*continued* ⟶

# Running a Load Through the Autoclave (concluded)

6. Close the door and start the unit. For automatic autoclaves, choose the cycle based on the type of load you are running. Consult the manufacturer's recommendations before choosing the load type.

7. For manual autoclaves, start the timer when the indicators show the recommended temperature and pressure.

8. Right after the end of the steam cycle and just before the start of the drying cycle, open the door to the autoclave slightly (between ¼ and ½ inch).

### Rationale

Opening the door more than ½ inch causes cold air to enter the autoclave, possibly resulting in excessive condensation in the chamber. This condensation would cause incomplete drying. Consult the manufacturer's recommendations regarding opening the door. Some automatic autoclaves do not require opening the door during the drying cycle.

9. Dry according to the manufacturer's recommendations. Packs and large items may require up to 45 minutes for complete drying.

10. Unload the autoclave after the drying cycle is finished. Do not unload any packs or instruments with wet wrappings, or the object inside will be considered unsterile and must be processed again.

### Rationale

Wet wrappings can transfer bacteria from your hands to the interior of the pack.

11. Unload each package carefully. Wear oven mitts to protect yourself from burns when removing wrapped packs. Use sterile transfer forceps to unload unwrapped individual objects.

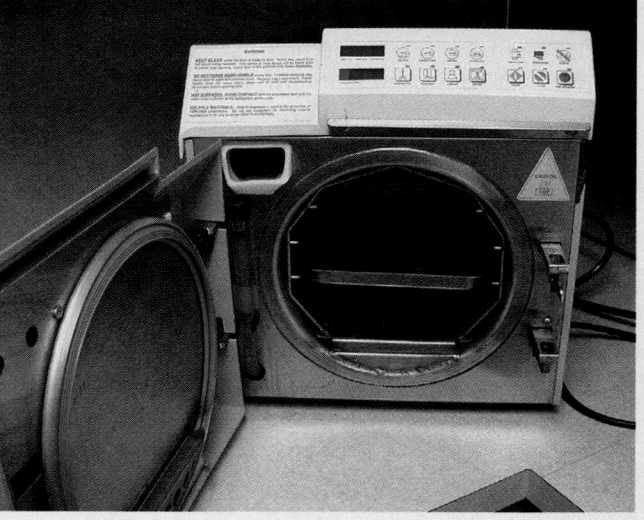

**Figure 20-11.** Properly loaded trays allow steam to reach all instruments and equipment.

12. Inspect each package or item, looking for moisture on the wrapping, underexposed sterilization indicators, and tears or breaks in the wrapping. Consider the pack unsterile if any of these conditions is present.

13. Place sterile packs aside for transfer to storage.

14. Place individual items that are not required to be sterile in clean containers.

15. Place items that must remain sterile in sterile containers, being sure to close the container covers tightly.

16. As you unload items, avoid placing them in an overly cool location because the cool temperature could cause condensation on the instruments or packs.

17. Remove gloves, dispose of them in the appropriate waste container, and wash your hands.

that change color when the correct temperature has been reached. Some also show when the proper temperature, pressure, and duration have occurred. Although it is generally acceptable to rely on these indicators as a guarantee of sterility, they are, in reality, only indicators that the load has been exposed to conditions that usually result in sterile surfaces. They do not guarantee that the contents of the autoclave are actually sterile.

Biological indicators are used as a quality control method to confirm that sterilization has occurred. These indicators contain bacterial spores and come in various forms including strips, disks, and ampules. Bacterial spores are used because they are more resistant to common sterilization processes than non-spore-forming organisms. The general procedure for using biological indicators is as follows:

- Place a biological indicator in a load to be sterilized.
- Place one biological indicator outside the autoclave as a positive control.
- Run the load as usual.

## CAUTION *Handle With Care*

### Interpreting the Results of a Biological Indicator

If you do not send the biological indicator to an outside lab, you may be asked to interpret the results. If the indicator exposed to the sterilization cycle is positive for bacterial growth, then sterilization has not occurred. The load should be held, the chemical indicators checked, and the biological indicator test repeated. If the second test is positive, have the sterilizer serviced. Once the sterilizer has been serviced, retest with three consecutive tests in an empty chamber. If all three tests are negative, the sterilizer can be returned to service. If the indicator exposed to the cycle shows no bacterial growth, you should check the growth of the positive control. There should be bacterial growth from the positive control because it has not been exposed to the sterilization cycle. It is important to note that if there is no growth on the positive control, you should repeat the quality control procedure with biological indicators from another manufactured lot number. The results of each biological indicator monitoring procedure should be recorded in the sterilization log.

Biological indicators should be used at the following times:

- If a new type of packaging material is used
- If you have a new autoclave
- After autoclave maintenance or repair
- On a weekly basis as a general quality control measure

---

- Place a biological indicator and positive control as recommended by the manufacturer or send to an outside lab for processing.
- Incubate as recommended by the manufacturer.

***Preventing Incomplete Sterilization.*** Although the autoclave is generally considered the simplest and most effective method for sterilizing instruments and equipment, certain pitfalls can cause incomplete sterilization. The four leading factors that cause incomplete sterilization are incorrect timing, insufficient temperature, overcrowding of packs, and inadequate steam levels. Once again, the manufacturer's guidelines provided with the autoclave unit are the best source of accurate information about how to operate it correctly.

***Timing Guidelines.*** After loading the autoclave, make sure the heating cycle lasts long enough to allow the steam to permeate all wrappings to reach the instruments and equipment inside. Timing for items to be sterilized should not be started until the unit has reached the proper temperature. Automatic autoclaves have preset timing for each load type. You should keep up with the amount of time an automatic autoclave takes to complete a cycle, noting any differences between loads. Large differences in the amount of time it takes to complete a load cycle should alert you to a problem with the autoclave. Although following timing guidelines helps ensure sterilization, you should also use sterilization indicators.

In general, place indicators in a sufficient number of places in the load so that you can be reasonably confident of the sterility of all items in the chamber. The following locations are suitable for indicator positioning:

- Within instrument packs
- On the outside of wrapped instrument packs
- Inside containers, especially those that cannot be positioned so that steam surrounds the item
- Near the air exhaust valve
- In any other areas into which steam might not be able to flow freely

If you have any doubt about the sterility of an instrument or piece of equipment, do not use it. Instead, put it aside for another cycle of sanitization, disinfection, and sterilization. The risks to patients and to you are too great to take chances.

***Temperature Guidelines.*** The length of the sterilization cycle is only one factor that has an impact on the final quality of autoclave operations. If the autoclave is manual, you must also be sure that the unit is operating at the correct temperature. Unit thermometers and sterilization indicators help confirm that correct temperatures have been reached.

Temperatures that are too high can cause problems as easily as those that are too low. If the temperature is too high inside the autoclave compartment, the steam does not have the correct level of moisture. The heat and moisture will not penetrate wrapped packs of instruments, and the result will be an unsterilized load.

If the temperature is too low, the steam contains too much moisture. Packs will be oversaturated, and the drying cycle will be insufficient. Wet packs can easily pick up contaminants from surfaces they touch after you unload them from the autoclave. Common causes of low temperature are failing to preheat the autoclave chamber, loading cold instruments into an overheated chamber, opening the unit door too wide during drying, and overfilling the water reservoir. Always make sure you are familiar with the manufacturer's recommendations before running a load through an autoclave.

***Overcrowding.*** Packs or instruments placed in too close proximity in the autoclave chamber may not be sterilized because of the inability of the steam to penetrate or reach all surfaces.

***Steam Level Guidelines.*** If the correct level of steam is not present during the autoclave cycle, items will not be sterile at the end of the cycle. It is vital that the unit force all air out of the chamber at the beginning of the sterilization cycle. It is also essential that you place items in the chamber in positions that will not cause formation of air pockets.

To help ensure proper operation of the unit, check all release valves and discharge lines to make sure they are free from obstruction. Clogged valves and lines may prevent elimination of all air from the chamber.

To prevent the formation of air pockets, load items in the autoclave so that the steam can circulate freely around all sides of the items. Place containers on their sides to avoid trapping air. Besides allowing the free flow of steam, careful positioning helps ensure that all items dry thoroughly before you remove them from the autoclave.

## Sterile Technique

Sterile technique requires strict adherence to a set order of procedures. If there is any interruption in this order, you must start the procedures again from the beginning. An object or area is considered either sterile or not sterile. If there is any question, you must consider the object or area contaminated. To prevent interruptions in the technique, you must also ensure that when objects touch one another, clean goes against clean, unclean goes against unclean, and sterile goes against sterile.

**Surgical Scrub.** The surgical scrub is of primary importance in surgical asepsis. Surgical scrub procedures are similar to those for aseptic hand washing, but there are several distinctions. Differences include the following:

- A sterile scrub brush is used instead of a nailbrush.
- Both hands and forearms are washed.
- The hands are kept above the elbows to prevent water from running from the arms onto washed areas.
- Sterile towels are used instead of paper towels.
- Sterile gloves are put on immediately after the hands are dried.

## Surgical Asepsis During a Surgical Procedure

Chapter 28 describes assisting with minor surgery. Several points concerning surgical asepsis, however, are introduced here. Before performing a surgical procedure, the doctor may ask you to help prepare the skin. Your goal is to remove as many microorganisms as possible from around the area that is to undergo surgery so that you reduce the chances of these organisms entering the surgical opening. The skin and body openings, particularly the nose, mouth, and perineum,

cannot be considered sterile. Nevertheless, the principles of aseptic technique require that you try to keep the area as contamination-free as possible.

Asepsis also involves keeping instruments and supplies sterile for use during the surgical procedure. After the sterile field has been created, handle items as little as possible to minimize the chance of contamination. Cover items that are not being used immediately with a sterile towel. If you are not wearing sterile gloves during a procedure (as when you are the only medical assistant and you must hand the doctor items from outside the sterile field), you must use transfer forceps to handle a sterile instrument. Transfer forceps look like big scissors or tweezers. Although the handles are not sterile, the tips that touch the instruments are.

If you are wearing sterile gloves, you handle sterile items directly and carefully avoid touching anything that is not sterile. Throughout the procedure, you are responsible for maintaining the sterile field (in this case, the area of surgery).

After the procedure, you continue using aseptic technique in caring for the patient's surgical wound. Typically, you need to apply dressings and keep the wound clean in an aseptic manner to prevent infection. You will also instruct the patient in how to care for the wound.

After you instruct the patient and guide the person out of the room, immediately place any supplies and disposable instruments that were used during the surgery into the appropriate **biohazardous waste containers.** These are leakproof containers that are color-coded red or labeled with a special biohazard symbol to show that they contain **biohazardous materials** (biological agents that can spread disease to living things). These containers are used to store and dispose of contaminated supplies and equipment in a way that preserves aseptic techniques and complies with the law.

## Surgical Asepsis After Surgical Procedures

After disposing of biohazardous waste, you must sanitize, disinfect, and sterilize reusable surgical instruments. You must also disinfect all work surfaces that were exposed to contamination. For this process, you must use bleach or a germ-killing solution approved by the U.S. government's Environment Protection Agency (EPA). If protective coverings on surfaces or equipment were exposed to contamination during a procedure, they must be replaced.

## Waste Disposal

The sanitization, disinfection, and sterilization processes generate some waste products. If you are resterilizing equipment whose shelf life has expired, the old wrappings should be considered unsterile and should be handled appropriately. Follow correct disposal procedures for biohazardous waste when discarding any supplies or equipment during the sterilization process.

# OSHA Blood-Borne Pathogens Standard and Universal Precautions

You must know the laws that require basic practices of infection control in a medical office. You must also know how to apply these laws in your office. Federal regulations related to infection control and asepsis were developed by the Department of Labor's **Occupational Safety and Health Administration (OSHA)** and described in the OSHA Blood-Borne Pathogens Standard of 1991. These laws protect health-care workers from health hazards on the job, particularly from accidentally acquiring infections. They also help protect patients and any other people who may come into the medical office from health hazards.

## OSHA Blood-Borne Pathogens Standard

To ensure that biohazardous materials do not endanger people or the environment, laws set forth in the OSHA Blood-Borne Pathogens Standard of 1991 dictate how you must handle infectious or potentially infectious waste generated during medical or surgical procedures. According to these rules, any potentially infectious waste materials must be discarded or held for processing in biohazardous waste containers. These wastes include the following:

- Blood products
- Body fluids
- Human tissues
- **Vaccines** (special preparations administered to produce immunity)
- Table paper, linen, towels, and gauze with body fluids on them
- Used scalpels, needles, sutures with needles attached, and other sharp instruments (known as sharps)
- Used gloves, disposable instruments, cotton swabs, and disposable applicators

Many medical offices today use only disposable paper gowns, drapes, coverings, and towels. Some offices, however, use cloth linens, which must be laundered. Certain rules apply to the laundering of cloth linens that are soiled with potentially infectious materials.

Medical offices use outside, licensed waste management services approved by the EPA to dispose of medical waste. A waste management service can provide instructions for preparing items before they are taken away.

The disposition and handling of contaminated sharps are of special concern because these instruments can easily puncture the skin and expose you to extremely dangerous viruses. Used sharps must never be bent, broken, recapped, or otherwise tampered with. After use, place them in a rigid, leak-proof, puncture-resistant biohazardous waste container for sharps. Disposable and reusable sharps are kept in separate containers. Metal basins containing disinfectant are often used to store reusable sharps until they can be processed. The outside waste management company may supply containers for the disposable items, sterilize them on its premises, and discard them in the city trash dump or incinerate them. See the Caution: Handle With Care section for a discussion of the guidelines you must follow when disposing of biohazardous waste and potentially infectious laundry waste.

OSHA's laws for hazardous waste disposal, as well as other OSHA regulations about measures to prevent the spread of infection, provide a margin of safety, ensuring that medical facilities meet at least the minimal criteria for asepsis. These laws include requirements for training personnel, keeping records, housekeeping, wearing protective gear, and other measures.

Although federal laws exist, individual states have some discretion in applying them. You should become familiar with the laws in your state to ensure that you are helping your medical office comply. Any outside cleaning service used by the office should be made aware of these standards as well. Penalties for failing to comply with regulations can be severe (see Table 20-1).

## Universal Precautions

OSHA requires medical professionals to follow specific "universal blood and body fluid precautions" as set forth by the Department of Health and Human Services' Centers for Disease Control and Prevention (CDC). These Universal Precautions prevent health-care workers from exposing themselves and others to infections. Following Universal Precautions means assuming that all blood and body fluids are infected with blood-borne pathogens. Universal Precautions apply to:

- Blood and blood products
- Human tissue
- Semen and vaginal secretions
- Saliva from dental procedures
- Cerebrospinal, synovial, pleural, peritoneal, pericardial, and amniotic fluids, which bathe various internal structures in the body
- Other body fluids, if visibly contaminated with blood or of questionable origin in the body

Breast milk, although not on the list of fluids covered by Universal Precautions, is generally treated as such because it has been shown that mothers can pass along the human immunodeficiency virus (HIV) to their infants through breast milk.

Hospitals now use **Standard Precautions,** which are a combination of Universal Precautions and rules to reduce the risk of disease transmission by means of moist body substances (known as Body Substance Isolation [BSI] guidelines). Standard Precautions apply to:

- Blood
- All body fluids, secretions, and excretions except sweat
- Nonintact skin
- Mucous membranes

**TABLE 20-1  Infectious Waste Disposal: Penalties for Not Following Regulations, as Set Forth by OSHA**

| Type of Violation | Characteristics of Violation | Penalties for Violation |
|---|---|---|
| Other than serious violation | Direct relationship to job safety and health but would probably not result in death or serious physical harm | Fine of up to $7,000 (discretionary) |
| Serious violation | Substantial probability that death or serious physical harm could result; employer knew, or should have known, of the hazard | Fine of up to $7,000 (mandatory) |
| Willful violation | Violation committed intentionally and knowingly | Fine of up to $70,000 with a $5,000 minimum; if violation resulted in death of employee, additional fine and/or up to 6 months' imprisonment |
| Repeated violation | Substantially similar (but not the same) violation found upon reinspection; not applicable if initial citation is under contest | Fine of up to $70,000 |
| Failure to correct prior violation | Initial violation was not corrected | Fine of up to $7,000 for each day the violation continues past the date it was supposed to stop |

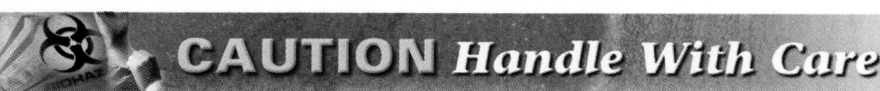

## CAUTION *Handle With Care*

## Proper Use of Biohazardous Waste Containers and Handling of Infectious Laundry Waste

Biohazardous waste containers are available in a variety of designs. Frequently, more than one design is used in the clinical setting. These containers are often provided by outside sterilization and waste management companies. Examples of biohazardous waste containers include:

- Bags or containers that are red or have a biohazardous waste label (for any material contaminated with blood or body fluids, such as used dressings or gloves)
- Boxes with biohazardous waste labels (sometimes lined with red bags and used for disposable gowns, examination table covers, and similar items that may be contaminated with blood or body fluids)
- Rigid, leakproof sharps containers that are red or have a biohazardous waste label (for lancets, needles, and other sharp objects)

Every biohazardous waste container has a lid that you must replace immediately after use. In addition, you may not overfill the container, and you must replace it when it is two-thirds full. All biohazardous waste containers must have a fluorescent orange or orange-red label with the biohazard symbol and the word *BIOHAZARD* in a contrasting color (Figure 20-12). Red bags or red containers may be substituted for containers with biohazardous waste labels.

You must follow these guidelines when handling hazardous waste.

- Always wear gloves.
- Place hazardous waste in the appropriate biohazardous waste container immediately or as soon as possible.
- Keep biohazardous waste containers close to the place where the waste material is generated.
- Keep the containers closed when not in use, close them before removing them from the area of use, and keep them upright to avoid any spills.
- If outside contamination of the primary container occurs, place that container in a secondary

*continued* ⟶

## Proper Use of Biohazardous Waste Containers and Handling of Infectious Laundry Waste *(concluded)*

container to prevent leakage during handling, processing, storage, and transport.

- Drop—do not push—intact contaminated needles into the biohazardous waste container for sharps.
- To avoid accidental puncture wounds, never break off, recap, reuse, or handle needles after use.
- If there is a danger of hazardous waste puncturing the primary container, place that container in a secondary container.
- Do not open, empty, or clean reusable sharps containers by hand.
- When they are two-thirds full, discard disposable sharps containers in large biohazardous waste containers.

When cleaning up spills, place the resulting contaminated material in a biohazardous waste bag. The bag must be leakproof on the sides and bottom and be closed tightly. Then place the plastic bag in a cardboard box also marked with the biohazard symbol. The outside waste management agency will pick up

the box for incineration before disposing of it in a public landfill.

Potentially infectious laundry waste must also be handled in a specific manner. OSHA has issued regulations for handling this type of waste. You must be sure to:

- Place contaminated laundry in a laundry bag that is red, marked with the biohazard symbol, or recognizable to facility employees as contaminated material to be handled using Universal Precautions (Figure 20-13).
- Pack any laundry to be transported so that it does not leak in transit.
- Have the laundry washed in a designated area on-site or at a professional laundry facility.

Any laundry service the medical office uses should abide by all OSHA regulations. For example, anyone handling laundry must wear gloves and handle contaminated materials as little as possible.

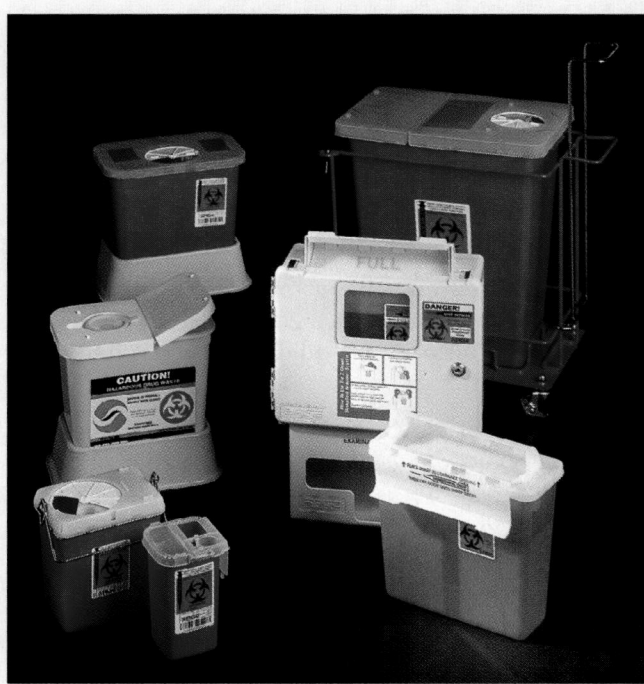

**Figure 20-12.** All biohazardous sharps containers must be rigid, leakproof, and labeled with the biohazard symbol.

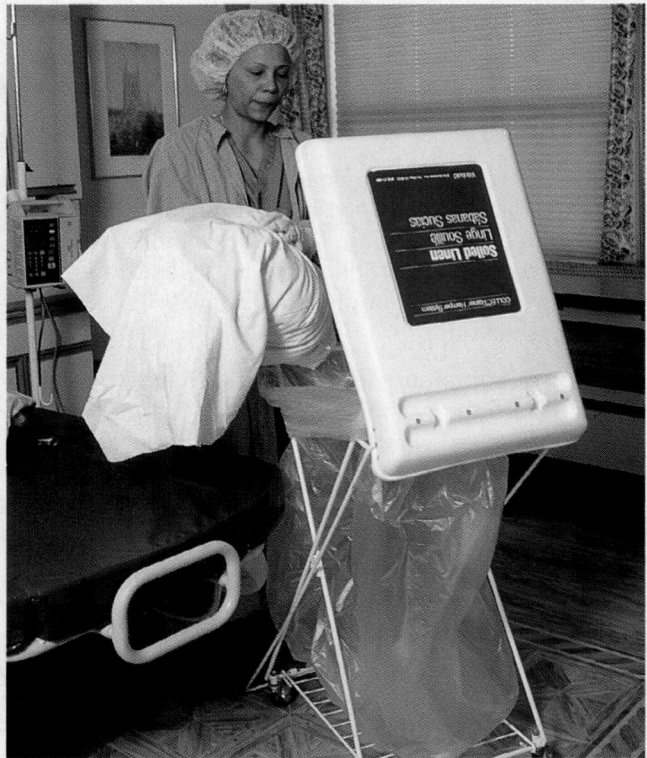

**Figure 20-13.** Place soiled linens and other laundry in an appropriate bag as soon as possible.

Standard Precautions are used in hospitals for the care of all patients. They are an important measure for preventing the transmission of disease in the hospital setting. In medical offices, Universal Precautions are used when dealing with patients. The application of Universal Precautions is expanding, in practice, to include all body fluids, secretions, excretions, and moist body surfaces.

As mentioned earlier, some types of pathogens can be transmitted when the host's infected blood comes in contact with another person's skin. Skin that has been broken from a needle puncture or other wound and mucous membranes, such as those lining the nose and throat, are the areas that need the most protection. If a patient's (or co-worker's) blood or body fluids come in contact with such areas, pathogens can be transferred from the patient's body to that of the medical worker.

OSHA outlines the routine safeguards to take when performing each medical procedure or task, depending on that task's level of risk. The degree of risk is determined by how much exposure to potentially infectious substances you are likely to encounter. When a procedure is explained, particular icons will be used to represent each of the OSHA guidelines. Figure 20-14 shows these icons.

OSHA divides tasks into the following three categories.

1. Category I tasks are those that expose a worker to blood, body fluids, or tissues or those that have a chance of spills or splashes. These tasks always require specific protective measures.

2. Category II tasks do not usually involve risk of exposure. Because they may involve exposure in certain situations, however, OSHA requires that precautions be taken.

3. Category III tasks do not require any special protection. These tasks, such as taking a patient's blood pressure, involve no exposure to blood, body fluids, or tissues. (Observe patients for open wounds before you touch them to perform such tasks.)

## Category I Tasks

A Category I task you might perform would be assisting with a minor surgical procedure in the office, such as the removal of a cyst. This procedure requires that you wash your hands before and after the procedure and that you wear protective gloves, a mask and protective eyewear or a face shield, and protective clothing. After the procedure, you must follow the guidelines for dealing with disposable and nondisposable sharp equipment and decontaminating work surfaces.

## Category II Tasks

A Category II task you might perform would be giving mouth-to-mouth resuscitation to a patient. Because blood is usually not visible in such situations, the task is not classified as Category I. Gloves are still recommended, however, although you may not have time to get them in an emergency. Because you will be exposed to saliva in such a procedure, OSHA recommends using disposable airway equipment and resuscitation bags (shown in Figure 20-15), which medical offices are required to supply.

OSHA recommends taking these precautions to decrease the risk of transmitting infectious diseases through mouth-to-mouth resuscitation. Of particular concern to health-care workers are HIV, which causes AIDS, and the hepatitis B virus (HBV).

AIDS damages the body's ability to fight disease, and is ultimately fatal in most instances. Hepatitis B is a highly contagious and potentially fatal disease that causes inflammation of the liver and sometimes liver failure. Health-care workers become infected with these viruses at work every year. Hepatitis B infection occurs far more frequently on the job than does HIV infection. (See Chapter 21 for detailed information on these and other blood-borne pathogens.)

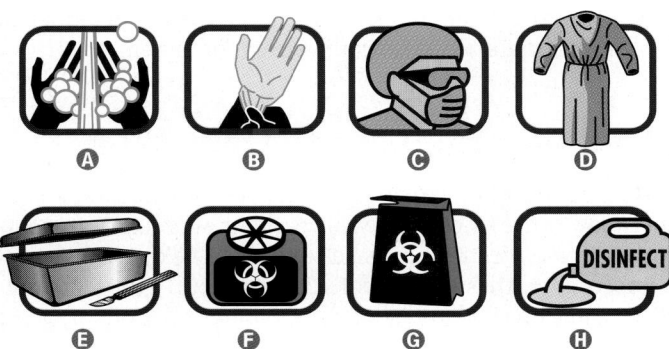

**Figure 20-14.** These icons will appear at the beginning of each Procedure to let you know which OSHA guidelines you should follow. They represent (A) hand washing, (B) gloves, (C) mask and protective eyewear or face shield, (D) laboratory coat or gown, (E) reusable sharps container, (F) sharps disposal, (G) biohazardous waste container, and (H) disinfection.

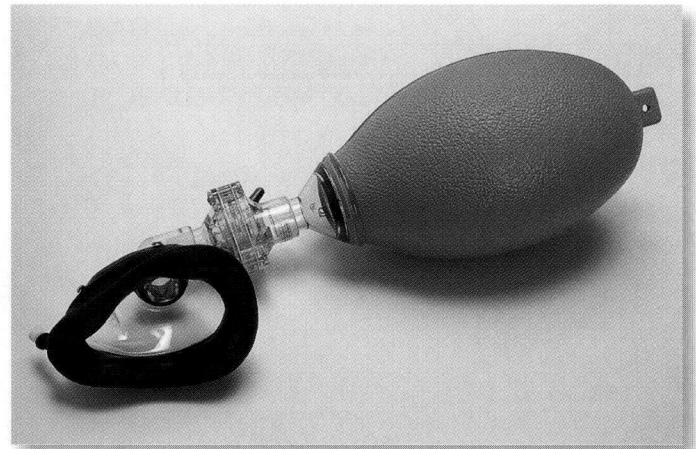

**Figure 20-15.** Resuscitation bags are sometimes used when a person requires mouth-to-mouth resuscitation. You must use one of these bags if blood is visible in the person's mouth or airway.

## Category III Tasks

A Category III procedure you may perform is giving a patient medicated nose drops. This task involves tilting the patient's head and holding the dropper above the patient's nostril. Although you must perform aseptic hand washing before and after the procedure, there are no other protective requirements. Some Category III tasks require no precautions. Examples of these tasks are instructing a patient in how to use a heating pad or how to take care of a cast for a broken leg.

## Personal Protective Equipment

Employers are required by law to supply **personal protective equipment (PPE)** at no charge to their employees. PPE is any type of protective gear worn to guard against physical hazards. Health-care workers require many kinds of personal protective equipment to do their jobs, including gloves, masks and protective eyewear or face shields, and protective clothing (Figure 20-16). During each procedure, keep in mind that the greater your chances of exposure to blood, the more protective equipment you need to wear.

**Gloves.** You must wear gloves for all procedures that involve exposure to blood, other body fluids, or broken skin. There are several kinds of gloves for different situations.

- Disposable gloves are worn once and then discarded. They cannot be used if they are torn, punctured, or otherwise damaged. Both examination and sterile gloves are disposable.
- Examination gloves are worn during procedures that do not require a sterile environment.
- Sterile gloves are used for sterile procedures such as minor surgery or urinary catheterization.
- Utility gloves (used when cleaning up) are stronger than disposable gloves and may be decontaminated

and reused if they show no signs of deterioration (including discoloration) after use.

**Masks and Protective Eyewear or Face Shields.** You must wear appropriate masks and protective eyewear or face shields for procedures in which your eyes, nose, and mouth may be exposed. These procedures are ones that have a potential for spraying or splashing blood, such as surgery or the collection or examination of blood.

**Protective Clothing.** If you are likely to have blood or body fluids sprayed or splashed on your clothing during a procedure, you must wear a protective laboratory coat, gown, or apron. You may also wear a hair covering and/or shoe coverings for such procedures. You should always have a change of work clothing available in the event that blood or body fluids penetrate your regular clothes around or through the protective clothing.

## OSHA Procedures for Postprocedure Cleanup

After a procedure, personnel in every medical office must follow specific steps to clean and decontaminate the environment. The cleanup steps that OSHA requires are as follows:

1. Decontaminate all exposed work surfaces with bleach or a germ-killing solution approved by the EPA.
2. Replace protective coverings on surfaces or equipment if they have been exposed.
3. Decontaminate receptacles, such as bins, pails, and cans, on a regular basis as part of routine housekeeping procedures.
4. Pick up any broken glass with tongs—never by hand—even when wearing gloves, because the sharp edges may cut the gloves and expose the skin to infecting organisms. Never use a vacuum to pick up broken glass.
5. Discard all potentially infectious waste materials in appropriate biohazardous waste containers.

## Applying the Law to Daily Work

In the course of daily work, you and other medical personnel may come in contact with patients who carry dangerous or fatal infectious disease. You are at risk for accidental exposure to these types of disease with every patient. Pathogens may be present in a patient's blood or other body fluids.

A patient or anyone who comes in contact with infectious waste generated by another patient or a health-care worker is at risk for infection. To minimize the risk of cross contamination, you need to become familiar with the OSHA regulations that describe the precautions medical office personnel must take in matters such as clothing, housekeeping, record keeping, and training.

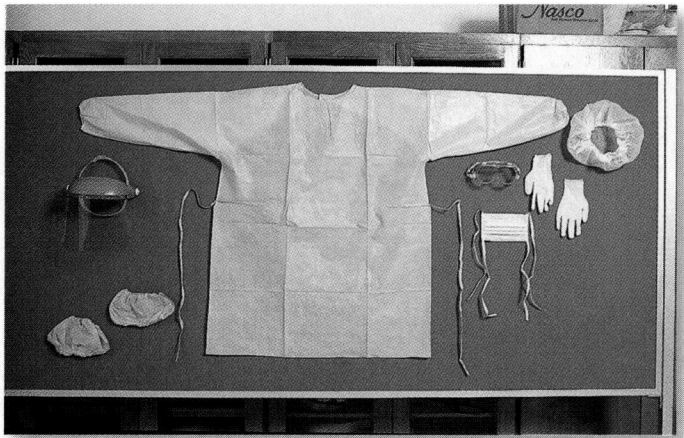

**Figure 20-16.** Health-care workers may need to use various types of personal protective equipment including gloves, masks and protective eyewear or face shields, gowns, and other protective clothing.

# Exposure Incidents

The OSHA Blood-Borne Pathogens Standard also specifies what to do in case of an exposure incident. An exposure incident is one in which a worker, despite all precautions, has reason to believe that he has come in contact with a substance that may transmit infection. Contact may occur when a medical worker accidentally sticks himself with a used needle. A puncture exposure incident is the most common kind of exposure.

The basic rules covering exposure incidents apply to all serious infections, such as HBV and HIV. The rules covering HBV also include vaccination.

When an exposure incident occurs, the physician or employer must be notified immediately. This prompt action is extremely important because quick and proper treatment can help prevent the development of many diseases, such as hepatitis B. Timely action can also prevent the worker from exposing other people to a potentially acquired infection. Reporting the incident helps to prevent the same type of accident from happening again.

After such an exposure, the employer must offer the exposed employee a free medical evaluation. The employer must refer the employee to a licensed health-care provider who can counsel the employee about what happened as well as about how to prevent the spread of any potential infection. The health-care provider also takes a blood sample and prescribes appropriate treatment. If the employee does not want to participate in the medical evaluation and treatment, he has the right to refuse it. If this occurs, the employee's refusal should be documented.

If an employee who has not received the HBV vaccination and is not known to be immune is exposed to any infected person, especially someone who is HBV-positive or at high risk, it is recommended that the employee be tested for HBV and receive the vaccination if necessary. This vaccination may prevent infection. When the source person's HBV status is unknown and the person does not wish to be tested, the employee should be tested. If the source person agrees to be tested, the law requires that the employee be informed of the test results. The employee may agree to give blood but not to be tested. In such a case, the blood sample must be kept for 90 days in case the employee later develops symptoms of HBV or HIV infection and decides to be tested then.

The health-care provider who performs the postexposure evaluation must give the employer a written report stating whether HBV vaccination was recommended and received and that the employee was informed of the results of any blood tests. Any additional information must be kept confidential.

# Other OSHA Requirements

OSHA also requires that all health-care workers who have occupational exposure to blood or other potentially infectious materials have the opportunity to receive the HBV vaccine, free of charge, as needed throughout employment. Within 10 days of a medical worker's starting a job, the doctor or employer is required to offer the worker the opportunity to receive this vaccination. The vaccine is recommended for all health-care workers *unless*:

- They have received it in the past.
- A blood test shows them to be immune to the virus.
- There are medical reasons for which the vaccine is contraindicated.

In most cases, the employee is permitted to decline the vaccination if he signs a form accepting all the conditions. (A few employers require HBV vaccination as a condition for employment.) Even if the health-care worker declines the vaccination when beginning employment, he still has the opportunity to receive the free vaccine and any necessary booster shots throughout his employment.

# Transmission from Health-Care Workers to Patients

There may be times when a health-care worker has a serious infection that could be transmitted to a patient. An infection acquired by a patient in a health-care facility is known as a **nosocomial infection.** OSHA has special recommendations for workers who perform procedures that could result in a patient's exposure to disease. Although the risk of a health-care worker's transmitting an infection to a patient is small if OSHA standards are followed, these additional precautions are advised for high-risk procedures. High-risk procedures include the following:

- Those that are thought to have caused the transmission of infection from a medical worker to a patient in the past
- Those that may carry a high risk of infection, such as oral, obstetric, and gynecologic procedures
- Those that involve needles, especially if a needle is in a body cavity or a body space that is difficult to see and the health-care worker's fingers are nearby (if the worker's skin was cut, the patient could be exposed to the worker's blood)

Workers who perform high-risk procedures should know their HIV and HBV status. HBV vaccination is strongly recommended. Also, workers who have skin conditions characterized by sores that secrete fluid should forgo direct patient care and the handling of equipment used for exposure-prone procedures until their condition has healed.

A member of the medical staff who is infected with HIV or HBV should not perform procedures that might result in exposure for the patient without the advice of an expert review panel. This panel could include the health-care worker's own physician, someone with expert knowledge about the transmission of infectious disease, a medical professional with expert knowledge about the procedures in question, public health officials, and a member of the infection-control committee of the institution, if applicable.

The panel advises the worker on whether procedures may be performed. The advice includes requiring the worker to inform potential patients of the infection before the procedure. The panel must otherwise protect the health-care worker's confidentiality.

Although great controversy has surrounded the subject of required testing of all health-care workers for HIV or HBV, no recommendations are in place for such testing. The risk of infection transmission from worker to patient is not considered great enough to justify the extensive resources that mandatory testing would require.

# Reporting Guidelines

The CDC requires reporting of certain diseases to the state or county department of health. This information, which is forwarded to the CDC, helps research epidemiologists control the spread of infection. Table 20-2 lists diseases that must be reported to the National Notifiable Disease Surveillance System of the CDC, through your state or county health department.

---

## TABLE 20-2  The Notifiable Disease Surveillance System

Acquired Immunodeficiency Syndrome (AIDS)

Anthrax

Arboviral neuroinvasive and non-neuroinvasive diseases

Botulism, foodborne

Botulism, infant

Botulism, other (wound and unspecified)

Brucellosis

Chancroid

*Chlamydia trachomatis,* genital infections

Cholera

Coccidiodomycosis

Cryptosporidiosis

Cyclosporiasis

Diphtheria

Ehrlichiosis, human granulocytic

Ehrlichiosis, human monocytic

Ehrlichiosis, human unspecified

Giardiasis

Gonorrhea

*Haemophilus influenzae,* invasive disease

Hansen disease (leprosy)

Hantavirus pulmonary syndrome

Hemolytic uremic syndrome, post-diarrhea

Hepatitis A

Hepatitis B

Hepatitis C

HIV infection

Influenza-associated pediatric mortality

Legionellosis

Lyme disease

Malaria

Measles

Meningococcal disease

Mumps

Pertussis

Plague

Poliomyelitis, paralytic

Psittacosis

Q fever

Rabies, animal

Rabies, human

Rocky Mountain spotted fever

Rubella

Rubella, congenital syndrome

Salmonellosis

Severe Acute Respiratory Syndrome-associated Coronavirus (SARS-CoV) disease

Shiga toxin-producing *Escherichia coli* (STEC)

Shigellosis

Smallpox

Streptococcal disease, invasive, Group A

Streptococcal toxic-shock syndrome

*Streptococcus pneumoniae,* drug resistant, invasive

*Streptococcus pneumoniae,* invasive in children < 5 years

Syphilis, all stages

Syphilis, congenital

Syphilitic stillbirth

Tetanus

Toxic-shock syndrome (other than Streptococcal)

Trichinellosis (Trichinosis)

Tuberculosis

Tularemia

Typhoid fever

Vancomycin-intermediate *Staphylococcus aureus* (VISA)

Vancomycin-resistant *Staphylococcus aureus* (VRSA)

Varicella (deaths only)

Varicella (morbidity)

Yellow fever

# Guideline for Isolation Precautions in Hospitals

In early 1996 the CDC issued the current Guideline for Isolation Precautions in Hospitals. If you work in a hospital, it is essential to understand and apply these precautions. You must always ensure that you create an environment that protects people from disease-causing microorganisms. The guideline includes the types of precautions needed and patients requiring these precautions. In addition to applying Standard Precautions, there are some infections that require the use of additional PPE. See Table 20-3 for a summary of selecting the appropriate PPE.

# Immunizations: Another Way to Control Infection

One of the necessary elements in the cycle of infection is the transmission of the pathogen to a susceptible host. You have already learned how to reduce the risk of infection by altering environmental conditions so that microorganisms find it difficult or impossible to survive. In addition, the risk of infection can be decreased by reducing the susceptibility of the host to infection. This reduction can be accomplished through **immunization,** which is the administration of a vaccine or a toxoid (a weakened toxin) to protect susceptible individuals from infectious diseases.

| TABLE 20-3 | Selecting Appropriate Personal Protective Equipment (PPE) | |
|---|---|---|
| **Infection** | **Precaution Type** | **Appropriate PPE** |
| Abscess | Contact | Gloves and gown |
| AIDS | Standard | Use appropriate PPE when exposed to blood or body fluids |
| Anthrax | Standard | Use appropriate PPE when exposed to blood or body fluids |
| Chickenpox | Airborne/Contact | Mask and goggles, or respirator and gloves |
| Diphtheria<br>• Cutaneous<br>• Pharyngeal | <br>Contact<br>Droplet | <br>Gloves and gown<br>Mask and goggles when working within 3 feet of patient |
| Gastroenteritis | Standard/Contact | Use appropriate PPE when exposed to blood or body fluids; avoid contact with fecal material by donning gloves and gown |
| Rotavirus | Contact | Gloves and gown |
| Hepatitis<br>• A<br>• B<br>• C<br>• E | <br>Contact<br>Standard<br>Standard<br>Standard | <br>Gloves and gown<br>Use appropriate PPE when exposed to blood or body fluids<br>Use appropriate PPE when exposed to blood or body fluids<br>Use appropriate PPE when exposed to blood or body fluids |
| Influenza | Droplet | Mask and goggles when working within 3 feet of patient |
| Measles | Airborne | Mask and goggles or respirator |
| Meningitis | Standard/Droplet | Use appropriate PPE when exposed to blood or body fluids; use mask and goggles when working within 3 feet of patient |
| Mumps | Droplet | Mask and goggles when working within 3 feet of patient |
| Pertussis | Droplet | Mask and goggles when working within 3 feet of patient |
| Poliomyelitis | Standard | Use appropriate PPE when exposed to blood or body fluids |
| Rubella | Droplet | Mask and goggles when working within 3 feet of patient |
| Scabies | Contact | Gloves and gown |
| Staphylococcal disease | Contact | Gloves and gown |
| Streptococcal disease | Contact/Droplet | Gloves, gown, mask, and goggles |
| Tuberculosis | Airborne | Mask and goggles or respirator |

When a healthy patient is vaccinated with a weakened strain of a virus, the patient's lymphocytes manufacture antibodies against that virus. These antibodies remain in the body, making it immune to that virus in the future. Live-virus vaccines are used to immunize against measles and poliomyelitis. Immunization with a related virus can also be effective against some diseases. For example, immunization with cowpox virus has completely eradicated the incidence of smallpox, a contagious disease that leaves permanent scars on the skin.

Killed-virus vaccines, which are used to immunize against influenza and typhoid fever, do not provide protection for as long a period as that provided by live-virus vaccines. Toxoids are used to produce active immunity against diseases such as tetanus and diphtheria.

## Immunization Recommendations

The Advisory Committee on Immunization Practices, the American Academy of Pediatrics, and the American Academy of Family Physicians jointly publish immunization schedules for children. The National Coalition for Adult Immunization (NCAI) publishes similar schedules for adults. You should be familiar with the current guidelines regarding these vaccination schedules. The pediatric schedule is shown in Figure 20-17. The adult schedule is shown in Figure 20-18.

**A**

### Recommended Immunization Schedule for Persons Aged 0–6 Years—United States, 2007

| Vaccine \ Age | Birth | 1 month | 2 months | 4 months | 6 months | 12 months | 15 months | 18 months | 19–23 months | 2–3 years | 4–6 years |
|---|---|---|---|---|---|---|---|---|---|---|---|
| Hepatitis B | HepB | HepB | | | | HepB | | | | HepB series | |
| Rotavirus | | | Rota | Rota | Rota | | | | | | |
| Diphtheria, tetanus, pertussis | | | DTaP | DTaP | DTaP | | DTaP | | | | DTaP |
| *Haemophilus influenzae* type b | | | Hib | Hib | Hib | Hib | | Hib | | | |
| Pneumococcal | | | PCV | PCV | PCV | PCV | | | | PCV PPV | |
| Inactivated poliovirus | | | IPV | IPV | | IPV | | | | | IPV |
| Influenza | | | | | | Influenza (yearly) | | | | | |
| Measles, mumps, rubella | | | | | | MMR | | | | | MMR |
| Varicella | | | | | | Varicella | | | | | Varicella |
| Hepatitis A | | | | | | HepA (2 doses) | | | | HepA series | |
| Meningococcal | | | | | | | | | | MPSV4 | |

| | Range of recommended ages | | Catch-up immunization | | Certain high-risk groups |
|---|---|---|---|---|---|

**B**

### Recommended Immunization Schedule for Persons Aged 7–18 Years—United States, 2007

| Vaccine \ Age | 7–10 years | 11–12 years | 13–14 years | 15 years | 16–18 years |
|---|---|---|---|---|---|
| Tetanus, diphtheria, pertussis | | Tdap | | Tdap | |
| Human papillomavirus | | HPV (3 doses) | | HPV series | |
| Meningococcal | MPSV4 | MCV4 | | MCV4 MCV4 | |
| Pneumococcal | | PPV | | | |
| Influenza | | Influenza (yearly) | | | |
| Hepatitis A | | HepA series | | | |
| Hepatitis B | | HepB series | | | |
| Inactivated poliovirus | | IPV series | | | |
| Measles, mumps, rubella | | MMR series | | | |
| Varicella | | Varicella series | | | |

**Figure 20-17.** This schedule shows recommended ages for various childhood immunizations.

# Recommended Adult Immunization Schedule—United States, October 2006–September 2007

Recommended adult immunization schedule, by vaccine and age group.

| Vaccine \ Age group | 19–49 years | 50–64 years | ≥65 years |
|---|---|---|---|
| Tetanus, diphtheria, pertussis (Td/Tdap) | 1-dose Td booster every 10 yrs | | |
| | Substitute 1 dose of Tdap for Td | | |
| Human papillomavirus (HPV) | 3 doses (females) | | |
| Measles, mumps, rubella (MMR) | 1 or 2 doses | 1 dose | |
| Varicella | 2 doses (0, 4–8 wks) | 2 doses (0, 4–8 wks) | |
| Influenza | 1 dose annually | 1 dose annually | |
| Pneumococcal (polysaccharide) | 1–2 doses | | 1 dose |
| Hepatitis A | 2 doses (0, 6–12 mos, or 0, 6–18 mos) | | |
| Hepatitis B | 3 doses (0, 1–2, 4–6 mos) | | |
| Meningococcal | 1 or more doses | | |

Recommended adult immunization schedule, by vaccine and medical and other indications.

| Vaccine \ Indication | Pregnancy | Congenital immunodeficiency; leukemia; lymphoma; generalized malignancy; cerebrospinal fluid leaks; therapy with alkylating agents, antimetabolites, radiation, or high-dose, long-term corticosteroids | Diabetes, heart disease, chronic pulmonary disease, chronic alcoholism | Asplenia (including elective splenectomy and terminal complement component deficiencies) | Chronic liver disease, recipients of clotting factor concentrates | Kidney failure, end-stage renal disease, recipients of hemodialysis | Human immunodeficiency virus (HIV) infection | Health-care workers |
|---|---|---|---|---|---|---|---|---|
| Tetanus, diphtheria, pertussis (Td/Tdap) | 1-dose Td booster every 10 yrs | | | | | | | |
| | | Substitute 1 dose of Tdap for Td | | | | | | |
| Human papillomavirus (HPV) | | 3 doses for women through age 26 years (0, 2, 6 mos) | | | | | | |
| Measles, mumps, rubella (MMR) | Contraindicated | 1 or 2 doses | | | | | | |
| Varicella | Contraindicated | 2 doses (0, 4–8 wks) | | | | | 2 doses | |
| Influenza | 1 dose annually | | 1 dose annually | 1 dose annually | | | | |
| Pneumococcal (polysaccharide) | 1–2 doses | 1–2 doses | | | | | | 1–2 doses |
| Hepatitis A | 2 doses (0, 6–12 mos, or 0, 6–18 mos) | | | 2 doses (0, 6–12 mos, or 0, 6–18 mos) | | | | |
| Hepatitis B | 3 doses (0, 1–2, 4–6 mos) | | | 3 doses (0, 1–2, 4–6 mos) | | | | |
| Meningococcal | 1 dose | | 1 dose | 1 dose | | | | |

Legend:
- For all persons in this category who meet the age requirements and who lack evidence of immunity (e.g., lack documentation of vaccination or have no evidence of prior infection)
- Recommended if some other risk factor is present (e.g., on the basis of medical, occupational, lifestyle, or other indications)
- Contraindicated

**Figure 20-18.** Adult immunizations are recommended for adults who did not receive vaccines as children and for older adults with chronic illnesses.

Many patients think of immunization requirements as existing only for children; however, there are also immunizations every adult should have. According to the NCAI, more than half of Americans older than age 50 are not properly immunized against two potent diseases: tetanus and diphtheria.

## Administering Immunizations

In many states, medical assistants may administer immunizations. Most immunizations are given as injections. (Chapter 38 describes the administration of various types of injections.) Some vaccines, such as live polio, are given orally.

Whether or not you administer vaccines, you must explain the need for immunization to patients as well as describe what side-effects, if any, they may experience. Common side effects of immunizations include soreness near the injection site, low-grade fever, and general malaise.

## Special Immunization Concerns

Patients who are young, pregnant, or elderly, as well as those who have a weakened immune system, may have special needs related to immunizations. Health-care workers have special immunization needs too.

**Pediatric Patients.**  Encourage parents to bring their children to the office at the recommended times for all immunizations. If a child has a fever, however, postpone the immunization until the fever has subsided. Do not postpone the visit if the child has an upper respiratory infection *without* a fever. Remember that the child does not need to restart a series of immunizations. He can simply receive the next scheduled immunization as soon as possible.

**Informed Consent.**  As with any drug, the physician may ask you to explain the benefits and risks of immunization. For a pediatric patient, provide this information to the parents. Explain that the side effects of immunizations are usually mild, such as a slight fever or soreness, and of short duration. Advise parents that the benefits of immunity greatly outweigh the risks. Then obtain informed consent for the child's immunization. Remember that religious beliefs may prohibit parents from consenting to immunizations for their child. Record this information in the patient's chart.

**Contraindications.**  Before administering a childhood immunization, check for any **contraindications** to its use. A contraindication is a symptom that renders use of a remedy or procedure inadvisable, usually because of risk. For example, pertussis vaccine must not be given to a child with a progressive neurological disorder. It also must not be administered to a child who developed seizures, persistent crying, or a fever of 104°F or higher after receiving a previous pertussis vaccine. In such a situation, the doctor would direct you to administer diphtheria and tetanus toxoids instead of diphtheria and tetanus toxoid and pertussis vaccine (DTP).

**Immunization Records.**  Under the National Childhood Vaccine Injury Act of 1988, you must record certain information about immunizations in a child's permanent medical record. Required information includes:

- The vaccine's type, manufacturer, and lot number
- The date of administration
- The name, address, and title of the health-care professional who administered the vaccine

You must also document:

- The administration site and route
- The vaccine's expiration date

Parents should maintain an accurate, up-to-date immunization record for each child. Each state issues an immunization record form, which may be available in languages other than English, depending on the state. You can obtain copies from your state's department of health. Complete a form after each child's first immunization. Instruct the parents to keep the form and bring it with the child for each subsequent immunization so that you can update the record.

Advise parents that this record is important to keep because it acts as proof of immunization, required by day-care centers, schools, the military, and other organizations. This record may also be helpful when parents consult another doctor, in case of emergency, or when moving to a new location.

**Pregnant Patients.**  Because pregnancy may increase a woman's susceptibility to diseases and because some maternal diseases can endanger the fetus, certain immunizations may be recommended during pregnancy. Other immunizations, such as that for rubella, however, should not be administered to pregnant women because they can cause fetal defects. In general, vaccines that are based on a live virus should not be given to pregnant patients.

Before administering any immunization or other drug to a pregnant patient, determine the fetal risks associated with it. One method is to find out the drug's pregnancy risk category. The FDA has established five categories to indicate the results of clinical tests performed on animals and humans:

- Category A indicates that there is no known risk to the fetus.
- Categories B, C, and D indicate some potential risk, which may be outweighed by the benefits of the drug.
- Category X indicates an unacceptable degree of risk to the fetus.

For a more detailed discussion of pregnancy risk categories, see Table 38-7 in Chapter 38. Each drug's package insert should indicate its pregnancy risk category and specific contraindications or precautions for taking the drug during pregnancy.

**Elderly Patients.**  Influenza and influenza-related pneumonia represent a serious health risk for patients older than age 65. Although elderly patients can be immunized against influenza each year and influenza-related pneumonia one time, they may have common misconceptions about vaccinations. They may worry about the expense, getting the disease from the vaccine, or the need for a vaccination when they do not feel ill.

Explain to patients who are concerned about the cost of vaccinations that if they are not enrolled in one of the many insurance plans that covers immunization, Medicare Part B covers the cost. For those worried about the potential side effects of immunization, describe the mild symptoms they may encounter, and emphasize that the symptoms are short-lived. You might also mention that compared to the potential dangers of contracting a serious infection, the symptoms are quite mild.

Because older patients are much more likely than younger patients to develop side effects as a result of immunizations, instruct older patients so that they recognize and immediately report any adverse effects. That way, the physician can treat elderly patients before their illness becomes severe.

**Immunocompromised Patients.** Patients who have an impaired or weakened immune system (are immunocompromised) include those with acquired immunodeficiency syndrome (AIDS) or other immune disorders and those undergoing chemotherapy. Infants may also be considered immunocompromised if they have mothers who are infected with HIV or have AIDS or an unknown immune status.

All immunizations affect the immune system. A patient with a compromised immune system can experience minimal to dangerous effects, depending on the vaccine. Before administration of any immunization, the physician should check the patient's medical history. If the patient is immunocompromised, the dosage may need to be adjusted or administration postponed.

Immunization for immunocompromised patients depends on exactly what disease is present. For example,

# Educating the Patient

## Disease Prevention

As a medical assistant, you can be influential in educating patients about ways to protect themselves from disease. Whenever you have the opportunity for patient education, you should stress the basic principles of hygiene and disease prevention.

- Wash hands frequently, especially before eating and after using the toilet, touching dirty objects, coming into contact with bodily fluids (including one's own), and touching doorknobs, railings, and handles
- Take a daily shower or bath, maintain daily dental care, and use clean clothes and bedding
- Thoroughly wash dirty drinking glasses, dishes, and utensils, especially when someone in the household is ill
- Use tissues when coughing or sneezing, and discard them properly after one use
- Maintain adequate light and ventilation in the home
- Routinely use a commercial disinfectant to clean rooms in the home, especially the bathroom and kitchen
- Use condoms if you have sexual intercourse with more than one partner or with people whose HIV or HBV status is unknown
- Adhere to immunization schedules
- Eat nutritious foods and keep physically fit

- Avoid stress
- Protect against exposure to potentially harmful insects or animals

To provide patients with the knowledge they need, you should educate them in the following subjects:

- Nutrition and diet
- Exercise and weight control
- Prevention of sexually transmitted diseases
- Smoking cessation
- Alcohol and drug abuse prevention and treatment
- Proper use of medications and prescribed treatments for an infection already acquired
- Stress-reduction techniques

The goal of patient education is to help patients take care of themselves. In fact, many patients expect this kind of education along with their treatment. Thus, you should encourage patients to play an active part in their own health care. A variety of patient education tools are available to help with this task. Charts, diagrams, brochures, videotapes, audiotapes, and anatomical models can be excellent teaching resources. You may find it helpful to develop or design some resources that deal with issues that are important to the patients you work with routinely.

inactive poliomyelitis vaccinations should be given to patients with altered immune systems, whereas the oral form that is based on the live virus can be given to patients with healthy immune systems. Also consider the immunization status of the patients' families and caregivers. All family members and caregivers of patients with AIDS should receive only inactive poliomyelitis vaccinations and should receive annual flu vaccinations.

**Health-Care Workers.** Health-care workers are at risk of contracting infectious diseases and should pay careful attention to their own immunization status. OSHA regulations require employers to offer medical workers vaccination against hepatitis B at no cost to employees. The CDC recommends that health-care workers receive three doses of hepatitis B vaccine. The first dose should be given at the start of employment, the second dose 1 to 2 months after the first, and the third 4 to 6 months after the second. Not all individuals who are vaccinated against hepatitis B acquire immunity. Your medical facility may require a hepatitis B titer after the three-dose hepatitis vaccine. You should check with your physician regarding your immune status. Health-care workers may choose to decline this service under certain circumstances, but if they do, a waiver must be signed and maintained in the personnel file. If the employee chooses to take the vaccine at a later date, it must be offered at no charge.

# Educating Patients About Preventing Disease Transmission

Educating patients about health promotion and disease prevention is an important part of your job. Patients with adequate knowledge can work to keep their defenses functioning properly. They can also avoid exposing themselves to infections and transmitting infections when they are ill.

In addition, they are more likely to have a successful recovery from illness.

In addition to educating patients about disease prevention, you will also need to educate them about disease treatment. Some patients do not follow their doctor's instructions, and they may prolong their illness or experience a relapse as a result. You will need to stress to patients the important role they play in their own treatment.

Your extensive interaction with patients and your key role in managing the office provide you with many opportunities for patient education. You will share the responsibility for educating patients with the doctor and other health-care personnel. On average, doctors spend 25% of their total office time providing information to, instructing, and counseling patients. Your role is to reinforce and explain the doctor's instructions. If you encounter patient concerns, questions, or problems that you are not equipped to deal with, refer them to the doctor.

# Summary

As a medical assistant you will be responsible for taking measures to prevent disease transmission in the medical office. You will accomplish this by applying principles of medical and surgical asepsis and by adhering to OSHA Blood-Borne Pathogens Standards. You will also follow CDC requirements for reporting cases of infectious disease, isolate patients when necessary, and choose appropriate PPE. You can play a vital role in reducing patient vulnerability by encouraging patients to maintain a correct immunization status and by remaining aware of special immunization concerns for certain patients.

## CASE STUDY *QUESTIONS*

Now that you have completed this chapter, review the case study at the beginning of the chapter and answer the following questions:

1. How might the patients have been infected?
2. What steps should the medical assistant have taken to prevent these infections?
3. How does the Blood-Borne Pathogens Standard apply to the medical assistant?
4. If the medical assistant did not observe the regulation, what penalties, if any, could be imposed by OSHA?

## Discussion Questions

1. A coworker responsible for autoclaving instruments is in a hurry to leave for the day; at the end of the autoclave sterilization cycle, the coworker does not allow time for the drying process. What significance, if any, does omitting the drying step have?
2. You are preparing to disinfect a tray of assorted equipment. At the bottom of the tray, you discover several pieces of gauze stained with what appears to be dried blood. What should you do with the instruments? What should you do with the gauze?
3. Identify several illnesses that must be reported to the state or county department of health. What might occur if you were to neglect reporting such illnesses?

## Critical Thinking Questions

1. You are taking the general history of a 13-year-old female patient. You discover that she never had a second measles-mumps-rubella (MMR) vaccination. What special considerations, if any, should be taken into account before administering the vaccination?
2. While unloading the autoclave you discover that some of the sterilization indicators in the center of the load are not activated (no color change has occurred). What actions should you take?
3. You notice that a coworker is not washing her hands between patients or before eating lunch. What steps should you take? How would you explain the importance of handwashing to your coworker?

## Application Activities

1. Prepare a receptacle of sanitized and disinfected instruments and equipment for steam autoclaving. Demonstrate the correct method for handling instruments with hinges or ratchets.
2. Load an autoclave with wrapped instrument packs and other equipment. Demonstrate the correct placement of open glass containers, plastic items, instrument packs, and a tray of loose instruments.
3. Work with another student to role-play a situation in which you explain the recommended immunizations for the following people: a 4-month-old baby, a 5-year-old boy who has never received any immunizations, a 15-year-old boy who has never had chickenpox, and an adult female who was born in 1958 and was never immunized for measles, mumps, and rubella.

## Virtual Fieldtrip

*Visit the McGraw-Hill Higher Education Medical Assisting website at www.mhhe.com/medicalassisting3 to complete the following activity:*

You have been asked to create an education program teaching patients about hand washing. After a brief discussion with your coworkers, you decide to start your search at the CDC website. Begin by searching the following topics:

- Hand hygiene
- Health promotion
- Clean hands save lives

Keep a journal of your trip. Include the following information:

- Trail Map (describe where your search led you)—This should include the URL of each link you found useful and a short synopsis of the information found at each link.
- Plan for how you will use this information in a patient education plan.

Open the CD and complete this chapter's practice activities, play the games, listen to the key terms, and test yourself with the interactive review. E-mail, print, and/or save your results to document your proficiency.

## CHAPTER 21

# HIV, Hepatitis, and Other Blood-Borne Pathogens

## KEY TERMS

- acquired immunodeficiency syndrome (AIDS)
- anergic reaction
- blood-borne pathogen
- chancre
- clinical drug trial
- enzyme-linked immunosorbent assay (ELISA) test
- hairy leukoplakia
- helper T cell
- human immunodeficiency virus (HIV)
- immunocompromised
- immunofluorescent antibody (IFA) test
- jaundice
- Kaposi's sarcoma
- mucocutaneous exposure
- percutaneous exposure
- terminal
- Western blot test

## MEDICAL ASSISTING COMPETENCIES

*In preparation for the certification examination, you should know the following areas of competence:*

| COMPETENCY | CMA | RMA |
|---|---|---|
| **Clinical** | | |
| Apply principles of aseptic techniques and infection control, including hand washing | X | X |
| Dispose of biohazardous materials | X | X |
| Practice Standard Precautions | X | X |
| Interview the patient to obtain and record the patient's history | X | X |
| Screen and follow up on patient test results | X | X |
| **General/Legal/Professional** | | |
| Identify and respond to issues of confidentiality by maintaining confidentiality at all times and following appropriate guidelines when releasing records or information | X | X |
| Be aware of and perform within legal and ethical boundaries | X | X |
| Determine the needs for documentation and reporting, and document accurately and appropriately | X | X |
| Provide patients with methods of health promotion and disease prevention | X | X |
| Identify community resources and information for patients and employers | X | X |
| Be impartial and show empathy when dealing with patients | | X |
| Use appropriate medical terminology | | X |

## CHAPTER OUTLINE

- Transmission of Blood-Borne Pathogens
- Universal Precautions
- Disease Profiles
- AIDS Patients
- Other Blood-Borne Infections
- Reporting Guidelines
- Patient Education
- Special Issues With Terminal Illness

# LEARNING OUTCOMES

After completing Chapter 21, you will be able to:

**21.1** Describe ways in which blood-borne pathogens can be transmitted.

**21.2** Explain why strict adherence to Universal Precautions is essential in preventing the spread of infection.

**21.3** Describe the symptoms of hepatitis and acquired immune deficiency syndrome (AIDS).

**21.4** List and describe the blood tests used to diagnose human immunodeficiency virus (HIV) infection.

**21.5** Identify chronic disorders often found in patients who have AIDS.

**21.6** Compare and contrast drugs used to treat AIDS/HIV infection.

**21.7** Describe the symptoms of infection by other common blood-borne pathogens.

**21.8** Describe the steps involved in reporting a communicable disease.

**21.9** Explain how to educate patients about minimizing the risks of transmitting blood-borne infections to others.

**21.10** Describe special issues you may encounter when dealing with patients who have terminal illnesses.

## Introduction

This chapter expands on the OSHA Blood-Borne Pathogen Standard and explains how you should reduce your risk of exposure to blood-borne pathogens. You will learn about **human immunodeficiency virus (HIV),** hepatitis, and other blood-borne infections; about reporting guidelines; and about educating patients on minimizing the risk of transmission. You will also be introduced to issues associated with terminal illnesses such as **acquired immune deficiency syndrome (AIDS).**

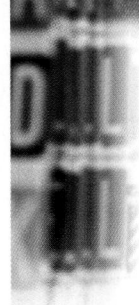

## CASE STUDY

An anxious 34-year-old nurse currently employed at the local hospital comes into the office with complaints of fatigue, stomach pain, and vomiting. While talking with the patient, you notice a yellowish color to her skin and eyes. The patient confides in you that the required vaccination for her job description was never administered. She also tells you that she had a needlestick injury a few weeks ago that she did not report. The physician diagnoses the patient with hepatitis.

As you read this chapter, consider the following questions:

1. What type of hepatitis does this patient probably have?
2. What are two medical terms for the yellowish discoloration you observed?
3. How long might the patient expect to suffer from the symptoms of the acute phase of the illness?
4. Could this disease have been prevented? If so, how?

## Transmission of Blood-Borne Pathogens

As discussed in Chapter 19, infectious diseases are spread through a cycle that involves transmission of pathogens from host to host. When you use medical and surgical asepsis and various techniques and procedures to sanitize, disinfect, and sterilize instruments, equipment, and surfaces, you help prevent the transmission of all types of pathogens. You also need to know about specific types of pathogens—how they are transmitted and what measures you can take to prevent their transmission. **Blood-borne pathogens** are disease-causing microorganisms carried in the host's blood. They are transmitted from one host to another through contact with infected blood, tissue, body fluids, or mucous membranes.

The Centers for Disease Control and Prevention (CDC) has identified specific substances that can serve as transmission agents for blood-borne diseases. (Although breast milk is not included, it has been implicated in the transmission of HIV. Breast-feeding is contraindicated for women who have HIV infection.) The following substances can serve as transmission agents:

- Blood
- Blood products (such as plasma)

- Human tissue
- Semen
- Vaginal secretions
- Saliva from dental procedures
- Cerebrospinal fluid (from around the brain and spinal cord)
- Synovial fluid (from joints and around tendons)
- Pleural fluid (from around the lungs)
- Peritoneal fluid (from the abdominal cavity)
- Pericardial fluid (from around the heart)
- Amniotic fluid (from the sac containing a fetus)

Some substances are not considered a viable means for transmitting blood-borne disease, even though they may transmit other types of disease. If any of these substances contain visible traces of blood, however, their status shifts because they may then serve as transmission agents for blood-borne diseases. The substances are as follows:

- Feces
- Nasal secretions
- Perspiration
- Sputum
- Tears
- Urine
- Vomitus
- Saliva

The growth cycle of pathogenic microorganisms requires a means of exit from the host. In the case of a blood-borne disease, the means of exit can be any of the substances identified as transmission agents or potential transmission agents. The cycle also requires a means of entrance into a new host. Blood-borne pathogens can be introduced into a new host through several routes, including:

- Needlesticks from needles used on an infected patient
- Cuts or abrasions on the skin of the uninfected person
- Any body opening of an uninfected person
- A transfusion with infected blood

## People at Increased Risk

People who are at increased risk for developing an infectious disease caused by blood-borne pathogens are those who come in contact with substances that may harbor the pathogens. Besides heath-care professionals, people in certain other careers are at increased risk for exposure to blood-borne pathogens, including members of these groups:

- Law enforcement officers
- Mortuary or morgue attendants
- Firefighters
- Medical equipment service technicians
- Barbers
- Cosmetologists

Of all the blood-borne microorganisms, the pathogens posing the greatest risk are two variants of the hepatitis virus (hepatitis B virus [HBV] and hepatitis C virus [HCV]) and HIV, which can lead to AIDS. The CDC records information about the occurrence of many blood-borne diseases, including AIDS/HIV infection and hepatitis. Table 21-1 shows reported cases of AIDS/HIV infection in heath-care workers to whom the virus was or may have been transmitted during the performance of their jobs.

## Researching the Spread of Infectious Diseases

Health-care workers across the country file reports on the incidence of infectious diseases, such as AIDS and hepatitis, to state health departments. These state health departments pass the information on to the CDC. Epidemiologists at the CDC use this information to research trends in the spread of infectious diseases. Their research into the trends and patterns of disease outbreaks helps identify effective disease control tactics and allocate resources to especially hard-hit areas.

## Universal Precautions

The most effective means of preventing the spread of HIV, hepatitis, and other blood-borne pathogens is to avoid contamination. As a medical assistant, you have a responsibility to help prevent infection in your patients, yourself, and your coworkers.

Following Universal Precautions, as required by the Department of Labor's Occupational Safety and Health Administration (OSHA), is critical to fulfillment of that responsibility. In recent years, the application of Universal Precautions has been broadened in medical offices to include all body fluids, secretions, excretions, and moist body surfaces. This broadening is more like the application of Standard Precautions, which must be used in hospitals. (See Chapter 20 for more information on Universal Precautions and Standard Precautions.) Your best course of action is to assume that every patient is contaminated with blood-borne pathogens. Procedure 21-1 explains how to apply Universal Precautions to prevent transmission of blood-borne pathogens during any procedure or treatment in your medical facility.

## Disease Profiles

You must understand infectious diseases, especially hepatitis and AIDS, to help prevent their spread. Because researchers continue to identify new diseases, you need to keep up-to-date on developments in the area of infectious diseases to perform your job effectively. This knowledge about diseases is useful to you for several reasons.

- You can identify symptoms that may indicate patients are infected with a blood-borne disease

## TABLE 21-1 Cases of Health-Care Workers With AIDS/HIV Infection

Health-care workers with documented and possible occupationally acquired AIDS/HIV infection, by occupation, reported through December 2001, United States[1]

| Occupation | Documented Occupational Transmission[2] Number | Possible Occupational Transmission[3] Number |
|---|---|---|
| Dental worker, including dentist | – | 6 |
| Embalmer/morgue technician | 1 | 2 |
| Emergency medical technician/paramedic | – | 12 |
| Health aide/attendant | 1 | 15 |
| Housekeeper/maintenance worker | 2 | 13 |
| Laboratory technician, clinical | 16 | 17 |
| Laboratory technician, nonclinical | 3 | – |
| Nurse | 24 | 35 |
| Physician, nonsurgical | 6 | 12 |
| Physician, surgical | – | 6 |
| Respiratory therapist | 1 | 2 |
| Technician, dialysis | 1 | 3 |
| Technician, surgical | 2 | 2 |
| Technician/therapist, other than those listed above | – | 9 |
| Other health-care occupations | – | 5 |
| **Total** | **57** | **139** |

[1]Health-care workers are defined as those persons, including students and trainees, who have worked in a health-care, clinical, or HIV laboratory setting at any time since 1978. See *MMWR* 1992; 41:823–25.

[2]Health-care workers who had documented HIV seroconversion after occupational exposure or had other laboratory evidence of occupational infection: 48 had percutaneous exposure, 5 had mucocutaneous exposure, 2 had both percutaneous and mucocutaneous exposures, and 2 had an unknown route of exposure. Forty-nine exposures were to blood from an HIV-infected person, 1 to visibly bloody fluid, 4 to an unspecified fluid, and 3 to concentrated virus in a laboratory. Twenty-four of these health-care workers developed AIDS.

[3]These health-care workers have been investigated and are without identifiable behavioral or transfusion risks; each reported percutaneous or mucocutaneous occupational exposures to blood or body fluids, or laboratory solutions containing HIV, but HIV seroconversion specifically resulting from an occupational exposure was not documented.

Source: Centers for Disease Control and Prevention.

- You can provide patients with education they can use to limit their risk of contracting such a disease
- You can identify habits your patients have that may increase their risk of spreading disease and educate them in different techniques to limit their risk

## Hepatitis

Hepatitis is a viral infection of the liver that can lead to cirrhosis and death. There are several hepatitis virus variants that differ in their means of transmission as well as in the presenting symptoms of infection. These variations include the following:

- Hepatitis A, caused by the hepatitis A virus (HAV). Hepatitis A is spread mainly through the fecal-oral route. People can be infected with HAV by drinking contaminated water, eating contaminated food, or having intimate contact with an infected person. HAV can spread in daycare settings when an attendant changes the diaper of an infected child, then helps another child with feeding before performing adequate hand washing. The disease is rarely fatal (the recovery rate is 99%), and there is a vaccine that prevents infection.
- Hepatitis B, which is the most common blood-borne hazard heath-care workers face. It is spread through contact with contaminated blood or body fluids and

# HIV/AIDS Instructor

*To gain medical assistant credentials, you must fulfill the requirements of either the American Association of Medical Assistants (for a Certified Medical Assistant) or the American Medical Technologists (for a Registered Medical Assistant). After obtaining your medical assistant certification or registration, you may wish to acquire additional skills in specialty areas through course work or on-the-job training. Although this course work or training may not lead to an additional certification or degree, it will enable you to expand your role in the medical office and advance your career as the demand for skilled health professionals increases.*

## Skills and Duties

An HIV/AIDS instructor educates people about HIV infection and AIDS. Trained and certified by the American Red Cross, the HIV/AIDS instructor presents factual information in an age-appropriate, nonjudgmental, and culturally sensitive manner. She educates the community about HIV transmission and prevention and personalizes the facts about HIV and AIDS. She also emphasizes the importance of showing compassion toward people who are living with HIV or whose family members, friends, or partners may be HIV-positive.

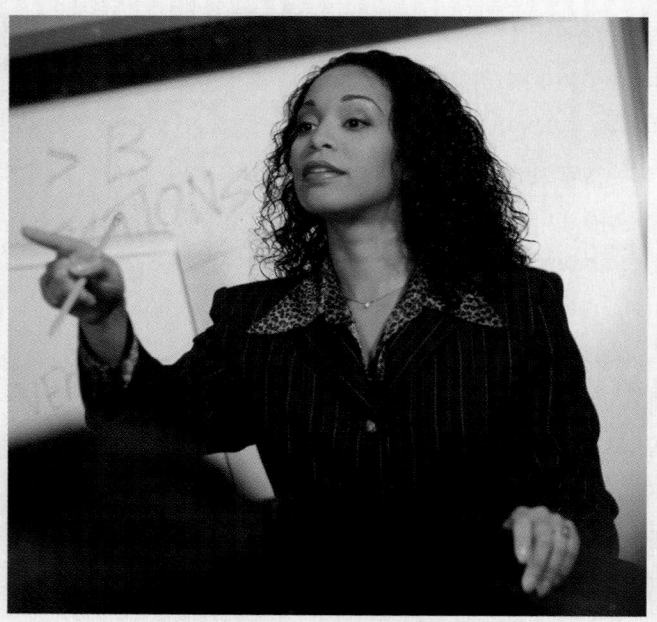

The HIV/AIDS instructor may be certified in a number of Red Cross programs, including:

- The Basic HIV/AIDS Program, which presents a variety of interactive educational activities to educate the community.
- The African American HIV/AIDS Program, which was developed by African American staff of the Red Cross in partnership with the National Urban League to present culturally affirming information.
- The Hispanic HIV/AIDS Program, which was developed by the Red Cross with national Hispanic organizations and is available in both Spanish and English.
- The Workplace HIV/AIDS Program, which is tailored for each specific work site and covers topics such as rights and responsibilities, disability laws, local resources, and other issues of interest to employers and employees.
- Act SMART, developed by the Red Cross and the Boys & Girls Clubs of America to provide prevention knowledge and skills through age-appropriate activities for people ages 6 through 17.

## Workplace Settings

HIV/AIDS instructors work in a variety of settings. They may run programs in schools, universities, offices, places of worship, community meeting rooms, clinics, hospitals, and people's homes.

## Education

To become an HIV/AIDS instructor, you must be trained and certified by your local American Red Cross chapter. There are no specific educational requirements to be eligible for the training. This is often an unpaid volunteer position.

More than 30,000 instructors have been trained in Red Cross HIV/AIDS programs. To date, instructors trained by the Red Cross have reached millions of people through HIV/AIDS education sessions. With the increasing awareness of AIDS and other sexually transmitted diseases, this field is expected to grow.

## Where to Go for More Information

The American Red Cross
HIV/AIDS Education, Health and Safety Services
8111 Gatehouse Road, 6th Floor
Falls Church, VA 22042
703-206-7180

# PROCEDURE 21.1

## Applying Universal Precautions

**Procedure Goal:** To take specific protective measures when performing tasks in which a worker may be exposed to blood, body fluids, or tissues

**OSHA Guidelines:**

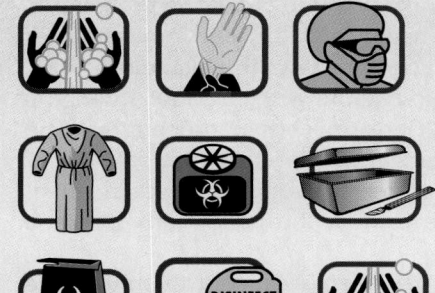

**Materials:** Items needed for the specific treatment or procedure being performed

**Method:**

1. Perform aseptic hand washing. (See Procedure 20-1 in Chapter 20.)
2. Put on gloves and a gown or a laboratory coat and, if required, eye protection and a mask or a face shield.
3. Assist with the treatment or procedure as your office policy dictates.
4. Follow OSHA procedures (outlined in Chapter 20) to clean and decontaminate the treatment area (Figure 21-1).
5. Place reusable instruments in appropriate containers for sanitizing, disinfecting, and sterilizing, as appropriate (see Chapter 20).
6. Remove your gloves and all personal protective equipment. Place them in waste containers or laundry receptacles, according to OSHA guidelines (see Chapter 20).
7. Wash your hands.

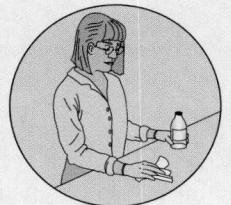 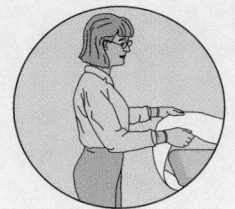 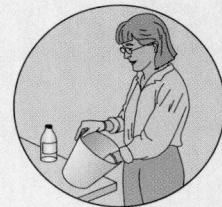 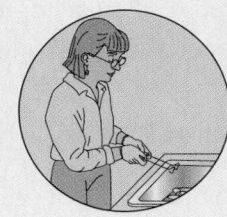 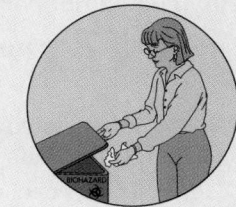

❶ Decontaminate exposed work areas.  ❷ Replace exposed protective coverings.  ❸ Decontaminate receptacles.  ❹ Pick up broken glass.  ❺ Discard infectious waste.

**Figure 21-1.** Follow these OSHA guidelines to clean and decontaminate the medical environment after each procedure or treatment.

through sexual contact. Most patients recover fully from HBV infection, but some patients develop chronic infection or remain carriers of the pathogen for the rest of their lives. Adults and children with hepatitis B who develop lifelong infections may experience serious health problems, including cirrhosis (scarring of the liver), liver cancer, liver failure, and death. Preventing the spread of the infection is the most effective means of combating the disease. Following Universal Precautions and receiving HBV vaccination are the most effective ways to control the spread of the infection.

- Hepatitis C (also referred to as non-A/non-B), which is also spread through contact with contaminated blood or body fluids and through sexual contact.

There is no cure for this variant, which has resulted in more deaths than hepatitis A and hepatitis B combined. Many people become carriers of hepatitis C without knowing it because they do not experience any symptoms of the virus. If the infection causes immediate symptoms, they often resemble the flu. Although treatment exists to suppress the virus, nothing can prevent or stop the virus from replicating. Over time, it is likely to damage the liver, causing cirrhosis, liver failure, and cancer. As with hepatitis B, preventing the spread of the infection is the best way to combat the disease.

- Hepatitis D (delta agent hepatitis), which occurs only in people infected with HBV. Delta agent infection may make the symptoms of hepatitis B more severe,

## CAUTION *Handle With Care*

## Preventing Transmission of Viruses in the Health-Care Setting

Certain procedures are thought to cause the transmission of infection from a medical worker to a patient. For example, skin-puncture injuries in medical workers are not uncommon. Therefore, many procedures involving needles are considered exposure-prone. If the worker's skin is cut or punctured, the patient could be exposed to the worker's blood.

The risk that a heath-care worker will transmit an infection to a patient is small, if proper precautions are taken. Workers participating in high-risk procedures, however, should take extra precautions. Workers with skin conditions characterized by sores that secrete fluid should forgo direct patient care and the handling of equipment used for exposure-prone procedures until the condition has healed. Workers performing high-risk procedures should know their HIV and HBV status. (HIV refers to the virus that causes AIDS; HBV refers to the hepatitis B virus.) HBV vaccination is strongly recommended.

A heath-care worker who is infected with HIV or HBV should not perform procedures that might result in exposure without the advice of an expert review panel. This panel might include the heath-care worker's own physician, someone with expert knowledge about the transmission of infectious disease, a medical professional with expert knowledge about the procedures in question, public health officials, and a member of the infection control committee of the institution.

The panel will advise the worker about when she will be allowed to perform certain procedures. The panel will require her to inform potential patients of the infection before the procedure. The panel must, however, otherwise protect the heath-care worker's confidentiality.

Although there has been great controversy on the subject, there are no recommendations in place for required testing of all heath-care workers for HIV or HBV because the risk of transmission from worker to patient is not considered great enough to justify the expense. Educational and training activities can help reinforce the extra precautions exposure-prone workers should take.

---

and it is associated with liver cancer. The HBV vaccine also prevents delta agent infection.

- Hepatitis E, caused by hepatitis E virus (HEV). Hepatitis E is transmitted by the fecal-oral route, usually through contaminated water. Chronic infection does not occur, but acute hepatitis E may be fatal in pregnant women.

**Risk Factors.** Risk factors for HBV and HCV infection are the same. Although both infections can be spread through sexual contact—and high-risk sexual activity is a risk factor for hepatitis—the main risk factor is working in an occupation that requires exposure to human blood and body fluids. Other risk factors include:

- Using intravenous drugs
- Having hemophilia, a disorder characterized by a permanent tendency to bleed and requiring blood transfusions
- Traveling internationally to areas with a high prevalence of hepatitis B
- Having received blood transfusions before screening for HBV/HCV was in place
- Receiving hemodialysis, a procedure in which toxic wastes are removed from a patient's blood
- Living with a partner who has hepatitis B or hepatitis C
- Having multiple sexual partners

**Risk in the Medical Community.** As described, the primary risk factor for HBV and HCV infection is occupational exposure to the virus. In fact, although exposure to HIV has received more publicity and causes the greatest fear, your risk of contracting hepatitis, particularly hepatitis B, is actually considerably greater. Studies show that the risk of contracting HIV from a single needlestick exposure is approximately 0.5%, whereas the risk of contracting hepatitis B from a single needlestick exposure varies from 6% to as much as 33%. Several variables are responsible for the broad range of measured risk in HBV infection, including the immune status of the recipient and the efficiency of the virus transmission.

**Progress of the Infection.** Infection with hepatitis is a multistage process. The stages are as follows:

1. The prodromal stage, in which patients may experience general malaise, specific symptoms such as nausea and vomiting, or no symptoms at all
2. The icteric, or **jaundice,** stage, characterized by yellowness of the skin, eyes, mucous membranes, and excretions (Figure 21-2), which usually appears 5 to 10 days after initial infection
3. The convalescent stage, which occurs after the two acute infection stages and can last from 2 to 3 weeks as symptoms gradually abate

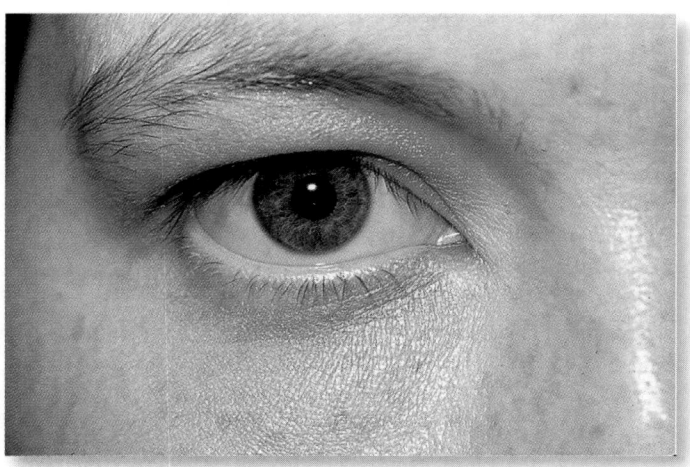

**Figure 21-2.** Jaundice is caused by excess bilirubin, which is produced in the liver and deposited throughout the body and which results in the yellow appearance of the patient's eyes and skin.

The acute illness lasts approximately 16 weeks for hepatitis B and hepatitis C. Although patients recover, they may remain infected with the virus for life.

**Symptoms.** People infected with hepatitis may show no symptoms, may experience such mild or subtle symptoms that they do not realize they are seriously ill, or may experience severe symptoms. When you treat patients with hepatitis infection, any of these signs and symptoms may be present:

- Jaundice
- Diminished appetite
- Fatigue
- Nausea
- Vomiting
- Joint pain or tenderness
- Stomach pain
- General malaise

**Diagnosis.** Diagnosis of hepatitis is made through an investigation of risk factors and exposure incidents as well as through several blood tests. Most of the blood tests indicate the presence of antigen-antibody systems that relate to infection by hepatitis. They can also be used to determine the stage of the disease.

**Preventive Measures.** The best prevention against hepatitis is avoiding contact with contaminated substances. Follow Universal Precautions when working with all patients, and be especially careful with patients who have unknown or hepatitis-positive status.

A vaccine is available to prevent HBV infection. In fact, OSHA has established guidelines that require your employer to offer you this vaccine at no charge. If you decline the offer, you must sign a waiver. Current standard medical practice recommends against declining the vaccine. (For more information on this vaccination, see Chapter 20.)

Vaccination against HBV does not protect you from other strains of hepatitis. There are currently no vaccines for HCV, for example.

In the past, HBV vaccination was recommended only for high-risk individuals, such as medical personnel, dialysis patients, homosexual men, and intravenous drug users. This program of vaccinating only selected individuals did not greatly reduce the incidence of infection. Today the CDC recommends routine vaccination for everyone.

If you are exposed to hepatitis B and have not been vaccinated, you can receive a postexposure inoculation of hepatitis B immune globulin (HBIG). HBIG is given in large doses during the 7-day period after exposure. Shortly after beginning the treatment, you would also receive HBV vaccination. The HBIG inoculation is also used for infants born to HBV-infected mothers.

## AIDS/HIV Infection

HIV is a virus that infects and gradually destroys components of the immune system. AIDS is the condition that results from the advanced stages of this viral infection.

Over a period of time and in most cases, HIV infection develops into AIDS, which results in death. The pathogen gradually destroys helper T cells. **Helper T cells** are white blood cells that are a key component of the body's immune system and that work in coordination with other white blood cells (B cells, macrophages, and so on) to combat infection.

The virus also attacks neurons, causing demyelination (destruction of the myelin sheath of a nerve), which results in neurological problems, including dementia. Most patients with AIDS acquire various opportunistic infections. Opportunistic microorganisms do not ordinarily cause disease in a person with a properly functioning immune system. Examples of opportunistic infections are *Pneumocystis carinii* pneumonia and oral candidiasis. More information regarding opportunistic infections is presented later in this chapter.

Virtually everyone is at risk for contracting AIDS. Although the initial outbreak of the disease in the United States appeared in the male homosexual population and currently homosexual and bisexual men comprise a large percentage of AIDS cases, the disease knows no limits. The incidence of HIV infection in homosexual men, however, has leveled off and even declined slightly in some areas of the United States. At the same time, the incidence of infection in heterosexual men and women and teenagers is increasing rapidly. The incubation period in adults is between 8 and 15 years, and the majority of adults with the disease are between the ages of 25 and 45.

**Risk Factors.** The greatest risk factor for contracting HIV infection is unprotected sexual activity. The virus can be found in blood, semen, and vaginal secretions and can be transmitted to an uninfected person through mucous membranes in the vagina, rectum, or mouth, especially if there are cuts or open sores in those areas. Some strains of the virus are more likely to infect the cells in the female reproductive tract (Langerhans cells). The HIV strain most common in the United States, however, targets the monocyte or lymphocyte white blood cells and is more prone to being passed along through anal sex and blood-to-blood contact.

The virus can also be spread by the sharing of needles used by intravenous drug users. The minute amount of blood left on a needle after injection provides an ample supply of the virus to transmit the infection to another host. Needles used in tattooing and piercing can also pose a risk. In all cases, needles should be new and sterile.

The virus can pass from mother to fetus during pregnancy, as well as to an infant during delivery or through breast-feeding. Not every infant born to an infected mother contracts the disease, and some infected infants have cleared the virus from their systems within a year after birth. Scientists are studying these children in an effort to determine how their immune systems allow them to escape infection altogether or to eradicate the virus after infection. Scientists suspect that either the immune systems of the infants in the study fought off an HIV invasion or the infants developed a permanent tolerance for it.

At one time the virus was also being spread through the nation's blood supply. Transmission was occurring through transfusion of HIV-contaminated blood products. This form of transmission has virtually stopped as a result of an aggressive screening program that began in 1985. All blood donations are tested for the virus, and contaminated donations are destroyed. People who received blood prior to 1986 (especially between 1978 and 1985) were at risk for coming down with AIDS. Because of the long incubation period of the virus (8 to 15 years), infected people may not have exhibited any symptoms of infection.

**Risk in the Medical Community.** Health-care workers have contracted HIV infection as a direct result of occupational activities (see Table 21-1). Investigations showed that infection in most of the cases occurred as a result of **percutaneous exposure,** that is, exposure through a puncture wound or needlestick. **Mucocutaneous exposure,** or exposure through a mucous membrane, resulted in infection in a few cases.

Further analysis identified that in most cases the infecting substance was HIV-infected blood. Concentrated virus cultures in the laboratory and visibly bloody body fluid caused a few of the cases.

**Progress of the Infection.** Current research has shown that development of AIDS occurs in three main stages:

1. Initial infection
2. Incubation period
3. Full-blown AIDS

Initial infection by the virus can occur years before any symptoms appear to arouse suspicions about HIV infection. In some cases, the initial infection is marked by severe flu-like symptoms. Identification of the initial infection, however, is almost always through hindsight. The virus attacks helper T cells during this initial phase.

During the initial phase of infection by HIV, the virus enters the cell, and the host cell produces multiple copies of the virus. As a result, helper T cells die or are disabled. The body's immune system responds to the attack at this point, cleansing the blood supply of the virus, and the virus enters an inactive phase.

The incubation period begins when the virus incorporates its genetic material into the genetic material of the helper T cells. The virus is trapped within the lymph system, and the host experiences few, if any, symptoms of the disease. Many doctors discover the infection in patients during this period when treating them for other illnesses. This incubation period, in which people are HIV-positive but do not have AIDS, generally lasts 8 to 15 years.

Sometime during the incubation period, HIV becomes active again and continues to attack and destroy helper T cells. As the number of helper T cells dwindles, the patient becomes more prone to opportunistic infections.

The threshold at which a patient is officially diagnosed with AIDS is the point at which there are 200 or fewer helper T cells per milliliter of blood. Once a person has full-blown AIDS—the third phase of infection— opportunistic infections take hold as the overall immune system undergoes deterioration. Neurons are destroyed, resulting in neurological problems, including dementia.

**Diagnosis.** The initial diagnosis may be accomplished through the use of a rapid HIV test. Rapid tests are available for testing whole blood, blood plasma, and oral fluids, and the results are available within 20 minutes. These tests are used for initial testing only. To know for certain whether a person is infected with HIV, that person must have a confirmatory blood test specifically for HIV infection. (All HIV testing is anonymous.)

The **enzyme-linked immunosorbent assay (ELISA) test** confirms the presence of antibodies developed by the body's immune system in response to an initial HIV infection. ELISA is only about 85% accurate because of cross-reactivity from other viruses. Therefore, positive specimens are confirmed by a different method—the **Western blot test** or the **immunofluorescent antibody (IFA) test.** These tests are more accurate because they are specific to individual viruses.

These HIV tests were first developed for use on blood samples, but the ELISA and Western blot tests can also be run on oral fluid samples obtained in the medical office. Positive results from two of the three HIV tests (ELISA plus one other) yield an accurate diagnosis in almost 100% of patients tested.

Home tests are available that involve an ELISA test followed by either a Western blot test or an IFA test if the ELISA results are positive. These tests are performed on a drop of the patient's blood, which is collected on a specially treated card. Patients are identified only by a number, which they use to obtain their test results. (Keep in mind that people who perform home tests may not report positive results to the proper authorities.) Patients should be made aware that not all home tests are Food and Drug Administration (FDA)-approved and may give false results. They should also know that if they are positive they will need medical care, including treatment and counseling.

In all cases involving testing for HIV, you must follow measures to ensure protection of the patient's confidentiality. Knowledge about a patient's test results should be limited to those who will be treating the patient and appropriate authorities as required by law. The patient's decision on whether or not to reveal test results to family and friends should be respected at all times.

**Symptoms.** HIV infection can cause a variety of problems as it progresses to AIDS. Patients with AIDS may complain of any of the following symptoms:

- Systemic complaints, such as weight loss, fatigue, fever, chills, and night sweats
- Respiratory complaints, such as sinus fullness, dry cough, shortness of breath, difficulty swallowing, and sinus drainage
- Oral complaints, such as gingivitis, oral lesions, and **hairy leukoplakia,** which is a white lesion on the tongue
- Gastrointestinal complaints, such as diarrhea and bloody stool
- Central nervous system (CNS) complaints, such as depression, personality changes, concentration difficulties, and confusion or dementia
- Peripheral nervous system complaints, such as tingling, numbness, pain, and weakness in the extremities
- Skin-related complaints, such as rashes, dry skin, and changes in the nail bed
- **Kaposi's sarcoma,** an unusual malignancy occurring in the skin and sometimes in the lymph nodes and organs manifested by reddish purple to dark blue patches or spots on the skin.

Because many other diseases can cause these symptoms, the occurrence of any one symptom is not necessarily indicative of AIDS. Be aware, however, that patients exhibiting a combination of symptoms should be tested. The two symptoms most indicative of AIDS are hairy leukoplakia and Kaposi's sarcoma.

**Preventive Measures.** The only way to prevent the spread of HIV infection is to avoid specific activities or to take safety precautions when engaging in these activities. Activities requiring preventive measures can be divided into three groups, based on the means of transmission of the disease:

1. Sexual contact
2. Sharing of intravenous needles
3. Medical procedures

***Prevention and Sexual Contact.*** The most effective method for preventing the spread of AIDS/HIV infection through sexual contact is to avoid high-risk sexual activity. Such high-risk activities or situations include:

- Having unprotected vaginal, oral, or anal sex, either homosexual or heterosexual, *unless* the individuals are involved in a long-term, monogamous relationship, they both have been tested and received negative results, and they have not engaged in any unsafe sexual activity 6 months before the test or anytime after the test
- Having multiple sexual partners, even when using protection against infection
- Experiencing a concurrent infection with another sexually transmitted disease

In addition, precautions must be taken when using a condom as a means of protection against infection. Proper use of a condom requires adherence to the following guidelines:

- A condom must be used every time the individual has sex and must never be reused.
- Only latex condoms provide protection against spread of the HIV pathogen. Lambskin condoms provide birth control only, not protection against disease.
- If lubrication is required, the lubricant must be water-based, not petroleum-based (such as petroleum jelly). Lubricants other than those specifically formulated for use with latex condoms can damage the condom, rendering it permeable and eliminating its usefulness as a barrier against disease.
- Condoms should be placed on the penis before any risk of leakage of seminal fluid occurs. Space should be left at the tip to act as a reservoir for ejaculated semen.
- Intercourse should not be attempted unless the penis is fully erect, and the penis should be withdrawn while it is still erect.
- The condom must remain in place from the beginning to the end of intercourse and should be held in place during withdrawal to prevent slippage. After withdrawal, the condom should be disposed of properly.

***Prevention and Intravenous Drug Use.*** Intravenous drug users are at risk for infection when they share needles. The most effective means of preventing the spread of the pathogen among drug users is to avoid sharing or reusing needles.

***Prevention and Medical Procedures.*** Preventing the spread of AIDS/HIV infection in the medical environment involves taking many precautions. You must take precautions to prevent the spread of infection between patients, between yourself and the patient, and when you are working with equipment, supplies, or instruments that may be contaminated.

Strict adherence to Universal Precautions (Standard Precautions in a hospital) when working with patients is the best method for preventing the spread of disease among patients and between the patient and you. You must use gloves whenever there is a risk of contact with blood, tissue, or body fluids, and you must dispose of gloves properly after use. (See Chapter 20 for specific disposal guidelines.)

You must wash your hands carefully and thoroughly between patients. Wear additional personal protective equipment in situations where there is a risk of being splashed or sprayed by blood or body fluids.

Although gloves and other personal protective equipment provide adequate protection in many situations, they provide only limited protection against injury. Be especially careful when handling pointed or sharp-edged instruments or equipment. Needles must be disposed of in a puncture-proof biohazardous waste container. Pick up broken glass with tongs, and dispose of it in a puncture-proof biohazardous waste container.

***Education as Prevention.*** As a medical assistant, you will encounter many opportunities to inform and educate patients about the dangers of HIV infection and AIDS, the ways in which the disease is spread, the ways in which it is not spread, and methods for preventing its spread. Use these opportunities to educate patients, because one of the best preventive measures is providing accurate and thorough information to people. For more information about HIV education resources, see Educating the Patient: Obtaining Information About AIDS and Hepatitis.

# AIDS Patients

Treating patients infected with HIV and those who have developed AIDS is one of today's most challenging areas of medicine. New research findings occur frequently and may change treatment and diagnostic procedures. Because HIV infection is nearly always fatal, patients—and their families and caregivers—usually experience extreme psychological stress.

## The AIDS Patient Profile

Although there are certain high-risk populations, such as intravenous drug users and homosexual men, virtually no one is immune to AIDS. Research evidence shows that HIV has been in the United States since approximately 1970. This conclusion is based on knowledge about the incubation period of the disease and the initial reports of *Pneumocystis carinii* pneumonia and Kaposi's sarcoma in homosexual men beginning in 1978. These diseases, which had been quite rare, are now considered hallmarks of HIV infection.

Because the infection seemed to occur exclusively in homosexual men, it was originally called gay-related infectious disease, or GRID. Rapidly, however, it became apparent that the disease could be passed not only through male-to-male sexual contact but also through blood transfusion, through the sharing of intravenous drug paraphernalia, through occupational exposure, through male-to-female sexual contact, through female-to-female sexual contact, and from mother to fetus as well as from mother to infant during breast-feeding.

As of December 1996, 22.6 million men, women, and children were HIV-infected worldwide. That number increased to approximately 40.3 million by the year 2005.

Homosexual men still constitute a large percentage of people with HIV infection and AIDS in the United States. Growth in infection of people in this group has slowed, however, as a result of educational campaigns and the population's adherence to "safer sex" practices. Data show that the disease occurs primarily among young people, especially those in large metropolitan areas. AIDS incidence rates for large metropolitan areas are approximately three times as high as rates for small metropolitan areas and nearly five times as high as rates in rural areas. Rural areas are, however, starting to show an increase in incidence.

Two groups of people who are contracting HIV infection in increasing numbers are intravenous drug users (especially African Americans and Hispanics in large metropolitan areas) and women. Because of the increase in infection among women, there has also been an increase in the number of infected children.

The CDC publishes a quarterly report, *The HIV/AIDS Surveillance Report,* which contains data about the incidence of HIV infection and AIDS nationwide. Information about age, gender, sexual orientation, race, occupation, residence, and source of infection are some of the facts collected in an effort to help epidemiologists generate an accurate picture of the patterns of the disease. Data also help identify the prevention programs most likely to succeed with a given population and help community leaders make decisions about the care of people with HIV infection and AIDS.

# Chronic Disorders of the AIDS Patient

The impaired immune system of the AIDS patient permits opportunistic infections, which further reduce the body's ability to fight off infection. These infections attack many different parts of the body (Figure 21-3).

One of the cornerstones of the care of patients who have AIDS is to prevent opportunistic infections and identify such infections as quickly as possible when they occur. Identifying malignancies, if they occur, is also of utmost importance. If you are familiar with the common disorders an AIDS patient faces, you will be better able to identify early signs of infection or malignancy and point them out to the doctor, in turn initiating early treatment, which is usually most effective. You can help patients who have been diagnosed with HIV to understand the risks they face as well as the measures best suited to preventing particular infections.

***Pneumocystis Carinii* Pneumonia.** The most common opportunistic infection in AIDS patients is *Pneumocystis carinii* pneumonia, or PCP. Nearly 75% of AIDS

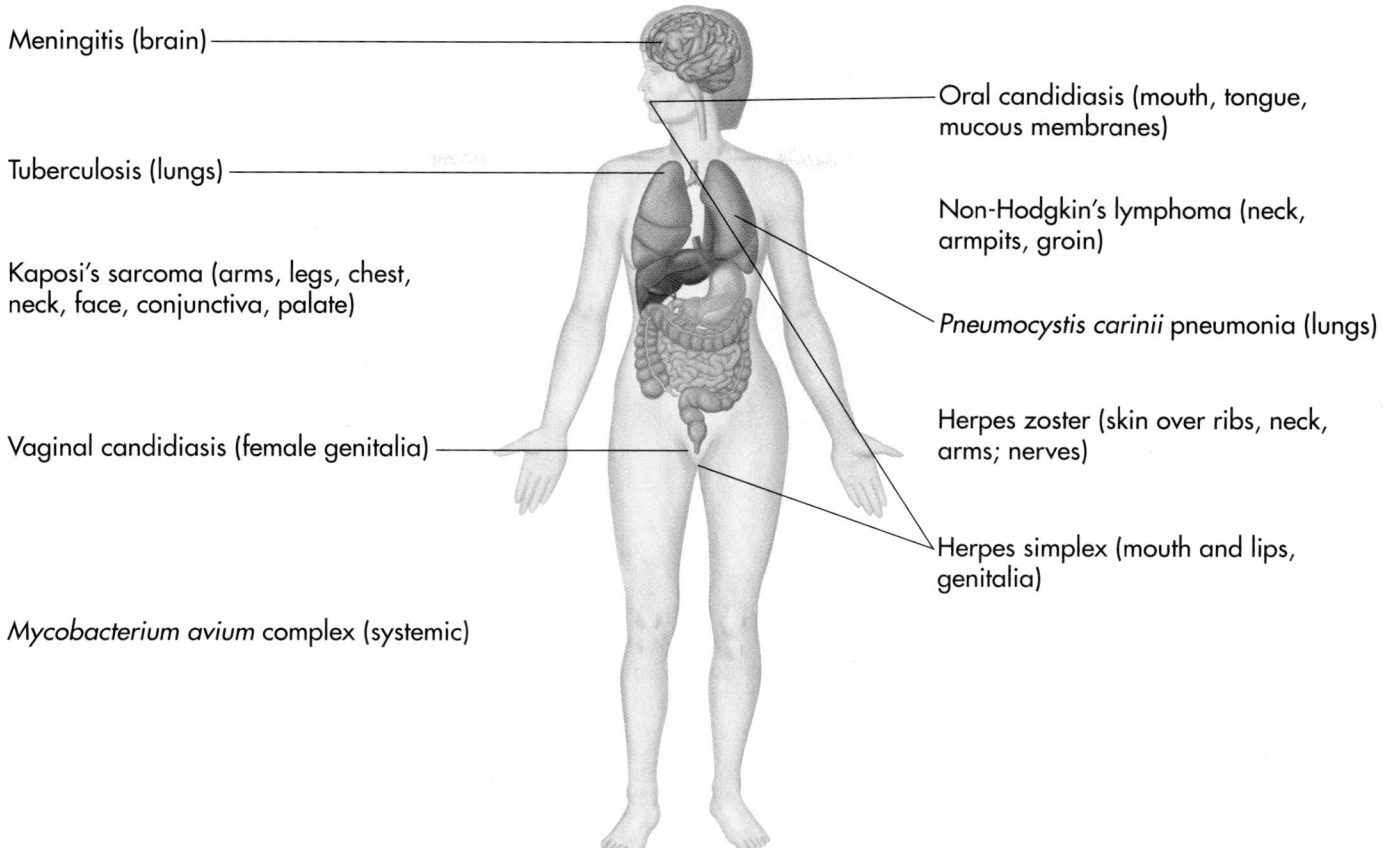

Meningitis (brain)

Oral candidiasis (mouth, tongue, mucous membranes)

Tuberculosis (lungs)

Non-Hodgkin's lymphoma (neck, armpits, groin)

Kaposi's sarcoma (arms, legs, chest, neck, face, conjunctiva, palate)

*Pneumocystis carinii* pneumonia (lungs)

Herpes zoster (skin over ribs, neck, arms; nerves)

Vaginal candidiasis (female genitalia)

Herpes simplex (mouth and lips, genitalia)

*Mycobacterium avium* complex (systemic)

**Figure 21-3.** The AIDS patient may contract a variety of opportunistic infections, which affect many different parts of the body.

patients experience this protozoal infection, with symptoms of fever, cough, and breathing difficulties. These symptoms are often very general, may not be very severe, and can be overlooked or attributed to other problems. Diagnosis is made through chest radiographs (x-ray film records of the chest), the Wright-Giesma sputum stain (substances that impart color so sputum can be studied), and bronchoalveolar lavage (a technique by which cells and fluid from alveoli, tiny sacs in the lungs, are removed for diagnosis).

AIDS patients should avoid contact with people who have colds or the flu. If contact is unavoidable, ill people should wear surgical masks to reduce the risk of spreading infection to AIDS patients. Everyone who comes in regular contact with AIDS patients should have a current flu immunization. Flu immunizations must be renewed every year.

Treatments for *Pneumocystis carinii* pneumonia can cause side effects. Some of the side effects are measurable only through laboratory tests, whereas some may be reported by the patient. Side effects include the following:

- Nausea
- Rash
- Hypotension (abnormally low blood pressure)
- Anemia
- Neutropenia (diminished number of neutrophils in the blood)
- Hepatitis
- Colitis (inflammation of the colon)
- Leukopenia (reduction in the number of leukocytes in the blood)

**Kaposi's Sarcoma.** Kaposi's sarcoma is a particularly aggressive form of tumor. Although it is uncommon in the general population (it is found in males averaging age 89 years in the Mediterranean Sea region), it is the most common HIV-related malignancy. Kaposi's sarcoma appears as reddish purple to dark blue skin lesions that are found anywhere on the body (Figure 21-4). They are usually first found on the arms and legs, then on the chest, neck, and face. The lesions may appear in areas such as the conjunctiva or the eyelids, between the toes, behind the ears, and on the palate.

Treatment for Kaposi's sarcoma includes chemotherapy. Chemotherapy may cause flu-like symptoms accompanied by fever.

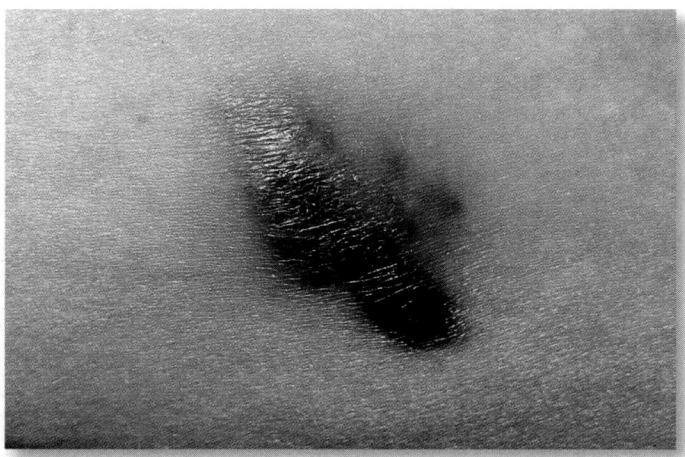

**Figure 21-4.** Kaposi's sarcoma is a rare form of skin cancer associated with AIDS.

**Non-Hodgkin's Lymphoma.** The second most common malignancy associated with HIV infection is non-Hodgkin's lymphoma (NHL). Because NHL can appear in multiple sites, it is difficult to predict the problems HIV-infected patients will encounter with it. The symptoms vary, depending on which, if any, opportunistic infections are present. Other considerations are the rate of tumor growth and the location of the malignancy.

**Tuberculosis.** Tuberculosis is often a curable disease when treatment regimens are followed exactly and completely. (See Chapter 19 for more information on tuberculosis.) There has, however, been a rise in the number of cases in recent years as a result of HIV infection and antibiotic resistance. HIV infection is by far the single largest risk factor for the development of tuberculosis infection into the active form of the disease. HIV infection reduces the effectiveness of the immune system and makes it possible for tuberculosis bacilli to multiply and spread infection more easily. AIDS patients who have symptoms of tuberculosis should receive the Mantoux skin test (intradermal TB test), a chest x-ray, and possibly a sputum culture. These tests are the only means of definitive diagnosis. AIDS patients should be tested yearly for tuberculosis infection. If they suspect they have been exposed to the pathogen through contact with a known or suspected source, they should undergo testing at the earliest opportunity.

The Mantoux skin test yields false negative results in some people with AIDS. In fact, as the number of helper T cells decreases, the more likely it is for patients to exhibit negative results. When two or more other antigens are combined with the tuberculin units used in the Mantoux test, a more accurate picture of infection emerges.

If patients do not respond to any of the substances injected for the test, they are considered to have an **anergic reaction.** An anergic reaction occurs when the body is unable to mount a normal response to invasion by a pathogen. Patients who respond to the other substances but not to the tuberculin units are considered free of tuberculosis infection.

People with AIDS who exhibit an anergic reaction to the test should be considered for preventive therapy designed to halt development of the tuberculosis infection into disease.

***Mycobacterium Avium Complex (MAC) Infection.*** *Mycobacterium avium* complex (MAC) is responsible for 97% of the nontuberculous bacterial infections in AIDS patients, although it is difficult to detect in these patients. Postmortem studies of AIDS patients indicate that the disease is undetected in more than 50% of cases. The pathogen can be acquired orally or through inhalation. Symptoms include the following:

- Systemic illness
- Fever
- Night sweats
- Fatigue
- Weight loss
- Diarrhea
- Stomach pain

**Meningitis.** The pathogens that cause many of the common opportunistic infections in patients with AIDS can result in several forms of meningitis. Diagnosis is often difficult because the presenting symptoms and laboratory results are not always consistent with those found in patients without compromised immune systems. Infection of the CNS in an AIDS patient can lead to AIDS dementia complex, in which the patient's mental and motor functions gradually and irreversibly decline.

**Oral Candidiasis.** More than half the patients diagnosed with AIDS develop oral candidiasis *(Candida albicans),* or thrush. The infection in an AIDS patient takes one of three primary forms:

1. Reddened, atrophic patches on the hard mucous membranes
2. Coating of the tongue
3. Patches on the tongue, soft palate, tonsils, and mucous membranes toward the cheek

**Vaginal Candidiasis.** Women who have AIDS are predisposed to vaginal candidiasis. Those who develop the infection often experience a severe case that is difficult to cure. Symptoms include these:

- Pruritus (extreme itching)
- Dysuria (painful or difficult urination)
- Labial excoriations (abrasions of the genital labia)
- Thick, adherent discharge

**Herpes Simplex.** One of the most common infections experienced by humans, herpes simplex virus (HSV), can manifest in a range of forms, from mild to life-threatening. People with compromised immune systems are especially at risk for infection by HSV. There are two forms of the virus: HSV-1 and HSV-2. HSV-2 is transmitted primarily through sexual exposure, whereas HSV-1 is transmitted primarily through exposure to oral secretions.

It is possible, however, for HSV-2 to be transmitted through oral contact and for HSV-1 to be transmitted sexually.

**Herpes Zoster.**   The herpes virus that causes chicken-pox may become dormant in the body and may return as shingles, or herpes zoster. Generally the patient experiences pain followed by the appearance of reddened, raised lesions on one side of the body. In a patient who has a healthy immune system, the lesions last from 3 to 5 days and clear up within 15 days, although it can take an additional month for the patient's skin to return to its preinfection condition. In a patient who is **immunocompromised** (having an impaired or weakened immune system), however, the formation of lesions can last as long as 2 weeks, and clearing may not occur for 21 to 28 days. Herpes zoster rarely proves fatal, even in immunocompromised patients.

## Treating Opportunistic Infections

The wide variety of opportunistic infections that may afflict AIDS patients makes treatment management a challenge. In some instances, drug side effects that patients with intact immune systems would easily tolerate pose major problems for the immunocompromised patient. Repeated episodes of infection can leave a patient allergic to treatment medication or with a tolerance to the medication, requiring higher and higher doses for effectiveness. The pathogen itself may mutate into a strain that is resistant to treatment. Treatment for one set of symptoms may conflict with treatment for another set or may exacerbate other symptoms.

## Testing Regulations

Currently the CDC does not recommend mandatory HIV testing for heath-care workers. Health-care professionals emphasize that a heath-care worker's chances of being infected by a patient are much higher than a patient's chances of being infected by a heath-care worker. Although there have been well-publicized incidents of infection from heath-care worker to patient, no required testing programs exist today. (Refer to Chapter 20 for additional precautions for avoiding transmission of disease from heath-care workers to patients.)

## Drug Treatments

A growing number of drugs are available for the treatment of HIV and AIDS. Billions of dollars are spent each year for research into HIV/AIDS treatments and vaccines. There is no cure for either of these diseases; however, pharmaceutical companies are making great strides in creating new drugs that slow the reproduction of the virus. A patient with HIV or AIDS is no longer limited to one or two therapies. Because more than 20 drugs are available for treatment, an individual with HIV or AIDS who has had no success with one regimen or treatment might find success with another. This is important for increasing life expectancy. Table 21-2 identifies different classifications of drugs currently approved by the FDA for the treatment of diseases associated with HIV infection and AIDS.

| TABLE 21-2   FDA-Approved Drugs for HIV/AIDS Infection (Antiretroviral Drugs) | | |
|---|---|---|
| **Classification** | **Generic Name** | **Major Side Effects** |
| **Fusion Inhibitor** Block viral entrance into the human cell | Fuzeon enfuvirtide (2003) | Bacterial pneumonia, allergic reaction, injection site infections |
| **Nonnucleoside Reverse Transcriptase Inhibitors (NNRTIs)** Block the ability of HIV to make copies of itself | Rescriptor delavirdine (1997) | Skin rash, eye inflammation, fever, joint or muscle pain, oral lesions, swelling |
| | Sustiva efavirenz (1998) | Skin rash, depression |
| **Nucleoside Reverse Transcriptase Inhibitors (NRTIs)** Block the ability of HIV to make copies of itself | 3TC lamivudine (1995) | Burning, numbness, pain, or tingling in the hands, arms, feet, or legs; fever, muscle aches, nausea, vomiting, skin rash |
| | Viread tenofovir disoproxil fumarate (2001) | Liver or kidney failure, lactic acidosis, pancreatitis |
| **Protease Inhibitors (PIs)** Block the ability of HIV to make copies of itself | Reyataz atazanavir (2003) | Jaundice, heart block, hyperglycemia, diarrhea, nausea; infection, hematuria |
| | Lexiva fosamprenavir (2003) | Severe rash, changes in body fat, increased cholesterol, hyperglycemia |

*Note:* Numbers in parentheses represent the date or dates the drugs were approved for the specified purpose.
*Source:* U.S. Department of Health and Human Services; Food and Drug Administration; and AIDSInfo.

**Treatment Goals.** The goals of drug treatment for HIV and AIDS include the following:

- Increasing the time between infection and symptomatic disease (AIDS)
- Improving the quality of life of those diagnosed with AIDS
- Reducing transmission of HIV to uninfected persons
- Reducing maternal-infant transmission
- Reducing the number of HIV-related deaths

**Treatment Guidelines.** Some basic guidelines for implementing HIV/AIDS treatment were developed by the Panel on Clinical Practices for Treatment of HIV Infection (the Panel). These guidelines include initial and follow-up testing of viral load and CD4 T cell count and drug resistance testing. Drug resistance testing is especially useful for patients who have failed initial therapy. Viral load and CD4 T cell counts are good indicators of the overall effectiveness of the treatment.

FDA-approved pharmaceutical agents used in the treatment of HIV/AIDS are divided into four classes: (1) fusion inhibitors, (2) nonnucleoside reverse transcriptase inhibitors (NNRTIs), (3) nucleoside reverse transcriptase inhibitors (NRTIs), and (4) protease inhibitors (PIs). Each of these classes of drugs has a different manner of working against the HIV virus. Fusion inhibitors block the entrance of the virus into the human cell. NNRTIs, NRTIs, and PIs all act to limit the HIV virus from making copies of itself, each acting in a slightly different way. All of these classes, used in combination, are important weapons in the arsenal of treatments used to combat HIV/AIDS.

The Panel recommends a combination of drug treatment called highly active anti-retroviral therapy (HAART). This therapy combines three or more HIV drugs. Taking three or more drugs has proven to be more effective than taking two or fewer, because viral load decrease is only temporary in those taking one or two HIV drugs. Treatment during pregnancy is the only exception to this. Because many HIV/AIDS drugs are contraindicated during pregnancy (with some exceptions), pregnant patients will be offered a single drug in order to limit passing HIV to their infants.

**Initiating Therapy.** When therapy should begin is an important decision that must be made by both the patient and the physician. To assist in making this decision, the Panel has made several recommendations. These recommendations are based on a combination of CD4 T cell count, viral load, and the presence or absence of symptoms. Starting therapy immediately is recommended if patients have severe symptoms (AIDS diagnosis) or if their CD4 T cell count is less than 200 cells/mm$^3$. The physician should consider treatment if the CD4 T cell count is between 200 and 350 cells/mm$^3$. In patients with a CD4 T cell count greater than 350 cells/mm$^3$, no symptoms, and a viral load greater than 55,000 copies/mL, observation of the patient is recommended with a delay of treatment. The

patient and physician should decide whether to take an aggressive approach or a conservative one. If a conservative approach is taken, the patient should have routine CD4 T cell and viral load counts.

***Delayed Treatment.*** There are advantages and disadvantages to delaying therapy. The benefits of delaying treatment include postponing drug-related adverse effects, delaying the development of drug resistance, and preserving treatment options for the future. The risks of delaying treatment include irreversible immune system damage and an increased risk of the patient transmitting HIV to others.

***Early Treatment.*** There are also advantages and disadvantages to beginning treatment early. The benefits of early treatment include the suppression of viral replication (that is, the spread of the virus within the patient's system), thus preserving immune function; a reduction in the risk of the patient's transmitting HIV to others; and helping the patient live symptom-free longer. The disadvantages of early treatment are:

- Development of drug toxicity
- Drug resistance and the subsequent transmission of drug-resistant HIV strains to others
- Adverse effects on the quality of life
- Loss of treatment options in the future

Each of these advantages and disadvantages must be carefully weighed by the patient and physician based on the patient's symptoms, lifestyle, and ability to comply with the treatment.

**Treating Complications.** In addition to treating the patient for the HIV virus, it is often necessary to treat the opportunistic infections and associated complications acquired by the patient. Individuals with a compromised immune system are more prone to bacterial, protozoal, viral, and fungal infections as well as to certain types of malignancies. See Table 21-2 for a list of drugs used in the treatment of these HIV- and AIDS-related complications.

**Continuing Research.** Researchers continue with their efforts to develop an effective vaccine. Until a vaccine is found, it is important to prevent new HIV infections and to effectively treat persons who are already infected. The U.S. Department of Health and Human Services has allocated billions of dollars for vaccine and treatment research, monitoring those with HIV/AIDS, caring for those who are infected, and fighting the disease on a global level. As a medical assistant, it is your responsibility to remain informed regarding new treatments and prevention methods and to assist in educating patients regarding these advances.

# Other Blood-Borne Infections

Hepatitis and HIV infections are the best known of the blood-borne pathogens you may encounter working in the medical field. There are also several other blood-borne diseases of which you should be aware. Some of these diseases pose particular risk to patients already infected with HIV. For this reason, you should advise HIV-positive patients about symptoms and preventive measures related to the diseases.

## Cytomegalovirus

People with compromised, or impaired, immune systems and infants (whose immune systems undergo additional development after birth) are especially at risk for cytomegalovirus (CMV). CMV is an extremely common infection. Blood tests show that nearly 80% of adults tested have antibodies for the virus. The presence of these antibodies indicates an infection at some point in the person's life. The infection rarely causes noticeable symptoms in adults with normal immune systems.

The disease sometimes takes a form similar to infectious mononucleosis in otherwise healthy adults; however, it may develop into severe lung disease in immunocompromised adults. Symptoms of the infection may include swollen glands, fever, and fatigue. Pregnant women can pass the disease on to their newborns. Infants with CMV present signs of jaundice, a rash, and low birth weight. In severe cases CMV can cause brain damage, mental retardation, deafness, blindness, and death.

## Erythema Infectiosum (Parvovirus B19)

Erythema infectiosum, or fifth disease, is a moderately contagious disease seen mainly in children and caused by human parvovirus B19. The term *fifth disease* was assigned to this "fifth" eruptive disease found in children in the late 1800s. (Sources vary on which diseases were considered first through fourth, but all include measles and rubella. Popular knowledge adds mumps and chickenpox to the list, while some more formal sources include scarlet fever and Dukes' disease.) The disease is characterized by the abrupt onset of a rash. The virus may be transmitted from mother to fetus, and although it does not cause birth defects, there is some risk of fetal death from infection. More severe signs of infection may be seen in immunocompromised patients.

## Human T-Cell Lymphotrophic Virus

Infection with the human T-cell lymphotrophic virus (HTLV-1) often appears in intravenous drug users, in people who have received multiple blood transfusions, and in the sexual partners, children, and household contacts of infected people. The virus attacks T cells, an important component of the body's immune system, by penetrating the cells and incorporating its genetic material into the cells' genetic material.

Some people who are infected with HTLV-1 show no symptoms, whereas others exhibit severe symptoms.

Infection with HTLV-1 most commonly leads to adult T-cell leukemia/lymphoma (ATLL), although patients can also contract disturbances of the spinal cord or partial paralysis.

Physical findings in cases of ATLL include skin lesions, disease of the lymph nodes, fever, abdominal distress, arthritis, and sometimes hypercalcemia (an excess of calcium in the blood). Diagnosis is confirmed when the virus is found in blood or other body tissues.

## Listeriosis

Listeriosis is an infectious disease caused by the bacterium *Listeria monocytogenes*. Once infected, an individual can pass the infection to others through contact with blood or blood products, and a pregnant woman can pass the infection to her fetus.

If the infection is passed to a fetus during the later stages of pregnancy, the infant may be stillborn. Infected infants who survive may develop meningitis, pneumonia, or septicemia (blood poisoning).

Symptoms in infected adults may include fever, shock, rash, and generalized aches, but most people do not notice any symptoms. The disease can rapidly cause death in elderly or immunocompromised patients through circulatory collapse.

Listeriosis is diagnosed by blood tests. If symptoms are present and the patient is at high risk, however, antibiotic therapy is sometimes initiated before positive identification of the pathogen.

## Malaria

Malarial infection is spread from person to person primarily through the bite of infected mosquitoes. There have also been cases of transmission from mother to fetus as well as from an infected to an uninfected person through an accidental needlestick. Malaria is mainly a tropical infection present in parts of Africa, Asia, and Central and South America.

The parasite usually enters the bloodstream through the mosquito's bite. It invades the liver, moving from there into red blood cells. Within a red blood cell, the parasite multiplies and eventually causes rupture of the cell. When the cell ruptures, new parasites are released to continue the cycle of infection, growth, rupture, and release. An infected person does not exhibit symptoms until several of these cycles have occurred. Symptoms are caused by the pigments released from the red blood cells and metabolic toxins from the parasites.

A 4- to 8-hour, three-part cycle marks infection with malaria. In the first stage of the cycle, the patient experiences shaking chills. In the second stage, the patient experiences high fever that spikes as high as 104°F or 105°F. The third stage is marked by excessive perspiration. The patient may also report nausea, vomiting, headache, and gastrointestinal symptoms and may exhibit an enlarged spleen and liver tenderness. Laboratory results will show normal or decreased white blood cell counts and decreased platelet count.

Avoidance of infection is the best means of preventing the spread of malaria. Once infected, most people recover from the disease if treated quickly. When malaria is suspected, blood tests are performed every few hours until the diagnosis is confirmed or another reason is discovered for the patient's symptoms.

## Syphilis

Syphilis is a sexually transmitted disease caused by the spirochete *Treponema pallidum.* A pregnant woman can pass this disease to her fetus. An affected infant experiences the most severe form of syphilis. An infant born with congenital syphilis may exhibit nail exfoliation (the nails falling off), hair loss, rhinitis (inflammation of the nose), lesions, anemia, failure to thrive, and paralysis of one or more limbs.

Syphilis in adults and adolescents occurs in the following three stages.

1. In the first stage, infection is indicated by the initial appearance of a painless ulcer, called a **chancre.** This ulcer may appear on the tongue, lips, genitalia, rectum, or elsewhere. In females, the chancre may not be visible, and the first stage could be missed.

2. Patients in the second stage may experience non-tender swelling of the lymph nodes. This stage may also include a generalized skin rash, fever, and the presence of mucous-membrane lesions. Condylomas (wartlike lesions of the skin) may appear in areas of moist skin.

3. The third stage may occur between several years and 2 or 3 decades after initial infection. During this stage, the patient may exhibit tumors of the skin, bones, and liver as well as CNS manifestations such as dementia, abnormal reflexes, and psychosis.

Between the first two stages and the final stage is a period of latency during which the patient exhibits no symptoms and appears to be disease-free. Blood tests will still show indications of infection, and treatment is usually administered in an effort to prevent the disease from reaching the late stage.

Identifying and treating syphilis in an HIV-positive individual are difficult tasks. Because the presence of the HIV pathogen alters the function of the immune system, test results that normally indicate the presence of syphilis may yield false-negative findings. Additional tests are required to confirm diagnosis. With the presence of HIV, the course of the syphilis infection may be accelerated, and the benefits of drug therapy to combat the infection may be reduced.

## Toxoplasmosis

The primary source of the pathogen *Toxoplasma gondii* is cat feces. Although undercooked meat products are

another source, most cases appear in people who have handled cat litter boxes. For that reason pregnant women and those with compromised immune systems, such as patients with AIDS, should not handle cat litter boxes.

Most people infected with toxoplasmosis experience no symptoms. Symptoms may, however, include fever, malaise, sore throat, rash, stiff neck, disease of the lymph nodes, and fatigue. A pregnant woman may pass the infection to her fetus, and the infection may result in spontaneous abortion, malformation, or retardation (depending on the trimester in which the organism enters). Infants who survive may also suffer from deafness, blindness, brain damage, and seizures. Diagnosis is confirmed through blood tests.

# Reporting Guidelines

Each state formulates requirements for reporting HIV infection and AIDS. That information is then sent to the Centers for Disease Control and Prevention. Table 21-3 lists states that require reporting of HIV infection by name of patient, states that accept anonymous reporting, and states that do not require reporting. Follow your employer's guidelines or procedures when you must report cases of HIV infection.

When you report a communicable disease, you must fill out a report form. Your state health department may have a different form for each reportable disease. You must obtain the correct form and a disease identification number from the health department every time you report a communicable disease. To fill out such a form, you need access to the following information:

- Disease identification (usually a code number as well as the name of the disease)
- Patient identification (including name, address, date of birth, sex, ethnic origin, and occupational or educational status) if required (as already noted, some states require only anonymous reporting of some diseases)
- Infection history (date of onset, vaccination history, laboratory results)
- Reporting-institution information (name of person completing report, title, contact information)

Each state and each medical facility have specific guidelines to which you must adhere when filling out such a form. Procedure 21-2 describes, in general, how to notify state and county agencies about reportable diseases.

Reporting guidelines must also be followed if a worker comes in contact with a substance that may transmit infection. These guidelines, which are explained in OSHA's Blood-Borne Pathogens Standard, include reporting exposure incidents to employers immediately. (See Chapter 20 for specific guidelines on handling exposure incidents.)

## TABLE 21-3  States' Reporting Guidelines for HIV Infection

| States Requiring Name-Based Reports | States Requiring Code-Based Reports[1] | States Requiring Name-to-Code-Based Reports[2] |
| --- | --- | --- |
| Alabama | California | Delaware |
| Alaska | District of Columbia | Maine |
| Arizona | Hawaii | Montana |
| Arkansas | Illinois | Oregon |
| Colorado | Kentucky | Washington |
| Connecticut | Maryland | |
| Florida | Massachusetts | |
| Idaho | Rhode Island | |
| Indiana | Vermont | |
| Iowa | | |
| Kansas | | |
| Louisiana | | |
| Michigan | | |
| Minnesota | | |
| Mississippi | | |
| Missouri | | |
| Nebraska | | |
| Nevada | | |
| New Jersey | | |
| New Mexico | | |
| New York | | |
| North Carolina | | |
| North Dakota | | |
| Ohio | | |
| Oklahoma | | |
| Pennsylvania | | |
| South Carolina | | |
| South Dakota | | |
| Tennessee | | |
| Texas | | |
| Utah | | |
| Virginia | | |
| West Virginia | | |
| Wisconsin | | |
| Wyoming | | |

[1]Code-Based Reporting: Coded identifiers are used in place of names.

[2]Name-to-Code-Based Reporting: Initially reported by name and then converted to a coded identifier.

*Note:* New Hampshire allows reporting to be either Name-Based or Code-Based. Georgia does not conduct follow-up reporting. HIV reporting is anonymous in Georgia.

*Source:* The Henry J. Kaiser Family Foundation, 2400 Sand Hill Road, Menlo Park, CA 94025; www.statehealthfacts.kff.org/.

# Notifying State and County Agencies About Reportable Diseases

**MICHIGAN DEPARTMENT OF PUBLIC HEALTH**
**Division of Disease Surveillance**

**ENTERIC ILLNESS CASE INVESTIGATION**
(Please check appropriate illness)

_____Shigellosis                          _____Giardiasis
_____Non-typhoid Salmonellosis            _____Amebiasis
_____Campylobacter enteritis

## CASE INFORMATION

Name: _____ Age or Birthdate: _____ Sex: _____ Race: _____

Address: _____ Phone: _____
       (Street)                (City)   (County)   (Zip)

Occupation:_____ *High Risk:   Y   N
          (What)               (Where)
     (If infant or student list school, nursery or day care center)

Attending                 Address or               Was the patient
Physician: _____ Phone:_____ hospitalized:   Y   N

Hospital: _____ Dates: _____
                                (Admission)          (Discharge)

Onset: _____ Date recovered: _____ Symptom Summary: _____

_____

Suspected Causative Agent: _____
(include species or serotype if known)

## HOUSEHOLD CONTACTS INFORMATION

| Name | Age | Family Relationship | Occupation | *High Risk<br>Y   N | Provide date of onset for all household members with concurrent similar illness |
|------|-----|---------------------|------------|----------------------|----------------------------------------------------------------------------------|
| 1) | | | | | |
| 2) | | | | | |
| 3) | | | | | |
| 4) | | | | | |
| 5) | | | | | |
| 6) | | | | | |
| 7) | | | | | |
| 8) | | | | | |
| 9) | | | | | |
| 10) | | | | | |

*"High Risk" = occupation as food handler, direct patient care worker, day care center worker or person attending day care or who is institutionalized. Stool specimens should be obtained on "high risk" cases and "high risk" household contacts as appropriate for the illness. Results may be recorded in Laboratory Information Section of this form (see over).

Name of the person who completed this form:_____ County:_____

Information obtained from: _____ Date:_____

Telephone Interview: _____ Home Visit: _____ Outbreak Investigation: _____

C-30 Rev. 10/83     AUTH: Act 368, P.A. 1978

**Figure 21-5.**   Some states have specific forms for use with particular communicable diseases or diseases of a certain type.

continued ⟶

# PROCEDURE 21.2

## Notifying State and County Agencies About Reportable Diseases (continued)

**Procedure Goal:** To report cases of infection with reportable disease to the proper state or county health department

**OSHA Guidelines:** This procedure does not involve exposure to blood, body fluids, or tissues.

**Materials:** Communicable disease report form, pen, envelope, stamp

**Method:**

1. Check to be sure you have the correct form. Some states have specific forms for each

reportable infectious disease or type of disease (Figure 21-5), as well as a general form (Figure 21-6). CDC forms may also be used for reporting specific diseases.

2. Fill in all blank areas unless they are shaded (generally for local health department use).

3. Follow office procedures for submitting the report to a supervisor or physician before sending it out.

4. Sign and date the form. Address the envelope, put a stamp on it, and place it in the mail.

### NON-HOUSEHOLD CONTACTS WITH A CONCURRENT SIMILAR ILLNESS

| Name | Approximate date of onset of symptoms | Address and/or Phone | Relationship to case (Nature of contact) |
|------|---------------------------------------|----------------------|------------------------------------------|
| 1) | | | |
| 2) | | | |
| 3) | | | |
| 4) | | | |
| 5) | | | |

### ADDITIONAL EXPOSURES OR COMMENTS

| | | | |
|---|---|---|---|
| Home Sewage System: | Municipal | Septic Tank | Other_____ |
| Home drinking Water Type: | Municipal | Private Well | Other_____ |

As appropriate for the illness, ask about meals eaten away from home, stores where groceries bought, brand of poultry, meat, dairy products consumed, overnight travel, recent foreign travel, group functions, exposure to raw milk, untreated water, animals, etc. within one incubation period before onset.

(shigellosis to 7 days, salmonellosis - up to 3 days, Campylobacter enteritis - up to 10 days)

Be specific, provide place name(s) and date(s).

### FOLLOW-UP FECAL CULTURE RESULTS FOR "HIGH RISK" CASE AND/OR CONTACTS.

| Name or Initials | Date(s) Obtained and Findings |
|------------------|-------------------------------|
| 1) | |
| 2) | |
| 3) | |
| 4) | |
| 5) | |

**Figure 21-5.** Continuation of form.

*continued* ⟶

| ARIZONA DEPARTMENT OF HEALTH SERVICES<br>COMMUNICABLE DISEASE REPORT<br>Important Instructions on Reverse Side<br>PLEASE PRINT OR TYPE | | County/IHS ID Number/Chapter | | State ID Number | |
|---|---|---|---|---|---|

| PATIENT'S NAME (Last) | (First) | DATE OF BIRTH | SEX<br>☐ Male<br>☐ Female | ETHNICITY<br>☐ Hispanic<br>☐ Non-Hispanic | |
|---|---|---|---|---|---|

| STREET ADDRESS | | CENSUS TRACT | CITY | RACE<br>☐ White<br>☐ Am. Indian<br>☐ Asian |
|---|---|---|---|---|

| COUNTY | STATE | ZIP CODE | PHONE NO. | ☐ Black<br>☐ Other<br>☐ Unknown |
|---|---|---|---|---|

| DIAGNOSIS OR SUSPECT REPORTABLE CONDITION | | | COUNTY USE ONLY:<br><br>LAB CONFIRMATION<br>DATE:_____ |
|---|---|---|---|

| DATE ONSET | DATE OF DIAGNOSIS | LAB RESULTS | ☐ Negative<br>☐ Positive |
|---|---|---|---|

PATIENT OCCUPATION OR SCHOOL    ☐ Not Done    ☐ Unknown

| PHYSICIAN OR OTHER REPORTING SOURCE | PHONE NUMBER | COUNTY USE ONLY:<br>☐ Confirmed case<br>☐ Probable case |
|---|---|---|

| STREET ADDRESS | CITY | STATE | ZIP CODE | ☐ Outbreak<br>Associated<br><br>☐ Ruled Out |
|---|---|---|---|---|

Original and 1st copy to County Health Department    ☐ CHECK IF ADDITIONAL FORMS ARE NEEDED  (Quantity)_____

---

## REPORTABLE DISEASES

Arizona Revised Statutes and Arizona Administrative Code require the following diseases to be reported to the County Health Department or Indian Health Services within 5 business days of diagnosis or treatment.

| | | | | |
|---|---|---|---|---|
| AIDS[3] | Cryptosporidiosis | Herpes Genitalis[3] | Plague* | Streptococcal diseases[1,2] |
| Amebiasis[1] | Dengue | HIV[3] | Poliomyelitis* | Syphilis[3] |
| Anthrax | Diphtheria* | Lead Poisoning[3] | Psittacosis | Tetanus |
| Aseptic meningitis | Ehrlichiosis | Legionellosis | Q Fever | Toxic Shock Syndrome |
| Botulism* | Encephalitis, viral | Leprosy | Rabies in humans* | Trichinosis |
| Brucellosis | Foodborne illness/ | Listeriosis | Relapsing fever | Tuberculosis[3] |
| Campylobacteriosis[1] | Waterborne illness* | Lyme Disease | Reye's Syndrome | Tuberculosis infection |
| Chancroid[3] | Giardiasis[1] | Malaria | Rocky Mt. spotted fever | in children <6 yrs of |
| Chlamydial infections | Gonorrhea[3] | Measles* | Rubella* | age |
| (genital)[3] | Haemophilus influenzae* | Meningococcal disease* | Congenital rubella syn. | Tularemia |
| Cholera* | Hemolytic Uremic Syndrome[1] | Mumps | Salmonellosis[1] | Typhoid Fever[1] |
| Coccidioidomycosis | Hepatitis A[1] | Pediculosis[2] | Scabies[2] | Typhus fever |
| Colorado tick fever | Hepatitis B, Delta Hepatitis | Pertussis* | Shigellosis[1] | Varicella |
| Conjunctivitis, acute[2] | Hepatitis Non-A, Non-B | Pesticide poisoning[3] | Staphylococcal disease[1,2] | Yellow Fever* |

*Telephone report required to the County Health Department or Indian Health Services within 24 hours.

[1] Report within 24 hours of diagnosis if in food handler.

[2] Outbreak reports only

[3] These conditions are reported on other forms, call 1-800-334-1540 for a supply

ADHS/DPS/OIDS/IDES-1 (Rev. 11-94)

**Figure 21-6.**  Each state has its own communicable disease report.

# Reflecting On . . . HIPAA

## HIPAA and Public Health

There may be times when you feel at odds about disclosing protected health information (PHI). It is sometimes necessary to disclose PHI in the interest of public health and safety. The HIPAA Privacy Rule permits the sharing of PHI for the purpose of protecting the public health. The Privacy Rule permits release of this information to legally authorized individuals and agencies as follows:

- Public health authorities
- Law enforcement agencies
- Organ procurement agencies
- Workers' compensation programs
- Research institutions

You may be asked by your physician to gather the necessary information from the patient's chart or complete a report form. Your office, as a covered entity, is required to disclose the minimum amount of information necessary to accomplish the specified goal. Although this information may be shared without prior patient authorization, you may need to review the HIPAA Guidelines and consult the office manager and physician for help determining what information is absolutely necessary.

The types of information that may be shared include:

- Reports of diseases
- Reports of injuries
- Reports of abuse, neglect, and domestic violence
- Information regarding disability
- Information used in health research
- Tissue and organ donation information
- Workers' compensation information
- Information regarding foodborne illness
- Information regarding problems with medical devices, drugs, and biological products

# Patient Education

Patient education is one of the most effective means of preventing disease transmission. As a medical assistant, you are in a pivotal position in relation to your patients. You can assess patients' understanding of their risk for infection, measures they must take to eradicate an infection (if possible), potential dangers posed by treatments, and methods for controlling an infection's spread. Staying up-to-date on new information will help you provide patients with effective, relevant education.

## Drug Trials

New drug treatments for HIV infection and AIDS are being tested every day. Some patients may be interested in information about clinical drug trials. **Clinical drug trials** are internationally recognized research protocols designed to evaluate the efficacy or safety of drugs and to produce scientifically valid results. According to your institution's protocol, you may be required to introduce certain patients to such programs or to monitor patients involved in drug trial programs. You can obtain information about drug trials from the AIDS Clinical Trials Information Service at 800-874-2572 or by visiting www.ClinicalTrials.gov.

## Patients With Special Concerns

You will be responsible for educating patients with a variety of needs and concerns. Some patients, particularly teenagers and patients about to be discharged from the hospital, may have specific concerns involving HIV and HBV infection.

## Teenagers

You may work with teenagers who have come in to obtain a means of birth control or receive treatment for sexually transmitted diseases (STDs). During the patient interview, you are in a position to educate the teenagers about the dangers of HIV and HBV infection. Most teenagers think that they are invincible and that disease happens only to "other people." You can effectively educate teenagers about HIV and HBV infection by helping them realize that disease can happen to anyone. Begin by establishing a trusting relationship with them and by providing them with facts rather than lectures or moral appeals. Figure 21-7 shows the various risk factors, or exposure categories, that are commonly implicated in the transmission of AIDS to male adolescents aged 13 to 19. Figure 21-8 provides similar information for females aged 13 to 19. In addition, the number of new HIV infections for male and female adolescents aged 13 to 19 can be found in Figure 21-9. Armed with data such as these, you can stress to teenage patients the importance of preventive behaviors in avoiding HIV infection (Figure 21-10).

**The Patient About to Be Discharged.** When a patient has been hospitalized with HBV or HIV infection, the disruption in his life often lingers long past the

HIV and AIDS Exposure Categories for Males Aged 13–24 (2005)

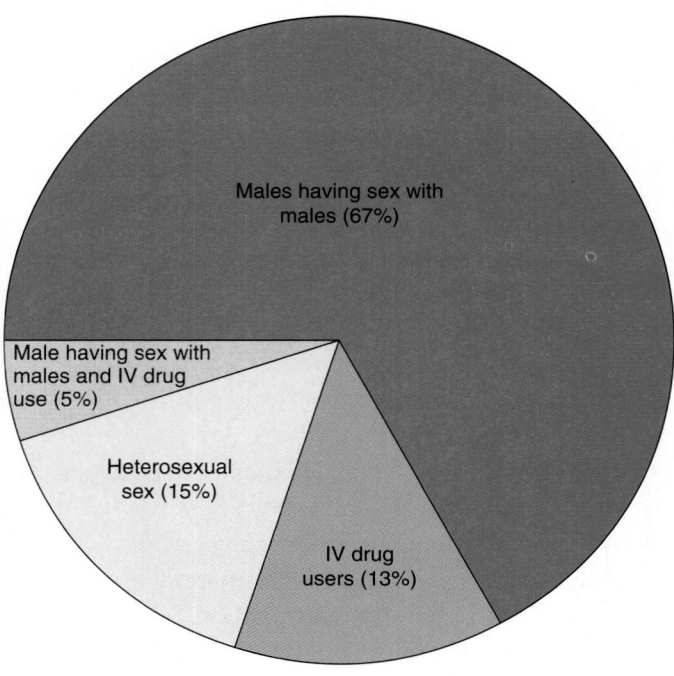

Males having sex with males (67%)

Male having sex with males and IV drug use (5%)

Heterosexual sex (15%)

IV drug users (13%)

**Figure 21-7.** These percentages provide insight into the types of exposure male teenagers should guard against.

HIV and AIDS Exposure Categories for Females Aged 13–24 (2005)

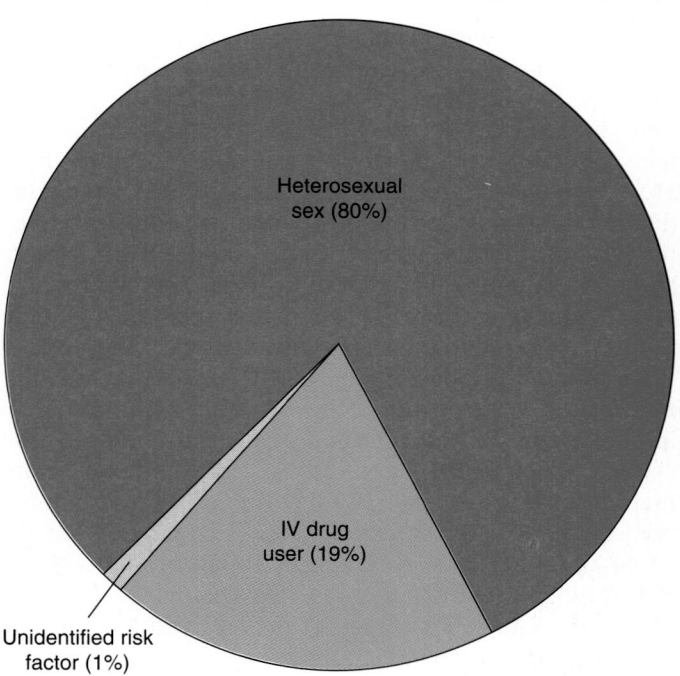

Heterosexual sex (80%)

IV drug user (19%)

Unidentified risk factor (1%)

**Figure 21-8.** Female teenagers face a greater risk of HIV infection from heterosexual contact than male teenagers do.

New HIV Diagnoses in Adolescents Age 13–19 (2004)

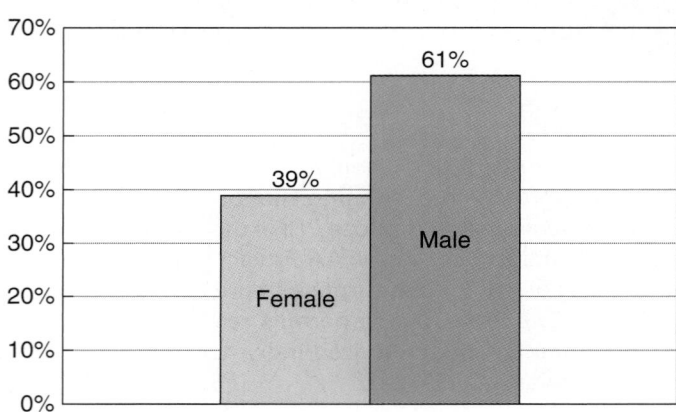

39% Female

61% Male

**Figure 21-9.** Male adolescents are at a higher risk of developing HIV than their female counterparts are.

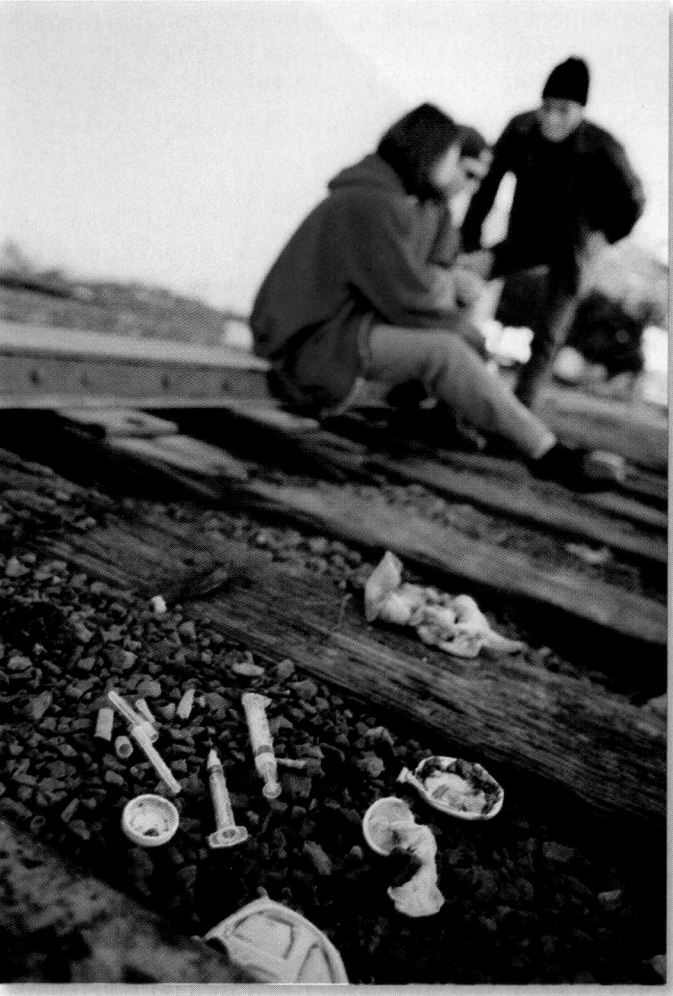

**Figure 21-10.** Teens should be educated about the variety of risks they may be exposed to and how to avoid them.

## Educating the Patient

### Obtaining Information About AIDS and Hepatitis

Some patients who have AIDS or hepatitis may want additional information about care options, drug treatments and clinical trials, prevention guidelines, risk factors, and therapy management. Many high-quality resources are available for these patients.

One of the best places to direct patients is to the Centers for Disease Control and Prevention, located in Atlanta, Georgia. The CDC offers a variety of services, such as the following:

- CDC National AIDS Clearinghouse (800-458-5231)
- CDC National AIDS Hotline (800-342-2437)
- AIDS Clinical Trials Information Service (800-874-2572)
- HIV/AIDS Treatment Information Service (800-448-0440)

- CDC Spanish AIDS Hotline (800-344-SIDA)
- CDC National Prevention Information Network (800-458-5231)

Patients who are comfortable using computers and who have access to the World Wide Web can find a variety of resources there. The website for the CDC (www.cdc.gov) is very comprehensive.

Many local support and resource organizations may also be available to the patient. Your local health department can assist you in finding these organizations. In your position you can serve both the patient, by helping him contact these organizations, and the organizations, by publicizing their efforts.

discharge date. He must make changes and continue some treatment when he goes home. Your job as a medical assistant is to make sure that the patient comes to the medical office for follow-up care, reports any adverse reactions to therapy or treatment, and knows which signs and symptoms to report to the doctor. You must also ensure that the patient knows what precautions to take to avoid transmitting the infection to others.

As part of the education process, the patient may request additional information from you, or you may need to provide information to the patient's family members or other caregivers. See the Educating the Patient section for suggestions on where to obtain information for patients and their families.

## Multicultural Concerns

Although you must be sensitive to and respectful toward patients from all backgrounds, you may need to target your education efforts toward certain groups. For example, according to the CDC's quarterly report, the incidence of HIV infection is increasing more in some groups than in others. Data in the report on the pattern of the disease can help you ascertain which groups need improved education. If you work with patients who are in these high-risk groups or who know people in them, you are in a unique position to provide them with information on preventive measures they can follow to avoid exposure to blood-borne pathogens. Because some patients may be reluctant to discuss sensitive subjects, be sure to have brochures available (in several languages) for them to take home and read.

## Special Issues With Terminal Illness

In this chapter you have learned about a variety of blood-borne diseases. One of these diseases is almost always fatal, and others may be fatal in certain situations. Just as you need to educate patients about preventing such diseases and about methods of treatment, you need to provide support and counsel to patients, their families, and their loved ones when they are informed that their illnesses are **terminal,** or fatal. You must understand something of people's reactions to a terminal diagnosis to help them cope with the situation.

Patients react to the idea of dying in different ways. Some are angry that death is coming to them. Others are grateful that relief from pain and suffering is near. Many terminal patients respond by denying that they are dying. After patients fully realize that they are going to die, depression is a common reaction. The only thing you can be certain of is that no two patients respond to a terminal diagnosis in exactly the same way.

You can help patients come to terms with the fact that they are going to die by:

- Supporting and accepting them no matter how they react
- Encouraging them to express their feelings and thoughts freely
- Communicating respect through your use of nonverbal communication, including your posture and touch

- Meeting reasonable needs and demands as quickly as possible
- Providing referrals to hospices, which offer a variety of services, including personal care for patients who are dying and emotional support for them and their families

## Summary

Infectious diseases are transmitted in many different ways. Medical and surgical asepsis and various techniques and procedures for sanitizing, disinfecting, and sterilizing instruments, equipment, and surfaces all help prevent disease transmission. Specific transmission methods dictate which approaches work best for which diseases. The focus of this chapter has been blood-borne transmission.

The transmission of blood-borne pathogens is a particular concern for medical assistants as well as for people in many other professions. The pathogens that pose the greatest risk are HIV, HBV, and HCV. Infection with these pathogens can result in death or chronic disease.

Your role as a medical assistant is to help prevent the spread of such infectious diseases. The preventive measures you will take at work include following Universal Precautions, watching patients for signs of infectious diseases, and educating patients about the risk factors associated with blood-borne diseases.

Information about infectious diseases changes constantly. You can best serve your patients and your employer if you keep up-to-date on research, advances in treatment, and general information. Your efforts with patient education may include information about preventive measures, drug trials, follow-up care, and hospices for terminally ill patients.

## CASE STUDY QUESTIONS

Now that you have completed this chapter, review the case study at the beginning of the chapter and answer the following questions:

1. What type of hepatitis does this patient probably have?
2. What are two medical terms for the yellowish discoloration you observed?
3. How long might the patient expect to suffer from the symptoms of the acute phase of the illness?
4. Could this disease have been prevented? If so, how?

## Discussion Questions

1. Describe the differences between the various forms of hepatitis and ways to prevent the transmission of each.
2. Discuss the various side effects of HIV/AIDS therapy and the challenges they pose to patient compliance.
3. Why do opportunistic infections pose such a risk to the HIV-infected patient?

## Critical Thinking Questions

1. During an interview, the patient asks you about HIV home testing. What information will you give the patient about these tests? Are there any cautions you should give the patient?
2. Accidental needlesticks are a risk to the medical community. What disease, HIV or hepatitis, is more likely to be contracted from an accidental needlestick from an infected patient? What can you do to protect yourself?
3. An HIV-positive patient mentions he will be traveling to a tropical part of Asia. What specific information should you give the patient about diseases in this area?

## Application Activities

1. Working in pairs, role-play a situation in which you are talking with a teenager about the risk factors of HBV, HCV, and HIV. Discuss ways a teen can avoid these risks. Have the class critique your performance.
2. Research your state's reporting guidelines for hepatitis and HIV. Report your findings to the class. Be sure to bring copies of any reporting forms so that your classmates can become familiar with them.
3. Identify resources in your area that a person might use if she is exposed to HIV. Explore what is available to patients at various points in the disease process. Prepare a brochure in which you identify the resources and what they provide.

## Virtual Fieldtrip

*Visit the McGraw-Hill Higher Education Medical Assisting website at www.mhhe.com/medicalassisting3 to complete the following activity:*

Using the recommended website, create an information sheet for your office that includes the following:

- Definition of a clinical trial
- Who can participate
- Benefits
- Risks
- How to search for clinical trials
- Current clinical trials for hepatitis and HIV occurring in your area

Open the CD and complete this chapter's practice activities, play the games, listen to the key terms, and test yourself with the interactive review. E-mail, print, and/or save your results to document your proficiency.

# Preparing the Exam and Treatment Areas

## KEY TERMS

accessibility
consumable
fixative
general physical exam
lubricant
occult blood
transcutaneous
absorption

## MEDICAL ASSISTING COMPETENCIES

*In preparation for the certification examination, you should know the following areas of competence:*

| COMPETENCY | CMA | RMA |
|---|---|---|
| **Clinical** | | |
| Apply principles of aseptic techniques and infection control, including hand washing | X | X |
| Perform sterilization techniques | X | X |
| Dispose of biohazardous materials | X | X |
| Practice Standard Precautions | X | X |
| Prepare and maintain exam and treatment areas | X | X |
| **General/Legal/Professional** | | |
| Perform risk management procedures | | X |
| Operate and maintain facilities, and perform routine maintenance of administrative and clinical equipment safely | X | X |
| Maintain the physical plant | | X |

## CHAPTER OUTLINE

- The Medical Assistant's Role in Preparing the Exam Room
- The Exam Room
- Cleanliness in the Exam Room
- Room Temperature, Lighting, and Ventilation
- Medical Instruments and Supplies
- Physical Safety in the Exam Room

## LEARNING OUTCOMES

After completing Chapter 22, you will be able to:

**22.1** Explain the medical assistant's role in preparing the exam room.
**22.2** Describe the layout and features of a typical exam room.
**22.3** Describe steps to prevent the spread of infection in the exam room.
**22.4** Explain how and when to disinfect exam room surfaces.

**22.5** Describe the importance of such factors as temperature, lighting, and ventilation in the exam room.

**22.6** Identify instruments and supplies used in a general physical exam, and tell how to arrange and prepare them.

**22.7** Explain how to eliminate hazards to physical safety in the exam room.

# Introduction

One of the most important tasks you encounter as a practicing medical assistant is the preparation of the exam room and treatment area. In this chapter you will learn about the common layouts of exam rooms; keeping the rooms clean and stocked with instruments and disposable and consumable supplies; maintaining the comfort of the room; and making the room safe for patients and coworkers. You will also be introduced to the requirements for accessibility established by the Americans With Disabilities Act.

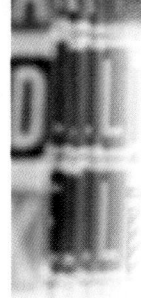

## CASE STUDY

As a medical assistant, you are reviewing the charts as you prepare for the next day's appointments, and you notice that a female patient who is scheduled for her routine gynecological checkup has a flag on her chart because she has bilateral cataracts.

As you read this chapter, consider the following questions:

1. What are bilateral cataracts, and why would this condition be a consideration when you come in contact with this patient?
2. What instruments should be assembled for the physician to use during the exam?
3. What disposable and consumable supplies may reasonably be anticipated for use?
4. What measures can you take to ensure the patient's comfort and safety?

# The Medical Assistant's Role in Preparing the Exam Room

When a patient enters an exam room, the patient expects to find it clean and neat. The doctor assumes that all medical instruments and supplies necessary for an exam or treatment are ready to use. Preparing the exam room for patients and doctors is your responsibility. You must keep this room not only spotlessly clean and in good order but also free from obstacles that might cause an accidental injury. Safety, efficiency, and comfort are the main concerns in the exam room.

# The Exam Room

The exam room is the area where the physician observes the patient, listens to the patient's description of symptoms, performs a general physical exam, and dispenses treatment. A physician performs a **general physical exam** to confirm a patient's health or diagnose a medical problem. Figure 22-1 shows a typical exam room.

# Number and Size of Rooms

The number of exam rooms in a medical office depends on the number of doctors who work there and on each doctor's patient load. Ideally, each doctor in a medical office

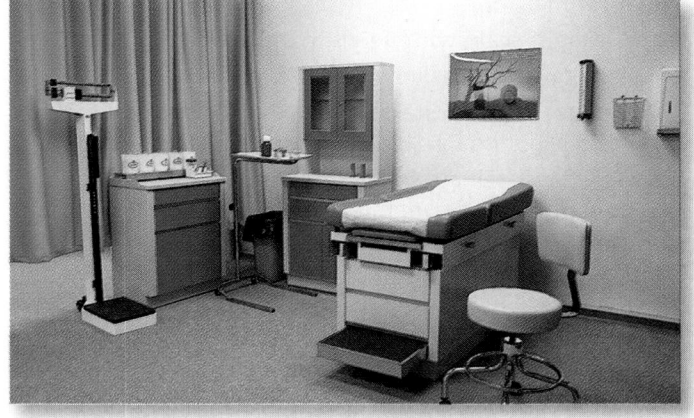

**Figure 22-1.** You are responsible for making sure the exam room is clean and orderly.

has at least two exam rooms for her or his exclusive use. A minimum of two rooms per doctor enables the medical assistant to prepare one room while the doctor examines a patient in the other room.

The customary size for an exam room is 8 by 12 feet. The room should be large enough to accommodate the doctor, the patient, and one assistant comfortably. At the same time, it should be small enough that instruments and supplies will be within easy reach. Doors and interior walls should be soundproofed to ensure privacy for patients.

Some exam rooms have dressing cubicles in one corner. Other rooms have screens in one corner, behind which the patient may disrobe. Regardless of a room's layout, you should provide privacy for patients whenever they need to disrobe and put on gowns.

A rack for the patient's medical records usually hangs on the wall directly outside the exam room or on the outside of the door. A light or other device on the wall or door may be used to signal that the room is occupied.

## Furnishings

Furnishings should be arranged for efficiency, the convenience of the physician, and the comfort of the patient. The examining table is the key piece of equipment in the exam room. It should be positioned in the center of the room or coming out from the wall. This arrangement allows the physician and an assistant to attend to the patient on at least three sides. The examining table usually contains a pullout step for the patient to use when getting onto the table. It may also contain drawers for storing instruments and table coverings.

Examining tables are usually adjustable to enable the patient to assume the various positions that the physical exam may require. The physician will probably tell you beforehand if you need to adjust the table in a particular way.

Most exam rooms also have a sink, a countertop, and a writing surface large enough to spread out the patient's records. Shelves, cupboards, and drawers store routine supplies such as dressings, adhesive tape, and bandages. The exam room may also include the following items:

- One or more chairs
- A rolling stool
- A weight scale with height bar
- A metal wastebasket with a lid
- Biohazardous waste containers for disposal of biohazardous materials (biological agents that can spread disease to living things)
- Puncture-proof containers for disposal of biohazardous sharps
- A high-intensity lamp
- Wall brackets for hanging instruments

## Special Features

The Americans With Disabilities Act of 1990 (ADA) requires that businesses, services, and public transportation provide "reasonable accommodations" for the disabled. To comply with this act, the exam room in a medical office must have features that make the area accessible to patients who use wheelchairs or who have visual or other types of physical impairments. **Accessibility** refers to the ease with which people can move in and out of a space. The ADA accessibility guidelines require the following:

- A doorway at least 36 inches (915 mm) wide to allow a person in a wheelchair to pass through
- A clearance space in rooms and hallways that is 60 inches (1525 mm) in diameter to allow a person in a wheelchair to make a 180-degree turn
- Stable, firm, slip-resistant flooring
- Door-opening hardware that can be grasped with one hand and does not require the twisting of the wrist to use
- Door closers adjusted to allow time for a person in a wheelchair to enter or exit through the door
- Grab bars in the lavatory

# Cleanliness in the Exam Room

As you learned in Chapter 20, you can follow specific measures to achieve medical asepsis and prevent the spread of pathogenic microorganisms in the medical office. These measures involve strict housekeeping standards and adherence to government guidelines.

A clean exam room is extremely important in preventing the spread of infectious diseases to patients and health-care workers. Part of your job is to carefully follow infection-control procedures in the medical office and to keep the exam room clean and neat.

## Infection Control

People with a variety of contagious diseases visit medical offices every day. The potential for the spread of infection is thus higher in medical offices than in most other places. For that reason, you must be especially careful to follow infection-control procedures at work. You can safeguard the health of staff members and patients by:

- Making hand washing a priority
- Keeping the examining table clean
- Disinfecting all work surfaces

**Hand Washing.** Clean hands are the first step in preventing infection transmission in the exam room. Wash your hands with disinfectant soap and warm water at the following times:

- At the beginning of the day
- Before and after having contact with each patient
- Before and after using gloves or performing any procedure

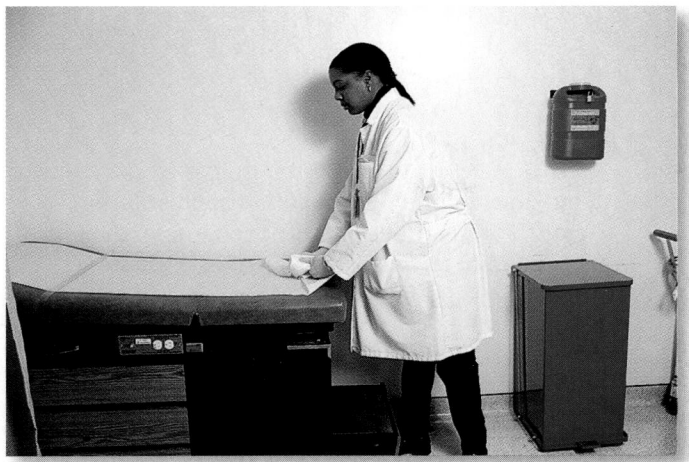

**Figure 22-2.** When you remove the cover from the examining table, roll it up tightly and quickly. Then carefully prepare it for disposal.

- Before handling clean or sterile supplies
- Before and after eating or taking a break
- Before and after using the bathroom
- After blowing your nose, coughing, or sneezing
- Before and after handling specimens or waste
- Before leaving for the day

After washing your hands, use a clean paper towel to handle faucets or doorknobs. The paper towel helps you avoid contaminating your clean hands with microorganisms. (See Procedure 20-1 in Chapter 20 for the steps in performing aseptic hand washing.)

**Examining Table.** The disposable paper that covers the examining table provides a barrier to infection during an exam. Always change the covering after each use (Figure 22-2). Your office might use precut lengths, or you might need to tear off a piece from a roll of paper. Cover pillows with fresh paper. Also, provide tissues or special wipes for patients who need to wipe away excess **lubricant** (a water-soluble gel used during an exam of the rectum or vaginal cavity) after certain procedures.

When you remove the used covering from the examining table, roll it up quickly and carefully. You should have a small, tight bundle of paper when you finish. Crumpling the paper haphazardly or shaking it in the air stirs up dust and microorganisms and can spread infection.

Dispose of used paper coverings soiled by body fluids, especially blood, in a biohazardous waste container. (Refer to Chapter 20 for specific guidelines for disposing of hazardous items.) Used coverings with no visible fluids may be disposed of according to the procedures established by your office. Place soiled linen cloths and pillowcases in biohazard-labeled bags for sending to a laundry for cleaning.

**Surfaces.** You are responsible for disinfecting work surfaces in the exam room, including the examining table,

sink, and countertop. As you learned in Chapter 20, disinfection involves exposing all parts of a surface to a disinfectant such as a 10% solution of household bleach in water or a product approved by the Environmental Protection Agency (EPA). Surfaces must be disinfected at the following times:

- After an exam or treatment during which surfaces have become visibly contaminated with tissue, blood, or other body fluids
- Immediately following accidental blood or body fluid spills or splatter
- At the end of your work shift

Clean and disinfect the toilet and sink in the patient lavatory, and inspect and disinfect reusable receptacles such as wastebaskets on a regular basis. In most offices these tasks are performed once a day. You must, however, follow the schedule established by your office. Procedure 22-1 describes how to disinfect work surfaces, floors, and equipment in the exam room. Replace protective coverings on equipment or surfaces that were exposed to blood, other body fluids, or tissue during the exam.

**Storage.** During the exam, you may need to collect biohazardous specimens, such as blood or urine, from the patient for testing. You are responsible for storing these specimens properly. See the Caution: Handle With Care section for guidelines to follow when storing biohazardous materials.

Storage of testing kits and specimens often involves refrigeration as a means of preservation. Adequate preservation requires maintaining careful control of the temperature in a refrigerator. Read the Caution: Handle With Care section for more information on preventing spoilage by controlling refrigerator temperature.

## Putting the Room in Order

After ensuring that the examining table is clean, all surfaces are properly disinfected, and all necessary items are stored, take time to straighten the exam room and put things in order. A neatly arranged room boosts patient confidence and supports the impression of a well-run office. It also contributes to the physical safety of patients and staff. Tasks include the following:

- Putting the rolling stool in its place
- Pushing in the examining-table step
- Returning supplies to containers
- Securing prescription pads and sample medications that may have been left out

## Housekeeping

Medical offices usually contract with a janitorial service for after-hours cleaning. Janitorial services perform general cleaning tasks such as emptying wastebaskets, vacuuming carpets, scrubbing floors, dusting furniture, washing windows, and cleaning blinds. To be sure that the service

# Guidelines for Disinfecting Exam Room Surfaces

**Procedure Goal:** To reduce the risk of exposure to potentially infectious microorganisms in the exam room

**OSHA Guidelines:**

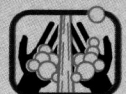 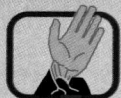 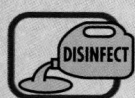

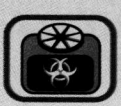 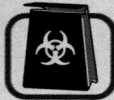 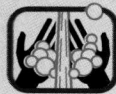

**Materials:** Utility gloves, disinfectant (10% bleach solution or EPA-approved disinfecting product), paper towels, dustpan and brush, tongs, forceps, clean sponge or heavy rag

**Method:**

1. Wash your hands and put on utility gloves.
2. Remove any visible soil from exam room surfaces with disposable paper towels or a rag.

*Rationale*

Removing visible soil first allows for better penetration of the disinfectant.

3. Thoroughly wipe all surfaces with the disinfectant.
4. In the event of an accident involving a broken glass container, use tongs, a dustpan and brush, or forceps to pick up shattered glass, which may be contaminated (Figure 22-3).

*Rationale*

Using your fingers to pick up broken glass puts you at risk for exposure to blood-borne pathogens.

5. Remove and replace protective coverings, such as plastic wrap or aluminum foil, on equipment if the equipment or the coverings have become contaminated. After removing the coverings, disinfect the equipment and allow it to air-dry. (Follow office procedures for the routine changing of protective coverings.)
6. When you finish cleaning, dispose of the paper towels or rags in a biohazardous waste receptacle. (This step is especially important if you are cleaning surfaces contaminated with blood, body fluids, or tissue.)
7. Remove the gloves and wash your hands.

8. If you keep a container of 10% bleach solution on hand for disinfection purposes, replace the solution daily to ensure its disinfecting potency (Figure 22-4).

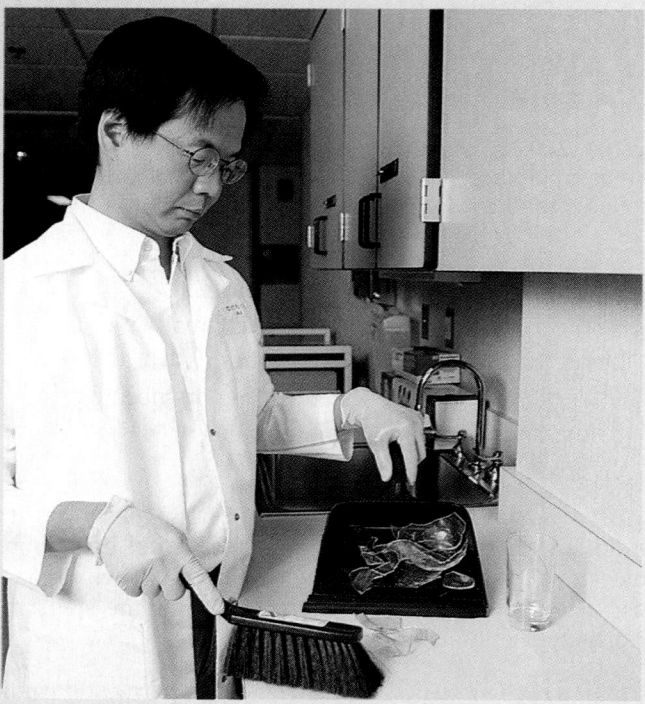

**Figure 22-3.** Because broken glass may be contaminated, never pick it up directly with your hands. Use a brush and dustpan, tongs, or forceps to clean it up.

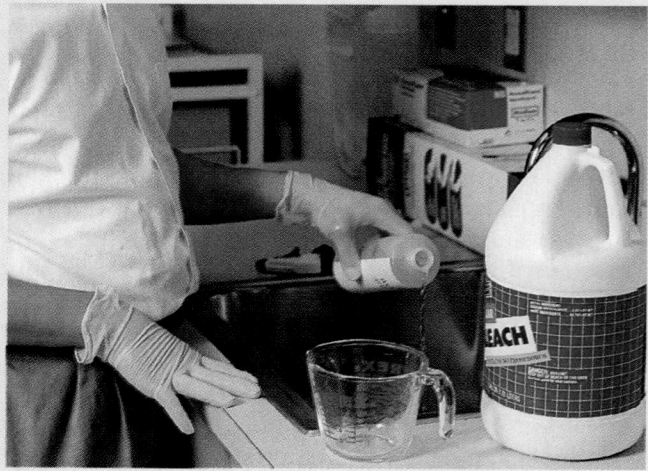

**Figure 22-4.** Replace the bleach solution each day to ensure its disinfecting potency.

## CAUTION *Handle With Care*

## Storing Biohazardous Materials

During a general physical exam, the physician may ask you to collect various types of specimens from the patient for testing in the laboratory. These specimens must be handled and stored properly because they have the potential to be biohazards. Exposure that can spread disease may occur through the following routes:

- Inhalation (breathing)
- Ingestion (swallowing)
- **Transcutaneous absorption** (absorption through a cut or crack in the skin)

Occupational Safety and Health Administration (OSHA) regulations require storing biohazardous materials separately from food and beverages. You must not place food and beverages in refrigerators, freezers, or cabinets where blood or other potentially infectious materials are present or put specimens in a refrigerator that is otherwise used to store food and beverages.

There are several reasons why it is dangerous to put food or beverages in the laboratory refrigerator. If a biohazardous substance is not clearly labeled and you are in a hurry, you might accidentally ingest it. There is always the possibility that containers of biohazardous substances might leak or spill or that residue from the hazardous material might not have been thoroughly cleaned from the outside of containers. This residue could lead to contamination of food or beverages.

OSHA regulations require that a warning label containing the biohazard symbol be clearly and securely posted on the outside of refrigerators, freezers, and cabinets where biohazardous materials are stored. The government also recommends keeping the laboratory refrigerator and the refrigerator for the employees' personal use in separate rooms. These measures help prevent employees from accidentally putting food and beverages in the wrong place.

OSHA regulations also prohibit medical personnel from doing any of the following activities in a room where potentially infectious materials are present:

- Eating
- Drinking
- Smoking
- Chewing gum
- Applying cosmetics
- Handling contact lenses
- Chewing pencils or pens
- Rubbing eyes

These work practice controls, like all OSHA regulations, represent safeguards to protect workers against the health hazards of blood-borne pathogens.

## CAUTION *Handle With Care*

## Refrigerator Temperature Control

Health inspectors visit medical facilities periodically to check that health and safety standards are being upheld. One of the first things they check is the temperature of refrigerators. To prevent spoilage or deterioration of testing kits, blood specimens, and other stored materials, the temperature of the laboratory refrigerator should be maintained between 36°F and 46°F (2°C and 8°C). Keep a thermometer in the laboratory refrigerator to monitor the temperature.

Similar guidelines apply to the refrigerator in the employee area. Food spoils quickly in a refrigerator if the temperature is not low enough. The temperature of the food refrigerator should be maintained between 32°F and 40°F (0°C and 4.4°C). In addition to monitoring the temperature, make sure that food is not stored in the refrigerator too long. All food containers—including brown bags containing lunches—should be dated and thrown out when their freshness has expired. You can prevent the growth of bacteria by wiping up food spills immediately and cleaning the interior and exterior of the refrigerator routinely.

Follow office procedures for the routine cleaning of both laboratory and food refrigerators and for the proper maintenance of the temperature of the refrigerators' contents while the refrigerators' interiors are cleaned. Specimens, for example, must be kept at a specific temperature at all times. For documentation purposes, keep a log of dates when the laboratory refrigerator is cleaned.

cleans and sanitizes all areas adequately, you need to work with your employer to develop and implement a cleaning schedule. Take into account the types of surfaces to be cleaned, the type of contamination present, and the tasks or procedures to be performed.

You may be responsible for assigning housekeeping chores to janitorial workers. If so, you will need to monitor their work and let the service know if there are any lapses in cleanliness. You may also do some housekeeping chores yourself, such as damp dusting an open shelf. Because dust harbors bacteria and allergens, it is important to keep the exam rooms as dust-free as possible.

# Room Temperature, Lighting, and Ventilation

No patient wants to sit in an exam room that looks unkempt. Nor do patients feel comfortable in a room that is cold, dimly lit, or stuffy. Adjusting the temperature, lighting, and ventilation is part of keeping the exam room in good order and fit for use.

## Room Temperature

Because patients may be wearing only a thin paper gown or drape while in the exam room, you must be sure the exam room is warm enough. Set the thermostat to maintain the temperature at approximately 72°F, and make sure there are no drafts from windows or doors. Patients often feel anxious while waiting for the doctor, and a warm room can help them relax.

## Lighting

Good lighting is required to make accurate diagnoses, to correctly carry out medical procedures, and to read orders and instructions. A well-lit room also helps prevent accidents.

Adjust room lights and blinds or drapes as necessary in preparation for an exam. If there is an exam lamp with a movable arm, be sure the arm is positioned appropriately. Replace all burned-out light bulbs as soon as possible.

## Ventilation

The air in the exam area should smell fresh and clean. From time to time, you may have to deal with offensive odors from urine, vomitus, body odors, or laboratory chemicals. First you must eliminate the source of the odor, especially if the source is potentially infectious or toxic. Then you can take steps to remove the odor.

Some exam rooms have a ventilation system with a filter that absorbs odors. If the rooms in your office do not, you may be able to turn on a high-speed blower to vent room air to the outside. In some cases an open window and a fan may be sufficient to freshen the air. Remember to check the room temperature after using fresh-air approaches to odor control.

If necessary, you can temporarily mask unpleasant odors with a room deodorizer or spray. Some sprays also help kill germs. Be careful that the room deodorizer you choose does not have a strong odor.

# Medical Instruments and Supplies

Doctors require various instruments and supplies to perform an exam or procedure. Instruments are tools or implements doctors use for particular purposes. Disposable instruments are often referred to as supplies.

You must maintain all instruments and supplies needed in the exam room. This responsibility involves the following three tasks:

1. Ordering and stocking all supplies needed for exams and treatment procedures
2. Keeping the instruments sanitized, disinfected, or sterilized (as appropriate) and in working order
3. Ensuring that all instruments and supplies are placed where the doctor can easily reach them

## Instruments Used in a General Physical Exam

Many of the instruments physicians use are made of fine-grade stainless steel and are reusable. Some of these instruments may have disposable parts.

Physicians also use a number of disposable instruments, such as curettes and needles, because these instruments are both convenient and sanitary. As discussed in Chapter 20, you must discard used disposable instruments and supplies according to OSHA guidelines. Place any such items contaminated with blood or other body fluids in biohazardous waste containers.

Commonly used instruments are shown in Figure 22-5.

- An anoscope is used to open the anus for an exam.
- An exam light provides an additional source of light during the exam. It is usually on a flexible arm to permit light to be directed to the area being examined.
- A laryngeal mirror reflects the inside of the mouth and throat for exam purposes.
- A nasal speculum is used to enlarge the opening of the nose to permit viewing. This type of speculum may consist of a reusable handle with a disposable speculum tip, or it may be a disposable one-piece unit.
- An ophthalmoscope is a lighted instrument that is used to examine the inner structures of the eye.
- An otoscope is used to examine the ear canal and the tympanic membrane. The otoscope consists of a light source, a magnifying lens, and an ear speculum. An otoscope may also be used to examine the nostrils and the anterior sinuses.

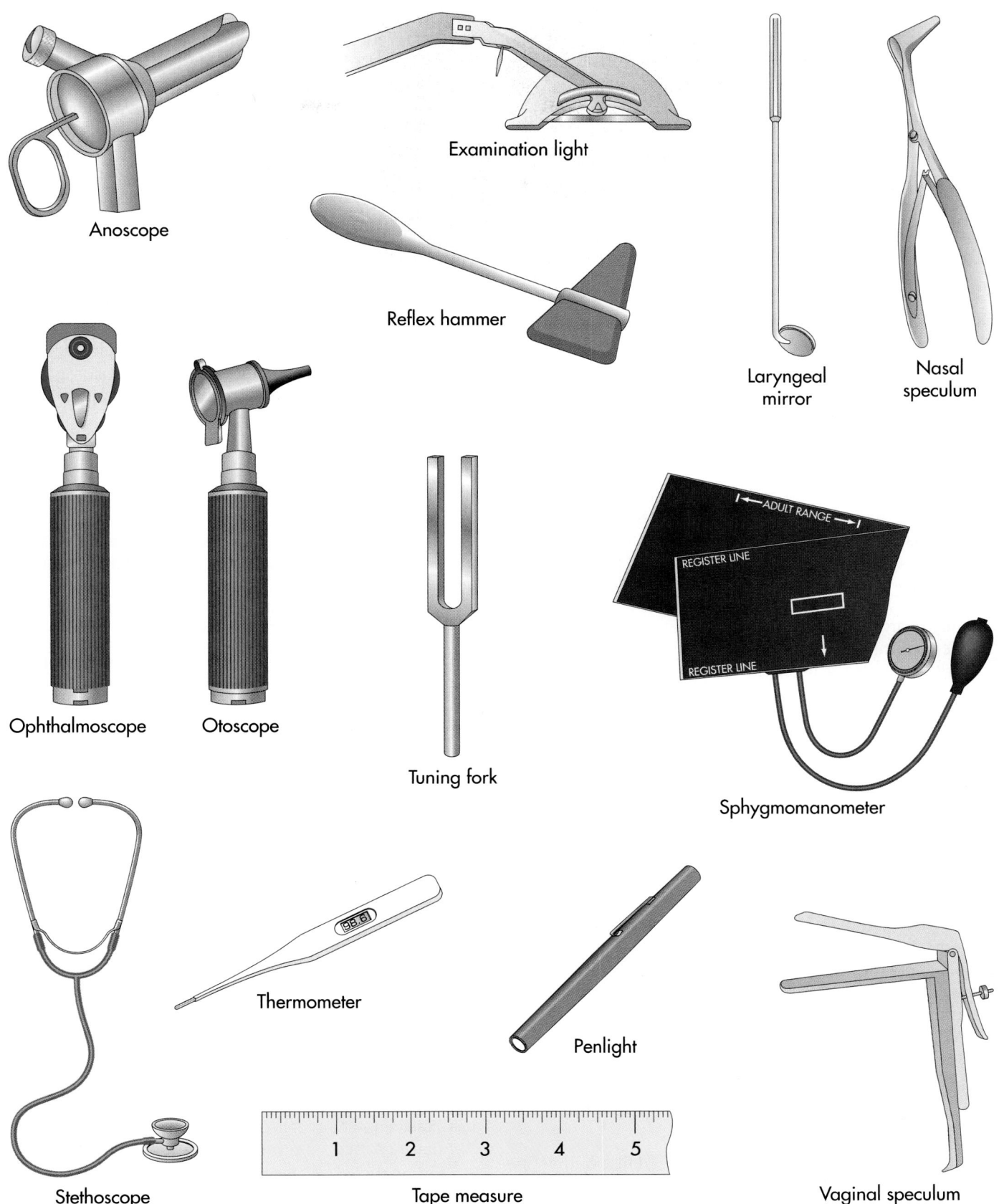

**Figure 22-5.** These instruments may be used in a general physical exam.

Anoscope

Examination light

Reflex hammer

Laryngeal mirror

Nasal speculum

Ophthalmoscope

Otoscope

Tuning fork

Sphygmomanometer

ADULT RANGE

REGISTER LINE

REGISTER LINE

Stethoscope

Thermometer

Tape measure

Penlight

Vaginal speculum

- A penlight is a small flashlight used when additional light is necessary in a small area. It may also be used to check pupil response in the eye.
- A reflex hammer has a hard-rubber triangular head. It is used to check a patient's reflexes.
- A sphygmomanometer is a piece of equipment used to measure blood pressure and is commonly referred to as a blood pressure cuff.
- A stethoscope is used to listen to body sounds. It is described in more detail in Chapter 24.
- A tape measure is a long, narrow strip of fabric, marked off in inches and sometimes in centimeters, used to measure size or development of an area or part of the body.
- A thermometer is used to measure body temperature.
- A tuning fork tests patients' hearing.
- A vaginal speculum is used to enlarge the vagina to make the vagina and the cervix accessible for visual exam and specimen collection.

**Inspecting and Maintaining Instruments.** Prior to the exam, make sure that all instruments are sanitized, disinfected, or sterilized (as appropriate) and that they are in good working order. (See Chapter 20 for a description of the types of instruments requiring sanitization, disinfection, or sterilization and of the methods used for each.) For example, test the lights on the otoscope and ophthalmoscope to make sure that the lights work. Place all rechargeable batteries in a battery charger when the instruments are not in use.

Medical instruments are expensive and are designed to work in precise ways. Read the manufacturers' directions so that you are familiar with the care and maintenance of various instruments. Routinely check instruments for chipping and rusting, and report to the doctor any instruments that need repair or replacement.

**Arranging Instruments.** The doctor must be able to find and reach instruments easily during an exam. You can assist by placing instruments in the same place for every exam or by arranging them in the order the doctor will use them.

Doctors usually begin a general physical exam by examining the patient's head and face and working down the body. They may want instruments placed in that order. Other doctors may have individual preferences about how they want instruments arranged. In any case, make certain you know each doctor's preferences.

With the exception of the stethoscope, which most doctors carry with them, instruments are kept in one of three places during an exam:

1. Mounted on the wall (sphygmomanometer, some otoscopes and ophthalmoscopes)
2. Set out on the countertop (penlight, reflex hammer, tape measure, tuning fork, thermometer, some otoscopes and ophthalmoscopes)
3. Set on a clean (or sterile, if appropriate) towel or tray (anoscope, laryngeal mirror, nasal speculum, vaginal speculum)

**Preparing Instruments.** You must prepare some instruments before they can be used. For example, you may need to warm a vaginal speculum by holding it under warm water just prior to the exam. You might warm the mirrored end of the laryngeal mirror with water or over an alcohol lamp. You can also spray it with a special spray that prevents fogging. Any time you will be handling instruments, you must first wash your hands. If the instruments are sterile, you must also wear sterile gloves.

**Cleaning Instruments.** After the exam, put used instruments in a container and take them to the cleaning area. Always handle instruments carefully, because mishandling can alter their precision. Dispose of supplies in the appropriate containers, and use approved procedures for sanitizing, disinfecting, and sterilizing reusable instruments and equipment. Refer to Table 22-1 for general guidelines on cleaning instruments. (See Chapter 20 for detailed information on this topic.)

## Supplies for a General Physical Exam

Supplies for a general physical exam may be either disposable or consumable. Figure 22-6 shows various types of supplies.

Disposable supplies are items that are used once and discarded. They include the following:

- Cervical scraper (a wooden scraper used to obtain samples of cervical secretions)
- Cotton balls
- Cotton-tipped applicators
- Curettes
- Disposable needles
- Disposable syringes
- Gauze, dressings, and bandages
- Glass slides
- Gloves, both sterile and exam (nonsterile) types
- Paper tissues
- Prepared paper slides used to test the stool for the presence of **occult blood** (blood not visible to the naked eye)
- Specimen containers
- Tongue depressors

**Consumable** supplies are items that can be emptied or used up in an exam. These items include the following:

- **Fixative** (a chemical spray used for preserving a specimen obtained from the body for pathologic exam)
- Isopropyl alcohol (for cleansing skin)
- Lubricant

As they do with instruments, doctors may have a preferred arrangement of supplies for the general physical exam. Figure 22-7 shows a typical arrangement of instruments.

## TABLE 22-1 General Guidelines for Cleaning Instruments

| Process | Guidelines* | Instruments |
|---------|-------------|-------------|
| Sanitization | • Use detergent, or as indicated by the manufacturer<br>• Applies to instruments that do not touch the patient or that touch only intact skin<br>• Disinfect these instruments with blood or body fluids | Ophthalmoscope<br>Otoscope<br>Penlight<br>Reflex hammer<br>Sphygmomanometer<br>Stethoscope<br>Tape measure<br>Tuning fork |
| Disinfection | • Use only EPA-approved chemical or a 10% bleach solution to kill infectious agents outside the body<br>• Applies to instruments that touch intact mucous membranes but do not penetrate the patient's body surfaces | Laryngeal mirror<br>Nasal speculum |
| Sterilization | • Use an autoclave or approved method to kill all microorganisms<br>• Applies to instruments that penetrate the skin or contact normally sterile areas of the body | Anoscope<br>Curette<br>Needle<br>Syringe<br>Vaginal speculum |

*Keep in mind that these guidelines are general. Each office may have its own methods and schedule for cleaning instruments, depending on the office's specialty.

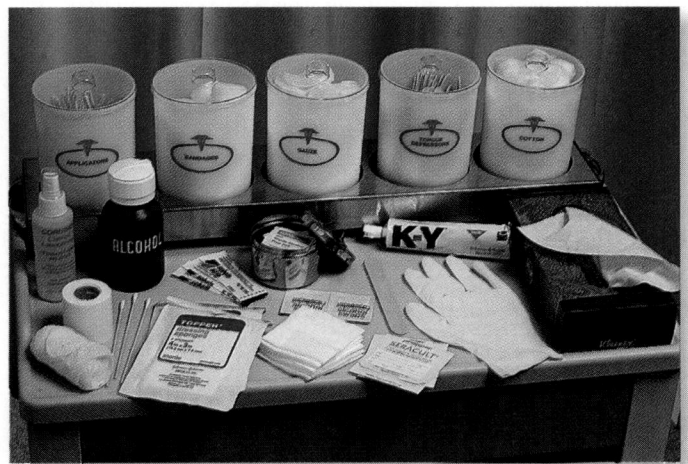

**Figure 22-6.** These supplies may be used in a general physical exam.

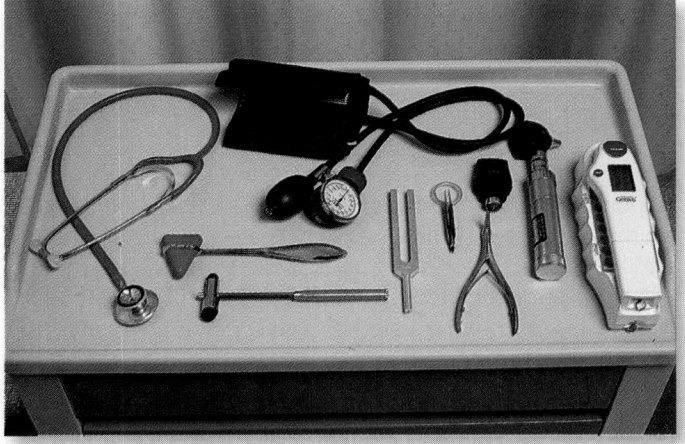

**Figure 22-7.** Arrange the instruments for a general physical exam so that they are convenient for the doctor.

Keep supplies such as prescription blanks, drugs (especially narcotics), and needles in a locked cabinet away from the patient exam areas. Make sure that patients do not have access to these items.

**Storing Supplies.** You can use the cabinets and drawers in the exam room to store nonperishable supplies. You should store every item in its own place so that you can find it quickly. You might even color-code or label drawers so that you can easily locate items. You should store supplies that come in various sizes, such as bandages, according to size. You need to routinely straighten and clean the insides of all cabinets and drawers in the exam room.

**Restocking Supplies.** To be sure you have a sufficient quantity of items on hand, order new supplies well in advance of needing them. A good guideline to follow is to order a new supply when the first half of a box, tube, or bottle has been used up. A record-keeping system will help you determine which supplies you need to restock most frequently and how long it takes for new supplies to arrive. The information you should keep track of to develop such a system includes the following:

- The types of supplies your office uses
- The quantities of each type of supply you use in a given amount of time, such as a month
- The frequency with which you must reorder particular supplies
- The names of various suppliers, along with the amount of time it takes to receive your orders

# Physical Safety in the Exam Room

Accidents can happen in the exam room. For example, patients and staff members can fall or cut themselves. You have an important responsibility to remove or correct hazards that might cause injury to patients, physicians, or staff members. This responsibility constitutes an integral part of a risk management plan.

## Maintaining a Safe Environment

It is easier to maintain a safe environment if you pay special attention to the following areas in the exam room:

- Floor
- Cabinets and drawers
- Furniture
- Cords and cables

**Floor.** You can take several measures to prevent falls. Wipe or mop up spills immediately. Clear the floor of dropped objects. If the floor is carpeted, make sure there are no snags or tears that could cause someone to trip and fall. Spilled medications, chemicals, and other substances pose a threat to young children, who may ingest anything they find on the floor. Destroy and dispose of medications that are accidentally dropped on the floor.

**Cabinets and Drawers.** Close overhead cabinet doors promptly after removing supplies. Leaving cabinet doors open can result in injury. In addition, an open cabinet door leaves supplies exposed to patients. Make sure drawers are kept closed so that no one bumps into them.

**Furniture.** Routinely inspect the furniture in the exam room and reception area. Make sure there are no rough edges or sharp corners on the examining table, countertop, chairs, or other furniture. If you are not authorized to repair or replace unsafe pieces of furniture, bring them to the attention of your supervisor.

**Cords and Cables.** Electrical cords and medical and office equipment cables should run along the walls and should be taped or fastened down securely. Replace tape on cords and cables when it becomes worn.

# Special Safety Precautions

Some patients, such as children and people with disabilities, may be particularly susceptible to accidents in your office. You need to take special precautions to ensure their safety.

**Children.** Keep sharp instruments out of the reach of children and store toxic items in high cabinets. Also, keep all medications and objects out of the reach of young children, because children are likely to pick up items and put them in their mouths and could choke or be poisoned.

If children's toys and books are kept in the reception area or exam room, make sure they are picked up when not in use and stored safely. Toys should be washable and made of safe materials. (Sanitize daily those toys that children put in their mouths; sanitize other toys weekly. If well children and sick children use the same reception area or exam room, sanitize and disinfect toys after sick children play with them.) Periodically check toys for sharp edges that might cause cuts. Make sure toys do not have small parts or pieces that could cause choking if swallowed. Figure 22-8 shows an appropriate toy for the medical office reception area or exam room.

**Patients With Physical Disabilities.** Patients with disabilities are more likely than other patients to fall. Some patients may use walkers or canes for support, whereas others may simply be unsteady on their feet. Patients with disabilities may need assistance disrobing prior to an exam or redressing afterward. For safety reasons, severely disabled patients should not be left alone in an exam room. You should check the office policies for guidelines regarding appropriate chaperones for patients with disabilities. Patients with vision impairments may have difficulty seeing obstacles, stairs, and other potential hazards. Safe flooring and handrails in the reception area, bathroom, hallways, and exam room help ensure the safety of patients with impaired mobility or vision.

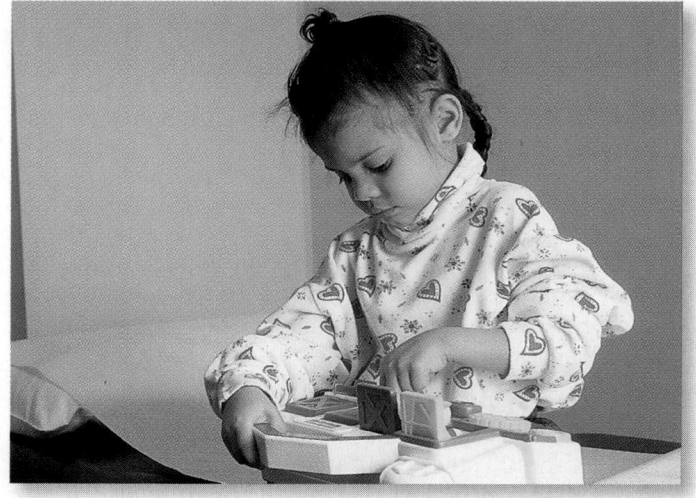

**Figure 22-8.** Toys provided must be safe for children of all ages.

# PROCEDURE 22.2

## Making the Exam Room Safe for Patients With Visual Impairments

**Procedure Goal:** To ensure that patients with visual impairments are safe in the exam room

**OSHA Guidelines:** This procedure does not involve exposure to blood, body fluids, or tissue.

**Materials:** Reflective tape, if needed

**Method:**

1. Make sure the hallway leading to the exam room is clear of obstacles.

   *Rationale*

   So that the patient does not trip over something unseen

2. Increase the amount of lighting in the room. Adjust the shades on windows in the room—if there are any windows—to allow for maximum natural light. Turn on all lights, especially those under cabinets, to dispel shadows.

   *Rationale*

   Many visually impaired individuals can see light and shadow. Allowing for maximum light increases the likelihood that the patient will see anything in her path.

3. Clear a path along which the patient can walk through the room. Make sure the chairs are out of the way. If there is a scale in the room, position it out of the path. If there is a step stool for the examining table, place it right up against the table.

4. Make sure the floor is not slippery.

5. Remove furniture that might be easily tipped over, such as a visitors' chair that is lightweight. If the physician will use an exam chair, push it out of the way.

6. Provide a sturdy chair with arms and a straight back to make it easier for the patient to sit down and stand up.

7. A wide strip of reflective tape will make the examining-table step visible for all patients. Apply it to the step's edge if tape is not there already. If your office uses a step stool instead of a step, make sure the tape on the stool is facing out.

8. Alert the patient to protruding equipment or furnishings.

9. Arrange the supplies for the patient, such as gowns or drapes, with the following guideline in mind: It is easier to see light objects against dark objects or dark objects against light objects than light objects against light objects or dark objects against dark objects. If, for example, there is a dressing cubicle, lay the light-colored gown or drape against a dark bench instead of hanging the gown or drape against a light wall.

   *Rationale*

   Visually impaired individuals can see objects more easily on a contrasting surface.

---

Procedure 22-2 explains how to make the exam room safe for visually impaired patients.

## Fire Safety

Fire is a safety hazard anywhere, but it is especially likely where there is sophisticated, high-voltage medical equipment—such as an x-ray machine. Any electrical instrument in the exam room, however, is a potential fire hazard. Other potentially hazardous items are gas tanks and flammable chemicals.

**Fire Prevention.** Be aware of anything that might cause a fire in the exam room. If you cannot correct the situation yourself, report the hazard to your supervisor.

Be alert to the following potential hazards:

- Frayed electrical wires, overloaded outlets, and improperly grounded plugs. These present a danger of electric

shock and fire. Contact a licensed electrician to remedy these problems.

- Materials that are extremely flammable, including alcohol and some disinfectants. Supplies such as paper table coverings can also ignite and spread flames quickly in the event of a fire. Check to make sure that all such items are stored and disposed of properly to minimize the fire danger. Flammable liquids should never be kept near a heat source. If you are not sure whether a chemical is flammable, read the manufacturer's label or Material Safety Data Sheet. (Material Safety Data Sheets are discussed in Chapter 32.)

- Smoking. Smoking should not be permitted anywhere in a medical facility. In addition to causing health problems, smoking is a fire hazard. "No Smoking" signs should be posted prominently throughout the office.

- Inoperative smoke detectors. Make sure that smoke detectors throughout the office are working properly. Replace batteries promptly. If smoke detectors are wired into the building's electrical system, report any malfunction to the building manager.

**In Case of Fire.** Despite the precautions that you and your coworkers take, a fire may break out. Be prepared to use fire safety equipment and to evacuate the building safely.

*Using Safety Equipment.* The number of fire extinguishers in the office depends on the size and number of rooms in the office. Regardless of the total number of extinguishers, you should locate an all-purpose fire extinguisher in or close to each exam room. Figure 22-9 shows how to operate a typical fire extinguisher. Have the fire extinguisher professionally serviced once a year to ensure its effectiveness. Each employee should learn how to use a fire extinguisher. OSHA recommends that employees know the "PASS" system:

- Pull the pin
- Aim at the base of the fire.
- Squeeze the trigger.
- Sweep side to side.

Posters with the "PASS" acronym are available from OSHA. You can also contact your local fire department for more information about fire safety training.

If there is a fire blanket in the exam room, be sure that you know how to use it and that it is stored so as to be easily accessible in an emergency. To use a fire blanket to smother burning clothing, wrap the victim in the blanket and roll him on the floor.

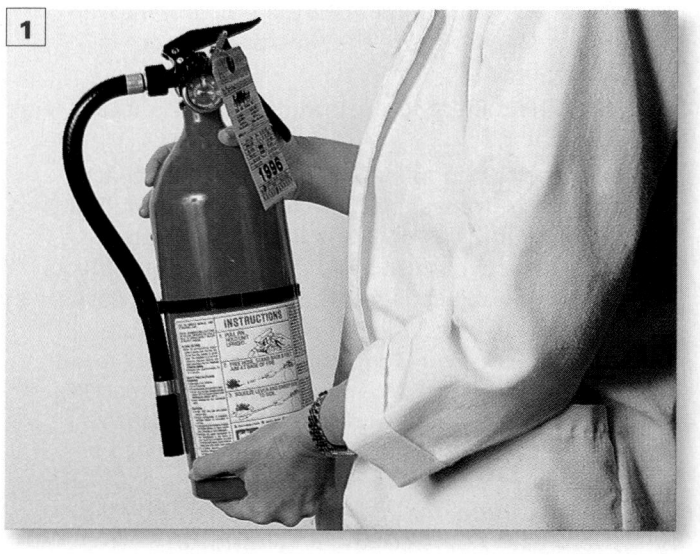

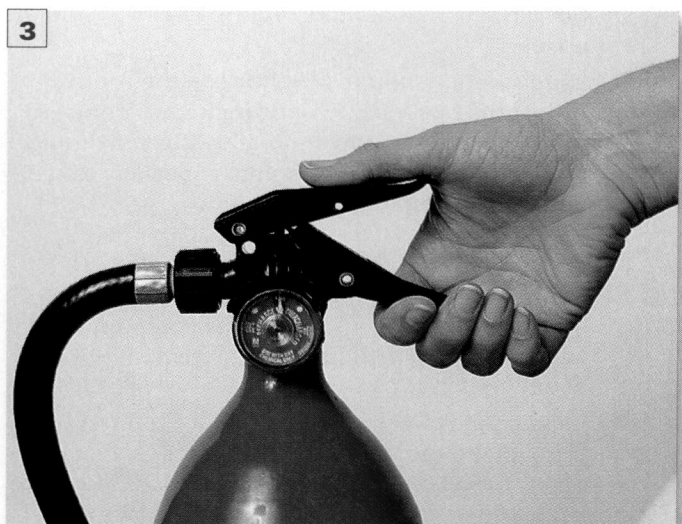

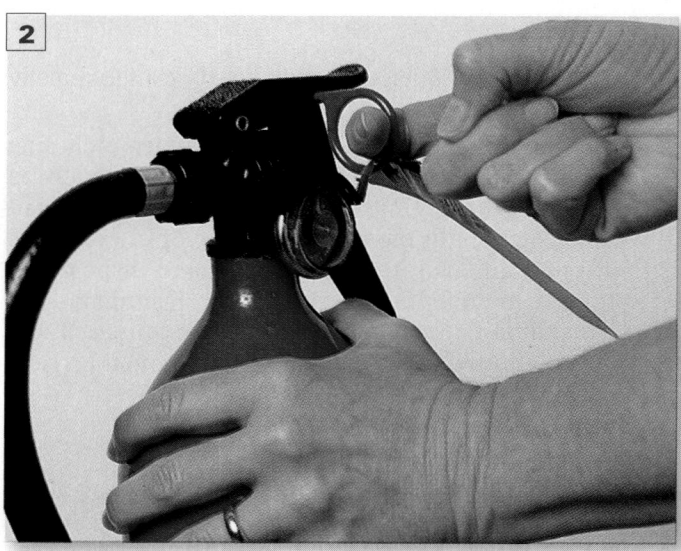

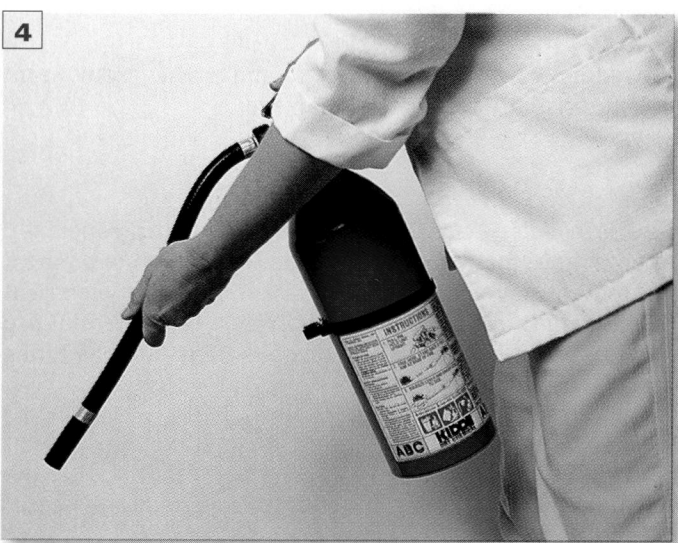

**Figure 22-9.** To use a fire extinguisher, (1) hold it upright, (2) remove the safety pin, (3) push the top handle down, and (4) direct the hose at the base of the fire.

***Planning an Evacuation Route.*** An evacuation route provides a safe way out of a building during an emergency. Learn the location of fire alarms, fire doors, and fire escapes in relation to the exam room. Use exit signs as a guide in unfamiliar areas of the building. Stage fire drills with your coworkers so that you can evacuate the facility and lead patients to safety. Plan what you will do if your route becomes blocked.

## Summary

Preparing the exam and treatment area for doctors and patients is part of your responsibility as a medical assistant. Room readiness involves making sure the room is clean, neat, and orderly and has adequate lighting, heat, and ventilation. You must select the instruments each doctor requires and make sure they are sanitized, disinfected, or sterilized (as appropriate) and ready for use. Room preparation also includes removing obstacles to physical safety, taking safety precautions, and following fire safety guidelines.

Your role in preparing the area is an important one for several reasons. First, you reduce the chance that infections will spread. Second, you help make the exam proceed efficiently. Third, you contribute to the comfort and safety of patients, doctors, and coworkers. Perform these tasks well, and you will inspire patients' confidence in the quality of the medical care provided at the facility.

# REVIEW

## CHAPTER 22

## CASE STUDY QUESTIONS

Now that you have completed this chapter, review the case study at the beginning of the chapter and answer the following questions:

1. What are bilateral cataracts, and why would this condition be a consideration when you come in contact with this patient?
2. What instruments should be assembled for the physician to use during the exam?
3. What disposable and consumable supplies may reasonably be anticipated for use?
4. What measures can you take to ensure the patient's comfort and safety?

## Discussion Questions

1. Inadequate hand washing has been identified as a primary cause for transmitting infections. List the circumstances in a medical office when you should wash your hands.
2. Describe each of the four steps in the "PASS" system.
3. Why is it important to keep the exam room neat and clean? What steps will you take to accomplish these tasks?

## Critical Thinking Questions

1. The Americans With Disabilities Act of 1990 enacted a provision for "reasonable accommodations" for accessibility for the disabled. Identify the accessibility guidelines, and explain why each is important.
2. Risk management is essential in the medical office. What types of problems can occur in the exam room, and what can you do to help prevent them?
3. The Occupational Safety and Health Administration mandates that biohazardous materials must be stored in a separate refrigerator. What is the rationale for this requirement?

## Application Activities

1. Make a checklist of steps for preparing the exam room. List tasks in the following categories: before/after an exam, daily, weekly, and monthly.
2. Create a fire safety program for a medical office. Present the program to the class. Have the class critique your plan.
3. Draw a floor plan of an exam room. Include the placement of furnishings and any special features the room might need. Be sure to include accommodations for individuals with disabilities. Present your floor plan to the class and lead a discussion about the layout of an exam room.

## Virtual Fieldtrip

*Visit the McGraw-Hill Higher Education Medical Assisting website at www.mhhe.com/medicalassisting3 to complete the following activity:*

Go to the OSHA website and search "Fire Safety." Navigate to the first three or four sites listed in the site. Keep notes of your search, including:

- The URL of each site visited
- A short synopsis of the information on the sites visited
- Whether the information applies to a medical office
- How the information can be used to develop a fire safety plan for a medical office

Open the CD and complete this chapter's practice activities, play the games, listen to the key terms, and test yourself with the interactive review. E-mail, print, and/or save your results to document your proficiency.

# SECTION 2

## ASSISTING WITH PATIENTS

# Interviewing the Patient, Taking a History, and Documentation

## MEDICAL ASSISTING COMPETENCIES

*In preparation of the certification examination, you should know the following areas of competence:*

| COMPETENCY | CMA | RMA |
|---|---|---|
| **Administrative** | | |
| Prepare, organize, and maintain medical records | X | X |
| **Clinical** | | |
| Perform telephone and in-person screening | X | X |
| Interview the patient to obtain and record the patient's history | X | X |
| **General/Legal/Professional** | | |
| Recognize and respond to verbal and nonverbal communications by being attentive and adapting communication to the recipient's level of understanding | X | X |
| Be aware of and perform within legal and ethical boundaries | X | X |
| Determine the needs for documentation and reporting, and document accurately and appropriately | X | X |
| Instruct individuals according to their needs | X | X |
| Provide patients with methods of health promotion and disease prevention | X | X |
| Serve as a liaison between the physician and others | | X |
| Interview effectively | | X |
| Use appropriate medical terminology | | X |

## KEY TERMS

addiction
chief complaint
mirroring
substance abuse
verbalizing

## CHAPTER OUTLINE

- The Patient Interview and History
- Your Role as an Observer
- Documenting Patient Information
- Recording the Patient's Medical History

## LEARNING OUTCOMES

After completing Chapter 23, you will be able to:

**23.1** Name the skills necessary to conduct a patient interview.

**23.2** Explain the procedure for conducting a patient interview.

**23.3** Recognize the signs of anxiety; depression; and physical, mental, or substance abuse.

**23.4** State the six Cs for writing an accurate patient history.

**23.5** Document on the patient's chart accurately.

**23.6** Obtain a patient history

**23.7** Identify parts of the health history form.

# Introduction

As a medical assistant, it is your job to prepare the patient and the patient's chart before the physician enters the exam room to examine the patient. You are the first contact with the patient in the exam room. How you conduct yourself during those first few moments can make a major difference in the patient's attitude and perception of the medical office. The patient must cooperate fully to provide the information the physician needs to diagnose and treat the patient successfully. Conducting the patient interview and recording the necessary medical history are essential to the practitioner's exam process.

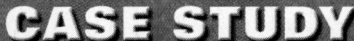

## CASE STUDY

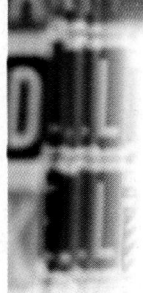

You are a medical assistant working at a busy office practice. You've been assigned to interview and obtain a history for a 75-year-old female who is hard of hearing. You will be required to chart the information you collect.

As you read this chapter, consider the following questions:

1. How can you ensure that the interview process goes smoothly?
2. Why is it important that you maintain a positive relationship with this patient?
3. What steps will you take to make sure all the documentation is completed correctly and accurately?

# The Patient Interview and History

The first step in the exam process is the patient interview. A well-conducted interview helps establish a beneficial relationship between you and the patient (Figure 23-1).

When a patient makes an office visit for a medical problem, you will ask the patient (or an attending family member) for specific pieces of information called data. These data include symptoms and the **chief complaint** (a subjective statement made by a patient describing the patient's most significant symptoms or signs of illness). Medicare and most insurers require this information. When a patient makes an office visit for a routine checkup, you will ask the patient about general health and lifestyle and about any changes in health status since the last visit.

The initial interview with the patient in the exam room is more than the process of filling out a standard form. It is an important communication tool that allows an exchange of information. The interview provides far more pertinent information than you and the physician could obtain from the standardized form alone.

A patient's medical and health history is the basis for all treatment rendered by the practitioner. The history provides information for research, reportable diseases, and insurance claims. The information contained on the chart becomes a legal record of the treatment rendered to the patient. It must be complete and accurate to be a good defense in case of legal action. All information regarding the patient should be documented precisely and accurately.

## Patient Rights, Responsibilities, and Privacy

It is important to remember that all the data you obtain are subject to legal and ethical considerations. Most states have adopted a version of the American Hospital Association's Patient's Bill of Rights, written in 1973 and revised

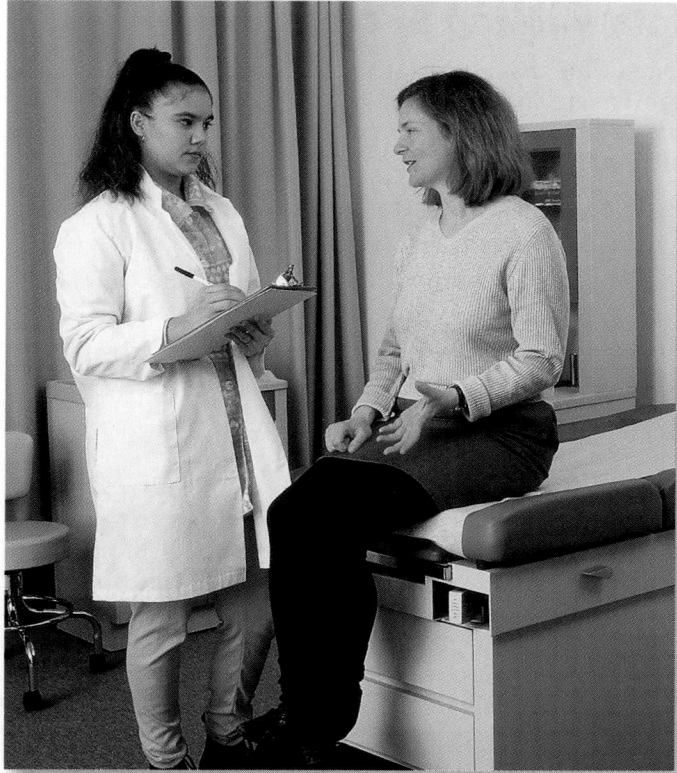

**Figure 23-1.** Encourage the patient to verbalize her concerns.

in 1992. Each state encourages health-care workers to be aware of and follow this document when caring for patients. The statement guarantees the patient's right to:

- Receive considerate and respectful care
- Receive complete and current information concerning his or her diagnosis, treatment, and prognosis
- Know the identity of physicians, nurses, and others involved with his or her care as well as know when those involved are students, residents, or trainees
- Know the immediate and long-term costs of treatment choices
- Receive information necessary to give informed consent prior to the start of any procedure or treatment
- Have an advance directive concerning treatment or be able to choose a representative to make decisions
- Refuse treatment to the extent permitted by law
- Receive every consideration of his or her privacy
- Be assured of confidentiality
- Obtain reasonable responses to requests for services
- Obtain information about his or her health care, be allowed to review his or her medical record, and to have any information explained or interpreted
- Know whether treatment is experimental and be able to consent or decline to participate in proposed research studies or human experimentation
- Expect reasonable continuity of care

- Ask about and be informed of the existence of business relationships between the hospital and others that may influence the patient's treatment and care
- Know which hospital policies and practices relate to patient care, treatment, and responsibilities
- Be informed of available resources for resolving disputes, grievances, and conflicts, such as ethics committees or patient representatives
- Examine his or her bill and have it explained, and be informed of available payment methods

Medical assistants should also know that patients have certain responsibilities when they seek medical care. Patients are responsible for:

- Providing information about past illnesses, hospitalizations, medications, and other matters related to their health status. If an incorrect diagnosis is made because a patient fails to give the physician the proper information, the physician is not liable.
- Participating in decision making by asking for additional information about their health status or treatment when they do not fully understand information and instructions.
- Providing health-care agencies with a copy of their written advance directive if they have one.
- Informing physicians and other caregivers if they anticipate problems in following a prescribed treatment.
- Following the physician's orders for treatment. If a patient willfully or negligently fails to follow the physician's instructions, that patient has little legal recourse.
- Providing health-care agencies with necessary information for insurance claims and working with the health-care facility to make arrangements to pay fees when necessary.

Additionally, in April of 2003, the enforcement of the Health Insurance Portability and Accountability Act (HIPAA) began. If this act is not followed, individual health-care workers can be subject to fines up to $250,000 and 10 years in jail. The privacy standards of this act ensure the following:

- Health-care facilities must provide patients with a written notice of their practices regarding the use and disclosure of all individually identifiable health information
- Health-care facilities may not use or disclose protected health information for any purpose that is not in the privacy notice
- Patient consent is required when protected information is used or disclosed for purposes of treatment, payment, or health operations
- Written authorization is required for other types of disclosures
- Hospitals must make the privacy notice available either prior to, or at the time of, the delivery of care

- A privacy notice must be posted in a clear and prominent location within the hospital facility

## Interviewing Skills

To conduct a successful patient interview and obtain history and health information, you will need to apply a variety of skills, including the following:

- Effective listening
- Being aware of nonverbal clues and body language
- Using a broad knowledge base
- Summarizing to form a general picture

**Effective Listening.** Listening attentively is one of the most important skills you will need for a successful interview. When you listen to what the patient is saying, you not only listen for details but also try to get an overall view of the patient's situation. As you become more experienced in conducting patient interviews, these skills will improve. One way to be a good listener is to hear, think about, and respond to what the patient has said. This technique is called active listening. Passive listeners simply sit back and hear. When you are an active listener, you pay attention and provide feedback. For example, you might repeat what the patient says in your own words or ask questions so that you understand details.

**Being Aware of Nonverbal Clues and Body Language.** Verbal communication is the asking and answering of questions. To conduct a successful interview, you must also be aware of nonverbal communication. The patient's tone of voice, facial expression, and body language are examples of nonverbal communication. These signs often communicate more than words could ever say. For example, a patient who has difficulty making eye contact may be embarrassed by some symptoms and may need your extra patience and encouragement to report symptoms fully. A child or adolescent may deny or exaggerate pain. Pay attention to the patient's facial expression and how much the patient guards the area in question.

**Using a Broad Knowledge Base.** To conduct a successful interview, you must have a broad knowledge base so that you can ask questions that will elicit the most meaningful information about the patient. You must take every opportunity to expand your knowledge base by learning more about medical terminology, symptoms, and diseases.

**Summarizing to Form a General Picture.** You will gather a variety of subjective and objective data as you conduct a patient interview. You must consider the relative importance of each piece of information so that you can summarize the data to formulate a general picture of the patient. It is always a good idea to repeat back a summary of information to the patient. This will ensure that all important data is recorded. Patients will sometimes forget to add something, and repeating the summary may jog their memory.

## Interviewing Successfully

One of the main goals of the patient interview is to give the patient an opportunity to fully explain in her own words the reason for the current office visit. These eight steps will help you conduct a successful interview.

1. Do your research before the patient interview
2. Plan the interview
3. Approach the patient and request the interview
4. Make the patient feel at ease
5. Conduct the interview in private without interruptions
6. Deal with sensitive topics with respect
7. Do not diagnose or give a diagnostic opinion
8. Formulate the general picture

**Doing Research Before the Patient Interview.** Before the interview, review the patient's medical record for history, medications, and chronic problems (for example, diabetes or high blood pressure). Note whether the patient has family problems that might have an impact on health issues. Make sure that all currently ordered diagnostic testing, laboratory work, and consultation results are in the chart. If you discover that you are missing a result, you have some time to retrieve it from the facility while the patient is in the office.

**Planning the Interview.** Develop a plan for the interview. Have a general idea of the questions you will ask. For example, if a patient is being treated for high blood pressure, you might ask about headaches or tinnitus (ringing in the ears), which are common signs of high blood pressure. Planning the interview helps you maintain your focus and ensures that you will obtain all the necessary information.

It is important to be organized before the interview takes place. Follow the office flow, for example, by recording the patient's height, weight and vital signs before you begin the interview with the patient. Make sure that you follow office policy on the types of information you will need to ask the patient during the interview. For example, some physicians prefer that you record the patient's medication list before the exam, whereas others prefer to record the medication list themselves. Planning for the types of information that you need to collect will save time for the visit itself.

**Approaching the Patient and Requesting the Interview.** Ask the patient whether you may pose some questions about the reason for the visit and the patient's current health situation. You may need to explain that the questions are necessary to plan the most effective care. It is more courteous to seek permission to ask questions than to say that you "need to take a history." Asking permission helps the patient feel more comfortable and emphasizes the importance of the interview process. It also makes the patient feel more like a participant in the medical care being provided.

**Making the Patient Feel at Ease.** Using certain words or phrases known as icebreakers can help set the stage for the interview. Icebreakers put the patient at ease and create a relaxed atmosphere. Examples of icebreakers include acknowledging the patient's reason for the visit, introducing yourself, or commenting about the weather. Icebreakers that also convey a sincere and sensitive interest in the patient are asking the patient how she prefers to be addressed or clarifying the pronunciation of a difficult name.

Another way to convey an image of a professional who is sensitive to the patient's needs is to sit with the patient and appear relaxed. By appearing relaxed, you help the patient relax and encourage a more open and comfortable interview. Eye contact is important when interviewing a patient. Sometimes patients will feel intimidated if they are forced to look up at you. If the patient sits in a chair, then it is best that you sit; if the patient sits on the examining table, then it is appropriate to stand while recording the visit.

**Conducting the Interview in Private Without Interruptions.** After setting the stage for the interview, ensure privacy by showing the patient to a private room or area or by closing the door if the patient is already in a private room. You can then begin to ask relevant questions. Some approaches are more effective than others, as shown in Table 23-1. Listening carefully to the patient's responses may lead you to ask questions other than those in your interview plan.

Developing a rapport with the patient is essential. Keep the atmosphere relaxed, do not rush, maintain eye contact, and use the patient's name in conversation. Avoid interruptions, such as taking phone calls and letting people walk in and out of the room. Make sure that you do not use "pet names" for your patients, such as "honey" or "sweetie." Doing so can offend some patients and sometimes can be misinterpreted as being insincere.

**Dealing With Sensitive Topics With Respect.** Sometimes you will have to ask patients questions about sensitive topics. Such topics may be related to sexuality, lifestyle, or behaviors that put a person at risk for diseases, such as those that are sexually transmitted. You must approach these topics gently so that the patient does not feel threatened by the questioning. You can show respect for the patient's rights and privacy by knowing when to stop. Both verbal and nonverbal clues can guide you in this area. It is also important to be conscious of your body language when dealing with sensitive subjects. You may find yourself exposed to situations that you do have any prior experience with and "shock" may register on your face.

**Avoiding Making a Diagnosis or Giving a Diagnostic Opinion.** Only the physician can make a diagnosis, based on the patient's symptoms and complaints. If the patient asks for your opinion about a diagnosis, explain that the physician should be asked about diagnoses. If pressed, you may need to say you are not able to give opinions about a diagnosis and the physician will answer any questions he or she may have. Never go beyond your scope of practice or job description.

**Formulating the General Picture.** Summarize the key points of the interview. Ask the patient whether he or she has questions or other information to add. You will be most successful with the interview process if you remain alert and organized but flexible. Procedure 23-1 demonstrates the proper approach to an interview.

# Your Role as an Observer

During the pre-exam stage of the office visit, you will gather most of your information through verbal and nonverbal communication. The nonverbal communication that occurs during the interview and history taking, however, sometimes reveals more about a patient than the patient's words. Listening attentively and observing the patient closely may help you detect a problem that might otherwise go unnoted.

## Anxiety

Anxiety is a common emotional response in patients. Some patients respond with anxiety to a specific fear, such as fear of pain. Others simply feel anxious when they are in an unfamiliar situation. For example, many patients have what is called "white coat syndrome," which is anxiety related to seeing a physician.

To recognize anxiety, you must understand that it varies from mild to severe. A patient with mild anxiety may have a heightened ability to observe and to make connections. A patient with severe anxiety has difficulty focusing on details, feels panicky, and is virtually helpless. A heightened focus or a lack of focus in a patient can hinder your ability to get the information and cooperation you need. When you observe signs of anxiety in a patient, make every effort to help her relax and release or reduce the anxious feelings. You may be able to help by allowing the patient to describe her feelings. If a patient becomes agitated while discussing a physical complaint, you may need to postpone talking about the matter until the patient is calmer. In either situation, give support in nonverbal ways by trying to make the patient as comfortable as possible. Give the patient time to respond and then wait quietly, provide privacy, make eye contact, and communicate at the level of the patient.

## Depression

Some symptoms of depression are the same as those of many common illnesses. Many patients with major depression develop great skill in hiding depression or are unaware they are suffering from it. Thus, depression may be difficult to recognize. Many patients, especially the elderly, have undiagnosed depression.

To recognize depression, you must be aware of common symptoms associated with the condition. Classic symptoms of depression are profound sadness and fatigue. In addition,

## TABLE 23-1   Methods of Collecting Patient Data

| Effective Methods | Characteristics |
|---|---|
| Asking open-ended questions | Requires more than a yes or no answer; allows the patient to more fully explain the situation, resulting in more relevant data. Instead of asking, "Do you have a cough?" ask, "Can you tell me about your symptoms?" |
| Asking hypothetical questions | Allows you to determine the patient's knowledge of the situation and whether it is accurate. For example, ask a patient who has been prescribed nitroglycerin for chest pain, "What would you do if you have chest pain?" |
| Mirroring patient's responses and verbalizing the implied | Allows nonthreatening ways for the patient to discuss the situation further and to provide underlying meaning. **Mirroring** means restating what the patient says in your own words. **Verbalizing** the implied means stating what you believe the patient is suggesting by his response. You might say, "So the pain started about 3 days ago and has been getting worse each day, and today it has not let up at all." |
| Focusing on patient | Shows the patient that you are really listening to what he is saying. You maintain eye contact (as culturally appropriate), assume a relaxed and open body posture, and use the proper responses. |
| Encouraging patient to take the lead | Motivates the patient to discuss or describe the situation in his own way. Ask a question such as "Where would you like to begin?" |
| Encouraging patient to provide additional information | Conveys sincere interest in the patient by continuing to explore topics in more detail when appropriate. You might ask the patient if he has experienced a symptom before or if he associates it with a change in routine. |
| Encouraging patient to evaluate his situation | Provides an idea of the patient's point of view about the situation; allows you to determine the patient's knowledge of the situation and possible fears. Ask the patient, "What do you think is going on here?" |

| Ineffective Methods | Characteristics |
|---|---|
| Asking closed-ended questions | Provides little information because closed-ended questions offer the patient little freedom to explain his answers. Closed-ended questions require only yes or no answers. |
| Asking leading questions | Leading questions suggest a desired response instead of the patient's true response. The patient tends to agree with such statements instead of elaborating on them. An example of a leading question is "You seem to be making progress, don't you agree?" This type of question limits the patient's response. |
| Challenging patient | The patient may feel you are disagreeing with what he is saying if you ask an emotional question or use a certain tone of voice. The patient may become defensive, which might block further communication. |
| Probing | Continuing to question a patient after he appears to have finished giving information can make him feel that you are invading his privacy. The patient may become defensive and withhold information. |
| Agreeing or disagreeing with patient | When you agree or disagree with a patient, it implies that the patient is either "right" or "wrong." This action can block further communication. |

a depressed person may have difficulty falling asleep at night or getting up in the morning. The depressed patient may suffer from loss of appetite, loss of energy, or both.

Depression seems to occur most frequently during late adolescence, in middle age, and after retirement. It is common in the elderly but is often mistaken for senility. If you observe any signs of depression, indicate them in the patient's chart and alert the physician.

Signs of depression, addiction, and substance abuse in adolescents can be difficult to distinguish. Signs of substance

# PROCEDURE 23.1

## Using Critical Thinking Skills During an Interview

**Procedure Goal:** To be able to use verbal and nonverbal clues and critical thinking skills to optimize the process of obtaining data for the patient's chart

**OSHA Guidelines:** This procedure does not involve exposure to blood, body fluids, or tissues.

**Materials:** Patient chart, pen with blue ink

**Method:**

### Example 1: Getting at an Underlying Meaning

1. You are interviewing a female patient with type 2 diabetes who has recently started insulin injections. She is in the office for a follow-up visit.
2. Use open-ended questions such as, "How are you managing your diabetes?"

#### Rationale

Open-ended questioning allows the patient to explain the situation in her own words and often provides more information than closed-ended questioning.

3. The patient states that she "just can't get used to the whole idea of injections."
4. To encourage her to verbalize her concerns more clearly, you can **mirror** her response, or restate her comments in your own words. For example, you might say, "You seem to be having some difficulty giving yourself injections."

#### Rationale

This response should encourage her to verbalize the specific area in which she is having problems such as loading the syringe, injecting herself, finding the time for the injections, and so on.

5. **Verbalize** the implied, which means that you state what you think the patient is suggesting by her response.

#### Rationale

Restating her response ensures you have understood.

6. After you determine the specific problem, you will be able to address it in the interview or note it in the patient's chart for the doctor's attention.

### Example 2: Dealing With a Potentially Violent Patient

1. You are interviewing a 24-year-old male patient who is new to the office. He appears agitated.

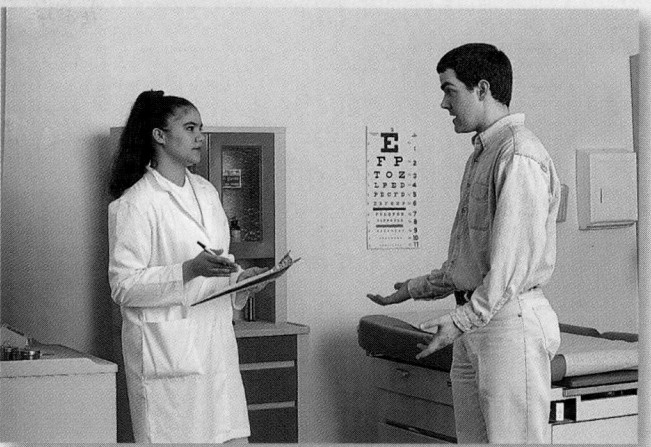

**Figure 23-2.** Do not try to handle a patient who may become violent by yourself. Ask for help from other staff members.

You ask his reason for seeing the doctor today.

2. The patient explains that he does not want to talk to "some assistant" about his problem. He just wants to see the doctor.
3. You say that you respect his wish not to discuss his symptoms but explain that you need to ask him a few questions so that the doctor can provide the proper medical care.

#### Rationale

The patient has the right to refuse to answer a question, even if it is a reasonable one.

4. The patient begins to yell at you, saying he wants to see the doctor and doesn't "want to answer stupid questions." (Figure 23-2).
5. The fact that the patient appears agitated and begins to raise his voice in anger should be a warning to you that he may become violent. It would be best not to handle this patient by yourself.
6. If you are alone with the patient, leave the room and request assistance from another staff member.

### Example 3: Gathering Symptom Information About a Child

1. A parent brings a 6-year-old boy to the office because the child is complaining about stomach pain.

*continued* ⟶

## Using Critical Thinking Skills During an Interview *(concluded)*

**2.** To gather the pertinent symptom information, ask the child various types of questions.

### Rationale

Talking to the child first allows him to feel that his view of the problem is important.

**a.** Can he tell you about the pain?

### Rationale

Open-ended questioning allows him to tell you about his problem in his own words.

**b.** Can he tell you exactly where it hurts (Figure 23-3)?

**c.** Is there anything else that hurts?

**3.** To confirm the child's answers, ask the parent to answer similar questions.

**4.** You should then ask the parent additional questions. Begin with an open-ended question, as above. Follow up with specific questions such as these.

**a.** How long has he had the pain?

**b.** Is the pain related to any specific event (such as going to school)?

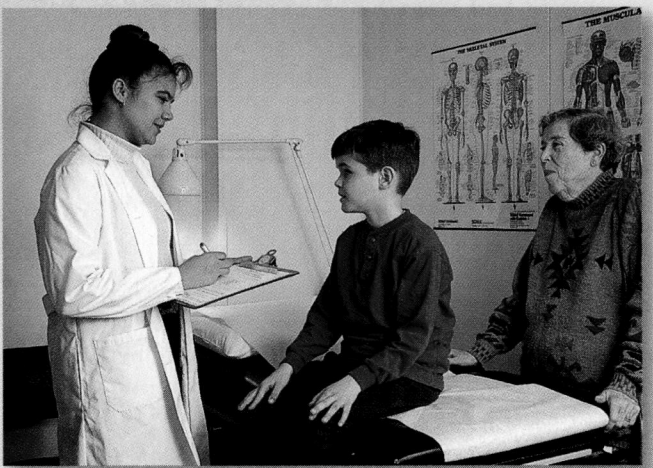

**Figure 23-3.** Gather any symptom information you can from a child. Then ask the parent or caregiver similar questions.

**5.** Ask the child to confirm the parent's answers. He may be able to provide additional information at this time.

# Reflecting On . . . Communication Issues

## Communicating With Professionalism

Your overall professionalism and poise can be a direct result of your verbal communication skills. If you use improper language skills, such as poor grammar or slang, or appear to have sloppy body language, you can give the patient the perception that you are not educated or intelligent. Your communication skills will have a direct impact on your career. Take care and pride in what and how you communicate. Think before you speak or react and you'll learn to avoid communication pitfalls.

abuse or addiction can be mistaken for depression. The reverse is also true. Sometimes all three conditions exist simultaneously. If you have any clues that point to one of these conditions in an adolescent patient, notify the physician immediately. For symptoms that may be signs of these disorders, see the Caution: Handle With Care section.

## Physical and Psychological Abuse

Abuse can involve people from all walks of life and of all ages. Abuse can be physical, psychological, or both. As a medical assistant, you are in a unique position to detect abuse in the patients you see. (See Chapter 26 for additional information related to child abuse, domestic violence, and elder abuse.)

Although you must not make hasty judgments, you may suspect abuse when a patient speaks in a guarded way. An unlikely explanation for an injury may also be a sign of abuse. There may be no history of the injury, or the history may be suspicious. In either case the following injuries may be signs of physical abuse:

- Head injuries and skull fractures
- Burns (especially those that appear to be deliberate, such as from a cigarette or an iron)
- Broken bones

# CAUTION *Handle With Care*

## Signs of Depression, Substance Abuse, and Addiction in Adolescents

Signs of depression, substance abuse, and addiction are often hard to distinguish in adolescents. Part of the difficulty is that adolescents are particularly skilled at hiding signs of all three disorders.

Various signs may indicate depression in an adolescent. One teenager may lose interest in or be unable to enjoy everyday activities. Another may sleep for long periods and have difficulty getting up in the morning, whereas yet another may sleep very little. Chronic fatigue or aches and pains may signal depression, as may trouble with concentration or school absenteeism. These signs may also indicate substance abuse or addiction.

It is important to know the difference between substance abuse and addiction. **Substance abuse** refers to the use of a substance, even an over-the-counter drug, in a way that is not medically approved. Inappropriate use includes such practices as using diet pills to stay awake or consuming large quantities of cough syrup that contains codeine. It also includes taking larger-than-prescribed doses of a medication. Substance abusers are not necessarily addicts, however.

**Addiction** refers to a physical or psychological dependence on a substance. Addiction usually involves a pattern of behavior that includes an obsessive or compulsive preoccupation with a substance and the security of its supply as well as a high rate of relapse after withdrawal.

As a medical assistant, you should not try to make a diagnosis. Quite probably an adolescent with one or more of these disorders will be uncooperative and refuse to answer relevant questions. You must be aware, however, of physical signs or behaviors that may be associated with depression, substance abuse, or addiction in an adolescent patient. The following signs or behaviors are important clues that you should report immediately to the doctor.

- The patient complains of altered eating habits or disturbed sleep patterns (either too much or too little sleep).
- The patient's weight has changed drastically (either up or down) since the previous office visit.
- The patient appears lethargic or sullen or exhibits radical mood changes.
- The patient has slurred speech.
- The patient appears to have illogical thought patterns.
- The patient appears to have needle tracks (anywhere on the body, especially on the arms or legs).
- The patient has pinpoint (highly constricted) pupils.

---

- Bruises (especially multiple bruises, those that are clearly in the shape of an object, and those in various stages of healing)

Although a patient can recover physically from abuse, the emotional and psychological scars may last a lifetime. Other signs of physical abuse (including sexual abuse and neglect) and signs of psychological abuse include the following:

- A child's failure to thrive
- Severe dehydration or underweight
- Delayed medical attention
- Hair loss
- Drug use
- Genital injuries

**Battered Women.** Women who are abused by their partners may come to the medical office with bruises or other injuries. Often they are afraid to discuss the problem.

A woman may fear that her partner will "get even" if she tells anyone about what happened. The woman may not feel strong enough emotionally to leave an abusing partner. If you suspect abuse, bring it to the physician's attention immediately. You or the physician, or the two of you together, may be able to convince the patient to seek help. Obtain the battered-woman hotline number for your area, and have it available for quick reference.

**Abused Children.** Children are often the targets of violence, much of which occurs in the home. In addition to being physically, emotionally, or sexually abused, children can be abused by being neglected. If you suspect child abuse, you must report it to the physician to contact the proper authorities. Keep the child abuse hotline number and numbers of local agencies for your area on file.

**The Abused Elderly.** Physical or mental disabilities can make elderly people dependent on others for care. When such care is perceived as a burden by the caregiver, elder abuse may occur. The disabilities that make an elderly person dependent can also leave him defenseless against abuse. Such a patient may have suspicious injuries or show signs of neglect. Find out whether there is an elder abuse hotline number for your area and, if so, keep it available for quick reference.

## Drug and Alcohol Abuse

Substance abuse and addiction to drugs or alcohol are serious social problems. Symptoms of substance abuse or addiction differ from drug to drug, as indicated in Table 23-2. Addiction, however, typically causes a gradual decline in the quality of someone's work or relationships. The patient may behave erratically, have frequent mood changes, suffer from loss of appetite, and be constantly tired.

Someone who is abusing alcohol may have no apparent signs or symptoms at first. As time goes on, however, that person may suffer from blackouts (failure to remember what happened while drinking) or may become secretive and guilty about drinking and deny that there is a problem. She may suffer from bruises, trembling hands, or chronic stomach problems. Even though the patient may feel she does not have a problem of substance abuse or addiction, members of the health-care team may recognize a problem. Then their job is to try to persuade the patient to seek help.

# Documenting Patient Information

Whenever you interview a patient, keep in mind that the patient chart is a legal document. The chart can be used as evidence in a court of law. Therefore, you must meet certain guidelines when recording data.

## TABLE 23-2 Symptoms Associated With Commonly Abused Drugs

| Drug Names/Type | Trade or Other Name | Symptoms, Effects |
|---|---|---|
| Amphetamines/stimulants | Benzedrine, Dexedrine, methamphetamine, black beauty, speed, uppers | Altered mental status, from confusion to paranoia; hyperactivity, then exhaustion; insomnia; loss of appetite |
| Anabolic steroids | Anadrol, Dianabol, Deca-durabotin, Depo-testosterone | Irritability, aggression, nervousness, male-pattern baldness |
| Barbiturates/sedatives | Amobarbital, phenobarbital, Butisol, secobarbital, yellow jackets, red birds | Slowed thinking, slowed reflexes, slowed respiration, loss of anxiety |
| Benzodiazepines/sedatives | Ativan, diazepam, Librium, Valium, downers, candy | Poor coordination, drowsiness, increased self-confidence |
| Cocaine/stimulant | Coke, snow, crack | Alternating euphoria and apprehension, intense craving for more of the drug |
| Ecstasy/psychoactive | Adam, XTC, MDMA | Confusion, depression, anxiety, paranoia, increase in heart rate and blood pressure |
| GHB/depressants | G, liquid ecstasy, georgia homeboy | Slow pulse and breathing, lowered blood pressure, drowsiness, poor concentration |
| Inhalants | Solvents: paint thinner; gases: aerosol, butane, or propane | Stimulation, intoxication, hearing loss, arm or leg spasms |
| LSD (lysergic acid diethylamine)/hallucinogen | Acid, microdot | Heightened sense of awareness, grandiose hallucinations, mystical experiences, flashbacks |
| Marijuana/cannabinoids/Hashish | Pot, grass, joint, reefer, weed, bone, buds, hash, boom | Altered thought processes, distorted sense of time and self, impaired short-term memory |
| Opium, morphine, codeine/opiate narcotics | Monkey, white stuff | Decreased level of consciousness, detachment, drowsiness, impaired judgment |
| PCP (phencyclidine)/hallucinogen | Angel dust | Decreased awareness of surroundings, hallucinations, poor perception of time and distance, possible overdose and death |

## The Six Cs of Charting

To help ensure that you record patient data accurately, you must follow the six Cs of charting. These guidelines are as follows.

1. *Client's words* must be recorded exactly. The doctor may uncover clues to use in diagnosing the patient's condition. Place quotation marks to indicate what the patient said.
2. *Clarity* is essential when you describe the patient's condition. You must use medical terminology and precise descriptions.
3. *Completeness* is required on all the forms used in the patient record.
4. *Conciseness* can save time and space when you are recording information.
5. *Chronological order* and dates on all entries in patient records are critical in the documentation of patient care. This information can also be used for legal questions regarding medical services. Most charts are arranged with the most recent information on top. This type of charting is known as *reverse chronological order*.
6. *Confidentiality* is essential to protect the patient's privacy. You cannot discuss a patient's records; forward them to another office, fax them, or show them to anyone except the doctor unless the patient gives you written permission to do so.

## Contents of Patient Charts

Each physician's office has its own forms and medical charts. All records, however, must contain the following standard information.

- The patient registration form carries the date of the patient's current visit and generally lists the patient's age, address, Social Security number, medical insurance, occupation, education, racial or ethnic background, marital status, number of children, and nearest relative. There is a section that allows the patient to indicate his or her preference about telephone contact, such as leaving messages, or relaying information to designated family members or friends. Make sure the patient understands the privacy information section and chooses the appropriate action.
- Patient medical history usually includes the chief complaint, history of the present illness, past medical history (including medical treatment, surgeries, known allergies, and current medications), family history, and social and occupational history (including diet, exercise, smoking, and use of alcohol or drugs). This section may also be used to record the results of a general physical exam. See Figure 23-4 for one example.
- Test results include those performed in the office and those received from other physicians, hospitals, or independent laboratories. Physicians may have tests run on a patient's blood, urine, or tissue samples to aid in their diagnoses. Figure 23-5 shows an example of a laboratory report of a panel of chemical tests on blood performed by an outside laboratory.

- Records from other physicians or hospitals are accompanied by a copy of the patient's written authorization to release the records.
- The physician's diagnosis and treatment plan are specific and detailed.
- Operative reports include a record of all procedures, surgeries, follow-up care, and additional notes the physician makes regarding the patient's case. Continuation forms can be used for additional information. Some medical offices also keep a separate log of telephone calls to and from the patient.
- Informed consent forms verify that the patient has understood the treatment offered and the possible outcomes or side effects of it. The patient signs the consent form but may withdraw consent if she decides to change or discontinue treatment.
- A discharge summary form is used when a patient is hospitalized. This form includes information that summarizes the reason the patient entered the hospital; tests, procedures, or operations performed in the hospital; medications administered; and the disposition, or outcome, of the case.
- Correspondence with or about the patient is marked or stamped with the date the document was received in the physician's office.

When recording information in the patient chart, be sure to date and initial every entry. This documentation makes it easy to tell which items you entered into the chart and which items others entered. The physician usually initials reports before they are filed to prove that she saw them.

## Methods of Charting

Various methods of charting are used on the medical record. Most methods are based on a series of steps to document the information. These steps are referred to as the SOAP method of documentation (Figure 23-6). Understanding the parts of SOAP will help you document information in a logical manner.

1. **Subjective** data. You obtain subjective data from conversation with the patient or an attending family member. Subjective data include thoughts, feelings, and perceptions, including the chief complaint. An example of subjective information is the patient's statement about his or her chief complaint: "I have an itchy red rash on my left hand that I noticed 3 days ago." The chief complaint should always be recorded in the patient's own words.
2. **Objective** data. Objective data are readily apparent and measurable; for example, vital signs or test results

## The Medical Center at Springfield
### Medical History

Name _____ Age _____ Sex _____ S M W D

Address _____ Phone _____ Date _____

Occupation _____ Ref. by _____

Chief Complaint _____

Present Illness _____

_____

_____

_____

_____

History —Military _____

　　　　—Social _____

　　　　—Family _____

　　　　—Marital _____

　　　　—Menstrual _____ Menarche _____ Para. _____ LMP _____

　　　　—Illness　Measles　Pert.　Var.　Pneu.　Pleur.　Typh.　Mal.　Rh. Fev.　Sc. Fev.　Diphth.　Other

　　　　—Surgery _____

　　　　—Allergies _____

　　　　—Current Medications _____

## Physical Examination

Temp. _____ Pulse _____ Resp. _____ BP _____ Ht. _____ Wt. _____

General Appearance _____ Skin _____ Mucous Membrane _____

Eyes: _____ Vision _____ Pupil _____ Fundus _____

Ears: _____

Nose: _____

Throat: _____ Pharynx _____ Tonsils _____

Chest: _____ Breasts _____

Heart: _____

Lungs: _____

Abdomen: _____

Genitalia: _____

Rectum: _____

Pelvic: _____

Extremities: _____ Pulses: _____

Lymph Nodes: _____ Neck _____ Axilla _____ Inguinal _____ Abdominal

Neurological: _____

Diagnosis: _____

_____

Treatment: _____

_____

Laboratory Findings:

Date _____ Blood _____

_____

Date _____ Urine _____

_____

**Figure 23-4.** Your office may have its own patient history form. This is a sample form.

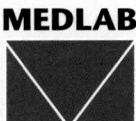

**MEDLAB**

266 Line Road
Montclair, Delaware 00956
800-555-4567

*Morris A. Turner, MD*

*C.L.I.A. #21-1862*

| WELLS, KARLA | 09/12/08 | 09/12/08 | 09/13/08 |
|---|---|---|---|
| Patient Name | Date Drawn | Date Received | Date of Report |

| F | 43 | | 23341 | 67294 |
|---|---|---|---|---|
| Sex | Age | | ID Number | Account Number |

Lisa W. Clark, MD
22 Landover Lane
Newark, Delaware 00964

| 166241809 | 897211 |
|---|---|
| Patient ID/Soc. Sec. Number | Specimen Number |

| TEST NAME | RESULT ABNORMAL | RESULT NORMAL | UNITS | REFERENCE RANGE |
|---|---|---|---|---|
| CHEM-SCREEN PANEL | | | | |
| GLUCOSE | | 76.0 | MG/DL | 65.0–115 |
| SODIUM | | 139.0 | MMOL/L | 134–143 |
| POTASSIUM | | 4.00 | MMOL/L | 3.60–5.10 |
| CHLORIDE | | 107.0 | MMOL/L | 96.0–107 |
| BUN | | 17.0 | MG/DL | 6.00–19.0 |
| BUN/CREATININE RATIO | | 14.2 | | |
| URIC ACID | | 4.30 | MG/DL | 2.20–6.20 |
| PHOSPHATE | | 2.40 | MG/DL | 2.40–4.50 |
| CALCIUM | | 9.50 | MG/DL | 8.60–10.0 |
| MAGNESIUM | | 1.75 | MEG/L | 1.40–2.00 |
| CHOLESTEROL | 237.0 | | MG/DL | 130–200 |
| CHOL. PERCENTILE | 90.0 | | PERCENTILE | 1.00–75.0 |
| HDL CHOLESTEROL | 41.0 | | MG/DL | 48.0–89.0 |
| CHOL./HDL RATIO | | 5.80 | | |
| LDL CHOL., CALCULATED | 175.0 | | MG/DL | 65.5–130 |
| TRIGLYCERIDES | | 104.0 | MG/DL | 00.0–200 |
| TOTAL PROTEIN | | 6.60 | GM/DL | 6.40–8.00 |
| ALBUMIN | | 4.10 | GM/DL | 3.70–4.80 |
| GLOBULIN | | 2.50 | GM/DL | 2.20–3.60 |
| ALB/GLOB RATIO | | 1.64 | | 1.10–2.10 |
| TOTAL BILIRUBIN | | 0.80 | MG/DL | 0.20–1.30 |
| DIRECT BILIRUBIN | | 0.15 | MG/DL | 0.00–0.20 |
| ALK. PHOSPHATASE | | 44.0 | UNITS/L | 25.0–125 |
| G-GLUTAMYL TRANSPEP. | | 8.00 | UNITS/L | 1.00–63.0 |
| AST (SGOT) | | 21.0 | IU/L | 1.00–40.0 |
| ALT (SGPT) | | 14.0 | IU/L | 1.00–50.0 |
| LD | | 134.0 | IU/L | 90.0–250 |
| IRON | | 130.0 | MCG/DL | 35.0–180 |

**Figure 23-5.** Laboratory reports provide physicians with valuable information about patients' health. Test results are accompanied by normal ranges appropriate for the laboratory's testing procedures.

## OUTLINE FORMAT PROGRESS NOTES

Patient Name _Hansen_ _Christopher_ _M._ Date of Birth _3_/_1_/_65_ Chart # _H234_
LAST | FIRST | MIDDLE

| Prob. No. or Letter | DATE | **S** Subjective | **O** Objective | **A** Assess | **P** Plans | Page _1_ |
|---|---|---|---|---|---|---|
| | 6/16/08 | Patient complaining of pain in lower right quadrant. Has been running fever of between 100.5° F and 101.3° F since Sunday morning. Has queasy feeling in stomach and has been unable to eat since yesterday morning. | | | | |
| | | | BP 125/75. Temperature 101.2° F. Abdominal exam revealed rebound tenderness and distension in lower right quadrant. | | | |
| | | | | Appendicitis | | |
| | | | | | 1. Admit to hospital | |
| | | | | | 2. Surgically remove appendix. | |

Signature _____

Start each Progress Note (Subjective, Objective, Assessment, and Plans) at the appropriate shaded column to create an outline form. Write through the intervening columns to the right margin of the page.

© 1976 BIBBERO SYSTEMS, INC., PETALUMA, CA        PROGRESS NOTES        TO REORDER CALL TOLL FREE: (800)BIBBERO (800 242-2376)
FORM # 26-7215-01

**Figure 23-6.** When you use the SOAP approach to documenting patient information, start each progress note at the appropriate shaded column to create an outline form. Write through the intervening columns to the right margin of the page.

and the physician's exam. An example of objective data is the exam of the rash by the physician.

3. **Assessment.** Assessment is the physician's diagnosis or impression of the patient's problem.

4. **Plan** of action. Options for treatment, the type of treatment chosen, medications, tests, consultations, patient education, and follow-up are included in a plan of action.

Three common methods for maintaining notes on a patient chart include:

1. Conventional or source-oriented medical records (SOMR). Information is arranged according to who supplied that data—the patient, the doctor, a specialist, or someone else. The medical form may have a space for patient remarks followed by a section for the doctor's comment.

2. Problem-oriented medical records (POMR). This method is used more extensively by large clinics or practices that may have more than one physician who may see the same patient. PMOR includes a problem list that is dated and numbers are assigned to each patient condition or problem. At the patient's initial visit, conditions or problems are identified by a number throughout the record until the problem is resolved. There are four components of the POMR:

- *Database.* This includes the patient's medical history, diagnostic and laboratory results, and physical exam reports. This is the foundation of the problem-oriented medical record.

- *Problem list.* Each patient condition or problem is listed individually, assigned a number, and dated.

- *Diagnostic and treatment plan.* Laboratory and other diagnostic tests are completed and the physician's treatment plan for the condition is documented.

- *Progress notes.* The physician enters notes on every condition or problem recorded on the problem list. Progress notes are entered chronologically and include the chief complaint, problems, conditions, treatments, and responses to treatment.

3. Computerized medical records. This method uses a combination of SOMR and POMR but provides accessibility by the physician or other health-care workers at any time from a computer terminal.

## Common Chart Terminology and Abbreviations

Most of the information that you collect verbally from a patient will be documented in the patient's medical record. Table 23-3 lists some of the most common abbreviations used in the medical chart.

To help reduce the amount of medical errors related to incorrect use of abbreviations, symbols, and acronyms, the Joint Commission on Accreditation of Healthcare Organizations (JCAHO) issued a list of abbreviations, acronyms, and symbols that should not be used. All medication orders, progress notes, consultation reports, operative

## TABLE 23-3 Common Medical Abbreviations

| | | | |
|---|---|---|---|
| Abortion | Ab | History of | H/O |
| Abnormal | Abnl | History and physical | H & P |
| Antibiotics | Abx | Left | L |
| Against medical advice | AMA | Right | R |
| Awake and oriented | A&O | Low back pain | LBP |
| As much as possible | AMAP | Low birth weight | LBW |
| Both | B | Last menstrual period | LMP |
| Biopsy | BX | No known allergies | NKA |
| Childhood diseases | CHD | Packs per day | PPD |
| Complains of | C/O | Range of motion | ROM |
| Cause of death | COD | Rule out | R/O |
| Chest x-ray | CXR | Shortness of breath | SOB |
| Date of birth | DOB | Sudden unexplained/unexpected death | SUD |
| Date of conception | DOC | Seizure | Sz |
| Digital rectal exam | DRE | Tonsillectomy and adenoidectomy | T & A |
| Follow-up | F/U | Years old | Y/O |
| Fracture | FX | Within normal limits | WNL |
| Growth and development | G & D | | |

reports, and clinical orders are subject to the "do not use" list. Table 23-4 provides a list of the most common "do not use" abbreviations, acronyms, and symbols.

# Recording the Patient's Medical History

A patient's medical history includes pertinent information about the patient and the patient's family. Age, previous illnesses, surgical history, allergies, medication history, and family medical history are key items.

When recording a patient history, you must do more than fill out the form (Figure 23-7). You must review the pieces of information, organize them, determine their importance, and document the facts. When you write your first histories, you may find it to be a lengthy process. When you become more experienced, however, you will be able to write histories more quickly. Whenever you write information on the chart you must consider its completeness and accuracy. For example, if a patient's chief complaint is pain in the left shoulder, you should probe the patient for some pertinent information. A

good interview technique is the "PQRST" Interview Technique. It will help you remember the types of questions that are appropriate for the condition.

**P: Provoke.** Provoke the patient to reveal the cause of the pain, such as:
- When did the pain start, and how long have you had the pain? (For example, the type of accident or injury, or the number of days or weeks, etc.)
- When does the pain occur? (For example, on movement, in the morning or evening, etc.)

**Q: Quality of pain.**
- Can you describe the pain? (For example, dull, aching, burning, sharp, etc.)
- Rate the pain on a scale of 1 to 10, with 10 being the worst. (A diagram is frequently used for this rating, as shown in Figure 23-8.)

**R: Region where the pain is located.**
- Where do you feel the pain?
- Does the pain move from one location to another?

**S: Signs and symptoms that accompany the pain such as nausea, redness, and swelling.**
- Is the area red or tender to the touch? Is there any swelling?

## TABLE 23-4 JCAHO "Do Not Use" Abbreviations, Acronyms, and Symbols

| Abbreviation | Potential Problem | Preferred Term |
|---|---|---|
| U (for unit) | Mistaken as zero, four, or cc | Write "unit" |
| IU (for international unit) | Mistaken as IV (intravenous) or 10 (ten) | Write "international unit" |
| Q.D., Q.O.D. (Latin abbreviation for once daily and every other day) | Mistaken for each other. The period after the Q can be mistaken for an "I" and the "O" can be mistaken for "I" | Write "daily" and "every other day" |
| Trailing zero (X.0 mg), Lack of leading zero (.X mg) | Decimal point is missed | Never write a zero by itself after a decimal point (X mg), and always use a zero before a decimal point (0.X mg) |
| MS<br>MSO₄<br>MgSO₄ | Confused for one another<br>Can mean morphine sulfate or magnesium sulfate | Write "morphine sulfate" or "magnesium sulfate" |
| μg (for microgram) | Mistaken for mg (milligrams) resulting in one thousand-fold dosing overdose | Write "mcg" |
| H.S. (for half-strength or Latin abbreviation for bedtime) | Mistaken for either half-strength or hour of sleep (at bedtime) q.H.S. mistaken for every hour. All can result in a dosing error. | Write out "half-strength" or "at bedtime" |
| T.I.W. (for three times a week) | Mistaken for three times a day or twice weekly, resulting in an overdose | Write "3 times weekly" or "three times weekly" |
| S.C. or S.Q. (for subcutaneous) | Mistaken as SL for sublingual, or "5 every" | Write "Sub-Q", "subQ", or "subcutaneously" |
| D/C (for discharge) | Interpreted as discontinue whatever medications follow (typically discharge meds). | Write "discharge" |
| c.c. (for cubic centimeter) | Mistaken for U (units) when poorly written. | Write "mL" for milliliters |
| A.S., A.D., A.U. (Latin abbreviation for left, right, or both ears)<br>O.S., O.D., O.U. (Latin abbreviation for left, right, or both eyes) | Mistaken for each other (e.g., AS for OS, AD for OD, AU for OU, etc.) | Write: "left ear," "right ear" or "both ears;" "left eye," "right eye," or "both eyes |

**T: Time of onset**

- When did you first notice the pain?
- Is the pain intermittent or continuous?
- How long does the pain last?

Providing this detailed information is important to the patient's care and treatment. In addition, you will need to chart other information prior to the physician visit. Figure 23-9 shows two types of forms used by the medical assistant and the licensed practitioner when seeing a patient. All information should be charted completely and accurately. Pay special attention to spelling. If you do not know how to spell a word, look it up or ask someone. Use only JCAHO-approved and recognized abbreviations. Many facilities have a written document identifying these abbreviations. Remember that the chart is a legal document; therefore, special attention to detail is required when charting. Many offices are transitioning from using black ink in charting to using blue ink. Blue ink is difficult to match in case an entry is altered.

## HEALTH HISTORY
(Confidential)

Name _____  Today's Date _____

Age _____  Birthdate _____  Date of last physical examination _____

What is your reason for visit? _____

**SYMPTOMS** Check (✓) symptoms you currently have or have had in the past year.

**GENERAL**
- ☐ Chills
- ☐ Depression
- ☐ Dizziness
- ☐ Fainting
- ☐ Fever
- ☐ Forgetfulness
- ☐ Headache
- ☐ Loss of sleep
- ☐ Loss of weight
- ☐ Nervousness
- ☐ Numbness
- ☐ Sweats

**MUSCLE/JOINT/BONE**
Pain, weakness, numbness in:
- ☐ Arms  ☐ Hips
- ☐ Back  ☐ Legs
- ☐ Feet  ☐ Neck
- ☐ Hands  ☐ Shoulders

**GENITO-URINARY**
- ☐ Blood in urine
- ☐ Frequent urination
- ☐ Lack of bladder control
- ☐ Painful urination

**GASTROINTESTINAL**
- ☐ Appetite poor
- ☐ Bloating
- ☐ Bowel changes
- ☐ Constipation
- ☐ Diarrhea
- ☐ Excessive hunger
- ☐ Excessive thirst
- ☐ Gas
- ☐ Hemorrhoids
- ☐ Indigestion
- ☐ Nausea
- ☐ Rectal bleeding
- ☐ Stomach pain
- ☐ Vomiting
- ☐ Vomiting blood

**CARDIOVASCULAR**
- ☐ Chest pain
- ☐ High blood pressure
- ☐ Irregular heart beat
- ☐ Low blood pressure
- ☐ Poor circulation
- ☐ Rapid heart beat
- ☐ Swelling of ankles
- ☐ Varicose veins

**EYE, EAR, NOSE, THROAT**
- ☐ Bleeding gums
- ☐ Blurred vision
- ☐ Crossed eyes
- ☐ Difficulty swallowing
- ☐ Double vision
- ☐ Earache
- ☐ Ear discharge
- ☐ Hay fever
- ☐ Hoarseness
- ☐ Loss of hearing
- ☐ Nosebleeds
- ☐ Persistent cough
- ☐ Ringing in ears
- ☐ Sinus problems
- ☐ Vision – Flashes
- ☐ Vision – Halos

**SKIN**
- ☐ Bruise easily
- ☐ Hives
- ☐ Itching
- ☐ Change in moles
- ☐ Rash
- ☐ Scars
- ☐ Sore that won't heal

**MEN only**
- ☐ Breast lump
- ☐ Erection difficulties
- ☐ Lump in testicles
- ☐ Penis discharge
- ☐ Sore on penis
- ☐ Other

**WOMEN only**
- ☐ Abnormal Pap smear
- ☐ Bleeding between periods
- ☐ Breast lump
- ☐ Extreme menstrual pain
- ☐ Hot flashes
- ☐ Nipple discharge
- ☐ Painful intercourse
- ☐ Vaginal discharge
- ☐ Other

Date of last menstrual period _____
Date of last Pap smear _____
Have you had a mammogram? _____
Are you pregnant? _____
Number of children _____

**CONDITIONS** Check (✓) conditions you have or have had in the past.

- ☐ AIDS
- ☐ Alcoholism
- ☐ Anemia
- ☐ Anorexia
- ☐ Appendicitis
- ☐ Arthritis
- ☐ Asthma
- ☐ Bleeding Disorders
- ☐ Breast Lump
- ☐ Bronchitis
- ☐ Bulimia
- ☐ Cancer
- ☐ Cataracts

- ☐ Chemical Dependency
- ☐ Chicken Pox
- ☐ Diabetes
- ☐ Emphysema
- ☐ Epilepsy
- ☐ Glaucoma
- ☐ Goiter
- ☐ Gonorrhea
- ☐ Gout
- ☐ Heart Disease
- ☐ Hepatitis
- ☐ Hernia
- ☐ Herpes

- ☐ High Cholesterol
- ☐ HIV Positive
- ☐ Kidney Disease
- ☐ Liver Disease
- ☐ Measles
- ☐ Migraine Headaches
- ☐ Miscarriage
- ☐ Mononucleosis
- ☐ Multiple Sclerosis
- ☐ Mumps
- ☐ Pacemaker
- ☐ Pneumonia
- ☐ Polio

- ☐ Prostate Problem
- ☐ Psychiatric Care
- ☐ Rheumatic Fever
- ☐ Scarlet Fever
- ☐ Stroke
- ☐ Suicide Attempt
- ☐ Thyroid Problems
- ☐ Tonsillitis
- ☐ Tuberculosis
- ☐ Typhoid Fever
- ☐ Ulcers
- ☐ Vaginal Infections
- ☐ Venereal Disease

**MEDICATIONS** List medications you are currently taking

**ALLERGIES** To medications or substances

Pharmacy Name _____  Phone _____

---

(All information is strictly confidential)

**FAMILY HISTORY** Fill in health information about your family.

| Relation | Age | State of Health | Age at Death | Cause of Death |
|---|---|---|---|---|
| Father | | | | |
| Mother | | | | |
| Brothers | | | | |
| | | | | |
| Sisters | | | | |
| | | | | |

**Check (✓) if your blood relatives had any of the following:**

| Disease | Relationship to you |
|---|---|
| Arthritis, Gout | |
| Asthma, Hay Fever | |
| Cancer | |
| Chemical Dependency | |
| Diabetes | |
| Heart Disease, Strokes | |
| High Blood Pressure | |
| Kidney Disease | |
| Tuberculosis | |
| Other | |

**PREGNANCY HISTORY**

| Year of Birth | Sex of Birth | Complications if any |
|---|---|---|
| | | |
| | | |

**HOSPITALIZATIONS**

| Year | Hospital | Reason for Hospitalization and Outcome |
|---|---|---|
| | | |
| | | |
| | | |
| | | |

Have you ever had a blood transfusion?  ☐ Yes  ☐ No
If yes, please give approximate dates. _____

**SERIOUS ILLNESS/INJURIES**

| | DATE | OUTCOME |
|---|---|---|
| | | |
| | | |
| | | |

**HEALTH HABITS** Check (✓) which substances you use and describe how much you use.

| | |
|---|---|
| Caffeine | |
| Tobacco | |
| Drugs | |
| Other | |

**OCCUPATIONAL CONCERNS**
Check (✓) if your work exposes you to the following:

| | |
|---|---|
| Stress | |
| Hazardous Substances | |
| Heavy Lifting | |
| Other | |

Your occupation: _____

I certify that the above information is correct to the best of my knowledge. I will not hold my doctor or any members of his/her staff responsible for any errors or omissions that I may have made in the completion of this form.

_____  _____
Signature  Date

_____  _____
Reviewed By  Date

---

**Figure 23-7.** The health history form must be complete and accurate. This sample form is started by the patient, then checked and completed by the medical assistant.

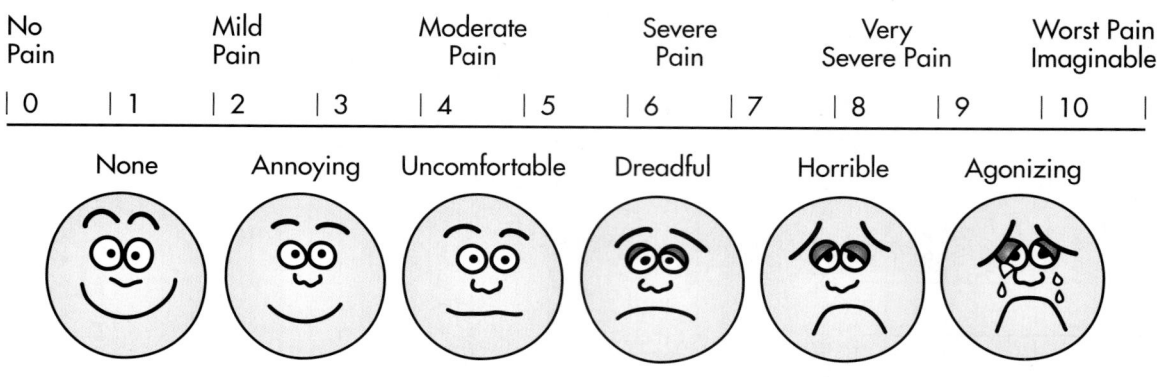

## Halifax Regional Medical Center
### Pain Management Is Our Concern
e 00964

| No Pain | Mild Pain | Moderate Pain | Severe Pain | Very Severe Pain | Worst Pain Imaginable |
|---|---|---|---|---|---|
| 0 | 1 | 2 3 | 4 5 | 6 7 | 8 9 | 10 |

| None | Annoying | Uncomfortable | Dreadful | Horrible | Agonizing |

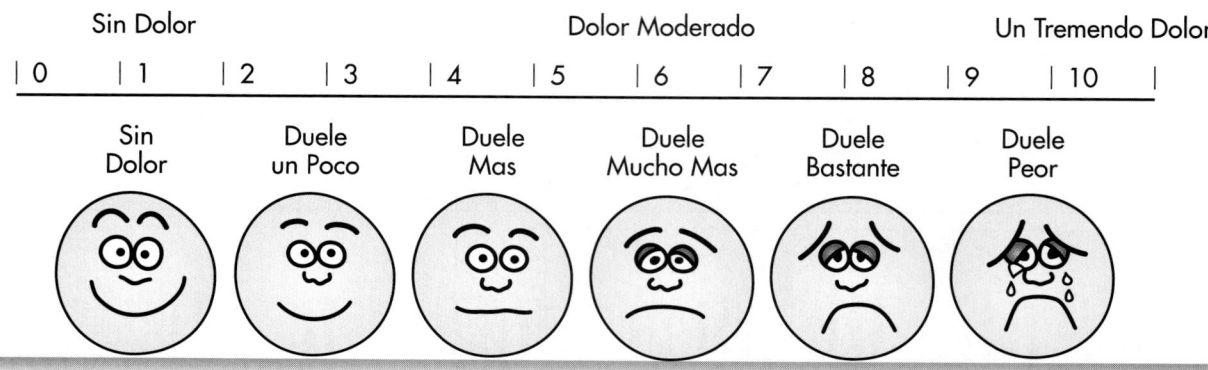

## El control del dolor es nuestra responsabilidad

| Sin Dolor | | Dolor Moderado | | Un Tremendo Dolor |
|---|---|---|---|---|
| 0 | 1 | 2 3 | 4 5 | 6 7 | 8 9 | 10 |

| Sin Dolor | Duele un Poco | Duele Mas | Duele Mucho Mas | Duele Bastante | Duele Peor |

**Figure 23-8.** Assessing a patient's pain, considered the fifth vital sign, is part of the interview and history-taking process. A chart similiar to this is used to make the process easier for the patient and the medical assistant.

## The Progress Note

Many offices use a variation of the progress note for established patients who are seen for routine follow-ups such as hypertension or arthritis (see Figure 23-6). The medical history form is primarily used for new patients who the physician is seeing for the first time. Some important guidelines to consider when using a progress note include:

- It must be arranged in reverse chronological order.
- Every entry must be initialed by the person making the entry.
- Entries most commonly made on progress notes include documentation for prescription refills, follow-up visits, telephone conversations with patients, appointment cancellations or no shows, and referrals and consultation efforts made by the office for the patient.

- The patient name must be recorded on every progress note along with any other identifying information such as birth date, Social Security number, or chart number.
- All entries must be dated.

Procedure 23-2 will guide you in how to use a progress note.

## Polypharmacy

Many patients will take a variety of different medications to treat several conditions, such as hypertension, elevated cholesterol, and diabetes. Some patients take several medications for the same condition, with each one treating a different aspect of the condition. Chapters 37 and 38 provide detailed information regarding various medications. During the patient interview, it is important to document current medications the patient is taking. The patient will often see several physicians

## Wildwood Medical Clinic
### Progress Notes

Name: *Carrie Shaw*  Chart #: *01769*

| DATE | |
|---|---|
| 10/12/08 | Patient c/o headache and cough X 3 days. HA is dull ache, pain scale 7/10 cough—non-productive. — H. Walton CMA |
| | |
| | |
| | |

Name *Jennifer Haddix*  DOB *12/05/84*  Date *08/28/08*

ALLERGIES: *Bee Stings, Penicillin*  Note

### Review of Systems

| Systems | NL | Note | Systems | NL | Note |
|---|---|---|---|---|---|
| Constitutional | | | Musculoskeletal | | |
| Eyes | | | Skin/breasts | | |
| ENT/mouth | | | Neurologic | | |
| Cardiovascular | | | Psychiatric | | |
| Respiratory | | | Endocrine | | |
| GI | | | Hem/lymph | | |
| GU | | | Allergy/immun | | |

| Current Medicines | Date | Current Diagnosis |
|---|---|---|
| ClaritinD prN<br>MVI Tqd<br>Ortho Novum 7/7/7<br>Tqd | | |

H: *5'7"?*  W: *140*  T: *97.8*  P: *88*  R: *20*

B/P Sitting *122/78* or Standing _____ Supine _____

Last Tetantus *06/12/03*

L.M.P. *08/20/08*

O2 Sat: *98%*  Pain Scale: *6/10*

Social Habits  Yes  No

Tobacco ___ ✓

Alcohol ✓ ooo

Rec. Drugs ___ ✓

CC: Ⓛ Shoulder pain X 3 days due to fall.
"Sharp pain that hurts when I move"

HPI:

**Figure 23-9.** These example forms are completed by the medical assistant prior to the physician visit. All information must be complete and accurate as shown.

or specialists, and it is important for your office to be up to date about the current treatments a patient is receiving.

Some offices may use a medication list for the physicians to record patient medication histories. In some cases, the medical assistant gathers the information for the current medication list. A helpful hint for organizing this task is to develop a form or card for the patient to use (if the office doesn't already have a form) and gather the initial medication history. Then instruct the patient to use the list and to have it updated by the other physicians that he or she sees. A drug reference guide or the Internet will assist you with the spelling of medications.

## The Health History Form

The medical office usually has a standard medical history form that is used for all patients. The specific arrangement and wording of items vary from office to office. The following sections contain brief descriptions of each of the parts of this form. Procedure 23-3 will assist in your practice of obtaining medical histories.

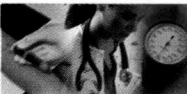

# PROCEDURE 23.2

## Using a Progress Note

**Procedure Goal:** To accurately record a chief complaint on a progress note

**OSHA Guidelines:** This procedure does not involve exposure to blood, body fluids, or tissues.

**Materials:** Progress note, patient chart, pen with blue ink

**Method:**

1. Wash your hands.
2. Review the patient's chart notes from the patient's previous office visit. Verify that all results for any previously ordered laboratory work or diagnostics are in the chart.

   ### Rationale
   Ensures that all reports have been reviewed by the physician.

3. Greet the patient and escort her to a private exam room.
4. Introduce yourself and ask the patient her name.

5. Using open-ended questions, find out why the patient is seeking medical care today.

   ### Rationale
   Asking open-ended questions such as "What is the reason for your visit today?" and "How long have you been feeling this way?" will encourage the patient to provide more details.

6. Accurately document the chief complaint on the progress note. Document vital signs. Initial the chart entry.
7. File the progress note in chronological order within the patient's chart.

   ### Rationale
   This ensures that the most current patient information is reviewed by the physician and the medical staff.

8. Thank the patient and offer to answer any questions she may have. Explain that the physician will come in soon to examine her.
9. Wash your hands.

# PROCEDURE 23.3

## Obtaining a Medical History

**Procedure Goal:** To obtain a complete medical history with accuracy and professionalism.

**OSHA Guidelines:** This procedure does not involve exposure to blood, body fluids, or tissues.

**Materials:** Medical history form, patient chart, pen with blue ink

**Method:**

1. Wash your hands.
2. Assemble the necessary materials. Review the medical history form and plan your interview.

   ### Rationale
   This saves time and improves the effectiveness of the visit, plus it will assist in determining the appropriate questions to ask.

3. Invite the patient to a private exam room and correctly identify the patient by introducing

yourself and asking his or her name and date of birth.

4. Explain the medical history form while maintaining eye contact. Make the patient feel at ease.
5. Using language that the patient can understand, ask appropriate questions related to the medical history form. Use open-ended questions. Listen actively to the patient's response.
6. Accurately document the patient's responses.
7. Thank the patient for his or her participation in the interview. Offer to answer any questions.
8. Sign or initial the medical history form and file it in the patient's chart.
9. Inform the physician that you are finished with the medical history according to the physician's office policy.
10. Wash your hands.

**Personal Data.** This information is obtained from the administrative sheet and includes the patient's name, Social Security number, birth date, and other basic data.

**Chief Complaint.** Abbreviated as CC, the chief complaint is the reason the patient came to visit the practitioner. It should be short and specific and should cover subjective and objective data.

**History of Present Illness.** This history includes detailed information about the chief complaint, including when the problem started and what the patient has done to treat the problem (including any medications taken). For example, a chief complaint might be "sore throat" and the history of the present illness would include when the sore throat started (e.g., 3 days ago), how severe the pain is on a scale of 1 to 10 (e.g., pain scale rating of 6 out of 10), and what treatments have been used (e.g., throat lozenges and four to six aspirin daily).

**Past Medical History.** The past medical history includes any and all health problems both present and past, including major illnesses and surgery. The past medical history would also include important information about medications and allergies. It should list any medications taken by the patient, including their dosages and the reasons for taking them. Over-the-counter and herbal medications should be considered as well. Known or suspected allergies to medications or other substances should be listed and clearly visible. Some facilities use a red sticker or other means on charts to identify allergies immediately.

**Family History.** This section includes information about the health of the patient's family members. Many times the family history can help lead a practitioner to the cause of a current medical problem. Obtain specific information about family members' current ages and medical conditions or, if deceased, their age at death and the cause. Ask open-ended questions about the siblings, parents, and grandparents. Because the death of a parent or sibling or the limited knowledge of an adopted child can be difficult to discuss, use great care and sensitivity when asking these questions.

**Social and Occupational History.** Information such as marital status, sexual behaviors and orientation, occupations, hobbies, and the use of chemical substances help determine a patient's risk for disease. Patients should be asked about their use of alcohol, tobacco, recreational drugs, or other chemical substances. Be aware that patients may feel uncomfortable or may refuse to provide certain information. Depending on the circumstances, you may ask the question later in the interview. For example, an adolescent child may not want to answer questions about his sexual behaviors in front of his parents. Occupational information regarding the patient's level of stress, exposure to hazardous substances, and heavy lifting may also be included here.

**Review of Systems.** Some of this information may be started by the patient but is completed by the practitioner. This systematic review of each of the body systems includes questions and an exam by the practitioner. The information is obtained in an orderly fashion but may vary depending on the physician or practitioner.

# Summary

As a medical assistant, you will play a key role in a patient's visit to the physician's office. Because you will begin the exam by interviewing the patient, you will set the tone of the visit. Keep in mind that some patients may be nervous or uncomfortable. It is important to make them feel at ease. Using interviewing skills effectively will help make the interview productive as well as comfortable for the patient. Taking a thorough history and using proper documentation methods will also allow you to ensure that patient records are complete and accurate. They will also help the practitioner to diagnose and treat the patient successfully.

# REVIEW

## CHAPTER 23

### CASE STUDY QUESTIONS

Now that you have completed this chapter, review the case study at the beginning of the chapter and answer the following questions:

1. How can you ensure that the interview process goes smoothly?
2. Why is it important that you maintain a positive relationship with this patient?
3. What steps will you take to make sure all the documentation is completed correctly and accurately?

### Discussion Questions

1. Explain the difference between subjective and objective data. Give examples of each type.
2. Describe the technique you would use to obtain accurate information from a pediatric patient.
3. What is the significance of each of the parts of the health history form?

### Critical Thinking Questions

1. A patient comes into the office with abdominal pain. On her chart is a notation that she is coming in with symptoms of appendicitis. What questions might you ask her to assist the doctor in determining whether her condition is appendicitis?
2. An adult woman brings her 89-year-old mother into the office for an annual physical. You notice that the elderly woman smells of urine and looks rather unkempt. She has lost 15 pounds since her last visit and she appears to be confused or disoriented. What observations should you make and what are some questions that you could ask the daughter and the patient? What kinds of assistance are available to this patient?
3. A 31-year-old male patient comes to the clinic after a fall that occurred at work. During the interview, he complains of pain in his left leg and right elbow. He is unable to describe what happened and says he just blacked out. What observations should you make, and what questions should you ask this patient?
4. While interviewing and recording the health history of a patient, you are required to list all the medications the patient is taking. The patient names several medications and provides the dosages; however, you cannot spell one of them and you are not sure about how to write the abbreviations for the dosages. What should you do?

### Application Activities

1. Have a partner assume the role of a patient who has come into the office with what appears to be low back pain. Conduct an interview using the PQRST technique and take a patient history.
2. With a partner, practice role-playing both effective and ineffective methods of collecting patient data. Create situations and questions that encourage and discourage communication. Compare and contrast the differences. Use Table 23-1 as a guideline.

### Virtual Fieldtrip

*Visit the McGraw-Hill Higher Education Medical Assisting website at www.mhhe.com/medicalassisting3 to complete the following activities:*

1. Explore the Internet to find resources for charting medical and health information. Find sites for medical abbreviations, medical terminology, and medications, and then create favorites or quick links from the browser on your computer for handy reference when writing in the patient's chart.
2. Research the Internet for a commonly abused recreational drug, and create a brief oral or written report. Visit the National Institute of Drug Abuse to begin your research. Include the following information in your report:
   a. The drug's street name
   b. How it affects the body both physically and psychologically
   c. The signs and symptoms of abuse
   d. How you would notice if a patient is abusing this drug

Open the CD and complete this chapter's practice activities, play the games, listen to the key terms, and test yourself with the interactive review. E-mail, print, and/or save your results to document your proficiency.

## CHAPTER 24

# Obtaining Vital Signs and Measurements

## MEDICAL ASSISTING COMPETENCIES

*In preparation for the certification examination, you should know the following areas of competence:*

| COMPETENCY | CMA | RMA |
|---|---|---|
| **Clinical** | | |
| Practice Standard Precautions | X | X |
| Obtain vital signs | X | X |
| Perform telephone and in-person screening | X | X |
| **General/Legal/Professional** | | |
| Respond to and initiate written communications by using correct grammar, spelling, and formatting techniques | X | X |
| Recognize and respond to verbal and nonverbal communications by being attentive and adapting communication to the recipient's level of understanding | X | X |
| Identify and respond to issues of confidentiality by maintaining confidentiality at all times and following appropriate guidelines when releasing records or information | X | X |
| Be aware of and perform within legal and ethical boundaries | X | X |
| Instruct individuals according to their needs | X | X |
| Provide patients with methods of health promotion and disease prevention | X | X |
| Operate and maintain facilities, and perform routine maintenance of administrative and clinical equipment safely | X | X |
| Use appropriate medical terminology | | X |
| Utilize computer software and electronic technology to maintain office systems | X | X |

## CHAPTER OUTLINE

- Vital Signs
- Body Measurements

## KEY TERMS

afebrile
antecubital space
apex
apical
apnea
auscultated blood pressure
axilla
brachial artery
bradycardia
calibrate
Celsius (centigrade)
Cheyne-Stokes respirations
Fahrenheit
febrile
hyperpnea
hyperpyrexia
hypertension
hypotension
meniscus
orthostatic hypotension
palpatory method
positive tilt test
postural hypotension
radial artery
rales
sphygmomanometer
stethoscope
tachycardia
tachypnea
temporal scanner
thermometer
tympanic thermometer

## LEARNING OUTCOMES

After completing Chapter 24, you will be able to:

**24.1** Recognize common terminology and abbreviations used in documenting and discussing vital signs.

**24.2** Describe the instruments used to measure vital signs and body measurements.

**24.3** Explain the procedure used to measure vital signs and body measurements.

# Introduction

Vital signs are one of the most important assessments you can make when preparing the patient to be examined by the practitioner. Temperature, pulse, respirations, and blood pressure give information about how a patient will adjust to changes within the body and in the environment. Changes in the vital signs can indicate an abnormality.

Measurements such as height, weight, and head circumference can indicate physical growth and development, especially in infants and children. These measurements are also used to evaluate health problems, such as obesity. Other measurements are also completed to evaluate a patient's condition. For example, you may need to measure the size of a wound or bruise or the diameter of an arm or leg. In all cases, you must be accurate when performing and recording vital signs and body measurements. The practitioner uses your results when making a diagnosis.

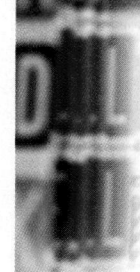

## CASE STUDY

A 68-year-old female has been a patient for 2 years at the clinic where you work as a medical assistant. She suffers from both hypertension and obesity and is taking a diuretic medication (HCTZ, or hydrochlorothiazide) daily.

As you read this chapter, consider the following questions:
1. Why is it essential for you to take accurate measurements of this patient?
2. How can you help ensure the accuracy of these measurements?

# Vital Signs

As a medical assistant, you will usually take the vital signs before the doctor examines the patient. Temperature, pulse, respiration, and blood pressure (vital signs) provide the doctor with information about the patient's overall condition.

Pre-exam procedures in some offices are performed in a general area outside the patient exam room. In other offices and in most pediatric offices, these measurements are taken in the exam room. In either case you typically take the measurements before the patient disrobes. Follow the standard procedure used in your office. Also be certain to follow the HIPAA regulations and provide for the privacy of your results.

## General Considerations

Vital signs are the primary indicators of a patient's overall general condition. Four vital signs are:

1. Temperature
2. Pulse
3. Respiration
4. Blood pressure

Assessment of pain, which was discussed in Chapter 23, can be considered the fifth vital sign. It is typically assessed at the same time as the other vital signs.

Vital signs are usually measured at every office visit. There is a standard range of values for each measurement, as shown in Table 24-1. Each patient has an individual baseline value that is normal for that patient. However, the difference between a patient's current values and normal values can help the physician in making a diagnosis. You must follow closely the guidelines from the Department of Labor's Occupational Safety and Health Administration (OSHA) for taking measurements of vital signs (Table 24-2). These guidelines are intended to prevent transmission of disease to or from the patient. They help protect the patient and you, plus keep the workplace safe.

## TABLE 24-1 Normal Ranges for Vital Signs*

| Vital Sign | Age | | | | |
|---|---|---|---|---|---|
| | 0–1 year | 1–6 years | 6–11 years | 11–16 years | Adult |
| **Temperature** | | | | | |
| Oral (°F) | 96–99.5 (less than 4 weeks) | 98.5–99.5 | 97.5–99.6 | 97.6–99.6 | 97.6–99.6 |
| Rectal (°F) | 99.0–100.0 | 99.0–100.0 | 98.5–99.6 | 98.6–100.6 | 98.6–100.6 |
| **Pulse** (beats per minute) | 80–160 | 75–130 | 70–115 | 55–110 | 60–100 |
| **Respirations** (per minute) | 26–40 | 20–30 | 18–24 | 16–24 | 12–20 |
| **Blood Pressure** (mm Hg) | | | | | |
| Systolic | 74–100 | 80–112 | 80–120 | 88–120 | <120 |
| Diastolic | 50–70 | 50–80 | 50–80 | 58–80 | <80 |

*Normal vital signs vary. Always compare your results with previous results taken on the patient.

## TABLE 24-2 OSHA Guidelines for Taking Measurements of Vital Signs

| Situation | OSHA Guidelines |
|---|---|
| Before and after all patient contact | Examination area cleaned according to OSHA standards Aseptic hand washing (Procedure 19-1 in Chapter 19) |
| Temperature by oral or rectal route Contact with patient with lesions Contact with patient suspect for infectious disease | Gloves worn Biohazard bags used for disposal of used thermometer sheaths, otoscope tips, alcohol swabs, dressings, and bandages |
| In presence of patient suspect for airborne infectious disease (particularly sneezing) | Mask worn Patient weighed, measured, and examined in room away from staff and other patients Protective clothing (laboratory coat, gown, or apron) worn Biohazard bags used as above |

# Temperature

When you take a patient's temperature, you will determine whether the patient is **febrile** (has a body temperature above the patient's normal range) or whether the patient is **afebrile** (has a body temperature at about the patient's normal range). A fever is usually a sign of inflammation or infection. An exceptionally high fever is known as **hyperpyrexia.** Body temperature varies based upon the time of day (usually higher at night due to exercise and food intake), the metabolism (the faster the metabolism or body processes, the higher the temperature), and the location where it is measured. You can take a temperature in one of five locations:

1. Mouth (oral)
2. Ear (tympanic)
3. Rectum (rectal)
4. Armpit, or **axilla** (axillary)
5. Temporal artery (temporal)

Temperature can be measured in degrees **Fahrenheit** (°F) or degrees **Celsius** (**centigrade; °C**). Table 24-3 gives equivalent values for these two temperature scales. Normal adult oral temperature is considered to be about 98.6°F or 37.0°C. See *Points on Practice* box to review formulas and example conversions.

Temperature is measured with either an electronic or disposable **thermometer.**

**Electronic Digital Thermometers.** Electronic digital thermometers are used frequently in medical offices. These thermometers provide a digital readout of the

## TABLE 24-3  Fahrenheit and Celsius Equivalents for Temperature

| °F | °C | °F | °C | °F | °C | °F | °C |
|---|---|---|---|---|---|---|---|
| 95.0 | 35.0 | 98.4 | 36.9 | 101.8 | 38.8 | 105.2 | 40.7 |
| 95.2 | 35.1 | 98.6 | 37.0 | 102.0 | 38.9 | 105.4 | 40.8 |
| 95.4 | 35.2 | 98.8 | 37.1 | 102.2 | 39.0 | 105.6 | 40.9 |
| 95.6 | 35.3 | 99.0 | 37.2 | 102.4 | 39.1 | 105.8 | 41.0 |
| 95.8 | 35.4 | 99.2 | 37.3 | 102.6 | 39.2 | 106.0 | 41.1 |
| 96.0 | 35.6 | 99.4 | 37.4 | 102.8 | 39.3 | 106.2 | 41.2 |
| 96.2 | 35.7 | 99.6 | 37.6 | 103.0 | 39.4 | 106.4 | 41.3 |
| 96.4 | 35.8 | 99.8 | 37.7 | 103.2 | 39.6 | 106.6 | 41.4 |
| 96.6 | 35.9 | 100.0 | 37.8 | 103.4 | 39.7 | 106.8 | 41.6 |
| 96.8 | 36.0 | 100.2 | 37.9 | 103.6 | 39.8 | 107.0 | 41.7 |
| 97.0 | 36.1 | 100.4 | 38.0 | 103.8 | 39.9 | 107.2 | 41.8 |
| 97.2 | 36.2 | 100.6 | 38.1 | 104.0 | 40.0 | 107.4 | 41.9 |
| 97.4 | 36.3 | 100.8 | 38.2 | 104.2 | 40.1 | 107.6 | 42.0 |
| 97.6 | 36.4 | 101.0 | 38.3 | 104.4 | 40.2 | 107.8 | 42.1 |
| 97.8 | 36.6 | 101.2 | 38.4 | 104.6 | 40.3 | 108.0 | 42.2 |
| 98.0 | 36.7 | 101.4 | 38.6 | 104.8 | 40.4 | | |
| 98.2 | 36.8 | 101.6 | 38.7 | 105.0 | 40.6 | | |

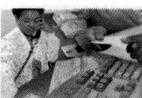

## Points on Practice

### Math for Measurements

When performing vital signs and measurements, certain basic math conversions may be required. You may need to convert a temperature from Fahrenheit (°F) to Celsius (°C) or weight from pounds (lb) to kilograms (kg). Review the following formulas and examples in preparation for practice:

**To convert °C to °F, use this formula:**
$$°F = (°C \times \tfrac{9}{5}) + 32$$
Example: Convert 37.6 °C to °F:
$$°F = (37.6 \times \tfrac{9}{5}) + 32$$
$$°F = \left(\tfrac{338.4}{5}\right) + 32$$
$$°F = 67.68 + 32$$
°F = 99.68 rounded to the nearest tenth equals 99.7

**To convert °F to °C, use this formula:**
$$°C = (°F - 32) \times \tfrac{5}{9}$$
Example: Convert 99.6 °F to °C
$$°C = (99.6 - 32) \times \tfrac{5}{9}$$
$$°C = 67.6 \times \tfrac{5}{9}$$
$$°C = \tfrac{338}{9}$$
°C = 37.55 rounded to the nearest tenth equals 37.6

**To convert kgs to lbs, use this formula:**
**lbs = kg × 2.205**
Example: Convert 52.4 kg to lbs
lbs = 52.4 × 2.205
lbs = 115.542 rounded to the nearest tenth equals 115.5

**To convert lbs to kgs, use this formula:**
**kg = lbs × 0.454**
Example: Convert 134 lbs to kg
kg = 134 × 0.454
kg = 60.836 rounded to the nearest tenths equals 60.8

patient's temperature (Figure 24-1). They are accurate, fast, easy to read, and comfortable for the patient. Separate probes and tips are available for oral or rectal use. Most units have an audible indicator, such as a beep, to let you know when the temperature has registered and is displayed.

Another type of electronic thermometer is the **tympanic thermometer.** It is designed for use in the ear, as shown in Figure 24-2. This thermometer measures infrared energy emitted from the tympanic membrane (eardrum). This energy is converted into a temperature reading. The tip is covered with a disposable sheath to prevent cross-contamination.

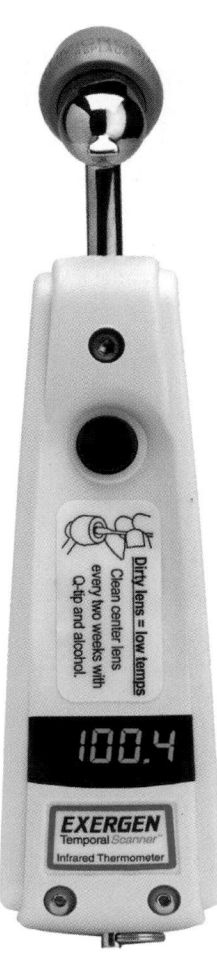

**Figure 24-3.** This Temporal Scanner is posted over the forehead to measure the temperature of the blood in the temporal artery.

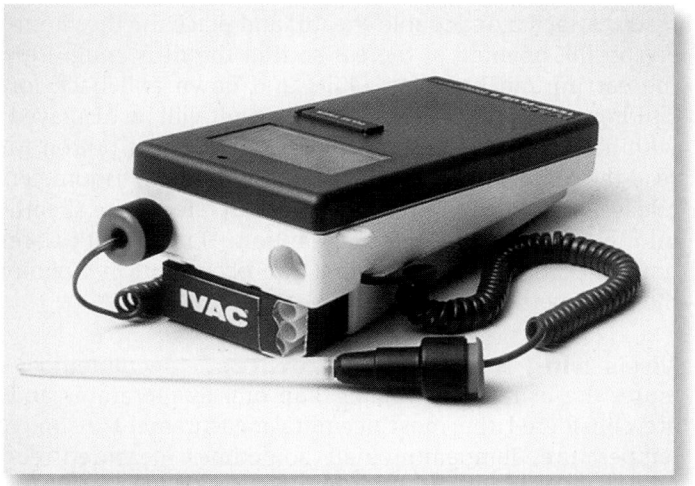

**Figure 24-1.** The electronic digital thermometer provides a digital readout of the patient's temperature.

A third type of electronic thermometer is a temporal scanner (Figure 24-3). This thermometer measures the infrared heat of the temporal artery and the temperature of the site where the temperature is taken. These two readings are synthesized and displayed on the screen.

**Disposable Thermometers.** Disposable, single-use thermometers are usually made of thin strips of plastic with specially treated dot or strip indicators (Figure 24-4). The indicators change color according to the temperature. This type of thermometer is used for oral and axillary or skin temperature measurements, particularly in children. Although not as accurate, disposable thermometers are useful for patients in their homes.

## Taking Temperatures

Using the proper instrument and technique provides the most accurate temperature readings and prevents the spread of infection. All temperature measurements

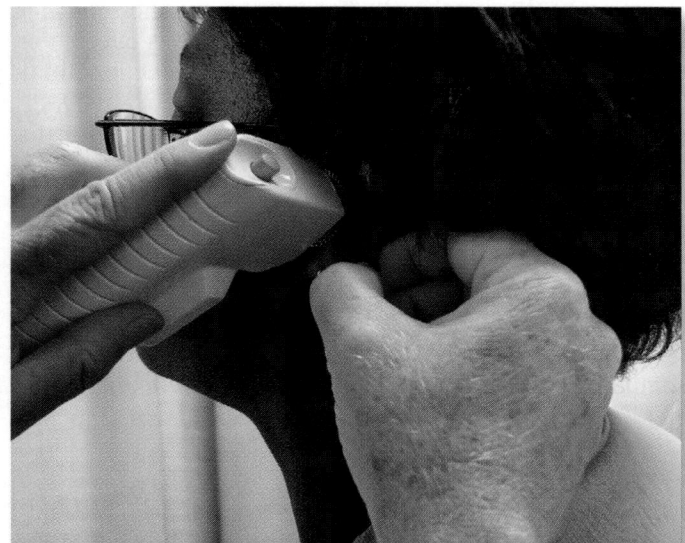

**Figure 24-2.** The tympanic thermometer measures infrared energy emitted from the tympanic membrane. The result, converted to body temperature, is displayed within seconds of insertion of the shielded tip into the ear.

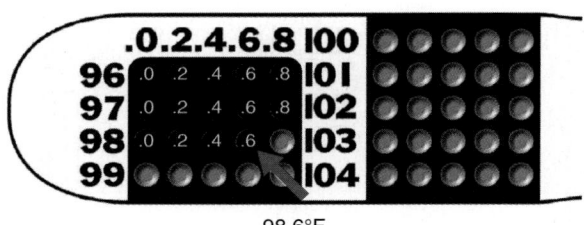

98.6°F

**A** NexTemp® thermometer after taking a normal temperature

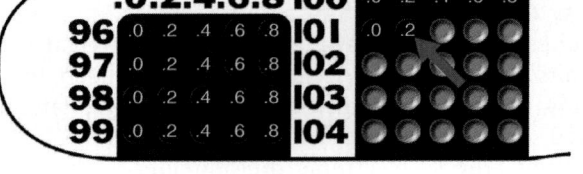

101.2°F

**B** NexTemp® thermometer after taking an elevated temperature

**Figure 24-4.** A disposable thermometer like this one is an accurate and convenient method for taking a temperature.

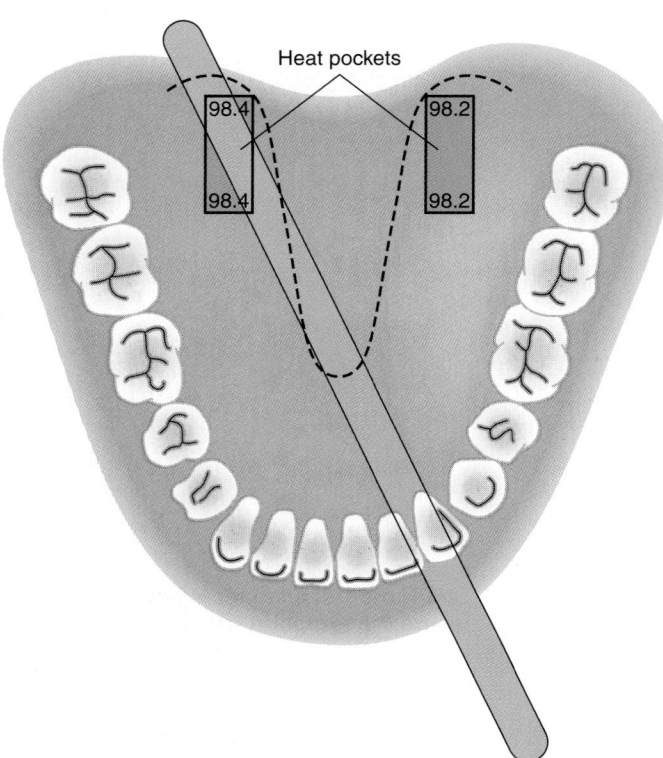

**Figure 24-5.** Placement of an oral thermometer. When taking an oral temperature, place the thermometer under the tongue to the side of the mouth as shown here.

should be recorded to the nearest one-tenth of a degree. The procedure for taking temperatures is described in Procedure 24-1.

**Measuring Oral Temperatures.** To take an oral temperature, make sure the patient is able to hold the thermometer in the mouth. The patient must also be able to breathe through the nose. Place the thermometer under the tongue in either pocket just off-center in the lower jaw (Figure 24-5). The patient should hold the thermometer with lips closed. Wait at least 15 minutes after a patient has been eating, drinking, or smoking before taking an oral temperature; otherwise, you may obtain an inaccurate result.

**Measuring Tympanic Temperatures.** Proper technique must be used when measuring a tympanic temperature. These thermometers are easy to use, and you

must follow manufacturers' instructions precisely. First, remove the thermometer from its recharging cradle, and then wait for the indicator light to show that the unit is ready. Attach a disposable sheath, and place the thermometer in the opening of the ear so that the fit is snug. Pull the ear up and back for adults and down and back for children. Press the button, and the result will be displayed within seconds. Be certain to press the correct button to read the temperature. Another button on the thermometer releases the sheath. You do not want to release the sheath into the patient's ear. See the Caution: Handle With Care box for potential problems that can occur with tympanic thermometers.

**Measuring Rectal Temperatures.** Rectal temperatures are usually 1°F higher than oral temperatures and are considered the most accurate measurement of body temperature. Temperatures are sometimes measured rectally in infants and adults in whom an oral temperature cannot be taken. Gloves are always worn and the patient is placed on his or her side. The left side is the preferred position because the rectum is angled in this direction. This position promotes comfort and prevents accidental puncture of the rectal wall. The bulb of the thermometer should be inserted slowly and gently until it is covered or until you feel resistance, at approximately 1 inch for adults and ½ inch for infants and small children. For safety, always hold the thermometer in place while taking the temperature.

**Measuring Axillary Temperatures.** To take an axillary temperature, first have the patient sit or lie down. Place the tip of the thermometer in the middle of the axilla, with the shaft facing forward. The patient's upper arm should be pressed against his side, and his lower arm should be crossed over the stomach to hold the thermometer in place. Make sure the tip of the thermometer touches skin on all sides of the probe.

**Measuring Temporal Temperatures.** The **temporal scanner** is a noninvasive and quick procedure for taking temperatures. You gently stroke the thermometer across the forehead crossing over the temporal artery. As with all electronic devices, check the manufacturer's instructions before using.

# PROCEDURE 24.1

## Measuring and Recording Temperature

**Procedure Goal:** To accurately measure the temperature of patients while preventing the spread of infection.

### OSHA Guidelines

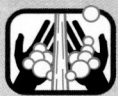  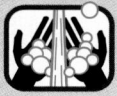

**Materials:** Thermometer, probe cover if required by thermometer, lubricant for rectal temperature, gloves, trash receptacle, patient's chart, and recording device

### Method:

1. Gather the equipment and make sure the thermometer is in working order.
2. Identify the patient and introduce yourself.
3. Wash your hands and explain the procedure to the patient.
4. Prepare the patient for the temperature
   a. Oral. If the patient has had anything to eat or drink, or has been smoking, wait at least 15 minutes before measuring the temperature orally.

      *Rationale*

      Inaccurate reading could result.

   b. Rectal. Have the patient remove the appropriate clothing; assist as needed. Have the patient lie on his or her left side and drape for comfort.

      *Rationale*

      Proper positioning is necessary for the patient's safety and comfort.

   c. Axillary. Assist the patient to expose the axilla. Provide for privacy and comfort. Pat dry the axilla.

      *Rationale*

      Perspiration or heavy deodorant prevents the thermometer from coming in direct contact with the skin.

   d. Temporal or Tympanic. Remove the patient's hat if necessary.

5. Prepare the equipment
   a. Prepare an electronic thermometer by inserting the probe into the probe cover if necessary.

      *Rationale*

      Probe covers are needed to prevent contamination of the probe.

   b. Prepare the disposable thermometer by removing the wrapper to expose the handle end. Avoid touching the part of the thermometer that goes in the mouth or on the skin.

      *Rationale*

      Touching the thermometer could interfere with an accurate reading.

   c. Prepare the temporal scanner by removing the protective cap and making sure the lens is clean.

      *Rationale*

      This will ensure accuracy of the reading.

6. Measure the temperature
   a. Oral. Place the thermometer under the tongue in the back of the mouth on one side. Have the patient hold it in place with his or her lips and tongue. Wait for the electronic thermometer to beep or indicate completion. For a disposable thermometer, wait at the required time, usually 60 seconds.

   b. Rectal. Put on gloves. Lubricate the thermometer tip. Raise the buttock to expose the anus with one hand and insert the thermometer into the anal canal, 1½ inches for adults and ½ to 1 inch for infants and children. Hold the thermometer securely in place until the indicator beeps or blinks.

      *Rationale*

      Injury could occur of the thermometer is inserted too far or if the patient moves during the procedure.

   c. Axillary. Place the thermometer into the axilla making sure the tip is in direct

*continued* ⟶

## Measuring and Recording Temperature *(continued)*

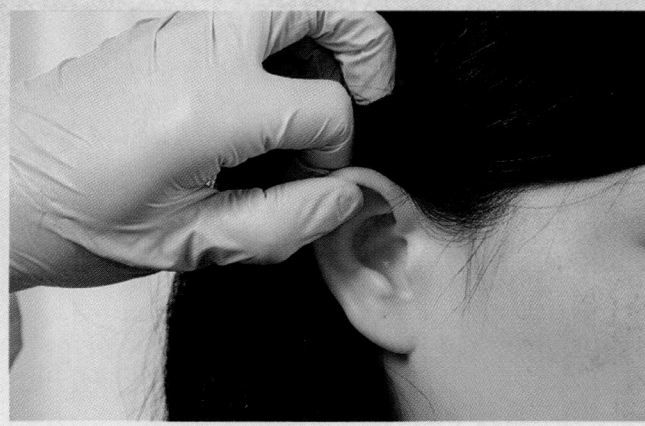

**A** Adult          **B** Child

**Figure 24-6.** When placing an aural thermometer, seal the ear canal by holding the pinna (outer ear) upward and outward for an adult (A) and downward and backward for a child (B).

contact with the top of the axilla and is touching skin on all skins. Hold the arm firmly against the body until the indicator light blinks or beeps or the proper amount of time has passed.

### Rationale

Ensures accuracy

**d.** Tympanic. Hold the outer edge of the ear (pinna) with your free hand. Gently pull the pinna up for adults and down for children (Figure 24-6 A–B). Insert the probe into the ear canal directed to the eardrum and sealing the ear canal. Press the scan button.

### Rationale

Ensures accuracy

**e.** Temporal. Position the probe flat on the center of the exposed forehead. Press and hold the SCAN button and then slide the thermometer straight across the forehead until it beeps and the red light blinks (Figure 24-7).

**7.** Remove and read the measurement in the display or on the thermometer. Discard the

disposable thermometer. Eject and discard the probe cover for an electronic thermometer. Replace the cap and/or place the thermometer into the charging base.

### Rationale

Contaminated items should be removed and the thermometer should be protected and charged until the next use.

**8.** Record the results. Chart by including the date and location where the temperature was taken. Oral: 98.6, Rectal: 99.6 R, Axillary; 97.6 Ax, Temporal: 97.6 Temp., Tympanic 97.6 Tymp.

### Rationale

The temperature varies depending upon the location and this location should be charted to ensure an accurate diagnosis.

**9.** Help the patient to replace clothing as necessary. Clear the area and provide for safety and comfort for the patient.

**10.** Wash your hands.

continued ⟶

# Measuring and Recording Temperature *(concluded)*

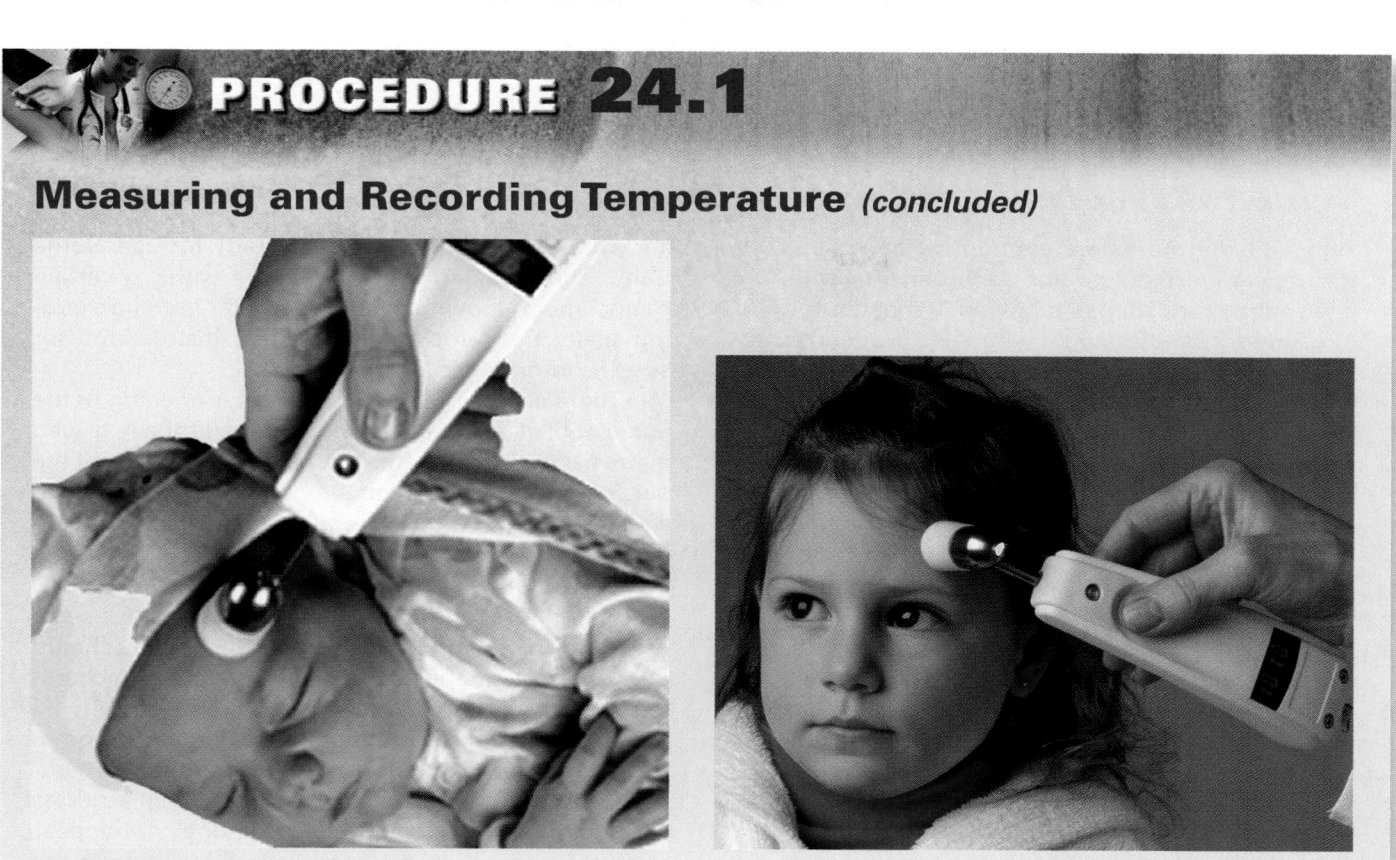

**Figure 24-7.** Temporal scanner in use.

**Special Considerations in Children.** Taking a child's or an infant's temperature can be a challenge. If the infant or child is likely to cry or become agitated, take the temperature last. Measure pulse, respiration, and blood pressure (if ordered) before you take the temperature to avoid having these measurements elevated because of the child's agitation.

Oral thermometers are not appropriate for children younger than 5 years of age because these children are too young to safely hold the thermometer in their mouths. Instead, take axillary, rectal, tympanic, or temporal temperatures. If you use a rectal thermometer, hold it in place until the temperature registers to prevent the thermometer from being expelled or injury to the patient. Tympanic and temporal thermometers are especially useful in pediatric offices because of their speed and safety.

## Pulse and Respiration

Pulse and respiration are related because the circulatory and respiratory systems work together. Pulse is measured as the number of times the heart beats in 1 minute. Respiration is the number of times a patient breathes in 1 minute. One breath, or respiration, equals one inhalation and one exhalation. Usually if either the pulse or respiration

rate is high or low, the other is also. The usual ratio of the pulse rate to the respiration rate is about 4:1 (for example, a pulse of 80 and a respiration of 20). In general, the younger the patient, the higher the normal pulse and respiration rate. Additionally, adult female rates tend to be faster than males. You should be familiar with these rates and how to perform the procedure. See Table 24-1 and Procedure 24-2.

**Pulse.** A pulse rate gives information about the patient's cardiovascular system. It is an indirect measurement of the patient's cardiac output or the amount of blood the heart is able to pump in one minute. If the pulse is abnormally fast (**tachycardia**), slow (**bradycardia**), weak, or irregular, the patient may have a medical problem.

Measure the pulse of adults at the **radial artery,** where it can be felt in the groove on the thumb side of the inner wrist. Press lightly on this pulse point with your fingers and not your thumb (a pulse is located in your thumb, and you may feel it instead of the patient's pulse). Count the number of beats you feel in 1 minute and note the rhythm and volume. The rhythm can be regular and irregular. The volume can be weak, strong, and bounding. Office policy may direct that you count the pulse for 30 seconds and multiply the results by 2 to obtain the beats per minute. If you take a pulse for less than 1 minute and notice the rhythm is

![BIOHAZARD] **CAUTION** *Handle With Care*

## Tympanic Thermometers: What You Need to Know

Tympanic thermometers are popular and useful with uncooperative patients and with patients who have been eating, drinking, or smoking. Tympanic temperatures are fast and accurate when performed properly. To prevent inaccurate readings, here is a summary of what you need to know.

### Why the Eardrum?

The eardrum is an ideal place to measure temperature because it shares the same blood supply with the hypothalamus, the organ that controls body temperature.

### How Do Tympanic Thermometers Work?

Tympanic thermometers convert the infrared energy, a type of heat energy emitted from the eardrum, into a temperature reading, usually within seconds. Most tympanic thermometers run on a rechargeable battery that must be recharged between uses.

### Where Problems Can Occur

The technique for taking a tympanic temperature may vary slightly, depending on which brand of thermometer you use. Most units have an indicator to let you know when the thermometer is ready for use. Some units require taking the temperature within a certain period after removing the thermometer from its charging base. Read the manufacturer's instructions for specific information.

There can be problems if the outer opening of the ear is not sealed completely when the probe is placed at the ear canal or the thermometer is not aimed at the eardrum. You may need to tug gently on the ear to position the thermometer properly and aim it at the eardrum.

If the thermometer has been charging for several hours before use, the initial reading may be inaccurately high. Therefore, some experts believe you should take two measurements on the first patient after charging the unit and record only the second reading.

Even with good technique, problems can sometimes occur. For example, excessive or impacted cerumen (earwax) or otitis media may prevent an accurate reading. If you obtain a reading that does not appear to match the patient's general condition, repeat the temperature measurement to be sure. It may also be necessary to use a different method.

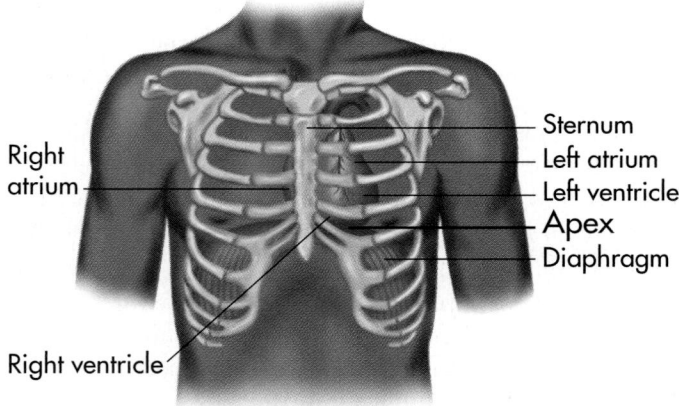

**Figure 24-8.** A stethoscope is used over the apex of the heart to listen for the pulse in patients in whom pulse is not otherwise detectable.

irregular or the pulse is weak or bounding, you must count for 1 full minute and document the irregularities.

Pulse sites other than the radial pulse may be used for various reasons. For example, in young children, the radial artery may be hard to feel. You may instead take the pulse at the **brachial artery,** which is in the bend of the elbow (the **antecubital space**) or on the inner side of the upper arm. If you cannot feel the brachial pulse, then take the pulse over the **apex** (the left lower corner) of the heart, where the strongest heart sounds can be heard. Count the **apical** pulse while you listen with a **stethoscope,** an instrument that amplifies body sounds. The apex is located in the fifth intercostal space between the ribs on the left side of the chest, directly below the center of the clavicle. Consult Figure 24-8 for placement of the stethoscope. You may also use other locations to take a pulse. Figure 24-9 shows the location of common pulse points.

**Electronic Pulse.** The pulse may be measured electronically using a device attached to the finger or sometimes the earlobe. Figure 24-10 shows one type of device used as part of an electronic blood pressure machine. A pulse oximeter machine, which measures the oxygen level of the blood, can also be used (Figure 24-11). When using these devices, be certain to attach the clip firmly to the finger or lobe. The clip uses an infrared light to measure the pulse and oxygen levels, so it works best when no nail polish is present on the patient's finger. The pulse reading and the oxygen saturation of the blood will display on the screen. If the pulse is outside the normal range (see Table 24-1), it should be taken again or performed manually. If the oxygen level is less than 92%, the patient should be asked to take deep breaths during the procedure to increase her oxygen level. An oxygen level below 92% that does not improve with deep breaths should be reported.

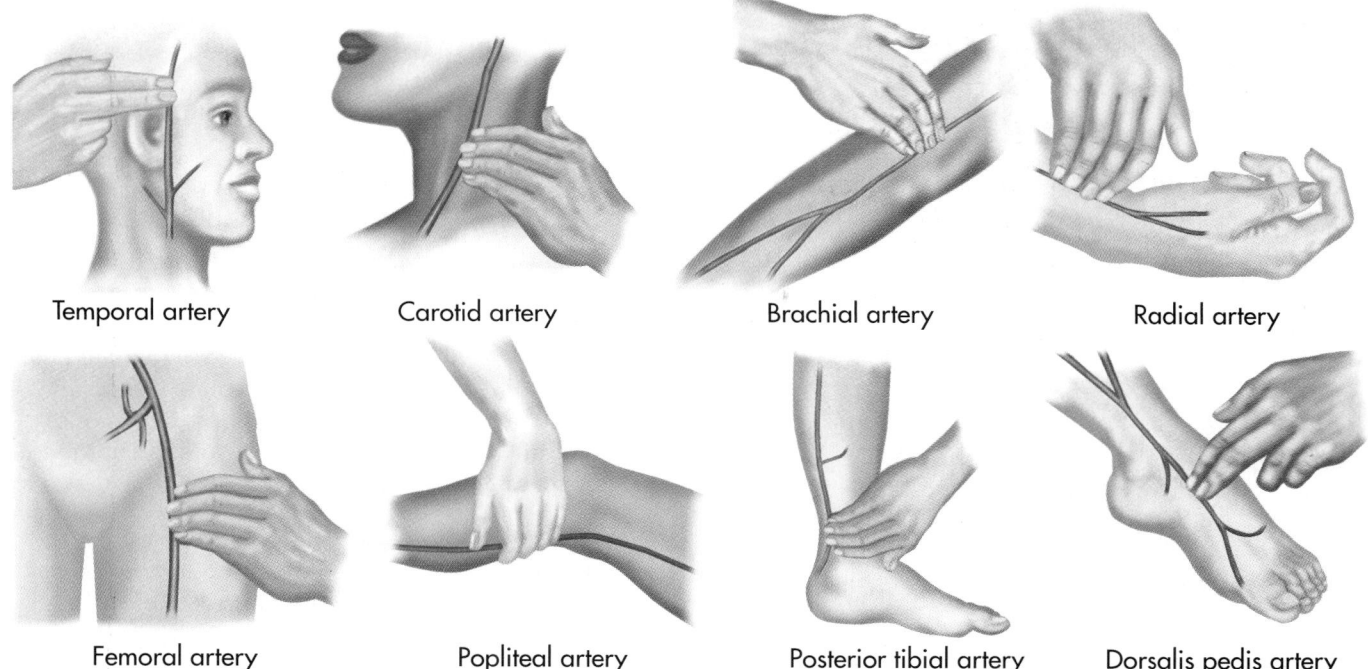

Temporal artery      Carotid artery      Brachial artery      Radial artery

Femoral artery      Popliteal artery      Posterior tibial artery      Dorsalis pedis artery

**Figure 24-9.** There are many locations on the body where major arteries are close enough to the surface to allow a pulse to be felt and counted.

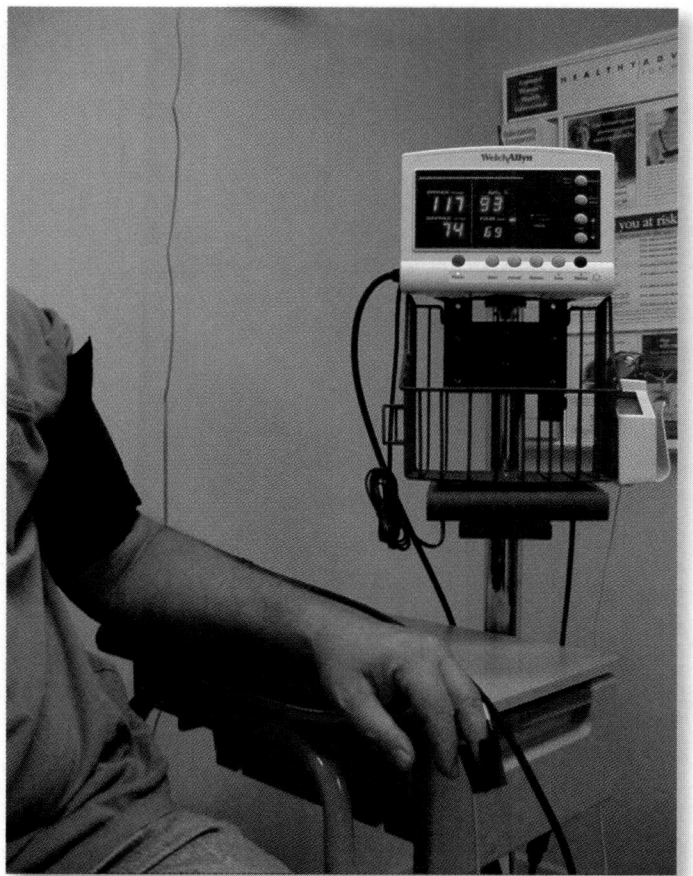

**Figure 24-10.** Pulse, blood pressure, and oxygen saturation can all be measured with this electronic blood pressure device.

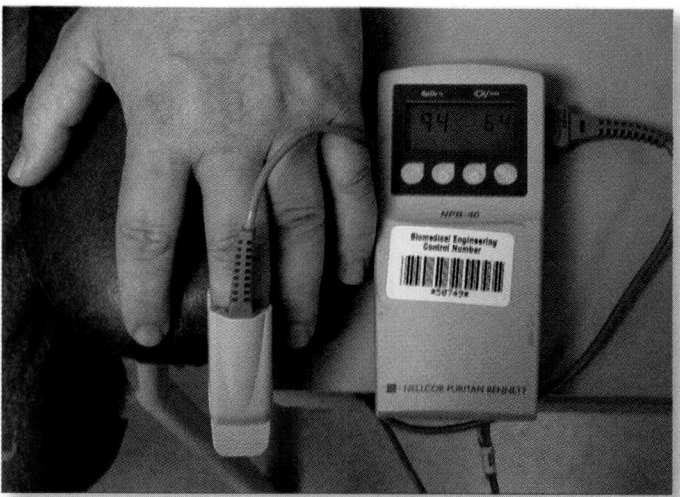

**Figure 24-11.** A pulse oximeter measures the pulse and oxygen saturation of the blood.

**Respiration.** Respiration rate indicates how well a patient's body is providing oxygen to tissues. The best way to check respiration is by watching, listening, or feeling the movement at the patient's chest, stomach, back, or shoulders. If you cannot see the chest movement, then place your hand over the patient's chest, shoulder, or abdomen and listen and feel for the movement of air.

Respirations may also be counted with a stethoscope. Place the stethoscope on one side of the spine in the middle of the back to count respirations. You need to count

**Obtaining Vital Signs and Measurements**     **513**

## Measuring and Recording Pulse and Respirations

**Procedure Goal:** To accurately measure the pulse and respiration of a patient while keeping the patient unaware the respirations are being counted.

### OSHA Guidelines

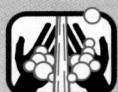 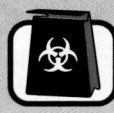 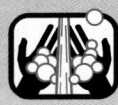

**Materials:** Watch with a second hand, patient's charts, and recording device.

### Method:

1. Gather the equipment and wash your hands.
2. Introduce yourself and identify the patient.
3. Explain the procedure saying, "I am going to take your vital signs. We'll start with your pulse first." Do not tell them you are counting the respirations.

   *Rationale*

   If the patient is aware you are counting respirations, he may unconsciously change his or her breathing rate.
4. Ask the patient to sit or lie in a comfortable position. Have the patient rest the arm on a table. The palm should be facing downward.
5. Position yourself so you can observe and/or feel the chest wall movements. You may want to lay the patient's arm over the chest to feel the respiratory chest movements.

6. Place two to three fingers on the radial pulse site. Find the radial bone on the thumb side of the wrist, then slide your fingers into the groove on the inside of the wrist to locate the pulse.
7. Count the pulse for 15 to 30 seconds if regular. Note the rhythm and volume. If irregular, count for a full minute. Remember or note the number if necessary.

   *Rationale*

   An irregular pulse is counted for a full minute to ensure accuracy and note abnormalities.
8. Without letting go of the wrist, observe and feel the respirations. Counting for one full minute. Observe for rhythm, volume, and effort.
9. Once you are certain of both numbers, release the wrist and record them. If the pulse was taken for less than one minute, obtain the number of beats per minute. Multiply the number of beats counted in 30 seconds by two or the number of beats counted in 15 seconds by 4.
10. Document results with the date and time. (Example: 6/18/08 P 88 regular and strong R 16 regular)
11. Report any findings that are a significant change from a previous result or outside the normal values as shown in Table 24-1.

---

respirations subtly because once the patient is aware that respiration is being measured, he may unintentionally alter his breathing. If using a stethoscope, tell the patient that you want to listen to his lungs. When you are not using a stethoscope, count the respirations while you have your hand on the pulse site.

Respirations are counted for one full minute in order to determine the rate, rhythm, and effort (quality). Counting for less than a minute may cause you to miss certain breathing abnormalities. The rhythm should be regular. The quality of effort should be normal, shallow, or deep. Irregularities such as hyperventilation (excessive rate and depth of breathing usually due to hysteria), dyspnea (difficult or painful breathing), **tachypnea** (rapid breathing), or **hyperpnea** (abnormally rapid or deep breathing) are indications of possible disease and should be noted. **Rales** (noisy) breathing can indicate constriction or blockage of bronchial passages. They may be noted in pneumonia, bronchitis, asthma, or other pulmonary diseases. **Cheyne-Stokes respirations** are characterized by periods of increasing and decreasing depth of respiration between periods of **apnea** (the absence of respiration). This pattern of breathing may be seen in patients with strokes, head injuries, brain tumors, and in patients with congestive heart failure.

# Blood Pressure

Blood pressure (also known as arterial blood pressure) is the force at which blood is pumped against the walls of the arteries. The standard unit for measuring blood pressure is millimeters of mercury (mm Hg). The pressure measured when the left ventricle of the heart contracts is known as the systolic pressure. The pressure measured when the heart relaxes is known as the diastolic pressure. The diastolic pressure indicates the minimum amount of pressure exerted against the vessel walls at all times.

Expected adult systolic readings are less than 120 mm Hg. Expected adult diastolic readings are less than 80 mm Hg. These values may increase with advancing age. A systolic reading between 121 and 140 mm Hg and a diastolic reading between 81 and 90 mm Hg is considered prehypertension. Over 140 mm Hg systolic and over 90 mm Hg diastolic is considered hypertension.

**Hypertension,** or high blood pressure, is a major contributor to heart attack and stroke. The doctor may ask a patient whose blood pressure is elevated to return for a checkup or blood pressure check. If the blood pressure remains elevated, the patient may be diagnosed with hypertension. **Hypotension,** or low blood pressure, is not generally a chronic health problem. Slightly low blood pressure may be normal for some patients and does not usually require treatment. Severe hypotension may be present with shock, heart failure, severe burns, and excessive bleeding.

## Blood Pressure Measuring Equipment.
Blood pressure is measured with an instrument called a **sphygmomanometer.** A sphygmomanometer consists of an inflatable cuff, a pressure bulb or automatic device for inflating the cuff, and a manometer to read the pressure. The three basic types of sphygmomanometers differ in how the pressure is displayed.

*Aneroid Sphygmomanometers.* Aneroid sphygmomanometers have a circular gauge for registering pressure. The needle on the gauge rotates as pressure rises. This type of sphygmomanometer is very accurate. Each measurement line indicates 2 mm Hg (Figure 24-12).

*Electronic Sphygmomanometers.* Electronic sphygmomanometers provide a digital readout of blood pressure on a lit display (Figure 24-13). Unlike aneroid sphygmomanometers, these devices do not require use of a stethoscope to determine blood pressure. They are easy to use, but can be costly. Accuracy can sometimes be an issue, so maintain the equipment according to the manufacturer's instructions. If you question the results of an electronic blood pressure measurement, take it again with an aneroid cuff.

*Mercury Sphygmomanometers.* Mercury sphygmomanometers contain a column of mercury. The mercury column rises with an increase in pressure as the cuff is inflated. Mercury sphygmomanometers may be wall-mounted units, tabletop units, or freestanding units on wheels.

### ANEROID BLOOD PRESSURE GAUGE

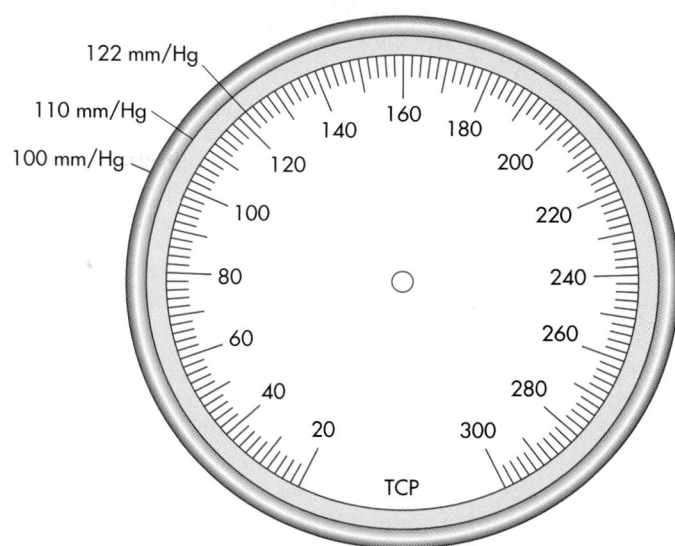

**Figure 24-12.** Each line on the aneroid gauge indicates 2 mm Hg. To prevent inaccuracies, look directly at this gauge when performing a blood pressure test.

Source: Borrowed from Kathryn Booth, *Health Care Science Technology: Career Technology,* 1st ed., Peoria, IL: Glencoe/McGraw-Hill, 2004.

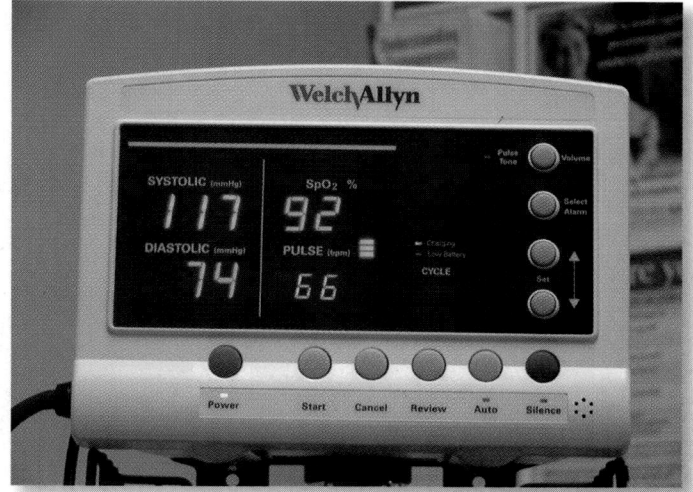

**Figure 24-13.** This electronic sphygmomanometer displays the patient's blood pressure, pulse, and oxygen saturation. If you question any of the results, repeat the test using a manual method.

Mercury instruments are used less frequently because the government has restricted the use of mercury due to its effects on the environment. Consequently, no new mercury sphygmomanometers are being manufactured.

## Calibrating the Sphygmomanometer.
To ensure that sphygmomanometers are working properly, you or a medical supply dealer must calibrate them regularly.

To **calibrate** means to standardize a measuring instrument. Mercury sphygmomanometers must be checked for faults, serviced, and calibrated every 6 to 12 months. Aneroid sphygmomanometers must be checked, serviced, and calibrated every 3 to 6 months. Follow the manufacturer's instructions for an electronic sphygmomanometer.

Do not use a sphygmomanometer unless you are certain it is calibrated because inaccurate readings can result. To calibrate, follow these steps.

- For a mercury sphygmomanometer, check that the **meniscus** (curve in the air-to-liquid surface of the specimen in the cylinder) of mercury on the mercury column rests at zero when you view it at eye level.
- For an aneroid sphygmomanometer, check that the recording needle on the dial rests within the small square at the bottom of the dial. To calibrate the dial, use a Y connector to attach the dial to a pressure bulb and a calibrated mercury manometer. Use the pressure bulb to elevate both manometer readings to 250 mm Hg. As you let the pressure fall, record both readings at four different points. The difference between paired readings should not exceed 3 mm Hg.

**The Stethoscope.** A stethoscope amplifies body sounds, making them louder. It consists of earpieces, binaurals, rubber or plastic tubing, and a chestpiece (Figure 24-14).

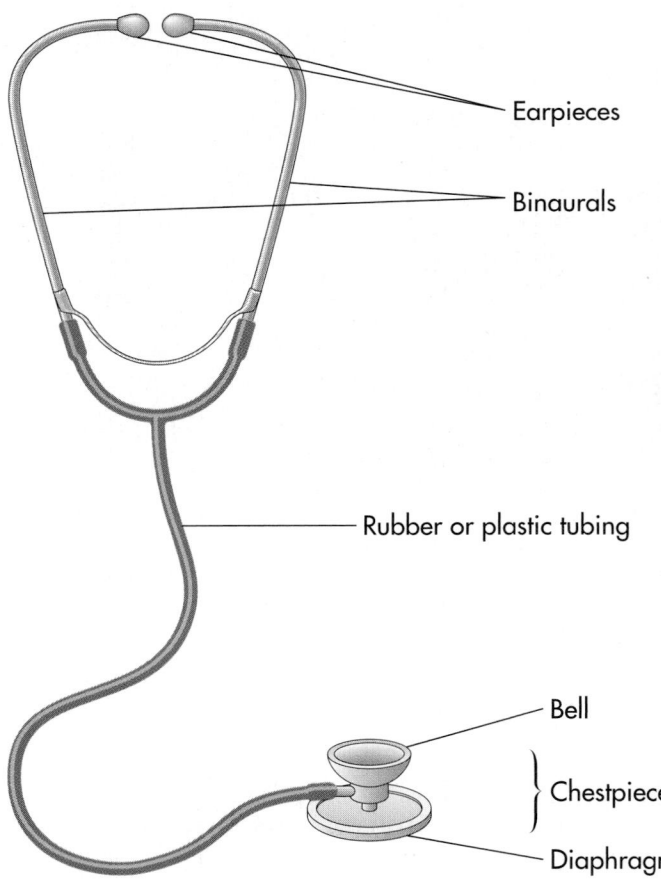

**Figure 24-14.** The stethoscope amplifies body sounds.

For best results the earpieces should fit snugly and comfortably in your ears. When placing them in your ears, face the angle of the earpiece up and forward for the best fit.

The chestpiece consists of two parts: the diaphragm and the bell. The diaphragm is the larger, flat side of the chestpiece. It is covered by a thin, plastic disk. The diaphragm must be placed firmly against the skin for proper amplification of sound. The diaphragm is best at amplifying high-pitched sounds, such as bowel and lung sounds.

The bell is the cone-shaped side of the stethoscope chestpiece. It must be held lightly against the skin to amplify sound. The bell is best at amplifying low-pitched sounds, such as vascular and heart sounds. With practice you may find you prefer to use one side rather than the other for various purposes.

**Measuring Blood Pressure.** To measure blood pressure, wrap the rubber cuff of the sphygmomanometer around the patient's upper arm, just above the pulse point of the brachial artery (Figure 24-15). This pulse point is located in the bend of the elbow, or the antecubital space. Inflate the cuff. Then while you release the air in the cuff, listen with the stethoscope. The cuff is usually inflated to 30 mm Hg above the palpatory result, or approximately 180 to 200 mm Hg. You will hear vascular sounds that will change. These sounds are also called Korotkoff sounds. They are produced by the obstruction and release of the arterial blood flow.

The first heartbeat you hear is the systolic pressure. As the pressure in the cuff is released, this strong heartbeat changes to a softer, muffled sound. The point at which the

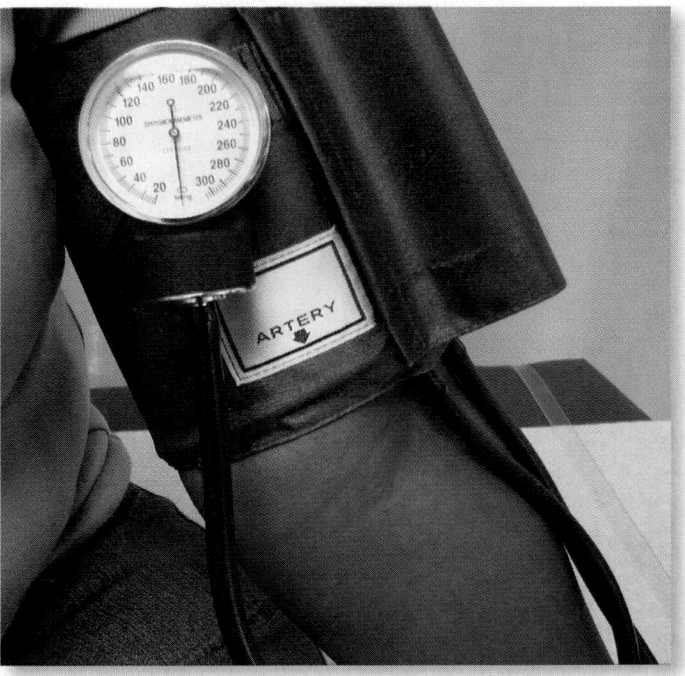

**Figure 24-15.** The blood pressure cuff should be one inch above the elbow with the center of the bladder directly above the brachial pulse.

sound disappears is the diastolic pressure. The patient's blood pressure reading is recorded as the numbers registered for the first and last sounds separated by a slash mark, as in BP 120/76. Although only the systolic and diastolic readings are usually recorded for adults, a third number may be included at times. For example, if there is a pressure difference greater than 10 mm Hg between the muffled sound and its disappearance, the blood pressure is recorded with all three sounds noted, such as 120/80/60. The process of taking blood pressure is described in Procedure 24-3.

## PROCEDURE 24.3

## Taking the Blood Pressure of Adults and Older Children

**Procedure Goal:** To accurately measure blood pressure in adults and older children

### OSHA Guidelines

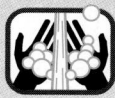 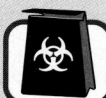 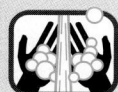

**Materials:** Aneroid or mercury sphygmomanometer, stethoscope, alcohol gauze squares, patient's chart, and black pen

### Method:

1. Gather the equipment and make sure the sphygmomanometer is in working order and is correctly calibrated.

   *Rationale*

   Calibration helps ensure an accurate result.

2. Identify the patient and introduce yourself.

3. Wash your hands and explain the procedure to the patient.

4. Have the patient sit in a quiet area. If she is wearing long-sleeved clothing, have her loosely roll up one sleeve. If she cannot, have her change into a gown.

5. Have the patient rest her bared arm on a flat surface so that the midpoint of the upper arm is at the same level as the heart.

   *Rationale*

   Doing so ensures an accurate reading.

6. Select a cuff that is the appropriate size for the patient. The bladder inside the cuff should encircle 80% of the arm in adults and 100% of the arm in children younger than the age of 13. If you are not sure about the size, use a larger cuff.

   *Rationale*

   The proper cuff size ensures an accurate reading.

7. Locate the brachial artery in the antecubital space.

8. Position the cuff so that the midline of the bladder is above the arterial pulsation. Then wrap and secure the cuff snugly around the patient's bare upper arm. The lower edge of the cuff should be 1 inch above the antecubital space, where the head of the stethoscope is to be placed.

   *Rationale*

   If the blood pressure cuff touches the stethoscope, it could interfere with your ability to hear.

9. Place the manometer so that the center of the aneroid dial or mercury column is at eye level and easily visible and so that the tubing from the cuff is unobstructed.

10. Close the valve of the pressure bulb until it is finger-tight.

11. Inflate the cuff rapidly to 70 mm Hg with one hand, and increase this pressure by 10 mm Hg increments while palpating the radial pulse with your other hand. Note the level of pressure at which the pulse disappears and subsequently reappears during deflation. This procedure, the **palpatory method,** provides an approximation of the systolic blood pressure to ensure an adequate level of inflation when the actual measurement is made.

12. Open the valve to release the pressure, deflate the cuff completely, and wait 30 seconds or remove and replace the cuff.

    *Rationale*

    If you do not deflate the cuff completely and wait, blood may pool in the artery and give a falsely high reading.

13. Place the earpieces of the stethoscope in your ear canals, and adjust them to fit snugly and comfortably. When placed in the ears, they should point up or toward the nose. Switch the stethoscope head to the diaphragm position. Confirm the setting by listening as you tap the stethoscope head gently.

*continued* ⟶

# Taking the Blood Pressure of Adults and Older Children *(concluded)*

**14.** Place the head of the stethoscope over the brachial artery pulsation, just above and medial to the antecubital space but below the lower edge of the cuff. Hold the stethoscope firmly in place between the index and middle fingers, making sure the head is in contact with the skin around its entire circumference.

### Rationale

Do not hold the stethoscope with the thumb, because the pulse of your thumb can interfere with the reading.

**15.** Inflate the bladder rapidly and steadily to a pressure 20 to 30 mm Hg above the level previously determined by palpation. Then partially open (unscrew) the valve, and deflate the bladder at 2 mm per second while you listen for the appearance of the Korotkoff sounds.

**16.** As the pressure in the bladder falls, note the level of pressure on the manometer at the first appearance of repetitive sounds. This reading is the systolic pressure.

**17.** Continue to deflate the cuff gradually, noting the point at which the sound changes from strong to muffled.

**18.** Continue to deflate the cuff, and note when the sound disappears. This reading is the diastolic pressure.

**19.** Deflate the cuff completely, and remove it from the patient's arm.

**20.** Record the numbers, separated by slashes, in the patient's chart. Chart the date and time of the measurement, the arm on which the measurement was made, the subject's position, and the cuff size when a nonstandard size is used.

### Rationale

The value recorded is an exact measurement of the **auscultated blood pressure,** meaning that it was determined by listening with a stethoscope.

**21.** Fold the cuff and replace it in the holder.

**22.** Inform the patient that you have completed the procedure.

**23.** Disinfect the earpieces and diaphragm of the stethoscope with gauze squares moistened with alcohol.

**24.** Properly dispose of the used gauze squares and wash your hands.

**Special Considerations in Adults.** Blood pressure is elevated during and just after exercise. If a patient has engaged in strenuous activity before the exam, you should wait 15 minutes before taking blood pressure measurements. This waiting period also applies to patients with ambulatory disabilities, to those who are obese, and to those who have a known blood pressure problem. If you ensure that patients have relaxed for 15 minutes before you measure their blood pressure, you should get an accurate reading.

Blood pressure may also be elevated when a patient is anxious or under stress. The patient may be aware that a blood pressure reading is high or low and upset about the reading. If the patient seems stressed or upset, allow him to rest for about 5 minutes before measuring his blood pressure. To help the patient relax, try to engage the person in conversation rather than calling attention to the fact that you are waiting to take his blood pressure. If the patient still appears anxious or under stress, take his blood pressure anyway, and make a notation for the physician (who may want to repeat the measurement later in the visit).

There are certain instances when you should not take a blood pressure measurement on a particular arm. Blood pressure should not be taken on an arm that is on the same side as a mastectomy (breast removal) or on an arm that has an injury, a blocked artery, or a device under the skin (implant) at the site. In such cases, use the other arm or the upper leg. Note the measurements and their locations in the patient's chart.

Be sure you use the proper size cuff when taking blood pressure. The bladder inside the cuff should encircle 80% to 100% the distance around the arm or leg. Although the standard adult cuff can be used for most adults, some may require the larger size. Using an improper size may result in an inaccurate reading.

**Special Considerations in Children.** Blood pressure in children or infants is not routinely measured at each visit. Instead, the measurement is taken on the order of the doctor. The procedure is the same as that for taking blood pressure in adults, except for these modifications.

1. Ideally, take the patient's blood pressure before performing other tests or procedures that may cause anxiety. In this way you can avoid a falsely high result.

2. Be sure to use the correct cuff size for the child or infant. The bladder width should not exceed two-thirds the length of the upper or lower arm. The bladder should cover three-fourths the circumference of the extremity.

3. Do not attempt to estimate an infant's blood pressure in the manner described in Procedure 24-3—the palpatory method usually cannot be used on an infant.

4. Inflate the pressure cuff to 20 mm Hg above the point at which the radial pulse disappears.

5. Deflate the cuff at a rate of 2 mm Hg per second.

6. You may continue to hear a heartbeat on a child or infant until the pressure reaches zero, so note when the strong heartbeat becomes muffled.

## Orthostatic or Postural Vital Signs

Orthostatic vital signs usually consist of taking the blood pressure and pulse. The vital signs are taken in different positions to assess for **orthostatic** or **postural hypotension.** This means that as the patient moves from a lying to standing position, the blood pressure becomes low and, as a result, the pulse increases. This usually indicates some sort of fluid loss or malfunctioning of the cardiovascular system, such as from vomiting, diarrhea, or prolonged bed rest.

Orthostatic vital signs are taken in three different positions. BP and pulse are taken with the patient lying down, then sitting up, and then standing. It is recommended to wait 2 to 5 minutes before taking the vital signs after repositioning to allow the body's systems to adjust. If there is an increase in the pulse rate of more than 10 bpm, and the blood pressure drops more than 20 points, then the patient is considered to have orthostatic hypotension. This is sometimes documented as a **positive tilt test.**

## Body Measurements

Certain measurements are obtained prior to the patient's being seen by the practitioner. These include height and weight for adults and older children, and weight, length, and head circumference for infants. Usually these measurements are taken before or after the vital signs, depending on the office policy. Depending on the patient, you may choose to take the patient's vital signs first. For example, if a patient may become upset about her weight, you should take her vital signs first so that the patient's vital signs will not be affected by the weight results. Follow the policy at your facility.

Measurements provide baseline values for a patient's current condition. Any extreme or abnormal changes may indicate a disease or disorder and should be noted for the practitioner. For children and adolescents, these measurements should be taken at each office visit, which allows the physician to follow growth and development. Many physicians use growth charts to compare a child's growth with that of other children the same age (Figure 24-16, p. 520).

These charts help physicians recognize possible growth and nutritional problems.

Measurements are also important in determining the extent of an injury or illness and certain treatment regimens. For example, dosages of certain medications are based on patient weight, or a wound or bruise may be measured to determine how well it is healing. These measurements may also be necessary for correct interpretation of certain diagnostic tests, such as electrocardiography. Metric conversions for weight and height measurements are given in Tables 24-4 and 24-5. To complete these conversions yourself, review the Points on Practice feature, Math for Measurements, on page 506.

## Measuring the Weight of Adults

An adult's weight is taken at each office visit. Weight should be listed in the patient's chart to the nearest quarter of a pound. The steps for weighing an adult are described in Procedure 24-4.

## Measuring the Height of Adults

The height of an adult should be measured at the patient's initial visit and whenever a complete physical exam is performed or at least yearly. Height should be measured to the nearest quarter of an inch. Measure the patient's height after weighing the patient. Most office scales have a height bar located in the center of the scale. This bar is calibrated in inches and quarter inches (Figure 24-17). The steps for measuring the height of an adult are described in Procedure 24-4.

## Measuring the Weight of Children and Infants

Children and infants are weighed at each office visit. Children who can stand may be weighed on an adult scale. If toddlers cannot remain still on an adult scale, weight may be determined by weighing an adult holding the toddler, then subtracting the weight of the adult.

Infants are weighed on infant scales, which typically measure pounds and ounces. Infant scales are sometimes built into a pediatric examining table. The steps for weighing children and infants are described in Procedure 24-5.

## Measuring the Height of Children and Infants

The height of children and the length of infants are measured at each office visit. Measure children in the same manner as you measure an adult. Some offices are equipped with height bars or wall charts that are separate from a

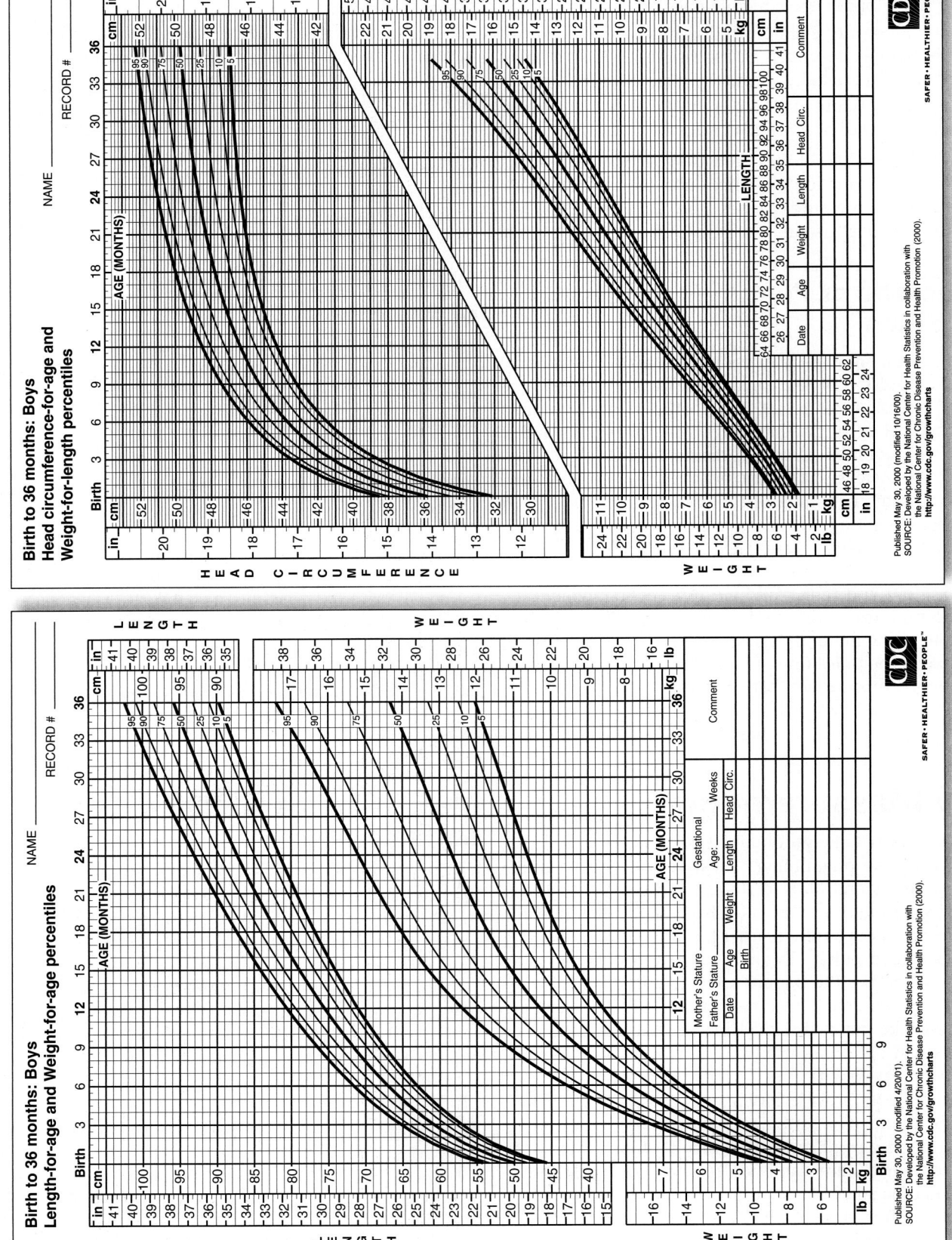

**Figure 24-16.** The curved lines on these growth charts are used to chart the growth for boys from birth to age 36

| TABLE 24-4 | Metric Conversions for Weight | | | | |
|---|---|---|---|---|---|
| lb | kg | lb | kg | lb | kg |
| 10 | 4.5 | 95 | 43.1 | 180 | 81.7 |
| 15 | 6.8 | 100 | 45.4 | 185 | 84.0 |
| 20 | 9.1 | 105 | 47.7 | 190 | 86.3 |
| 25 | 11.4 | 110 | 49.9 | 195 | 88.5 |
| 30 | 13.6 | 115 | 52.2 | 200 | 90.8 |
| 35 | 15.9 | 120 | 54.5 | 205 | 93.1 |
| 40 | 18.2 | 125 | 56.8 | 210 | 95.3 |
| 45 | 20.4 | 130 | 59.0 | 215 | 97.6 |
| 50 | 22.7 | 135 | 61.3 | 220 | 99.9 |
| 55 | 25.0 | 140 | 63.6 | 225 | 102.2 |
| 60 | 27.2 | 145 | 65.8 | 230 | 104.4 |
| 65 | 29.5 | 150 | 68.1 | 235 | 106.7 |
| 70 | 31.8 | 155 | 70.4 | 240 | 109.0 |
| 75 | 34.1 | 160 | 72.6 | 245 | 111.2 |
| 80 | 36.3 | 165 | 74.9 | 250 | 113.5 |
| 85 | 38.6 | 170 | 77.2 | | |
| 90 | 40.9 | 175 | 79.5 | | |

Note: kg = lb × 0.454; lb = kg × 2.205. Conversions are rounded to nearest tenth.

| TABLE 24-5 | Metric Conversions for Height | | | | |
|---|---|---|---|---|---|
| in | cm | in | cm | in | cm |
| 20 | 51 | 42 | 107 | 62 | 157 |
| 22 | 56 | 44 | 112 | 64 | 163 |
| 24 | 61 | 46 | 117 | 66 | 168 |
| 26 | 66 | 48 | 122 | 68 | 173 |
| 28 | 71 | 50 | 127 | 70 | 178 |
| 30 | 76 | 52 | 132 | 72 | 183 |
| 32 | 81 | 54 | 137 | 74 | 188 |
| 34 | 86 | 56 | 142 | 76 | 193 |
| 36 | 91 | 58 | 147 | 78 | 198 |
| 38 | 97 | 60 | 152 | 80 | 203 |
| 40 | 102 | | | | |

Note: cm = in × 2.54; in = cm × 0.394. Conversions are rounded to nearest whole number.

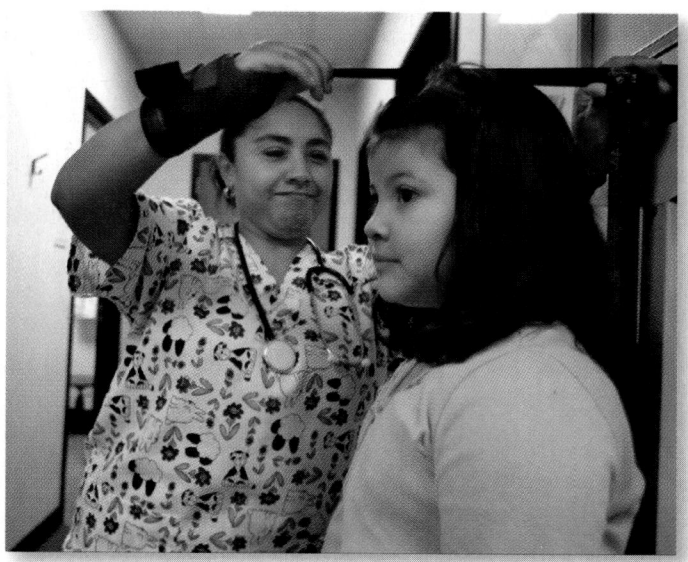

**Figure 24-17.** The scale with attached height bar is used for measuring the height and weight of children and adults.

scale. Use these devices in the same way as those that are attached to a scale.

Measure infants while they are lying down. In this instance you are measuring length instead of height. Some pediatric examining tables have a built-in bar for measuring length. You can also use a tape measure or yardstick. The steps for measuring the height of a child or the length of an infant are described in Procedure 24-5.

## Measuring the Head Circumference of Infants

The circumference of an infant's head is an important measure of growth and development and is used to evaluate diseases such as hydrocephalus or excessive cerebrospinal fluid in the cranial cavity, which causes enlargement of the head. You may be asked to perform or assist with this measurement (Figure 24-18) when you measure the infant's length. The steps for measuring the circumference of an infant's head are described in Procedure 24-5.

## Other Body Measurements

In some facilities, you may be asked to obtain other body measurements. For example, if a patient has edema (swelling) of an arm or leg, you might be asked to measure the diameter. You should measure both arms or legs to determine the difference in size. If a patient has a wound, bruise, or other injury, you may need to measure its length and width to evaluate the healing process. Additionally, sometimes an infant will need his chest circumference measured, or an adult would require a measurement around his abdomen, which is known as abdominal girth.

# PROCEDURE 24.4

## Measuring Adults and Children

**Procedure Goal:** To accurately measure weight and height of adults and children

### OSHA Guidelines

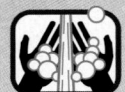  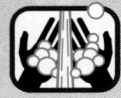

**Materials:** For an adult or older child, adult scale with height bar, disposable towel; for toddler, adult scale with height bar or height chart, disposable towel

### Method:

#### Adult or Older Child: Weight

1. Identify the patient and introduce yourself.
2. Wash your hands and explain the procedure to the patient.
3. Check to see whether the scale is in balance by moving all the weights to the left side. The indicator should be level with the middle mark. If not, check the manufacturer's directions and adjust it to ensure a zero balance. If you are using a scale equipped to measure either kilograms or pounds, check to see that it is set on the desired units and that the upper and lower weights show the same units.

   *Rationale*

   Proper functioning of the scale ensures an accurate result.

4. Place a disposable towel on the scale or have the patient leave their socks on.

   *Rationale*

   Prevents cross-contamination of the scale from various patients' feet.

5. Ask the patient to remove her shoes, if that is the standard office policy.

   *Rationale*

   Follow the policy and use the same procedure for all visits for consistency of results.

6. Ask the patient to step on the center of the scale, facing forward. Assist as necessary.
7. Place the lower weight at the highest number that does not cause the balance indicator to drop to the bottom.

   *Rationale*

   To ensure accuracy.

8. Move the upper weight slowly to the right until the balance bar is centered at the middle mark, adjusting as necessary.

   *Rationale*

   To ensure accuracy.

9. Add the two weights together to get the patient's weight.
10. Record the patient's weight in the chart to the nearest quarter of a pound or tenth of a kilogram.
11. Return the weights to their starting positions on the left side.

#### Adult or Older Child: Height

12. With the patient off the scale, raise the height bar well above the patient's head and swing out the extension.

    *Rationale*

    Doing so prevents hitting the patient with the extension bar.

13. Ask the patient to step on the center of the scale and to stand up straight and look forward.

    *Rationale*

    Standing straight is necessary for accuracy.

14. Gently lower the height bar until the extension rests on the patient's head.
15. Have the patient step off the scale before reading the measurement.

    *Rationale*

    To better visualize the height measurement.

16. If the patient is fewer than 50 inches tall, read the height on the bottom part of the ruler; if the patient is more than 50 inches tall, read the height on the top movable part of the ruler at the point at which it meets the bottom part of the ruler. Note that the numbers increase on the bottom part of the bar and decrease on the top, moveable part of the bar. Read the height in the right direction.
17. Record the patient's height.
18. Have the patient put her shoes back on, if necessary.
19. Properly dispose of the used towel and wash your hands.

#### Toddler: Weight

1. Identify the patient and obtain permission from the parent to weigh the toddler.

*continued* ⟶

## Measuring Adults and Children *(concluded)*

2. Wash your hands and explain the procedure to the parent.

3. Check to see whether the scale is in balance, and place a disposable towel on the scale or have the patient wear shoes or socks, depending upon the policy of the facility.

4. Ask the parent to hold the patient and to step on the scale. Follow the procedure for obtaining the weight of an adult.

5. Have the parent put the child down or hand the child to another staff member.

### Rationale

This is done to find the difference between the two weights.

6. Obtain the parent's weight.

7. Subtract the parent's weight from the combined weight to determine the weight of the child.

8. Record the patient's weight in the chart to the nearest quarter of a pound or tenth of a kilogram.

### Toddler: Height

9. Measure the child's height in the same manner as you measure adult height, or have the child stand with his back against the height chart. Measure height at the crown of the head.

10. Record the height in the patient's chart.

11. Properly dispose of the towel (if used) and wash your hands.

### Rationale

Doing so prevents infection.

---

## Measuring Infants

**Procedure Goal:** To accurately measure weight and length of infants and infant head circumference.

### OSHA Guidelines

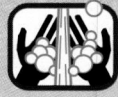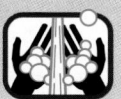

**Materials:** Pediatric examining table or infant scale, cardboard, pencil, yardstick, tape measure, disposable towel

### Method:

#### Weight

1. Identify the patient and obtain permission from the parent to weigh the infant.

2. Wash your hands and explain the procedure to the parent.

3. Ask the parent to undress the infant.

### Rationale

The infant's clothing and diaper can affect the results.

4. Check to see whether the infant scale is in balance, and place a disposable towel on it.

### Rationale

Balancing the scale ensures accuracy.

5. Have the parent place the child face up on the scale (or on the examining table if the scale is built into it). Keep one hand over the infant at all times and hold a diaper over a male patient's penis to catch any urine the infant might void.

### Rationale

Keeping one hand over the infant can prevent a fall, and holding a diaper over a male patient's penis prevents contamination of yourself and the weighing area from urine.

6. Place the lower weight at the highest number that does not cause the balance indicator to drop to the bottom.

### Rationale

Doing so ensures accuracy.

7. Move the upper weight slowly to the right until the balance bar is centered at the middle mark, adjusting as necessary.

### Rationale

Doing so ensures accuracy.

*continued* ⟶

### Measuring Infants (concluded)

8. Add the two weights together to get the infant's weight.

9. Record the infant's weight in the chart in pounds and ounces or to the nearest tenth of a kilogram.

10. Return the weights to their starting positions on the left side.

#### Length: Scale With Length (Height) Bar

11. If the scale has a height bar, move the infant toward the head of the scale or examining table until her head touches the bar.

12. Have the parent hold the infant by the shoulders in this position.

13. Holding the infant's ankles, gently extend the legs and slide the bottom bar to touch the soles of the feet.

#### Rationale

The legs are held to ensure the correct length will be measured.

14. Note the length and release the infant's ankles.

15. Record the length in the patient's chart.

#### Length: Scale or Examining Table Without Length (Height) Bar

16. If neither the scale nor the examining table has a height bar, have the parent position the infant close to the head of the examining table and hold the infant by the shoulders in this position.

17. Place a stiff piece of cardboard against the crown of the infant's head, and mark a line on the towel or paper, or hold a yardstick against the cardboard.

18. Holding the infant's ankles, gently extend the legs and draw a line on the towel or paper to mark the heel, or note the measure on the yardstick.

#### Rationale

The legs are held to ensure the correct length will be measured.

19. Release the infant's ankles and measure the distance between the two markings on the towel or paper using the yardstick or a tape measure.

20. Record the length in the patient's chart.

#### Head Circumference

Measurement of head circumference may be performed at the same time as weight and length, or it may be part of the general physical exam.

21. With the infant in a sitting or supine position, place the tape measure around the infant's head at the forehead.

22. Adjust the tape so that it surrounds the infant's head at its largest circumference.

23. Overlap the ends of the tape, and read the measure at the point of overlap.

24. Remove the tape, and record the circumference in the patient's chart.

25. Properly dispose of the used towel and wash your hands.

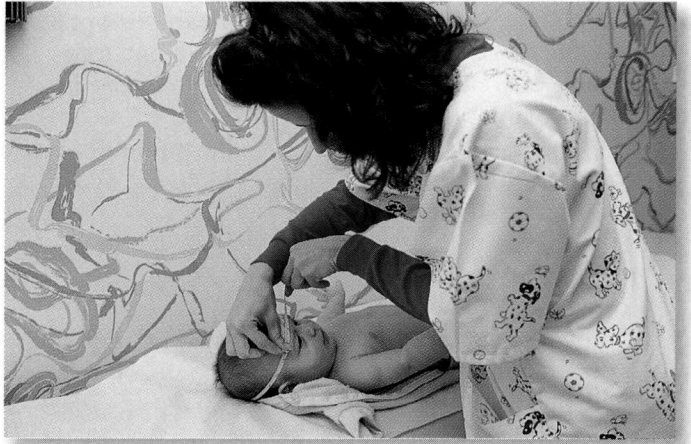

**Figure 24-18.** The medical assistant uses a flexible tape to measure the circumference of an infant's head.

## Summary

One of your duties as a medical assistant will be to measure and record the patient's vital signs, weight, and height. Gathering this information is crucial to the outcome of the patient's visit. Remember that the physician relies on these data as they appear on the chart from visit to visit and when making a diagnosis. Using the proper techniques and the same equipment each and every time you measure a patient's weight, height, and vital signs will help you to provide information that is precise and accurate.

## CASE STUDY *QUESTIONS*

Now that you have completed this chapter, review the case study at the beginning of the chapter and answer the following questions:

1. Why is it essential for you to take accurate measurements of this patient?
2. How can you help ensure the accuracy of these measurements?

## Discussion Questions

1. What are the pros and cons of using growth charts when charting children's growth?
2. Compare and contrast the different types of sphygmomanometers.
3. Compare and contrast the different types of thermometers.

## Critical Thinking Questions

1. A 45-year-old patient comes to the clinic for a follow-up appointment regarding her elevated blood pressure. Prior to seeing the patient, you note on her chart that her last blood pressure reading was 152/90 and her weight was 295 pounds. What measurement should you first take for this patient and why?
2. You take the pulse and blood pressure of a 68-year-old male with an electronic sphygmomanometer and note the following results: BP 169/98, P 104. Are these within normal limits for this patient? If not, what should you do?
3. Describe how you would perform vital signs and measurements on an uncooperative child or crying infant.
4. Describe how you might obtain height and weight measurements of a patient who is deaf.

## Application Activities

1. Pair up with a classmate and practice measuring each other's weight and height.
2. Measure the weight and temperature of at least five people and convert the measurements between pounds and kilograms and the Celsius and Fahrenheit temperature scales. Use the formula provided in the Points on Practice box on page 506. When completing this activity, be certain to show all your calculations.
3. Practice measuring vital signs of several classmates. Compare your measurements with others to verify accuracy.

## Virtual Fieldtrip

*Visit the McGraw-Hill Higher Education Medical Assisting website at www.mhhe.com/medicalassisting3 to complete the following activities:*

1. Take a virtual field trip to the National Heart, Lung, and Blood Institute or American Heart Association using the Web links provided on the McGraw-Hill website. Research the site to determine methods of preventing and treating high blood pressure (hypertension). Use the information to develop a teaching plan for a patient with hypertension.
2. Take a virtual field trip to the Centers for Disease Control. For the patient noted below, find and print copies of the following growth charts: Head Circumference for Age, Weight for Length, Length for Age, and Weight for Age. Then chart the measurements provided.

    18-month-old girl:  Length—30¼ inches
    Weight—23½ lbs.
    Head Circumference—18 inches

Open the CD and complete this chapter's practice activities, play the games, listen to the key terms, and test yourself with the interactive review. E-mail, print, and/or save your results to document your proficiency.

# Assisting With a General Physical Exam

## KEY TERMS

auscultation
clinical diagnosis
culture
differential diagnosis
digital exam
fenestrated drape
inspection
kyphosis
manipulation
mensuration
nasal mucosa
palpation
patient compliance
percussion
prognosis
quadrants
SARS (severe acute
    respiratory syndrome)
symmetry

## MEDICAL ASSISTING COMPETENCIES

*In preparation for the certification examination, you should know the following:*

| COMPETENCY | CMA | RMA |
| --- | --- | --- |
| **Clinical** | | |
| Dispose of biohazardous materials | X | X |
| Practice Standard Precautions | X | X |
| Prepare the patient for and assist the physician with routine and specialty exams, treatments, and minor office surgeries | X | X |
| **General/Legal/Professional** | | |
| Determine the needs for documentation and reporting, and document accurately and appropriately | X | X |
| Demonstrate knowledge of and monitor current federal and state health-care legislation and regulations; maintain licenses and accreditation | X | X |
| Instruct individuals according to their needs | X | X |
| Provide patients with methods of health promotion and disease prevention | X | X |
| Be impartial and show empathy when dealing with patients | | X |
| Serve as a liaison between the physician and others | | X |

## CHAPTER OUTLINE

- The Purpose of a General Physical Exam
- The Role of the Medical Assistant
- Safety Precautions
- Preparing the Patient for an Exam
- Exam Methods
- Components of a General Physical Exam
- Completing the Exam

# LEARNING OUTCOMES

After completing Chapter 25, you will be able to:

25.1 State the purpose of a general physical exam.

25.2 Describe the role of the medical assistant in a general physical exam.

25.3 Explain safety precautions used during a general physical exam.

25.4 Outline the steps necessary to prepare the patient for an exam.

25.5 Describe how to position and drape a patient in each of the ten common exam positions.

25.6 Explain ways to assist patients from different cultures, patients with disabilities, pediatric patients, and pregnant women.

25.7 Identify and describe the six examination methods used in a general physical exam.

25.8 List the components of a general physical exam.

25.9 Explain and perform the procedures for vision screenings.

25.10 Explain and perform the procedures for hearing screenings.

25.11 Explain the special needs of the elderly for patient education.

25.12 Identify ways to help a patient follow up on a doctor's recommendations.

# Introduction

Whether a patient comes for a regular checkup or to have a problem diagnosed and treated, the physical exam is the first step in the process for the physician or practitioner. During the physical exam, the medical assistant must make the patient comfortable and assist the physician as necessary. A skilled medical assistant who is sensitive to patient needs plus proficient in performing these skills can create an atmosphere that results in a positive outcome for the patient during the physical exam.

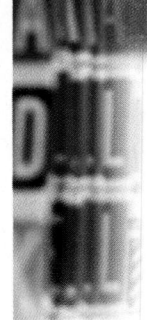

## CASE STUDY

A 50-year-old male patient who cannot speak English comes for a general physical exam. You must prepare the patient for the exam, including proper positioning, explain each component of the exam, and assist the physician as necessary.

As you read this chapter, consider the following questions:
1. English is the only language you speak. How can you provide adequate explanation?
2. How can you prevent embarrassment when preparing the patient for the exam?
3. During what parts of the exam do you expect to provide assistance for the physician?

# The Purpose of a General Physical Exam

Physicians perform general physical exams for two purposes. The first is to examine a healthy patient to confirm an overall state of health and to provide baseline values for vital signs and measurements. The second is to examine a patient to diagnose a medical problem.

To confirm a patient's health status, physicians usually perform exams on a routine basis, such as once a year. Some exams are done to fulfill a requirement before an individual starts school, begins a new job, or starts an exercise program.

To diagnose medical problems, physicians usually focus on a particular organ system, as indicated by the patient's chief complaint. Because organ systems are so interdependent, however, physicians generally perform an overall physical exam even when a specific medical problem exists.

During a general physical exam, physicians check all the major organs and body systems. They can determine much about a patient's general condition of health from the exam. If appropriate, they also try to make a **clinical diagnosis,** a diagnosis based on the signs and symptoms of a disease. A sign is objective information that can be detected by a person other than the affected person. Some examples of signs are blood in the stool or a bloody nose.

A symptom is subjective information supplied by the patient. Anxiety, back pain, abdominal pain, and fatigue are examples of symptoms. Only the patient can perceive these sensations.

It is helpful for the physician to evaluate symptoms and signs to diagnose the causes of health problems and disease. The physician also considers the signs and symptoms to monitor the status of diagnosed disorders, such as treatment medications, to determine the effectiveness and the development of side effects.

After forming an initial diagnosis of a patient's problem, physicians may order laboratory or other diagnostic tests. These tests are done to confirm a clinical diagnosis or to rule out other possible disorders. These additional steps are necessary when a patient has symptoms that may indicate more than one condition. Determining the correct diagnosis when two or more diagnoses are possible is called making a **differential diagnosis.**

Laboratory and diagnostic tests may also aid physicians in developing a **prognosis,** or a forecast of the probable course and outcome of the disorder and the prospects of recovery. In addition, such tests help physicians formulate a treatment plan or appropriate drug therapy. Physicians may ask to have these tests repeated as part of the follow-up evaluation of a patient's progress.

# The Role of the Medical Assistant

Your job as a medical assistant is to assist both the doctor and the patient during the general physical exam. Your presence enables the doctor to perform his exam as efficiently and professionally as possible. Patients benefit from your positive and caring attention; you contribute to their confidence in the care they receive.

As described in Chapter 23, the process begins when you first have contact with the patient. You interview the patient, write an accurate history, determine vital signs, and measure weight and height. You then assist the doctor during the exam.

Generally, your responsibilities include ensuring that all instruments and supplies are readily available to the doctor during the exam. You also ensure that the patient is physically and emotionally comfortable during the exam. It is important to observe the patient for signs that indicate distress or the need for assistance. Elderly patients, who may have physical limitations or special needs, often require extra time and attention.

# Safety Precautions

As you prepare for and assist with a general physical exam, you will use a variety of safety measures. Some of these are outlined by the Department of Labor's Occupational Safety and Health Administration (OSHA). OSHA standards and guidelines (detailed in Chapter 20) are designed to protect employees and make the workplace safe.

The Department of Health and Human Services' Centers for Disease Control and Prevention (CDC) establishes the guidelines intended to protect both patients and health-care professionals in the medical office and the hospital setting. (These guidelines are also discussed in Chapter 20.) Taken together, these safety measures help protect you, the physician, and the patient from disease transmission.

Safety measures that you must take before, during, and after a general physical exam include the following.

1. Perform a thorough hand washing before and after contact with each patient and before and after each procedure. Procedure 20-1 in Chapter 20 describes how to perform aseptic hand washing. Additionally, according to OSHA standards, you can use an approved waterless, alcohol-based hand cleaner between patients if no gross contamination or visible soilage is on your hands.

2. Wear gloves whenever there is a possibility that you may come in contact with blood, body fluids, nonintact skin, or moist surfaces (during the exam of the patient or when handling specimens). Refer to Chapter 20 for details on personal protective equipment.

3. Wear a mask in the presence of a patient suspected of having an infectious disease that is transmitted by airborne droplets, such as **severe acute respiratory syndrome (SARS)** or tuberculosis (TB) (Table 25-1).

4. Patients with highly contagious infectious diseases, such as diphtheria or chickenpox, must be examined under isolation precautions, such as in a private room. Wear personal protective equipment during contact. For more information on isolation guidelines, see Chapter 20. (Because infectious diseases are common in children, you are most likely to deal with them in a pediatrician's office.)

5. Discard in biohazardous waste containers all disposable equipment and supplies that come in contact with a patient's blood or body fluids. See Chapter 20 for guidelines on the proper disposal of biohazardous waste.

6. Clean and disinfect the exam room following the exam of each patient. Refer to Chapter 22 for information on cleanliness in the exam room.

7. Sanitize, disinfect, and sterilize equipment, as appropriate, after the exam of each patient. Chapter 20 describes these procedures in detail.

# Preparing the Patient for an Exam

You can help prepare patients for exams by making sure that they are comfortable and know what to expect. It is easier for the doctor to obtain an accurate assessment of a patient's condition when the patient is emotionally and physically prepared.

| TABLE 25-1 | Infectious Diseases Transmitted by Airborne Droplets | |
|---|---|---|
| **Viral Infections** | **Bacterial Infections** | |
| Chickenpox | Epiglottitis (caused by *Haemophilus influenzae* type B) | |
| Diphtheria | Meningitis | |
| Herpes zoster (shingles) | Pertussis (whooping cough) | |
| Meningitis | Pneumonia | |
| Mumps | Tuberculosis | |
| Pneumonia | | |
| Rabies | | |
| Rubella (German measles) | | |
| Rubeola (measles) | | |
| Severe acute respiratory syndrome (SARS) | | |

Note: Health-care professionals should use masks when coming in contact with patients suspected of having any of these diseases.

## Emotional Preparation

To prepare patients, begin by explaining exactly what will occur during the exam. Use simple, direct language that patients can understand. Describe what patients can expect to feel and how their cooperation can contribute to the success of the procedure.

Emotional preparedness is particularly important when dealing with children. They deserve to have the same sort of information and reassurance as adults. To involve children in the exam process, you might allow them to inspect the blunt instruments. Speak to them calmly during the procedure, and praise them when they are cooperative.

Infants and toddlers are likely to be afraid of you because you are a stranger. Approach these children slowly, smile, and use a gentle voice. Children of preschool age are sometimes uncooperative and challenging. In such cases remain calm, perform the procedures quickly, and restrain the child (with assistance from the parent) when appropriate. To prevent children from getting injured, watch them at all times.

If you are a male medical assistant, a female doctor may ask you to remain in the room when she examines a male patient. Likewise, if you are a female medical assistant, a male doctor may ask you to remain in the room when he examines a woman. These measures are for the protection of both the patient and the doctor. Such policies depend on the standard procedures in each medical practice or facility.

## Physical Preparation

To ensure that the patient is physically prepared before the doctor enters the exam room, give the patient an opportunity to empty his bladder or bowels. If a urine specimen is needed, it should be collected at this time. That way the patient will be more comfortable during the exam.

When the patient is ready, ask him to disrobe and put on an exam gown or cover himself with a drape. The extent of disrobing depends on the type of exam and the doctor's preference. If the doctor requests a gown for the patient, show the patient how to put on the gown. Include specific instructions on whether the gown should open in the back or front and whether it should be left open or tied. Leave the exam room while the patient disrobes to give him privacy, unless he needs and requests assistance.

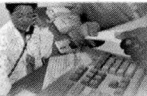

## Points on Practice

## Patient Modesty and Comfort

Imagine what it feels like to visit a doctor for the first time for a gynecological exam. You are asked to disrobe completely and wait for the physician. You are given a paper gown and a drape. As you disrobe and put on the gown, you notice that it is very small, it doesn't fit you, and it's beginning to tear.

In order to ensure patient comfort, make sure that a variety of sizes are available for patient use. Use your critical thinking skills when selecting a patient gown. Your patient will remember this gesture and appreciate your consideration.

# Positioning and Draping

During the exam, the patient may need to assume a variety of positions. These positions facilitate the physician's exam of certain areas of the body. The physician will indicate which positions are needed for specific exams. You will help the patient assume these positions. To protect yourself from injury when positioning a patient, always follow the basic rules of good body mechanics. These include lifting with your strongest muscles including your legs and arms rather than your back, keeping your feet apart, and bending from the hip and knees. Some positions are embarrassing or physically uncomfortable for some patients. If you perceive embarrassment, explain the need for the position, and help the patient assume the position when necessary. Help minimize the time a patient spends in any embarrassing or uncomfortable position.

If a patient is physically uncomfortable in a position, you may be able to ease the discomfort by using a small pillow to support part of the body. You may have to help the patient maintain a position during the exam. Always try to make the patient as comfortable as possible.

When you need to make changes in the patient's position, do so gradually. If your office is equipped with an examining table that can be adjusted automatically, learn to use the controls efficiently to maximize patient comfort. Always tell the patient what movement to expect.

When patients have assumed the correct position, cover them with an appropriate drape. Drapes vary in size. Make sure you choose one that will help keep the patient warm and maintain privacy. You will position drapes differently depending on the exam position and the parts of the patient's body that the physician examines.

## Exam Positions

The positions commonly used during a medical exam include the following:

- Sitting
- Supine (recumbent)
- Dorsal recumbent
- Lithotomy
- Trendelenburg's
- Fowler's
- Prone
- Sims'
- Knee-chest
- Proctologic

**Sitting.** In the sitting position, the patient sits at the edge of the examining table without back support (see Figure 25-1A). The physician examines the patient's head, neck, chest, heart, back, and arms. While the patient is in the sitting position, the physician evaluates the patient's ability to fully expand the lungs. She then checks the upper body parts for **symmetry,** the degree to which one side is the same as the other. In this position the drape is placed across the patient's lap for men or across the patient's chest and lap for women.

If a patient is too weak to sit unsupported, another position is necessary. One possible alternative is the supine position.

**Supine (Recumbent).** In the supine, or recumbent, position, the patient lies flat on the back (Figure 25-1B). (*Supine* means "lying down faceup"; *recumbent* means "lying down." Either term is used to describe this position.) This is the most relaxed position for many patients. A doctor can examine the head, neck, chest, heart, abdomen, arms, and legs when a patient is in the supine position. The patient is normally draped from the neck or underarms down to the feet.

The supine position may not be comfortable for patients who become short of breath easily. Also, patients with a back injury or lower-back pain may find it uncomfortable. You can make these patients more comfortable by placing a pillow under their heads and under their knees. Some patients, however, may need to be placed in the dorsal recumbent position.

**Dorsal Recumbent.** In the dorsal recumbent position, the patient lies faceup, with his back supporting all his weight. (The term *dorsal* refers to the back.) This position is the same as the supine position, except that the patient's knees are drawn up and the feet are flat on the table, as shown in Figure 25-1C. The physician may examine the head, neck, chest, and heart while a patient is in this position. The patient is normally draped from the neck or underarms down to the feet.

Patients who have leg disabilities may find the dorsal recumbent position uncomfortable or even impossible. On the other hand, patients who are elderly or have painful disorders such as arthritis or back pain may find the dorsal recumbent position more comfortable than the supine position because the knees are bent. This position is sometimes used as an alternative to the lithotomy position when patients have severe arthritis or joint deformities.

**Lithotomy.** The lithotomy position is used during exam of the female genitalia. In this position, the patient lies on her back with her knees bent and her feet in stirrups attached to the end of the examining table. You may need to help the patient place her feet in the stirrups. She should then slide forward to position her buttocks near the edge of the table, as shown in Figure 25-1D.

Many women are embarrassed and physically uncomfortable in this position, so you should not ask a patient to remain in this position any longer than necessary. Use a large drape that covers the patient from the breasts to the ankles. Placing the drape with one point or corner between the legs will make the exam easier in this position.

A patient with severe arthritis or joint deformities in the hips or knees may have difficulty assuming the lithotomy position. She may be able to place only one leg in the

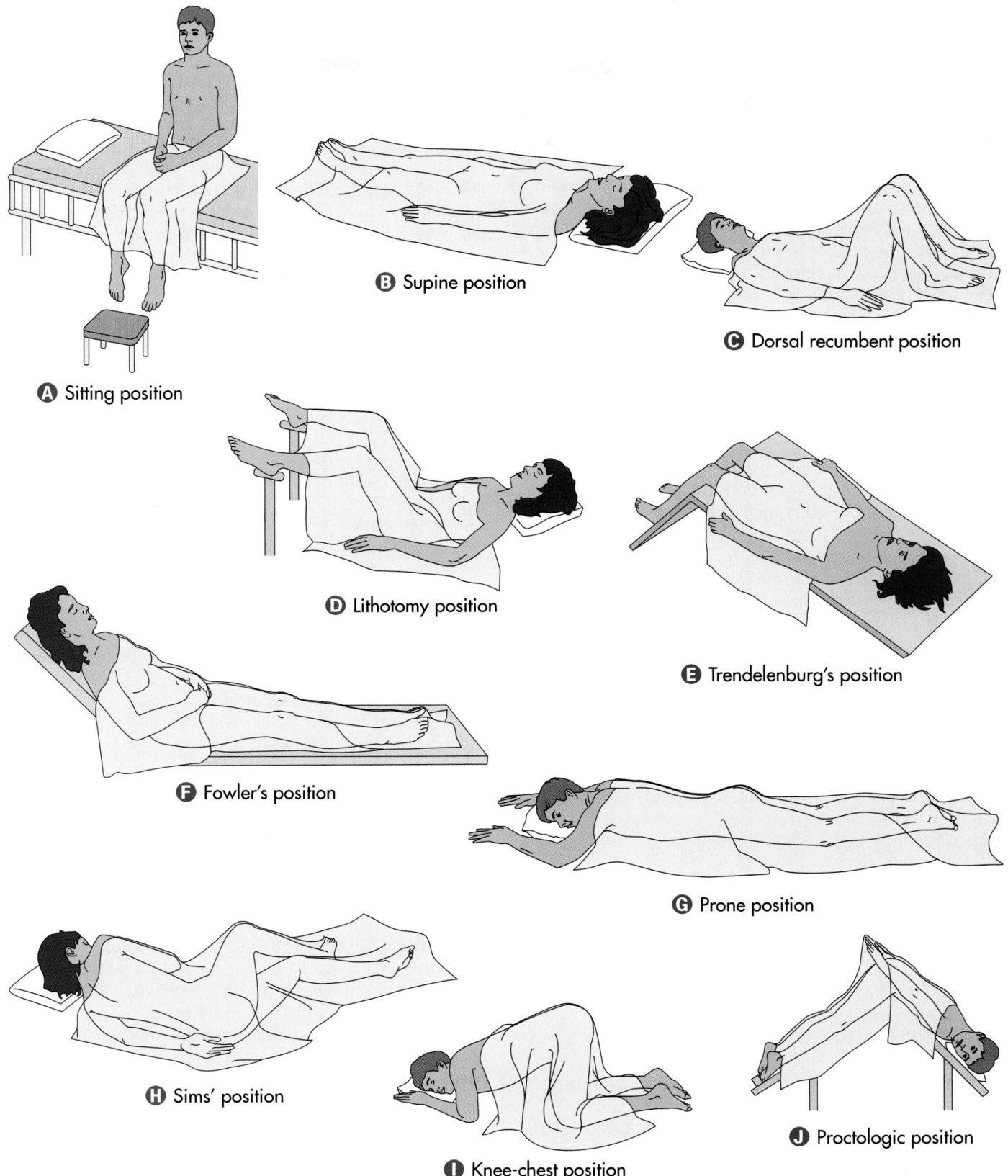

**A** Sitting position

**B** Supine position

**C** Dorsal recumbent position

**D** Lithotomy position

**E** Trendelenburg's position

**F** Fowler's position

**G** Prone position

**H** Sims' position

**I** Knee-chest position

**J** Proctologic position

**Figure 25-1.** These positions may be used during the general physical examination.

stirrup, or she may need your assistance in separating her thighs. An alternative position for such a patient is the dorsal recumbent position. Other patients who may have difficulty with the lithotomy position are those who are obese or in the late stages of pregnancy.

**Trendelenburg's.** In Trendelenburg's position, the patient is supine on a tilted table with the head lower than the legs. Some tables have flexible positioning so that the patient's legs can be bent with the feet lower than the knees, as shown in Figure 25-1E. Although physicians do not generally use this position for physical exams, they use it in certain surgical procedures or emergencies. If this position is necessary on a standard examining table, you can place the patient with the feet at the head of the table and then raise the head. This position may be used for a patient with low blood pressure or a patient experiencing shock. It cannot be used for patients who have a head injury, however. The drape is typically positioned from the neck or underarms down to the knees.

**Fowler's.** In Fowler's position, the patient lies back on an examining table on which the head is elevated, as shown in Figure 25-1F. Although the head of the table can be raised to a 90-degree angle, the most common position is a 45-degree angle. The doctor may examine the head, neck, and chest areas while the patient is in this position. The patient is usually draped from the neck or underarms down to the feet.

Fowler's position is one of the best positions for examining patients who are experiencing shortness of breath or individuals with a lower-back injury.

**Prone.** In the prone position, the patient is lying flat on the table, facedown. The patient's head is turned to one side, and his arms are placed at his sides or bent at the elbows, as shown in Figure 25-1G. The patient is normally draped from the upper back to the feet.

With the patient in this position, the physician can examine the back, feet, or musculoskeletal system. The prone position is unsuitable for women in advanced stages of pregnancy, obese patients, patients with respiratory difficulties, or the elderly.

**Sims'.** In Sims' position, the patient lies on the left side. The patient's left leg is slightly bent, and the left arm is placed behind the back so that the patient's weight is resting primarily on the chest. The right knee is bent and raised toward the chest, and the right arm is bent toward the head for support, as shown in Figure 25-1H. The patient is draped from the upper back to the feet.

Sims' position is used during anal or rectal exams and may also be used for perineal and certain pelvic exams. Patients with joint deformities of the hips and knees may have difficulty assuming this position.

**Knee-Chest.** In the knee-chest position, the patient is lying on the table facedown, supporting the body with the knees and chest. The patient should have the thighs at a 90-degree angle to the table and slightly separated. The head is turned to one side, and the arms are placed to the side or above the head, as shown in Figure 25-1I. The patient may need your assistance to assume this position correctly and to maintain it during the exam.

The knee-chest position is used during exams of the anal and perineal areas and during certain proctologic procedures. Some patients—those who are pregnant, obese, or elderly—have difficulty assuming this position. An alternative that puts less strain on the patient and is easier to maintain is the knee-elbow position. This position is the same as the knee-chest position except that the patient supports body weight with the knees and elbows rather than the knees and chest. In either of these two positions, the patient is commonly covered with a **fenestrated drape,** in which a special opening provides access to the area to be examined.

**Proctologic.** The proctologic position may be used as an alternative to the Sims' or knee-chest position. In the proctologic position, also called the jackknife position, the patient is bent at the hips at a 90-degree angle. The patient can assume this position by standing next to the examining table and bending at the waist until the chest rests on the table. If an adjustable examining table is available, the patient can assume the position by lying prone on the table, which is then raised in the middle with both ends pointing down. This places the patient at the correct 90-degree angle, as shown in Figure 25-1J. In either variation of this position, the patient is draped with a fenestrated drape, as in the knee-chest position.

The steps for placing patients into these positions are described in Procedure 25-1.

# Special Considerations: Patients from Different Cultures

During your career you will come in contact with patients from many different cultures. A **culture,** in this sociological sense, is defined as a pattern of assumptions, beliefs, and practices that shape the way people think and act. Avoid the temptation to stereotype an individual or group on the basis of a single patient's behavior. Stereotyping can lead to incorrect judgments, which may influence the care you provide to patients. Avoid making judgments about patients or cultural groups on the basis of your experience with other patients or with your own family and friends.

Patients from different cultures may never have had a medical exam by a physician and may not know what to expect. These patients may be more modest than other patients and may have a greater need for privacy. They may not want the physician to examine certain areas of their bodies. Procedure 25-2 describes techniques you can use to ensure effective communication with patients from other cultures while meeting their privacy needs.

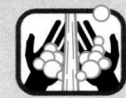

# PROCEDURE 25.1

## Positioning the Patient for an Exam

**Procedure Goal:** To effectively assist a patient in assuming the various positions used in a general physical exam

**OSHA Guidelines**

**Materials:** Adjustable examining table or gynecologic table, step stool, exam gown, drape

### Method:

1. Identify the patient and introduce yourself.
2. Wash your hands.
3. Explain the procedure to the patient.
4. Provide a gown or drape if the physician has requested one, and instruct the patient in the proper way to wear it after disrobing. Allow the patient privacy while disrobing, and assist only if the patient requests help.

### Rationale

Taking an extra minute to explain to the patient how to wear the gown will make the visit more efficient and the patient more comfortable.

5. Explain to the patient the necessary exam and the position required.
6. Ask the patient to step on the stool or the pullout step of the examining table. If necessary, assist the patient onto the examining table.
7. Assist the patient into the required position:

a. Sitting. Do not use this position for patients who cannot sit unsupported.

b. Supine (Recumbent). Do not use this position for patients with back injuries, low back pain, or difficulty breathing. Place a pillow or other support under the head and knees for comfort, if needed.

c. Dorsal Recumbent. This position may be difficult for someone with leg disabilities. It may be used for patients when lithotomy is difficult.

d. Lithotomy. This position is used to examine the female genitalia, with the patient's feet placed in stirrups. Assist as necessary. The patient's buttocks should be near the edge of the table. Drape the client with a large drape to help prevent embarrassment.

e. Trendelenburg. This position is a supine position with the patient's head lower than her feet. It is used infrequently in the physician's office but may be necessary for low blood pressure or shock.

f. Fowler's. Adjust the head of the table to the desired angle. Help the patient move toward the head of the table until the patient's buttocks meet the point at which the head of the table begins to incline upward (Figures 25-2 and 25-3).

g. Prone. This position is when the patient lies face down. It is not used for later stages of pregnancy, obese patients, patients with

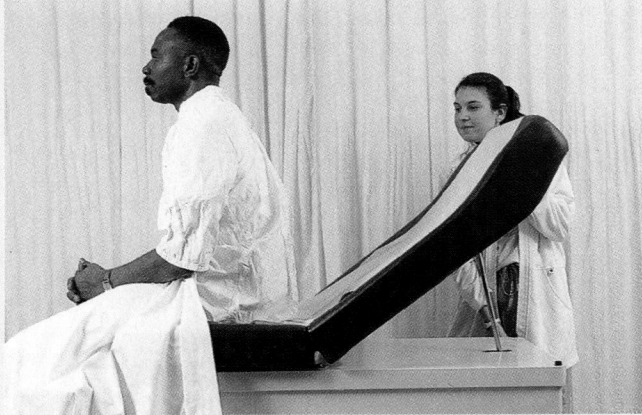

**Figure 25-2.** Adjust the head of the examination table to a 45-degree angle.

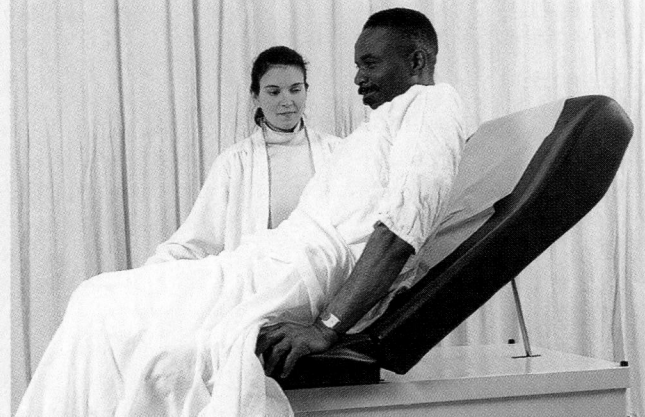

**Figure 25-3.** Encourage the patient to slide back until the buttocks meet the point at which the head of the table begins to incline upward.

*continued* ⟶

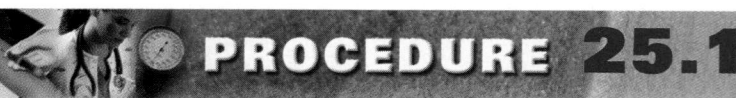
# Positioning the Patient for an Exam (concluded)

respiratory difficulty, or certain elderly patients.

**h.** Sims'. In this position, the patient lies on her left side with her left leg slightly bent and her left arm behind her back. Her right knee is bent and raised toward her chest and her right arm is bent toward her head. This position may be difficult for patients with joint deformities.

**i.** Knee-Chest. This position is difficult for patients to assume. The patient is face down, supporting his weight on his knees and chest or an alternative knee-elbow position. This position is used for rectal and perineal exams. Keep the patient in this position for the shortest amount of time possible.

**j.** Proctologic. This position is also used for rectal and perineal exams. In this position, the patient bends over the examining table with his chest resting on the table.

**8.** Drape the client to prevent exposure and avoid embarrassment. Place pillows for comfort as needed.

### Rationale
The patient's comfort and safety are mandatory.

**9.** Adjust the drapes during the exam.

**10.** On completion of the exam, assist the client as necessary out of the position and provide privacy as the client dresses.

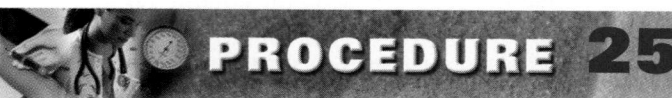
# Communicating Effectively With Patients from Other Cultures and Meeting Their Needs for Privacy

**Procedure Goal:** To ensure effective communication with patients from other cultures while meeting their needs for privacy

**OSHA Guidelines:** This procedure does not involve exposure to blood, body fluids, or tissues.

**Materials:** Exam gown, drapes

**Method:**

### Effective Communication

**1.** When it is necessary to use a translator, direct conversation or instruction to the translator.

### Rationale
Translators will reduce the risk of litigation and improve patient outcomes.

**2.** Direct demonstrations of what to do, such as putting on an exam gown, to the patient.

**3.** Confirm with the translator that the patient has understood the instruction or demonstration.

**4.** Allow the translator to be present during the exam if that is the patient's preference.

**5.** If the patient understands some English, speak slowly, use simple language, and demonstrate instructions whenever possible.

### Meeting the Need for Privacy

**1.** Before the procedure, thoroughly explain to the patient or translator the reason for disrobing. Indicate that you will allow the patient privacy and ample time to undress.

**2.** If the patient is reluctant, reassure him that the physician respects the need for privacy and will look at only what is necessary for the exam.

### Rationale
Some patients from certain cultures are embarrassed when exposed.

**3.** Provide extra drapes if you think doing so will make the patient feel more comfortable.

**4.** If the patient is still reluctant, discuss the problem with the physician; the physician may be able to negotiate a compromise with the patient.

**5.** During the procedure, ensure that the patient is undraped only as much as necessary.

**6.** Whenever possible, minimize the amount of time the patient remains undraped.

## Special Considerations: Patients With Disabilities

As a medical assistant, you will come in contact with patients with physical disabilities. These patients will have different strengths and weaknesses. They will also vary in their ability to ambulate (move from place to place). Many patients with physical disabilities require the use of devices such as wheelchairs, canes, or walkers or other special equipment that permits or enhances mobility.

Depending on the extent of their disability, these patients may require extra assistance in preparing for a general physical exam. You may need to help them disrobe, move from a mobility device to the examining table, and assume certain positions on or off the examining table. At all times you should ask another staff member for assistance if you are not sure whether you can safely move or lift a patient on your own. Procedure 25-3 outlines the steps you would take to transfer a patient from a wheelchair to the examining table.

## Special Considerations: Children

No matter what type of office you work in, you will probably deal with children at times. You will base your choice of an exam position for children on each child's age and ability to cooperate. Although young infants are usually examined on an examining table, older infants and toddlers may need to be examined while held on a parent's lap. Some toddlers may cooperate while standing on the examining table with a parent nearby. Preschool children can usually be placed on the examining table if a parent is nearby. Regardless of their position, watch children at all times to prevent injury.

When examining young children, doctors typically perform percussion and auscultation first, because children are more likely to be calm and quiet at the outset. Doctors always examine painful areas last. Doctors may examine older children's genitalia last, because after a certain age children tend to find such an exam embarrassing.

## Special Considerations: Pregnant Women

When a pregnant patient needs a general physical exam, remember that she has several special needs. Some positions (such as the prone or lithotomy positions) are not recommended for a pregnant patient, especially during late stages of pregnancy. Other positions may be difficult or impossible for a pregnant woman to achieve. Procedure 25-4 outlines steps you can take to ensure that a pregnant woman's needs are addressed during an exam.

## Exam Methods

There are six methods for examining a patient during a general physical exam. These methods enable the physician to gather important information about the patient's condition, and they are normally performed in the following sequence:

1. Inspection
2. Palpation
3. Percussion
4. Auscultation
5. Mensuration
6. Manipulation

# PROCEDURE 25.3

## Transferring a Patient in a Wheelchair and Preparing for an Exam

**Procedure Goal:** To assist a patient in transferring from a wheelchair to the examining table safely and efficiently

**OSHA Guidelines**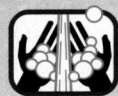

**Materials:** Adjustable examining table or gynecologic table, step stool (optional), exam gown, drape

**Method:** Never risk injuring yourself; call for assistance when in doubt. As a rule you should not attempt to lift more than 35% of your body weight.

### Preparation Before Transfer

1. Identify the patient and introduce yourself.
2. Wash your hands.
3. Explain the procedure in detail.
4. Position the wheelchair at a right angle to the end of the examining table. This position reduces the distance between the wheelchair and the end of the examining table across which the patient must move.
5. Lock the wheels of the wheelchair.

#### Rationale
To prevent the wheelchair from moving during the transfer.

*continued* ⟶

# Transferring a Patient in a Wheelchair and Preparing for an Exam *(continued)*

6. Lift the patient's feet and fold back the foot and leg supports of the wheelchair.

7. Place the patient's feet on the floor. The patient should have shoes or slippers with nonskid soles. Place your feet in front of the patient's feet.

*Rationale*

These actions prevent the patient from slipping.

8. If needed, place a step stool in front of the table, and place the patient's feet flat on the stool.

## Transferring the Patient by Yourself

9. Face the patient, spread your feet apart, align your knees with the patient's knees, and bend your knees slightly.

*Rationale*

If you lift while bending at the waist instead of bending your knees, you can cause serious injury to your back.

10. Have the patient hold on to your shoulders.

11. Place your arms around the patient, under the patient's arms (Figure 25-4).

12. Tell the patient that you will lift on the count of 3, and ask the patient to support as much of his own weight as possible (if he is able).

13. At the count of 3, lift the patient.

14. Pivot the patient to bring the back of the patient's knees against the table.

15. Gently lower the patient into a sitting position on the table. If the patient cannot sit unassisted, help him move into a supine position (Figure 25-5).

16. Move the wheelchair out of the way.

17. Assist the patient with disrobing as necessary, providing a gown and drape.

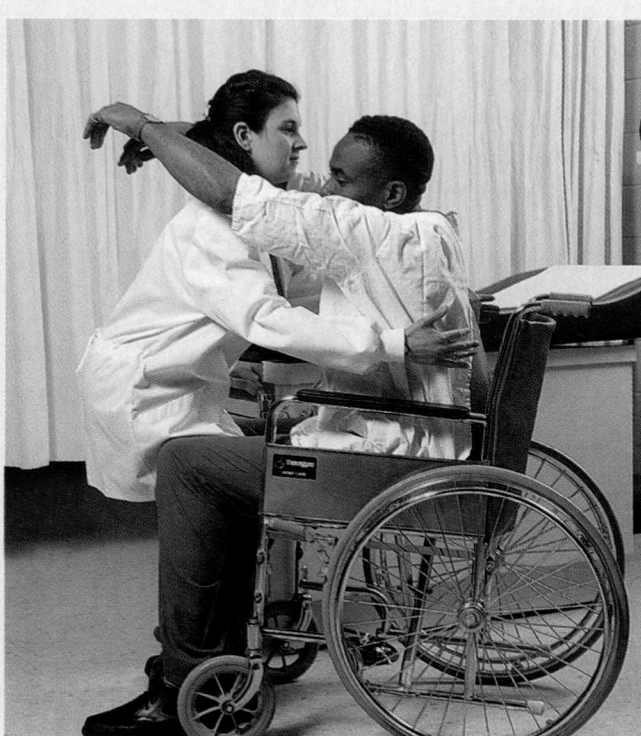

**Figure 25-4.** Align your knees, slightly bent, with the patient's knees. Have the patient hold on to your shoulders while you place your arms around the patient, under the patient's arms.

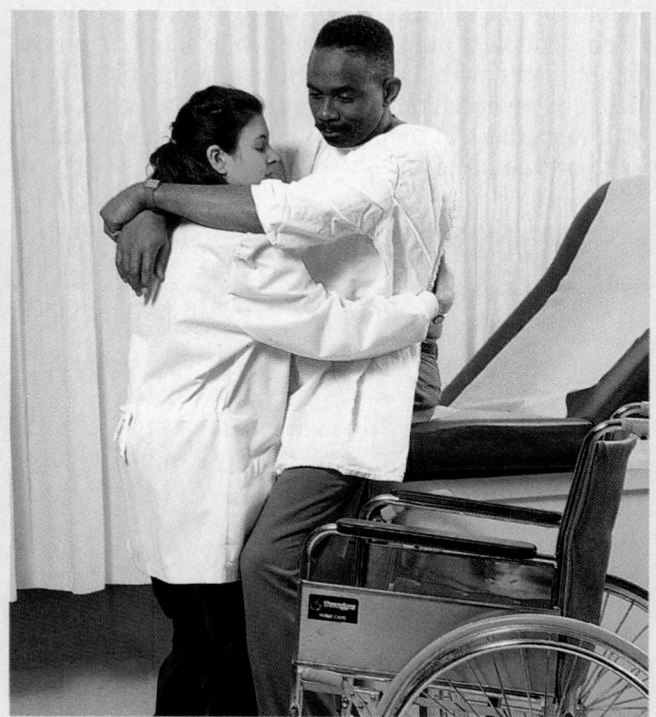

**Figure 25-5.** When you have lifted the patient, pivot him to bring the back of the knees against the table. Gently lower the patient into a sitting position, or into a supine position if the patient cannot sit unassisted.

*continued* →

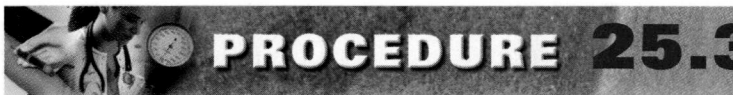

# PROCEDURE 25.3

## Transferring a Patient in a Wheelchair and Preparing for an Exam *(concluded)*

### Transferring the Patient With Assistance

9. Working with your partner, both of you face the patient, spread your feet apart, position yourselves so that one of each of your knees is aligned with the patient's knees, and bend your knees slightly.

#### Rationale
If you lift while bending at your waist instead of bending your knees, you can cause serious injury to your back.

10. Have the patient place one hand on each of your shoulders and hold on.

11. Each of you places your outermost arm around the patient, one under each of the patient's arms. Then interlock your wrists (Figure 25-6).

12. Tell the patient that you will lift on the count of 3, and ask the patient to support as much of his own weight as possible (if he is able).

13. At the count of 3, you should lift the patient together.

14. The stronger of the two of you should pivot the patient to bring the back of the patient's knees against the table.

15. Working together, gently lower the patient into a sitting position on the table. If the patient cannot sit unassisted, help him move into a supine position (Figure 25-7).

16. Move the wheelchair out of the way.

17. Assist the patient with disrobing as necessary, providing a gown and drape.

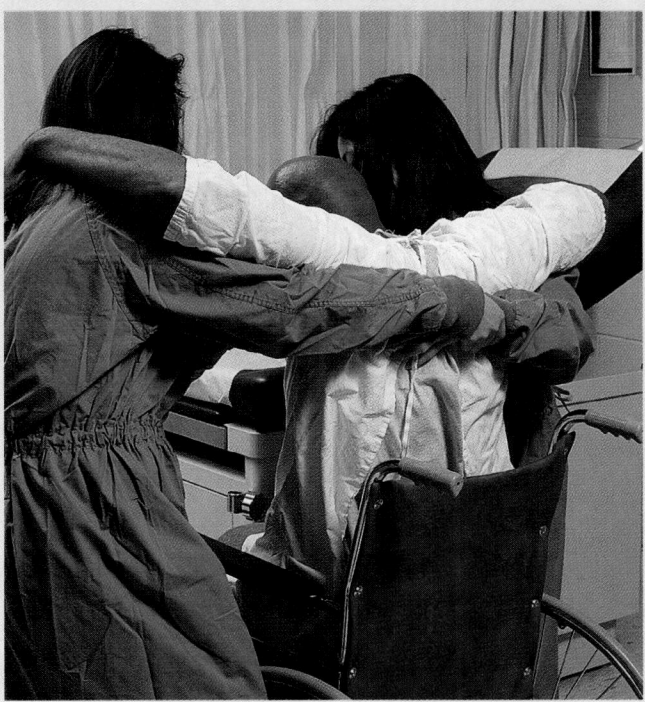

**Figure 25-6.** If you have an assistant, have the patient place one hand on each of your shoulders. Each of you should place your outermost arm around the patient, under one of the patient's arms. Interlock your wrists and, together, lift the patient.

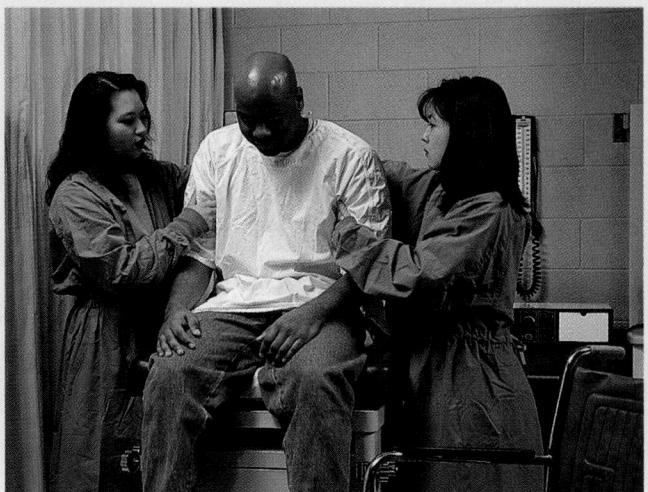

**Figure 25-7.** The stronger of the two of you should pivot the patient to bring the back of the patient's knees against the table. Gently lower the patient into a sitting position, or a supine position if the patient cannot sit unassisted.

## PROCEDURE 25.4

## Meeting the Needs of the Pregnant Patient During an Exam

**Procedure Goal:** To meet the special needs of the pregnant woman during the general physical exam

**OSHA Guidelines**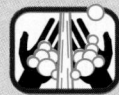

**Materials:** Patient education materials, examining table, exam gown, drape

**Method:**

### Providing Patient Information

1. Identify the patient and introduce yourself.
2. Assess the patient's need for education by asking appropriate questions and having the patient describe what she already knows about the information you are providing.
3. Provide any appropriate instructions or materials.
4. Ask the patient whether she has any special concerns or questions about her pregnancy that she might want to discuss with the physician.
5. Communicate the patient's concerns or questions to the physician; include all pertinent background information on the patient.

### Rationale

Maintains your scope of practice and ensures the patient receives correct information.

### Ensuring Comfort During the Exam

1. Identify the patient and introduce yourself.
2. Wash your hands.
3. Explain the procedure to the patient.

4. Provide a gown or drape, and instruct the patient in the proper way to wear it after disrobing. (Allow the patient privacy while disrobing, and assist only if she requests help.)
5. Ask the patient to step on the stool or the pullout step of the examining table.
6. Assist the patient onto the examining table.

### Rationale

Pregnant women may need assistance during the later stages of pregnancy.

7. Keeping position restrictions in mind, help the patient into the position requested by the physician.
8. Provide and adjust additional drapes as needed.
9. Keep in mind any difficulties the patient may have in achieving a certain position; suggest alternative positions whenever possible.
10. Minimize the time the patient must spend in uncomfortable positions.

### Rationale

Make sure that the physician has all supplies and equipment for the exam before it begins.

11. If the patient appears to be uncomfortable during the procedure, ask whether she would like to reposition herself or take a break; assist as necessary.
12. To prevent pelvic pooling of blood and subsequent dizziness or hyperventilation, allow the patient time to adjust to sitting before standing after she has been lying on the examining table.

## Inspection

**Inspection** is the visual exam of the patient's entire body and overall appearance. During inspection the physician assesses posture, mannerisms, and hygiene. The physician also inspects parts of the body for size, shape, color, position, symmetry, and the presence of abnormalities such as rashes or growths. You can help the physician perform the inspection by making sure that good lighting is available and that the patient's body parts are properly exposed.

## Palpation

The doctor uses **palpation** (touch) extensively in the general physical exam. During palpation the doctor assesses characteristics such as texture, temperature, shape, and the presence of vibrations or movements. The doctor may palpate superficially (on the skin surface), or she may palpate with additional pressure. She uses extra pressure when assessing characteristics of underlying tissues and organs. Depending on the characteristic the doctor is measuring, she may perform palpation using the fingertips, one hand, two hands (bimanual), or the palm of the hand.

# Percussion

**Percussion** involves tapping or striking the body to hear sounds or feel vibrations. Physicians use percussion to determine the location, size, or density of a body structure or organ under the skin. For example, physicians use percussion to determine whether the lungs contain air or fluid.

The physician may perform percussion by striking the body directly with one or two fingers. More commonly, however, he performs indirect percussion by placing one finger of one hand on the area and striking it with a finger from the other hand.

# Auscultation

**Auscultation** is the process of listening to body sounds. Doctors use auscultation to detect the flow of blood through an artery. Doctors perform auscultation extensively in the general exam to assess sounds from the heart, lungs, and abdominal organs. They use a stethoscope to hear most of these sounds.

# Mensuration

**Mensuration** is the process of measuring. In addition to the measurements you take before the exam—weight and height—you may need to take other measurements during the exam. For example, measurements may be done to monitor the growth of the uterus during pregnancy or to note the length and diameter of an extremity. You will usually use a tape measure or small ruler to take measurements.

# Manipulation

**Manipulation** is the systematic moving of a patient's body parts. Physicians may palpate an area of the body while manipulating it to check for abnormalities that affect movement. Physicians often use manipulation to determine the range of motion (ROM) of a joint.

# Components of a General Physical Exam

Each physician performs the general physical exam in a certain order. Most physicians begin by assessing the patient's overall appearance and the condition of the patient's skin, nails, and hair. They usually then proceed with the exam in the following order, using the exam methods described in the previous section:

1. Head
2. Neck
3. Eyes
4. Ears
5. Nose and sinuses
6. Mouth and throat
7. Chest and lungs
8. Heart
9. Breasts
10. Abdomen
11. Genitalia
12. Rectum
13. Musculoskeletal system
14. Neurological system

Learn the standard order that the physicians in your facility follow when performing the general exam. You should also be familiar with the components of the exam and the instruments and supplies needed for each component (see Table 25-2 and Figure 25-8). Instruments and supplies are discussed in detail in Chapter 22 and should include the following basic items:

- Penlight
- Otoscope/ophthalmoscope
- Vision chart
- Color vision chart
- Audiometer
- Nasal speculum
- Gloves
- Tongue depressor
- Stethoscope
- Vaginal speculum
- Lubricant
- Tape measure

Certain parts of the exam are your responsibility, and you should know how to perform them. You should also understand the physician's responsibilities.

Part of the medical assistant's role in the general exam is to ensure that the patient is as comfortable as possible. You can do this by helping to protect the patient's modesty as much as you can. For example, when the physician removes a drape or gown to expose an area for inspection, watch the patient for signs of embarrassment. If you notice any such signs, do your best to keep the patient covered without hindering the physician's exam. The steps for assisting the doctor with a general physical exam are outlined in Procedure 25-5.

## General Appearance

The physician usually begins the exam by reviewing the patient's general appearance and noting whether the patient appears to be in good health and of an acceptable weight. The physician also notes whether the patient appears to be distressed or in pain and assesses the level of the patient's alertness. Then the physician examines the patient's skin, nails, and hair.

**Skin.** The physician may prefer to examine all of the patient's skin at one time or to look at certain areas of skin while examining specific body parts. The physician notes

## TABLE 25-2 Components and Materials of a General Physical Exam

| Component | Materials Required* |
|---|---|
| General appearance (skin, nails, hair) | No special materials needed |
| Head | No special materials needed |
| Neck | No special materials needed |
| Eyes and vision** | Penlight, ophthalmoscope, vision and color vision charts |
| Ears and hearing** | Otoscope, audiometer |
| Nose and sinuses | Penlight, nasal speculum |
| Mouth and throat | Gloves, tongue depressor |
| Chest and lungs | Stethoscope |
| Heart | Stethoscope |
| Breasts | No special materials needed |
| Abdomen | Stethoscope |
| Genitalia (women) | Gloves, vaginal speculum, lubricant |
| Genitalia (men) | Gloves |
| Rectum | Gloves, lubricant |
| Musculoskeletal system | Tape measure |
| Neurological system | Reflex hammer, penlight |

*Gloves should always be worn if your hands will come in contact with the patient's nonintact skin, blood, body fluids, or moist surfaces or if the patient is suspected of having an infectious disease.

**Procedures performed alone by the medical assistant are described in Chapter 26; all other listed procedures are performed by a physician with help from a medical assistant.

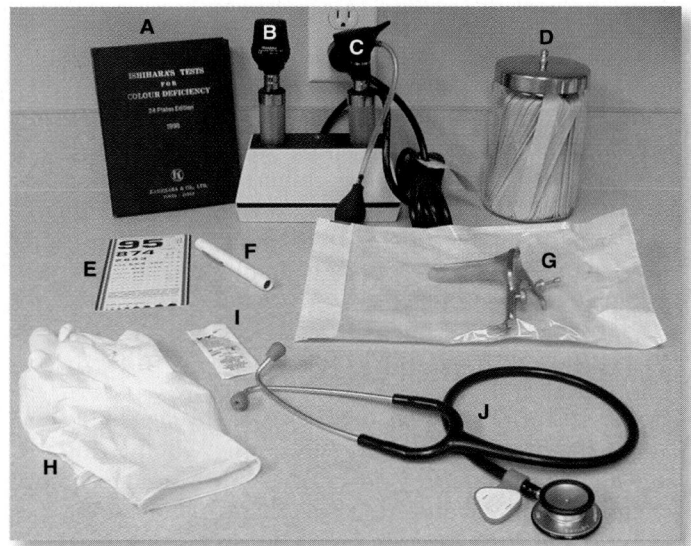

**Figure 25-8.** Some common instruments and supplies for the general physical examination are: (A) color vision chart, (B) ophthalmoscope, (C) otoscope, (D) tongue blades, (E) near vision chart, (F) penlight, (G) vaginal speculum, (H) gloves, (I) lubricant, and (J) stethoscope.

the color, texture, moisture level, temperature, and elasticity of the skin. The condition of the skin is a good indicator of overall health. If the physician notices any lesions, she wears gloves to prevent possible transmission of microorganisms. The physician may also request that a specimen be taken from a lesion or wound for later exam to determine the infecting microorganism.

**Nails.** When the physician examines the patient's nails, he looks at both the nails and the nail beds. The condition of the nails may indicate poor nutrition, disease, infection, or injury. If applicable, remind the patient to remove nail cosmetics prior to the appointment.

**Hair.** The physician notes the patient's pattern of hair growth and the texture of the hair on the patient's scalp and on the rest of the body. Sudden hair loss or changes in hair growth may be indicators of an underlying disease.

## Head

After reviewing the patient's general appearance, the doctor examines the patient's head. He looks for any abnormal condition of the scalp or skin, puffiness around the eyes or lips or in other areas of the face, or any abnormal growths.

# PROCEDURE 25.5

## Assisting With a General Physical Exam

**Procedure Goal:** To effectively assist the physician with a general physical exam

### OSHA Guidelines

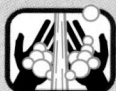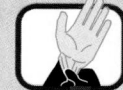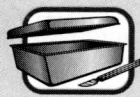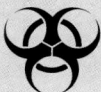

**Materials:** Supplies and equipment will vary depending on the type and purpose of the exam and the physician's practice preferences. Supplies may include the following: Gown, drape, adjustable examining table, gloves, laryngeal mirror, lubricant, nasal speculum, otoscope and ophthalmoscope, pillow, reflex hammer, tuning fork, sphygmomanometer, stethoscope, tape measure, tongue depressors, penlight

### Method:

1. Wash your hands and adhere to standard precautions throughout the procedure.

   *Rationale*

   Safe, aseptic technique greatly reduces the transmission of an infectious disease.

2. Gather and assemble the equipment and supplies.

3. Arrange the instruments and equipment in a logical sequence for the physician's use.

4. Greet and properly identify the patient using at least two patient identifiers.

   *Rationale*

   To prevent treatment errors.

5. Obtain the patient's weight and height (with shoes removed).

6. Obtain a urine specimen before the patient undresses for the exam.

7. Explain the procedure and exam to the patient.

   *Rationale*

   This builds the patient's confidence with the office, and prepares the patient physically and emotionally.

8. Review the patient's medical history with the patient if office policy requires it.

9. Obtain blood specimens or other laboratory tests per the chart or verbal order.

10. Obtain vital statistics per the physician's preference.

11. Provide the patient with an appropriate gown and drape, and explain where the opening for the gown is placed.

12. Obtain the ECG if ordered by the physician.

13. Assist patient to a sitting position at the end of the table with the drape placed across his or her legs.

14. Inform the physician that the patient is ready, and remain in the room to assist the physician.

15. You may be asked to shut off the light in the exam room to allow the patient's pupils to dilate sufficiently for a retinal exam.

16. Hand the instruments to the physician as requested.

17. Assist the patient to a supine position and drape him or her for an exam of the front of the body.

18. If a gynecological exam is needed, assist and drape the patient in the lithotomy position.

19. If a rectal exam is needed, assist and drape the patient in the Sims' position.

20. Assist the patient to a prone position for a posterior body exam.

21. When the exam is complete, assist the patient to a sitting position and ask the patient to sit for a brief period of time.

    *Rationale*

    Some patients experience dizziness when they first sit up.

22. Ask the patient if he or she needs assistance in dressing.

23. Dispose of contaminated materials in an appropriate container.

24. Remove the table paper and pillow covering, and dispose of them in the proper container.

25. Disinfect and clean counters and the examining table with a disinfectant.

26. Sanitize and sterilize the instruments, if needed.

27. Prepare the room for the next patient by replacing the table paper, pillow case, equipment, and supplies.

28. Document the procedure.

## Neck

To check the neck, the doctor palpates the patient's lymph nodes, thyroid gland, and major blood vessels. Enlarged lymph nodes may be a sign of infection or a blood cancer. An enlarged thyroid gland may indicate thyroid disease. The doctor also checks the neck for symmetry and range of motion.

## Eyes

The physician examines the patient's eyes—particularly the eyelids and conjunctiva—for the presence of disease or abnormalities. She checks eye muscles by observing the patient's ability to follow the movement of a finger. She checks the pupils for their response to light (the pupils should contract—become smaller—when a penlight is directed toward them). Then she uses an ophthalmoscope to examine the patient's retinas and other internal structures of the eyes. You may be required to perform various vision tests either before or after the general physical exam.

## Ears

The doctor checks the patient's outer ears for size, symmetry, and the presence of lesions, redness, or swelling. Using an otoscope, he then examines the inner structures of the patient's ears. The doctor may ask you to assist in keeping the patient's head still during the otoscopic exam, particularly when the patient is a young child. Although this procedure is usually painless, patients with an ear infection may find it uncomfortable or painful.

The doctor checks the patient's ear canals for redness, drainage, lesions, foreign objects, or the presence of excessive cerumen (a waxy secretion from the ear, also known as earwax). During the most important part of the exam of the ears, the doctor assesses the color, shape, and reflectiveness of the eardrums. If an eardrum bulges outward or reflects light abnormally, the middle ear could be infected.

One of your responsibilities may be to perform various hearing tests either before or after the general physical exam.

## Nose and Sinuses

When examining the nose, the physician checks for the presence of infection or allergy. She uses a penlight to view the color of the **nasal mucosa** (lining of the nose) and notes any discharge, lesions, obstructions, swelling, or inflammation. A mucosa that is red or swollen and is accompanied by a yellowish discharge usually indicates an infection. A pale, swollen mucosa accompanied by a clear discharge indicates an allergy. When examining adults, the physician uses the nasal speculum to view the structures of the nose.

The physician may use palpation to check for tenderness in a patient's sinuses. Tenderness is an indication of inflammation or swelling.

## Mouth and Throat

The doctor checks the condition of the patient's mouth to get a general impression of overall health and hygiene. Using a tongue depressor to draw back the patient's cheeks, the doctor examines the lining of the cheeks, the underside of the tongue, and the floor of the mouth. Changes in color or any lesions in these areas may indicate possible infection or oral cancer. The doctor also assesses the condition of the teeth and gums. When examining children, she counts the number of teeth. Most doctors leave this part of the exam of infants and toddlers until last, because children of this age tend to resist opening their mouths.

The doctor examines the patient's throat carefully because it is a common site of infection. She uses a tongue depressor to press the patient's tongue down and out of the way while asking the patient to say "ah." This procedure allows the doctor to view the throat and tonsils more clearly while checking them for redness or swelling, which can indicate the presence of infection.

## Chest and Lungs

The physician usually assesses the patient's chest and lungs while the patient sits at the end of the examining table. When the patient is examined in this position, the chest can expand to its maximum capacity. Typically, the physician removes the patient's gown or lowers the drape from the waist up. Then he asks the patient to breathe normally or to take deep breaths. A patient who becomes dizzy during deep breathing may be hyperventilating. Hyperventilation is overly deep breathing that leads to a loss of carbon dioxide in the blood. You can help by having the patient breathe into a paper bag. If no bag is available, the patient can breathe into cupped hands. With your help the patient should recover quickly.

The physician inspects the patient's chest from the back, side, and front. He checks its shape, symmetry, and postural position and looks for the presence of any type of deformity. Postural abnormalities such as **kyphosis** often occur in the elderly. Frequently, especially in elderly women, these abnormalities are caused by osteoporosis, the loss of bone density. This bone density loss causes the patient to have a rounded back, or "humpback."

The physician also palpates the chest and performs percussion to check for the presence of fluid or a foreign mass in the lungs. The physician then uses a stethoscope to auscultate the chest from the back, side, and front. He listens to the lung sounds during both normal and deep breathing. The stethoscope allows him to hear abnormal breathing that may result from such disorders as bronchitis, asthma, or pneumonia.

## Heart

The doctor usually examines the patient's heart and vascular system at the same time as, or immediately after, the lung exam. He may palpate the area first to locate the correct anatomical landmarks for placing the stethoscope. He may use percussion to check the size of the heart. The patient should not speak while the physician auscultates the heart sounds with the stethoscope. The physician notes the rate, rhythm, intensity, and pitch of the heart.

## Breasts

During a general physical exam, every woman should have a complete breast exam. Breast cancer is the most common cancer in women. Because growths are also possible in men's breasts, doctors should perform a breast exam on all patients.

The doctor begins the exam with the patient in a sitting position. The doctor asks the patient to hold her arms at her sides while he inspects the breasts for symmetry, contour, masses, and retracted areas. The doctor then asks the patient to raise her arms above her head while he palpates the lymph nodes under her arms.

Next, the doctor asks the patient to lie down and place her hand under her head on the first side to be examined. The doctor may ask you to place a small pillow or folded towel under the patient's shoulder blade on the same side. This procedure allows the breast tissue to flatten evenly against the chest wall, permitting easier palpation. The doctor then palpates the breast in a circular, systematic manner to check for lumps, examines the areola and nipple, and then repeats the procedure on the other side.

When examining male patients, the doctor palpates the patient's breasts and lymph nodes in the same manner that he does with his female patients. The doctor also checks the breasts of his male patients for lesions or swelling.

## Abdomen

The physician examines the patient's abdomen while the patient is in a supine position with arms down at the sides. The abdominal muscles should be completely relaxed for this part of the exam. The physician may ask you to place a small pillow under the patient's head or knees (or both) to keep the abdomen relaxed. If the patient is wearing a gown, it is raised to just under the breasts. If the patient is draped, the drape must be lowered to just above the genitalia to allow a complete view of the area. A separate drape should be placed to cover a female patient's breasts.

The order of exam methods for the abdomen is different from the order for other areas. The physician begins with inspection and auscultation, followed by percussion and palpation. Following this order allows the physician to listen to bowel sounds before palpating the abdominal organs. Palpation of this area can change bowel sounds in such a way that the physician could misdiagnose a patient's condition.

The physician must assess the abdomen thoroughly, because there are many organs in the abdominal cavity. The physician describes observations based on a system of landmarks that map out the abdominal region. The

abdomen is typically divided into four equal sections, or **quadrants,** as shown in Figure 25-9. Some physicians divide the abdomen into nine sections, similar to a tick-tack-toe board, as shown in Figure 25-10.

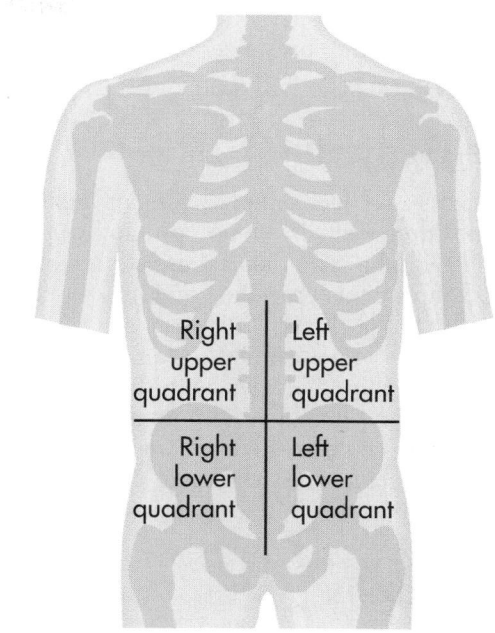

**Figure 25-9.** The abdomen is typically divided into four equal sections, or quadrants.

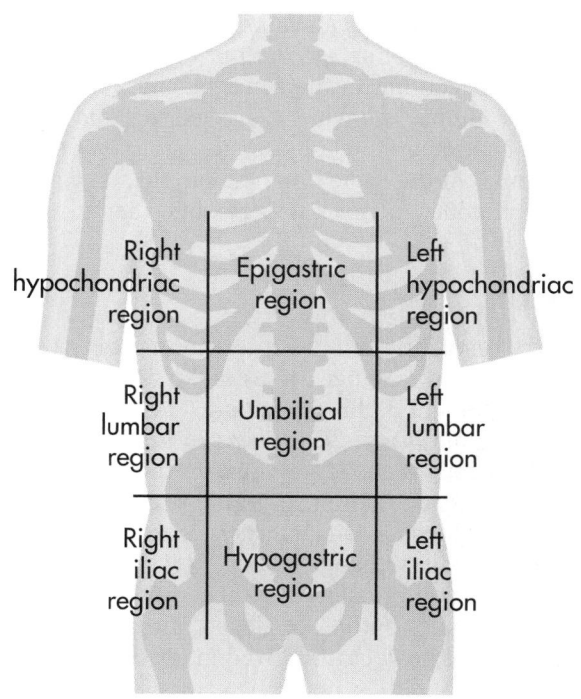

**Figure 25-10.** Some physicians divide the abdomen into nine sections, similar to a tic-tac-toe board.

If the physician has not assessed the skin in this area already, she begins with an inspection of the abdominal skin's color and surface and follows with an inspection of the shape and symmetry of the abdomen. She then uses auscultation to check bowel and vascular sounds and uses percussion to note the size and position of the organs. Lastly, she uses palpation to check muscle tone and to determine the presence of any tenderness or masses.

## Female Genitalia

Female patients may feel self-conscious or anxious in the lithotomy position—which is most commonly used during exam of the genitalia. The medical assistant may help the patient relax during this procedure and may assist patients in maintaining the position.

If the doctor who performs the exam is male, a female medical assistant should always be in the room to protect both the patient and doctor from potential lawsuits. This type of exam may be performed by a specialist or by a primary care physician. The procedure for a gynecologic exam is described in detail in Chapter 26.

## Male Genitalia

During the exam of the genitalia, men may be just as embarrassed or uncomfortable as women may be. If the physician who is performing the assessment is female, a male medical assistant should be in the room to protect both the patient and physician from potential lawsuits.

The procedure begins with the patient in the supine position. The physician puts on gloves and visually inspects the patient's penis for signs of infection or structural abnormalities, palpating any lesions. The physician then examines the scrotum in the same manner, palpating the testicles for lumps. The patient is asked to stand while the physician checks for any bulges in the groin that may indicate a hernia. At the same time, the physician palpates the local lymph nodes to check for any abnormality.

## Rectum

The doctor usually examines the rectum after examining the genitalia. You may need to assist an adult patient into a dorsal recumbent or Sims' position. The doctor normally examines a child when the child is in the prone position and inspects only the external areas of the rectum.

In adults the doctor uses a **digital exam** to palpate the rectum for lesions or irregularities. Doctors recommend that patients older than age 40 have a yearly digital exam for early detection of colorectal cancer. For this exam the doctor puts on a clean pair of gloves. You assist by applying lubricant to the doctor's gloved index finger before the exam begins. As with exam of the genitalia, patients often find a digital exam of the rectum embarrassing and uncomfortable.

After performing the procedure, the doctor may request that any stool found on the glove be tested for the presence of occult blood using a guiac-based fecal occult blood test. The presence of occult blood in the stool is a possible indication of colorectal cancer or gastrointestinal bleeding. This test—often called by its brand name, Hemoccult or Seracult test—involves placing a sample of stool on a special cardboard slide. You assist by presenting the slide to the doctor. To produce an accurate test, three consecutive bowel movements are tested; this sample is usually the first. After the exam you may be responsible for instructing the patient on how to collect the additional two samples. The procedure is outlined on the package of the occult blood-testing kit.

After the rectal exam, offer the patient the opportunity to clean the anal area before you adjust the drape. Dispose of gloves and soiled materials in a biohazardous waste container.

## Musculoskeletal System

If the physician did not examine the patient's back during the chest exam, he does so during the musculoskeletal assessment. The physician checks for good posture from the back and side. He may ask the patient to walk so that he can assess her gait. The physician always asks a child to bend at the waist so that he can check for the presence of scoliosis, a lateral curvature of the spine.

During the musculoskeletal assessment, the physician determines range of motion, the strength of various muscle groups, and body measurements. The physician also examines the arms, hands, legs, and feet for any lesions, deformities, or circulatory problems.

The physician checks a patient's range of motion to detect joint deformities and to learn whether the patient has any limitations in movement caused by an injury or other conditions, such as arthritis. Checking a patient's range of motion also allows the physician to follow a patient's progress during recovery from an injury or surgery.

As part of the assessment of a child's health, the physician asks the child to perform certain tasks, such as walking a straight line and balancing or hopping on one foot. The physician uses these tasks to evaluate the child's development and coordination and to provide the physician with information about the functioning of the child's neurological system.

## Neurological System

The doctor's neurologic assessment includes an evaluation of the patient's reflexes, mental and emotional status (including intelligence, speech, and behavior), and sensory and motor functions. The doctor often performs the neurologic assessment at the same time as the musculoskeletal assessment because both systems are involved in movement and coordination.

The doctor may incorporate certain aspects of the neurologic assessment into other parts of the exam. For example, testing how a patient's pupils react to light is part of an eye exam, but because this test also examines the patient's light reflex, the test includes a neurological assessment as well.

The doctor checks the patient's reflexes to assess both sensory and motor nerve pathways at different areas of the spinal cord. To check reflexes, the doctor uses a reflex hammer to tap tendons in different areas of the patient's body.

Most exams of children also include an intellectual assessment, in which the doctor asks the child general questions appropriate to the child's age. Doctors may also test the mental status and memory of older adults to detect disorders such as senility and Alzheimer's disease in patients who show signs of confusion or complain of memory loss.

# Completing the Exam

After the physician completes the exam, you should help the patient into a sitting position. Then allow the patient to perform any necessary self-hygiene measures.

## Additional Tests or Procedures

Before the patient dresses, check to see whether the physician has ordered any additional tests or procedures that are more conveniently performed while the patient is undressed. These tests might include taking body fat measurements or blood samples or preparing the patient for a diagnostic or therapeutic procedure, such as an x-ray or physical therapy session. The physician may also ask you to perform other procedures. Some of these procedures, which are covered in other chapters, include the following:

- Cold or heat therapy (Chapter 29)
- Applying a bandage (Chapter 30)
- Performing Clinical Laboratory Improvement Amendments (CLIA)–waived laboratory tests, such as a reagent strip urinalysis (Chapter 34)
- Collecting culture specimens (Chapters 33, 34, and 35)
- Administering an injection (Chapter 38)
- Applying a topical medication (Chapter 38)

If the physician has not ordered any additional procedures—or if wearing clothing does not interfere with the procedures ordered—the patient may dress. Help the patient get off the examining table, and allow her to dress in privacy. Make sure she knows you are available to assist if she needs help dressing.

The physician may ask you to perform other tests and procedures that can be done after the patient has dressed, including these procedures, which are discussed in detail where noted:

- Otic or ophthalmic irrigation (Chapter 38)
- Administration of certain medications (Chapter 38)
- Pulmonary function tests (Chapter 39)

# Screening for Visual Acuity

Many physicians will require a visual acuity exam as a component of the physical exam. Visual acuity screenings are a common procedure that medical assistants perform in physician offices. The Snellen chart is the most common screening for distance visual acuity. The Jaegar chart is the most common screening for near vision and the Ishihara book is the most common for color vision screening. In addition to performing the visual screening procedures, the medical assistant must observe for any actions by the patient to indicate visual difficulties, such as squinting, or leaning forward, and slow responses during the screening. Refer to Procedure 25-6 for the correct method to perform vision screening tests.

**Special Considerations.** Certain patients may need special attention when having vision tests. For example, children may be uncooperative or unable to follow directions. To encourage cooperation, show the child the chart you will be using before you begin the test. Point to the symbols and read them aloud once so the child knows the proper term for each symbol. Most physicians use pictorial charts when they start screening a child's vision at the 4-year or 5-year checkup. You can provide assistance during the test by guiding the child through each step in the procedure or by covering the child's eye. Watch the child closely for signs that she is having difficulty seeing the chart. Examples of signs include straining, squinting, blinking or watering of the eyes, and puckering of the face.

If a child has difficulty following directions, enlist the parent's or guardian's help. He may be able to explain or interpret information for the child more effectively than you can. Ask the parent if he has ever observed signs of vision problems in his child. For example, does the child rub her eyes frequently, blink a great deal, or hold books very close to her face? Be sure to note the answers in the child's chart so the physician is aware of them.

A patient with dementia or Alzheimer's disease may also require special attention during a vision test. Before the test, encourage a family member to stay with the patient so he is more comfortable. During the test, use simple language to explain the procedure and demonstrate whenever possible. Proceed through the exam slowly, one step at a time. Because the patient's memory and language skills may be impaired, you may need to repeat directions many times and help him name a particular object. If he appears to have trouble with one part of the exam, proceed to another part and return later to the part that was difficult for him.

# Performing Vision Screening Tests

**Objectives:** To screen a patient's ability to see distant or close objects, to determine contrast sensitivity, or to detect color blindness

## OSHA Guidelines

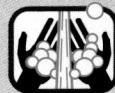  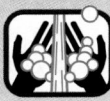

**Materials:** Occluder or card; alcohol; gauze squares; appropriate vision charts to test for distance vision, near vision, and color blindness

## Method:

### Distance Vision

1. Wash your hands, identify the patient, introduce yourself, and explain the procedure.

2. Mount one of the following eye charts at eye level: Snellen letter or similar chart (for patients who can read); Snellen E, Landolt C, pictorial, or similar chart (for patients who cannot read) (Figures 25-11 and 25-12). If using the Snellen

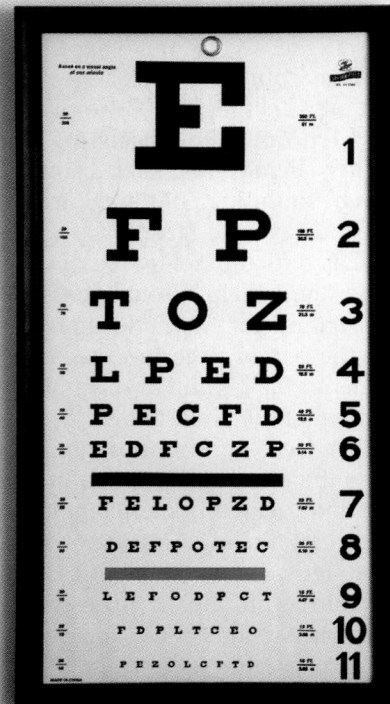

**Figure 25-11.** The Snellen letter chart is used to test the ability to see objects that are relatively far away.

letter chart, verify that the patient knows the letters of the alphabet. With children or nonreading adults, use demonstration cards to verify that they can identify the pictures or direction of the letters.

### Rationale

If the patient does not understand the instructions, the results will not be accurate.

3. Make a mark on the floor 20 feet away from the chart.

4. Have the patient stand with the heels at the 20-foot mark or sit with the back of the chair at the mark.

5. Instruct the patient to keep both eyes open and not to squint or lean forward during the test.

### Rationale

Closing one eye, squinting, or leaning will lead to inaccurate results.

6. Test both eyes first, then the right eye, and then the left eye. (Different offices may test in a different order. Follow your office policy.) Refer to Figure 25-13.

### Rationale

Following office policy leads to consistency in the results of all medical records.

7. Have the patient read the lines on the chart (or identify the picture/direction), beginning with the 20-foot line. If the patient cannot read this line, begin with the smallest line the patient can read. (Some offices use a pointer to select one symbol at a time in random order to prevent patients from memorizing the order. It is common to start with children at the 40- or 30-foot line, or larger if low vision is suspected, and proceed to the 20-foot line.)

8. Note the smallest line the patient can read or identify. (When testing children, note the smallest line on which they can identify three out of four or four out of six symbols correctly.)

9. Record the results as a fraction (for example, O.U. 20/40 –1 if the patient misses one letter on a line or O.U. 20/40 –2 if the patient misses two letters on a line).

10. Show the patient how to cover the left eye with the occluder or card. Again, instruct the patient

*continued →*

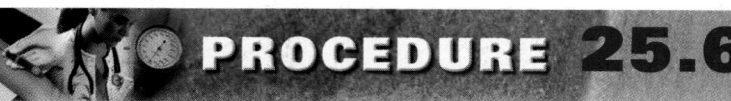
# Performing Vision Screening Tests *(continued)*

to keep both eyes open and not to squint or lean forward during the test.

**11.** Have the patient read the lines on the chart.

**12.** Record the results of the right eye (for example, Right Eye 20/30).

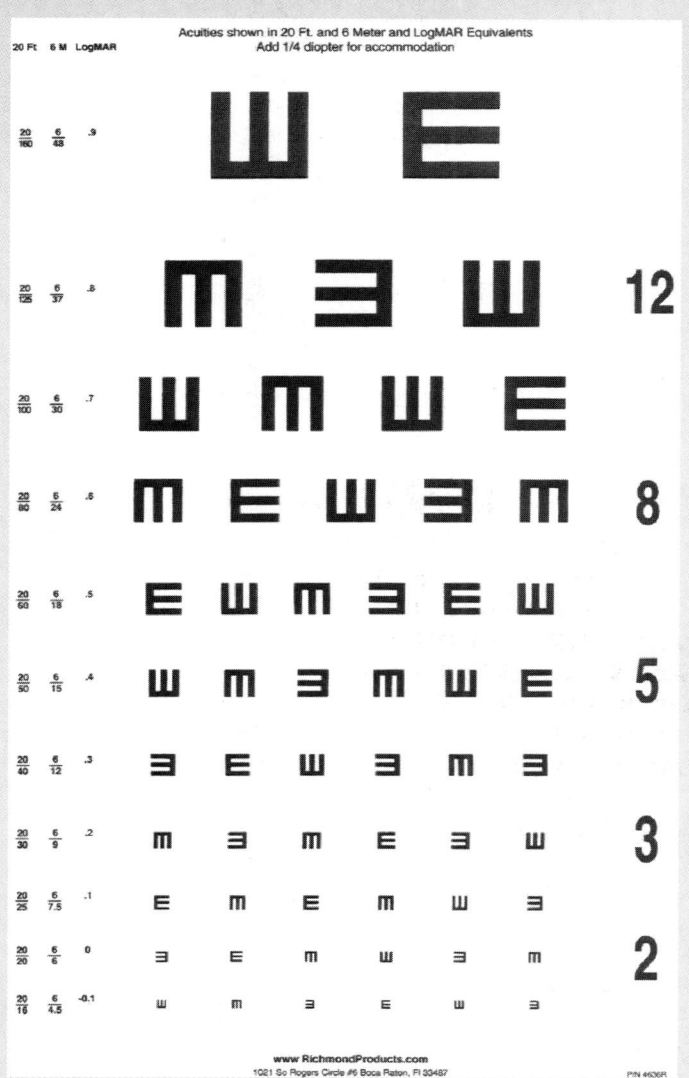

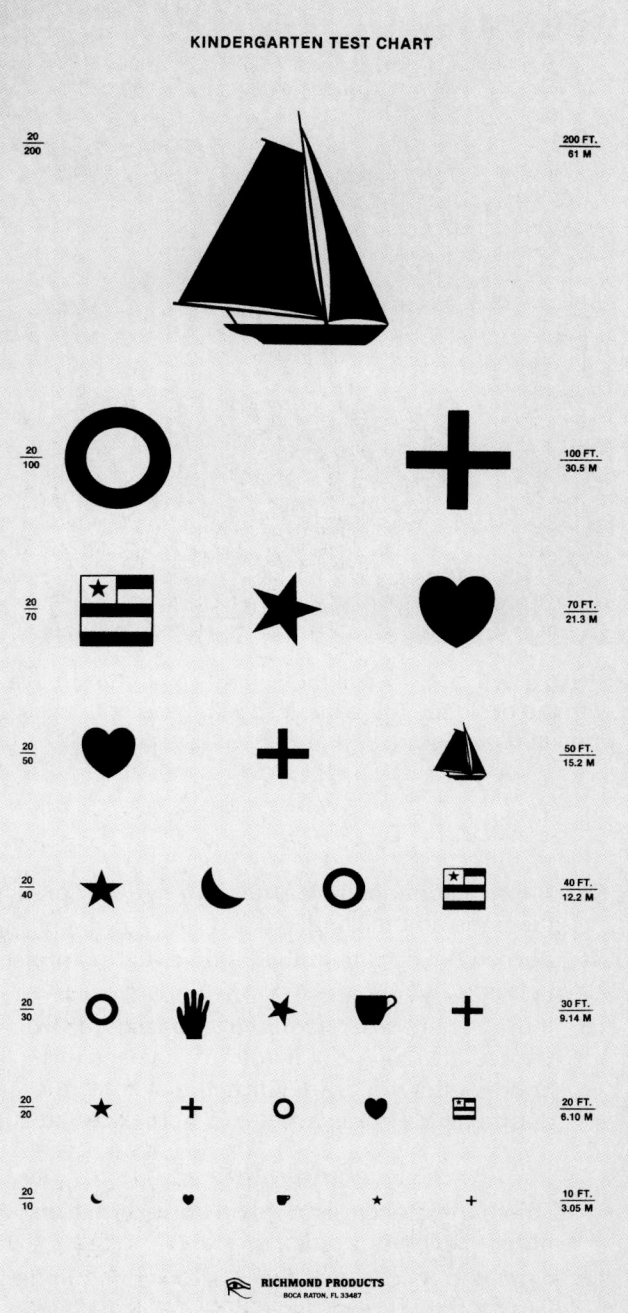

**Figure 25-12.** The Snellen E eye chart (left) or a pictorial eye chart (right) is used to test the vision of children and nonreading adults. (Reprinted with permission of Richmond Products, Inc.)

*continued* ⟶

## Performing Vision Screening Tests *(continued)*

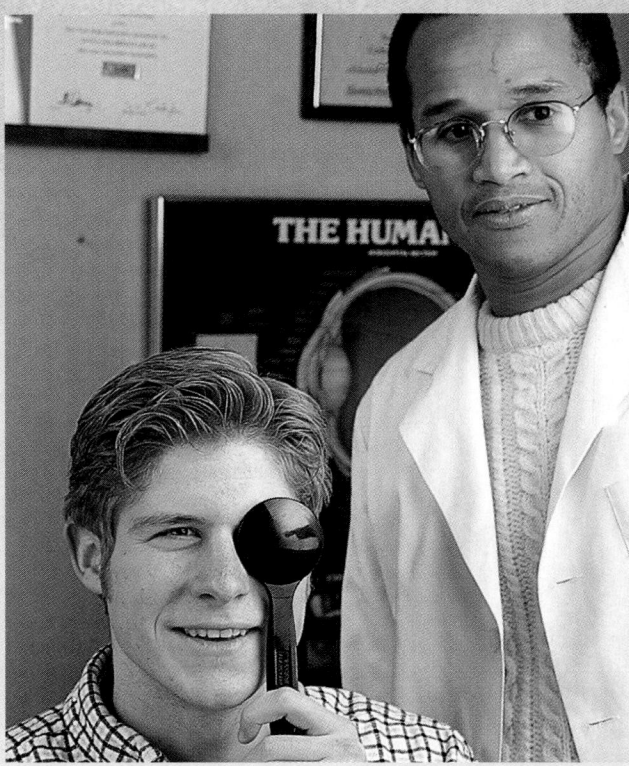

**Figure 25-13.** Have the patient cover the left eye with the occluder. The patient should keep both eyes open and not squint.

13. Have the patient cover the right eye and read the lines on the chart.

14. Record the results of the left eye (for example, Left Eye 20/20).

15. If the patient wears corrective lenses, record the results using $\overline{cc}$ ( if your office uses this abbreviation for "with correction") in front of the abbreviation (for example, $\overline{cc}$ both eyes. 20/20).

### Rationale

For charting accuracy, vision correction must be noted using your office format.

16. Note and record any observations of squinting, head tilting, or excessive blinking or tearing.

17. Ask the patient to keep both eyes open and to identify the two colored bars, and record the results in the patient's chart.

18. Clean the occluder with a gauze square dampened with alcohol.

19. Properly dispose of the gauze square and wash your hands.

### Rationale

Maintain principles of aseptic technique at all times.

### Near Vision

1. Wash your hands, identify the patient, introduce yourself, and explain the procedure.

2. Have the patient hold one of the following at normal reading distance (approximately 14 to 16 inches): Jaeger, Richmond pocket, or similar chart or card (Figures 25-14 and 25-15).

3. Ask the patient to keep both eyes open and to read or identify the letters, symbols, or paragraphs.

### Rationale

If both eyes are not open, results may not be accurate.

4. Record the smallest line read without error.

5. If the card is laminated, clean it with a gauze square dampened with alcohol.

6. Properly dispose of the gauze square and wash your hands.

### Rationale

Maintain principles of aseptic technique at all times.

### Color Vision

1. Wash your hands, identify the patient, introduce yourself, and explain the procedure.

2. Hold one of the following color charts or books at the patient's normal reading distance (approximately 14 to 16 inches): Ishihara, Richmond pseudoisochromatic, or similar color-testing system (Figure 25-16).

3. Ask the patient to tell you the number or symbol within the colored dots on each chart or page.

4. Proceed through all the charts or pages.

5. Record the number correctly identified and failed with a slash between them (for example, 13 passed/1 failed).

*continued* ⟶

# Performing Vision Screening Tests (continued)

V = .50 D.

The fourteenth of August was the day fixed upon for the sailing of the brig Pilgrim, on her voyage from Boston round Cape Horn, to the western coast of North America. As she was to get under way early in the afternoon, I made my appearance on board at twelve o'clock in full sea-rig, and with my chest, containing an outfit for a two or three years voyage,

which I had undertaken from a determination to cure, if possible, by an entire change of life, and by a long absence from books and study, a weakness of the eyes which had obliged me to give up my pursuits, and which no medical aid seemed likely to cure. The change from the tight dress coat, silk cap and kid gloves of an undergraduate at Cambridge, to the

V = .75 D.

loose duck trousers, checked shirt and tarpaulin hat of a sailor, though somewhat of a transformation, was soon made, and I supposed that I should pass very well for a Jack tar. But it is impossible to deceive the practiced eye in these matters; and while I supposed myself to be looking as salt as Neptune himself, I was, no doubt, known for a landsman by every one on board, as soon as I hove in sight. A sailor has a peculiar cut to his clothes, and a way of wear-

V = 1.  D.

ing them which a green hand can never get. The trousers, tight around the hips, and thence hanging long and loose around the feet, a superabundance of checked shirt, a low-crowned, well-varnished black hat, worn on the back of the head, with half a fathom of black ribbon hanging over the left eye, and a peculiar tie to the black silk neckerchief, with sundry other *details*, are signs the want of which betray the beginner at once.

V = 1.25 D.

Beside the points in my dress which were out of the way, doubtless my complexion and hands would distinguish me from the regular *salt*, who, with a sun-browned cheek, wide step and rolling gait, swings his bronzed and toughened hands athwartships half open, as though just to ready to grasp a rope. "With all my imperfections

V = 1.50 D.

on my head," I joined the crew, and we hauled out into the stream and came to anchor for the night. The next day we were employed in preparation for sea, reeving and studding-sail gear, crossing royal yards, putting on chafing gear, and taking on board our powder. On the

V = 1.75 D.

following night I stood my first watch. I remained awake nearly all the first part of the night, from fear that I might not hear when I was called; and when I went on deck, so great were my ideas of the importance of my trust, that I

V = 2.  D.

walked regularly fore and aft the whole length of the vessel, looking out over the bows and taffrail at each turn, and was not a little surprised at the unconcerned manner in which the billows turned up their

Your glasses are of value to you only as they accurately interpret your prescription and this only as they are fitted and serviced in accordance with these needs. They are a therapeutic device.

 **RICHMOND PRODUCTS**
BOCA RATON, FL 33487

No. 11974 R

**Figure 25-14.** This near-vision chart is used to test the ability to see objects at a normal reading distance. (Reprinted with permission of Richmond Products, Inc.)

*continued* ⟶

## Performing Vision Screening Tests *(concluded)*

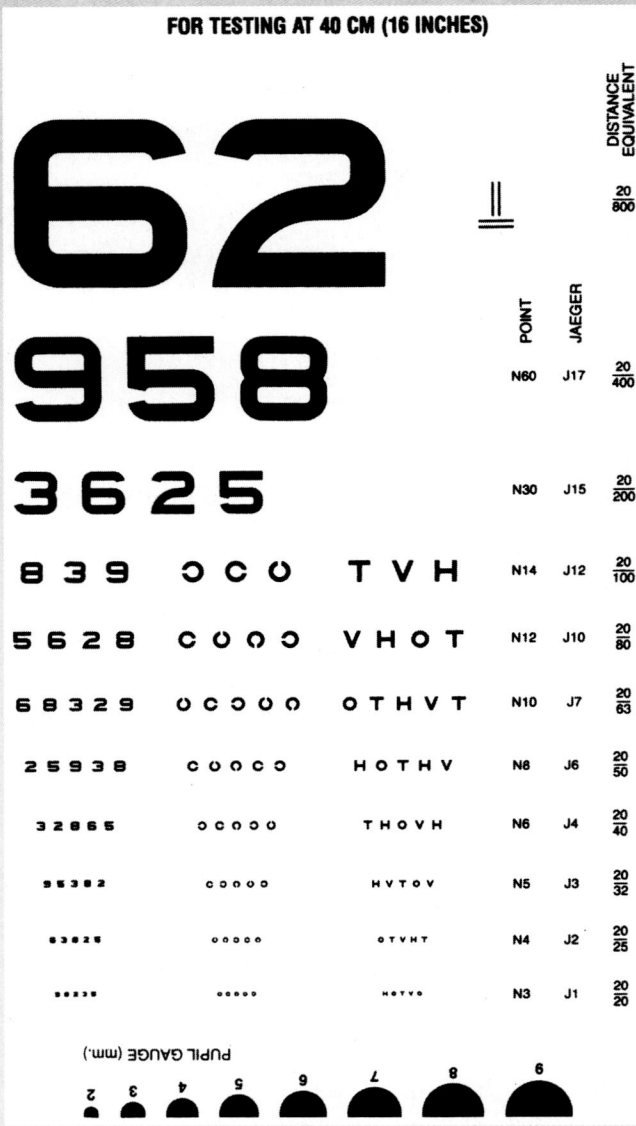

**FOR TESTING AT 40 CM (16 INCHES)**

**Figure 25-15.** The Richmond pocket vision screener is also used to test near vision. (Reprinted with permission of Richmond Products, Inc.)

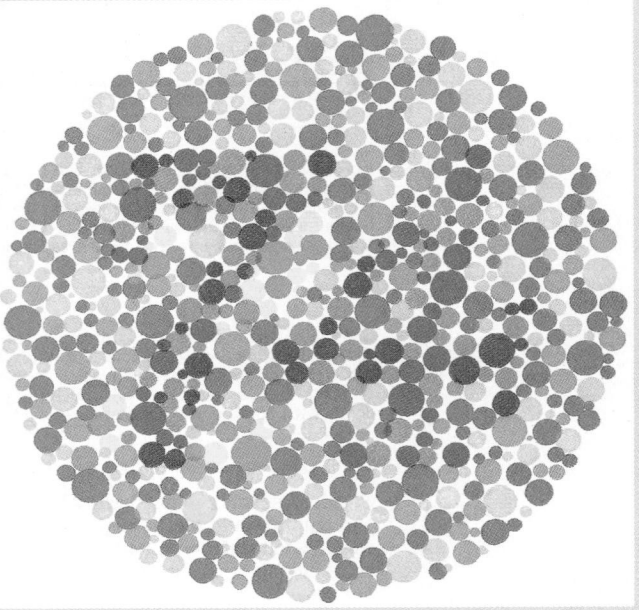

**Figure 25-16.** The Richmond pseudoisochromatic color chart is used to test a person's ability to see colors. (Reprinted with permission of Richmond Products, Inc.)

6. If the charts are laminated, clean them with a gauze square dampened with alcohol.
7. Properly dispose of the gauze square and wash your hands.

*Rationale*

Maintain principles of aseptic technique at all times.

## Auditory Acuity

The physician may order a hearing acuity test after the exam based on the observations made during the exam or by the subjective information supplied by the patient. An audiometer is a common electronic hearing acuity device and is available in several models that can be simple or complex to operate, depending on the model (Figure 25-17). Procedure 25-7 details the steps for measuring auditory acuity.

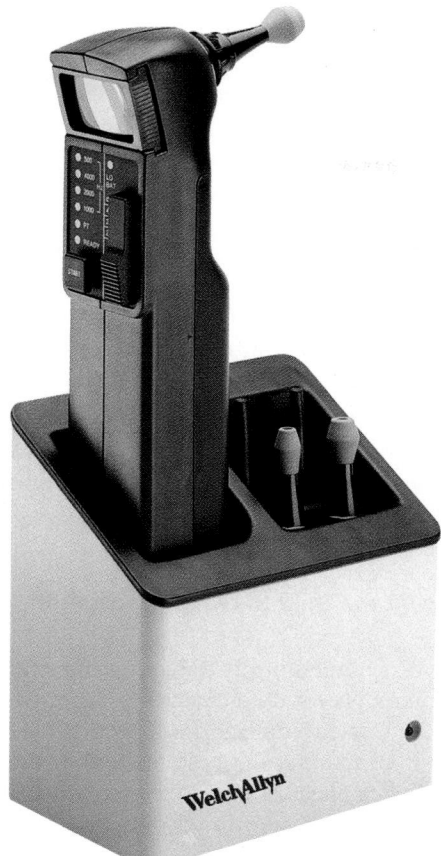

**Figure 25-17.** This type of simple audiometer can be found in many physicians' offices.

## Patient Education

The general physical exam provides you with the opportunity to assess the patient's educational needs. Basing your findings on the patient's interview, history, and exam, you can identify areas in which the patient may benefit from additional education.

Pay special attention to educating patients about risk factors for disease. For example, women are often instructed about the risk factors for breast cancer. The risk factors include being older than 50 (many physicians recommend that women older than 40 have a mammogram every 2 years and that women older than 50 have one every year), having a family history of breast cancer, having the first child after age 30, never being pregnant, and beginning to menstruate at an early age.

The physician may also request that you teach patients how to administer certain medications or how to perform self-help or diagnostic techniques, such as a breast self-exam, at home (see the Educating the Patient section). These procedures may involve collecting samples for occult blood testing or urine testing, applying cold or hot packs, or instilling eyedrops. It is important to teach the patient the correct way to perform a diagnostic test. If a specimen is incorrectly obtained, the test results will be inaccurate.

Regardless of the type of instruction, be sure that you address patients at a language level they can understand without talking down to them. To ensure that they understand fully, ask patients to repeat each instruction and to perform each demonstration as you give it to them.

# PROCEDURE 25.7

## Measuring Auditory Acuity

**Objective:** To determine how well a patient hears

**OSHA Guidelines**

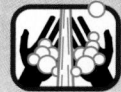  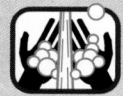

**Materials:** Audiometer, headset, graph pad (if applicable), alcohol, gauze squares

**Method:**

### Adults and Children

1. Wash your hands, identify the patient, introduce yourself, and explain the procedure.
2. Clean the earpieces of the headset with a gauze square dampened with alcohol.

### Rationale
Maintain aseptic technique at all times.

3. Have the patient sit with his back to you.
4. Assist the patient in putting on the headset, and adjust it until it is comfortable.
5. Tell the patient he will hear tones in the right ear.
6. Tell the patient to raise his finger or press the indicator button when he hears a tone.
7. Set the audiometer for the right ear.
8. Set the audiometer for the lowest range of frequencies and the first degree of loudness (usually 15 decibels). (When using automated audiometers, follow the instructions printed in the user's manual.)

*continued* ⟶

## Measuring Auditory Acuity (concluded)

9. Press the tone button or switch and observe the patient.

10. If the patient does not hear the first degree of loudness, raise it two or three times to greater degrees, up to 50 or 60 decibels.

11. If the patient indicates that he has heard the tone, record the setting on the graph.

12. Change the setting to the next frequency. Repeat steps 9, 10, and 11.

13. Proceed to the mid-range frequencies. Repeat steps 9, 10, and 11.

14. Proceed to the high-range frequencies. Repeat steps 9, 10, and 11.

15. Set the audiometer for the left ear.

16. Tell the patient that he will hear tones in the left ear, and ask him to raise his finger or press the indicator button when he hears a tone.

17. Repeat steps 8 through 14.

18. Set the audiometer for both ears.

19. Ask the patient to listen with both ears and to raise his finger or press the indicator button when he hears a tone.

20. Repeat steps 8 through 14.

21. Have the patient remove the headset.

22. Clean the earpieces with a gauze square dampened with alcohol.

23. Properly dispose of the used gauze square and wash your hands.

### Rationale
Maintain aseptic technique at all times.

### Infants and Toddlers

1. Identify the patient and introduce yourself.

2. Wash your hands.

3. Pick a quiet location.

4. The patient can be sitting, lying down, or held by the parent.

5. Instruct the parent to be silent during the procedure.

6. Position yourself so your hands are behind the child's right ear and out of sight.

### Rationale
You want the child to respond to sound, not to sight.

7. Clap your hands loudly. Observe the child's response. (Never clap directly in front of the ear because this can damage the eardrum. As an alternative to clapping, use special devices, such as rattles or clickers, which may be available in the office to generate sounds of varying loudness.)

8. Record the child's response as positive or negative for loud noise.

9. Position one hand behind the child's right ear, as before.

10. Snap your fingers. Observe the child's response.

11. Record the response as positive or negative for moderate noise.

12. Repeat steps 6 through 11 for the left ear.

## CAUTION *Handle With Care*

## Helping Patients With Suspected Breast Cancer

If the physician detects a suspicious lump in a patient's breast during the general physical exam, your main concern is to help the patient remain calm. Although most suspicious lumps are not cancerous, the patient is likely to be anxious and upset about the finding. The best thing you can do for her is to schedule her for a mammogram as soon as possible.

### Preparing the Patient for a Mammogram
To alleviate some of the patient's fears, explain exactly what a mammogram is. Give the patient the following information.

1. A mammogram is a special type of x-ray of the breast that is used to detect cancer and other abnormalities of the breast.

*continued* ⟶

## Helping Patients With Suspected Breast Cancer *(concluded)*

2. A technician specially trained in performing mammography will position the patient's breast along a flat plastic plate. A second plate will be brought into position and pressure will be applied for about 20 to 30 seconds to flatten the breast (to obtain a clearer x-ray) while the x-ray is taken. This will be done in two directions (planes) for each breast.

3. Mammography is generally not a painful procedure, but some women may find it uncomfortable. Many professionals suggest that patients avoid scheduling a mammogram during the week prior to a menstrual period to reduce potential discomfort.

4. The mammography appointment normally takes ½ to 1 hour. The actual mammography takes only about 15 minutes.

5. Because the patient will have to undress from the waist up, she should wear a separate top and slacks or a skirt rather than a dress.

6. The patient should have no creams, powders, or deodorants on her breasts or underarms when the mammography is performed because chemicals in these preparations can produce misleading images in the mammogram.

7. If the patient has films from previous mammograms, it is important for the radiologist to see the films for a comparison study. If you schedule a mammogram, make sure you instruct the patient to obtain previous mammogram films prior to the screening if the films are located in a facility other than the one scheduled.

Answer any questions the patient has, and provide patient education materials related to mammography and breast disease. Reassure her that most lumps are not cancerous.

If your office refers patients to a particular facility that you are familiar with, give the patient an idea of how long she can expect to wait for the results. Ensure her that she will be notified as soon as the physician receives the report. You may want to schedule a follow-up visit at this time, based on when results are expected.

Because this is a difficult time for a patient, you should be as supportive as possible. You can help the patient cope by showing your concern and giving her prompt attention. Tell the patient that if she has any questions at all, she should call the physician.

---

(For additional patient education tips related to specialty exams, refer to Chapters 26 and 27.) Give patients written instructions that they can refer to at home.

## Special Problems of the Elderly

The elderly often have a greater need for patient education than do younger patients because certain diseases are common in older patients. Moreover, the elderly frequently are not aware of these diseases or of advances in their treatment. Here are some common problems of the elderly:

- Incontinence
- Depression
- Lack of information on preventive medicine
- Lack of compliance when taking medications

**Incontinence.** Physicians estimate that most patients who suffer from incontinence (involuntary leakage of urine) can be helped. Because most people are too embarrassed to ask for help or are unaware of possible solutions, however, only 1 out of 12 persons actually seeks help for the condition.

**Depression.** Depression is common in the elderly, but many of the symptoms of depression mimic those of other conditions. You can help elderly patients—and their families—recognize the signs of depression. Knowing what to look for may help patients seek help sooner than they otherwise would and receive prompt diagnosis and treatment. See the Caution: Handle With Care section for a discussion of symptoms and treatment of depression in the elderly.

**Lack of Information on Preventive Medicine.** Many of the elderly are still not aware of the concept of preventive medicine (measures taken to prevent illness). Many come from environments in which people went to a doctor only when they were very ill. Thus, they do not realize the importance of preventive measures such as regular checkups and yearly digital rectal exams to detect colorectal cancer. Older women often do not recognize the need for regular mammograms and Pap smears to detect cancers of the breast and cervix.

Use any educational tools available to you to make elderly patients more aware of these disorders and the importance of preventive measures. If you reinforce

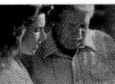

# How to Perform a Breast Self-Exam

You may be responsible for reinforcing patient education about monthly breast self-exam (BSE), which can be instrumental in the early detection of breast cancer. Figure 25-18 shows the steps suggested by the National Cancer Institute for performing this procedure.

Check the office policy to see which of several methods it recommends for teaching BSE. One approach uses the following steps.

1. Explain the purpose of BSE.

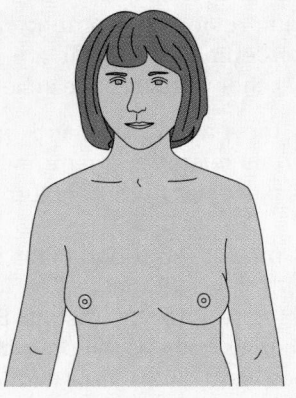
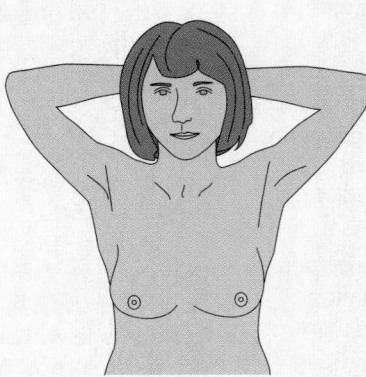

❶ Stand before a mirror. Inspect both breasts for anything unusual such as any discharge from the nipples or puckering, dimpling, or scaling of the skin.

The next two steps are designed to emphasize any change in the shape or contour of your breasts. As you do them, you should be able to feel your chest muscles tighten.

❷ Watching closely in the mirror, clasp your hands behind your head, and press your hands forward.

❸ Next, press your hands firmly on your hips, and bow slightly toward your mirror as you pull your shoulders and elbows forward.

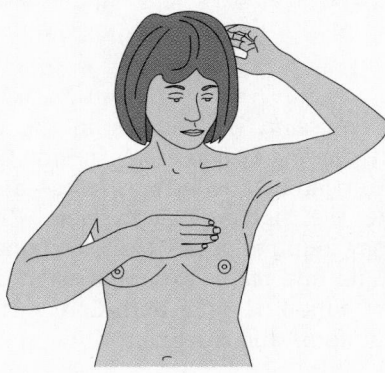
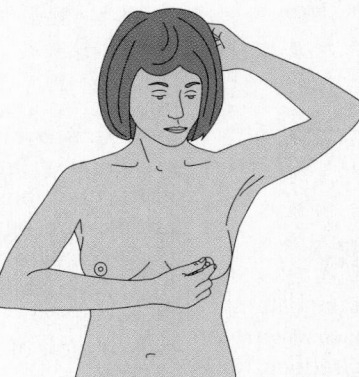
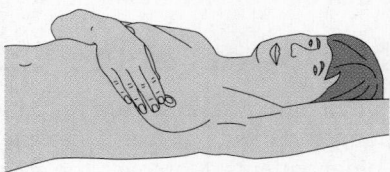

Some women do the next part of the exam in the shower because fingers glide over soapy skin, making it easy to concentrate on the texture underneath.

❹ Raise your left arm. Use three or four fingers of your right hand to explore your left breast firmly, carefully, and thoroughly. Beginning at the outer edge, press the flat part of your fingers in small circles, moving the circles slowly around the breast. and the underarm, including the underarm itself. Feel for any unusual lump or mass under the skin.

❺ Gently squeeze the nipple and look for a discharge. (If you have any discharge during the month—whether or not it is during BSE—see your doctor.) Repeat steps 4 and 5 on your right breast.

❻ Steps 4 and 5 should be repeated lying down. Lie flat on your back with your left arm over your head and a pillow or folded towel under your left shoulder. This position flattens the breast and makes it easier to examine. Use the same circular motion described earlier. Repeat the examination on your right breast.

**Figure 25-18.** The National Cancer Institute includes these instructions and illustrations in the brochure *Breast Exams: What You Should Know* (NIH Publication No. 90-2000).

*continued* ⟶

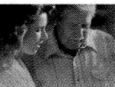
## How to Perform a Breast Self-Exam *(concluded)*

2. Assist the patient to the standing position, and instruct her to use a large mirror to view the breasts during this part of the procedure.

3. Explain to the patient what she should look for when inspecting her breasts while standing.

4. Demonstrate the positioning of arms and hands for this visual inspection: first, her arms at her sides; then, her arms raised and her hands clasped behind her head; finally, her arms lowered with her hands on her hips.

5. Demonstrate, on the patient's breast, how to perform the small rotary motions with the flat pads of the fingers from the outer rim (including the armpit and collarbone area) toward the nipple. (Synthetic breast models are available that may be helpful in teaching the proper technique.)

6. Demonstrate how to inspect the nipples.

7. Ask the patient to practice the procedure.

8. Observe the patient's self-exam technique. (If the patient is reluctant to examine herself in front of you, have her repeat the highlights of the procedure.)

9. Assist the patient to lie down, with a small pillow or folded towel under the shoulder on the side to be examined.

10. Repeat steps 5 through 8.

11. Suggest that the patient mark her calendar for a monthly reminder to perform the exam 1 week after the onset of menses.

12. Give the patient educational materials that explain how to perform BSE.

Make sure the patient knows that she should perform BSE around the same date of each month—after her period ends, if she is still menstruating. (At this time the breasts are most normal and least swollen and lumpy.) You must also emphasize that BSE is not a substitute for mammograms or regular breast exam by a doctor. Early cancer detection depends on the performance of all three types of breast exam.

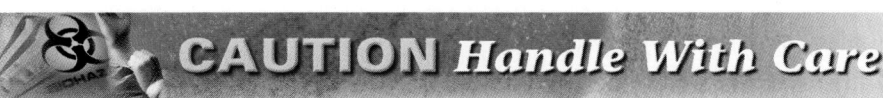

# CAUTION *Handle With Care*

## Helping Elderly Patients With Depression

Depression is a common problem among elderly people. Studies published by the National Institutes of Health (NIH) indicate that at least 5% of elderly people attending primary care clinics suffer from depression. For elderly people in nursing homes, that percentage rises to between 15% and 25%. The NIH also indicates that only about 10% of elderly people who need treatment for depression ever receive it. Additionally, the NIH considers depression in people age 65 and older to be a major public health concern. Suicide is more common among the elderly than any other age group.

One reason for this low rate of treatment is that many older people—and their families—believe that depression is a normal consequence of growing old. Older people may experience the deaths of a spouse and siblings; they have to adjust to retirement and, possibly, loneliness. They may have to deal with a relocation. They may suffer economic hardship and are likely to experience a variety of physical ailments. Because of these circumstances, doctors and family may miss the signs of depression.

### Recognizing the Symptoms

There is, unfortunately, no specific diagnostic test for depression, so a diagnosis must be made on the basis of symptoms. The symptoms of depression in the elderly are similar to those in other age groups and include the following:

- Decreased ability to enjoy life or to show an interest in activities or people
- Slow thinking, indecisiveness, or difficulty in concentrating
- Increased or decreased appetite

*continued* ⟶

## CAUTION *Handle With Care*

### Helping Elderly Patients with Depression *(concluded)*

- Increased or decreased time spent sleeping
- Recurrent feelings of worthlessness
- Loss of energy and motivation
- Exaggerated feelings of sadness, hopelessness, or anxiety
- Recurrent thoughts of death or suicide

The failure to realize that symptoms such as these indicate an illness prevents many older people from seeking help. Yet there is evidence that treatment for depression in the elderly can be highly effective.

#### Treatment for Depression

Treatment for depression generally combines a course of antidepressant drugs with psychotherapy. Older people generally respond to antidepressants more slowly than younger people do, so older people may not experience relief until more than 6 weeks after starting treatment. For this and other reasons, compliance in taking medications for depression is a problem with elderly people. Many of them do not understand depression and the importance of taking medications

as prescribed. They may also be frightened by the idea of taking medication for a mental problem.

Psychotherapy aims to help older people talk through their anxieties, develop coping skills, and improve the quality of their lives. Again, compliance is a problem. Many older people are unwilling to admit that they have a mental-health problem and refuse to follow up on referrals to mental-health professionals.

#### Benefits of Treatment

Elderly people who follow a course of treatment for depression benefit in a number of ways. They gain:

- Relief from many of the symptoms associated with depression
- Relief from some of the pain and suffering associated with physical ailments
- Improved physical, mental, and social well-being

Health-care providers can play a significant role in recognizing symptoms of depression in the elderly and in encouraging them to get the treatment they need.

---

the doctor's recommendations with education, you increase the chance that patients will heed the advice they are given.

**Lack of Compliance When Taking Medications.** Some elderly people need several medications, and many of them find it difficult to keep track and take the right medication at the right time. You can help by telling elderly patients about available medication reminder boxes, timers, or medication organizers. These devices can help ensure **patient compliance** (obedience in following the physician's orders). Patient compliance helps patients remain healthier and get well faster.

## Follow-Up

After the exam, you must help the patient follow up on all of the doctor's recommendations. Follow-up may include these actions:

1. Scheduling the patient for future visits at the office
2. Making outside appointments for certain diagnostic tests, such as mammograms or other radiologic procedures, or for therapeutic procedures, such as physical therapy
3. Helping the patient and the patient's family plan for home nursing care after an illness or a surgical procedure

---

## Reflecting On . . . HIPAA

### Involving Family Members in Patient Care

Family-centered medicine is a mainstream patient care model that is adopted in many health-care facilities. Involving family members in treatment decisions increases positive patient outcomes. Make sure to review the patient demographic form to see if family members are designated by the patient to discuss his or her medical record. Talk to elderly patients about the importance of involving family members in their care.

4. Helping the patient obtain help from community or social service organizations, such as adult day care, counseling, or meal programs

Follow-up appointments can vary depending on the outcome of the patient visit. Patient follow-up can be scheduled to review diagnostic testing or laboratory results and to discuss possible treatment methods for any abnormal test results. Another type of follow-up visit is to monitor previous treatments for conditions that have been diagnosed, such as hypertension or diabetes.

During the follow-up exam, it is important to make sure that the patient preparation is appropriate for the type of exam scheduled. For example, it is not necessary for a patient to disrobe for a follow-up exam for hypertension. Use your critical thinking skills and follow office procedures for correctly preparing patients for the various types of patient visits.

Patient follow-up is particularly crucial for patients suspected of having breast cancer. You have an important responsibility to track patients who have suspicious findings on a breast exam. See the Caution: Handle With Care section for an explanation of the steps you can take to help such patients. Patients may file medical malpractice suits if doctors fail to diagnose breast cancer. In fact, this is one of the most frequent causes of malpractice suits.

## Summary

The general physical exam provides substantial information about a patient's overall health status and assists the physician in making a diagnosis, prognosis, and treatment plan. The general physical exam is the cornerstone of medical care.

The physician uses a number of assessment methods to gather information during the exam. Although one common order of exam is presented in this chapter, you should learn the order preferred by the physician(s) you assist. Be aware, too, that a physician may change the order of an exam to accommodate the needs of a particular patient.

During the exam, your first priority as a medical assistant is to address the comfort, privacy, and educational needs of the patient. You must also anticipate the needs of the physician throughout the procedure. In addition, you must be aware of the special needs of children, pregnant women, and the elderly and the areas in which patient education is likely to be needed.

# REVIEW

## CHAPTER 25

## CASE STUDY QUESTIONS

Now that you have completed this chapter, review the case study at the beginning of the chapter and answer the following questions:

1. English is the only language you speak. How can you provide adequate explanation?
2. How can you prevent embarrassment when preparing the patient for the exam?
3. During what parts of the exam do you expect to provide assistance for the physician?

## Discussion Questions

1. What is the main role of the medical assistant during a general physical exam?
2. In what ways do children and the elderly present special problems during or after a general physical exam?
3. What patient teaching opportunities arise from a general physical exam?
4. What signs or clues would occur during a physical exam that would prompt a physician to order a hearing acuity screening?

## Critical Thinking Questions

1. Discuss the different types of exams that may be performed while the patient is placed in the following exam positions:
   a. Lithotomy
   b. Sims'
   c. Dorsal recumbent
   d. Supine
   e. Prone
2. Discuss the components of the general physical exam and list the equipment and supplies needed for each of the following:
   a. Eyes
   b. Ears
   c. Mouth and throat
   d. Genitalia

3. When the general physical exam in complete, the physician often will order additional tests or procedures. What types of procedures or tests might be ordered?
4. An elderly patient arrives at the clinic for a physical exam. She is using a walker, has weakness and arthritis in her legs, and is hard of hearing. You need to place her in position for an exam of the head, neck, chest, and heart. What should you do?
5. A Spanish-speaking 5-year-old child arrives at your clinic for a physical in preparation for school. The mother is with the child and speaks and understands very little English. You must prepare the child for the exam, and no interpreter is available. What should you do?

## Application Activities

1. With a partner, practice assisting each other in assuming the various exam positions and in placing drapes properly.
2. Role-play with a partner, with one student taking the role of the medical assistant and the other the role of a patient. The student acting as the medical assistant should explain to the patient how to perform a BSE. Switch roles so that each student role-plays both parts.
3. Using an Ishihara book, work in pairs, obtaining a color vision screening on each other and document it accurately.

## Virtual Fieldtrip

*Visit the McGraw-Hill Higher Education Medical Assisting website at www.mhhe.com/medicalassisting3 to complete the following activity:*

Research one of the following topics and design a patient education program, including information on lifestyle changes, current treatments, and preventative measures to be taken by the patient.

- Breast cancer
- Women's cardiac health

Open the CD and complete this chapter's practice activities, play the games, listen to the key terms, and test yourself with the interactive review. E-mail, print, and/or save your results to document your proficiency.

# SECTION 3

## SPECIALTY PRACTICES AND MEDICAL EMERGENCIES

# Assisting With Exams in the Basic Specialties

## MEDICAL ASSISTING COMPETENCIES

*In preparation for the certification examination, you should know the following areas of competence:*

| COMPETENCY | CMA | RMA |
|---|---|---|
| **Clinical** | | |
| Apply principles of aseptic techniques and infection control, including hand washing | X | X |
| Dispose of biohazardous materials | X | X |
| Practice Standard Precautions | X | X |
| Obtain vital signs | X | X |
| Prepare the patient for and assist the physician with routine and specialty exams, treatments, and minor office surgeries | X | X |
| Maintain medication and immunization records | X | X |
| Screen and follow up on patient test results | X | X |
| **General/Legal/Professional** | | |
| Recognize and respond to verbal and nonverbal communications by being attentive and adapting communication to the recipient's level of understanding | X | X |
| Be aware of and perform within legal and ethical boundaries | X | X |
| Instruct individuals according to their needs | X | X |
| Provide patients with methods of health promotion and disease prevention | X | X |
| Conduct work within scope of education, training, and ability | | X |
| Be impartial and show empathy when dealing with patients | | X |
| Interview effectively | | X |

## CHAPTER OUTLINE

- The Medical Assistant's Role in Specialty Exams
- Internal Medicine
- Pediatrics
- Obstetrics and Gynecology

# LEARNING OUTCOMES

After completing Chapter 26, you will be able to:

**26.1** Briefly describe the medical specialties of internal medicine, pediatrics, and obstetrics and gynecology.

**26.2** Describe the types of exams and diagnostic tests performed in each of these specialties and the medical assistant's role in them.

**26.3** List and describe some common diseases and disorders seen in these medical specialties and typical treatments for them.

**26.4** Identify common signs of domestic violence and child abuse.

**26.5** Describe the medical assistant's role in assisting with a cervical biopsy.

# Introduction

Specialty exams are usually performed by specialists. Specialists are physicians, such as pediatricians and gynecologists, who have taken additional training beyond medical school and their required residencies to become board-certified in their respective specialties. Physicians who wish to become board-certified must pass rigorous exams in their chosen specialty and be elected by the board for that specialty.

As a medical assistant, you may be employed to assist with exams in the basic specialties. This chapter introduces you to the basic specialties of internal medicine, pediatrics, and obstetrics and gynecology. You will learn about the types of exams and diagnostic tests used in these specialties and about the common diseases and disorders seen in these specialties. You will also learn to watch for the signs of domestic violence and child abuse.

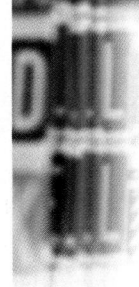

## CASE STUDY

After working for a year in the office of a general practice physician, you want a chance to increase your knowledge and skills. There are three opportunities available to you: an internal medicine practice, a pediatrician's office, and an obstetrics and gynecology clinic. Because you are looking for change, you must first learn about the types of patients and procedures you might encounter in these facilities.

As you read this chapter, consider the following questions:

1. What kind of patients would you see in each of these offices?
2. What additional duties and procedures would you perform?

# The Medical Assistant's Role in Specialty Exams

Different and additional duties may be required of the medical assistant working in basic specialties. These duties and procedures are based on your education, training, and certification. They are also based on your state's medical practice act. A **medical practice act** is a law that defines the exact duties that physicians and other health-care personnel may perform. It determines the ways that you can assist in exams, procedures, and diagnostic tests. It also determines which of these tasks you can perform alone. For example, many states have acts that give physicians the right to delegate certain clinical procedures to medical assistants and other qualified health professionals. A medical assistant is allowed to perform clinical procedures only under the supervision of the physician or other licensed health-care professional who is granted the right and who delegates the specific clinical procedures to the medical assistant. Because state laws vary, you will need to know the scope of practice for medical assistants in the state where you work.

If you work for a specialist, she may have her own rules regarding exams, procedures, and diagnostic tests with which she permits assistance. The physician may want to perform some procedures alone, with only minimal assistance from you. She may need more assistance with other procedures. She may ask you to perform some procedures on your own.

You must have a thorough understanding of basic anatomy and physiology of various body systems to perform procedures alone and to communicate effectively with patients. You must also be familiar with the specific exams and steps for the procedures in the specialty in which you are employed. Acquiring this knowledge will help you become a valuable member of your practice.

## Providing Emotional Support

You will often deal with a variety of diseases and disorders in a specialty setting. Patients' illnesses may be acute, chronic, or both. **Acute** means that a disease's onset and progress is rapid, as in acute appendicitis. An illness that lasts a long time or recurs frequently is referred to as **chronic,** such as chronic osteoarthritis. Patients may have strong reactions to acute or chronic illness, including fear, defensive behavior, and frustration with physical limitations. Your empathy and support will help patients identify and cope with their feelings and behaviors.

## Providing Patient Education

Patients do not generally visit specialists as frequently as they do a general practitioner, and they may have more questions during a general physical exam. Therefore, communicating effectively with patients and providing educational materials will be one of your primary responsibilities. You will explain the functioning of the appropriate body system and the purpose of and preparation for specific exam procedures and tests. You will also teach patients how to perform prescribed home-care regimens. Remember that just giving patients a brochure may not be enough. Make sure the patient knows what is necessary and has an opportunity to ask questions.

# Internal Medicine

Internal medicine is the specialty of an internist, who diagnoses and treats disorders and diseases of the body's internal organs. The internist is often the first doctor to see a patient with a complaint. Internists treat medical problems with medicine, either alone or in combination with other modalities (therapeutic agents). In some cases, an internist refers the patient to a doctor in one of the internal medicine subspecialties.

## Assisting With the Physical Exam

An internist's physical exam is usually conducted in the same way as is the general physical exam described in Chapter 25. Some of your responsibilities will include gathering information and preparing patients for a physical exam. You may also use this opportunity to detect possible substance abuse, domestic violence, or elder abuse. These topics were introduced in Chapter 23.

**Detecting Substance Abuse.** You should be alert for signs of substance abuse when you assist with an exam. Signs of substance abuse vary, depending on the type of drug and the individual's response to it. In general, signs you can observe are as follows:

- Alcohol: depressed pulse rate, respiration, and blood pressure; slurred speech; odor of alcohol on breath; reduced coordination and reflexes; poor vision and depth perception
- Cocaine and amphetamines: excitation, increased pulse rate and blood pressure, increased respiration and body temperature, dilated pupils, loss of appetite
- Hallucinogens such as LSD and angel dust: hallucinations, poor perception of time and distance, severe panic, violent and bizarre behavior
- Inhalants such as nitrous oxide and household solvents: muscle weakness, hearing loss, changes in heart rate, nausea, dizziness
- Marijuana: reddening of the eyes, increased heart rate, heightened appetite, muscular weakness
- Narcotics such as codeine and morphine: drowsiness, depressed respiration, constricted pupils, nausea, vomiting, constipation
- Sedatives such as barbiturates: nausea, slurred speech, drunken behavior without odor of alcohol

If you see any of these signs of substance abuse in a patient, inform the physician. Also inform the physician if you find such indications in someone who works in your office. If your state requires reporting suspected substance abuse by health-care workers, be sure you know the procedure for doing so.

**Detecting Domestic Violence.** During a physical exam, you and the internist are in a position to detect signs of domestic violence. It is crucial that you bring to the doctor's attention any clues you notice during the initial interview. The doctor can then use your observations to examine and question the patient for possible internal injuries. See the Caution: Handle With Care section for guidelines on dealing with this issue.

**Detecting Elder Abuse.** It is difficult to detect elder abuse. There is no uniform and comprehensive definition of this type of abuse, and bruises from falls and other accidents can be mistaken for abuse. Also, the signs of neglect can be similar to the signs of some chronic medical conditions.

There are three basic categories of elder abuse: domestic elder abuse, institutional elder abuse, and self-neglect, or self-abuse. Elders can be abused physically, sexually, or psychologically. Elders may also be neglected, abandoned, or exploited materially or financially. Elders may even choose to neglect or abuse themselves. More than one type of abuse can occur simultaneously. Elder abuse occurs in all racial, socioeconomic, and religious groups. However, most victims are older women with chronic illness or disabilities. Risk factors or situations that increase the possibility of elder abuse include

- History of alcoholism, drug abuse, or violence in the family
- History of mental illness in the abuser or victim

- Isolation of the victim from family members and friends other than the abuser
- Recent stressful events affecting the abuser or victim

You can assist the doctor by taking a careful history. Ask the patient about living arrangements, social contact, and emotional stress. Try to note the interaction between caregiver and patient. If you suspect abuse, inform the doctor. He will then be able to direct the physical exam toward possible internal injuries, malnutrition, or lack of cognitive ability. Signs of neglect include the following:

- Foul odor from the patient's body
- Poor skin color
- Inappropriate clothing for the season
- Soiled clothing
- Extreme concern about money

You can increase your awareness by consulting the guidelines for diagnosis and treatment of elder abuse and neglect published by the American Medical Association (AMA). Most states require doctors who suspect elder abuse or neglect to report their concerns to a designated office. Early intervention usually results in better living arrangements for both the patient and the caregiver.

## Diagnostic Testing

Based on a patient's physical exam, an internist may order a number of diagnostic tests. As a medical assistant in an internist's office, you must be familiar with commonly ordered tests. They include urine and blood tests, radiologic tests, bacterial cultures, electrocardiograms (ECGs), and pulmonary function tests (PFTs), all of which are discussed in later chapters. Descriptions of a few specific diagnostic tests follow.

**Radiologic Tests.** The physician orders a radiologic test to confirm or rule out a diagnosis. The choice of radiologic procedure depends on the suspected problem. Internists order plain films (roentgenograms or x-rays), computed tomography (CT) scans, magnetic resonance imaging (MRI), ultrasound, and radionuclide imaging (also known as nuclear imaging). Radiologic procedures are discussed in detail in Chapter 40.

Although you will not perform radiologic procedures, the physician will expect you to set up appointments and explain procedures to the patient. You may need to explain what kinds of preparations the patient must make prior to the test. Be sure to ask the radiologic facility about the requirements for the specific type of test.

*Chest X-Ray.* Internists may order a chest x-ray, which can reveal respiratory and cardiac disorders such as pneumonia, tuberculosis, or cardiomegaly (enlarged heart). It may also reveal abnormal masses in the upper thoracic region.

*Venography and Venous Ultrasonography.* Venography and venous ultrasonography are tests used to rule out deep vein thrombosis (DVT). A patient has DVT when there is a thrombus, or blood clot, in the veins. This occurs most often in the larger veins of the lower leg or thigh. If the thrombus becomes dislodged and travels in the bloodstream, it is known as an embolus. This moving blood clot can obstruct a blood vessel, causing an **embolism.** An embolism can be fatal, depending on its location. Risk factors for DVTs are poor circulation, vein injury, prolonged bed rest, recent surgery or childbirth, irregular blood coagulation, and use of oral contraceptives.

For a venogram, a contrast medium is injected into a vein, and x-rays are taken of the veins. Venous ultrasonography uses inaudible sound waves that bounce off liquid (in this case, blood) to form a two-dimensional

---

### CAUTION *Handle With Care*

## Detecting Domestic Violence

Physicians and medical assistants are in a position to detect signs of domestic violence. These signs can be seen in unusual bruising or injuries that the patient may try to hide or excuse. You may hear signs in a patient's tone of voice or choice of words during a conversation in the office or over the telephone. Many times patients who are abused blame themselves.

You play an important role in noticing these signs, and you must inform the physician of any signs that you detect. You must also create a supportive office environment where the patient can seek help. Encourage the physician to join the American Medical Association's National Coalition of Physicians Against Family Violence, if she is not already a member. This organization provides posters—which

often help patients feel encouraged to discuss domestic violence—in addition to pamphlets and other information.

Reporting suspected domestic violence is mandatory in some states. You should have a folder that contains lists of the phone numbers for domestic violence hotlines, women's shelters, and other helpful resources. You can offer the following general guidelines to women.

- Ignoring the problem never works—silence does not help anyone.
- Understand that abusive family members may not be able to help themselves.
- Call for help if a physical threat exists.

image. Internists generally prefer venous ultrasonography to venography because it is noninvasive.

# Diseases and Disorders

Internists treat a variety of diseases and disorders. Some of the most common include diseases of aging, infectious diseases, and sexually transmitted diseases.

**Diseases of Aging.** The elderly constitute a large percentage of patients in an internal medicine practice. Many of the serious disorders frequently seen in the elderly are discussed in Chapter 27. They include hypertension, coronary artery disease, and diabetes mellitus. Other disorders, such as constipation, diarrhea, and osteoporosis—while not serious for young and middle-aged adults—can create major problems for the elderly.

*Constipation-Diarrhea Cycle.* The cycle of constipation followed by diarrhea occurs when people's diets lack the fiber and liquids to maintain healthy bowel function and they use harsh laxatives to treat their constipation. The patient then complains of diarrhea and asks for antidiarrheal medication, which in turn causes constipation again. Encourage elderly patients to eat more high-fiber foods, such as cereals, fruits, and vegetables, and to increase their fluid intake.

*Hyperlipidemia.* Hyperlipidemia is a condition in which cholesterol levels are above normal. It is not just a disease of the elderly, but it can cause serious problems for older people. High cholesterol levels can lead to atherosclerosis, the accumulation of fatty deposits along the inner walls of arteries (Figure 26-1). These deposits, along with other substances in the blood, can form an atherosclerotic plaque. This plaque can narrow the opening in an artery to the point of obstructing blood flow. Atherosclerosis is a primary cause of cardiovascular disease and stroke.

Your role as a patient educator is vital to helping people with high cholesterol levels. Take every opportunity to teach patients about eating foods with lower amounts of cholesterol (see Chapter 36). Provide patients with printed materials on cholesterol, available from the AMA and other sources. The doctor may also prescribe medication to lower cholesterol in patients when diet modification and exercise are not adequate.

*Osteoporosis.* Osteoporosis is an endocrine and metabolic disorder of the musculoskeletal system. The condition is common in the elderly and is more common in women than in men. It is characterized by a loss of bone mass, which results in fractures. The disorder may be caused by inadequate calcium consumption, estrogen deficiency, or alcoholism. Prevention methods include regular exercise, a diet high in calcium (perhaps including supplemental calcium), and hormone replacement therapy in women who are menopausal or postmenopausal (Figure 26-2).

*Alzheimer's Disease.* Alzheimer's disease is a severely debilitating brain disorder. Warning signs include changes in personality, mood, or behavior; recent memory loss and an increase in forgetfulness; decreased ability to perform familiar

**Figure 26-1.** High cholesterol can lead to atherosclerosis. Help patients reduce their cholesterol through proper diet and exercise, along with medication, if prescribed.
Source: McGraw-Hill's Digital Asset Library.

Cholesterol crystals

Fat

Damaged area

Intima

Smooth muscle cells

Lumen of vessel

Media

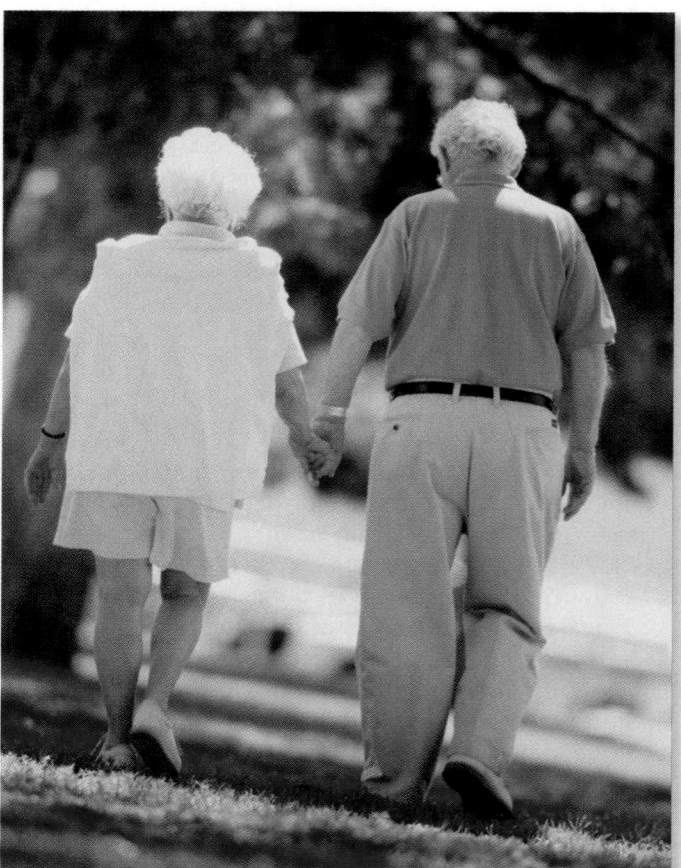

**Figure 26-2.** Regular exercise helps prevent osteoporosis.

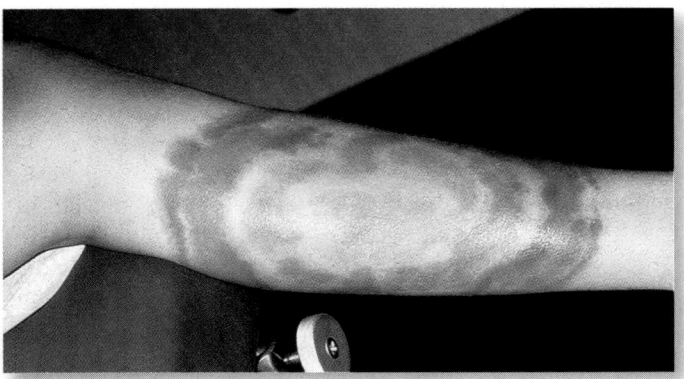

**Figure 26-3.** A bull's-eye rash is a symptom of the first stage of Lyme disease.

tasks; difficulty with use of language and abstract thinking; decreased powers of judgment; and disorientation to time or place. Because there is no cure, the primary role of caregivers is to provide comfort and safety to the patient.

**Infectious Diseases.** An internist is usually the primary physician for treating infectious diseases. Most of the infectious diseases discussed in Chapters 19 and 21 are treated by either an internist or a pediatrician. Descriptions of other common infectious diseases follow.

*Lyme Disease.* Lyme disease is a serious infection caused by a spirochete bacterium carried by the deer tick. When the condition is diagnosed early, treatment with antibiotics is effective. Diagnosis is difficult, however, because symptoms can occur in any order or overlap.

The first symptom of Lyme disease is often the appearance of a raised, red dot at the site of the tick bite. A circular rash may surround the bite (Figure 26-3). In many cases, however, the bite goes unnoticed. Headache, fever, and fatigue develop, followed by muscle aches and inflammation of the joints. Left untreated, the disease can progress to arthritis and heart and neurologic problems.

When a tick bite is reported, tell the patient to save the tick and place it in a plastic bag. It should be taken to a U.S. Department of Agriculture Extension Office for identification. A tick identified as a deer tick will be tested for the presence of the spirochete bacterium. Even if the tick tests positive for Lyme disease bacteria, the risk of the patient contracting the disease is not great if the tick was removed from the patient within 24 hours. Your main role in dealing with Lyme disease is patient education. Many doctors' offices display pamphlets or posters to show patients how to prevent and recognize symptoms of Lyme disease.

*Pneumonia.* Pneumonia is an acute infection of the lung tissue caused by bacteria or viruses. It often occurs in conjunction with a chronic weakening illness. Symptoms range from coughing, sputum production, and chest pain to chills and fever. It is treated with bed rest, antibiotics, adequate fluids, respiratory support measures, and pain medication.

*Rabies.* Rabies is a virus transmitted to humans by a bite from a mammal, such as a dog, cat, or bat. A patient who has been bitten by an animal that may be rabid should receive a rabies vaccination, which is a series of injections. Dogs, cats, and people who are at risk for exposure to the virus should have the vaccination at regular intervals. Patients must be vaccinated during the incubation period, before symptoms appear. Symptoms are nonspecific at onset and include malaise, fatigue, anxiety, or insomnia. Later there are neurologic symptoms. After symptoms have occurred, nearly 100% of people who are infected with rabies die.

*Staphylococcal and Streptococcal Infections (Staph and Strep).* Staphylococci and streptococci are common bacteria, with many species occurring naturally in the body. When the body's resistance is low, however, these bacteria can cause infections, such as strep throat, skin abscess, impetigo, and pneumonia. Antibiotics are the standard treatment for staphylococcal and streptococcal infections. Because these organisms become resistant to antibiotics, however, researchers are constantly working to develop effective new drugs. Always stress to patients the importance of finishing the entire course of prescribed medication. Otherwise the patient will not receive enough of the drug to kill the organism, and the organism will build up a resistance to the antibiotic.

**Sexually Transmitted Diseases.** Sexually transmitted diseases (STDs)—diseases acquired through sexual contact with an infected person—are also infectious diseases. The number and severity of these diseases, their high incidence, and the great amount of misinformation about them warrant a discussion apart from other infectious diseases. (AIDS is discussed in Chapter 21.) Internists, infectious disease specialists, pediatricians, urologists, and gynecologists are all involved in the diagnosis and treatment of STDs.

*Patient Education About STDs.* Your role as an educator is vital in dealing with patients who have STDs. Some patients may be hesitant to ask for information. Providing educational materials in the exam room will help answer their questions and put them at ease. These materials deal with sensitive or embarrassing topics, and the patient's privacy must be maintained. Printed materials are available from several medical agencies and should be provided to your patients. In addition, you must educate patients about prevention and treatment of STDs. The Educating the Patient section provides more information on this topic.

*Common Types of STDs.* Your role in assisting the doctor in the treatment of STDs will involve emphasizing to the patient the importance of completing the course of therapy and avoiding sexual contact while the infection is still active. Sexual partners must also be treated to avoid reinfection. Several types of STDs are fairly common.

Candidiasis is a yeast infection. It is not a true STD but is included with the STDs because the infection can be transmitted between sexual partners. Symptoms include severe genital itching, redness and swelling of the vaginal or vulval tissue, light yellow or white patches (usually cheesy or curd-like) on the vagina, and vaginal discharge. The infection is treated with an antimycotic (antifungal) drug.

Chlamydia usually produces symptoms of discharge and uncomfortable urination, although it may be asymptomatic, particularly in women. Untreated, the disease can cause scarring of the fallopian tubes and eventual infertility. Diagnosis is made by aspirating pus from the urethra of men, the endocervix of women, or other infected tissue and having it examined in a laboratory. Chlamydia is treated with antibiotics.

Genital herpes is a type of herpes virus. Symptoms include blister-like sores on the genitalia, difficult urination, swelling of the legs, fatigue, and a general ill feeling. Because this disease is cyclical, symptoms disappear and reappear periodically. Although there is no cure for genital

herpes, an antiviral drug can reduce or suppress the symptoms. Herpes may be transmitted to the fetus during pregnancy or delivery. It is often fatal to an infant.

Genital warts and human papilloma virus (HPV) are found on or in men and women. Patients may generally be asymptomatic, but some have burning and itching in the genital area. Some types of HPV have been shown to increase the risk of cancer of the vulva, vagina, and cervix. There is no treatment for the virus after infection occurs. However, a vaccine is currently being tested to prevent certain types of HPV. HPV symptoms usually disappear within 6 to 18 months in a person with a normal immune system. However, even though the symptoms subside, the virus remains present in the patient.

Gonorrhea causes inflammation of the genitalia, with a greenish yellow discharge from the cervix, sore throat, anal discharge, swollen glands, and lower abdominal

## Educating the Patient

## Teaching Patients About Sexually Transmitted Diseases

You must provide complete and detailed information with a nonjudgmental and supportive attitude when you teach patients about STDs. Begin with the principle that all STDs are preventable. The key to prevention is avoiding sexual activities in which blood, semen, or vaginal secretions pass from one person to another.

There are various levels of protection in connection with STDs. The only absolute methods of "safe sex" are abstinence (no sex) and masturbation (self-stimulation). The next level is mutual monogamy, in which partners have sex only with each other. Emphasize that monogamy provides protection from STDs only if neither partner has an STD when the relationship begins. A final level of prevention applies to people who do not practice abstinence or mutual monogamy but wish to protect themselves and others from STDs. The following measures provide some protection.

- Use a latex condom and spermicide for every act of intercourse. (Use a latex condom during vaginal, oral, or anal sex.)
- Use only water-based lubricants with latex condoms. (Oil- and petroleum-based lubricants can break down latex, causing the condom to tear or break.)
- Know all your sexual partners, and discuss STD prevention with them.
- Have a physician regularly screen you for STDs because many people, especially men, have no signs when they are infected.

- Consult a physician if any signs of STDs develop, such as a blister, sore, discharge, rash, or abdominal pain.

Encourage patients to ask questions and discuss any concerns they have. Explain the need to make follow-up appointments with a physician if appropriate.

Teaching a patient who has been diagnosed with an STD how to treat or manage the disease is especially important. Make sure the patient understands all directions and the necessity for treatment. Bacterial infections such as chlamydia, gonorrhea, and syphilis can be cured with antibiotics as long as the patient takes all the medication in the prescribed manner. Viral infections such as AIDS, genital herpes, and genital warts cannot be cured, although they can be treated and managed to differing degrees.

Emphasize to patients with an STD that they should avoid all sexual contact until the infection has been treated completely. Many STDs can be spread through any type of genital contact, including vaginal intercourse, anal sex, and oral sex. Herpes can be spread through kissing if there are herpes sores in the mouth. Encourage patients to inform each person with whom they had sexual contact that they have contracted an STD. Explain that unless all sexual partners are treated successfully, the disease will pass back and forth indefinitely.

You can reinforce your education efforts by providing patients with materials on the prevention and treatment of STDs. Keep a variety of pamphlets, books, and other resources in your office to help patients cope with and manage STDs.

| TABLE 26-1 | Common Diseases and Disorders Treated by Internists | |
|---|---|---|
| **Condition** | **Description** | **Treatment** |
| **Anemia** | Results from deficiency of iron or vitamins, such as folic acid and vitamin $B_{12}$; can also result from loss of blood (acute blood loss anemia); body's cells do not get enough oxygen, resulting in fatigue, listlessness, pallor, inability to concentrate, difficulty breathing on exertion | Oral supplements of appropriate vitamin or iron; if caused by acute blood loss, blood transfusion |
| **Arthritis** | Chronic inflammatory disease of tissues of joints; symptoms include pain and stiffness in joints | Medication to reduce inflammation and pain; surgery in severe cases |
| **Gout** | Metabolic disease involving acute joint pain, most commonly in the big toe at night; caused by overproduction or retention of uric acid | Medication and diet restrictions to decrease production of uric acid and promote its excretion |
| **Hypertension** | An elevation of blood pressure over 140 systolic and 90 diastolic. There are often no symptoms or symptoms are mild. | Medications to reduce blood pressure. Diet restrictions to reduce fat and sodium and lose weight. Increase exercise to lose weight and strengthen heart. |
| **Peptic ulcer** | Lesion of mucous membrane of esophagus, stomach, or duodenum (first section of small intestine); symptoms include heartburn, vomiting, and dull, gnawing pain or burning sensation in area | Medication and diet restrictions to reduce amount and acidity of gastric juices; stress reduction; surgery in severe cases |

pain. Treatment is with antibiotics such as penicillin or tetracycline.

Trichomoniasis symptoms in women include inflammation of the genital area and an abundant white or yellow vaginal discharge with a foul odor. (It is usually asymptomatic in men.) The infection is diagnosed by inspecting a specimen of the discharge under the microscope. The condition is usually treated with a course of antibiotics.

**Other Diseases and Disorders.** Internists may diagnose and treat other diseases and disorders, including anemia, arthritis, gout, and peptic ulcer (Table 26-1). They may also refer patients to a physician in one of the highly specialized areas.

# Pediatrics

A pediatrician specializes in the health care of children, monitoring their development and diagnosing and treating their illnesses. Just as with internal medicine, there are subspecialties of pediatrics, such as surgery and oncology. To be a good pediatric medical assistant, you must first like children of all ages. If you do, you will be better able to relate to them and to communicate with them effectively.

Parent or caregiver education, adherence to immunization schedules (see Chapter 20), and child abuse detection are primary areas of responsibility for medical assistants who work in pediatrics. You will also assist with

the physical exam and treatment of the pediatric patient. Your role as liaison in these areas between caregiver and physician will be an important one.

## Assisting With a Pediatric Physical Exam

Many of the exam procedures for a pediatric patient are the same as those for an adult. While you prepare the child or adolescent for exam, you might discuss with the parent, caregiver, or child such topics as eating habits, sleep patterns, daily activities, immunization schedules, and toilet training. This discussion will provide important clues to possible abnormal mental, physical, emotional, or social development. Topics such as STDs and drugs and alcohol may be appropriate for you to discuss with an adolescent. Point out potential problems to the doctor.

Be mindful of adolescents' sensitivity toward rapid growth and physical, sexual, and social development when you prepare them for exam. Adolescents and preadolescents often feel awkward and self-conscious about being examined. They may also prefer to dress alone and to be alone with the doctor.

Some children are afraid of going to the doctor's office. You can help relieve a child's fear by calmly explaining procedures before they occur, giving the reason for each procedure, and being cheerful and mindful of a

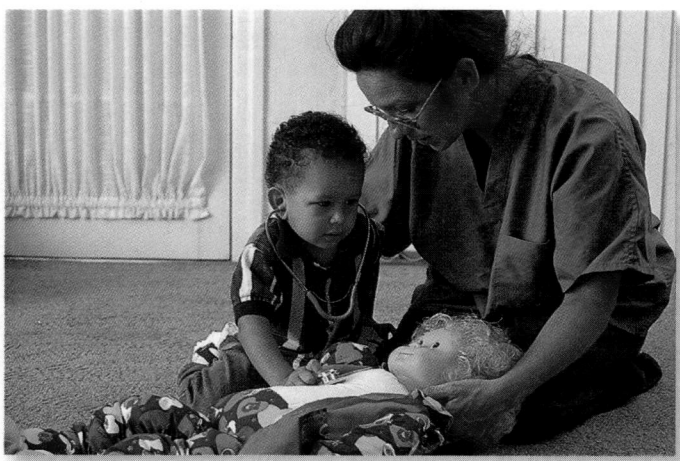

**Figure 26-4.** Providing a pediatric patient with a diversion may help lessen the child's fear.

child's feelings. Allowing a child to examine some of the instruments may also lessen fear (Figure 26-4). If a patient is physically resistant to exam, you may need to call for assistance from the doctor or caregiver, or the child may need to be restrained.

Try to speak in terms aimed at the child's age level, and kneel if necessary to make eye contact with the child. Treat the child with respect and provide positive reinforcement when a child is cooperative. Avoid making light of crying or pain. Make a game out of some aspect of a procedure, and provide a small token reward at the end of a visit. For infants, a gentle approach, such as talking quietly and holding them comfortingly, is helpful.

**Examining the Well Child.** Parents should bring their infants and children to the pediatrician for regular checkups and growth monitoring. The American Academy of Pediatrics recommends the following frequency:

- Infants need seven well-baby exams during their first year, at these intervals: 2 weeks, 1 month, 2 months, 4 months, 6 months, 9 months, 1 year.
- Children in the second year of life should have checkups at 15 and 18 months.
- From the age of 2, children should have checkups every year.

Follow Universal Precautions and prepare for the physical exam the same way you would for an adult, except for draping and positioning. Ask the parent of an infant or toddler to remove all the child's clothing except the diaper because the child should be nude for the exam. Then keep the child covered until the physician enters the exam room.

An infant or toddler may be crying during the exam. To assist the physician in hearing chest sounds with a stethoscope, ask the parent to allow the child to suck on a pacifier to quiet the crying. Feeding the child during the exam is not encouraged because stomach sounds interfere with clear auscultation.

Parents play a more active role during the exam of infants and toddlers than they play during the exam of older children. You or the parent may assist the child into position during the exam, or the physician may allow the parent to hold the child. Distracting infants and toddlers with mobiles, shiny surfaces, or toys may help the exam go more smoothly.

**Detecting Child Abuse or Neglect.** Child abuse is an all-too-common and potentially fatal problem. Whenever a child comes to the office, you should watch for any signs of serious problems in the relationship between the parent or caregiver and the child. Also notice any signs of physical injury, such as unexplained bruises or burns. Any suspicious lesion on a child's genitalia should prompt an investigation of sexual abuse. Possible signs of neglect include a dirty or neglected appearance, hunger, extreme sadness or fear, and an inability to communicate. Note any suspicions in the chart, and report them to the doctor before he sees the patient. The doctor will respond to your information by examining the child for clues to indicate the following:

- Internal injuries: tenderness when palpated or auscultated
- Malnutrition: tooth discoloration, unhealthy gums or skin color
- Lack of cognitive ability: dulled neurologic responses

Studies show that certain risk factors are usually present in parents who abuse their children. Some risk factors are stress, single parenthood, inadequate knowledge of normal developmental expectations, lack of family support, family hostility, financial problems, and mental health problems. Other risk factors include prolonged separation of parent and child, ambivalent feelings toward the child, and a mother younger than 16 years. Additional risk factors include an unhealthy or unsafe home environment, inappropriate supervision, substance abuse, a parental crime record, a negative attitude toward pregnancy, and a history of parents having been abused.

Intervention, such as home visits by nurses, can significantly lower the rate of child abuse. Managed care systems may provide this service as part of their postpartum program. These nurses provide information on normal child growth and development and routine health needs, serve as informational support persons, and refer families to appropriate services when they require assistance.

You are legally responsible for reporting suspected child abuse or neglect. Contact the child protection agency in your community. Post the appropriate telephone number in your office.

**Examining for Growth Abnormalities.** Pediatricians look for any sign of growth abnormality during routine well-child visits. Physicians compare a child's physical, intellectual, and social signs to charts showing national averages. In general, physicians look for signs that the child is in the appropriate stage of growth for her age. Growth can be divided into five stages.

***Stages One and Two: The First and Second Years.*** In-fancy, the first year of life, is marked by the development of strength and coordination of the trunk, head, and limbs. Intellectual growth primarily involves receiving information through the senses and performing motor (physical) functions in response to the environment. In the second year of life, the child develops fine motor skills (involving control of smaller muscles, such as those in the fingers) and manual dexterity. Sociologically, the child develops some independence and begins to test parental limits.

***Stage Three: Ages 3 to 5 Years.*** During ages 3 to 5 years, the child develops physical skills of muscle coordination and both large motor skills (involving control of larger muscles, such as those in the arms and legs) and fine motor skills. Intellectually, the child observes and copies older children and adults without fully understanding them. The child also learns to initiate play with others and begins to make requests of family members.

***Stage Four: Age 6 Years to Puberty.*** The fourth stage occurs from approximately age 6 to **puberty,** the period of adolescence when a person begins to develop sexual traits. Muscle coordination and fine and large motor skills develop further. The child begins to get involved in scholastic and extracurricular activities. The child also develops an identity, based partially on both intellectual and physical skills, and learns how to achieve goals in the environment.

***Stage Five: Adolescence.*** Physical growth and development in the teenage years are centered on normal sexual change. Girls usually begin puberty between 8 and 14 years of age; boys begin between 9½ and 16, on average. Menarche, the onset of menstruation, usually occurs about 2½ years after the onset of puberty. The beginning of nocturnal emissions of seminal fluid signals sexual maturation in boys. This awareness of sexuality is accompanied by concern with body image. Intellectually, adolescents are able to understand abstract concepts and think about themselves in terms of the past and future. The process of developing independence, a personal identity, and future plans is also important during this time of life.

**General Eye Exam.** As part of the general exam, the pediatrician examines the interior of the child's eyes with an ophthalmoscope. You will probably perform the visual acuity test (Figure 26-5). Make a game of covering the child's eye if the child resists this part of the procedure. Watch for signs of visual difficulty during the test, such as tilting the head in a certain direction, blinking, squinting, or frowning. If the caregiver brought the child in specifically for a vision test, record in the child's chart whatever symptoms the caregiver mentions.

**General Ear Exam.** A pediatric ear exam is important because so many children have ear infections or upper respiratory infections involving the ear. Because children's eustachian tubes are more horizontal than those of adults, fluid collects more easily in the tubes and can promote bacterial growth. The tubes are also short and connected

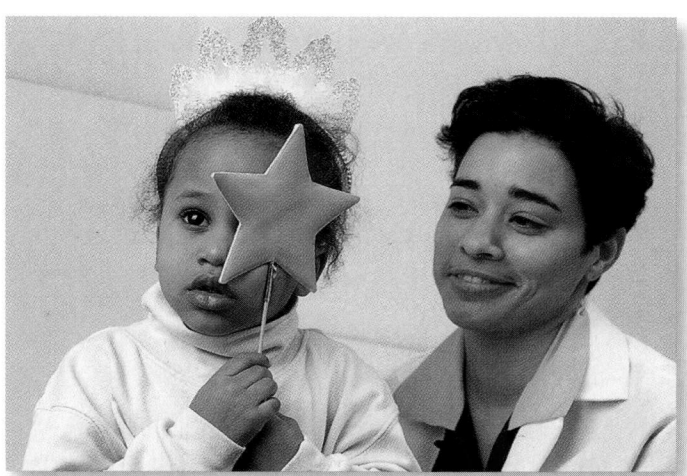

**Figure 26-5.** Making a game out of the visual acuity test helps put a child at ease.

to the throat. Any upper respiratory infections can easily travel to the ear.

# Diagnostic Testing

Many adult diagnostic procedures are also used for children. The pediatrician uses the same laboratory tests and radiologic tests. He performs some diagnostic tests in the office.

Because streptococcal infection can be especially serious in a child, some pediatricians perform a rapid test for the presence of streptococcal bacteria so they can immediately start the appropriate medical treatment. If the test is positive, the physician begins treatment with antibiotics specifically for this type of bacteria.

Some physicians believe the rapid strep test is not always reliable. To confirm a negative test result, these physicians also do a throat culture. A throat culture can determine which of the streptococcal bacteria is present or whether other organisms are causing the symptoms. The results can indicate a possible change in medication. The method for obtaining a throat culture is outlined in Chapter 33. You may also be required to collect a pediatric urine specimen. This process is described in Procedure 34-2 in Chapter 34. Additionally, collecting blood may be part of your responsibility. This procedure is discussed in Chapter 35.

# Immunizations

Immunizations are usually given during routine office visits (Figure 26-6). Public health authorities recommend a schedule (see Chapter 20) for immunizing children against diseases such as hepatitis B, diphtheria, tetanus, pertussis (whooping cough), poliomyelitis, measles, mumps, rubella (German measles), chickenpox, and *Haemophilus influenzae* type B (Hib). Many vaccines have largely eliminated the threat of these once-prevalent, life-threatening diseases.

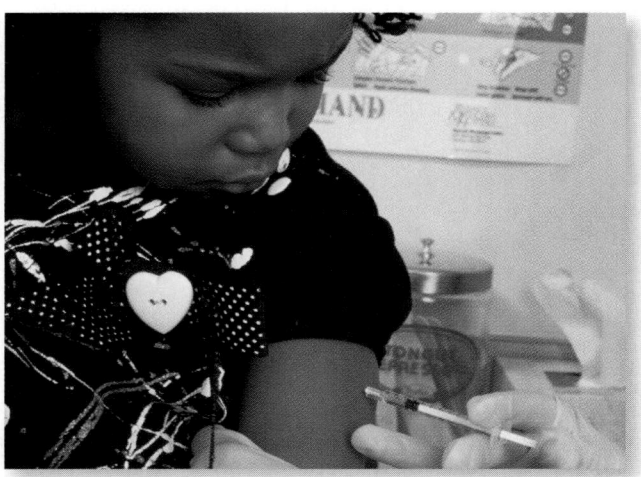

**Figure 26-6.** Immunizations are part of routine well-child visits in a pediatric practice.

The first vaccine, for hepatitis B, is given to a newborn the day after birth. Some vaccines require a series of doses to give immunity. Booster doses may be required for a particular vaccine at a later age. Most vaccinations may be administered even if the child has a mild illness. A child with a fever less than 104.9°F may still be vaccinated. The physician will make the decision to vaccinate a child who is ill based on the disease and the severity of the symptoms. The Centers for Disease Control and Prevention (CDC) recommends that physicians take every reasonable opportunity to vaccinate a child, assuring the child will receive the protection he needs.

As a medical assistant, you will play a vital role in the immunization process. Your duties may include:

- Ensuring proper vaccine storage
- Administering the vaccine correctly
- Keeping careful immunization records, including the vaccine type, the date of vaccination, and the vaccine lot number
- Educating parents about the benefits and risks of vaccines
- Scheduling follow-up visits at the appropriate time based on the immunization schedule

You might be required to give more than two vaccinations in a single visit. Careful site selection is important when giving multiple injections. Refer to Chapter 37 for more information regarding selecting an injection site.

## Pediatric Diseases and Disorders

If you work in a pediatric office, you should know the signs and symptoms of common childhood diseases. Some diseases, including chickenpox, influenza, measles, mumps, rubella, scarlet fever, and tetanus, are described in Chapter 19. Other common diseases are outlined in Table 26-2. Many common disorders found in children are not specific diseases. Upper respiratory infections, including colds and viral influenza, occur frequently among children. It is important not to make assumptions regarding diagnosis or treatment. When reported symptoms include fever, sore throat, runny nose, and earache, any number of conditions could be the cause. Encourage the parent to bring the child to the office. You should, however, tell the doctor as soon as possible when a child has an extremely high fever. The doctor may want the child to go to an emergency room. Do not recommend aspirin for fever in children. The use of aspirin in children has been associated with Reye syndrome, a potentially fatal disease of the central nervous system (CNS) and liver. Acetaminophen (Tylenol) or ibuprofen is preferred for treating fever in children. You should check with the doctor before recommending any fever-reducing medication.

Some less common diseases and disorders can be found in children. You need to be aware of the basic symptoms and the treatments for these disorders.

**AIDS.** Most childhood cases of human immunodeficiency virus (HIV) infection are transmitted from a mother to her infant. When a woman is HIV-positive and remains untreated, her baby has a 25% to 33% chance of being infected. Babies born to HIV-positive mothers receiving treatment have a less than 2% chance of being infected. All babies born to HIV-positive mothers have HIV antibodies that are detectable through testing at birth. The antibodies persist for a period of 15 to 18 months, but not all such babies remain permanently infected. AIDS has no cure, but treating the pregnant woman and newborn child with antiviral agents has been shown to lower the rate of HIV infection in the child.

**Juvenile Rheumatoid Arthritis.** Juvenile rheumatoid arthritis (JRA) is an autoimmune disease of the joints that occurs in children aged 16 or younger. The symptoms of JRA include swelling, pain, and stiffness of the joints. The knees, hands, and feet are most commonly affected. The severity of the disease ranges from mild to severe and may affect the eyes and internal organs. A child with JRA will have periods of remission (a lessening of symptoms) and flare-up (a worsening of symptoms). JRA is diagnosed based on the severity of symptoms, specific laboratory tests, and x-rays. Treatment of this disease includes nonsteroidal anti-inflammatory drugs (NSAIDs), disease-modifying anti-rheumatic drugs (DMARDs), corticosteroids, biologic agents, and physical therapy.

As a medical assistant, your role in caring for children with JRA includes emphasizing the value of exercise and physical therapy, stressing the importance of taking medications as directed, and offering assistance by providing patient education brochures and information regarding local support groups and organizations.

**Attention Deficit Hyperactivity Disorder and Learning Disabilities.** Attention deficit hyperactivity disorder (ADHD) and learning disabilities (LD) are found in children, adolescents, and adults. These disorders can cause gross motor disability, inability to read or write, hyperactivity, distractibility, impulsiveness, and

## TABLE 26-2  Common Pediatric Diseases and Disorders

| Condition | Description | Treatment |
|---|---|---|
| Head lice | Small insects easily spread among children by head-to-head contact and by sharing objects such as combs and hairbrushes; lice live on scalp and lay eggs strongly attached to hair shafts; symptoms include itchy scalp; identify by locating crawling lice or nits (eggs) attached to hair; examine parted hair carefully at scalp and bottom of hair strands | Antilice shampoo or 1% permethrin cream rinse; removal of eggs with fine-tooth comb; disinfection of clothing, bedding, and washable toys by machine washing and drying in hot cycles or by dry cleaning; tight bagging for 30 days of items that cannot be washed; disinfection of combs and brushes (used for hair) by washing in shampoo |
| Herpes simplex virus (HSV) | In children virus causes cold sore blisters on or near mouth; diagnosis made by inspecting lesions; first stage (2–12 days before appearance of blister) involves tingling and itching sensations; later blister ruptures and forms yellow crust; outbreak takes about 3 weeks to heal completely | Application of ice cube to blister, which may promote faster healing; ointments to alleviate cracking and discomfort; avoidance of sun exposure because it may trigger outbreak |
| Impetigo | Highly contagious dermatologic disease caused by staphylococcal, sometimes streptococcal, bacteria; transmitted by direct contact; causes inflammation and pustules, which are small lymph-filled bumps that rupture and become encrusted before healing; frequently seen around mouth and nostrils | Avoidance of scratching lesions and sharing utensils, towels, bed linens, or bath or pool water that could cause further transmission; careful washing of affected areas two to three times per day to keep lesions clean and dry; topical antibacterial cream |
| Infectious conjunctivitis ("pink eye") | Highly contagious streptococcal or staphylococcal bacterial infection of conjunctiva of eye; transmitted by direct contact; causes redness, pain, swelling, discharge; usually begins in one eye and spreads to other | Avoidance of scratching eyes and sharing utensils, towels, or bed linens that could cause further transmission; warm compresses to relieve discomfort; antibiotic drops or ointment |
| Pinworms | Parasites transmitted by swallowing worm eggs, by touching something that infected person has touched, or by putting infested sand or dirt into mouth; when eggs hatch in body, worms attach to intestinal lining; mature females travel to areas just outside rectum to lay eggs, which causes itching | Medication usually given to whole family to treat and prevent further infestation |
| Ringworm | Contagious fungal infection involving scalp, groin, feet, or other areas of body, causing flat, dry, and scaly or moist and crusty lesions; lesions develop into clear center with outer ring; when scalp is affected, may cause bald patches | Oral and topical antifungal medication; isolation to prevent spreading; frequent changing of towels, bedding, with no sharing with others in family; caution that child not use others' combs or brushes |
| Streptococcal sore throat ("strep throat") | Contagious disease caused by streptococcal bacteria and spread by droplet; complications include progression to rheumatic fever (with arthritis, nephritis, and inflammation of endocardium, or inner lining of heart); symptoms include headache, high fever, vomiting, and extremely painful, swollen, and red or white sore throat; causes difficulty swallowing | Streptococci-specific antibiotics given as soon as possible; because of potential complications, therapy based on the practitioner's experience is sometimes given without confirmed diagnosis from throat culture; antibiotics are adjusted with confirmation of infecting organism; possible hospitalization in acute cases |

generally disruptive behavior. ADHD encompasses all conditions formerly identified as hyperactivity, or hyperkinesis, and attention deficit. LD encompasses a wide range of conditions that interfere with learning, including dyslexia (reading problems), dysgraphia (writing problems), and dyscalculia (math problems).

ADHD is misunderstood, misdiagnosed, and overdiagnosed in children. Some physicians fail to recognize ADHD as a cause of academic, social, and emotional problems. Others are quick to attribute too many such problems to ADHD. When ADHD is the correct diagnosis, methylphenidate hydrochloride (Ritalin) and other drugs may alleviate the symptoms but not without risk of adverse effects, such as insomnia, increased heart rate and blood pressure, and interference with growth rate. Successful treatment usually requires a combination of drug and behavioral therapies and educational, psychological, and emotional support tailored to the child.

**Cerebral Palsy.** Cerebral palsy, a birth-related disorder of the nerves and muscles, is the most frequent crippling disease in children. It is caused by brain damage that occurs before, during, or shortly after birth or in early childhood. Signs of spastic cerebral palsy (the most common form) include hyperactive tendon reflexes, rapid alteration between muscular contraction and relaxation, permanent muscle shortening, and underdevelopment of extremities. Among people who have this disease, 40% are mentally retarded, 25% have seizures, and 80% have impaired speech. There is no known cure, but the effects of the disorder can be alleviated with physical therapy, speech therapy, orthopedic surgery, splints, skeletal muscle relaxants, and anticonvulsant medication.

**Congenital Heart Disease.** Congenital heart disease is caused by a cardiovascular malformation in the fetus before birth. If the fetus survives, the newborn is usually small. The defect may be so small, however, that it may not be recognized until days, months, or even years later. Some patients have such a mild case of the disease that no treatment is necessary. Others require only low-risk surgery. In still others, major high-risk surgery is necessary. Many patients diagnosed with the problem are treated with antibiotics to avoid secondary infections.

A cardiovascular defect can be caused by genetic mutations (changes in the genes), maternal infections (such as rubella or cytomegalovirus), maternal alcoholism, or maternal insulin-dependent diabetes. Blue lips and fingernails, signs of cyanosis in a newborn, are obvious indications of a cardiac defect.

**Down Syndrome.** Down syndrome is a genetic disorder resulting from one extra chromosome in each of the millions of cells formed during development of the fetus. It is the most common chromosomal abnormality in humans. Down syndrome is not caused by any parental behavior, such as diet or activity. The estimated risk for a Down syndrome birth increases, however, as maternal age increases. Down syndrome is characterized by

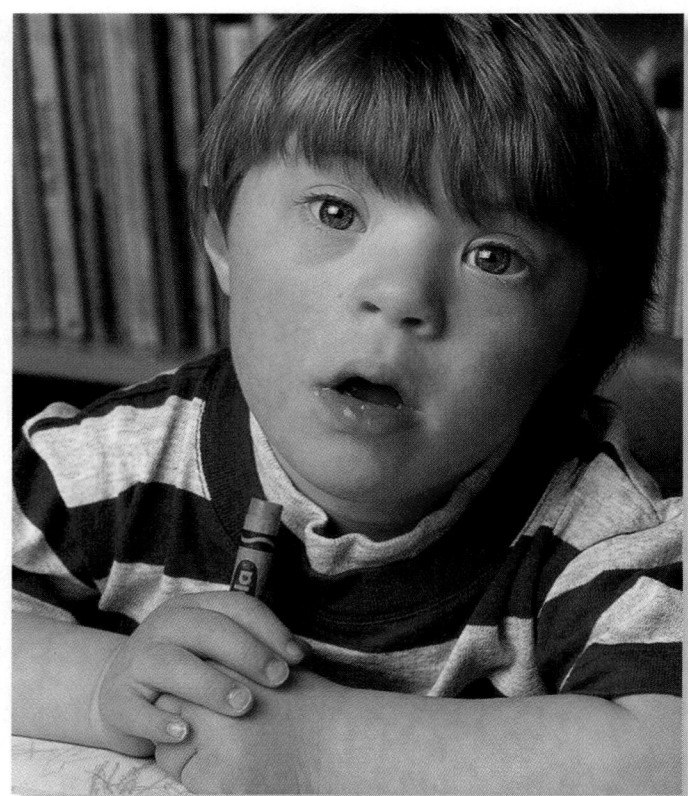

**Figure 26-7.** A child with Down syndrome usually has distinct facial features.

low muscle tone, which can be alleviated with physical therapy. Characteristic facial features are also evident (Figure 26-7). These include broad face, flattened nasal bridge, narrow nasal passages (increasing the risk of congestion), slanting eyes (vision problems are common), and small teeth and ears. Mental retardation, which can range from mild to severe, is also a characteristic of Down syndrome.

**Hepatitis B.** Infection with the hepatitis B virus (HBV) can lead to a serious and chronic infection of the liver. A child can carry the virus for years and only later develop liver failure or liver cancer. The virus can be transmitted across the placenta or during birth if the mother is infected. The disease may also be transmitted sexually, by blood transfusion, or by direct contact. It is frequently seen among drug abusers who share needles. Immunization is available, and children should be immunized starting the day after birth. Children who have not been immunized should begin to receive the series of immunizations for protection from infection.

**Respiratory Syncytial Virus.** The respiratory syncytial virus (RSV) is a major cause of lower respiratory disease in infants and young children. RSV is most often seen in the winter and spring as outbreaks of pneumonia, bronchiolitis, and tracheobronchitis. It is highly contagious, and reinfection is common. Treatment is difficult because the infection is viral rather than bacterial. Antibiotics are thus effective for treating only the possible secondary infections that develop during or after contracting RSV. You may be asked to obtain nasal smears to assist in the diagnosis of RSV. More information about collecting specimens is found in Chapter 33.

**Sudden Infant Death Syndrome.** Sudden infant death syndrome (SIDS)—formerly known as crib death—is the sudden death of an infant that remains unexplained after all other possible causes have been carefully ruled out. Most SIDS cases occur before the infant is 6 months of age. Victims appear to be healthy and are more likely to be male than female. SIDS occurs during sleep. Some factors that may put babies between the ages of 1 week and 1 year at high risk have been identified:

- Exposure to smoke in utero and to secondhand smoke after birth
- Being overheated
- A prone or side sleeping position
- Soft sleeping surfaces
- Being born prematurely
- A low birth weight
- Receiving little or no prenatal care

The National Sudden Infant Death Foundation has local chapters for parents whose babies have died of the syndrome. Counseling and information are available through local health organizations. Support groups are very helpful to the parents of a SIDS infant. Recommend and refer families when necessary.

**Spina Bifida.** Spina bifida is a defect of spinal development that results when tissues fail to close properly around the spinal cord during the first trimester of pregnancy. Neurologic symptoms are common because the spinal cord is not fully protected by the bony and connective tissues of the spine. These symptoms may vary with the severity of the defect, ranging from foot weakness and bladder or bowel problems to paralysis of the lower extremities and mental retardation. The skin over the spinal cord often has a depression, tuft of hair, or port wine stain when the defect is not readily apparent.

The treatment and outcome of spina bifida are based on the extent of damage. Surgical closure or implants are sometimes required. Unfortunately, the neurologic conditions cannot be reversed.

**Viral Gastroenteritis.** Gastroenteritis is an inflammation of the stomach and intestines. Gastroenteritis caused by a virus may be called the flu, traveler's diarrhea, or food poisoning. Viral gastroenteritis usually subsides within 1 to 2 days. It can be serious in young children, however, because it can cause extreme fluid loss that results in dehydration and electrolyte imbalances.

Symptoms include fever, nausea, abdominal cramping, diarrhea, and vomiting. Gastroenteritis is treated with bed rest, increased fluid intake, dietary modifications (usually only clear liquids), and medication for vomiting

and diarrhea if necessary. Antibiotics may be prescribed if evidence of bacterial involvement is present.

## Patient and Caregiver Education for Pediatric Patients

Patients and caregivers in a pediatrician's office usually have many questions. You will be able to answer some of the questions yourself, sparing valuable time for the pediatrician. Helpful brochures and booklets are available from the American Academy of Pediatrics. You should obtain the current list of publications and encourage your employer to order what the office needs.

# Obstetrics and Gynecology

An obstetrician/gynecologist (OB/GYN) specializes in the female reproductive system. Physicians who focus on caring for women during pregnancy and childbirth are called obstetricians. Physicians who treat other conditions of the female reproductive system are called gynecologists.

As a medical assistant in an OB/GYN office, you will need to be familiar with the female reproductive system and its functions, including pregnancy, fertility, and menopause. You need to know about the common diagnostic tests and procedures performed in this specialty. You must also be familiar with the common diseases and disorders in obstetrics and gynecology, be prepared to answer patients' questions, and provide patient education materials.

## Assisting With the Gynecologic Physical Exam

An annual gynecologic exam is recommended for all women age 18 and older. The exam is intended to provide an overview of a woman's health and to provide the opportunity for important cancer-screening exams and tests. A female medical assistant should be in the exam room during the physical exam to assist a male doctor and to provide legal protection. Your role during the exam is similar to that for the general physical exam.

Ask the patient to empty her bladder; if a urine specimen is needed, it should be collected at this time. Provide the patient with a gown before the exam, and give her privacy while she changes. When you interview her, discuss her gynecologic and general health, and inquire about any changes in appetite, weight, or emotional status. Also find out the date of her last menstrual period. Then have her sit on the examining table while you check her vital signs.

**The Physician's Interview.** The gynecologic physical exam is more than an internal pelvic exam. It is an evaluation of the patient's total health and a review of factors that could be an indication of possible cancer or STDs. The physician asks questions about the patient's menstrual cycle and about any abnormal discharge or discomfort during sexual intercourse. The physician also listens to the patient's heart and lungs before beginning the gynecologic exam.

**Breast Exam.** The physician examines the patient's breasts and underarm areas to check for abnormal lumps that could be cancerous. Your role as patient educator is crucial. Patients must understand the need for regular breast exams. When interviewing the patient and after the exam, emphasize the breast cancer detection guidelines of the American Cancer Society and National Cancer Institute:

1. Beginning at age 40, all women should be encouraged to have a mammogram every year. Mammography should begin earlier in patients with a strong family history of breast cancer.
2. Women should have breast exams during their annual routine checkups at least every 3 years for women ages 20 to 39 and yearly for women 40 and older.
3. Women should do breast self-exam (BSE) monthly.

These guidelines emphasize the importance of education and awareness of the patient.

While reviewing the patient's chart, the physician checks to see when the last mammogram was performed. He may also ask the patient whether she knows how to perform a BSE and whether she is performing it monthly. If needed, he may ask you to instruct the patient in performing the BSE. The teaching technique for the BSE is found in the Educating the Patient section on page 554 of Chapter 25.

**Pelvic Exam.** During the pelvic exam, the doctor checks the external genitalia, cervix, vaginal wall, internal reproductive organs, and rectum. Exam methods include palpation and inspection with a **speculum,** an instrument that expands the vaginal opening to permit viewing of the vagina and cervix. The doctor wears gloves and may use a lubricant for patient comfort.

Your role is to assist the patient into position, with her feet in the stirrups of the examining table and her buttocks at the end of the table. Drape her so that only the area between the thighs is exposed. Assist the doctor by having gloves and instruments ready for use and by applying lubricant, if indicated, to the doctor's gloved fingers. You may also warm the speculum for the patient's comfort. Be prepared to provide reassurance and explanation to a patient who appears to be uncomfortable or nervous. Encourage her to breathe deeply to help relax the pelvic muscles and reduce discomfort. See Procedure 26-1 for further instructions on how to assist with a gynecological exam.

After checking the vagina and cervix and while the speculum is still in place, the doctor will most likely take a Pap smear (Papanicolaou smear) (Figure 26-8). She may also take a sample for testing with potassium hydroxide (KOH). In this test, KOH is added to a cervical smear on a glass slide. The KOH helps dissolve epithelial cells and mucus, thus improving visualization of any fungus that might be present. The doctor then removes the speculum

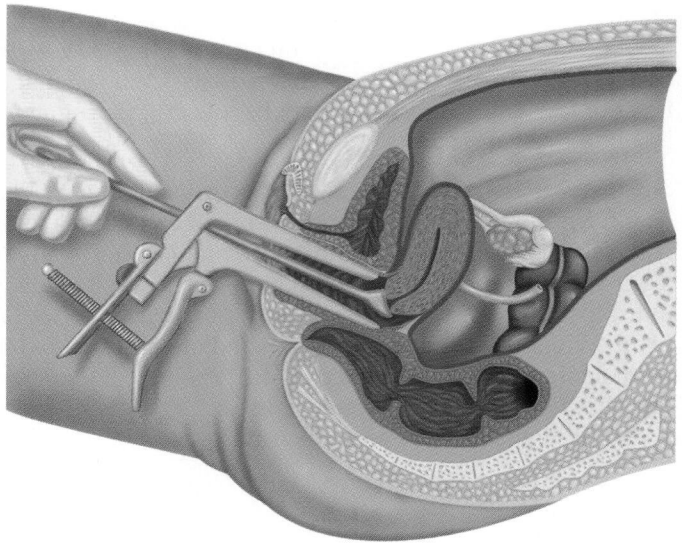

**Figure 26-8.** A speculum is used to expand the vaginal opening to help view the vagina and cervix.

and begins the bimanual phase of the exam. She will ask for your assistance in removing the examining gloves, putting on new gloves, and lubricating two fingers. Placing those fingers in the vagina and using the other hand to palpate the abdomen, the doctor assesses the position of the uterus. She may then place a lubricated finger in the rectum and palpate for abnormal growths with the other hand by pressing on the lower abdomen.

When the doctor completes the exam, she usually asks the patient if she has any questions or concerns. Ask the patient whether she has additional questions after the doctor leaves the exam room. You may need to provide written information in addition to answering the patient's questions orally.

The medical assistant in many OB/GYN offices provides handouts describing female anatomy and recommended female screening procedures. Printed materials are available from a variety of sources, including the AMA, government agencies, and pharmaceutical companies. The website of the National Women's Health Information Center is an excellent resource.

## Life Cycle Changes

Women experience physical changes as a result of maturation. The two distinct changes that occur as part of the life cycle involve menstruation and menopause.

**Menstruation.** Menstruation is a woman's normal cycle of preparation for conception (the union of egg and sperm that initiates pregnancy). The normal age range of menarche, the beginning of menstruation, is 10 to 15 years of age. Each month (averaging every 28 days) the endometrium, which lines the uterus, is shed in vaginal bleeding. If the woman becomes pregnant, this shedding does not

## Assisting With a Gynecological Exam

**Procedure Goal:** To assist the physician and maintain the client's comfort and privacy during a gynecological exam

### OSHA Guidelines

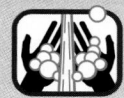 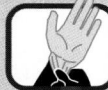 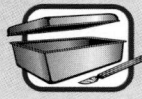 

**Materials:** Gown and drape, vaginal speculum, specimen collection equipment, including cervical brush, cervical broom, and/or scraper, cotton-tipped applicator, potassium hydroxide solution (KOH), exam gloves, tissues, laboratory requisition, water-soluble lubricant, examining table with stirrups, exam light, microscopic slide(s), thin-layer collection vial, tissues, spray fixative, pen and pencil

### Method:

1. Gather equipment and make sure all items are in working order. Correctly label the slide and/or the collection vials.

   *Rationale*

   Slides or vials should be properly labeled to avoid confusing one patient's sample with another's.

2. Identify the patient and explain the procedure. The patient should remove all clothing, including underwear, and put the gown on with the opening in the front.

3. Ask the patient to sit on the edge of the examining table with the drape until the physician arrives.

4. When the physician is ready, have the patient place her feet into the stirrups and move her buttocks to the edge of the table. This is the lithotomy position.

   *Rationale*

   Putting the patient in the lithotomy position too early can cause the patient to experience back and leg cramps.

5. Provide the physician with gloves and an exam lamp as she examines the genitalia by inspection and palpation.

6. Pass the speculum to the physician. To increase patient comfort, you may place it in warm water before handing it to the physician. Water-based lubricant is not recommended prior to the Pap smear because it may interfere with the test results.

7. For the Pap (Papanicolaou) smear, be prepared to pass a cotton-tipped applicator and cervical brush, broom, or scraper for the collection of the specimens. Have the labeled slide or vial available for the physician to place the specimen on the slide. Depending on the physician, the specimen collected, the method of collection, and the method of preparation, two or more slides or collection vials may be necessary. They may be labeled based on where the specimen was collected: endocervical E, vaginal V, and cervical C.

8. Once the specimen is on the slide, a cytology fixative must be applied immediately. A spray fixative is common, and it should be held 6 inches from the slide and sprayed lightly with a back and forth motion. Allow the slide to dry completely.

   *Rationale*

   The fixative holds the cells in place until a microscopic exam is performed.

   Cells collected for thin-layer preparation should be washed into the collection vial and transported to an outside lab for processing and analysis.

9. After the physician removes the speculum, a digital exam is performed to check the position of the internal organs. Provide the physician with additional lubricant as needed.

10. Upon completion of the exam, help the patient switch from the lithotomy position to a supine or sitting position.

11. Provide tissues or moist wipes for the patient to remove the lubricant, and ask the patient to get dressed. Assist as necessary or provide for privacy. Explain the procedure for communicating the laboratory results.

12. After the patient has left, don gloves and clean the exam room and equipment. Dispose of the disposable speculum, specimen collection devices, and other contaminated waste in a biohazardous waste container.

13. Store the supplies, straighten the room, and discard the used exam paper on the table.

14. Prepare the laboratory requisition slip, and place it and the specimen in the proper place for transport to an outside laboratory.

15. Remove your gloves and wash your hands.

## CAUTION *Handle With Care*

## Guidelines for Cervical Specimen Collection and Submission

In order to ensure that the cervical specimen collected is adequate for optimal screening, the American Society of Cytopathology has certain clinical guidelines. As a medical assistant, you will be responsible for helping the physician implement these guidelines. These include:

- Collecting patient information:
  - Scheduling a patient appointment about 2 weeks after the patient's last menstrual period
  - Instructing patients not to douche, use tampons, foams, or jellies, or have sexual intercourse 48 hours prior to test
  - Completing a Lab Requisition Form, which includes the following information:
    - Patient name (note any recent name changes)

- Date of birth
- Menstrual status (last menstrual period, hysterectomy, etc.)
- Any patient risk factors
- Specimen source
- Completing a specimen label:
  - Glass slide
    - Label the frosted end of the slide with the patient's first and last name
    - Include additional identifier, such as patient record number
  - Liquid samples
    - Complete all requested information on label and affix to vial

---

occur, and the woman misses her menstrual period. Note the last menstrual period (LMP) for each patient in her chart at each visit. A period lasts an average of 5 days, with durations of 3 to 7 days considered normal. Menstrual cycles are prompted by changes in hormonal (estrogen and progesterone) levels.

**Menopause.** Menopause is the cessation of the menstrual cycle. Menopause is a natural occurrence, not a disease or disorder. Several stages surround menopause. Premenopause is the time period before menopause, during which the menstrual periods may be irregular. The time just before and after menopause is called perimenopause. During perimenopause a woman may experience irregular periods, hot flashes, and vaginal dryness, all caused by changing levels of estrogen. Because hormonal change is occurring, the woman may experience mood swings or other psychological changes.

Menopause can also be brought on by the surgical removal of the uterus and ovaries (see the discussion of hysterectomy in this chapter). The symptoms and treatment are the same as those of naturally occurring menopause.

A woman entering menopause may feel embarrassed to discuss her symptoms with you. Reassure her not only that it is a natural occurrence but also that there are ways to make menopause more comfortable.

## Diagnostic Tests and Procedures

The physician uses a number of diagnostic tests, including urine and blood tests (described in Chapters 34 and 35). Many OB/GYN offices have their own small laboratories for immediate results, especially for pregnancy-related tests.

**Pregnancy Test.** Pregnancy tests are done on a specimen of blood or urine (the patient's first urine of the morning). These tests detect whether or not the hormone human chorionic gonadotropin (HCG), which is produced during pregnancy, is present. A variety of testing kits are available, including over-the-counter urine self-test kits that the patient can use at home.

These tests are not foolproof; false-positives and false-negatives do occur. An abnormal pregnancy can result in a lower level of HCG, not detectable by the tests. Urine specimens that contain blood, protein, or drugs can also give a false-positive result. False-negatives may result from testing too early or from a urine specimen that is too dilute. The tests are also subject to human error. The physician confirms pregnancy after taking the patient's history, performing an exam, and ordering a pregnancy test.

**Tests for STDs.** The doctor diagnoses and treats STDs by taking bacterial and tissue cultures, examining lesions, ordering blood tests, and discussing the patient's history, as appropriate for the specific disease. Some facilities do not permit the release of these results, even to the parents of a minor, without the patient's written consent. Be sure you are familiar with your state's regulations regarding the reporting of STDs to the state epidemiology department.

**Radiologic Tests.** Several radiologic tests are used in obstetrics and gynecology. The gynecologist uses x-ray, ultrasonography, CT scan, and MRI. X-rays are avoided when a patient is pregnant. If it is crucial for a pregnant woman to have an x-ray, a lead apron must

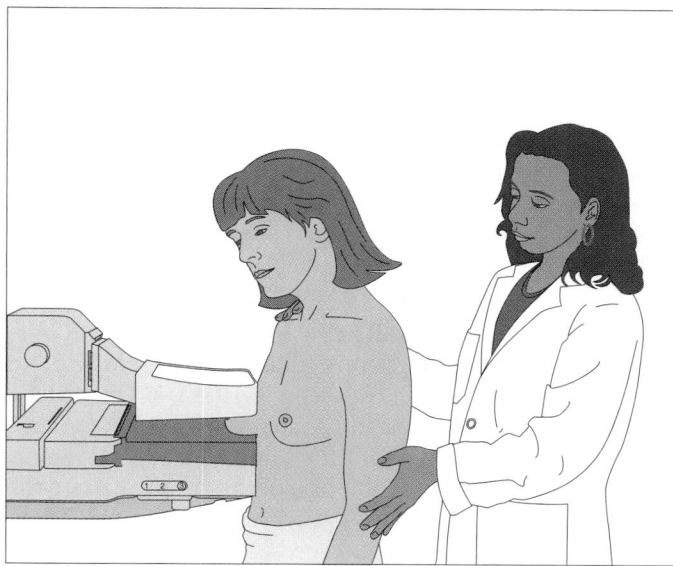

**Figure 26-9.** Mammography consists of two views of each breast and is achieved by compressing the breast between the radiography plates.

cover her abdomen, and she must be made aware that the x-ray could possibly cause an abnormality in the fetus. You will usually schedule the appointment for radiologic tests. Tell the patient when and where to go for the test, and answer her questions about the procedure. Medical assistants need further training to assist with x-ray procedures.

*Hysterosalpingography.* Hysterosalpingography is an x-ray exam of the fallopian, or uterine, tubes and the uterus that uses a contrast medium, such as dye or air. Because the procedure is quite uncomfortable, the physician may prescribe a sedative.

*Mammogram.* A mammogram is a low-dose x-ray of the breast, taken with a special mammogram camera. It can detect cancer about 2 years before it can be palpated with BSE. A first, or baseline, mammogram is taken when a woman is between the ages of 35 and 40 for later comparison.

A patient should schedule mammography for the week after her menstrual period, when the breasts are most normal and least swollen. The procedure involves compressing the breast to obtain a clear x-ray (Figure 26-9). Tell the patient that although the procedure is uncomfortable, it is usually not painful. The patient should avoid wearing perfume, deodorant, or body powders on the day of the exam because they can cause false readings.

**Fetal Screening.** Tests for determining the health of an unborn child are performed on many women. Some, such as an ultrasound, may be performed routinely. Other tests are used only for women whose unborn babies are at high risk of having birth defects. Fetal screening tests can indicate the presence of several birth defects, including Down syndrome and spina bifida. The doctor will consider the patient's age and medical history

and the age of the unborn baby when ordering fetal screening tests.

*Alpha Fetoprotein.* Alpha fetoprotein (AFP) is a protein produced by the unborn child that normally passes into the blood of the mother. A blood test determines whether the AFP level in the blood is normal. Too little or too much AFP in the blood can indicate a fetal abnormality known as a neural tube defect. A neural tube defect is a developmental abnormality of the brain or spinal cord. AFP is also measured in amniotic fluid collected by amniocentesis. The doctor may order a blood test known as a triple screen or triple test.

In addition to AFP, maternal levels of human chorionic gonadotropin and estriol are tested. The test is used to detect neural tube defects and is a better indicator of Down syndrome than AFP alone. This test is generally done between the 15th and 22nd weeks of pregnancy.

*Ultrasound.* Ultrasound translates the echoes of sound waves into a picture of an internal part of the body. The picture or image is called a sonogram, and it can help identify and diagnose cysts and tumors in the abdominal cavity or obstructions of the urinary tract. Ultrasound is painless and safe to use on pregnant women to determine fetal size and position. It is also used to guide a physician in performing amniocentesis.

A patient who is going to have an ultrasound exam during early pregnancy should be instructed not to urinate before the test, because a full bladder allows a better view of the uterus. The patient is asked to lie on an examining table, and a gel or lotion is applied to enhance sound wave conduction and reduce friction of the transducer on the skin (Figure 26-10).

**Diagnostic and Therapeutic Procedures.** Many surgical OB/GYN procedures require the use of needles or other instruments to obtain tissue or amniotic fluid samples. Some procedures are used for obstetric reasons only; others may be used gynecologically and obstetrically.

*Amniocentesis.* Amniocentesis is a procedure performed when a genetic or metabolic defect is suspected in a fetus. The test involves removing a small amount of amniotic fluid, which surrounds the fetus, from the uterus. The doctor inserts a needle, which is guided with ultrasonography, through the anesthetized lower abdominal wall. Fetal skin cells obtained from the fluid are then grown in a culture and examined for chromosomal abnormalities. The level of AFP may also be measured in amniotic fluid.

*Biopsy.* Biopsy is the surgical removal of tissue for later microscopic exam. It is the most accurate and, in some cases, the only way to diagnose breast and other cancers. Biopsy of the endometrium, which is the mucous membrane lining the uterus, may help the doctor diagnose uterine cancer and show whether ovulation is occurring.

It may also indicate whether infection, polyps, or abnormal cells are present. If a patient's Pap smear indicates abnormal cells, a cervical or endocervical biopsy

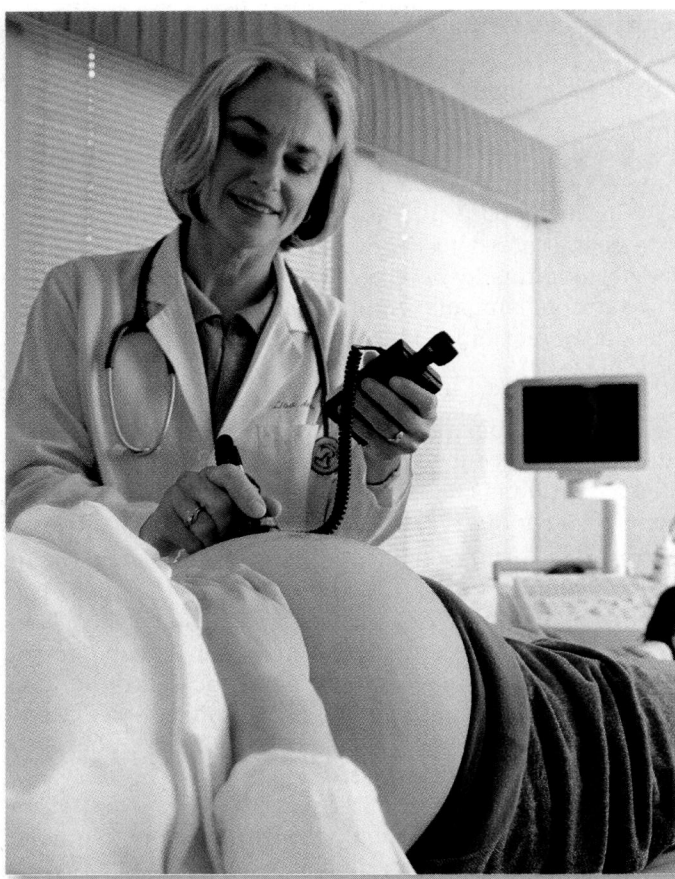

**Figure 26-10.** An ultrasound technician lightly rubs the transducer over a pregnant woman's abdomen to reveal the anatomy of her fetus.

may be performed to rule out or diagnose cervical cancer. Procedure 26-2 explains how to assist with a cervical biopsy.

To assist with these biopsies, you must have knowledge of the female anatomy, the order of procedure, and the instruments used. You will also need to instruct patients about having an escort, appropriate clothing, and any special dietary restrictions. A careful medical history must be obtained to screen for problems such as possible allergic reactions. The day before the biopsy, you might call the patient to confirm the appointment and address any concerns.

A biopsy is considered minor surgery and consequently requires observance of Universal Precautions and sterile technique. Depending on the extent and site of the biopsy, the patient may be given sedation or local anesthesia. During the procedure you may be responsible for clipping excess material from sutures (stitches) and any other special assistance the doctor requests. You must place the biopsy specimen in a sterile, solution-filled container provided by the laboratory. You may assist with or perform the cleaning and bandaging of the site after the procedure.

***Colposcopy.*** **Colposcopy** is the exam of the vagina and cervix with an instrument called a colposcope. Assisting with the colposcopy procedure is similar to assisting with

a cervical biopsy. The physician first cleanses the cervix with saline solution. She then cleanses the cervix with acetic acid, which makes abnormal tissue appear white. The physician inserts the colposcope into the vagina and uses the attached magnifying lens to identify abnormal cells, such as cancerous or precancerous cells.

This procedure is often performed prior to a biopsy after results of a Pap smear show the presence of abnormal cells. The abnormal cells may not be cancerous but may be caused by infection or medication.

***Dilation and Curettage (D&C).*** A D&C consists of widening the opening of the cervix (dilation) and scraping the uterine lining (curettage). Reasons for the D&C procedure include assessing the size and shape of the uterus, removing polyps and fibroids from the endometrium, obtaining endometrial specimens for biopsy, performing an abortion, and completing an incomplete miscarriage. Other diagnoses for which a D&C may be performed include abnormal uterine bleeding, abnormal menstrual bleeding, postcoital bleeding, spotting between periods, postmenopausal bleeding, and an imbedded intrauterine device (IUD).

The procedure is usually performed in a hospital or outpatient surgical facility. Tell the patient she will need to have someone take her to and from the facility. Inform the patient that she will have anesthesia before the doctor performs a routine pelvic exam. The doctor then swabs the vagina with an antiseptic and inserts a speculum. After dilating the cervix, the doctor uses a curette to remove a portion of the endometrium to assess the texture. Both cervical and endometrial tissue may be sent to a laboratory for examination. Exploration of the uterine cavity and removal of any abnormal growths complete the procedure.

Instruct the patient not to have intercourse, take tub baths, or use tampons for 1 week after the procedure. She should also avoid strenuous activity.

***Fine-Needle Aspiration.*** During fine-needle aspiration the physician uses a fine needle to remove by vacuum a sample of tissue from a cyst, lump, or tumor of the breast. This procedure may be used instead of mammography to diagnose breast disorders in pregnant patients, thus avoiding the use of radiation. Patients with fibrocystic breast disease (involving multiple cystic lumps within the breast tissue) may have needle aspiration of a cyst followed by replacement of the cystic fluid with a steroid to prevent recurrence.

***Hysterectomy.*** A hysterectomy is the surgical removal of the uterus. If surgery includes removal of one or both fallopian tubes, it is called a hysterosalpingectomy. Surgical removal of the uterus, the fallopian tubes, and the ovaries is called a hysterosalpingo-oophorectomy. A hysterectomy or a related surgery may be performed for the following reasons: cervical or endometrial cancer; severe endometriosis; unusual bleeding; a leiomyoma, or fibroid; defects of pelvic supports; pregnancy-related problems; and pelvic adhesions or other causes of uterine pain not controllable by other methods.

# PROCEDURE 26.2

## Assisting With a Cervical Biopsy

**Procedure Goal:** To assist the physician in obtaining a sample of cervical tissue for analysis

### OSHA Guidelines

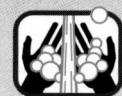 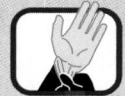 
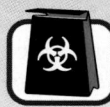 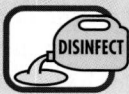 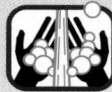

**Materials:** Gown and drape, tray or Mayo stand, disposable cervical biopsy kit (disposable forceps, curette, and spatula in a sterile pack), transfer forceps, vaginal speculum, biopsy specimen container, clean basin, sterile cotton balls, sterile gauze squares, sanitary napkin

### Method:

1. Identify the patient and introduce yourself.
2. Look at the patient's chart, and ask the patient to confirm information or explain any changes. Specific patient information you need to ask about and note in the chart includes the following:
   - Date of birth and Social Security number (verify that you have the correct chart for the correct patient)
   - Date of last menstrual period
   - Method of contraception, if any
   - Previous gynecologic surgery
   - Use of hormone replacement therapy or other steroids
3. Describe the biopsy procedure to the patient, noting that a piece of tissue will be removed to diagnose the cause of her problem. Explain that it may be painful but only for the brief moment during which tissue is taken.
4. Give the patient a gown, if needed, and a drape. Direct her to undress from the waist down and to wrap the drape around herself. Tell her to sit at the end of the examining table.
5. Wash your hands and put on exam gloves.
6. Using sterile method, open the sterile pack to create a sterile field on the tray or Mayo stand, and arrange the instruments with transfer forceps. Add the vaginal speculum and sterile supplies to the sterile field.

### Rationale
The instruments and supplies must stay sterile because this is an invasive procedure.

7. When the physician arrives in the exam room, ask the patient to lie back, place her heels in the stirrups of the table, and move her buttocks to the edge of the table.

### Rationale
Placing the patient in the lithotomy position too early can cause the patient's back and legs to cramp.

8. Assist the physician by arranging the drape so that only the genitalia are exposed, and place the light so that the genitalia are illuminated.
9. Use transfer forceps to hand instruments and supplies to the physician as he requests them. You may don sterile gloves and hand the physician supplies and instruments directly. When he is ready to obtain the biopsy, tell the patient that it may hurt. If she seems particularly fearful, instruct her to take a deep breath and let it out slowly.
10. When the physician hands you the instrument with the tissue specimen, place the specimen in the specimen container and discard the instrument in the appropriate container.
11. Label the specimen container with the patient's name, the date and time, cervical or endocervical (as indicated by the physician), the physician's name, and your initials.
12. Place the container and the cytology laboratory requisition form in the envelope or bag provided by the laboratory.
13. When the physician has removed the vaginal speculum, place it in the clean basin for later sanitization, disinfection, and sterilization. Properly dispose of used supplies and disposable instruments.
14. Remove the gloves and wash your hands.
15. Tell the patient that she may get dressed. Inform her that she may have some vaginal bleeding for a couple of days, and provide her with a sanitary napkin. Instruct her not to take tub baths or have intercourse and not to use tampons for 2 days. Encourage her to call the office if she experiences problems or has questions.

Inform the patient that a procedure of this type is major surgery that requires hospitalization. It also requires preadmission urine and blood tests, cleansing enemas, and shaving of the pelvic area. Normal activities, including sexual intercourse, can usually be resumed within a few weeks.

Premenopausal women who have hysterectomies or hysterosalpingectomies may begin menopause sooner than they otherwise would have. Premenopausal women who have hysterosalpingo-oophorectomies will experience menopause immediately after the surgery. Some doctors prescribe hormone replacement therapy to help alleviate menopausal symptoms.

*Laparoscopy.* A laparoscope is a long tubular instrument. It contains fiber-optic threads that illuminate the organs and a lens that resembles a small telescope. A physician can use the laparoscope to view the internal female organs. Laparoscopy is used to help determine the cause of infertility, to obtain tissue samples, to remove abnormal growths, and to surgically sterilize a patient. It is also used in the treatment of ectopic pregnancies, endometriosis, and laparoscopy-assisted hysterectomy.

The patient is anesthetized before a tube is inserted into a small incision in or near the navel. Carbon dioxide or another gas is pumped into the abdomen to spread the organs apart and thereby make them easier to see. The patient's body is then tilted with her head lower than her hips to allow the intestines to move away from the lower abdomen. This positioning permits a clearer view of the ovaries, uterus, and fallopian tubes.

*Pap Smear.* A Pap smear is used to determine the presence of abnormal or precancerous cells. As discussed earlier, during a pelvic exam, cells from the cervix, endocervix, and vagina are smeared on a special, properly labeled slide. They are then sprayed with a fixative and sent to a laboratory for microscopic analysis. The test results are classified according to level of abnormality, using the standardized Bethesda system (Table 26-3).

**TABLE 26-3    The Bethesda System for Classification of the Papanicolaou Smear**

| Classification | What It Means | Tests and Treatments That May Be Included |
|---|---|---|
| Negative | No intraepithelial lesion or malignancy | Continue routine Pap smears |
| ASC—atypical squamous cells, which may present in one of two types: | ASC—Abnormalities in the squamous cells, which are the thin, flat cells on the cervix | |
| ASC-US—atypical squamous cells of undetermined significance | ASC-US—Considered a mild abnormality; may be related to HPV infection | Repeat the Pap smear; sometimes changes can go away without treatment |
| ASC-H—atypical squamous cells that cannot exclude a high-grade squamous intraepithelial lesion | ASC-H—May be at risk of being precancerous | HPV testing; repeat Pap test; colposcopy and biopsy; administer estrogen cream |
| AGC—atypical glandular cells (mucus-producing cells) | Glandular cells do not appear normal, but it is uncertain what the changes mean | Colposcopy and biopsy; endocervical curettage |
| AIS—endocervical adenocarcinoma in situ | Precancerous cells are found in the glandular tissue | Colposcopy and biopsy; endocervical curettage |
| LSIL—low-grade squamous intraepithelial lesion  May also be called mild dysplasia or cervical intraepithelial neoplasia-1 (CIN-1) | Early changes in cells and an area of abnormal tissue; mild abnormalities caused by HPV infection | Colposcopy and biopsy |
| HSIL—high-grade squamous intraepithelial lesion  May also be called moderate dysplasia, severe dysplasia, CIN-2, CIN-3, or carcinoma in situ (CIS) | Marked changes in the size and shape of the abnormal (precancerous) cells; a higher likelihood of progressing to invasive cancer | Colposcopy and biopsy; endocervical curettage; further treatment with cryotherapy, laser therapy, conization, or hysterectomy |

## Points on Practice

### Pap Smear Technologies

Obtaining accurate pap smear results is an important tool in the successful treatment of cervical cancer. A false-negative test occurs when abnormal cells are not detected. This can occur as a result of the following:

- Too many cells left on the sampling device (brush, broom, or spatula)
- Too many cells piled on top of one another on the slide
- Epithelial cells hidden by extraneous material (blood, mucus, etc.)

A false-negative result could cause a delay in treatment of a year of more, depending on the timing of the next Pap smear.

In an effort to reduce false-negative Pap smear readings, advances in the processing methods of cytologic specimens have been developed. The thin-layer preparation of cells is a liquid-based sampling technique. The physician collects cervical cells in much the same way as for traditional Pap smears, using a brush or broom-like device. Once collected, the cells are suspended in a liquid-preserving medium rather than being smeared directly onto a glass slide. The cells are then sent to an outside laboratory where they are fil-tered or centrifuged and placed on a slide in a thin layer. This method has been shown to produce samples that are more accurately interpreted by cytotechnologists. A cytotechnologist is a health-care professional who uses a microscope to examine cells for changes that might indicate the presence of cancer. The advantages of thin-layer preparation over conventional specimen preparation include the following:

- Artifacts caused by air drying are reduced because cells are placed in a fixative solution immediately.
- The possibility of hidden cells is reduced because cells are placed on the slide in a single layer.
- Blood and cellular debris are removed from the field of view because they are washed away or filtered out.
- The fluid left over after the thin-layer slide preparation may be used for additional testing (e.g., DNA testing for human papilloma virus)

If your office uses a thin-layer cell preparation system, make sure you read and follow all instructions for handling specimens. These instructions can be found in the package inserts for the individual tests.

# Pregnancy

Pregnancy progresses in three stages. These stages are referred to as trimesters, and each lasts for 3 months. Figure 26-11 shows the developing fetus during each stage of growth.

**First Trimester.** After conception, the resulting cell begins to divide. This cluster of cells, the embryo, is implanted in the uterine wall about 36 hours after fertilization. Implantation initiates the embryonic period, during which most of the organ systems develop. The embryonic period lasts 8 weeks, after which the embryo is called a fetus. Week 12 marks the end of the first trimester, or one third of the pregnancy.

**Second Trimester.** Fine, soft hair (lanugo) appears on the shoulders, back, and head of the fetus during the fourth month. By the 20th week fetal movement may be felt, and the pregnant woman begins to show fullness in the abdomen. There are identifiable periods of fetal sleep and wakefulness as the second trimester ends at the completion of the sixth month.

**Third Trimester.** The last trimester encompasses the most noticeable period of growth, both in the fetus and in the mother. By the end of 30 weeks, the fetus has assumed a head-down position and has a 50% chance of survival if it is born at this time. The fetus is said to have come full term after it is approximately 9 months (40 weeks) old.

**Nägele's Rule.** To estimate the delivery date for a pregnant woman, most doctors use Nägele's rule. Begin with the first day of the patient's last menstrual period, subtract 3 months, and add 7 days plus 1 year. If, for example, the first day of the last menstrual period was June 30, 2008, subtracting 3 months would give you March 30, 2008. After the addition of 7 days plus 1 year, April 6, 2009, would be the estimated delivery date.

**Prenatal Care.** Pregnant women need to be particularly attentive to nutrition, exercise, medical monitoring, and childbirth classes. They should avoid using tobacco, alcohol, and drugs. Normal manifestations during pregnancy include morning sickness (usually in the first trimester), weight gain, urinary frequency, fatigue, depression, constipation, and swollen hands and feet.

You may perform or assist with routine tests for pregnant women, or you may send them to an outside laboratory. These tests may include the complete blood count (CBC), Rh-antibody determination, blood typing, Pap smear, urinalysis, and hematocrit. Others may include tests for syphilis, hepatitis B antibodies, HIV, and chlamydia.

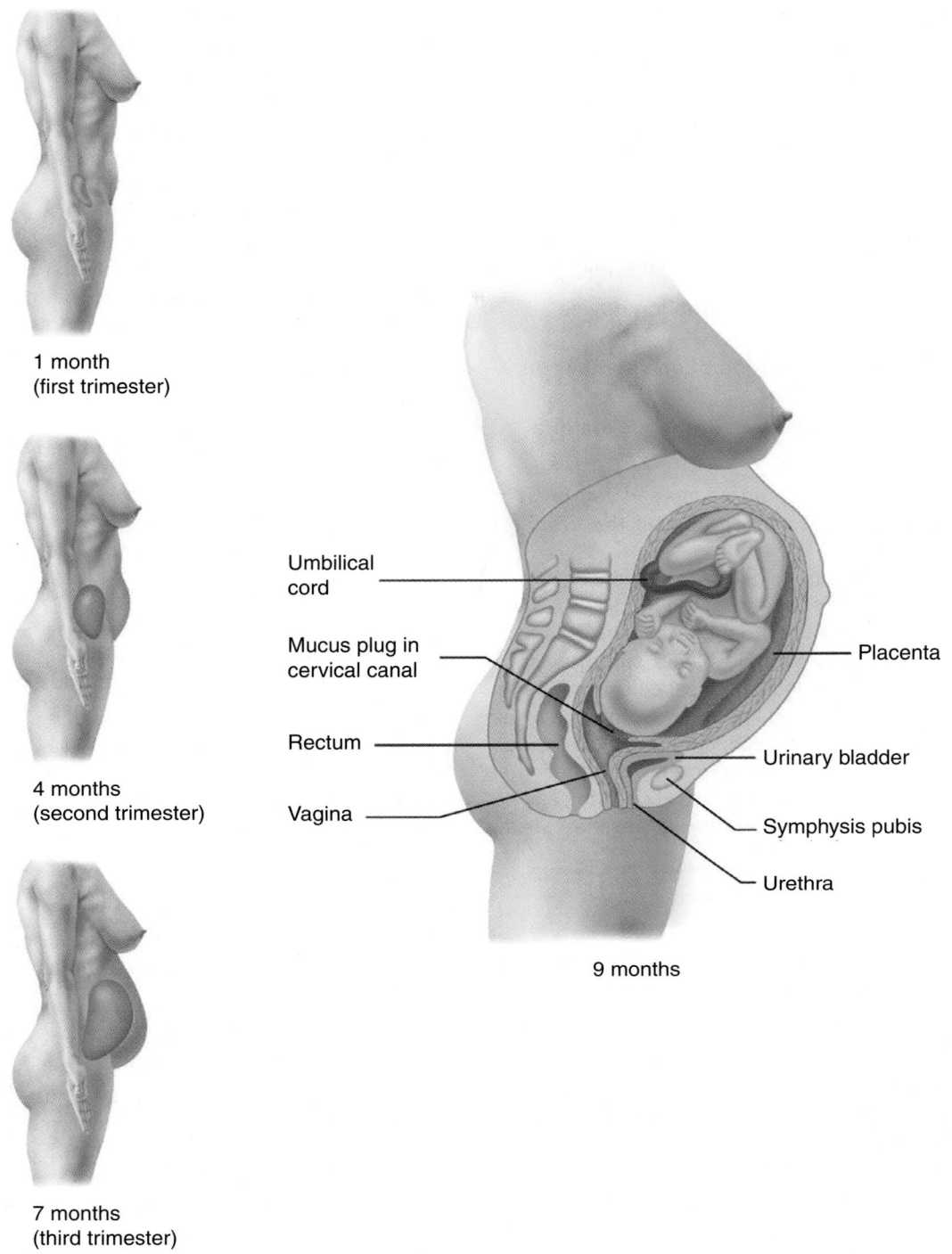

1 month
(first trimester)

4 months
(second trimester)

7 months
(third trimester)

Umbilical cord

Mucus plug in cervical canal

Rectum

Vagina

Placenta

Urinary bladder

Symphysis pubis

Urethra

9 months

**Figure 26-11.** The fetus develops over the course of three trimesters.
Source: McGraw-Hill's Digital Asset Library.

***Assisting With Prenatal Care.*** You will play an important role in encouraging the obstetric patient to have regular checkups and to take proper care of herself. You will also help teach and support both parents throughout the pregnancy. You must document all information given to or taken from the patient.

Providing information on the effects of using drugs or alcohol during pregnancy is particularly important. Alcohol, for example, crosses the placental barrier and directly affects fetal development. Drinking alcohol during pregnancy can cause fetal alcohol syndrome (FAS). This syndrome may include fetal growth deficiencies, mental retardation or learning disabilities, heart defects, cleft palate, a small head, a small brain, and deformed limbs. There is no known safe level of alcohol consumption during pregnancy. You can help prevent FAS by teaching all pregnant patients about the potential effects of alcohol on their unborn babies. If a pregnant patient who is an alcoholic expresses a desire to stop drinking, inform the physician, who may wish to discuss admission to an alcoholic rehabilitation program with her.

You may also refer the patient to Alcoholics Anonymous or a similar community group for assistance. Drug use during pregnancy poses similar problems for a woman's developing fetus.

When assisting with routine prenatal patient visits, you may:

1. Ask the patient about any problems and record any symptoms she reports.
2. Ask the patient to empty her bladder and obtain a urine specimen in the cup you provide.
3. Weigh the patient and note her weight in the chart.
4. Perform the reagent urine test (chemical analysis) and note the results in her chart.
5. Give the patient a drape and ask her to undress from the waist down if the physician will be performing an internal exam.
6. Assist the patient to the examining table. Take her vital signs. Record them in her chart.
7. Assist the physician as needed with the exam. Provide the flexible centimeter tape measure and Doppler, an instrument used to listen to fetal heartbeat.
8. Assist the patient from the examining table after the exam.

***Prenatal Care by the Doctor.*** The doctor carefully monitors the progress of a pregnancy. She watches blood pressure, weight changes, and urinalysis results for possible signs of preeclampsia. Increased blood pressure (hypertension), unusual weight gain because of edema, and protein in the urine are signs of this serious complication of pregnancy. The doctor examines urine specimens for possible urinary tract infections (UTIs) and occasionally asks for other laboratory tests, such as a CBC. She may prescribe special vitamins and iron as dietary supplements.

**Labor.** Changes occur in the mother's body chemistry when the fetus is ready to be born. These changes signal the release of the hormone oxytocin, which initiates labor. The first stage of labor is marked by regular contractions and cervical dilation. The second stage is characterized by complete cervical dilation and the entrance of the head (or buttocks if it is a breech birth) into the vagina. Further contractions and the mother's bearing down push the baby into the birth canal and out of the mother's body. The last contractions push out the placenta and its membranes (afterbirth), attached to the baby with the umbilical cord. This is the third and final stage of labor.

**Delivery.** At birth a newborn's average weight and length are 7.5 lb and 20 inches. The baby's mouth and nose are suctioned to clear them of mucus. Crying indicates that the baby is breathing on her own. The lungs inflate, and the color of the skin changes from bluish to normal. The physician clamps, ties, and cuts the umbilical cord and presents the baby to the mother.

If the pregnant woman cannot deliver the baby vaginally, the physician may deliver the baby by performing an operation known as a cesarean section. Several conditions may require a cesarean section, such as a large baby in a breech position. To perform a cesarean section, the physician makes a series of incisions. First the skin, underlying muscles, and abdomen are opened. Then the uterus is opened, and the infant is removed.

**Newborn Function Testing.** The newborn is assessed at 1 and 5 minutes after delivery for cardiovascular, respiratory, and neurologic function. This is known as the Apgar test. The tests are repeated until the infant's condition stabilizes. With the Apgar test, the baby's heart rate, respiratory effort, muscle tone, reflex irritability, and color are each evaluated with a score of 0, 1, or 2. The best possible Apgar rating is 10 (five evaluations with a score of 2). A score of 7 to 9 is adequate; 4 to 6 indicates that treatment and close observation are warranted; below 4 requires immediate treatment.

**Breast-Feeding.** Human milk is the preferred form of nutrition for an infant. Colostrum, the first milk the mother produces after delivery, is rich in antibodies that provide passive natural immunity to the baby as well. Breast-feeding is economical and convenient. There is no need to buy or make formula or wash bottles and nipples. Breast milk is always available to the baby at the correct temperature.

A woman's success at breast-feeding depends largely on her desire to breast-feed, her satisfaction with it, and her available support systems. You can support patients who choose to breast-feed by providing them with pamphlets and other written materials. Emphasize how essential the mother's nutritional intake is, and explain that she needs to follow a high-protein, high-calorie diet. Patients who need help may be referred to lactation consultants or support groups such as the La Leche League.

# Contraception

Couples who want to prevent pregnancy practice contraception. The type of contraception chosen is based on variables such as price, convenience, effectiveness, and side effects. The only method that is 100% effective is abstinence. Contraceptive methods include the following:

- The birth control pill is a daily oral contraceptive. Synthetic hormones in the pills inhibit ovulation.
- The birth control patch is placed on the lower abdomen or buttocks. It is replaced once a week for 3 weeks, then no patch is used the 4th week.
- Injection is a method in which a synthetic hormone is administered every 3 months to inhibit ovulation.
- A condom is worn on the penis or inserted into the vagina to serve as a barrier to sperm.
- Spermicidal foam, cream, jelly, and vaginal suppositories contain spermicides (sperm-killing chemicals). They are inserted into the woman's vagina.
- A diaphragm is a dome-shaped rubber cup prescribed to fit over the patient's cervix and used with spermicide to provide a barrier to sperm.

- A vaginal contraceptive ring is inserted by the woman for 3 weeks and then removed for 1 week.
- A cervical cap is similar to a diaphragm, except that it covers a smaller area of the woman's cervix.
- An IUD is a small piece of plastic or metal that fits inside the uterus and inhibits fertilization or implantation. Insertion of an IUD is performed by a doctor.
- Sterilization is a surgical procedure. A man can have a vasectomy, in which the doctor removes a section of each tube that carries sperm from each testicle to the penis. A female can have her fallopian tubes cut or blocked.
- Periodic abstinence (sometimes called the rhythm method) involves refraining from sexual intercourse when a woman is fertile and likely to become pregnant.
- Withdrawal consists of withdrawing the penis from the vagina before ejaculation occurs.
- Postcoital pills taken to prevent implantation of the embryo in the uterus must be taken within 72 hours of having unprotected sex.

Contraception information should be obtained and provided to patients as required. The Planned Parenthood Federation, the National Library of Medicine, and the FDA are valuable resources.

## Infertility

Infertility is the inability of a couple to conceive a child. Physicians usually test both the man and woman for infertility. Depending on the cause of the problem, the physician may treat the man, the woman, or both.

If you work in an OB/GYN office, the physicians may test couples for fertility and provide them with treatments or options so they can have children. In such an office you should be familiar with basic infertility tests and treatments. You may need to explain procedures to couples, assist with tests or treatments, and provide emotional support and encouragement.

Tests to determine the cause of infertility in a woman examine whether ovulation occurs, whether the fallopian tubes are clear of obstruction, whether the uterus is healthy enough to support the implantation and growth of a fetus, and whether the woman is healthy enough to maintain pregnancy. Tests to determine the cause of infertility in a man examine whether the sperm are healthy and numerous enough to fertilize an egg.

Various treatments and options are available for the infertile couple. You must be aware of the current methods used by the physician with whom you are employed.

## Diseases and Disorders

Many of the diseases and disorders encountered in the OB/GYN practice have been mentioned in the context of the procedures in this chapter. Table 26-4 outlines common obstetric and gynecologic diseases and disorders.

| TABLE 26-4 | Common Obstetric and Gynecologic Diseases and Disorders | |
| --- | --- | --- |
| **Condition** | **Description** | **Treatment** |
| Cancer | Common occurrence in cervix, endometrium (uterus), ovaries; cells divide uncontrollably, eventually forming tumor or other growth of abnormal tissue; most often seen in women between the ages of 50 and 60; symptoms differ for each type of cancer | Surgery (hysterectomy), radiation, chemotherapy, hormones; for ovarian cancer, surgical removal of all reproductive organs, affected lymph nodes, appendix, and some muscle tissue, followed by chemotherapy (to extend survival time) |
| Ectopic pregnancy | Fertilized egg unable to move out of fallopian tube into uterus for implantation; patient experiences pain within a few weeks of conception; can be fatal | Surgery to remove embryo from fallopian tube before tube ruptures |
| Endometriosis | Endometrial tissue present outside uterus, usually in pelvic area; not life-threatening but may cause sterility; symptoms include abnormal menstruation and pain (sometimes severe) in lower abdominal area and back | Hormone therapy, hysterectomy for severe cases, endometrial ablation (1-day surgery, alternative to hysterectomy), leuprolide acetate injection |
| Fibroids, or leiomyomas | Common, benign, smooth tumors of muscle cells (not fibrous tissue) grouped in uterus; symptoms include excessive menstruation and bloating; diagnosis by bimanual examination and ultrasound | Surgery for severe cases |
| Fibrocystic breast disease | Benign, fluid-filled cysts or nodules in breast; sometimes confused with malignant growths in breast until complete diagnostic tests performed; symptoms include pain and tenderness | Depending on severity, vitamin E supplements, hormones, compresses, analgesics, aspiration, biopsy; restricted caffeine intake |

| TABLE 26-4 | Common Obstetric and Gynecologic Diseases and Disorders *(concluded)* | |
|---|---|---|
| **Condition** | **Description** | **Treatment** |
| Menstrual disturbances | May be (1) amenorrhea (absence of menstruation), (2) dysmenorrhea (painful menstruation), (3) menorrhagia (excessive amount of menstrual flow or prolonged period of menstruation), or (4) metrorrhagia (bleeding between menstrual periods) | Treatment according to symptoms; analgesics; possibly D & C; for severe cases, hysterectomy |
| Ovarian cysts | Sacs of fluid or semisolid material, usually benign and without symptoms; occur anytime between puberty and menopause; extensive ovarian cysts may cause pelvic discomfort, lower back pain, and abnormal bleeding | Analgesics and bed rest if severe pain; hormone therapy; surgery, usually reserved for cysts that rupture or are large enough to put pressure on surrounding organs |
| Pelvic inflammatory disease (PID) | Acute, chronic infection of reproductive tract; causes include untreated STDs, such as gonorrhea and chlamydia, and organisms such as staphylococci and streptococci; symptoms include vaginal discharge, fever, and general discomfort | Antibiotics |
| Pelvic support problems | Abnormal weakening of vaginal tissue, unusual increase in abdominal pressure, congenital weakening (weakness since birth); symptoms include urine leakage, pelvic heaviness ("bottom falling out"), pain or discomfort in pelvic area, pulling or aching feeling in lower back, abdomen, or groin | Kegel or perineal exercises to strengthen muscles, insertion of pessary (device to hold pelvic organs in place), surgery to repair muscles |
| Polyps | Red, soft, and fragile growths, with slender stem attachment, sometimes found on mucous membranes of cervix or endometrium; may cause pain | Depending on size and shape, may be removed in office or hospital |
| Premenstrual dysphoric disorder (PMDD) | A severe form of premenstrual syndrome that affects 5% of women; symptoms have a very disrupting effect on the patient's life; screening tests and physician evaluation are necessary for diagnosis | Medications, including antidepressants, antianxiety drugs, analgesics, hormones, and diuretics; exercise, relaxation, diet modification, vitamins, minerals, and herbal preparations are also useful |
| Premenstrual syndrome (PMS) | Symptoms include swelling, bloating, weight gain, breast tenderness, headaches, and mood shifts 1 week to 10 days before menstruation | Vitamins, diuretics, hormones, oral contraceptives, tranquilizers, other medications; stress-reduction methods as needed; restricted intake of dietary sodium, alcohol, and caffeine |
| Sexual function disorders | Interruption or lack of sexual response cycle (excitement, plateau, orgasm, and resolution); unhealthy view of one's feelings about oneself as a woman and feelings toward sex; sometimes caused by painful intercourse, abusive partner, unrealistic demands on oneself, or menopause | Counseling (for both woman and partner) to teach relaxation, effective communication, and identification of cycle stages and natural responses |
| Vaginitis | Inflammation of vagina caused by bacteria, viruses, yeasts, or chemicals in sprays, douches, or tampons; symptoms include itching, redness, pain, swelling | Treatment prescribed according to cause; avoiding douches, tampons, tight pants, wiping from back to front; sometimes avoiding sex during treatment |

# Summary

Many specialties provide you with opportunities for rewarding and challenging work as a medical assistant. You might enjoy working in the specialty of internal medicine, assisting doctors who diagnose and treat disorders and diseases of the body's internal organs. In such a practice, you might help detect possible substance abuse. You could perform or assist with diagnostic testing such as urine and blood tests and bacterial cultures. You might educate patients on diseases of aging, infectious diseases, and STDs.

Pediatrics might provide interesting and satisfying work, especially if you like working with children. Your primary responsibilities would involve educating parents or caregivers, preparing children for exam, and detecting child abuse. Specific duties might include assisting in regular checkups and performing a throat culture to test for strep. Your role as an educator could involve providing facts on sudden infant death syndrome to parents or giving pamphlets on learning disabilities to caregivers.

Obstetricians and gynecologists are specialists who treat conditions of the female reproductive system, care for pregnant women, and deliver babies. Assisting in this specialty might involve preparing women for a pelvic exam, assisting with a cervical biopsy, and providing support to infertile couples. You would also be responsible for providing information to pregnant women about prenatal care.

Medical assisting positions in the basic specialties usually involve a wide range of responsibilities and tasks. You will find many opportunities to develop your skills and interests if you work in one of these medical specialties.

## CASE STUDY QUESTIONS

Now that you have completed this chapter, review the case study at the beginning of the chapter and answer the following questions:

1. What kind of patients would you see in each of these offices?
2. What additional duties and procedures would you perform?

## Discussion Questions

1. You are the medical assistant to an internist. As you are preparing a patient for an exam, the patient describes some symptoms that sound as if they could be part of an STD. What should you say? What should you not say?
2. What would you say to a child who is afraid to go into the exam room? How could you make her more comfortable?
3. What are the benefits of the thin-layer preparation technique for pap smears?

## Critical Thinking Questions

1. A patient calls because he has found a small tick behind his son's ear. What would you advise him to do?
2. A mother calls your office and tells you her son is scheduled to come in for routine immunizations but he has a mild cold. What should you tell the patient?
3. A patient comes in with slurred speech and behavior that suggests intoxication. What types of substances might this patient be abusing? How might you differentiate between them?
4. An elderly female patient arrives at your facility and makes the following statement regarding her recent change in living arrangements: "I miss my old friends. Since I moved in with my niece, she does not let me have company. We talk too loud, she says, and we have nothing worthwhile to say." What should you do?
5. A 2-month-old infant arrives at the client for a well-child visit. During the exam by the physician, the infant is crying and agitated. What should you do?

## Application Activities

1. A woman who is in her eighth month of pregnancy tells you she is thinking about breast-feeding her baby but can't decide. Prepare a pamphlet of information you can give the patient.
2. Instruct another student in how to prevent STDs. Be sure to encourage the student to ask questions. Then ask the student to evaluate your teaching technique.
3. Create a list of potential subjects to discuss with a patient who comes in for a routine exam with a gynecologist—first for a 16-year-old girl and then for a middle-aged woman.

## Virtual Fieldtrip

*Visit the McGraw-Hill Higher Education Medical Assisting website at www.mhhe.com/medicalassisting3 to complete the following activity:*

Using websites provided by your instructor or searching the Internet for additional sites, create a teaching brochure for a disease or disorder presented in this chapter. Obtain a sample brochure to use as a guideline for your creation, but do not use the same topic. Place the data in a word processing or presentation program. Use graphics and clip art to make your brochure interesting and appealing to the patient. Print your completed brochure for evaluation.

Open the CD and complete this chapter's practice activities, play the games, listen to the key terms, and test yourself with the interactive review. E-mail, print, and/or save your results to document your proficiency.

# CHAPTER 27

# Assisting With Highly Specialized Exams

## KEY TERMS

angiography

arthroscopy

balloon angioplasty

cardiac catheterization

cholecystography

colonoscopy

computed tomography

coronary artery bypass
 graft (CABG)

echocardiography

electroencephalography

electromyography

endoscopy

fracture

intradermal test

magnetic resonance
 imaging (MRI)

myelography

ophthalmoscope

patch test

positron emission
 tomography (PET)

proctoscopy

refraction exam

scratch test

sigmoidoscopy

slitlamp

stent

stress test

whole-body skin
 examination

Wood's light examination

## MEDICAL ASSISTING COMPETENCIES

*In preparation for the certification examination, you
should know the following areas of competence:*

| COMPETENCY | CMA | RMA |
|---|---|---|
| **Clinical** | | |
| Apply principles of aseptic techniques and infection control, including hand washing | X | X |
| Dispose of biohazardous materials | X | X |
| Practice Standard Precautions | X | X |
| Interview the patient to obtain and record the patient's history | X | X |
| Prepare and maintain exam and treatment areas | X | X |
| Prepare the patient for and assist the physician with routine and specialty exams, treatments, and minor office surgeries | X | X |
| **General/Legal/Professional** | | |
| Instruct individuals according to their needs | X | X |
| Provide patients with methods of health promotion and disease prevention | X | X |
| Conduct work within scope of education, training, and ability | | X |

## CHAPTER OUTLINE

- The Medical Assistant's Role in Specialty Exams
- Allergy
- Cardiology
- Dermatology
- Endocrinology
- Gastroenterology
- Neurology
- Oncology
- Ophthalmology
- Orthopedics
- Otology
- Surgery
- Urology

# LEARNING OUTCOMES

After completing Chapter 27, you will be able to:

**27.1** Briefly describe the medical specialties of allergy, cardiology, dermatology, endocrinology, gastroenterology, neurology, oncology, ophthalmology, orthopedics, otology, surgery, and urology.

**27.2** Describe the types of exams and diagnostic tests performed in each of these specialties and the medical assistant's role in these exams and tests.

**27.3** Identify and describe the most common diseases and disorders seen in these medical specialties and typical treatments for them.

**27.4** Describe the medical assistant's duties in performing a scratch test.

**27.5** Describe the medical assistant's role in assisting with a sigmoidoscopy.

**27.6** Outline the medical assistant's responsibilities in preparing the ophthalmoscope for use.

**27.7** Describe the medical assistant's role in assisting with a needle biopsy.

## Introduction

Many physicians choose to specialize within various fields. As a medical assistant, you may be employed in a role to assist with specialized exams. This chapter introduces you to many of the specialties, their diseases and disorders, the types of exams involved, and how the medical assistant can assist with diagnostic testing by collecting and processing specimens. Certain specialized tests and how to correctly administer them are also included in this chapter.

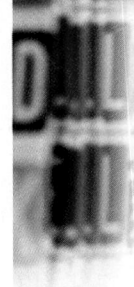

## CASE STUDY

A young, apparently healthy 35-year-old male has a consultation appointment with a cardiologist today in the office where you work as a medical assistant. When he presents to the office, he complains of a recent onset of shortness of breath and an unexplained swelling (edema) of the lower extremities. As part of the screening process, the physician orders an electrocardiogram (ECG), which shows abnormalities. The patient states that he had some dental work done approximately 2 weeks before the symptoms of shortness of breath and edema began. Because the ECG was abnormal, the physician asks you to schedule a stress test with Doppler studies for later in the week. The diagnosis on the chart is to rule out a suspected cardiomyopathy.

As you read this chapter, consider the following questions:

1. What was the purpose of the ECG?
2. What special instructions should be provided to the patient when scheduling him for the stress test and Doppler studies?
3. What educational requirements should you meet in order to conduct these tests with the physician present?

## The Medical Assistant's Role in Specialty Exams

You learned about exams in a number of basic medical specialties in Chapter 26. This chapter discusses exams that are highly specialized. Physicians working in these areas focus on one body system (such as the skin) or even on a single type of disease (such as cancer) or medical intervention (such as surgery).

Although the exams and procedures differ from specialty to specialty, as a medical assistant you will be expected to perform certain tasks wherever you are employed. You will, for example, perform general administrative and clinical tasks. You will assist with exams and procedures and perform certain procedures on your own. It is important that you understand the anatomy and physiology of various body systems as well as the specific exam and procedural steps for each specialty area.

Another responsibility will be communicating with and educating patients. Certain concerns and questions are common to patients within a specialty area. Being prepared to address these concerns and questions will allow you to help patients effectively and fulfill a vital role on the medical team.

# Allergy

An allergist specializes in diagnosing and treating allergies. Allergies involve inappropriate immune system responses to substances that are normally harmless. During an allergic reaction, inflammation and tissue damage occur. The substances that cause allergic reactions are called allergens. Common allergens include certain foods (such as eggs and nuts), pollens, medications, insect venom, and animal saliva or dander. Allergic reactions may show themselves locally—with a skin rash or nasal congestion—or may manifest themselves throughout the body.

The most severe kind of allergic reaction is anaphylaxis, or anaphylactic shock, which is life-threatening. Symptoms of anaphylaxis include respiratory distress, difficulty in swallowing, pallor, and a drastic drop in blood pressure that can lead to circulatory collapse. When anaphylaxis occurs, immediate medical intervention is needed to save the patient's life. Chapter 30 addresses emergency medical intervention in anaphylaxis.

## Allergy Exams

An allergy exam involves a medical history and, usually, several diagnostic tests. You may assist with these tests or perform them yourself under a physician's supervision. Skin tests, for example, involve introducing solutions containing suspected allergens onto or just below the skin. Any reaction is observed and assessed.

As an allergist's medical assistant, you will need to understand the function of the immune system and how allergies are commonly treated. Allergy treatments include allergen avoidance, medications, and desensitization to a substance by means of injections. Part of your job will be to encourage patients to make necessary lifestyle changes to avoid allergens. You will also help them adhere to regimens of injections or medication.

## Allergy Testing

Three tests are commonly performed in the allergist's office. They are the scratch test, the intradermal test, and the patch test. The radioallergosorbent test is performed in a laboratory.

**Scratch Test.**   A **scratch test** is performed to test the patient for specific allergies. Extracts of suspected allergens are applied to the patient's skin, usually on the arms or back. One site is always a negative control—a solution like the one used to carry the allergens but containing no allergen is applied. Then the skin is scratched to allow the extracts to penetrate. Procedure 27-1 describes how to perform a scratch test using sterile needles or lancets. Some allergists prefer to use multiple applicators that allow the tester to apply allergens to and puncture the skin in several places at once, as shown in Figure 27-1.

Be sure to let the patient know that the procedure may cause some discomfort and that itching afterward can be

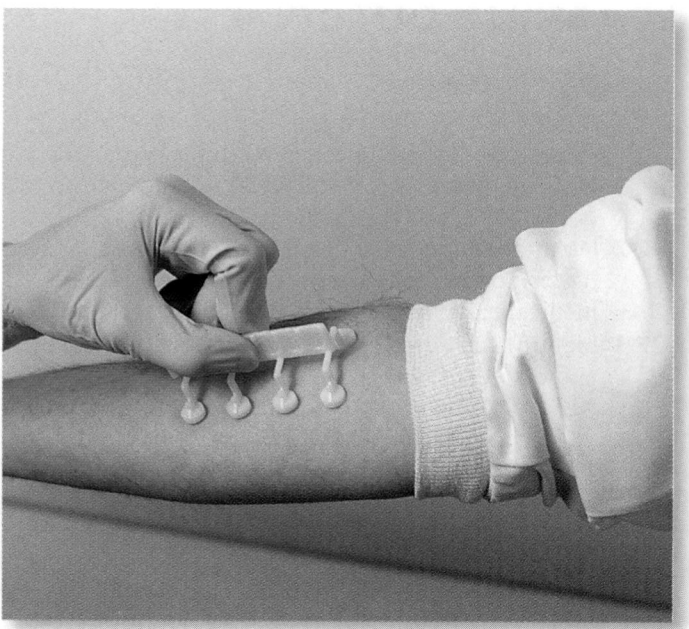

**Figure 27-1.**   A multiple applicator allows the medical assistant to apply several allergens at one time.

relieved with cold packs. The doctor interprets the test results. Because a delayed reaction is possible, the doctor may wish to recheck the scratch sites in 24 hours. When the results of the scratch test are inconclusive, another test, such as an intradermal test, may be ordered.

**Intradermal Test.**   The **intradermal test** is performed by introducing dilute solutions of allergens into the skin of the inner forearm or upper back with a fine-gauge needle. The intradermal test is more sensitive than the scratch test. A small blister, also known as a wheal, which is filled with the introduced fluid, appears on the skin over the injection site. The allergic reaction time is about 15 to 30 minutes, although some substances may cause delayed reactions. If no reaction appears, the test can be repeated with a more concentrated solution to confirm the result. If a severe reaction occurs, the doctor will order epinephrine to be administered.

The tuberculin test, or purified protein derivative (PPD) test, is a type of intradermal skin test. In most offices today it is administered with a needle and syringe. (In the past this test was administered using a disposable device consisting of a disk with tines and was called a tine test.) An extract from the tubercle bacillus is injected into the skin. The results are read in 48 to 72 hours. Raising and hardening of the skin around the area (induration), rather than redness alone, indicate a positive reaction.

**Patch Test.**   You perform a **patch test** by placing a linen or paper patch on uninvolved skin and then using a dropper to soak the patch with the suspected allergen (Figure 27-2). Cellophane or another occlusive material, usually covered with an adhesive patch, is then applied over the linen or paper patch. The test is used to discover the cause of contact dermatitis.

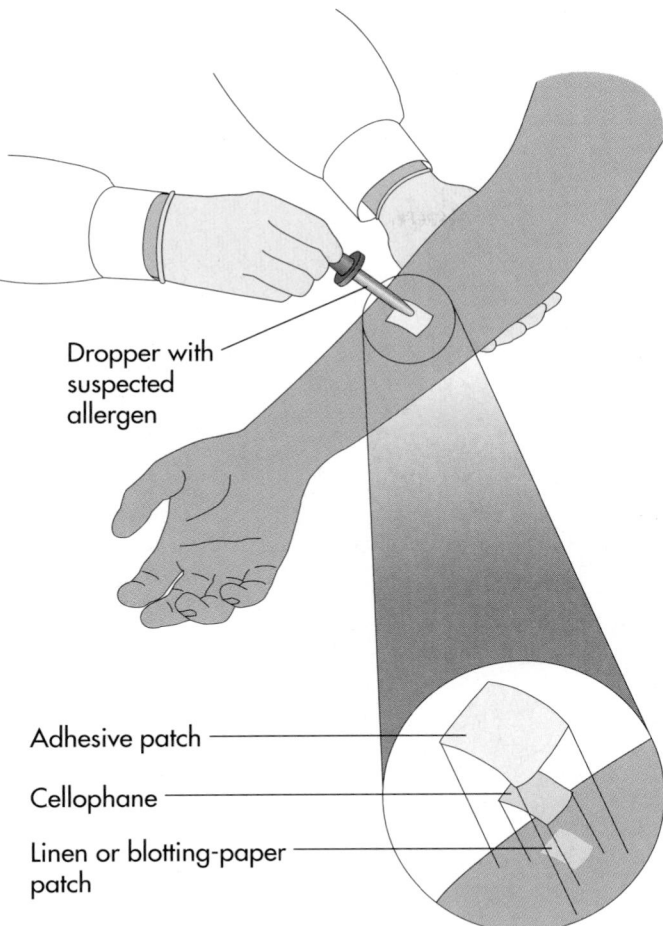

**Dropper with suspected allergen**

**Adhesive patch**

**Cellophane**

**Linen or blotting-paper patch**

**Figure 27-2.** A patch test is usually done on the arm and is read in 48 hours.

**Radioallergosorbent Test (RAST).** The RAST measures blood levels of antibodies to specific allergens. You obtain a blood sample from the patient and send it to a laboratory. There the blood serum is exposed to suspected allergens, and the levels of antibodies are measured. This test usually provides more information than skin testing but is more expensive.

# Cardiology

A physician specializing in heart diseases and disorders is called a cardiologist. To assist a cardiologist, you must be familiar with the structure of the cardiovascular system and the typical exams and measurements associated with it. You also need to know about common heart diseases and their treatments.

Many of the diagnostic tests performed in this specialty, including electrocardiography and stress testing, are described in detail in Chapter 39. Imaging techniques, such as x-rays and echocardiography, may also be employed. You will assist with or perform some of these tests. Because managing a heart condition often involves many lifestyle changes, your role in educating the patient about topics such as diet and exercise will be especially important. You will also provide emotional support to patients with serious illnesses.

## Cardiology Exams

A general cardiovascular exam usually begins with cardiac auscultation to obtain a blood pressure reading and an evaluation of overall cardiac health. The cardiologist also palpates the heart and chest wall and the vessels in the extremities to detect abnormal vibrations, pulses, swelling, or temperature. In addition, an electrocardiogram may be obtained.

## Educating the Patient

### Creating a Dust-Free Bedroom

Patients with household dust allergies will need to reduce their dust exposure as much as possible. One way they can do this is to keep their bedroom as clean as possible. You can help patients with this task by providing them with information about effective dust control. The National Institute of Allergy and Infectious Diseases suggests the following:

- Prepare the room by removing all contents, cleaning and scrubbing all woodwork, removing carpeting (if possible), and closing doors and windows
- Maintain the room by cleaning it thoroughly once a week. This includes floors, the tops of

doors, and windowsill and frames. Use a special vacuum filter and wash any curtains often.

- Keep the bed and bedding as dust free as possible by encasing box springs and mattress in a dust-proof cover and washing all bed clothes in 130°F water.

Additionally, it is important to keep furniture in the room to a minimum, use furnace air filters (high-efficiency particulate absorption, or HEPA, filters are best), avoid stuffed animals, and keep pets out of the bedroom.

# PROCEDURE 27.1

## Performing a Scratch Test

**Procedure Goal:** To determine substances to which a patient has an allergic reaction

### OSHA Guidelines

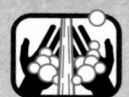 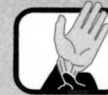 
 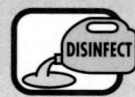 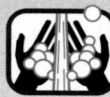

**Materials:** Disposable sterile needles or lancets, allergen extracts, control solution, cotton balls, alcohol, timer, adhesive tape, ruler, cold packs or ice bag

### Method:

1. Wash your hands and assemble the necessary materials.
2. Identify the patient and introduce yourself.
3. Show the patient into the treatment area. Explain the procedure and discuss any concerns. Confirm whether the patient followed pretesting procedures (discontinuing antihistamines, etc.)

*Rationale*

Antihistamines and steroids may interfere with the test.

4. Put on exam gloves and assist the patient into a comfortable position.
5. Swab the test site, usually the upper arm or back, with an alcohol prep pad.
6. Identify the sites (if more than one) with adhesive-tape labels (Figure 27-3).

*Rationale*

The sites must be easily identified so that you can record reactions to individual antigens

7. Apply small drops of the allergen extracts and control solution onto the test site at evenly spaced intervals, about 1½ to 2 inches apart.
8. Open the package containing the first needle or lancet, making sure you do not contaminate the instrument.

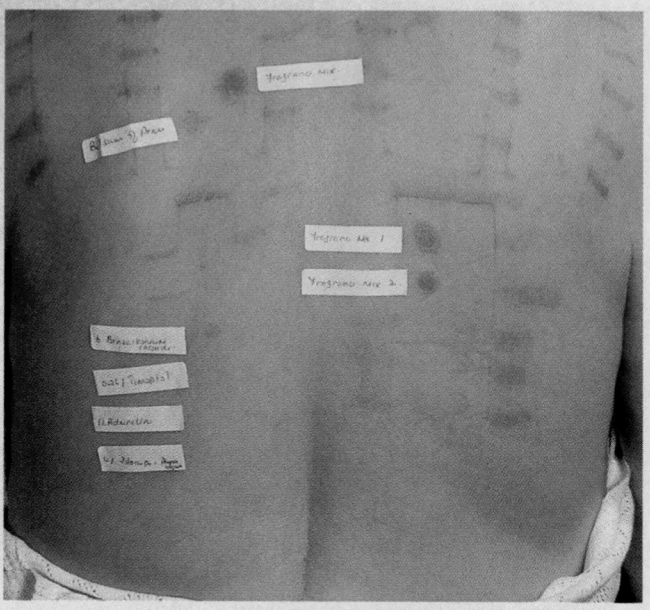

**Figure 27-3.** Label each site with the name of the allergen or an accepted abbreviation.

9. Using a new sterile needle or lancet for each site, scratch the skin beneath each drop of allergen, no more than ⅛-inch deep.
10. Start the timer for the 20-minute reaction period.
11. After the reaction time has passed, cleanse each site with an alcohol prep pad. (Do not remove identifying labels until the doctor has checked the patient.)
12. Examine and measure the sites (Figure 27-4).
13. Apply cold packs or an ice bag to sites as needed to relieve itching.
14. Record the test results in the patient's chart, and initial your entries.
15. Properly dispose of used materials and instruments.
16. Clean and disinfect the area according to OSHA guidelines.
17. Remove the gloves and wash your hands.

*continued* ⟶

## Performing a Scratch Test *(concluded)*

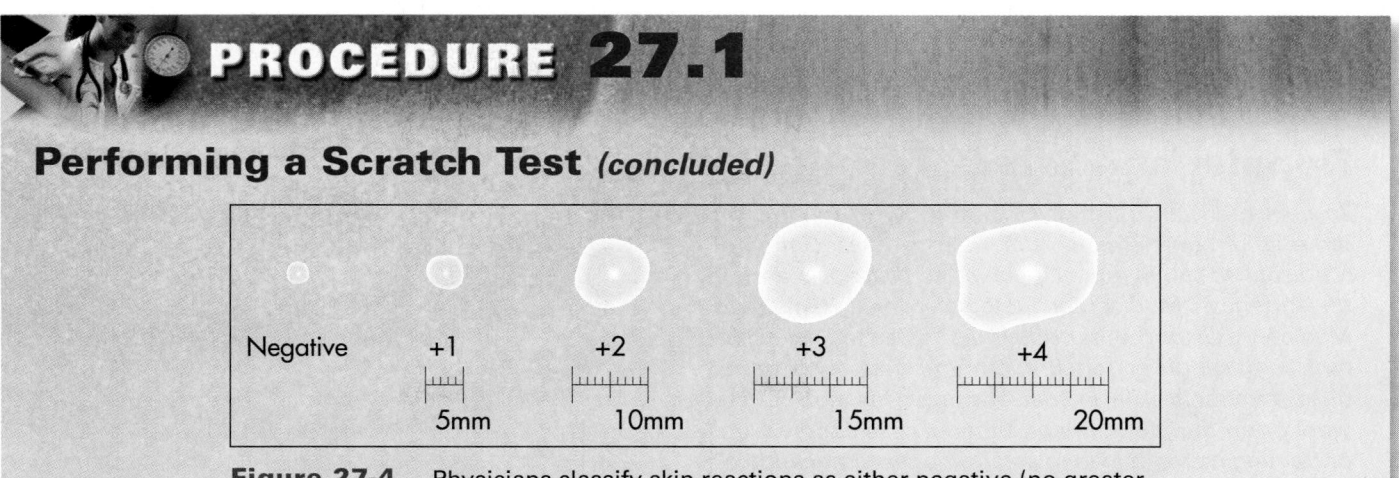

**Figure 27-4.** Physicians classify skin reactions as either negative (no greater than the reaction to the control) or positive. Positive reactions are rated on a scale of +1 to +4, depending on the size of the wheal.

**Electrocardiogram.** An electrocardiogram (abbreviated ECG or EKG) provides a measurement of the electrical activity of the heart. Electrocardiography is a painless, safe diagnostic test that is a routine part of a cardiovascular exam. Electrodes are placed on the skin in particular areas of the chest and limbs. The heart's electrical activity is shown as a tracing on a strip of graph paper. (ECG is fully described in Chapter 39.)

*Stress Test.* An ECG is usually obtained in one of two ways. A resting ECG is performed while the patient is lying down. A **stress test** involves recording an ECG while the patient is exercising on a stationary bicycle, treadmill, or stair-stepping ergometer. This test measures the patient's response to a constant or increasing workload. Part of your job may involve keeping the equipment properly maintained and calibrated. You may also be responsible for administering the test itself. A doctor should always be present, however, because of the risk of cardiac crisis.

Before the test the patient has a screening appointment with the doctor, during which you take a careful medical history and explain pretest requirements. On the day of the test, be sure the patient has followed pretest directions, such as abstaining from smoking or consuming alcohol, and has signed the proper consent form.

The patient is prepared as for an ECG by having the electrodes attached to the skin. Show the patient how to use the ergometric device. If the device is a treadmill, show the patient how to step on and off it and how to use the metal railing for balance. (Exercise electrocardiography, or stress testing, is further described in Chapter 39.)

A type of stress test called the stress thallium ECG is performed by injecting the radioisotope thallium ($^{201}$Tl) into the patient's veins at the time of peak stress. The patient is checked several minutes later to find out how much thallium has been taken up by the heart. Damaged areas do not take up the thallium as rapidly as healthy areas do.

*Holter Monitor.* The Holter monitor is an ECG device that includes a small cassette recorder, allowing readings to be taken over a specific period of time. Electrodes are attached to the patient's chest wall in the physician's office. The patient wears a recording device on a belt or sling (Figure 27-5). The patient returns home, and the device monitors heart activity for 24 hours. (Ambulatory electrocardiography, or Holter monitoring, is fully described in Chapter 39.)

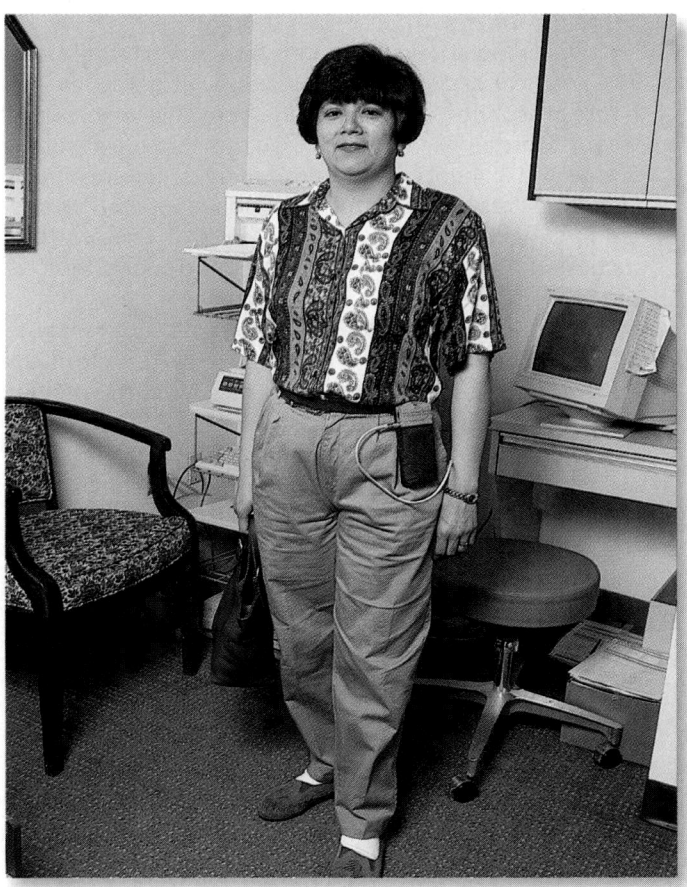

**Figure 27-5.** A Holter monitor allows the doctor to assess heart function during periods of normal activity.

## Doppler and Stress Testing

*To gain medical assistant credentials, you must fulfill the requirements of either the American Association of Medical Assistants (for a Certified Medical Assistant) or the American Medical Technologists (for a Registered Medical Assistant). After obtaining your medical assistant certification or registration, you may wish to acquire additional skills in specialty areas through course work or on-the-job training. Although this course work or training may not lead to an additional certification or degree, it will enable you to expand your role in the medical office and advance your career as the demand for skilled health professionals increases.*

### Skills and Duties

Doppler and stress testing are two procedures that help physicians diagnose cardiac problems. The Doppler test uses an ultrasound transducer, a device that emits and receives ultrasonic waves, to provide a sound wave image of blood flow. The stress test monitors the effect of physical activity on a person's heart. Both procedures can be performed by a medical assistant with appropriate training.

The Doppler test takes between 5 and 10 minutes. The medical assistant applies a special gel to the patient's chest. The gel facilitates the transmission of sound waves. The medical assistant then moves the transducer across the patient's chest, producing a picture on the Doppler screen. This picture can be videotaped or copied in still photographs for later viewing. The assistant records the results of the session and reports them to the physician.

To perform a stress test, the medical assistant uses an electrocardiograph, a machine that monitors the electrical activity of the heart and records the activity as an electrocardiogram (ECG) on special graph paper. The medical assistant attaches metal electrodes (sensors) from the electrocardiograph to the patient's chest, arms, and legs. A baseline ECG of the patient's heartbeat at rest is then obtained.

The patient then exercises on a treadmill or bicycle, with the level of difficulty increasing every 2 to 3 minutes. The medical assistant monitors the patient's blood pressure and ECG and stops the test as soon as the patient experiences fatigue, breathlessness, chest pain, or unusual ECG readings. (A physician is always present during a stress test to deal with cardiac emergencies.) After the test is completed, the assistant records the patient's vital signs. Medical assistants who specialize in Doppler and stress testing may also maintain the

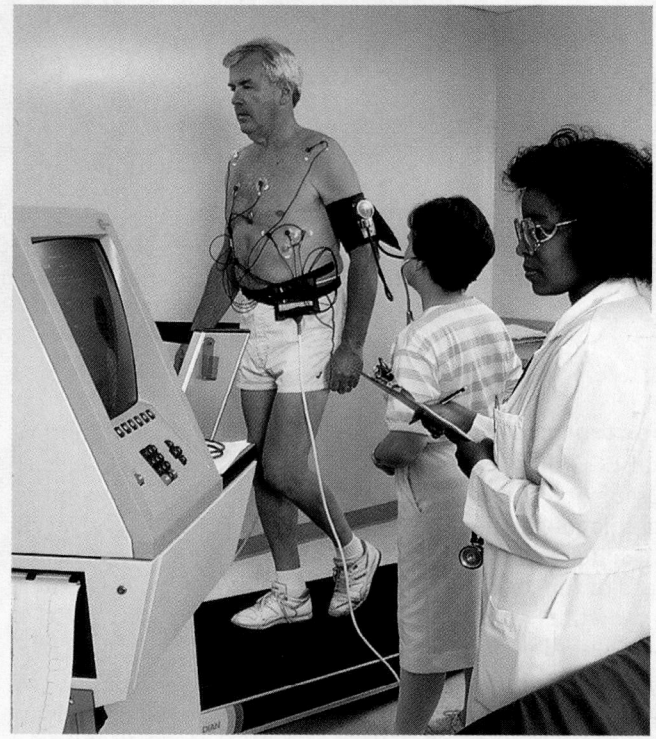

equipment, schedule appointments, type test results and physician instructions, and maintain patient files.

### Workplace Settings

Most medical assistants who perform Doppler and stress tests work in a hospital or cardiologist's office. Some medical assistants may perform these tests in clinics, rehabilitation centers, and managed care facilities.

### Education

Medical assistants interested in Doppler and stress testing must, at minimum, have a high school diploma. Many medical assistants who specialize in stress testing are trained on the job, a process that takes between 8 and 16 weeks. In addition, some colleges and hospitals offer a 1-year certificate program for stress testing.

To perform Doppler testing, medical assistants must receive additional education. Many colleges offer 2-year programs specializing in noninvasive technology, which features tests such as the Doppler.

Although the job outlook for this area is good, the demand for a technician who performs only these tests

*continued* ⟶

## Career Opportunities

### Doppler and Stress Testing *(concluded)*

may not be high. Health-care professionals who have other skills in addition to training in Doppler and stress testing will find the greatest demand for their services.

**Where to Go for More Information**

American College of Cardiology
9111 Old Georgetown Road
Bethesda, MD 20814
(301) 897-5400

American Medical Association
Division of Allied Health Education and
    Accreditation
515 North State Street, Chicago, IL 60610
(312) 464-5000

American Society for Cardiovascular Professionals
120 Falcon Drive, Unit 3
Fredericksburg, VA 22408
(540) 891-0079

## Radiography and Imaging Techniques

Various radiography techniques are used in cardiology. Chest x-rays can reveal conditions such as cardiac enlargement. In radionuclide studies, the patient ingests or is injected with a radioactive contrast medium, often referred to as a dye. X-rays are then taken. For example, fluoroscopy studies are x-ray exams in which a contrast medium is injected and pictures of the heart in motion are projected onto a closed-circuit television screen. A venogram allows evaluation of the deep veins of the legs. **Angiography** is an x-ray examination of a blood vessel after the injection of a contrast medium. The test, performed in a hospital, usually evaluates the function and structure of one or more arteries.

Ultrasound, a noninvasive diagnostic method, is also used in cardiology. Doppler ultrasonography tests the body's main blood vessels for conditions such as weaknesses in vessel walls or blocked arteries. With the use of a handheld probe, sound waves are transmitted through the skin and are reflected by the blood cells moving through the blood vessels.

**Echocardiography** tests the structure and function of the heart through the use of reflected sound waves, or echoes. Sound waves of an extremely high frequency are projected through the chest wall into the heart and are reflected back through a mechanical device. The echoes, which are recorded on paper or video, can indicate conditions such as structural defects and fluid accumulation (Figure 27-6).

Heart magnetic resonance imaging (MRI) is a diagnostic procedure that uses strong magnets and radio waves to produce images of the heart. This procedure is noninvasive and does not use ionizing radiation, so it is safer than other imaging techniques. Detailed pictures of the heart and heart vessels can be obtained using heart MRI.

**Cardiac catheterization** is a diagnostic method in which a catheter (a slender, hollow tube) is inserted into a vein or artery in the right or left arm or leg and passed through the blood vessels into the heart. The cardiologist can use this method to take blood samples for analysis,

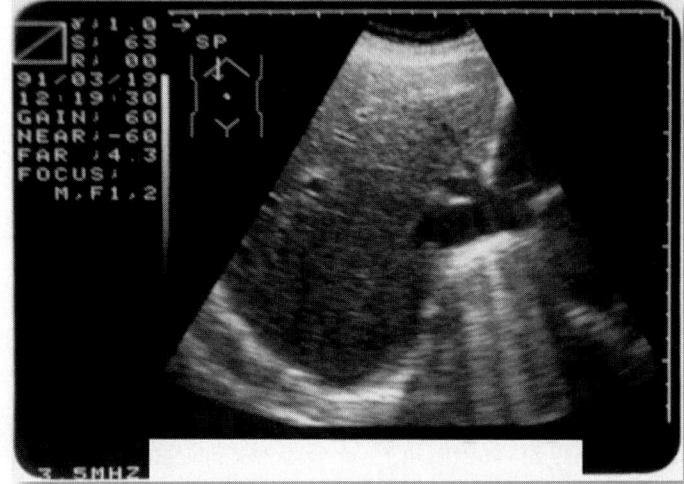

**Figure 27-6.** An echocardiograph shows the structures and function of the heart.

measure the pressure in the heart's chambers, and view the heart's motions with the aid of fluoroscopy. During the cardiac catheterization, the physician may choose to perform a **balloon angioplasty** to open partially blocked coronary arteries. This procedure involves passing a slender, hollow tube through the artery at the site of the blockage. The balloon at the end of the tube is inflated, compressing the blockage and widening the artery. A metal mesh tube known as a **stent** may also be placed in the artery in order to keep it open. If the blockage is extensive, the patient may need surgery known as **coronary artery bypass graft (CABG)**. This surgery involves bypassing the blockage with a vessel taken from another area. All of these procedures are performed in the hospital.

## Cardiac Diseases and Disorders

All of these diagnostic tests are used to reveal heart diseases and disorders. Table 27-1 lists the types of diseases and disorders you may encounter in a cardiologist's office.

## TABLE 27-1 Types of Cardiovascular Diseases and Disorders

| Category of Disease/Disorder | Common Conditions | Treatment |
|---|---|---|
| Arterial/vascular disorders | Aneurysms: abnormal dilation of artery wall caused by area of weakness | Medication, surgery |
| | Arteriosclerosis: thickening or hardening of arterial wall | Medication, lifestyle and diet management, surgery |
| | Atherosclerosis: accumulation of deposits along inner walls of arteries, obstructing blood flow | Medication, lifestyle and diet management, surgery |
| | Hypertension: persistent high blood pressure; systolic pressure greater than 120 mm Hg, diastolic pressure greater than 80 mm Hg | Medication, lifestyle and diet management, stress management |
| | Varicose veins: distended veins in the legs caused by weakening of vein walls and failure of one-way valves inside veins | Wearing of elastic stockings, weight loss, elevation of legs, weight control, surgery |
| Cardiomyopathy: disease of heart muscle causing fatigue, breathing problems, and leading to heart failure | Dilated cardiomyopathy: dilated heart chambers | Medication, heart transplant surgery |
| | Hypertrophic cardiomyopathy: thickening of heart walls and narrowing of chambers | Medication, heart transplant surgery |
| | Restrictive cardiomyopathy: decrease in elasticity and narrowing of heart chambers | Medication, heart transplant surgery |
| Coronary artery disease: condition involving partial or complete blockage of major coronary arteries that surround heart | Angina pectoris: disorder caused by reduced blood supply to heart muscle | Medication, rest, lifestyle management |
| | Myocardial infarction: death of heart tissue because of oxygen deprivation | Medication, oxygen administration, rest, lifestyle management |
| Dysrhythmias: disorders of heartbeat | Atrial fibrillation: uncoordinated atrial contractions, resulting in diminished cardiac output | Medication, cardioversion (delivery of electric shock to myocardium, or heart muscle) |
| | Conduction delays or blocks: problems with transmission of electrical impulses in heart | Medication, implantation of pacemaker |
| | Tachycardia: rapid heartbeat (more than 100 beats per minute) | Medication, diet management |
| Heart failure | Congestive heart failure: inability of heart to pump blood effectively, causing fluid to build up in tissues and lungs | Medication, diet management, rest |
| Inflammations: infections of heart tissue, often caused by systemic infections | Endocarditis: inflammation of heart lining, including valves | Medication, surgery to repair or replace valves |
| | Myocarditis: inflammation of myocardium, or heart muscle | Specific treatment for underlying cause, medication, rest |
| | Pericarditis: inflammation of pericardium (tissue sac covering heart) | Medication, rest |
| Valvular diseases: disorders in which heart valves do not open or close fully | Aortic stenosis: narrowing of aortic valve opening, restricting blood flow | Surgical replacement of valve |
| | Mitral stenosis: narrowing of mitral valve opening, restricting blood flow | Medication, rest, surgical repair or replacement of valve |
| | Mitral valve prolapse: condition in which a portion of mitral valve falls into left atrium during systole | Medication (usually antibiotic prophylaxis to prevent subacute bacterial endocarditis) |

# Dermatology

Dermatologists diagnose and treat skin diseases and disorders such as acne, eczema, and skin cancer. Some skin conditions involve only the skin itself; others are a sign of disease elsewhere in the body.

To assist in a dermatologist's office, you must understand the basic elements of dermatologic exams and procedures. You should develop familiarity with skin disorders and their treatments. You also need to understand the terminology used to describe skin lesions, as outlined in Table 27-2.

Assisting with positioning and draping during a skin examination and taking skin scrapings or wound cultures might be among your duties in a dermatologist's office. You might also perform procedures such as administering sunlamp treatments and applying topical medications. You will also instruct patients about caring for a skin condition or wound site at home.

## Dermatology Exams

During a **whole-body skin examination,** the dermatologist examines the visible top layer of the entire surface of the skin, including the scalp, the genital area, and the areas between the toes. The physician uses a magnifying lens and a bright light to look for lesions, especially suspicious

## TABLE 27-2 Skin Lesions

| Type of Lesion | Appearance | Type of Lesion | Appearance |
|---|---|---|---|
| Macule: flat, discolored spot on skin (less than 1 cm in diameter), such as freckle or flat mole | | Bulla: large vesicle (more than 1 cm in diameter), such as burn blister | |
| Papule: firm, raised lesion (less than 1 cm in diameter), such as wart or raised mole | | Pustule: raised lesion containing pus, such as acne or impetigo pustule | |
| Nodule: raised, firm lesion larger and deeper than papule, such as sebaceous cyst | | Ulcer: depression in skin formed when skin layers are destroyed, such as pressure sore | |

*continued* ⟶

**TABLE 27-2** *Skin Lesions (concluded)*

| Type of Lesion | Appearance | Type of Lesion | Appearance |
|---|---|---|---|
| Vesicle: small skin elevation (less than 1 cm in diameter) filled with clear fluid, such as blister | 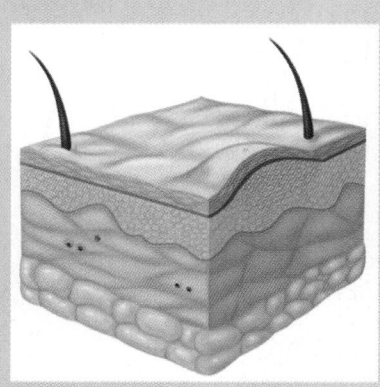 | Tumor: solid abnormal mass of cells larger than 1 cm | 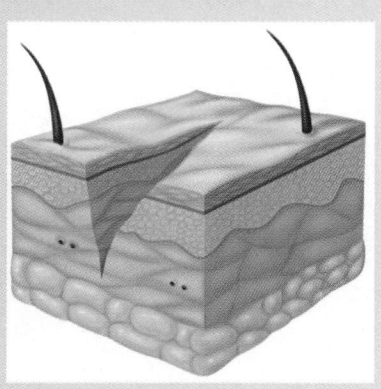 |
| Wheal: temporary elevation of skin caused by swelling, as with hives or insect bites, or by administration of an intradermal injection | | Fissure: crack in skin, such as fissure caused by athlete's foot | |

moles or precancerous growths. The physician may photograph or sketch a lesion to aid in detecting future changes.

Your role in this exam includes preparing patients and helping them into the proper position before examining each skin area. During the exam, drape patients to protect their privacy as much as possible while exposing the area to be examined. The physician may also ask you to take photographs or make sketches of lesions.

Another type of dermatologic exam is the **Wood's light examination,** in which the physician inspects the patient's skin under an ultraviolet lamp in a darkened room. This examination highlights certain abnormal skin characteristics and aids in diagnosis. The dermatologist may also perform more limited, focused exams to evaluate specific skin conditions or disorders.

## Dermatologic Conditions and Disorders

The condition of the skin plays a large part in a person's appearance. Patients with skin disorders, therefore, may worry about their attractiveness to and acceptance by others. Allow patients to express their anxieties; in return, provide encouragement about the course and outcome of their treatment.

**Acne Vulgaris.** Acne vulgaris, also called acne, is an inflammation of the follicles of the skin's sebaceous (oil)

glands. It causes skin eruptions of pimples, blackheads, and cysts, mainly on the face but sometimes on the back or other areas. Acne occurs most frequently in adolescents but can affect adults as well. Its ultimate cause is unknown, but it is thought to involve a hormonal dysfunction that creates excess skin oil (sebum). The sebum hardens at the follicle openings, closing off the flow of skin secretions and causing eruptions.

Medications, either topical or oral, do not cure acne; rather, the treatments help to manage the outbreaks and are based on the type of acne diagnosed. Most often, medications used for treatment include those that:

- Help to unplug pores and stop them from getting plugged with oil
- Kill bacteria, such as antibiotics
- Reduce the amount of sebum produced
- Reduce the effects of hormones contributing to the acne

Retinoic acid cannot be used by patients who are pregnant or likely to become pregnant, because retinoic acid damages the fetus.

Patients need to understand the prescribed treatment regimen and its requirements, such as avoiding sun overexposure if vitamin A products are being used. You may also be asked to instruct patients in proper skin cleansing and care.

**Contact Dermatitis.**   Contact dermatitis is a skin inflammation that can be caused by irritants as diverse as rough fabrics, cosmetics, pollen, or plants such as poison ivy or poison oak. Symptoms include redness, itching, edema, and lesions.

Treatment of contact dermatitis depends on the cause and type of lesions. Anti-inflammatory medications may be applied to the skin, or antihistamines may be taken internally. Corticosteroids are prescribed for severe inflammation. The dermatologist may wish to use a patch test to determine whether a condition is caused by a specific allergen. If such a cause is found, the patient should be taught how to avoid that substance and what to do after accidental exposure.

**Psoriasis.**   Psoriasis is a skin disease characterized by patches of red, thickened skin with silver scales. These patches are mostly found on the knees, elbows, scalp, face, palms, and soles of the feet. The condition is more common in adults than in children. To diagnose psoriasis, the physician will usually take skin scrapings for microscopic examination. Treatment includes topical creams and ointments, light therapy, and systemic and combination therapies.

**Ringworm.**   Ringworm, or tinea, is a term for various fungal infections that most often affect the feet (athlete's foot, or tinea pedis), groin (jock itch, or tinea cruris), and scalp (tinea capitis). Ringworm produces flat lesions on the body that are dry and scaly or moist and crusty. These lesions eventually develop a clear center with an outer ring, for which these infections are named. When ringworm appears on the scalp, it creates small lesions and scaly bald patches.

Ringworm is treated with topical antifungal medications and, when an infection is well established, oral medications. Ringworm is contagious, so instruct the infected individual in how to prevent contamination. The person should not share bedding, combs, towels, or other personal items with anyone until the infection is gone.

**Moles.**   A mole (nevus) is a raised or unraised brown, black, or tan spot on the skin, with even coloring, a round or oval shape, and clear borders. It is usually less than 6 mm in diameter. It may be present at birth, but most appear during childhood or adolescence. Most moles are harmless; in fact, everyone has some. Because moles have the potential to become malignant, however, they must be monitored for bleeding, itching, or changes in color, size, shape, or texture. Some people choose to have a harmless mole removed because it is cosmetically unappealing or because it is in a place especially vulnerable to injury.

**Skin Cancer.**   One of the most serious conditions treated in a dermatologist's office is skin cancer. Skin cancer can appear in the form of basal cell carcinomas, squamous cell carcinomas, and malignant melanomas. Overexposure to the sun is a risk factor for all these types of skin cancer. Other triggers include x-rays, irritants, various chemical carcinogens, and the presence of premalignant lesions. The following people have a higher-than-average risk of developing skin cancer: those who have had severe, blistering sunburns in their teens or 20s; those who have fair skin and hair and light-colored eyes; and those who work outdoors.

Basal cell carcinomas are malignant lesions that occur most often on areas exposed to the sun, such as the face and neck. Basal cell carcinomas are the most common malignant tumor in Caucasians. The lesions look like small, waxy craters with rolled borders (Figure 27-7).

Squamous cell carcinomas also appear on sun-exposed areas. The lesions often look ulcerated or have a crust (Figure 27-8). They invade deeper into the skin and

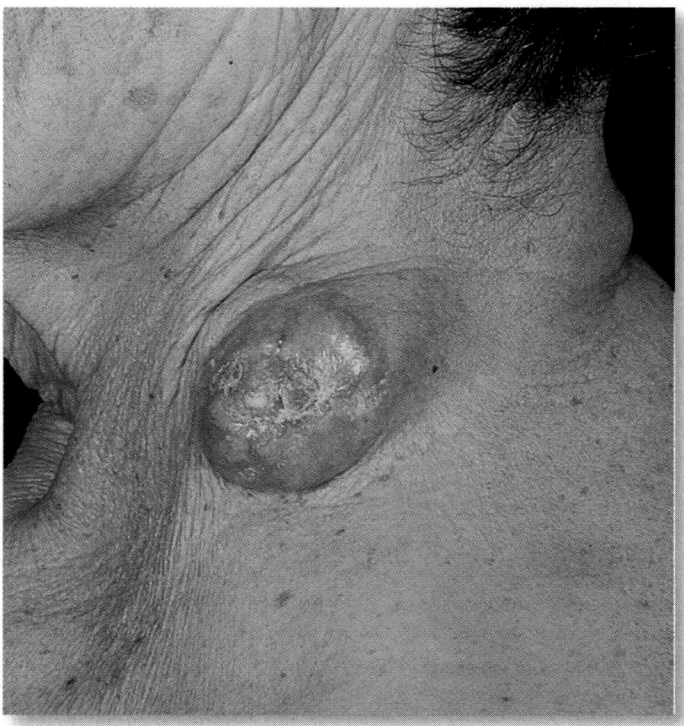

**Figure 27-7.**   Left untreated, basal cell carcinomas can damage bones or blood vessels.

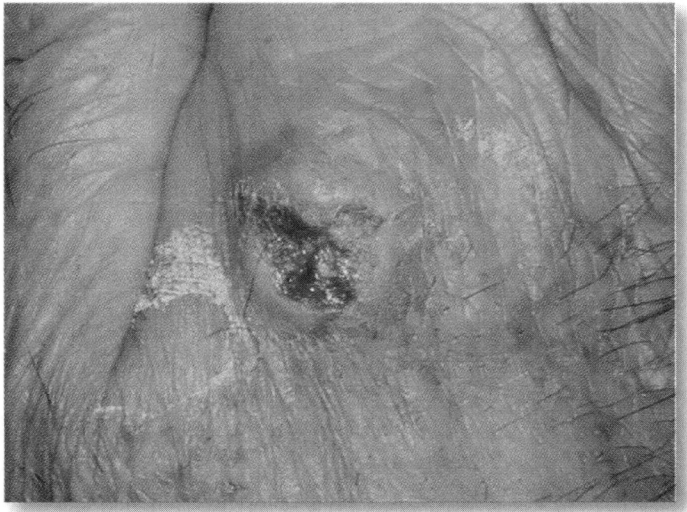

**Figure 27-8.**   Repeated injury to an area, as well as sun exposure, is a risk factor for squamous cell carcinoma.

**Assisting With Highly Specialized Exams**      **599**

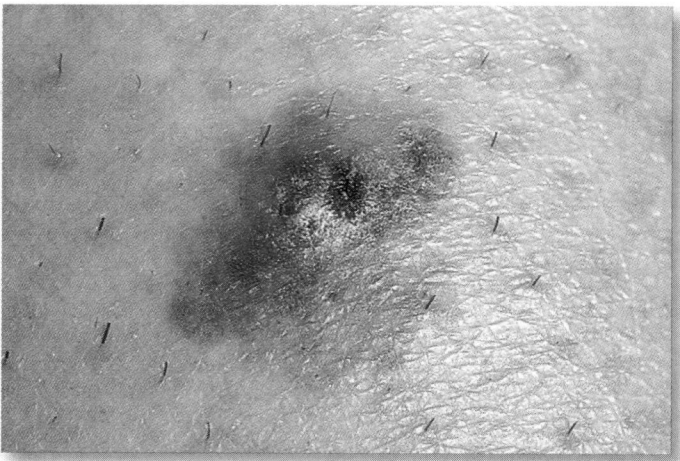

**Figure 27-9.** Early diagnosis is critical in successfully treating malignant melanoma.

have a greater tendency to spread to other areas of the body than do basal cell carcinomas.

Malignant melanomas, which originate in cells that produce the pigment melanin, are the most dangerous type of skin cancer (Figure 27-9). Malignant cells may spread through the bloodstream or lymphatic system to the liver, lungs, and other parts of the body. A sudden or continuous change in the appearance of a mole may signal melanoma. Early diagnosis is critical for successful treatment.

Treatments for skin cancer vary with the type of cancer and its extent. Treatments include surgery, electrosurgery, cryosurgery, radiation therapy, and chemotherapy.

**Warts.** Warts (verrucae) are benign skin tumors that result from a viral skin infection. If a wart is scratched open, the virus may spread by contact to another part of the body or to another person. There are several kinds of warts. Common warts are raised, rounded, flesh-colored lesions that usually occur on the hands and fingers. Plantar warts appear on the soles of the feet. Venereal warts appear on the genitalia and anus and are transmitted through sexual contact.

Treatment depends on the type of wart. Some warts go away without treatment. Physicians often remove warts by burning or freezing the wart tissue. Instruct the patient to keep the wart removal site clean and dry until a scab forms or the wart falls off in a few days.

**Other Conditions and Disorders.** The following conditions may also be diagnosed and treated in a dermatologist's office:

- Eczema: skin inflammation that may be an allergic response to allergens, such as chemicals or foods
- Impetigo: highly contagious bacterial skin infection
- Psoriasis: chronic noninfectious disease that manifests itself in itching lesions covered with scales
- Herpes zoster: acute viral infection of nerves under the skin, often called shingles; causes painful skin eruptions
- Scabies: contagious skin disease caused by a mite; causes intense itching

# Endocrinology

Endocrinologists treat diseases and disorders of the endocrine system, which includes glands that regulate and coordinate the systems of the body. Hormonal imbalances can affect the basic processes of growth, metabolism, and reproduction. In the endocrinologist's office you will assist with exams as well as collect specimens for analysis.

## Endocrine Exams

Before an exam you will take a thorough medical history. The physician will assess the patient's skin condition, weight, and cardiac functioning for clues about illness. Most of the endocrine glands are located deep within the body; only the thyroid, the testes, and, to some extent, the ovaries can be examined with palpation or auscultation. Therefore, diagnostic urine and blood tests are essential. You may be asked to collect a urine specimen or draw blood (see Chapters 34 and 35). Other diagnostic tools used in endocrinology include radiologic tests such as x-rays and iodine scans.

An endocrinologist will perform a complete physical exam, including palpation of the thyroid gland. In a thyroid scan the patient receives an oral or intravenous (IV) dose of radioactive iodine, and the thyroid is x-rayed as the material is absorbed. Ultrasound can also be employed to view glands or detect tumors. Urine and blood may be tested for the presence of glucose or hormones.

## Endocrine Diseases and Disorders

An endocrine disorder commonly treated by endocrinologists is diabetes mellitus. This name is used for several related disorders characterized by hyperglycemia, an elevated level of glucose in the blood. When blood sugar is abnormally low, the condition is called hypoglycemia. Normally, the glucose level is regulated by insulin, a hormone secreted by the pancreas. A deficiency of insulin or a resistance to it interferes with the metabolism of carbohydrates, proteins, and fats, raising the glucose level in the blood. The symptoms of diabetes are often subtle and include frequent urination, excessive thirst, extreme hunger, unexplained weight loss, fatigue, and blurry vision.

Type I diabetes, an autoimmune disorder of the pancreas, is usually diagnosed in childhood or early adulthood. An autoimmune disorder occurs when the body's own immune system attacks itself. With type I diabetes, the body does not produce enough insulin as a result of damage to the pancreas. People with type I diabetes need to take insulin injections daily.

Type II diabetes, the most common form of diabetes, is generally diagnosed in adults. However, childhood diagnosis is on the rise. The risk factors for type II diabetes include:

- Obesity
- Inactivity
- Family history of diabetes
- Previous history of gestational diabetes

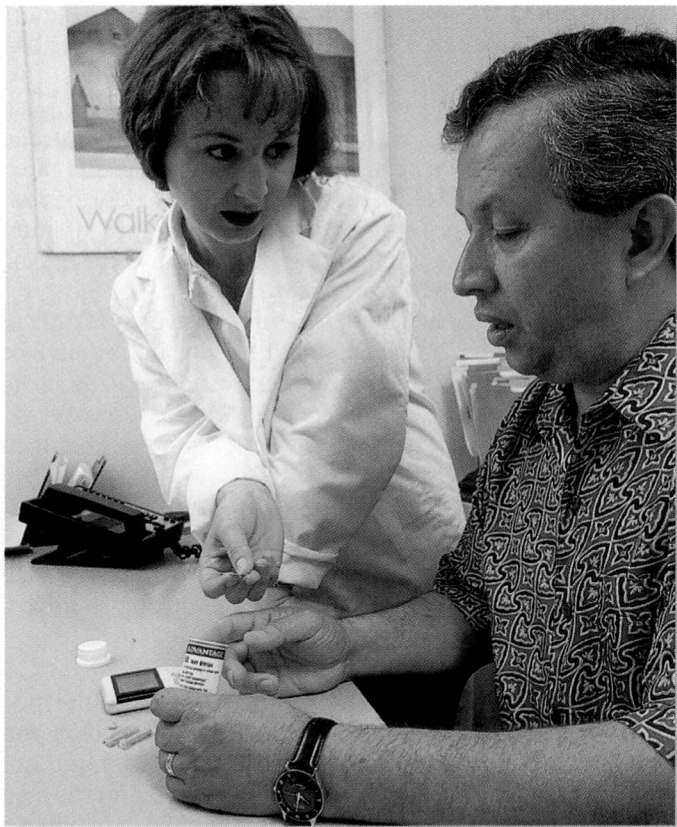

**Figure 27-10.** Patients with diabetes can use a glucometer to monitor their own blood glucose levels.

Type II diabetes is managed with blood glucose self-monitoring, diet, exercise, and, if necessary, oral medications or insulin.

Gestational diabetes occurs only during pregnancy. Diabetes screening is recommended during the 24th and 28th weeks of pregnancy. Women with gestational diabetes must control blood sugar levels in order to reduce the risk to the fetus. This is accomplished through self-monitoring of blood glucose, diet, exercise, and, if necessary, insulin injections (Figure 27-10).Careful management of diabetes can reduce the risk of long-term secondary complications, including:

- Blindness
- Heart disease
- Kidney failure
- Nerve damage
- Amputations

No mater the type of diabetes, the goal is basically the same: Keep blood sugar levels within a normal range, eat a healthy diet, exercise regularly, and see your health-care provider regularly.

**Thyroid Gland Dysfunctions.** Several of the most common endocrine system disorders occur when there is a dysfunction of the thyroid gland. These disorders include hypothyroidism, hyperthyroidism, and goiter.

***Hypothyroidism.*** Hypothyroidism is characterized by decreased activity of the thyroid gland and underproduction of the hormone thyroxine. This shortage can cause cretinism in children, with resulting mental and physical retardation. Underproduction of thyroxine in adults results in myxedema. Patients with this condition have fatigue, low blood pressure, dry skin and hair, facial puffiness, and goiter. Treatment for hypothyroidism consists of thyroid hormone supplements.

***Hyperthyroidism.*** Hyperthyroidism, also called Graves disease, is characterized by increased thyroid gland activity. Too much thyroxine is produced, and the patient has anxiety, irritability, elevated heart rate and blood pressure, tremors, and weight loss despite an increased appetite. Sometimes hyperthyroidism causes the patient's eyes to protrude, a condition known as exophthalmos. Treatment includes the administration of radioactive iodine, antithyroid drugs, or surgery to remove part or all of the thyroid gland. Many patients require supplemental thyroid hormones following treatment for a hyperactive thyroid.

***Goiter.*** An enlarged thyroid gland, commonly called a goiter, is usually caused by a deficiency of iodine in the diet. Iodine is found in seafood, iodized salt, and vegetables grown in soil containing iodine. Without this mineral the thyroid gland enlarges in an attempt to produce more thyroid hormones. Treatment usually involves the administration of iodine.

# Gastroenterology

Gastroenterologists diagnose and treat disorders of the entire gastrointestinal (GI) tract, from the mouth to the anus, as well as the liver and pancreas. (Proctologists treat disorders of the rectum and anus only.)

A patient who sees a GI specialist has usually been referred by a family doctor, internist, or pediatrician who suspects a GI problem requiring additional expertise. You will need to understand the basic elements of GI exams and procedures to assist in a gastroenterologist's office. You must also be familiar with common GI disorders, their treatments, and the terminology used to describe them.

In a gastroenterologist's office you will tell patients how to prepare for exams, whether in the office, a radiology facility, or a hospital. You will order informational brochures and make them available to patients. You will also be prepared to answer patient questions.

## Gastrointestinal Exams

The gastroenterologist's examination of the patient's GI tract covers the mouth (lips, oral cavity, and tongue), the abdomen and lower thorax, the lower sigmoid colon, the rectum, and the anus. Your role as a medical assistant will be to prepare the equipment and the patient.

Depending on the patient's symptoms, the physician may perform an invasive exam procedure during the patient's first visit. Formerly, such procedures were performed only in hospitals or special medical facilities. Now many GI specialists' offices are equipped for these procedures and the management of possible resulting emergencies.

You must provide reassurance during exams and help patients be as comfortable as possible. Your duties during the procedures will vary according to your state's scope of practice and the physician for whom you work. Instruct patients in advance to arrange for someone to drive them to and from the exam. After a procedure in which patients have had a local anesthetic at the back of the throat, caution them to avoid eating until the drug has been eliminated from the body. Otherwise, they could choke or aspirate food particles into the trachea.

**Endoscopy.** **Endoscopy** generally refers to any procedure in which a scope is used to visually inspect a canal or cavity within the body. Several endoscopic exams are performed with a flexible fiber-optic tube that has a lighted instrument on the end. These exams provide direct visualization of a body cavity and provide a means for collecting tissue biopsies and removing polyps, as in the colon. Endoscopy helps diagnose tumors, ulcers, structural abnormalities, and other problems. It is particularly useful in performing procedures that formerly would have required an incision, such as removing stones from the bile duct.

*Peroral Endoscopy.* Peroral endoscopy involves inserting the scope by way of the mouth (Figure 27-11). The patient is sedated, and the gag reflex is inhibited with a local anesthetic. The peroral endoscopic procedures include panendoscopy (esophagus, stomach, and duodenum), esophagoscopy (esophagus only), gastroscopy (stomach only), and duodenoscopy (duodenum only).

*Colonoscopy.* **Colonoscopy,** which is performed by inserting a colonoscope through the anus, can provide direct visualization of the large intestine. The gastroenterologist uses this procedure to determine the cause of diarrhea, constipation, bleeding, or lower abdominal pain.

Patient preparation is designed to clear the colon of fecal material so that the colon can be seen clearly.

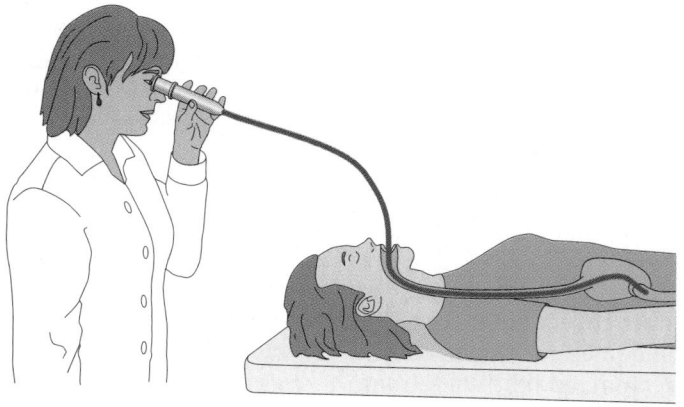

**Figure 27-11.** To perform peroral endoscopy, the physician inserts a scope into the patient's mouth.

Instruct patients to follow a liquid diet for 24 to 48 hours before the procedure. Patients should take a prescribed cathartic on the two evenings prior to the colonoscopy. Instruct patients to use one or more prepackaged enema preparations on the night before and the day of the procedure. (Alternatively, provide patients a prepared electrolyte solution to consume over a 2- to 4-hour period. During this time patients should keep a record of their intake, output, and symptoms. Tell patients to expect diarrhea and possibly mild cramps.)

Immediately before the procedure, instruct patients to empty the bladder. Patients should be given a sedative or an analgesic before undergoing the procedure. Patients lie in the Sims' position as the scope is guided through the large intestine. The doctor may manipulate the abdomen to facilitate passage of the scope.

*Proctoscopy.* **Proctoscopy** is an examination of the lower rectum and anal canal. After an initial digital exam, the proctoscopy is performed with a 3-inch instrument called a proctoscope. This exam can detect hemorrhoids, polyps, fissures, fistulas, and abscesses.

*Sigmoidoscopy.* **Sigmoidoscopy** is similar to colonoscopy, except that only the sigmoid area of the large intestine (the S-shaped segment between the descending colon and the rectum) is examined. Sigmoidoscopy is an important part of many complete physical exams and is performed by many general practitioners and internists. It aids in diagnosing colon cancer, ulcerations, polyps, tumors, bleeding, and other lower intestinal problems.

Patient preparation involves using one or two prepackaged enemas either the night before or the morning of the procedure, depending on the doctor's instructions. The method for assisting the doctor during a sigmoidoscopy is described in Procedure 27-2. The sigmoidoscope, a lighted instrument with a magnifying lens, allows the doctor to see and to examine the mucous membrane of the sigmoid colon.

## Diagnostic Testing

Common diagnostic tests in this specialty include analysis of the contents of the stomach, analysis of a stool specimen, and urine and blood tests. Gastroenterologists sometimes use imaging techniques, such as x-rays, ultrasound, radionuclide imaging, computed tomography (CT), and magnetic resonance imaging (MRI).

**Laboratory Tests.** A GI specialist may order laboratory analysis of stomach contents (obtained by gastric lavage) to determine the presence of bacteria or gastric bleeding. The physician may also request blood or urine tests. Another important test for GI specialists is the occult blood test, in which the feces are analyzed for occult, or hidden, bleeding from the intestinal tract. (This test is discussed in Chapter 25.)

**Radiologic Exams.** Most GI radiologic exams are not performed in an office, but you should know enough about them to answer patients' questions. Generally, these exams are performed in a hospital x-ray laboratory or an

# PROCEDURE 27.2

## Assisting With a Sigmoidoscopy

**Procedure Goal:** To assist the doctor during the examination of the rectum, anus, and sigmoid colon using a sigmoidoscope

**OSHA Guidelines**

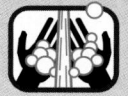 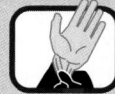 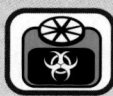
 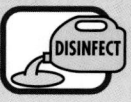 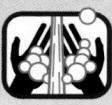

**Materials:** Sigmoidoscope, suction pump, lubricating jelly, drape, patient gown, tissues

**Method:**

1. Wash your hands and assemble and position materials and equipment according to the preference of the doctor.
2. Test the suction pump.
3. Identify the patient and introduce yourself.
4. Show the patient into the treatment room. Explain the procedure and discuss any concerns the patient may have.
5. Instruct the patient to empty the bladder, take off all clothing from the waist down, and put on the gown with the opening in the back.
6. Put on exam gloves and assist the patient into the knee-chest or Sims' position. Immediately cover the patient with a drape.

7. Use warm water to bring the sigmoidoscope to slightly above body temperature; lubricate the tip.

   *Rationale*
   To ensure patient comfort

8. Assist as needed, including handing the doctor the necessary instruments and equipment.
9. Monitor the patient's reactions during the procedure, and relay any signs of pain to the doctor.
10. Clean the anal area with tissues after the exam.
11. Properly dispose of used materials and disposable instruments.
12. Remove the gloves and wash your hands.
13. Help the patient gradually assume a comfortable position.

    *Rationale*
    The patient should sit up slowly so that he does not become faint.

14. Instruct the patient to dress.
15. Put on clean gloves.
16. Sanitize reusable instruments and prepare them for disinfection and/or sterilization, as necessary.
17. Clean and disinfect the equipment and the room according to OSHA guidelines.
18. Remove the gloves and wash your hands.

---

outpatient facility. You may be responsible for scheduling tests at such facilities for patients. You can help prepare the patient in general terms for these exams; however, the patient should discuss specific preparation with personnel from the radiologic facility.

***Cholecystography.*** **Cholecystography** is a gallbladder function test performed by x-ray with a contrast agent. The patient swallows tablets of the contrast agent the night before the test. X-rays taken 12 to 14 hours later should show the contrast agent in the gallbladder. The patient then swallows a substance high in fat, which should make the gallbladder contract and empty the contrast agent into the duodenum. If the contrast agent is not taken up by the gallbladder or if the gallbladder does not contract properly, the doctor can determine whether there is bile duct obstruction or gallstones.

***Ultrasound.*** Ultrasound is used commonly for diagnosing problems in the gallbladder, pancreas, spleen, and liver.

The patient should have nothing to eat or drink after midnight of the night before and on the morning of the exam. Some gastroenterologists may perform ultrasound exams in the office.

***Barium Swallow.*** The barium swallow (also called an upper GI series) is used to detect abnormalities in the esophagus, stomach, and small intestine. The patient swallows a liquid containing barium, an insoluble contrast agent. This material is viewed using fluoroscopy (moving x-ray images) as the liquid is swallowed and passes into the stomach. X-ray films are taken at frequent intervals to record the diagnostic images. The patient is asked to move into various positions while the barium is tracked through the small intestine. To prepare for this test, the patient should have nothing to eat or drink after midnight of the night before and on the morning of the procedure.

***Barium Enema.*** A barium enema (also called a lower GI series) is used to detect abnormalities in the large

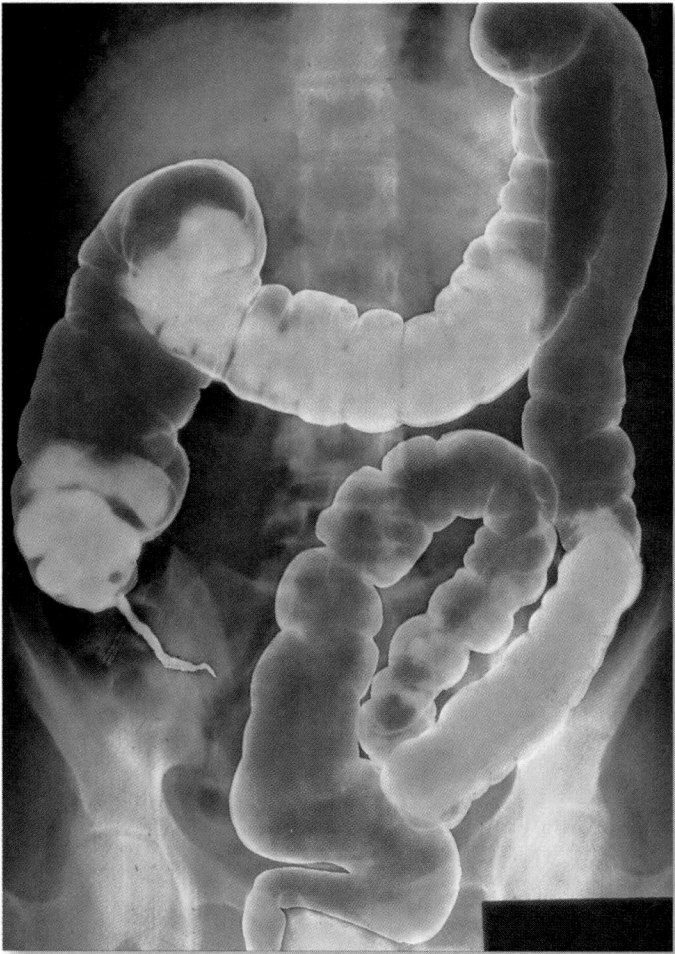

**Figure 27-12.** During a barium enema, the barium is tracked on x-rays.

intestine. Barium is given as an enema in this test. A balloon-like tube is inflated in the rectum during the x-ray, and the patient is asked to move into various positions to ensure that the barium is distributed completely (Figure 27-12).

Patients must eat no meats or vegetables for 1 to 3 days before the test to avoid incorrect indications on the x-ray. For 24 hours before the test, they must also follow a liquid diet, which includes drinking special liquid laxative preparations and more than a quart of water. The staff at the facility performing the test instructs patients about the specific steps, but the intent is to cleanse the colon completely.

*Radionuclide Imaging.* Radiology subspecialists who are trained in nuclear medicine perform nuclear medicine studies with radionuclide imaging. The patient is first injected with a radioactive substance, then waits a prescribed length of time for the radioactive substance to be taken up by the body part that is being imaged. The patient is scanned or photographed with a special gamma camera, which can read the radioactive areas to determine abnormalities in their composition. This technique is commonly used for liver, spleen, thyroid, and bone scans.

## Gastrointestinal Diseases and Disorders

The level of discomfort from GI disorders can be misleading in relation to severity. There may be severe pain with intestinal gas, which is not serious, whereas there is virtually no pain in the initial stage of appendicitis, which is potentially life-threatening. Be sure that your notes are accurate and complete when a patient reports GI symptoms. Note the level of the patient's pain and whether over-the-counter (OTC) drugs have been administered. Common diseases and disorders treated by a GI specialist are outlined in Table 27-3.

## Neurology

Neurologists diagnose and treat diseases and disorders of the central nervous system (CNS) and associated systems. Nervous system injuries or diseases can result in loss of sensation, loss or impairment of voluntary movement, seizures, or mental confusion.

Your duties in a neurologist's office include assisting with exams by readying equipment for use, positioning the patient, and handing the doctor tools and other items. You may be asked to perform parts of these exams. You may also assist with certain diagnostic tests, such as electroencephalography. Your responsibilities will include instructing and educating patients and their families about procedures, disorders, and treatments.

| TABLE 27-3 | Common Gastrointestinal Diseases and Disorders | |
|---|---|---|
| **Condition** | **Description** | **Treatment** |
| Abdominal hernia | Weakness of abdominal wall muscle with outpouching, caused by heavy lifting; exacerbated by general lack of muscle tone; usually asymptomatic except for outpouching; severe pain may indicate complication of strangulated hernia, causing lack of blood supply | Surgery to repair muscle |

*continued* ⟶

## TABLE 27-3 Common Gastrointestinal Diseases and Disorders *(concluded)*

| Condition | Description | Treatment |
|---|---|---|
| Anal fissure | Ulcer in anal wall; symptoms include painful defecation with burning; may develop into fistula (abnormal duct to rectum) | Dependent on extent, may include surgery to repair |
| Cholecystitis | Inflammation of gallbladder; may be caused by intolerance to fatty foods, gallstones, or bacterial infection; symptoms include pain, nausea, diarrhea | Avoidance of fatty foods for intolerance; lithotripsy (noninvasive shock waves) to break up stones; antibiotic for bacterial infection |
| Cholelithiasis | Formation of gallstones from cholesterol in bile; symptoms include pain, nausea, diarrhea; complications include secondary bacterial infection | Lithotripsy, antibiotics to prevent secondary infection |
| Colitis | Inflammation of colon caused by bacteria, food intolerance, anxiety, or emotional disorder; symptoms include cramping, pain, diarrhea or bloody diarrhea with mucus or pus, fever, malaise, weight loss, nausea; complications include life-threatening infection or blood poisoning, liver damage, hemorrhoids, anemia, arthritis | Diet modification (clear liquid for acute phase), medication, psychotherapy, fluid replacement, surgery for severe cases; surgery may include insertion of elimination tube (colostomy tube) for temporary or permanent elimination of solid waste |
| Constipation | Hard feces or stools, decrease in frequency of or ability to have bowel movements, complication of fecal impaction | Diet modification, stool-softener medication, enemas, surgery if necessary for impaction |
| Diarrhea | Abnormally frequent and watery bowel movements caused by bacterial or viral infection or food poisoning, complication of dehydration with fluid-electrolyte imbalance | Diet modification, antibiotics for bacterial infection, medication to prevent dehydration |
| Diverticulitis | Inflammation of diverticulum, usually in colon; symptoms may be absent, may include abdominal pain | Diet modification, surgery possible for severe cases |
| Gastritis | Inflammation of stomach lining, causing excess secretion of gastric acids and bloating; numerous causes | Diet modification, drug therapy |
| Gastroesophageal reflux | Gastric acid rising into esophagus due to abnormal valve function; causes heartburn; symptoms may be similar to those of angina, dysphagia (inability to swallow) | Diet modification (including eating small meals), antacids, upright eating, remaining upright for several hours after eating, surgery (rarely) |
| Hemorrhoids | Enlargement of veins in rectal or anal area, may protrude from anus; symptoms include itching, pain, red blood with defecation | Diet modification, surgery |
| Hiatal hernia | Protrusion of stomach through diaphragm defect into thorax; symptoms similar to those of gastroesophageal reflux plus pain | Diet therapy with small and frequent meals, exercise, upright eating, medication |
| Stomatitis (canker sores) | Sore gums or other oral areas caused by herpes virus or acidic body chemistry; exacerbated by emotional distress, foods high in acid; symptoms include ulcerations (canker sores) with burning, sometimes swelling | Bland diet, avoidance of stress, medicated mouth rinses, topical anesthetic |

## Neurologic Exams

The neurologist evaluates five categories of neurologic function in a complete exam:

1. Cognitive function (mental status)
2. Cranial nerves
3. Motor system
4. Reflexes
5. Sensory system

Cognitive function can be assessed by observing general appearance and grooming as well as by asking patients specific questions. The neurologist also determines the status of the cranial nerves, which affect smell and taste, eye movements, hearing, voice quality, facial expression, and facial mobility. The physician may, for example, ask patients to close their eyes and then identify familiar smells. The neurologist observes patients' faces for symmetry of movement and tests visual and auditory acuity. The physician assesses motor ability by testing coordination, observing gait, and determining muscle strength. Finally, the neurologist tests patients' reflexes and examines the function of the sensory system in areas of tactile sensation, pain and temperature sensitivity, and awareness of vibration. You are likely to assist the physician in completing these exams, and you may perform certain components yourself.

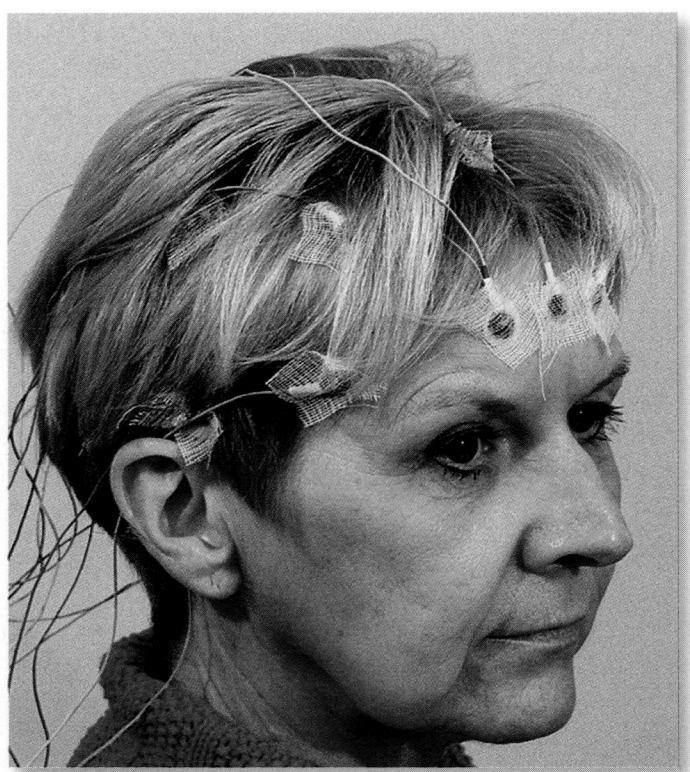

**Figure 27-13.** EEG electrodes are attached to the patient's forehead and scalp.

## Diagnostic Testing

Common diagnostic tests in neurology include electroencephalography and various radiologic tests. You may assist in performing these tests. Many tests are done at a site apart from the physician's office. In such cases you will need to schedule the procedures, instruct patients about pretest preparations, and educate them about the procedure and what to expect.

**Electroencephalography.** **Electroencephalography** records the electrical activity of the brain on a strip of graph paper. The tracing is an electroencephalogram (EEG). Electrodes are attached to the patient's scalp, and readings are taken while the patient is at rest and engaged in specific activities (Figure 27-13). An EEG can be used to detect or examine conditions such as tumors, seizure disorders, or brain injury. You may assist with electrode placement or, after training, obtain the EEG on your own.

**Imaging Procedures.** Several imaging techniques are used as neurological diagnostic tools. Types of procedures include angiograms, brain scans, CT, MRI, myelography, and skull x-rays.

***Cerebral Angiography.*** Cerebral angiography (or angiogram) is a radiologic study of the cerebral blood vessels. After a contrast medium is injected into an artery, x-rays are taken to visualize the cerebral blood vessels.

***Brain Scan.*** A brain scan is performed by injecting the patient with radioisotopes and, after a period of time, using a scanner to detect the material. The radioisotopes tend to gather in areas of abnormality, such as tumors or abscesses.

***Computed Tomography.*** **Computed tomography,** often called a CT scan, is a radiographic exam that produces a three-dimensional, cross-sectional view of the brain. Often one scan is done without a contrast medium. Then a contrast medium is injected for greater clarity. CT scans can help diagnose a wide range of conditions, including tumors, blood clots, and brain swelling.

***Magnetic Resonance Imaging.*** **Magnetic resonance imaging (MRI)** is a viewing technique that enables physicians to see areas inside the body without exposing the patient to x-rays or surgery. The procedure, which takes 30 to 60 minutes, requires the patient to lie still on a padded table that is moved into a tunnel-like structure (Figure 27-14). A powerful magnetic field produces an image of internal body structures.

***Positron Emission Tomography.*** **Positron emission tomography,** often called a **PET** scan, studies the blood flow and metabolic activity in the brain to help physicians identify certain neurological and CNS disorders. These disorders include Parkinson's disease, multiple sclerosis, Alzheimer's disease, transient ischemic attack (TIA), amyotrophic lateral sclerosis (ALS), Huntington's disease, epilepsy, stroke, and schizophrenia.

***Myelography.*** **Myelography** is an x-ray visualization of the spinal cord after the injection of a radioactive contrast medium or air into the spinal subarachnoid space

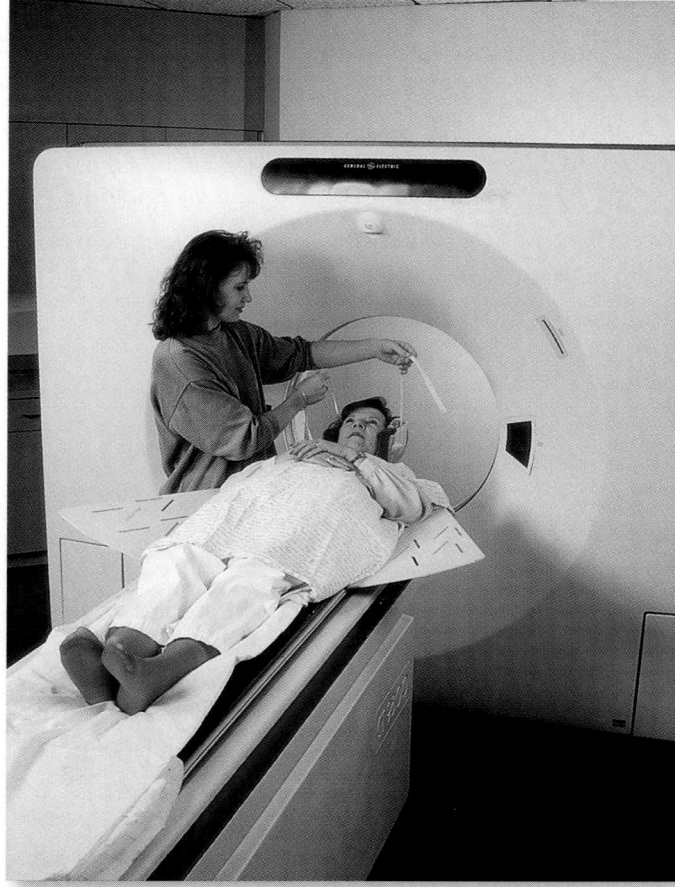

**Figure 27-14.** Magnetic resonance imaging is used to diagnose disorders in many specialties.

(between the second and innermost of three membranes that cover the spinal cord). This test can reveal tumors, cysts, spinal stenosis, or herniated disks.

*Skull X-Ray.* Skull x-rays may be used to detect breaks in the skull. They can also be used to locate tumors.

**Other Tests.** Other diagnostic tests do not involve imaging techniques. They include lumbar puncture and electromyography. A lumbar puncture, or spinal tap, involves collecting a sample of cerebrospinal fluid (CSF). A needle is inserted between two lumbar vertebrae and into the subarachnoid space. The collected fluid is sent to a laboratory for analysis. This test is used to diagnose infection, to measure CSF pressure, and to check for blood cells and proteins in the fluid.

**Electromyography** is used to detect neuromuscular disorders or nerve damage. Needle electrodes are inserted into some of the patient's skeletal muscles. When the muscles contract, a monitor records the nerve impulses and measures conduction time.

## Neurologic Diseases and Disorders

Common diseases of the neurologic system are described in Table 27-4. Trauma can also cause damage to the nervous system. Traumatic injuries can result in loss of

sensation and voluntary motion. Paralysis on one side of the body, as a result of damage to the opposite side of the brain, is called hemiplegia. Paraplegia involves motor or sensory loss in the lower extremities. Paralysis of the arms, legs, and muscles below the place where the spinal cord is damaged is called quadriplegia.

Patients with acquired immunodeficiency syndrome (AIDS) may exhibit specific neurologic symptoms related to their disease. These include:

- Meningitis caused by a fungal infection
- Encephalopathy (degenerative effect on the brain), resulting in headaches, difficulty concentrating, and apathy
- Peripheral neuropathies (disorders of the peripheral nerves) that result in pain or changes in gait

## Oncology

An oncologist specializes in the detection and treatment of tumors and cancerous growths. The term cancer refers to a number of oncologic diseases that affect different body systems. All cancers are characterized by the uncontrolled growth and spread of abnormal cells. A tumor is a lump of abnormal cells. Tumors are classified as benign or malignant. Benign tumors contain abnormal cells, but the cells do not invade and actively destroy surrounding tissue. Malignant tumors contain cells that grow uncontrollably, invading and actively destroying the tissue around them. Malignant, or cancerous, growths are capable of metastasis, the transfer of abnormal cells to body sites far removed from the original tumor. When cells become malignant, the process is called carcinogenesis.

You will encounter patients with a variety of medical conditions in an oncologist's office. You must be aware of the various types of cancer, what their symptoms are, and how they are treated (Table 27-5). Part of your job will involve preparing patients for the side effects of cancer treatment and helping patients deal with them. Patient and family education and support are essential.

## Diagnostic Testing

Cancer is detected and diagnosed through a variety of procedures. You will schedule some of these tests and provide pretest instructions and explanations to patients. You may obtain blood specimens for some tests and assist in other diagnostic procedures, including:

- X-rays
- CT scan
- MRI
- Blood tests, especially those to detect tumor markers, such as carcinoembryonic antigen (CEA) (increased levels of CEA indicate a variety of cancers), CA125, and CA15-3

## TABLE 27-4 Common Diseases of the Neurological System

| Condition | Description | Treatment |
|---|---|---|
| Alzheimer's disease | Disabling disease that usually affects elderly people; involves dementia and deterioration of physical function | Frequent stimulation to possibly help slow deterioration, medications that may slow progression of some symptoms |
| Bell's palsy | Suddenly occurring cranial nerve disease that causes weakness or paralysis on one side of face | Usually resolves without treatment in 1 to 8 weeks |
| Encephalitis | Inflammation of brain tissue usually caused by viral infection; symptoms include fever, headache, vomiting, stiff neck, drowsiness | Medication, rest |
| Epilepsy | Disease caused by misfiring of nerve groups in brain, resulting in seizures | Medication |
| Herpes zoster | Disease caused by virus that causes chickenpox; symptoms include painful blisters that form along path of one or more nerves | Medication to relieve pain |
| Meningitis | Inflammation of meninges (membranes covering brain and spinal cord) caused by bacterial or viral infection; symptoms include fever, chills, stiff neck, headache, vomiting | Medication such as antibiotics and drugs to reduce swelling |
| Migraine headaches | Severe headaches caused by vascular disturbance and characterized by pain, nausea, and sometimes visual disturbances | Medication |
| Multiple sclerosis | Degenerative disease of central nervous system that results in visual problems, muscle weakness, paralysis | Anti-inflammatory medications used during attacks |
| Neuritis | Inflammation of one or more nerves; symptoms include severe pain and discomfort or paralysis of affected area | Medication and rest |
| Parkinson's disease | Progressive neurological disease, causing symptoms of muscular rigidity and tremors | Medication to relieve symptoms |
| Sciatica | Inflammation of sciatic nerve causing pain in back of thigh and down leg | Medication to relieve pain, rest, heat applications |

- Ultrasonography
- Biopsy, the removal of a sample of fluid or tissue from a growth (see the discussion of surgery as a medical specialty later in this chapter)

## Cancer Treatment

Cancer treatments fall into three general categories: surgery, radiation therapy, and chemotherapy. Often a combination of these treatment methods is used. All methods damage healthy as well as cancerous cells. The success of treatment depends on many factors, and recovery varies greatly from patient to patient.

**Surgery.** Surgical removal of all or part of the tumor and some surrounding tissue is one method of cancer treatment. It is most effective when the tumor appears to be contained within a particular organ or is localized in an area of the skin. Surgery is often followed, however, by either radiation therapy or chemotherapy.

**Radiation Therapy.** Radiation therapy uses radiation to kill and stop the growth of tumor cells. It is often used in conjunction with surgery or chemotherapy. Radiation therapy is effective because radiation has the most damaging effect on cells that are undergoing rapid division, such as cancer cells.

**Chemotherapy.** Chemotherapy is also used in conjunction with other therapies. Chemotherapy uses strong anticancer drugs to kill malignant cells. As with radiation therapy, rapidly dividing cells, such as cancer cells, are most strongly affected by these medications.

## TABLE 27-5 Common Cancers by Body System

| Body System | Symptoms | Treatment |
|---|---|---|
| **Skeletal System** | | |
| Osteosarcoma: malignant lesion, usually in femur, tibia, or humerus | Pain and swelling, central hardened portion with softer edges, possible pathologic fracture | Radiation and chemotherapy to minimize tumor, surgery |
| Chondrosarcomas: malignant tumors of cartilage | Dull pain and swelling | Radiation and chemotherapy to minimize tumor, surgery |
| **Nervous System** | | |
| Malignant gliomas: tumors of brain and brainstem | Headache, vomiting, changes in sensation or personality | Surgery, radiation, chemotherapy |
| **Endocrine System** | | |
| Thyroid cancer | Nodules on thyroid gland | Surgery, radiation |
| Pancreatic cancer | Weight loss, abdominal pain, jaundice; very lethal form of cancer | Surgery, chemotherapy with radiation |
| **Circulatory System** | | |
| Leukemia: several diseases involving abnormal overproduction of cells in bone marrow | Fatigue, paleness, repeated infections | Chemotherapy, bone marrow transplants |
| Lymphoma: cancers of lymph system; divided into Hodgkin's lymphoma and non-Hodgkin's lymphoma | Enlarged lymph nodes, itching, fever, weight loss | Chemotherapy, radiation |
| **Respiratory System** | | |
| Lung cancer | Often no early symptoms; later, new cough or cold that lingers; chest, shoulder, and/or back pain; wheezing and shortness of breath; hoarseness; coughing up blood; swelling in the face and neck; difficulty in swallowing; weight loss and anorexia; increased fatigue; recurrent respiratory infections | Surgery, radiation, chemotherapy |
| **Digestive System** | | |
| Oral cancer: cancer of mouth or throat | May begin with painless sore or mass; later, difficulty chewing or swallowing | Surgery, radiation, chemotherapy |
| Esophageal cancer | Often no early symptoms; later, difficulty swallowing, regurgitation of food | Surgery, radiation, chemotherapy |
| Stomach cancer | Indigestion, weight loss, nausea | Surgery, chemotherapy |
| Liver cancer | Abdominal pain, fatigue, jaundice | Surgery, liver transplant |
| Colorectal cancer | Changes in bowel habits, blood in stools, rectal or abdominal pain | Surgery combined with radiation or chemotherapy |

*continued* ⟶

## TABLE 27-5  Common Cancers by Body System (concluded)

| Body System | Symptoms | Treatment |
| --- | --- | --- |
| **Urinary System** | | |
| Bladder cancer | Urinary frequency or urgency, blood in urine | Surgery, chemotherapy |
| Kidney cancer | Back or abdominal pain, blood in urine | Surgery, radiation, chemotherapy |
| **Reproductive System** | | |
| Cervical cancer | Usually none, possible painless vaginal bleeding; abnormal Pap smear (Papanicolaou smear) | Surgery, radiation, chemotherapy |
| Endometrial cancer: cancer of uterine lining | Postmenopausal bleeding | Surgery, radiation, chemotherapy |
| Ovarian cancer | Usually none, possible abdominal pain | Surgery, radiation, chemotherapy |
| Breast cancer | Lump or thickening in breast, changed appearance, discharge | Surgery, radiation, chemotherapy |
| Prostate cancer | Often none; possible difficult, frequent, or painful urination | Surgery, radiation, chemotherapy |
| Testicular cancer | Lump in testicle | Surgery, radiation, chemotherapy |

## TABLE 27-6  Chemotherapy Drugs

| Category | Mechanism of Action | Examples |
| --- | --- | --- |
| Alkylating agents | Hinder cell division | Chlorambucil, cyclophosphamide |
| Antimetabolites | Interfere with folic acid and nucleic acid synthesis | Methotrexate, fluorouracil |
| Antibiotics | Break DNA strands | Actinomycin, bleomycin |
| Antimitotic agents | Affect cell division | Vinblastine, paclitaxel |

There are a variety of chemotherapy drugs available, each with slightly different mechanisms of action. Table 27-6 outlines the major categories of chemotherapy drugs, their mechanism of action, and some examples in each category. These drugs can be used alone or in combination depending on the type of cancer being treated. Although it is unlikely that you will prepare or administer anticancer drugs, you need to be aware that they are highly toxic. General protective guidelines must be followed whenever there is risk of contact with the drugs or patients' body fluids. Measures include wearing complete personal protective equipment and properly handling and disposing of materials contaminated with body fluids.

# Ophthalmology

An ophthalmologist treats the eyes and related tissues. Chapter 25 discussed vision screening tests and procedures that might be encountered in a general physician's office. Some eye exams and procedures will also be performed in an ophthalmologist's office. The most common eye disorders that an ophthalmologist treats are visual defects, which are often correctable with eyeglasses or contact lenses. Ophthalmologists also treat eye injuries and remove foreign bodies from the eye. More serious disorders, such as cataracts and glaucoma, require medication or surgery. In an ophthalmologist's

# PROCEDURE 27.3

## Preparing the Ophthalmoscope for Use

**Procedure Goal:** To ensure that the ophthalmoscope is ready for use during an eye exam

**OSHA Guidelines:** This procedure does not involve exposure to blood, body fluids, or tissues.

**Materials:** Ophthalmoscope, lens, spare bulb, spare battery

**Method:**

1. Wash your hands.
2. Take the ophthalmoscope out of its battery charger. In a darkened room, turn on the ophthalmoscope light.
3. Shine the large beam of white light on the back of your hand to check that the instrument's tiny lightbulb is providing strong enough light (Figure 27-15).
4. Replace the bulb or battery if necessary. (The battery is located in the ophthalmoscope's handle.)

5. Make sure the instrument's lens is screwed into the handle. If it is not, attach the lens.

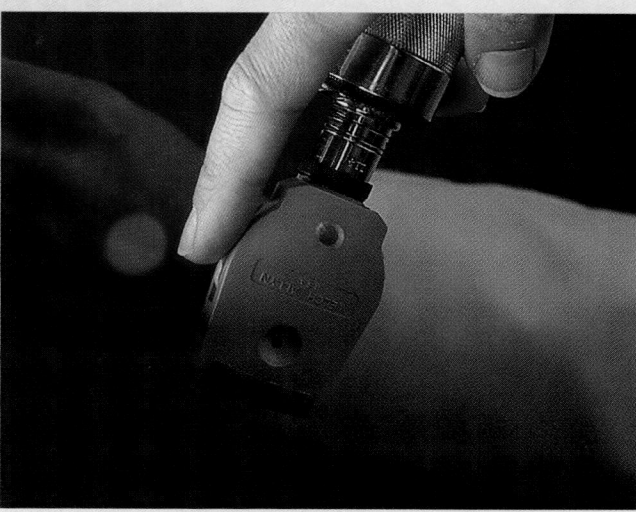

**Figure 27-15.** Shine the ophthalmoscope light on your hand to check the strength of the beam.

---

office you may perform some of the procedures that involve measuring various aspects and functions of the eye, such as visual acuity, color vision, and intraocular pressure.

## Ophthalmic Exams

An ophthalmologist performs an eye exam by inspecting the interior of the patient's eyes, including the retina, optic nerve, and blood vessels. The physician uses an **ophthalmoscope,** a handheld instrument with a light, to view the inner eye structures. You will maintain and prepare this instrument for the physician's use, as described in Procedure 27-3.

An ophthalmologist also tests the patient's visual fields. The visual field is the entire area visible to the eye when the patient looks at an object straight ahead. Visual fields are assessed by the confrontation method. The doctor stands or sits about 2 feet in front of the patient. The patient covers one eye, and the doctor closes her own opposite eye. (This makes the visual fields of the two individuals roughly the same.) Then the doctor moves a pencil or other object into the patient's horizontal or vertical visual field, asking the patient to say "Now" when the object comes into view. Defects in field of vision are noted. Convergence of the eyes is tested by bringing the handheld object to the patient's nose as the eyes focus on it.

The ophthalmologist also routinely tests for glaucoma with the aid of a tonometer (Figure 27-16). The tonometer measures intraocular pressure, shown by the eyeball's resistance to indentation. Your role is to explain the procedure to the patient, instill anesthetizing eyedrops into the patient's eyes when required, assist the patient into position, and hand the doctor the instruments.

The eye exam may also include a **refraction exam** to verify the need for corrective lenses. Normally, the lens and other parts of the eye work together to focus images on the retina. When errors of refraction exist, images are focused incorrectly, causing conditions such as farsightedness and nearsightedness. A refraction exam is performed with a retinoscope or a Phoroptor, the trademark name for a device that contains many different lenses. The doctor has the patient look through a succession of lens combinations to find out which one creates the clearest image (Figure 27-17).

Another instrument the ophthalmologist may use during the exam is the **slitlamp.** This instrument consists of a magnifying lens combined with a light source. It is used to examine the anterior structures of the eye including the eyelids, iris, lens, and cornea. Patients rest their chin on the device's chin rest and stare straight ahead while the doctor shines a narrow beam (slit) of light into the eye and looks at the eye through the instrument's lens.

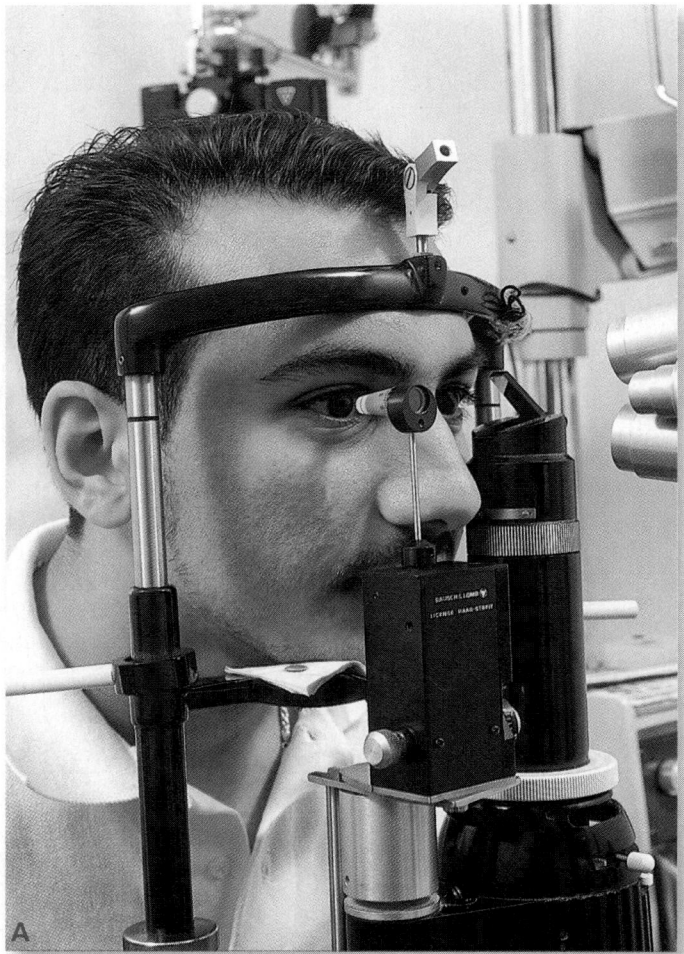

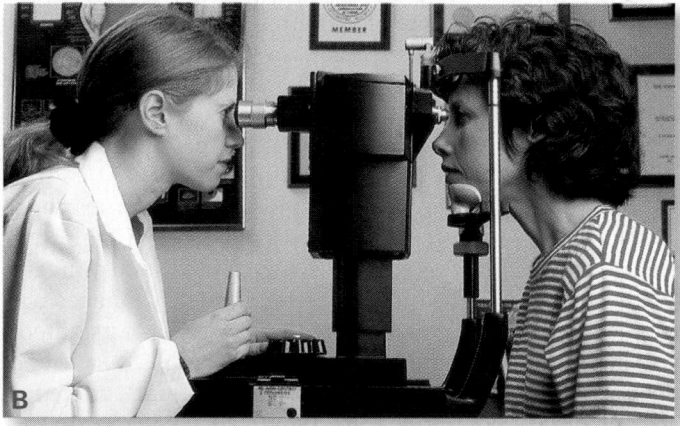

**Figure 27-16.** Two types of tonometers are: (A) the applanation tonometer, which actually touches the eyeball during assessment; and (B) the noncontract, or air-puff, tonometer, which directs a puff of air at the cornea.

## Eye Diseases and Disorders

An ophthalmologist treats a wide range of eye diseases and disorders. Some, such as a sty or conjunctivitis, do not greatly affect vision and may be treated by a general practitioner. Others affect the internal workings of the eye and require the attention of a specialist.

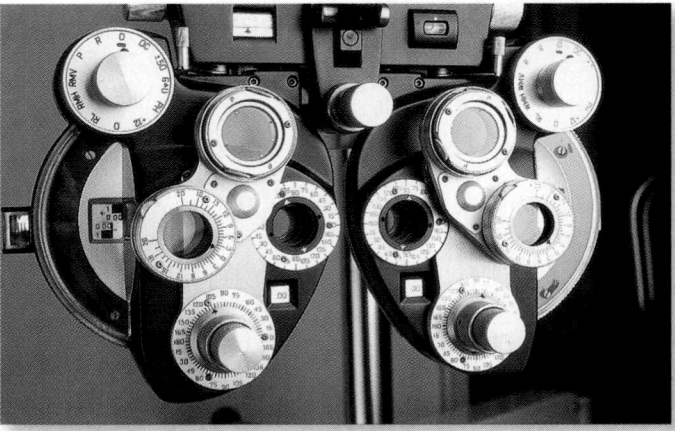

**Figure 27-17.** The Phoroptor helps the ophthalmologist assess errors of refraction.

**Disorders of External Eye Structures.** Some disorders affect external eye structures. These structures include the eyelid and the eyelashes.

*Blepharitis.* Blepharitis is a chronic inflammation of the edges of the eyelid, more common in older individuals than in younger people. It can be caused by infection or by the same skin condition that causes dandruff. Symptoms include red, swollen eyelids with scaling or crusting of skin at the edges. The patient's eyes may be irritated and itchy. Proper eye care and hygiene often clear up the condition successfully. Antibiotic creams may be necessary in severe cases.

*Ptosis.* Ptosis is a drooping of the upper eyelid in which the lid partially or completely covers the eye. It is caused by weakness of or damage to the muscle that raises the eyelid or by problems with the nerve that controls the muscle. Often no treatment is required, although surgery may be performed if the condition interferes with vision or if the patient is concerned about appearance.

*Sty.* A sty (external hordeolum) is the result of an infection of an eyelash follicle. A red, painful swelling appears on the edge of the eye and typically forms a white head of pus. The head bursts and drains before it heals in about a week. Applying warm, moist compresses to the sty may help it drain sooner.

**Disorders of Structures at the Front of the Eye.** Another group of disorders affects structures at the front of the eye. These structures include the conjunctiva and the cornea.

*Conjunctivitis.* Conjunctivitis, or pinkeye, is an inflammation of the conjunctiva caused by allergy, an irritant, or infection. It is a common disorder that is annoying but normally not serious.

Allergic conjunctivitis occurs when a person has an allergic reaction to pollen, makeup, or other substance. The symptoms are itchy, red eyes. The doctor may prescribe medication to relieve troublesome symptoms and suggest avoidance of the trigger whenever possible.

Conjunctivitis may also be caused by irritants such as dust, smoke, wind, pollutants, and excessive glare.

Infectious conjunctivitis can be caused by either a bacterial or a viral infection. Both forms are easily spread and have symptoms including redness and a gritty feeling in the eye. Bacterial infections typically produce pus, which may form a crust on the eye during sleep. Viral infections usually produce a watery discharge. Although eye irrigation or saline drops may be used to soothe eyes affected by either type of infection, only bacterial infections are treated with antibiotic drops or ointment.

Because you may not know the cause of a patient's conjunctivitis (allergies, irritants, bacteria, viruses), take precautions to avoid spreading infection. As with any potentially infectious disease, use Universal Precautions in medical settings. Wear appropriate personal protective equipment when dealing with any patient who has conjunctivitis.

***Corneal Ulcers and Abrasions.*** Ulcers (lesions) on the cornea may be the result of injury, infection, or both. An injury such as an abrasion (scratch) on the cornea can become infected with bacteria, viruses, or fungi. The symptoms of a corneal ulcer include pain or discomfort and unclear vision. Treatment consists of antibiotic eyedrops or ointments and use of an eye patch.

## Disorders Involving Internal Eye Structures.
Another group of disorders affects structures inside the eye. Cataracts, for example, affect the lens. Glaucoma can damage several internal eye structures.

***Cataracts.*** Cataracts are cloudy or opaque areas in the normally clear lens of the eye. Cataracts develop gradually, blocking the passage of light through the eye. The result is a progressive loss of vision in one or both eyes. In severe cases you can actually see the cloudy lens through the pupil of the eye (Figure 27-18).

Cataracts are more common in the elderly than in younger people because the lens deteriorates with aging.

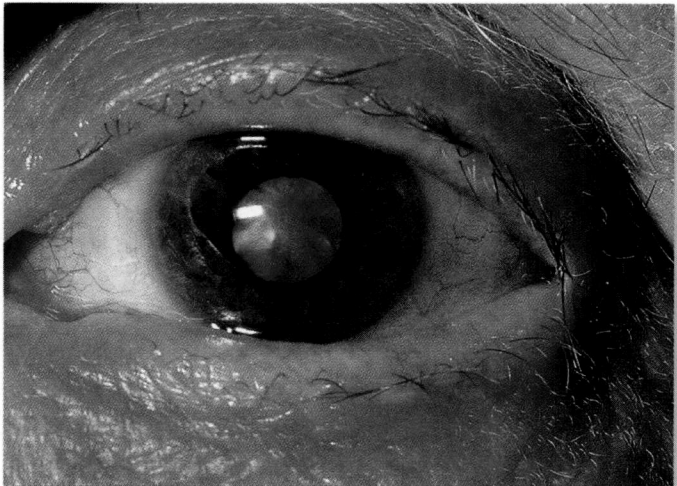

**Figure 27-18.** The lens of an eye with a cataract has a clouded appearance.

Cataracts can also be caused by iritis, injury, ultraviolet radiation, or diabetes. Some cataracts are congenital. Cataracts are treated by surgically removing the lens and using an artificial lens in its place. The artificial lens may be in the form of special eyeglasses, special contact lenses, or an intraocular lens inserted at the time of cataract surgery.

***Glaucoma.*** Glaucoma is a condition in which fluid pressure builds up inside the eye. This pressure damages the internal structures of the eye and gradually destroys vision. Glaucoma is the second leading cause of blindness in the United States and the first cause among African Americans.

Aqueous humor is produced by capillaries in the ciliary body. This fluid circulates between the lens and the cornea. The fluid drains out of this area through the angle formed by the iris and the cornea. The aqueous humor diffuses into a vascular channel (Schlemm's canal) that encircles the cornea where it meets the sclera. The aqueous humor then returns to the systemic circulation (the circulation of the blood to body tissues).

In a patient with glaucoma, the fluid drains out of the eye too slowly or fails to drain at all. The result is a buildup of intraocular pressure. Retinal nerve fibers are damaged and blood vessels are destroyed, leading to loss of vision and possible blindness.

Glaucoma is treated with medication that reduces pressure in the eye. Drops, pills, or both may be prescribed to reduce the production of aqueous humor. A procedure called an iridotomy is sometimes performed. This procedure is a type of laser surgery in which a small hole is created in the iris that allows the excess fluid to drain. If the surgery is not effective, an iridectomy (removal of part of the iris) is done to create a larger opening in the iris to allow drainage.

***Iritis.*** Iritis, also known as uveitis, is an inflammation of the iris and sometimes the ciliary body. White blood cells from the inflamed area and protein that leaks from small blood vessels float in the aqueous humor. The symptoms of iritis are pain or discomfort in one or both eyes; pain may be worse in bright light. The eye is red, and loss of vision may occur. Left untreated, iritis can lead to other complications, such as glaucoma and cataracts. Iritis is treated with anti-inflammatory drops or ointment.

## Disorders of the Retina.
Several serious disorders affect the retina, the internal layer of the back of the eye. These disorders include retinal detachment, diabetic retinopathy, and macular degeneration.

***Retinal Detachment.*** Retinal detachment occurs when the retina separates from the underlying choroid layer. When this separation occurs, vision is damaged.

Retinal detachment is rare; however, it is more common as people age. Early symptoms of detachment include flashes of light or floating black shapes, both of which can occur as the hole in the retina forms. Patients occasionally describe their field of vision as being like a window shade that has been pulled down. Peripheral vision is lost as the retina detaches. Vision becomes progressively blurred as detachment continues.

When detected early, a hole can be "sealed" so that the retina does not detach. If the retina has already detached, some vision can often be restored with new surgical and laser treatments.

***Diabetic Retinopathy.*** Diabetic retinopathy is a complication of diabetes. People who have had diabetes for a long time or who do not keep their condition under control experience damage to small blood vessels that supply the retina. The vessels initially leak fluid, which distorts vision. As the disease progresses, fragile new blood vessels grow on the retina and bleed into the vitreous humor. Scar tissue may also form on the retina. The result is loss of vision. The damage usually cannot be repaired, but the disorder can be controlled to prevent further loss of vision.

***Macular Degeneration.*** The macula is the area of the retina responsible for the central area of a person's visual field. For unknown reasons the macula begins to deteriorate as some individuals age. Macular degeneration causes loss of vision in the center of an image; peripheral vision remains intact. Macular degeneration is the leading cause of blindness among the elderly in the United States.

Loss of sharp vision occurs very gradually and without pain. One of the first signs is difficulty in reading. The loss of vision often appears as a dark spot in the center of the field of vision. If macular degeneration is detected early, laser surgery may restore some vision or prevent further loss.

**Disorders Involving Eye Movement.** Normally, both eyes move together when people look at objects. Strabismus is the name for a deviation of one eye. Strabismus in young children is caused by misaligned or unbalanced eye muscles. A condition called amblyopia may occur as the misaligned eye becomes "lazy." The brain tends to ignore what the lazy eye sees; if the condition is not treated, vision will be affected in this eye. Treatment involves putting a patch over the fully working eye to force the child to use the other eye. Eyeglasses may be used along with the patch. In some cases surgery on the eye muscle is required.

Strabismus in adults usually results from problems with the nerves connecting the brain and the eye muscles or with the muscles themselves. Conditions that can cause such problems include diabetes, high blood pressure, brain injury, muscular dystrophy, and inflammation of certain cerebral arteries. Treatment depends on the cause of the condition.

**Refractive Disorders.** Refraction refers to the way light from objects is focused through the eye to form an image on the retina. The normal eye focuses light exactly at the retina, producing a clear image (Figure 27-19). In

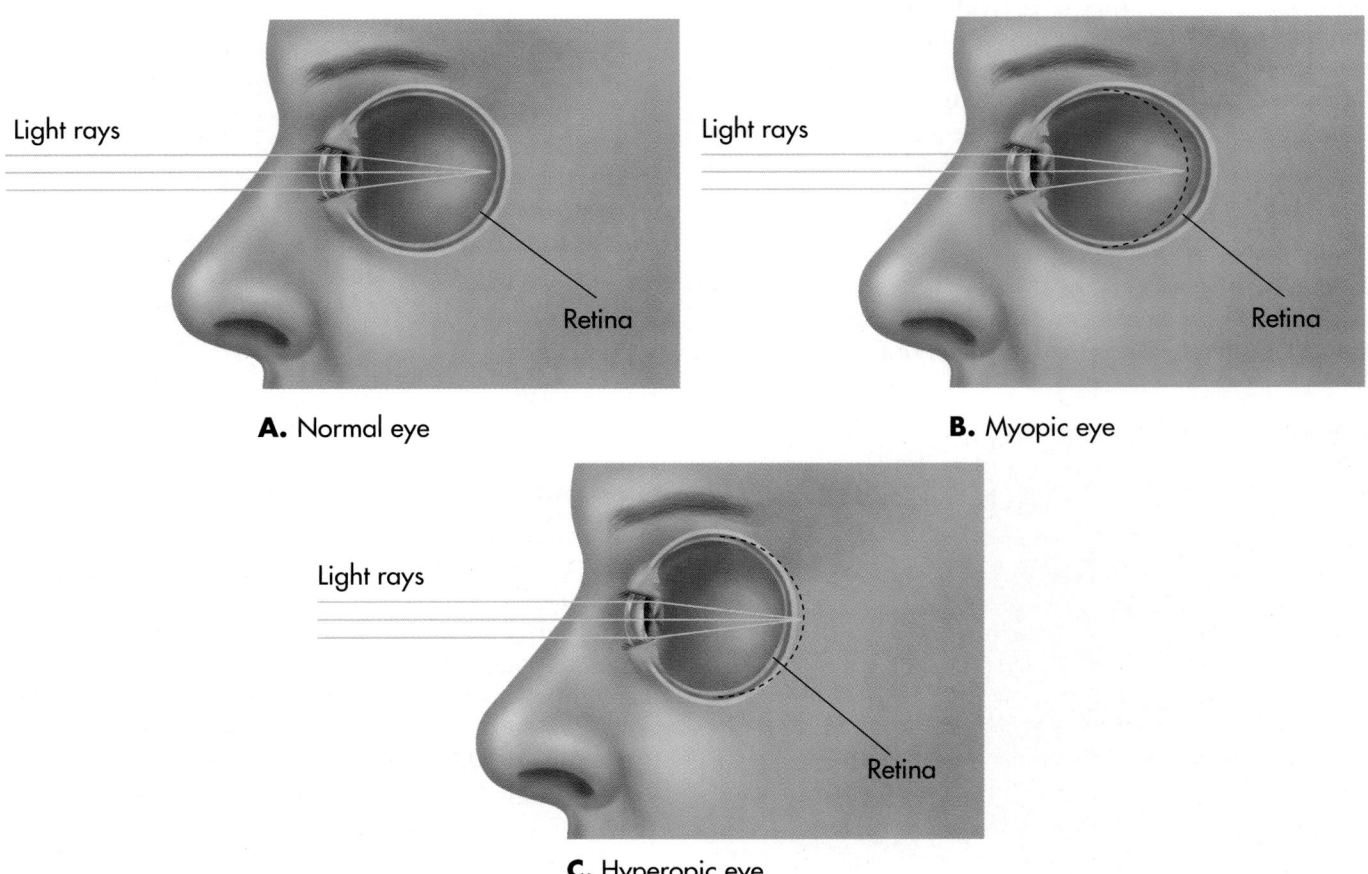

**A.** Normal eye

**B.** Myopic eye

**C.** Hyperopic eye

**Figure 27-19.** (A) In the normal eye, light rays are focused directly on the retina. (B) With myopia, an elongated eyeball causes light rays to be focused in front of the retina. (C) With hyperopia, a shortened eyeball cases light rays to be focused behind the retina.

some people the eye focuses light either in front of or behind the retina, so the image is not clear. The problem may be the result of an abnormal shape of the eye or to abnormal focusing of the light by the cornea and lens. The four most common refractive disorders are nearsightedness, farsightedness, presbyopia, and astigmatism.

*Myopia (Nearsightedness).* Myopia is the condition in which images of distant objects come into focus in front of the retina (Figure 27-19). This condition occurs if the eye is too long or if the cornea and lens bend light rays more than normally. Nearby objects are usually seen clearly, but objects far away are unclear.

Nearsightedness is corrected with eyeglasses or contact lenses that have inwardly curving (concave) lenses. The lenses correct the bending of light rays so that they focus on the retina. Surgical and laser techniques are also used to correct myopia by changing the shape of the cornea.

*Hyperopia (Farsightedness) and Presbyopia.* Hyperopia, or hypermetropia, causes images to come into focus behind the retina (Figure 27-19). The eyeball may be too short, or the cornea and lens may bend light rays less than normally. Faraway objects are usually seen clearly, but nearby objects are unclear. Young eyes can compensate for the problem by a process known as accommodation. The ciliary muscles contract during accommodation, thickening the lens and increasing its convexity. These changes allow the image to come into focus on the retina.

Patients with mild farsightedness may have no symptoms or may have blurred vision. They may have symptoms of eyestrain (an aching in the eye) because the ciliary muscles are overworked. Farsightedness is corrected with eyeglasses or contact lenses that have outwardly turning (convex) lenses. Aging usually causes the ciliary muscles to weaken, so a person may need stronger eyeglasses over time.

Presbyopia is a condition that most commonly affects people starting in their mid-40s. Older eyes tend to lose the ability to accommodate because the lens becomes more rigid. As a result, images come into focus behind the retina, as they do with farsightedness. Individuals find they must hold reading materials farther away to see them clearly. Corrective lenses are used to treat this condition.

*Astigmatism.* Sometimes vision is distorted because the cornea is unevenly curved. This condition is called astigmatism. Astigmatism may cause vertical or horizontal lines to appear out of focus. It can occur along with either nearsightedness or farsightedness. Astigmatism is treated with lenses that correct the unevenness of the cornea.

A surgical vision-correcting treatment for myopia is laser vision correction or LASIK. The procedure, which is done on an outpatient basis under local anesthesia, involves reshaping the cornea with a special laser. After LASIK surgery, 70% of patients have normal vision. A very small percentage of patients have postsurgical complications that cause their vision to worsen. Patients may still need to wear glasses to correct presbyopia.

# Orthopedics

Orthopedics is the medical specialty focusing on disorders, injuries, and diseases of the muscular and skeletal systems. The two systems are so interdependent that they are sometimes referred to as the musculoskeletal system, especially by orthopedists. In the office of an orthopedist, you will be asked to assist with general exams. Other responsibilities may include assisting with x-rays, helping with casting, applying hot or cold treatments (discussed in Chapter 29), and educating patients about therapy regimens. You must be knowledgeable about the musculoskeletal system and its common disorders and treatments.

## Orthopedic Exams and Procedures

An orthopedist uses inspection, palpation, and a variety of diagnostic tests to assess the structure and function of the musculoskeletal system. The patient is asked to stand, walk, and perform several range-of-motion exercises. In these maneuvers the patient moves a joint in a variety of ways; the doctor usually measures the degree of mobility with a device called a goniometer. A complete exam takes some time, and you may need to help drape, position, or physically support the patient, especially if the patient is elderly or incapacitated. You may also be responsible for instructing the patient about care for a musculoskeletal condition, including how to perform therapeutic exercises.

Orthopedists use a variety of diagnostic tests. As in most other specialties, x-rays play a vital role in diagnosis. They are especially useful in determining the nature and extent of a bone injury. Other common radiographic exams in the orthopedic specialty include the following:

- CT scan
- MRI
- Angiography (for affected vascular structures)
- Myelography (for spinal disorders)
- Diskography (for intervertebral disk disorders)
- Arthrography (for joint disorders)
- Bone scans

More information about diagnostic radiology is covered in Chapter 40.

**Arthroscopy** enables the orthopedist to see inside a joint, usually the knee or shoulder, with an arthroscope. This tubular instrument includes an optical system; when the tube is inserted into the joint, it can be visualized (Figure 27-20). Arthroscopy is used to give the physician a closer look at conditions such as injuries and degenerative joint diseases and to guide surgical procedures.

Bone and muscle biopsies may be performed to detect disorders such as bone infection and muscle atrophy. Electromyography is another diagnostic tool used in this specialty. An orthopedist may also order urine and blood tests to detect levels of substances such as calcium or phosphorus.

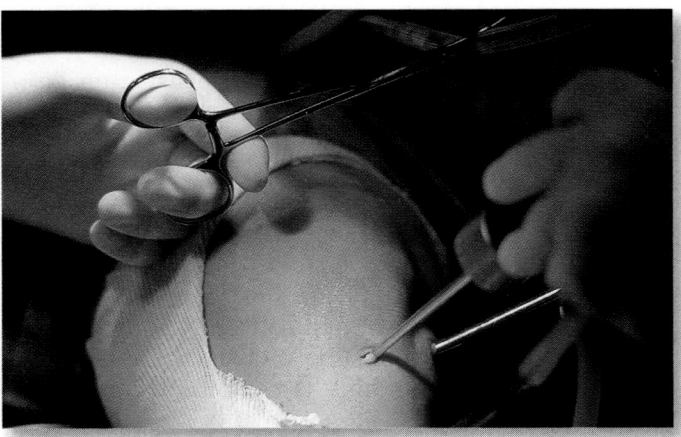

**Figure 27-20.** Arthroscopy can be used for diagnosis as well as biopsy and surgical repair.

Joint replacement surgery is often used to treat knee and hip joints severely damaged by arthritis or injury. Hip replacement may be indicated in cases of severe arthritis pain, femoral neck fractures, or hip joint tumors. Knee pain that does not respond to medications or physical therapy or a knee that is damaged by severe arthritis may indicate the need for knee replacement. Both surgeries require that the damaged joint be removed and an artificial joint inserted in its place. Physical therapy is usually started soon after surgery. Most patients fully recover in 3 to 12 months.

## Orthopedic Diseases and Disorders

Table 27-7 lists many of the diseases and disorders you will encounter in an orthopedic specialty. Back pain, especially lower back pain, is a common disorder. It can

| TABLE 27-7 | Common Diseases and Disorders of the Musculoskeletal System | |
|---|---|---|
| **Condition** | **Description** | **Treatment** |
| Arthritis | Inflammation of joints—rheumatoid or degenerative (osteoarthritis); rheumatoid arthritis causes joint stiffness and soreness, pain, and swelling and may lead to deformity; osteoarthritis produces pain, stiffness, and possible enlargement of bones, without deformity | Anti-inflammatory medications, application of heat, rest, exercise, occupational and physical therapy, surgery such as joint replacement (arthroplasty) |
| Bursitis | Inflammation of one or more bursae (sacs surrounding joints); symptoms include pain (especially on movement), restricted motion, and swelling | Anti-inflammatory medications |
| Carpal tunnel syndrome | Compression of median nerve, causing wrist pain and numbness | Rest and occupational adjustments, splinting of wrists, injection of corticosteroids, surgical decompression of nerve |
| Dislocation | Displacement of bones at joint so that parts that are supposed to make contact no longer come together; occurs most often to fingers, shoulder, knee, and hip | Relocation, or shifting bones back into place; anti-inflammatory medications |
| Herniated intervertebral disk (HID) | Protruding contents of disk compress nerve roots and cause severe pain | Rest, traction, physical therapy, muscle relaxants, surgery |
| Osteomyelitis | Infection of bone; principal symptom is pain | Antibiotics and analgesics, surgery |
| Osteoporosis | Metabolic disorder that causes decreased bone mass; bones become brittle and fracture easily | Exercise, dietary supplements, hormone therapy, drug therapy (alendronate) |
| Paget's disease | Chronic condition that causes bone deformities and affects 2% to 3% of people older than age 50 | Exercise, dietary supplements, hormone therapy, drug therapy (alendronate) |
| Scoliosis | Abnormal curving of spine | Back brace, surgery |
| Sprain | Injury to ligament caused by joint overextension; symptoms include pain, swelling, and discoloration | Rest, support, application of cold, anti-inflammatory medications |
| Tendonitis | Inflammation of tendon | Rest, support, anti-inflammatory medications |

have many causes, including muscle strain, osteoarthritis, and the presence of a tumor. The orthopedist determines the nature of the problem based on the symptoms and diagnostic x-rays and CT scans. Treatments include the application of heat, administration of analgesics or muscle relaxants, exercise therapy, special braces, and traction.

Another condition that is commonly encountered in the orthopedist's office is a **fracture,** or break in a bone. Fractures and their treatment are discussed in Chapter 30.

# Otology

An otologist treats diseases and disorders of the ears. Procedures common to this specialty are sometimes performed by other physicians as well, especially general practitioners, internists, and allergists. Chapter 25 discussed auditory acuity and the procedures that might be done in a general practitioner's office. Some ear exams are performed in an otologist's office too. You may assist with or perform auditory screening, and you may help with diagnostic tests such as tympanometry. Otology specialists whose practices include problems affecting the nose and throat are called otorhinolaryngologists.

## Common Disorders of the Outer Ear

Several disorders affect the external parts of the ear. These include cerumen impaction, otitis externa, and pruritus.

**Cerumen Impaction.** A condition called cerumen impaction occurs when the ear canal becomes blocked by a buildup of cerumen (earwax). The symptoms include a feeling that the ear is stopped up, partial hearing loss, ringing in the ear, and, occasionally, pain. The wax can be softened with special, eardrops, and irrigation can be performed to remove the wax.

**Otitis Externa.** Otitis externa is an infection of the outer ear, usually caused by bacteria or fungi. The infection can be localized, as with a boil or abscess, or the entire ear canal lining can be affected. Fungal infections are common in swimmers because of persistent moisture in the ear canal.

Symptoms of otitis externa include itching, pain, and pus in the ear. This infection is sometimes treated with a combination of an antibiotic or antifungal agent and an anti-inflammatory medication.

**Pruritus.** A common problem in the elderly is pruritus, or itching, of the ear canal. Because the sebaceous glands produce less wax with aging, the ear becomes dry and itchy. Dryness can be overcome by a regular routine of lubricating the ear canal with a few drops of mineral oil.

## Common Disorders of the Middle Ear

Middle ear disorders involve the eardrum and the chamber behind it. They include otitis media, mastoiditis, otosclerosis, and ruptured eardrum.

**Otitis Media.** Otitis media is an inflammation of the middle ear characterized by a buildup of fluid. It is most commonly referred to as an ear infection.

**Mastoiditis.** The mastoid bone is located just behind the ear. It is connected to the middle ear by air cells, or sinuses, in the bone. Sometimes, if left untreated, an infection in the middle ear can spread to the mastoid bone through these air cells. Although mastoiditis is fairly rare, it may be serious because the mastoid air cells are close to the organs of hearing, important nerves, the covering of the brain, and the jugular vein. Severe cases of mastoiditis may require removal of the affected bone.

**Otosclerosis.** Otosclerosis occurs when bone tissue grows abnormally around the stapes, or stirrup (the innermost of the three tiny bones that connect the eardrum and the inner ear). This overgrowth of tissue prevents the stapes from transmitting sound vibrations to the inner ear. The result is hearing loss that involves one or both ears. The condition is often hereditary.

Symptoms of otosclerosis include gradual loss of hearing and tinnitus (described in the next section). Surgery to replace the stapes can restore or improve hearing in almost 90% of patients with otosclerosis. Alternatively, a hearing aid may improve hearing for some patients.

**Ruptured Eardrum.** The eardrum may become ruptured in several ways: by a sharp object, an explosion, a blow to the ear, or a severe middle ear infection. Sometimes the eardrum is ruptured by a sudden change in air pressure, as might occur when flying in an airplane or diving. Symptoms include pain, partial hearing loss, and a slight discharge or bleeding. The symptoms typically last only a few hours. A ruptured eardrum usually heals on its own in 1 to 2 weeks, but the doctor may prescribe an antibiotic or the use of a temporary patch to prevent infection.

## Common Disorders of the Inner Ear

Disorders of the inner ear, or labyrinth, affect the cochlea and the semicircular canals. They include labyrinthitis, Ménière's disease, presbycusis, and tinnitus.

**Labyrinthitis.** Labyrinthitis is an infection of the labyrinth, most commonly caused by a virus. Because the labyrinth includes the semicircular canals, which are involved in balance, this infection causes symptoms of dizziness or vertigo. The room may appear to spin, and any movement exacerbates the sensation, sometimes to the point of nausea and vomiting. Although disturbing, labyrinthitis disappears on its own within 1 to 3 weeks. The patient may need to rest in bed for a few days, and medication can be given for symptoms.

**Ménière's Disease.** Ménière's disease is caused by increased fluid in the labyrinth. The pressure of the fluid disturbs the sense of balance and may even rupture the labyrinth wall or damage the cochlea with its hearing receptors. One or both ears may be affected. Symptoms of this disorder include vertigo, nausea, vomiting, distorted hearing, and tinnitus. Some people may suffer hearing loss ranging from mild to severe. Medications may be used to combat vertigo, nausea, and vomiting. Other treatments that help some people include using diuretics and following a low-sodium diet.

**Presbycusis.** Presbycusis is a type of sensorineural hearing loss. This disorder involves a gradual deterioration of the sensory receptors in the cochlea, leading to gradual loss of hearing. It is the most common form of hearing loss in older adults, affecting about 25% of people by the age of 60 or 70. Men are affected more often than women. Typically both ears are affected, and the patient has difficulty hearing high-pitched tones as well as normal conversation. Presbycusis is thought to be caused by factors such as prolonged exposure to loud noise, infection, injury, certain medications, and some diseases. Hearing loss can be treated effectively, however, with a hearing aid.

**Tinnitus.** Tinnitus is more commonly called a ringing in the ears. It can, however, take several forms, including a buzzing, whistling, or hissing sound. The most common causes of tinnitus are damage to the hearing receptors from noise or toxins, age-related changes in the organs of the ear, and use of aspirin. Tinnitus can affect people at any age but is more common as people get older. If tinnitus becomes chronic, the patient may find relief by listening to music or other distracting sounds or by using a device similar to a hearing aid that masks the noise with more pleasant sounds.

# Surgery

Surgery is used to treat a variety of diseases and disorders. Surgery may be performed to repair wounds and broken bones or to repair or remove diseased or injured tissues, organs, and limbs. Some surgeons specialize in one field, such as ophthalmology or cardiology, and others are general surgeons.

Assisting a general or specialty surgeon requires familiarity with body systems. You should also understand presurgical procedures such as patient education, operating room preparation, and skin preparation; surgical assisting procedures such as maintaining asepsis; and postsurgical responsibilities such as decontaminating the operating room and dressing wounds.

A relatively simple surgical procedure is a tissue biopsy. There are several types of biopsies. A surgeon performs an incisional, or open, biopsy by making an incision and removing a piece of tissue. A needle biopsy is performed by removing tissue with a needle inserted into the growth or area through the skin. A surgeon performs needle aspiration by removing fluid from a lump or cyst with a needle. You may be asked to assist during these types of surgery. Procedure 27-4 describes the steps in assisting with a needle biopsy.

During a biopsy, Universal Precautions and sterile technique must be maintained. Always place the specimen in a prepared, labeled container provided by the laboratory. Transport it according to laboratory instructions, attaching the proper accompanying forms. After the biopsy you might assist with or perform the cleaning and bandaging of the site.

# Urology

A urologist diagnoses and treats disorders and diseases of the urinary system in both males and females as well as the male reproductive system. Urologists also perform surgical procedures such as hernia repairs and vasectomies. A vasectomy is a sterilization procedure for men in which a section of each vas deferens is removed.

In a urologist's office, you would assist with general exams; collect and process urine, blood, and other specimens; obtain cultures; and participate in patient education about conditions as well as about presurgical and postsurgical care. You must understand the urinary system and the diseases and disorders you are likely to encounter.

## Urology Exams

You must be thorough when you take a patient's history for a urologist. Much information about urinary problems is obtained by questioning the patient about changes in frequency or urgency of urination, difficulty or pain with urination (dysuria), and incontinence. The physical exam usually includes palpation of the kidneys and bladder and visual inspection of the external genitalia. Women are examined in the lithotomy position, and men are usually seated when the exam begins.

During examination of the male reproductive system, the urologist inspects and palpates the patient's penis and scrotum. The genitalia are usually examined with the patient standing and the chest and abdomen draped. The doctor usually examines the inguinal region for a hernia and, in men over 40, checks the prostate gland. This gland is examined by digital insertion into the rectum.

The doctor instructs the patient as needed in performing a regular testicular self-exam (TSE). This instruction, discussed in the Educating the Patient section, may also be your responsibility.

# PROCEDURE 27.4

## Assisting With a Needle Biopsy

**Procedure Goal:** To remove tissue from a patient's body so that it can be examined in a laboratory

**OSHA Guidelines**

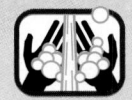 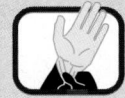 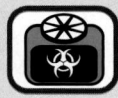
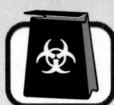 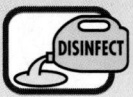 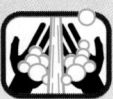

**Materials:** Sterile drapes, tray or Mayo stand, antiseptic solution, cotton balls, local anesthetic, disposable sterile biopsy needle or disposable sterile syringe and needle, sterile sponges, specimen bottle with fixative solution, laboratory packaging, sterile wound-dressing materials

**Method:**

1. Identify the patient and introduce yourself; instruct the patient as needed.
2. Wash your hands and assemble the necessary materials.
3. Prepare the sterile field and instruments.
4. Put on exam gloves.
5. Cleanse the biopsy site. Prepare the patient's skin.

### Rationale

To reduce the possibility of infection.

6. Remove the gloves, wash your hands, and put on clean exam gloves.
7. Assist the doctor as she injects anesthetic.
8. During the procedure, help drape and position the patient.
9. If you will be handing the doctor the instruments, remove the gloves, perform a surgical scrub, and put on sterile gloves.
10. Place the sample in a properly labeled specimen bottle, complete the laboratory requisition form, and package the specimen for immediate transport to the laboratory.

### Rationale

The specimen must be properly labeled and accompanied by a completed laboratory requisition form to ensure that the specimen is not lost and the appropriate tests are completed in the lab.

11. Dress the patient's wound site.
12. Properly dispose of used supplies and instruments.
13. Clean and disinfect the room according to OSHA guidelines.
14. Remove the gloves and wash your hands.

## Diagnostic Testing

Urologists sometimes use imaging techniques, such as CT scans and MRIs. Pyelography is an x-ray of the kidney area with an iodine-based contrast agent. It is used to diagnose renal (kidney-related) disorders. Urologists also use several other diagnostic techniques.

**Urine and Blood Tests.** Urinalysis is the most common test ordered in a urology practice. Urine can be tested for the presence of bacteria, blood, and other substances. Blood testing is also done for a variety of reasons, including monitoring for dysfunctions of the prostate gland and for certain sexually transmitted diseases (STDs).

**Semen Analysis and Smears.** Semen samples may be obtained to determine fertility or to evaluate the success of a vasectomy. The patient usually collects these samples at home, but you may be required to provide a

container, written instructions, and laboratory paperwork. Smears are used in diagnosing infections.

**Cystometry.** Cystometry is used to measure urinary bladder capacity and pressure. Using a catheter passed through the urethra, the doctor fills the bladder with carbon dioxide gas. The test results are examined to diagnose disorders of bladder function.

**Cystoscopy.** In cystoscopy the physician examines the walls of the bladder and urethra by visualization and inspection. A special viewing instrument, called a cystoscope, is used for this procedure. The cystoscope is inserted into the bladder through the urethra.

**Testicular Biopsy.** Testicular biopsy, a hospital procedure, involves obtaining a tissue sample of a mass for laboratory examination. The patient will need your emotional support because he will most likely be very anxious about the nature of the lump.

## Testicular Self-Exam

Testicular cancer is rare, but when it occurs, it usually affects men between the ages of 29 and 35. The American Cancer Society recommends that all men perform a monthly testicular self-exam (TSE) from age 15 onward to increase the chances of early detection. Although testicular cancer is one of the most curable cancers, early detection is vital to its treatment.

A man who perceives an abnormality during TSE should be examined by a physician right away. TSE should be performed after a warm shower or bath, when scrotal skin is relaxed.

1. The man first observes the testes for changes in appearance, such as swelling. He then manually examines each testicle, gently rolling it between the fingers and thumbs of both hands to feel for hard lumps (see Figure 27-21).
2. After examining each testicle, the man should locate the area of the epididymis and spermatic

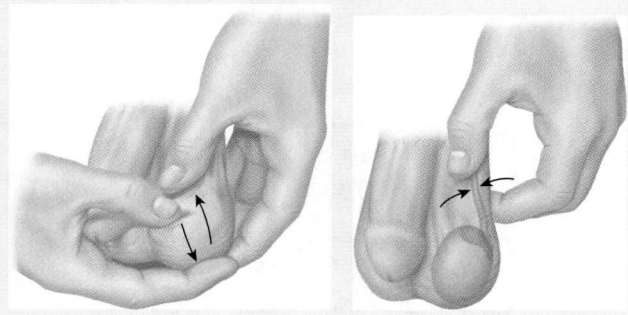

**Figure 27-21.** Males from age 15 onward should perform a monthly testicular self-exam.

cord. This area can be felt as a cordlike structure originating at the top back of each testicle.

Warning signs of testicular cancer include a heavy or dragging feeling in the groin, enlargement of one testicle, and a dull ache in the groin.

## Urologic Diseases and Disorders

Diagnostic tests are used to identify a variety of urologic diseases and disorders. If you work in a urologist's office, you will probably encounter many of these conditions.

**Cystitis.** Cystitis is an inflammation of the urinary bladder resulting from a bacterial infection. Among women, who are more prone to this disorder than are men, the most common cause is the bacterium *Escherichia coli*. In men the infection is usually related to a separate condition such as prostatitis or epididymitis. The symptoms of cystitis are bladder spasms, fever, nausea and vomiting, chills, lower back pain, and pain on voiding (dysuria). Diagnosis of cystitis is confirmed through urinalysis, and the condition is treated with antibiotics. Female patients should be taught to wipe and cleanse the perineal area from front to back to prevent bacteria from the rectum from infecting the urethra.

**Epididymitis.** Epididymitis is a bacterial infection of the epididymis. It causes pain, swelling, and sometimes fever. It is treated with rest and antibiotic medications.

**Hydrocele.** Hydrocele is the name for excess fluid in the scrotum. It is usually caused by infection of the epididymis or testes. In other cases it results from a congenital defect or occurs after injury. The fluid may be aspirated to relieve discomfort.

**Impotence.** Impotence is the inability either to achieve or to maintain an erection. The cause may be physical, as when it results from cardiovascular or endocrine disease, or it may be a side effect of some medication such as certain diuretics and chemotherapy agents. The cause may also be psychological or emotional. In at least half the cases, a combination of physical and emotional factors is involved. Treatment depends on the cause or causes and may include medication, counseling, or surgical procedures.

**Kidney Stones.** Kidney stones occur when chemical substances in the urine form crystals in the kidney, ureter, or bladder. If kidney stones cannot pass through the ureter, they can cause excruciating pain. Although some stones pass, large stones often must be removed surgically or broken up by means of sound waves (lithotripsy) or laser techniques.

**Prostatic Hypertrophy.** Prostatic hypertrophy, or enlargement of the prostate gland, occurs most commonly in men over 50. Hypertrophy may constrict the urethra, causing difficulty in urinating and repeated urinary infections. Medications to reduce the hypertrophy and surgery are common treatments.

**Prostatitis.** Prostatitis is an inflammation of the prostate, usually bacterial. Symptoms are pain on urination and, often, fever. Patients are instructed to avoid sitting for long periods. Treatments include antibiotic medications and sitz baths.

**Prostate Cancer.** Prostate cancer is the most common type of cancer among men. Often no symptoms are evident. Sometimes a nodule may be felt on palpation of the prostate; if the growth is large enough, problems with urination may occur. A blood test known as a prostate-specific antigen (PSA) is used for screening in men over 50 years of age; an abnormal elevation of the PSA could indicate prostate cancer. Treatment options include radiation therapy and removal of the prostate.

**STDs.** Urologists also diagnose and treat STDs. These diseases are discussed in Chapter 26.

**Urethritis.** Urethritis is an inflammation of the urethra. Like cystitis, it is usually caused by bacterial infection and requires similar, if not the same, treatment. Urethritis frequently accompanies cystitis.

# Summary

As a medical assistant, you will find interesting and stimulating work in a specialty medical practice. Each specialty has precise requirements for knowledge and skills that are particular to that field of practice. All medical specialties require that you have a firm foundation in and understanding of basic principles and procedures.

You will need to familiarize yourself with the anatomy and physiology relevant to the specialty in which you work. You will assist with highly specialized exams, diagnostic testing, and modes of treatment. By working to understand the diseases and disorders common to the specialty you choose, you will develop the ability to better educate patients and respond to their concerns.

# REVIEW

## CASE STUDY QUESTIONS

Now that you have completed this chapter, review the case study at the beginning of the chapter and answer the following questions:

1. What was the purpose of the ECG?
2. What special instructions should be provided to the patient when scheduling him for the stress test and Doppler studies?
3. What educational requirements should you meet in order to conduct these tests with the physician present?

## Discussion Questions

1. Discuss what tips you would give a patient with allergies about keeping a dust-free room.
2. What common dermatologic conditions may be presented in a dermatologist's office?
3. What categories of neurologic function are included in a complete exam?

## Critical Thinking Questions

1. List the types of diagnostic testing used in gastroenterology and explain why the tests may be requested by the physician.
2. Identify the common cancers by body system. Of these, which cancer has the most limited symptomology? Explain your answer.
3. Why is it important that the physician be present during a patient's cardiac stress test?

## Application Activities

1. Using a gauze square that you moisten with water, perform the patch test procedure on another student. Have the other student critique your technique.
2. Create a patient information brochure about colonoscopy. Include information about what the patient should do before the procedure and what he should expect during the procedure.
3. Gather information and make a presentation to the class on resources available in your community to help families and patients affected by one of the following diseases: Alzheimer's disease, breast cancer, multiple sclerosis, rheumatoid arthritis, or AIDS.

## Virtual Fieldtrip

*Visit the McGraw-Hill Higher Education Medical Assisting website at www.mhhe.com/medicalassisting3 to complete the following activity:*

Search the U.S. Food and Drug Administration (FDA) website for information regarding the risks and benefits of LASIK surgery. Create a table of these risks and benefits. Consider if you are a likely candidate for this surgery. Why or why not?

Open the CD and complete this chapter's practice activities, play the games, listen to the key terms, and test yourself with the interactive review. E-mail, print, and/or save your results to document your proficiency.

# Assisting With Minor Surgery

## MEDICAL ASSISTING COMPETENCIES

*In preparation for the certification examination, you should know the following areas of competence:*

| COMPETENCY | CMA | RMA |
|---|---|---|
| **Clinical** | | |
| Apply principles of aseptic techniques and infection control, including hand washing | X | X |
| Perform sterilization techniques | X | X |
| Dispose of biohazardous materials | X | X |
| Practice Standard Precautions | X | X |
| Interview the patient to obtain and record the patient's history | X | X |
| Prepare and maintain exam and treatment areas | X | X |
| Prepare the patient for and assist the physician with routine and specialty exams, treatments, and minor office surgeries | X | X |
| Apply pharmacology principles to prepare and administer oral and parenteral (excluding IV) medications as directed by the physician | X | X |
| **General/Legal/Professional** | | |
| Recognize and respond to verbal and nonverbal communications by being attentive and adapting communication to the recipient's level of understanding | X | X |
| Be aware of and perform within legal and ethical boundaries | X | X |
| Determine the needs for documentation and reporting, and document accurately and appropriately | X | X |
| Explain general office policies and procedures | X | X |
| Instruct individuals according to their needs | X | X |
| Exercise efficient time management | | X |
| Conduct work within scope of education, training, and ability | | X |
| Serve as a liaison between the physician and others | | X |
| Interview effectively | | X |
| Use appropriate medical terminology | | X |

## KEY TERMS

abscess
anesthesia
anesthetic
approximate
biopsy specimen
cryosurgery
debridement
dressing
electrocauterization
floater
formalin
incision
inflammatory phase
intraoperative
laceration
ligature
maturation phase
Mayo stand
medical asepsis
needle biopsy
onychectomy
postoperative
preoperative
proliferation phase
puncture wound
sterile field
sterile scrub assistant
surgical asepsis
suture
topical
vial

# CHAPTER OUTLINE

- The Medical Assistant's Role in Minor Surgery
- Surgery in the Physician's Office
- Instruments Used in Minor Surgery
- Asepsis

- Preoperative Procedures
- Intraoperative Procedures
- Postoperative Procedures

# LEARNING OUTCOMES

After completing Chapter 28, you will be able to:

**28.1** Define the medical assistant's role in minor surgical procedures.

**28.2** Describe types of wounds and explain how they heal.

**28.3** Describe special surgical procedures performed in an office setting.

**28.4** List the instruments used in minor surgery and describe their functions.

**28.5** Describe and contrast the procedures for medical and sterile asepsis in minor surgery.

**28.6** Describe the medical assistant's duties in preparing to assist in minor surgery.

**28.7** Describe the medical assistant's duties in preparing a patient for surgery.

**28.8** Describe the types of local anesthetics for minor surgery and the medical assistant's role in their administration.

**28.9** Describe the duties of the medical assistant as a floater and as a sterile scrub assistant.

**28.10** Describe the medical assistant's duties in the postoperative period.

# Introduction

Minor surgical procedures are frequently performed in ambulatory care settings and office practices. As a medical assistant, you must be knowledgeable of the types of procedures performed where you are employed. You need to know how to prepare the patient for surgery, assist the practitioner during surgery, and care for the patient after surgery. Because all types of surgery require surgical asepsis, discussed in Chapter 20, a working knowledge of this technique is mandatory. Assisting with minor surgery requires a variety of duties and skills.

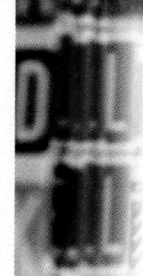

## CASE STUDY

You work in a dermatology clinic, and one of your patients is a 35-year-old female who is scheduled to have a wart removed from her left hand. Her boyfriend is with her to drive her home. She appears apprehensive and wants to know exactly what is going to happen.

As you read this chapter, consider the following questions:
1. How could you reduce the patient's apprehension?
2. What would you say to her before the physician arrives to perform the minor surgery?

# The Medical Assistant's Role in Minor Surgery

Medical assistants play an important role in all aspects of minor surgical procedures. You will perform administrative tasks prior to the patient's surgery, including completing forms for insurance and obtaining signed informed consent from the patient. You will explain basic aspects of the surgical procedure and answer the patient's questions. Informing the doctor of all current prescription and over-the-counter (OTC) medications that the patient is currently taking is also an administrative task. Finally, you will make sure the patient knows how to follow the appropriate presurgical instructions.

You will perform many tasks directly related to the surgical procedure. You will make sure the surgical room is clean, neat, and properly lit. You will see that all the equipment, instruments, and supplies the doctor will use are clean, disinfected or sterilized, and properly arranged. You may also function as an unsterile assistant, ensuring the safety and comfort of the patient during the procedure and performing other duties. At other times you may directly assist with the surgical procedure in a sterile capacity.

Following the surgical procedure, you will help dress the wound and perform other postoperative patient care, making sure the patient is not experiencing ill effects from the surgery or local anesthetic. You will educate the patient about wound care and proper procedures to follow after surgery and make sure the patient has safe transportation home. You will also clean the room and prepare it for the next patient.

# Surgery in the Physician's Office

Minor surgical procedures are those that can be safely performed in the physician's office or clinic without general anesthesia. **Anesthesia** is a loss of sensation, particularly the feeling of pain. An **anesthetic** is a medication that causes anesthesia. A general anesthetic affects the entire body, whereas a local anesthetic affects only a particular area. Minor surgical procedures typically involve the use of a local anesthetic in the form of an injection or a cream applied to the skin.

Minor surgical procedures are performed for many reasons. Sometimes the purpose is to diagnose an illness or to repair an injury. Other procedures may be elective, or optional. Removal of a wart, skin tag (a small outgrowth of skin, occurring frequently on the neck as people get older), or other small growth for cosmetic reasons is an elective procedure. Some of the common minor surgical procedures you may assist the doctor with include the following:

- Repair of a laceration
- Irrigation and cleaning of a puncture wound
- Wound debridement
- Removal of foreign bodies
- Removal of small growths
- Removal of a nail or part of a nail
- Drainage of an abscess
- Collection of a biopsy specimen
- Cryosurgery
- Laser surgery
- Electrocauterization

# Common Surgical Procedures

Many surgical procedures are routinely performed in a doctor's office. You may perform some of these procedures on your own. For example, you may change dressings for surgical wounds, and under doctor's orders you may remove sutures (commonly called stitches) or staples after wounds have healed. Any procedure that requires an **incision** (a surgical wound made by cutting into body tissue) must be performed by a doctor.

**Draining an Abscess.** An **abscess** is a collection of pus (white blood cells [WBCs], bacteria, and dead skin cells) that forms as a result of infection. A protective lining can form around an abscess and prevent it from healing. In such a case, the physician may make an incision in the lining of the abscess. The physician may allow the abscess to drain on its own or will insert a drainage tube.

**Obtaining a Biopsy Specimen.** A **biopsy specimen** is a small amount of tissue removed from the body for examination under a microscope. Most biopsies involve cutting the tissue. A **needle biopsy** uses a needle and syringe to aspirate (withdraw by suction) fluid or tissue cells. (Procedure 27-4 in Chapter 27 describes how to assist with a needle biopsy.) All specimens must be placed in a preservative, most commonly a 10% **formalin** solution (a dilute solution of formaldehyde), to prevent changes in the tissue.

**Caring for Wounds.** A wound is any break in the skin. The break may be accidental or intentional, as from a surgical procedure. There are several types of accidental wounds. A **laceration** is a jagged, open wound in the skin that can extend down into the underlying tissue. The jagged edges may have to be cut away before the wound is closed. A **puncture wound** is a deep wound caused by a sharp object. (See Chapter 30 for further information on types and care of accidental wounds.) Both surgical and accidental wounds require special care to prevent infection. Proper wound care that promotes healing without infection is discussed in the Caution: Handle With Care section.

*Cleaning a Wound.* The first step in preventing a nonsurgical wound from becoming infected is careful cleansing. The wound must be thoroughly cleaned with soap and water. Then it must be irrigated with sterile saline solution or sterile water that is applied with a syringe and needle.

**Debridement,** the removal of debris or dead tissue from the wound, may be necessary to expose healthy tissue. There are a number of wound debridement methods the doctor may use:

- Surgical—cutting away tissue with scalpel and scissors
- Chemical—using special compounds to dissolve tissue

## Surgical Technologist

*To gain medical assistant credentials, you must fulfill the requirements of either the American Association of Medical Assistants (for a Certified Medical Assistant) or the American Medical Technologists (for a Registered Medical Assistant). After obtaining your medical assistant certification or registration, you may wish to acquire additional skills in specialty areas through course work or on-the-job training. Although this course work or training may not lead to an additional certification or degree, it will enable you to expand your role in the medical office and advance your career as the demand for health professionals increases.*

### Skills and Duties

The surgical technologist, sometimes called a surgical technician or operating room technician, is a vital member of the surgical team. He assists surgeons, nurses, and other surgical staff before, during, and after an operation.

Prior to an operation the technologist sets up the operating room. He sterilizes and prepares instruments and supplies and arranges them for the surgical staff. He also checks all operating room equipment to make sure the machines are fully functional.

The surgical technologist also prepares the patient for surgery. He washes the surgical site and shaves the area if necessary. He then transports the patient to the operating room and lifts her to position her on the table, requesting assistance if needed. He may apply antiseptic to the incision site and arrange sterile drapes around the site to create a sterile field. He may also help surgeons, nurses, and staff scrub up and dress in their gowns, gloves, and masks.

During the operation the surgical technologist observes vital signs, checks charts, and passes instruments and supplies to nurses and surgeons. He wears a mask and other personal protective equipment during the operation. He also may operate the lights, suction machines, or diagnostic equipment and help prepare specimens for transport to the laboratory or apply dressings to the patient's wound.

Following the operation the technologist lifts and transfers the patient to the recovery room, requesting assistance if needed. He then cleans and disinfects the operating room, restocking supplies as needed.

### Workplace Settings

Surgical technologists typically work in hospital operating rooms. Some surgical technologists also work in clinics, surgery centers, or physicians' and dentists' offices where outpatient surgery is performed. A few are employed privately by surgeons who use their own surgical teams for specialized work.

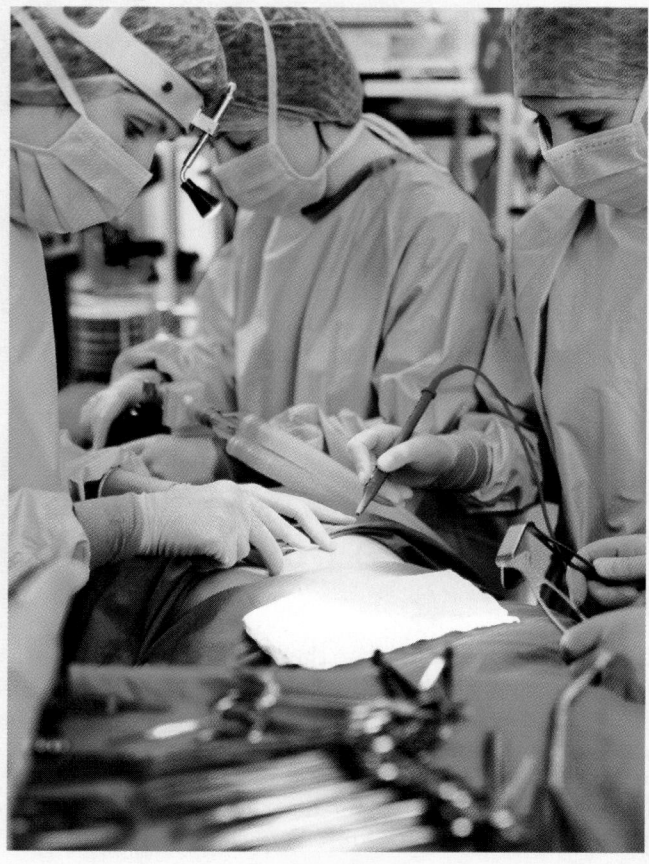

Surgical technologists usually work a standard 40-hour week. They may also be placed on call for emergencies during nights and weekends.

### Education

The Commission on Accreditation of Allied Health Education Programs recognizes more than 400 programs for surgical technologists. Programs are offered by colleges and universities, hospitals, vocational schools, and the military. They range from 9 months to 2 years in duration and offer the graduate a certificate, diploma, or associate degree.

After graduating from a program, surgical technologists may voluntarily take an examination to receive professional certification from the Liaison Council on Certification for the Surgical Technologist. Certification must be renewed every 4 years.

### Where to Go for More Information

Association of Surgical Technologists
6 West Dry Creek Circle
Littleton, CO 80120
(303) 694-9130

- Mechanical—applying a dressing that sticks to the wound, removing dead tissue when the dressing is removed or irrigating the wound with sterile saline
- Autolytic—applying a special dressing that helps the body's natural fluids dissolve dead tissue

***Wound Healing.*** It is important to know how a wound heals so that you can care for it properly. A wound heals in three phases: inflammatory phase, proliferation phase, and maturation phase. During the initial phase, or **inflammatory phase,** bleeding is reduced as blood vessels in the affected area constrict. Platelets, clotting factors, and WBCs play an important role in this phase. They seal the wound, clot the blood that has seeped into the area, and remove bacteria and debris from the wound. The wound contracts under the clot or scab that forms.

During the second phase, or **proliferation phase,** new tissue forms. Skin cells at the edges of the wound begin to move together to close off the wound. The scab that often forms over a wound actually slows down this movement of skin cells. The edges of the wound do eventually come together and form a continuous layer, closing off the wound.

The **maturation phase** (the third phase) involves the formation of scar tissue. Scar tissue is important for closing large, gaping, or jagged wounds. The continuous layer of skin cells formed during the second phase becomes thicker and pushes off the scab, leaving a scar. Scar tissue contains no nerves or blood vessels and lacks the resilience of skin.

The proliferation phase is sped up if the edges of an incision or nonsurgical wound are **approximated**—brought together so the tissue surfaces are close. This intervention protects the area from further contamination and minimizes scab and scar formation. Small wounds can be held together with butterfly closures, sterile strips, or adhesive. Skin adhesive is a special type of glue used for closing small wounds. Larger wounds or those subject to strain may require suturing or stapling.

***Closing a Wound.*** **Sutures** are surgical stitches used to close a wound. Suture materials, or **ligature,** can be either absorbable or nonabsorbable. The body breaks down absorbable sutures, so they do not require removal after the wound has healed. They are typically made of catgut (a sterile strand made of collagen fibers usually obtained from sheep or cow intestines). If a wound is particularly deep, the doctor may need to suture in layers, from inside to outside. In this case absorbable sutures are used for the inner suturing. Removable (nonabsorbable) sutures are generally used for the outside layer. Nonabsorbable ligature must be removed after wound healing is well under way. Nonabsorbable sutures may be made of silk, nylon, or polyester. Suture materials come in thicknesses ranging from size 11-0 (smallest) to size 7 (largest). The needle is already attached to most prepackaged ligature.

Staples may be used to bring the edges of a wound together if there is considerable stress on the incision. For example, a long and deep surgical wound or a wound across the leg would have a strong tendency to gape open if not firmly secured. Surgical staples look somewhat like ordinary staples. They are inserted into the skin with a disposable staple unit.

## Special Minor Surgical Procedures

Some types of minor surgical procedures require special surgical instruments. These procedures include laser surgery, cryosurgery, and electrocauterization. They all remove excess or abnormal tissue, as in the case of warts or skin lesions. These procedures usually require surgical aseptic technique because they break the integrity of the skin.

**Laser Surgery.** A laser emits an intense beam of light that is used to cut away tissue. Laser surgery is sometimes preferred over conventional surgery because it causes less damage to surrounding healthy tissue than does conventional surgery. Laser surgery also promotes quick healing and helps prevent infection.

When a laser is used in an office setting, close blinds and shades to keep out stray light. Remove any items that could catch fire if they came in contact with the laser beam. Cover any shiny or reflective surfaces. Make sure that everyone in the room, including the patient, wears special safety goggles to protect the eyes. Post a standard laser warning placard in the entryway to the room, per Occupational Safety and Health Administration (OSHA) regulations.

Position, drape, and prepare the patient as you would for conventional surgery. Place gauze around the surgical site, and assist the physician with administration of a local anesthetic if requested. The physician uses the laser to vaporize the unwanted tissue; vaporized tissue is cleared away by the vacuum hose portion of the unit (see Figure 28-1). You may be asked to apply

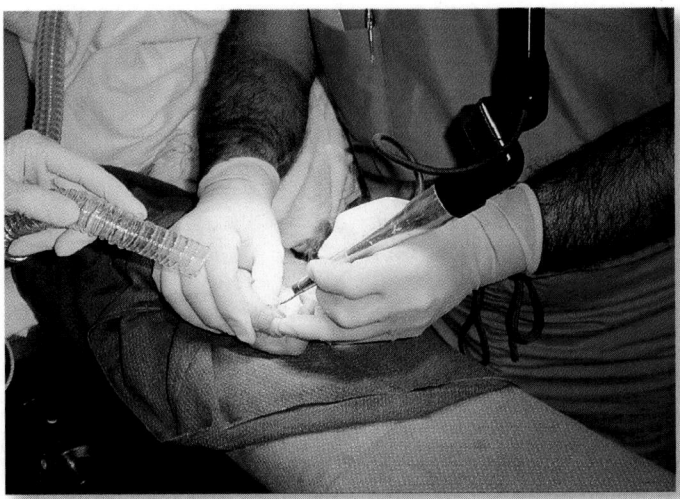

**Figure 28-1.** Suction eliminates vaporized tissue as a physician uses a laser to remove a wart from a patient's hand.

# CAUTION *Handle With Care*

## Conditions That Interfere With Fast, Effective Wound Healing

The goals for treating both surgical and nonsurgical wounds are similar: they are to heal the wound without infection and to preserve normal skin function and appearance. Nonsurgical wounds often involve conditions that do not promote fast, effective healing. In these cases the wound requires special attention to ensure good results.

Many types of nonsurgical wounds may contain foreign material that can lead to infection. For example, a child may have a deep laceration from landing on a dirty, broken bottle when falling off a bicycle. These types of wounds always need vigorous cleaning. Some may need debridement.

Wounds heal better when the edges are brought closely together, or approximated. Jagged edges in a laceration make approximation harder. It is also difficult to approximate crushed tissue, as you would see with fingers closed in a car door. Crushing disrupts a tissue's blood supply by rupturing blood vessels throughout the affected area. A physician might debride this type of wound with a scalpel to remove severely damaged tissue and achieve a clean wound edge before suturing.

After a surgical or nonsurgical wound is closed and sutured, it is essential to keep the wound clean and dry to help prevent infection. Infection delays the healing process and can have other serious consequences.

A sutured wound heals more quickly and smoothly when no scab forms because the migrating skin cells encounter no barrier to their movement. Proper postoperative care, including daily cleaning with soap and water or a mild antiseptic, keeps a wound scab-free. Although skin cells migrate across the space of a wound more easily in a somewhat moist environment, a wet wound offers the ideal conditions for bacteria to grow and cause infection. Covering a wound with antiseptic ointment and a clean, dry dressing keeps the wound slightly moist yet helps prevent infection.

Wound healing may be delayed in a number of instances not directly related to the surgery or injury. The presence of any of the following conditions can put a patient at risk for wound-healing problems. Wounds in such patients may require extra attention and care.

- **Poor circulation.** This condition results in inadequate supplies of nutrients, blood cells, and oxygen to the wound, all of which delay the healing process.
- **Aging.** Physiologic changes that occur with age can decrease a person's resistance to infection.
- **Diabetes.** Patients with diabetes experience changes in the walls of their arteries that result in poor circulation to peripheral tissues. These patients may also have a decreased resistance to infection.
- **Poor nutrition.** Patients who are undernourished, particularly those who are deficient in protein or vitamin C, do not have the physiologic resources for vigorous healing.
- **High levels of stress.** An increase in stress-related hormones can decrease resistance to infection.
- **Weakened immune system.** Patients who are on certain medications or who have certain chronic diseases may have weakened immune systems, putting them at increased risk of infection.
- **Obesity.** When someone is obese, the circulation directly under the skin is often poor, leading to slow healing.
- **Smoking.** Nicotine constricts the blood vessels in the skin, reducing circulation to the area of the wound and slowing healing.

---

pressure to control any bleeding. Clean the wound with an antiseptic, and apply a sterile dressing. Give the patient the normal instructions on wound care, including the recommendation to protect the site from exposure to the sun.

**Cryosurgery.** The use of extreme cold to destroy unwanted tissue is called **cryosurgery.** Cryosurgery is often used to remove skin lesions and lesions on the cervix. Before cryosurgery inform the patient that an initial sensation of cold will be followed by a burning sensation. Instruct the patient to remain as still as possible to prevent damage of nearby tissue.

The doctor may freeze the tissue by touching it with a cotton-tipped applicator dipped in liquid nitrogen or by spraying it with liquid nitrogen from a pressurized can. Sometimes a special cryosurgical instrument is used, most often during surgery on the cervix.

Make the patient aware that more than one freezing cycle may be necessary. A local anesthetic is usually not required because the cold itself reduces sensation in the area. After the procedure, the area is cleaned with an antiseptic, and a sterile dressing may be applied. An ice pack may be applied to reduce swelling, and pain relievers may be given for pain.

Reassure the patient that some pain, swelling, or redness is normal after a cryosurgical procedure. Encourage the patient to use ice and pain relievers as necessary. Let the patient know that a large, painful, bloody blister may form. Left undisturbed, the blister usually ruptures in about 2 weeks. It should be left intact to promote healing and prevent infection. The patient should call the doctor if a blister becomes too painful. Be sure to provide the patient with complete wound-care instructions.

**Electrocauterization.** **Electrocauterization** is a technique whereby a needle, probe, or loop heated by electric current destroys the target tissue. A physician may use this technique to remove growths such as warts, to stop bleeding, and to control nosebleeds that either will not subside or continually recur.

Several types of electrocautery units are in use. Some are small, often handheld, units powered by battery or by ordinary household electric current. Other, larger units are designed for countertop placement or for mounting on a wall. Some units use disposable probes, whereas others employ reusable ones.

With certain units, a grounding pad or plate is placed somewhere on the patient's body (or under it) during the procedure. This grounding completes the circuit and prevents electric shock to the patient, the physician, and staff members. Reassure the patient that grounding causes no discomfort.

A local anesthetic may be administered before the procedure. A scab or crust generally forms over the area. Healing may take 2 to 3 weeks. General wound-care instructions are appropriate for this procedure, except that a dressing may be omitted to keep the area drier.

# Instruments Used in Minor Surgery

The type of minor surgical procedure determines which surgical instruments are used. Surgical instruments have specific purposes and may be classified by function.

## Cutting and Dissecting Instruments

Cutting and dissecting instruments have sharp edges and are used to cut (incise) skin and tissue. Figure 28-2 illustrates some of the basic cutting and dissecting instruments you will encounter. You must be careful when cleaning, sterilizing, and storing these instruments to avoid injuring yourself and to protect the instruments' sharp edges.

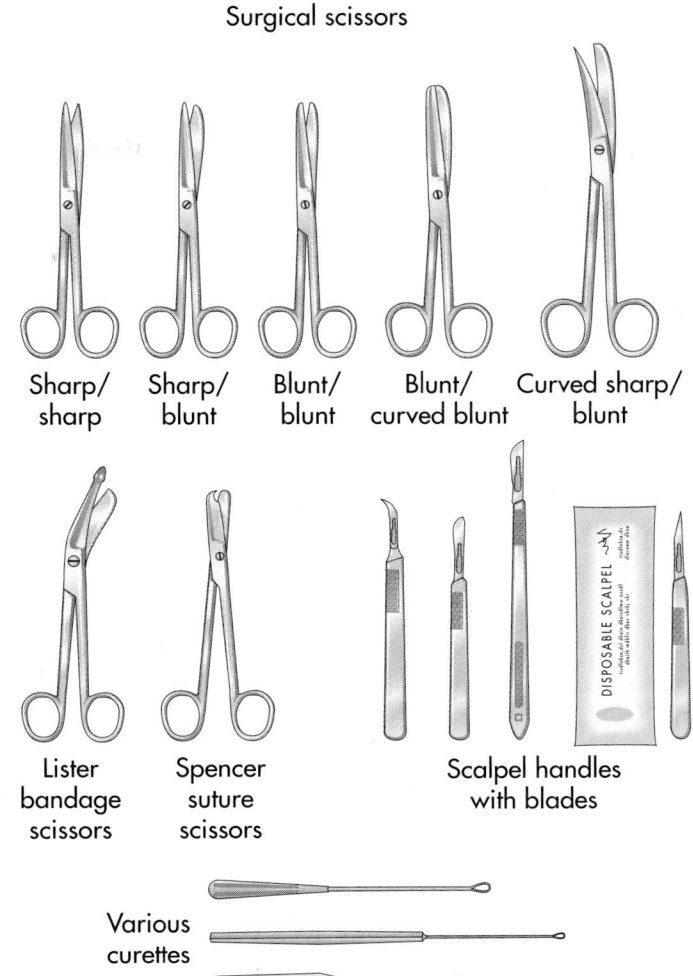

Surgical scissors

Sharp/ sharp — Sharp/ blunt — Blunt/ blunt — Blunt/ curved blunt — Curved sharp/ blunt

Lister bandage scissors — Spencer suture scissors — Scalpel handles with blades — DISPOSABLE SCALPEL

Various curettes

**Figure 28-2.** These are typical cutting and dissecting instruments used in minor surgical procedures.

**Scalpels.** A scalpel consists of a handle that holds a disposable blade. Scalpel handles are either reusable or disposable and vary in width and length. A scalpel's specific use determines the shape and size of its blade. General-purpose scalpels have wide blades and a straight cutting surface. A no. 15 blade is the most common one for performing minor procedures.

**Scissors.** Surgical scissors come in various sizes. They may be straight or curved and have either blunt or pointed tips. Tissue scissors must be sharp enough to cut without damaging or ripping surrounding tissue. Suture scissors have blunt points and a curved lower blade. The lower blade is inserted under the suture material to cut it. Bandage scissors are used to remove dressings. They have a blunt lower blade so that the skin next to the dressing is not injured. Clippers are scissor-like instruments used for cutting nails or thick materials.

**Curettes.** The doctor uses a curette for scraping tissue. Curettes come in a variety of shapes and sizes. They consist of a circular blade—actually a loop—attached to a rod-shaped handle. The blade is blunt on the outside and sharp on the inside. The inner part of the blade may also be serrated. Serrated blades may be used to take Pap smears (Papanicolaou smears) and to perform ear irrigations where a large amount of cerumen has accumulated.

# Grasping and Clamping Instruments

Special instruments are used for grasping and clamping tissue. Grasping instruments are used to hold surgical materials or to remove foreign objects, such as splinters, from the body. Clamping instruments are used to apply pressure and close off blood vessels. They are also used to hold tissue and other materials in position. Figure 28-3 shows some common grasping and clamping instruments.

**Forceps.** Forceps are instruments that are most often used to grasp or hold objects. Grasping types are usually shaped like tweezers and include thumb forceps and tissue forceps. Thumb forceps, also called smooth forceps, vary in shape and size. The blades of thumb forceps are tapered to a point and have small grooves at the tip. Tissue forceps (serrated forceps) have one or more fine teeth at the tips of the blades. When closed, these forceps hold tissue firmly. Holding forceps have handles with ratchets that lock the teeth in a closed position. Dressing, or sponge, forceps have ridges to hold a sponge or gauze when it is used to absorb body fluids.

**Hemostats.** The most commonly used surgical instruments are hemostats. These surgical clamps vary in size and shape. Hemostats are typically used to close off blood vessels. The serrated jaws of hemostats taper to a point. Like holding forceps, hemostats have handles that lock on ratchets, holding the jaws securely closed.

**Towel Clamps.** Towel clamps are used to keep towels in place during a surgical procedure. This stability is important in maintaining a sterile field.

# Retracting, Dilating, and Probing Instruments

Retracting instruments are used to hold back the sides of a wound or incision. Dilating and probing instruments may be used to enlarge, examine, or clear body openings, body cavities, or wounds. The shapes of these instruments vary with their functions. Some typical retracting, dilating, and probing instruments are shown in Figure 28-4.

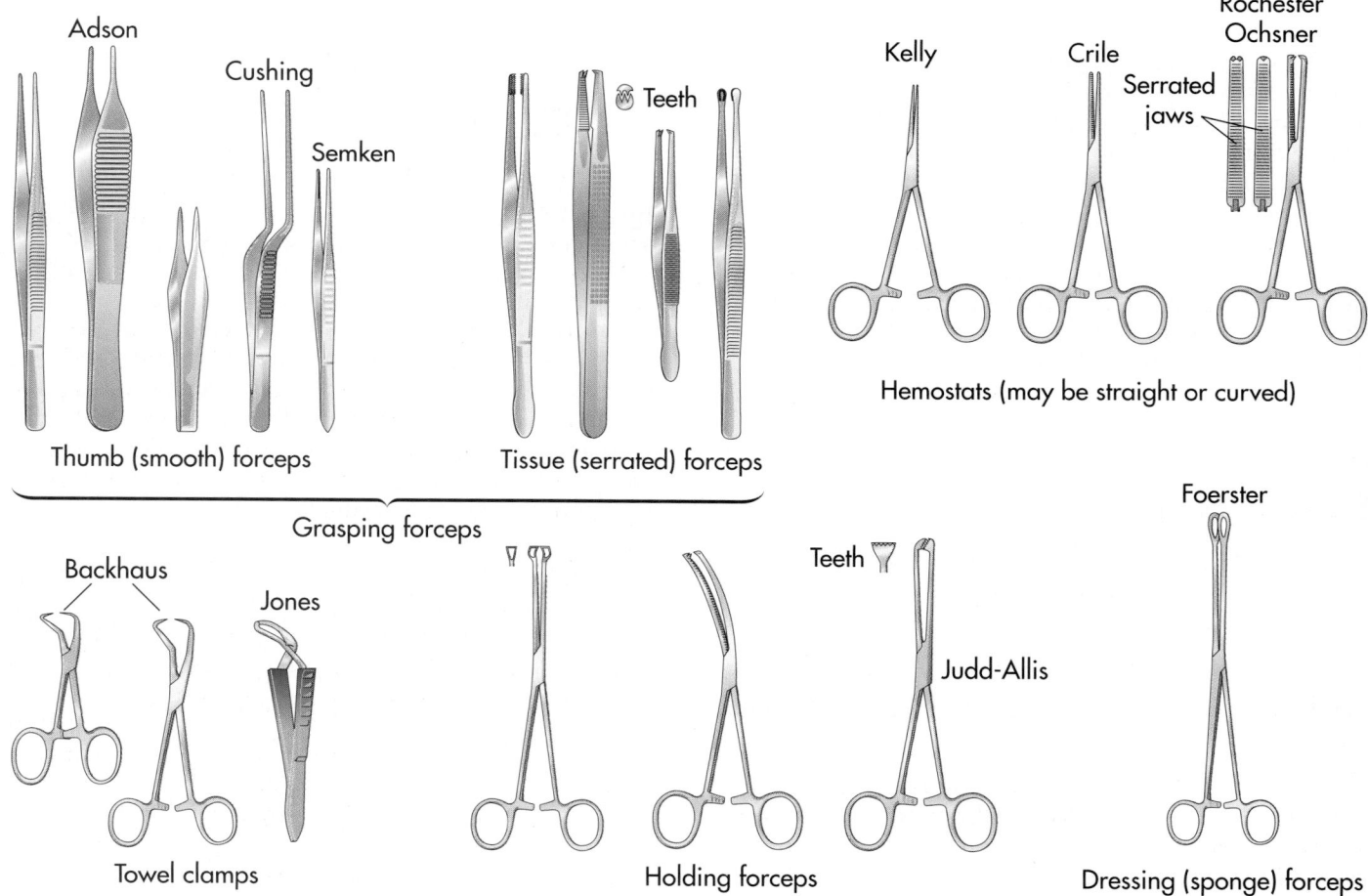

**Figure 28-3.** These are typical grasping and clamping instruments used in minor surgical procedures.

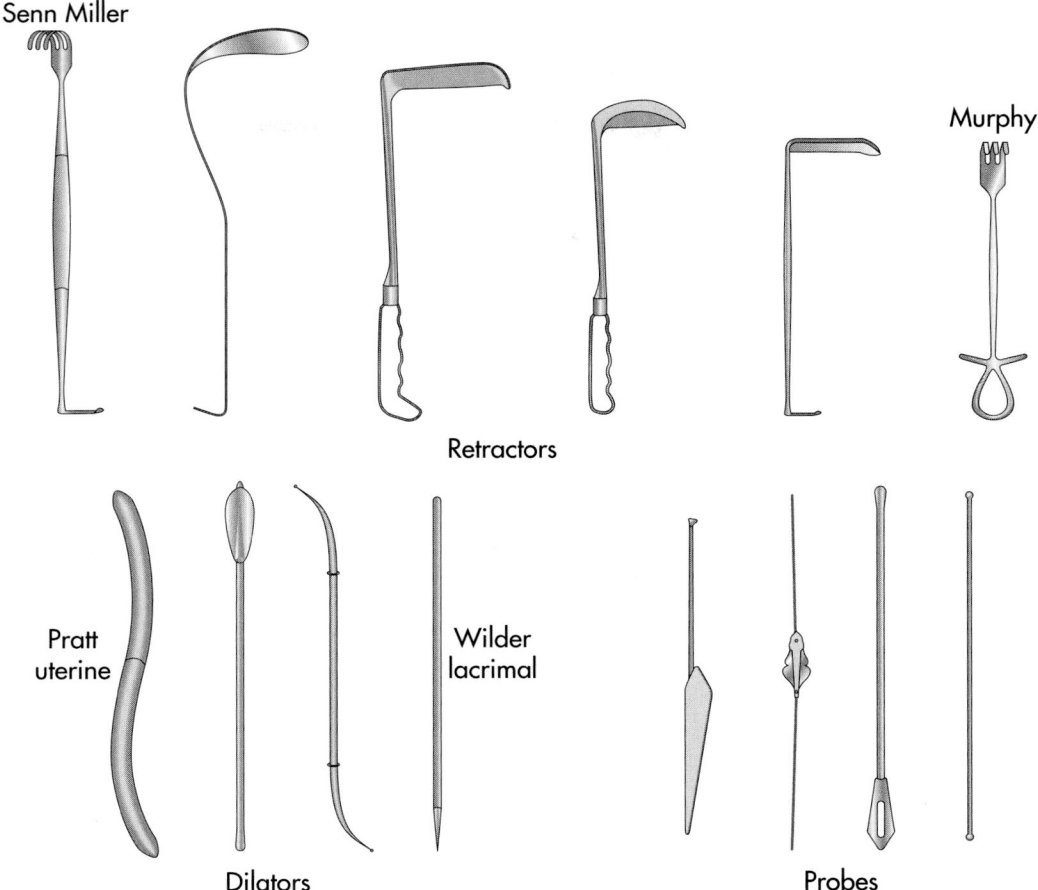

Senn Miller

Murphy

Retractors

Pratt
uterine

Dilators

Wilder
lacrimal

Probes

**Figure 28-4.** These are typical retracting, dialating, and probing instruments used in minor surgical procedures.

**Retractors.** The use of retractors allows greater access to and a better view of a surgical site. Some retractors must be held open by hand, whereas others have ratchets or locks to keep them open.

**Dilators.** Dilators are slender, pointed instruments. They are used to enlarge a body opening, such as a tear duct.

**Probes.** A surgical probe is a slender rod with a blunt tip shaped like a bulb. Probes are used to explore wounds or body cavities and to locate or clear blockages.

## Suturing Instruments

Suturing instruments are used to introduce suture materials into and retrieve them from a wound. Some carry the suture material, whereas others manipulate the suture carriers. Examples of suturing instruments are shown in Figure 28-5.

**Suture Needles.** Surgical suture needles carry suture material, also called ligature, through the tissue being sutured. They are either pointed or blunt at one end. They may have an eye at the other end to hold suture materials. Ligature often comes prepackaged with the needle already

connected. Prepackaged suture needles with attached ligature have no eye and produce less trauma to the tissue being sutured than do suture needles with eyes.

Suture needles may be straight, or they may be curved to allow deeper placement of sutures. Taper point needles (needles that taper into a sharp point) are used to suture tissues that are easily penetrated. They create only very small holes, thus minimizing leakage of tissue fluids. Cutting needles (needles that have at least two sharpened edges) are used on tough tissues that are not easily penetrated, such as skin.

Several measurements are used to determine the size of a surgical needle. Needle length is the distance from the tip to the end, measuring along the body of the needle. Chord length is the straight-line distance from the tip to the end of the needle. (Chord length is not the same as needle length in curved needles.) The radius of a curved needle is determined by mentally continuing the curve of the needle into a full circle and finding the distance from the center of the circle to the needle body. The diameter is the thickness of the needle. Needle size generally corresponds to the size of suture material used. Smaller needles are used for delicate procedures, such as eye surgery or repairing a facial laceration. Larger needles are used

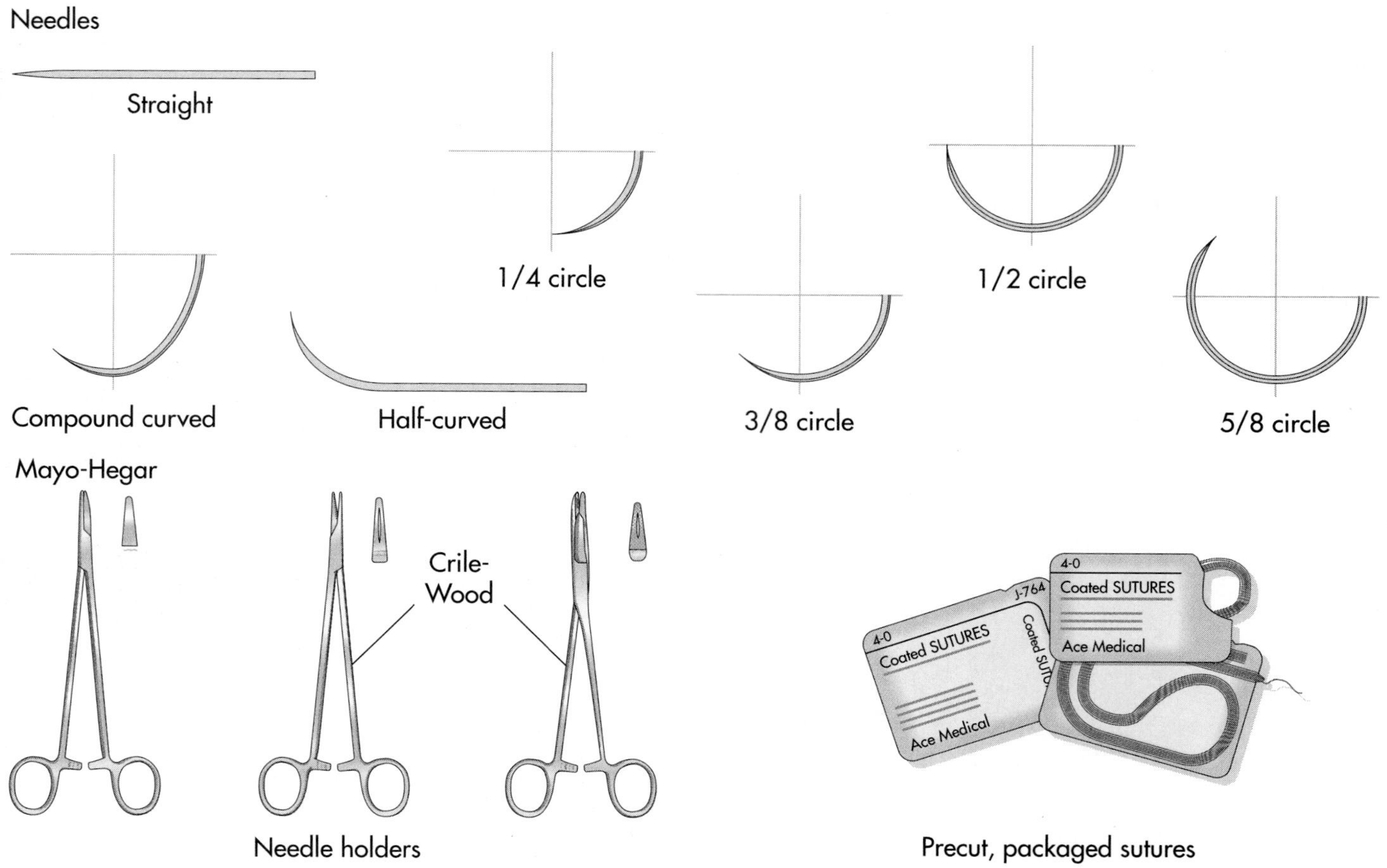

Needles

Straight

1/4 circle

1/2 circle

Compound curved          Half-curved

3/8 circle                          5/8 circle

Mayo-Hegar

Crile-
Wood

Needle holders

Precut, packaged sutures

4-0 Coated SUTURES
Ace Medical

4-0 Coated SUTURES
Ace Medical

**Figure 28-5.**   These are typical suturing instruments.

for suturing wounds of less delicate parts of the body, such as the hands or legs.

**Needle Holders.**   Curved suture needles require special instruments to hold, insert, and retrieve them during suturing. Most needle holders look like hemostats with short, sturdy jaws.

## Syringes and Needles

Sterile syringes and needles are used to inject anesthetic solutions, withdraw fluids, or obtain biopsy specimens. The size of the syringe and needle varies with the intended use. For example, a needle used to perform a biopsy is generally larger than needles used for most injections. (Syringes and needles used for injections are discussed and illustrated in Chapter 38.) Both syringes and needles are provided in individual sterile envelopes.

## Instrument Trays and Packs

All the surgical instruments needed for a specific procedure are usually assembled beforehand. They are then sterilized together in a pack. Certain surgical supplies necessary for the procedure (such as gauze) are included in the pack because they, too, must be sterile. Surgical

trays can be quickly set up with these instrument packs. Individually wrapped items may also be added as needed.

These are common types of instrument trays:

• Laceration repair tray (see Figure 28-6)
• Laceration repair with debridement tray

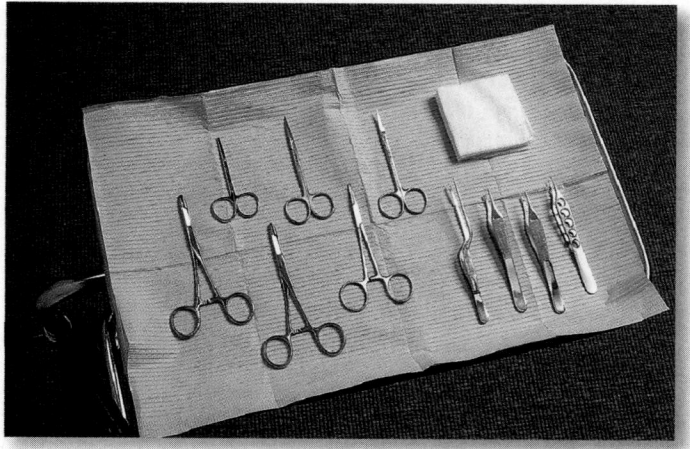

**Figure 28-6.**   This laceration tray contains scissors, several pairs of forceps, a needle holder, suture material, and sterile gauze.

- Incision and drainage tray
- Foreign body or growth removal tray
- **Onychectomy** (nail removal) tray
- Vasectomy (male sterilization procedure) tray
- Suture removal tray
- Staple removal tray

# Asepsis

Maintaining asepsis during surgical procedures is always a priority. It is critical to the health and safety of both the patient and the health-care professional. The two levels of aseptic technique, medical asepsis (clean technique) and surgical asepsis (sterile technique), are described in detail in Chapter 20. You will use both levels of asepsis when assisting with minor surgery.

## Medical Asepsis

**Medical asepsis** involves procedures to reduce the number of microorganisms and thus prevent the spread of disease. These procedures do not necessarily eliminate microorganisms. Hand washing is always the first line of defense against spreading disease. The use of antimicrobial agents (agents that kill microorganisms or suppress their growth) and personal protective equipment are also part of medical asepsis. Other practices include proper handling and disposal of sharps and biohazardous materials.

**Personal Protective Equipment.** Personal protective equipment, or PPE, includes all items used as a barrier between the wearer and potentially infectious or hazardous medical materials. PPE includes gloves, gowns, and masks and protective eyewear or face shields (Figure 28-7). OSHA regulations regarding PPE are discussed in detail in Chapter 19.

Gloves are of particular importance during surgical procedures. You should wear properly sized latex or vinyl gloves during any procedure that might expose you to potentially infectious or hazardous materials. (Gloves that are too big can catch on instruments or equipment and cause accidents.) When you wear gloves, you also protect the patient from any infectious organisms on your hands.

Both vinyl and latex gloves can prevent contamination of the hands with bacteria. Many health-care institutions prefer latex gloves. However, the incidence of latex allergy among health-care professionals has grown. Allergic reactions to latex can range from a skin rash to shock and even death. Many health-care institutions are switching to less allergenic latex gloves, such as low-powder and powderless varieties. The powder in the gloves, which makes them easier to put on, is one of the primary sources of latex allergy. The latex protein that causes the allergy mixes with the powder. When the gloves are removed, the powder containing the latex protein becomes airborne and is inhaled.

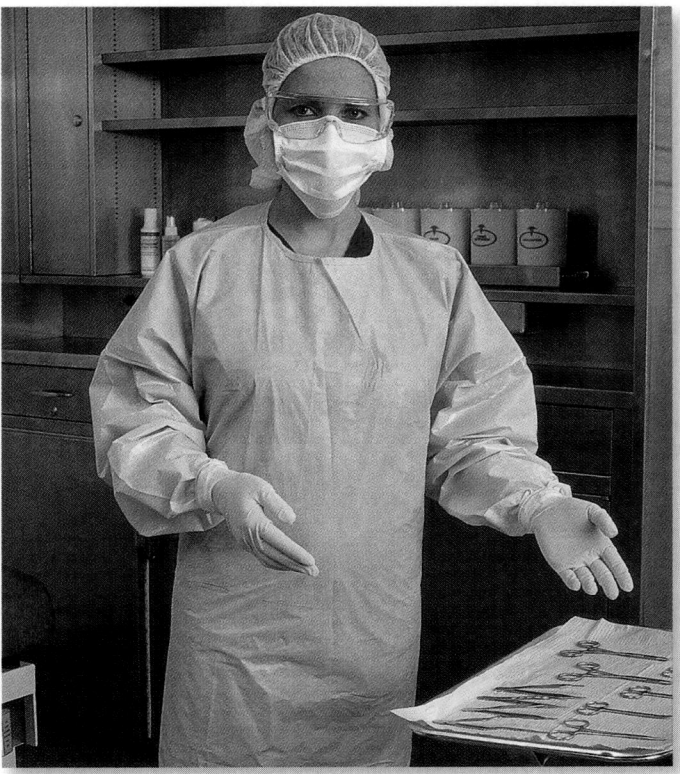

**Figure 28-7.** Personal protective equipment provides a barrier between infections or hazardous medical materials and the wearer.

Other steps to prevent latex allergy include changing gloves frequently, thoroughly drying hands after washing, and frequently applying lotion to the hands. If you notice symptoms of a latex allergy, you should consider consulting an allergist. You should also discuss your symptoms with your supervisor, who will recommend that you switch to hypoallergenic or vinyl gloves. If you have an allergy, the health-care facility where you are employed is required to provide nonlatex gloves for your use.

**Sharps and Biohazardous Waste Handling and Disposal.** Sharp medical and surgical instruments have great potential for transmitting infection through cuts and puncture wounds. Used scalpels, needles, syringes, and other sharp objects should be disposed of in a puncture-resistant sharps container.

All items other than sharps that have come in contact with tissue, blood, or body fluids must be disposed of in a leakproof plastic bag or container. The container must either be red or be labeled with the orange-red biohazard symbol. The proper procedure for handling and disposing of sharps and biohazardous waste is discussed in detail in Chapter 20.

## Surgical Asepsis

In contrast to medical asepsis, the purpose of **surgical asepsis** is to eliminate all microorganisms. Surgical asepsis does not just reduce the quantity of microorganisms but

## CAUTION *Handle With Care*

### Rules for Sterile Technique

A sterile field is an area used during a surgical procedure that is free of microorganisms. To maintain sterility throughout the procedure, follow the surgical technique and adhere to these rules:

1. The contact of a sterile area or article with a nonsterile article renders it nonsterile.

2. If there is a doubt about the sterility of an article or area, it is considered nonsterile.

3. Unused, opened sterile supplies must be discarded or resterilized.

4. Packages are wrapped or sealed in such a way that they can be opened without contamination.

5. The edges of wrappers (1-inch margin) covering sterile supplies, the outer lips of bottles, or flasks containing sterile solutions are not considered sterile.

6. When a sterile surface or package becomes wet, it is considered contaminated.

7. Reaching over a sterile field when you are not wearing sterile clothing contaminates the area.

8. When wearing sterile gloves, keep your hands between your shoulders and your waist to maintain sterility.

9. Even in a sterile gown, your back is considered contaminated; do not turn your back on a sterile field.

---

completely eliminates them. View the Caution: Handle With Care section that contains rules for sterile technique.

Common procedures involving sterile technique that you will be expected to perform include the following:

- Creating a sterile field
- Adding sterile items to the sterile field
- Performing a surgical scrub
- Putting on sterile gloves
- Sanitizing, disinfecting, and sterilizing equipment

**Creating a Sterile Field.** A **sterile field** is an area free of microorganisms that will be used as a work area during a surgical procedure. Always be aware that in the following instances the sterile field is considered to become contaminated and must be redone:

- An unsterile item touches the field
- Someone reaches across the field
- The field becomes wet
- The field is left unattended and uncovered
- You turn your back on the field

The sterile field is often set up on a **Mayo stand,** a movable stainless steel instrument tray on a stand. You should adjust the stand so the tray is above waist level. Remember, items placed below waist level are considered contaminated. Before beginning, disinfect the Mayo stand with 70% isopropyl alcohol, and allow it to dry.

To create the sterile field, cover the stand with two layers of sterile material. This material can be sterile disposable drapes, separately sterilized muslin towels, or the muslin towels that the surgical instruments are wrapped in before autoclaving to produce office-sterilized sterile instrument packs. Commercially prepared sterile instrument packs, usu-

ally with disposable paper wrappings, are also used to create a sterile field. Procedure 28-1 describes how to prepare a sterile field and how to open sterile packages.

When assembling the necessary supplies, place all unsterile items that may be used during the procedure outside the sterile field. Unsterile items include items that are sterile on the inside but not on the outside, such as a sterile gauze pack or sterile liquid such as alcohol, saline, or peroxide inside an unsterile bottle. Unsterile supplies should be arranged on a counter away from the sterile field. A typical arrangement of unsterile items used in surgery is shown in Figure 28-8. If you place an unsterile item within the sterile field, the field is no longer sterile and you must repeat the entire process.

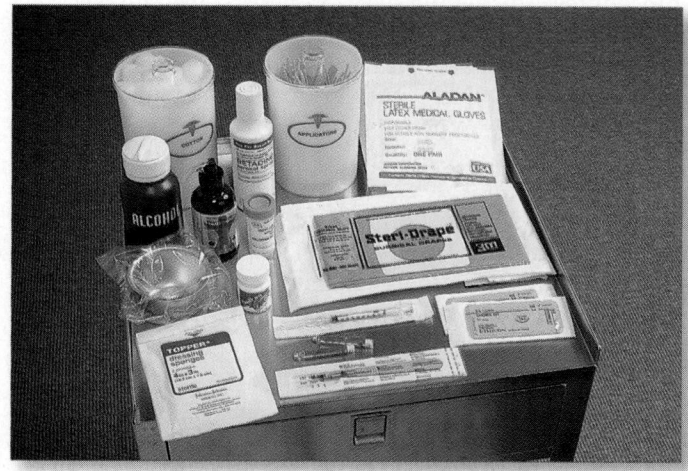

**Figure 28-8.** For each surgical procedure, unsterile surgical supplies must be gathered and arranged in an area separate from the sterile field.

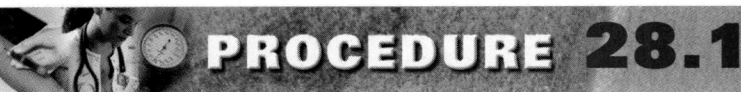

# PROCEDURE 28.1

## Creating a Sterile Field

**Procedure Goal:** To create a sterile field for a minor surgical procedure

**OSHA Guidelines:** This procedure does not involve exposure to blood, body fluids, or tissues.

**Materials:** Tray or Mayo stand, sterile instrument pack, sterile transfer forceps, cleaning solution, sterile drape, additionally packaged sterile items as required

**Method:**

1. Clean and disinfect the tray or Mayo stand.
2. Wash your hands and assemble the necessary materials.
3. Check the label on the instrument pack to make sure it is the correct pack for the procedure.
4. Check the date and sterilization indicator on the instrument pack to make sure the pack is still sterile (Figure 28-9).

### Rationale

Using a pack that is out of date puts the patient at risk for post-surgical infection.

5. Place the sterile pack on the tray or stand, and unfold the outermost fold away from yourself.
6. Unfold the sides of the pack outward, touching only the areas that will become the underside of the sterile field.

### Rationale

Touching the inside of the pack will contaminate the sterile field.

7. Open the final flap toward yourself, stepping back and away from the sterile field (Figure 28-10).

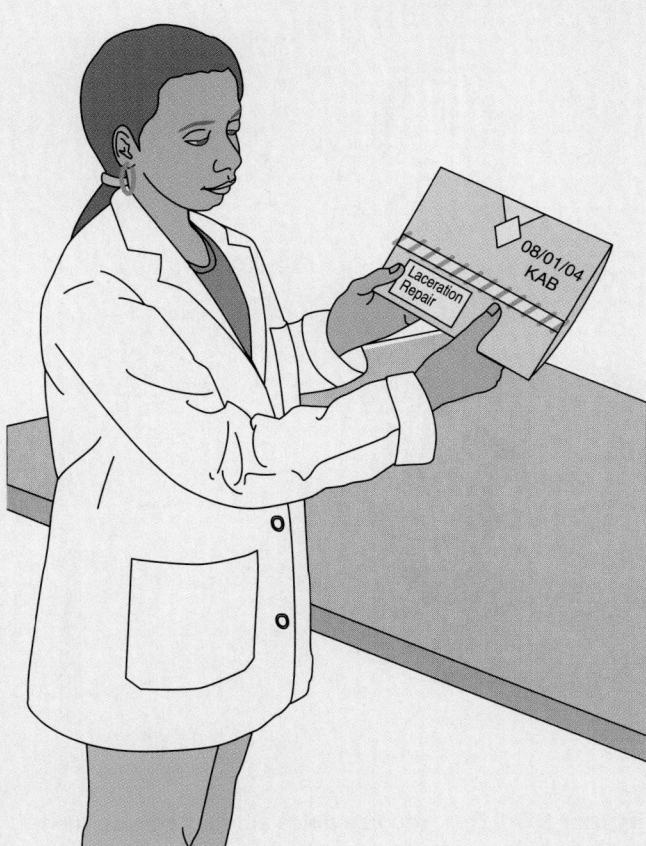

**Figure 28-9.** Before you open it, confirm that you have the correct instrument pack and that it has not expired.

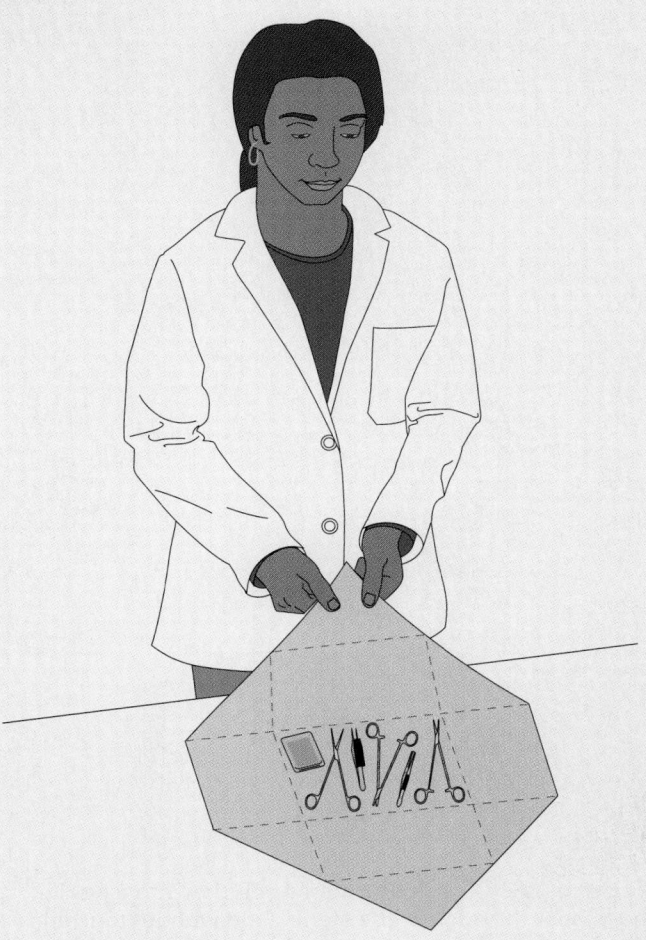

**Figure 28-10.** The fully open instrument pack constitutes a sterile field.

*continued* ⟶

## Creating a Sterile Field *(concluded)*

8. Place additional packaged sterile items on the sterile field.

   • Ensure that you have the correct item or instrument and that the package is still sterile.

   • Stand away from the sterile field.

   • Grasp the package flaps and pull apart about halfway.

   • Bring the corners of the wrapping beneath the package, paying attention not to contaminate the inner package or item.

   • Hold the package over the sterile field with the opening down; with a quick movement, pull the flap completely open and snap the sterile item onto the field.

9. Place basins and bowls near the edge of the sterile field so you can pour liquids without reaching over the field (Figure 28-11).

   *Rationale*
   Reaching over the field may drop contaminants in the field.

10. Use sterile transfer forceps if necessary to add additional items to the sterile field (Figure 28-12).

11. If necessary, don sterile gloves after a sterile scrub to arrange items on the sterile field.

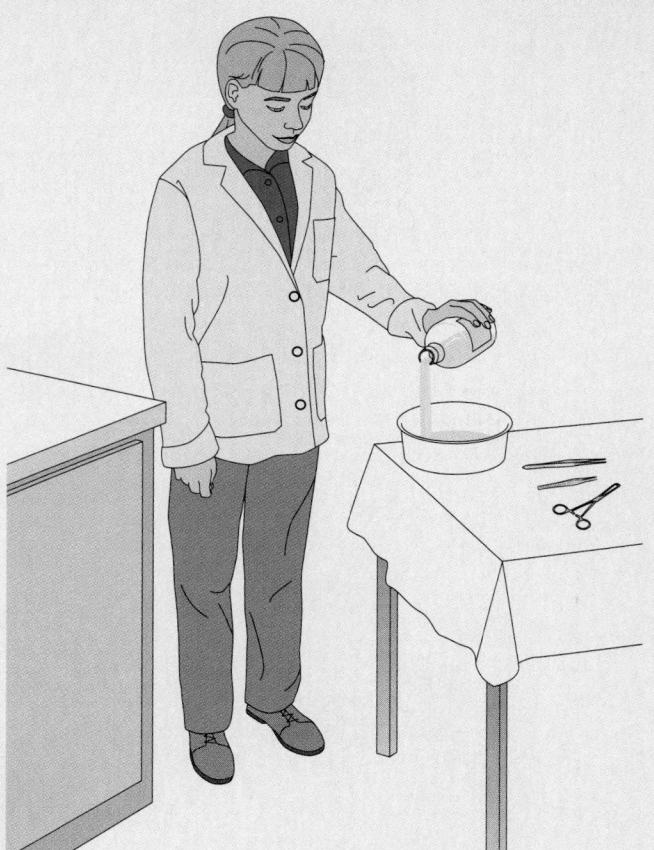

**Figure 28-11.** Pour a sterile solution into a sterile bowl near the edge of the sterile field without touching the rim of the bowl, splashing the solution, or reaching over the field.

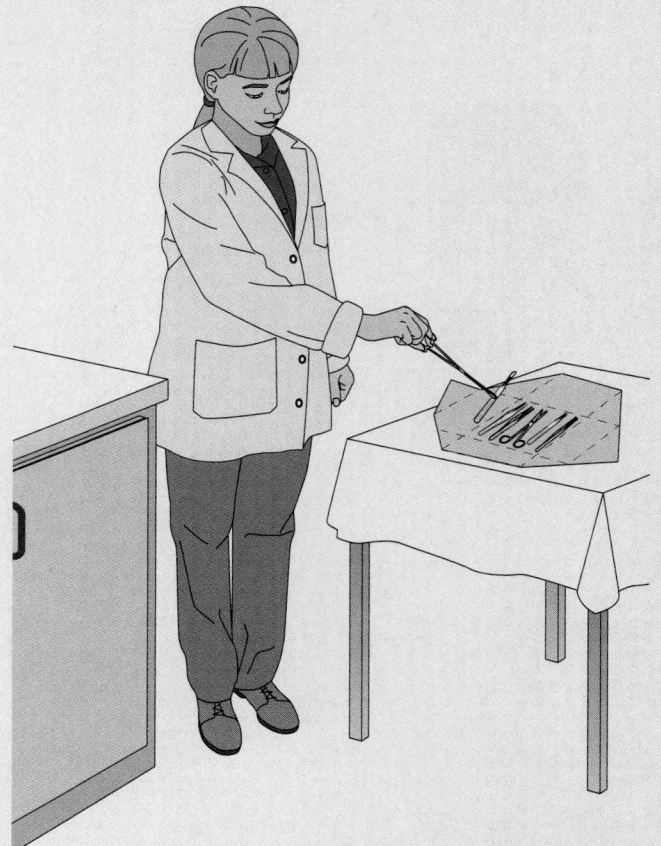

**Figure 28-12.** You can place sterile items on the sterile field by using transfer forceps.

**Adding Sterile Items to the Sterile Field.** The outer 1 inch of the sterile field is considered contaminated. Therefore, before you add sterile items to the sterile field, carefully plan where you will place the instruments so that they are within the sterile field.

***Instruments and Supplies.*** If you have used sterile disposable drapes or separately sterilized muslin towels to create the sterile field, you will need to add the necessary instruments. Stand away from the sterile field, and open the sterile instrument pack in the manner described in Procedure 28-1. Place the pack on a counter or hold it open in your hand. Transfer and arrange the instruments on the sterile field with sterile transfer forceps (see Figure 28-12). Avoid reaching across the sterile field.

If you must add other items to the field, open them using the same method. Stand away from the sterile field. As you unwrap the item, gather the corners of the wrapping beneath it. You can place the contents on the sterile field by using sterile transfer forceps or by using the sterile inside of the wrapping to prevent your hands from touching the item. Place basins or bowls near the edge of the sterile field so you can pour liquids without reaching over the field.

Some instruments are sterilized individually in autoclave bags, and sterile supplies are often prepackaged. Stand away from the sterile field as you open an individual bag or package. You can pull the flaps of the packaging partway apart, then snap (remove from position by a sudden movement) the item onto the sterile field from a distance of 8 to 12 inches. Alternatively, you can use sterile forceps to grasp and place the items in the sterile field.

***Pouring Sterile Solutions.*** Sterile solutions are often required during the surgical procedure to rinse or wash the wound. Sterile solutions can be added to the sterile field after the sterile instruments. Several sterile solutions are commonly used during minor surgical procedures. These include sterile water and physiological (normal) saline (0.9% sodium chloride).

Bottles of these sterile solutions come in a variety of sizes. You should choose the smallest size that will meet the solutions needed during the procedure. Using the smallest size possible minimizes the cost because unused solutions must be discarded.

When pouring a solution, cover the label on the bottle with the palm of your hand to keep the label dry. Pour a small amount of the liquid into a liquid waste receptacle to clean the lip of the bottle. As you pour the solution into a sterile bowl on the field, hold the bottle at an angle so that you do not reach over the sterile area (see Figure 28-11). Hold the bottle fairly close to the bowl without touching it. Pour the contents slowly to avoid splashing the drape, which would contaminate the field.

When a sterile solution bottle is opened and may be used again during the procedure, do not let any unsterile object touch the inside of its cap. To accomplish this, place the cap on a clean location with the sterile inside of the cap facing down.

**Performing a Surgical Scrub and Donning Sterile Gloves.** If you assist in a surgical procedure, you must perform a surgical scrub and wear sterile surgical gloves. You may wonder why a surgical scrub is necessary if you are planning to wear sterile gloves. The answer is that there is always the possibility that a glove may be punctured. If the skin is as clean as possible, the risk of contamination from a punctured glove is minimized. Nevertheless, if a glove is damaged during a sterile procedure, you must consider anything touched by that glove to be contaminated. Contaminated items must be resterilized or replaced before you continue.

A surgical scrub removes microorganisms more effectively than does routine hand washing. Routine hand washing removes bacteria present on the skin's surface, whereas the surgical scrub removes bacteria in deeper layers of the skin—where the hair follicles and oil-producing glands are. Procedure 28-2 describes the process.

Sterile gloves are required for many procedures. You don sterile gloves after you perform the surgical scrub. The process is described in Procedure 28-3.

Remember that once you are wearing sterile gloves, you may touch only the items in the sterile field. Therefore, you must remove any drape covering the sterile instrument tray before you glove. Sterile gloves provide a small margin of safety in preventing contamination. You must keep your movements controlled and precise to work within that margin to protect the sterile area.

**Sanitizing, Disinfecting, and Sterilizing Equipment.** Many supplies used in a doctor's office are disposable. Most surgical instruments, however, are made of steel and are reusable. Preparing surgical instruments for reuse involves cleaning them with soap and water (a process called sanitization), then disinfecting and/or sterilizing them, depending on how the equipment will be used. (These procedures are described more fully in Chapter 20.)

# Preoperative Procedures

You must complete a number of steps before a surgical procedure. The steps include performing various preliminary duties, preparing the surgical room, and physically preparing the patient for surgery.

## Preliminary Duties

You will perform several preliminary tasks before the surgery. They include providing **preoperative** (prior to surgery or "preop") instructions to the patient, completing various administrative tasks, and easing the patient's fears.

**Preoperative Instructions.** When a patient is scheduled for a minor surgical procedure in the doctor's office, you must explain the preoperative instructions. You should also be prepared to answer the patient's questions about the procedure and about possible risks. The patient

# Performing a Surgical Scrub

**Procedure Goal:** To remove dirt and microorganisms from under the fingernails and from the surface of the skin, hair follicles, and oil glands of the hands and forearms

**OSHA Guidelines:** This procedure does not involve exposure to blood, body fluids, or tissues.

**Materials:** Dispenser with surgical soap, sterile surgical scrub brush or sponge, sterile towels

**Method:**

1. Remove all jewelry and roll up your sleeves to above the elbow.
2. Assemble the necessary materials.
3. Turn on the faucet using the foot or knee pedal.
4. Wet your hands from the fingertips to the elbows. You must keep your hands higher than your elbows.

*Rationale*

This prevents water from running down your arms and contaminating the washed area.

5. Under running water, use a sterile brush to clean under your fingernails.
6. Apply surgical soap, and scrub your hands, fingers, areas between the fingers, wrists, and forearms with the scrub sponge, using a firm circular motion (Figure 28-13). Follow the manufacturer's recommendations to determine appropriate length of time, usually 2 to 6 minutes.

*Rationale*

Scrubbing all surfaces dislodges microorganisms so that they may be rinsed away.

7. Rinse from fingers to elbows, always keeping your hands higher than your elbows (Figure 28-14).
8. Thoroughly dry your hands and forearms with sterile towels, working from the hands to the elbows (Figure 28-15).

*Rationale*

Using sterile towels prevents recontaminating your hands.

9. Turn off the faucet with the foot or knee pedal. Use a clean paper towel if a foot or knee pedal is not used.

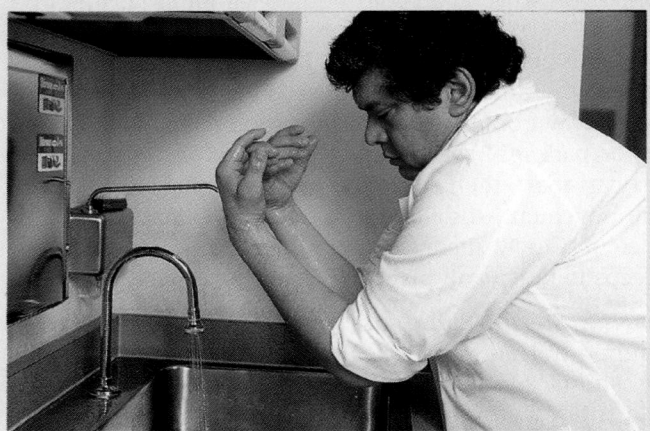

**Figure 28-14.** Keep your hands above your elbows while rinsing from fingertips to elbows.

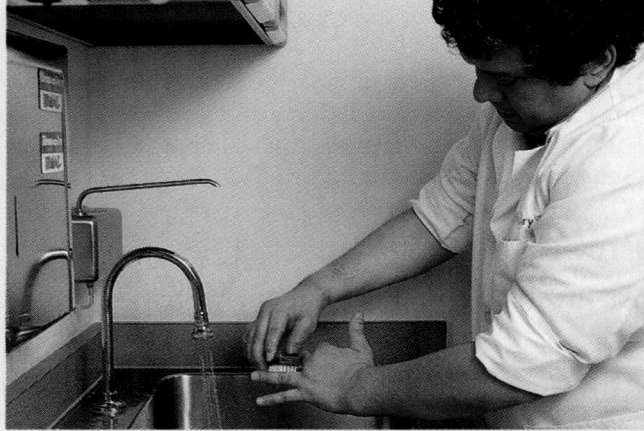

**Figure 28-13.** Use the scrub brush to work the surgical soap into your fingers, then your wrists, and then your forearms with a firm, circular motion.

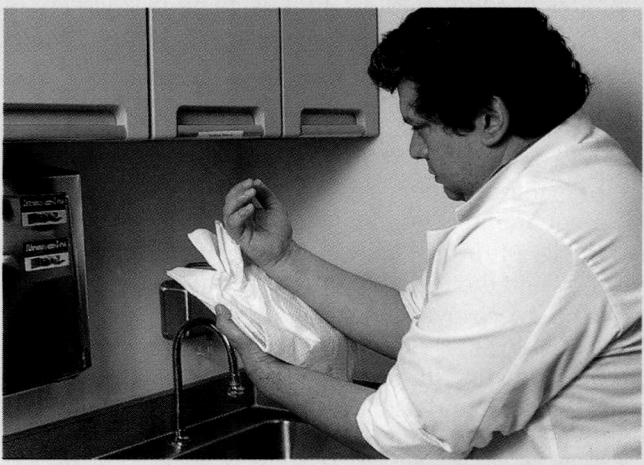

**Figure 28-15.** Dry your hands thoroughly before carefully drying your forearms.

# Donning Sterile Gloves

**Procedure Goal:** To don sterile gloves without compromising the sterility of the outer surface of the gloves

**OSHA Guidelines:** This procedure does not involve exposure to blood, body fluids, or tissues.

**Materials:** Correctly sized, prepackaged, double-wrapped sterile gloves

**Method:**

1. Obtain the correct size gloves.
2. Check the package for tears, and ensure that the expiration date has not passed.

   *Rationale*

   A torn package should be considered unsterile.
3. Perform a surgical scrub.
4. Peel the outer wrap from gloves and place the inner wrapper on a clean surface above waist level (Figure 28-16).
5. Position gloves so the cuff end is closest to your body.
6. Touch only the flaps as you open the package.

   *Rationale*

   Touching the inside of the package could contaminate the gloves.
7. Use instructions provided on the inner package, if available.

8. Do not reach over the sterile inside of the inner package.
9. Follow these steps if there are no instructions:
   a. Open the package so the first flap is opened away from you.
   b. Pinch the corner and pull to one side.
   c. Put your fingertips under the side flaps and gently pull until the package is completely open.
10. Use your nondominant hand to grasp the inside cuff of the opposite glove (the folded edge). Do not touch the outside of the glove. If you are right-handed, use your left hand to put on the right glove first, and vice versa.

    *Rationale*

    Grabbing the inside of the gloves allows you to put it on without contaminating the outside of the gloves.
11. Holding the glove at arm's length and waist level, insert the dominant hand into the glove with the palm facing up. Don't let the outside of the glove touch any other surface (Figure 28-17).
12. With your sterile gloved hand, slip the gloved fingers into the cuff of the other glove.

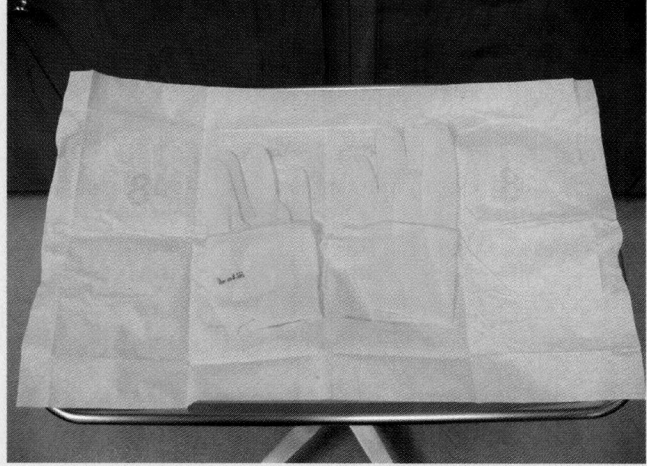

**Figure 28-16.** You must put these sterile gloves on without reaching across the sterile surfaces of the gloves or the sterile inner wrap of the pack.

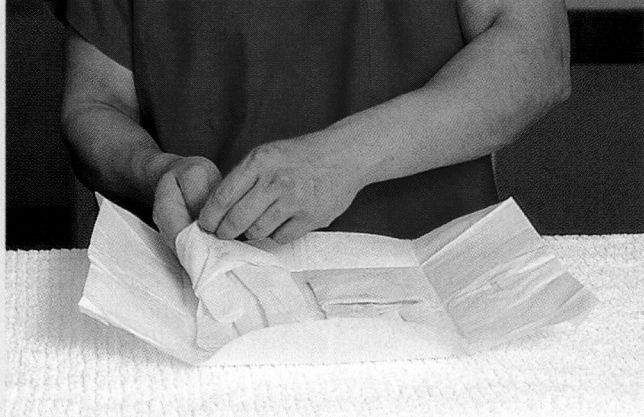

**Figure 28-17.** Your palm should face up as you slide your dominant hand into the first glove.

*continued* ⟶

## Donning Sterile Gloves *(concluded)*

**13.** Pick up the other glove, touching only the outside. Don't touch any other surfaces (Figure 28-18).

**14.** Pull the glove up and onto your hand. Ensure that the sterile gloved hand does not touch skin (Figure 28-19).

**15.** Adjust your fingers as necessary, touching only glove to glove.

**16.** Do not adjust the cuffs because your forearms may contaminate the gloves.

**17.** Keep your hands in front of you, between your shoulders and waist. If you move your hands out of this area, they are considered contaminated.

**18.** If contamination or the possibility of contamination occurs, change gloves.

**19.** Remove gloves the same way you remove clean gloves, by touching only the inside.

### Rationale
Touching only the inside of the gloves reduces exposure to the patient's blood and body fluids.

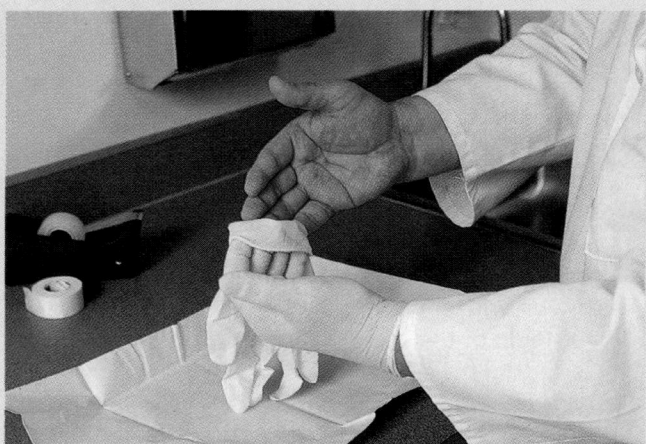

**Figure 28-18.** Your gloved fingers secure the remaining glove while you slip it over your nondominant hand.

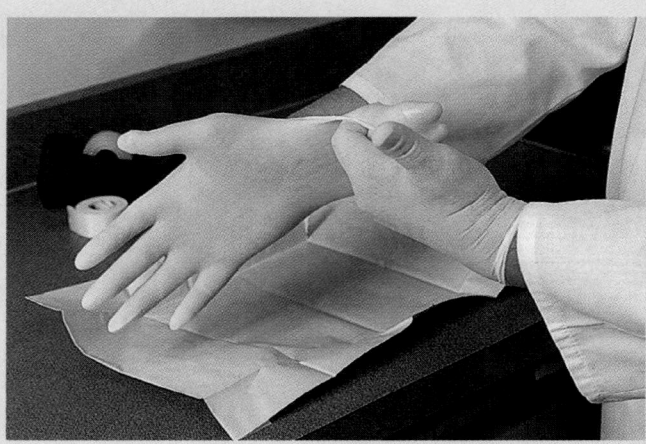

**Figure 28-19.** Unfold the cuff over your arm while touching only the sterile surface of the glove.

---

may ask you, rather than the doctor, such questions or may need clarification of information provided by the doctor.

A patient may need to follow certain dietary and fluid restrictions before a minor surgical procedure. Not eating or drinking for a specific period of time is a common restriction. There may also be restrictions on what medications a patient may take, because of the administration of an anesthetic during the procedure. You will need to tell non–English-speaking patients to bring along a family member or other interpreter who can help them understand the forms they must sign and their instructions.

You should instruct the patient to wear either comfortable, loose-fitting clothes that will not interfere with the procedure or clothing that can be removed easily. In most cases patients also need to arrange for someone to drive them home after a procedure and stay with them for 24 hours after the procedure.

**Administrative and Legal Tasks.** You must ensure that all the necessary paperwork is completed before surgery. Routine administrative tasks include completing the required insurance forms and obtaining prior authorization from the patient's insurance company.

Make absolutely certain that the patient reads, understands, and signs the surgical consent form. The patient needs a clear understanding of what to expect during and after the surgery to give informed consent as required by law. Sometimes surgery is performed on a child or a patient with limited understanding of legal documents. In such cases the consent form must be signed by the patient's parent or legal guardian.

Failure to obtain the necessary paperwork prior to a surgical procedure can cause serious legal problems. The doctor and other staff members could be held legally liable if problems were to develop during or after the procedure.

It is common practice to call the patient the day before the surgery to confirm the appointment. This call also provides a chance to ensure that the patient follows the preoperative instructions. You may be responsible for making this call.

**Easing the Patient's Fears.** Knowing what to expect during and after a surgical procedure will ease patients' fears. This information allows them to plan their daily activities and, if necessary, to arrange for help at home during the recovery period.

Some offices may have educational materials such as brochures, fact sheets, or videotapes about the procedure the patient will undergo. The availability of such materials varies with the practice specialty and the frequency with which the procedure is performed. You may assist in preparing or acquiring these materials if your office's policy includes such participation for medical assistants. This type of information may increase patient compliance with the pre- and postoperative instructions.

Much of a patient's fear about a surgical procedure can be overcome if you spend sufficient time before the procedure explaining what to expect. Be prepared to answer the patient's questions honestly, calmly, and confidently. Your calm and knowledgeable manner will reassure the patient. If the answer to a question requires experience or knowledge beyond your own, pass the question on to the doctor.

# Preparing the Surgical Room

Prior to surgery the doctor should inform you of specific instructions concerning patient preparation. He will also tell you what special equipment or supplies are necessary for the procedure.

Because patients are likely to feel anxious before a procedure, it is best to have everything ready in the surgical room before you escort the patient into the room. Make sure the room is clean, neat, and free of waste from previous procedures. The examining table should have been cleaned and disinfected, and surface barriers (table paper and pillow covers) should have been changed.

Check to see that there is adequate lighting. Make sure that all equipment and supplies necessary for the procedure are available. Check the date and sterilization indicator on sterilized packs and supplies. Sterile packs are typically considered unsterile if more than 1 month has passed since they were originally sterilized.

You will then wash your hands and prepare the sterile field as outlined in Procedure 28-1. The sterile field and the instruments should be draped with a sterile towel.

# Preparing the Patient

Just before the surgery, various concerns must be addressed and procedures completed in sequence. The initial tasks are followed by gowning and positioning the patient and preparing the patient's skin for surgery.

**Initial Tasks.** Before leading the patient into the surgical room, find out whether he has followed the presurgical instructions. Restrictions on food and fluid intake are of particular concern. It is also important to ask what medications the patient is taking and whether he has taken that day's dosage.

Measure the patient's vital signs. Ask if there are any symptoms or problems the doctor should know about before the surgery. If any unusual signs or symptoms are present, notify the doctor. The doctor will want to examine the patient before proceeding.

Check the chart for medication orders, such as pain medication or a tranquilizer to calm the patient. Medications should be administered at this time so that they will take effect before surgery.

**Gowning and Positioning the Patient.** Some procedures require the patient to disrobe and put on a gown to expose the surgical site. If this is the case, you should offer to assist, if appropriate, or leave the room while the patient changes. You should then help the patient onto the table and into the position required for the procedure. You may use one or more small pillows to make the patient as comfortable as possible. Then adequately drape the patient to retain body heat and preserve personal dignity.

Sterile drapes are also used to create a sterile field on a patient's body around the surgical site. Drapes come in a variety of sizes and styles. A fenestrated drape has a round or slitlike opening cut out in the center to provide access to the surgical site.

**Surgical Skin Preparation.** Proper preparation of the patient's skin before surgery reduces the number of microorganisms and the risk of infection. The prepared area should extend 2 inches beyond the surgical field—the area exposed in the center of the fenestrated drape. This extra margin allows for draping without contaminating the field.

*Cleaning the Area.* Before proceeding with the surgical skin preparation, wash your hands and put on exam gloves. Place a plastic-backed drape under the surgical site to absorb any liquids. Clean the site first with antiseptic soap and sterile water, using forceps and gauze sponges dipped in the solution. Begin at the center of the surgical site, and work outward in a firm, circular motion (Figure 28-20). Discard the gauze sponge after each complete pass. Clean in concentric circles until you cover the full preparation area. Continue the process, repeating as necessary, for at least 2 minutes or the amount of time specified in the office's procedure manual. Cleaning takes more time if a wound is dirty or contains foreign materials. When procedures are performed on a hand or foot, clean the entire hand or foot.

*Removing Hair from the Area.* Depending on office policy, you may be required to remove hair from the surgical site. Shaving often causes many small wounds on the skin, which increases the risk of infection, and is not recommended. Some experts feel that hair should not be commonly used, but chlorhexidine gluconate (Hibiclens) or benzalkonium chloride (Zephiran Chloride) may also be used, particularly if the patient is allergic to iodine. Swab an area 2 inches larger than the surgical field with the antiseptic solution in a circular outward motion, starting at the surgical site. This is the same motion that is used for cleaning the surgical site. For surgery on a hand or foot, swab the entire hand or foot. Allow the antiseptic to air-dry; do not pat it dry—that would remove some of the solution's antiseptic properties.

When the area is dry, treat it as a sterile field. Instruct the patient not to touch the area. Cover the area with a sterile fenestrated drape, from front to back. Avoid reaching over the field. At this point notify the physician that the patient is ready. Then prepare yourself to assist with the surgery.

# Intraoperative Procedures

**Intraoperative** procedures are procedures that take place during surgery. You may be asked to perform a wide variety of unsterile and sterile tasks during surgery, such as preparing local anesthetic for the doctor, monitoring the patient, processing specimens, and handing instruments to the doctor. The doctor may also ask you to explain to the patient step by step what will be done next during the procedure.

## Administering a Local Anesthetic

Before beginning the surgical procedure, the physician will administer a local anesthetic. Some local anesthetics are injected. An injected anesthetic is packaged in a sterile **vial** (a small glass bottle with a self-sealing rubber stopper). Other local anesthetics come in a cream, gel, or spray form. These anesthetics are **topical** (applied directly to the skin) and affect only the area to which they are applied.

Lidocaine (Xylocaine) is the most commonly used anesthetic. It is often used as a topical gel anesthetic. Tetracaine hydrochloride (Pontocaine), a long-acting anesthetic, is injected.

The physician administers the local anesthetic by injection or by applying it directly to the skin. The choice of administration method depends on how invasive or painful the procedure is likely to be.

**Topical Application.** Anesthetic gels, creams, and sprays may be used topically in certain surgical procedures. A topical anesthetic is useful when the pain will be mild or when only the upper layers of the skin are affected. It is common to use such agents to anesthetize the area of a small laceration prior to suturing. Sometimes an anesthetic cream is applied before a local anesthetic is injected. This application reduces or eliminates the pain caused by the injection. A topical anesthetic must usually remain on the skin for 10 to 15 minutes for the area to become sufficiently anesthetized.

**Injections.** If a local anesthetic is to be injected, it is typically administered after the skin is prepared but before the patient is draped. In some cases, however, the anesthetic

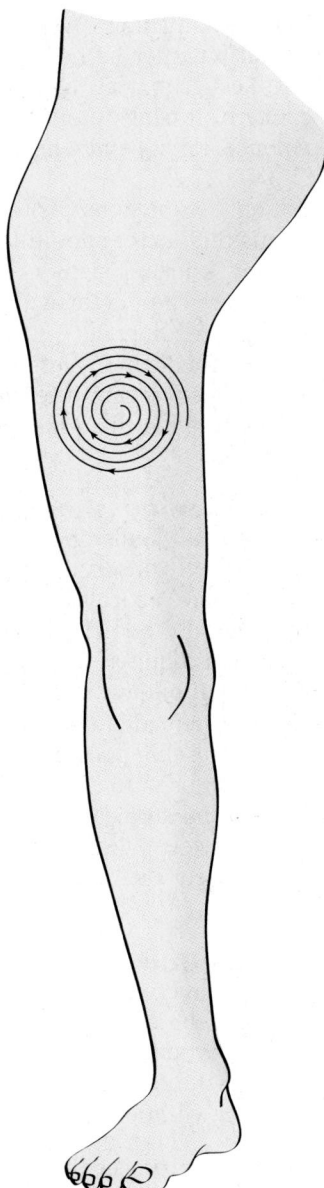

**Figure 28-20.** Clean the surgical site with antiseptic soap and sterile water. Begin at the center of the surgical site, and work outward in a firm, circular motion. Clean in a circular, outward pattern 2 inches larger than the surgical field.

Source: From Medical Assisting, Administrative & Clinical Competencies 4th edition by KEIR/WISE/KREBS, © 1998. Reprinted with permission of Delmar Learning, a division of Thomson Learning: www.thomsonrights.com. Fax 800-730-2215.

removed unless it is thick enough to interfere with surgery. If this is the case, hair may be trimmed with scissors or electric trimmers or smoothed out of the way. This should be done immediately before surgery.

*Applying the Antiseptic.* Next apply antiseptic solution to the area. Antiseptics are agents that are applied to the skin to limit the growth of microorganisms and to help prevent infection. Povidone iodine (Betadine) is most

is injected prior to skin preparation to allow time for it to take effect. In either case it is important to note the time of anesthetic administration in the patient's chart.

If the doctor is already wearing sterile gloves, you may be asked to assist in administering the anesthetic. Administering anesthetic is an unsterile task because the outside of the vial is unsterile. When performing this task, follow proper procedure to protect the sterility of the doctor's gloves and the anesthetic solution.

First check the label of the anesthetic vial two times to confirm that it is the correct solution. Clean the vial's rubber stopper with a 70% isopropyl alcohol solution, and leave the pad on top of the stopper. Present the requested needle and syringe to the doctor by peeling half the outer wrapper away and allowing the doctor to remove them from the wrapper.

Remove the pad from the rubber stopper, and hold the vial so the doctor can verify that it is the proper medication. Turn the vial upside down, and hold it securely around the base, without touching the sterile stopper. Be sure to hold the vial in front of you at shoulder height. Because significant force will be necessary to push the needle through the rubber stopper, you should brace the wrist of the hand holding the vial with your free hand. Hold the vial firmly so the doctor can withdraw the anesthetic from it (Figure 28-21). Check the vial a third time to confirm it is the correct solution.

### Potential Side Effects of the Anesthetic.
You should inform the patient of possible reactions to the anesthetic medication. Although rare, reactions may include dizziness, loss of consciousness, seizures, or cardiac arrest. Adverse reactions can occur if the anesthetic dose is too high or if it is absorbed too quickly. They can also occur if the patient is taking other medications that should not be mixed with the anesthetic. It is vital to document all medications (including OTC ones) that the patient is taking at the time of the surgery.

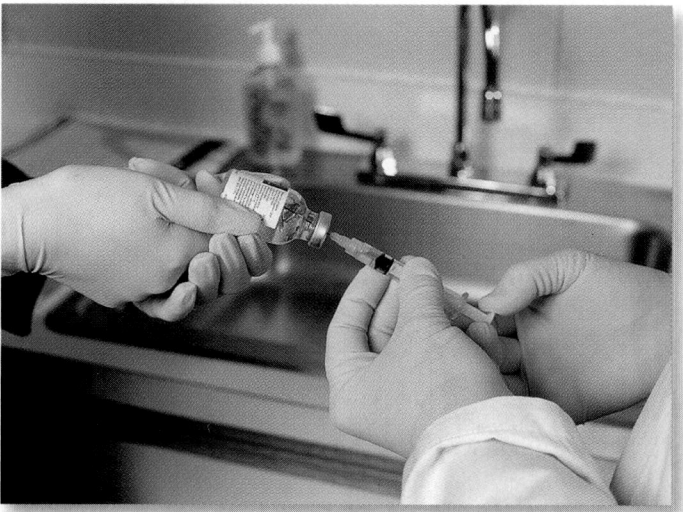

**Figure 28-21.** You must hold the anesthetic vial firmly to allow the physician to puncture the rubber stopper with the needle.

### Use of Epinephrine.
Epinephrine is a sterile solution that is sometimes injected along with an anesthetic. Epinephrine constricts the blood vessels, making them narrower. This constriction reduces bleeding and prolongs the action of the local anesthetic. Epinephrine is used if the site of surgery is an area with many small blood vessels that are expected to bleed profusely (such as the head). Reducing bleeding makes it easier to see and to repair the wound. (Epinephrine should be used with caution, however, in patients with heart disease or respiratory disease.)

When epinephrine is combined with the anesthetic to reduce bleeding, it prolongs the anesthesia because epinephrine slows the rate at which anesthetic spreads into the tissue. This effect may or may not be desirable. Epinephrine should not be used in areas such as the fingers, toes, nose, or ears, where it could also compromise the local blood supply. There is some concern that epinephrine may increase wound infection rates.

## Assisting the Physician During Surgery

Your role in surgical assisting depends on the type of surgery and the physician's preference. You may assist the physician in one of two capacities. You may serve as a **floater,** an unsterile assistant who is free to move about the room and attend to unsterile needs. Alternatively, you may serve as a **sterile scrub assistant,** who assists in handling sterile equipment during the procedure. The duties are different for the two functions.

### The Floater.
First the surgical room is set up and the patient is prepared. If you are assisting as a floater (sometimes called a circulator), you will perform a routine hand wash and put on exam gloves. Remember that you cannot touch sterile items in the sterile field because you have not performed a surgical scrub and are not wearing sterile gloves. Procedure 28-4 outlines the tasks performed by a floater (unsterile assistant).

*Monitoring and Recording.* One of the most important duties of a floater is to monitor the patient during the procedure. You must measure vital signs regularly and observe the patient for reactions to the anesthetic. Record all observations in the patient's chart. Also write down any information or notes the doctor requests. You must keep a record of time, including when the anesthetic is administered, when the procedure begins, and when the procedure is completed.

*Processing Specimens.* When you serve as a floater during surgery, the doctor may ask you to receive and process specimens for laboratory examination. Most tissues are placed in a 10% formalin solution to preserve them before they are sent to the laboratory. If the container is not prefilled, half-fill the specimen container with the formalin solution ahead of time. Remove the lid of the specimen container without touching the rim. Hold the container out toward the doctor so she can place the tissue directly into it without contaminating the sample (Figure 28-22).

# Assisting as a Floater (Unsterile Assistant) During Minor Surgical Procedures

**Procedure Goal:** To provide assistance to the doctor during minor surgery while maintaining clean or sterile technique as appropriate

**OSHA Guidelines**

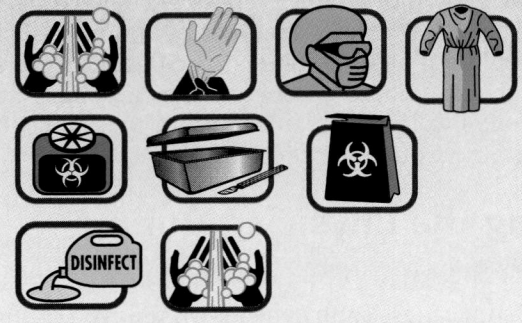

**Materials:** Sterile towel, tray or Mayo stand, appropriate instrument pack(s), needles and syringes, anesthetic, antiseptic, sterile water or normal saline, small sterile bowl, sterile gauze squares or cotton balls, specimen containers half-filled with preservative, suture materials, sterile dressings and tape

**Method:**

1. Perform routine hand washing and put on exam gloves.
2. Monitor the patient during the procedure; record the results in the patient's chart.
3. During the surgery, assist as needed.
4. Add sterile items to the tray as necessary.

5. Pour sterile solution into a sterile bowl as needed.
6. Assist in administering additional anesthetic.
   a. Check the medication vial two times.
   b. Clean the rubber stopper with an alcohol pad (write the date opened when using a new bottle); leave pad on top.
   c. Present the needle and syringe to the doctor.
   d. Remove the alcohol pad from the vial, and show the label to the doctor.
   e. Hold the vial upside down, and grasp the lower edge firmly; brace your wrist with your free hand.

   *Rationale*
   This firmly supports the vial to sustain the force of the needle being inserted into the rubber stopper.
   f. Allow the doctor to fill the syringe.
   g. Check the medication vial a final time
7. Receive specimens for laboratory examination.
   a. Uncap the specimen container; present it to the doctor for the introduction of the specimen.
   b. Replace the cap and label the container.
   c. Treat all specimens as infectious.
   d. Place the specimen container in a transport bag or other container.
   e. Complete the requisition form to send the specimen to the laboratory.

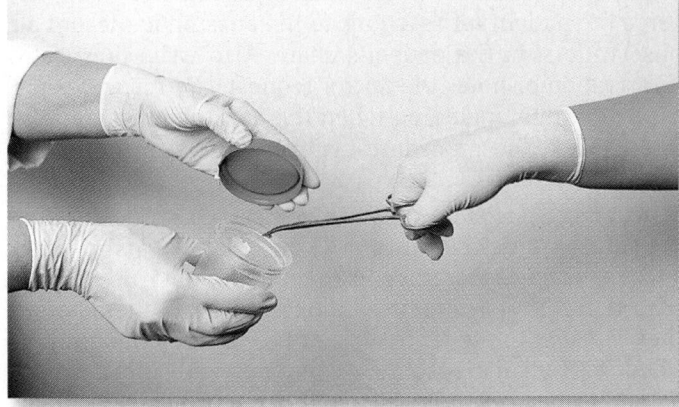

**Figure 28-22.** Be sure to hold the specimen container so that the doctor can place the tissue in it without touching the rim or the outside of the container with the tissue.

The container should be labeled with the following information:

- The patient's name and the doctor's name
- The date and time of collection
- The body site from which the specimen was obtained
- Your initials

If more than one specimen is obtained from a patient, place each specimen in a separate container. Label each container with the necessary information, along with a number to indicate the order in which the specimens are obtained (no. 1, no. 2, and so on). You will also fill out a laboratory requisition slip to send along with the specimen(s). Specimen containers should be red in color or labeled with the biohazard symbol. Specimen

# PROCEDURE 28.5

## Assisting as a Sterile Scrub Assistant During Minor Surgical Procedures

**Procedure Goal:** To provide assistance to the doctor during minor surgery while maintaining clean or sterile technique as appropriate

### OSHA Guidelines

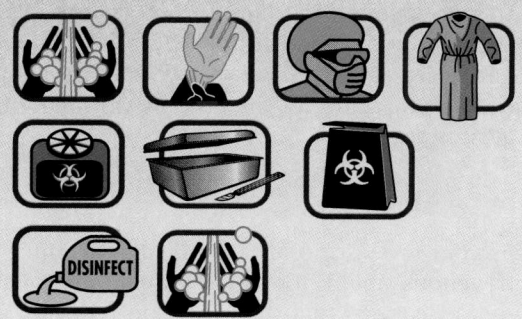

**Materials:** Sterile towel, tray or Mayo stand, appropriate instrument pack(s), needles and syringes, anesthetic, antiseptic, sterile water or normal saline, small sterile bowl, sterile gauze squares or cotton balls, specimen containers half-filled with preservative, suture materials, sterile dressings and tape

### Sterile Scrub Assistant

1. Perform a surgical scrub and put on sterile gloves. (Remember to remove the sterile towel covering the sterile field and instruments before gloving.)

   #### Rationale
   You will be handling sterile instruments.

2. Close and arrange the surgical instruments on the tray.

   #### Rationale
   They should be quickly and easily located.

3. Prepare for swabbing by inserting gauze squares into the sterile dressing forceps.
4. Pass the instruments as necessary.
5. Swab the wound as requested.
6. Retract the wound as requested.
7. Cut the sutures as requested.

---

containers should be placed in specially designed bags for transport.

***Other Duties.*** As a floater, you may also be asked to perform a number of other duties, including these:

- Assisting with the injection of additional anesthetic
- Adding additional sterile items to the sterile tray
- Pouring sterile solutions
- Keeping the surgical area clean and neat during the procedure
- Repositioning the patient as necessary
- Adjusting lighting

**The Sterile Scrub Assistant.** When you serve as a sterile scrub assistant, you perform a surgical scrub and wear sterile gloves. You may be asked to perform a variety of tasks under sterile conditions. Remember not to touch unsterile items after putting on sterile gloves. Procedure 28-5 outlines the tasks performed by a sterile scrub assistant.

***Handling Instruments.*** Your first duty as a sterile scrub assistant is, typically, to close the instruments on the sterile tray because they are normally left in the open position during sterilization. Your next duty is to rearrange the instruments on the tray. Instruments should be arranged in the order in which they will be used or according to the doctor's preference. Instruments are generally used in the following sequence:

- Cutting instruments
- Grasping instruments
- Retractors
- Probes
- Suture materials
- Needle holders and scissors

Prepare for swabbing by placing several sterile gauze squares in the dressing forceps. They will then be ready when needed. As the sterile scrub assistant, you will be asked to pass instruments to the doctor during the procedure. You must hold instruments so that the doctor can grasp them safely and securely, and will not need to reposition them in her hands. At the same time, the instruments must be handled properly to maintain their sterility.

When passing scissors and clamps, hold them by the hinge (Figure 28-23). You will have a clear view of the tip of the instrument, and the doctor will have full use of the handles. Firmly slap the instrument handles into the doctor's extended palm. The doctor's hand will close around the handles as a reflex action to the slapping. This technique reduces the risk of dropping an instrument. If the scissors or clamp is curved, the curve should follow the same curve as the doctor's hand.

When passing a scalpel, hold it above and just behind the cutting edge of the blade so the doctor can grasp the

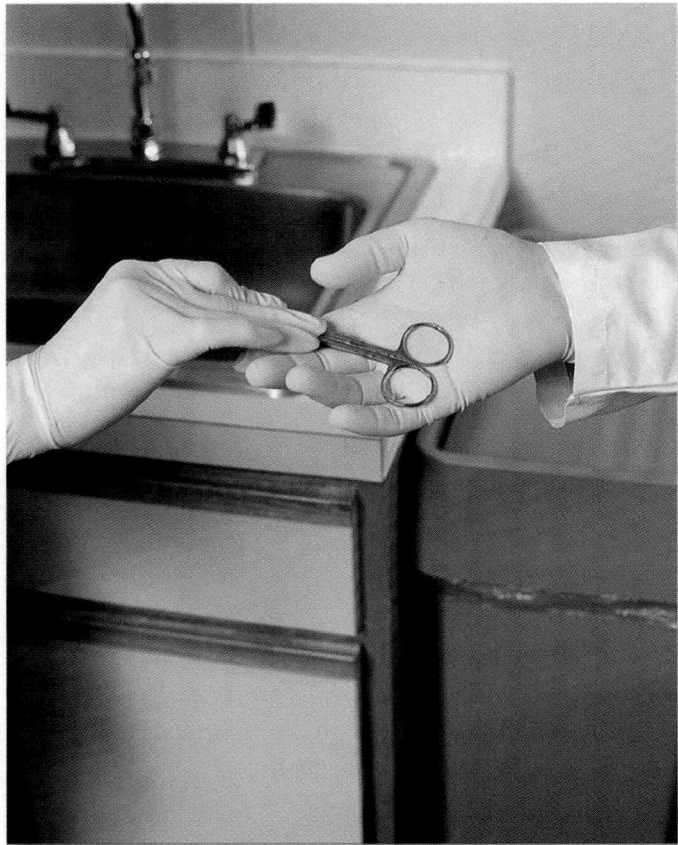

**Figure 28-23.** Holding the scissors by the hinge, slap the handles into the doctor's hand.

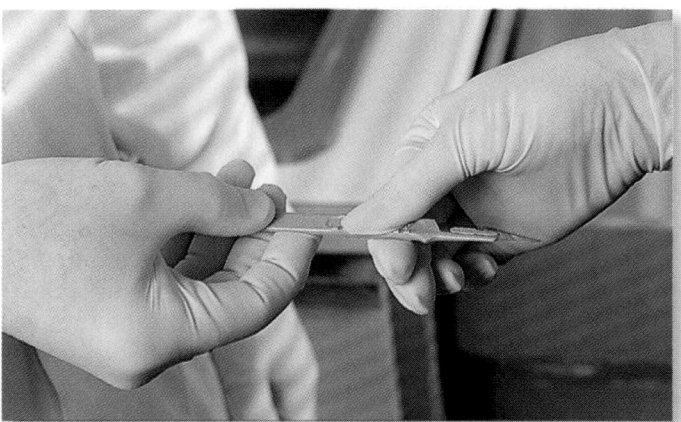

**Figure 28-24.** Hold a scalpel above and just behind the cutting edge as you pass the handle into the palm of the doctor's hand.

entire handle (Figure 28-24). Pass a needle holder with suture material so that the needle is pointing up, and hold the end of the suture material with your other hand to prevent the material from becoming tangled in the handles.

*Other Duties.* As a sterile scrub assistant, you may also be asked to swab fluids from a wound or to retract the edges of a wound to help the doctor view the area. While the doctor is closing the wound, you may be required to

cut the suture material after each stitch. The doctor may not verbalize every request to you. With practice and after experience with a particular doctor, you will learn how to respond to the doctor's actions.

When cutting suture materials, leave ⅛ inch of the material above the knot. This excess material prevents the suture from coming untied. It also leaves the material short enough so that it does not bother the patient.

# Postoperative Procedures

You will be responsible for the patient's **postoperative** ("postop") follow-up after the surgical procedure. Your duties may include immediate care of the patient, proper cleaning of the surgical room, and follow-up care of the patient. Procedure 28-6 outlines the tasks performed after a minor surgical procedure.

## Immediate Patient Care

Patient care is your top priority as a medical assistant. Except for intravenous medications, you will administer postoperative medications that the physician requests for the patient. You will also ensure that the patient remains lying down on the examining table for the prescribed length of time after the procedure. During this period, continue to monitor the patient's vital signs, and watch for adverse reactions. It is important to document your observations in the patient's chart.

**Dressing the Wound.** You may also dress the wound during the monitoring period. **Dressings** are sterile materials used to cover an incision. They serve a number of functions. They protect the wound from further injury and keep the wound clean, thus preventing infection. Dressings also reduce bleeding, absorb fluid drainage, reduce discomfort to the patient, speed healing, and reduce the possibility of scarring. Gauze dressings are the most common type of dressings and come in a variety of sizes and shapes.

Before dressing the wound, put on clean exam gloves. Clean the site with povidone iodine (Betadine), and allow it to dry. If ordered by the physician, apply antibiotic ointment over the wound. Place the sterile dressing over the site, and secure it appropriately.

**Bandaging the Wound.** It may be necessary to apply a bandage (a clean strip of gauze or elastic material) over the dressing to help hold it in place. Bandages may also be used to improve circulation, to provide support or reduce tension on a wound or suture and prevent it from reopening, or to prevent movement of that area of the body. Adhesive tape may also be used for these purposes. Some patients are allergic to the adhesive, but most tapes are now hypoallergenic. The patient is usually more comfortable after a bandage or adhesive tape has been applied.

**Postoperative Instructions.** After the procedure, provide oral postoperative instructions to the patient. You may do this during the monitoring part of the postoperative

# PROCEDURE 28.6

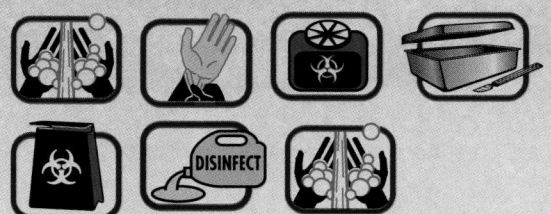

## Assisting After Minor Surgical Procedures

**Procedure Goal:** To provide assistance to the doctor during minor surgery while maintaining clean or sterile technique as appropriate

### OSHA Guidelines

**Materials:** Examination gloves, antiseptic, tray or Mayo stand, sterile dressings and tape

### Method:

1. Monitor the patient.
2. Put on clean exam gloves, and clean the wound with antiseptic.
3. Dress the wound.

#### Rationale

To protect the wound

4. Remove the gloves and wash your hands.
5. Give the patient oral postoperative instructions in addition to the release packet.

#### Rationale

The patient will need to understand wound care, medication use, and diet instructions for proper healing.

6. Discharge the patient.
7. Put on clean exam gloves.
8. Properly dispose of used materials and disposable instruments.
9. Sanitize reusable instruments and prepare them for disinfection and/or sterilization as needed.
10. Clean equipment and the exam room according to OSHA guidelines.
11. Remove the gloves and wash your hands.

---

period or afterward. These instructions include guidelines for pain management and instructions for wound care. Postoperative information also includes dietary or activity restrictions, if any, and when to come in for a follow-up appointment. It is a good idea to ask patients to repeat what you say so that you know they understand the information.

Instructions should be provided in writing as part of a complete postoperative information packet. You may be asked to help prepare or update packet materials, especially if you routinely assist patients as they recover from minor surgery. A postoperative information packet might include the following information:

- Proper wound-care instructions
- Suggestions for pain relief and reduction of swelling, such as medications and hot or cold packs
- Dietary restrictions
- Activity restrictions
- Timing for a follow-up appointment or an appointment card

Wound-care instructions include details on dressing changes, keeping the wound clean, recognizing signs of infection, and protecting the wound. The instructions may vary depending on the depth and size of the wound. In general, the bandage should be removed after the first 24 hours or if it becomes soaked with blood, wet, or dirty. A wet dressing allows bacteria and other contaminants to enter the wound. In most cases, the wound may be cleaned

with soap and water after 24 to 48 hours. Once cleaned, gently dry the incision and cover with a clean, dry bandage. The doctor may ask the patient to use an antibiotic ointment on the wound site.

You should teach the patient about the signs of infection. For more information, see Educating the Patient: When to Call the Doctor About a Wound. Encourage the patient to protect the incision from sun exposure for the first 6 months; doing so helps prevent the incision line from becoming darker than the surrounding skin.

The length of time it takes for a wound to heal varies with the site, the patient's age, and the severity of the wound. Each patient therefore needs specific instructions on how long to continue with the dressings and when to return for suture or staple removal. He or she may also need specific information about limiting activities.

**Patient Release.** Notify the doctor when the patient is stabilized and ready to leave. The doctor may want to further observe and instruct the patient. Be sure to offer assistance if the patient needs help getting dressed.

Then help the patient check out. Schedule the next appointment for the patient. Make sure the patient has the correct discharge packet. Confirm arrangements to transport the patient home. Finally, assist the patient to the car or other transport if this is part of office procedure.

If a patient insists on driving himself home, enter this information on the chart. Indicate the time and have the patient initial the entry. This documentation is important

# Educating the Patient

## When to Call the Doctor About a Wound

Whether a wound is post-surgical or from an accident, it is important for patients to know when they should call the doctor. Understanding when a wound needs medical attention can reduce the instances of scarring and infection. You can help by teaching them what to look for when they have a wound. Patients with any wounds should call the office if they have any of the following:

- Jagged or gaping edges
- A face wound

- Limited movement in the area of the wound
- Tenderness or inflammation at the wound site
- Purulent drainage
- A fever greater than 100°F
- Red streaks near the wound
- A puncture wound
- Bleeding that does not stop after 10 minutes of pressure
- Sutures coming out on their own or too early

for legal reasons. It would clarify liability should an accident occur as a result of a reaction to the surgery or the anesthetic.

## Surgical Room Cleanup

If there is time during the monitoring period, begin to clean up the surgical area. If time is not available then, perform the cleanup routine after the patient has been released.

Until the reusable instruments can be cleaned, place them in a disinfectant soak. A reusable sharps container is generally used for this purpose for surgical instruments. Place disposable waste in the sharps or biohazardous waste container. Clean the counters, examining table, and trays according to OSHA guidelines by disinfecting them. A 10% chlorine bleach solution, which is one part household bleach to nine parts water, is commonly used. Disinfect small pieces of nonsurgical equipment (stethoscopes, thermometers, and so on) with 70% isopropyl alcohol. Replace paper table and pillow covers at this time, along with necessary supplies.

## Follow-Up Care

During a follow-up appointment the physician examines the patient's surgical wound. You may be asked to change the dressing or remove the wound closures.

Typically, suture or staple removal takes place 5 to 10 days after minor surgery. The sutures or staples are ready for removal when a clean, unbroken suture line is observed. There should be no scabs, no seepage from the wound, and no visible opening. Any of these signs may indicate unhealed areas. Suture removal is described in Procedure 28-7. Staple removal is similar, except that staple removal forceps, rather than forceps and scissors, are used to remove the staples.

# PROCEDURE 28.7

## Suture Removal

**Procedure Goal:** To remove sutures from a healing wound while maintaining sterile technique and protecting the integrity of the closed wound

### OSHA Guidelines

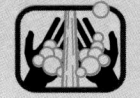 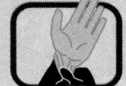 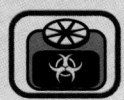 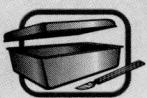
 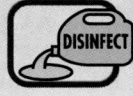 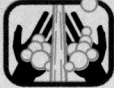

**Materials:** Tray or Mayo stand, suture removal pack (suture scissors and thumb forceps), sterile towel, antiseptic solution, hydrogen peroxide (3%), two small sterile bowls, sterile gauze squares, sterile strips or butterfly closures, sterile dressings and tape

### Method:

1. Clean and disinfect the tray or Mayo stand.
2. Wash your hands and assemble the necessary materials.

*continued* ——→

# Suture Removal *(continued)*

3. Check the date and sterilization indicator on the suture removal pack.

### Rationale

You must ensure that the pack has been subjected to a sterilization procedure and has not expired.

4. Unwrap the suture removal pack, and place it on the tray or stand to create a sterile field.

### Rationale

You need to maintain a sterile field so that you do not contaminate the wound.

5. Unwrap the sterile bowls and add them to the sterile field.

6. Pour a small amount of antiseptic solution into one bowl, and pour a small amount of hydrogen peroxide into the other bowl.

7. Cover the tray with a sterile towel to protect the sterile field while you are out of the room.

8. Escort the patient to the exam room and explain the procedure.

9. Perform a routine hand wash, remove the towel from the tray, and put on exam gloves.

10. Remove the old dressing.

    a. Lift the tape toward the middle of the dressing to avoid pulling on the wound.

    b. If the dressing adheres to the wound, cover the dressing with gauze squares soaked in hydrogen peroxide. Leave the wet gauze in place for several seconds to loosen the dressing.

    c. Save the old dressing for the doctor to inspect.

11. Inspect the wound for signs of infection.

12. Clean the wound with gauze pads soaked in antiseptic, and pat it dry with clean gauze pads.

13. Remove the gloves and wash your hands.

14. Notify the doctor that the wound is ready for examination.

### Rationale

The doctor should determine if the sutures should be removed.

15. Once the doctor indicates that the wound is sufficiently healed to proceed, put on clean exam gloves.

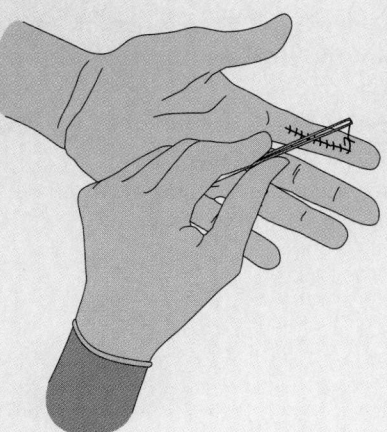

**Figure 28-25.** Without pulling on the wound, lift the suture knot away from the skin to make room for the suture scissors.

16. Place a square of gauze next to the wound for collecting the sutures as they are removed.

17. Grasp the first suture knot with forceps.

18. Gently lift the knot away from the skin to allow room for the suture scissors (Figure 28-25).

19. Slide the suture scissors under the suture material, and cut the suture where it enters the skin (Figure 28-26).

### Rationale

This minimizes the amount of exposed suture that travels beneath the skin during removal.

20. Gently lift the knot up and toward the wound to remove the suture without opening the wound (Figure 28-27).

21. Place the suture on the gauze pad, and inspect to ensure that the entire suture is present.

### Rationale

Sutures inadvertently left in place may cause an infection.

22. Repeat the removal process until all sutures have been removed.

23. Count the sutures and compare the number with the number indicated in the patient's record (Figure 28-28).

24. Clean the wound with antiseptic, and allow the wound to air-dry.

*continued* ⟶

## Suture Removal *(concluded)*

25. Dress the wound as ordered, or notify the doctor if the sterile strips or butterfly closures are to be applied.
26. Observe the patient for signs of distress, such as wincing or grimacing.
27. Properly dispose of used materials and disposable instruments.
28. Remove the gloves and wash your hands.
29. Instruct the patient on wound care.
30. In the patient's chart, record pertinent information, such as the condition of the wound and the type of closures used, if any.
31. Escort the patient to the checkout area.
32. Put on clean gloves.
33. Sanitize reusable instruments and prepare them for disinfection and/or sterilization as needed.
34. Clean the equipment and exam room according to OSHA guidelines.
35. Remove the gloves and wash your hands.

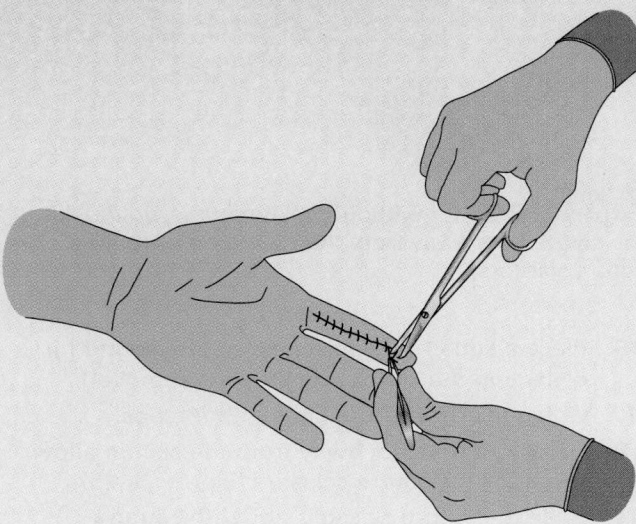

**Figure 28-26.** Cut the suture material as close as possible to its entry point in the skin.

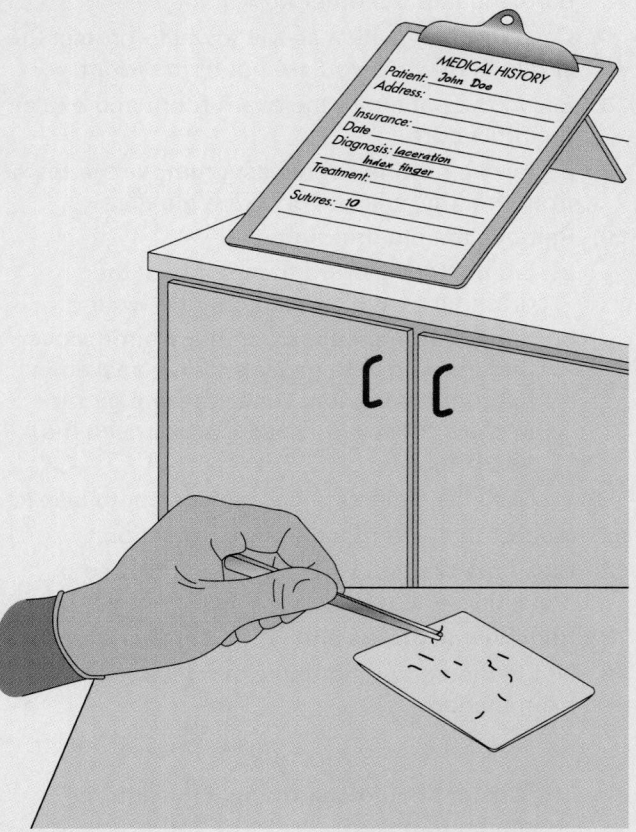

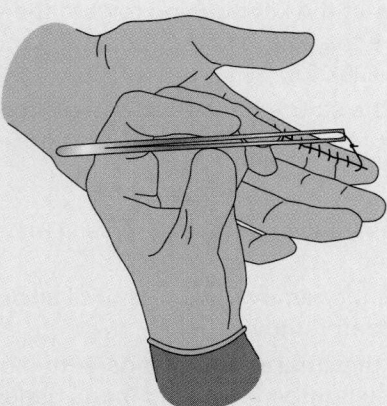

**Figure 28-27.** Remove the suture by lifting the knot up and toward the wound.

**Figure 28-28.** Compare the number of sutures removed with the recorded number of sutures placed.

# Summary

As the doctor's assistant in minor surgical procedures, you perform many functions. Your responsibilities during the patient's preoperative and postoperative care, however, are just as important.

Before surgery, you provide the patient with preoperative instructions, make sure the necessary administrative and legal forms are completed, help prepare the patient emotionally, and set up the surgical room. You then confirm that the patient has followed all preoperative instructions and physically prepare the patient for surgery.

During the procedure, you follow proper medical and surgical aseptic techniques. Your actual responsibilities vary with the role you play as a floater or a sterile scrub assistant for a particular surgery. At all times you ensure the safety and comfort of the patient and are knowledgeable enough to function as the doctor's "right hand" during the procedure.

After the surgery, you provide the postoperative patient with care and instruction that will help ensure prompt healing. Finally, you clean the surgical room and prepare it for the next procedure.

# REVIEW

## CHAPTER 28

## CASE STUDY *QUESTIONS*

Now that you have completed this chapter, review the case study at the beginning of the chapter and answer the following questions:

1. How could you reduce the patient's apprehension?
2. What would you say to her before the physician arrives to perform the minor surgery?

## Discussion Questions

1. Explain the stages of wound healing and the benefit of approximation.
2. List five different categories of surgical instruments by function, give an example of each, and describe how instruments in each category are used.
3. List six conditions that put patients at risk for wound healing problems and discuss how each condition might delay healing.

## Critical Thinking Questions

1. The physician asks you to add additional sterile saline to the sterile field during a surgical procedure. As an unsterile assistant, describe what steps you will take to accomplish this.
2. Explain the procedure you would follow if you were functioning as a sterile scrub assistant and your glove was punctured while you were handling instruments during a surgical procedure.
3. Explain how to make sure that a patient has understood the postoperative instructions for wound care.
4. After a surgical procedure, explain the steps you will take to prepare the room for the next patient.
5. A patient will need to have a minor surgical procedure done next week at your clinic. What administrative tasks must you perform before the procedure?

## Application Activities

1. Choose a minor surgical procedure and create a staff information poster about that procedure. Include a brief description of the procedure, the preoperative instructions, the necessary instruments and supplies, and the postoperative instructions.
2. Working with one or two classmates, practice opening a sterile pack and creating a sterile field. Practice adding additional instruments and a sterile bowl to the sterile field. Offer suggestions to each other for improving your techniques.
3. Create a specimen container label for use in your office. Make sure you leave space for all necessary information.
4. With a partner, practice preparing a site for surgery. Obtain the necessary equipment to clean the site, apply antiseptic, and drape. Follow the procedure steps carefully, paying close attention to your cleaning technique. Be certain to use concentric circles. Practice various surgical sites, and evaluate each other's technique. Note: You may choose not to use actual soap and antiseptic for practice in order to avoid irritation.

## Virtual Fieldtrip

*Visit the McGraw-Hill Higher Education Medical Assisting website at www.mhhe.com/medicalassisting3 to complete the following activity:*

Use the Centers for Disease Control and Prevention (CDC)'s Infection Control in Healthcare Settings website. Search for infection control guidelines for surgical site infections available on this page. Briefly describe the guidelines, including the date the guidelines first appeared and the last update or modification. Summarize the contents of the guidelines.

Open the CD and complete this chapter's practice activities, play the games, listen to the key terms, and test yourself with the interactive review. E-mail, print, and/or save your results to document your proficiency.

# Assisting With Cold and Heat Therapy and Ambulation

## MEDICAL ASSISTING COMPETENCIES

*In preparation for the certification examination, you should know the following areas of competence:*

| COMPETENCY | CMA | RMA |
|---|---|---|
| **Administrative** | | |
| Schedule and oversee appointments | X | X |
| **Clinical** | | |
| Apply principles of aseptic techniques and infection control, including hand washing | X | X |
| Interview the patient to obtain and record the patient's history | X | X |
| Prepare and maintain exam and treatment areas | X | X |
| Prepare the patient for and assist the physician with routine and specialty exams, treatments, and minor office surgeries | X | X |
| **General/Legal/Professional** | | |
| Be aware of and perform within legal and ethical boundaries | X | X |
| Determine the needs for documentation and reporting, and document accurately and appropriately | X | X |
| Instruct individuals according to their needs | X | X |
| Provide patients with methods of health promotion and disease prevention | X | X |
| Project a positive attitude | | X |
| Be a "team player" | | X |
| Conduct work within scope of education, training, and ability | | X |
| Interview effectively | | X |
| Use appropriate medical terminology | | X |
| Understand allied health professions and credentialing | | X |

## KEY TERMS

cryotherapy
diathermy
erythema
fluidotherapy
gait
goniometer
hydrotherapy
mobility aid
physical therapy
posture
range of motion (ROM)
therapeutic team
thermotherapy
traction

## CHAPTER OUTLINE

- General Principles of Physical Therapy
- Cryotherapy and Thermotherapy
- Hydrotherapy
- Exercise Therapy
- Traction
- Mobility Aids
- Referral to a Physical Therapist

# LEARNING OUTCOMES

After completing Chapter 29, you will be able to:

29.1 Explain how medical assistants might assist with some forms of physical therapy.

29.2 Describe ways to test joint mobility, muscle strength, gait, and posture.

29.3 Discuss the benefits of cold and heat therapies.

29.4 List contraindications to cold and heat therapies.

29.5 Identify various cold and heat therapies.

29.6 Demonstrate how to perform cold and heat therapies.

29.7 Describe hydrotherapy methods.

29.8 Identify several methods of exercise therapy.

29.9 Compare different methods of traction.

29.10 Demonstrate how to teach a patient to use a cane, a walker, crutches, and a wheelchair.

## Introduction

Applying cold and heat therapy and assisting patients with ambulation are common responsibilities of a medical assistant. These activities are part of the field of physical therapy. For a full program of physical therapy, a physician generally refers a patient to a licensed physical therapist. However, a physician may request that you assist with some forms of physical therapy, including:

- Applying cold and heat
- Teaching basic exercises
- Demonstrating how to use a cane, walker, and crutches
- Demonstrating how to use a wheelchair
- Discussing with the patient specific therapies for use at home

## CASE STUDY

While on vacation, a 28-year-old male had a mountain biking accident that resulted in a broken leg and other injuries. He went to the local emergency room for treatment and was instructed to follow up with his primary care physician on arriving home. Three days after the accident, he presents in your office with crutches and a cast on his left leg. Using the crutches, he stumbles and almost falls as you ask him back to the exam area. You also notice a dry, crusted, bloody injury on his left forearm.

As you read this chapter, consider the following questions:

1. What type of teaching do you think this patient will need?
2. What type of therapy may be necessary for the crusted bloody injury on his forearm, and how would you perform it?

## General Principles of Physical Therapy

**Physical therapy** is a medical specialty for the treatment of musculoskeletal, nervous, and cardiopulmonary disorders. A physical therapist uses a variety of treatments, including cold, heat, water, exercise, massage, and traction. Some physical therapy regimens combine two or more treatments. Exercising in a pool, for example, combines the use of water and exercise. In addition, the physical therapist actively promotes patient education and rehabilitation programs.

Physical therapy benefits patients in several ways. It restores and improves muscle function, builds strength, increases joint mobility, relieves pain, and increases circulation. Physical therapy is used to treat various disorders, including

arthritis, stroke, lower back pain, muscle spasms, muscle injuries or diseases, pressure sores, skin disorders, and burns.

### Assisting Within a Therapeutic Team

Many people who require physical therapy are recovering from traumatic injuries or dealing with chronic illnesses. They may therefore be receiving therapeutic attention from several different specialists. Physicians, nurses, medical assistants, and other specialists who work with patients dealing with chronic illness or recovery from major injuries make up a **therapeutic team.** When you work with such patients, your responsibilities may include:

- Coordinating the patient's schedule of sessions with different specialists

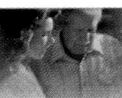

# Educating the Patient

## Specialized Therapies and Their Benefits

Health-care professionals recognize the contribution of specialized therapies to a patient's recovery. Because many people do not know about these specialized therapies, you may be called on to explain them to patients. You can educate patients about potential benefits of art therapy or other specialized therapies. When specialized therapies are ordered, patients will be more at ease if they know what to expect. You can help when necessary by explaining the following types of therapies and their advantages.

- In art therapy, patients learn to express themselves visually through drawing, painting, and sculpture. Art therapy aids both physical and mental healing; provides a recreational outlet; improves mobility and fine motor coordination; provides an outlet for expressing fears or other emotions that patients may be unaware of or unable or unwilling to express verbally; helps relieve anxiety; allows patients to focus on something other than their physical condition; and encourages patients to take better care of themselves. To aid in the art therapy process, encourage patients to relax and give this approach time to work. Although the benefits of art therapy may be evident immediately, they are just as likely to be perceived only after the course of therapy is well under way.

- In music therapy, patients listen to and create music to calm their nerves and to alleviate anxiety. This therapy is often used with surgical patients and patients with chronic pain.
- In dance therapy, patients participate in dance to improve balance, flexibility, strength, and quality of life.
- In writing therapy, patients express themselves through a chosen form of writing such as poetry or a journal.
- In crafts therapy, patients express themselves by using a variety of media to create handiworks.
- In pet therapy, patients play with, groom, or walk a pet. Pets provide companionship and the opportunity to nurture.
- In aquatic therapy, patients swim in a therapeutic pool equipped with a ramp and a lift so that it is accessible to all. Many patients who cannot walk when on land can move their legs remarkably well in water.
- In horticultural therapy, patients work with plants and flowers to bring beauty into their daily lives and to help improve their balance, strength, memory, and socialization skills.
- In equestrian therapy, patients ride horses to help develop strength, coordination, and muscle tone and to improve balance.

---

- Making referrals, as directed by the physician
- Explaining a specialist's treatment approach to the patient
- Communicating the physician's findings to the specialist
- Documenting the specialist's treatments and findings for the physician
- Reinforcing the specialist's instructions for the patient
- Answering the patient's questions

To fulfill these responsibilities, you must have a working knowledge of therapy techniques. If, for example, the physician refers a patient to an art therapist, you would set up an art therapy appointment and explain in general terms what the patient can expect. The Educating the Patient section offers basic information about various specialized therapies.

Besides learning the basic information you need to know about physical therapy, you will want to keep up-to-date on emerging techniques. You may want to become proficient in some of these new techniques. By expanding your knowledge and skills, you increase your value as a member of the therapeutic team.

## Assisting With Patient Assessment

Before the doctor prescribes physical therapy, she assesses the patient's physical abilities and condition. She inspects and palpates the patient's joints and muscles and tests the patient's joint mobility, muscle strength, gait, and posture. You will typically assist with these tests. In some cases the doctor may direct you to perform them.

**Joint Mobility Testing.** People usually assume that their joints are mobile until stiffness or injury limits them. When a patient complains of these difficulties, the doctor may ask you to assist in testing range of motion. **Range of motion (ROM)** is the degree to which a joint is able to move, measured in degrees with a protractor device called

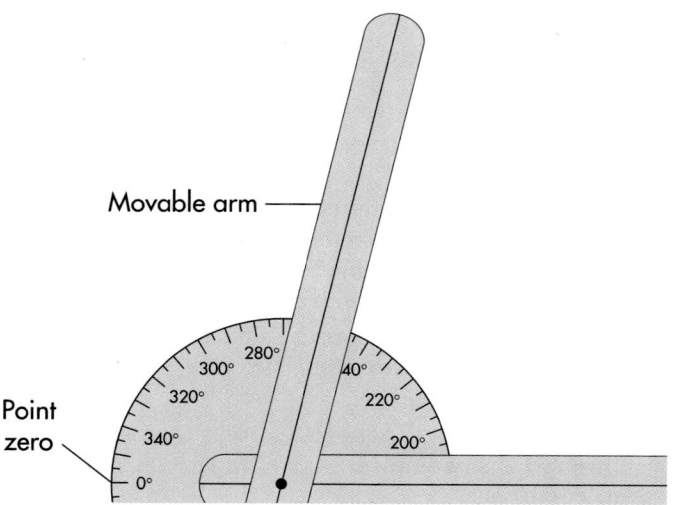

Movable arm

Point zero

280°
300°
320°
340°
0°
40°
220°
200°

**Figure 29-1.** A universal goniometer is a protractor with a movable pointer that measures degrees of joint movement.

a universal **goniometer** (Figure 29-1). The measurement of joint mobility is known as goniometry, a noninvasive test that is frequently performed in doctors' offices and that requires the patient to move each major joint in various ways. The specific movements that are evaluated are described in Table 29-1 and Figure 29-2. The doctor may ask you to assist with goniometry. After special training, you may be asked to perform goniometry. When performing goniometry, you measure the joints from the head to the feet, comparing each joint measurement with a standard measurement (in degrees of movement) for that joint.

**Muscle Strength Testing.** The physician tests muscle strength to determine the amount of force the patient is able to exert with a muscle or group of muscles. This test is usually done at the same time as ROM testing. It may be performed by the physician with your assistance, or once you have had special training, the physician may ask you to perform it yourself.

| TABLE 29-1 | Range of Motion Movements Measured by Goniometry | |
|---|---|---|
| **Term** | **Description** | **Example** |
| Abduction | Movement away from midline of body or movement away from axis of limb | Raising arm straight out to side |
| Adduction (opposite of abduction) | Movement toward midline of body or movement toward axis of limb | Lowering raised arm down to side |
| Circumduction | Circular movement of body part | Performing arm circles |
| Dorsiflexion | Upward or backward movement of body part | Flexing foot—toes pointing upward |
| Eversion | Outward movement of body part | Moving ankle—sole of foot turning outward |
| Extension | Movement that spreads apart two body parts or that opens joint | Straightening leg after being in bent-knee position |
| Flexion (opposite of extension) | Movement that brings together two body parts or that closes joint | Bending leg at knee |
| Inversion (opposite of eversion) | Inward movement of body part | Moving ankle—sole of foot turning inward |
| Plantar flexion (opposite of dorsiflexion) | Downward movement of body part | Flexing foot—toes pointing downward |
| Pronation | Twisting movement that brings palm face down | Turning wrist so palm faces down |
| Rotation | Movement of body part around axis | Turning head from side to side |
| Supination (opposite of pronation) | Rotating movement that brings palm facing upward | Turning wrist so that palm faces upward |

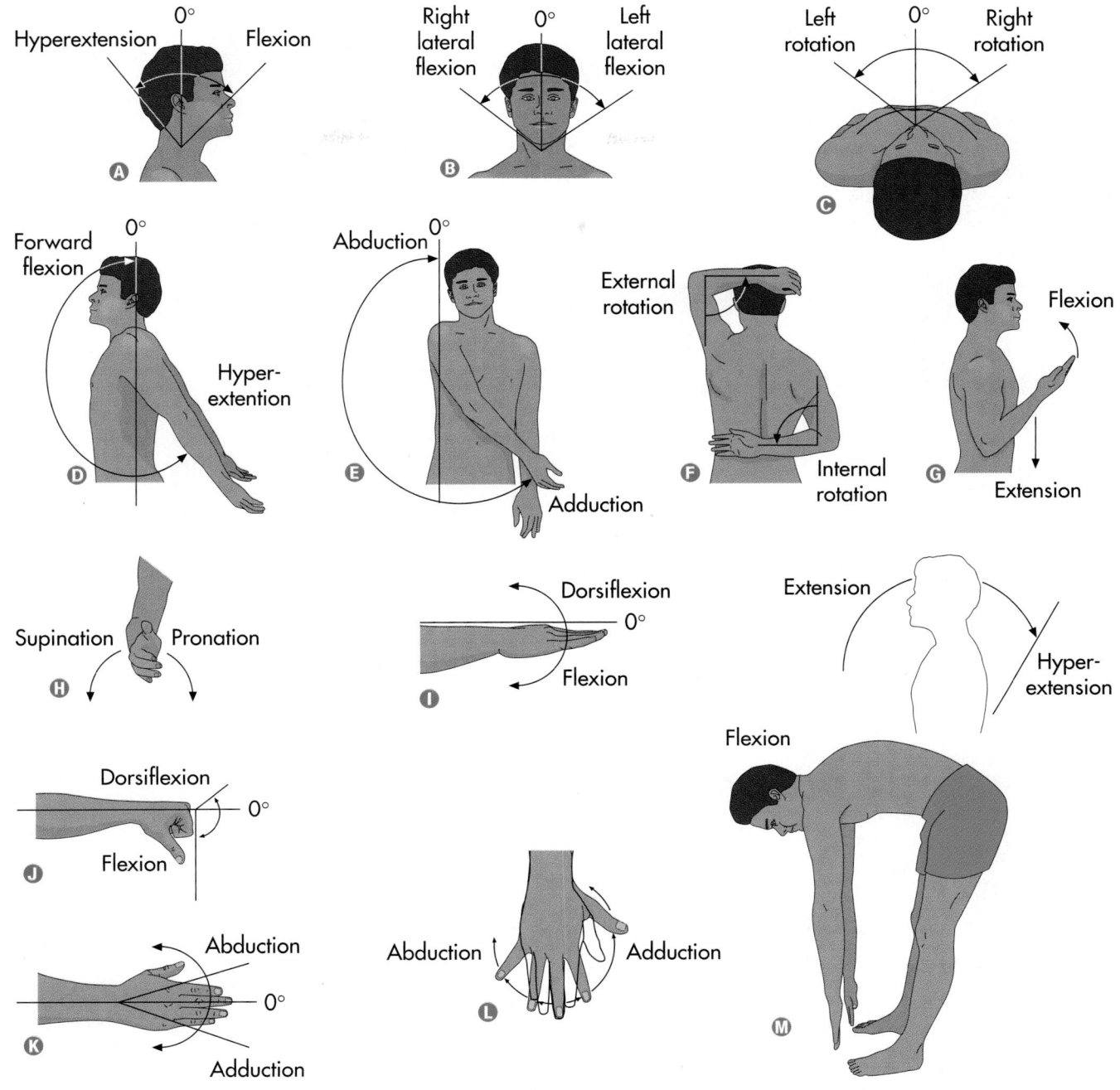

**Figure 29-2.** When you measure joint ROM, begin at the head and work down to the feet. (*continued*)

Like the ROM test, the muscle strength test is usually done from head to foot. The patient is asked to resist the pressure that you or the physician applies to each muscle or group of muscles (usually near a joint). Strength is rated according to a five-point scale.

Typically, a patient can move a joint a certain distance and can easily resist the pressure you apply. The patient usually has equal strength on both sides of the body. If the patient has weakness, however, a medical problem may be indicated. The physician must be made aware of weaknesses so that he can use this information to develop a treatment plan.

**Gait Testing.** **Gait** is the way a person walks. Generally, a physician or physical therapist assesses a patient's gait. To do so, the physician asks the patient to walk away, turn around, and walk back. Assessment of gait includes an appraisal of the patient's length of stride, balance, coordination, direction of knees (inward or outward), and direction of feet (inward or outward).

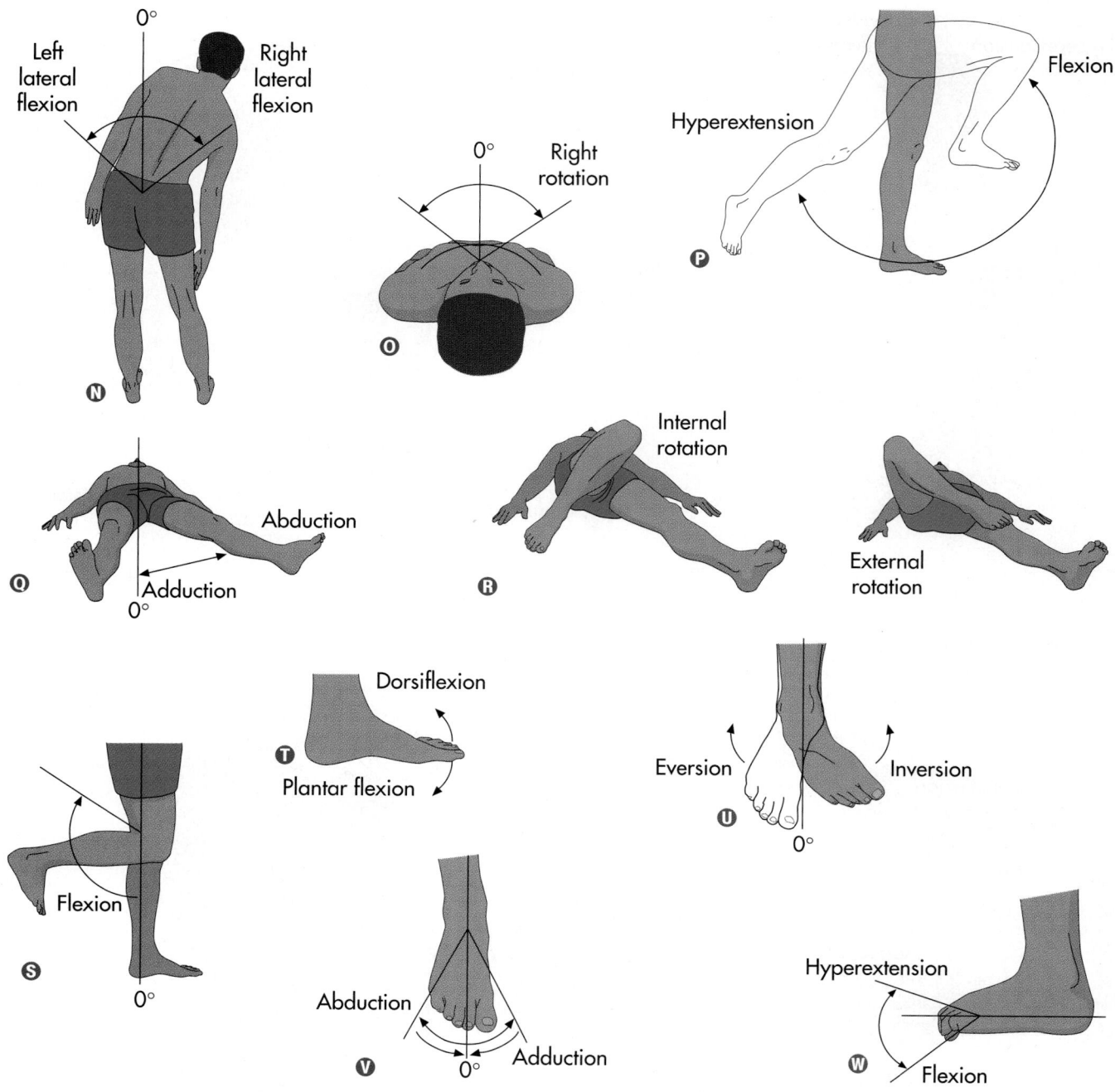

**Figure 29-2.** *(concluded)*

**Posture Testing.** **Posture** is body position and alignment. The doctor assesses posture by looking at the patient's spinal curve from the sides, back, and front. Normally, the thoracic spine has a convex (outward) curve, and the lumbar spine has a concave (inward) curve. The doctor also notes the symmetry of alignment of the shoulders, knees, and hips.

To assess alignment and degree of straightness of the spine, the doctor asks the patient to bend at the waist and let the arms dangle freely. To assess knee position, the doctor asks the patient to stand with both feet together to determine whether the knees are at the same height, facing forward, and symmetrical.

# Cryotherapy and Thermotherapy

Applying cold to a patient's body for therapeutic reasons is called **cryotherapy.** This type of therapy can be administered in a number of ways. Treatments may be dry or wet, and they may be chemical or natural. Examples of dry cold applications are ice bags and ice packs. Wet cold applications include cold compresses and ice massage.

Applying heat to a patient's body for therapeutic reasons is called **thermotherapy.** As with cryotherapy, thermotherapy can be administered in a variety of ways. Examples of devices used in dry heat treatments are electric heating pads, hot-water bottles, and heat lamps. Moist heat treatments include hot soaks and the use of hot compresses and hot packs.

## Factors Affecting the Use of Cryotherapy and Thermotherapy

To choose a cold or heat therapy for a patient, the physician considers the therapy's purpose, the location and condition of the affected area, and the patient's age and general health. After choosing a therapy, the physician may direct you to apply the cold or heat treatment and to teach the patient and family how to continue the therapy at home.

Performed correctly, cold and heat therapies generally promote healing. These therapies can, however, cause side effects in some patients. Therefore, you need to exercise caution when applying the therapies. Cold therapy can cause damage to underlying nerves and tissues if applied incorrectly or for too long. Heat therapy can cause burns to the skin and underlying tissues if incorrectly applied. Monitor the patient carefully for signs of tissue damage. These signs include extreme blanching, redness, or blistering of the skin. You also need to be aware of conditions that contraindicate (make inadvisable) cold or heat therapies. Table 29-2 summarizes circumstances that warrant precautions or contraindications for the therapies as well as possible side effects. When performing any cold or heat therapy, you should consider the age of the patient, treatment location, patient problems with circulation or sensation, and individual temperature tolerance.

**Age.** Age is an important consideration because young children and elderly patients usually are more sensitive than others to cold and heat. When administering cryotherapy or thermotherapy, stay with the patient during its application to check the patient's skin frequently for excessive paleness or redness.

**Treatment Location.** Thin-skinned areas that are usually covered with clothing (such as the back, chest, and abdomen) are more sensitive to cold and heat therapies than other areas, such as the face and hands. Use caution around any broken skin (as with a wound), because it is susceptible to further tissue damage from cryotherapy or thermotherapy.

**Circulation or Sensation Impairment.** Patients with diabetes or cardiovascular disease may have impaired circulation or sensory perception. These impairments may prevent such patients from sensing that a treatment is too cold or too hot. These patients require close monitoring during cryotherapy or thermotherapy. Carefully observe their skin to determine the treatment's therapeutic effect.

**Temperature Tolerance.** Tolerance of temperature extremes varies greatly from person to person. Some people are unusually sensitive to cold or to heat. Listen carefully to patients for any indication of temperature intolerance during treatment. Cases of intolerance should be reported to the physician, who may decide to change the treatment.

## Principles of Cryotherapy

The application of cryotherapy causes blood vessels to constrict and involuntary muscles of the skin to contract. These physiologic responses can have the following results:

- Prevention of swelling by limiting edema, or fluid accumulation in body tissue
- Control of bleeding by constricting blood vessels
- Reduction of inflammation by slowing blood and fluid movement in the affected area
- Provision of an anesthetic effect for pain by reducing inflammation
- Reduction of pus formation by inhibiting microorganism activity
- Lowering of body temperature

| TABLE 29-2 | Contraindications, Precautions, and Side Effects Related to Cold and Heat | | |
|---|---|---|---|
| **Therapy** | **Precautions** | **Contraindications** | **Side Effects** |
| Dry and moist cold applications | Poor circulation, extreme age or youth, arthritis, impaired sensation (insensitivity to cold) | Severe circulatory problems, inability to tolerate weight of device, pain caused by application (more common with moist cold) | Numbness, pain, very pale or bluish skin, blood clots (rare) |
| Dry and moist hot applications | Impaired kidney, heart, or lung functions; arteriosclerosis and atherosclerosis; impaired sensation (insensitivity to heat); extreme age or youth; pregnancy | Possibility of hemorrhage; malignancy; acute inflammation, such as appendicitis; severe circulation problems; pain caused by weight of device | Burns (especially with heat lamps), increased respiratory rate, lowered blood pressure |

## Administering Cryotherapy

Cryotherapy is highly effective in alleviating swelling, pain, inflammation, and bleeding caused by various types of injuries. For best results, cryotherapy should be used frequently (about 20 minutes every hour) for the first 48 hours after an injury. As cold is applied, the skin becomes cool and pale because blood vessels constrict, decreasing the blood supply to the area. The decreased blood supply also reduces tissue metabolism, oxygen use, and waste accumulation.

**Dry Cold Applications.** Dry cold applications include ice bags, ice collars, and chemical ice packs. An ice bag is a rubber or plastic bag with a locking lid. An ice collar is a rubber or plastic kidney-shaped bag that is specially curved to fit around the back of the neck. A chemical ice pack is usually a flat plastic bag containing a semifluid chemical (Figure 29-3). Ice packs come in various sizes and types. Some are disposable, whereas others can be stored in a freezer and reused. The chemical prevents them from freezing solid, allowing them to be molded to the area to be treated. Chemical ice packs may require squeezing or shaking to activate the cooling action. Most packs remain cold for 30 to 60 minutes. Some ice packs come with a soft covering; others must be wrapped in a cloth before they are applied to the skin.

**Wet Cold Applications.** Wet cold applications include cold compresses and ice massage. A cold compress is a cloth or gauze pad moistened with ice water. It may be used to treat the pain associated with a toothache, tooth extraction, eye injury, or headache. The ice used in ice massage may be a cube wrapped in a plastic bag or water frozen in a paper cup. The combination of the cold temperature and the motion of the massage can provide therapeutic relief for the localized pain resulting from a sprain or strain. Although cold causes muscles to contract, the pain-relieving effect can help a patient relax. The procedure for administering cryotherapy is outlined in Procedure 29-1.

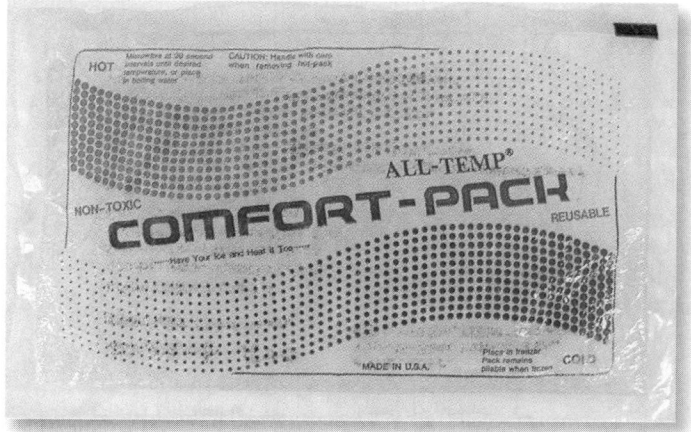

**Figure 29-3.** This chemical pack can be frozen, boiled, or microwaved for cold or heat therapy.

## Principles of Thermotherapy

The application of thermotherapy causes blood vessels to dilate (expand), which increases the blood supply to the area. Increased blood supply brings about an increased tissue metabolism that carries oxygen and nutrients to the cells of the area being treated. Increased metabolism carries toxins and wastes away from the cells. During thermotherapy, the treated skin becomes warm and develops **erythema** (redness) as the capillaries in the deep layers of the skin fill with blood. These physiologic responses can have the following results:

- Relief of pain and congestion
- Reduction of muscle spasms
- Muscle relaxation
- Reduction of inflammation
- Reduction of swelling by increasing the fluid absorption from the tissues

## Administering Thermotherapy

Thermotherapy is highly effective in relieving pain, congestion, muscle spasms, and inflammation and promoting muscle relaxation. However, if heat is applied for too long, it may increase skin secretions that soften the skin and lower resistance. Heat that is too extreme can burn the skin or increase edema. Always monitor patients receiving thermotherapy, particularly children and elderly patients. The three basic types of thermotherapy are dry heat, moist heat, and diathermy. The general principles for administering the following types of thermotherapy are outlined in Procedure 29-2.

**Dry Heat Therapies.** There are several types of dry heat therapy. They include the use of chemical hot packs, heating pads, hot-water bottles, heat lamps with infrared or ultraviolet bulbs, and fluidotherapy.

***Chemical Hot Pack.*** A chemical hot pack is a disposable, flexible pack of chemicals that becomes hot when you activate it by kneading or slapping it. After activating the pack, cover it with a cloth, and place it on the patient's skin in the area being treated. Chemical hot packs are pliable and conform to body contours. For best results, follow the manufacturer's directions.

***Heating Pad.*** A heating pad is a flat pad with electrical coils between layers of soft fabric. When turned on, the coils provide localized heat. The physician should specify the heating pad temperature (low, medium, or high) and the length of time the pad should be applied.

Before applying a heating pad, cover it with a pillowcase or towel, check to be sure the cord is not frayed, and plug it into an electrical outlet. Make sure the patient's skin is dry. Then turn on the pad, and set the temperature selector switch to the specified temperature. The patient should never lie on top of a heating pad because burns could result.

# PROCEDURE 29.1

## Administering Cryotherapy

**Procedure Goal:** To reduce pain and swelling by safely and effectively administering cryotherapy

### OSHA Guidelines

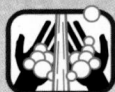  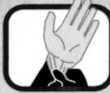

**Materials:** Gloves, cold application materials required as ordered: ice bag, ice collar, chemical cold pack, washcloth or gauze squares, or ice

### Method:

1. Double-check the physician's order. Be sure you know where to apply therapy, and how long it should remain in place.
2. Identify the patient, and explain the procedure and its purpose. Ask if the patient has any questions.
3. Have the patient undress and put on a gown, if required; provide privacy or assistance as needed.
4. Wash your hands and put on gloves.
5. Position the patient comfortably and drape appropriately.

   *Rationale*

   The patient should be able to relax during the therapy.

6. Prepare the therapy as ordered.
   - Ice bag or collar
     a. Prior to use, check the ice bag or collar for leaks.
     b. Fill the ice bag or collar two-thirds full with ice chips or small ice cubes. Compress the container to expel any air and then close it.

     *Rationale*

     Ice will not conform to the patient if there is air in the bag.

     c. Dry the bag or collar completely and cover it with a towel. This will absorb moisture and provide comfort.
   - Chemical ice pack
     a. Check the pack for leaks.

     *Rationale*

     To avoid chemical coming in contact with the patient.

   b. Shake or squeeze the pack to activate the chemicals, or use a cold chemical pack taken from a refrigerator or freezer.

   *Rationale*

   Pack will not be cold if it is not activated.

   c. Cover the pack with a towel.

   *Rationale*

   To keep the patient comfortable and avoid cold burn.
   - Cold compress
     a. Place the washcloth or gauze squares under a stream of running water.
     b. Wring them out.
     c. Rewet at frequent intervals.

7. Place the device on the patient's affected body part. If you are using a compress, place an ice bag on it, if desired, to keep it colder longer.
8. Ask the patient how the device feels.

   *Rationale*

   To prevent cold burn of the skin.

9. Explain that the cold is of great benefit, although it may be somewhat uncomfortable.
10. Leave the device in place for the length of time ordered by the physician. Periodically check the skin for color, feeling, and pain. If the area becomes excessively pale or blue, numb, or painful, remove the device and have the physician examine the area. For cold application using ice, limit application time to 20 minutes.

    *Rationale*

    To reduce the possibility of cold burn.
11. Remove the application and observe the area for reduced swelling, redness, and pain. If the patient has a dressing, replace it at this time.
12. Help the patient dress, if needed.
13. Remove equipment and supplies, properly discarding used disposable materials sanitize, disinfect, and/or sterilize reusable equipment and materials as needed.
14. Remove the gloves and wash your hands.
15. Document the treatment and your observation in the patient's chart. If you teach the patient or the patient's family how to use the device, document your instructions.

# PROCEDURE 29.2

## Administering Thermotherapy

**Procedure Goal:** To administer thermotherapy safely and effectively

### OSHA Guidelines

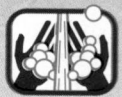  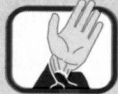

**Materials:** Gloves, towels, blanket, heat application materials required for order: chemical hot pack, heating pad, hot-water bottle, heat lamp, container and medication for hot soak, container and gauze for hot compress

### Method:

1. Double-check the physician's order. Be sure you know where to apply therapy, the proper temperature for the application, and how long it should remain in place.

2. Identify the patient, and explain the procedure and its purpose. Ask if the patient has any questions.

3. Have the patient undress and put on a gown, if required; provide privacy or assistance as needed.

4. Wash your hands and put on gloves.

5. Position the patient comfortably and drape appropriately.

   *Rationale*
   The patient should be able to relax during the therapy.

6. If the patient has a dressing, check the dressing for blood and change as necessary. Alert the physician and ask if treatment should continue.

   *Rationale*
   If the wound is actively bleeding, heat application could cause increased bleeding.

7. Check the temperature by touch and look for the presence of adverse skin conditions (excessive redness, blistering, or irritation) on all applications before and during the treatment.

   *Rationale*
   To avoid patient burn injuries

8. As necessary, reheat devices or solutions to provide therapeutic temperatures and then reapply them.

9. Prepare the therapy as ordered.
   - Chemical hot pack
     a. Check the pack for leaks.

        *Rationale*
        To avoid chemical coming in contact with the patient.

     b. Activate the pack. (Check manufacturer's directions.)

        *Rationale*
        The pack will not get hot if it is not activated.

     c. Cover the pack with a towel.
   - Heating pad
     a. Turn the heating pad on, selecting the appropriate temperature setting.
     b. Cover the pad with a towel or pillowcase.
     c. Make sure the patient's skin is dry, and do not allow the patient to lie on top of the heating pad.

        *Rationale*
        To avoid burns.
   - Hot-water bottle
     a. Fill the bottle one-half full with hot water of the correct temperature—usually 110°F to 115°F. Use a thermometer. The physician can provide information on the ideal temperature water that should be used, which will depend on the area being treated.
     b. Expel the air and close the bottle.

        *Rationale*
        The bottle should conform to the body part.

     c. Cover the bottle with a towel or pillowcase.

        *Rationale*
        To avoid burns.
   - Heat lamp
     a. Place the lamp 2 feet to 4 feet away from the treatment area. (Check manufacturer's directions.)
     b. Follow the treatment time as ordered.

*continued* ⟶

# Administering Thermotherapy *(concluded)*

- Hot soak
  - **a.** Select a container of the appropriate size for the area to be treated.
  - **b.** Fill the container with hot water that is no more than 110°F. Use a thermometer. Add medication to the container if ordered.
- Hot compress
  - **a.** Soak a washcloth or gauze in hot water. Wring it out.
  - **b.** Frequently rewarm the compress to maintain the temperature.

**10.** Place the device on the patient's affected body part, or place the affected body part in the container. If you are using a compress, place a hot-water bottle on top, if desired, to keep it warm longer.

**11.** Ask the patient how the device feels. During any heat therapy, remember that dilated blood vessels cause heat loss from the skin and that this heat loss may make the patient feel chilled. Be prepared to cover the patient with sheets or blankets.

**12.** Leave the device in place for the length of time ordered by the physician. Periodically check the skin for redness, blistering, or irritation. If the area becomes excessively red or develops blisters, remove the patient from the heat source and have the physician examine the area.

**13.** Remove the application and observe the area for inflammation and swelling. Replace the patient's dressing if necessary.

**14.** Help the patient dress, if needed.

**15.** Remove equipment and supplies, properly discarding used disposable materials, and sanitize, disinfect, and/or sterilize reusable equipment and materials as needed.

**16.** Remove the gloves and wash your hands.

**17.** Document the treatment and your observation in the patient's chart. If you teach the patient or the patient's family how to use the device, document your instructions.

*Hot-Water Bottle.* A hot-water bottle is a flat, flexible, plastic or rubber bottle with a stopper. Fill the bottle with hot water, using a thermometer to make sure the water temperature does not exceed 125°F. For children under the age of 2 years and for elderly patients, the temperature should range from 105° to 115°F. For older children, a safe temperature is 115° to 125°F. Fill the bottle halfway; then compress it to expel air. The half-filled bottle can conform to the area to be treated. A half-filled bottle is also lighter than a full one and therefore more comfortable for the patient. Cover the bottle with a cloth or pillowcase before you apply it.

After you apply the hot-water bottle, check with the patient to make sure the temperature is not too hot. Check the temperature frequently, and replace the hot water as needed. Each time you remove the bottle, check the patient's skin to make sure that it is merely warm to the touch.

*Heat Lamp.* A heat lamp uses an infrared or ultraviolet bulb to provide heat. When the lamp is turned on, infrared rays heat and penetrate the skin's surface to a depth of 3 to 5 millimeters. To avoid burning the skin, place an infrared heat lamp 2 to 4 feet from the area being treated. Treatment usually lasts for 20 to 30 minutes or as directed by the physician.

Although ultraviolet rays produce little heat, they can burn the skin and damage the eyes. They are used to kill bacteria and to promote vitamin D formation. Ultraviolet rays stimulate epithelial cells and cause blood vessels to overfill, increasing the skin's defenses against bacterial infections. Ultraviolet lamps are used to treat psoriasis, pressure sores, and wound infections.

Before recommending the use of an ultraviolet lamp, the physician assesses the patient's sensitivity and determines the treatment duration. Treatments typically range from 30 seconds to a few minutes. The duration is usually increased in 10-second intervals. Because ultraviolet rays can burn the skin, monitor the patient closely. Do not leave the room during the treatment. Both you and the patient must wear goggles to prevent harm to the eyes.

*Fluidotherapy.* **Fluidotherapy** is a relatively new technique for stimulating healing, particularly in the hands and feet. The patient places the affected body part in a container of glass beads that are heated and agitated with hot air. Although the therapy is dry, its effect is similar to that of a therapy using water.

**Moist Heat Applications.** Moist heat is often used to increase circulation and decrease pain to specific areas of the body, especially muscles and tendons. Moist heat applications include hot soak, hot compress, hot pack, and paraffin bath.

**Hot Soak.** With hot-soak therapy, the patient places the affected body part—usually an arm or leg—in a container of plain or medicated water that has been heated to no more than 110°F. A hot soak should last about 15 minutes.

**Hot Compress.** A compress is a piece of gauze or cloth suitable for covering a small area. After soaking the compress in hot water, wring it out and apply it to the area to be treated. Keep the compress warm either by placing a hot-water bottle on top of it or by frequently rewarming the compress in hot water.

**Hot Pack.** A hot pack is a large canvas bag filled with heat-retaining gel that is used on a large body area. Like a hot compress, a hot pack retains heat after being placed in hot water.

**Paraffin Bath.** A paraffin bath is a receptacle of heated wax and mineral oil. It is used to reduce pain, muscle spasms, and stiffness in patients with arthritis and similar disorders. The patient's affected area is dipped repeatedly into the mixture until the area is covered with a thick coat of wax. The wax remains on the area for about 30 minutes and then is peeled off. Particularly useful for joints, the paraffin bath has the added benefit of leaving the skin warm, flexible, and soft. Some erythema may result.

**Alternating Hot and Cold Packs.** A physician may order application of a hot pack followed by a cold pack. This increases circulation to the area by dilating and constricting the blood vessels. Be sure to apply the hot pack first. Applying the cold pack first can numb the skin and keep the patient from recognizing that a hot pack is too hot. This can result in serious skin burns.

**Diathermy.** **Diathermy** is a type of heat therapy in which a machine produces high-frequency waves that achieve deep heat penetration in muscle tissue. The heat helps decrease joint stiffness, dilate blood vessels, relieve muscle spasms, and reduce discomfort from sprains and strains. Three types of diathermy are ultrasound, shortwave, and microwave. Equipment for these therapies is continually being improved. Be sure to familiarize yourself with the manufacturer's instructions regarding the specific equipment in your office.

**Ultrasound.** Ultrasound is the most common type of diathermy. It projects high-frequency sound waves that are converted to heat in muscle tissue. This type of diathermy is used to treat sprains, strains, and other acute ailments.

Ultrasound diathermy may be administered by rubbing a gel-covered transducer over the skin in circular patterns. It may also be administered to a body part under water. Do not use ultrasound in areas where bones are near the skin's surface, because it could cause bone damage.

**Shortwave.** Shortwave diathermy uses radio waves that travel through the body between two condenser plates and are converted to heat in the tissues. This type of diathermy is used to treat acute, subacute, and chronic inflammation. Treatment duration typically ranges from 20

to 30 minutes. Do not use shortwave diathermy on a patient who has a pacemaker.

**Microwave.** Microwave diathermy uses microwaves to provide heat deep in body tissues. Contraindications include use on patients with pacemakers, use in combination with wet dressings, or use in high dosages on patients with swollen tissue. Also, never use microwave diathermy near metal implants, because the reaction between metal and microwaves could cause burns.

# Hydrotherapy

**Hydrotherapy** is the use of water to treat physical problems. It is typically performed in the physical therapy department of a hospital, in an outpatient clinic, or at home. Common forms of hydrotherapy include the use of whirlpools and contrast baths and underwater exercises.

## Whirlpools

Whirlpools are tanks in which water is agitated by jets of air under pressure. Whirlpools vary in size from small (capable of accommodating only one body part) to very large (capable of accommodating a wheelchair or full-body submersion). The action of the agitated water in a whirlpool generates a hydromassage, which relaxes muscles and increases circulation. Whirlpools are also used to cleanse and debride (remove foreign matter and dead tissue from) the skin of patients with wounds, ulcers, or burns.

## Contrast Baths

Contrast baths are separate baths, one filled with hot water and the other with cold water. The patient alternately moves the treated body part quickly from one bath to the other. This treatment induces relaxation, stimulates improved circulation (which speeds up healing), and results in greater mobility.

## Underwater Exercises

Underwater exercises are usually performed in a warm swimming pool. They are prescribed for patients with joint injuries, burns, and arthritis. Because the water's buoyancy takes pressure off the joints, underwater exercises are particularly useful for patients with painful or limited movement. Combined with the movement of the water around the body, the exercises promote relaxation and increased circulation.

# Exercise Therapy

For many patients, exercise is as important as medications or other treatments. Exercise offers both preventive and therapeutic benefits. As a patient ages, exercise helps promote flexibility, mobility, muscle tone, and strength. Exercise is a primary treatment for fractures, arthritis, and some

# Physical Therapist Assistant

*To gain medical assistant credentials, you must fulfill the requirements of either the American Association of Medical Assistants (for a Certified Medical Assistant) or the American Medical Technologists (for a Registered Medical Assistant). After obtaining your medical assistant certification or registration, you may wish to acquire additional skills in specialty areas through course work or on-the-job training. Although this course work or training may not lead to an additional certification or degree, it will enable you to expand your role in the medical office and advance your career as the demand for skilled health professionals increases.*

## Skills and Duties

A relatively new profession, physical therapist assisting was first developed in the late 1960s because of the overwhelming interest in the potential of physical therapy in rehabilitation. The goal of physical therapy is to restore or increase physical movement and strength. A physical therapist assistant helps patients improve their physical function when it has been impaired by injury, disease, birth defects, or other causes. Physical therapist assistants often work as part of a team of therapeutic specialists, which may include physicians, physical therapists, occupational therapists, and sometimes social workers.

Working under the supervision of a physical therapist, the assistant carries out the treatments and exercises prescribed by the therapist. She may administer cold and heat therapy, massage, or ultraviolet light to decrease pain and relax muscles. In addition, she helps the patient perform physical exercises to build muscle strength and stamina and to increase mobility. When helping patients exercise, the physical therapist assistant often works in swimming pools or with gym equipment, such as stationary bicycles, weights, and parallel bars. She may take measurements, such as vital signs or range of motion, to help evaluate patients' progress.

The physical therapist assistant may also fit assistive devices for patients who have lost limbs or need mobility training. She routinely teaches them how to use and care for wheelchairs, walkers, braces, and artificial arms and legs. In all cases she records patients' progress for the physical therapist to evaluate. In addition, the physical therapist assistant may perform administrative office work, such as scheduling therapy sessions and maintaining records, and may prepare both equipment and patients for therapy.

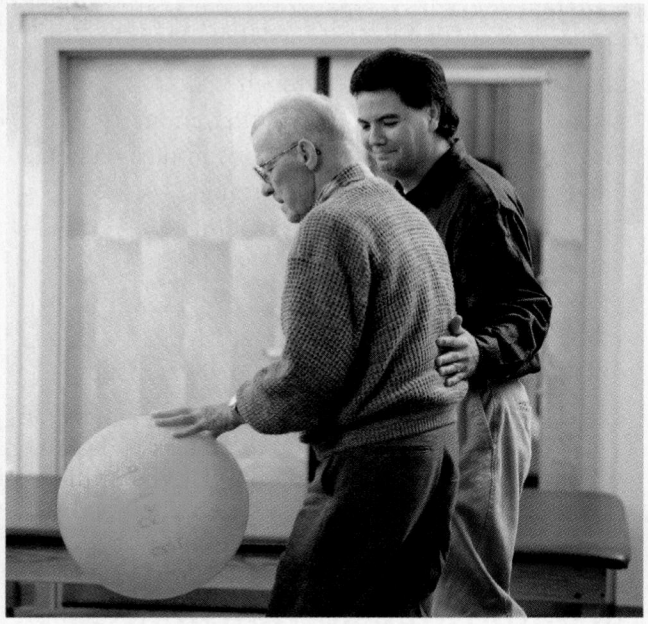

Because the job can be physically demanding, people entering this career should be physically fit. Good communication skills are also important.

## Workplace Settings

Physical therapist assistants most often work in hospitals and rehabilitation centers. They may also work in nursing homes, physicians' offices, or clinics. Most work 40-hour weeks, although some are employed part-time.

## Education

A physical therapist assistant requires less education than a physical therapist. In most states she must complete an accredited 2-year associate degree program at a junior or community college. In 36 states physical therapist assistants must also become licensed by passing a written examination. License renewal differs from state to state.

## Where to Go for More Information

American Physical Therapy
Association/Foundation for Physical Therapy
1111 North Fairfax Street
Alexandria, VA 22314
(703) 684-2782

National Rehabilitation Association
633 South Washington Street
Alexandria, VA 22314
(703) 836-0850

respiratory disorders; it can minimize symptoms or help slow disease progression. For patients who have had surgery, stroke, burns, or amputation, regular exercise therapy can help prevent problems caused by inactivity.

A doctor orders exercise therapy for many reasons. Exercise improves or restores general health and is especially therapeutic when a patient is weak from illness. Explain to patients that exercise will help them to:

- Improve muscle tone and strength
- Regain range of motion (ROM) after an injury
- Prevent ROM from diminishing in chronic conditions
- Prevent or correct physical deformities
- Promote neuromuscular coordination
- Improve circulation
- Relieve stress
- Lower cholesterol levels
- Aid in the resumption of normal daily activities

Exercise therapy is commonly used for treating sports injuries. Exercise therapy for injured athletes is described in the Educating the Patient section. This type of therapy focuses primarily on regaining muscle strength and flexibility in the injured area.

## Role of the Medical Assistant

As a medical assistant, you may have several roles in exercise therapy. As an information resource for the patient and family, you must understand various types of exercise programs and the patient's specific treatment plan. You may also serve as a source of support and encouragement when exercise programs are long and difficult. You may, for example, assist with ROM exercises and teach the patient and family how to perform them at home.

When teaching patients about exercises, give them illustrations of the exercises. Include with each illustration written instructions on the number of times to perform the exercise, as prescribed by the doctor.

After demonstrating each exercise, have patients perform it while you watch and give direction. Patients are more likely to perform exercises properly at home if they can perform them correctly in your presence. It is also helpful for patients' caregivers or family members to watch and perform the exercises to become familiar with them.

## Types of Exercise

Before a patient begins an exercise program, the doctor evaluates the patient's heart and lung function and overall physical condition. The doctor adjusts the level of exercise accordingly and may prescribe other forms of physical therapy, such as cryotherapy, thermotherapy, or hydrotherapy. Careful preparation by the doctor and patient before beginning a program of exercise therapy helps prevent injuries. Some measures to prevent and treat common exercise therapy problems are outlined in Table 29-3. A doctor may also refer a patient to a physical therapist, who will develop an exercise program specifically for that patient. Types of exercises in therapeutic programs include active mobility, passive mobility, aided mobility, active resistance, isometric, and ROM.

**Active Mobility Exercises.** Active mobility exercises are self-directed exercises that the patient performs without assistance. Their purpose is to increase muscle strength and function. They often require equipment such as a stationary bicycle or a treadmill.

**Passive Mobility Exercises.** In passive mobility exercises, the physical therapist or a machine moves a patient's body part. The patient does not actively assist in these exercises. Patients who require passive mobility exercises may have neuromuscular disability or weakness. Passive mobility exercises can help retain patients' ROM and improve their circulation.

**Aided Mobility Exercises.** Aided mobility exercises are self-directed exercises. The patient performs them with the aid of a device such as an exercise machine or a therapy pool. Aided mobility exercises help retain or increase patients' ROM.

**Active Resistance Exercises.** In active resistance exercises, the patient works against resistance (counterpressure). Resistance is provided manually by the therapist or mechanically by an exercise machine. These exercises increase the patient's muscle strength.

| TABLE 29-3 | Preventing and Treating Common Problems of Exercise Therapy | |
|---|---|---|
| **Problem** | **Prevention Methods** | **Treatment** |
| Muscle strain | Beginning with gentle warm-up exercises | Rest and application of heat followed by ice |
| Muscle aches | Keeping track of number of repetitions and amount of weight (resistance), if used; increasing number of repetitions or amount of weight slowly | Rest, soaking in hot bath to relieve aches |
| Impatience with slowness of progress | Discussing expectations with patient; setting realistic goals with patient; stressing necessity of avoiding recurrent injury, which would prolong recovery | Creation of goal sheet, noting small successes as therapy progresses |

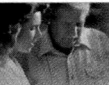

# Educating the Patient

## The Injured Athlete

The risk of injury is associated with most sports, but some sports carry a greater risk of serious injury than others. Many sports-related injuries affect joints—in the neck, shoulders, elbows, wrists, hands, knees, ankles, and feet.

You may be called on to educate injured athletes and to start them on the road to recovery. To do so, you need to understand the mind of the athlete. Why do many athletes get injured in the first place? Here are some reasons.

- The sport they participate in has a high injury rate.
- They return to a sport before their injuries are completely healed.
- They become impatient with a physical therapy regimen.
- They do not work at gradual muscle strengthening.

When does your job begin? After diagnosing the injury, the physician will probably refer the athlete to a sports medicine center or other physical therapy setting, where an individualized program will be set up. As a medical assistant, you will often be responsible for counseling an athlete about the physical therapy program she will be entering. Here are some basic rules that you can communicate.

- Follow the physical therapy regimen set up by the physician or physical therapist—even if it is tedious or time consuming.
- Use only the equipment specified by the therapist: free weights, weight-training equipment, stationary bike, other aerobic equipment, or swimming pool. The physical therapist recommends the designated equipment based on the type of injury. Using other equipment could cause further injury or interfere with healing.
- Do not rush the therapy in an attempt to recover more quickly.
- Work slowly to strengthen muscles and improve flexibility.
- Continue exercises at home as instructed.
- Be patient.

Explain to the athlete how the physical therapy program will be presented. Knowing what to expect from the physical therapist can improve the athlete's compliance. Here are some explanations you might offer.

- The therapist will demonstrate exercises and then watch you perform them.
- The therapist may increase the number of repetitions or the amount of resistance (weight) but probably not both at the same time.
- The therapist will provide handouts illustrating the exercises, along with instructions on how to perform them.
- The therapist may provide an activity log to help you chart your progress.

An athlete who is impatient with a physical therapy regimen and returns to a sport before an injury has completely healed has an increased risk of repeated injury. Impress on the athlete the importance of the physical therapy process. Emphasize the need for gradual strengthening and healing over a period of time. To help the athlete in the long run, focus on recovery from injury and on the need to prevent recurrent injury.

**Isometric Exercises.** During isometric exercises, the patient relaxes and then contracts the muscles of a body part while in a fixed position. Isometric exercises can maintain the patient's muscle strength when a joint is temporarily or permanently immobilized.

**ROM Exercises.** ROM exercises move each joint through its full range of motion. These exercises should be done slowly and gently. Doing them too quickly or too soon after an injury can cause pain, fracture, or bleeding into the joint. For this reason a physical therapist assesses the patient and determines a recommended regimen of ROM exercises. You may be asked to educate the patient and caregiver or family about the regimen.

ROM exercises are typically prescribed after a joint injury. The physical therapist may recommend that the joint be moved in its full range of motion three times, twice a day. ROM exercises are also recommended for elderly people, to improve circulation and muscle function. The therapist will prescribe one of two types of ROM exercises for patients:

1. Active range of motion exercises: performed by the patient without assistance
2. Passive range of motion exercises: performed by the patient with the help of another person or a machine

Active and passive ROM exercises do not build muscle strength but do improve flexibility and mobility. Typical ROM exercises are illustrated in Figure 29-4.

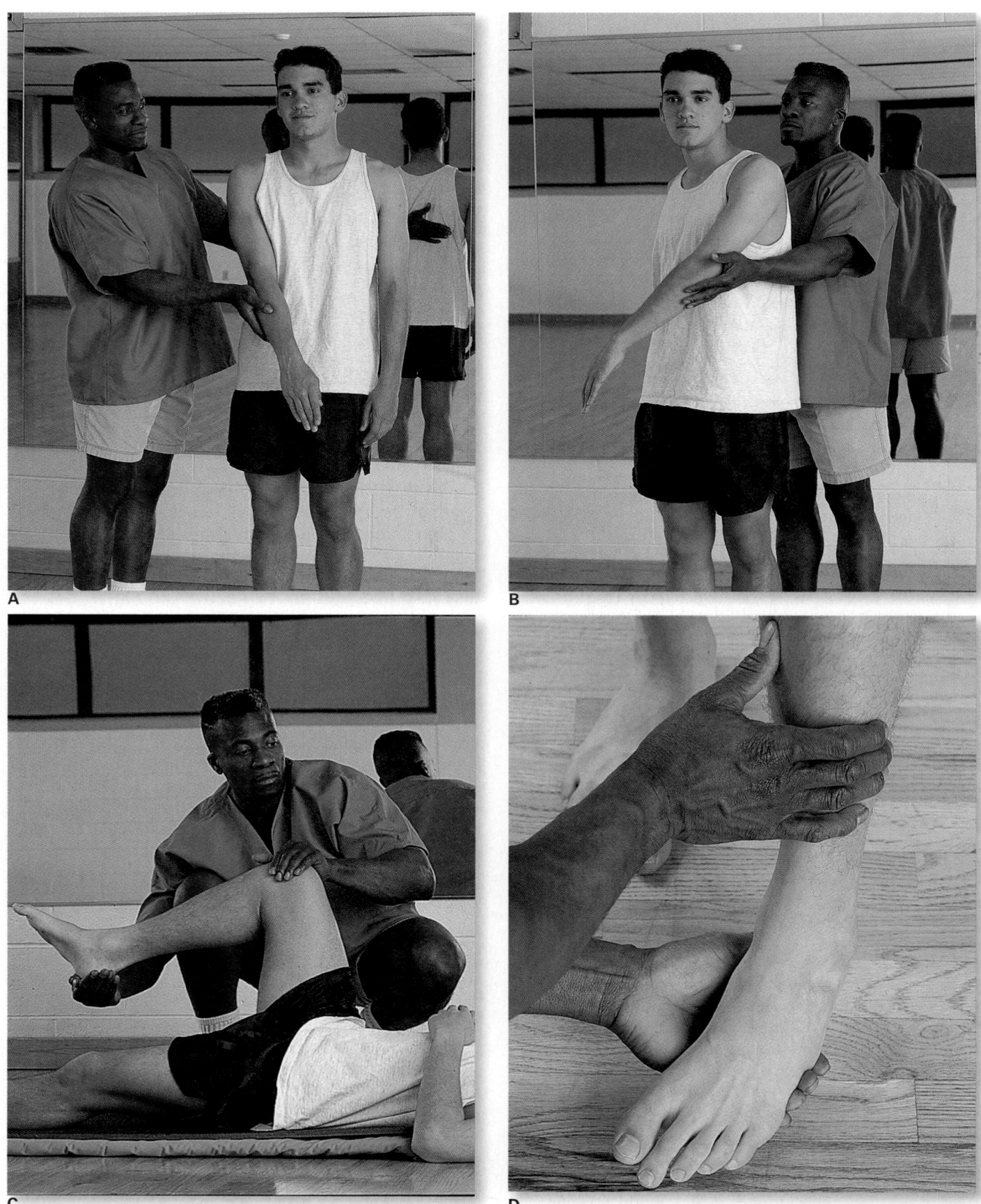

**Figure 29-4.** A medical assistant helps a patient perform typical ROM exercises: (A) shoulder abduction, (B) back rotation, (C) hip flexion, and (D) toe abduction.

## Occupational Therapist Assistant

*To gain medical assistant credentials, you must fulfill the requirements of either the American Association of Medical Assistants (for a Certified Medical Assistant) or the American Medical Technologists (for a Registered Medical Assistant). After obtaining your medical assistant certification or registration, you may wish to acquire additional skills in specialty areas through course work or on-the-job training. Although this course work or training may not lead to an additional certification or degree, it will enable you to expand your role in the medical office and advance your career as the demand for skilled health professionals increases.*

### Skills and Duties

Occupational therapy assisting programs were first accredited by the American Occupational Therapy Association in 1958. The goal of occupational therapy is to improve an injured person's ability to perform her daily activities both at home and in the workplace. Occupational therapist assistants work under the supervision of occupational therapists. They are involved with the rehabilitation of persons with mental, physical, emotional, and developmental disabilities. An occupational therapist assistant helps people learn to compensate for their physical disabilities, thus increasing their independence.

Occupational therapist assistants work as a part of a therapeutic team including physicians, occupational therapists, and physical therapists. They may be involved in performing home and workplace evaluations to help patients adapt to new ways of performing tasks. They assist in training patients in the use of adaptive equipment, including wheelchairs, bathtub transfer devices, and grasping, holding, dressing, reaching, and carrying devices. They often help implement and monitor patient exercise programs developed by an occupational therapist.

The job can be physically demanding, requiring lifting, stooping, kneeling, and standing. People wishing to enter this career should be physically fit. Good communication and teamwork skills are also important.

### Workplace Settings

Occupational therapist assistants work in hospitals, outpatient clinics, rehabilitation facilities, and nursing care facilities. Most work 40-hour weeks, although some are employed part-time.

### Education

An occupational therapist assistant requires less education than an occupational therapist. In most states, he must complete an accredited 2-year associate degree or certificate program at a community college or technical college. Most states require national certification. An occupational therapist assistant who passes the national certification examination is titled a Certified Occupational Therapist Assistant.

### Where to Go for More Information

American Occupational Therapy Association
4720 Montgomery Lane
Bethesda, MD 20824
301-652-2682

## Electrical Stimulation

Electrical stimulators deliver controlled amounts of low-voltage electric current to motor and sensory nerves to stimulate muscles. Electrical stimulation helps prevent atrophy in muscles that cannot move voluntarily by causing the muscles to contract involuntarily (on impulse) and relax. Frequent and regular electrical stimulation also aids in healing injured joints and in revitalizing muscles.

Electrical stimulation can help retrain a patient to use injured muscles by creating a perceivable connection between the stimulus (muscle movement) and the area of the brain that controls those muscles. If a limb does not function because of injury or disease, this therapy can give the patient hope that injured muscles are not dead. Hope often encourages a patient to work harder and to cooperate in the physical therapy regimen, which can be long and arduous. Electrical stimulation units that patients can wear are being developed for people with spinal cord injuries to help them retrain affected muscles.

## Traction

**Traction** is the pulling or stretching of the musculoskeletal system to treat fractured bones and dislocated, arthritic, or other diseased joints. It is traditionally performed by a therapist in a specially equipped setting. A physical therapist may set up traction in the patient's home and visit regularly to ensure that the equipment is used and maintained properly. Traction may be used to:

- Create and maintain proper bone alignment
- Reduce or prevent joint stiffening and abnormal muscle shortening
- Correct deformities

- Relieve compression of vertebral joints
- Reduce or relieve muscle spasms

Although you will not be setting up or performing traction, you should know about its types and uses. This information will prepare you to answer basic questions from patients and family members.

## Manual Traction

The physical therapist performs manual traction by using his hands to pull a patient's limb or head gently. Pulling stretches the muscles and separates the joints, allowing for greater motion and less stiffening. Manual traction is used with patients who have muscle spasms, stiffness, and arthritis.

## Static Traction

To perform static traction (also called weight traction), the therapist places a patient's limb, pelvis, or chin in a harness. The harness is then attached to weights through a system of pulleys. This type of traction is commonly used to relieve muscle spasms.

## Skeletal Traction

Skeletal traction is performed in inpatient facilities on patients whose injuries require long traction time and heavy weights. During surgery, a surgeon inserts pins, wires, or tongs into bones. After surgery, the pins, wires, or tongs are attached to pulleys and weights to provide continuous traction.

## Mechanical Traction

Mechanical traction uses a special device that intermittently pulls and relaxes a prescribed body part, for example, the neck. The therapist sets the time intervals between contractions and relaxations. Mechanical traction is used to promote relaxation.

# Mobility Aids

**Mobility aids** (also called mobility assistive devices) include canes, walkers, crutches, and wheelchairs. These devices are designed to improve patients' ability to ambulate, or move from one place to another.

The appropriate aid depends on the patient's disability, muscle coordination, strength, and age. The patient may need a device temporarily—perhaps crutches after a sprain—or permanently—such as a wheelchair in the case of permanent paralysis.

## Canes

Canes come in several styles, including standard, tripod, and quad-base (Figure 29-5). All styles are lightweight, made of wood or aluminum, and have a rubber tip or tips at the bottom. They provide support and help patients

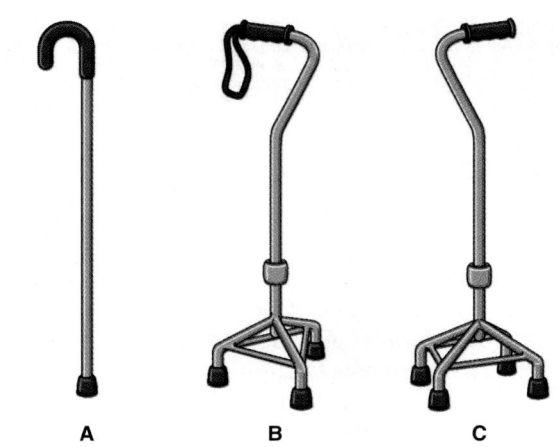

**Figure 29-5.** Shown here are three types of canes: (A) standard, (B) tripod, and (C) quad-base.
Source: Borrowed from McGraw-Hill *Health Care Science Technology* by Booth, 2004.

maintain balance. Canes are especially useful for patients with weaknesses on one side of the body (possibly due to a stroke), joint disability, or neuromuscular defect.

A standard cane is best for a patient who needs only a small amount of support. Its curved handle is convenient, allowing the patient to hang it from a pocket or a doorknob. When the patient uses a standard cane, however, the curved handle concentrates most of the patient's weight in one small area of the hand. To avoid stressing the hand in this way, some standard canes have a T-shaped handle, which distributes pressure on the hand more evenly. Tripod canes have three legs, and quad-base canes have four. The multiple legs create a wide base of support, making them more stable than a standard cane. Tripod and quad-base canes can stand alone, freeing up the patient's hands when she sits down. These canes are bulkier and more difficult to pick up and put down than a standard cane, however. Both styles have T-shaped handles.

After determining the most suitable cane for the patient, the physical therapist adjusts the cane's height. When the cane is the correct height, the patient's elbow is flexed at 20 degrees to 25 degrees, and the patient stands tall while using the cane (instead of leaning on it for support). The therapist makes sure that the handle is the right size for the patient's hand and instructs the patient on how to use the cane. If directed, you may do the teaching or reinforce it, as discussed in Procedure 29-3.

## Walkers

A walker is an aluminum frame that is open on one side and has four widely placed legs with rubber tips (Figure 29-6). The legs are adjustable for various heights. Some models are designed to fold up for storage. To use a walker, the patient stands within the frame and leans on the upper bar, which has a handgrip on each side. The frame is lightweight, so it is easy for most patients to use.

## PROCEDURE 29.3

# Teaching a Patient How to Use a Cane

**Procedure Goal:** To teach a patient how to use a cane safely

**OSHA Guidelines:** This procedure does not involve exposure to blood, body fluids, or tissues.

**Materials:** Cane suited to the patient's needs

**Method:**

### Standing from a Sitting Position

1. Instruct the patient to slide his buttocks to the edge of the chair.
2. Tell the patient to place his right foot slightly behind and inside the right front leg of the chair and his left foot slightly behind and inside the left front leg of the chair. (This provides him with a wide, stable stance.)
3. Instruct the patient to lean forward and use the armrests or seat of the chair to push upward. Caution the patient not to lean on the cane.
4. Have the patient position the cane for support on the uninjured or strong side of his body as indicated.

### Walking

1. Teach the patient to hold the cane on the uninjured or strong side of her body with the tip(s) of the cane 4 to 6 inches from the side and in front of her strong foot. Remind the patient to make sure the tip is flat on the ground.

   *Rationale*
   To reduce the risk of the patient falling.

2. Have the patient move the cane forward approximately 8 inches and then move her affected foot forward, parallel to the cane.

3. Next have the patient move her strong leg forward past the cane and her weak leg.
4. Observe as the patient repeats this process.

### Ascending Stairs

1. Instruct the patient to always start with his uninjured or strong leg when going up stairs.
2. Advise the patient to keep the cane on the uninjured or strong side of his body and to use the wall or rail, if available, for support on the weak side. If a rail is not available, the patient may need assistance for safety.
3. After the patient steps on the strong leg, instruct him to bring up his weak leg and then the cane.
4. Remind the patient not to rush.

### Descending Stairs

1. Instruct the patient to always start with her weak leg when going down stairs.
2. Advise the patient to keep the cane on the uninjured or strong side of her body and to use the wall or rail, if available, for support on the weak side. If a rail is not available, the patient may need assistance for safety.
3. Have the patient use the uninjured or strong leg and wall or rail to support her body, put the cane on the next step, and bend the strong leg as she lowers the weak leg to the next step.
4. Instruct the patient to step down with the strong leg.

### Walking on Snow or Ice

Suggest that the patient try a metal ice-gripping cane or a ski pole. These can be dug into the snow or ice to prevent slipping. Instruct the patient to avoid walking on ice unless absolutely necessary.

---

Typically, a walker is used by older patients who are too weak to walk unassisted or who have balance problems. The walker is designed to give these patients a sense of stability as they ambulate. In tight spaces or in areas with throw rugs, however, a walker may be difficult to manage. A patient who is too weak to pick up the walker may use a walker on wheels. Wheeled walkers have brakes for safety. Patients should never slide a walker that does not have wheels because the movement could easily result in a fall.

A physical therapist selects a walker that suits the patient's abilities and height. A walker should reach the patient's hipbone. See Table 29-4 for more information about different types of walkers. Although the physical therapist usually trains the patient in the use of a walker, you may be asked to do this, or you may need to reinforce the information presented in Procedure 29-4.

## Crutches

Crutches allow a patient to walk without putting weight on the feet or legs by transferring that weight to the arms. Crutches are made of aluminum or wood. Aluminum crutches are lighter and usually more expensive than those made of wood. Pediatric crutches are available for children. The two basic types of crutches are axillary and Lofstrand. Procedure 29-5 provides the steps for teaching patients how to use crutches.

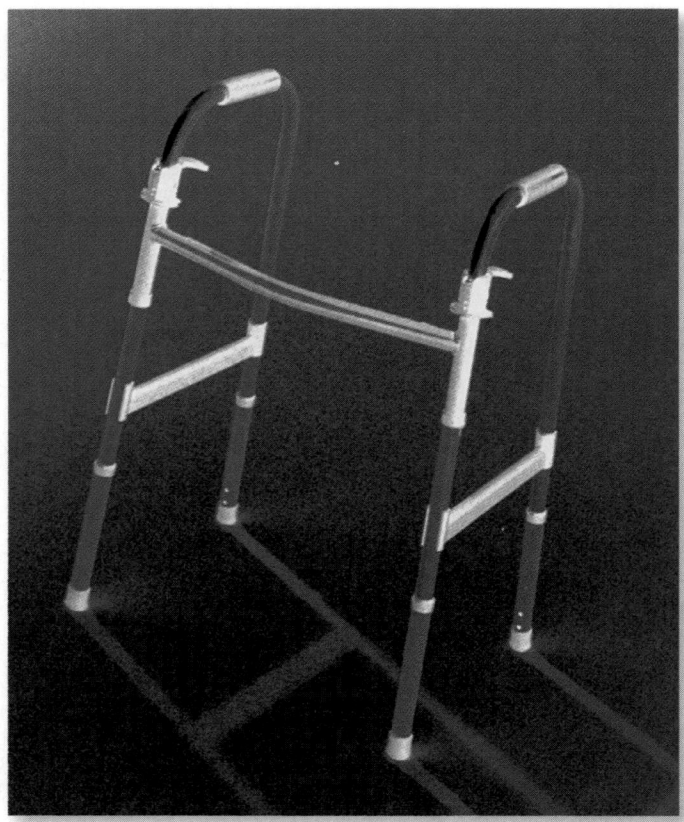

**Figure 29-6.** A standard walker.

Axillary crutches reach from the ground to the armpit. Each crutch has a rubber tip on the bottom to prevent slipping. This type of crutch is designed for short-term use by patients with such injuries as a sprained ankle.

Lofstrand, or Canadian, crutches reach from the ground to the forearm, and each one has a rubber tip on the bottom to prevent slipping. For additional support, this type has a handgrip extension attached at a 90-degree angle and a metal cuff that fits securely around the patient's forearm. Lofstrand crutches are geared for long-term use by patients with such disorders as paraplegia (Figure 29-7).

**Measuring the Patient for Crutches.** To prevent back pain and nerve injury to the armpits and palms, crutches must be measured to fit each patient. Axillary crutches that are too long can put pressure on nerves in the armpit, causing a condition called crutch palsy (muscle weakness in the forearm, wrist, and hand). They can also force the patient's shoulders forward, causing strain on the back and making ambulation difficult. Crutches that are too short force the patient to bend forward during ambulation, causing back pain or imbalance, which can lead to falls.

Before a patient who uses crutches leaves the office, make sure the crutches fit properly and that the patient is comfortable walking with them. To confirm that the fit is correct, check for the following conditions.

- The patient is wearing the type of shoes he will wear when walking.
- The patient is standing erect with feet slightly apart.

| TABLE 29-4 Types of Walkers | | | |
|---|---|---|---|
| **Walker** | **Features** | **Advantages** | **Disadvantages** |
| Standard | No wheels, adjustable legs | Very stable on flat surfaces; easier to use than crutches | Requires upper body strength to use |
| Standard folding | No wheels, sides fold in | Easy to transport and store | Requires upper body strength to use, requires pressing a tab to release and fold |
| Rolling | Front wheels | Requires less upper body strength to use | Not as stable as standard walker |
| Rolling with brakes | Front wheels and brakes | Disengages wheels when weight from upper body is applied | Not as stable as standard walker |
| Three wheel rolling with brakes | Bicycle style hand brakes | Better maneuverability; folds for transport or storage | Requires better balance than other walkers |
| Reciprocal | Each side of walker moves alternately | Allows for more natural gait | Requires better balance and coordination than other walkers; catches on some floor surfaces |

## PROCEDURE 29.4

# Teaching a Patient How to Use a Walker

**Procedure Goal:** To teach a patient how to use a walker safely

**OSHA Guidelines:** This procedure does not involve exposure to blood, body fluids, or tissues.

**Materials:** Walker suited to the patient's needs

**Method:**

*Walking*

1. Instruct the patient to step into the walker.
2. Tell the patient to place her hands on the handgrips on the sides of the walker.
3. Make sure the patient's feet are far enough apart so that she feels balanced.

### Rationale

A wider base provides for better balance.

4. Instruct the patient to pick up the walker and move it forward about 6 inches.
5. Have the patient move one foot forward and then the other foot.
6. Instruct the patient to pick up the walker again and move it forward. If the patient is strong enough, explain that she may advance the walker after moving each leg rather than waiting until she has moved both legs.

*Sitting*

1. Teach the patient to turn his back to the chair or bed.
2. Instruct the patient to take small, careful steps and to back up until he feels the chair or bed at the back of his legs.
3. Instruct the patient to keep the walker in front of himself, let go of the walker, and place both his hands on the arms or seat of the chair or on the bed.
4. Teach the patient to balance himself on his arms while lowering himself slowly to the chair or bed.
5. If the patient has an injured or affected leg, he should keep it forward while bending his unaffected leg and lowering his body to the chair or bed.

*Ascending and Descending Stairs*

If a patient needs to use a walker on stairs, refer him to a physical therapist for additional training.

---

- The crutch tips are positioned 2 to 4 inches in front of the patient's feet and 4 to 6 inches to the side of each foot.
- The axillary supports allow 2 to 3 finger-widths between supports and armpits. (Use wing nuts and bolts to adjust crutches.)
- The handgrips are positioned to create 30-degree flexion at the elbows. (Use wing nuts and bolts to adjust; use a goniometer to check flexion.) See Figure 29-8.

**Crutch Gaits.** To teach a patient how to stand and walk with crutches, you must learn the crutch gaits, or walks. First show the patient the standing, or tripod, position. To do this, have the patient stand erect and look straight ahead. The patient should place the crutch tips 4 to 6 inches in front of her feet and 4 to 6 inches away from the side of each foot. See Figure 29-9.

To determine the proper gait for a patient, you will make a preteaching assessment of the patient's muscle coordination and physical condition. In general, instruct a patient to use a slow gait in crowded areas or when feeling tired. The patient can use a faster gait in open places or when feeling more energetic. Using various gaits and speeds enables the patient to exercise different muscle groups and improve overall conditioning.

**Four-Point Gait.** The four-point gait is a slow gait used only when a patient can bear weight on both legs. Because this gait has three points of contact with the ground at all times, it is stable and safe. It is especially useful for patients with leg muscle weakness, spasticity, or poor balance or coordination. To teach this gait, have the patient start in the tripod position. Then outline the following steps, as illustrated in Figure 29-10.

1. Move the right crutch forward.
2. Move the left foot forward to the level of the left crutch.
3. Move the left crutch forward.
4. Move the right foot forward to level of the right crutch.

**Three-Point Gait.** The three-point gait is used when a patient cannot bear weight on one leg but can bear full weight on the unaffected leg. This gait allows the patient's weight to be carried alternately by the crutches and by the unaffected leg. It is appropriate for amputees, patients with tissue or musculoskeletal trauma (such as

# Teaching a Patient How to Use Crutches

**Procedure Goal:** To teach a patient how to use crutches safely

**OSHA Guidelines:** This procedure does not involve exposure to blood, body fluids, or tissues.

**Materials:** Crutches suited to the patient's needs

**Method:**

1. Verify the physician's order for the type of crutches and gait to be used.

2. Wash your hands, identify the patient, and explain the procedure.

3. Elderly patients or patients with muscle weakness should be taught muscle strength exercises for their arms.

4. Have the patient stand erect and look straight ahead.

5. Tell the patient to place the crutch tips 2 to 4 inches in front of and 4 to 6 inches to the side of each foot.

6. When instructing a patient to use an axillary crutch, make sure the patient has a 2-inch gap between the axilla and the axillary bar and that each elbow is flexed 25 degrees to 30 degrees.

*Rationale*

To reduce the incidence of nerve injury to the axilla

7. Teach the patient how to get up from a chair:

   a. Instruct the patient to hold both crutches on his affected or weaker side.

   b. Have the patient slide to the edge of the chair.

   c. Tell the patient to push down on the arm or seat of the chair on his stronger side and use his strong leg to push up. If indicated, keep the affected leg forward.

   d. Advise the patient to put the crutches under his arms and press down on the hand grips with his hands.

8. Teach the patient the required gait. Which gait the patient will use depends on the muscle strength and coordination of the patient. It also depends on the type of crutches, the injury, and the patient's condition. Check the physician's orders, and see Figures 29-10 and 29-11 for examples.

9. Teach the patient how to ascend stairs:

   a. Start the patient close to the bottom step, and tell her to push down with her hands.

   b. Instruct the patient to step up on the first step with her good foot.

   c. Tell the patient to lift the crutches to the same step and then lift her other foot. Advise the patient to keep her crutches with her affected limb.

   d. Remind the patient to check her balance before she proceeds to the next step.

10. Teach the patient how to descend stairs:

    a. Have the patient start at the edge of the steps.

    b. Instruct the patient to bring his crutches and then the affected foot down first. Advise the patient to bend at the hips and knees to prevent leaning forward, which could cause him to fall.

    c. Tell the patient to bring his unaffected foot to the same step.

    d. Remind the patient to check his balance before he proceeds. In some cases, a handrail may be easier and can be used with both crutches in one hand.

11. Give the patient the following general information related to the use of crutches:

    a. Do not lean on crutches.

    b. Report to the physician any tingling or numbness in the arms, hands, or shoulders.

    c. Support body weight with the hands.

    d. Always stand erect to prevent muscle strain.

    e. Look straight ahead when walking.

    f. Generally, move the crutches not more than 6 inches at a time to maintain good balance.

    g. Check the crutch tips regularly for wear; replace the tips as needed.

    h. Check the crutch tips for wetness; dry the tips if they are wet.

    i. Check all wing nuts and bolts for tightness.

    j. Wear flat, well-fitting, nonskid shoes.

    k. Remove throw rugs and other unsecured articles from traffic areas.

    l. Report any unusual pain in the affected leg.

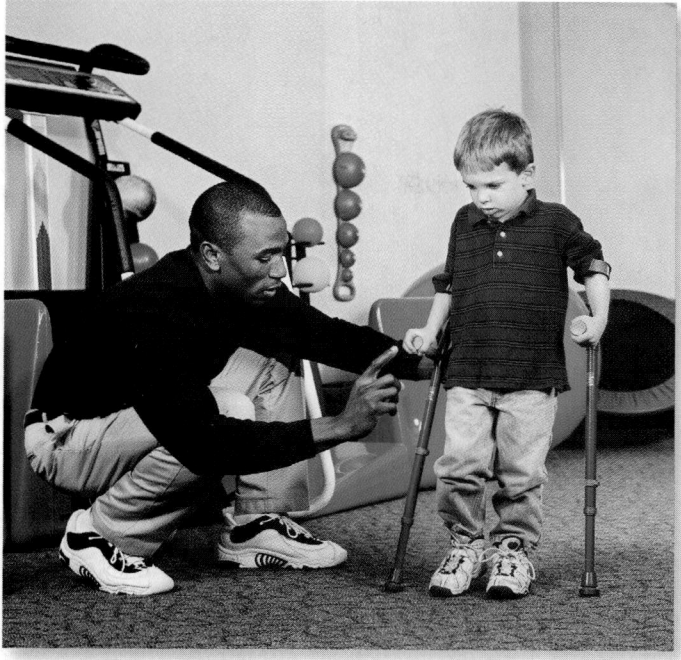

**Figure 29-7.** A child using Lofstrand crutches.

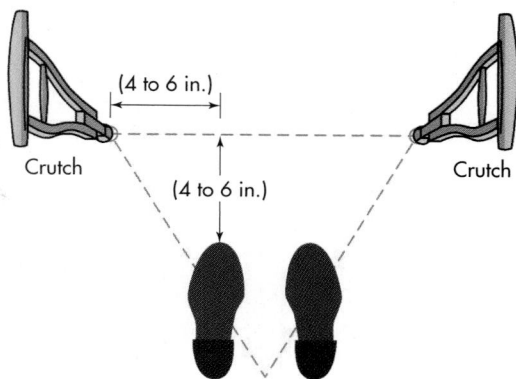

**Figure 29-9.** This is the correct beginning position for the patient's feet and crutches when you are teaching a patient to walk with crutches.

Source: Borrowed from McGraw-Hill *Health Care Science Technology* by Booth, 2004.

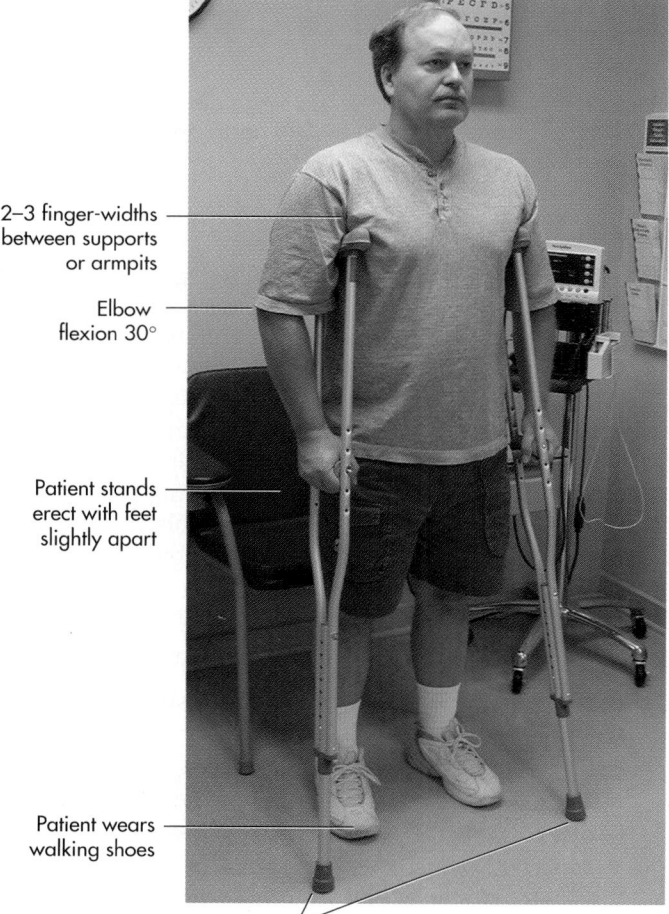

2–3 finger-widths between supports or armpits

Elbow flexion 30°

Patient stands erect with feet slightly apart

Patient wears walking shoes

Crutch tips 2 to 4 inches in front of and 4 to 6 inches to each side

**Figure 29-8.** Use these guidelines when measuring a patient for crutches.

a fractured or sprained leg), and those recovering from leg surgery. The patient must have good muscle coordination and arm strength, however. To teach this gait, have the patient start in the tripod position. Then give the patient the following instructions, as illustrated in Figure 29-10B.

1. Move both crutches and the affected leg forward.
2. Move the unaffected leg forward while weight is balanced on both crutches.

***Two-Point Gait.*** The two-point gait is faster than the four-point gait and is used by patients who can bear some weight on both feet and have good muscle coordination and balance. To teach this gait, have the patient start in the tripod position. Then outline the following steps, as illustrated in Figure 29-10C.

1. Move the left crutch and the right foot forward at the same time.
2. Move the right crutch and the left foot forward at the same time.

***Swing Gaits.*** Patients with severe disabilities, such as leg paralysis or deformity, may use one of two swing gaits: the swing-to gait or the swing-through gait (Figure 29-11A and B). To teach the swing-to gait, have the patient start in the tripod position. Then outline the following steps.

1. Move both crutches forward at the same time.
2. Lift the body and swing to the crutches.
3. End with the tripod position again.

To teach the swing-through gait, have the patient start in the tripod position. Then go over the following steps.

1. Move both crutches forward.
2. Move the body and swing past the crutches.

**Assisting With Cold and Heat Therapy and Ambulation**

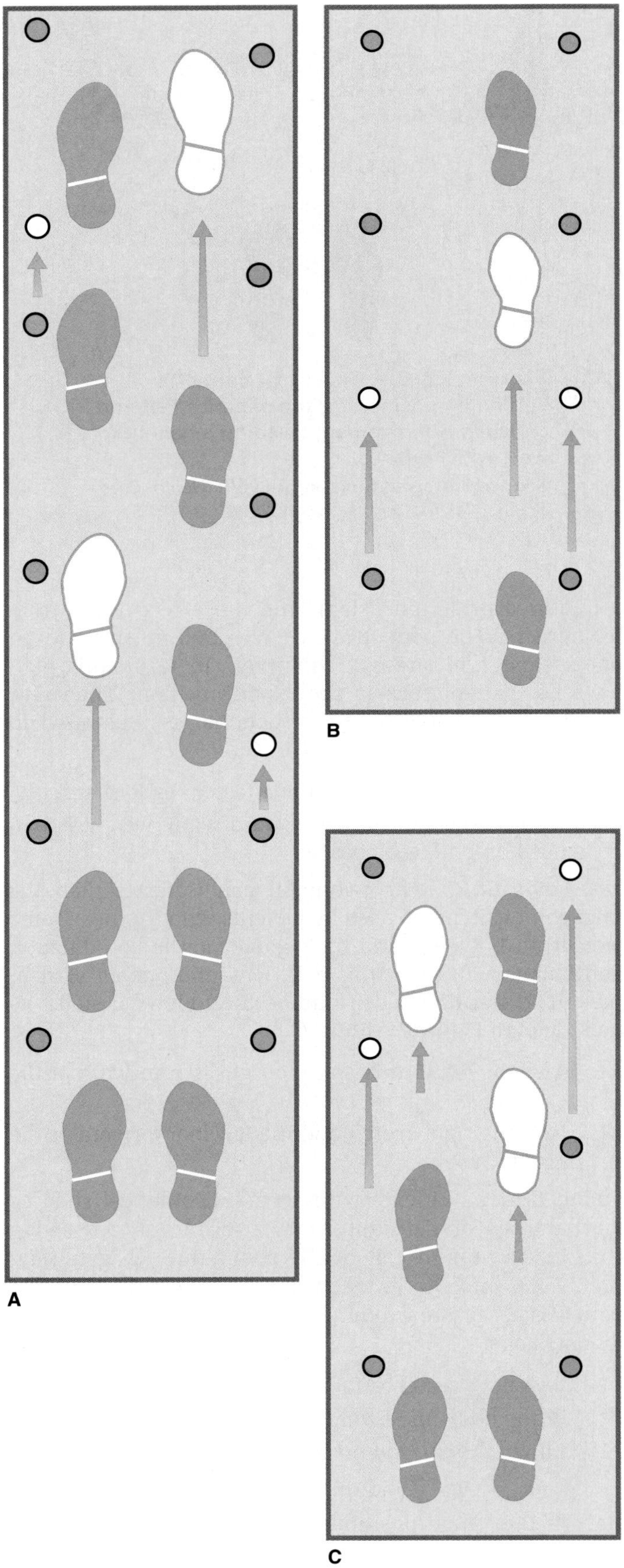

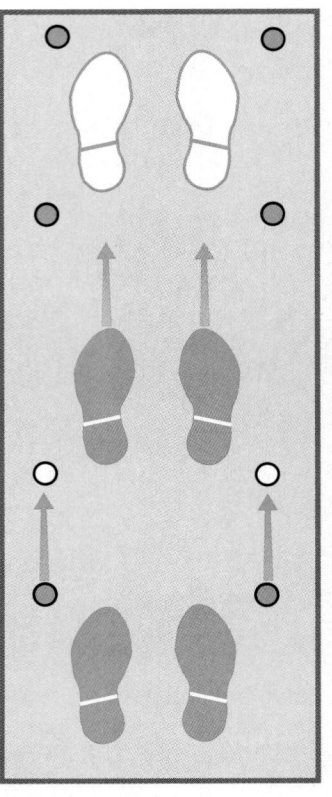

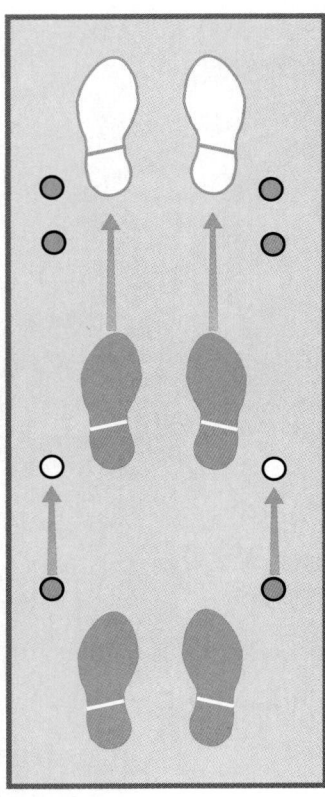

**Figure 29-11.** Patients with severe disabilities may walk with crutches using (A) the swing-to gait or (B) the swing-through gait.

## Wheelchairs

Wheelchairs range from small, folding models to large, motorized ones. Depending on the patient's disability and the length of time the wheelchair will be needed, the physical therapist will select an appropriate wheelchair.

When patients come to the medical office in a wheelchair, the doctor may not be able to examine them adequately if they remain in their wheelchair. If this is the case, you will be responsible for transferring the patients from the wheelchair to the examining table and back to the wheelchair after the exam. To ensure their safety and yours, follow the steps in Procedure 25-3 in Chapter 25. Here are some reminders on preventing injury.

- Ask for help if the patient is weak, heavy, or unstable.
- Explain to the patient the steps of transfer you will use.
- Before starting the transfer, make sure that the wheelchair is in the locked position and that the patient is sitting at the front of the wheelchair seat.
- When you lift, use the large muscles in your thighs, which are stronger than your back muscles.
- When lifting, bend from the knees and keep your back straight.
- Count to 3 and enlist the patient's help on the count of 3.

**Figure 29-10.** Crutch gaits include (A) a four-point gait, (B) a three-point gait, and (C) a two-point gait.

# Referral to a Physical Therapist

If the doctor refers the patient to a physical therapist or other specialist, you may be asked to contact the specialist directly or to give the patient a written order and information about contacting the specialist. Keep a file with information about the therapists that your office uses. In the file, note the forms and information each therapist requires. If you speak to the therapist, be sure to inform the doctor and to document the referral in the patient's chart. The therapist may be an independent practitioner or may be employed by a hospital, clinic, or home health-care agency.

In addition to physical therapy, some patients may decide to try alternative therapies, such as acupuncture, chiropractic, or biofeedback training. Although some doctors believe that alternative therapies provide some benefits, such as pain relief, many doctors do not. See Chapter 31 for information about a variety of alternative therapies.

# Summary

Physical therapy is a medical specialty that helps patients who have musculoskeletal and neurologic disorders. It produces therapeutic effects through physical and mechanical processes, patient education, and rehabilitation programs.

Before prescribing physical therapy, the physician must assess a patient's joint mobility, muscle strength, gait, and posture. Depending on the patient's needs, the physician may decide to include cryotherapy, thermotherapy, or hydrotherapy in the physical therapy program. The physician or physical therapist may also recommend exercise therapy, massage, or traction. If the patient has difficulty with ambulation, the physical therapist may indicate a mobility aid such as a cane, a walker, crutches, or a wheelchair.

As a medical assistant, you may be asked to help a patient with cryotherapy or thermotherapy, range of motion (ROM) exercises, hydrotherapy, and other treatments. You may also need to teach a patient how to use mobility aids. Working directly with patients to help alleviate their pain and improve their mobility will reward you with immediate and long-term satisfaction.

# REVIEW

## CHAPTER 29

### CASE STUDY QUESTIONS

Now that you have completed this chapter, review the case study at the beginning of the chapter and answer the following questions:

1. What type of teaching do you think this patient will need?
2. What type of therapy may be necessary for the crusted bloody injury on his forearm, and how would you perform it?

### Discussion Questions

1. Identify three conditions that can be treated with cryotherapy, and give two examples of dry cold applications and two examples of wet cold applications.
2. Discuss four ways physical therapy benefits patients.
3. Discuss three types of walkers and the advantages and disadvantages of each.

### Critical Thinking Questions

1. Your patient's physical therapist has prescribed hydrotherapy three times a week. Although the patient can drive, he tells you that he cannot keep his appointments because his wife has Alzheimer's disease and should not be left alone. How could you help solve this problem?
2. When teaching patients how to use a walker, what changes to their home environment would you suggest to ensure their safety?
3. While administering cryotherapy to a patient, she complains of a burning and tingling sensation. What should you do?
4. A 76-year-old man arrives at the clinic using a walker. As he enters the exam room, you notice that he is pushing the walker and not lifting it. What should you do?
5. You notice a patient using crutches is leaning down on her underarms. What should you tell the patient?

### Application Activities

1. With a partner, prepare and apply one type of cryotherapy and one type of thermotherapy to each other. Check the treatments after 5, 10, and 20 minutes. Evaluate the skin, and report how it looks and feels. Evaluate your partner's technique.
2. Review with a classmate the benefits of exercise therapy. Review three types of exercise and the use of each type.
3. Measure crutches for three different classmates. Teach each one a different gait. Then have a classmate measure crutches for you and teach you a gait.

### Virtual Fieldtrip

*Visit the McGraw-Hill Higher Education Medical Assisting website at www.mhhe.com/medicalassisting3 to complete the following activity:*

Use the National Library of Medicine's reference website and complete the following activities:

Search the words "rehabilitation + art therapy" and find out more about art therapy. Answer the following questions:

1. What is art therapy?
2. What types of disorders are treated with art therapy?
3. Where do art therapists work?

Open the CD and complete this chapter's practice activities, play the games, listen to the key terms, and test yourself with the interactive review. E-mail, print, and/or save your results to document your proficiency.

## CHAPTER 30

# Medical Emergencies and First Aid

## MEDICAL ASSISTING COMPETENCIES

*In preparation for the certification examination, you should know the following areas of competence:*

| COMPETENCY | CMA | RMA |
|---|---|---|
| **Clinical** | | |
| Apply principles of aseptic techniques and infection control, including hand washing | X | X |
| Dispose of biohazardous materials | X | X |
| Practice Standard Precautions | X | X |
| Recognize emergencies; perform first aid and CPR | | X |
| **General/Legal/Professional** | | |
| Recognize and respond to verbal and nonverbal communications by being attentive and adapting communication to the recipient's level of understanding | X | X |
| Be aware of and perform within legal and ethical boundaries | X | X |
| Provide patients with methods of health promotion and disease prevention | X | X |
| Identify community resources and information for patients and employers | X | X |

## KEY TERMS

automated external defibrillator (AED)

bioterrorism

cast

chain of custody

concussion

contusion

crash cart

dehydration

dislocation

epistaxis

hematemesis

hematoma

hyperglycemia

hypoglycemia

hypovolemic shock

palpitations

recovery position

septic shock

splint

sprain

strain

stroke

ventricular fibrillation (VF)

## CHAPTER OUTLINE

- Understanding Medical Emergencies
- Preparing for Medical Emergencies
- Accidental Injuries
- Common Illnesses
- Less Common Illnesses
- Common Psychosocial Emergencies
- The Patient Under Stress
- Educating the Patient
- Disasters
- Bioterrorism

# LEARNING OUTCOMES

After completing Chapter 30, you will be able to:

**30.1** Discuss the importance of first aid during a medical emergency.

**30.2** Describe the purpose of the emergency medical services (EMS) system and explain how to contact it.

**30.3** List items found on a crash cart or first-aid tray.

**30.4** List general guidelines to follow in emergencies.

**30.5** Compare various degrees of burns and their treatments.

**30.6** Demonstrate how to help a choking victim.

**30.7** Demonstrate cardiopulmonary resuscitation (CPR).

**30.8** Demonstrate four ways to control bleeding.

**30.9** List the symptoms of heart attack, shock, and stroke.

**30.10** Explain how to calm a patient who is under extreme stress.

**30.11** Discuss ways to educate patients about ways to prevent and respond to emergencies.

**30.12** Describe your role in responding to natural disasters and those caused by humans.

# Introduction

Emergencies of all types can occur when you are working as a medical assistant. Patients may come to your facility with an acute illness or an injury. You may have to handle a phone call from a patient who has an urgent physical or psychological problem. Additionally, you could experience a disaster—anything from a simple office fire to a bomb threat or bioterrorism. As a medical assistant you must be prepared to determine the urgency and handle any emergency that arises. Remember to stay calm and think through each situation in order to respond appropriately and create the best outcome.

## CASE STUDY

While you are working as a medical assistant in a busy office practice, the following three things occur at the same time:

1. You have a telephone call waiting for you; a woman wants to speak to you regarding her 4-year-old daughter. According to the administrative assistant, who took the call, the daughter has a fever of 103°F, and the mother wants to know how much acetaminophen or aspirin she can give her.

2. A 56-year-old male in room 2 comes out of the room to tell you that his chest is hurting and he is having difficulty breathing.

3. Three patients are waiting to be seen, and you have only the patient in room 2 ready for the physician. The other two exam rooms are empty.

As you read this chapter, consider each situation and determine the order in which you will respond. Explain your decisions.

# Understanding Medical Emergencies

A medical emergency is any situation in which a person suddenly becomes ill or sustains an injury that requires immediate help by a health-care professional. Your prompt action in a medical emergency could prevent permanent disability or even death.

You may see life-threatening medical emergencies in the health-care setting. For example, a patient in the waiting room may have chest pains that could indicate a heart attack is imminent. You may see emergencies that are not life-threatening, such as a coworker sustaining a minor injury on the job. You may also encounter emergencies outside the office. For example, a family member might cut a finger while using a kitchen knife, or a patron in a restaurant might choke on a piece of food. Your quick response is vital in all of these situations.

In or out of the office, a medical emergency may require you to perform first aid. First aid is the immediate care given to someone who is injured or suddenly becomes ill, before complete medical care can be obtained. Prompt and appropriate first aid can:

- Save a life
- Reduce pain
- Prevent further injury

- Reduce the risk of permanent disability
- Increase the chance of early recovery

Because most emergencies do not occur in a medical office, your role in patient education is critical. The more you teach patients about first aid and the proper way to respond to emergencies, the better equipped they will be to handle accidental injuries and illnesses.

# Preparing for Medical Emergencies

How well prepared you are for an emergency can mean the difference between life and death for a patient. You must be able to perform procedures quickly and correctly. Keeping your skills up-to-date will enable you to handle medical emergencies effectively.

Just as important is your ability to ensure that the medical office where you work is ready to handle whatever emergencies arise. This preparedness will depend on your own organizational skills and knowledge of community resources.

## Preparing the Office

You must first establish with the doctor which duties are expected of you and of other office personnel in case of an emergency and determine what resources are available. One of your most important allies will be the local emergency medical services (EMS) system. An EMS system is a network of qualified emergency services personnel who use community resources and equipment to provide emergency care to victims of injury or sudden illness.

**Posting Emergency Telephone Numbers.** Although the telephone number for the local EMS system is 911 in many parts of the country, some areas may not have 911 service. Post the area's EMS system telephone number at every telephone and on the **crash cart** (the rolling cart of emergency supplies and equipment) or first-aid tray. Every office employee should know this number. If the community has no EMS system, post the telephone number of the local ambulance or rescue squad. You should also post the telephone numbers of the nearest fire company, police station, poison control center, women's shelter, rape hotline, and drug and alcohol center.

When you call the EMS system for medical assistance and transport, speak clearly and calmly to the dispatcher. Be prepared to provide the following information:

- Your name, telephone number, and location
- Nature of the emergency
- Number of people in need of help
- Condition of the injured or ill patient(s)
- Summary of the first aid that has been given
- Directions on how to reach the location of the emergency

| TABLE 30-1 | Contents of a First Aid Kit |
| --- | --- |

- Absorbent cotton (sterile)
- Adhesive tape
- Airway or mouthpiece
- Analgesics, such as aspirin or acetaminophen
- Antiseptic solution or spray
- Antiseptic wipes
- Calamine lotion
- Chemical cold packs
- Diphenhydramine (Benadryl®)
- Disposable gloves
- Elastic bandages in various sizes
- Emergency blanket
- First aid book or information card
- Glucose tablets or sugar source
- Personal protective equipment (PPE): gloves, mask and goggles or face shield, gown, shower cap, booties, pocket mask or mouth shield
- Plastic bags
- Premoistened towelettes or hand cleaner
- Scissors
- Splints in various sizes
- Sterile gauze pads in various sizes
- Sterile rolls of gauze
- Sterile saline solution
- Sunscreen
- Triangular bandage
- Tweezers
- Waterproof flashlight with extra batteries

Do not hang up until the dispatcher gives you permission to do so.

**Common Emergency and First-Aid Supplies.** The crash cart or tray contains basic drugs, supplies, and equipment for medical emergencies. Most crash carts also contain a first-aid kit with supplies for managing minor injuries and ailments. Table 30-1 lists the usual items in a first-aid kit. The actual contents of the crash cart or tray may vary slightly from practice to practice. Become familiar with these contents and know where they are located in the office. Procedure 30-1 describes how to check and restock the essential items on a crash cart.

## Guidelines for Handling Emergencies

A medical emergency requires you to take certain steps. You are not responsible for diagnosing or providing medical care other than first aid. You are expected, however, to note the presence of serious conditions that threaten the patient's life. Then take appropriate action, but perform only those procedures that you have been trained to perform.

# PROCEDURE 30.1

## Stocking the Crash Cart

**Procedure Goal:** To ensure that the crash cart includes all appropriate drugs, supplies, and equipment needed for emergencies

**OSHA Guidelines:** This procedure does not involve exposure to blood, body fluids, or tissues.

**Materials:** Protocol for or list of crash cart items, crash cart

**Method:**

1. Review the office protocol for or list of items that should be on the crash cart.
2. Verify each drug on the crash cart, and check the amount against the office protocol or list. Restock those that were used, and replace those that have passed their expiration date.

### Rationale

Drugs on the crash cart should be available in quantities sufficient for use during an emergency. A drug that is out of date is of no use in an emergency.

Some typical crash cart drugs are listed here:

- Activated charcoal
- Atropine
- Dextrose 50%
- Diazepam (Valium)
- Digoxin (Lanoxin)
- Diphenhydramine hydrochloride (Benadryl)
- Epinephrine, injectable
- Furosemide (Lasix)
- Glucagon
- Glucose paste or tablets
- Insulin (regular or a variety)
- Intravenous dextrose in saline and intravenous dextrose in water
- Isoproterenol hydrochloride (Isuprel), aerosol inhaler and injectable
- Lactated Ringer's solution
- Lidocaine (Xylocaine), injectable
- Methylprednisolone tablets
- Nitroglycerin tablets
- Phenobarbital, injectable
- Phenytoin (Dilantin)

- Saline solution, isotonic (0.9%)
- Sodium bicarbonate, injectable
- Sterile water for injection

3. Check the supplies on the crash cart against the list. Restock items that were used, and make sure the packaging of supplies on the cart has not been opened.

### Rationale

Items on the cart must be available and ready for use at the time of an emergency.

Some typical crash cart supplies are listed here:

- Adhesive tape
- Constricting band or tourniquet
- Dressing supplies (alcohol wipes, rolls of gauze, bandage strips, bandage scissors)
- Intravenous tubing, venipuncture devices, and butterfly needles
- Personal protective equipment
- Syringes and needles in various sizes

4. Check the equipment on the crash cart against the list, and examine it to make sure that it is in working order. Restock equipment that is missing or broken.

### Rationale

There is no time during an emergency to make sure equipment works.

Some typical crash cart equipment is listed here:

- Airways in assorted sizes
- Ambu-bag, a trademark for a breathing bag used to assist respiratory ventilation
- **Automated external defibrillator** (electrical device that shocks the heart to restore normal beating)
- Endotracheal tubes in various sizes
- Oxygen tank with oxygen mask and cannula

5. Check miscellaneous items on the crash cart against the list, and restock as needed. Some typical miscellaneous crash cart items are listed here:

- Orange juice
- Sugar packets

**Patient Emergencies.** Assess the situation and surroundings to determine whether it is safe for you to assist. If safe, put on the appropriate personal protective equipment (PPE), such as gloves. Next, do an initial assessment to detect and immediately correct any life-threatening problems of the airway, breathing, and circulation. Corrections of life-threatening problems are essential to survival. There are six steps in the initial assessment: (1) form a general impression of the patient, (2) determine the patient's level of responsiveness, (3) assess the airway, breathing, and circulation status of the patient, sometimes referred to as the ABCs, (4) determine the priority or urgency of the patient's condition, (5) conduct a focused exam, and (6) document a history. Procedure 30-2 provides guidelines for performing these six steps.

**Telephone Emergencies.** Sometimes a patient or a patient's family member calls the medical office with an emergency. If you are responsible for handling telephone calls, be prepared to triage the injuries by telephone. Triaging is the classification of injuries according to severity, urgency of treatment, and place for treatment.

To handle emergency calls, follow the practice's telephone triage protocols. For example, if a parent calls to say her daughter has broken her arm and the child's bone is visible, tell her to call the local EMS system for immediate care and transport to the hospital. If, however, a parent calls to say her son swallowed half a bottle of baby bath, tell her to remain calm and give her the telephone number of the poison control center. Depending on circumstances, you may offer to make the necessary telephone call yourself.

Adhere to the following general guidelines in any emergency situation.

- Stay calm
- Reassure the patient
- Act in a confident, organized manner

**Personal Protection.** Whenever you administer first aid and emergency treatment, try to reduce or eliminate the risk of exposing yourself and others to infection. Follow Standard Precautions and assume that all blood and body fluids are infected with blood-borne pathogens. To protect yourself and others, take the following basic precautions. Include PPE in your first-aid kit at work and at home. Standard PPE includes gloves, goggles and mask or face shield, gown, cap, and booties. A pocket mask or mouth shield provides personal protection when you perform rescue breathing. Plan to use specific PPE based on the condition of the patient. Table 30-2 provides examples of PPE to use in various emergency situations. When in doubt, wear more PPE than you may think is called for.

Wear gloves if you expect hand contact with blood, body fluids, mucous membranes, torn skin, or potentially contaminated articles or surfaces. In addition, if you have any cuts or lesions, wear PPE over the affected area.

Minimize splashing, splattering, or spraying of blood or other body fluids when performing first aid. If blood or other body fluids splash into your eyes, nose, or mouth, flush the area with water as soon as possible.

Wash your hands thoroughly with soap and water after removing the gloves. Also wash other skin surfaces that have come in contact with blood or other body fluids. Do not touch your mouth, nose, or eyes, and do not eat or drink after providing emergency care until you have washed your hands thoroughly. If you have been exposed to blood or other body fluids, be sure to tell the doctor. You may need postexposure treatment.

**Documentation.** Document all office emergencies in the patient's chart. Be sure to include your assessment, treatment given, and the patient's response. If the patient was transported to another facility, record the location. Include the date and time with the documentation, as well as your signature and credentials.

# Accidental Injuries

No matter where you encounter an emergency, your knowledge and certifications should enable you to provide first aid for the patient until a physician or EMT arrives. To help you become familiar with how to handle various emergency situations, the following sections present accidental injuries, common illnesses, and less common illnesses.

Accidental injuries that may call for emergency medical intervention include the following:

- Bites and stings
- Burns
- Choking
- Ear trauma
- Eye trauma
- Falls
- Fractures, dislocations, sprains, and strains
- Head injuries
- Hemorrhaging
- Multiple injuries
- Poisoning
- Weather-related injuries
- Wounds

## Bites and Stings

Dog and cat bites and bee, wasp, and hornet stings are fairly common. Less common are snakebites and spider bites, which you are more likely to encounter in certain parts of the country, such as Florida or the Southwest, than in other areas.

**Animal Bites.** An animal bite may bruise the skin, tear it, or leave a puncture wound. A wound that tears the skin should be seen by a doctor and will need to be

# PROCEDURE 30.2

## Performing an Emergency Assessment

**Procedure Goal:** To assess a medical emergency quickly and accurately

**OSHA Guidelines**

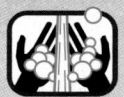 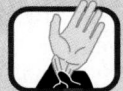 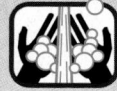

**Materials:** Patient's chart, pen, gloves

**Method:**

1. Put on gloves.
2. Form a general impression of the patient, including his level of responsiveness, level of distress, facial expressions, age, ability to talk, and skin color.
3. If the patient can communicate clearly, ask what happened. If not, ask someone who observed the accident or injury.
4. Assess an unresponsive patient by tapping on his shoulder and asking, "Are you OK?" If there is no response, proceed to the next step.

### Rationale

You must know if a patient is unresponsive before proceeding. The patient's responsiveness will determine if you need to assess their airway.

5. Assess the patient's airway. If necessary, open the airway by using the head tilt–chin lift maneuver. Give two breaths of 1 second each.
6. Assess the patient's breathing. If the patient is not breathing, then perform rescue breathing.
7. Assess the patient's circulation. Determine if the patient has a pulse. Is there any serious external bleeding? Perform CPR as needed (Procedure 30-8). Control any significant bleeding (Procedure 30-5).
8. If all life-threatening problems have been identified and treated, perform a focused exam. Start at the head and perform the following steps rapidly, taking about 90 seconds.
   a. Head: Check for deformities, bruises, open wounds, tenderness, depressions, and swelling. Check the ears, nose, and mouth for fluid, blood, or foreign bodies.
   b. Eyes: Open the eyes and compare the pupils. They should be the same size.
   c. Neck: Look and feel for deformities, bruises, depressions, open wounds, tenderness, and swelling. Check for a medical alert bracelet or necklace.
   d. Chest: Look and feel for deformities, bruises, open wounds, tenderness, depressions, and swelling.
   e. Abdomen: Look and feel for deformities, bruises, open wounds, tenderness, depressions, and swelling.
   f. Pelvis: Look and feel for deformities, bruises, open wounds, tenderness, depressions, and swelling.
   g. Arms: Look and feel for deformities, bruises, open wounds, depressions, tenderness, and swelling. Compare the arms for any differences in size, color, or temperature.
   h. Legs: Look and feel for deformities, bruises, open wounds, depressions, tenderness, and swelling. Compare the legs for any differences in size, color, or temperature.
   i. Back: Look and feel for deformities, bruises, open wounds, depressions, tenderness, and swelling. Feel under the patient for pools of blood.

### Rationale

Pools of blood indicate rapid hemorrhage.

9. Check vital signs and observe the patient for pallor (paleness) or cyanosis (a bluish tint). If the patient is dark-skinned, observe for pallor or cyanosis on the inside of the lips and mouth.

### Rationale

A patient's status may change quickly. Checking vital signs often will alert you to any changes in the patient's condition.

10. Document your findings and report them to the doctor or emergency medical technician (EMT).
11. Assist the doctor or EMT as requested.
12. Dispose of biohazardous waste according to OSHA guidelines.
13. Remove your gloves and wash your hands.

## TABLE 30-2 Personal Protective Equipment for Emergencies

| Equipment | Conditions for Use | Sample Emergencies Requiring Equipment |
|---|---|---|
| Gloves | Chance of contact with blood or other body secretion or excretion during emergency | Open wound, eye trauma |
| Goggles and mask or face shield and possible head cover | Chance of blood or other body secretion or excretion being splattered, coughed, or sprayed onto the mucus membranes of the eyes, mouth, or nose | Bleeding, vomiting, most emergency care for small children (because of squirming) |
| Gown and possible booties | Chance of contact with excessive bleeding or secretion and excretion | Childbirth, severe nosebleed |
| Pocket mask or mouth shield | Needed for CPR or rescue breathing | Heart attack, respiratory arrest |

reported to the police, animal control officer, and local health department. If the animal can be found, it should be checked for rabies. Then, depending on the animal's rabies vaccination status, the animal may need to be quarantined. If the animal is a probable carrier of rabies and cannot be found, the doctor may administer antirabies serum to the patient as a precaution.

Dogs, cats, skunks, squirrels, raccoons, bats, and foxes are more likely to carry rabies than are other animals. Hamsters, gerbils, guinea pigs, and mice are rarely infected by the rabies virus.

Human bites can raise concerns about transmitting the human immunodeficiency virus (HIV) or hepatitis B virus. HIV can be transmitted only if the bite breaks the skin and if the biter has bleeding gums. Hepatitis B virus may be transmitted by a human bite that punctures the skin. In this case a series of three injections is required to immunize against hepatitis B.

Immediate care for bites calls for washing the area thoroughly with antiseptic soap and water. (If the bite caused a puncture wound, try to make it bleed to flush out bacteria. Then wash the area with soap and water.) Apply an antibiotic ointment and a dry, sterile dressing. The doctor will administer tetanus toxoid if the patient has not received it in the last 7 to 10 years.

**Insect Stings.** Insect stings are merely a nuisance to most patients. The site of the sting can become red, swollen, itchy, and painful. If the patient was stung by a honeybee, you must first remove the stinger, because it still has the ability to release venom. Remove the stinger by scraping the skin with a credit card or other flat, hard, sharp object. Be careful not to release more venom. Avoid using your fingers or tweezers, because squeezing the stinger may force more venom into the wound. (If you cannot remove the stinger, call the physician.) Wash the skin with soap and water. After the stinger is removed, apply ice to the site, 10 minutes on and 10 minutes off, to reduce the pain and swelling.

A sting can be deadly to a patient who is allergic to the insect venom, because anaphylaxis can develop. The symptoms of and treatment for anaphylaxis are described later in this chapter.

**Snakebites.** Poisonous snakes in the United States include rattlesnakes, water moccasins (or cottonmouths), copperheads, and coral snakes. Because snakes are cold-blooded, they often lie on rocks to warm themselves. Most bites occur when a person steps onto, sits down on, or reaches over or between rocks where a snake is sunning itself.

The bites of most poisonous snakes produce similar symptoms: one or two puncture marks, pain, and swelling at the site; rapid pulse; nausea; vomiting; and perhaps unconsciousness and seizures. If possible, get a description of the snake so the EMS team or the hospital can procure the proper antivenin (a substance that counteracts the snake poison) ahead of time. Snakebites are dangerous, but with proper intervention, they rarely lead to death.

If a patient has been bitten by a snake that may be poisonous, call a doctor or the EMS system. If the patient must walk, have him walk slowly to prevent dispersion of the poison through the circulation. To care for a poisonous snakebite while you await help, keep the patient calm, and remove rings, watches, or tight clothing in the area. If possible, immobilize the injured part and position it below heart level. Do not apply ice or a tourniquet, and do not cut or suction the wound.

**Spider Bites.** Only two types of spiders in the United States are a serious threat to health: the black widow spider, which has a red hourglass mark on its abdomen, and the brown recluse spider, which has a violin-shaped mark on its head. The black widow bite causes swelling and pain at the site as well as nausea, vomiting, rigid abdomen, fever, rash, and difficulty breathing or swallowing. The brown recluse bite causes severe swelling and tenderness and, eventually, ulceration along the nerve closest to the location of the bite.

You are not expected to classify spiders and their bites accurately. Therefore, any patient bitten by a spider must be seen by a physician. To care for a patient with a spider bite, wash the area thoroughly with soap and water. Apply an ice pack to the area to reduce swelling and pain. If possible, keep the area below heart level to prevent the poison from spreading. Healing of the bite can sometimes take several months.

# Burns

Burns involve tissue injury that occurs from heat, chemicals, electricity, or radiation. Be sure that you teach patients about emergency treatment for burns as well as any follow-up care prescribed by the physician.

## Types of Burns

***Thermal Burns.*** Thermal burns may be caused by contact with hot liquids, steam, flames, radiation, and excessive heat from fires or hot objects. Call the EMS team immediately for victims of such burns. To stop the burning process, use water to cool a burning substance, or use a wet cloth or blanket to put out the fire.

***Chemical Burns.*** Chemical burns are more likely to affect workers at chemical or industrial facilities than individuals in the home. To treat this type of burn, first remove the cause of the burn. Take care not to come into contact with the chemical. Brush off any excess dry chemical and remove any clothing contaminated with the chemical. Gently flood the area with cool water for at least 15 minutes. Cover the area with a dry sterile dressing. If the burn is severe, call EMS to transport the patient to the hospital. Monitor the patient carefully for signs of shock.

***Electrical Burns.*** Electrical burns are injuries from exposure to electrical currents, including lightning. These burns occur at the site where the electricity enters the body and where the current exits the body and enters the ground. Along the current's pathway, extensive tissue damage can occur from heat followed by chemical changes to nerve, muscle, and heart tissue. Call the EMS team immediately for these types of injuries.

**Classifications of Burns.** The severity of a burn is determined by the depth and extent of the burn area, the source of the burn, the age of the patient, body regions burned, and other patient illnesses and injuries. When classifying burns, use the categories *minor, moderate,* and *major.* These categories take into account all the factors that determine severity. For example, a burn might be considered minor although it damages all skin layers if it affects only a small area of one leg on an otherwise healthy person. A major burn includes any burn in children younger than age 2, electrical burns, burns complicated by fractures or serious trauma, and burns on the hands, face, feet, or perineum.

Burns classified according to the depth of skin damage are called superficial, partial thickness, and full thickness (Figure 30-1). In a superficial burn, formally called a first-degree burn, the epidermis is damaged and the skin is reddened. Blisters result from a second-degree burn, in which part of the dermis is destroyed. A third-degree burn damages all the skin layers.

***Superficial (First-Degree) Burns.*** A superficial burn causes pain and makes the surrounding skin turn red. It is equivalent to a sunburn. Treat first-degree burns by applying cold-water

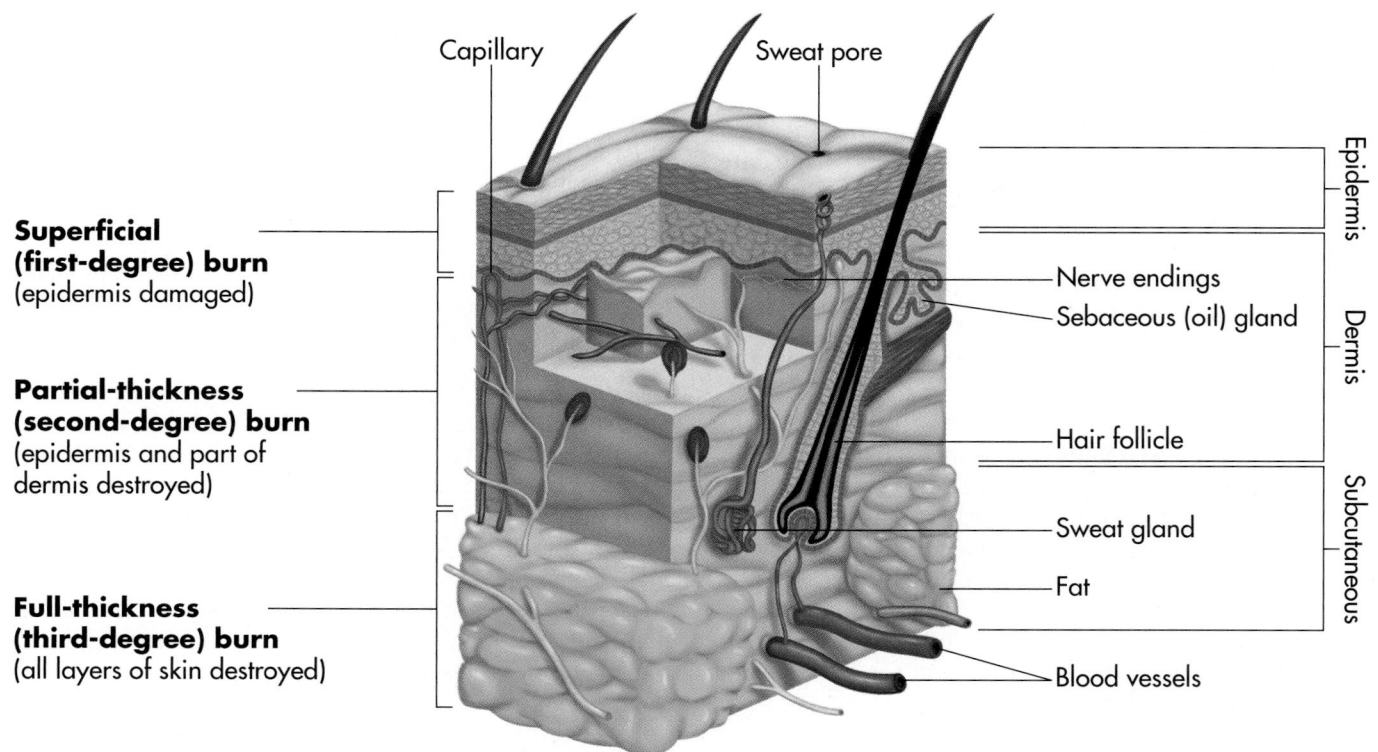

**Figure 30-1.** The depth of skin damage is one factor used to determine the severity of burns.

dressings or by immersing the affected area in cold water. Gently pat the area dry, and apply a dry, sterile dressing. Do not use greasy ointments, butter, or other substances because they prevent oxygen from reaching the wound and will have to be scrubbed off before any treatment can be administered. Scrubbing would be very painful.

*Partial-Thickness (Second-Degree) Burns.* Partial thickness burns extend deeper into the skin than first-degree burns. They cause blistering along with pain and redness. Immerse second-degree burns in cold water until the pain subsides. Then gently pat the area dry, taking care not to break blisters, and apply a dry, sterile dressing. Do not apply antiseptic ointment unless the doctor orders it. If the arms or legs are affected, elevate them to reduce swelling.

*Full-Thickness (Third-Degree) Burns.* Full-thickness burns, such as those received in a fire, involve all layers of skin and demand immediate emergency medical assistance. While you wait for the EMS team, do not remove charred or adhered clothing from the patient. Cover the burns and adhered clothing with thick, sterile dressings. If the hands, arms, or legs are burned, elevate them above the heart. Keep the patient warm and provide reassurance. Check to see whether the patient is suffering from smoke inhalation. Signs of smoke inhalation include difficulty breathing (often accompanied by coughing), smoky-smelling breath, or black residue in the patient's mouth and nose. If any of these signs are present, gently move the patient into a sitting position and monitor her breathing. Third-degree burns are usually not painful at first because of nerve damage.

**Estimating the Extent of the Burn.** Various methods are used to estimate the extent of the burn area (Figure 30-2). To calculate the amount of skin surface burned on an adult, use the rule of nines. This rule assigns each of the following areas 9% of the body surface: the head and neck, each upper limb, the chest, the abdomen, the upper back, the lower back and buttocks, the front of each lower limb, and the back of each lower limb. These areas make up 99% of the body's surface. The genital region is the remaining 1%. The figures to use when making calculations in children and infants are shown in Figure 30-2.

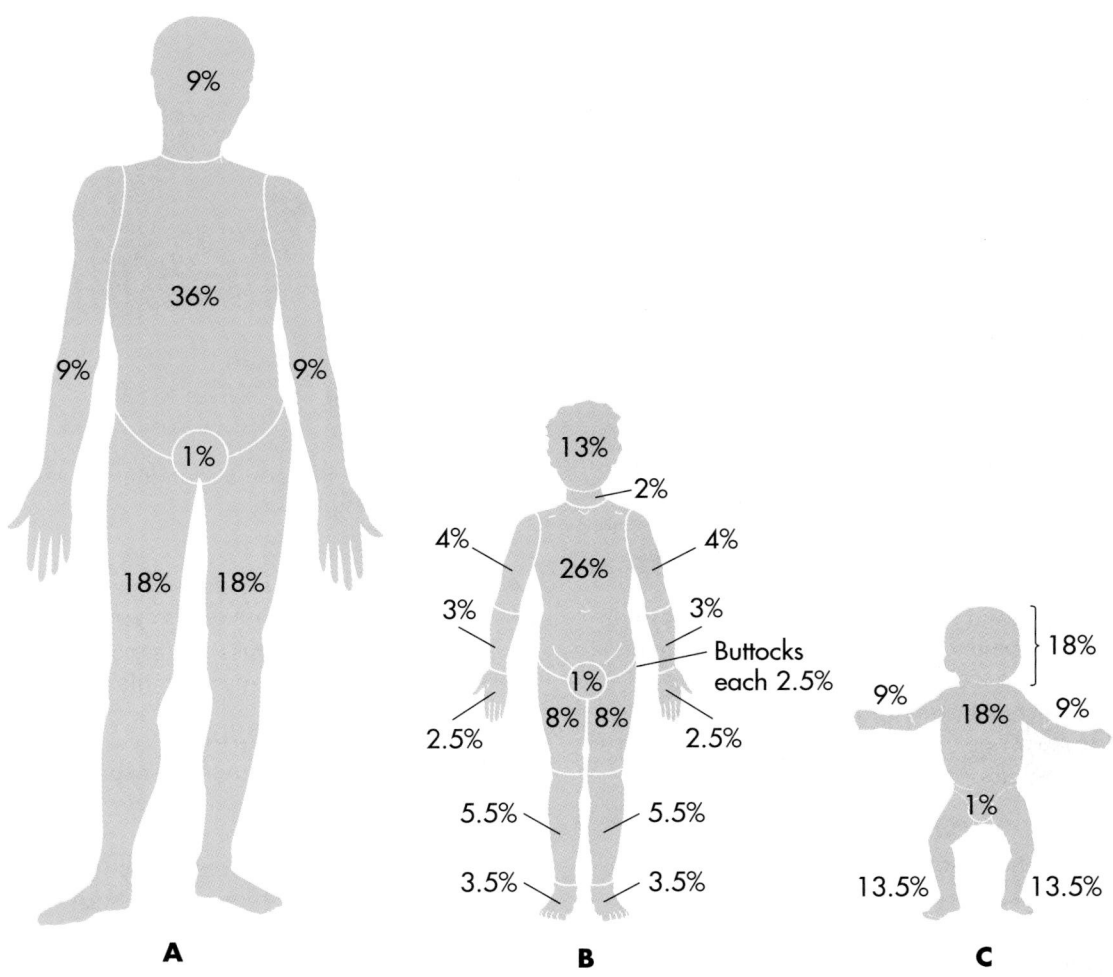

**Figure 30-2.** (A) Use the rule of nines to calculate the percentage of body surface affected by burns in adults. Except for the genital region, percentage figures combine front and back surfaces. (B) In children, use the percentages based on the Lund and Browder chart. These numbers take into account that children's body proportions differ from those of adults. (C) In infants, the rule of nines is used. These numbers take into account an infant's different body properties.

## Choking

Choking occurs when food or a foreign object blocks a person's trachea, or windpipe. The main symptom of a choking emergency is the inability to speak. A choking person who cannot talk may give the universal sign of choking—a hand up to the throat and a fearful look. If you see someone giving the universal sign, be prepared to act promptly.

Procedure 30-3 provides guidelines for assisting an adult or a child who is responsive and choking. The American Heart Association generally considers anyone between the ages of one and eight years old a child. Procedure 30-4 provides the guidelines for assisting an infant who is responsive and has a foreign body airway obstruction. An infant is defined by the American Heart Association as any child younger than the age of 1 year.

## PROCEDURE 30.3

### Foreign Body Airway Obstruction in a Responsive Adult or Child

**Procedure Goal:** To correctly relieve a foreign body from the airway of an adult or child

**OSHA Guidelines:** This procedure does not involve exposure to blood, body fluids, or tissues.

**Materials:** Choking adult or child patient
*Caution: Never perform this procedure on someone who is not choking.*

**Method:**

1. Ask, "Are you choking?" If the answer is "Yes," indicated by a nod of the head or some other sign, ask, "Can you speak?" If the answer is "No," tell the patient that you can help. A choking person cannot speak, cough, or breathe, and exhibits the universal sign of choking. If the patient is coughing, observe him closely to see if he clears the object. If he is not coughing or stops coughing, use abdominal thrusts.

2. Position yourself behind the patient. Place your fist against the abdomen just above the navel and below the xiphoid process.

3. Grasp your fist with your other hand, and provide quick inward and upward thrusts into the patient's abdomen (Figure 30-3).

   *Rationale*

   The thrust should be sufficient to move enough air from the lungs so that the object can be displaced from the airway.

   Note: If a pregnant or obese person is choking, you will need to place your arms around the chest and perform thrusts over the center of the breastbone (Figure 30-4).

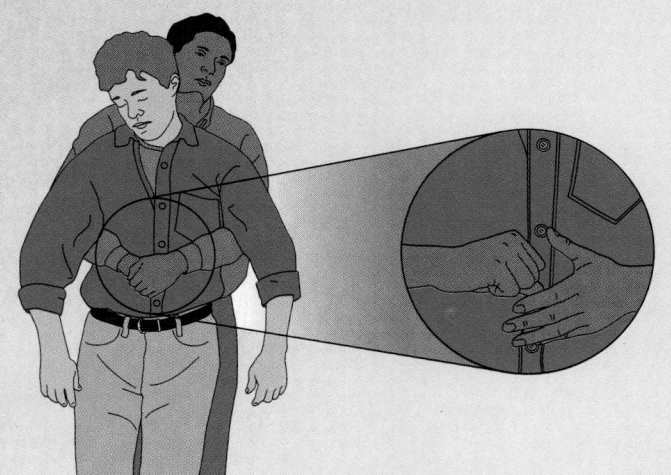

**Figure 30-3.** Perform abdominal thrusts on a conscious choking victim.

4. Continue the thrusts until the object is expelled or the patient becomes unresponsive.

5. If the patient becomes unresponsive, call EMS and position the patient on his back.

   *Rationale*

   A patient who becomes unresponsive is most likely not getting the necessary amount of oxygen to the brain.

6. Open his mouth by grasping both the tongue and lower jaw between your thumb and fingers and pull up the lower jawbone.

7. Look into the mouth. If you see the foreign body, remove it using your index finger. Do not perform any blind finger sweeps on a child (Figure 30-5).

*continued* ⟶

## Foreign Body Airway Obstruction in a Responsive Adult or Child *(concluded)*

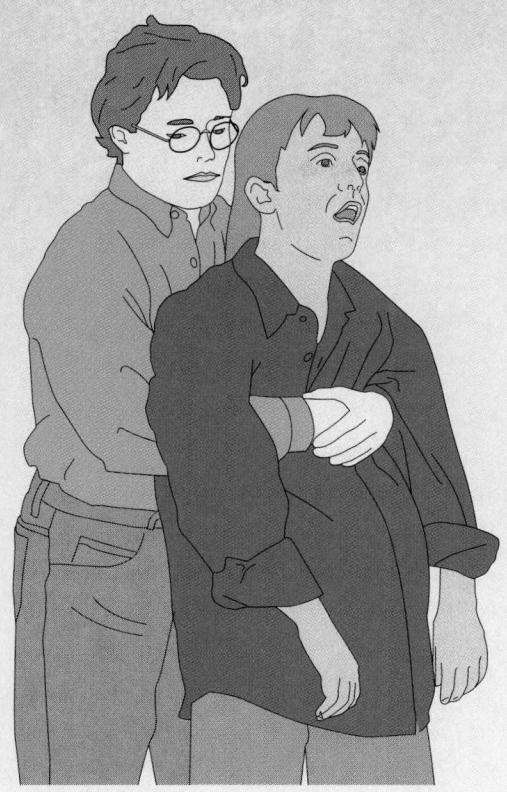

**Figure 30-4.** Use a chest thrust for a choking victim who is pregnant or obese.

8. Open the airway and look, listen, and feel for breathing. If the patient is not breathing, attempt a rescue breath. Observe the chest. If it does not rise with the breath, reposition the airway and administer another rescue breath. If the chest does not rise after the second attempt, assume that the airway is still blocked and begin CPR (Procedure 30-8).

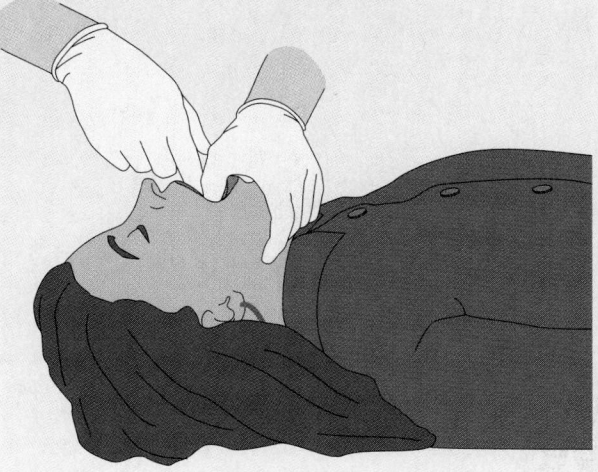

**Figure 30-5.** Use a finger sweep to remove a foreign object from the mouth. Do not perform a blind finger sweep on children or infants.

## Foreign Body Airway Obstruction in a Responsive Infant

**Procedure Goal:** To correctly relieve a foreign body from the airway of an infant

**OSHA Guidelines:** This procedure does not involve exposure to blood, body fluids, or tissues.

**Materials:** Choking infant
*Caution: Never perform this procedure on an infant who is not choking.*

**Method:**

1. Assess the infant for signs of severe or complete airway obstruction, which include:

   a. Sudden onset of difficulty in breathing.
   b. Inability to speak, make sounds, or cry.
   c. A high-pitched, noisy, wheezing sound, or no sounds while inhaling.
   d. Weak, ineffective coughs.
   e. Blue lips or skin.

2. Hold the infant with his head down, supporting the body with your forearm. His legs should straddle your forearm and you should support his jaw and head with your hand and fingers. This is best done in a sitting or kneeling position (Figure 30-6).

*continued* ⟶

## Foreign Body Airway Obstruction in a Responsive Infant (concluded)

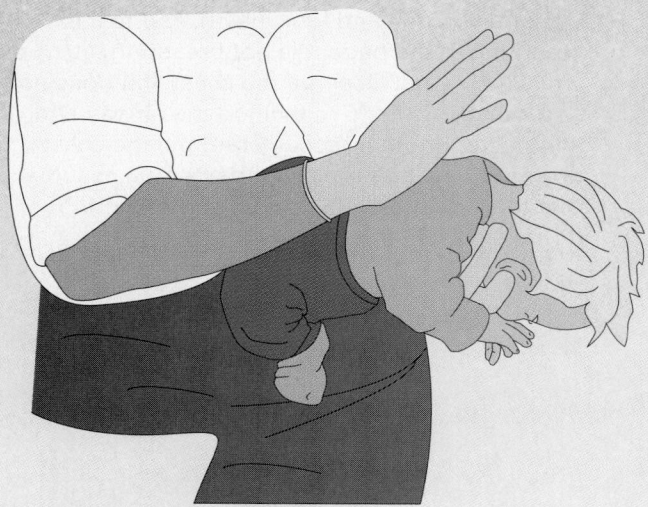

**Figure 30-6.** Use back blows for a choking infant.
Source: *Glencoe Health Care Science Technology*, Booth 2004, p. 113, Figure 4-21.

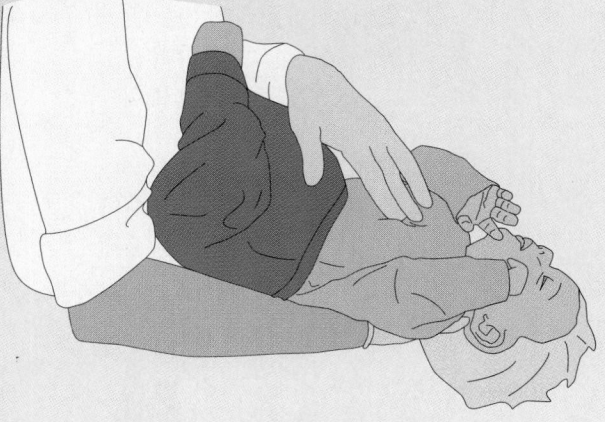

**Figure 30-7.** Keep the infant's head and neck supported.

3. Give up to five back blows with the heel of your free hand, as shown in Figure 30-6. Strike the infant's back forcefully between the shoulder blades. At any point, if the object is expelled, discontinue the back blows.

### Rationale

Effective back blows may successfully dislodge the object. Having the infant's head down will allow the object to fall out.

4. If the obstruction is not cleared, turn the infant over as a unit, supporting the head with your hands and the body between your forearms (Figure 30-7).

5. Keep the head lower than the chest and perform five chest thrusts.

### Rationale

Chest thrusts will force air out of the lungs, helping dislodge the object.

Place two fingers over the breastbone (sternum), above the xiphoid. Give five quick chest thrusts about ½ to 1 inch deep. Stop the compressions if the object is expelled.

6. Alternate five back blows and five chest thrusts until the object is expelled or until the infant becomes unconscious. If the infant becomes unconscious, call EMS or have someone do it for you.

7. Open the infant's mouth by grasping both the tongue and the lower jaw between the thumb and fingers, and pull up the lower jawbone. If you see the object, remove it using your smallest finger. Do not use blind finger sweeps on an infant.

### Rationale

A blind finger sweep may push the object deeper into the airway.

8. Open the airway and attempt to provide rescue breaths. If the chest does not rise, reposition the airway (both head and chin) and try to provide another rescue breath.

9. If the rescue breaths are unsuccessful, begin CPR. Hold the infant, supporting her body with your forearm and her head with your hand and fingers. Deliver 30 chest compressions about ½ to 1 inch deep.

10. Open the infant's mouth and look for the foreign object. If you see an object, remove it with your smallest finger.

11. Open the airway and attempt to provide rescue breaths. If the chest does not rise, continue CPR until the doctor or EMS arrives.

## Ear Trauma

Treat any cut or laceration to the ear by lightly applying a bandage, with even pressure, over the injury. It may be possible to reattach a severed ear surgically. Carefully wrap the severed ear in a sterile dressing secured with a self-adherent gauze bandage. Then wrap the ear in plastic, label it, and place it in an ice chest or over an ice pack so that it is kept chilled but is not in direct contact with the ice. Send it with the patient to the hospital.

## Eye Trauma

Depending on its severity, eye trauma may require no more than an ice pack, or it may require hospital care. Eye trauma may result from a fall, a blow to the eye, or a wound from a pointed object. Whatever the cause, you should carefully examine the eye to the best of your ability and notify the physician of the patient's condition.

Eye injuries are commonly caused by foreign objects in the eye. Tiny specks cause tearing and can be painful. To remove them, use moistened sterile gauze or a tissue. Do not use a cotton ball, because it may leave behind cotton wisps that can irritate the eye. If an object has penetrated the eye, do not try to remove it. Seek medical attention immediately.

## Falls

If a patient falls from a chair or an examining table and cannot get up, call for help. Do not move the patient until the physician or an EMT examines him. Instruct the patient not to move his head, neck, or back if injuries to those areas are suspected. If possible, have someone hold the patient's neck to stabilize it until the physician or EMT arrives. Move the patient only in a life-threatening situation, such as if the building is on fire. Arrange for transport to the hospital, and document the fall and injury in the patient's chart.

If the fall results in only a bump, apply ice and observe for bruises and swelling. Give the patient time to collect himself. Be sure to notify the doctor, who should examine the patient. Then document the fall, the injury, and the treatment in the patient's chart.

Falls are not limited to the physician's office, of course. Follow these procedures wherever you encounter someone who has fallen.

## Fractures, Dislocations, Sprains, and Strains

A fracture is a break in a bone. Fractures are categorized in several ways (Figure 30-8). Complete fractures go across the entire bone; incomplete fractures go through only part of the bone. Comminuted fractures are those in which the bone has broken into several fragments. In a greenstick fracture, the bone is bent, but only one side is fractured. Greenstick fractures occur most often in children because their bones are still soft and pliable. A fracture is closed if it does not cause a break in the skin. In open fractures, the bone breaks through the skin.

A **dislocation** is the displacement of a bone end from the joint. Both fractures and dislocations usually result from accidents or sports injuries. They can cause pain, tenderness, loss of function, deformity, swelling, and discoloration. The injury is usually diagnosed by x-ray.

Treatment of fractures and dislocations depends on factors such as the nature of the injury and the patient's age and physical condition. The basic emergency steps are:

1. Keep the person calm and limit his movement.
2. Assess him for any other injuries.
3. Notify the doctor or call EMS if needed.
   - Do not try to move the person until the doctor or EMS arrives.
4. If the skin is broken, cover with a sterile dressing.
5. Immobilize the extremity with a splint or sling (Figure 30-9).
   - Use rolled up newspaper, strips of wood, etc.
   - Immobilize the joint above and below the injury.
   - Immobilize the bone in the position it is found.
   - Do not try to put the bone back in place.
6. Place an ice pack on the affected area.
7. Monitor him for signs of shock.
8. Assess for signs of lack of circulation in the injured limb including pale or blue skin, loss of feeling, and tingling in the area.

Immobilization is sometimes provided by the application of a splint or cast. The purpose of both splints and casts is to keep an injured body part in place and protect it as it heals. A **splint** is an appliance used for conditions that do not require rigid immobilization or, as a temporary measure, for those in which swelling is anticipated. A **cast** is a rigid, external dressing, usually made of plaster or fiberglass, which is molded to the contours of the body part to which it is applied. You may assist the physician with the application of a cast (Figure 30-10). You may also educate the patient about these basic elements of cast care.

- Report any of the following to the physician immediately: pain, swelling, discoloration of exposed portions, lack of pulsation and warmth, or the inability to move exposed parts
- Keep the casted extremity elevated for the first day
- Avoid indenting the cast until it is completely dry
- Check the movement and sensation of the visible extremities frequently
- Restrict strenuous activities for the first few days
- Avoid allowing the affected limb to hang down for any length of time
- Do not put anything inside the cast
- Keep the cast dry
- Follow the physician's orders regarding restrictions of activities

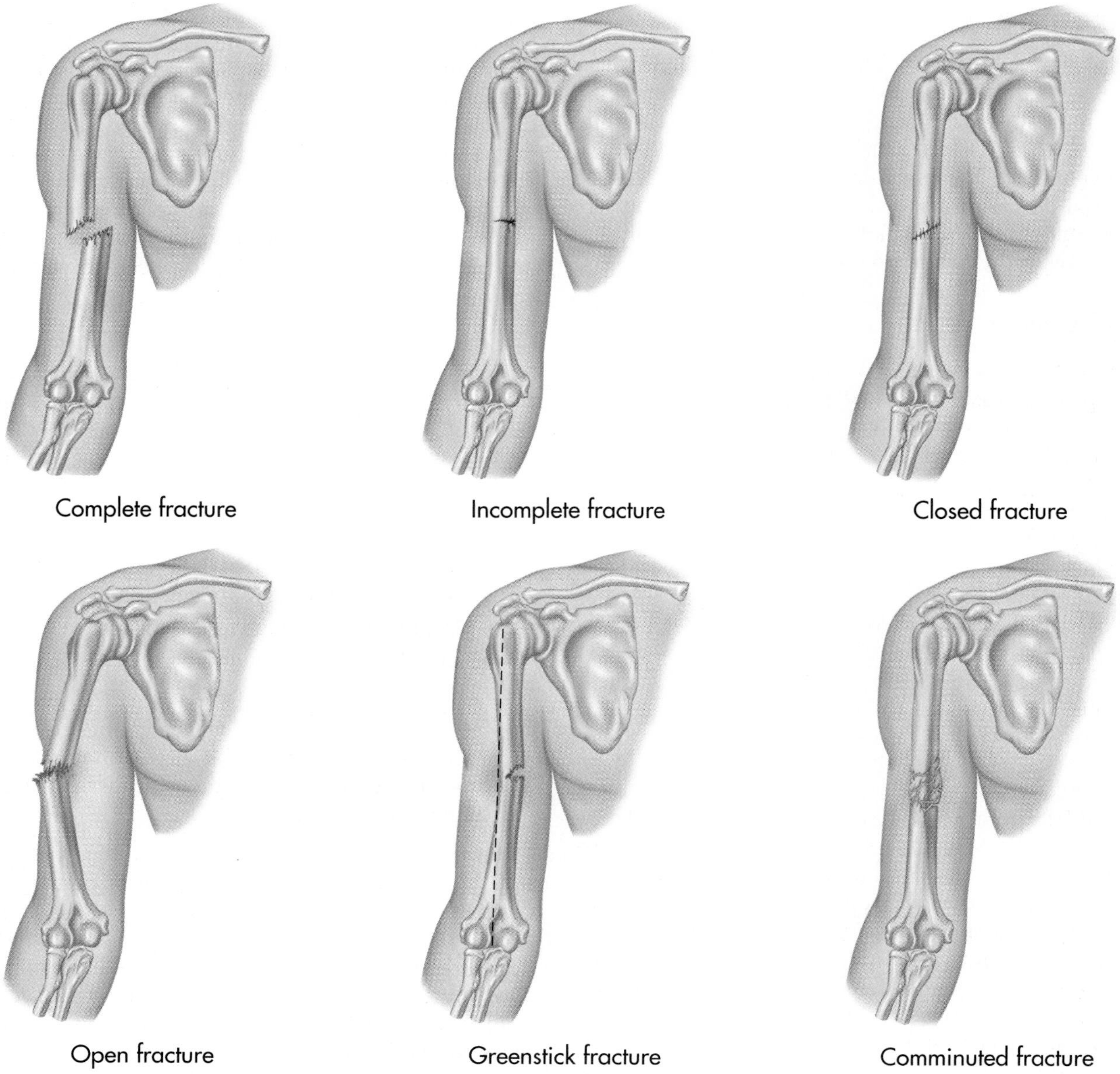

Complete fracture

Incomplete fracture

Closed fracture

Open fracture

Greenstick fracture

Comminuted fracture

**Figure 30-8.** These illustrations show various types of fractures.

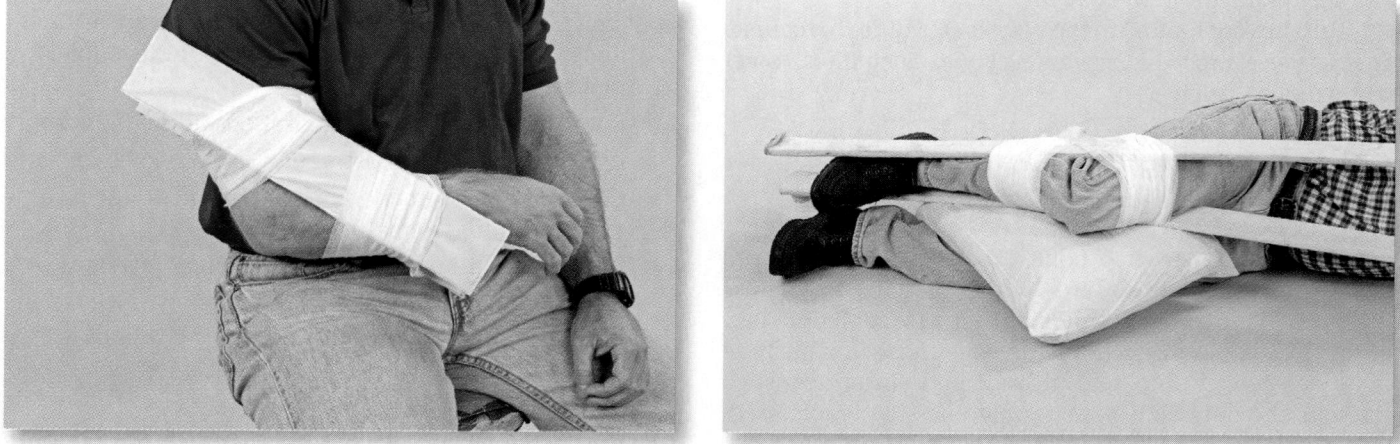

**Figure 30-9.** When using a splint, make sure you immobilize above and below the injured joint.

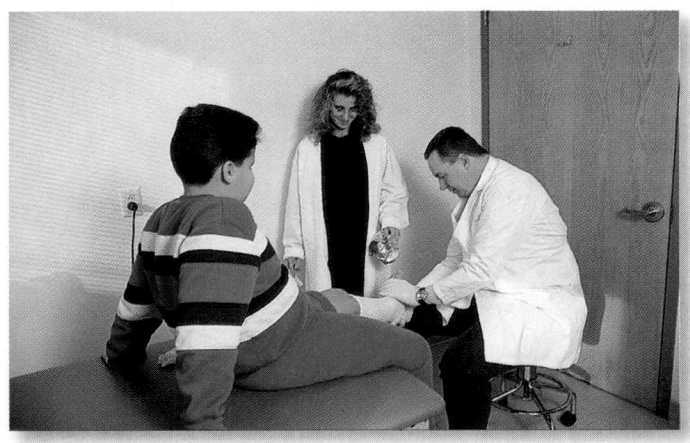

**Figure 30-10.** Patients should be instructed to keep the cast dry and to notify the physician if they have pain or unusual sensations.

Sprains and strains often result from sports injuries and accidents. A **sprain** is an injury characterized by partial tearing of a ligament that supports a joint, such as the ankle. A sprain may also involve injuries to tendons, muscles, and local blood vessels and contusions of the surrounding soft tissue. A **strain** is a muscle injury that results from overexertion. For example, back strain may occur when a person carries a heavy load.

Symptoms of a sprain include swelling, tenderness, pain during movement, and local discoloration. If you suspect a sprain, splint the joint, apply ice, and call the EMS system if needed. Inform the patient that an x-ray may be required to confirm that there is no fracture. A strain causes pain on motion. In most cases it should be examined by a physician, who may prescribe rest, application of heat, and a muscle relaxant.

## Head Injuries

Head injuries include concussions, contusions, fractures, intracranial bleeding, and scalp hematomas and lacerations. Some head injuries can be life-threatening and require immediate medical attention.

**Concussion.** A **concussion** is a jarring injury to the brain. It is the most common type of head injury. Someone who has a concussion may lose consciousness. Temporary loss of vision, pallor (paleness), listlessness, memory loss, or vomiting can also occur. Symptoms may disappear rapidly or last up to 24 hours. A concussion may produce slow intracranial bleeding. Teach the patient and the patient's family basic precautions after this type of injury. See the Educating the Patient section for more information on concussions.

**Severe Head Injuries.** Contusions, fractures, and intracranial bleeding cause symptoms similar to, but more profound than, symptoms of concussions. Symptoms to look for are leakage of clear or bloody fluid from the ears

## Educating the Patient

### Concussion

Because a concussion can cause intracranial bleeding, handle gently a patient who is being treated for this type of injury. If bleeding is slow, it might take up to 24 hours to produce symptoms. Because intracranial bleeding may require brain surgery, use the following patient education guidelines to help ensure patient safety after a concussion.

- Inform the patient that the first 24 hours after the injury are the most critical.
- Tell the patient to refrain from strenuous activity, to rest, and to return to regular activity gradually. Instruct the patient to avoid using pain medicines other than acetaminophen, unless the drugs are approved by the physician.
- Advise the patient to eat lightly, especially if nausea and vomiting occur.
- Tell a family member to check on the patient every few hours. The family member should make sure the patient knows his own name, his location, and the name of the family member.

- Instruct the family member to call for medical assistance immediately if the patient exhibits any of these warning signs:
  - Any symptom that is getting worse, such as headaches, sleepiness, or nausea, including nausea that doesn't go away
  - Changes in behavior, such as irritability or confusion
  - Dilated pupils (pupils that are bigger than normal) or pupils of different sizes
  - Trouble walking or speaking
  - Drainage of bloody or clear fluids from ears or nose
  - Vomiting
  - Seizures
  - Weakness or numbness in the arms or legs
  - A less serious head injury in a patient taking blood thinners or who has a bleeding disorder such as hemophilia

# Controlling Bleeding

**Procedure Goal:** To control bleeding and minimize blood loss

## OSHA Guidelines

**Materials:** Clean or sterile dressings

## Method:

1. If you have time, wash your hands and put on exam gloves, face protection, and a gown.

### Rationale

To protect yourself from splatters, splashes, and sprays

2. Using a clean or sterile dressing, apply direct pressure over the wound.

3. If blood soaks through the dressing, do not remove it. Apply an additional dressing over the original one.

### Rationale

Removing the dressing may dislodge a clot and cause more bleeding.

4. If possible, elevate the body part that is bleeding.

5. If direct pressure and elevation do not stop the bleeding, apply pressure over the nearest pressure point between the bleeding and the heart (Figure 30-11). For example, if the wound is on the lower arm, apply pressure on the brachial artery. For a lower-leg wound, apply pressure on the femoral artery in the groin.

6. When the doctor or EMT arrives, assist as requested.

7. After the patient has been transferred to a hospital, properly dispose of contaminated materials.

8. Remove the gloves and wash your hands.

9. Document your care in the patient's chart.

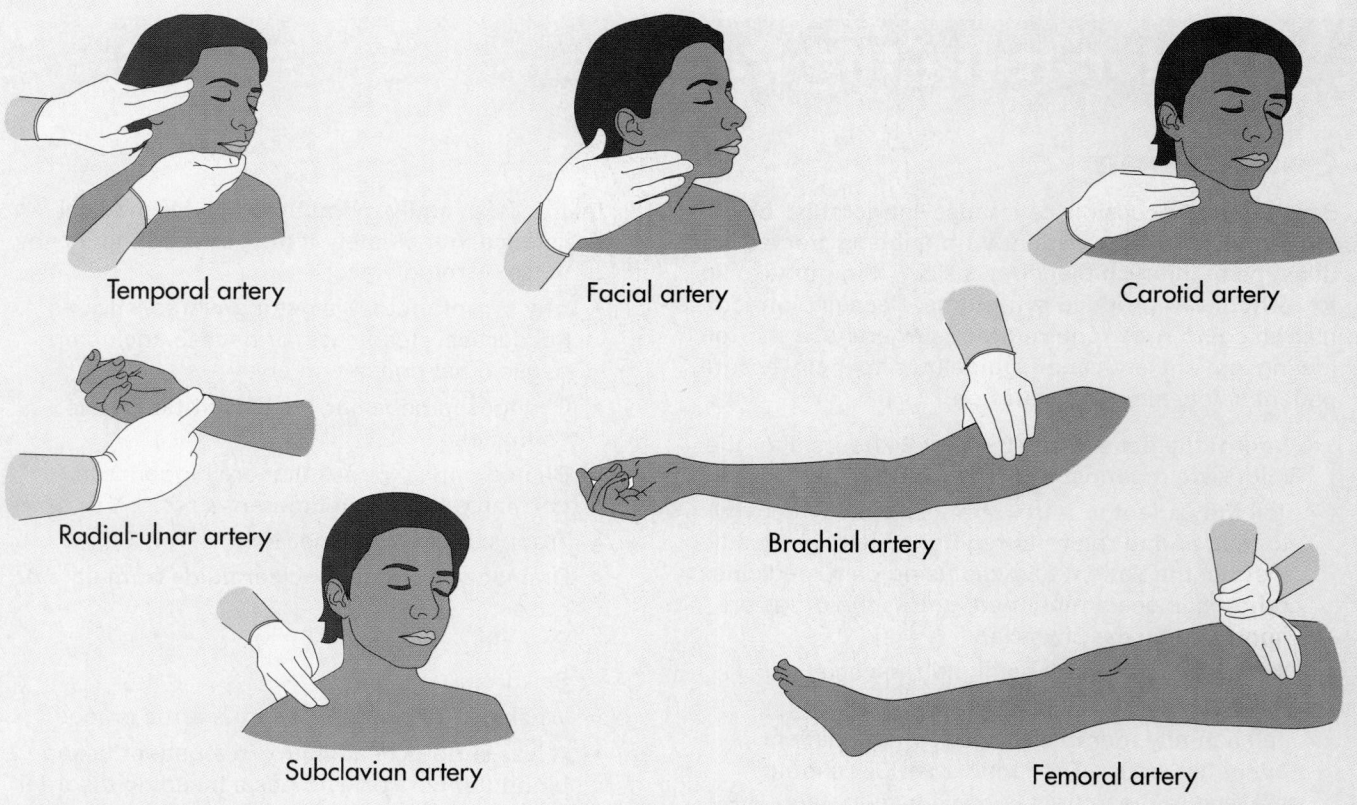

Temporal artery

Facial artery

Carotid artery

Radial-ulnar artery

Brachial artery

Subclavian artery

Femoral artery

**Figure 30-11.** Apply pressure on these pressure points to stop bleeding.

or nose, seizures, and respiratory arrest. A patient with a severe head injury requires immediate hospitalization. Your priority is to maintain the patient's airway and to begin CPR if needed.

**Scalp Hematomas and Lacerations.** A **hematoma** is a swelling caused by blood under the skin. A scalp hematoma causes a bump on the head. This swelling can be reduced by applying ice immediately after the injury. Because blood vessels in the scalp are close to the skin, scalp lacerations often bleed profusely and look worse than they really are. Apply direct pressure to stop bleeding from a scalp laceration, wash the area with soap and water, and apply a dry, sterile dressing over the area.

# Hemorrhaging

Hemorrhaging (heavy or uncontrollable bleeding) is generally the result of an injury. It may also be caused by an illness. The first-aid treatment remains the same in both cases. Bleeding can be internal or external. When administering first aid to a patient who may have internal bleeding, cover the patient with a blanket for warmth, keep the patient quiet and calm, and get medical help immediately.

Control external bleeding to prevent rapid blood loss and shock. Use direct pressure, apply additional dressings as needed, elevate the bleeding body part, and put pressure over a pressure point, as described in Procedure 30-5 and as illustrated in Figure 30-11. Then transport the patient to an emergency care facility.

As a last resort, if medical help is more than an hour away, you may need to use a tourniquet (Figure 30-12) to save a person's life. You apply a tourniquet over the main pressure point just above the wound and tighten the tourniquet until the bleeding stops. If you apply a tourniquet, make sure you write the application time on the tourniquet or the patient's forehead. Many people do not recommend applying a tourniquet in any situation because it may be difficult to judge when a person's life is at stake. Keep in mind that application of a tourniquet to a person's limb almost surely leads to loss of the limb.

# Multiple Injuries

Sometimes a patient sustains more than one type of injury—for example, an arm fracture, head injury, lacerations, and internal bleeding. Multiple injuries often result from a car accident or a fall. If you need to assist a patient with multiple injuries, assess the ABCs and perform CPR if needed. Then call (or have someone else call) the EMS system or the physician. Once you have ensured an open airway, breathing, and circulation, perform first aid for the most life-threatening injuries first.

# Poisoning

A poison is a substance that produces harmful effects if it enters the body. Poisoning is serious and it can result in

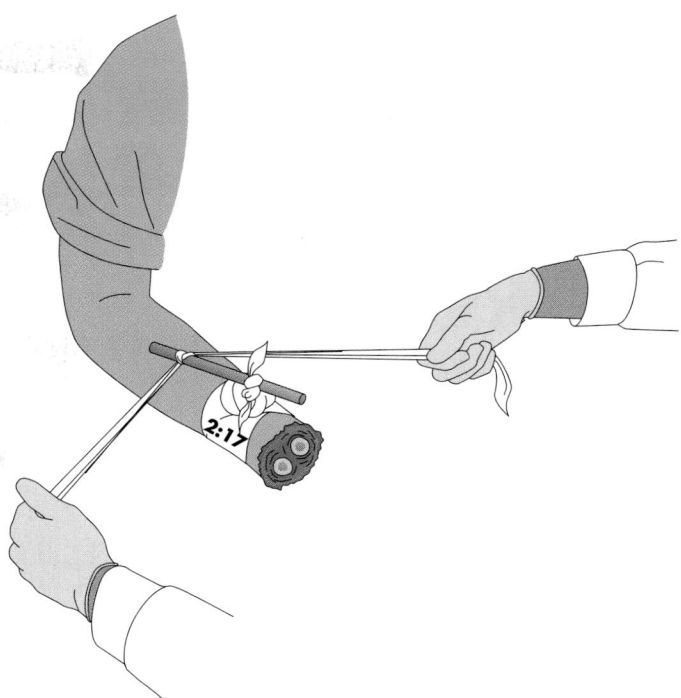

**Figure 30-12.** Apply a tourniquet only as a last resort, that is, if bleeding cannot be stopped and the patient is likely to die as a result.

death or permanent injury if immediate medical care is not provided.

In addition to being able to handle a poisoning emergency, you need to educate patients in how to do the same. You should teach them about the symptoms of and treatment for the different types of poisoning. Provide them with pamphlets that describe the procedures to follow and stickers with the telephone number of the regional poison control center.

The majority of accidental poisonings happen to children younger than the age of 5. Young children are not necessarily put off by strong smells or burning sensations when they swallow something. Common causes of poisoning in children are household cleaning products, household plants, and medications. Poisons can also be caused by improperly prepared or contaminated food. These types of poisons are ingested, or swallowed.

Poisoning that results from coming in contact with plants, such as poison ivy, poison sumac, and poison oak, is common and generally fairly minor. This type of poisoning is referred to as absorbed poisoning. It can be serious, however, if the poisoning occurs over a large surface of the body.

Poisons can also be inhaled. This situation occurs when a person inhales a poisonous gas such as carbon monoxide or the fumes from burning poisonous plants.

**Ingested Poisons.** Poison that is swallowed remains in the stomach only a short time. Most of it is absorbed while in the small intestine. Symptoms of poisoning include abdominal pain and cramping; nausea; vomiting; diarrhea; odor, stains, or burns around or in the mouth; drowsiness; and unconsciousness. You should also suspect poisoning if packages containing poisonous substances are near a person who has one or more of these symptoms.

It is extremely important to call a poison control center (if available), hospital emergency room, doctor, or the EMS system for instructions if you think a patient has swallowed a poison. When you call, you will need to know the following:

- The patient's age
- The name of the poison
- The amount of poison swallowed
- When the poison was swallowed
- Whether or not the person has vomited
- How much time it will take to get the patient to a medical facility

Poisons vary in their toxicity. Some cause damage right away, whereas others cause damage several hours later. If the patient is alert and not having convulsions, follow these steps.

1. Call the regional poison control center.
2. If directed by the poison control center, induce vomiting with syrup of ipecac.
3. Seek immediate medical attention.

Do not induce vomiting unless directed by a medical authority. The patient may have ingested a strong acid, alkali, or petroleum product, such as chlorine bleach or gasoline. These products may cause further damage to the throat and esophagus during vomiting. If you do not know what the patient ingested, never induce vomiting.

Turn the patient on her left side. This position delays stomach emptying by several hours and prevents aspiration if the patient vomits. Take both poison container and vomited material to the hospital for inspection.

Food poisoning, another type of ingested poisoning, can occur when bacteria produce toxins in food. Botulism, for example, results from eating improperly canned or preserved foods that have been contaminated with the bacterium *Clostridium botulinum*. Symptoms appear within 12 to 36 hours after eating contaminated food. Initial symptoms include dry mouth, sore throat, weakness, vomiting, and diarrhea.

Food poisoning is often difficult to detect because the signs and symptoms vary greatly. A patient with food poisoning usually has abdominal pain, nausea, vomiting, gas, frequent bowel sounds, and diarrhea. Chills, joint pain, and excessive sweating may also occur. If you suspect that a patient has food poisoning, call the poison control center and arrange for immediate transport to the hospital.

**Absorbed Poisons.** Most people have had the red, itchy rash that results from contact with poison ivy, poison sumac, or poison oak. In some people, however, the rash may be accompanied by a generalized swelling, burning eyes, headache, fever, and abnormal pulse or respirations.

To treat a patient who has come in contact with an absorbed poison, call the regional poison control center. Have the patient immediately remove all contaminated clothing. Then wash the affected skin thoroughly with soap and water, drench it with alcohol, and rinse well. To help relieve symptoms, apply wet compresses soaked with calamine lotion. Also suggest baths in colloidal oatmeal or applications of a paste made from 3 teaspoons baking soda and 1 teaspoon water to soothe the itching. If the rash is severe, the doctor may prescribe a corticosteroid ointment. Tell the patient to seek medical assistance if a fever or swelling develops.

**Inhaled Poisons.** A patient may inhale poisons by breathing air contaminated by chemicals in the workplace or by a malfunctioning stove or furnace in the home. The patient may not realize she has been exposed to a poisonous gas until symptoms arise. Even then, a patient may merely suspect the flu because some symptoms of inhalation poisoning mimic those of influenza. Common symptoms include headache, tinnitus (ringing in the ears), angina (chest pain), shortness of breath, muscle weakness, nausea, vomiting, confusion, and dizziness, followed by blurred or double vision, difficulty breathing, unconsciousness, and cardiac arrest. Also, a patient who has facial burns may have sustained an inhalation injury.

To treat poisoning by inhalation, first get the patient into fresh air. Have someone call the EMS system or the regional poison control center. Loosen tight-fitting clothing and wrap the patient in a blanket to prevent shock. Check the patient's ABCs and begin CPR if needed.

Carbon monoxide is a major cause of inhalation poisoning in the home. It is a colorless and odorless natural gas produced by incomplete combustion of organic fuels, such as coal, wood, or gasoline. Carbon monoxide is especially dangerous in closed spaces because, when inhaled, it replaces oxygen in the blood. If you suspect carbon monoxide poisoning, look for clues in the environment such as a malfunctioning furnace or a car engine left running in a closed space such as a garage.

Mild carbon monoxide poisoning can cause headache and flulike symptoms without fever. Moderate poisoning may cause tinnitus, drowsiness, severe seizures, coma, and cardiopulmonary problems. Because the gas is odorless, people are often unaware they are being poisoned. They may fall asleep, lapse into unconsciousness, and die.

## Weather-Related Injuries

Exposure to extreme cold, extreme heat, and the sun's damaging rays can cause weather-related injuries. These injuries may require emergency medical attention.

**Hypothermia.** Hypothermia occurs when a person loses more body heat than he or she can produce, resulting in a body temperature below 95°F. It is caused by exposure to cold. Hypothermia most often occurs in the very old or very young, or in chronically ill or malnourished individuals. People who are outdoors with insufficient clothing in the winter or who get wet in cold weather are more likely to suffer from hypothermia.

Symptoms of hypothermia include lethargy, loss of coordination, confusion, and uncontrollable shivering. If the person's body temperature is extremely low, the person may stop shivering. If untreated, hypothermia can result in cardiac arrest and coma.

Treat hypothermia by moving the person inside if possible and covering him with blankets. If he is wet, remove his wet clothing. If he is confused or unconscious, monitor his breathing and call the EMS system. If he is awake and alert, give him warm liquids. Do not give him alcoholic liquids.

**Frostbite.** When body tissues are exposed to below-freezing temperatures, frostbite can occur. Frostbite causes ice crystals to form between tissue cells, and these crystals enlarge as they extract water from the cells. Frostbite also causes obstruction to the blood supply in the form of blood clots. This aspect of frostbite prevents blood from flowing to the tissues and causes additional, severe damage to cells.

Symptoms of frostbite include white, waxy, or grayish yellow skin. The affected body part feels cold, tingling, and painful. The skin surface may feel crusty and the underlying tissue soft in comparison. If the frostbite is deep, the body part may feel cold and hard and not be sensitive to pain. Blisters may appear after rewarming.

Treat frostbite by wrapping warm clothing or blankets around the affected body part or placing it in contact with another body part that is warm. Do not rub or massage the affected area or you may cause further damage to the frozen tissue. Call for medical assistance. If you are in a remote area, use the wet rapid rewarming method. This method involves placing the affected part in warm (100°F to 104°F) water. Hot water should be added at regular intervals to keep the temperature of the bath stable. As an alternative method, you can heat the affected area with warm compresses. Continue rewarming for 20 to 40 minutes. After the affected area becomes soft, place dry, sterile gauze between skin surfaces, such as between the toes or the fingers or between the ear and the side of the head. Do not massage the skin or break blisters.

**Heatstroke.** Heatstroke results from prolonged exposure to high temperatures and humidity. This condition may lead to excessive loss of fluids (dehydration) and insufficient blood in the circulatory system (hypovolemic shock). High body temperature can damage tissues and organs throughout the body. If untreated, the patient will die. People most susceptible to heatstroke are children, the elderly, athletes, and patients who are obese, are diabetic, or have circulatory problems or other chronic illnesses.

Symptoms of heatstroke include hot, dry skin; high body temperature; altered mental state; rapid pulse; rapid breathing; dizziness; and weakness. If you suspect that a patient has heatstroke, check the patient's ABCs, and call the EMS system. Move the patient to a cool place, and remove outer clothing unless it is made of light cotton or other light fabric. Also, cool the patient with any means available, such as gentle spraying with a hose, movement to an air-conditioned place, vigorous fanning, or application of a wet sheet. If the humidity is above 75%, place ice packs on the patient's groin and armpits. Stop cooling when the patient's mental state improves. Keep the patient's head and shoulders slightly elevated.

**Sunburn.** Do not dismiss a sunburn as trivial. It is a burn that can cause redness, tenderness, pain, swelling, blisters, and peeling skin. It can lead to skin damage or cancer later in life.

Soak sunburned skin in cool water to help reduce the heat. Apply cold compresses, and later calamine lotion, to bring relief from the burning sensation. Have the patient elevate the legs and arms to prevent swelling. The patient should also drink plenty of water and take a pain reliever.

Educate the patient about the importance of using sunscreen and reapplying it every 2 to 3 hours when outdoors. Advise the patient to stay out of direct sunlight between 10:00 A.M. and 2:00 P.M., because the sun's rays are strongest during that period.

# Wounds

A wound is an injury in which the skin or tissues under the skin are damaged. Wounds can be either open or closed. Figure 30-13 shows the various types of wounds.

**Open Wounds.** An open wound is a break in the skin or mucous membrane. Types of open wounds include incisions, lacerations, abrasions, and punctures.

*Incisions and Lacerations.* An incision is a clean and smooth cut, such as that from a kitchen knife. A laceration has jagged edges, as may result when a child steps on a piece of broken glass in the sand at the beach. Care of minor incisions and lacerations involves controlling bleeding by covering the wound with a clean or sterile dressing and applying direct pressure. After the bleeding stops, clean and dress the wound. Procedure 30-6 explains how to clean minor wounds. Teach the patient the importance of keeping the wound clean and checking for signs of infection, such as heat, redness, pain, and swelling.

If the wound is deep and involves muscle, tendons, the face, the genitals, the mouth, or the tongue, control the bleeding with direct pressure to the wound (with a sterile dressing or clean cloth held against its surface), elevation, and use of pressure points. Contact the doctor and, if necessary, the EMS system.

*Amputations.* If a fingertip or toe is completely or nearly severed, quick action may increase the likelihood that it can be saved. You should elevate the injured extremity, cover the digit with a dry dressing, and immobilize the hand or foot. Retrieve the severed digit, wrap it in gauze, put it in a plastic bag, put the bag on ice, and send the part with the patient to the hospital.

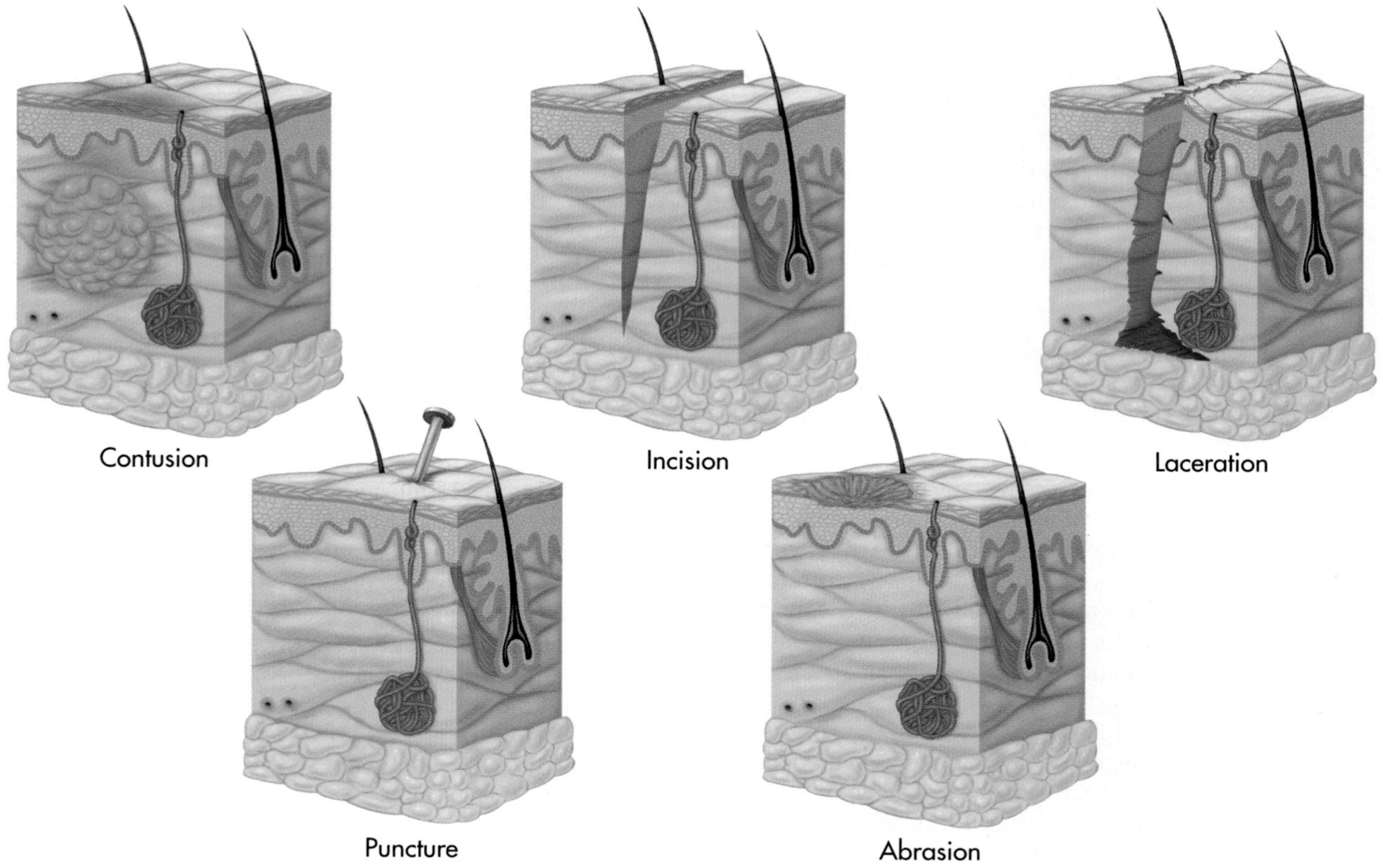

Contusion

Incision

Laceration

Puncture

Abrasion

**Figure 30-13.** Different types of wounds produce different degrees of tissue damage.

## PROCEDURE 30.6

### Cleaning Minor Wounds

**Procedure Goal:** To clean and dress minor wounds

**OSHA Guidelines**

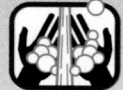 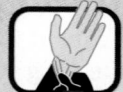  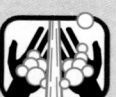

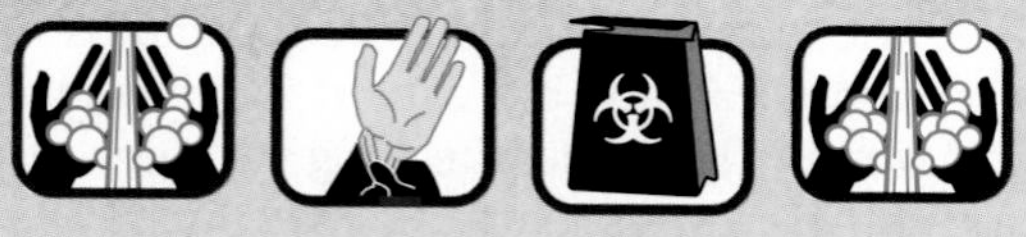

**Materials:** Sterile gauze squares, basin, antiseptic soap, warm water, sterile dressing

**Method:**

1. Wash your hands and put on exam gloves.
2. Dip several gauze squares in a basin of warm, soapy water.
3. Wash the wound from the center outward.

*Rationale*
To avoid bringing contaminants from the surrounding skin into the wound

Use a new gauze square for each cleansing motion.

4. As you wash, remove debris that could cause infection.
5. Rinse the area thoroughly, preferably by placing the wound under warm, running water.

*Rationale*
Running water will wash away debris.

6. Pat the wound dry with sterile gauze squares.
7. Cover the wound with a dry, sterile dressing. Bandage the dressing in place.
8. Properly dispose of contaminated materials.
9. Remove the gloves and wash your hands.
10. Instruct the patient on wound care.
11. Record the procedure in the patient's chart.

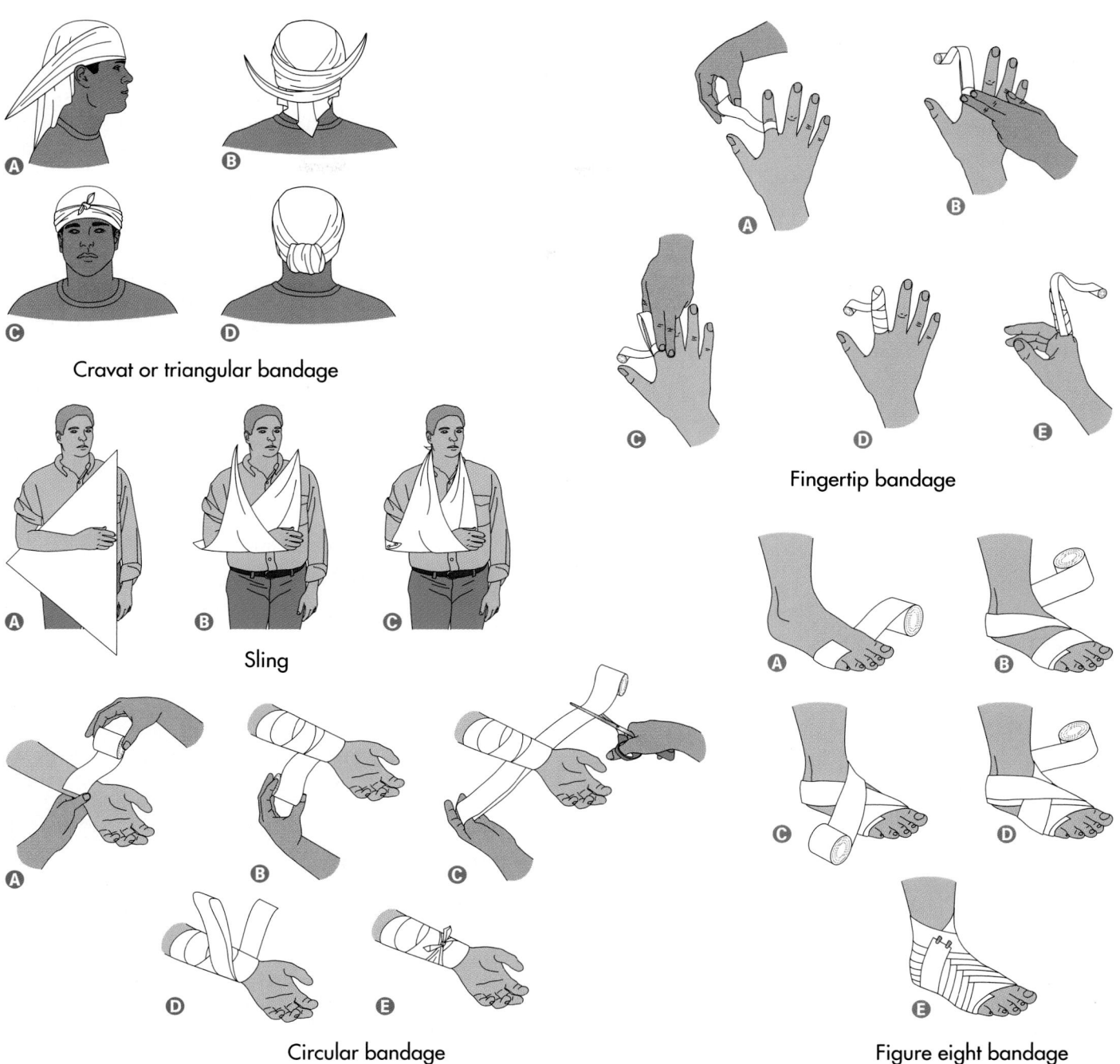

Cravat or triangular bandage

Sling

Circular bandage

Fingertip bandage

Figure eight bandage

**Figure 30-14.** Apply a bandage, as needed, to a wound.

*Abrasions.* An abrasion is a scraping of the skin, as when someone slides across gravel during a softball game. Abrasions require washing with soap and water. Be sure to remove all the dirt and debris to prevent tattooing (dark discoloration under the skin). Minor abrasions do not need a dressing or bandage, but large ones do. Various types of bandaging are shown in Figure 30-14. As with any wound, teach the patient to watch for signs of infection.

*Punctures.* A puncture wound is a small hole created by a piercing object, such as a bullet, knife, nail, or animal tooth. Puncture wounds are a potential breeding ground for tetanus bacteria, because the bacteria can live and thrive in the absence of oxygen. Rinse the wound under running water for 15 minutes. Then clean the wound with soap and water, and apply a dry, sterile dressing. If the patient has not had a tetanus toxoid immunization in the past 7 to 10 years, inform the physician so that one can be ordered.

**Closed Wounds.** A closed wound is an injury that occurs inside the body without breaking the skin. Closed wounds, which are usually called **contusions** (bruises), are caused by a blunt object striking the tissue. This action produces broken blood vessels and internal, localized bleeding (hematoma) below the area that has been struck.

Treat such a wound with cold compresses to reduce swelling. The affected area will turn from black and blue to green to yellow as blood pigments oxidize. Inform the patient that these color changes are part of the normal healing process.

# Common Illnesses

A variety of common illnesses frequently call for emergency medical intervention. As a patient educator, you can help ensure that patients recognize the symptoms of these illnesses and know when to call for medical assistance. Teaching patients the importance of following physician's orders for follow-up care is also your responsibility. Common illnesses include the following:

- Abdominal pain
- Asthma
- Dehydration
- Diarrhea
- Fainting
- Fever
- Hyperventilation
- Nosebleed
- Tachycardia
- Vomiting

## Abdominal Pain

Acute abdominal pain that occurs suddenly and is accompanied by fever may indicate an emergency that requires surgery. The pain may involve spasmodic contractions. It may feel knifelike or ache dully, and it may be localized or may radiate. The location of the pain gives clues to its cause. Acute pain in the right upper quadrant, for example, may signal a gallbladder attack. Pain in the right lower quadrant may indicate appendicitis.

Other causes include internal hemorrhage, intestinal perforation or obstruction, peptic ulcer, and hernia. In women, pelvic pain can indicate a gynecologic problem. Obviously, trauma to the area, such as wounds or blows, can produce acute abdominal pain.

While waiting for patient transport, have the patient lie on his back with his knees flexed (unless there is a wound or swelling in the abdomen). This position lets the abdominal muscles relax. Keep the patient quiet and warm, and act calm and concerned. Do not give anything by mouth, and keep an emesis basin handy in case the patient vomits. Do not apply heat to the abdomen because heat may exacerbate inflammation. Monitor the patient's pulse and consciousness, and check for signs of shock.

## Asthma

Asthma is a common disorder caused by spasmodic narrowing of the bronchi. It is often an inherited tendency—that is, several members of one family may suffer from it.

A patient who is having an acute attack wheezes, coughs, and is short of breath. She may become frightened and feel as if she cannot get enough air. If you suspect an asthma attack, check the patient's ABCs, and notify the doctor at once. You may assist the patient in using a respiratory inhaler if she carries one with her. If directed, administer a mini-nebulizer treatment with a bronchodilator (drug that opens the bronchi), such as albuterol (Proventil) or epinephrine.

## Dehydration

**Dehydration** results from a lack of adequate water in the body. The body's fluid intake is not sufficient to meet its fluid needs. Severe dehydration can result from vomiting, excessive heat and sweating, diarrhea, or lack of food or fluid intake. The following are symptoms of dehydration:

- Extreme thirst
- Tiredness
- Light-headedness
- Abdominal or muscle cramping
- Confusion (especially in elderly people)

Perform the following steps to administer first aid to a dehydrated person.

1. Move the victim into the shade or to a cool area.
2. To replace lost fluids, give the victim frequent, small amounts of decaffeinated fluids.
3. If symptoms persist or are accompanied by nausea, diarrhea, or convulsions, call for the EMS system or a physician.

## Diarrhea (Acute)

Acute diarrhea can be caused by an intestinal infection, food poisoning, a bowel disorder, or the side effects of medication. Severe diarrhea causes dehydration and dangerous electrolyte imbalances that can lead to shock. Symptoms of shock include rapid pulse, low blood pressure, and pale, clammy skin.

Help the patient lie on his back and elevate his legs. Report the patient's condition to the doctor. As directed, prepare to assist in administering intravenous fluids to correct dehydration and restore electrolytes and to draw blood for testing.

## Fainting (Syncope)

Fainting, or syncope, is a partial or complete loss of consciousness. It usually follows a decrease in the amount of blood flow to the brain. Before fainting, patients may feel weak, dizzy, cold, or nauseated. They may perspire or look pale and anxious.

If you are with a patient who feels as if she is going to faint, tell her to lower her head between her legs and to breathe deeply. Stay with her until the feeling passes. If the patient is having difficulty breathing or faints, lay her flat on her back with her feet slightly elevated. Loosen tight clothing and apply a cold cloth to her face. Observe the patient carefully, monitoring her breathing and level of consciousness. Observe for weakness in her arms and legs. Let her rest for at least 10 minutes after she regains full consciousness. Notify the physician that the patient fainted.

If your efforts do not revive a patient who has fainted, call the physician and the EMS system. The patient may be slipping into a coma.

## Fever

Fever is a common clinical sign that often indicates infection. Mild or moderate fever can accompany a cold or an upset stomach. It can usually be managed with aspirin, ibuprofen, or acetaminophen. A fever of 106°F or higher (hyperthermia) is dangerous, however, because irreversible brain damage can occur if the fever is not lowered immediately.

If a patient's temperature is dangerously high, you must proceed at once to check the other vital signs and the level of consciousness. Notify the doctor and be prepared to start rapid cooling measures. Place ice packs on the groin and axilla, or give the patient a tepid sponge bath. If the patient is a child, be prepared to manage seizures (discussed later in this chapter). Do not give a child with a fever aspirin unless directed by a physician.

## Hyperventilation

Some patients who are under a great deal of stress lack the skills to deal with the stress effectively. They may seem anxious, frazzled, and more emotional than average patients. Patients under stress may begin to hyperventilate, or breathe too rapidly and too deeply. This breathing disturbs the normal balance of oxygen and carbon dioxide in the blood, and the carbon dioxide concentration falls below normal levels. Patients who are hyperventilating may also feel light-headed and as if they cannot get enough air. In addition, they may have chest pain and feel apprehensive.

Move a hyperventilating patient to a quiet area. Have the patient sit quietly and visualize a calm and serene environment, such as a beach or the mountains. With a calm and soothing voice, coach the patient to take slow, normal breaths.

## Nosebleed

Nosebleed, or **epistaxis,** can occur for a variety of reasons. They include blowing the nose too hard, local irritation or dryness, frequent sneezing, fragile or superficial blood vessels, high blood pressure, a blow to the nose, and a foreign body in the nose. Nosebleeds are common in children, especially at night.

Treat a nosebleed by having the patient sit up with the head tilted forward to prevent blood from running down the back of the throat. Next, have the patient gently pinch the nostrils shut at the bottom for at least 5 minutes. If that does not stop the bleeding, apply an ice pack or cold compress to the nose and face, and continue to pinch the nostrils. If the bleeding cannot be controlled, arrange for transport to the office or to a hospital for cauterization or nasal packing.

## Tachycardia

Tachycardia is a rapid heart rate, generally in excess of 100 beats per minute. A patient with tachycardia may report having **palpitations,** unusually rapid, strong, or irregular pulsations of the heart. He may feel as if his heart is pounding. Help the patient lie down, take his vital signs, and, if instructed, obtain an electrocardiogram (ECG). (Electrocardiography is discussed in Chapter 39.) If tachycardia is accompanied by low blood pressure and light-headedness, notify the physician immediately. These symptoms indicate that the patient could faint or go into shock. Remain with the patient and keep him calm.

## Vomiting

Vomiting is a symptom common to many disorders, ranging from food poisoning to various infections. When severe, it can lead to dehydration and dangerous changes in electrolyte levels, especially in patients who are very young, very old, or diabetic or who also have diarrhea. Because these problems can be severe, notify the doctor and provide appropriate care. Procedure 30-7 describes how to provide emergency care for a patient who is vomiting.

## Less Common Illnesses

Even though some illnesses are less common than those previously discussed, you should still be familiar enough with them so that you can handle them effectively if a physician or EMT is not immediately available. Educate patients about symptoms they may encounter that require emergency medical intervention as well as about the importance of follow-up care when they are recovering from such illnesses. Less common illnesses that may require emergency medical intervention include the following:

- Anaphylaxis
- Bacterial meningitis
- Diabetic emergencies
- Gallbladder attack
- Heart attack
- Hematemesis
- Obstetric emergencies
- Respiratory arrest
- Seizures

## PROCEDURE 30.7

### Caring for a Patient Who Is Vomiting

**Procedure Goal:** To increase comfort and minimize complications, such as aspiration, for a patient who is vomiting

**OSHA Guidelines**

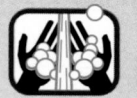 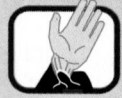 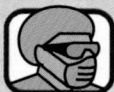
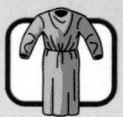 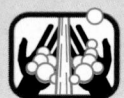

**Materials:** Emesis basin, cool compress, cup of cool water, paper tissues or a towel, and (if ordered) intravenous fluids and electrolytes and an antinausea drug

**Method:**

1. Wash your hands and put on exam gloves and other PPE.

2. Ask the patient when and how the vomiting started and how frequently it occurs. Find out whether she is nauseated or in pain.

3. Give the patient an emesis basin to collect vomit. Observe and document its amount, color, odor, and consistency. Particularly note blood, bile, undigested food, or feces in the vomit.

4. Place a cool compress on the patient's forehead to make her more comfortable. Offer water and paper tissues or a towel to clean her mouth.

5. Monitor for signs of dehydration, such as confusion, irritability, and flushed, dry skin. Also monitor for signs of electrolyte imbalances, such as leg cramps or an irregular pulse.

6. If requested, assist by laying out supplies and equipment for the physician to use in administering intravenous fluids and electrolytes. Administer an antinausea drug if prescribed.

7. Prepare the patient for diagnostic tests if instructed.

8. Remove the gloves and wash your hands.

---

- Shock
- Stroke
- Toxic shock syndrome
- Viral encephalitis

## Anaphylaxis

Anaphylaxis, or anaphylactic shock, is a severe, often life-threatening allergic reaction. The reaction can be immediate or delayed up to 2 hours. It happens to people who have become sensitized to certain substances. For example, it can result from eating a type of food, being stung by an insect, or taking a particular type of medication, such as penicillin.

The first sign of anaphylaxis usually comes from the patient's skin. It becomes itchy, turns red, feels hot, and develops hives. The face may also become puffy. The throat may swell so that the patient has trouble breathing and swallowing and feels as if he has a "lump in the throat." Other symptoms include pallor, perspiration, and a weak, rapid, irregular pulse. If you detect these symptoms or if the patient becomes restless, has a headache, or says that his throat feels as if it is closing up, take the following steps immediately.

Check the patient's ABCs and then notify the doctor. As directed, administer epinephrine, oral antihistamines, and oxygen, and help the patient sit up. After the patient receives epinephrine, monitor his vital signs every 2 to 3 minutes. Note skin color and monitor the airway. If he does not recover quickly, arrange for immediate transport to the hospital.

When severely allergic patients stabilize, the doctor prescribes an epinephrine autoinjector for patients to carry with them. You are responsible for teaching patients how to use this device. See the Educating the Patient section in Chapter 38 for directions.

Because of the possibility of anaphylaxis, a patient who has just received any type of injection should routinely be kept in the office for 20 to 30 minutes of observation. This procedure reduces the possibility that an allergic reaction to the medication will occur while the patient is unattended.

A less severe allergic reaction to drugs or certain foods may cause sneezing, itching, slight swelling of the skin, rash, or hives. This type of reaction can usually be controlled with diphenhydramine hydrochloride (Benadryl) or another antihistamine. The patient should be monitored closely, however, to make sure the condition does not progress to anaphylaxis.

# Bacterial Meningitis

Bacterial meningitis is almost always a complication of another bacterial infection, such as otitis media (middle ear infection) or pneumonia. Therefore, first find out whether the patient currently has or recently has had a bacterial infection. The signs of bacterial meningitis are fever, chills, headache, neck stiffness, and vomiting. If the patient has these signs and then develops a fever of 102°F, becomes less alert, has altered respirations, or experiences seizures, the infection has progressed to a dangerous state.

If these signs are present, assess the patient's ABCs and notify the physician of the change in the patient's condition. Expect to arrange for transport to the hospital, where the patient will be treated with intravenous antibiotics.

# Diabetic Emergencies

Diabetes is a fairly common disorder of carbohydrate metabolism (see Chapter 27). The body needs insulin, a hormone secreted by the pancreas, to use blood sugar to fuel body cells. Insulin secretion is impaired in patients with diabetes.

You can teach patients who have diabetes or who are at risk for diabetes how to recognize early signs of **hypoglycemia** (low blood sugar) and **hyperglycemia** (high blood sugar) before these conditions become medical emergencies. Symptoms of hypoglycemia include dizziness; headache; hunger; weakness; full, rapid pulse; and pallor. Symptoms of hyperglycemia include dry mouth, intense thirst, muscle weakness, and blurred vision. You should also be familiar with the signs and symptoms of the two most common diabetic emergencies you will encounter: insulin shock and diabetic coma.

**Insulin Shock.** Insulin shock is basically very severe hypoglycemia, in which a patient has too little sugar in the blood. Insulin shock occurs when insulin levels are so high that they move too much sugar from the blood into cells. Symptoms include rapid pulse; shallow respiration; hunger; profuse sweating; pale, cool, clammy skin; double vision; tremors; restlessness; confusion; and possibly fainting. Insulin shock can usually be corrected with administration of some form of sugar (candy, juice, or regular soda for a conscious patient or a sprinkle of table sugar on the tongue for an unconscious patient). If the cause of a diabetic emergency is unknown, give sugar. Patients will improve quickly if the cause is insulin shock and will not be harmed if the cause is diabetic coma, provided they are then transported to the hospital.

**Diabetic Coma.** Diabetic coma is the end result of severe hyperglycemia, in which a patient has too much sugar in the blood. It occurs when insulin levels are insufficient to move blood sugar into body cells. Its symptoms include rapid, deep gulping breaths; flushed, warm, dry skin; thirst; acetone breath (a sweet or fruity odor from the mouth); and disorientation or confusion. If you suspect diabetic coma, notify the doctor at once, and expect to arrange transport to the hospital.

# Gallbladder Attack (Acute)

A classic acute gallbladder attack occurs after a person eats a high-fat meal rich in cholesterol. The patient may wake up in the night with acute abdominal pain (gallbladder colic) in the right upper quadrant. The pain is caused by inflammation of the gallbladder, usually related to gallstones obstructing the cystic duct, through which bile is secreted by the gallbladder. The pain may radiate to the back between the shoulder blades or be localized in the epigastric region (the upper central region of the abdomen) and the front chest area. The attack may be accompanied by nausea and vomiting. The pain is usually so severe that the patient seeks medical attention; many patients think they are having a heart attack.

Gallbladder attacks caused by gallstones are more common among women who are older than age 40 and obese, and the frequency of attacks increases with age (especially after age 65). Diagnosis is usually made with the help of ultrasonography. The patient may require surgery to remove the gallbladder.

# Heart Attack

A heart attack, or myocardial infarction (MI), occurs when the blood flow to the heart is reduced as a result of blockage in the coronary arteries or their branches. Chest pain is the cardinal symptom of a heart attack. The patient may describe the pain as crushing, burning, heavy, aching, or like that of indigestion. The pain may radiate down the left arm or into the jaw, throat, or both shoulders. It may be accompanied by shortness of breath, sweating, nausea, and vomiting. The patient may be pale and have a feeling of doom. If you cannot easily detect pallor (paleness) because the patient has dark skin, check the patient's inner lip for paleness. Elderly patients may experience atypical symptoms of a heart attack, such as jaw pain, because responses to pain diminish during the aging process. The pain of a heart attack is not relieved by nitroglycerin.

If you think a patient is having a heart attack, notify the physician and EMS system immediately. Do not let the patient walk. Loosen tight clothing and have the patient sit up to aid breathing. The physician may order you to administer oxygen at 4 to 6 liters per minute; make sure that no one in the area is smoking. Stay with the patient, observe the ABCs, and begin CPR if required (Procedure 30-8). If directed, obtain an ECG. Take apical and radial pulses, as instructed by the physician. Be prepared to obtain medication from the crash cart or use a defibrillator if required.

# CPR Instructor

*To gain medical assistant credentials, you must fulfill the requirements of either the American Association of Medical Assistants (for a Certified Medical Assistant) or the American Medical Technologists (for a Registered Medical Assistant). After obtaining your medical assistant certification or registration, you may wish to acquire additional skills in specialty areas through course work or on-the-job training. Although this course work or training may not lead to an additional certification or degree, it will enable you to expand your role in the medical office and advance your career as the demand for skilled health professionals increases.*

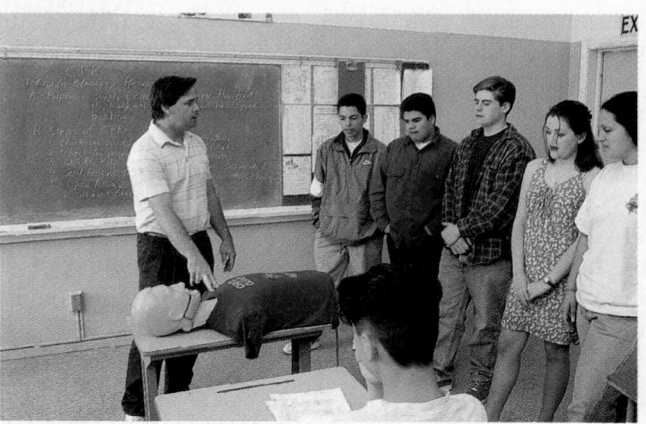

## Skills and Duties

A CPR (cardiopulmonary resuscitation) instructor provides people with the knowledge and skills necessary to help save a person's life in an emergency. He teaches his students how to:

- Call for help.
- Help sustain life.
- Reduce pain.
- Minimize the consequences of injury or sudden illness until professional medical help arrives.

To teach a CPR class, an instructor must plan and coordinate the course in conjunction with a local American Red Cross unit or American Heart Association affiliate. He demonstrates the appropriate skills to his students and observes their technique. He then provides constructive feedback as they learn skills and make decisions regarding the appropriate action to take in an emergency.

The instructor is responsible for identifying participants who are having difficulty with the skills. He must develop effective strategies to help these students meet the course objectives. At the end of the course, the CPR instructor submits completed course records to the local American Red Cross chapter or American Heart Association affiliate.

## Workplace Settings

CPR instructors teach classes in a variety of settings, including schools and universities, community rooms, camps, religious institutions, and medical clinics. Some employers, such as operators of swimming pools, camps, and day-care facilities, may require CPR instruction as a condition of employment.

## Education

To be certified as a CPR instructor by the Red Cross, you must be at least 17 years old. In addition, you must complete two Red Cross courses. The first, the instructor candidate training course, provides instruction in teaching methods, evaluation, and reporting. After completing this course, you will be awarded an instructor candidate training certificate, which qualifies you to take the first aid and CPR instructor course. You must then pass a written test with a grade of 80% or better to gain certification. CPR instructors must teach one class every 2 years for recertification from the Red Cross.

The American Heart Association also provides training for CPR instructors. You must first pass the basic life support course for health-care providers, which teaches CPR skills. You then must take the instructor course, which covers teaching methods. After passing the instructor course, you must co-teach a CPR class with an experienced instructor, who will monitor your performance. You will then become an approved instructor. CPR instructors affiliated with the American Heart Association are required to teach a minimum of two classes a year. The association has no minimum age to become an instructor.

CPR instructors may be paid or work as volunteers. There is no specific salary range for the job.

## Where to Go for More Information

American Heart Association
National Center
7272 Greenville Avenue
Dallas, TX 75231-4596
(800) 242-8721, or call your local center

American Red Cross
2025 E Street, NW
Washington, DC 20006
(202) 303-4498, or call your local chapter

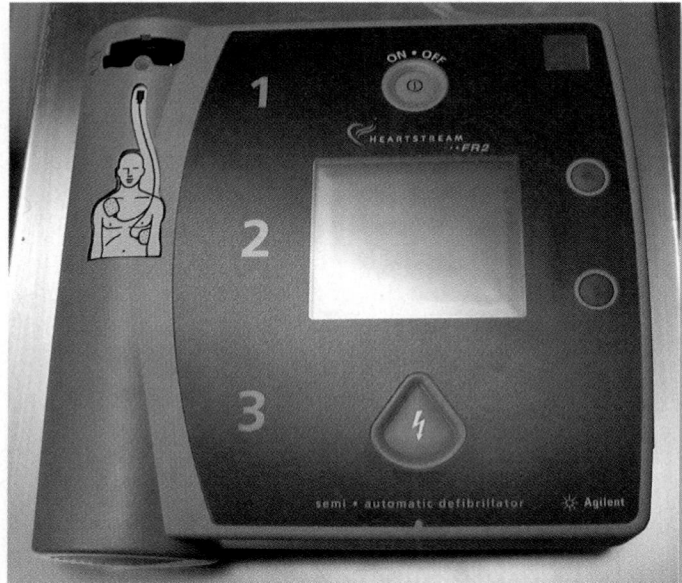

**Figure 30-15.** An automated external defibrillator delivers an electric current to the heart to stop a chaotic rhythm such as ventricular defibrillation.

**Ventricular fibrillation (VF)** is an abnormal heart rhythm. It is the most common cause of cardiac arrest. During VF the heart's rhythm becomes chaotic and the heart does not pump blood. The treatment for VF is defibrillation using a medical device called a defibrillator. This device works by delivering an electrical shock to the heart, which interrupts the chaotic rhythm. Defibrillators are effective only if used within minutes of the patient's collapse. An automated external defibrillator (AED) is a computerized defibrillator programmed to recognize VF and other lethal heart rhythms (Figure 30-15). These devices are found in many public places, including airports, but may also be used at the clinic where you are employed.

To use an AED, attach the adhesive electrode pads to the client's chest in a specific arrangement as determined by the manufacturer. Look at the illustration on the electrode's packing or machine. Activate the AED, and it will analyze the rhythm of the heart and determine if a shock is required. Pressing the "Shock" button will deliver an electrical charge to the patient's heart by way of the AED's electrode wires, which are attached to the chest.

In order to use an AED, you must be properly trained. Training is included as part of the CPR courses of the American Red Cross and the American Heart Association. Obtaining CPR and first aid certification will be an asset to you as a medical assistant.

## Hematemesis

**Hematemesis** is the vomiting of blood. A patient who vomits bright red blood may have a gastrointestinal disorder, such as a bleeding ulcer. A patient who vomits blood that looks like coffee grounds may have slow bleeding into the stomach.

Quickly check the vital signs of a patient with hematemesis. If pulse and breathing are rapid and blood pressure is low, the patient may be going into shock. Notify the doctor immediately, and get the crash cart to help the doctor start an intravenous line to replace lost fluid. Then call the EMS system.

## Obstetric Emergencies

If you work in an obstetric practice, you may see emergencies that are unique to this specialty. Although the physician handles most obstetric emergencies, you can assist by asking the patient specific questions about her problem so that the physician can decide what treatment is necessary.

Set up written protocols to handle these situations. For example, if the patient calls from home and reports gushing vaginal bleeding, your protocol may be to call the EMS system for her and tell her to lie down with her feet elevated. If the patient has a miscarriage, have her bring the expelled tissue with her to the office or hospital.

If you work in an obstetrician's office, you must also know how to assist a physician with an emergency childbirth. If there is no physician present when the emergency occurs, however, whether it is inside or outside the office, summon help and begin the procedure on your own. Never try to delay delivery when a birth is imminent. Procedure 30-9 describes how to assist with an emergency childbirth.

## Respiratory Arrest

Respiratory arrest, or lack of breathing, is usually preceded by symptoms of respiratory distress. Symptoms include difficulty breathing, rapid breathing, palpitations, racing pulse, high or low blood pressure, sweating, pale or bluish skin, and decreasing level of consciousness. If a patient shows these symptoms, notify the doctor right away. If the patient develops respiratory arrest, have someone call the doctor and the EMS system while you perform CPR as described in Procedure 30-8.

## Seizures

A seizure, or convulsion, is a series of violent and involuntary contractions of the muscles. Seizures are usually related to brain malfunctions that can result from diseased or injured brain tissues. A seizure may be caused by high fever, epilepsy (a brain disorder that causes seizures with varying severity), meningitis, diabetic states, and many other medical problems.

Follow this emergency care for seizure patients.

1. Remove objects that may cause injury.
2. Place the patient on the floor or the ground. If possible, position him on his side with his head turned to the side to help keep the airway open and unobstructed

# Performing Cardiopulmonary Resuscitation (CPR)

**Procedure Goal:** To provide ventilation and blood circulation for a patient who shows none

## OSHA Guidelines

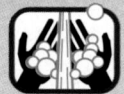 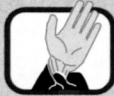 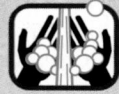

**Materials:** Mouth shield, or if not in the office, a piece of plastic with a hole for the mouth

## Method:

1. Check responsiveness.
   - Tap shoulder.
   - Ask "Are you OK?"
2. If patient is unresponsive, call 911 or the local emergency number or have someone place the call for you.

### Rationale

Quick response from EMS increases the patient's chances of survival.

3. Open the patient's airway.
   - Tilt the patient's head back, using the head tilt–chin lift maneuver (Figure 30-16).

### Rationale

Simply opening the airway may cause the patient to start breathing again.

4. Check for breathing.

- Place your ear next to the patient's mouth, turn your head, and watch the chest.
- Look for the chest to rise and fall, listen for sounds coming out of the mouth or nose, and feel for air movement.
- If the patient is breathing and you do not suspect a spinal injury, place him in the **recovery position:**
  - Kneel beside the patient and place the arm closest to you straight out from the body.

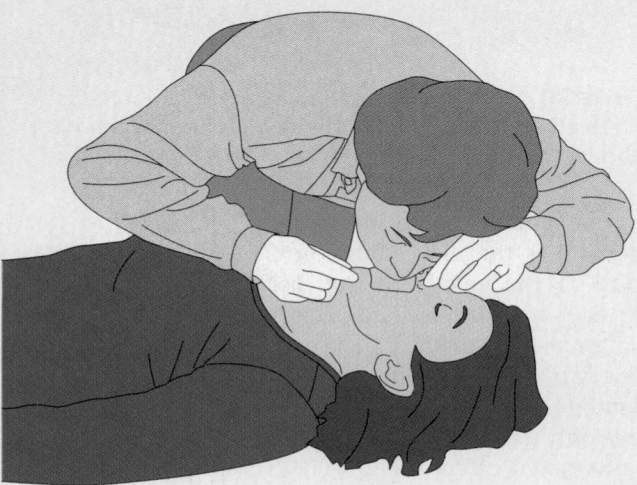

**Figure 30-17.** Perform mouth-to-mouth rescue breathing.

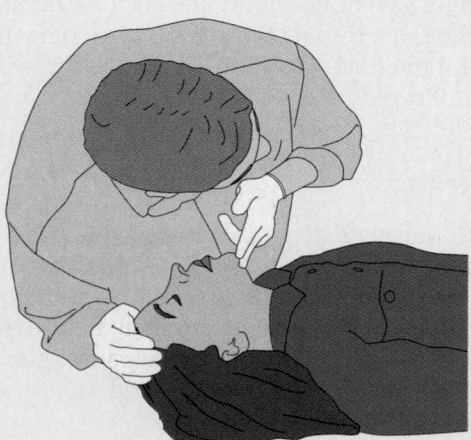

**Figure 30-16.** Use the head tilt–chin lift maneuver to open an airway.

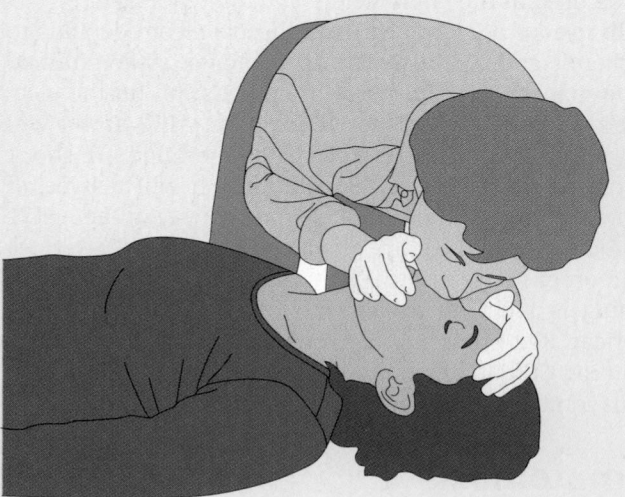

**Figure 30-18.** Use mouth-to-nose breathing if mouth-to-mouth breathing is not possible.

*continued* ⟶

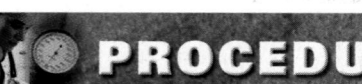

# PROCEDURE 30.8

## Performing Cardiopulmonary Resuscitation (CPR) *(continued)*

Position the far arm with the back of the hand against the patient's near cheek.

- Grab and bend the patient's far knee.
- Protecting the patient's head with one hand, gently roll him toward you by pulling the opposite knee over and to the ground.

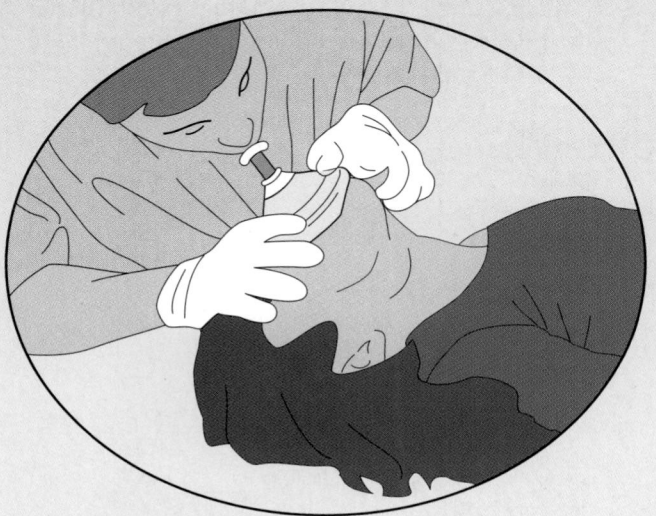

**Figure 30-19.**   The side or the head technique can be used when performing mouth-to-mask ventilations.

Source: *Glencoe Health Care Science Technology,* Booth 2004, p. 98.

- Position the top leg to balance the patient onto his side.
- Tilt his head up slightly so that the airway is open. Make sure that his hand is under his cheek. Place a blanket or coat over the person, and stay close until help arrives.
- If the patient is not breathing or has inadequate breathing, position the patient on his back and give two rescue breaths, each one second long. Each breath should cause the chest to rise. When giving rescue breaths, use one of three methods:

   **a.** Mouth-to-mouth or mouth-to-nose rescue breathing (Figures 30-17 and 30-18):
   - Place your mouth around the patient's mouth and pinch the nose, or close the patient's mouth and place your mouth around the patient's nose.
   - Deliver two slow breaths. Use a face shield.

   **b.** Mouth-to-mask device (Figure 30-19).

   **c.** Bag-mask ventilation (Figure 30-20). Ensure the adequate rise and fall of the patient's chest. If his chest does not rise,

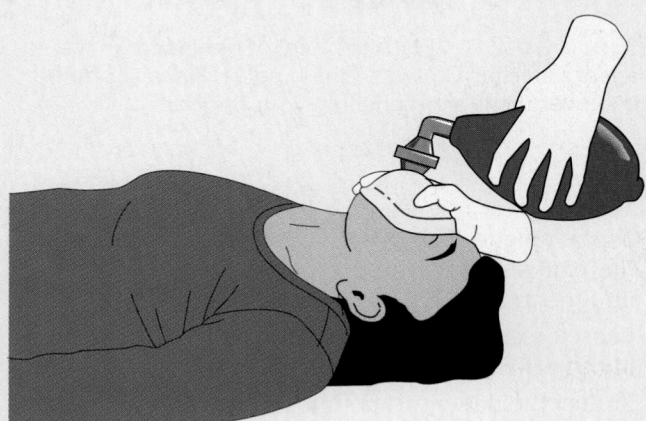

**Figure 30-20.**   When using the bag-mask ventilation, circle the top edges of the mask with your thumb and index finger and use your other three fingers to lift the jaw and open the airway.

Source: *Glencoe Health Care Science Technology,* Booth 2004, p. 101, Figure 4-8.

*continued* ⟶

# Performing Cardiopulmonary Resuscitation (CPR) *(concluded)*

reposition the airway and try again. If on the second attempt the chest does not rise, your patient may have an airway obstruction. See Procedure 30-3.

5. Place the heel of one hand on the patient's sternum between the nipples. Place your other hand over the first, interlacing your fingers (Figure 30-21).

6. Give 30 chest compressions one and one half to two inches deep. You should compress the chest hard and fast (100 compressions per minute) (Figure 30-22).

*Rationale*

Rapid chest compression increases the likelihood of blood reaching the brain and other vital tissues.

Give two breaths.

7. Continue cycles of 30:2 until the patient begins to move, an AED is available, qualified help arrives, or you are too exhausted to continue.

8. If the patient starts moving, check for breathing. If the patient is breathing adequately, put him in the recovery position and monitor him until the doctor or EMS arrives.

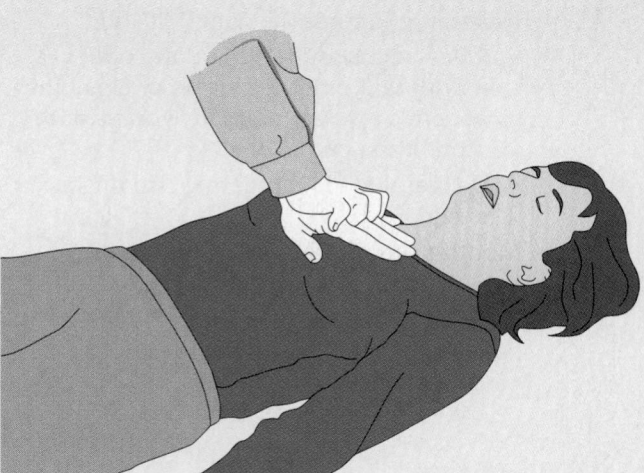

**Figure 30-21.** Place the heel of one hand on the patient's sternum between the nipples. Place your other hand over the first, interlacing your fingers.

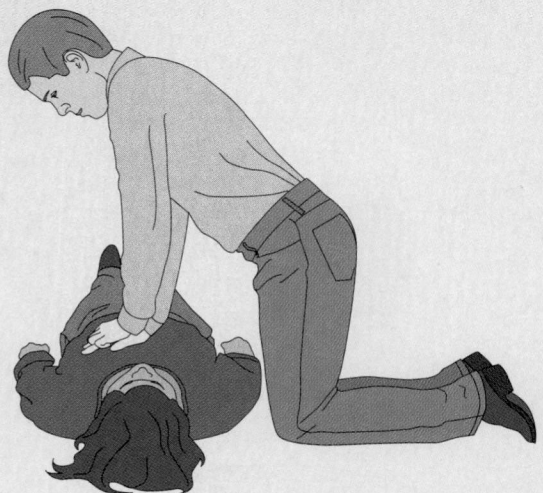

**Figure 30-22.** Align your shoulders directly over the victim's sternum, with your elbows locked.

by the tongue. This position is especially important if the patient vomits, to prevent aspiration of vomitus into the lungs.

3. Loosen restrictive clothing, and never place anything in the patient's mouth.

4. Protect the patient from injury, but do not try to hold him still during convulsions.

5. After convulsions end, keep the patient at rest, positioned for drainage from the mouth.

6. Make sure the patient is breathing. If he is not, begin rescue breathing or CPR.

7. Take vital signs and monitor respirations closely.

8. Move the patient to an exam room, or have him taken to a medical facility.

# Shock

Generally speaking, shock is a life-threatening state associated with failure of the cardiovascular system. It can bring to a stop all normal metabolic functions. This condition prevents the vital organs from receiving blood.

Early symptoms of shock include restlessness; irritability; fear; rapid pulse; pale, cool skin; and increased respiratory rate. Treat a patient in shock by elevating the feet 8 to 12 inches. If you suspect a head injury, however, keep the patient flat. Monitor the patient's ABCs and take steps to control bleeding. If the patient is chilly, wrap the patient in a blanket. Call the EMS system.

Several types of shock are possible. Anaphylactic shock, or anaphylaxis, is usually associated with an

# PROCEDURE 30.9

## Assisting With Emergency Childbirth

**Procedure Goal:** To assist in performing an emergency childbirth

### OSHA Guidelines

**Materials:** Clean cloths, sterile or clean sheets or towels, two sterile clamps or two pieces of string boiled in water for at least 10 minutes, sterile scissors, plastic bag, soft blankets or towels

### Method:

1. Ask the woman her name and age, how far apart her contractions are (about two per minute signals that the birth is near), if her water has broken, and if she feels straining or pressure as if the baby is coming. Alert the doctor or call the EMS system.

2. Help remove the woman's lower clothing.

3. Explain that you are about to do a visual inspection to see if the baby's head is in position. Ask the woman to lie on her back with her thighs spread, her knees flexed, and her feet flat. Examine her to see if there is crowning (a bulging at the vaginal opening from the baby's head) (see Figure 30-23).

4. If the head is crowning, childbirth is imminent. Place clean cloths under the woman's buttocks, and use sterile sheets or towels (if they are available) to cover her legs and stomach.

5. Wash your hands thoroughly and put on exam gloves. If other PPE is available, put it on now.

6. At this point the physician would begin to take steps to deliver the baby, and you would position yourself at the woman's head to provide emotional support and help in case she vomited. If no physician is available, position yourself at the woman's side so that you have a constant view of the vaginal opening.

7. Talk to the woman and encourage her to relax between contractions while allowing the delivery to proceed naturally.

8. Position your gloved hands at the woman's vaginal opening when the baby's head starts to appear.

### Rationale
To support and guide the infant's head as it is expelled
   Do not touch her skin.

9. Place one hand below the baby's head as it is delivered. Spread your fingers evenly around the baby's head.

### Rationale
To support the baby's head so that it does not touch the mother's anal area.

   Use your other hand to help cradle the baby's head (see Figure 30-24). Never pull on the baby.

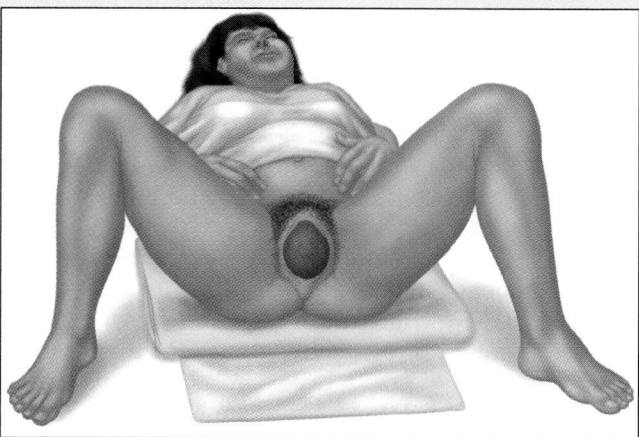

**Figure 30-23.** Crowning occurs when part of the baby's head becomes visible with each contraction.

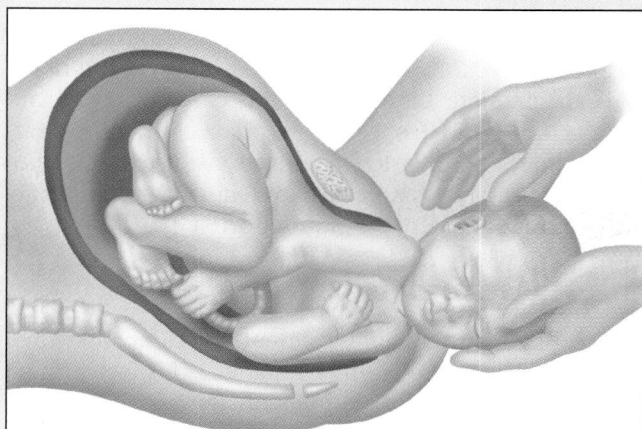

**Figure 30-24.** Support the baby's head with one hand while using the other hand to cradle the baby's head.

*continued* ⟶

## Assisting With Emergency Childbirth *(concluded)*

10. If the umbilical cord is wrapped around the baby's neck, gently loosen the cord and slide it over the baby's head.

11. If the amniotic sac has not broken by the time the baby's head is delivered, use your finger to puncture the membrane. Then pull the membranes away from the baby's mouth and nose.

*Rationale*

So that the baby can breathe.

12. Wipe blood or mucus from the baby's mouth with a clean cloth.

13. Continue to support the baby's head as the shoulders emerge. The upper shoulder will deliver first, followed quickly by the lower shoulder.

14. After the feet are delivered, lay the baby on his side with the head slightly lower than the body. Keep the baby at the same level as the mother until you cut the umbilical cord.

15. If the baby is not breathing, lower the head, raise the lower part of the body, and tap the soles of the feet. If the baby is still not breathing, begin rescue breathing and CPR.

16. To cut the cord, wait several minutes, until pulsations stop. Use the clamps or pieces of string to tie the cord in two places.

17. Use sterilized scissors to cut the cord in between the placement of the two clamps or pieces of string.

18. Within 10 minutes of the baby's birth, the placenta will begin to expel. Save it in a plastic bag for further examination.

19. Keep the mother and baby warm by wrapping them in towels or blankets. Do not touch the baby any more than necessary.

20. Massage the mother's abdomen just below the navel every few minutes to control internal bleeding.

21. Arrange for transport of the mother and baby to the hospital.

---

allergic reaction, as previously discussed. Hypovolemic shock and septic shock are two other types of shock.

**Hypovolemic Shock.** **Hypovolemic shock** results from insufficient blood volume in the circulatory system. It occurs after an injury that causes major fluid loss. Hemorrhage or burns can cause this type of fluid loss. Patients with hypovolemic shock must be transported to an emergency facility immediately.

**Septic Shock.** **Septic shock** results from massive, widespread infection that affects the ability of the blood vessels to circulate blood. Common causes are urinary tract infection (UTI) (especially in older adults), postpartum infection, and a variety of infections in patients with immunosuppression (as caused by chemotherapy or acquired immunodeficiency syndrome [AIDS]).

## Stroke (Brain Attack)

A **stroke,** or cerebrovascular accident (CVA), occurs when the blood supply to the brain is impaired. This impairment may cause temporary or permanent damage, depending on how long the brain cells are deprived of oxygen.

A minor stroke can cause headache, confusion, dizziness, tinnitus, minor speech difficulties, personality changes, weakness of the limbs, and memory loss. A major stroke typically produces loss of consciousness, paralysis on one side of the body, difficulty swallowing, loss of bladder and bowel control, slurred or garbled speech, and unequal pupil size.

If a patient has a stroke in the office, notify the physician at once, and call the EMS system. Maintain the patient's airway by turning the head toward the affected side to allow secretions to drain out rather than be aspirated. Loosen tight clothing. If directed by the physician, monitor vital signs and administer oxygen.

## Toxic Shock Syndrome

Toxic shock syndrome (TSS) is an acute infection caused by the bacterium *Staphylococcus aureus*. The toxin produced by the bacterium can enter the body through a break in the skin or through the uterus. Although the infection is most common in menstruating women who are using tampons at the time of onset, the link between tampon use and TSS is unclear.

TSS symptoms include high fever, intense muscle aches, vomiting, diarrhea, headache, bouts of violent shivering, vaginal discharge, red eyes, and a decreased level of consciousness. A sign specific to TSS is a deep red rash on the palms of the hands and the soles of the feet. This skin then sloughs off. A menstruating patient with these symptoms should be instructed to remove the tampon immediately and replace it with a sanitary napkin.

TSS is treated with intravenous antibiotics and fluids. The patient will require hospitalization.

## Viral Encephalitis

Viral encephalitis is a severe inflammation of the brain caused directly by a virus or secondary to a complication resulting from a viral infection. Viral encephalitis may result from an epidemic, or it may arise sporadically. This condition requires accurate identification and prompt treatment. Symptoms develop suddenly, beginning with fever, headache, and vomiting. They quickly progress to stiff neck and back, decreased level of consciousness (from drowsiness to coma), and paralysis and seizures.

The level of consciousness must be monitored frequently in a patient with viral encephalitis. Prepare the patient for treatment with antiviral drugs, and arrange for transport to a hospital for a lumbar puncture and other diagnostic tests.

# Common Psychosocial Emergencies

You will probably encounter psychosocial emergencies in the medical office at some point. These may result from drug or alcohol abuse, spousal abuse, child abuse, or elder abuse. Handle these situations as you were directed in Chapters 23 and 26. If you encounter patients who have overdosed on drugs, exhibit violent behavior, mention suicide, or have been raped, follow the specific clinical responsibilities described in this section.

You may also be responsible for referring patients with psychosocial emergencies to resources in the community. Some of these resources are listed in Table 30-3.

A patient who is overdosing on drugs can suffer serious medical problems and can even die. If a patient who has taken an overdose is brought to the medical office, call the EMS system immediately, and arrange for transport to the hospital.

Patients on drugs may become violent during withdrawal from the substance or while under the influence. If, at any time, a patient becomes aggressive or threatening, follow office protocol for handling violent behavior. The protocol should state when to call the police, how to document the incident, and when to notify the insurance carrier.

During a psychosocial emergency, a patient may tell you he is so depressed that he has thought about killing himself. Allow the patient to talk freely. Listen carefully without interrupting. Whenever a patient mentions suicide or talks about life in ways that make you suspect suicidal tendencies, discuss your suspicions with the physician. Take comments on suicide seriously, no matter how casual they may seem.

Victims of rape may be of any age and either gender, but more than 90% are women. If a patient says she has been raped, provide privacy. Limit the number of people who ask her questions. She may feel traumatized, embarrassed, and fearful. Do not make her go through the office routine at this time.

If the physician asks you to speak to the patient, explain to her that you are legally required to contact the police so that they can file a report. The patient can decide later whether she wishes to press charges.

Contact the local rape hotline, and request that a rape counselor come to the office to stay with the patient during the exam and police report procedures. The physician should be familiar with state laws for collecting specimens and the protocol for caring for a rape victim.

The procedure of ensuring that a specimen is obtained from the victim and is correctly identified, that the specimen is under the uninterrupted control of authorized personnel, and that the specimen has not been altered or replaced is called establishing **chain of custody.** This procedure is required for medicolegal issues such as evidence of rape as well as for drug tests for illicit drug use. If the chain between the victim and the specimen cannot be proved to have remained unbroken, the specimen must be considered invalid.

The first link in the chain of custody is collecting the specimen. Semen specimens are commonly collected for typing in a rape exam. Other samples collected from the victim's body and clothing may include hair and skin that can help identify the offender.

Proper specimen identification is important. Without it, the chain of custody is broken at the beginning. If you are responsible for collecting the specimen, you must be sure the specimen is collected from the correct patient and that no one tampers with it. The chain of custody form (see Figure 30-25) must be completed correctly, and the patient may be required to sign or initial the form as well.

Multiple copies of the form are used as a safeguard system. One copy, usually the original, accompanies the specimen in a sealed envelope. Another copy is attached to the outside of the envelope so that each person who handles the specimen can initial the form. A third copy is usually retained in the patient's file.

These general procedures help maintain an intact chain of custody. Always refer to your office's procedures to make sure you are meeting all relevant requirements.

# The Patient Under Stress

In emergency situations, patients and family members are under a great deal of stress. You must realize that people react differently to emergency situations. You can learn how to detect signs of extreme stress by being alert for patients whose behavior varies from that previously observed or who cannot focus or follow directions.

Your role during many emergency situations may be to keep victims and their families and friends calm. You can promote calmness by listening carefully and giving your full attention. Your first priority, at all times, is the victim's well-being. If he is very distraught, for example, hold his hand while the doctor examines him. If one of his

## TABLE 30-3 Resources for Patient Assistance

| Resource | Contact Information |
|---|---|
| Al-Anon and Alateen | 888-4AL-ANON (425-2666)<br>WSO@al-anon.org<br>www.al-anon.alateen.org |
| Alcoholics Anonymous | 212-870-3400<br>PO Box 459, New York, NY 10163<br>www.alcoholics-anonymous.org |
| Child Abuse Hotline | 800-4-A-CHILD, 800-422-4453, or 480-922-8212<br>Fax: 480-922-7061<br>15757 N. 78th Street,<br>Scottsdale, AZ 85260<br>www.childhelpusa.org |
| Mothers Against Drunk Driving (MADD) | 800-GET-MADD (438-6233)<br>MADD National Office, 511 E. John Carpenter Frwy,<br>Suite 700, Irving, TX 75062<br>www.madd.org |
| Narcotics Anonymous | 818-773-9999<br>Fax: 818-700-0700<br>World Service Office in Los Angeles<br>PO Box 9999, Van Nuys, CA 91409<br>www.na.org |
| National Institute for Alcohol Abuse and Alcoholism (NIAAA) | 5635 Fishers Lane, MSC 9304<br>Bethesda, MD 20892-7003<br>www.niaaa.nih.gov |
| National Coalition Against Domestic Violence | 800-799-SAFE (7233)<br>www.ncadv.org |
| National Council on Child Abuse and Family Violence | 202-429-6695<br>FAX: 831-655-3930<br>1025 Connecticut Ave. NW, Suite 1000<br>Washington, DC 20036<br>info@NCCAFV.org,<br>www.nccafv.org |
| National Domestic Violence Hotline | 800-799-SAFE (7233)<br>www.ndvh.org |
| National Families in Action Drug Information Center | 404-248-9676<br>Fax: 404-248-1312<br>2957 Clairmont Road NE, Suite 150, Atlanta, GA 30329<br>www.nationalfamilies.org |
| National Institute on Drug Abuse | 301-443-1124<br>6001 Executive Boulevard, Room 5213,<br>Bethesda, MD 20892-9561<br>Information@lists.nida.nih.gov<br>www.nida.nih.gov |
| National Organization for Victim Assistance | 800-TRY-NOVA (879-6682)<br>Courthouse Square, 510 King Street,<br>Suite 424, Alexandria, VA 22314<br>www.try-nova.org |
| Students Against Destructive Decisions | 877-SADD-INC (723-3462)<br>Fax: 508-481-5759<br>255 Main Street, Marlborough, MA 01752<br>www.sadd.org |

# CHAIN OF CUSTODY FORM

**MADISON CLINICAL LABORATORY**

195 North Parkway
Madison, WA 90869
(608) 555-3030

SPECIMEN I.D. NO:

## STEP 1—TO BE COMPLETED BY COLLECTOR OR EMPLOYER REPRESENTATIVE.

Employer Name, Address, and I.D. No.:        OR        Medical Review Officer Name and Address:

_____        _____

_____        _____

_____        _____

Donor Social Security No. or Employee I.D. No.: _____

Donor I.D. verified:    ❐ Photo I.D.    ❐ Employer Representative _____
                                                                    Signature

Reason for test: (check one)    ❐ Preemployment    ❐ Random    ❐ Postaccident
                                ❐ Periodic    ❐ Reasonable suspicion/cause
                                ❐ Return to duty    ❐ Other (specify)

Test(s) to be performed: _____    Total tests ordered: ☐

Type of specimen obtained:    ❐ Urine    ❐ Blood    ❐ Semen    ❐ Other (specify)
                            *Submit only one specimen with each requisition.*

## STEP 2—TO BE COMPLETED BY COLLECTOR.

For urine specimens, read temperature within 4 minutes of collection.
Check here if specimen temperature is within range.    ❐ Yes, 90°–100°F/32°–38°C
Or record actual temperature here: _____

## STEP 3—TO BE COMPLETED BY COLLECTOR.

Collection site: _____    Address _____

City _____    State _____    Zip _____    Phone _____

Collection date: _____    Time: _____    ❐ a.m.    ❐ p.m.

I certify that the specimen identified on this form is the specimen presented to me by the donor identified in step 1 above, and that it was collected, labeled, and sealed in the donor's presence.

Collector's name: _____    Signature of collector _____

## STEP 4—TO BE INITIATED BY DONOR AND COMPLETED AS NECESSARY THEREAFTER.

| Purpose of change | Released by Signature | Received by Signature | Date |
|---|---|---|---|
| A. Provide specimen for testing | | | |
| B. Shipment to Laboratory | | | |
| C. | | | |

Comments:

## STEP 5—TO BE COMPLETED BY THE LABORATORY:

Specimen package seal(s) intact when received in lab?    ❐ Yes    ❐ No. If no, explain.
Laboratory receiver's initials _____

Copy 1 - Original - Must accompany specimen to laboratory.

**Figure 30-25.**   The chain of custody form provides documentation that specific specimen collection safeguards have been followed.

relatives is crying and causing him to become emotional, suggest that the relative do something to help—for example, fill out paperwork in another room.

You may face special challenges when communicating with victims during emergencies. Victims may not speak your language, or they may have a visual or hearing impairment. In such instances, follow these guidelines.

- Use gestures throughout the process for non–English-speaking victims. Continue to speak, however, because they may be able to understand some English.
- Tell patients who have visual impairments what you are going to do before you do it, and maintain voice and touch contact while caring for them.
- Ask patients who have hearing impairments whether they can read lips. If they can, speak slowly to them and never turn away while you are speaking. If they cannot read lips, communicate by writing and using gestures. At all times try to remain face to face and keep direct physical contact.

## Educating the Patient

During minor medical emergencies, after major emergencies have been resolved, and during routine office visits, you can educate patients about ways to prevent and handle various medical emergencies. For example, you might tell them how to contact the local American Red Cross office, post notices of upcoming classes that the Red Cross offers, and encourage patients and family members to learn basic first aid. You might also develop a first-aid kit checklist and make it available to patients and families.

Make sure that all family members, including children, are familiar with the local EMS system and know how to contact it in an emergency. Suggest that families keep emergency numbers by the telephone. In addition, teach parents how to childproof their home for children of various ages. Remember that childproofing differs for different children—for example, for children who can crawl as opposed to children who can walk.

Provide brief, easy-to-read handouts to reinforce the information you present to patients. Prepare handouts in multiple languages if you provide care for non–English-speaking patients. Find and use patient education resources for the types of patients seen by the practice. For example, if you work in an obstetric office, obtain educational materials for pregnant and postpartum patients from companies that provide pregnancy-related products. Ask company representatives what materials are available. Many companies provide free videos and booklets.

## Disasters

Your skills in dealing with emergencies, including first-aid and CPR training, will be an enormous help to your community in the event of a disaster. To be fully effective, you must also be familiar with standard protocols for responding to disasters. Table 30-4 shows ways that you can help in certain types of disasters. You may even want to participate in fire or other disaster drills to familiarize yourself with emergency procedures.

## Bioterrorism

**Bioterrorism** is the intentional release of a biologic agent with the intent to harm individuals. The Centers for Disease Control and Prevention (CDC) defines a biologic agent as a weapon when it is easy to disseminate, has a high potential for mortality, can cause a public panic or social disruption, and requires public health preparedness. There are numerous

| TABLE 30-4 | Assisting in a Disaster |
|---|---|
| **Type of Disaster** | **Action to Take** |
| Weather disaster, such as a flood or hurricane | • Report to the community command post.<br>• Have your credentials with you.<br>• Receive an identifying tag or vest and assignment.<br>• Accept only an assignment that is appropriate for your abilities. Expect to be part of a team.<br>• Document what medical care each victim receives on each person's disaster tag. |
| Office fire | • Activate the alarm system.<br>• Use a fire extinguisher if the fire is confined to a small container, such as a trash can.<br>• Turn off oxygen.<br>• Shut windows and doors.<br>• Seal doors with wet cloths to prevent smoke from entering.<br>• If evacuation is necessary, proceed quietly and calmly. Direct ambulatory patients and family members to the appropriate exit route. Assist patients who need help leaving the building. |

biologic agents identified as weapons, including anthrax, tularemia, smallpox, plague, and botulism. The CDC maintains an Internet site with current information about identified biologic agents at www.bt.cdc.gov.

Physicians' offices will be on the front lines should a biologic agent be intentionally released. It will be up to physicians and their staff to sound the alarm to public officials that something may be amiss. Physicians and medical assistants should be vigilant about cases that present themselves as well as common trends in syndromes. Be on the lookout for unusual patterns in affected patients. Indications of a bioterrorist attack might include many patients having been in the same place at the same time or an unusual distribution for common illnesses, such as an increase in chickenpox-like illness in adults that might be smallpox.

If you suspect that bioterrorism is responsible for an illness, report your suspicions to the physician. It is the responsibility of your facility to immediately contact the local public health department. The information about the patient should be recorded, and appropriate tests should be performed. The laboratory should be notified of the potential for bioterrorism. Additionally, consultations with specialists and discussions of all findings are necessary when bioterrorism is suspected. The following is a list of clues of a bioterroristic attack as defined by the American College of Physicians—American Society of Internal Medicine.

- Unusual temporal or geographic clustering of illness
- Unusual age distribution of common disease, such as an illness that appears to be chickenpox in adults but is really smallpox
- A large epidemic with greater caseloads than expected, especially in a discrete population
- More severe disease than expected
- Unusual route of exposure
- A disease that is outside its normal transmission season or is impossible to transmit naturally in the absence of its normal vector
- Multiple simultaneous epidemics of different diseases
- A disease outbreak with health consequences to humans and animals
- Unusual strains or variants of organisms or antimicrobial resistance patterns

In any disaster, you may be asked to perform triage. When you perform triage, you give each injured victim a tag that classifies the person as emergent (needing immediate care), urgent (needing care within several hours), nonurgent (needing care when time is not critical), or dead. The triage process is outlined in Procedure 30-10.

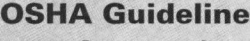

## PROCEDURE 30.10

## Performing Triage in a Disaster

**Procedure Goal:** To prioritize disaster victims

### OSHA Guidelines

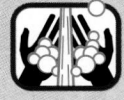 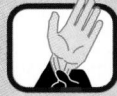  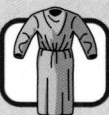

**Materials:** Disaster tag and pen

### Method:

1. Wash your hands and put on exam gloves and other PPE if available.
2. Quickly assess each victim.
3. Sort victims by type of injury and need for care, classifying them as emergent, urgent, nonurgent, or dead.

### Rationale

Sorting the victims allows for rapid treatment based on need.

4. Label the emergent patients no. 1, and send them to appropriate treatment stations immediately. Emergent patients, such as those who are in shock or who are hemorrhaging, need immediate care.

5. Label the urgent patients no. 2, and send them to basic first-aid stations. Urgent patients need care within the next several hours. Such patients may have lacerations that can be dressed quickly to stop the bleeding but can wait for suturing.

6. Label nonurgent patients no. 3, and send them to volunteers who will be empathic and provide refreshments. Nonurgent patients are those for whom timing of treatment is not critical, such as patients who have no physical injuries but who are emotionally upset.

7. Label patients who are dead no. 4. Ensure that the bodies are moved to an area where they will be safe until they can be identified and proper action can be taken.

# Summary

A medical emergency can occur anywhere—in a doctor's office, at home, in a restaurant, or on the street. The more you learn about handling each type of medical emergency, the more valuable your contributions to the situation become. You can make a substantial, positive difference in the health and lives of people who face medical emergencies to which you respond.

Always notify the doctor or the local EMS system when you encounter a medical emergency. Do not, at any time, perform procedures you have not been trained to do. Use common sense, assess the situation and the patient's condition, and provide first aid until a doctor or EMT arrives.

Patients having a medical emergency are often under extreme stress. Remember to stay calm and communicate clearly. Communicating with non–English-speaking patients and those with visual or hearing impairments requires special skills. You can develop these skills through educational and training programs you seek out or during routine office visits with these patients.

You may not be present when medical emergencies occur, so patients need to know how to respond to emergency circumstances. Take every opportunity to educate patients about preventing and responding to medical emergencies. Remember to draw on community resources when you provide information or support to patients and their families. There will always be opportunities to expand your knowledge, skills, and network for dealing with medical emergencies in your medical assisting work.

## CASE STUDY *QUESTIONS*

Now that you have completed this chapter, review the case study at the beginning of the chapter. Consider each situation and determine the order in which you will respond. Explain your decisions.

### Discussion Questions

1. What PPE should you keep in a first-aid kit?
2. How would you assist a person who was bleeding from accidental injuries if you had no personal protective equipment with you?
3. Why should you be certified in first aid and CPR?
4. A 26-year-old is being seen in your office for a dog bite on the hand. What should you ask her?
5. Your daughter is going to the lake for the weekend. What tips can you give her about avoiding getting sunburned?

### Critical Thinking Questions

1. A 27-year-old male patient with diabetes comes to the office for treatment of an upper respiratory infection. While in the waiting room, he begins to sweat profusely and becomes restless and confused. What should you do and why?
2. Your 2-year-old has swallowed some cleaning solution you were using to clean the kitchen floor. What should you do?
3. A 39-year-old female patient has visited your office many times. Today, however, you notice that she is disheveled and anxious. After you greet her, she describes general, nonspecific complaints in a sad, tired tone of voice. What should you do?
4. While attending the office picnic, one of your coworkers gets stung by a bee. What should you do?

## Application Activities

1. On a classmate or mannequin, demonstrate first aid for someone who is having a seizure. Have the class critique your technique.
2. Demonstrate on a classmate how to stop bleeding from a large laceration on the lower arm. Switch roles and critique each other's technique.
3. With two other students, role-play calling the EMS system. Have one student act as the EMS dispatcher and the other provide a description of an emergency situation and then a critique of your performance.
4. With a partner, practice applying bandages to each other. Use Figure 30-14 as a reference. After each bandage is applied, check it for correctness, and check the skin color and circulation of each area bandaged.

## Virtual Fieldtrip

*Visit the McGraw-Hill Higher Education Medical Assisting website at www.mhhe.com/medicalassisting3 to complete the following activity:*

Research the CDC Bioterrorism website. Write a report about how you can use this site to better prepare your office for the possibility of a bioterrorist attack.

Open the CD and complete this chapter's practice activities, play the games, listen to the key terms, and test yourself with the interactive review. E-mail, print, and/or save your results to document your proficiency.

# CHAPTER 31

# Complementary and Alternative Medicine

## KEY TERMS

acupressure
acupuncture
adjustment
allopathy
alternative medicine
aromatherapy
Ayurveda
bioelectromagnetic-based
    therapies
biofeedback
biofield therapies
chiropractor
complementary and
    alternative medicine
    (CAM)
complementary medicine
conventional medicine
dietary supplement
disclaimer
health fraud
homeopathic medicine
hypnosis
integrative medicine
magnetic therapy
massage
meditation
meridian
moxibustion
National Center for
    Complementary and
    Alternative Medicine
    (NCCAM)
naturopathic medicine

## MEDICAL ASSISTING COMPETENCIES

*In preparation for the certification examination, you should know the following:*

| COMPETENCY | CMA | RMA |
|---|---|---|
| **General/Legal/Professional** | | |
| Recognize and respond to verbal and nonverbal communications by being attentive and adapting communication to the recipient's level of understanding | X | X |
| Be aware of and perform within legal and ethical boundaries | X | X |
| Demonstrate knowledge of and monitor current federal and state health-care legislation and regulations; maintain licenses and accreditation | X | X |
| Instruct individuals according to their needs | X | X |
| Provide patients with methods of health promotion and disease prevention | X | X |
| Identify community resources and information for patients and employers | X | X |
| Exhibit initiative | | X |
| Adapt to change | | X |
| Conduct work within scope of education, training, and ability | | X |
| Be impartial and show empathy when dealing with patients | | X |
| Serve as a liaison between the physician and others | | X |
| Receive, organize, prioritize, and transmit information appropriately | | X |

## KEY TERMS *(Concluded)*

| | | |
|---|---|---|
| placebo effect | remedy | traditional Chinese medicine (TCM) |
| qi | standardization | |
| reflexology | therapeutic touch | yoga |
| Reiki | | |

# CHAPTER OUTLINE

- What Is CAM?
- Types of CAM
- Patients Seeking CAM Therapy
- Insurance and CAM
- Regulation of CAM Therapies
- Health Fraud

# LEARNING OUTCOMES

After completing Chapter 31, you will be able to:

**31.1** Define CAM.

**31.2** Compare complementary and alternative medicine to conventional medicine.

**31.3** Discuss how CAM and conventional medicine are used together.

**31.4** Identify various types of complementary and alternative medicine.

**31.5** Describe how a medical assistant may use his or her knowledge of CAM.

**31.6** Explain why patients and health-care practitioners are turning to complementary treatments.

**31.7** Discuss insurance and payment for CAM treatments.

**31.8** Explain how CAM is regulated.

**31.9** Describe health fraud.

# Introduction

The use of complementary and alternative medicine (CAM) is on the rise. People are becoming more aware of complementary therapies and alternatives to traditional treatments and medications. More than one-third of the population older than the age of 18 uses some form of CAM to help them relieve problems and promote wellness. Sometimes people turn to complementary and alternative medicine when they are unable to find relief from their problems using traditional treatments. Sometimes physicians and other health-care practitioners use a combination of traditional and complementary treatments to provide the best care for their patients. This chapter will discuss complementary and alternative medicine and how, as a medical assistant, you will most likely encounter them.

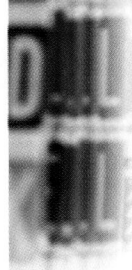

## CASE STUDY

You will be working directly with a new physician that has been hired at your facility. On the day you meet her she says, "I plan to use more complementary medicine in my practice here. Because you will be working with my patients, I would like you to know more about it." You are not really sure what complimentary medicine is, so you set out to find out more about it.

As you read this chapter, consider the following questions:

1. What is CAM?
2. What types of therapies are included in CAM?
3. How and when would you use your knowledge of CAM in your career as a medical assistant?

# What Is CAM?

**Complementary and alternative medicine (CAM)** is a group of practices and products that are not necessarily considered to be part of conventional medicine. **Conventional medicine,** also known as **allopathy,** is the common and usual practice of physicians and other allied health professionals, such as physical therapists, psychologists, medical assistants, and registered nurses. Complementary and alternative medicine includes numerous practices such as acupuncture, massage, chiropractic, Ayurveda, or Chinese medicine, and dietary supplement use. See Table 31-1, Examples of Complementary and Alternative Medicine. Although complementary and alternative medicines are defined together, they do differ. **Complementary medicine** is used with conventional medicine. For example, a complementary therapy is using **aromatherapy** to help lessen a patient's discomfort following surgery. **Alternative medicine** is used in place of conventional medicine. A patient may decide to use a special diet to treat cancer instead

## TABLE 31-1 Examples of Complementary and Alternative Medicine

| Type of Therapy | Description |
| --- | --- |
| Acupressure | The use of pressure, applied by hand, to various areas of the body in order to restore balance |
| Acupuncture | A practice of inserting needles into various areas of the body to restore balance |
| Aromatherapy | The use of essential oils, extracts, or essences from flowers, herbs, and trees to promote health and well-being |
| Ayurveda | A system of medicine originating in India that uses herbal preparations, dietary changes, exercises, and meditation to restore health and promote well-being |
| Biofeedback | A process in which an individual learns how to control involuntary body responses to promote health and treat disease |
| Chiropractic medicine | Adjustments of the spine that are made to relieve pressure and/or pain |
| Dietary supplements | Vitamins, minerals, herbals, and other substances taken by mouth without a prescription to promote health and well-being |
| Homeopathy | A system of medicine that uses remedies in an attempt to stimulate the body to recover itself |
| Hypnosis | A trance-like state usually induced by another person to access the subconscious mind and promote healing |
| Magnetic therapy | A practice in which magnets are placed on the body to penetrate and correct the body's energy fields |
| Massage | The use of pressure, kneading, stroking, and touch to alleviate pain and promote healing through relaxation |
| Meditation | A state in which the body is consciously relaxed and the mind becomes calm and focused |
| Naturopathy | A system of medicine that relies upon the healing power of the body and supports that power through various health-care practices such as nutrition, lifestyle, and exercise |
| Reflexology | A manual therapy to the feet and/or hands in which pressure is applied to reflex "zones" mapped out on the feet and hands |
| Reiki | The use of visualization and touch to balance energy flow and bring healthy energy to affected body parts |
| Therapeutic touch | The use of touch to detect and correct a person's energy fields, thus promoting healing and health |
| Traditional Chinese medicine (TCM) | Ancient system of medicine originating in China that involves preparations from herbal and animal sources to treat illness. This type of medicine includes various treatments such as acupuncture and acupressure |
| Yoga | A series of poses and breathing exercises that provide awareness of the unity of a person's whole being (physical and spiritual) |

of undergoing surgery, radiation, or chemotherapy that has been recommended by a conventional doctor.

Although scientific evidence exists regarding some CAM therapies, there are still many questions about others. Scientific research is continually in progress to answer questions regarding the safety and effectiveness of complementary and alternative therapies. The list of what is considered to be CAM changes continually. Additionally, what your patient understands about CAM and its uses will also vary greatly.

As therapies are proven to be safe and effective and are adopted into conventional health care, another type of medicine, called **integrative medicine,** has evolved. Integrative medicine essentially combines mainstream medical therapies and the CAM therapies for which there is some high-quality scientific evidence of safety and effectiveness.

# Types of CAM

There are various types of CAM and they share similarities with each other:

- A focus on individualized treatments, good nutrition, and preventive health practices
- Treatment of the whole person
- Promotion of self-care and self-healing
- Recognition of the spiritual nature of the individual

CAM is constantly changing. From the time this chapter was written to your reading it, specifics about CAM may have changed. Research is ongoing and new discoveries are made frequently. This section will provide some basic details about the types of CAM. For the most current information, you may want to consult the Internet and the links provided on the Online Learning Center that accompanies this book. The **National Center for Complementary and Alternative Medicine (NCCAM)** would be a good place to start looking for the latest research and updates to CAM.

The NCCAM classifies CAM therapies into five categories:

- Alternative Medical Systems
- Mind-Body Interventions
- Biologically Based Therapies
- Manipulative and Body-Based Methods
- Energy Therapies

## Alternative Medical Systems

Alternative medical systems are complete systems of theory and practice that have evolved apart from conventional medicine. For example, two types of alternative medical systems that have developed in Western cultures are homeopathic medicine and naturopathic medicine. Two systems of medicine from non-Western cultures include traditional Chinese medicine and Ayurveda.

**Homeopathic Medicine.** **Homeopathic medicine** (homeopathy) is the practice of treating the syndromes and conditions that constitute disease with remedies that have produced similar syndromes and conditions in healthy persons. The principles of homeopathy were discovered by Samuel Hahnemann, a German physician, in the early 1800s. Homeopathic medicine is based upon the Latin principle *similia similibus curentur,* which translated means, "Let likes cure likes." A homeopath, or a physician who practices homeopathy, uses substances made from various plants, minerals, or animals in extremely small doses to stimulate the sick person's natural defenses in an attempt to stimulate the body to recover itself. The medicines are individually chosen based upon their ability to cause symptoms similar to those experienced by the patient when given in large doses.

A **remedy** or homeopathic medicine is a substance that produces the same symptoms that it is given to treat. A medicine is homeopathic only if it is taken based upon the similar nature of the medicine to the illness. A homeopathic remedy is meant to stimulate the immune system to help the body recover and cure the illness.

Homeopathy looks at individuals and not at diseases. For example, each of us suffers a cold in his or her unique way. Homeopathy looks for the one substance that will cure the individual case. The person with a cold, characterized by slow onset, aching, loss of appetite, chills, and a desire to be left alone, will need a different remedy than the person whose cold comes on a bit quicker and is characterized by intense sneezing, a runny nose that burns the upper lip, a desire for hot drinks, and a bone-chilling coldness. Both are colds, but they are expressed differently and, therefore, are treated with different homeopathic remedies.

Training for homeopathy is offered through diploma programs, certificate programs, short courses, and correspondence courses. Most homeopathic medicine practiced in the United States is done with another health-care practice such as conventional medicine, naturopathy, chiropractic, dentistry, acupuncture, or veterinary medicine. (Yes, homeopathy is also used to treat animals.) Homeopathic training is also part of medical school training in naturopathy, which we will discuss later. Laws about what is required to practice homeopathy vary among states.

## Educating the Patient

### CAM Therapies

As a medical assistant, you should be aware of the scope of practice regarding educating patients about CAM therapies. Your state and place of employment regulate what therapies you may assist with and what questions you may answer. In most cases, you should refer the patient's specific questions about CAM therapy to a licensed practitioner. You may provide additional information to the patient in the form of approved printed literature or web links as allowed by your place of employment. The information in this chapter is meant to introduce you to CAM and is not meant as a resource for answering patients' specific questions about CAM treatments.

## TABLE 31-2 Homeopathic Remedies Used for Common Ailments

| Remedy Name | Common Name | Effect | Common Use |
|---|---|---|---|
| Allium cepa | Onion | Causes tearing of the eyes and dripping of the nose | Common cold and hay fever |
| Arnica | Mountain daisy | Reduces pain and helps speed healing | Trauma and sports injury |
| Chamomilla | Chamomile | Aids in sleep and produces calm | Irritable infant from colic or teething |
| Hypericum | St. John's wort | Suspected to prevent nerve cells in the brain from reabsorbing serotonin, a chemical that improves the feeling of well-being | Depression and shooting nerve pain |
| Ignatia | St. Ignatius bean | Trembling, agitation | Grief, anxiety, and depression |
| Magnesia phosphorica | Phosphate of magnesia | Reduces cramps | Menstrual cramps |
| Nux vomica | Poison nut | Increases appetite and stimulates peristalsis | Overeating and too much alcohol, constipation |
| Pulsatilla | Windflower | Antispasmodic alternative and diaphoretic | Disorders of the mucous membranes of the respiratory and digestive tract |
| Rhus tox | Poison ivy | Pain upon motion, burning, itchy, swelling, and painful blistered skin | Itching, red swollen skin, joint or muscle ailments, sprains and strains |

Usually it can be employed by those whose degree entitles them to practice medicine in that state. States such as Nevada and Arizona have their own state board of homeopathic medicine.

As a medical assistant, you may work with a homeopath or other practitioner who practices homeopathy. Patients usually undergo a very lengthy first visit so that the practitioner can take an in-depth assessment. This assessment is critical to guide the selection of one or more homeopathic remedies. During follow-up visits, patients report how they are responding to the remedy or remedies, which will help the practitioner make decisions about further treatment.

Your duties in the office of a homeopath may be similar to other medical office duties, with some exceptions. To prepare for employment in this area of CAM, it is useful to have a working knowledge of commonly used remedies. The U.S. Food and Drug Administration (FDA), an agency of the federal government, requires that these remedies meet certain legal standards for strength, quality, purity, and packaging. Homeopathic remedies must list the indications or reason for use on the label along with the ingredients, dilutions, and instructions for safe use.

Homeopathic remedies are derived from natural substances that come from plants, minerals, or animals. Remedies go through the process of *potentization*, in which the original substance is diluted in factors of 10 or 100. It goes through this process multiple times and after each dilution

it is strongly shaken. Remedies are sold in liquid, pellet, and tablet forms. See Table 31-2 for a brief description of some common homeopathic remedies.

**Naturopathic Medicine.** **Naturopathic medicine,** also known as naturopathy, relies upon the healing power of the body to establish, maintain, and restore health. Practitioners work with the patient with a goal of supporting this power through the use of treatments such as the following:

- Nutrition and lifestyle counseling
- Dietary supplements
- Medicinal plants
- Exercise
- Homeopathy
- Other treatments from traditional Chinese medicine

Naturopathic medicine is considered primary health care and includes the diagnosis, treatment, and prevention of illness. A licensed naturopathic physician (ND) attends a 4-year graduate level naturopathic medical school and is educated in all of the same basic sciences as an MD In addition to these sciences, an ND also studies holistic and nontoxic approaches to therapy that emphasize disease prevention and wellness. In addition to a medical curriculum, the naturopathic physician must complete 4 years of training in clinical nutrition, acupuncture, homeopathic medicine, botanical medicine, psychology, and counseling.

According to the American Association of Naturopathic physicians, the ND is recognized as a medical expert in natural therapies. They practice and research complementary medicine by combining many therapies. As a medical assistant, you will find these practitioners emphasize treatments and lifestyle changes that will allow the patient to restore and maintain health and prevent illness. Once again, a basic knowledge of the various therapies practiced by the ND is an essential part of the medical assistant's duties. Keep in mind that not all practitioners of naturopathic medicine are licensed. Each state differs and you should be aware of the regulations for naturopathic medicine in the state where you are employed.

**Traditional Chinese Medicine.** Incredibly, **traditional Chinese medicine (TCM)** dates back to 200 B.C. in written form. TCM is the current term for an ancient system of health care from China that, through historic and political forces, has become CAM. Other countries such as Korea, Japan, and Vietnam have their own unique version of medicine based upon TCM. TCM includes some practices you may already know about, including herbs, acupuncture, and massage.

The basis of TCM is the concept of balanced **qi** (pronounced "chee"), or vital energy. This vital energy (qi) flows throughout the body. Qi regulates a person's spiritual, emotional, mental, and physical balance. It is influenced by the opposing forces of yin and yang. Yin, which is characterized as negative energy, represents the cold, slow, or passive principle. Yang, which is characterized as positive energy, represents the hot, excited, or active principle. An imbalance of yin and yang leads to blockage in the flow of qi (or vital energy) and of blood along energetic pathways known as **meridians** (Figure 31-1). Disease results from the disrupted flow of qi, which results in yin and yang becoming imbalanced. Practitioners help unblock qi and promote energy and blood flow in the meridians of patients in an attempt to bring the body back into harmony and wellness.

*Acupuncture.* **Acupuncture** is practiced separately or as part of TCM. The acupuncturist focuses on the medical history, nutritional habits, and environmental factors of the patient. The acupuncturist also takes the pulse of many different meridians and examines the tongue closely for shape and color variations. During treatment, the acupuncturist inserts thin, hollow needles under the skin to balance the flow of qi in the body. The needles are inserted in specific locations where the meridians or channels come close to the skin's surface. The acupuncturist may twirl, raise, rotate, or vibrate the needles to achieve the desired effects.

There are varying types of acupuncture. One type, electro-acupuncture, is done by applying a very small amount of electrical current through the acupuncture needles. This method is generally used to relieve or prevent pain. There is no danger of electrical shock to the patient.

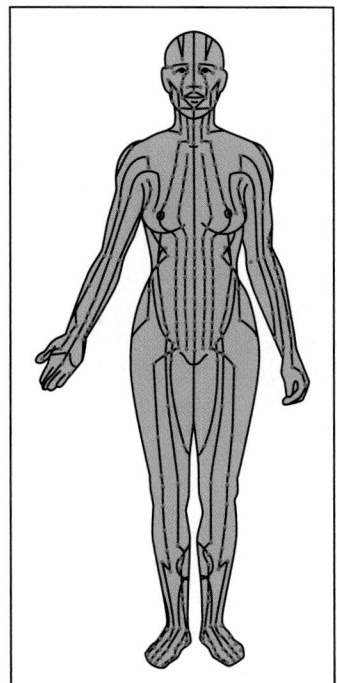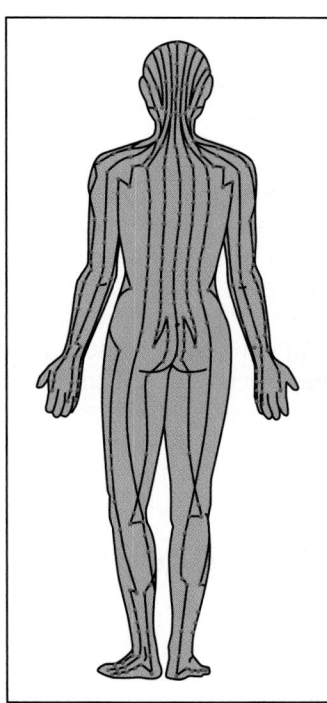

**Figure 31-1.** Meridians are pathways for blood flow in the body that are treated as part of traditional Chinese medicine to restore the body's harmony and wellness.
Source: Booth: *Health Care Science Technology*, Figure 21-4, page 692.

The amount of electricity going through the needles is very small, but the frequency of the current can vary. High-frequency electrical current has been used successfully to block the pain of surgery without the use of anesthesia.

**Moxibustion** and **acupressure** are two other types of acupuncture treatment. During moxibustion, the acupuncturist applies heat to the places where the needles are inserted. This may be done to increase the effectiveness of the acupuncture treatment. Moxibustion is used to treat conditions such as arthritis, bronchial asthma, bronchitis, and certain kinds of paralysis. Acupressure is performed without needles. The points along the meridians are stimulated using an instrument or finger pressure.

**Ayurveda.** **Ayurveda** has been practiced primarily in India for 5000 years. It is a holistic system of medicine that aims to provide guidance regarding food and lifestyle so that healthy people can stay healthy and people with health challenges can improve their health. Ayurveda has several unique aspects, including the following:

- Its recommendations are specific to each person regarding which foods and lifestyle he or she should follow in order to be completely healthy.
- Everything in Ayurveda is validated by observation, inquiry, direct examination, and knowledge derived from ancient texts.
- It understands that there are energetic forces that influence nature and human beings. These forces, called

Tridoshas, assist with the creation of the various tissues of the body and remove any unnecessary waste products from the body. Tridoshas also influence all movements, transformations, sensory functions, and many of the other activities in the human body and mind.

Ayurvedic practices include dietary recommendations and herbal remedies. They emphasize the use of body, mind, and spirit in disease prevention and treatment. Some of the primary Ayurvedic treatments include diet, exercise, meditation, herbs, massage, exposure to sunlight, and controlled breathing. In India, Ayurvedic treatments have been developed for various diseases, including diabetes, cardiovascular conditions, and neurologic disorders. Individuals in the United States practice Ayurveda and some of their therapies are considered very useful.

## Mind-Body Interventions

Mind-body interventions are techniques used to enhance the mind's capacity to affect bodily functions and symptoms. Techniques such as yoga, hypnosis, meditation, prayer, mental healing, biofeedback, and creative therapies such as art, dance, and music therapy are mind-body therapies that are considered CAM. These techniques are used to enhance each person's capacity for self-knowledge and self-care.

Two types of mind-body techniques that used to be considered CAM are now part of traditional medicine. These are support groups and cognitive-behavioral therapy. Scientific research has documented the benefits of both of these types of therapy. Thus, it is common practice for a patient to join a support group for many types of illness and recovery, such as cancer or alcoholism. Cognitive-behavioral therapy helps individuals discover behavior and thought patterns that lead to emotional distress. It has been found to be very useful for treating depression and other mental disorders.

The roots of mind-body interventions began with traditional Chinese medicine and Ayurveda more than 2000 years ago. Hippocrates, the father of modern medicine, recognized the moral and spiritual aspects of healing. He believed that treatment could occur only by considering attitude and environmental influences, and using natural remedies. As technology developed in Western culture, with things like the stethoscope, microscope, and blood pressure cuff, personal belief and emotion were given less consideration during health care. It wasn't until the 1920s that the physician began to re-emphasize the connection between emotion and physical responses within the body.

What we know as the **placebo effect** was discovered during World War II. When the pain medicine morphine was in short supply, wounded soldiers were given saline instead, without their knowledge. The physician, Henry Beecher, MD, discovered that much of the pain was controlled just by the soldiers' belief that they received morphine. Later, research by the same physician showed that up to 35% of a therapeutic response to any medical treatment was the result of belief. The placebo effect is still being debated, yet its discovery helps support the use of mind-body interventions.

Mind-body interventions are the most commonly used types of CAM. One-third of the population uses some type of mind-body intervention. Many problems, such as coronary artery disease (CAD) and chronic arthritis pain, are being treated successfully with mind-body interventions. As a medical assistant, you must be aware of the types of mind-body interventions that the practitioner may employ or the patient may practice. You must also be respectful of the mind-body treatments chosen by patients, even if they do not reflect your own beliefs.

Regardless of the varieties of religious affiliations, prayer is the most widely practiced form of mind-body intervention. More than 50% of the population use prayer as a method of healing. In addition to prayer, some other common types of mind-body intervention include yoga, meditation, hypnosis, and biofeedback.

**Yoga.** The term **yoga** means union. The aim of yoga is the awareness of the unity of our whole being. It is basically a series of poses and breathing exercises. Supporters of yoga believe that the spine nourishes the central nervous system (CNS) and the condition of the spine is critical for our physical and emotional well-being. Yoga postures exercise the spine and stimulate the lymphatic system, helping to remove toxins from the body. When toxins accumulate, they may cause pain and stiffness in the muscles and joints. The physical postures, breathing exercises, and meditation practices of yoga have been proven to reduce stress, lower blood pressure, regulate heart rate, and even slow the aging process.

**Meditation.** **Meditation** usually refers to a state in which the body is consciously relaxed and the mind is allowed to become calm and focused. Several religions include ritual meditation and prayer; most of the popular systems of meditation include various forms of Christian, Jewish, and Muslim meditation. Meditation is often similar to prayer and worship, in which the goal is spiritual insight and new understanding. However, meditation itself need not be a religious or spiritual activity.

Meditation is said to balance a person's physical, emotional, and mental states. It has been used as an aid in treating stress, anxiety, and pain management, and as part of an overall treatment for other conditions including hypertension and heart disease. Research shows that meditation decreases the heart rate, respiratory rate, oxygen consumption, and even blood pressure.

**Hypnosis.** Hypnosis dates back more than 200 years, yet in recent years has gained popularity. **Hypnosis** is a sleep- or trance-like state usually induced by another person. During hypnosis, the individual retains awareness of the presence of the hypnotist and has a heightened state of suggestibility, relaxation, and imagination. The hypnotist can access the person's subconscious mind and help the person relax or calm the conscious mind. Calming the conscious mind helps the individual change habits, access a suppressed memory, decrease pain, or cure illness.

There are various uses for hypnosis. One common use for hypnosis is to help individuals change habits that are affecting their health. For example, a hypnotist may reprogram the subconscious mind to help a person reduce his or her need for smoking or overeating. Hypnotism might also be used to help patients overcome pain or cure illness. For example, after training by a hypnotist, a patient suffering from migraines might be taught to hypnotize himself in order to reduce stress and the symptoms that cause these headaches. Hypnosis might also be used to help individuals overcome fear or access memories of past events.

**Biofeedback.** **Biofeedback** is another type of mind-body therapy aimed at helping individuals achieve the best level of awareness for a variety of situations. A biofeedback specialist uses a variety of monitoring procedures and equipment to teach the individual to control involuntary body responses. These involuntary responses include things such as brain activity, blood pressure, muscle tension, and heart rate. Once an individual learns to recognize and control these responses, the techniques can be used to treat a wide range of mental and physical health problems. For example, controlling responses might help prevent a panic attack, control a migraine, or cure incontinence. There are numerous conditions that might be treated with biofeedback. Additionally, biofeedback is said to help improve overall health and a sense of well-being.

# Biologically Based Therapies

Biologically based CAM therapies use substances found in nature, such as herbs, foods, and vitamins. Some examples include dietary supplements, herbal products, and the use of other natural but as yet scientifically unproven therapies.

Dietary and herbal products are clearly becoming mainstream treatments for patients. As our population ages, individuals are looking for ways to stay young, remain or become thin, sleep and think better, and, in general, maintain an optimal state of health. Many of them are turning to dietary and herbal supplements in hopes of meeting their goals.

As a medical assistant, you should have up-to-date information about dietary and herbal products to help yourself and your patients make informed decisions about using them. You should be able to provide patients with reliable resources for information about dietary and herbal products. However, remember to refer a patient with specific questions to the practitioner.

**Dietary Supplements.** **Dietary supplements** were defined by Congress in 1994 as products that:

- Are intended to supplement a diet
- Contain one or more dietary ingredients, such as vitamins, minerals, herbs, or other substances

- Are intended to be taken by mouth
- Are labeled as a dietary supplement

There is one important difference between dietary supplements and medications. Medications must meet approval of the FDA prior to being marketed and sold. (The FDA is a government agency that regulates the quality of food and drugs sold in the United States.) Manufacturers of drugs must provide scientific documentation of the effectiveness of a drug before it can be marketed. On the other hand, manufacturers of dietary supplements do not have to provide evidence of effectiveness or safety. (Of course, they are not permitted to market or sell a product that is proven unsafe.) However, once a supplement is marketed the FDA must prove that the product is not safe to have it taken from the market. For example, the dietary supplement made from ephedrine alkaloids (ephedra) was on the market to assist with weight loss and claimed to enhance sports performance. After research, the FDA found that it presented significant and unreasonable health risks as marketed and issued a regulation prohibiting its sale and advised consumers to stop taking the product.

Dietary supplements are not standardized between batches or among manufacturers. **Standardization** is a process that ensures the consistency and quality of each batch of supplement that is produced. Thus, the amount and quality of a dietary supplement may differ between batches by one manufacturer or between the same supplement made by two manufacturers. In contrast, medications approved by the FDA must be standardized and will always be consistent between batches and manufacturers.

The FDA does require that certain information appear on the labels of dietary supplements. Dietary supplements may include claims on their labels that describe the effect of a substance in maintaining the body's normal structure or function. It may not imply that the product treats or cures a disease. For example a label might state, "Promotes healthy joints and bones." The FDA does not review or authorize this claim, so the manufacturer is required to also place a **disclaimer** on the product. This disclaimer is a statement indicating that the claims have not been evaluated by the FDA. For example, the disclaimer for the claim above would be: "This statement has not been evaluated by the Food and Drug Administration. This product is not intended to diagnose, treat, cure or prevent disease." See Figure 31-2 for an example of a label that meets the FDA's labeling requirements.

Dietary supplements include vitamins, minerals, herbals, and other substances. Vitamins and minerals are necessary for proper nutrition and a recommended daily amount has been established by the FDA. Frequently, people take vitamin and mineral supplements, especially when their diet lacks a variety of foods. These necessary vitamins and minerals are discussed in more detail in Chapter 36, Nutrition and Special Diets.

Many individuals take certain vitamins and minerals in an amount greater than recommended to improve health or prevent illness. This is sometimes called megadose

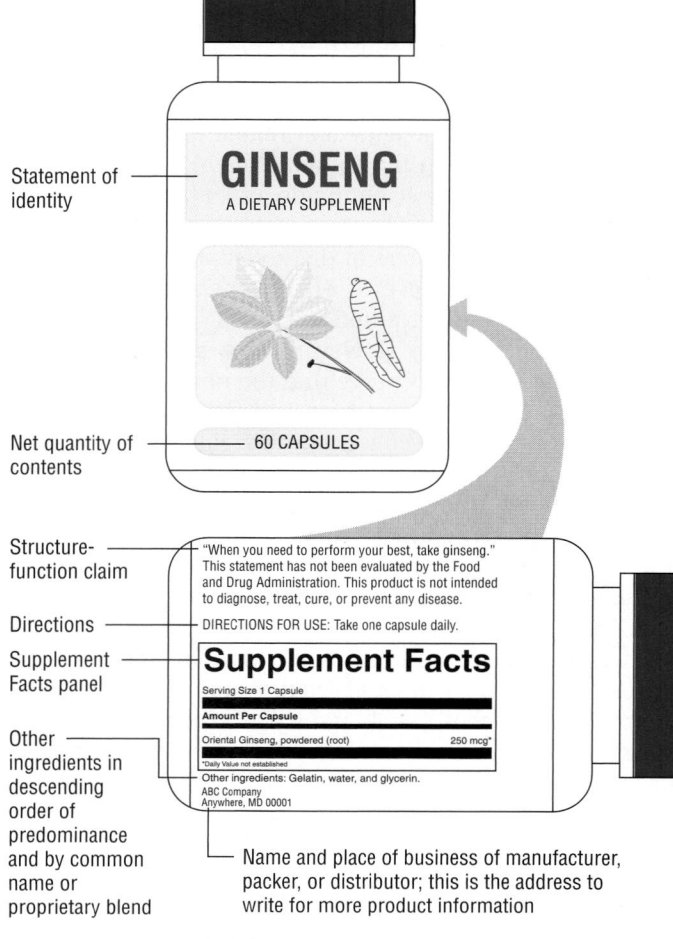

**Anatomy of the New Requirements for Dietary Supplement Labels (Effective March 1999)**

Statement of identity

Net quantity of contents

Structure-function claim

Directions

Supplement Facts panel

Other ingredients in descending order of predominance and by common name or proprietary blend

**GINSENG**
A DIETARY SUPPLEMENT

60 CAPSULES

"When you need to perform your best, take ginseng." This statement has not been evaluated by the Food and Drug Administration. This product is not intended to diagnose, treat, cure, or prevent any disease.

DIRECTIONS FOR USE: Take one capsule daily.

**Supplement Facts**
Serving Size 1 Capsule

**Amount Per Capsule**

Oriental Ginseng, powdered (root)       250 mcg*

*Daily Value not established

Other ingredients: Gelatin, water, and glycerin.
ABC Company
Anywhere, MD 00001

Name and place of business of manufacturer, packer, or distributor; this is the address to write for more product information

**Figure 31-2.** The Food and Drug Administration provides specific guidelines for the information found on a dietary supplement label.

vitamin and/or mineral therapy. Megadose vitamins and minerals are generally taken in amounts at least 10 times greater than the recommended daily allowance (RDA).

Herbals and other substances do not have a recommended amount established by the FDA. These are taken for specific effects to improve health or treat illness.

As a medical assistant, you should have a working knowledge of dietary supplements, their uses, and their possible adverse reactions or interactions. Patients should report all dietary supplements they take along with their medications. Tables 31-3 and 31-4 provide information about common dietary supplements, including examples of megadose vitamin and mineral therapy.

## Manipulative and Body-Based Methods

Manipulative and body-based CAM methods are based on manipulation and/or movement of one or more parts of the body. The two most common types include **massage** therapy and chiropractic manipulation. In fact, some research indicates that visits to chiropractors and massage therapists combined represent about 50% of all visits to CAM practitioners. Some other types of manipulative and body-based methods include:

- **Reflexology.** A manual therapy of the foot and/or hand in which pressure is applied to "reflex" zones and points mapped out on the feet or hands. (See Figure 31-3). Related to massage therapy, reflexology is gaining popularity.
- Alexander technique. This therapy educates patients, providing them with guidance about ways to improve posture and movement, and to use muscles efficiently.

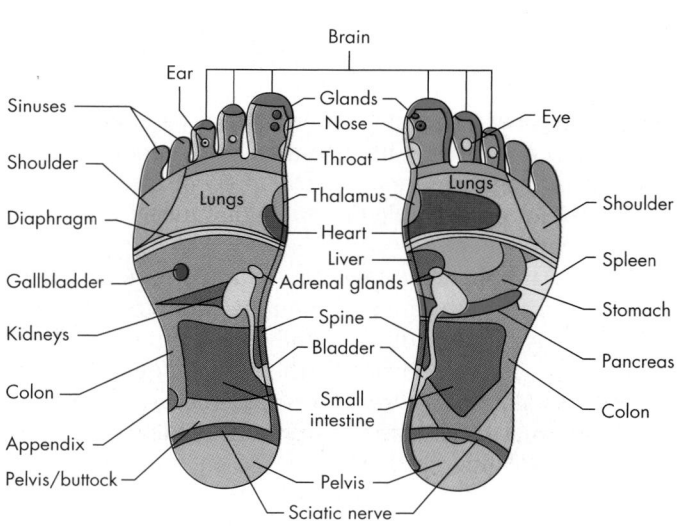

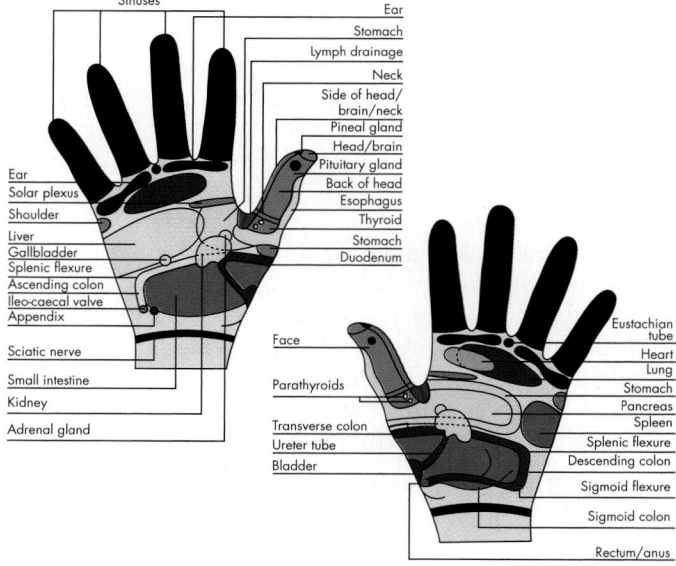

**Figure 31-3.** Hand and foot map used in reflexology. Each part of the foot and hand has a corresponding body part. Treatment to the hand and/or foot promotes healing in the area noted on this map.

## TABLE 31-3  Common Dietary Supplements–Vitamins and Minerals

| Common Name | Megadose Amount (per Day) | Claims/Benefits | *Possible* Health Hazard from Megadose Therapy |
|---|---|---|---|
| Vitamin A | 25,000 or more international units (IUs) | Antioxidant that protects cells from free radicals that can cause chronic diseases | Birth defects, bone abnormalities, and severe liver disease |
| Vitamin B$_6$ | More than 100 milligrams | Treats asthma and cardiovascular disease | Balance difficulties, nerve injury causing changes in touch sensation |
| Niacin | Slow-released doses of 500 mg or more or immediate-release doses of 750 mg or more | Decreases cholesterol | Stomach pain, vomiting, bloating, nausea, cramping, diarrhea, liver disease, muscle disease, eye damage, and heart injury |
| Selenium | 800 to 1000 micrograms (mcg) | Reduces cancer risk | Tissue damage of the hair, nails, liver, nervous system, and teeth |
| Beta carotene | More than 1.5 to 1.8 mg | Improves the body's chemical reactions to dangerous free radicals, with health-promoting effects such as preventing lung cancer or heart disease for ex-smokers | Lung cancer, death |
| Vitamin E | More than 400 to 1000 IUs | Improves the body's chemical reactions to dangerous free radicals, with health-promoting effects such as preventing lung cancer or heart disease for ex-smokers. | Increased blood coagulation, stroke, and death |
| Vitamin C | More than 100 mg | Improves the body's chemical reactions to dangerous free radicals, with health-promoting effects such as preventing lung cancer or heart disease for ex-smokers | Gastrointestinal distress and kidney stones |
| Vitamin D | More than 2.5 mg | Treats tuberculosis, rheumatoid arthritis, and skin disorders | Bone demineralization, tendonitis, and skeletal pain; potential heart and kidney damage |
| Folic acid | More than 1000 mg | Reduces the risk of heart disease | Without known adverse effects |

- Bowen technique. A gentle massage of muscles and tendons over acupuncture and reflex points.
- Craniosacral therapy. A form of massage that uses gentle pressure on the plates of the patient's skull.
- Feldenkrais method. Group classes and hands-on lessons that are designed to improve the coordination of the whole person through comfortable, effective, and intelligent movement.
- Rolfing. Deep tissue massage.

- Trager bodywork. Slight rocking and shaking of the patient's trunk and limbs in a rhythmic fashion.
- Tui Na. Application of pressure with the fingers and thumb, and manipulation of specific points on the body, known as *acupoints*.

**Massage.** The practice of massage uses pressure, kneading, stroking, vibration, and tapping to positively affect the health and well-being of patients. Massage helps

## TABLE 31-4 Dietary Supplements—Herbals and Other Substances

| Common Name | Uses/Claims | Side Effects | Precautions/Comments |
|---|---|---|---|
| Anabolic steroids | Promote growth of skeletal muscles and the development of male sexual characteristics; used to improve sports performance | Men: reduced sperm production, shrinking of the testicles, male-pattern baldness, breast development<br>Women: masculinization, breast size and body fat decrease, coarse skin, clitoris enlargement, deepened voice | Can also cause short stature, heart enlargement or heart attacks, cancer, rage, mania, or delusions. Many side effects are irreversible. Addiction is possible. Withdrawal causes depression. |
| Black cohosh | Manages symptoms of menopause, such as hot flashes; lowers cholesterol | Stomach discomfort, headaches, heaviness in the legs, nausea, dizziness, increased perspiration, reduced pulse, visual disturbances | Should not be taken by pregnant women or those with breast cancer |
| Cartilage (bovine and shark) | Cancer | Fatigue, nausea, fever, dizziness, bad taste in the mouth, scrotal swelling, constipation, vomiting, low blood pressure, cramping and/or bloating | Can cause an abnormally high level of calcium in the blood |
| Coenzyme Q10 | Treats cancer and Parkinson's disease | Mild insomnia, rash, nausea, fatigue | May interact with medications that lower cholesterol and blood sugar |
| Colloidal silver products | Treat infections and cancer | Argyria (bluish-gray color of skin because of excess silver), seizures, stomach distress, headaches, fevers, kidney damage, fatigue, and skin irritation | May interfere with the absorption of penicillamine, quinolones, tetracyclines, and thyroxine |
| Cranberry | Relieves the symptoms of and reduces the risk of urinary tract infections | Diarrhea | Excessive amounts may result in cramping and diarrhea |
| Echinacea | Aids in wound healing, stimulates immune function | Nausea, vomiting, unpleasant taste, abdominal pain, diarrhea | May shorten the duration of the common cold<br>May help prevent viral infection, although less effective |
| Essiac/Flor-Essence | Relieve pain, detoxify the body, strengthen the immune system, reduce tumor size | Nausea and vomiting, increased bowel movements, frequent urination, swollen glands, skin blemishes, flu-like symptoms, slight headaches | May increase tumor formation |
| Garlic | Lowers blood sugar and cholesterol levels, exhibits antiseptic and antibacterial activity | Strong odor, burning of the mouth and esophagus, nausea, sweating, lightheadedness | To be used cautiously by patients taking anticoagulant and/or antiplatelet agents<br>May interact with anticoagulant and/or antiplatelet agents (use cautiously)<br>*continued* —→ |

**TABLE 31-4** **Dietary Supplements—Herbals and Other Substances** *(continued)*

| Common Name | Uses/Claims | Side Effects | Precautions/Comments |
|---|---|---|---|
| Ginger | Decreases nausea and vomiting, decreases cholesterol, stimulates circulation, decreases cough; used as flavoring; acts as a fungicide, pesticide | High doses may cause drowsiness and decreased platelet aggregation | Use caution in patients taking anticoagulant and/or antiplatelet agents. |
| Ginseng | Increases mental and physical capacity for work, relieves fatigue, enhances the immune system | Nervousness, agitation, breast nodules, vaginal bleeding, hypoglycemia | Interacts with anticoagulants, loop diuretics, and antipsychotic drugs |
| Gingko | Increases circulation, improves memory, relieves anxiety or stress, alleviates tinnitus, improves the symptoms of asthma | Headache, dizziness, palpitations, rash, allergy, nausea, vomiting | Avoid in pregnancy and lactation. Seeds contain toxin associated with seizures and death. Discontinue 2 weeks prior to surgical or dental procedure to prevent increased bleeding |
| Glucosamine Chondroitin | Treats osteoarthritis by reducing pain and slowing down joint cartilage damage | Elevated blood sugar | Dosages vary greatly among manufacturers. Glucosamine should be avoided in patients who are allergic to shellfish. Diabetics and people using blood thinners should use with caution. |
| Kava | Relieves the symptoms associated with stress; exhibits sedative activity | Skin rash, visual disturbances, risk of dependence | Contraindicated in pregnancy, lactation, and patients who have depression. Enhances the effect of other sedatives. Not to be used while driving or operating heavy machinery. Use should be limited to three months. |
| Melatonin | Sleep disorders | None noted with short-term use | Long-term use is not suggested |
| Milkthistle | Protects the liver from damage and hepatitis C | Allergic reactions, stomach upset, nausea, diarrhea | None noted |
| Mistletoe extracts | Increases uterine and intestinal motility; provides anticancer activity | Allergy, toxic syndrome (nausea, delirium, bradycardia, hypertension, hallucinations, diarrhea) | All parts of the plant are toxic and may cause cardiac arrest. |

*continued* ⟶

## TABLE 31-4  Dietary Supplements—Herbals and Other Substances (concluded)

| Common Name | Uses/Claims | Side Effects | Precautions/Comments |
|---|---|---|---|
| Methylsulfonyl-methane (MSM) | Relieves stomach upset, improves immune system function, relieves musculoskeletal pain and arthritis | None reported | Possible vision problems |
| Omega-3 fatty acids | Improve heart health; reduce hypertension; improve rheumatoid arthritis, lupus, Raynaud's disease, and other autoimmune diseases, depression; prevent cancer | Possible fishy aftertaste, flatulence, diarrhea | Intake is especially important in pregnancy. Use with caution in patients who bruise or bleed easily or are taking heparin or warfarin. |
| Reishi/Lingzhi | Improves immunity; anti-inflammatory; treats cancer, liver disease, AIDS, and high blood pressure | Dizziness, itchiness, and thirst resulting from increased defecation and urination | Reishi is the Japanese name and Lingzhi is the Chinese name; comes from the mushroom Ganoderma Lucidum |
| SAMe (S-adeno-sylmethionine) | May enhance mood and help manage the symptoms of osteoarthritis, fibromyalgia, liver disorders, migraine headache, and insomnia | Nausea, vomiting | Avoid use in patients with bipolar disorder, as the agent may trigger a manic phase |
| Saw palmetto | Relieves symptoms of benign prostatic hypertrophy | Nausea | Contraindicated in pregnancy. May interfere with the metabolism of hormones. |
| Soy | Prevents hot flashes and symptoms of menopause | Menstrual changes, stomach upset, diarrhea | Use with caution in patients with thyroid conditions |
| St. John's wort | May enhance mood and have inhibitory effects on viruses | Dry mouth, dizziness, constipation, photosensitivity, confusion, insomnia, nervousness | Products vary in content. Avoid use with tricyclic antidepressants, selective serotonin reuptake inhibitors (SSRIs), and monoamine oxidase (MAO) inhibitors. |
| Tea (green) | Lowers cholesterol levels; may decrease the risk of cancer; prevents cavities | Agitation, nervousness, insomnia, allergic reactions | Use may impair iron metabolism. Avoid use in individuals sensitive to caffeine. |
| Valerian | Insomnia | Drowsiness | Avoid use with other sedative-hypnotic agents. |

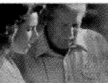

# Educating the Patient

## Using Dietary Supplements

Frequently, patients choose to take various types of dietary supplements in addition to their prescribed medications. These may include vitamins, minerals, or any other type of over-the-counter (OTC) supplements. When asked about medications, in many cases, the patient neglects to mention supplements taken because they may not have been prescribed by a physician. You should teach the patient the importance of reporting any and all supplements that they take in addition to prescribed medications. Encourage them to bring the bottles when visiting the clinic and ask specific questions about the amount they are taking. Check the bottle for the exact dose and record all information in the patient's chart. Because supplements can interact with prescribed medications, all medications and dietary supplements should be included on the chart. Table 31-5 provides just a few examples of dietary supplement-drug interactions.

**TABLE 31-5  Examples of Dietary Supplement-Drug Interactions**

| Dietary Supplements | Drug Type | Interaction |
| --- | --- | --- |
| Garlic, gingko, ginger | Antiplatelet agents, anticoagulants | Increased risk of bleeding |
| St. John's wort | Antidepressants | Increased blood pressure |
| Kava, valerian | Sedatives, benzodiazepines | Increased sedative effects |
| Ginseng | Decongestants, sympathomimetics | Increased nervousness, insomnia, agitation, palpitations |

the patient relax and counteracts the effects of stress. During massage, the heart rate and blood pressure are lowered and blood circulation and lymph flow are increased. Massage helps reduce pain caused by tight muscles and helps relax muscle spasms.

Massage benefits the mind as well as the body: It helps improve concentration, promotes restful sleep, and helps the mind relax. Many patients find that they handle daily stresses better when they have regular massage. People who get massages on a regular basis find that they are not ill as often or as severely and that they feel less stressed and tense. Some patients notice their muscles beginning to tighten and are aware that if they get a massage, it will decrease muscle tension before it becomes severe.

Certain types of massage are part of TCM. For example, *Shiatsu* and acupressure are types of massage that use finger pressure. They are based on the theory of qi from TCM. Practitioners of this type of massage believe that blocked meridians cause physical discomfort, and the finger pressure of shiatsu applied to specific meridian points releases the blockage and balances energy flow. Shiatsu is generally done on a mat on the floor rather than on a massage table. There are more than 200 other types of massage. Three of the more common types include Swedish, neuromuscular, and seated massage.

***Swedish Massage.***   Swedish massage is one of the best-known and most frequently taught massage techniques. It stimulates circulation and lymph flow with five basic strokes that manipulate the soft tissues of the body. The strokes include pétrissage (kneading), effleurage (stroking), tapotement (percussion), vibration, and friction. Oils and/or lotions are used to reduce friction on the patient's skin. One type of Swedish massage is done immediately after exercise on warm muscles. Another type is a stress-reduction massage that is done with the same basic strokes on patients who have not been exercising (Figure 31-4).

***Neuromuscular Massage.***   Neuromuscular massage is applied to specific muscles and helps release tension and knots, relieve pain and release pressure on nerves, and increase blood flow. Trigger point therapy is one type of neuromuscular massage in which strong finger pressure is applied to trigger points in the muscles.

***Seated Massage.***   Shiatsu and Swedish techniques may be used to provide massage to a patient who is fully clothed and seated in a specially designed massage chair. This type of massage is very popular for short massages focused on the back and the neck. The therapist can easily provide massage for clients in a business or commercial setting, such as an airport or a shopping mall (Figure 31-5).

**Chiropractic Medicine.**   Chiropractic manipulation involves adjustments of the joints of the spine, as well as other joints and muscles. A **chiropractor** treats people who are ill or in pain without using prescription drugs or surgery. Chiropractors believe that the body has a natural

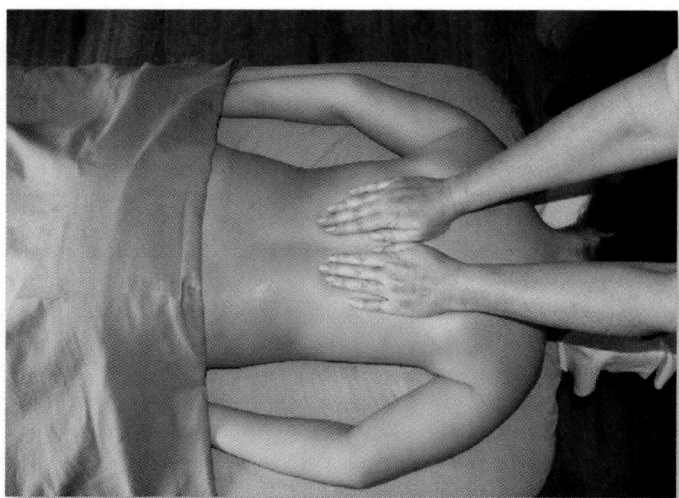

**Figure 31-4.** An example of Swedish massage. Massage uses kneading, pressure, stroking, and human touch to alleviate pain and promote healing through relaxation.

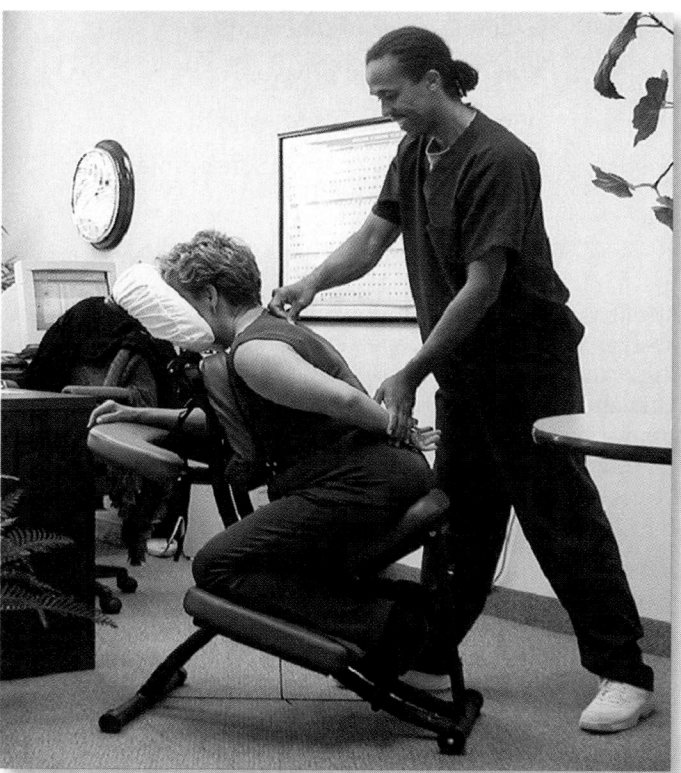

**Figure 31-5.** Seated massage is a very popular type of CAM therapy practiced at airports, shopping malls, and businesses.

power to heal itself. They use manual treatments, physical therapy treatments, exercise programs, nutritional advice, and lifestyle modification to help correct the problem that causes the pain. The manual treatments they use are called **adjustments.**

Chiropractors focus their treatment on the patient's spine. The spinal nerves relay messages from the brain and spinal cord to the rest of the body and return messages back to the brain. When a vertebrae of the spine is subluxated (has lost its proper position in relationship to vertebrae above and below it), it can restrict the function of the spinal nerves. A chiropractic adjustment is a manual treatment to re-align the vertebra and restore the function of the spinal nerves. Some chiropractors adjust using a mechanical tool, such as an activator. Some chiropractors adjust with gentle pressure or by relaxing muscles so the vertebra realigns without force. During the adjustment, the patient may hear a popping sound. As a medical assistant, it may be your responsibility to inform the patient this may occur.

People who come to a chiropractor frequently have pain in their back, arm(s), neck, shoulder(s), or leg(s), or they may have frequent headaches. Spinal adjustments, exercise, early return to activities, and OTC pain medications have been very effective for treating these conditions. Chiropractic care has been found to be effective in treating other problems that may occur as a result of spinal subluxation that interferes with nerve function. These include respiratory problems and digestive disorders.

Most chiropractors have a medical assistant to help them care for patients. Their duties will be similar to those performed in a medical physician's office. When a patient visits a chiropractor, the doctor will do an examination and take a history. The chiropractor asks many of the same questions about health problems that a medical doctor asks: illnesses, surgeries, and current symptoms. The chiropractor also asks questions about lifestyle, medications, nutrition, stress, and exercise. Chiropractors also evaluate past or recent trauma to the neck and spine, such as from falls, car accidents, and sports injuries.

Chiropractors take x-rays, perform muscle testing, and analyze posture to make their diagnosis. In some states, the medical assistant may assist with the x-ray process. Chiropractors do not diagnose in the same way as medical doctors; rather, their diagnosis is based on which vertebrae are subluxated and in which direction they have tilted or twisted. The chiropractor then develops a treatment plan based on these findings. The treatment plan generally requires several visits per week for several weeks or months. Because this treatment does not involve prescription drugs or surgery, the body needs time for healing and correction to occur.

When the patient returns for follow-up visits, the chiropractor will adjust the areas of the spine that are subluxated (Figure 31-6). Some chiropractors use heat, ultrasound, gentle traction, or massage therapy prior to the adjustment. These therapies help relax the tight muscles around the spine so the vertebra moves easily and the adjustment lasts longer. As a medical assistant, you may assist the chiropractor with any of these types of therapies.

Chiropractors often see patients who are not ill or in pain. After an acute condition has been successfully treated, patients may return for maintenance care. This means that the chiropractor checks the spine to be sure that no subluxations exist. (A subluxation can be present without causing any symptoms, so the chiropractor checks

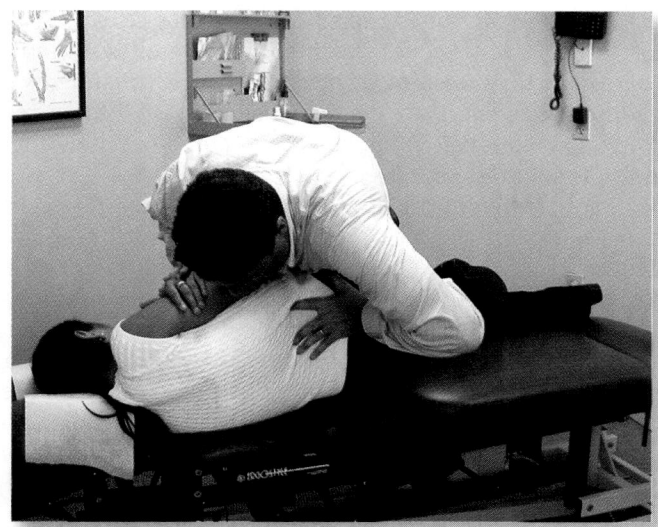

**Figure 31-6.** A chiropractor performs manual adjustment on the spine to realign the vertebrae and relieve pain and pressure.

for problems before they become illnesses or cause pain.) Chiropractors see patients frequently at the beginning of treatment for an acute problem, and then may see them for years for maintenance care. Thus, it is common for the chiropractor and his or her medical assistant to have a close relationship with their patients.

## Energy Therapies

Energy therapies involve the use of energy fields. There are essentially two types: bioelectromagnetic-based therapies and biofield therapies. **Bioelectromagnetic-based therapies** use the measurable energy fields in such things as magnetic therapy, millimeter wave therapy, sound energy therapy, and light therapy. **Biofield therapies** are intended to affect energy fields that surround and penetrate the human body. These energy fields have not yet been scientifically proven.

**Bioelectromagnetic-Based Therapies.** Electricity and magnetic energy exists in the body. Electromagnetic therapy is used to balance the electromagnetic fields (EMFs). When the EMFs are out of balance, they disrupt the body's chemical makeup and result in disease and illness. Although as of this writing no scientific evidence has proven this theory, the use of bioelectromagnetic therapy is common for things such as cancer, pain, stress, insomnia, and infection. The most common type of bioelectromagnetic-based therapy is magnetic therapy.

*Magnetic Therapy.* **Magnetic therapy** involves the use of magnets of varying sizes and strengths that are placed on the body to relieve pain or treat disease. The principle of magnetic therapy is based upon the fact that cells and tissues in the human body give off electromagnetic impulses. The belief is that the presence of illness disrupts these fields. Using magnets with various energy fields to penetrate the body corrects the disturbance and restores health to the affected tissue or system.

Magnets can be attached to a wrist, elbow, knee, ankle, foot, waist, or lower back. They may be thin metal bands, attached to jewelry, or attached with adhesive. They may even be embedded in a pillow, shoes, or mattress pad. The amount and length of time of treatment vary, depending upon the condition.

Although the FDA considers magnetic therapy to be without medical value, it also considers it to be relatively harmless and therefore does not regulate its use. Because it is a noninvasive, drug-free form of treatment, it has few or no side effects. However, this type of therapy should not be used by someone with a cardiac pacemaker or defibrillator.

**Biofield Therapies.** Biofield therapies manipulate the energy field believed to surround the body by applying pressure and/or manipulating the body by placing the hands in, or through, these fields. Two examples include Reiki and therapeutic touch.

*Reiki.* **Reiki** is one type of biofield therapy. Reiki is based on the principle of qi, discussed earlier (Figure 31-7). Reiki is believed to have Tibetan and Buddhist origins. Reiki practitioners use visualization and touch to balance the patient's energy flow and to bring healing energy to specific organs and glands. The practitioner serves as a channel for the life energy, which promotes emotional and physical healing.

*Therapeutic Touch.* **Therapeutic touch** is based on an ancient therapy called the laying on of hands. It was reconceived in the early 1970s by a registered nurse (RN). Essentially, the hands are used to direct human energies to help or heal someone who is ill. Practitioners of this therapy detect and manipulate the patient's energy field through a series of steps. Although little scientific evidence exists about the effectiveness of this therapy, supporters of the practice state there are over 100,000 practitioners in the United States. Therapeutic touch is sometimes practiced in conjunction with massage. Many individuals utilize therapeutic touch to improve their health and well-being.

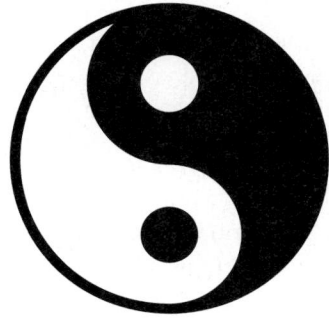

**Figure 31-7.** The theory of qi. The figure represents a perfectly balanced yin and yang. In qi, these two forces must be balanced in order for the body to be in harmony.
Source: Booth: *Health Care Science Technology,* Figure 21-9, page 695.

# Patients Seeking CAM Therapy

Although many conventional medicine practitioners are incorporating CAM into their treatment of patients, it should be noted that this is not always the case. Some physicians choose not to use CAM therapies because they consider them to be untested and unproven. In some cases, they may discourage patients from seeking, using, or continuing to use these treatments. Patients do have the right to make their own choice regarding the use of CAM treatments and the use of CAM by patients is increasing.

CAM approaches and therapies are more common in recent years for a variety of reasons. Patients are seeking agents and treatments to manage their health problems that are less expensive, have fewer side effects, and are more accessible than traditional medical interventions. Additionally, an increase in spirituality, personal growth, and environmentalism has sparked the growth in CAM practices. Many individuals also practice CAM therapies as part of preventive health care. No matter the reason, the growth in the use of CAM therapies is remarkable.

The failure of traditional medical interventions to treat certain diseases and conditions is considered one of the largest reasons for the increased use of CAM. Traditional medicine offers little to patients with chronic debilitating conditions such as cancer, chronic pain, and HIV. These patients tend to be the most frequent users of CAM. After trying conventional medicine with no cure or even relief, patients turn to CAM. In some cases, individuals use CAM to treat the side effects of conventional medicine's treatment.

Cancer patients frequently use at least two CAM therapies. These include things such as spiritual approaches, relaxation, exercise, lifestyle, diet, and nutritional supplements. When asked, patients using these therapies consistently believed that CAM helped improve their quality of life and their ability to cope with life's stress and illness. In general, the concept of maintaining overall wellness to cope with the stress of cancer and cancer treatments is very popular. There are medical facilities that treat cancer using conventional, complementary, and alternative therapies as standard practice.

Pain frequently motivates a patient to use CAM. Patients with chronic back or neck pain are often seen at a chiropractor's office. Chiropractors who treat pain tend to retain a larger portion of their patients than traditional practitioners. Other types of pain, such as headache and arthritis, may cause a patient to use a CAM therapy such as massage or acupuncture. Many individuals with pain prefer to use CAM therapy to treat the pain rather than take pain medications to mask the pain. Given the possibility of addiction to pain medication, CAM therapy is frequently considered a better long-term treatment for chronic pain.

HIV infection will frequently cause a patient to seek CAM therapies. HIV patients commonly use high doses of vitamin C and E, multiple vitamin and mineral supplements, and garlic to combat their illness. A smaller portion of HIV patients use marijuana to treat weight loss, nausea, and vomiting. HIV patients also tend to visit their CAM practitioner more frequently than their traditional medicine practitioner. Patients with HIV are frequently looking for ways to cope with the chronic illness and CAM helps provide that means.

# Insurance and CAM

Although CAM therapies are becoming increasingly popular with both patients and practitioners, in general, insurance companies are not following suit. Many therapies, such as chiropractic care, massage, and acupuncture, are increasingly recognized as useful; however, most insurance plans do not offer substantial, if any, coverage for these treatments. Insurance companies are providing some benefits

## Reflecting On . . . Cultural Issues

### Ethnic Differences in CAM Usage

An individual's culture may have an effect on the type and amount of CAM therapy used by a patient. Surveys discussed in the White House Commission on Complementary and Alternative Medicine Policy (WHCCAMP) indicate the following:

- About one-half of the Mexican-American and Hispanic populations use CAM at least one time a year, including things such as herbal medicine, spiritual healing techniques, and traditional healers.

- Native Americans use herbal medicine, spiritual healing techniques, and traditional healers at a higher rate than the general population.

As a medical assistant, you should be respectful to patients of all cultures who use any type of CAM, even if you do not accept or agree with its use for yourself. Every patient has a right to choose his or her own therapy.

for alternative therapies. Yet these plans do not always cover alternative therapies; they may just offer a limited amount of coverage and often put restrictions on the coverage. In response to the need for CAM health insurance coverage, some unique alternative health insurance companies and insurance policies have become available.

Both state and federal lawmakers have become interested in the practice, availability, and reimbursement of CAM. In 1997, 137 laws addressing access and reimbursement of CAM were enacted in 41 states. In 1998, 91 laws were enacted in 39 states. By the end of 2000, 38 states required insurers to offer chiropractic coverage and seven required acupuncture coverage. One state, Alaska, requires coverage of naturopathy. New laws on both the state and federal levels are being proposed and enacted on a continuing basis.

Even with current laws regarding CAM, the lack of clear research and data documenting the effectiveness of CAM treatments has prevented insurance companies from paying for many of them. Insurance companies do not want to pay for services that do not document scientific evidence of effectiveness.

Consumers usually only receive reimbursement for treatments that cure, not those that heal. Curing refers to eliminating a disease physiologically while healing focuses on moving toward wholeness, growth, and a greater balance at physical, mental, social, and emotional levels. Insurance companies emphasize the physiological or biochemical responses to treatments, not the emotional, psychological, or spiritual effects. Thus, treatment for healing rather than curing an illness is usually not coverable.

Some studies show that although reliance on conventional medicine does not disappear when patients turn to CAM, trips to traditional physicians may decrease. Also, patients who have access to alternative therapies may become more concerned with prevention and may not use as many expensive traditional treatments. For example,

nutritional therapy may be used to reduce weight, thus preventing cardiovascular disease. Therefore, CAM therapies may have the potential to decrease overall health-care costs. However, with lack of data to support this information, again, little or no insurance payments are made for these alternative therapies.

CAM insurance coverage is a positive step for CAM practitioners, patients, and other supporters. As more CAM therapies are accepted, researched, and practiced, insurance companies should increase their coverage of such therapies. Currently, CAM practitioners, such as chiropractors, acupuncturists, and others, may be covered by insurance.

Insurance coverage for CAM therapies will vary from state to state and from insurance company to insurance company. It is also expected that, in time, more CAM therapies will be reimbursed. As a medical assistant, it is your responsibility to be knowledgeable of the CAM treatments performed at your facility, including whether or not it is covered by health insurance. If no payment from insurance is expected, payment at the time the services are completed is usually expected from the patient.

# Regulation of CAM Therapies

With the increased consumer use of CAM, the scope of practice and licensure of CAM practitioners has been and continues to be of concern. Laws vary and are usually designed to protect health-care consumers. Because of concerns regarding the safety and efficacy of CAM, Congress established the Office of Alternative Medicine (OAM) at the National Institutes of Health (NIH) in 1992. Its goal was to conduct research on complementary and alternative therapies. In 1999, this office became the National Center for Complementary and Alternative Medicine (NCCAM). NCCAM conducts and supports CAM research

## Points on Practice

### Understanding CAM and Insurance

To assist your patients and practitioners, discover the laws about CAM insurance coverage in your area. In addition to calling the insurance company directly, there are two resources for your use. First, there is likely to be one or more national professional associations for practitioners of that treatment. For example, there are associations for chiropractors and naturopathic physicians. These organizations frequently monitor insurance coverage and reimbursement for their specialty. You can try an Internet search for the specific type of practitioner, and then search their website for information about possible insurance reimbursement.

As a second resource for CAM insurance coverage, each of the 50 states, as well as the District of Columbia and the four U.S. territories, has an agency that regulates the insurance industry, enforces insurance laws, and assists consumers. This agency is often called the office of the state insurance commissioner. Although the specific service each office provides varies by state, they all handle consumer inquiries. Contact your commissioner's office to determine requirements in your state for insurance coverage of a specific CAM treatment.

and provides CAM information to health-care providers and the public. Its four primary areas of focus are:

- Research of CAM therapies through grants and clinical trials
- Training and career development for current or future CAM practitioners
- To develop and hold conferences and educational programs that provide information about CAM therapies
- Integration of scientifically proven CAM practices into conventional medicine, including support for health-care curriculums

## WHCCAMP

In March, 2000, Congress created the White House Commission on Complementary and Alternative Medicine Policy (WHCCAMP). Its purpose was to develop legislative and administrative policy recommendations regarding CAM practices and products. The final report of the Commission was published in late March 2002. It has 29 recommendations and included things such as:

- Increased funding for research
- Increased communication between CAM and conventional medical practitioners
- Increased availability of CAM practitioners
- The provision of quality CAM products to the U.S. consumer
- The encouragement and support of state review and evaluation of CAM practitioners
- Insurance coverage options for safe and effective CAM interventions

This policy was clearly a step in support of CAM. With its implementation, research and legislation is continually being conducted regarding various CAM therapies and practices. Most importantly, the federal government is helping to ensure the safe and effective integration of complementary and alternative health practices and products, thus protecting the health-care consumer.

# Health Fraud

**Health fraud,** as defined by the FDA, is "articles of unproven effectiveness that are promoted to improve health, well-being, or appearance." The unproven articles may be such things as drugs, devices, foods, or cosmetics for human or animal use. Health fraud is basically a deception or trickery related to health prevention or care for profit. It is practiced by individuals or organizations that play on the emotions and desperation of people in order to profit.

Health fraud promoters often target people who are overweight or have serious incurable conditions, including multiple sclerosis, diabetes, Alzheimer's disease, cancer, HIV and AIDS, and arthritis. Hoping to find a cure, improve their health, or just look better, people fall victim

to products and devices that do nothing more than cheat them out of their money and steer them away from useful, proven treatments. In many cases, the products and/or devices could possibly do more harm than good.

The FDA and the Federal Trade Commission (FTC) share responsibility for the regulation of health fraud products. The FTC regulates the advertising of health fraud products. Its mission is to enforce laws and prevent advertising practices that are unfair or deceptive, thus providing consumers with enough information to exercise informed choices. The FDA regulates safety, manufacturing, and product labeling. It scientifically evaluates and monitors claims in labeling, such as package inserts and accompanying literature.

## Health Claims

Claims on labeling that are not medically or scientifically proven must be accompanied by a disclaimer. As described earlier in this chapter, nonproven claims about dietary supplements are not evaluated by the FDA and must include a disclaimer.

The FDA does allow certain scientifically based claims to be made in labeling food and supplements. These claims include FDA-approved claims that show a strong link, based on scientific evidence, between a food substance and a disease or health condition. These approved claims can state only that a food substance reduces the risk of certain health problems, not that it can treat or cure a disease. Two examples of FDA-approved claims allowed in food and supplement labeling are:

- *The vitamin folic acid may reduce the risk of neural tube defect-affected pregnancies.*
- *Calcium may reduce the risk of the bone disease osteoporosis.*

See Table 31-6 for some additional FDA-approved claims. Each of these claims must follow the guidelines and requirements as established by the FDA Center for Food Safety and Applied Nutrition.

## Recognizing Health Fraud

As a medical assistant, you should be aware of how to recognize health fraud. This knowledge will not only help you make wise decisions about your own health care but provide you with suggestions for your patients. As a medical assistant, patients frequently ask you about health care and products. You should suggest they discuss the care or product with the practitioner at your facility. However, the following are some general suggestions to help you or the patient determine possible health fraud:

- Check with the Better Business Bureau or attorney general's office to see if any complaints have been made against the product or manufacturer.
- Check with the appropriate health-care group. For example, if a practice or product claims to cure cancer,

## TABLE 31-6 FDA-Approved Health Claims*

| Approved Claim | Example Claim Statement |
| --- | --- |
| Calcium and osteoporosis | Regular exercise and a healthy diet with enough calcium help teens and young, adult white and Asian women maintain good bone health and may reduce their high risk of osteoporosis later in life. |
| Sodium and hypertension | Diets low in sodium may reduce the risk of high blood pressure, a disease associated with many factors. |
| Dietary fat and cancer | The development of cancer depends on many factors. A diet low in total fat may reduce the risk of some cancers. |
| Dietary saturated fat and cholesterol, and the risk of coronary heart disease | Although many factors affect heart disease, diets low in saturated fat and cholesterol may reduce the risk of this disease. |
| Fiber-containing grain products, fruits, and vegetables, and cancer | Low-fat diets rich in fiber-containing grain products, fruits, and vegetables may reduce the risk of some types of cancer, a disease associated with many factors. |
| Fruits, vegetables, and grain products that contain fiber, particularly soluble fiber, and the risk of coronary heart disease | Diets low in saturated fat and cholesterol and rich in fruits, vegetables, and grain products that contain some types of dietary fiber, particularly soluble fiber, may reduce the risk of heart disease, a disease associated with many factors. |
| Fruits and vegetables, and cancer | Low-fat diets rich in fruits and vegetables (foods that are low in fat and may contain dietary fiber, Vitamin A, or Vitamin C) may reduce the risk of some types of cancer, a disease associated with many factors. Broccoli is high in Vitamin A and C, and it is a good source of dietary fiber. |
| Folate and neural tube defects | Healthful diets with adequate folate may reduce a woman's risk of having a child with a brain or spinal cord defect. |
| Dietary sugar alcohol and dental caries | Full claim: Frequent between-meal consumption of foods high in sugars and starches promotes tooth decay. The sugar alcohols in [*name of food*] do not promote tooth decay.<br><br>Shortened claim (on small packages only): Does not promote tooth decay |
| Soluble fiber from certain foods and the risk of coronary heart disease | Soluble fiber from foods such as [*name of soluble fiber source, and, if desired, name of food product*], as part of a diet low in saturated fat and cholesterol, may reduce the risk of heart disease. A serving of [*name of food product*] supplies __ grams of the [*necessary daily dietary intake for the benefit*] soluble fiber from [*name of soluble fiber source*] necessary per day to have this effect. |
| Soy protein and the risk of coronary heart disease | (1) 25 grams of soy protein a day, as part of a diet low in saturated fat and cholesterol, may reduce the risk of heart disease. A serving of [*name of food*] supplies __ grams of soy protein.<br><br>(2) Diets low in saturated fat and cholesterol that include 25 grams of soy protein a day may reduce the risk of heart disease. One serving of [*name of food*] provides __ grams of soy protein. |
| Plant sterol/stanol esters and the risk of coronary heart disease | (1) Foods containing at least 0.65 gram per serving of vegetable oil sterol esters, eaten twice a day with meals for a daily total intake of at least 1.3 grams, as part of a diet low in saturated fat and cholesterol, may reduce the risk of heart disease. A serving of [*name of food*] supplies __ grams of vegetable oil sterol esters.<br><br>(2) Diets low in saturated fat and cholesterol that include two servings of foods that provide a daily total of at least 3.4 grams of plant stanol esters in two meals may reduce the risk of heart disease. A serving of [*name of food*] supplies __ grams of plant stanol esters. |

*continued* ⟶

## TABLE 31-6 FDA-Approved Health Claims* (concluded)

| Approved Claim | Example Claim Statement |
|---|---|
| Whole grain foods and the risk of heart disease and certain cancers | Diets rich in whole grain foods and other plant foods and low in total fat, saturated fat, and cholesterol may reduce the risk of heart disease and some cancers. |
| Potassium and the risk of high blood pressure and stroke | Diets containing foods that are a good source of potassium and that are low in sodium may reduce the risk of high blood pressure and stroke. |

*Adapted from the FDA Center for Food Safety, "A Food Labeling Guide, Appendix C."

check with the American Cancer Society for more information.

- Contact the FDA by phone or through their website. The FDA and the NCCAM provides alerts and advisories on their respective websites.

- Remember, if the claim seems too good to be true, it probably is not true. For example, claims that indicate they can help you lose 20 pounds without diet or exercise or cure diabetes are probably not true and should be questioned.

- If the product or practice is unproven, it is best to get a second opinion from a medical specialist.

- Talk to friends and family members. Be aware of "secret cures or treatments."

## Summary

Complementary and alternative medicine is therapy and products outside the scope of traditional or conventional medicine. Complementary medicine is used in conjunction with conventional medicine. Alternative medicine is typically used as a replacement for conventional medicine. A new type of medicine called integrative medicine has emerged when conventional medicine and scientifically proven CAM therapies are used together.

There are five classifications for CAM. They include alternative medical systems, mind-body interventions, biologically based therapies, manipulative and body-based methods, and energy therapies. Each of these classifications has various types of products and therapies associated with it. Patients seeking CAM may be looking for low-cost products and services that help to maintain health and prevent disease so they turn to CAM. Other patients are turning to CAM for additional options. Health-care practitioners are using many types of complementary therapy as they become accepted and, in many cases, scientifically proven.

A basic understanding of CAM therapies, insurance reimbursement, and health fraud are important aspects of the medical assistant's role.

The NCCAM conducts and supports CAM research and provides CAM information to health-care providers and the public. State and federal laws have been enacted to help regulate CAM and more laws and regulations are expected as research is conducted. Staying abreast of these laws and current health fraud information is mandatory in this changing health-care environment.

## CASE STUDY QUESTIONS

Now that you have completed this chapter, review the case study at the beginning of the chapter and answer the following questions:

1. What is CAM?
2. What types of therapies are included in CAM?
3. How and when would you use your knowledge of CAM in your career as a medical assistant?

## Discussion Questions

1. What the pros and cons of using complementary and alternative medicine?
2. Compare and contrast the five areas of CAM therapy. Explain which area of CAM therapy you prefer and why.

## Critical Thinking Questions

1. A 23-year-old female states that she is taking the following dietary supplements: saw palmetto, Omega-3 fatty acids, and cranberry capsules. What do you know about these three dietary supplements and what should you do?
2. A patient tells you he is using a miracle cure for his diabetes. What should you say or do?
3. Which of the following practitioners would see a patient for a longer period of time and why: an orthopedic surgeon or a chiropractor?

## Application Activities

1. Contact your state's office of the insurance commissioner and determine what types of CAM are covered by insurance in your state.
2. Visit the offices of different types of local CAM practitioners and interview them to find out more about their services.

## Virtual Fieldtrip

*Visit the McGraw-Hill Higher Education Medical Assisting website at www.mhhe.com/medicalassisting3 to complete the following activities:*

1. Visit the National Center for Complementary and Alternative Medicine website and find the article called "10 Things to Know About Evaluating Medical Resources on the Web." Read and review the information and create a patient brochure, a bulletin board, or a collage that can be used in a physician's office for patient education.
2. The U.S. FDA and the National Center for Complementary and Alternative Medicine provide *alerts and advisories* for CAM therapies. Review their websites and search for the latest postings. Then create patient alert posters, a collage, or a bulletin board for a physician's office.

Open the CD and complete this chapter's practice activities, play the games, listen to the key terms, and test yourself with the interactive review. E-mail, print, and/or save your results to document your proficiency.

# SECTION 4

## PHYSICIAN'S OFFICE LABORATORY PROCEDURES

# Laboratory Equipment and Safety

## MEDICAL ASSISTING COMPETENCIES

*In preparation for the certification examination, you should know the following areas of competence:*

| COMPETENCY | CMA | RMA |
|---|:---:|:---:|
| **Clinical** | | |
| Apply principles of aseptic techniques and infection control, including hand washing | X | X |
| Dispose of biohazardous materials | X | X |
| Practice Standard Precautions | X | X |
| **General/Legal/Professional** | | |
| Recognize and respond to verbal and nonverbal communications by being attentive and adapting communication to the recipient's level of understanding | X | X |
| Be aware of and perform within legal and ethical boundaries | X | X |
| Determine the needs for documentation and reporting, and document accurately and appropriately | X | X |
| Demonstrate knowledge of and monitor current federal and state health-care legislation and regulations; maintain licenses and accreditation | X | X |
| Perform risk management procedures | X | X |
| Perform an inventory of supplies and equipment | | X |
| Operate and maintain facilities, and perform routine maintenance of administrative and clinical equipment safely | X | X |
| Utilize computer software and electronic technology to maintain office systems | X | X |
| Perform quality control procedures | X | X |
| Conduct work within scope of education, training, and ability | | X |

## KEY TERMS

10× lens
artifact
biohazard symbol
centrifuge
Certificate of Waiver tests
compound microscope
control sample
hazard label
objectives
ocular
oil-immersion objective
optical microscope
photometer
physician's office laboratory (POL)
proficiency testing program
qualitative test response
quality assurance program
quality control program
quantitative test result
reagent
reference laboratory
standard

# CHAPTER OUTLINE

- The Role of Laboratory Testing in Patient Care
- The Medical Assistant's Role
- Use of Laboratory Equipment
- Safety in the Laboratory
- Quality Assurance Programs
- Communicating With the Patient
- Record Keeping

# LEARNING OUTCOMES

After completing Chapter 32, you will be able to:

**32.1** Describe the purpose of the physician's office laboratory.

**32.2** List the medical assistant's duties in the physician's office laboratory.

**32.3** Identify important pieces of laboratory equipment.

**32.4** Operate a microscope.

**32.5** Identify the regulatory controls governing procedures completed in the physician's office laboratory.

**32.6** Identify measures to prevent accidents.

**32.7** Describe the goal of a quality assurance program in a physician's office laboratory.

**32.8** Identify the medical assistant's record-keeping responsibilities.

**32.9** Describe correct waste disposal procedures.

**32.10** Describe the need for quality assurance and quality control programs.

**32.11** Maintain accurate documentation, including all logs related to quality control.

**32.12** List common reference materials to consult for information on procedures performed in the physician's office laboratory.

**32.13** Communicate with patients regarding test preparation and follow-up.

# Introduction

Laboratory testing of patients' specimens is an integral component of patient care. Medical assistants often find a role in the clinical laboratory setting, in either the physician's office or a hospital setting. This chapter will introduce you to various types of common laboratory equipment and their use. You will learn about safety in the laboratory mandated by Occupational Safety and Health Administration (OSHA) regulations and steps to aid in preventing accidents. A discussion of the Clinical Laboratory Improvement Amendments of 1988 (CLIA '88) and this law's impact on the laboratory setting is included in this chapter for your understanding of quality assurance, quality control procedures, and required record keeping.

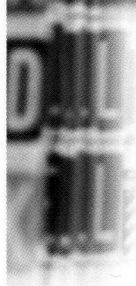

## CASE STUDY

You have been employed as a medical assistant in a physician's office for approximately a year, and part of your duties include the performance of waived laboratory tests in the POL. The POL is supervised by a pathologist and is also staffed by a full-time medical laboratory technologist. When you arrive at the office one morning, you are informed by the office manager that the laboratory technologist has called in sick and that you will have to take over the performance of the moderate-complexity testing in addition to the waived testing. You have never been trained for the moderate-complexity testing, you do not know how to operate the instruments for this testing, nor are you familiar with the proper quality control procedure.

As you read this chapter, consider the following questions:

1. What is a POL?
2. What enactment regulates laboratories, personnel, and the testing they perform?
3. What is the difference between waived testing and moderate-complexity testing?
4. Does quality control have an impact on laboratories? If so, how?
5. Should you perform the testing as requested? Why or why not?

# The Role of Laboratory Testing in Patient Care

Laboratory analysis of blood, urine, or other body fluids and substances provides three kinds of information about a patient. First, regular monitoring through laboratory tests, such as those that are part of an annual exam, can help a physician identify possible diseases or other problems. Second, specific tests can help confirm or contradict a physician's initial diagnosis. Third, laboratory testing can help a physician determine and monitor the proper dosage of a patient's medication.

## Kinds of Laboratories

Some physicians prefer to have all laboratory tests performed by a **reference laboratory,** a laboratory owned and operated by an organization outside the practice. Other physicians choose to have some tests completed by the reference laboratory and some completed in the office in the **physician's office laboratory (POL).**

There are advantages and disadvantages to each method of managing laboratory analyses. Reference laboratories often have technological resources beyond those available in the POL. Using a reference laboratory frees a physician's staff from testing duties and allows more time for patient care. Furthermore, some managed care companies have contracts with laboratory companies that require their subscribers to use a specific reference laboratory. On the other hand, processing tests in the POL produces quicker turnaround and eliminates the need for the patient to travel to other test locations.

## The Purpose of the Physician's Office Laboratory

Office policy determines which tests, if any, will be performed at your location and which tests will be performed by a reference laboratory. A POL, such as the one shown in Figure 32-1, is responsible for accurate and timely processing of routine tests, usually involving blood or urine, and for reporting test results to the physician. (A reference laboratory offers a complete range of tests in all specialties and subspecialties: cytology, toxicology, immunology, blood banking, urinalysis, histology, serology, chemistry, microbiology, and hematology.)

A POL usually processes chemical analyses, hematologic tests, microbiologic tests, and urinalyses. Chemical analyses are performed on blood and its components, urine, and other body fluids. Hematologic tests usually use samples of whole blood to identify problems with the count, size, or shape of blood cells that could indicate disease. Microbiologic tests examine blood, urine, sputum, reproductive fluids, and fluids from wounds to identify the presence of pathogenic organisms such as bacteria, viruses, fungi, protozoans, and parasites. Semen may be examined microscopically to determine sperm levels, appearance, and

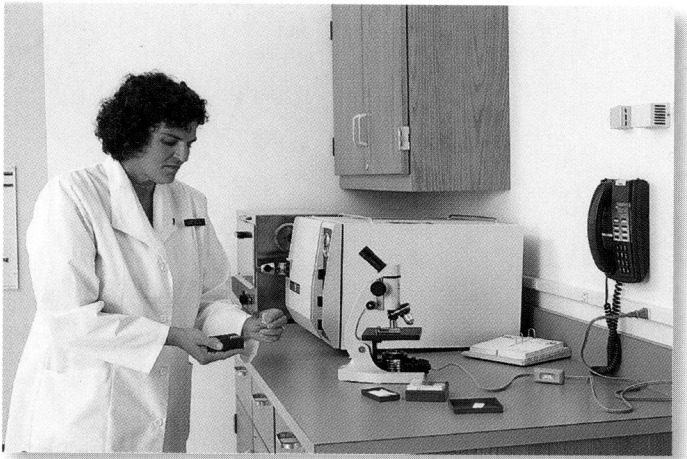

**Figure 32-1.** A physician's office laboratory (POL) may be simple or elaborate, depending on what tests the office performs.

motility. Urinalysis includes chemical analysis of the urine sample, analysis of its physical characteristics, and microscopic examination of the sample to detect disease states.

## The Medical Assistant's Role

As a medical assistant, you may be responsible for processing tests done in the POL, including preparing the patient for the test, collecting the sample, completing the test, reporting the results to the physician, and communicating information about the test from the physician to the patient. Your role in the POL requires you to integrate a great deal of information to serve both the physician and the patient effectively. You will need to master the following subjects:

- Use of laboratory equipment
- Regulations governing laboratory practices and procedures
- Precautions for accident prevention
- Waste disposal requirements
- Housekeeping and maintenance routines
- Quality assurance and control procedures
- Technical aspects of specimen collection and test processing, including expected results
- Communication with patients
- Reporting of test results to the physician
- Record keeping of test specimens, procedures, and results
- Inventory and ordering of equipment and supplies
- Use of reference materials in the POL
- Screening and follow-up of test results

## Use of Laboratory Equipment

Learning to use a specific piece of equipment may take the form of on-the-job training, or you may attend training programs conducted by manufacturers' representatives at

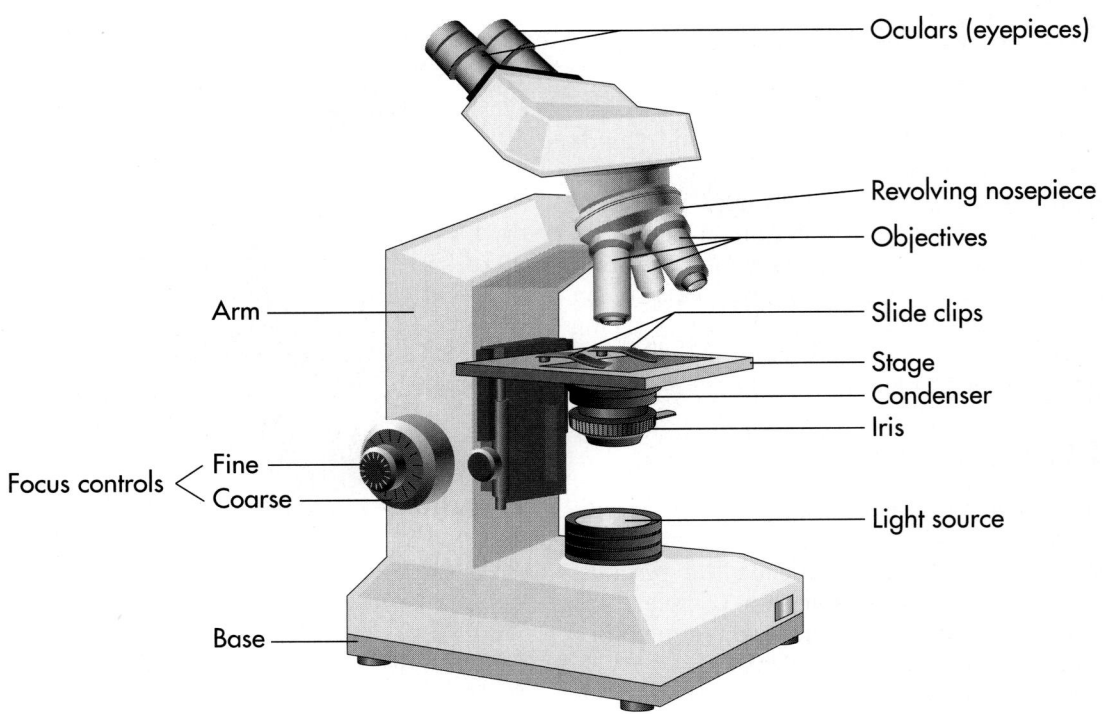

**Figure 32-2.** The microscope is the most heavily used piece of equipment in a POL.

Labels in figure:
- Oculars (eyepieces)
- Revolving nosepiece
- Objectives
- Slide clips
- Stage
- Condenser
- Iris
- Light source
- Arm
- Focus controls { Fine / Coarse
- Base

your location or at their training centers. You must be familiar with the operation of common laboratory equipment. You may routinely use the following equipment:

- Autoclave
- Centrifuge
- Microscope
- Electronic equipment and software
- Equipment used for measurement

## Autoclave

A steam autoclave is used to sterilize, or eradicate all organisms on, the surfaces of instruments and equipment before they are used on a patient or in testing procedures. Use of the autoclave is discussed in Chapter 20.

## Centrifuge

A **centrifuge** is a device for spinning a specimen at high speed until it separates into its component parts. The centrifuge in a POL is generally used to separate whole blood samples into blood components or to prepare urine samples for examination. Use of a centrifuge is described in greater detail in Chapter 34.

## Microscope

The instrument used most often in a POL is the microscope. Common uses of the microscope are the examination of blood smears and identification of microorganisms in body fluid samples.

The usual microscope in a POL is an **optical microscope** (Figure 32-2). An optical microscope uses light, concentrated through a condenser and focused through the object being examined, to project an image. Most optical microscopes in POLs are **compound microscopes,** which use two lenses to magnify the image created by the condensed light.

You must be able to operate an optical microscope correctly. First you need to become familiar with the component parts.

**Oculars.** The **oculars** are the eyepieces through which you view the image. A microscope is either monocular, with a single eyepiece, or binocular, with two eyepieces. You can adjust the oculars on a binocular microscope to compensate for differences in visual acuity between your right and left eyes. You can also adjust the distance between oculars to match the distance between your eyes. The ocular contains a magnifying lens that usually magnifies an image ten times. Such a lens is called a **10× lens.**

**Objectives.** Just below the ocular or oculars, the **objectives** are mounted on a swivel base called the *nosepiece.* An objective contains another magnifying lens. Generally, microscopes used in the POL have a three-piece objective system. An objective is moved into position directly under the ocular when needed.

Two of the objectives are dry objectives; this means there is air space between the specimen under examination and the objective. Condensed light passes through the specimen and the air space above the specimen as it travels toward the objective lens. These dry objectives are

# Clinical Laboratory Technicians

*To gain medical assistant credentials, you must fulfill the requirements of either the American Association of Medical Assistants (for a Certified Medical Assistant) or the American Medical Technologists (for a Registered Medical Assistant). After obtaining your medical assistant certification or registration, you may wish to acquire additional skills in specialty areas through course work or on-the-job training. Although this course work or training may not lead to an additional certification or degree, it will enable you to expand your role in the medical office and advance your career as the demand for skilled health professionals increases.*

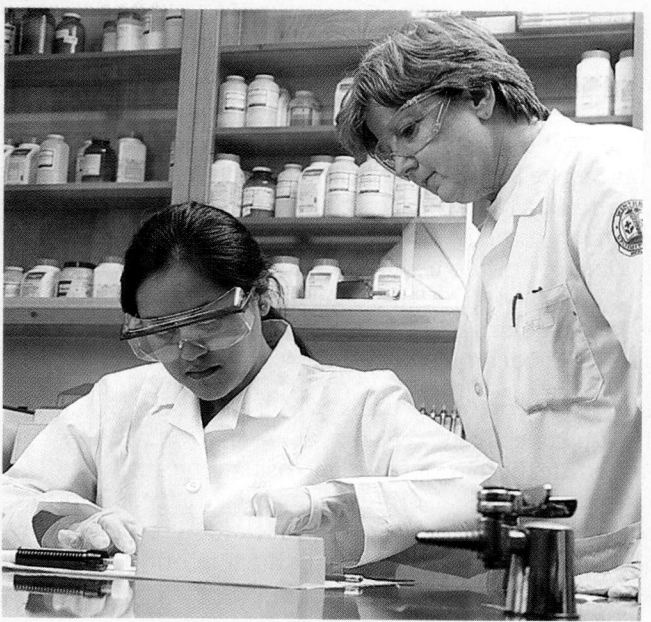

## Skills and Duties

A clinical laboratory technician conducts laboratory tests on specimens of body fluids and tissue. Samples may be tested to diagnose disease, to develop new treatments to combat disease, or to evaluate the success of existing treatments. A clinical laboratory technician works under the supervision of a medical laboratory technologist or physician.

The technician uses sophisticated laboratory equipment to collect, process, and analyze samples of body fluids. The assistant may prepare slides of the samples for viewing under the microscope or may separate components within the samples for further testing. As part of the testing process, the technician labels all samples and fills out reports of the analyses for the physician.

The range of tests performed by a particular clinical laboratory technician will vary, depending on the type of laboratory. For example, a technician who works in a small rural laboratory may perform a wide variety of tests, whereas a technician working in a large reference laboratory may only perform tests of a single type. Some procedures require specialized knowledge and training. A clinical laboratory technician's education and experience will determine the complexity of the tests that may be performed.

## Workplace Settings

Clinical laboratory technicians usually work in a hospital, clinic, or research center. An increasing number are also finding work at medical laboratories that run tests for hospitals and physicians. Clinical laboratory technicians usually work a standard 40-hour week, although hospital laboratories sometimes require some evening and weekend shifts.

## Education

A clinical laboratory technician must have a high school diploma or the equivalent. Some assistants acquire their additional training on the job, but most are trained in a certified program. The National Accrediting Agency for Clinical Laboratory Sciences accredits more than 450 training programs, which range in length from 1 to 2 years, at vocational schools and community colleges. In some cases students may be able to combine courses in medical assisting with a liberal arts program to gain an associate's degree in medical laboratory technology.

Certification as a clinical laboratory assistant is not required, but it is helpful in getting a job and advancing to other positions. In addition, some states require that clinical laboratory assistants, along with all other laboratory staff, be licensed or registered.

## Where to Go for More Information

American Medical Technologists
710 Higgins Road
Park Ridge, IL 60068
(847) 823-5169

American Society of Clinical Pathologists
2100 West Harrison Street
Chicago, IL 60612
(312) 738-1336

National Accrediting Agency for Clinical
    Laboratory Sciences
8410 West Bryn Mawr Avenue, Suite 670
Chicago, IL 60631
(773) 714-8880

low- and high-power lenses, usually 10× and 40×, respectively. When the low-power objective lens is combined with the ocular lenses, the total magnification factor is 100× (10× times 10×). The high-power lens and ocular lenses yield a magnification factor of 400×.

The third objective is an **oil-immersion objective.** It is designed to be lowered into a drop of immersion oil placed directly above the prepared specimen under examination. This design eliminates the air space between the microscope slide and the objective, where some of the light scatters beyond the objective. Placing the end of the objective in oil reduces the loss of light. A much sharper, brighter image results, allowing for greater magnification. An oil-immersion objective has a magnification factor of 100×. Combined with the ocular lenses, the total magnification factor is 1000×. The oil-immersion objective is used for specimens that need extreme magnification, such as blood smears and bacteriological slides.

**Arm and Focus Controls.** The ocular(s) and objectives, collectively referred to as the body tube, are attached to the base of the microscope by the arm. The microscope arm is also the location of the focus controls. There are two focus controls: coarse and fine. These controls move the body tube up and down to bring into focus the object being examined.

**Stage and Substage.** The objectives and oculars are focused on a specimen placed on the stage of the microscope. The stage is the platform on which rests the specimen slide, held in place by metal clips. Under the stage is the substage containing the condenser, which concentrates the light being directed through the sample, and the iris. The iris is a diaphragm that opens and closes like the shutter of a camera to increase or decrease the amount of light illuminating the specimen. The stage is controlled by the stage mechanisms, which control left-right and forward-backward movements of the stage, allowing you to examine different areas of the specimen without reseating the slide.

**Light Source.** Under the stage and substage assemblies is the light source. Most POL microscopes use a built-in electric light source, and most of these are equipped with controls that allow you to adjust the light intensity. In place of a built-in light source, older microscopes use a mirror, which gathers and focuses light from a microscope lamp onto the specimen.

**Specimen Slides and Coverslip.** Although the specimen slide is not technically part of the microscope assembly, it is necessary for using the microscope. All specimens must be placed on slides. Many specimens also require a coverslip, or cover glass. The slide and coverslip support and position the specimen. They also prevent contamination of the microscope by the specimen. Specimens that are to be stained or immersed in oil, such as blood smears, do not require coverslips.

**Using an Optical Microscope.** To use an optical microscope, you must be able to focus it using each of the three objectives. Procedure 32-1 describes how to operate an optical microscope correctly.

You will also be responsible for the proper care and maintenance of the optical microscope in your office. Related concerns and techniques are described in the Caution: Handle With Care section.

## Electronic Equipment and Software

Electronic equipment is used in the POL because it is more accurate, safer, and more efficient than manual methods; generally requires little maintenance; and does not require extensive training prior to its use. A wide variety of tasks, such as cell counting, and complex chemical analyses, are performed with electronic equipment. There are a variety of clinical laboratory software systems available. These systems are used to create and maintain clinical data, making remote access and tracking between facilities easier. Manufacturers' instructions for operation and maintenance must be followed to ensure safety, efficiency, and reliable results.

A **photometer,** which measures light intensity, is a basic electronic component of many pieces of analytic laboratory equipment. A handheld glucometer (Figure 32-8), for example, contains a photometer that measures reflected light. A glucometer is used by patients with diabetes and by clinical personnel to monitor blood glucose levels.

## Equipment Used for Measurement

Precise measurement is critical in the POL because it produces accurate test results. Much of the measurement required in the POL is built into the electronic equipment or premeasured kits you will use. You still must perform various measurements, however, when blood, semen, urine, and other body fluids are analyzed using manual tests. Some reagents also require measuring.

Metric system units are commonly used in the POL. For information on metric system weight, height, and temperature measurements, see Chapter 24. To learn how to convert between measurement systems, see Chapter 38.

A variety of equipment is used to provide accurate measurements. You must take these measurements carefully for them to be of value in the final test results. Other types of measuring equipment include:

- Pipettes, either mechanical or manual, which are used to measure small amounts of liquids
- Volumetric or graduated flasks or beakers, which are used to measure the relatively large amounts of liquids necessary for reagents
- A hemocytometer, which is a slide calibrated to the exact measurements needed to count blood cells and sperm under a microscope
- Thermometers, generally in degrees centigrade, which are used to provide legal documentation that refrigerators, bacterial incubators, and other appliances maintain the precise temperature range required for accurate laboratory work

# PROCEDURE 32.1

## Using a Microscope

**Procedure Goal:** To correctly focus the microscope using each of the three objectives for examination of a prepared specimen slide

### OSHA Guidelines

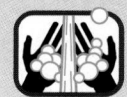 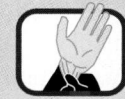 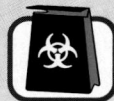
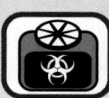 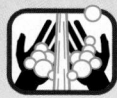

**Materials:** Microscope, lens paper, lens cleaner, prepared specimen slide, immersion oil, tissues

### Method:

1. Wash your hands and put on exam gloves.

2. Remove the protective cover from the microscope. Examine the microscope to make sure that it is clean and that all parts are intact.

3. Plug in the microscope and make sure the light is working. If you need to replace the bulb, refer to the manufacturer's guidelines. (Be sure to note bulb replacements in the maintenance log for the microscope.) Turn the light off before cleaning the lenses.

4. Clean the lenses and oculars with lens paper. Avoid touching the lenses with anything except lens paper. Pay careful attention to the oculars. They are easily dirtied by dust and eye makeup. If a lens is particularly dirty, use a small amount of lens cleaner. Oil-immersion lenses are prone to oil buildup if not cleaned properly. Too much lens cleaner, however, can loosen the cement that holds the lens in place.

*Rationale*
The lenses must be clean to reduce artifacts.

5. Place the specimen slide on the stage. Slide the edges of the slide under the slide clips to secure the slide to the stage (Figure 32-3).

6. Adjust the distance between the oculars to a position of comfort.

7. Adjust the objectives so that the low-power (10×) objective points directly at the specimen slide, as shown in Figure 32-4. Before swiveling the objective assembly, be sure you have sufficient space for the objective. Recheck the distance between the oculars, making sure the

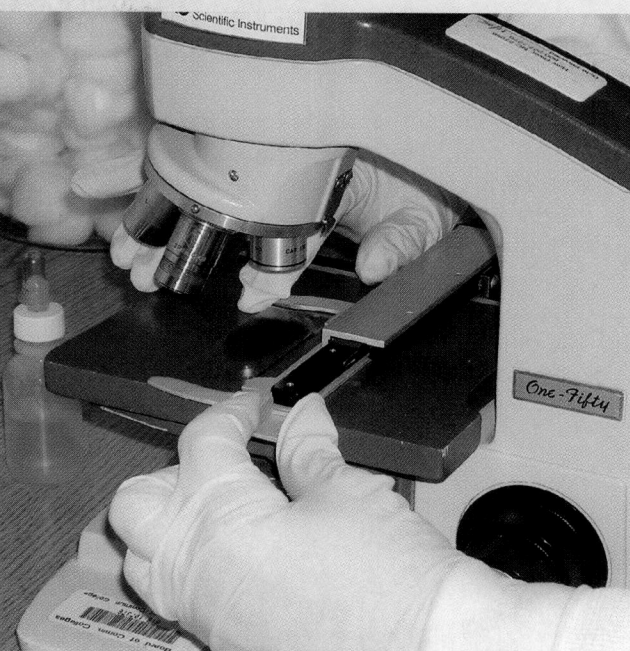

**Figure 32-3.** Carefully secure the specimen slide on the stage of the microscope.

field you see through the eyepieces is a merged field, not separate left and right fields. Raise the body tube by using the coarse adjustment control, and lower the stage as needed.

*Rationale*
If the objective assembly is too close to the stage, you may hit the specimen slide and crack it. The specimen is then contaminated and cannot be used. The objective may also be damaged.

8. Turn on the light and, using the iris controls, adjust the amount of light illuminating the specimen so that the light fills the field but does not wash out the image. (At this point you are not examining the specimen image for focus but adjusting the overall light level.)

9. Observe the microscope from one side, and slowly lower the body tube to move the objective closer to the stage and specimen slide. This adjustment is shown in Figure 32-5. If you used the stage controls to lower the stage away from the objectives, you may also need to adjust those controls. Again, take care not to

*continued* ⟶

## Using a Microscope *(continued)*

strike the stage with the objective. The objective should almost meet the specimen slide but not touch it.

10. Look through the oculars and use the coarse focus control to slowly adjust the image. If necessary, adjust the amount of light coming through the iris.

11. Continue using the fine focus control to adjust the image. When the image is correctly focused, the specimen will be clearly visible, and the field illumination will be bright enough to show details but not so bright that it is uncomfortable to view or washed out.

12. Switch to the high-power (40×) objective. Use the fine focus controls to view the specimen clearly.

### Rationale

Using the coarse adjustment could cause lens damage if the lens touches the slide.

13. Rotate the objective assembly so that no objective points directly at the stage and specimen slide. You will now have enough room to apply a drop of immersion oil to the slide. (Only dry slides, without coverslips, are used with the oil-immersion objective.)

14. Apply a small drop of immersion oil to the specimen slide, as shown in Figure 32-6.

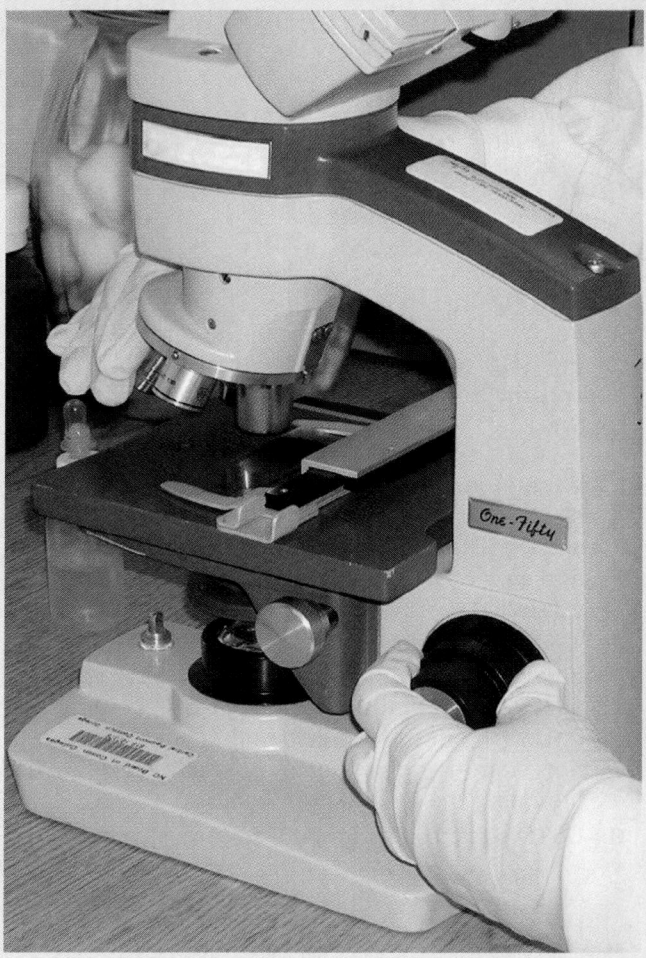

**Figure 32-4.** Move the low-power objective into position above the specimen slide.

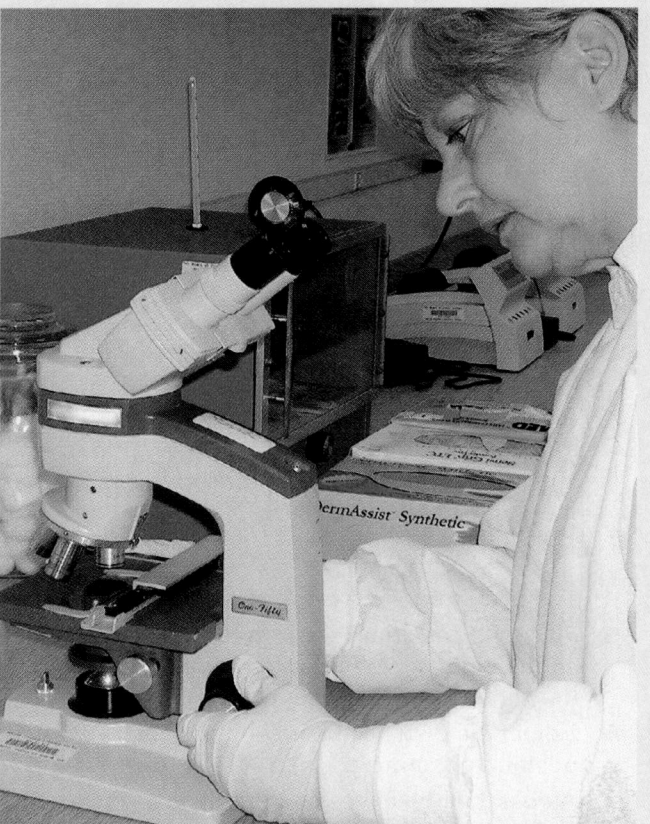

**Figure 32-5.** When lowering the objective toward the stage and specimen slide, observe the microscope from the side to be sure you do not hit the stage with the objective and crack the slide.

*continued* ⟶

## Using a Microscope *(concluded)*

15. Gently swing the oil-immersion (100×) objective over the stage and specimen slide so that it is surrounded by the immersion oil.

16. Examine the image and adjust the amount of light and focus as needed. Only use the fine focus adjustment with this objective. To eliminate air bubbles in the immersion oil, gently move the stage left and right.

17. After you have examined the specimen as required by the testing procedure, lower the stage and raise the objectives.

18. Remove the slide. Dispose of it or store it as required by the testing procedure. If you must dispose of the slide, be sure to use the appropriate biohazardous waste container. If you must store the slide, remove the immersion oil with a tissue.

19. Turn off the light. Unplug the microscope if that is your laboratory's standard operating procedure.

20. Clean the microscope stage, ocular lenses, and objectives (Figure 32-7). Be careful to remove all traces of immersion oil from the stage and oil-immersion objective.

21. Rotate the objective assembly so that the low-power objective points toward the stage. Lower the objective so that it comes close to but does not rest on the stage.

22. Cover the microscope with its protective cover. Check the work area to be sure you have cleaned everything correctly and disposed of all waste material.

23. Remove the gloves and wash your hands.

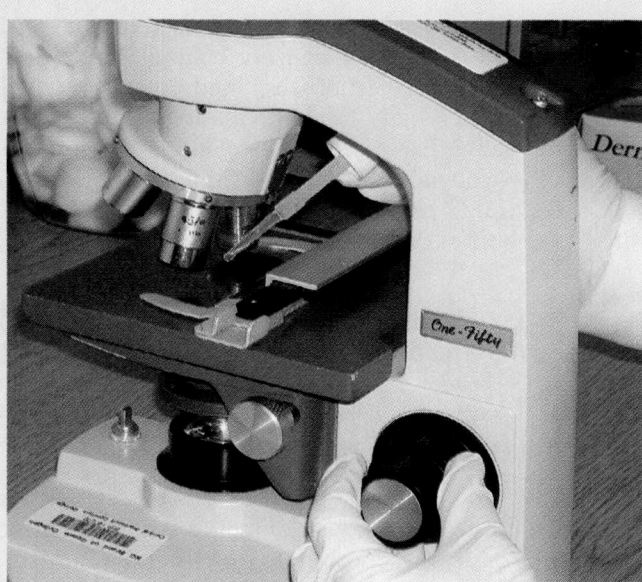

**Figure 32-6.** Place a small drop of immersion oil directly on the dry specimen.

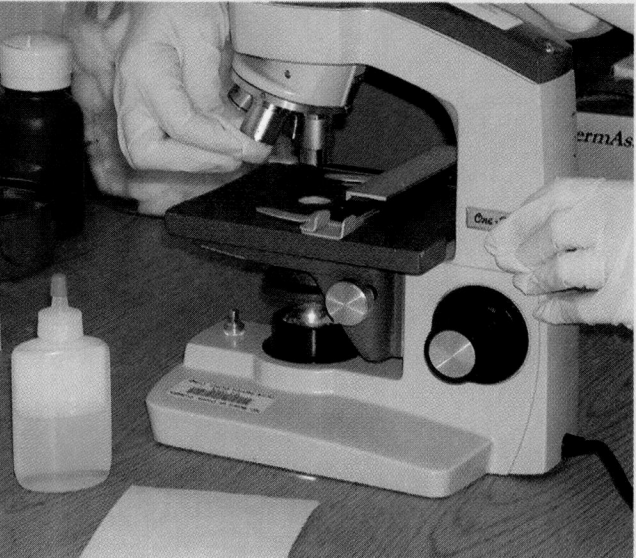

**Figure 32-7.** You need to remove all traces of immersion oil when you clean the microscope stage, ocular lenses, and objectives.

# Safety in the Laboratory

Safety is a primary concern in any laboratory environment. It is especially important in a physician's office laboratory because patients as well as laboratory workers may be at risk. For your own protection, as well as that of patients and coworkers, you must always be aware of and observe guidelines for laboratory safety.

# Occupational Safety and Health Administration

The Occupational Safety and Health Administration (OSHA) was created within the Department of Labor as a result of legislation passed in 1970 (the Occupational Safety and Health Acts) to protect the safety of employees in the workplace. OSHA's duties include the creation and

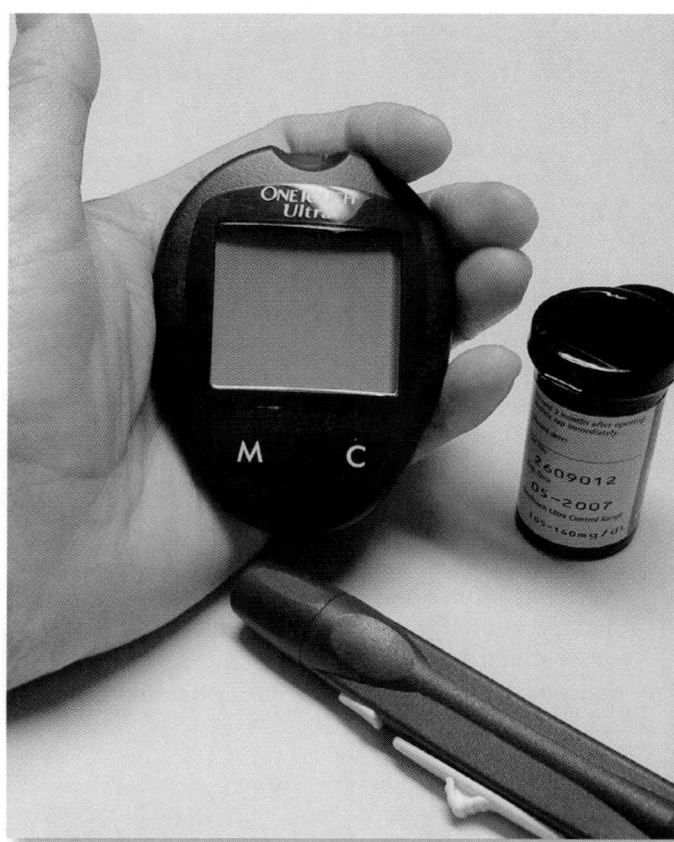

**Figure 32-8.** A handheld glucometer translates the amount of reflected light into the level of glucose in a blood sample.

enforcement of both general safety standards and standards for specific industries and operations. In general, if a specific standard exists, its guidelines must be followed, but if no specific standard has been developed, the "general duty clause" takes effect. This clause requires an employer to maintain a workplace free from hazards that are recognized as likely to cause death or serious injury. OSHA also acts to enforce guidelines developed by the Centers for Disease Control and Prevention (CDC), in particular the guidelines for Standard Precautions. Copies of these guidelines can be obtained from many sources, including local OSHA offices; the CDC in Atlanta, Georgia; many industrial organizations throughout the country; and the Internet.

Important regulations or guidelines with which you should be familiar as you work as a medical assistant include the following:

- Standard Precautions
- Hazard Communication Standard
- OSHA Bloodborne Pathogens Standard
- Hazardous Waste Operations and Emergency Response Final Rule
- Needlestick Safety and Prevention Act

**Standard Precautions.** As discussed in Chapter 20 and elsewhere, the general concept behind Standard Precautions is to assume that all blood, blood products, human tissue, and body fluids (including semen, vaginal secretions, saliva from dental procedures, cerebrospinal fluid (CSF), synovial fluid, pleural fluid, peritoneal fluid, pericardial fluid, and amniotic fluid) are contaminated with blood-borne pathogens.

## CAUTION *Handle With Care*

### Care and Maintenance of the Microscope

The microscope is the workhorse of the POL. For it to provide trouble-free service, however, it must be well cared for. Dust, oil, and other contaminants cause major problems with microscopes. Careless cleaning and haphazard storage will also eventually cause problems. These problems may include mechanical difficulties with the microscope or contamination of the specimen being examined. Foreign objects visible through a microscope, but unrelated to the specimen, are called **artifacts** and may be misinterpreted when the specimen is examined.

Clean the microscope after each use. Inspect the body tube, arm, and stage to make sure they are free from dust and other contaminants. Clean the ocular and objective lenses with lens paper, not tissue or other products. Tissue fibers are a common artifact. The eyepiece is an area in which skin oil, dust, and eye makeup may collect, posing a risk of disease transmission and making images difficult to see. Use lens-cleaning products according to the manufacturer's guidelines. Excess amounts of these products may dissolve the cement holding the lenses in place, rendering the microscope useless.

When not in use, the microscope should be stored under its plastic cover. If there is a power cord, wrap it loosely around the base, and secure it with a twist tie or elastic band. Lower the low-power objective close to the stage and center the stage.

If the microscope must be moved, hold it by the arm, and support it under the base. Never carry a microscope with one hand or by just the arm. Carry the cord so that it does not dangle and pose a tripping hazard. Place the microscope on a sturdy table or bench, away from the edge.

It has become common practice in the medical office to use Standard Precautions when handling all body fluids, excretions, and secretions. If you have any doubt about whether you need to take precautions, take them. Even though some substances do not present a risk of transmitting blood-borne pathogens, they may present a high risk of transmitting bacteria, viruses, or parasites. Follow these guidelines.

- Wear gloves when handling all body fluids, secretions, and excretions.
- Change gloves every time you move from patient to patient as you collect specimens for testing.
- Wash your hands immediately after removing used gloves.
- Wear other protective gear such as eye protection and face masks during procedures in which there is a risk that droplets or spray may come in contact with your eyes, nose, or mouth.
- Take special care to avoid injury from sharp or pointed instruments or equipment. Although gloves protect you from surface exposure to potentially infected substances, they offer little protection against exposure from needlesticks or cuts. Never use needles or other sharp instruments unnecessarily.
- Use only recommended instruments and equipment. A once common laboratory technique that has been discontinued is the use of a mouth pipette (a type of calibrated glass or plastic straw) to transfer specimens. Under no circumstances should you use a mouth pipette to transfer blood from one collection device to another.
- Take care to prevent spills and splashes when transporting specimens to the laboratory and when moving specimens in the laboratory.
- If a work surface becomes contaminated because of spilling or splashing, disinfect the area completely, using an approved solution such as 10% bleach, before beginning any other procedure.
- Dispose of waste products carefully and correctly.
- Be sure to remove protective gear before leaving the laboratory.

**Hazard Communication Standard.** The Hazard Communication Standard requires that employees receive training regarding workplace hazards, including how to interpret documentation about hazardous substances that pose an exposure threat. Hazardous materials must be correctly labeled, and employees must have access to information about the materials. The information must include the measures that employees can take to protect themselves against harm from these substances.

*Biohazard Labels.* All containers used to store waste products, blood, blood products, or other specimens that may be contaminated with blood-borne pathogens are considered biohazardous. They must be clearly marked with the **biohazard symbol,** as shown in Figure 32-9. The biohazard symbol label must be bright orange-red and clearly lettered

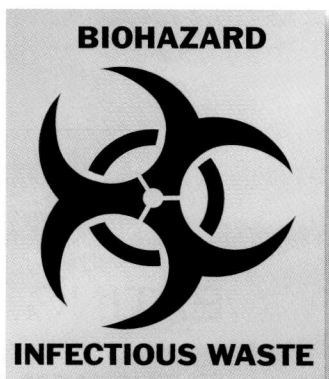

**Figure 32-9.** The biohazard symbol identifies material that has been exposed to potentially contaminated substances such as blood, blood products, or other body fluids.

so that no one can mistake the meaning of the warning. Labels should be securely attached to containers.

In addition to individual biohazard labels that identify particular containers, warning signs must be posted in the laboratory itself. These signs, such as the one shown in Figure 32-10, identify the presence of biohazardous material and list important safeguards to follow.

*Material Safety Data Sheets.* Material Safety Data Sheets (MSDSs) contain information about hazardous chemicals or other substances. A sample MSDS is shown in Figure 32-11. Each MSDS must contain the following information about the product it describes:

- Substance name, as it appears on the container label
- Chemical name(s) of each ingredient
- Common name(s) of each ingredient
- Chemical characteristics of the product (boiling point, specific gravity, melting point, appearance, odor)
- Physical hazards posed by the product (fire, vapor pressure)
- Health hazards posed by the product (carcinogenicity [ability to cause cancer], routes and methods of entry, signs and symptoms of exposure)
- Guidelines for safe handling of the substance
- Emergency and first-aid procedures to be followed in the event of exposure

*Hazard Labels.* In addition to the MSDS, each hazardous substance must be identified with a hazard label. A **hazard label** is a shortened version of the MSDS that is permanently affixed to the substance container. OSHA requires that a hazard label display the name of the material contained, either trade or chemical, and a brief statement of the hazardous effects of the chemical. They do not specify a system of colors or numbers that require special training to identify a product. If you encounter a label with a color-coded, numbered system, consult the manufacturer for a description of the specific labeling system. Different manufacturers use slightly different labeling systems. A sample hazard label is shown in Figure 32-12.

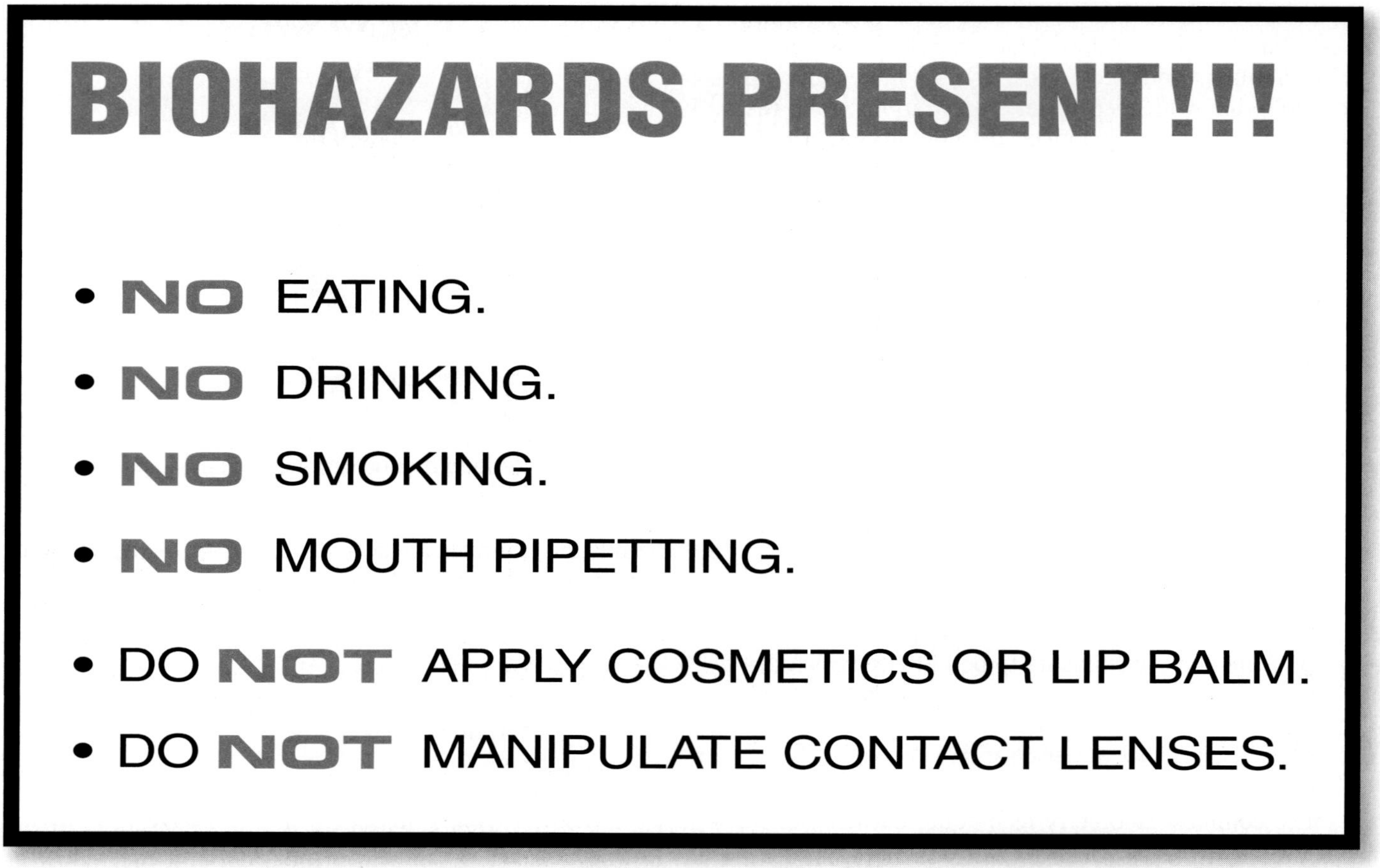

# BIOHAZARDS PRESENT!!!

- **NO** EATING.

- **NO** DRINKING.

- **NO** SMOKING.

- **NO** MOUTH PIPETTING.

- DO **NOT** APPLY COSMETICS OR LIP BALM.

- DO **NOT** MANIPULATE CONTACT LENSES.

**Figure 32-10.** The biohazard warning sign alerts personnel to the presence of potentially contaminated substances and advises them about safety guidelines.

**OSHA Bloodborne Pathogens Standard.** The OSHA Bloodborne Pathogens Standard identifies methods for reducing the risk of transmission of blood-borne pathogens, specifically the hepatitis B virus (HBV) and the human immunodeficiency virus (HIV). HIV is the virus that causes acquired immunodeficiency syndrome (AIDS). The standard identifies laboratory procedures that must be followed to prevent occupational exposure. It also describes the procedure that must be followed in the event of exposure to one of these viruses. To be in compliance with this standard, an employer must meet the following requirements.

- A written OSHA Exposure Control Plan must be created and updated annually or whenever procedures that require exposure to potentially contaminated material are added or changed. The plan must be available to all employees and to authorized OSHA authorities.

- Training must be provided to all employees describing the documentation mandated by the standard. This documentation includes the symptoms, methods of transmission, and epidemiology of infectious diseases caused by blood-borne pathogens. Employees must also be instructed in the use of personal protective equipment, Universal Precautions, and engineering controls designed to prevent exposure. Procedures to follow in the event of exposure or emergency situations must also be part of the training.

- The employer must make hepatitis B vaccine available at no charge to all employees who are at risk for occupational exposure. Employees must either receive the vaccination or decline it in writing. The employer must maintain documentation of vaccinations and refusals. Employees who initially decline the vaccine are free to reverse their decision at any point during their employment.

**Hazardous Waste Operations and Emergency Response Final Rule.** OSHA regulations also extend to the disposal of waste products generated during laboratory procedures. Hazardous waste products include the following:

- Blood
- Blood products
- Body fluids
- Body tissues
- Cultures
- Vaccines, killed or attenuated (live but weakened)
- Sharps
- Gloves

# WAVICIDE-01

## MATERIAL SAFETY DATA SHEET

Date Issued:

### SECTION 1    IDENTIFICATION

**Manufacturers Name and Address:** Wave Energy Systems, Inc.
25 Mansard Court
Wayne, NJ 07470

**Phone:** 1-800-252-1125
**Fax:** (201) 633-1023

**Product Name:** WAVICIDE-01 (2.5% aqueous glutaraldehyde solution)

**Product Code:** 0104 (case of 4 gallons) or 0112 (case of 12 quarts)

**Product Type/General Information:** Chemical Sterilant/Disinfectant

**EPA Registration Number:** 15136-1

**Chemical Name:** (active ingredient) 2.5% glutaraldehyde

*The New Jersey Poison Control Center has been provided information for use in medical emergencies involving this product. Call 1-800-962-1253.*

**Hazardous Chemicals:** Glutaraldehyde
**Routes of entry:** Inhalation ✓  Skin/Eye ✓  Ingestion ✓

**PRECAUTIONARY LABELING**
(HMIS Rating System)
Health                3
Flammability          0
Reactivity            0
Physical Hazard:      None

### SECTION 2    HAZARDOUS INGREDIENTS/IDENTITY INFORMATION

WAVICIDE-01 contains the following hazardous ingredients at concentrations greater than 1.0%:

| CHEMICAL COMPONENTS | CAS% | % w/v | OSHA PEL | ACGIH TLV |
|---|---|---|---|---|
| Glutaraldehyde (active ingredient) | 111-30-8 | 2.5 | 0.2 ppm[1] | 0.2 ppm |

WAVICIDE-01 contains no hazardous ingredients listed as carcinogens or potential carcinogens by the National Toxicology Program (NTP), International Agency on Cancer (IARC) or OSHA, and present at a concentration greater than 0.1%:

[1] The OSHA Permissible Exposure Level (PEL) for glutaraldehyde was invalidated in 1992 by court order. However, the PEL may remain valid in some OSHA approved state plans, and also can be enforced by federal OSHA under its General Duty Clause.

### SECTION 3    PHYSICAL/CHEMICAL CHARACTERISTICS

**Boiling Point:** 100°C/212°F
**Specific Gravity:** 1.005 - 1.013
**Vapor Pressure:** 16.9 mm Hg
**Melting point:** N/A
**Vapor Density:** 1.1 (air = 1)
**Freezing Point:** 0°C/32°F (same as water)

**Evaporation Rate:** 0.81 (Butyl Acetate = 1)
**Solubility (H₂O):** Complete
**Appearance & Color:** A clear, slightly yellow liquid with typical aldehyde odor and added lemon scent.
**pH:** Approximately 6.30
**Molecular Weight:** 100.11 (glutaraldehyde)
**Odor Threshold:** 0.04 ppm, detectable (ACGIH)

### SECTION 4    FIRE AND EXPLOSION HAZARD DATA

**Flash Point (Test Method):** None (Tag Closed Cup ASTM D 56)
**Special Fire Fighting Procedures:** Self-Contained Breathing Apparatus (SCBA) and protective clothing should be worn when fighting chemical fires.
**Unusual Fire and Explosion Hazards:** None known          **Extinguishing Media:** Carbon dioxide, foam, dry chemical.

### SECTION 5    REACTIVITY DATA

**Stability:** Stable ✓   Unstable          **Hazardous Polymerization:** May Occur   Will Not Occur ✓

**Hazardous Decomposition Products:** Thermal decomposition may produce carbon dioxide and/or carbon monoxide.

**Conditions and Materials to Avoid:** Alkaline (pH > 10) and acidic (pH < 3) materials catalyze an aldol-type condensation (exothermic but not expected to be violent). Avoid High temperatures above 40°C/104°F and or evaporation of H₂O.

**Figure 32-11.**  This two-page Material Safety Data Sheet (MSDS), as required by OSHA, contains important information about each hazardous substance used in the POL.

Source: Courtesy of Wave Energy Systems, Inc., Wayne, NJ. (continued)

## SECTION 6     HEALTH HAZARD DATA

Routes of Entry:   Inhalation. ✓    Skin. ✓   Ingestion. ✓   Eyes. ✓

**Signs and Symptoms Associated With Overexposure (one-time or repeated):**

Ingestion:   May cause irritation and possibly chemical burns of the mouth, throat, stomach and esophagus. May produce discomfort in the mouth, throat, chest and abdomen, nausea, vomiting, diarrhea, dizziness, faintness, drowsiness, thirst and weakness.

Eyes:   Solution contact may cause damage, including severe corneal injury, which could permanently impair vision if prompt first-aid and medical treatment are not obtained. Vapors may cause stinging sensation in the eye with excess tear production, blinking, and redness of the conjuntiva.

Skin:   Direct solution contact may cause skin irritation or aggravation of an existing dermatitis. May also cause skin to turn a harmless yellow or brown color.

Inhalation:   Vapor is irritating to the respiratory tract. May cause stinging sensations in the nose and throat, chest discomfort and tightening, difficulty with breathing and headache. May also aggravate pre-existing asthma and pulmonary disease.

**Emergency and First Aid Procedure:**

Ingestion:   DO NOT INDUCE VOMITING. Drink large quantities of water and call a physician immediately
NOTE TO PHYSICIAN: Probable mucosal damage from oral exposure may contraindicate the use of gastric lavage.

Eyes:   Immediately flush eyes with water and continue washing for at least 15 minutes. Obtain medical attention immediately, and follow up with an ophthalmologist.

Skin:   Immediately remove contaminated clothing and flush skin with soap and water for a minimum of 15 minutes. If irritation persists, seek medical attention. Wash or discard contaminated clothing.

Inhalation:   Remove to fresh air. Give artificial respiration if not breathing. If breathing is difficult, oxygen may be given by qualified personnel. If irritation persists, seek medical help.

**Medical Conditions Generally Aggravated by Overexposure:**   See above.

## SECTION 7     PRECAUTIONS FOR SAFE HANDLING AND USE

**Steps to be Taken if Material is Released or Spilled:** Wear suitable protective equipment, including nitrile gloves, chemically resistant gown or apron, and protective eyewear (safety glasses or shield). A full face respirator , or half-face respirator with gas proof goggles, both worn with organic vapor cartridges, is recommended for small spills. A respirator is essential for large spills, or if you experience discomfort watery eyes, nasal or respiratory irritation) due to inadequate ventilation. For small spills of 1 gallon or less, gather up a bucket, household ammonia, and a sponge or mop. Don protective equipment and mix approximately 1 cup of ammonia with 1 cup of water in the bucket. Mop or sponge the ammonia mixture into the spill until thoroughly combined (about 2 minutes). Wipe or mop up resulting mixture and discard down the drain with a copious amount of water. Rinse bucket, mop or sponge with water, and give spill area a final wipe or mop with fresh water. Re-rinse all equipment, and allow spill area to dry. For large spills of more than 1 gallon, remove people from immediate spill area, and isolate until cleaned up. Don protective equipment including an organic vapor cartridges. Contain spill with absorbent material, ie. towels. Add approximately 228 grams of sodium bisulfite powder per gallon of WAVICIDE-01 spilled (aqueous sodium hydroxide and ammonium will also neutralize glutaraldehyde). With a sponge, mix neutralizing chemical into spill, and allow 5 minutes for deactivation to occur. Discard resulting mixture according to your facility's waste disposal guidelines. Mop spill area with fresh water. Rinse out all equipment (bucket, mop, towels) with large amounts of water. If paper towels were used, dispose of in a tightly closed trash bag. Let spill area dry, and if possible increase ventilation. Once glutaraldehyde odor is below allowable levels (TLV), the area may be released from isolation.

**Waste Disposal Method:** Dispose of WAVICIDE-01 after 30 days of re-use, or the MEC Indicator shows the solution is below it's minimum effective concentration (1.7% w/v), which ever is sooner. This may be accomplished by pouring solution down drain in accordance with state and local regulations. Flush with a large quantity of water. Do not reuse empty containers. Rinse thoroughly with water and dispose of in trash.

**Precautions to be Taken in Handling and Storing:** WAVICIDE-01 should be stored in it's original sealed container at controlled room temperature (15°C/50°F to 30°C/85°F).

**Precautionary Labeling:** Avoid contact with eyes, prolonged and repeated contact with skin, and contamination with food.

## SECTION 8     TRANSPORATATION DATA & ADDITIONAL INFORMATION

| | | | | |
|---|---|---|---|---|
| **Proper Shipping Name:** 2.5% Glutaraldehyde Solution | **DOT (ground):** Not regulated | **IATA (air):** Not Regulated | **IMO (ocean):** Not Regulated |
| **Hazard Class:** None | **Labels:** None needed | **Packaging:** None | **ID#:** None | **Special Instructions:** None | **Reportable Quantity:** None |

## SECTION 9     CONTROL MEASURES

**Eye Protection:** Safety glasses, goggles or face shield recommended when working with WAVICIDE-01. An eye wash, and full face respirator with organic vapor cartridges or half face respirator with gas proof goggles and organic vapor cartridges should be available for emergency situations.

**Ventilation:** WAVICIDE-01 should be used in closed containers with tight fitting lids. The working area should be large enough with ventilation necessary to keep the level of atmospheric glutaraldehyde below the Threshold Limit Value (TLV). If the solution vapors are irritating to eyes and nose, the TLV is probably being exceeded, and additional ventilation may be necessary. A fume hood or self contained fume absorber may be appropriate for this purpose. Any ventilation should pull fumes away from worker and towards the floor.

**Skin Protection:** Nitrile gloves and a chemical resistant gown or apron should be worn when working with WAVICIDE-01. Rubber boots may be needed to contain large spills.

**Respiratory Protection:** None required if glutaraldehyde vapor levels are below the TLV. A full face respirator with organic vapor cartridges or SCBA should be available for emergencies.

## SECTION 10     SPECIAL REQUIREMENTS

None

**Figure 32-11.**   Material Safety Data Sheet (concluded)

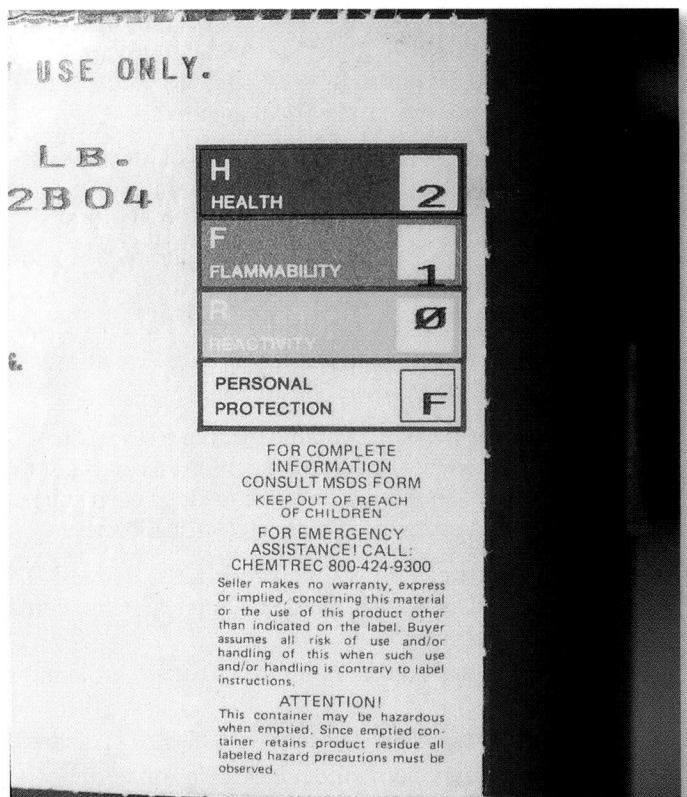

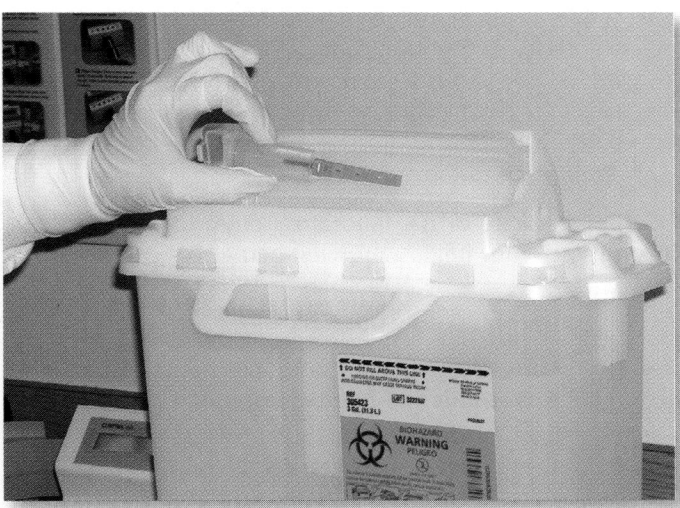

**Figure 32-12.** A hazard label is a condensed version of the MSDS and displays important information about a substance. It must be permanently affixed to the substance container.

- Specula
- Inoculating loops
- Paper products contaminated with body fluids

Hazardous waste must be disposed of in properly constructed and labeled containers. Containers for sharps must be puncture-proof, leak-resistant, and rigid (Figure 32-13). Needles should be dropped into the sharps container without bending, breaking, or recapping them and with as little extra handling as possible. Other waste must be placed in plastic bags clearly labeled to identify the infectious contents. All biohazardous waste containers should be placed as close as possible to the area in which the waste is generated. This last procedure is followed to reduce the risk of spillage on the way to the disposal container.

**Needlestick Safety and Prevention Act.** In response to the Needlestick Safety and Prevention Act, which was signed into law in November 2000, OSHA revised the Bloodborne Pathogens Standard. The additional provisions to the standard are:

- Health-care employers must evaluate new safety-engineered control devices on an annual basis and implement the use of devices that reasonably reduce the risk of needlestick injuries

**Figure 32-13.** A sharps disposal container is a receptacle for used needles, lancets, specimen slides, and other disposable pointed or edged instruments, supplies, and equipment.

- Health-care facilities must maintain a detailed log of sharps injuries that are incurred from contaminated sharps
- Health-care employers must solicit input from employees involved in direct patient care to identify, evaluate, and implement engineering and work practice controls

## Accident Prevention Guidelines

Work in the POL exposes you to hazards of four main types: physical, fire and electrical, chemical, and biologic. The following safeguards reduce the risk in one or more of these hazard categories. For example, by handling chemical containers carefully and correctly, you protect yourself from harmful chemical exposure as well as from physical injury from broken glass or other materials.

**Physical Safety.** There are many ways to ensure physical safety in the laboratory. You must understand and apply all the appropriate safeguards. Because accidents can happen, however, post emergency numbers in multiple locations throughout the laboratory. Once each quarter, make sure the numbers are accurate and up-to-date.

Some safeguards come under the heading of common sense. Their application requires no special knowledge.

- Walk, do not run, in the laboratory. Be careful when carrying objects through the laboratory, especially when approaching blind corners.
- Close all cabinet and closet doors and all desk and worktable drawers.
- Never use damaged equipment or supplies, such as cracked or chipped glassware.
- Do not overextend your reach when attempting to grasp supplies. Use only approved equipment, such as stepladders or stools, to reach high shelves. Do not climb onto chairs, desks, or tables to reach anything.

- When lifting an object, squat close to the object. Keep your back straight but not rigid. Lift the item by pushing up with your legs, not by pulling with your back. Hold the load firmly with both hands, close to your body. If necessary, put on a back-support belt before attempting to move heavy loads.

Being aware of the laboratory environment will help you protect your health and well-being. For example:

- Adjust your seat to the correct position to prevent back strain.
- If you are using a computer, take frequent breaks to reduce eyestrain and hand cramping.
- Do not eat or drink in the laboratory, and do not store food there. Never use laboratory supplies, such as beakers or flasks, for eating or drinking.
- Do not put anything in your mouth while working in the laboratory. (Some people have a habit of chewing on the end of their pencils, for example.)
- Do not apply makeup or lip balm or insert contact lenses in the laboratory.
- Familiarize yourself with the location of the first-aid kit. If you are responsible for the kit in your area, check it weekly to make sure that it is adequately stocked with supplies and that expiration dates on medications have not passed.
- Familiarize yourself with the location and operation of the emergency eyewash and shower stations.

Wear appropriate protective gear and clothing in the laboratory. Use heat-resistant mitts or gloves to prevent burns. Wear sturdy, low-heeled, closed-toe shoes with rubber soles to prevent injury if you drop or spill something and to avoid slipping. Do not wear dangling jewelry or loose clothing that could get caught in laboratory equipment. Keep hair pulled back or covered for the same reason.

When you work with laboratory equipment, always follow manufacturers' guidelines. For example, wait for centrifuges to stop spinning before you open them.

Many laboratory materials and supplies require special handling and precautions.

- Store caustic chemicals and other hazardous substances below eye level to reduce the risk of upsetting the container and spilling the substance into your eyes.
- Do not attempt to grasp bottles, jars, or other containers if your hands or the containers are wet.
- Close containers immediately after use.
- Clean up spills immediately. If the floor is wet, either dry it or use appropriate warning devices to alert others to the hazard.
- Clean up broken glass with a broom. Do not handle the debris. If the material is biohazardous, use tongs or forceps to pick up the glass. Package the pieces in a sturdy container with a label identifying the contents.

**Fire and Electrical Safety.** The equipment and materials used in the POL make it especially vulnerable to fire and electrical hazards. It is critical for you to know how to respond to a fire or electrical accident.

- Familiarize yourself with the location of all fire extinguishers and fire blankets in the laboratory. Review the floor plan, noting the location of fire exits.
- Make sure you know how to operate the fire extinguishers.
- Participate in all office fire drills.
- Familiarize yourself with the location of circuit breakers and emergency power shutoffs.

It is, of course, never acceptable to smoke in the laboratory. Keep your area clear of clutter such as boxes or empty storage containers. Such materials can feed, or even start, a fire. The following safeguards reduce electrical hazards.

- Avoid using extension cords. If they must be used, be sure the circuit is not overloaded. Tape extension cords to the floor to avoid tripping.
- Repair or replace equipment that has a broken or frayed cord.
- Dry your hands before working with electrical devices.
- Do not position electrical devices near sinks, faucets, or other sources of water. Be sure electrical cords do not run through water.

Work in the laboratory may sometimes require that you use a flame. Special precautions are essential in such circumstances.

- If you must use an open flame, extinguish it immediately after use.
- When using an open flame, be careful to keep your hair, clothing, and jewelry away from the flame source.
- If you must use a chemical in a procedure that requires an open flame, double-check the MSDS to identify the level of risk of fire for that chemical. If necessary, bring a fire extinguisher to the area in which you will be working.
- Never lean over an open flame.
- Never leave an open flame unattended.
- Turn off gas valves immediately after use. If you must use an open flame in the vicinity of a gas valve, always double-check to be sure the gas is off. Make sure there is adequate ventilation.

**Chemical Safety.** Familiarize yourself with the MSDS and hazard label of every chemical you will use during a procedure. If the MSDS indicates the need for special equipment or conditions to use a chemical safely, be sure you meet the requirements before beginning to work with the substance. General precautions as you prepare include the following:

- Wear protective gear to prevent harm to your skin or damage to your clothing. (Be sure to remove the protective gear before leaving the laboratory.)

- Always carry chemical containers with both hands as you gather supplies.
- Make sure you work in an area that is properly ventilated.

When you are ready to begin work, adhere to these guidelines.

- If you must smell the chemicals you are using, do not hold them directly under your nose. Instead, hold them a few inches away, and fan air across them and toward your nose.
- Work inside a fume hood if the chemical vapor is hazardous.
- Wear a personal ventilation device when working with certain chemicals, as specified by the MSDS.
- Never combine chemicals in ways not specifically required in test procedures.
- Mouth pipetting is prohibited at all times.
- If you are combining acids with other substances, always add the acid to the other substance. Adding substances to acid increases the risk of splashing.
- If you encounter a spill of an unknown chemical substance, do not pour any other chemicals on it. Clean it up following strict hazardous waste control procedures. Never touch an unknown substance with your bare hands.

**Biologic Safety.** You will work with test specimens that may be contaminated with blood-borne or other pathogens. Treat every specimen as if it were contaminated.

- Follow Standard Precautions.
- If you have any cuts, lesions, or sores, do not expose yourself to potentially contaminated material. Consult your supervisor if you have any doubt about whether you can safely perform test procedures.
- Wash your hands before and after every procedure and whenever you come in contact with a potentially contaminated substance.
- Wear gloves at all times. Use other protective gear as appropriate to prevent exposing your eyes, nose, and mouth to potentially contaminated material.
- Mouth pipetting is prohibited at all times. Use specially made rubber suction bulbs to draw specimens mechanically.
- Work in a biologic safety cabinet (similar to a fume hood) when completing procedures that are likely to generate droplet sprays or splashes of potentially contaminated material.
- When transferring a blood specimen from a collection tube to another container, cover the tube stopper with an absorbent pad or a commercial stopper remover to prevent spray or splatter from the tube. Do not rock the stopper back and forth, because this could cause the tube to break. Always remove the stopper by opening it away from your face so that the vapor pressure flows away from you. Place the stopper on a sterile gauze pad while you work with the collection tube. Do not allow the stopper to come in contact with other work surfaces. Keep the collection tube stoppered unless you are actively using it.
- Establish clean and dirty areas in the laboratory. Place all used instruments and equipment in the dirty area for sanitization, disinfection, and sterilization.
- Disinfect your work area at least once a day with a 10% bleach solution or a germ-killing solution approved by the Environmental Protection Agency (EPA). If a spill occurs, immediately disinfect the work area.
- Dispose of waste products immediately.
- Dispose of needles in the appropriate sharps container. Do not bend, break, or recap a used needle, and never reuse a disposable needle.
- If an instrument or piece of equipment must be serviced, be sure it has been decontaminated first.
- If you use a bleach solution for disinfection, change it daily.

**Accident Reporting.** Despite all precautions, accidents still occur in the laboratory. Armed with an understanding of the materials with which you are working and basic first-aid procedures, you should be able to deal with most emergencies. Your office should also have written procedures to follow in the event of an accident. Familiarize yourself with the procedures beforehand so that you will know what to do if an accident occurs.

Your first responsibility is to ensure your safety and that of your colleagues and patients. If someone is injured as a result of an accident, administer first aid if required, and take steps to ensure that appropriate health-care personnel take charge of the injured person.

If exposure to spilled chemicals or other substances does not pose a threat, clean up the spill. Take precautions to prevent any of the spilled substances from coming in contact with your skin or clothes. Use appropriate cleaning products for spilled chemicals. Do not touch broken pieces of glass with your hands. Use tongs or a broom and dustpan to pick up the pieces.

Disinfect the surfaces on which the substance spilled. Soaking surfaces with a 10% bleach solution, made fresh each day, is usually sufficient to remove any contamination from blood, blood products, or body fluids.

Report the accident to your supervisor or other personnel as required by your office's policies. If the accident involves exposure to blood or blood products, OSHA regulations require that several steps be followed:

1. Immediate cleaning of the area, including disinfection of contaminated surfaces and sterilization of contaminated instruments and equipment
2. Notification of a designated emergency contact, as identified in your office's safety manual
3. Documentation of the incident on a form similar to that shown in Figure 32-14, including the names of all parties involved, the names of witnesses, a

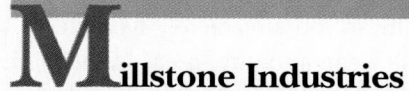

# Millstone Industries

## Central State Division
## Incident Report

Name of Injured Employee _____

Department _____ Job Title _____

Supervisor _____

Date of Accident _____ Time _____

Nature of Injury _____

Was injured acting in a regular line of duty? _____

Was first aid given? _____ By whom? _____

Was designated emergency contact notified? _____

Did injured receive medical treatment?_____

Was injured tested for infection? _____ If no, why not? _____

Did injured go to ER? _____ Other? _____

Did injured leave work? _____ Date _____ Hour _____ A.M. P.M.

Did injured return to work?_____ Date _____ Hour _____ A.M. P.M.

Other Parties Involved _____

Names of Witnesses _____

Describe where and how accident occurred. _____

_____

_____

What, in your opinion, caused the accident? _____

_____

Has anything been done to prevent a similar accident? _____

_____

Has the hazard causing the injury been reported by telephone or in writing? _____

_____

| _____ | _____ |
| Date | Employee's Signature |

| _____ | _____ |
| Date | Supervisor's Signature |

## IF TREATMENT IS NEEDED, TAKE THE ORIGINAL AND DUPLICATE OF THIS FORM TO THE EMERGENCY ROOM.

. . . . . . . . . . . . . . . . . . . . . . . . . . . . . . . . . . . . . . . . . . . . . . . . . . . . . . . . . . . . . .

### This part for Employee Health Office use only

Was incident investigated? _____

Has injured had follow-up medical care? _____

Comments _____

_____

*Original copy to Employee Health Office*       *Duplicate copy to supervisor*

**Figure 32-14.** In the event of an accident or exposure incident in the POL, OSHA regulations require completion of an incident report form.

description of the incident, and a record of medical treatments given to those involved

4. Medical evaluation and follow-up exam of the employees involved

5. Written evaluation of the medical condition of the involved individuals as well as testing for infection, provided that such testing does not violate confidentiality regulations

## Housekeeping

There is a high risk of serious contamination in the laboratory. Laboratory housekeeping duties are designed to reduce the risk of disease transmission. Great care must be taken to ensure that these duties are done correctly and regularly. Guidelines to ensure good operating procedures and to reduce the risk of infection are as follows:

- Refer to your office's written policies and procedures to ensure that you are performing housekeeping duties correctly and according to schedule.
- Immediately clean up spills or splashes of potentially contaminated material. Depending on the material, you may need to use special hazardous waste control products, such as those shown in Figure 32-15. Be sure to dry the area if appropriate, or clearly indicate that the area is still wet.

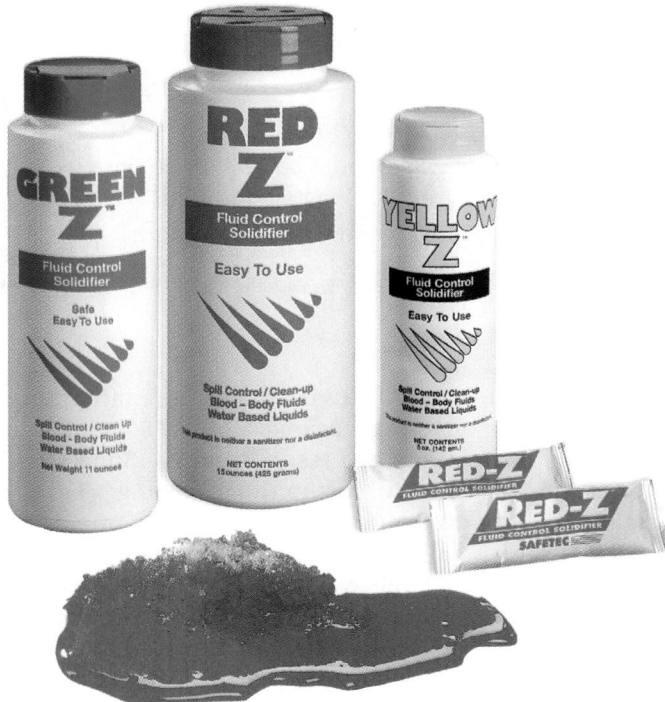

**Figure 32-15.** Certain substances require cleanup with specially formulated products such as these.

- Clean laboratory equipment immediately after use. Contaminants often become hard to remove if they are left on for a long time.
- Dispose of waste products carefully and correctly. Use extreme caution when handling and disposing of sharps. Procedure 32-2 describes how to dispose of biohazardous waste properly.

# Quality Assurance Programs

The operation of a POL can have a significant impact on the health of the patients who depend on the medical practice for care. Accurate testing of specimens from patients is a primary concern. A **quality assurance program** is designed to monitor the quality of the patient care that a medical laboratory provides. It also helps to ensure the safety of laboratory workers. An effective quality assurance program should be a written plan that includes both internal and external reviews of procedures. It serves to assess the quality of the tests performed in a clinical laboratory based on a set of written standards and procedures.

## Clinical Laboratory Improvement Amendments

In response to public concern over the accuracy of laboratory tests, Congress enacted the Clinical Laboratory Improvement Amendments of 1988 (CLIA '88). This law placed all laboratory facilities that conduct tests for diagnosing, preventing, or treating human disease or for assessing human health under federal regulations administered by the Health Care Financing Administration (HCFA) and the CDC. State governments have the ability to implement their own standards, which must be at least as stringent as federal standards. If your state has its own standards, your office will operate under those standards. The state health department provides information about which standards to follow in a given locale.

CLIA '88 has had a major impact on office laboratories. Because of the complexity of the regulations and the expense required to meet them, many doctors have closed their laboratories or sharply reduced the number of tests they perform. Several attempts have been made to change the federal legislation, including an effort to exempt POLs from the regulations. As the health-care debate continues, you may see changes in laboratory operations as a result of changes in CLIA '88 regulations.

As updated and implemented in 1992, CLIA '88 standards apply to four areas of laboratory operation: standards, fees, enforcement, and accreditation programs. Most of the regulations relate to laboratory standards. The specific standards that must be met depend on the test. Tests have been divided into three categories, based on complexity. They are Certificate of Waiver tests; tests of moderate complexity; and tests of high complexity.

# PROCEDURE 32.2

## Disposing of Biohazardous Waste

**Procedure Goal:** To correctly dispose of contaminated waste products, including sharps and contaminated cleaning and paper products

### OSHA Guidelines

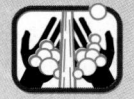 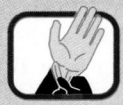 
 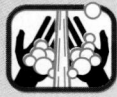

**Materials:** Biohazardous waste containers, gloves, waste materials

### Method:

To dispose of sharps or other materials that pose a danger of cutting, slicing, or puncturing the skin:

1. While wearing gloves, hold the article by the unpointed or blunt end.
2. Drop the object directly into an approved container. (If you are using an evacuation system, do not unscrew the needle. Drop the entire system with the needle attached and the safety device engaged into the receptacle.) The container should be puncture-proof, with rigid sides and a tight-fitting lid.

#### Rationale

To avoid needlestick injuries

3. If you are disposing of a needle, do not bend, break, or attempt to recap the needle before disposal. If the needle is equipped with a safety device, activate the device immediately, and drop the entire assembly into the sharps container.

#### Rationale

Bending, breaking, or recapping increases your risk of needlestick injury.

4. When the container is two-thirds full, replace it with an empty container.

#### Rationale

Overfilling a container puts you at risk for needlestick injury.

5. Depending on your office's procedures, the container and its contents may be sterilized before further disposal, or they may be collected by an authorized waste management agency.
6. Remove the gloves and wash your hands.

To dispose of contaminated paper waste:

1. While wearing gloves, deposit the materials in a properly marked biohazardous waste container. A standard biohazardous waste container has an inner plastic liner, either red or orange and marked with the biohazard symbol, and a puncture-proof outer shell, also marked with the biohazard symbol.
2. If the container is full, secure the inner liner and place it in the appropriate area for biohazardous waste.

#### Rationale

Biohazardous waste must be held in an area separate from regular waste and trash.

3. Remove the gloves and wash your hands.

---

**Certificate of Waiver Tests.** The **Certificate of Waiver tests,** as listed in Table 32-1, are laboratory tests defined as follows.

- The tests pose an insignificant risk to the patient if they are performed or interpreted incorrectly
- The procedures involved are simple and accurate to such a degree that the risk of obtaining incorrect results is minimal
- The tests have been approved by the Food and Drug Administration (FDA) for use by patients at home

If laboratory management decides to perform these tests only, the office may apply for a Certificate of Waiver. When the certificate is granted, the laboratory is exempt from meeting various CLIA '88 standards that apply to the other two test categories. Such laboratories, however, are subject to the following: (1) random inspections to ensure that laboratories operating under a Certificate of Waiver are performing only those tests that qualify for the waiver and (2) investigation of the laboratory if there is any reason to believe the laboratory is not operating safely or if there have been complaints against the laboratory. See the feature Caution: Handle With Care: Operating a Reliable Certificate of Waiver Laboratory for more information about good lab practice.

## TABLE 32-1 Certificate of Waiver Tests

| | |
|---|---|
| **Urine tests** | Urinalysis by dipstick (reagent strip) or tablet reagent (nonautomated) for bilirubin, glucose, hemoglobin, ketone, leukocytes, nitrite, pH, protein, specific gravity, and urobilinogen |
| | Ovulation (visual color comparison tests) |
| | Pregnancy (visual color comparison tests) |
| | Home-screening tests for drugs (opioids, cocaine, methamphetamines, cannabinoids) |
| | Nicotine detection tests |
| | Urine chemistry analyzer for microalbumin and creatinine (semi-quantitative) |
| | Tumor-associated antigen for bladder cancer (using devices approved by the FDA for home use) |
| | Catalase |
| **Blood tests** | Erythrocyte sedimentation rate (ESR), nonautomated |
| | Hemoglobin by copper sulfate, nonautomated |
| | Spun microhematocrit |
| | Blood glucose (using devices approved by the FDA for home use) |
| | Hemoglobin by single analyte instruments, automated |
| | Prothrombin time |
| | Ketones in whole blood, over-the-counter test only |
| | Total cholesterol, high-density lipoprotein (HDL), low-density lipoprotein (LDL), and triglycerides |
| | Hemoglobin A1c |
| | Lactate in whole blood |
| | Lead in whole blood |
| | Thyroid-stimulating hormone, rapid test |
| | Mononucleosis rapid test |
| | *Helicobacter pylori* rapid antibody test |
| | Lyme disease antibodies |
| | HIV antibody test |
| **Fecal tests** | Fecal occult blood |
| **Saliva tests** | Alcohol in saliva |
| **Nasal smear tests** | Influenza A and B antigens |
| **Vaginal smear tests** | *Trichomonas vaginals* antigens |
| | Vaginal pH |
| **Throat swab tests** | Strep A antigens |
| | Influenza A and B |
| **Semen** | Sperm concentration, home screening |

# CAUTION *Handle With Care*

## Operating a Reliable Certificate of Waiver Laboratory

CLIA requires that Certificate of Waiver laboratories obtain a certificate of waiver, pay biennial certificate fees, and follow manufacturers' test instructions. They also require that Certificate of Waiver laboratories submit to random inspections and investigation if indicated. CLIA does not require laboratory personnel to have any specific qualifications or training. In addition, quality control procedures and routine quality assessment are not required by CLIA. Although waived tests are simple to perform and interpret, they may have serious consequences if done incorrectly. Patient care decisions are often made based on the outcome of waived tests.

In order to help ensure quality testing procedures and reduce patient error, the Clinical Laboratory Improvement Advisory Committee (CLIAC) has made several recommendations for good practice in a Certificate of Waiver laboratory. These recommendations include laboratory management considerations and testing procedures before, during, and after the test. To ensure that you are operating a reliable laboratory, follow these recommendations:

### Laboratory Management and Personnel

- Designate the person who will be responsible for laboratory supervision. This person is usually a physician or someone with enough laboratory experience to make decisions about testing.
- Follow all applicable federal, state, and local regulations.
- Perform waived tests only.
- Follow manufacturer's instructions in the package insert.
- Do not make modifications to the instructions.
- Allow random inspections by authorized agencies such as the Centers for Medicare and Medicaid Services (CMS).
- Establish a laboratory safety plan that follows OSHA guidelines.
- Have a designated area that has adequate space and conditions.

- Have enough personnel in the lab and train them appropriately.
- Have written documentation of each test performed.

### Before the Test

- Confirm written test orders.
- Establish a procedure for patient identification.
- Give patients pre-test instructions and determine whether they have followed these instructions.
- Collect specimens according to package insert instructions.
- Label specimens appropriately.
- Never use expired reagents of test kits.

### During the Test

- Perform quality control testing as indicated in the package insert.
- Correct any problem discovered during quality control testing before testing patient samples.
- Establish a policy for frequency of control testing.
- Carefully follow all test-timing recommendations.
- Interpret test results using product inserts as a guide.
- Record test results according to your office policy.

### After the Test

- Report test results to the physician in a timely manner.
- Follow package insert recommendations for follow-up or confirmatory testing.
- Follow OSHA regulations for disposing of biohazardous waste.
- Participate in quality assurance assessment programs:
  - Internal assessment—Perform routine, in-house testing to ensure the accuracy of a test.
  - External assessment—Voluntary inspection of your facility by an outside agency

**Tests of Moderate Complexity.** Tests of moderate complexity make up approximately 75% of all tests performed in the laboratory. Among these tests are blood cell counts and cholesterol screening. Test procedures falling into this category include studies involving bacteriology, mycobacteriology, mycology, parasitology, virology, immunology, chemistry, hematology, and immunohematology.

A laboratory that performs moderate-complexity testing must be run by a pathologist who has an MD or PhD degree. Technicians performing the tests must have training beyond the high school level as defined by CLIA '88

## Quality Control Daily Log

| Name of Unit | Glucose Control Solution | Strip Lot No./ Exp. Date | Low Control Value 35–65 mg/dL | High Control Value 175–235 mg/dL | Analyzed By | Date | Remedial Action Taken If Control Values Abnormal | Retest After Remedial Action Taken |
|---|---|---|---|---|---|---|---|---|
| XYZ Glucometer | Check-strip control solution | Lot 851 10/15/99 | 39 mg/dL | 230 mg/dL | MSM | 1/17/99 | | |
| Mitchell Drugs Glucometer | Check-strip control solution | Lot 851 10/15/99 | 50 mg/dL | 267 mg/dL | MSM | 1/17/99 | Machine cleaned | 220 mg/dL high value |
| XYZ Glucometer | Check-strip control solution | Lot 851 10/15/99 | Unable to read | Unable to read | LMC | 1/18/99 | Battery changed | 38 mg/dL low 198 mg/dL high |
| Mitchell Drugs Glucometer | Check-strip control solution | Lot 851 10/15/99 | 45 mg/dL | 226 mg/dL | LMC | 1/18/99 | | |

**Figure 32-16.** The quality control log shows the completion of every quality control check conducted on a piece of equipment.

regulations. All personnel must participate in a quality assurance program for laboratory procedures, and the laboratory is subject to periodic unannounced inspections and proficiency testing.

**Tests of High Complexity.** Tests of high complexity include more complicated tests in the specialties and subspecialties, including any test in clinical cytogenics, histopathology, histocompatibility, and cytology; and any test not yet categorized by the CMS. Manufacturers' guidelines for testing products are often the best source for discovering the CMS determination for a test. The CMS publishes a directory of all moderate- and high-complexity tests.

Like a laboratory that conducts moderate-complexity tests, a laboratory that conducts high-complexity tests is subject to inspection, proficiency testing, and participation in a quality assurance program, and it must be headed by a medical doctor or a scientist who has a PhD degree. Testing procedures can be performed only by qualified laboratory personnel, whose training exceeds that provided by high schools and is defined by CLIA '88 regulations. Medical assistants will need additional training and education to perform moderate- and high-complexity tests. See the Career Opportunities feature, Clinical Laboratory Technicians, for more information about additional training.

## Components of Quality Assurance

Every quality assurance program must include the following components, in a measurable and structured system, to satisfy CLIA '88 requirements:

- Quality control
- Instrument and equipment maintenance
- Proficiency testing
- Training and continuing education
- Standard operating procedures documentation

## Quality Control and Maintenance

A **quality control program** is one component of a quality assurance program. The focus of the quality control program is to ensure accuracy in test results through careful monitoring of test procedures. To be in compliance with quality control standards, a laboratory must follow certain procedures.

**Calibration.** Testing equipment must be calibrated regularly, in accordance with manufacturers' guidelines. Calibration ensures that the equipment is operating correctly. Each calibration must be recorded in a quality control log, such as the one shown in Figure 32-16. Calibration routines are performed on a set of standards. A **standard** is a specimen, like the patient specimens you would normally process with the equipment, except that the value for each standard is already known. The calibration procedure requires that the test equipment yield the correct results for the standards supplied. If the equipment does not yield the expected results, it must be adjusted until the expected results are obtained. Calibration routines are run on the standards alone, never with patient samples. They are used exclusively to ensure that the equipment is performing according to manufacturers' specifications. Check the manufacturer's instructions to determine how often the equipment should be calibrated. Some equipment requires that trained service personnel perform the calibration.

**Control Samples.** **Control samples** are similar to standards in that they are specimens like those taken from a patient and have known values. Unlike standards, however, control samples are used every time before a patient sample is processed. Using a control sample serves as a check on the accuracy of the test. If the control tests do not fall within the manufacturer's prescribed ranges, patient samples are not analyzed, which prevents erroneous results.

| Urine Reagent Strip Control Log | | | | | | | | | Control Solution | | Exp. Date _____ | | Lot # _____ | |
|---|---|---|---|---|---|---|---|---|---|---|---|---|---|---|
| Reagent Strip Lot # & Exp. Date | Test | Specific Gravity | pH | Protein | Glucose | Ketone | Bilirubin | Blood | Nitrite | Urobi-linogen | Control Test Date | Remedial Action Taken If Reading Is Abnormal | Retest Date | Technician Initials |
| | Reagent Strip Expected Range | | | | | | | | | | | | | |
| | Test Results | | | | | | | | | | | | | |
| | Reagent Strip Expected Range | | | | | | | | | | | | | |
| | Test Results | | | | | | | | | | | | | |

**Figure 32-17.** The reagent control log shows the quality testing performed on every batch or lot of reagent products.

The control samples for certain laboratory procedures show normal (negative) and abnormal (positive) results. Generally, positive and negative control samples are used with tests that yield a **qualitative test response** (the substance being tested for is either present or absent).

Other control samples are formulated to show when results fall within a normal range. These samples are used for tests that yield **quantitative test results** (the concentration of a test substance in a specimen). At least two control samples containing different concentrations of the test substance should be run for quantitative tests.

**Reagent Control.** Control samples or standards are also run every time you open a new supply of testing products, such as staining materials, culture media, and reagents. **Reagents** are chemicals or chemically treated substances used in test procedures. A reagent is formulated to react in specific ways when exposed under specific conditions. One example of a reagent is the chemically coated strip used in blood glucose monitoring. A visual change on the reagent strip (also called a dipstick) occurs in the presence of glucose in a blood sample.

To ensure the quality of reagents, you should keep a reagent control log. If a defective reagent test is identified, it can be tracked to its source. A sample reagent control log is shown in Figure 32-17. Running controls on a routine basis gives you information about the equipment and the reagents used during the test. If a control consistently yields unexpected results (for example a positive control yields a negative result), you should check the reagents first and then the equipment calibration.

**Maintenance.** Testing instruments and equipment must be properly maintained, and all maintenance procedures must be documented. Follow manufacturers' guidelines for performing instrument and equipment maintenance. A maintenance log provides a complete record of all work performed on an instrument or a piece of equipment (Figure 32-18).

# Acme Medical Supplies
## Equipment Maintenance Record

**Practice** _____ Russo and Russo Medical Associates
**Name of Equipment** _____ Acme Microscope Model ABC-123
**Location** _____ Lab _____ **Purchase Date** _____ 12/1/08

| Date | Cleaning | Maintenance/Repair | Technician Initials |
|---|---|---|---|
| 6/5 | Microscope | Cleaned | CJC |
| 6/11 | Microscope high objective | Cleaned | DWM |
| 6/14 | Microscope | Changed bulb | CJC |
| 6/16 | Microscope eyepiece | Lens cover replaced | CJC |
| 6/17 | Microscope high objective | Cleaned | CJC |

**Figure 32-18.** A maintenance log must be kept for every piece of laboratory equipment. All work done on the equipment must be recorded in the log.

![BIOHAZARD symbol] **CAUTION** *Handle With Care*

## Troubleshooting Problems in a Physician's Office Laboratory

Working in a physician's office laboratory can be exciting and challenging. Part of your job as a medical assistant is to make sure that the tests you perform are accurate. Occasionally, you will encounter a piece of equipment that is not working or test results and controls that are consistently too high or too low. You will need to troubleshoot these problems to determine their cause. Troubleshooting is a thorough and logical investigation for the cause of a problem. You must eliminate possible causes of the problem one at a time. The general steps to troubleshooting a piece of equipment or test kit are:

- Have a written procedure for troubleshooting tests and equipment.
- Recognize the problem (controls give clues to possible problems).
- Think about possible causes.
- Start with the simplest cause first.
- Document your findings.
- Call your service company after you have checked everything you know to check.

When troubleshooting equipment, follow these steps:

- Check the power source at the machine, the wall outlet, the breaker box, or the battery.

- Check the equipment manual for troubleshooting information.
- Reboot the equipment by turning it off, waiting a few minutes, and then turning it back on.
- Check the service log for the date of the last maintenance.
- If you are able to repair the problem, run controls to verify the problem is fixed before testing patient samples.

When troubleshooting a test kit, follow these steps:

- Read the package insert to verify you have performed the test correctly.
- Check to make sure you have used the correct reagents or test strips.
- Check the dates on the reagents or test strips to make sure they are not outdated.
- Make sure you are using the proper sample for the test.
- Repeat the test using control samples.
- If the controls are correct, repeat the test with the patient sample.

---

*Troubleshooting.* You may need to investigate the cause of a problem with a piece of equipment or a test. To do this, you should take a systematic approach to rule out the cause of the problem. For more information regarding investigating equipment and test malfunctions, see the Caution: Handle With Care feature, Troubleshooting Problems in a Physician's Office Laboratory.

**Documentation.** A quality control program depends first on careful adherence to procedures designed to identify problems with equipment calibration, errors in testing procedures, and defective testing supplies. The second component of a quality control program is the careful documentation of all procedures. Besides maintaining the quality control log, the reagent control log, and the equipment maintenance log, you will also complete the following records as part of a quality control program:

- Reference laboratory log, which lists specimens sent to another laboratory for testing

- Daily workload log, which shows all procedures completed during the workday

## Proficiency Testing

All laboratories that perform moderate- and high-complexity tests as identified by CLIA '88 must participate in a proficiency testing program. **Proficiency testing programs** measure the accuracy of test results and adherence to standard operating procedures. Generally, proficiency tests include two parts: (1) a control sample from the proficiency testing organization engaged by your laboratory and (2) forms that must be completed to record the steps in the testing procedure. The control sample is processed normally, under the same conditions as any patient sample. The results, the forms, and sometimes the control samples are returned to the proficiency testing organization, which then informs your office of whether it has passed or failed the test. A passing mark means that your laboratory can continue to perform that particular test. A failing mark can mean that your laboratory must discontinue that test and possibly other tests as well.

## Training, Continuing Education, and Documentation

One of your employer's responsibilities is to provide opportunities for employee training and continuing education. Another is to provide written reference materials and documentation for all procedures conducted in the POL. Your responsibility is to consult reference materials and take part in available training to keep your skills sharpened and up to date.

It may seem unnecessary to refer to written instructions for procedures that you do many times a day. Changes can be made in a procedure for many reasons, however, and you must be aware of these changes. Here are some reference materials with which you should be familiar:

- Material Safety Data Sheets
- Standard operating procedures
- Safety manuals
- Equipment manufacturers' user or reference guides
- Clinical Laboratory Technical Procedure Manuals
- Regulatory documentation (OSHA standards, CLIA '88 requirements)
- Maintenance and housekeeping schedules

## Filling Out a Laboratory Requisition Form

As a medical assistant, it is your responsibility to ensure that the laboratory requisition form is properly completed. Missing information can lead to improper testing or lost results. The completed form should be included with the specimen collected or sent with the patient to the laboratory. Be sure to include the following information on all requisitions:

- Patient's full name, sex, date of birth, and address
- Patient's insurance information
- Physician's name, address, and phone number
- Source of the specimen
- Date and time of the specimen collection
- Test(s) requested
- Preliminary diagnosis
- Any current treatment that might affect the results

See Figure 32-19 for a sample laboratory requisitions form.

# Communicating With the Patient

In your job as a medical assistant, you will be involved with patients before they submit samples for laboratory testing, during the specimen collection procedure, and

after the physician has interpreted the test results. It is your responsibility to ensure that patients understand what is expected of them every step of the way.

## Before the Test

Certain tests require patients to prepare by fasting or restricting fluid intake. It is your duty to explain test preparations. Use simple, nontechnical language and check with patients to be sure they understand the information. In some cases providing a written instruction sheet may be helpful.

Explaining the reason for the preparation can help ensure compliance or unearth potential problems. For example, if you explain to a patient that he is to refrain from drinking anything for a particular period, he might ask whether that includes the water he uses to take a certain medication. You can then make sure the patient receives the answers he will need for carrying out the physician's orders in light of his own circumstances.

If you are the person who collects specimens, you need to determine whether patients have correctly completed the required test preparations. Test results are invalid in some cases if patients fail to follow test preparation guidelines. When preparations have not been completed correctly, discuss the situation with the physician or other appropriate staff member as required by your office to determine whether the specimen should still be collected. If the specimen is not collected, document the reason the test was not carried out as requested. Review the guidelines for specimen collection with the patient, and schedule another appointment if appropriate.

## During Specimen Collection

Before collecting a specimen, you must first be sure you have the right patient. Proper patient identification is an essential part of good laboratory practice. You do not want to collect a blood sample from someone who only needs a urinalysis. Patients do not always understand the tests they are having. It is up to you to make sure you have the right patient and are performing the test as it is ordered.

The instructions you deliver to patients during specimen collection vary with the nature of the specimen. Always deliver instructions clearly and in language patients can understand. Do not assume that patients do not need to hear the instructions, even if they have had the test before. Explain what you must do and what patients must do before moving to each new step in the process.

Patients are understandably nervous during many collection procedures. In addition to communicating technical information, you should provide any helpful advice that may make the test easier. Also provide reassurance as appropriate. For example, if a patient asks whether the blood-drawing procedure is painful, explain that a sharp stick or stinging sensation may be experienced

| LAB USE ONLY | Laboratory Name & Address | Requesting Physician Information |
|---|---|---|
| Acct # | | |
| DATE | | Address |
| TIME | | |

| Patient Information | | | | | |
|---|---|---|---|---|---|
| Patient Name (Last) | (First) | (MI) | Date of Birth / / | Phone Number | |
| Address | City, State | Zip | Phone Number | | |
| Patient I.D. Number | Responsible Party (Last) | (First) | (Phone) | Male | |
| | | | | Female | |
| Social Security Number | Physician | | | Date Time Specimen Collection | |

**Bill: Check One**
Our account    Medicare
Insurance Co./Patient

*Complete the Following Information for Billing a Patient and/or a Third Party Agency*

| Policy Holder Name | Policy Holder Address: | Relation |
|---|---|---|
| | Policy Holder Phone Number: | Self    Spouse    Child Other _____ |
| Insurance Co. Name | Address Insurance Co. | City , State, Zip |
| Employer | | |
| Policy          Group # | PATIENT or GUARDIAN SIGNATURE: | DATE: |

## CHECK DESIRED TESTS          PLEASE PROVIDE ICD=9-CM#

| √ | ORGAN DISEASE PANELS, BLOOD | ICD-9 | √ | TEST, BLOOD | ICD-9 | √ | TEST, BLOOD | ICD-9 | √ | TEST, URINE | ICD-9 |
|---|---|---|---|---|---|---|---|---|---|---|---|
| | ACUTE HEP. A,B,C | | | ESR | | | WBC with diff | | | U/A Routine | |
| | BASIC METABOLIC | | | EBV | | | PT | | | | |
| | THYROID | | | FBS | | | PTT | | | | |
| | ELECTROLYTES | | | Grp A β-hem strep | | | Bleeding time | | | | |
| | HEPATIC FUNCTION | | | Hgb | | | PCO$_2$ | | | | |
| | LIPID PROFILE | | | Hct | | | PO$_2$ | | | | |
| | RENAL FUNCTION | | | HgbA1c | | | CO$_2$ | | | | |
| | **TEST, BLOOD** | | | HIV antibodies | | | HCO$_3$ | | | **MICROBIOLOGY** | |
| | ACE | | | Insulin | | | Ca$^{++}$ | | | AFB culture | |
| | ADH | | | Iron | | | Cl$^-$ | | | C & S | |
| | ALT | | | Ketone bodies | | | | | | Chlamydia screen | |
| | AFP | | | LD | | | | | | Endocervical culture | |
| | Amylase | | | pH | | | | | | GC screen | |
| | Acetone | | | Phenylalanine | | | | | | Gram stain | |
| | AST | | | K$^+$ and Na$^+$ | | | **TEST, URINE** | | | O & P | |
| | Bilirubin | | | Proteins, Albumin | | | Cys | | | Strep A culture | |
| | BUN | | | Proteins, Fibrinogen | | | CrCl | | | Throat culture | |
| | CEA | | | PSA | | | Glucose | | | Urine culture | |
| | Calcium, total | | | RBC | | | HCG | | | Viral culture | |
| | Carbon dioxide, total | | | Sickle cells | | | UBG | | | Wound culture | |
| | Cholesterol, total | | | TSH | | | UFC | | | | |
| | Cholesterol, HDLs | | | T3 | | | UK | | | | |
| | Cholesterol, LDLs | | | T4 | | | UNA | | | | |
| | CK | | | Uric Acid | | | Uosm | | | | |
| | CMV | | | WBC | | | UUN | | | | |

**Figure 32-19.** The laboratory requisition form must be accurately completed.

when the needle is inserted but that no pain should be felt after that. Let the patient be your guide in determining how much information to provide. Some people want to know every detail, whereas others prefer to know as little as possible.

One important aspect of communicating with patients about testing procedures is your nonverbal communication skills. Even if you deliver accurate technical information and answer every question patients have, there can still be a breakdown in communication if your nonverbal signals do not support your verbal message. Follow these guidelines to ensure that your nonverbal actions are helping, not hindering, the communication process.

- Strike a balance between a strict, businesslike attitude and overly familiar friendliness. Your actions must impress on the patient that you are well informed about the procedure involved and that you care about the patient's understanding of it.
- Treat the patient with respect. Address the patient by name, using the appropriate courtesy title unless you have been invited to use the patient's first name or the patient is a child. Provide privacy during specimen collection. Privacy needs may be met by using a separate room or contained area for drawing blood, for example; a private bathroom is best for collecting urine specimens.
- Recognize that the patient may be under stress because of the test procedure or the pending results. Some patients may be familiar with the test procedures, but others may not know what to expect. You may need to repeat instructions or explain what you are doing more than one time. Remain calm and patient—never be abrupt or condescending.
- Direct your attention to the patient, particularly during a procedure that might be uncomfortable, such as drawing blood. Unless an emergency develops, pay attention to nothing else at that time.

## After Specimen Collection

If the patient must follow particular guidelines after you collect the specimen, explain them. Commonly, posttest instructions deal with care of venipuncture sites, signs and symptoms of infection, additional or continuing dietary restrictions, and the schedule for further testing if it is necessary.

## When the Test Results Return

When you receive the test results, do not communicate them to the patient but to the doctor. Only the doctor is qualified to interpret test results for the patient. Your role in reporting results comes after the doctor examines the test information and prepares a report. Sometimes the doctor discusses the results with the patient. At other times you will be asked to convey the test results to the patient along with instructions from the doctor. Answer only those patient questions that are within the range of your knowledge and experience. If the patient needs more information than you can provide, refer the patient to the doctor.

## Record Keeping

The importance of accurate and complete record keeping can be summed up in one statement: If it is not written down, it was not done. This motto applies to all your duties as a medical assistant. Besides recording information about quality control and equipment maintenance, you may be called on to handle inventory control, record test results in patient records, and keep track of every specimen that passes through your hands. You may need to use standard abbreviations for measures when recording test results. Table 32-2 provides a list of common abbreviations used in the laboratory.

| TABLE 32-2 | Abbreviations for Common Laboratory Measures |
|---|---|
| cm = centimeter | |
| $cm^3$ = cubic centimeter | |
| dL = deciliter | |
| fl oz = fluid ounce | |
| g = gram | |
| L = liter | |
| lb = pound | |
| m = meter | |
| mcg = microgram | |
| mg = milligram | |
| mL = milliliter | |
| mm = millimeter | |
| mm Hg = millimeters of mercury | |
| oz = ounce | |
| pt = pint | |
| QNS = quantity not sufficient | |
| QS = quantity sufficient | |
| qt = quart | |
| U = unit | |
| wt = weight | |

## Inventory Control

You will be responsible for taking inventory of equipment and supplies to ensure that the POL never runs out of them. To do so, you will keep a list of items that are used routinely and reordered systematically. Establish a regular schedule for counting items in the POL, perhaps every week. Then estimate when you will probably need to reorder an item—and put the date on your calendar.

## Patient Records

When recording test results, it is your responsibility to identify unusual findings. Many offices require that out-of-range test results be circled or underlined in red. Follow the procedure established by your office. Test results are not communicated to the patient until the physician has had the opportunity to review the information. The physician usually initials or otherwise marks the records after examining them.

## Specimen Identification

All specimens must be clearly identified with the patient's name, the patient's identification code if your office uses one, the date and time the specimen was collected, the initials of the person who collected the specimen, the physician's name, and other information as required by the test procedure or your office. If you encounter an unidentified or incorrectly identified specimen, you must make an effort to track it to its source. The specimen will probably be discarded or destroyed, however, because there is no guarantee that it was identified correctly. Even if you do manage to identify it, it may have been compromised in some way.

## Summary

The physician's office laboratory offers many opportunities for interesting and satisfying work in your role as a medical assistant. Those opportunities carry with them the responsibility to maintain and improve your technical skills; to stay abreast of technological, legislative, and regulatory developments; to take every precaution to prevent the transmission of disease and the occurrence of accidents or emergency situations; and to seek ways to improve the quality of patient care.

Keeping a level head and applying common sense will go a long way toward making your work in the laboratory efficient and accurate. Take time to do a procedure correctly the first time. Be systematic in your approach to investigating equipment and testing problems and their causes. Avoid shortcuts—they lead to mistakes and lost time.

The quantity of information you will need to learn, integrate, and convey to the patient through your actions and educational efforts may be daunting at first. As you gain understanding and confidence in your skills, however, much of it will become routine.

# REVIEW

## CHAPTER 32

### CASE STUDY QUESTIONS

Now that you have completed this chapter, review the case study at the beginning of the chapter and answer the following questions:

1. What is a POL?
2. What enactment regulates laboratories, personnel, and the testing they perform?
3. What is the difference between waived testing and moderate-complexity testing?
4. Does quality control have an impact on laboratories? If so, how?
5. Should you perform the testing as requested? Why or why not?

### Discussion Questions

1. Identify five common physical hazards in the laboratory and the steps you can take to eliminate them.
2. Discuss the importance of giving patients pretest instructions.
3. A common instrument used in laboratories is a microscope. Identify the component parts of a microscope.
4. What information must be included on MSDSs for chemicals?
5. Describe the steps you would take to troubleshoot a piece of equipment that is not working.

### Critical Thinking Questions

1. While you are holding a vial of blood, it slips out of your hand and breaks. What should you do?
2. How could a physician's office laboratory be more advantageous than a reference laboratory? What advantages does a reference laboratory afford?
3. While performing a test using a reagent test kit, you notice that the positive control yields a negative result. What action should you take?
4. What nonverbal communication techniques can you use when you are instructing patients during the specimen collection process?

### Application Activities

1. Examine a prepared slide under a microscope. With a partner, practice bringing the slide specimen into focus with each objective. Partners should check each other's work.
2. Obtain a Material Safety Data Sheet, and review the information on it. Explain to another student what hazards the substance poses, what measures can be taken to avoid injury from the substance, and what steps should be taken in the event of an accident.
3. Demonstrate how you would care for a microscope after its use.

### Virtual Fieldtrip

*Visit the McGraw-Hill Higher Education Medical Assisting website at www.mhhe.com/medicalassisting3 to complete the following activity:*

Search the FDA Office of In Vitro Diagnostic Device Evaluation and Safety website for information about safety tips for laboratorians.

- What type of information can be found on this site?
- How can you use this information to improve your laboratory?

Open the CD and complete this chapter's practice activities, play the games, listen to the key terms, and test yourself with the interactive review. E-mail, print, and/or save your results to document your proficiency.

## CHAPTER 33

# Introduction to Microbiology

## MEDICAL ASSISTING COMPETENCIES

**In preparation for the certification examination, you should know the following areas of competence:**

| COMPETENCY | CMA | RMA |
|---|---|---|
| **Clinical** | | |
| Apply principles of aseptic techniques and infection control, including hand washing | X | X |
| Dispose of biohazardous materials | X | X |
| Practice Standard Precautions | X | X |
| Obtain specimens for microbiological testing, including throat specimens and wound cultures | X | X |
| Instruct patients in the collection of fecal specimens | X | X |
| Perform selected CLIA-waived tests (e.g., "kit tests") | X | X |
| Perform microbiology testing | X | X |
| Screen and follow up on patient test results | X | X |
| **General/Legal/Professional** | | |
| Determine the needs for documentation and reporting, and document accurately and appropriately | X | X |
| Perform risk management procedures | | X |
| Operate and maintain facilities, and perform routine maintenance of administrative and clinical equipment safely | X | X |
| Perform quality control procedures | X | X |

## CHAPTER OUTLINE

- Microbiology and the Role of the Medical Assistant
- How Microorganisms Cause Disease
- Classification and Naming of Microorganisms
- Viruses
- Bacteria
- Protozoans
- Fungi
- Multicellular Parasites
- How Infections Are Diagnosed
- Specimen Collection
- Transporting Specimens to an Outside Laboratory
- Direct Examination of Specimens
- Preparation and Examination of Stained Specimens
- Culturing Specimens in the Medical Office
- Determining Antimicrobial Sensitivity
- Quality Control in the Medical Office

## KEY TERMS

- acid-fast stain
- aerobe
- agar
- anaerobe
- antimicrobial
- bacillus
- coccus
- colony
- culture
- culture and sensitivity (C&S)
- culture medium
- etiologic agent
- facultative
- fungus
- gram-negative
- gram-positive
- Gram's stain
- KOH mount
- microbiology
- mold
- mordant
- O&P specimen
- parasite
- protozoan
- qualitative analysis
- quality control (QC)
- quantitative analysis
- smear
- spirillum
- stain
- vibrio
- virus
- wet mount
- yeast

# LEARNING OUTCOMES

After completing Chapter 33, you will be able to:

**33.1** Define microbiology.

**33.2** Describe how microorganisms cause disease.

**33.3** Describe how microorganisms are classified and named.

**33.4** Explain how viruses, bacteria, protozoans, fungi, and parasites differ and give examples of each.

**33.5** Describe the process involved in diagnosing an infection.

**33.6** List general guidelines for obtaining specimens.

**33.7** Describe how throat culture, urine, sputum, wound, and stool specimens are obtained.

**33.8** Explain how to transport specimens to outside laboratories.

**33.9** Describe two techniques used in the direct examination of culture specimens.

**33.10** Explain how to prepare and examine stained specimens.

**33.11** Describe how to culture specimens in the medical office.

**33.12** Explain how cultures are interpreted.

**33.13** Describe how to perform an antimicrobial sensitivity determination.

**33.14** Explain how to implement quality control measures in the microbiology laboratory.

# Introduction

Humans are surrounded by tiny living organisms invisible to the naked eye. For the most part, these microorganisms cause no problems; however, when they are pathogenic in nature or are displaced from their natural environment, they can cause infections and disease. This chapter addresses the different life forms of microorganisms and how they may be identified; it also teaches you the proper collection technique for common types of specimens. You will learn about the processes involved in identifying microorganisms, the types of culture media used for these processes, how antimicrobial testing is done, and how quality control fits into ensuring reliable patient results.

## CASE STUDY

You awoke this morning with a scratchy sore throat and slight fever. You decide to go to work at the doctor's office because you don't really feel that bad, but as the morning progresses, so do your symptoms. You ask the doctor for permission to have a throat culture obtained, and with approval, you ask another medical assistant to collect the specimen. While the specimen is being collected, you can't help but notice that the swab touches your lips and tongue, but not the back of your throat. The rapid strep test is negative, so the doctor does not prescribe any medication for you. The next morning when you arise, you feel much worse and have a temperature of 102.8°F. When you return to the office, the doctor briefly examines you and decides to repeat the test; this one is properly collected and the results come back as positive for strep throat. You are then prescribed antibiotics and sent home to rest.

As you read this chapter, consider the following questions:

1. What is the proper technique for collecting a throat specimen?
2. Why do you think the first test result came back as negative?
3. What organism is responsible for causing strep throat?
4. What complications may have developed if you had not had another throat culture obtained and been prescribed antibiotics?

# Microbiology and the Role of the Medical Assistant

**Microbiology** is the study of microorganisms—simple forms of life that are microscopic (visible only through a microscope) and are commonly made up of a single cell. Microorganisms are found everywhere. Some microorganisms are normally found on the skin and within the human body; they are called normal flora. They do not typically cause disease. Instead, they perform a number of important functions. For example, microorganisms in the intestines produce vitamins and help digest food. They also help protect the body from infection.

Many microorganisms cause infections. These microorganisms are referred to as pathogenic, or disease-causing. Infections can be mild, as in the case of the common cold.

Infections can, however, sometimes lead to serious conditions. The proper diagnosis and treatment of infections are essential to restoring good health.

You may assist the physician in performing a number of microbiologic procedures that aid in diagnosing and treating infectious diseases. The types of microbiologic procedures you may be required to perform in the medical office include obtaining specimens or assisting the physician in doing so, preparing specimens for direct examination by the physician, and preparing specimens for transportation to a microbiology laboratory for identification.

Some physicians' offices have their own laboratories and are equipped to perform certain microbiology procedures. If you work in such an office, you may be required to perform additional microbiologic procedures.

# How Microorganisms Cause Disease

Anton van Leeuwenhoek first observed single-celled organisms through a microscope more than 300 years ago. It was not until much later, however, that microorganisms were identified as the cause of disease, through the works of scientists such as Louis Pasteur and Robert Koch.

Microorganisms can cause disease in a variety of ways. They may use up nutrients or other materials needed by the cells and tissues they invade. Microorganisms may damage body cells directly by reproducing themselves within cells, or the presence of microorganisms may make body cells the targets of the body's own defenses. Some microorganisms produce toxins, or poisons, that damage cells and tissues. Infecting microorganisms, or toxins they produce, may remain localized or may travel throughout the body, damaging or killing cells and tissues. The resulting symptoms include local swelling, pain, warmth, and redness along with generalized symptoms of fever, tiredness, aches, and weakness. Infection by certain organisms may also cause skin reactions, gastrointestinal upset, or other symptoms.

Pathogenic organisms can be transmitted from one person to another in one of two ways:

1. Through direct person-to-person contact, such as touching

2. Through indirect contact, as with vectors, contaminated objects, droplets expelled in the air, or contaminated food or drink

The microorganisms that make up normal flora, in addition to intact skin and mucous membranes, act as a barrier against infection by certain pathogens. Even these protective microorganisms, however, can cause infection if they invade other areas of the body.

# Classification and Naming of Microorganisms

There are many different types of microorganisms, several of which can cause disease. Scientists classify microorganisms on the basis of their structure. Common classifications of microorganisms include the following:

- Subcellular, which consist of hereditary material, either deoxyribonucleic acid (DNA) or ribonucleic acid (RNA), surrounded by a protein coat
- Prokaryotic, which have a simple cell structure with no nucleus and no organelles in the cytoplasm
- Eukaryotic, which have a complex cell structure containing a nucleus and specialized organelles in the cytoplasm

Table 33-1 lists the characteristics that distinguish these classifications as well as the types of microorganisms found in the classifications. Types of microorganisms include the following:

- Viruses
- Bacteria
- Protozoans
- Fungi
- Multicellular parasites

These types may be further divided into special groups that share certain characteristics. For example, within the bacteria are the special groups, mycobacteria and rickettsiae, within each of which the members share distinct characteristics.

| TABLE 33-1 Classifications of Microorganisms | | |
|---|---|---|
| **Classification** | **Characteristics** | **Examples** |
| Subcellular | Noncellular<br>Nucleic acid surrounded by protein coat | Viruses |
| Prokaryotic cells | Simple structure<br>Single chromosome<br>No organelles | Bacteria |
| Eukaryotic cells | Highly structured<br>Nucleus and cytoplasm<br>Organelles | Protozoans, fungi, parasites |

Specific microorganisms are named in a standard way, using two words. The first word refers to the genus (a category of biologic classification between the family and the species) to which the microorganism belongs. The second word refers to the particular species of the organism. Each species represents a distinct kind of microorganism. For example, within the bacteria is the *Staphylococcus* genus. Then within that genus are various species such as *Staphylococcus aureus* and *Staphylococcus epidermidis*. Although the two bacteria belong to the same genus, they differ greatly in their ability to cause disease. The first letter of the genus is always capitalized, and the species name is always written in all lowercase letters.

# Viruses

**Viruses** are among the smallest known infectious agents. They cannot be seen with a regular microscope. Viruses are a simpler life form than the cell, consisting only of nucleic acid surrounded by a protein coat, as shown in Figure 33-1. Because of this fact, viruses can live and grow only within the living cells of other organisms.

Many viruses cause disease in people. Viruses are the cause of many of the common illnesses and conditions seen frequently in the medical office, including the common cold, influenza, chickenpox, croup, hepatitis, mononucleosis, and warts. Other illnesses caused by viruses are acquired immunodeficiency syndrome (AIDS), mumps, rubella, measles, encephalitis, and herpes. Vaccines are available to protect people from many of these viruses.

# Bacteria

Bacteria are single-celled prokaryotic organisms that reproduce very quickly and are one of the major causes of disease. Under the right conditions—the right temperature, the right nutrients, and moisture—bacterial cells can double in number in 15 to 30 minutes. This rapid reproduction is one reason why untreated infections can be dangerous.

## Classification and Identification

There are many different kinds of bacteria and many ways to identify them. Bacteria can be classified according to their shape, their ability to retain certain dyes, their ability

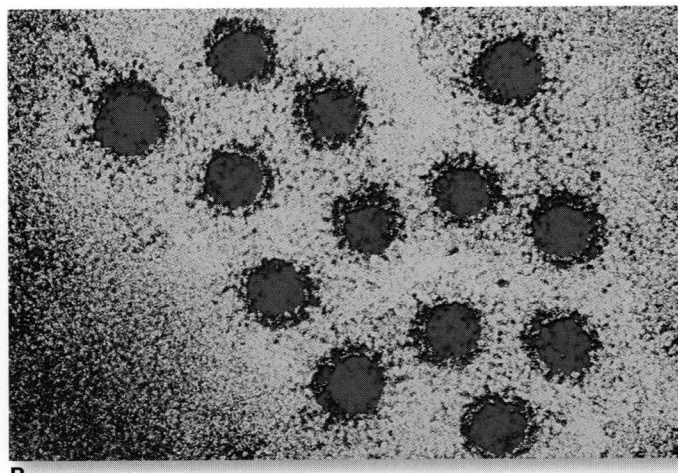

**B**

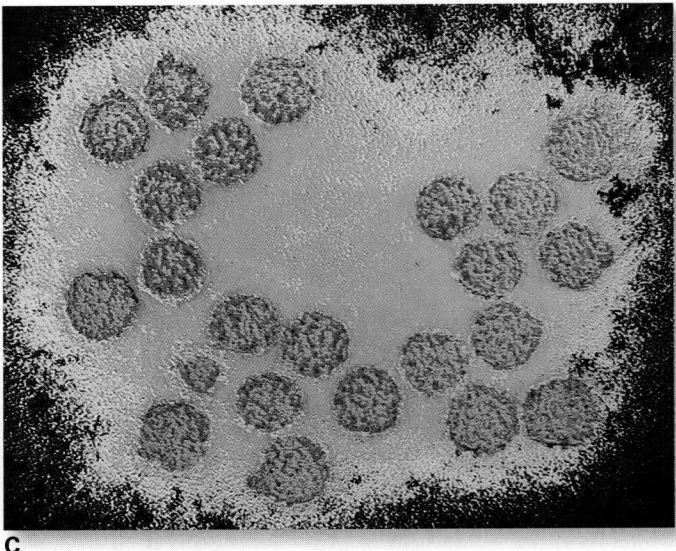

**C**

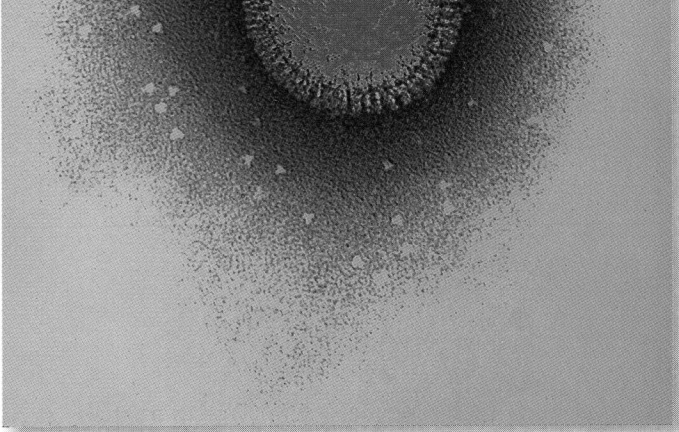

**A**

**Figure 33-1.** The three types of viral diseases often seen in medical offices are: (A) influenza, (B) hepatitis, and (C) warts.

## TABLE 33-2  Some Major Groups of Bacteria

### Gram-Positive Bacteria

| Shape | Characteristic | Genus | Species |
|---|---|---|---|
| Spherical, round, or ovoid | Grow in clusters<br>Grow in chains | Staphylococcus<br>Streptococcus | aureus, epidermidis<br>pyogenes, pneumoniae |
| Straight rod | Are aerobic<br>Are anaerobic | Bacillus<br>Clostridium | subtilis<br>botulinum, tetani |

### Gram-Negative Bacteria

| Shape | Characteristic | Genus | Species |
|---|---|---|---|
| Spherical, round, or ovoid | Are aerobic | Neisseria | meningitidis, gonorrhoeae |
| Straight rod | Are aerobic | Pseudomonas<br>Haemophilus | aeruginosa<br>influenzae |
| | Are facultative | Escherichia<br>Salmonella<br>Shigella | coli<br>typhi<br>dysenteriae |
| Comma | Are facultative | Vibrio | cholerae |
| Spiral | Move by undulating | Treponema | pallidum |

### Other Groups

| Shape | Characteristic | Genus | Species |
|---|---|---|---|
| Straight, curved, or branched rod | Are acid-fast | Mycobacterium | tuberculosis |
| Variable | Have no rigid cell wall<br>Are intracellular parasites | Mycoplasma<br>Rickettsia | pneumoniae<br>rickettsii |
| Spherical, round, or ovoid | Are intracellular parasites | Chlamydia | trachomatis |

to grow with or without air, and certain biochemical reactions. Table 33-2 lists some representatives of the major groups of bacteria, with distinguishing characteristics and a few examples.

**Shape.** The most common way to classify bacteria is according to their shape. A **coccus** (plural, cocci) is spherical, round, or ovoid; a **bacillus** (plural, bacilli) is rod-shaped; a **spirillum** (plural, spirilla) is spiral-shaped; and a **vibrio** (plural, vibrios) is comma-shaped. Figure 33-2 illustrates the four shapes.

- Cocci can be further divided into three types. Staphylococci are grapelike clusters of cocci commonly found on the skin. One species of this microorganism causes a variety of infections, including boils, acne, abscesses, food poisoning, and a type of pneumonia. Diplococci are pairs of cocci. The causative agents for gonorrhea and some forms of meningitis are diplococci. Streptococci are cocci that grow in chains. These microorganisms are responsible for infections such as strep throat, certain types of pneumonia, and rheumatic fever.

- Bacilli, or rod-shaped bacteria, are responsible for a wide variety of infections, including gastroenteritis, tuberculosis, pneumonia, whooping cough, urinary tract infections (UTIs), botulism, and tetanus.

- Spirilla, or spiral-shaped bacteria, are responsible for infections such as syphilis and Lyme disease.

- Vibrios, or comma-shaped bacteria, are responsible for diseases such as cholera and some cases of food poisoning.

**Ability to Retain Certain Dyes.** In addition to their shape, bacteria are commonly classified by how they react to certain stains. A **stain** is a solution of a dye or group of dyes that imparts a color to microorganisms. The most common staining procedure in use today is the **Gram's stain,** a method of staining that differentiates bacteria according to the chemical composition of their cell walls. This procedure is often performed in the medical office. Another important stain is the **acid-fast stain,** a staining procedure for identifying bacteria with a waxy cell wall. The bacteria that cause tuberculosis can be stained with this procedure.

**Introduction to Microbiology**     **775**

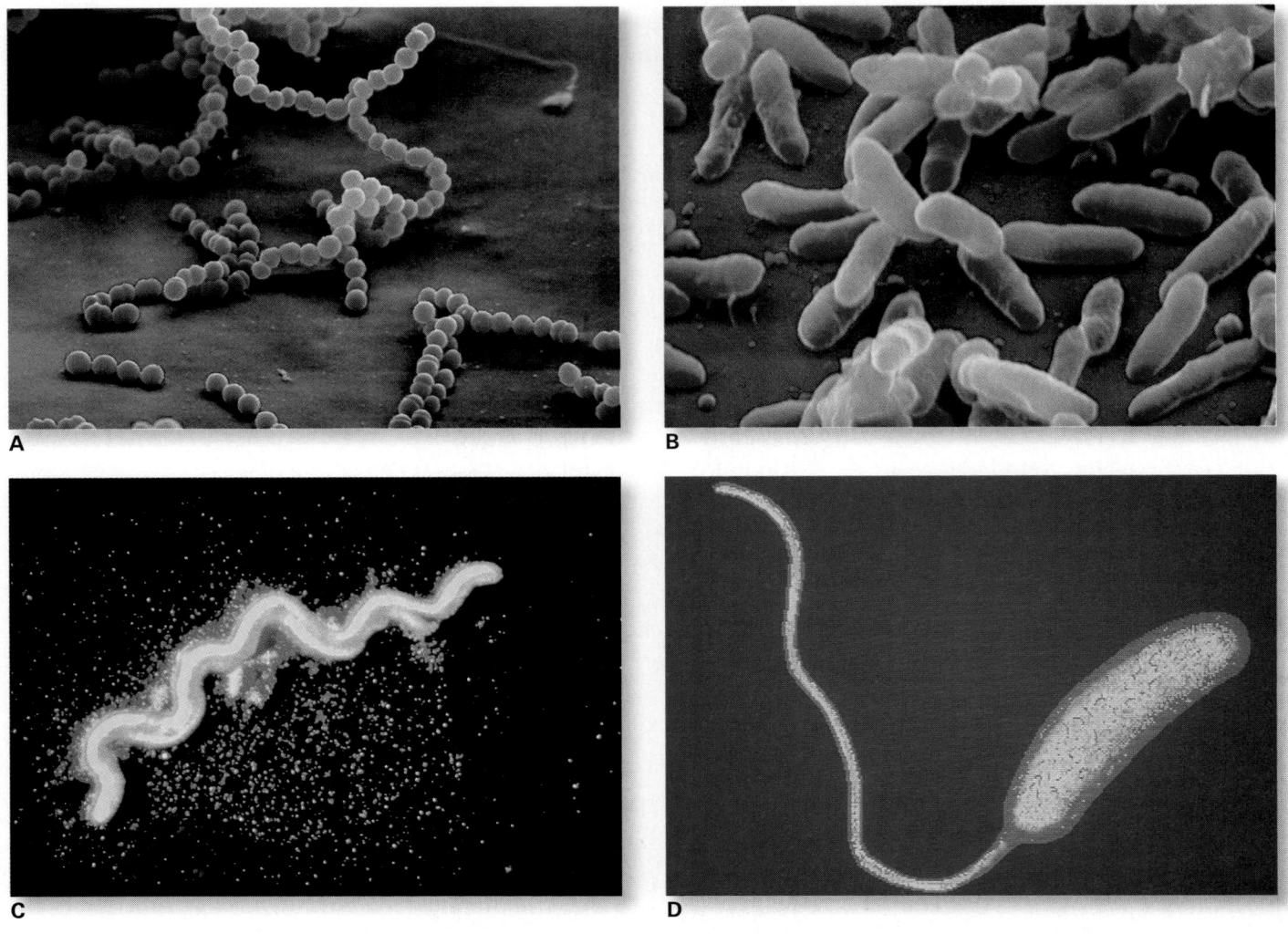

**Figure 33-2.** The four bacterial classifications by shape are: (A) coccus, (B) bacillus, (C) spirillum, and (D) vibrio.

**Ability to Grow in the Presence or Absence of Air.** Bacteria that grow best in the presence of oxygen are referred to as **aerobes.** Those that grow best in the absence of oxygen are referred to as **anaerobes.** Organisms that can grow in either environment are referred to as being **facultative.** Although most common bacteria are aerobes, many of the bacteria that make up the normal flora of the body are anaerobes. Not surprisingly, anaerobes are often responsible for infections within the body.

**Biochemical Reactions.** Many closely related bacteria can be differentiated from one another only by certain biochemical reactions that occur within the bacterial cell. One way to identify a particular bacterial strain is to look at what type of sugars the bacteria can grow on.

## Special Groups of Bacteria

Several groups of bacteria have certain characteristics that set them apart from most other bacteria. These include the mycobacteria, rickettsiae, chlamydiae, and mycoplasmas.

**Mycobacteria.** Mycobacteria are rod-shaped bacilli with a distinct cell wall that differs from that of most bacteria. Certain types of mycobacteria cause disease in humans. For example, *Mycobacterium tuberculosis* causes the respiratory disease tuberculosis, and *Mycobacterium leprae* causes leprosy.

**Rickettsiae.** Rickettsiae are very small bacteria that can live and grow only within other living cells. Rickettsiae are commonly found in insects such as ticks and mites but may be transmitted to humans through bites. Rickettsiae are responsible for diseases such as Rocky Mountain spotted fever and typhus.

**Chlamydiae.** Chlamydiae are organisms that differ from other bacteria in the structure of their cell walls. Like rickettsiae, they can live and grow only within other living cells. In humans, chlamydiae can cause venereal disease, eye disease, certain types of pneumonia, and certain types of heart disease.

**Mycoplasmas.** Mycoplasmas are small bacteria that completely lack the rigid cell wall of other bacteria. These bacteria cause a variety of human diseases, including venereal disease and a form of pneumonia.

# Protozoans

**Protozoans** are single-celled eukaryotic organisms that are generally much larger than bacteria. Protozoans are found in soil and water, and most do not cause disease in people. Certain protozoans are pathogenic, however, and cause diseases such as malaria (see Figure 33-3), amebic dysentery (a type of diarrhea), and trichomoniasis vaginitis (a type of venereal disease). Protozoal diseases are a leading cause of death in developing countries because the lack of proper sanitation in some areas promotes their spread. These diseases are also common in patients with depressed immune systems.

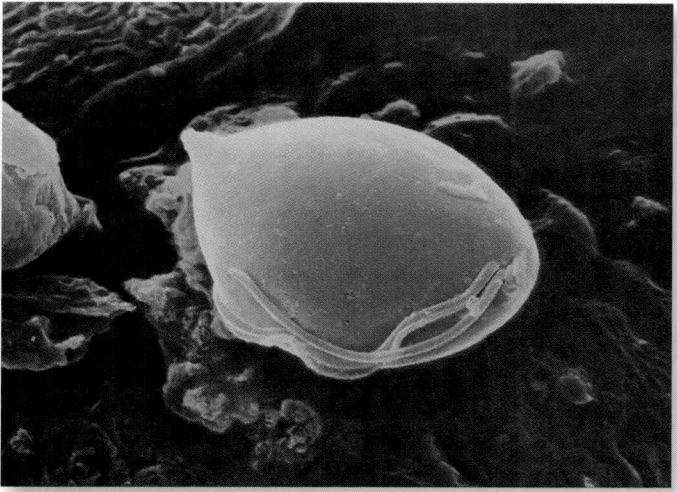

**Figure 33-3.** The protozoan *Trichomonus vaginalis* causes a veneral disease in humans.

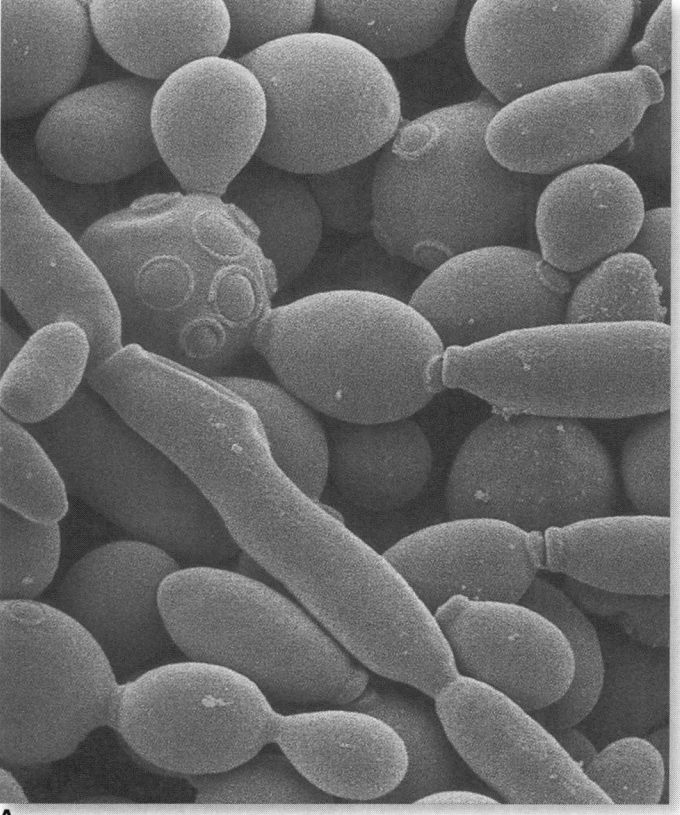

# Fungi

A **fungus** (plural, fungi) is a eukaryotic organism that has a rigid cell wall at some stage in the life cycle. Fungi that grow mainly as single-celled organisms that reproduce by budding are referred to as **yeasts,** whereas fungi that grow into large, fuzzy, multicelled organisms that produce spores are called **molds.** Figure 33-4 shows the differences between these two types of fungi.

Most fungi do not cause disease in humans. Of those that do, the majority produce superficial infections such as athlete's foot (tinea pedis), ringworm, thrush, and vaginal yeast infections. Fungi can produce serious, life-threatening illness, however, when they infect the body's internal tissues. This kind of infection can occur when patients have a depressed immune system, as in patients who are undergoing treatment for cancer and patients with AIDS.

# Multicellular Parasites

A **parasite** is an organism that lives on or in another organism and uses that other organism for its own nourishment, or for some other advantage, to the detriment of the host organism. Viruses, rickettsiae, chlamydiae, and some protozoans are parasitic. Multicellular organisms can also be parasitic, and some of these organisms are microscopic during all or part of their lives. An infection caused by a parasite is called an infestation. Multicellular parasites

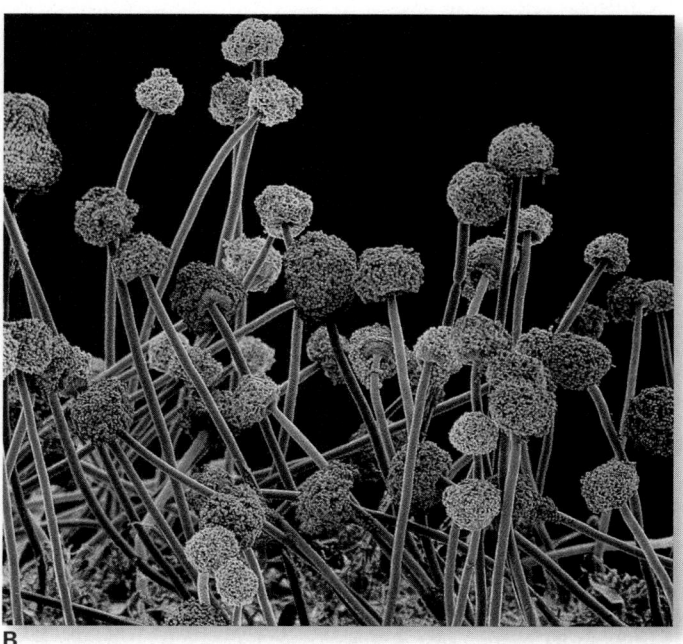

A B

**Figure 33-4.** Because fungi lack the ability to make their own food, they depend on other life forms. (A) Single-celled fungi are called yeasts. (B) Multicelled fungi are called molds.

that cause human disease include certain worms and insects, as illustrated in Figure 33-5.

## Parasitic Worms

People can be infected with a parasitic worm by ingesting its eggs or an immature form of the worm or by having the parasite penetrate the skin. As with the protozoans, infestation

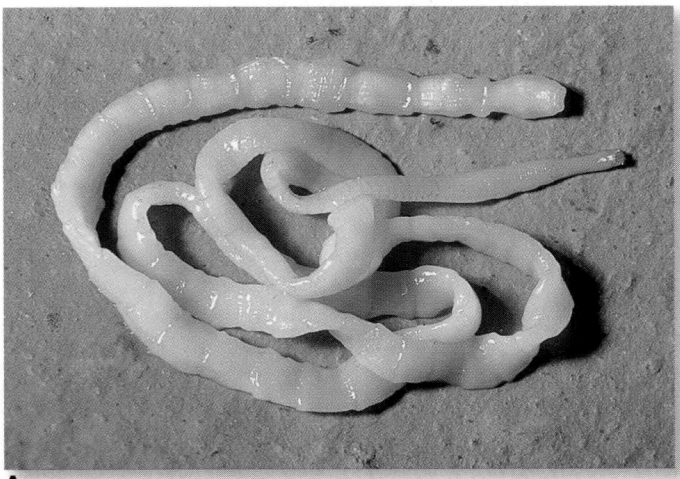

A

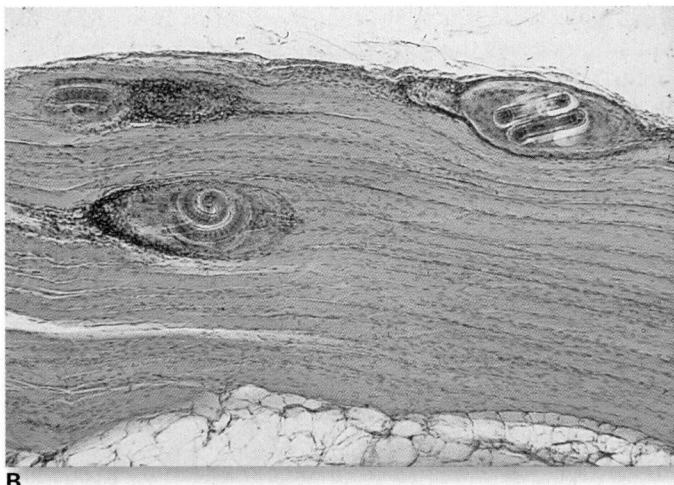

B

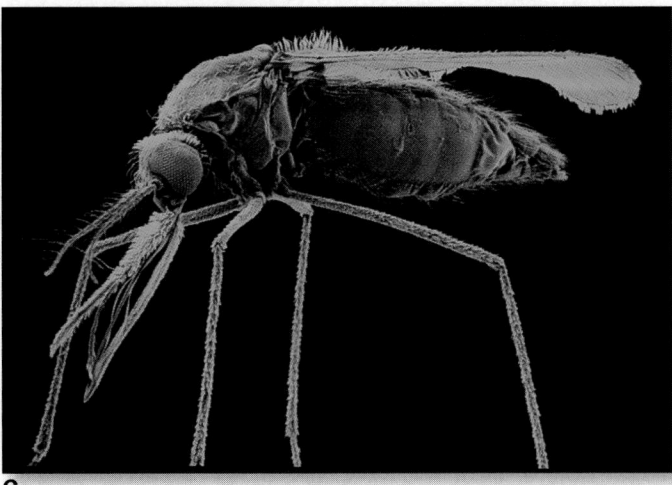

C

by these parasites is more common in developing nations that have poor sanitation.

Worms that infect people include roundworms, flatworms, and tapeworms. Roundworms can occur in the intestines, as in the case of pinworms, a common infection in children. Other roundworms, such as *Trichinella*, are found in muscle tissue. *Trichinella spiralis*, which causes the infection trichinosis, enters the human body in infected meat eaten raw or insufficiently cooked. People may also get flatworms and tapeworms by eating undercooked meats. A trained medical professional must inspect a patient's stool for the presence of the parasite or its eggs to diagnose an intestinal infection with a parasitic worm.

## Parasitic Insects

Insects that can bite or burrow under the skin include mosquitoes, ticks, lice, and mites. These insects spread many viral, bacterial (including rickettsial), and protozoal diseases.

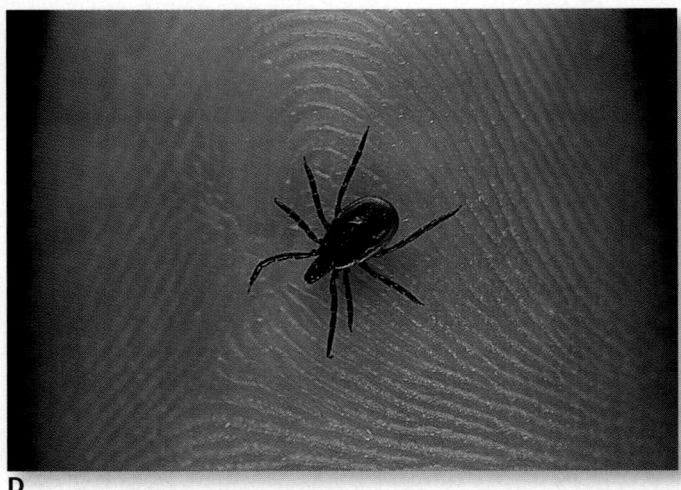

D

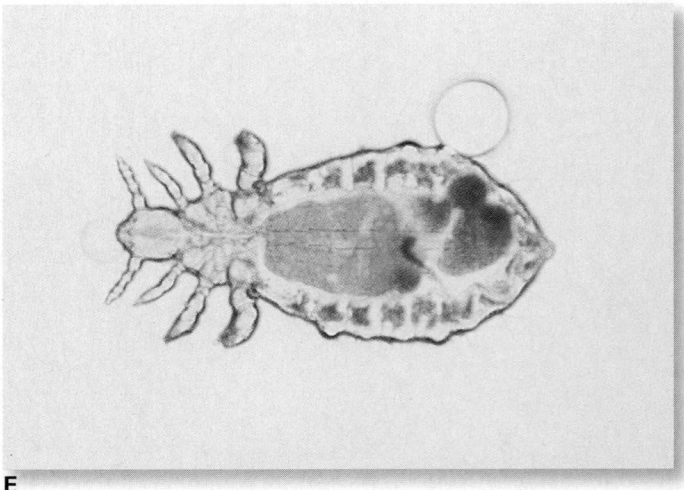

E

**Figure 33-5.** Parasitic worms, such as (A) tapeworms and (B) *Trichinella*, cause disease in humans when they are ingested. Parasitic insects, such as (C) mosquitoes, (D) deer ticks, and (E) mites, cause disease by biting or burrowing into the skin.

The causative organisms can live in the insects' bodies and enter people's bodies when they are bitten by the insects. Such diseases include Lyme disease, malaria, Rocky Mountain spotted fever, and encephalitis. Lice are small insects that live on hair and skin and feed on blood. Scabies infestations are caused by mites that burrow under the skin.

# How Infections Are Diagnosed

To assist with the diagnosis and treatment of an infection, you must work closely with other members of the medical team. The basic steps in diagnosis and treatment are summarized in Figure 33-6.

## Step 1. Examine the Patient

When a patient comes into the office with signs or symptoms that suggest an infection, begin by taking the patient's vital signs and noting the patient's complaints. On the basis of these findings and examination of the patient, the doctor can make a presumptive, or tentative, clinical diagnosis.

In many cases signs and symptoms of a particular infection are so characteristic of the disease that the doctor need not perform additional tests to reach a diagnosis. An example might be a case of chickenpox or mumps. At other times, however, the doctor needs to gather additional information to confirm a diagnosis and determine the cause.

## Step 2. Obtain One or More Specimens

To determine the cause of an infection, you may need to obtain material from one or more areas of the patient's body. Label each specimen properly and include with it the physician's presumptive diagnosis. If the sample is to be transported to an outside laboratory, ensure that it is transported in such a way that any pathogenic organisms remain alive (and safely contained) during transit.

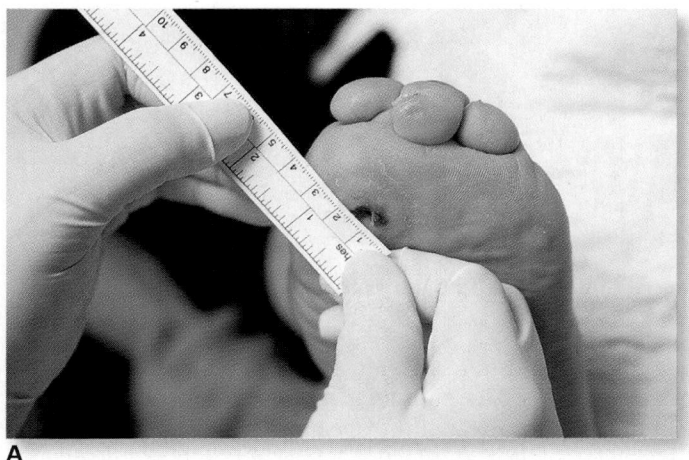

A

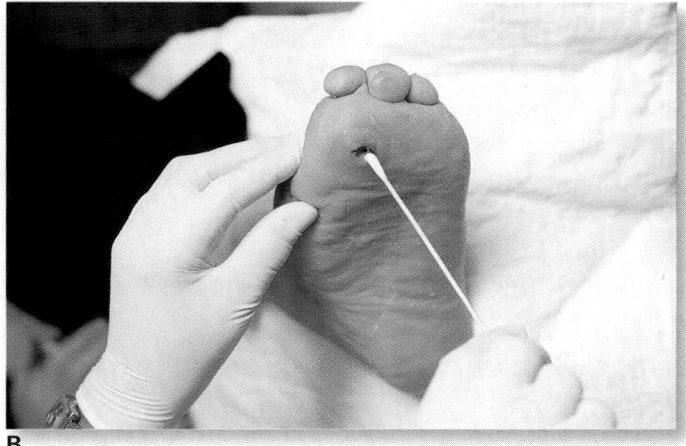

B

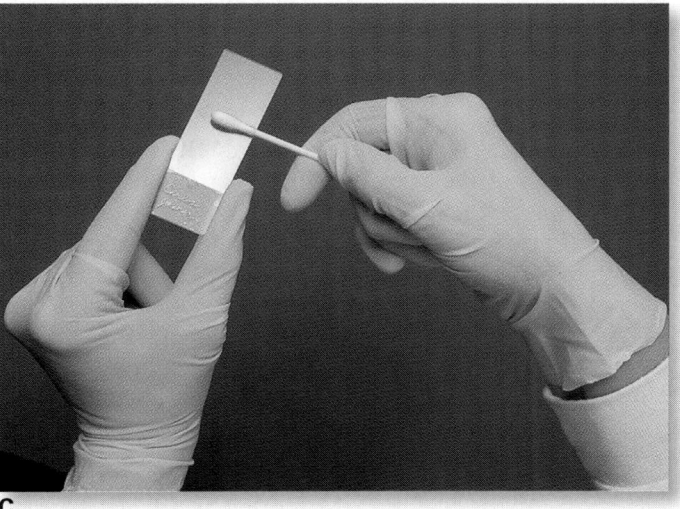

C

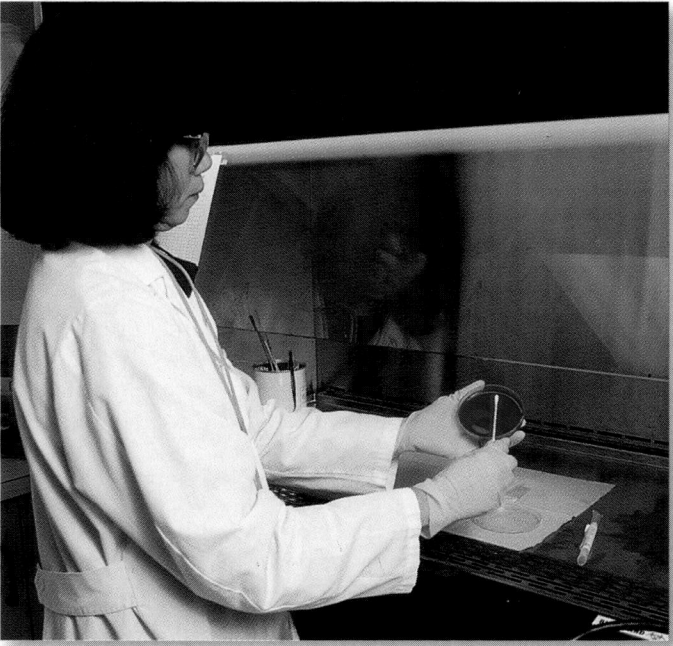

D

**Figure 33-6.** The steps in diagnosis and treatment of an infection: (A) Examine the patient. (B) Obtain one or more specimens. (C) Examine the specimen directly, by wet mount or smear. (D) Culture the specimen. *(continued)*

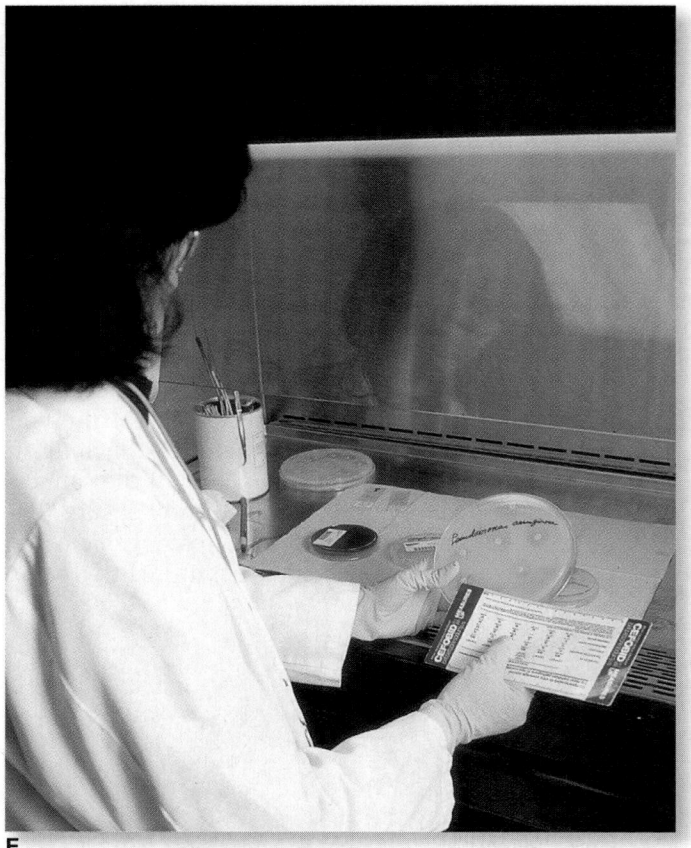
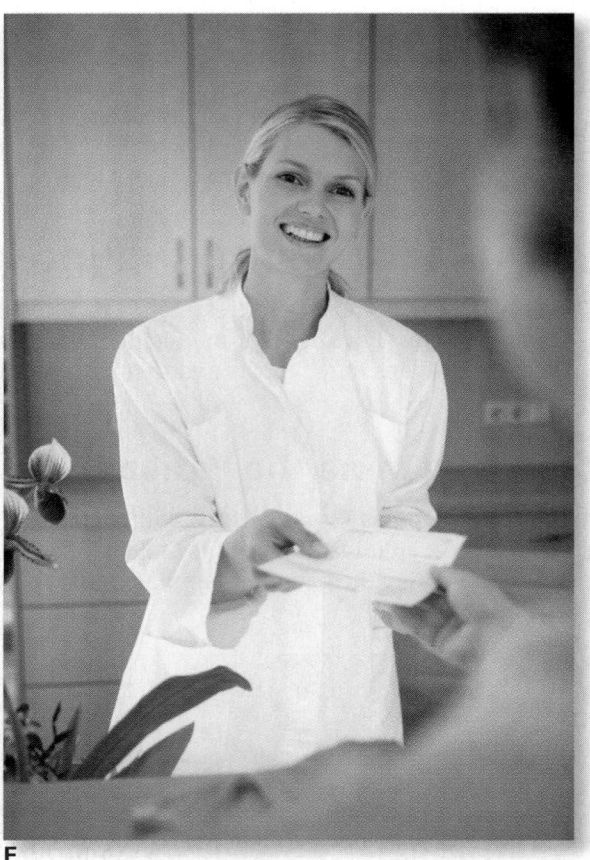

E

F

**Figure 33-6.** *(concluded)*
(E) Determine the culture's antibiotic sensitivity. (F) Treat the patient as ordered by the physician.

## Step 3. Examine the Specimen Directly

You must sometimes obtain more than one specimen from each site. The doctor or specially trained laboratory or microbiology personnel will then directly examine one specimen under the microscope. The specimen may be viewed in one of two ways:

1. As a **wet mount,** a preparation of a specimen in a liquid that allows the organisms to remain alive and mobile while they are being identified

2. As a **smear,** in which a specimen is spread thinly and evenly across a slide

If you make a smear, allow it to dry, and treat or stain it as ordered before it is examined microscopically. In some cases direct examination allows the doctor to make a presumptive diagnosis of the offending microorganism.

## Step 4. Culture the Specimen

If the physician still needs a more definitive identification of the microorganism, you may perform a **culture,** in which a sample of the specimen is placed in or on a substance that allows microorganisms to grow. A **culture medium** is a substance that contains all the nutrients a particular type of microorganism needs. Most media come in the form of a semisolid gel. The particular medium is chosen according to the site from which the specimen was obtained and the suspected cause of infection. After you inoculate (place a sample of the specimen in or on) the medium, place it in an incubator (a chamber that can be set to a specific temperature and humidity) to allow the microorganism to grow.

The culture is examined visually and microscopically after a specified time, and a preliminary identification is made. The physician sets up additional tests to confirm the identification of the microorganism that has been isolated from the specimen. See Table 33-3 for information on specific microbial diseases and the body systems they affect. Most microbiology laboratories and some physicians' office laboratories are equipped to grow routine bacterial cultures and some fungal cultures. Physicians' office laboratories, in particular, may have to send out other types of cultures, such as virus cultures, to a specialized laboratory for identification.

## Step 5. Determine the Culture's Antibiotic Sensitivity

In many cases of bacterial infection, a **culture and sensitivity (C&S)** is performed. This procedure involves culturing a specimen and then testing the isolated

| | | **TABLE 33-3** | **Microbial Diseases** | |
|---|---|---|---|---|
| **System** | **Disease** | **Causative Organism** | **Route of Transmission** | **Signs and Symptoms** |
| Integumentary System | Anthrax | *Bacillus anthracis* | Inhalation or ingestion of spores; consumption of contaminated food | Fever, chills, night sweats, cough, shortness of breath, fatigue, muscle aches, sore throat |
| | Skin infections | *Staphylococcus aureus* | Direct contact of individuals colonized or infected with this bacteria; hand hygiene is the single most important step in controlling spread of these bacteria | Minor: pimples, boils Major: septicemia, surgical wound infection, necrotizing fasciitis |
| | Chickenpox | *Varicella-zoster virus* | Droplets spread through coughing and sneezing | Skin rash of blister-like lesions, usually on the face, scalp, or trunk |
| Respiratory System | Pneumonia | *Haemophilus influenzae Streptococcus pneumoniae Mycoplasma pneumoniae* | Direct contact with respiratory droplets | Fever, decreased breath sounds, shortness of breath, increased heart rate (tachycardia), increased respiratory rate (tachypnea) |
| | Legionellosis • Legionnaire's disease (severe form) • Pontiac fever (mild form) | *Legionella pneumophila* | Breathing water mists contaminated with *Legionella* bacteria (spa, air conditioner, shower) | Fever, chills, and a cough; muscle aches, headache, tiredness, loss of appetite, and occasionally diarrhea |
| | Tuberculosis | *Mycobacterium tuberculosis* | Respiratory droplet spread | Bad cough that lasts longer than 2 weeks, pain in the chest, coughing up blood or sputum (phlegm from deep inside the lungs), weakness, fatigue, weight loss, no appetite, chills, fever, and night sweats |
| | Pertussis | *Bordetella pertussis* | Contact with respiratory droplets | Typically manifested in children with paroxysmal spasms of severe coughing, whooping, and post-tussive vomiting |
| | Diphtheria | *Corynebacterium diphtheriae* | Person-to-person spread through respiratory tract secretions | Sore throat; low-grade fever; adherent membrane of the tonsils, pharynx, or nose; neck swelling |

*continued* ⟶

## TABLE 33-3 Microbial Diseases *(continued)*

| System | Disease | Causative Organism | Route of Transmission | Signs and Symptoms |
|---|---|---|---|---|
| Respiratory System | Influenza | Influenza A and B virus | Respiratory droplet spread | Fever (usually high), headache, extreme tiredness, dry cough, sore throat, runny nose, and muscle aches; gastrointestinal symptoms include nausea, vomiting, and diarrhea |
| | Common cold | Rhinoviruses | Respiratory droplet spread | Runny nose; sneezing; sore throat; mild, hacking cough |
| | Severe acute respiratory syndrome (SARS) | SARS-associated coronavirus (SARS-CoV) | Close person-to-person contact | High fever (temperature greater than 100.4°F [38.0°C]), headache, overall feeling of discomfort, body aches, dry cough, pneumonia |
| Gastrointestinal System | Salmonellosis | *Salmonella enteritidis* | Consumption of contaminated food (raw eggs, chicken, or beef) | Fever, abdominal cramps, and diarrhea beginning 12 to 72 hours after consuming a contaminated food or beverage |
| | Typhoid fever | *Salmonella typhi* | Fecal oral | Sustained high fever (103°F–104°F), weakness, stomach pains, headache, loss of appetite |
| | *E.coli* diarrhea | *Escherichia coli* O157:H7 | Eating contaminated foods (ground beef, raw milk) | Severe bloody diarrhea and abdominal cramps |
| | Cholera | *Vibrio cholerae* | Drinking contaminated water or eating contaminated food | Severe disease characterized by profuse watery diarrhea, vomiting, leg cramps, dehydration, and shock |
| | Botulism | *Clostridium botulinum* | Consuming improperly canned food contaminated with botulinum | Double vision, blurred vision, drooping eyelids, slurred speech, difficulty swallowing, dry mouth, and muscle weakness |
| | Mumps | Mumps virus (paramyxovirus) | Airborne and direct contact with infected respiratory droplets | Fever, headache, muscle ache, and swelling of the lymph nodes close to the jaw |
| | Hepatitis A Hepatitis B Hepatitis C | Hepatitis A virus Hepatitis B virus Hepatitis C virus | Hepatitus A: fecal oral Hepatitus B: blood and body fluids Hepatitus C: blood and body fluids | Symptoms are similar for each: Jaundice, fatigue, abdominal pain, loss of appetite, nausea, diarrhea, fever, joint pain, dark urine |

*continued* ⟶

**TABLE 33-3** **Microbial Diseases** *(continued)*

| System | Disease | Causative Organism | Route of Transmission | Signs and Symptoms |
|---|---|---|---|---|
| Genitourinary System | Chlamydia | *Chlamydia trachomatis* | Sexual contact | Usually silent; can have mild symptoms of abnormal vaginal discharge or a burning sensation when urinating |
| | Gonorrhea | *Neisseria gonorrhea* | Sexual contact | Mucopurulent endocervical or urethral exudate |
| | Syphilis | *Treponema pallidum* | Sexual contact; can be passed to the fetus from an infected woman | Single sore, usually firm, round, small, and painless, that appears at the spot where syphilis entered the body |
| | Genital herpes | Herpes simplex viruses type 1 (HSV-1) and type 2 (HSV-2) | HSV-1: oral and genital contact HSV-2: sexual contact | Genital sores, flu-like symptoms including fever and swollen glands |
| Nervous System | Meningitis | *Neisseria meningitides Streptococcus pneumoniae Haemophilus influenzae* | Direct contact with respiratory secretions from a carrier | High fever, headache, stiff neck, nausea, vomiting, photophobia, confusion, and sleepiness |
| | Toxoplasmosis | *Toxoplasma gondii* | Accidental ingestion of cat feces, ingestion of contaminated raw or undercooked meat or contaminated water | Swollen lymph glands or muscle aches and pains that last for a month or more |
| | Poliomyelitis | Polioviruses 1, 2, and 3 | Person-to-person, fecal or oral | Ranges from asymptomatic to symptomatic, including acute flaccid paralysis, quadriplegia, respiratory failure, and, rarely, death |
| | Rabies | Rabies virus | Bite of a rabid animal | Fever, headache, confusion, sleepiness, or agitation |
| Blood and Immune System | Plague | *Yersinia pestis* | Flea-borne from infected rodents to humans; respiratory droplets from cats and humans with pneumonic plague | Bubonic plague: enlarged, tender lymph nodes, fever, chills, and prostration Septicemic plague: fever, chills, prostration, abdominal pain, shock, and bleeding into skin and other organs Pneumonic plague: fever, chills, cough, and difficulty breathing; rapid shock |

*continued* ⟶

**TABLE 33-3** **Microbial Diseases** *(concluded)*

| System | Disease | Causative Organism | Route of Transmission | Signs and Symptoms |
|---|---|---|---|---|
| Blood and Immune System | Rocky Mountain spotted fever | *Rickettsia rickettsii* | Tick-borne ixodid ticks infected with *R. rickettsii* | Fever, nausea, vomiting, severe headache, muscle pain, lack of appetite, rash, abdominal pain, joint pain, and diarrhea |
| | Lyme disease | *Borrelia burgdorferi* | Tick-borne deer ticks infected with *Borrelia burgdorferi* | Fever, headache, fatigue, and myalgia |
| | Mononucleosis | Epstein-Barr virus | Contact with saliva of infected person | Fever, sore throat, and swollen lymph glands |
| | HIV/AIDS | Human immunodeficiency virus | Blood and body fluids | The following *may be* warning signs of infection with HIV: rapid weight loss; dry cough; recurring fever or profuse night sweats; profound and unexplained fatigue; swollen lymph glands in the armpits, groin, or neck; diarrhea that lasts for more than a week; white spots or unusual blemishes on the tongue, in the mouth, or in the throat; pneumonia; red, brown, pink, or purplish blotches on or under the skin or inside the mouth, nose, or eyelids; memory loss, depression, and other neurologic disorders |
| | Malaria | *Plasmodium: P. falciparum, P. vivax, P. ovale,* or *P. malariae* | Mosquito-borne from Anopheles mosquito infected with *P. malariae* | Fever and influenza-like symptoms, including chills, headache, myalgias, and malaise |

Source: Centers for Disease Control, Health Topics A to Z. Atlanta, Georgia, 2003. http://www.cdc.gov/health/default.htm

bacterium's susceptibility (sensitivity) to certain antibiotics. The results help the doctor determine which antibiotics might be most effective in treating the infection.

## Step 6. Treat the Patient as Ordered by the Physician

On the basis of identification of the microorganism and antibiotic sensitivity, if determined, the physician can prescribe an **antimicrobial.** This agent, which kills microorganisms or suppresses their growth, should help clear up the patient's

infection. Table 33-4 gives some examples of common diseases and the antimicrobial agents used to treat them.

## Specimen Collection

Perhaps the most important step in isolating and identifying a microorganism as the cause of an infection is collecting the specimen. If you do not collect the specimen properly, the organism may not grow in culture so that it can be identified. The result may be an untreated infection. Furthermore, if the specimen becomes contaminated

## TABLE 33-4   Common Antimicrobial Drugs and their Uses

| Infectious Agent | Typical Infection | Some Drugs of Choice |
|---|---|---|
| **Bacteria** | | |
| Gram-Positive Cocci | | |
| *Staphylococcus aureus* | Abscess, skin, toxic shock | Penicillin, vancomycin, cephalosporin |
| *Streptococcus pyogenes* | Strep throat, rheumatic fever | Penicillin, cephalosporin, erythromycin |
| Gram-Positive Rods | | |
| *Corynebacterium* | Diphtheria | Erythromycin, penicillin |
| Acid-Fast Rods | | |
| *Mycobacterium* | Tuberculosis | Isoniazid, rifampin, pyrazinamide |
| Gram-Negative Cocci | | |
| *Neisseria gonorrhoeae* | Gonorrhea | Ceftriaxone, quinolones, spectinomycin |
| Gram-Negative Rods | | |
| *Escherichia coli* | Sepsis, diarrhea, urinary tract infection | Cephalosporin, quinolone, |
| *Haemophilus influenzae* | Meningitis | Cefotaxime, ceftriaxone |
| *Pseudomonas* | Opportunistic lung and burn infections | Ticarcillin, aminoglycoside |
| Spirochetes | | |
| *Borrelia* | Lyme disease | Ceftriaxone, doxycycline |
| *Treponema pallidum* | Syphilis | Penicillin, tetracycline |
| Mycoplasma | | |
| *Mycoplasma pneumoniae* | Pneumonia | Erythromycin, azithromycin, clarithromycin |
| **Fungi** | | |
| *Candida albicans* | Candidiasis | Amphotericin B, fluconazole |
| *Pneumocystis carinii* | Pneumonia (PCP) | SxT, pentamidine |
| **Protozoa** | | |
| *Giardia lamblia* | Giardiasis | Quinacrine, metronidazole |
| *Trichomonas vaginalis* | Trichomoniasis | Metronidazole |
| **Helminths** | | |
| Schistosoma | Schistosomiasis | Praziquantel, metrifonate |
| **Viruses** | | |
| Herpes virus | Genital herpes, oral herpes, shingles | Acyclovir, ganciclovir |
| Orthomyxovirus | Type A influenza | Amantadine, rimantadine |

during collection and the contaminant is mistakenly identified as the cause of the infection, the patient may receive incorrect or even harmful therapy.

In addition to vaginal specimens (discussed in detail in Chapter 26), the most common types of culture specimens involve the following:

- Throat
- Urine
- Sputum
- Wound
- Stool

## Specimen-Collection Devices

To help ensure optimal recovery of microorganisms, you must use the appropriate collection device or specimen container. This container is usually provided by the laboratory where the specimen is going to be analyzed. Special collection devices are available for the collection of sputum, urine, and stool specimens, as shown in Figure 33-7. These containers are designed with large openings to allow collection of the specimen with minimal chance of contamination. They also have tight-fitting caps to prevent leakage and contamination.

**Sterile Swabs.** The most common device for obtaining cultures is the sterile swab. They vary in the absorbent

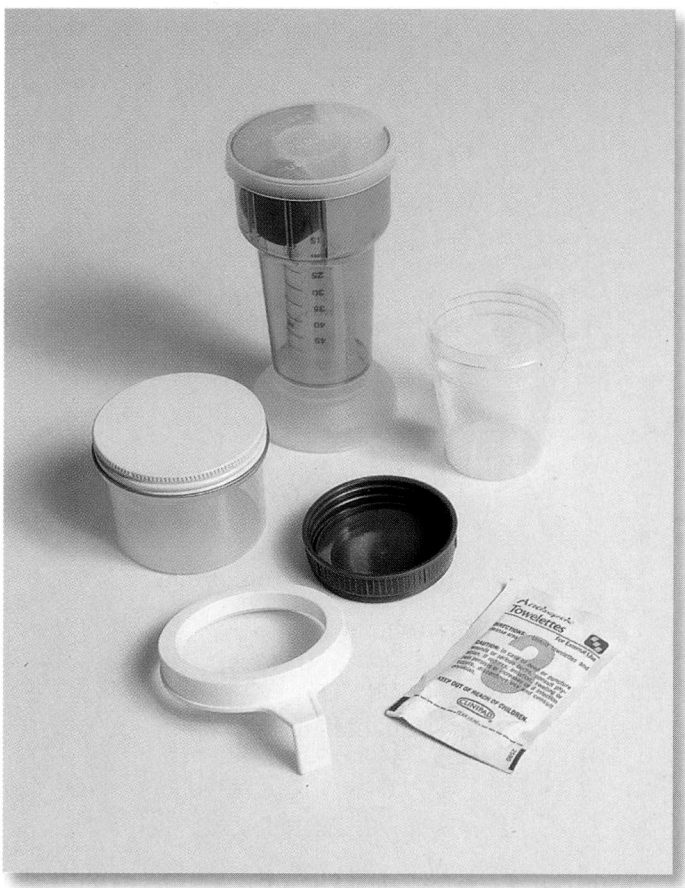

**Figure 33-7.** You may use specially designed collection containers to collect sputum, urine, and stool specimens.

material at the tip and in the composition of the shaft (Figure 33-8).

Although cotton is absorbent, it is no longer used for culture swabs because natural chemicals in cotton inhibit the growth of certain microorganisms. Polyester, rayon, or calcium alginate fibers are preferred. Most swabs used to collect routine specimens have a wooden or plastic shaft for rigidity. There are also swabs with a small tip and a flexible wire shaft made especially for culturing hard-to-reach areas and obtaining pediatric specimens. Some collection containers contain two swabs—one for a culture and one for a smear.

## Collection and Transport Systems

Sterile, self-contained systems for obtaining and transporting specimens are commercially available from many suppliers. The CULTURETTE Collection and Transport System, manufactured by Becton Dickinson Microbiology Systems of Sparks, Maryland, is a well-known example. The unit, shown in Figure 33-9, contains a polyester swab and a small,

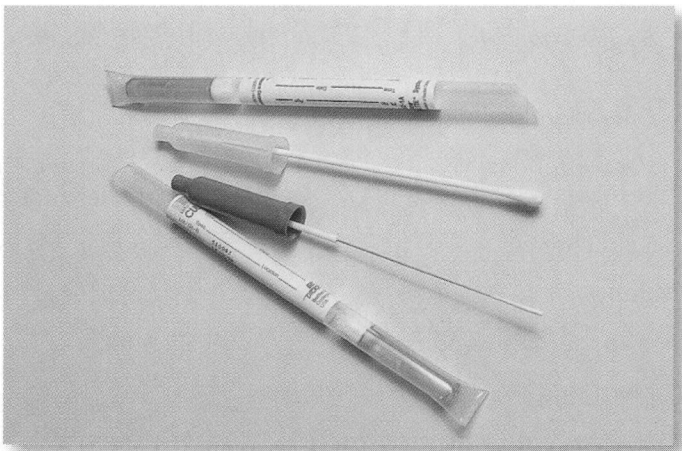

**Figure 33-8.** Sterile swabs vary in size and in material.

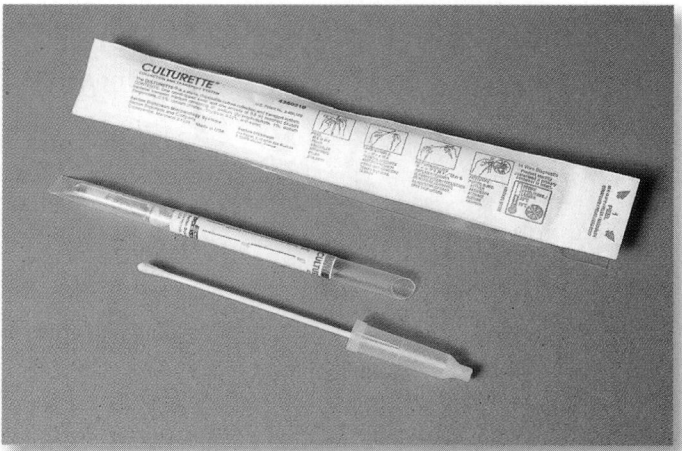

**Figure 33-9.** The CULTURETTE is used to obtain and transport microbiologic specimens to outside laboratories.
Source: Courtesy of Becton Dickinson Microbiology Systems.

thin-walled vial of transport medium in a plastic sleeve. If a specimen will not be tested within 30 minutes after it is obtained, the swab is replaced in the sleeve, and the vial is crushed between the thumb and the index finger. The moisture and nutrients provided by the transport medium help keep the bacteria alive during transport to the laboratory.

Several collection systems are also available for culturing anaerobic organisms. These systems provide a means of generating an oxygen-free environment so that the anaerobic organisms remain viable (alive and able to reproduce) during transport.

## Specimen-Collection Guidelines

To collect specimens properly, you should follow a number of general guidelines.

- Obtain the specimen with great care to avoid causing the patient harm, discomfort, or undue embarrassment. If patients are to collect specimens on their own, give them clear, detailed instructions along with the proper container.

- Collect the material from a site where the organism is most likely to be found and where contamination is least likely to occur. For example, the best location to obtain a specimen for diagnosing strep throat is at the back of the throat in the area of the tonsils. A properly collected sputum specimen should contain mucus that is coughed up from the respiratory tract, but it should not contain saliva, which is a contaminant.

- Obtain the specimen at a time that allows optimal chance of recovery of the microorganism. Knowledge of the infectious disease process allows the doctor to determine the best time to collect a specimen. For example, certain viruses are more readily isolated during the early, symptomatic stage of an illness.

- Use appropriate collection devices, specimen containers, transport systems, and culture media to ensure optimal recovery of microorganisms. The purpose of such equipment and materials is to preserve the viability of any microorganisms so that they will grow in culture. Special collection devices are available for certain body areas or suspected pathogens.

- Obtain a sufficient quantity of the specimen for performing the requested procedures. If, for example, both a culture and a direct examination of a swabbed specimen will be done, you must collect two specimens. Each procedure requires its own sample.

- Obtain the specimen before antimicrobial therapy begins. If the patient is already taking an antibiotic, note this fact on the laboratory request form, or ask the doctor whether you should obtain the specimen.

After correctly collecting the specimen, you must label the container and include the appropriate requisition form. The label should contain the following information:

- Patient's name and identification number (if appropriate)

- Source (collection site) of the specimen
- Date and time of collection
- Doctor's name
- Your initials (if you obtained the specimen)

The requisition form should include the following information:

- Patient's name, address, and identification number
- Patient's age and gender
- Patient's insurance billing information
- Type and source of the microbiologic specimen (for example, discharge from wound, big toe)
- Date and time of microbiologic specimen collection
- Test requested
- Medications the patient is currently receiving
- Doctor's presumptive diagnosis
- Doctor's name, address, and phone number
- Special instructions or orders

## Throat Culture Specimens

A microbiologic procedure frequently performed in a medical office is obtaining a throat culture. The doctor may request a culture on patients with signs or symptoms of an upper respiratory, throat, or sinus infection. Identification of the microorganism responsible for the infection allows the doctor to treat the patient as effectively as possible.

In most cases the doctor wants to determine whether the patient has strep throat, an infection caused by the bacterium *Streptococcus pyogenes,* a group A streptococcus. It is particularly important to diagnose and treat this infection because, left untreated, strep throat can lead to complications such as rheumatic fever. Rheumatic fever is an inflammation of the heart tissue that occurs more frequently in school-age children than in any other population.

When you obtain a throat culture specimen, you must avoid touching any structures inside the mouth, because this will contaminate the specimen. The correct technique for obtaining a throat culture specimen is outlined in Procedure 33-1.

Many doctors order rapid strep tests done if strep is suspected. Antigen-antibody test kits for strep are available in a variety of brands. They provide immediate indications of the presence of the strep antigen on a throat swab, sparing the patient the expense and waiting period associated with having a culture done.

If your office does not culture microbiologic specimens, you need to use a sterile collection system to obtain the specimen. If your office has the equipment to perform its own cultures, use a sterile swab and inoculate a culture plate directly with the swab. Specimens to be evaluated in the office should be cultured immediately after collection.

## Obtaining a Throat Culture Specimen

**Procedure Goal:** To isolate a pathogenic microorganism from the throat or to rule out strep throat

**OSHA Guidelines**

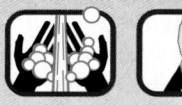 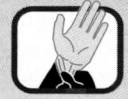   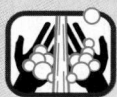

**Materials:** Tongue depressor, sterile collection system or sterile swab plus blood agar culture plate

**Method:**

1. Identify the patient, introduce yourself, and explain the procedure.

2. Assemble the necessary supplies; label the culture plate if used.

3. Wash your hands and put on examination gloves and goggles and a mask or a face shield.

*Rationale*

The patient may cough while you swab the throat.

4. Have the patient assume a sitting position. (Having a small child lie down rather than sit may make the process easier. If the child refuses to open the mouth, gently squeeze the nostrils shut. The child will eventually open the mouth to breathe. Enlist the help of the parent to restrain the child's hands if necessary.)

5. Open the collection system or sterile swab package by peeling the wrapper halfway down; remove the swab with your dominant hand.

6. Ask the patient to tilt back her head and open her mouth as wide as possible.

7. With your other hand, depress the patient's tongue with the tongue depressor.

8. Ask the patient to say "Ah."

9. Insert the swab and quickly swab the back of the throat in the area of the tonsils (Figure 33-10), twirling the swab over representative areas on both sides of the throat. Avoid touching the uvula, the soft tissue hanging from the roof of the mouth, the cheeks, or the tongue.

*Rationale*

Touching these areas will contaminate the specimen.

10. Remove the swab and then the tongue depressor from the patient's mouth.

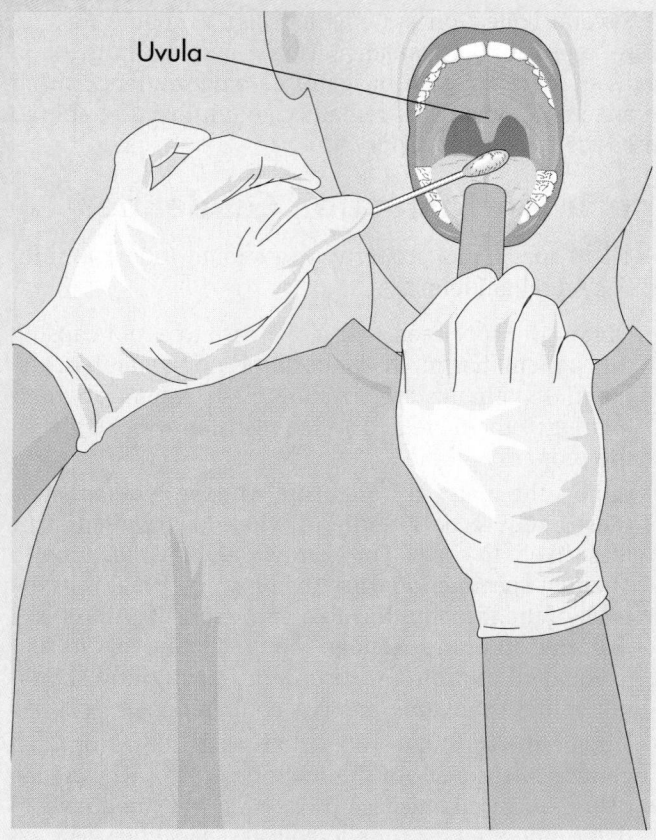

**Figure 33-10.** When obtaining a throat culture specimen, swab the back of the throat in the area of the tonsils on each side, taking care to avoid touching the uvula.

11. Discard the tongue depressor in a biohazardous waste container.

To transport the specimen to a reference laboratory:

12. Immediately insert the swab back into the plastic sleeve, being careful not to touch the outside of the sleeve with the swab.

*Rationale*

To keep the microorganisms alive during transport

13. Crush the vial of transport medium to moisten the tip of the swab (Figure 33-11).

14. Label the collection system and arrange for transport to the laboratory.

*continued →*

## Obtaining a Throat Culture Specimen *(concluded)*

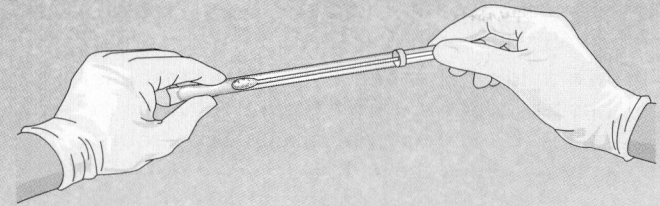

**Figure 33-11.** The transport medium released from the crushed capsule keeps microorganisms alive while in transit to the laboratory for culturing.

To prepare the specimen for evaluation in the physician's office laboratory:

12. Immediately inoculate the culture plate with the swab, using a back-and-forth motion.

13. Discard the swab in a biohazardous waste container.
14. Place the culture plate in the incubator.

To use the specimen for a quick strep screening test:

12. Collect a throat culture specimen using the swab provided in the quick strep test kit.
13. Follow manufacturer's instructions in the test kit. Confirm that the controls worked as expected.
14. Dispose of biohazardous materials according to OSHA guidelines.

When finished with all specimens:

15. Remove the gloves and wash your hands.
16. Document the procedure in the patient's chart.

## Urine Specimens

To minimize contaminants in urine specimens, it is important to obtain a clean-catch midstream specimen. You must process urine specimens within an hour of collection or refrigerate them to prevent continued bacterial growth. (Collection of urine specimens for culturing is discussed in detail in Chapter 34.)

## Sputum Specimens

To obtain sputum specimens, have the patient expectorate (cough up) mucus from the lungs into a wide-mouthed specimen container. Beforehand, instruct the patient to avoid contaminating the specimen with saliva. If sputum specimens are not cultured right away, they should be refrigerated.

Observe Standard Precautions whenever you handle sputum samples. Wear a face shield or mask and goggles when collecting such a specimen, especially if the patient is coughing. Even when tuberculosis is not suspected, the potential for transmission of this type of bacteria always exists.

## Wound Specimens

You usually obtain specimens from infected wounds and lesions by swabbing. The procedure is similar to that of a throat culture. Be sure you obtain representative material from a deep area and a surface area of the wound without contaminating the swab by touching areas outside the site.

## Stool Specimens

If the physician suspects that the patient has certain diseases, such as cancer or colitis or bacterial, protozoal, or parasitic infections, you may need to obtain stool specimens. The collection technique varies with the suspected microorganism. Although both you and the patient may be embarrassed to discuss instructions for collecting stool specimens, do not let this interfere with proper specimen collection. For more information about stool sample collection, see the Educating the Patient feature, Collecting a Stool Sample.

**Suspected Bacterial Infection.** Bacterial infections caused by species of the *Shigella* or *Salmonella* genus can cause loose, bloody, or mucus-tinged stools. A doctor who suspects that a patient has one of these types of infections may request that a stool specimen be obtained for culture.

Successful recovery of these pathogenic bacteria from a stool specimen depends on timely inoculation of special culture media. The doctor may request obtaining a sample in the office whenever possible to avoid delay in processing the specimen. Several types of culture media promote the growth of intestinal pathogens while suppressing the growth of other microorganisms.

**Suspected Protozoal or Parasitic Infection.** In cases of a suspected protozoal or parasitic infection, the physician may request what is known as an **O&P specimen,** short for an ova and parasites specimen. This type of stool sample is examined for the presence of certain forms of protozoans or parasites, including their eggs (ova).

When a physician requests an O&P test, obtain both a fresh and a preserved stool specimen. A fresh specimen is examined both macroscopically and microscopically for the presence of microorganisms. A preserved specimen is also necessary because certain forms of these organisms are destroyed within a short time after leaving the body and may not be detected in the fresh specimen. You must

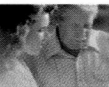

# Educating the Patient

## Collecting a Stool Sample

Patients must collect stool specimens properly so they are not contaminated with urine or water from the toilet, both of which can lead to inaccurate results. If the sample is contaminated, it will have to be collected again.

There are a number of ways a patient can collect a stool specimen. What works for one patient may not work for another. Obtaining stool specimens from young children can also be challenging. Educate patients to collect samples:

- On a clean paper plate
- In a clean waxed-paper carton
- In a container
- On collection tissue that you provide
- On plastic wrap draped loosely over the back half of the toilet seat with enough material to form a collection pocket in the middle

- In a plastic hat-like device placed on the toilet under the seat or placed underneath a child
- In a child's diaper lined with plastic that has been positioned toward the back and rolled up to make a dam, which helps keep urine from contaminating the sample

After collecting the sample, have the patient:

- Use a tongue depressor to place a portion of the sample in a specimen container with a tight-fitting lid.
- Transport the specimen to the office or laboratory as soon as possible.
- Refrigerate the specimen if transport will be delayed.

always obtain a preserved specimen when stool samples are sent to an outside laboratory.

Special stool collection kits are available. They contain a specimen container for a fresh sample along with vials of two types of preservatives, formalin (a dilute solution of formaldehyde) and polyvinyl alcohol (PVA). Instruct the patient to place the stool sample in the specimen container and to mix portions of the specimen in each of the preservative vials. The laboratory will examine all specimens for the presence of microorganisms.

When a physician suspects that a patient has a protozoal or parasitic infection, he will request that a series of at least three stool specimens be examined. Three specimens are required because different diagnostic forms of the microorganism may be present in the stool at different times. The presence of the microorganism could be missed with only one sample. Because certain medications can interfere with detection of these microorganisms, the patient may be asked to refrain from using medications such as antidiarrheal compounds, antacids, and mineral oil laxatives for at least a week before samples are obtained.

## Transporting Specimens to an Outside Laboratory

Many physicians' offices do not perform microbiologic testing. They choose to send their culture specimens to an outside laboratory. In addition, many specialized microbiologic procedures cannot be performed routinely in the office laboratory and must be sent out. One example of a specialized procedure is a virus culture. Culturing and identifying viruses require special techniques and equipment that are almost never found in a physician's office laboratory. Culturing a specimen for bacteria such as chlamydia is also a procedure that requires special techniques.

## Your Main Objectives

When you collect and transport a microbiologic specimen to an outside laboratory, you have three main objectives:

1. To be sure you follow the proper collection procedures and use the proper collection device. Most laboratories have specific directions for sample collection and packaging that you must follow. A laboratory may even provide specific containers in which to collect and transport samples. If you collect or package any specimens improperly, the laboratory may not accept them for testing. Improperly packaged specimens could be contaminated or no longer viable.

2. To maintain the samples in a state as close to their original as possible. You must take specific steps to prevent them from deteriorating.

3. To protect anyone who handles a specimen container from exposure to potentially infectious material. To do so, ensure that the specimen container has a tight-fitting lid. As extra protection against leakage, place the specimen container in a secondary container or zipper-type plastic bag. The laboratory usually provides such a bag.

# PROCEDURE 33.2

## Preparing Microbiologic Specimens for Transport to an Outside Laboratory

**Procedure Goal:** To properly prepare a microbiologic specimen for transport to an outside laboratory

### OSHA Guidelines

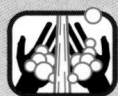 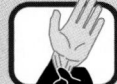  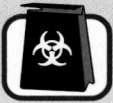 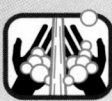

**Materials:** Specimen-collection device, requisition form, secondary container or zipper-type plastic bag

### Method:

1. Wash your hands and put on examination gloves (and goggles and a mask or a face shield if you are collecting a microbiologic throat culture specimen).
2. Obtain the microbiologic culture specimen.
   a. Use the collection system specified by the outside laboratory for the test requested.
   b. Label the microbiologic specimen-collection device at the time of collection.
   c. Collect the microbiologic specimen according to the guidelines provided by the laboratory and office procedure.

   *Rationale*

   To ensure that the specimen is correctly collected and handled

3. Remove the gloves and wash your hands.

4. Complete the test requisition form.
5. Place the microbiologic specimen container in a secondary container or zipper-type plastic bag.

   *Rationale*

   To prevent contaminating anyone who handles the specimen during transport

6. Attach the test requisition form to the outside of the secondary container or bag, per laboratory policy.
7. Log the microbiologic specimen in the list of outgoing specimens.

   *Rationale*

   So that you can follow up on lab tests sent to outside laboratories

8. Store the microbiologic specimen according to guidelines provided by the laboratory for that type of specimen (for example, refrigerated, frozen, or 37°C).
9. Call the laboratory for pickup of the microbiologic specimen, or hold it until the next scheduled pickup.
10. At the time of pickup ensure that the carrier takes all microbiologic specimens that are logged and scheduled to be picked up.
11. If you are ever unsure about collection or transportation details, call the laboratory.

## Methods of Transportation

Specimens that are to be tested by an outside laboratory may be transported there in one of three ways:

1. During regularly scheduled daily pickups by the laboratory
2. During an as-needed pickup by the laboratory
3. Through the mail

Pickup by the laboratory is the most reliable and timely method of transporting microbiologic specimens. Although each laboratory has its own procedure, the general steps for preparing specimens for transport to a laboratory are outlined in Procedure 33-2.

## Sending Specimens by Mail

There may be times when you must send a specimen through the mail to a special reference laboratory for a test that is not normally done by a local laboratory. The U.S. Postal Service accepts a package containing microbiologic specimens as long as the total volume of specimen material is less than 50 milliliters and it is packaged under strict regulations specified by the U.S. Public Health Service.

When sending specimens through the mail, pack them securely with adequate cushioning material to prevent breakage and leakage. Leakage can not only contaminate the specimen but also put mail handlers at risk of contamination with infectious materials. The proper technique for packaging and labeling microbiologic specimens is outlined by the Centers for Disease Control and Prevention (CDC) and shown in Figure 33-12.

Securely close the primary culture container, and surround it with enough absorbent packing material to absorb the entire fluid contents if the container were to leak. Place these items together in a secondary container, commonly a metal container with a screw-top or snap-on lid. Then place the secondary container in an outer shipping carton made of cardboard or Styrofoam.

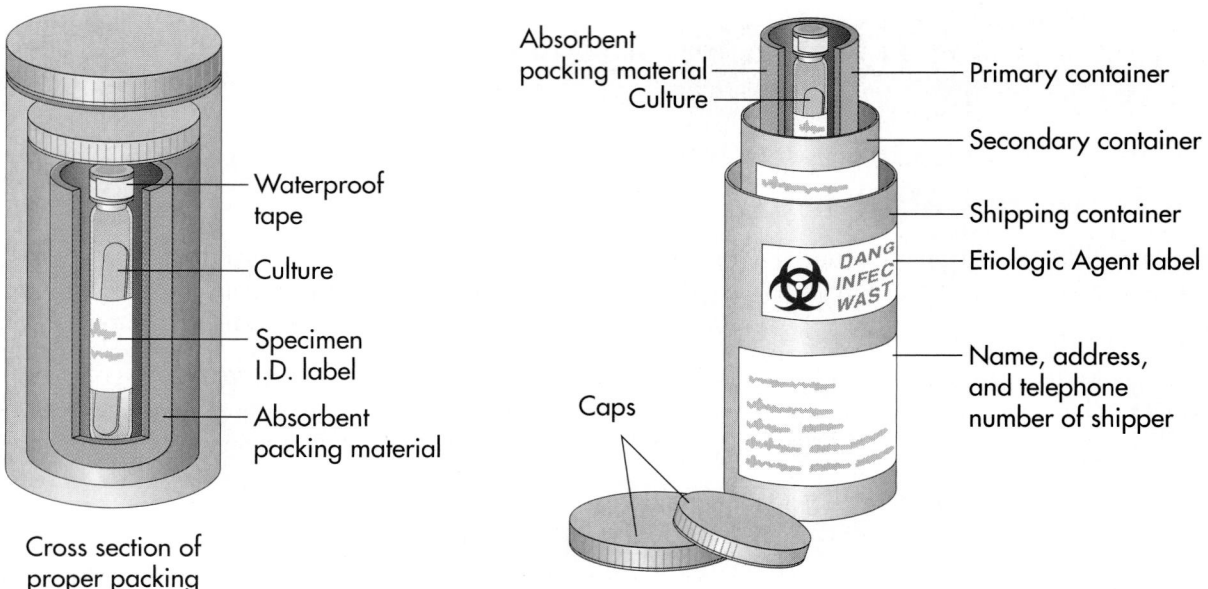

**Figure 33-12.** When packaging and labeling a specimen for mail delivery, you must follow the procedures set by the CDC, based on U.S. Public Health Service regulations.

In addition to the address label, microbiologic specimens sent through the mail must have an Etiologic Agent label affixed to the package, as shown in Figure 33-12. This label uses the biohazard symbol to alert the mail carrier as to the nature of the contents. The term **etiologic agent** refers to a living microorganism or its toxin that may cause human disease.

# Direct Examination of Specimens

At times, the physician may directly examine the specimen under a microscope to detect the presence of microorganisms or to identify them. The physician may perform this procedure in the office to get the information needed to initiate treatment immediately.

Two types of procedures that allow direct examination of microbiologic specimens are preparing wet mounts and preparing potassium hydroxide (KOH) mounts. You may be required to perform these procedures as part of your duties.

## Wet Mounts

A wet mount permits quick identification of many microorganisms. Wet mounts are easy to prepare.

1. Wearing examination gloves, mix a small amount of the specimen with a drop of normal saline (0.9% sodium chloride [NaCl] solution) on a glass slide.
2. Apply a coverslip over the mixture.
3. Provide the doctor with the slide for direct examination under the microscope.

If you obtain a specimen from a body site that is normally sterile, detection of microorganisms on a wet mount immediately tells the doctor whether there is infection.

Wet mounts are also useful in determining whether a microorganism is motile, or able to move, which helps in identifying the microorganisms.

## Potassium Hydroxide (KOH) Mounts

A **KOH mount** is a type of mount used when a physician suspects that a patient has a fungal infection of the skin, nails, hair, or vagina. It is difficult to visualize a fungus directly in these types of specimens because the body produces a tough, hard protein called keratin that often masks any fungus present. The chemical potassium hydroxide (KOH) is added to the specimen to dissolve the keratin and allow visualization of any fungus.

To prepare a KOH mount, follow these steps.

1. Wearing examination gloves, suspend the specimen in a drop of 10% KOH on a glass slide.
2. Apply a coverslip.
3. Allow the specimen to sit at room temperature for 30 minutes to dissolve the keratin.
4. Provide the physician with the slide to examine for microscopic evidence of fungal structures.

# Preparation and Examination of Stained Specimens

Although wet mounts are a useful tool for detecting microorganisms, microorganisms and their structures can be seen more clearly when you stain them with a dye or group of dyes. As with wet mounts and KOH mounts, the doctor can make a quick, tentative diagnosis with stained specimens. A stained specimen also enables the doctor to differentiate between types of infections, such as bacterial and yeast infections, or between bacterial infections of one type and another. Stains also help doctors identify microorganisms that have grown on culture plates.

## Preparation of Smears

The first step in staining a microbiologic specimen is to prepare a smear. To do so, simply apply a small amount of the specimen to a glass slide. Allow the sample to dry, and briefly heat the slide to "fix" the sample to the slide so that it does not wash off during the staining process. The steps in preparing a specimen smear are described in detail in Procedure 33-3.

## Gram's Stain

The stain that is most frequently used for microscopic examination of bacteriologic specimens is the Gram's stain. A Gram's stain is a moderate-complexity test that you can perform in the medical office. The steps for performing a Gram's stain are outlined in Procedure 33-4.

A Gram's stain involves performing a series of staining and washing steps on the heat-fixed smear. First, apply a purple stain called crystal violet (also known as gentian violet) to the smear. After washing the slide in water, apply iodine. The iodine acts as a **mordant,** a substance that can intensify or deepen the response of a specimen to a stain. Iodine helps bind the dye to the bacterial cell wall.

## PROCEDURE 33.3

## Preparing a Microbiologic Specimen Smear

**Procedure Goal:** To prepare a smear of a microbiologic specimen for staining

**OSHA Guidelines**

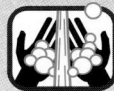 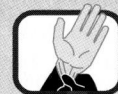  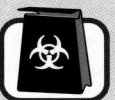 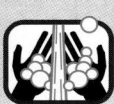

**Materials:** Glass slide with frosted end, pencil, specimen swab, Bunsen burner, forceps

**Method:**

1. Wash your hands and put on exam gloves.
2. Assemble all the necessary items.
3. Use a pencil to label the frosted end of the slide with the patient's name.
4. Roll the specimen swab evenly over the smooth part of the slide, making sure that all areas of the swab touch the slide (Figure 33-13).

   *Rationale*

   To make sure a representative specimen is transferred to the slide

5. Discard the swab in a biohazardous waste container. (Retain the microbiologic specimen for culture as necessary or according to office policy.)
6. Allow the smear to air-dry. Do not wave the slide to dry it.

   *Rationale*

   So that you do not spread pathogens or contaminate the slide

7. Heat-fix the slide by holding the frosted end with forceps and passing the clear part of the slide, with the smear side up, through the

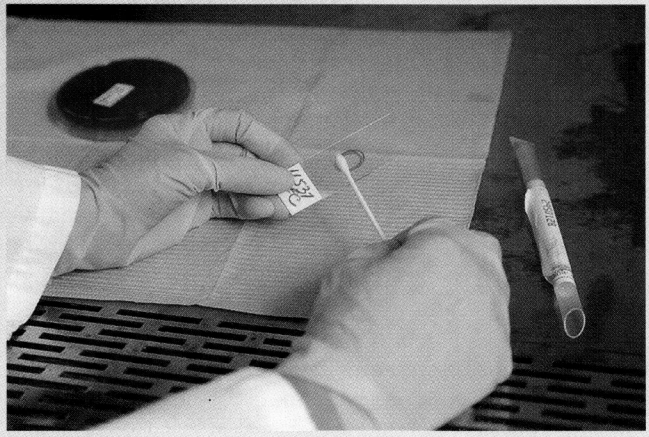

**Figure 33-13.** Rolling the swab ensures that representative microorganisms collected on it are deposited on the slide.

flame of a Bunsen burner three or four times. (Your office may use an alternate procedure for fixing the slide, such as flooding the smear with alcohol, allowing it to sit for a few minutes, and either pouring off the remaining liquid or allowing the smear to air-dry. Chlamydia slides come with their own fixative.)

   *Rationale*

   The specimen must be fixed to the slide to prevent washing the microorganism off during staining or handling

8. Allow the slide to cool before the smear is stained.
9. Return the materials to their proper location.
10. Remove the gloves and wash your hands.

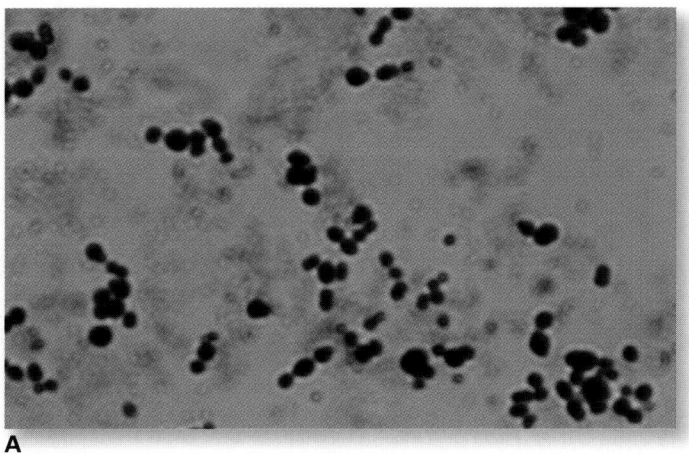
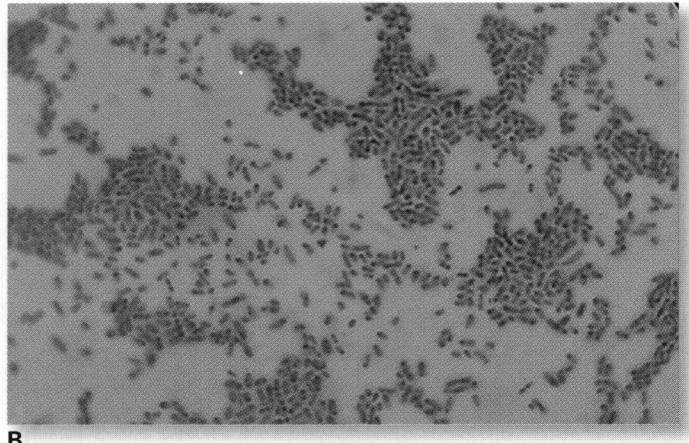

**Figure 33-14.** (A) Gram-positive organisms appear blue or violet after staining. (B) Gram-negative organisms appear red.

After washing the slide again in water, apply a decolorizing solution (alcohol or acetone-alcohol). Certain bacterial species retain the purple dye even after the decolorizer is added. These bacteria appear blue or violet and are referred to as being **gram-positive.**

Other bacteria lose their purple color when the decolorizer is added. To allow the physician to visualize these bacteria, apply a red counterstain (safranin) to the smear. Bacteria that lose the purple color and pick up the red color of the safranin are referred to as being **gram-negative.** Figure 33-14 illustrates gram-positive and gram-negative bacteria. It is important that you follow each step in the gram stain process carefully to reduce the likelihood of misidentifying the microorganisms.

On the bases of a bacterium's staining characteristics and the shape and arrangement of cells, the physician can make a presumptive identification of an organism. For example, clusters of cocci that appear gram-positive typically suggest an infection with staphylococci.

Besides bacteria, other types of microorganisms, such as protozoans and parasites, can often be visualized with the Gram's stain. Because the Gram's stain is typically not the best type of stain for these microorganisms, however, the physician may order another type of stain.

# Culturing Specimens in the Medical Office

If your medical office is equipped with a laboratory and if you have the necessary on-the-job training or additional courses, you may be required to culture certain specimens. It is, however, becoming more common for doctors' offices to send specimens to outside laboratories because of Clinical Laboratory Improvement Amendments of 1988 (CLIA '88) guidelines and the additional requirements concerning personnel and administrative work.

Culturing involves placing a sample of the specimen on or in a specialized culture medium. This medium contains nutrients that enable microorganisms such as bacteria and fungi to grow. The medium is placed in an incubator set at 37°C (body temperature), the optimal temperature for growth. As the microorganism multiplies, a **colony**—a distinct group of the organisms—can be seen on the surface of the culture medium. The microorganism is identified according to the colony appearance, its staining characteristics, and certain biochemical reactions. A microorganism's biochemical reactions are determined by their growth on specific types of culture media.

## Culture Media

Culture media come in liquid, semisolid, and solid forms. In the medical office you will most likely work with a semi-solid. The medium contains **agar,** a gelatin-like substance derived from seaweed that gives the medium its consistency. This form of medium comes commercially prepared in culture plates—round, covered glass or plastic dishes also called petri dishes.

When using petri dishes, handle them only on the outside, so that they do not become contaminated. You can avoid introducing contaminants by storing the petri dishes with the agar side up. Use the palm of your hand to pick up the agar-containing part of the dish when you are ready to inoculate it with a specimen.

**Types of Media.** Many different types of semisolid media are commercially available. The type of medium used for culturing depends on the type of suspected organism and the site from which the specimen is obtained. Some types allow the growth of only certain kinds of bacteria while inhibiting the growth of others. These types are referred to as selective media. Selective media are commonly used for specimens that normally contain bacteria, such as stool or vaginal samples.

Other types of media support the growth of most organisms and are referred to as nonselective media. The most common type of culture medium used in the laboratory is blood agar, a nonselective medium. Blood agar gets its red color from sheep's blood. Comparing the growth of a specimen on selective and nonselective media often provides important information about the microorganisms present.

You will typically use a blood agar plate when you culture a throat swab specimen. The organism that causes strep throat (*Streptococcus pyogenes*) can be identified when it grows on blood agar because it destroys the blood cells in the agar, leaving a clear zone surrounding each colony. This process of red blood cell destruction is referred to as hemolysis.

**Special Culture Units.** Small physicians' office laboratories often use commercial culture units with specific culturing purposes. Units for performing rapid urine

# PROCEDURE 33.4

## Performing a Gram's Stain

**Procedure Goal:** To make bacteria present in a specimen smear visible for microscopic identification

### OSHA Guidelines

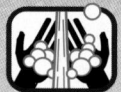 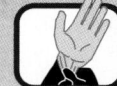 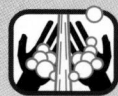

**Materials:** Heat-fixed smear, slide staining rack and tray, crystal violet dye, iodine solution, alcohol or acetone-alcohol decolorizer, safranin dye, wash bottle filled with water, forceps, blotting paper or paper towels (optional)

### Method:

1. Assemble all the necessary supplies.
2. Wash your hands and put on examination gloves.
3. Place the heat-fixed smear on a level staining rack and tray, with the smear side up.
4. Completely cover the specimen area of the slide with the crystal violet stain (Figure 33-15A). (Many commercially available Gram's stain solutions have flip-up bottle caps that allow you to dispense stain by the drop. If the stain bottle you are using does not have an attached dropper cap, use an eyedropper.)
5. Allow the stain to sit for 1 minute; wash the slide thoroughly with water from the wash bottle (Figure 33-15B).

#### Rationale
Washing the slide after 1 minute stops the staining process and prevents over- staining of the specimen.

6. Use the forceps to hold the slide at the frosted end, tilting the slide to remove excess water.
7. Place the slide flat on the rack again, and completely cover the specimen area with iodine solution (Figure 33-15C).

8. Allow the iodine to remain for 1 minute; wash the slide thoroughly with water (Figure 33-15D).

#### Rationale
The iodine helps increase cell staining.

9. Use the forceps to hold and tilt the slide to remove excess water.
10. While still tilting the slide, apply the alcohol or decolorizer drop by drop until no more purple color washes off (Figure 33-15E). (This step usually takes 10 seconds to 30 seconds.)

#### Rationale
The decolorizing step is essential for differentiation between gram-positive and gram-negative bacteria.

11. Wash the slide thoroughly with water (Figure 33-15F); use the forceps to hold and tip the slide to remove excess water.
12. Completely cover the specimen with safranin dye (Figure 33-15G).
13. Allow the safranin to remain for 1 minute; wash the slide thoroughly with water (Figure 33-15H).

#### Rationale
To counter-stain the specimen so that gram-negative organisms can be visualized

14. Use the forceps to hold the stained smear by the frosted end, and carefully wipe the back of the slide to remove excess stain.
15. Place the smear in a vertical position and allow it to air-dry. (The smear may be blotted lightly between blotting paper or paper towels to hasten drying {Figure 33-15I}. Take care not to rub the slide, or the specimen may be damaged.)
16. Sanitize and disinfect the work area.
17. Remove the gloves and wash your hands.

*continued* ⟶

## Performing a Gram's Stain *(concluded)*

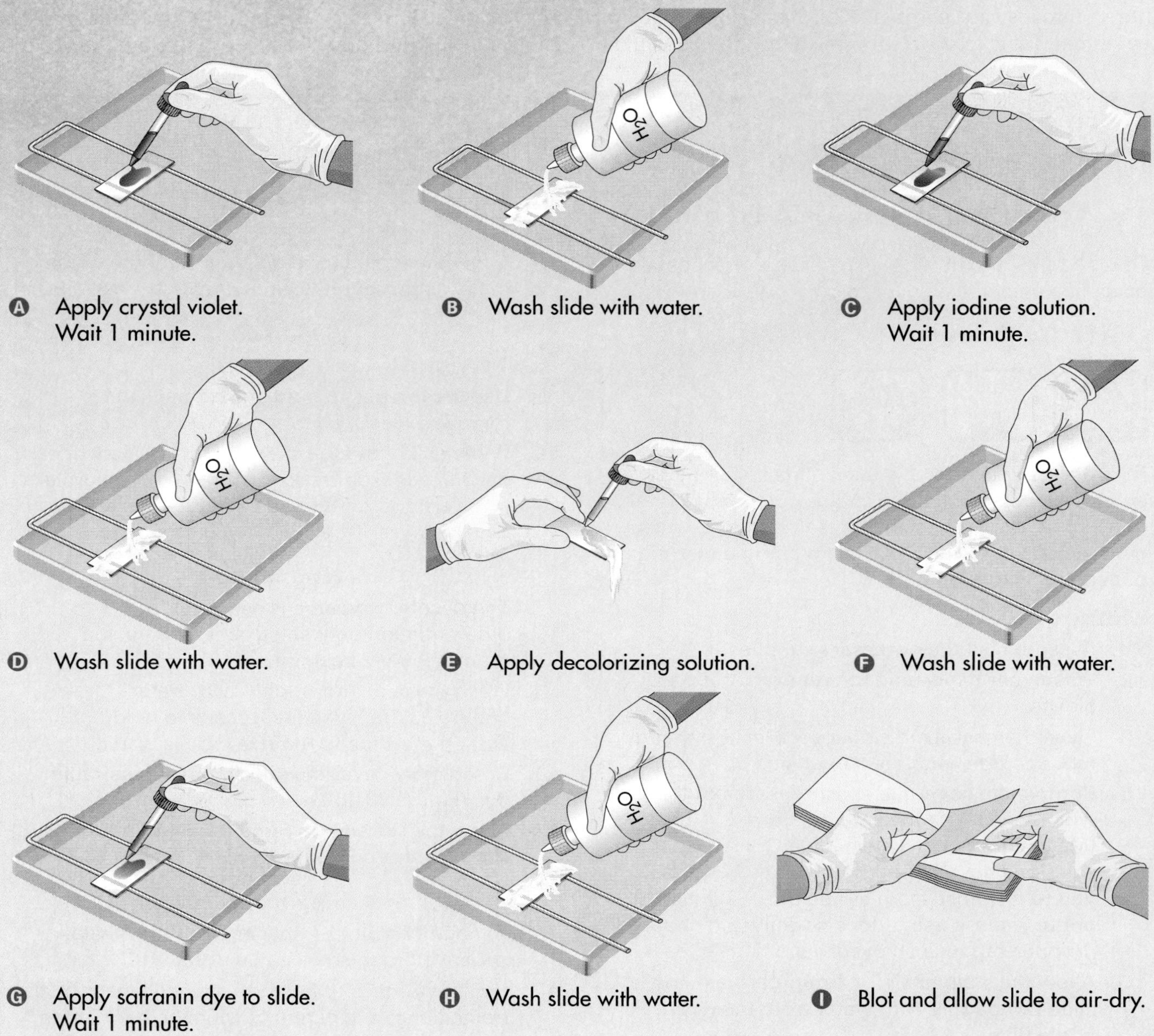

**Ⓐ** Apply crystal violet. Wait 1 minute.

**Ⓑ** Wash slide with water.

**Ⓒ** Apply iodine solution. Wait 1 minute.

**Ⓓ** Wash slide with water.

**Ⓔ** Apply decolorizing solution.

**Ⓕ** Wash slide with water.

**Ⓖ** Apply safranin dye to slide. Wait 1 minute.

**Ⓗ** Wash slide with water.

**Ⓘ** Blot and allow slide to air-dry.

**Figure 33-15.** The procedure for performing a Gram's stain on a microbiologic specimen involves covering the specimen with a series of stains, water washes, and alcohol in a specific order, for precise periods of time.

culture, such as Uricult (manufactured by Orion Diagnostica, Somerset, New Jersey), are typical. Uricult consists of a small vial that has a double-sided paddle attached to a screw-on top (Figure 33-16). Each side of the paddle contains a different type of medium on its surface. To culture a urine specimen, simply dip the media paddle into the clean-catch midstream urine specimen or catheterized specimen, coating both sides of the paddle. Then remove the paddle from the specimen, screw it into the vial, and place it upright in the incubator for 18 to 24 hours. If bacteria are present, they will grow on the surfaces of the media. Other units for culturing urine, throat specimens, vaginal specimens, and blood are also simple to use. These units usually enable you to obtain an estimate of the

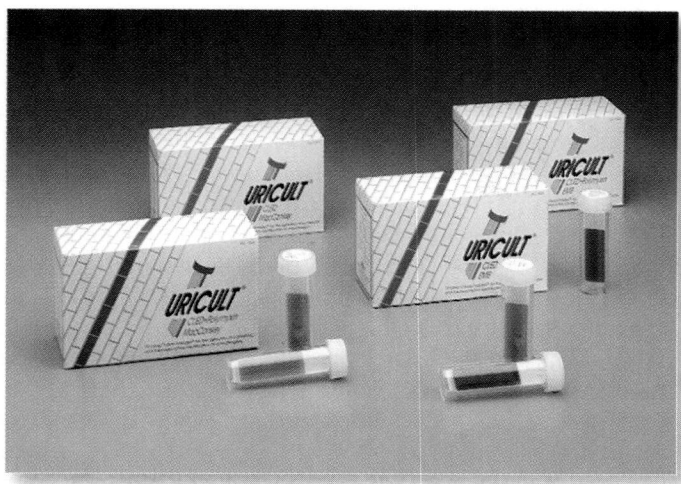

**Figure 33-16.** One common urine culture device consists of a lid and attached double-sided paddle that screws into a vial.

number of bacteria in the sample in addition to identifying the bacteria.

# Inoculating a Culture Plate

Inoculating a culture plate involves transferring some or all of the specimen onto the plate. Before inoculating a plate, label it on the bottom (agar side) rather than the lid, because the lid can be lost or switched. Label the plate with the patient's name, doctor's name, source of the sample, date and time of inoculation, and your initials. You can apply a label or write the information with a grease pencil or permanent marker.

In the case of a specimen swab, inoculate the plate by streaking the swab across the plate. Bacterial colonies can be identified by their appearance. This determination of the type of pathogen is referred to as a **qualitative analysis** of the specimen.

To perform a qualitative analysis of a specimen such as urine, introduce only a small portion of the specimen

onto the plate. A calibrated inoculating loop is used for this purpose. A loop is a small circle of wire or plastic attached to a long handle. When this loop is dipped into the specimen, a small specific amount of liquid can be transferred to the plate. There are different sizes of calibrated loops that deliver different volumes of fluid.

In addition, you may need to perform a separate determination of the number of bacteria present in specimens such as urine. This determination is referred to as a **quantitative analysis.** A quantitative analysis is important with a specimen such as urine because a few bacteria may contaminate a urine sample during collection. A true infection is confirmed by the presence of a certain number of bacteria; any number beneath this level is typically considered contamination.

**Inoculating for Qualitative Analysis.** To inoculate an agar plate for qualitative analysis, perform the first pass with a culture swab (as with a throat culture) or an inoculating loop (as with a urine culture). If you use a culture swab, roll and streak it back and forth across an area covering roughly one-third of the culture plate to deposit the microorganisms. When using an inoculating loop, spread the material by streaking the loop across one-third of the plate in the same back-and-forth pattern. Figure 33-17 shows the correct pattern for inoculating a plate.

Because there may be a great many microorganisms in the specimen, you need to streak the inoculated (first-pass) area with a sterile loop to separate out individual colonies that can be identified on the remaining areas of the culture plate. Unless you use a sterile disposable loop, first sterilize the loop by heating it in a bacterial loop incinerator until it glows red. Allow the loop to cool, and pass it once across the inoculated area of the plate to pick up a small number of microorganisms. Then streak it in a back-and-forth pattern over the second one-third of the plate. Next, sterilize the loop again, pass it once across the second inoculated area of the plate, and streak

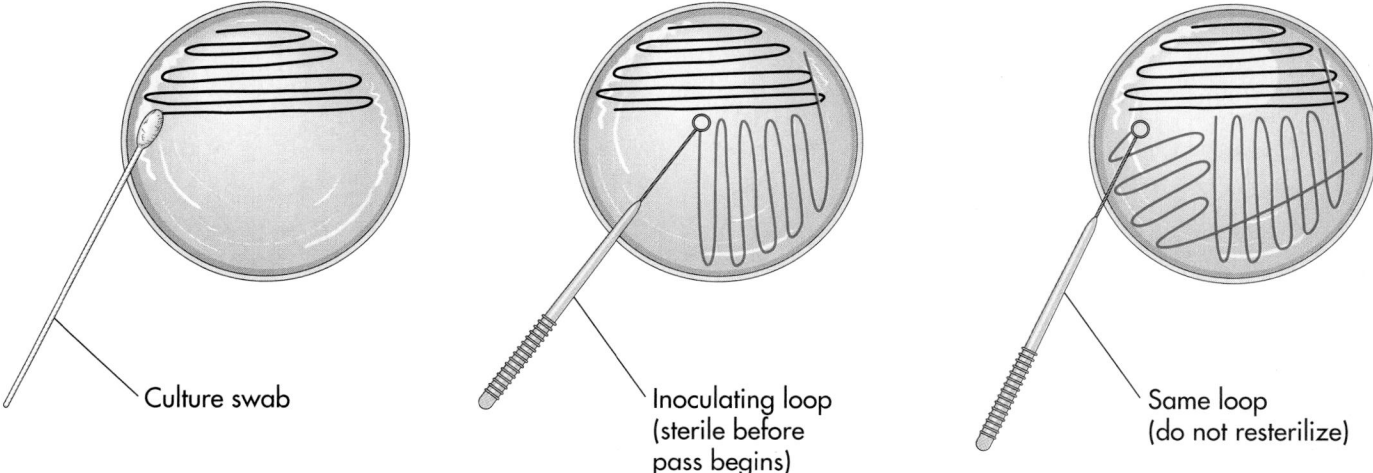

Culture swab

Inoculating loop (sterile before pass begins)

Same loop (do not resterilize)

**Figure 33-17.** When inoculating a plate for qualitative analysis, roll and streak the culture swab or inoculating loop of specimen material across one-third of the surface of the culture plate. Begin the next pass with a sterile loop.

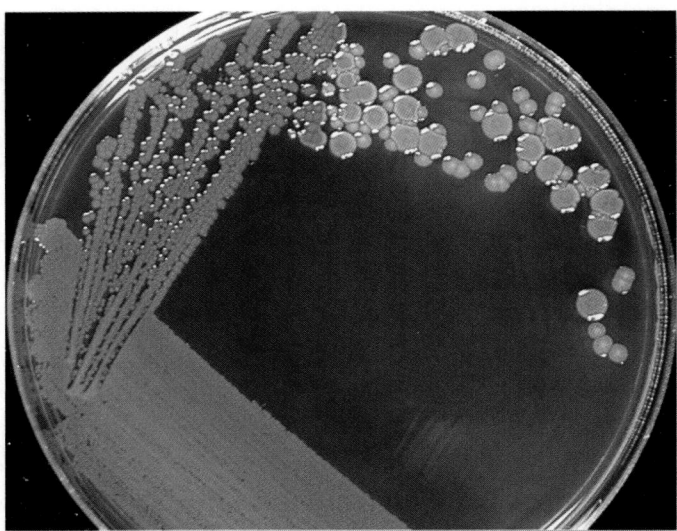

**Figure 33-18.** You can see individual colony-forming units in the last third of an inoculated culture plate.

it back and forth over the last one-third of the plate. Each successive pass serves to reduce the concentration of the microorganisms. This procedure allows isolated colonies, or colony-forming units, to be observed in the area of the last pass of the loop, as Figure 33-18 shows.

For throat cultures, the physician may simply want you to screen the sample to see whether streptococcal organisms are present. You may not need to use a loop to spread the microorganisms; the swab will be sufficient, as described in Procedure 33-1, when preparing the specimen for screening.

**Inoculating for Quantitative Analysis.** To perform a quantitative analysis of a urine specimen, use a calibrated loop to withdraw a portion of urine from the sample. The circle on a calibrated loop is a precise size that picks up an exact volume of liquid when it is dipped into the specimen. For example, calibrated loops may allow you to pick up either 0.01 or 0.001 milliliter of liquid.

When you perform a quantitative analysis, be sure the urine specimen is well mixed before taking the sample. Mixing is required because the microorganisms may settle to the bottom of the specimen cup. Sterilize, cool, and dip the calibrated loop into the sample. Transfer the entire volume to the surface of an agar plate by making a single streak down the center of the plate. Next spread the specimen evenly across the plate at a right angle to the initial streak, using the same loop (without sterilizing it). Turn the plate and spread the material again, at a right angle to the last streak, over the entire surface. Figure 33-19 illustrates this technique.

After the microorganisms are allowed to grow for 24 hours, estimate the number of microorganisms by counting the number of colonies that appear on the surface of the plate. For example, if you use a 0.001 milliliter calibrated loop to streak the plate and 50 colonies grow, multiply the 50 colonies by 1000 to obtain the number of colonies per milliliter. In this case you would estimate that there are 50,000 colony-forming units per milliliter of urine. You must be especially careful that your counts and calculations are correct so that the doctor has accurate information on which to base a diagnosis.

## Incubating Culture Plates

After inoculating a plate, place it in an incubator set at 95°F to 98.6°F (human body temperature) to allow the bacteria to grow. Plates are always incubated with the agar side up, so that any moisture that collects in the plate will fall on the inside of the lid and not on the growing surface of the agar. How long plates are allowed to grow varies

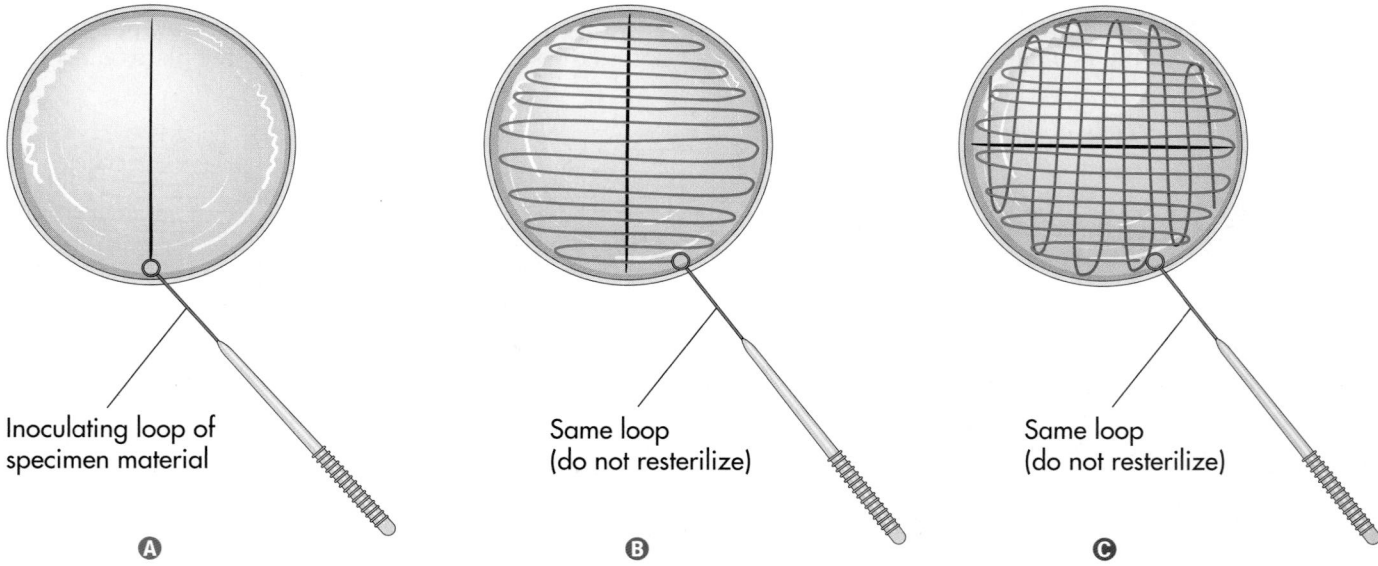

**Ⓐ** Inoculating loop of specimen material

**Ⓑ** Same loop (do not resterilize)

**Ⓒ** Same loop (do not resterilize)

**Figure 33-19.** When inoculating a plate for quantitative analysis, (A) streak the loop down the center of the plate. Next, (B) streak the loop at right angles to the first inoculation. Then, (C) turn the plate 90°, and streak the entire surface once more.

with the type of culture. Most bacteria grow sufficiently within 24 hours, but some require 48 hours. Fungi typically take longer to grow than bacteria and may grow at a slightly lower temperature (95°F to 96.8°F).

## Interpreting Cultures

After incubation, cultures are assessed for growth and are interpreted. Pathogens may be identified at this time. This process requires considerable skill and practice because pathogens must often be differentiated from normal flora. This step may be performed by the physician, a microbiologist, or a technician who has been properly trained to do so through on-the-job training or additional course work. The Points on Practice section discusses the types of qualifications and training you need to interpret cultures.

The process of interpreting a culture typically involves several determinations. The characteristics of the colonies growing on the agar are noted, along with their relative numbers. In addition, any changes in the media surrounding the colonies are noted, because these changes may reflect certain characteristics of the microorganism.

The physician decides at this point whether additional procedures are required. In the case of a throat culture, the presence of colonies of a characteristic shape, size, and

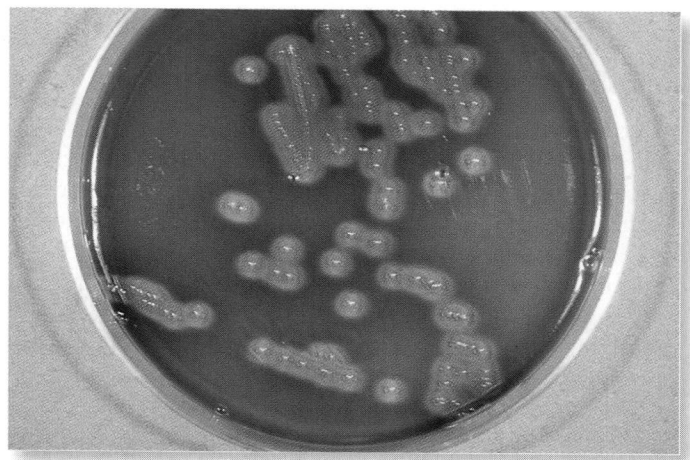

**Figure 33-20.** A positive strep throat culture contains distinctive colonies surrounded by areas of hemolysis.

color, surrounded by areas of hemolysis, suggests strep throat, as shown in Figure 33-20. A Gram's stain and determination of bacterial shape may be all that is necessary for a confirmed diagnosis. Many cultures, however, require additional biochemical and, in some cases, serologic tests for definitive identification of the pathogen.

## Points on Practice

## Obtaining Additional Training in Microbiology

Identifying microorganisms in culture specimens requires considerable skill and practice. In a microbiology laboratory, these tests may be performed by medical technologists (MTs), medical laboratory technicians (MLTs), or other health professionals, including medical assistants who have received special training.

These classifications differ in the amount of education and training required. Medical technologists, also called clinical laboratory scientists, must earn a bachelor's degree and undergo 1 year of clinical training. Medical laboratory technicians must have completed a 2-year program at an accredited college (or the equivalent amount of course work), be a graduate of an accredited professional school or armed forces school, or hold certification in another related field while completing specific on-the-job training. Certification for both MTs and MLTs requires successful completion of a national certifying examination. In addition to certification, some states require MTs and MLTs to obtain a state license to work in a laboratory.

As part of their training, MTs and MLTs routinely receive instruction in microbiology. They also learn the clinical laboratory skills involved in identifying

microorganisms. As part of your current medical assistant curriculum, you are learning the basic principles of microbiology and some of the techniques of specimen collection and processing. To be able to perform microbiologic tests, such as sensitivity tests, and interpret cultures of specimens, however, you would need additional training.

You can learn these types of skills and advance your career by taking part in the continuing education programs your office has to offer. Local colleges or schools of allied health may also offer clinical microbiology courses. Such a course will enable you to become proficient in performing microbiologic identification. All laboratories, including those in the doctor's office, require employees to participate in a proficiency testing program, according to guidelines set forth by the Clinical Laboratory Improvement Amendments of 1988 (CLIA '88).

Developing clinical skills in the area of microbiology can be challenging and satisfying. These skills will contribute to your office's efficiency and ability to provide high-quality patient care. Additional training in microbiology will also enhance your career by making you more valuable to any medical practice or facility.

# Determining Antimicrobial Sensitivity

After a particular bacterial (or sometimes fungal) pathogen is identified, the organism's sensitivity (also called susceptibility) to several different antimicrobial agents must be determined. This information enables the doctor to choose an agent for treating the infection that is likely to be effective in curing it. If your office does not perform antimicrobial sensitivity tests but, instead, receives reports on them from reference laboratories, the results are reported as sensitive (no growth), intermediate (little growth), or resistant (overgrown).

Performing an antimicrobial sensitivity test involves taking a sample of the isolated pathogen, suspending it in a small amount of liquid medium, and streaking it evenly on the surface of a culture plate. Small disks of filter paper containing various antimicrobial agents are placed on top of the inoculated agar plate. Although this step can be done manually using sterile forceps, a special dispenser that is often used places all the disks down at once (Figure 33-21).

The plate is then incubated at 98.6°F, and the results are evaluated the following day. If a particular antimicrobial agent is effective against the microorganism, there will be a clear zone around the disk, indicating that the growth was inhibited in the area of the agent, as seen in Figure 33-22. If there is growth right up to the disk, it means that the agent is not effective against the organism. Each zone is measured in millimeters and compared to a standard chart to determine the degree of effectiveness of the antimicrobial agent. The doctor uses these results to choose an effective antimicrobial agent to treat the patient.

Many bacterial identification systems are now available as automated systems. These systems are used at most larger institutions and reference laboratories. They require special instrumentation that has the capability to

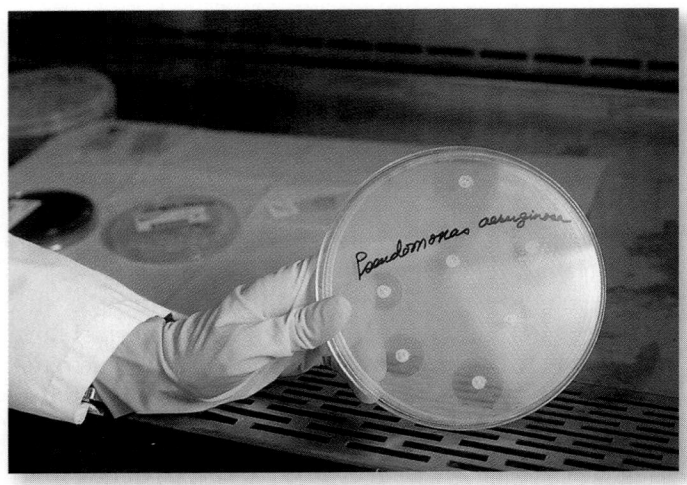

**Figure 33-22.** The effectiveness of different antimicrobial agents against an organism is apparent when an antimicrobial sensitivity test is performed.

identify the organism. This instrumentation also determines the antibiotic susceptibility, a procedure known as MIC (minimum inhibitory concentration). This susceptibility testing is performed in special welled plates that test the organism against an antibiotic dilution to determine the minimum antibiotic concentration that is required to inhibit bacterial growth.

# Quality Control in the Medical Office

Medical offices are required to have a **quality control (QC)** system in place, which is an ongoing system to evaluate the quality of medical care being provided. Although quality is sometimes difficult to define, most people would agree that high-quality care involves achieving the best possible medical outcome for each patient while attending to both the patient's and the family's needs. Quality control in the medical office provides an objective means of defining, monitoring, and correcting potential problems that affect the quality of care. Quality control is covered in more detail in Chapter 32.

## Quality Control in the Microbiology Laboratory

Quality control is necessary in several areas in a microbiology laboratory. All media, staining solutions, and reagents (chemicals and chemically treated substances used in test procedures) should be evaluated frequently for effectiveness. Media must also be evaluated for sterility. Equipment such as refrigerators, freezers, and incubators should be properly maintained, cleaned, and checked for accuracy of temperature. The essential components of a quality control program as established by the College of American Pathologists are outlined in the Points on Practice section.

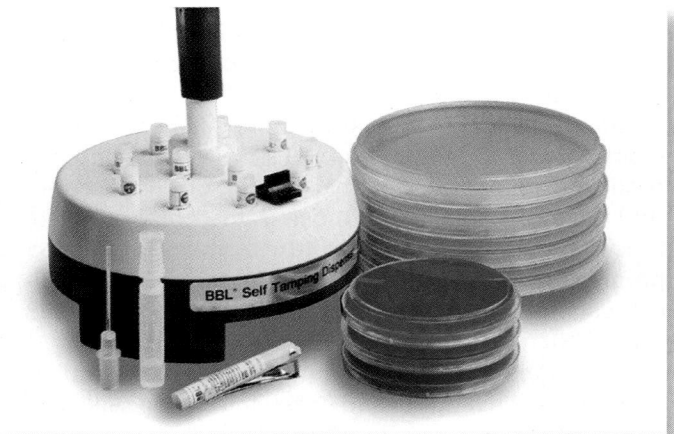

**Figure 33-21.** Antimicrobial disk dispensers simplify placement of antimicrobial disks, help ensure that each disk contains a single antimicrobial agent, and reduce the probability of contaminating the culture.

## The Impact of CLIA '88

In addition to an internal quality control program, all laboratories must incorporate the appropriate policies and procedures to comply with CLIA '88. (See Chapter 32 for a full discussion of CLIA '88.) A substantial part of these requirements involves proper documentation of laboratory policies and procedures, materials, and personnel qualifications and training. If a laboratory has a good quality control program in place, it is likely that the required guidelines are already being followed.

In addition, any laboratory that performs certain procedures must enroll and participate in an approved proficiency testing program. A proficiency testing program monitors the quality of a laboratory's test results. The procedures in a microbiology laboratory that require proficiency testing include those classified as moderately complex or highly complex. An example of a moderately complex procedure is performing a culture and sensitivity test.

Proficiency testing involves culturing, identifying, and determining the sensitivity of blind specimen samples, that is, samples that are unknown to laboratory personnel. The results are then checked for accuracy. If you perform these types of procedures in the medical office, you may be asked to participate in the proficiency testing program.

## Points on Practice

### Guidelines for a Quality Control Program in a Microbiology Laboratory

To maintain the highest possible standards of patient care and safety, all facets of a medical laboratory must be checked and monitored. The essential components of a quality control program in a microbiology laboratory include the following:

- Developing an up-to-date procedures manual. This manual is one of the most important documents in the laboratory. The procedures manual directs day-to-day activities and ensures that proper procedures are followed. It should include all general policies, regulations, and procedures, including those involving quality control and the transport of specimens to outside laboratories. The manual should be placed in a binder and kept in a location where all employees can refer to it. At least once a year, the laboratory director or supervisor should update and revise the manual.

- Monitoring laboratory equipment. A quality control program should include a preventive maintenance program for all laboratory equipment to ensure proper functioning. All equipment should be checked and cleaned at regular intervals. Temperatures of refrigerators, freezers, heating blocks, water baths, and incubators should be checked daily with an accurate standardized thermometer. Autoclaves should be tested each week with a spore strip to check sterility, and pH meters must be tested for accuracy using pH-calibrating solutions. A tachometer should be used to check the revolutions per minute of serology rotators and centrifuges. (All centrifuges must have lids.) Safety hoods should be checked two to four times per year to make certain that they permit adequate air flow. The results of all quality control tests should be documented each time a test is performed.

- Monitoring media, supplies, and reagents. Media should be periodically checked for sterility and the ability to grow certain strains of stock organisms. Stains and reagents should also be checked with control organisms to ensure accurate results. Each culture tube, plate of medium, and reagent should be labeled as to its content and its preparation and expiration dates.

- Ensuring qualified personnel. Only qualified personnel should be hired, and employees should be offered an effective continuing education program. All personnel should be given the opportunity to learn new skills. This procedure benefits the laboratory and can also help advance employees' careers. Proficiency testing of blind samples may be used as teaching exercises and should be made available to all interested personnel.

- Ensuring adequate space. One issue of quality control and safety in the laboratory that is often overlooked is the allocation of sufficient work space for personnel. A minimum of 100 square feet of work space for each full-time equivalent employee is recommended. Safety and high-quality performance are enhanced when there is sufficient space to perform each task.

# Summary

A variety of microorganisms can cause infection. They are a major cause of disease in humans. As a medical assistant, you play an important role in the diagnosis and treatment of infection.

Collecting a microbiologic specimen is the most important step in diagnosing an infection. To ensure accurate results, you must use the correct collection device and technique. Then you must process the specimen or transport it to the laboratory in a timely manner to enable recovery of microorganisms.

The process of identification often begins when the doctor examines the fresh or stained specimen. Most specimens are cultured and incubated, and the resultant growth is evaluated. The antibiotic sensitivity of an isolated pathogen can then be determined to aid the doctor in making treatment decisions.

Quality control in the microbiology laboratory is an important factor in ensuring high-quality medical care. The focus and attention you bring to this part of your work will pay handsome dividends in terms of patient care, laboratory safety, and personal satisfaction. Developing your clinical skills will be an asset to the office and will allow you to advance in your career.

## CASE STUDY *QUESTIONS*

Now that you have completed this chapter, review the case study at the beginning of the chapter and answer the following questions:

1. What is the proper technique for collecting a throat specimen?
2. Why do you think the first test result came back as negative?
3. What organism is responsible for causing strep throat?
4. What complications may have developed if you had not had another throat culture obtained and been prescribed antibiotics?

## Discussion Questions

1. What are the different classifications of microorganisms, and how do the classifications differ?
2. List the common sites from which cultures may be obtained.
3. What guidelines should you follow when collecting a specimen?

## Critical Thinking Questions

1. Gram's stain is a procedure performed to stain bacteria for microscopic examination. What are the reagents used to perform this test? Identify the staining characteristics of gram-positive and gram-negative organisms.
2. What should you do to minimize contamination of a urine specimen?
3. Why are cotton-tipped swabs no longer used as sterile specimen collection devices?

## Application Activities

1. With your instructor's approval, practice performing a throat culture on a partner.
2. Use one of your throat culture specimens to inoculate a blood agar plate. Incubate the culture and observe the appearance of normal throat flora.
3. Prepare a specimen swab for transport to an outside laboratory.

## Virtual Fieldtrip

*Visit the McGraw-Hill Higher Education Medical Assisting website at www.mhhe.com/medicalassisting3 to complete the following activity:*

Use the CDC GetSmart: Know When Antibiotics Work website to answer these questions:

1. What is antibiotic resistance?
2. How can health-care providers help prevent the spread of antibiotic resistance?
3. What role does antimicrobial sensitivity testing play in reducing antibiotic resistance?

Open the CD and complete this chapter's practice activities, play the games, listen to the key terms, and test yourself with the interactive review. E-mail, print, and/or save your results to document your proficiency.

# Collecting, Processing, and Testing Urine Specimens

## KEY TERMS

- anuria
- bilirubinuria
- cast
- catheterization
- clean-catch midstream urine specimen
- crystal
- drainage catheter
- enzyme immunoassay (EIA)
- first morning urine specimen
- glycosuria
- hematuria
- hemoglobinuria
- myoglobinuria
- nocturia
- oliguria
- phenylketonuria (PKU)
- proteinuria
- random urine specimen
- refractometer
- splinting catheter
- supernatant
- timed urine specimen
- 24-hour urine specimen
- urinalysis
- urinary catheter
- urinary pH
- urine specific gravity
- urobilinogen

## MEDICAL ASSISTING COMPETENCIES

*In preparation for the certification examination, you should know the following areas of competence:*

| COMPETENCY | CMA | RMA |
|---|---|---|
| **Clinical** | | |
| Apply principles of aseptic techniques and infection control, including hand washing | X | X |
| Dispose of biohazardous materials | X | X |
| Practice Standard Precautions | X | X |
| Instruct patients in the collection of a clean-catch midstream urine specimen | X | X |
| Perform selected CLIA-waived tests (e.g., "kit tests") | X | X |
| Perform urinalysis | X | X |
| Screen and follow up on patient test results | X | X |
| **General/Legal/Professional** | | |
| Determine the needs for documentation and reporting, and document accurately and appropriately | X | X |
| Perform risk management procedures | | X |
| Instruct individuals according to their needs | X | X |
| Provide patients with methods of health promotion and disease prevention | X | X |
| Operate and maintain facilities, and perform routine maintenance of administrative and clinical equipment safely | X | X |
| Perform quality control procedures | X | X |

## CHAPTER OUTLINE

- The Role of the Medical Assistant
- Anatomy and Physiology of the Urinary System
- Obtaining Specimens
- Urinalysis

# LEARNING OUTCOMES

After completing Chapter 34, you will be able to:

**34.1** Describe the characteristics of urine, including its formation, physical composition, and chemical properties.

**34.2** Explain how to instruct patients in specimen collection.

**34.3** Identify guidelines to follow when collecting urine specimens.

**34.4** Describe proper procedures for collecting various urine specimens.

**34.5** Explain the process of urinary catheterization.

**34.6** List special considerations that may require you to alter guidelines when collecting urine specimens.

**34.7** Explain how to maintain the chain of custody when processing urine specimens.

**34.8** Explain how to preserve and store urine specimens.

**34.9** Describe the process of urinalysis and its purpose.

**34.10** Identify the physical characteristics present in normal urine specimens.

**34.11** Identify the chemicals that may be found in urine specimens.

**34.12** Identify the elements categorized and counted as a result of microscopic examination of urine specimens.

# Introduction

The routine analysis of a urine specimen is a simple, noninvasive diagnostic test that provides a health-care provider with a window to a patient's health. Many significant conditions may be noted with the assessment of the physical, chemical, and microscopic examinations of a patient's specimen. This chapter reviews the function of the urinary system and the formation of urine. You will learn about various types of urine specimens and how to properly instruct or assist patients with the collection of these specimens. Additionally, you will learn how to correctly process a specimen, including a random specimen and a chain of custody drug screen. You will learn to identify normal and abnormal constituents of urine samples and what may cause these abnormal elements to be present in a specimen.

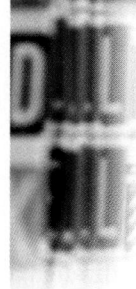

## CASE STUDY

As a medical assistant, you are performing reagent chemical strip analyses on patient specimens when you discover a specimen that is more than 2 hours old and has been sitting at room temperature during this time. When you remove the lid from the container, you smell a foul, ammonia-like odor. The chemical strip indicates positive protein, positive nitrite, and positive bacteria. The microscopic analysis reveals four bacteria but no evidence of white blood cells.

As you read this chapter, consider the following questions:

1. What is the maximum length of time that a urine specimen should be left at room temperature? If analysis cannot be performed within that maximum length of time, how should the specimen be handled?
2. An ammonia-like or foul odor associated with a specimen ordinarily indicates what condition or disease?
3. Does the chemical analysis confirm your suspicion associated with the odor?
4. Given the circumstances, can you trust the results on this specimen?

# The Role of the Medical Assistant

You will help collect, process, and test urine specimens. To perform your duties, you need to know about the anatomy and physiology of the kidneys, how urine is formed, and what its normal contents are. This information will help you collect various specimen types, process them, and perform urinalysis on them. Dealing with a variety of patient groups who require special care, including elderly patients and pediatric patients, will also be an important part of your job as a medical assistant.

Although you will not generally be dealing with blood-borne pathogens when obtaining and processing urine specimens, you will deal with potentially infectious body waste. For this reason you must take precautions to

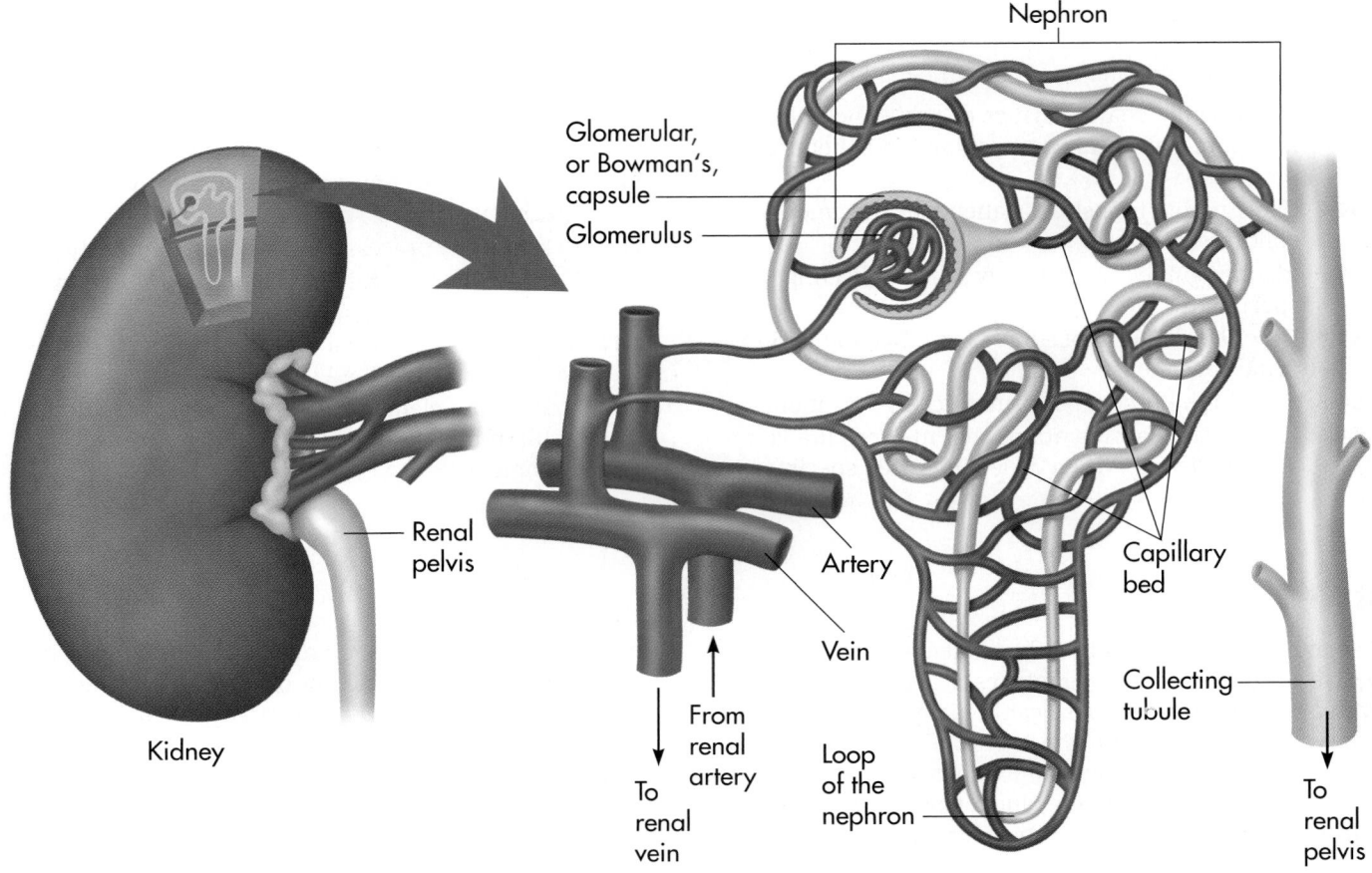

Figure 34-1. Urine is formed in the nephron, a long tubular structure, during a complex filtering process.

protect yourself, the patient, and others in the environment from transmitting disease-causing microorganisms. Most medical offices use Standard Precautions when dealing with urine. (See Chapters 20 and 21 for detailed information on these precautions.) During all procedures you must be sure to wear adequate personal protective equipment (PPE), handle and dispose of specimens properly, dispose of used supplies and equipment properly, and sanitize, disinfect, and/or sterilize all reusable equipment.

# Anatomy and Physiology of the Urinary System

The urinary system comprises two kidneys, two ureters, a bladder, and a urethra. The kidneys are located behind the peritoneum on either side of the lumbar spine. They remove excess water from the body and waste products from the blood in the form of urine. The urine then drains through the ureters and into the urinary bladder. The urinary bladder stores urine until it leaves the body through the urethra. The ureters, bladder, and urethra make up the urinary tract.

# Formation of Urine in the Kidney

Urine formation is essentially a filtering process that occurs in the nephrons. Nephrons are the functional units of the kidney (Figure 34-1). Each kidney contains about a million nephrons, each of which is capable of forming urine.

Glomerular filtration occurs as blood moves through a tight ball of capillaries called the glomerulus. The glomerular capsule (Bowman's capsule) surrounds the glomerulus. Filtered fluid collects in this capsule, which is the functional beginning of the nephron. A capillary bed surrounds the winding tubule that makes up the rest of the nephron structure. Reabsorption of water, nutrients, and some electrolytes returns these substances to the blood as the filtered fluid passes through the long tubule. Other electrolytes and some additional substances are secreted from the blood into the tubule. Urine is the fluid that flows out of the nephron into the collecting tubule, passes through the funnel-shaped renal pelvis, leaves the kidney, and is carried down the ureter to the bladder.

The specific function of the nephron is to remove certain end products of metabolism from the blood plasma. Because the nephron allows for reabsorption of water and

## TABLE 34-1 Abbreviations Common to Urine Analysis and Testing

| | | | |
|---|---|---|---|
| ADH | antidiuretic hormone | RBCs | red blood cells |
| BIL; bili; BR | bilirubin | SPG; sp gr; sp.gr. | specific gravity |
| BJP | Bence Jones proteins | U/A | urinalysis |
| Ca | calcium | UBG | urobilinogen |
| CC | clean catch (urine) | U/C | urine culture |
| CCMS | clean catch, midstream (urine) | UC | urinary catheter |
| CL VOID | clean voided specimen (urine) | UC&S | urine culture and sensitivity |
| CrCl | creatinine clearance | UcaV | urinary calcium volume |
| CSU | catheter specimen (urine) | UCRE | urine creatinine |
| Cys | cysteine | UFC | urinary free cortisol |
| CYS | cystoscopy | UK | urine potassium |
| EMU | early morning urine(s) | Una | urinary sodium |
| HCG; hcg; hCG | human chorionic gonadotropin | Uosm | urine osmolarity |
| IVP | intravenous pyelogram | UTI | urinary tract infection |
| K | potassium | UUN | urinary urea nitrogen |
| pH | hydrogen ion concentration | UV | urinary volume |
| PKD | polycystic kidney disease | Vol | volume |
| PKU | phenylketonuria | WBCs | white blood cells |

some electrolytes back into the blood, the nephron also plays a vital role in maintaining normal fluid balance in the body.

## Physical Composition and Chemical Properties

Urine is made up of 95% water and 5% waste products and other dissolved chemicals. Components other than water include urea, uric acid, ammonia, calcium, creatinine, sodium, chloride, potassium, sulfates, phosphates, bicarbonates, hydrogen ions, urochrome, urobilinogen, a few red blood cells, and a few white blood cells. If a patient is taking any drugs that are excreted renally, the drugs may also show up in the urine. Urine in males may contain a few sperm cells. Table 34-1 provides a list of abbreviations commonly used in urine analysis and testing.

# Obtaining Specimens

It is essential to collect, store, and preserve urine specimens in ways that do not alter their physical, chemical, or microscopic properties. You must follow guidelines each time you obtain specimens and instruct patients in the proper guidelines to follow.

## General Collection Guidelines

When you collect urine specimens from patients, follow these guidelines.

- Make sure you are following the procedure that is specified for the urine test that will be performed.
- Use the type of specimen container indicated by the laboratory. If a patient must bring in a specimen, be sure that the container is provided by the physician's office or that the container is appropriate for the testing protocol. If you provide the patient with a container that contains a preservative, make sure the appropriate warning labels are attached. You should also warn the patient that the additive may contain acid and they should take care not to spill the acid on themselves.
- Label the specimen container before giving it to the patient or on receipt of a container that the patient provides. Include the patient's name, the physician's name, the date and time of collection, and the initials of the person collecting the sample. Label the side of the specimen container, not the lid, because lids may be lost or switched.
- If the patient is having an invasive test, such as catheterization, always explain the procedure to the patient completely, using simple, clear language.

- If you are assisting in the collection process, wash your hands before and after the procedure, and wear gloves during the procedure.
- Complete all necessary paperwork, recording the collection in the patient's chart and making sure you use the correct request slip for the test that has been ordered.

In many instances, patients need to collect a urine specimen at home. It is your responsibility to give patients instructions for obtaining the specific type of specimen. In addition, provide them with the following general instructions.

- Urinate into the container indicated by the laboratory. In most instances urinate into a widemouthed, throwaway, spouted specimen container as instructed. Do not add anything to the container except the urine.
- If the collection container contains liquid or powdered preservative, do not pour it out.
- If any of the preservative spills on you, wash the area immediately and contact the physician's office.
- Always refrigerate the labeled collection container or keep it in a cooler or pail filled with ice.
- Be sure to keep the lid on the container.

## Specimen Types

Many different tests are performed on urine. You may need to obtain different types of specimens for different tests. The specimens may be used from quantitative analysis or qualitative analysis. A quantitative analysis is a test that measures the amount of a specific substance in the urine. A qualitative analysis simply measures the presence of a substance in urine. Specimens vary in two ways: in the method used to collect them and in the time frame in which they are collected.

Whenever you collect a specimen, you must follow the steps in the procedure exactly—or have the patient follow them exactly. Quality assurance is essential in the physician's office laboratory. As discussed in Chapter 32, control samples must be used every time you test patient specimens. These are the types of urine specimens:

- Random
- First morning
- Clean-catch midstream
- Timed
- 24-hour

**Random Urine Specimen.** The **random urine specimen** is the most common type of sample. It is a single urine specimen taken at any time of the day. A random urine specimen is collected in a clean, dry container. If the doctor is requesting that a culture be done on the specimen, provide the patient with a sterile container.

If the collection of a random urine specimen is to be done at the doctor's office, supply the patient with a urine specimen container. Show the patient to the bathroom, and ask the patient to void a few ounces of urine into the specimen cup and to leave the cup on the sink. Retrieve the specimen when the patient leaves the bathroom and attach a properly completed label and requisition slip. Transport the specimen to the laboratory immediately. Urine specimens should be processed within 1 hour of collection. If this is not possible, refrigerate the specimens. Before processing refrigerated specimens, however, allow them to come to room temperature. If specimens will be shipped to an outside laboratory, chemical preservatives are added.

If patients are to collect a random urine specimen at home, have them use the container indicated by the laboratory. Either provide patients with a urine specimen container or instruct them to use a clean, widemouthed glass jar with a tight-fitting lid. Explain that a household dishwasher provides hot enough water to disinfect a jar adequately. Tell patients to refrigerate specimens until they bring them to the doctor's office and to keep them cool during transport.

**First Morning Urine Specimen.** The **first morning urine specimen** is collected after a night's sleep. This type of specimen contains greater concentrations of substances that collect over time than do specimens taken during the day. A urine specimen container or clean, dry jar is used to collect the urine as per the laboratory's request.

**Clean-Catch Midstream Urine Specimen.** The **clean-catch midstream urine specimen,** sometimes referred to as mid-void, may be collected and submitted for culturing to identify the number and the types of pathogens present. The presence of clinical symptoms or unexplained bacteria in a urinalysis specimen is an indication for urine culture. This method is not like other urine tests in which urine is simply voided into a specimen container. Instead, the clean-catch midstream method requires special cleansing of the external genitalia to avoid contamination by organisms residing near the urethral meatus (the external opening of the urethra). Voiding a small amount of urine into the toilet prior to collecting the midstream specimen flushes the normal flora out of the distal urethra to prevent possible contamination of the specimen. The only other way to obtain a specimen without this type of contamination is through catheterization, a procedure not routinely recommended because of the risk of infection. Procedure 34-1 describes how to collect a clean-catch midstream urine specimen and how to instruct patients to perform this technique.

**Timed Urine Specimen.** A physician may order a **timed urine specimen** to measure a patient's urinary output or to analyze substances (see also the discussion of the 24-hour urine specimen). First determine whether the required time period means that the patient must collect the specimen at home. If so, provide the patient with the proper collection container; written instructions on the process, including preservation of the specimen; and the following oral instructions.

- Discard the first specimen
- Then collect *all* urine for the specified time (2 to 24 hours)

# Collecting a Clean-Catch Midstream Urine Specimen

**Procedure Goal:** To collect a urine specimen that is free from contamination

## OSHA Guidelines

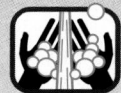 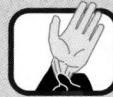 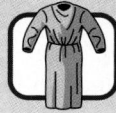 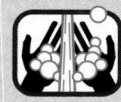

**Materials:** Dry, sterile urine container with lid; label; written instructions (if the patient is to perform procedure independently); antiseptic towelettes

## Method:

1. Confirm the patient's identity and be sure all forms are correctly completed.

2. Label the sterile urine specimen container with the patient's name, ID number, date of birth, the physician's name, the date and time of collection, and the initials of the person collecting the specimen.

When the patient will be completing the procedure independently:

3. Explain the procedure in detail. Provide the patient with written instructions, antiseptic towelettes, and the labeled sterile specimen container.

4. Confirm that the patient understands the instructions, especially not to touch the inside of the specimen container and to refrigerate the specimen until bringing it to the physician's office.

### Rationale

Touching the inside of the container will introduce microorganisms into the container and can interfere with the test results. The specimen should be refrigerated to keep bacteria from growing and causing a false-positive result.

When you are assisting a patient:

3. Explain the procedure and how you will be assisting in the collection.

4. Wash your hands and put on exam gloves.

When you are assisting in the collection for female patients:

5. Remove the lid from the specimen container, and place the lid upside down on a flat surface.

6. Use three antiseptic towelettes to clean the perineal area by spreading the labia and wiping from front to back. Wipe with the first towelette on one side and discard it. Wipe with the second towelette on the other side and discard it. Wipe with the third towelette down the middle and discard it. To remove soap residue that could cause a higher pH and affect chemical test results, rinse the area once from front to back with water.

### Rationale

The area must be thoroughly cleaned so that microorganisms from the vulva do not contaminate the specimen.

7. Keeping the patient's labia spread to avoid contamination, tell her to urinate into the toilet. After she has expressed a small amount of urine, instruct her to stop the flow.

### Rationale

So that microorganisms are washed away from the urethral opening

8. Position the specimen container close to but not touching the patient.

9. Tell the patient to start urinating again. Collect the necessary amount of urine in the container. (If the patient cannot stop her urine flow, move the container into the urine flow and collect the specimen anyway.)

10. Allow the patient to finish urinating. Place the lid back on the collection container.

11. Remove the gloves and wash your hands.

12. Complete the test request slip, and record the collection in the patient's chart.

When you are assisting in the collection for male patients:

5. Remove the lid from the specimen container, and place the lid upside down on a flat surface.

6. If the patient is circumcised, use an antiseptic towelette to clean the head of the penis. Wipe with a second towelette directly across the urethral opening. If the patient is uncircumcised, retract the foreskin before cleaning the penis. To remove soap residue that could cause a higher pH and affect chemical test results, rinse the area once from front to back with water.

### Rationale

The area must be thoroughly cleaned so that microorganisms from the head of the penis do not contaminate the specimen.

*continued* ⟶

## Collecting a Clean-Catch Midstream Urine Specimen (concluded)

7. Keeping an uncircumcised patient's foreskin retracted, tell the patient to urinate into the toilet. After he has expressed a small amount of urine, instruct him to stop the flow.

    *Rationale*

    So that microorganisms are washed away from the urethral opening

8. Position the specimen container close to but not touching the patient.

9. Tell the patient to start urinating again. Collect the necessary amount of urine in the container. (If the patient cannot stop his urine flow, move the container into the urine flow and collect the specimen anyway.)

10. Allow the patient to finish urinating. Place the lid back on the collection container.

11. Remove the gloves and wash your hands.

12. Complete the laboratory request form, and record the collection in the patient's chart.

---

- Be sure the urine does not mix with stool or toilet paper
- Keep the sample refrigerated until returning it to the physician's office or laboratory

**24-Hour Urine Specimen.** A **24-hour urine specimen** is collected over a 24-hour period and is used to complete a quantitative and qualitative analysis of one or more substances, such as sodium, chloride, and calcium. You need to instruct the patient in the proper collection process. If an outside laboratory will be testing the specimen, you will receive protocols for collection, preservation, and transport. See the Educating the Patient section for specific information on the 24-hour collection process.

## Catheterization

A **urinary catheter** is a sterile plastic tube inserted to provide urinary drainage. Such a catheter may be inserted into the kidney, the ureter, or the bladder. **Catheterization** is the procedure during which the catheter is inserted. Catheterization is performed for various reasons, including to:

- Relieve urinary retention
- Obtain a sterile urine specimen from a patient
- Measure the amount of residual urine in the bladder to determine how much urine remains after normal voiding (Patient voids and is then catheterized; more than 50 milliliters is considered abnormal.)
- Obtain a urine specimen if the patient cannot void naturally
- Instill chemotherapy as a treatment for bladder cancer
- Empty the bladder before and during surgery and before some diagnostic exams

There are two primary types of urinary catheters:

1. **Drainage catheters,** which are used to withdraw fluids and include an indwelling urethral (Foley) catheter

placed in the bladder, a retention catheter in the renal pelvis, a ureteral catheter, a catheter for drainage through a wound that leads to the bladder (cystostomy tube), and a straight catheter to collect specimens or instill medications

2. **Splinting catheters,** which are inserted after plastic repair of the ureter and must remain in place for at least a week after surgery

Catheterization is not routinely recommended because it can introduce infection. Some states do not permit medical assistants to perform catheterization, and in most health-care institutions, only a physician or nurse can insert or withdraw a catheter. Check the protocol in your state. If you cannot perform the procedure, you may be asked to assemble the necessary supplies and to assist the physician during it.

Catheterization performed in a physician's office is usually done for diagnostic purposes. Specially prepared catheterization kits are available that contain all necessary instruments and supplies. These kits include a sterile instrument pack that is used to create a sterile field for the procedure.

If a patient is incontinent, the physician may use a bladder-drainage catheter to help drain the bladder and keep the patient dry. Another type of drainage catheter, the ureteral, is inserted into the ureter to help drain urine.

The indwelling urethral (Foley) catheter is designed to stay in place within the bladder (Figure 34-2). It consists of two tubes, one inside the other. The inside tube is connected to a balloon, which is filled with water or air to keep the catheter from slipping out of the bladder. Urine travels through the bladder and drains from the outside tube into a soft plastic container. The physician may order a leg bag to attach to the patient's thigh. The bag is anchored to the leg by two bands placed around the thigh. Make sure the bag is positioned so that there is no tension on the catheter tube. To prevent back-flow into the patient's bladder, the container must always be lower than the bladder.

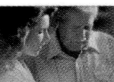
# Educating the Patient

## How to Collect a 24-Hour Urine Specimen

When a patient needs to collect a 24-hour urine specimen, you must explain the procedure thoroughly and provide explicit written instructions. Be sure the patient understands that she must collect all her urine over the 24-hour period.

Provide the patient with a labeled sterile urine container with a lid. Tell her that at the start of the observation period (usually early in the morning), she should void and discard that specimen. Then every time she voids for the next 24 hours, she must collect the entire amount in the sterile container.

Tell the patient that the urine will be tested for substances that are released sporadically into the urine. Thus, it is extremely important to avoid using a bedpan, urinal, or toilet tissue, which could retain the substances for which the test is being done. Instead, the patient should urinate directly into a small collection container and then pour the urine into the large urine specimen container. Explain that the small container must be sanitized between uses with soap and warm water.

Explain that the large specimen container may have a preservative in it to prevent contamination and other alterations in the specimen. Instruct the patient to keep the specimen covered and in the refrigerator when not in use during the collection period. Emphasize the need to deliver the specimen to the doctor's office or laboratory as soon as possible after the 24-hour period is over, keeping the specimen cool during transport.

## Special Considerations

When you obtain a urine specimen from a patient or take a history of a patient who may have a urinary problem, you need to consider the patient's sex, condition, and age. Some patients may require special care during collection procedures.

**Special Considerations in Male and Female Patients.** Depending on the test, you may need to alter guidelines for collecting urine specimens from a male or female patient. For example, Procedure 34-1 describes how to assist in collecting a clean-catch urine specimen from a female patient and from a male patient. In addition, when you take a medical history on a male or female patient, you

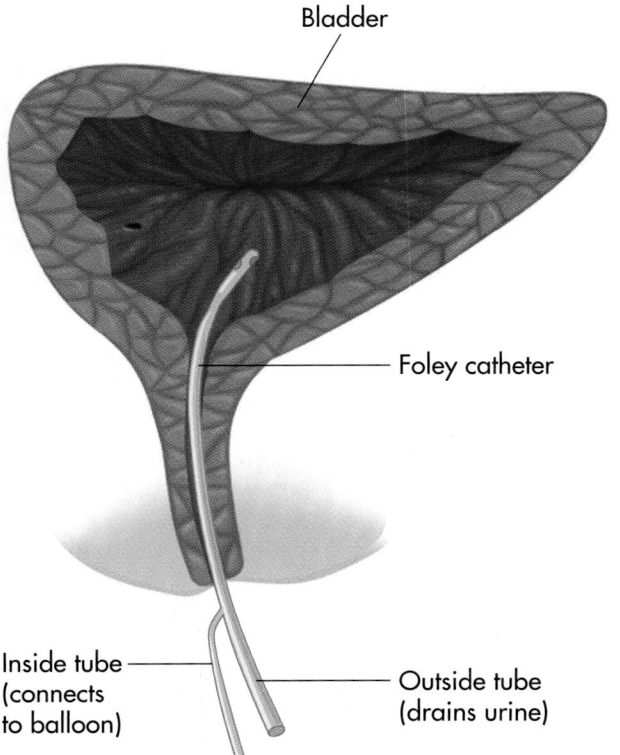

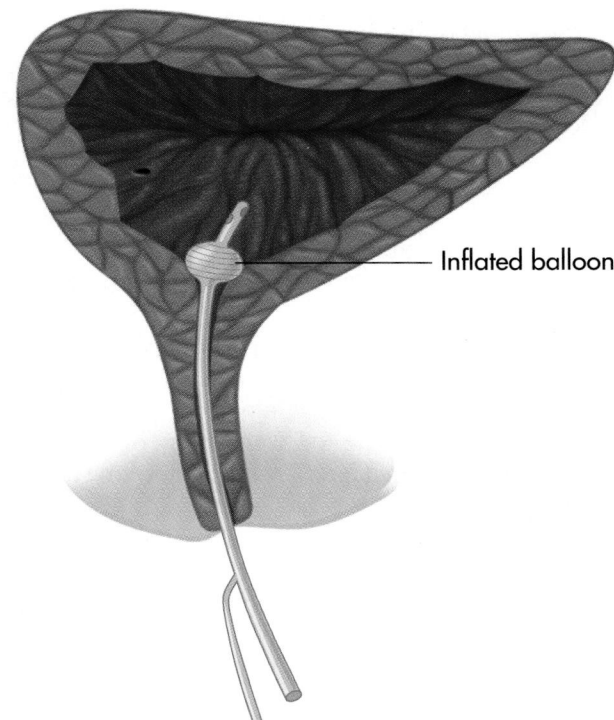

Bladder

Foley catheter

Inside tube (connects to balloon)

Outside tube (drains urine)

Inflated balloon

**Figure 34-2.** A Foley catheter stays in place within the bladder and has a collection container that is emptied periodically.

will need to ask particular questions as part of your assessment. For example, if a female patient leaks urine when laughing or coughing, she may have bladder dysfunction, which would affect collecting a 24-hour urine specimen.

### Special Considerations in Pregnant Patients.
Pregnant women normally have increased urinary frequency. They may also be prone to urinary tract infections. At each prenatal visit pregnant women must have their urine checked for abnormal levels of glucose (a screening test for diabetes) and abnormal levels of protein (a screening test for preeclampsia or renal problems).

Ask a pregnant patient whether she has any pain during urination or in the kidney area. A positive response may indicate a urinary tract infection or kidney stones. Also ask about urine leakage and whether she has previously been pregnant. Leakage may occur in a woman who has had multiple births, because the pressure of the fetus on the bladder or delivery of the baby may have weakened the patient's bladder control. Additionally, ask whether any of the babies were delivered by forceps, which can injure urinary and genital structures.

### Special Considerations in Elderly Patients.
When you collect urine specimens from elderly patients, you must consider several points.

- Bladder muscles weaken with age, often leading to incomplete bladder emptying and chronic urine retention, which can cause urinary tract infection, **nocturia** (excessive nighttime urination), and incontinence. Incontinence can interfere with collecting a 24-hour urine specimen.
- Weakening of the supports of the uterus may cause it to prolapse (work its way down the vaginal canal). The uterus pulls with it the vaginal walls, bladder, and rectum. This weakening, which is often the result of several childbirths, may not occur until a woman is postmenopausal. Symptoms include pressure, incontinence, and urinary retention. Normal activities, such as walking up the stairs, can aggravate the problem. This condition can interfere with collecting a 24-hour specimen.
- Find out whether the patient ever loses bladder control. If so, ask whether it occurs suddenly or whether a feeling of intense pressure precedes it. These symptoms can be a sign of weakening of the bladder muscles, which can interfere with collecting a 24-hour specimen.
- Keep in mind that some elderly patients need assistance in providing a urine specimen. For example, you may have to accompany the patient to the bathroom and hold the specimen container. (Wash your hands before and after doing so, and wear gloves while providing this help.)
- If necessary, offer repeated explanations or reminders about the procedure or the specimens that need to be provided.

### Special Considerations in Pediatric Patients.
When you collect a urine specimen from a pediatric patient, involve the child (if age-appropriate) and the parents or guardians. Explain the procedure thoroughly and ask specific questions, including the following.

- If the child is in diapers, ask whether there is a problem of persistent diaper rash. (Rash may indicate a change in urine composition because of renal dysfunction.)
- Is the child excessively thirsty? (In this case the patient may not be taking in enough fluids for the amount of urine being excreted. Excessive thirst, combined with increased urinary frequency and volume, is symptomatic of diabetes.)
- Has the child experienced any difficulty urinating or a urine stream change? (These signs may suggest an obstruction in the urinary tract.)
- Does the child cry when urinating? (If so, the child may have pain or burning on urination, which can indicate a urinary tract infection.)
- If the child is in diapers, ask how many diapers are wet each day. Has the number changed recently? (Responses to these questions can rule out or confirm a urine volume change. For example, a child with a fever and increased perspiration might experience decreased urine volume.)
- Has the child experienced deterioration in bladder control, such as bed-wetting (enuresis)? (The child may be under stress or may have a small bladder capacity or a urinary tract infection.)
- If the child is having problems with toilet training and is older than 4 years old, ask whether the child learned to sit, stand, and talk at the age-appropriate times. (If so, the child may have a urinary system dysfunction.)

When you collect a urine specimen from a child who is toilet-trained, follow the same procedures as for an adult. If the child is an infant or not toilet-trained, however, follow the steps outlined in Procedure 34-2.

## Establishing Chain of Custody

Occasionally you may need to obtain urine specimens for drug and alcohol analysis. When you do so, you must establish a proper chain of custody.

The general approach to establishing a chain of custody is described in Chapter 30. Because of the medicolegal issues involved, it is important to follow the procedure exactly. If you alter the procedure at any point, you have broken the chain. Also, because supplying a specimen for drug or alcohol testing could be self-incriminating, it is important to thoroughly explain the procedure to donors and have them sign a consent form (Figure 34-4). The consent form may be a part of the chain of custody form (CCF), or it may be a separate

# PROCEDURE 34.2

## Collecting a Urine Specimen from a Pediatric Patient

**Procedure Goal:** To collect a urine specimen from an infant or a child who is not toilet-trained

**OSHA Guidelines**

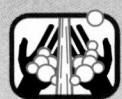 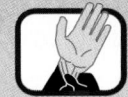 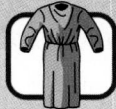 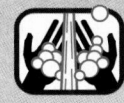

**Materials:** Urine specimen bottle or container, label, sterile cotton balls, soapy water, sterile water, plastic disposable urine collection bag

**Method:**

1. Confirm the patient's identity and be sure all forms are correctly completed.

2. Label the urine specimen container with the patient's name, ID number, and date of birth, the physician's name, the date and time of collection, and your initials.

3. Explain the procedure to the child (if age-appropriate) and to the parents or guardians.

4. Wash your hands and put on exam gloves.

5. Have the parents pull the child's pants down and take off the diaper.

6. Position the child with the genitalia exposed.

7. Clean the genitalia. For a male patient, wipe the tip of the penis with a soapy cotton ball, and then rinse it with a cotton ball saturated with sterile water. Allow to air-dry. For a female patient, use soapy cotton balls to clean the labia majora from front to back, using one cotton ball for each wipe. Again, use cotton balls saturated in sterile water to rinse the area, and allow it to air-dry.

### Rationale

The area must be thoroughly cleaned so that microorganisms from the head of the penis or vulva do not contaminate the specimen.

8. Remove the paper backing from the plastic urine collection bag, and apply the sticky, adhesive surface over the penis and scrotum (in a male

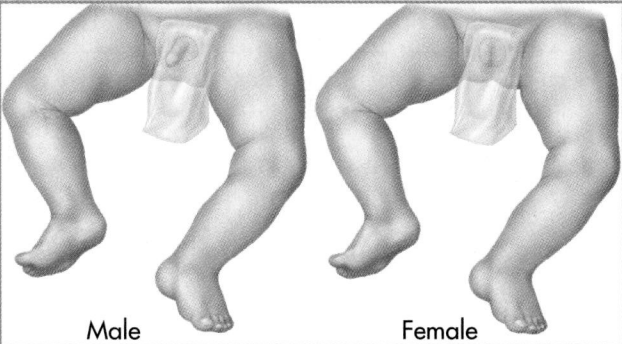

**Figure 34-3.** When you apply a pediatric urine bag, make sure there are no leaks.

patient) or vulva (in a female patient), as shown in Figure 34-3. Seal tightly to avoid leaks. Do not include the child's rectum within the collection bag or cover it with the adhesive surface.

9. Diaper the child.

10. Remove the gloves and wash your hands.

11. Check the collection bag every half-hour for urine. You must open the diaper to check; do not just feel the diaper.

### Rationale

The diaper should not be wet, and feeling the diaper without looking could dislodge the bag.

12. If the child has voided, wash your hands and put on exam gloves.

13. Remove the diaper, take off the urine collection bag very carefully so that you do not irritate the child's skin, wash off the adhesive residue, rinse, and pat dry.

14. Diaper the child.

15. Place the specimen in the specimen container and cover it.

16. Remove the gloves and wash your hands.

17. Complete the laboratory request form, and record the collection in the patient's chart.

form. The consent form states the purpose of the test and gives you permission to collect the specimen, prepare it for transport to the laboratory for analysis, and release the results to the agency requesting the test. Distribute copies of the CCF to the medical review officer, laboratory, patient, collector, and employer or other requesting party.

Inform the patient that medication (both prescription and nonprescription), drugs, and alcohol will show up in the test results. Encourage the patient to list on the consent form or CCF all substances consumed in the last 30 days, including what was taken and how much.

The chain of custody form, described in Chapter 30 (Figure 30-25), indicates the source of the urine sample.

**Crossroads Medical Center**
Newfield, New Jersey 07655-3213
201-555-4000

**Drug Screen Consent Form**

A urine drug test is required by_____ as part of your pre-employment screening. Please provide us with a list of all medications that you are presently taking.

_____

_____

_____

_____

I understand that my prospective or continued employment is contingent on a successful screening.
Date: _____     Signature:_____
Witness: _____

**Figure 34-4.** A consent form is a legal requirement when urine is collected for drug testing.

This form verifies that the patient whose name is on the CCF and consent forms is the same person who provided the sealed specimen sent to the laboratory. Follow Procedure 34-3 when collecting a urine sample for drug or alcohol testing.

## Preservation and Storage

Proper preservation and storage of specimens are essential. Changes that affect the chemical and microscopic properties of urine occur in urine kept at room temperature for more than 1 hour. Such changes invalidate certain test results. If you leave a specimen unpreserved by any means for more than 1 hour, changes occur in the urine that affect the results of all urine testing—physical, chemical, and microscopic.

Refrigeration is the most common method for storing and preserving urine. It prevents bacterial growth in a specimen for at least 24 hours. Refrigeration can cause other changes in the urine, however, that may affect the physical characteristics of sediment and specific gravity. Bringing the specimen back to room temperature before testing will correct these problems. You can use chemical preservatives to preserve specimens, especially 24-hour specimens or those that must be sent a long distance to a laboratory.

## Urinalysis

**Urinalysis** is the evaluation of urine by various types of testing methods to obtain information about body health and disease. Urinalysis consists of three types of testing:

* Physical
* Chemical
* Microscopic

There are normal values for all tests done on urine. The normal value for a specific substance may be negative or none, normal, or it may be a range in concentration. Urine test results within normal ranges indicate health and normality. Table 34-2 identifies normal values for a variety of urine tests. Because a urine test is a screening test, all abnormal values must be followed up with a confirmatory test.

Urinalysis is done as part of a general physical exam to screen for certain substances or to diagnose various medical conditions (Table 34-3). For example, daily urine output provides a picture of renal function. With adequate fluid intake, the average adult daily urine output is 1250 milliliters per 24 hours. When total intake and output measurements are not approximately equal, urinary tract dysfunction may be the cause.

# PROCEDURE 34.3

## Establishing Chain of Custody for a Urine Specimen

**Procedure Goal:** To collect a urine specimen for drug testing, maintaining a chain of custody

### OSHA Guidelines

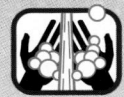 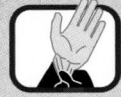 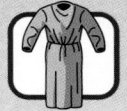 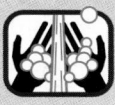

**Materials:** Dry, sterile urine container with lid; chain of custody form (CCF); two additional specimen containers

### Method:

1. Positively identify the patient. (Complete the top part of CCF with the name and address of the drug testing laboratory, the name and address of requesting company, and the Social Security number of the patient. Make a note on the form if the patient refuses to give her Social Security number.) Ensure that the number on the printed label matches the number at the top of the form.

2. Ensure that the patient removes any outer clothing and empties her pockets, displaying all items.

### Rationale

So that the patient does not bring anything into the room to adulterate the specimen, resulting in a false-negative result

3. Instruct the patient to wash and dry her hands.

4. Instruct the patient that no water is to be running while the specimen is being collected. Tape the faucet handles in the *off* position and add bluing agent to the toilet.

### Rationale

So that the patient cannot warm a specimen brought in from another source and has no water available to dilute the specimen

5. Instruct the patient to provide the specimen as soon as it is collected so that you may record the temperature of the specimen.

6. Remain by the door of the restroom.

7. Measure and record the temperature of the urine specimen within 4 minutes of collection. Make a note if its temperature is out of acceptable range.

### Rationale

To determine that the patient voided the specimen and did not bring it from an outside source

8. Examine the specimen for signs of adulteration (unusual color or odor).

9. *In the presence of the patient,* check the "single specimen" or "split specimen" box. The patient should witness you transferring the specimen into the transport specimen bottle(s), capping the bottle(s), and affixing the label on the bottle(s).

### Rationale

To maintain the chain of custody

10. The patient should initial the specimen bottle label(s) *after* it is placed on the bottle(s).

### Rationale

To maintain the chain of custody

11. Complete any additional information requested on the form, including the authorization for drug screening. This information will include:
    - Patient's daytime telephone number
    - Patient's evening telephone number
    - Test requested
    - Patient's name
    - Patient's signature
    - Date

12. Sign the CCF; print your full name, and note the date and time of the collection, and the name of the courier service.

13. Give the patient a copy of the CCF.

14. Place the specimen in a leakproof bag with the appropriate copy of the form.

15. Release the specimen to the courier service.

16. Distribute additional copies as required.

The urinary system works with other body systems to help the body function normally. Therefore, a disorder in another body system can affect urinary function. For example, the kidneys interact with the nervous system to help regulate blood pressure and control urination. Thus, a nervous system disorder can affect the circulatory and urinary systems. The cardiovascular system delivers blood to the kidneys for filtration, and the kidneys regulate fluid balance, which helps maintain circulation of blood and myocardial function. A cardiovascular system disorder can allow blood to be delivered to the kidneys at a pressure inadequate for filtration, which would affect urinary system function.

# TABLE 34-2    Standard Urine Values

## Physical Characteristics

| Test | Normal Values |
| --- | --- |
| Color | Pale yellow to yellow |
| Clarity | Clear–slightly turbid |

## Reagent Strip Test

| Test | Normal Values |
| --- | --- |
| Bilirubin | Negative |
| Blood | Negative |
| Glucose | Negative |
| Ketone bodies (Acetone) | Negative |
| Leukocytes | Negative |
| Nitrites | Negative |
| pH | 4.5–8.0 |
| Protein | Negative–trace |
| Specific gravity | 1.002–1.028 |
| Urobilinogen | 0.3–1.0 E. U. |

## Microscopic Examination

| Test | Normal Values |
| --- | --- |
| Bacteria | Negative |
| Casts | |
| Epithelial cell | Negative |
| Granular | Negative |
| Hyaline | Few |
| Red blood cell | Negative |
| Waxy | Negative |
| White blood cell | Negative |
| Crystals | |
| Amorphous phosphates | Normal |
| Calcium carbonate | Normal |
| Calcium oxalate | Normal |
| Cholesterol | Negative |
| Cystine | Negative |
| Leucine | Negative |
| Sulfonamide | Negative |
| Triple phosphate | Normal |
| Tyrosine | Negative |
| Uric acid | Normal |

## Microscopic Examination

| Test | Normal Values |
| --- | --- |
| Epithelial cells | |
| Renal | Negative |
| Squamous, adult females | Moderate |
| Squamous, adult males | Few |
| Transitional | Rare |
| Mucus | Rare–few |
| Protozoa | Negative |
| Red blood cells | 0–3/high-power field |
| White blood cells | 0–8/high-power field |
| Yeast | Few |

## 24 Hour

| Test | Normal Values |
| --- | --- |
| 5HIAA | 2–8 mg |
| Albumin (quantitative) | 10–140 mg/L |
| Ammonia | 140–1500 mg |
| Calcium (quantitative) | 100–300 mg |
| Catecholamines, total | <100 mcg |
| Chloride | 110–120 mEq |
| Cortisol | 10–100 mcg |
| Creatine, nonpregnant women/men | <100 mg |
| Creatine, pregnant women | ≤12% of creatinine |
| Creatinine, men | 1.0–1.9 g |
| Creatinine, women | 0.8–1.7 g |
| Cystine and cysteine | <38.1 mg |
| Glucose, quantitative | 50–500 mg |
| Phosphorus | 0.4–1.3 g |
| Potassium | 25–120 mEq/L |
| Protein (Bence Jones) | Negative |
| Sodium | 80–180 mEq |
| Urea nitrogen | 6–17 g |
| Uric acid | 0.25–0.75 g |
| Urobilinogen, quantitative | 1.0–4.0 mg |
| Volume, adult females | 600–1600 mL |
| Volume, adult males | 800–1800 mL |
| Volume, children | 3–4 times adult rate/kg |

*Note*: Individual laboratories may have slightly different reference values. Consult the reference values provided by the lab performing the test.

## TABLE 34-3  Common Urine Tests According to Clinical Condition

| Clinical Condition or Suspected Disease | Types of Urine Testing |
|---|---|
| Acidosis | Reagent strip* for pH <br> Specific gravity |
| Alkalosis (metabolic, respiratory) | Reagent strip* for pH <br> Specific gravity |
| Diabetes mellitus | Odor (fruity) <br> Microscopic examination for fatty, waxy casts <br> Reagent strip* for ketonuria, glycosuria <br> Specific gravity |
| Drug abuse | Gas chromatography; mass spectrometry** |
| Genitourinary infections (prostatitis, urethritis, vaginitis) | Cultures for bacteria, yeasts, parasites <br> Microscopic examination for bacteria, RBCs |
| Human immunodeficiency virus (HIV) | Culture for virus (antibiotic added to kill bacteria) <br> Other tests as indicated by specific symptoms |
| Hypercalcemia | Microscopic examination for calcium oxalate crystals <br> Specific gravity |
| Hypertension | Microscopic examination for casts (hyaline, RBC) <br> Specific gravity |
| Infectious diseases (bacterial) or other inflammatory diseases | Color and odor <br> Cultures for bacteria, yeasts, viruses <br> Microscopic examination for bacteria, WBCs, RBC casts (in severe cases) <br> Reagent strip* for bacteria <br> Turbidity |
| Metabolic disorders (except diabetes mellitus) | Color <br> Microscopic examination for cystine crystals <br> Reagent strip* for ketonuria, fructosuria, galactosuria, pentosuria, pH |
| Nephron disorders (nephrotic syndrome, glomerulonephritis, nephrosis, nephrolithiasis, pyelonephritis) | Color <br> Microscopic examination for casts (epithelial, fatty, waxy, RBC), RBCs <br> Reagent strip* for proteinuria <br> Specific gravity <br> Turbidity |
| Phenylketonuria | Color <br> Reagent strip* for pH |
| Poisoning (arsenic, cadmium, lead, mercury) | Color <br> Mass spectrometry** |
| Polycystic kidney disease | Proteinuria <br> Urinary volume |
| Pregnancy | Reagent strip* for human chorionic gonadotropin (HCG) |

*continued* ⟶

| Clinical Condition or Suspected Disease | Types of Urine Testing |
|---|---|
| Renal infections (acute glomerulonephritis, nephrotic syndrome, pyelonephritis, pyogenic infection) | Color<br>Microscopic examination for epithelial cells (especially with tubular degeneration), numerous casts (granular, hyaline, WBC), RBCs, WBCs<br>Radioimmunoassay (RIA)**<br>Reagent strip* for bacteria, albumin<br>Specific gravity<br>Turbidity<br>Urinary volume |
| Renal disease, renal failure, severe renal damage, acute renal failure, renal tubular degeneration | Microscopic examination for epithelial cells (especially with tubular degeneration), numerous casts (hyaline, fatty, waxy, RBC)<br>Reagent strip* for proteinuria (albumin), pH<br>Specific gravity<br>Turbidity<br>Urinary volume |
| Sickle cell anemia | RBC casts |
| Starvation, dietary imbalance, extreme change in diet, dehydration | Color<br>Odor (fruity)<br>Reagent strip* for ketonuria<br>Specific gravity |
| Urinary tract infection or mild inflammation (cystitis, pyelonephritis) | Color and odor<br>Cultures for bacteria, yeasts, viruses<br>Microscopic examination for bacteria, WBC casts, RBCs, WBCs<br>Reagent strip* for bacteria, albumin, pH<br>Specific gravity<br>Turbidity |
| Urinary obstruction (tumor, trauma, inflammation) | Color<br>Microscopic examination for RBCs<br>Specific gravity<br>Urinary volume |

*Federal listings of waived tests refer to these as dipstick tests.

**Drug screening and some other common urine tests must be performed by a forensic laboratory or other laboratory capable of performing gas chromatography, mass spectrometry, and radioimmunoassay.

## Physical Examination and Testing of Urine Specimens

The first step in urinalysis is the visual examination of physical characteristics. Prior to starting the physical examination, it is essential to check the specimen for proper labeling. As part of quality assurance, examine it to make sure there is no visible contamination and that no more than 1 hour has passed since collection (or since the sample was refrigerated and brought back to room temperature). These physical characteristics are examined:

- Color and turbidity
- Volume
- Odor
- Specific gravity

**Color and Turbidity.** Normal urine ranges from pale yellow (straw-colored) to dark amber. The color, which comes from a yellow pigment called urochrome, depends

## TABLE 34-4　Urine Color and Turbidity: Possible Causes

| Color and Turbidity | Pathologic Causes | Other Causes |
| --- | --- | --- |
| Colorless or pale straw color (dilute) | Diabetes, anxiety, chronic renal disease | Diuretic therapy, excessive fluid intake (water, beer, coffee) |
| Cloudy | Infection, inflammation, glomerular nephritis | Vegetarian diet |
| Milky white | Fats, pus | Amorphous phosphates, spermatozoa |
| Dark yellow, dark amber (concentrated) | Acute febrile disease, vomiting or diarrhea (fluid loss or dehydration) | Low fluid intake, excessive sweating |
| Yellow-brown | Excessive RBC destruction, bile duct obstruction, diminished liver-cell function, bilirubin | |
| Orange-yellow, orange-red, orange-brown | Excessive RBC destruction, diminished liver-cell function, bile, hepatitis, urobilinuria, obstructive jaundice, hematuria | Drugs (such as pyridium, rifampin), dyes |
| Salmon pink | | Amorphous urates |
| Cloudy red | RBCs, excessive destruction of skeletal or cardiac muscle | |
| Bright yellow or red | RBCs (hemorrhage, myoglobin, hemoglobin), excessive destruction of skeletal or cardiac muscle, porphyria | Beets, drugs (such as phenazopyridine hydrochloride), dyes (such as food coloring and contrast media) |
| Dark red, red-brown | Porphyria, RBCs (menstrual contamination, hemorrhage, hemoglobin), blood from previous hemorrhage | |
| Green, blue-green | Biliverdin, *Pseudomonas* organisms, oxidation of bilirubin | Vitamin B, methylene blue, asparagus (for green) |
| Green-brown | Bile duct obstruction | |
| Brownish black | Methemoglobin, melanin | Drugs (levodopa) |
| Dark brown or black | Acute glomerulonephritis | Drugs (nitrofurantoin, chlorpromazine, iron preparations) |

on food or fluid intake, medications (including vitamin supplements), and waste products present in the urine. In general, a pale color indicates dilute urine, and a dark color indicates concentrated urine.

You will assess urine for turbidity, or cloudiness, by noting whether the urine is clear, slightly cloudy, cloudy, or very cloudy. Typically, urine is clear, although cloudy urine does not always indicate an abnormal condition.

The color of urine and any turbidity that is present can reveal medical conditions that require treatment. Table 34-4 provides more information on variations in urine color and turbidity and the possible causes or sources of these variations. Both pathologic (resulting from disease) and nonpathologic causes are noted.

**Volume.**　Normal urine volume, or output, varies according to the patient's age. Normal adult urine volume is 600 to 1800 milliliters per 24 hours (average of 1250 milliliters per 24 hours). Infants and children have smaller total urine volumes, although they produce more urine per unit of body weight. Urine volume is typically measured on a timed specimen (such as a 24-hour urine specimen) rather than a random specimen.

**Oliguria,** insufficient production (or volume) of urine, occurs in such conditions as dehydration, decreased fluid intake, shock, and renal disease. The absence of urine production is called **anuria.** Renal or urethral obstruction and renal failure can cause anuria.

**Odor.**　Although the odor of urine is not typically recorded or considered a significant indicator of disease, it can provide clues about the body's condition. The odor of normal, freshly voided urine is distinct but not unpleasant and is sometimes characterized as aromatic. After urine has been standing for a while, bacteria in the specimen decompose the urea, which causes an odor similar to ammonia.

Diseases, the presence of bacteria, and particular foods (such as asparagus and garlic) can cause changes in urine odor. For example, in the presence of urinary tract infections, urine is foul-smelling, and in patients with uncontrolled diabetes, the smell is characterized as fruity (because of the presence of ketones). Phenylketonuria, a congenital metabolic disease, produces a strange, "mousy" odor in an infant's wet diaper.

**Specific Gravity.** Urine specific gravity is a measure of the concentration or amount of substances dissolved in urine. Because the kidneys remove metabolic wastes and other substances from the blood, the specific gravity of the urine they produce is an indicator of kidney function. The physician's office laboratory uses any of two methods to determine specific gravity:

1. Refractometer
2. Reagent strip (dipstick)

Specific gravity is a relative measure that is always compared to a standard. The standard for liquids is distilled water, which contains no dissolved substances.

$$\text{Specific gravity} = \frac{\text{weight of sample}}{\text{weight of distilled water}}$$

The specific gravity of distilled water is 1.000. You use special equipment to test for specific gravity (Figure 34-5).

The normal range of urine specific gravity is 1.002 to 1.028. Specific gravity fluctuates throughout the day in response to fluid intake. A first morning urine specimen normally has a higher specific gravity than a specimen provided later in the day. An increase in urine specific gravity indicates that the kidneys cannot properly dilute the urine. The urine then becomes more concentrated, causing it to darken. Increased specific gravity may indicate such conditions as a urinary tract infection, dehydration (for example, from fever, vomiting, or diarrhea), adrenal insufficiency, hepatic disease, or congestive heart failure. A decrease in the specific gravity of urine causes a lighter than normal urine color, may indicate that the kidneys cannot properly concentrate the urine, and may suggest such conditions as over-hydration (excess fluid in the body), diabetes insipidus, chronic renal disease, or systemic lupus erythematosus.

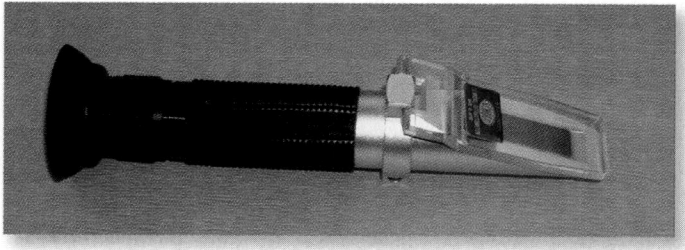

**Figure 34-5.** Specific gravity is commonly determined using a refractometer or reagent strips.

*Refractometer Measurement.* A **refractometer** is an optical instrument that measures the refraction, or bending, of light as it passes through a liquid. The degree of refraction, or refractive index, is proportional to the amount of dissolved material in the liquid. You must calibrate a refractometer each day with distilled water by setting the instrument at 1.000 with the set screw. Two standard solutions (solutions of known specific gravity) are also used to ensure accuracy. Advantages of using a refractometer to measure urine specific gravity are that the process takes little time and requires little urine. Only a drop of urine is used for this determination. Procedure 34-4 describes how to measure specific gravity with a refractometer.

*Reagent Strip Measurement.* You may use special reagent strips, or dipsticks, to test for specific gravity. Test pads along these plastic strips contain chemicals that react with substances in the urine and change color in precise ways. The reagent strip container includes a color chart for interpreting color changes on the test pads. When you evaluate urine specific gravity in this way, keep in mind that this type of test depends on precisely timed intervals identified by the manufacturer. Follow all directions exactly. Procedure 34-5 describes how to perform a reagent strip test.

## Chemical Testing of Urine Specimens

As a medical assistant, you may be asked to perform chemical tests on urine. Prior to performing chemical tests, always check for proper identification on the urine specimen to be tested. Chemical testing is usually done with reagent strips. It can also be performed with certain automated machines that use photometry.

The doctor orders chemical testing of urine to determine the status of body processes such as carbohydrate metabolism, liver or kidney function, or acid-base balance. Other reasons for chemical testing include determining the presence of drugs, toxic environmental substances, or infections.

**Testing With Reagent Strips.** As already described in the discussion of specific gravity, reagents (on plastic strips) are chemicals that react with a particular substance in urine and change color in precise ways. These changes indicate the presence of that substance and the amount or concentration of the substance in the urine specimen. For example, when a reagent strip is used to test for ketones, the reacted color on the strip will correspond either to a specific concentration of ketone bodies, such as acetoacetic acid, or to no ketones present.

Reagent strips are used to test urine for a number of substances. In addition to ketones, these substances include nitrite, pH, blood, bilirubin, glucose, specific gravity, protein, and leukocytes.

There are numerous trade names for urine reagent strips, or dipsticks (for example, Multistix and Chemstrip). Not all reagents are reactive for the same chemicals. You

# PROCEDURE 34.4

## Measuring Specific Gravity With a Refractometer

**Procedure Goal:** To measure the specific gravity of a urine specimen with a refractometer

### OSHA Guidelines

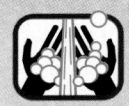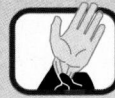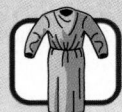
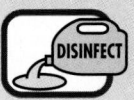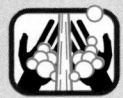

**Materials:** Urine specimen, refractometer, dropper, laboratory report form

### Method:

1. Wash your hands and put on exam gloves.
2. Check the specimen for proper labeling, and examine it to make sure that there is no visible contamination and that no more than 1 hour has passed since collection (or since the specimen has been removed from the refrigerator and brought back to room temperature).
3. Swirl the specimen.

#### Rationale

To mix the specimen thoroughly

4. Confirm that the refractometer has been calibrated that day. If not, you must calibrate it with distilled water. You must also use two standard solutions as controls to check the accuracy of the refractometer. Follow steps 6 through 11, using each of the three samples in place of the specimen. Clean the refractometer and the dropper after each use, and record the calibration values in the quality control log.

#### Rationale

To ensure that the refractometer is standardized prior to testing the specimen

5. Open the hinged lid of the refractometer.
6. Draw up a small amount of the specimen into the dropper.

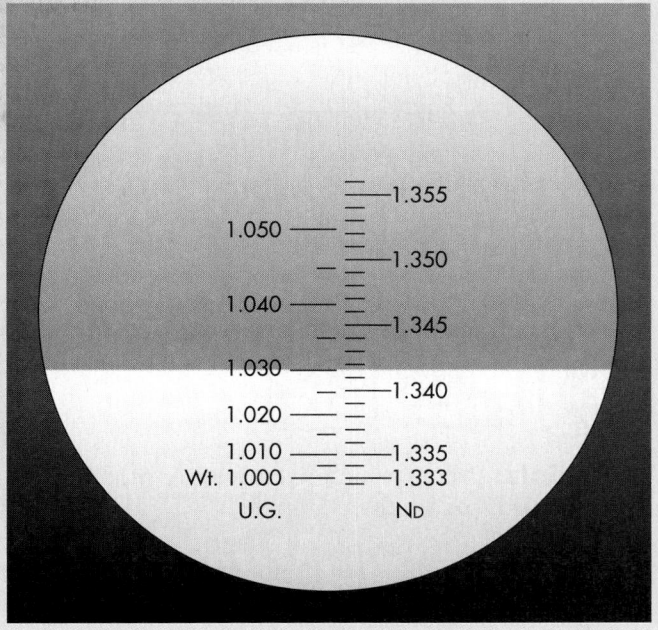

**Figure 34-6.** A refractometer uses light refraction to measure specific gravity.

7. Place one drop of the specimen under the cover.
8. Close the lid.
9. Turn on the light, and look into the eyepiece of the refractometer. As the light passes through the specimen, the refractometer measures the refraction of the light and displays the refractive index on a scale on the right with corresponding specific gravity values on the left (see Figure 34-6).
10. Read the specific gravity value at the line where light and dark meet.
11. Record the value on the laboratory report form.
12. Sanitize and disinfect the refractometer and the dropper. Put them away when they are dry.
13. Clean and disinfect the work area.
14. Remove the gloves and wash your hands.
15. Record the value in the patient's chart.

must choose the appropriate strip according to the chemical test requested. All reagent strips are used once and discarded.

Follow the exact directions that come with the reagent strips to ensure accurate results. For quality assurance, take these basic precautions: Keep strips in tightly closed containers in a cool, dry area. Never remove them from the container until immediately before testing. Never touch the pads on the strip with your fingers or gloved hands. Examine strips for discoloration before use; discard discolored strips. Check the expiration date on the bottle; do not use strips that have expired. Use strips within 6 months of

# PROCEDURE 34.5

## Performing a Reagent Strip Test

**Procedure Goal:** To perform chemical testing on urine specimens (This test is used to screen for the presence of leukocytes, nitrite, urobilinogen, protein, pH, blood, specific gravity, ketones, bilirubin, and glucose.)

### OSHA Guidelines

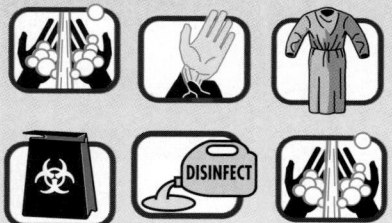

**Materials:** Urine specimen, laboratory report form, reagent strips, paper towel, timer

### Method:

1. Wash your hands and put on personal protective equipment.

2. Check the specimen for proper labeling and examine it to make sure that there is no visible contamination. Perform the test as soon as possible after collection. Refrigerate the specimen if testing will take place more than 1 hour later. Bring the refrigerated specimen back to room temperature prior to testing.

3. Check the expiration date on the reagent strip container and check the strip for damaged or discolored pads.

   *Rationale*

   To ensure the reagent strip is still valid

4. Swirl the specimen.

   *Rationale*

   To mix the specimen thoroughly

5. Dip a urine strip into the specimen, making sure each pad is completely covered. Briefly tap the

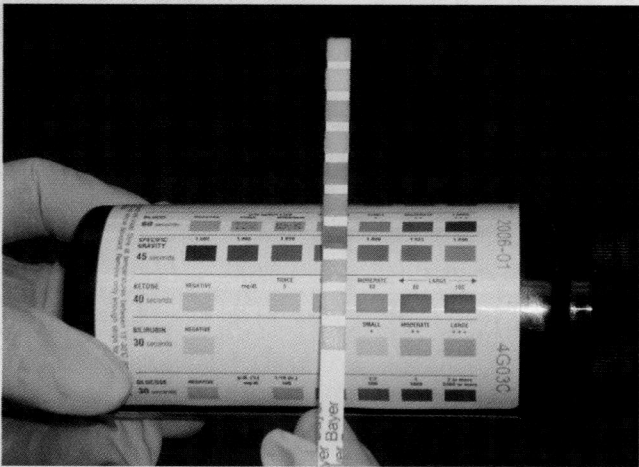

**Figure 34-7.** Read the reagent strip by the time indicated in the manufacturer's instructions.

strip sideways on a paper towel. *Do not blot* the test pads.

   *Rationale*

   Excess urine could migrate to the other pads and alter the test results

6. Read each test pad against the chart on the bottle at the designated time. Note: It is important to read each pad at the appropriate time. Most reagent strip results are invalid after 2 minutes (Figure 34-7).

   *Rationale*

   Test pads read at inappropriate times will yield inaccurate results

7. Record the values on the laboratory report form.

8. Discard the used disposable supplies.

9. Clean and disinfect the work area.

10. Remove your gloves and wash your hands.

11. Record the result in the patient's chart.

opening the container. Every time you open a new supply of reagents, run control samples to check for proper operation. Write the date opened on the bottle.

Although the process is essentially the same for all reagent strip tests, there are variations in time intervals before reading results. Some reagent strips are designed to test for several substances at once. The basic procedure

for using reagent strips for chemical tests can be found in Procedure 34–5.

***Ketone Bodies.*** Ketone bodies (or ketones) are intermediary products of fat and protein metabolism in the body. They include acetone, acetoacetic acid, and beta-hydroxybutyric acid. Only the first two substances can be determined by a reagent strip test. Normally, there are no ketones in urine. The presence of ketones in the urine may indicate that a patient is following a low-carbohydrate diet, or it may indicate that the patient has a condition such as starvation, excessive vomiting, or diabetes mellitus. Because ketones evaporate at room temperature, be sure to test urine immediately or cover the specimen tightly and refrigerate it until testing can be done.

*pH.* **Urinary pH** is a measure of the degree of acidity or alkalinity of the urine. Determination of pH can provide information about a patient's metabolic status, diet, medications being taken, and several conditions. The normal pH of freshly voided urine ranges from 5.0 to 8.0. The average urine pH is 6.0, which is slightly acidic. A pH of 7.0 is neutral, a lower pH is acidic, and a higher one is alkaline. Patients with alkaline urine may have such conditions as urinary tract infection or metabolic or respiratory alkalosis. Those with acidic urine may have such conditions as phenylketonuria or acidosis. Reagent strip, or dipstick, tests on both urine and blood are used to measure pH in the body. (See Chapter 35 for information on blood tests for pH.)

*Blood.* A patient who has blood in the urine may be menstruating, have a urinary tract infection, or have trauma or bleeding in the kidneys. To test for blood in urine, use a reagent strip that reacts with hemoglobin. There are two indicators on the strip. One is for nonhemolyzed blood, the other for hemolyzed blood.

Colors on the strip range from orange through green to dark blue and may indicate **hematuria** (the presence of blood in the urine) caused by cystitis; kidney stones; menstruation; or ureteral, bladder, or urethral irritation. The presence of free hemoglobin in the urine is known as **hemoglobinuria,** a rare condition caused by transfusion reactions, malaria, drug reactions, snakebites, or severe burns. Injured or damaged muscle tissue—such as occurs in crushing injuries, myocardial infarction, muscular dystrophy, or injuries during contact sports—can cause **myoglobinuria** (the presence of myoglobin in the urine). Reagent strip testing does not distinguish between these two conditions.

*Bilirubin and Urobilinogen.* When hemoglobin breaks down, it converts into conjugated bilirubin in the liver and then to urobilinogen in the intestines. Presence of the bile pigment bilirubin in the urine **(bilirubinuria)** is one of the first signs of liver disease or conditions that involve the liver. When bilirubin is present, urine turns yellow-brown to greenish orange. You usually use a reagent strip to test for bilirubin. If the reagent strip test is positive, a confirmatory test called an Ictotest® is usually performed. The Ictotest® is a reagent tablet test that is more sensitive than the reagent strip test.

Although **urobilinogen** is present in the urine in small amounts, elevated levels of this colorless compound formed in the intestines may indicate increased red blood cell destruction or liver disease. Lack of urobilinogen in the urine may suggest total bile duct obstruction, as a result of which urobilinogen is not formed in the intestines or reabsorbed in the circulation. To test for urobilinogen, you use reagent strips.

Testing for either bilirubin or urobilinogen must be performed on a fresh urine specimen. Bilirubin decomposes rapidly in bright light to form biliverdin, which is not detected by the reagent strip test for bilirubin. Urobilinogen breaks down to urobilin on standing.

*Glucose.* Glucose is present in patients with normal urine, but only in small quantities not detectable by the reagent strip test for glucose. **Glycosuria** (the presence of significant glucose in the urine) is common in patients with diabetes. Blood is more commonly tested for glucose than urine is, because reagent strip tests may show false-negative results when used for testing urine.

*Protein.* Although a small amount of protein is excreted in the urine every day, an excess of protein in the urine **(proteinuria)** usually indicates renal disease. Proteinuria is also common in pregnant patients or after heavy exercise.

*Nitrite.* The presence of nitrite in the urine suggests a bacterial infection of the urinary tract. The test is not definitive, however, because some bacteria cannot convert nitrate to nitrite. Also, if an insufficient number of bacteria are present in the urine or if the urine has not incubated long enough in the bladder for a reaction to take place, a negative nitrite test can occur. The best urine specimen to test for nitrites is the first morning specimen.

When testing for urinary nitrite, you must test the urine immediately or refrigerate the specimen. Bacteria can multiply in a specimen that is allowed to sit at room temperature, thus causing a false-positive test result. Bacteria can also further metabolize the nitrite already produced, thus causing a false-negative result.

*Leukocytes.* Leukocytes appear in the urine in urinary tract or renal infections. Use strip tests for leukocyte esterase, a chemical seen when leukocytes are present, to test for leukocytes.

**Other Types of Chemical Testing.** There are other types of chemical tests that may be performed on urine specimens. They generally involve testing for electrolytes and osmolality. Because these tests are performed in an outside laboratory rather than in a physician's office laboratory, you do not need to know the steps in each procedure.

*Phenylketones.* The presence of phenylketones in a patient's urine indicates **phenylketonuria (PKU),** a genetically inherited disorder in which the body cannot properly metabolize the nutrient phenylalanine. This disorder causes phenylketones to accumulate in the bloodstream, resulting in mental retardation. PKU can be treated successfully by limiting the dietary intake of phenylalanine, which makes up 5% of all natural protein, from early infancy. Although urine can be tested for the presence of phenylketones, blood testing is routine for newborns before discharge, at least 24 hours after birth.

*Pregnancy Tests.* Pregnancy testing is based on detecting the hormone secreted by the placenta. The name of the hormone is human chorionic gonadotropin, or HCG. The levels of HCG vary throughout pregnancy: they usually peak at about 8 weeks; they drop to lower levels in the second trimester; and then detectable levels recur in the last trimester. Many commercial pregnancy tests are manufactured for use in the clinical setting and at home. These tests are sensitive, easy to perform and interpret, and give quick results. Most tests are now designed as an **enzyme immunoassay (EIA)** test, which always involves an antigen, an antibody specific for the antigen, and a second antibody conjugated to an enzyme. Newer technologies have been developed that are called membrane EIAs; in these tests, most of the reagents are incorporated into an absorbent membrane in a plastic case. Using either urine or serum, a sample is added through a chamber window where it migrates through the membrane and combines with the reagents to produce a reaction. Although the technology used in the design of these tests is quite complex, the actual test itself is easy to set up and interpret (Procedure 34-6). The tests are all designed with a control feature incorporated into the reagent pack for quality assurance of the test results.

***Urine Tests for the Presence of STDs.*** In response to increasing numbers of sexually transmitted diseases, the CDC recommends that all sexually active females

# PROCEDURE 34.6

## Pregnancy Testing Using the EIA Method

**Procedure Goal:** To perform the enzyme immunoassay in order to detect HCG in the urine (or serum) and to interpret results as positive or negative

**OSHA Guidelines**

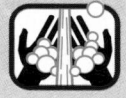 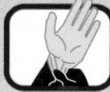 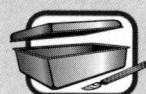
 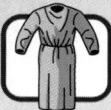

**Materials:** Gloves, urine specimen, timing device, surface disinfectant, pregnancy control solutions, pregnancy test kits

**Method:**

1. Wash your hands and put on exam gloves.
2. Gather the necessary supplies and equipment.
3. If materials have been refrigerated, allow all materials to reach room temperature prior to conducting the testing.
4. Label the test chamber with the patient's name or identification number; label one test chamber for a negative and positive control.
5. Apply the urine (or serum) to the test chamber per the manufacturer's instructions.

*Rationale*

Different tests may have slightly different instructions.

6. At the appropriate time, read and interpret the results (Figure 34-8).

*Rationale*

Most tests are invalid after 10 minutes.

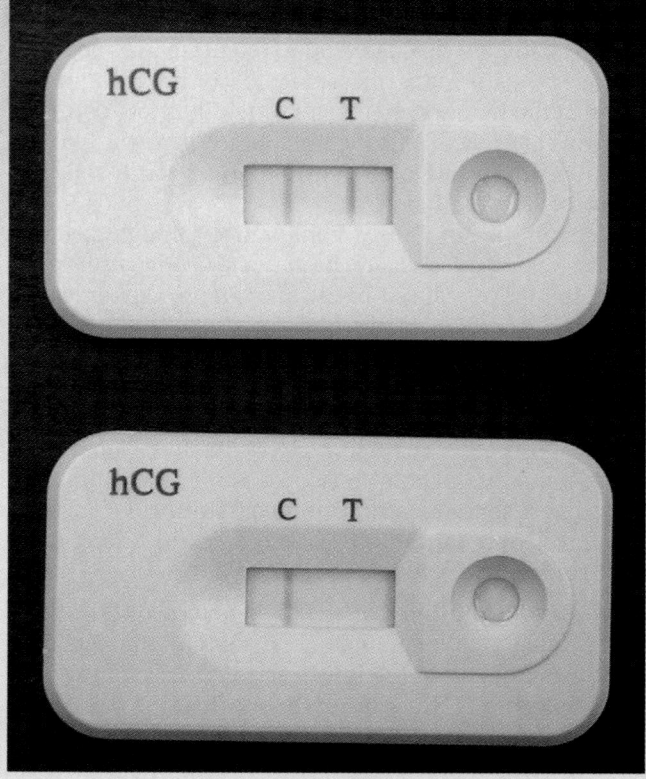

**Figure 34-8.** A positive pregnancy test (top) and a negative control (bottom).

7. Document the patient's results in the chart; document the quality control results in the appropriate log book.
8. Dispose of used reagents in a biohazard container.
9. Clean the work area with a disinfectant solution.
10. Wash your hands.

between the ages of 15 and 25 be screened annually for chlamydia. To accomplish this, several tests called nucleic acid amplification tests (NAATs) have recently been developed. These tests utilize urine samples to detect the presence of nucleic acid. Patients infected with either *Chlamydia trachomatis* or *Neisseria gonorrhoeae* will have nucleic acid in their urine. By amplifying nucleic acids specific to chlamydia and gonorrhea, the test can detect the presence of very small numbers of bacteria.

These tests have several advantages:

- Sample collection is noninvasive and easily collected.
- The tests are highly specific.
- The tests are highly sensitive. As little as one copy of bacterial nucleic acids can be detected in a urine specimen.
- Organisms do not have to be living to be detected.
- The tests are good screening tools for asymptomatic patients.

The tests also have some disadvantages:

- The tests are expensive.
- No living organisms remain for use in a follow-up culture. Therefore, positive tests must be confirmed by culture from an endocervical or urethral swab.

## Microscopic Examination of Urine Specimens

A microscopic examination of a urine sediment may be performed to view elements only visible with a microscope. You will use a centrifuge to obtain sediment for analysis. A centrifuge spins test tubes containing fluid at speeds that cause heavier substances in the fluid to settle to the bottom of the tubes.

During microscopic examination, elements that are categorized and counted include the cells, casts, crystals, yeast, bacteria, and parasites that form sediment (precipitate) after urine is centrifuged. You may use the KOVA System®, manufactured by Hycor Biomedical, Irvine, California, to prepare urine sediment for microscopic examination. When you use the KOVA System®, the sediment is evenly distributed to four calibrated chambers before the microscopic elements are counted. Procedure 34-7 describes how to process a urine specimen for microscopic examination of sediment.

**Cells.** High-power magnification is used to classify and count cells. Three types of cells are found in urine (Figure 34-9):

- Epithelial cells
- White blood cells
- Red blood cells

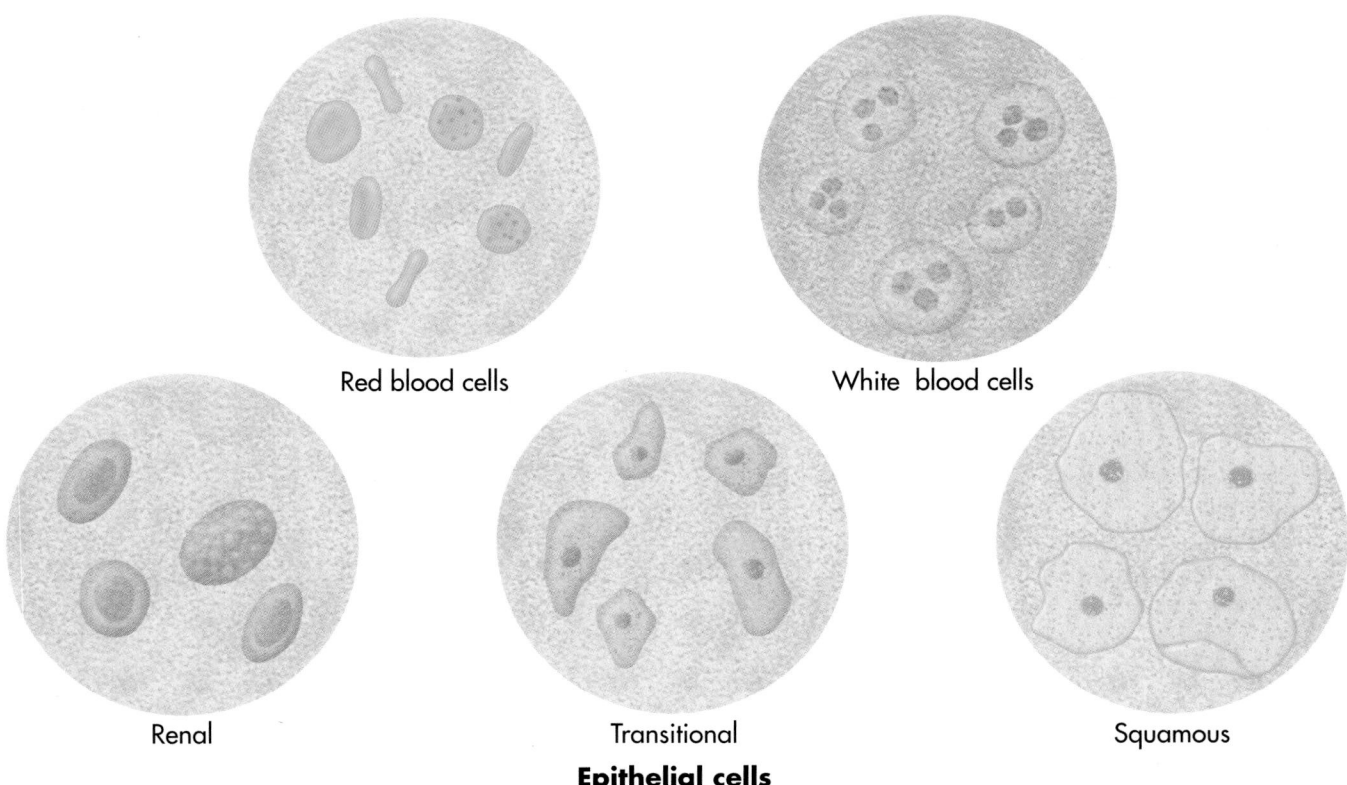

Red blood cells

White blood cells

Renal

Transitional

Squamous

**Epithelial cells**

**Figure 34-9.** The number and types of cells found in urine constitute important diagnostic information about a patient's condition.

# Processing a Urine Specimen for Microscopic Examination of Sediment

**Objective:** To prepare a slide for microscopic examination of urine sediment

**OSHA Guidelines**

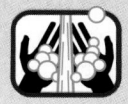 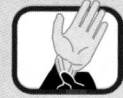 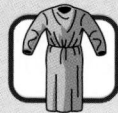
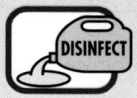 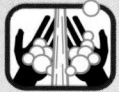

**Materials:** Fresh urine specimen, two glass or plastic test tubes, water, centrifuge, tapered pipette, glass slide with coverslip, microscope with light source, laboratory report form

**Method:**

1. Wash your hands and put on exam gloves.

2. Check the specimen for proper labeling, and examine it to make sure that there is no visible contamination and that no more than 1 hour has passed since collection (or since the specimen has been removed from the refrigerator and brought back to room temperature).

3. Swirl the urine specimen.

   *Rationale*

   To mix the specimen thoroughly

4. Pour approximately 10 mL of urine into one test tube and 10 mL of plain water into the balance tube (Figure 34-10).

5. Balance the centrifuge by placing the test tubes on either side (Figure 34-11).

   *Rationale*

   An unbalanced tube could "walk" or wobble off the table

6. Make sure the lid is secure, and set the centrifuge timer (Figure 34-12) for 5 to 10 minutes.

   *Rationale*

   Spinning the urine will force the solids (cells, casts, and crystals) to the bottom of the tube

7. Set the speed as prescribed by your office's protocol (usually 1500 to 2000 revolutions per minute) and start the centrifuge.

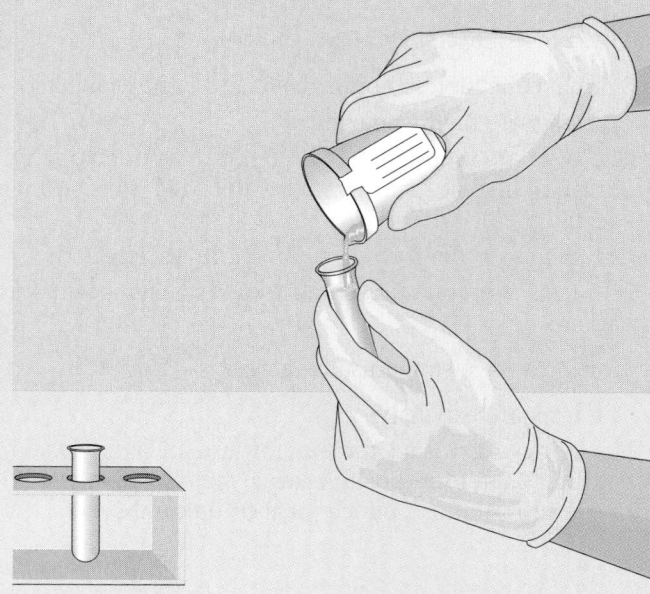

**Figure 34-10.** Fill one test tube with approximately 10 mL of urine and the other with 10 mL of water.

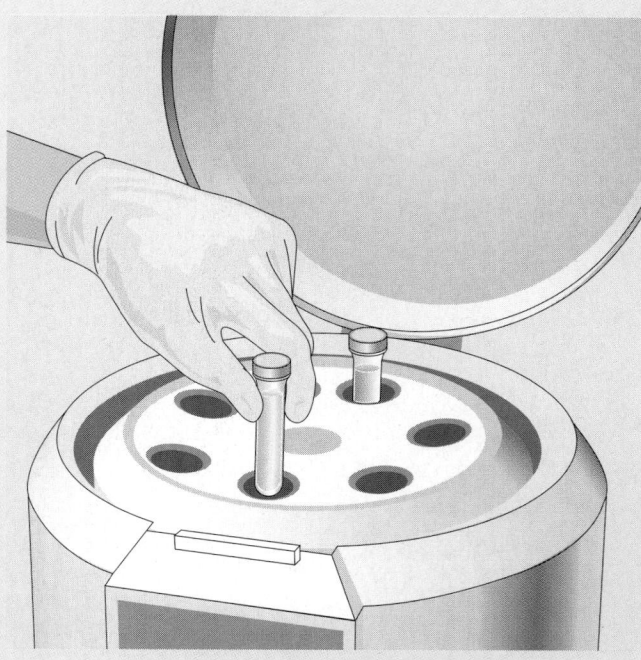

**Figure 34-11.** The centrifuge must be balanced by placing one test tube on each side.

*continued* ⟶

## Processing a Urine Specimen for Microscopic Examination of Sediment (concluded)

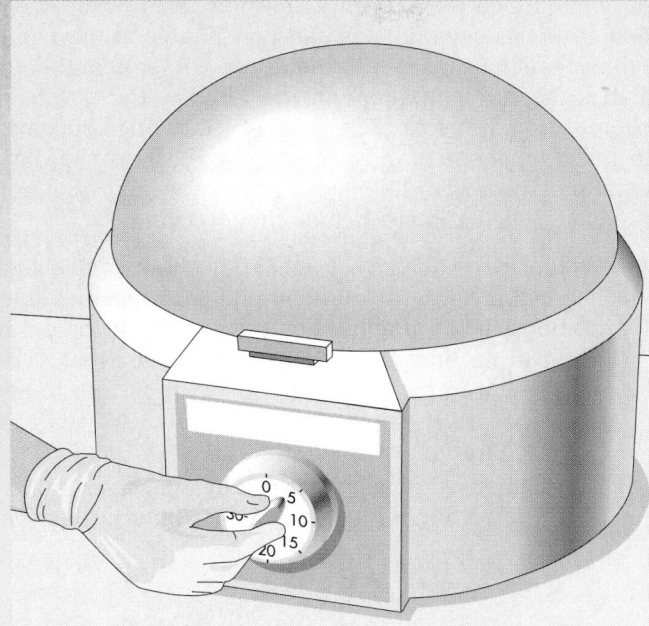

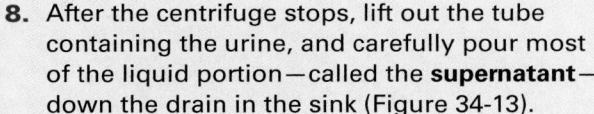

**Figure 34-12.** Set the centrifuge timer for 3 to 5 minutes.

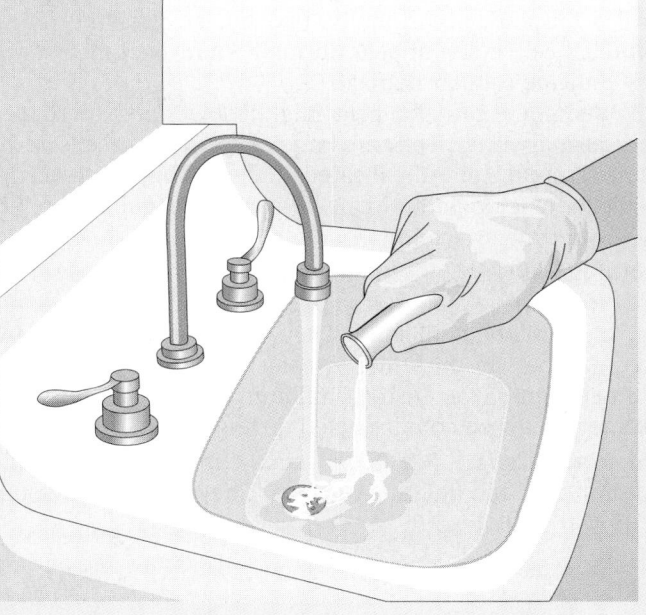

**Figure 34-13.** Make sure you do not lose any sediment when you pour off the urine.

8. After the centrifuge stops, lift out the tube containing the urine, and carefully pour most of the liquid portion—called the **supernatant**—down the drain in the sink (Figure 34-13).

9. A few drops of urine should remain in the bottom of the test tube with any sediment. Mix the urine and sediment together by gently tapping the bottom of the tube on the palm of your hand.

### Rationale
To resuspend the solid material

10. Use the tapered pipette to obtain a drop or two of urine sediment. Place the drops in the center of a clean glass slide.

11. Place the coverslip over the specimen, allow it to settle, and place it on the stage of the microscope.

12. Correctly focus the microscope as directed in Procedure 32-1.

*Note:* Most medical assistants are trained to perform this procedure only up to this point. After this, the physician usually examines the specimen. You may, however, be asked to clean the items after the

examination is completed. The remaining steps are provided for your information.

13. Use a dim light and view the slide under the low-power objective. Observe the slide for casts (found mainly around the edges of the coverslip) and count the casts viewed.

14. Switch to the high-power objective. Identify the casts. Identify any epithelial cells, mucus, protozoa, yeasts, and crystals. Adjust the slide position so that you can view and count the cells, protozoa, yeasts, and crystals from at least ten different fields. Turn off the light after the examination is completed.

15. Record the observations on the laboratory report form.

16. Properly dispose of used disposable materials.

17. Sanitize and disinfect nondisposable items; put them away when they are dry.

18. Clean and disinfect the work area.

19. Remove the gloves and wash your hands.

20. Record the observations in the patient's chart.

***Epithelial Cells.*** Epithelial cells are classified as renal, transitional, or squamous. Renal epithelial cells can be round to oval and have a large, oval, and sometimes eccentric nucleus. Although a few of these cells appear normally in urine, several may indicate tubular damage in the kidneys.

Transitional epithelial cells line the urinary tract from the renal pelvis (the beginning of the ureter) to the upper portion of the urethra. They can be round to oval and may have a tail and, occasionally, two nuclei. Like the renal epithelial cell, a few appear normally in urine, but several may indicate tubular damage.

Squamous epithelial cells line the lower portion of the genitourinary tract. They are large, flat, irregular cells with a small, round, centrally located nucleus. They often occur in sheets or clumps and can be easily recognized under low-power magnification.

***White Blood Cells.*** White blood cells are larger than red blood cells, have a granular appearance, and usually contain a multilobed nucleus. They are typically found in large numbers in the urine (greater than the normal zero to 8 per high-power field) if inflammation is present or if the specimen was contaminated during collection.

***Red Blood Cells.*** Red blood cells can be pale, round, nongranular, and flat or biconcave. They have no nucleus and enter the urinary tract during inflammation or injury. From zero to three red blood cells per high-power field in urine is normal. Numerous red blood cells may indicate a variety of problems, however, including urinary infection, obstruction, inflammation, trauma, or tumor.

**Casts.** **Casts,** which are cylinder-shaped elements with flat or rounded ends, form when protein from the breakdown of cells accumulates and precipitates in the kidney tubules and is washed into the urine. The protein then assumes the size and shape of the tubules. Casts differ in composition and size (Figure 34-14). Classified according to their appearance and composition, casts can indicate renal pathologic conditions or can be caused by strenuous exercise. Types of casts include the following:

- Hyaline casts, which are pale, transparent, and shaped like cylinders, with rounded ends and parallel sides. Composed of protein, they form because of diminished urine flow through individual nephrons. They are present in patients with kidney disease or in people who have exercised strenuously. A few casts observed in the urine is normal.

- Granular casts, which resemble hyaline casts and can also result from kidney disease or strenuous exercise.

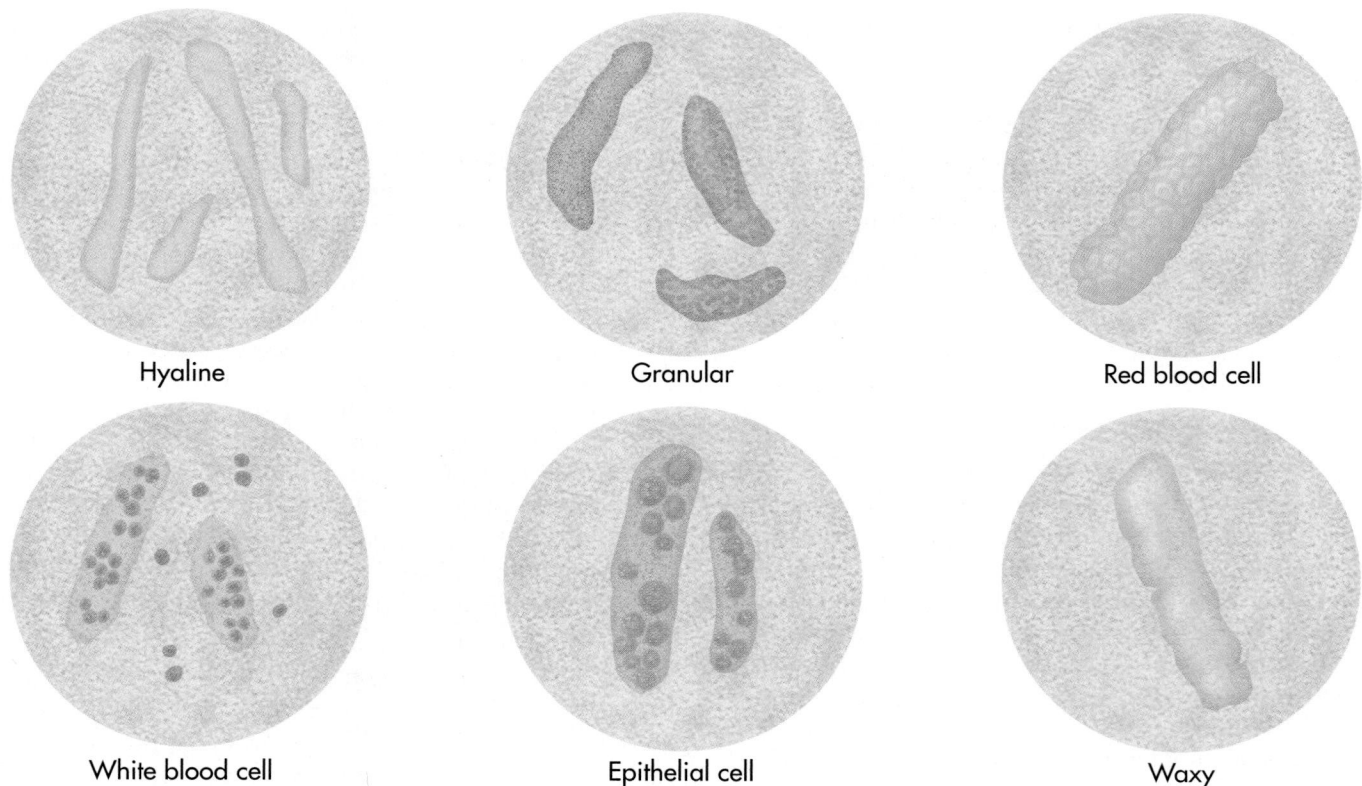

| Hyaline | Granular | Red blood cell |
| White blood cell | Epithelial cell | Waxy |

**Figure 34-14.** Casts, which are shaped like cylinders with flat or rounded ends, are formed when protein accumulates in the kidney tubules and is washed into the urine.

## Preventing Urinary Tract Infections

Millions of people are treated each year for urinary tract infections (UTIs). Women are more likely to develop UTIs than men. These infections occur most often when microorganisms from the colon or vagina enter the urethra. Once the microorganisms enter the urethra, they begin to multiply and can enter the bladder, ureters, and kidneys if left untreated.

Certain medical conditions can increase the risk of getting a UTI, including an enlarged prostate, diabetes, or kidney stones. Individuals who require frequent or permanent catheterization also have an increased risk of UTIs.

Sometimes individuals with UTIs have no symptoms. More often, the symptoms include frequent urinary urgency and frequency and pain and burning during urination. Women may feel a sensation of pressure above the pubic bone. Men occasionally have a full feeling in the rectum. Patients may notice that their urine is cloudy or blood-tinged.

There are some steps women can take to help prevent UTIs. These include:

- Drinking plenty of water
- Avoiding holding urine
- Wiping from front to back after a bowel movement
- Avoiding baths, and showering only
- Cleansing the genital area prior to and after intercourse
- Voiding immediately after intercourse
- Avoiding scented douches and feminine sprays
- Wearing underwear with a cotton crotch

---

The granules are believed to come from degeneration of cellular inclusions.

- Red blood cell casts, which always indicate an abnormality and are hyaline casts with embedded red cells. Because of the red blood cells, these casts sometimes appear brown.
- White blood cell casts, which are hyaline casts with leukocytes. These casts typically have a multilobed nucleus and may indicate pyelonephritis, which is an inflammation of the kidney and renal pelvis.
- Epithelial cell casts, which contain embedded renal tubular epithelial cells and indicate excessive kidney damage. Causes include shock, renal ischemia, heavy-metal poisoning, certain allergic reactions, and nephrotoxic drugs. These casts are often confused with white blood cell casts.
- Waxy casts, which are rare, yellow, glassy, brittle, smooth, and homogeneous structures with cracks or fissures and squared or broken ends. These casts occur with severe renal disease.

**Crystals.** **Crystals**, naturally produced solids of definite form, are commonly seen in urine specimens, especially those permitted to cool. They usually do not indicate a significant disorder, except when found in large numbers in patients with kidney stones and in a few pathologic conditions (such as hypercalcemia and some inborn errors of metabolism). Figure 34-15 shows common crystals found in urine specimens. Because different substances tend to crystallize in urine that is acidic and in urine that is alkaline, or basic, it is important to determine the pH of a patient's urine before you try to identify any crystals that are present.

**Yeast Cells.** Yeast cells, which are usually oval and may show budding, may be confused with red blood cells. Yeast cells in urine sediment are associated with genitourinary tract infection, external genitalia contamination, vaginitis, urethritis, and prostatitis. These cells are also commonly seen in the urine of patients with diabetes.

**Bacteria.** Although a few bacteria are normally found in urine, urinary tract infection may be indicated if the urine has bacteria along with a putrid odor and numerous white blood cells.

Tips for preventing bladder infections are found in Educating the Patient: Preventing Urinary Tract Infections. Bacteria under high-power magnification appear rod- or cocci-shaped.

**Parasites.** The presence of parasites in sediment may signal genitourinary tract infection or external genitalia contamination. The most common urinary parasite, *Trichomonas vaginalis* (a pear-shaped protozoan with four flagella), is typically found in vaginal disorders but may also appear in males. When a urine specimen is cooled, *Trichomonas* organisms die.

# Crystals found in acid urine

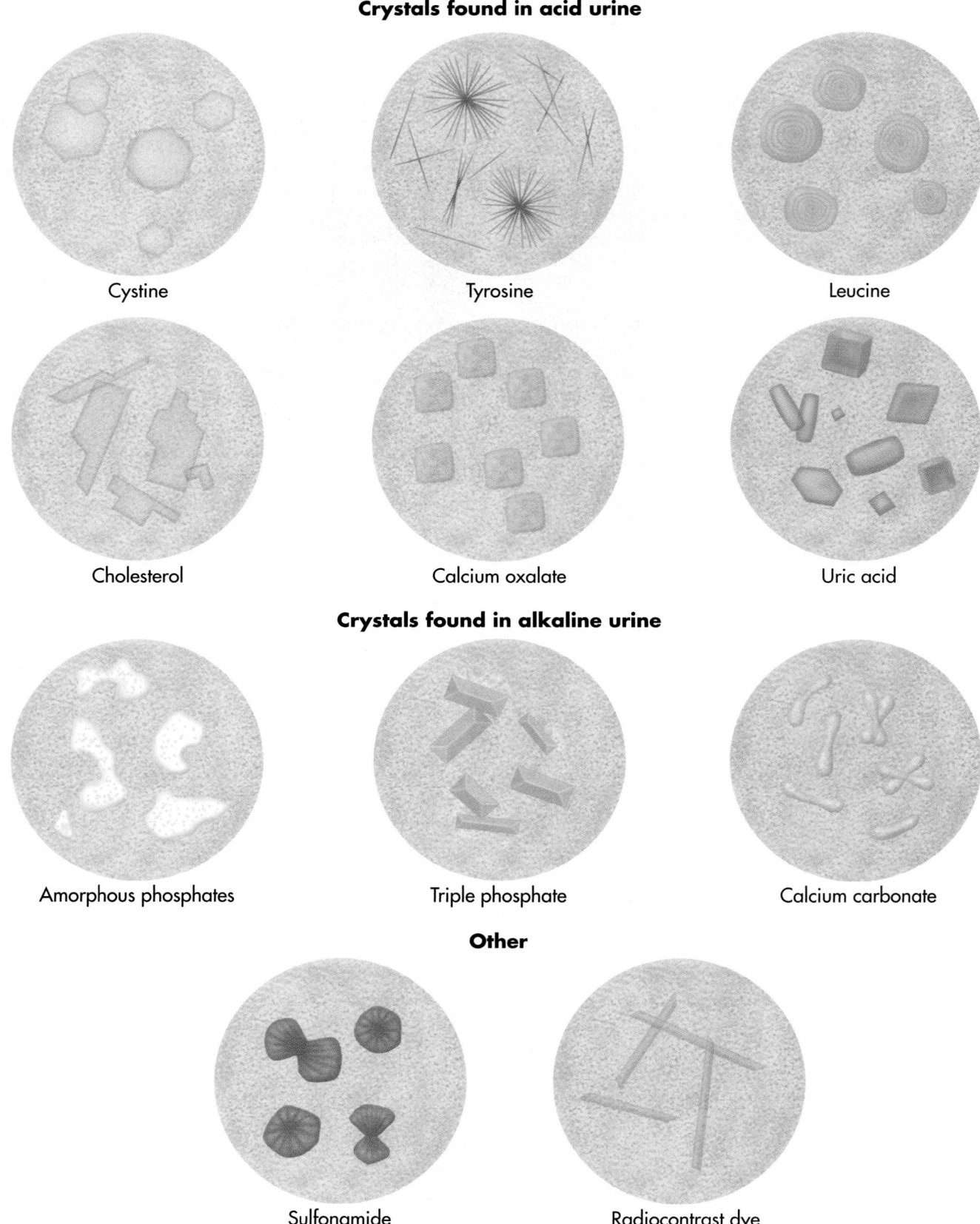

Cystine

Tyrosine

Leucine

Cholesterol

Calcium oxalate

Uric acid

# Crystals found in alkaline urine

Amorphous phosphates

Triple phosphate

Calcium carbonate

# Other

Sulfonamide

Radiocontrast dye

**Figure 34-15.**  You should be able to identify common crystals in urine and what they mean.

# Summary

The volume and physical, chemical, and microscopic characteristics of urine provide a great deal of information about a patient's health. Although invasive collection methods are sometimes necessary, routine urine specimens can be obtained by noninvasive, painless means. Urinalysis is the most common diagnostic test performed in doctors' offices.

You will have a substantial role in collecting, processing, and testing urine specimens. You will need to understand the urinary tract system and the basic characteristics of urine, including how it is formed, its physical composition, its chemical properties, and its microscopic characteristics.

Assisting patients and instructing them in the procedures required to collect different types of specimens are important aspects of your job. You must understand the purposes and procedures for collecting random specimens, first morning specimens, clean-catch midstream specimens, timed specimens, and 24-hour specimens. Throughout all collecting and processing procedures, you must practice quality assurance and employ precautions to avoid spreading disease-causing microorganisms.

When obtaining and processing specimens, you need to follow general guidelines as well as take into account special considerations for specific groups of patients. You are responsible for ensuring that specimens are preserved and stored so that they are not contaminated or otherwise altered.

You may perform some tests on urine and prepare urine specimens for evaluation by the doctor. In either case you must be able to distinguish between normal and abnormal findings concerning the physical, chemical, and microscopic characteristics of urine.

Urinalysis provides important information to the doctor. You play a significant role in seeing that the specimen has been properly collected, processed, and tested, so that the information obtained from the analysis is useful and accurate.

# REVIEW

CHAPTER **34**

## CASE STUDY QUESTIONS

Now that you have completed this chapter, review the case study at the beginning of the chapter and answer the following questions:

1. What is the maximum length of time that a urine specimen should be left at room temperature? If analysis cannot be performed within that maximum length of time, how should the specimen be handled?
2. An ammonia-like or foul odor associated with a specimen ordinarily indicates what condition or disease?
3. Does the chemical analysis confirm your suspicion associated with the odor?
4. Given the circumstances, can you trust the results on this specimen?

## Discussion Questions

1. In the collection of a clean-catch midstream urine specimen, what purposes are served by the external cleansing of the genitalia and the voiding the first part of the specimen?
2. List the physical characteristics of a urine sample that should be observed during routine urinalysis. What would you look for in each characteristic?
3. When collecting a urine specimen for a drug screen, why is it important both to tape faucets in the *off* position so that they cannot be turned on and also to put bluing agent in the toilet?

## Critical Thinking Questions

1. Why is it important to ask a patient about urinary incontinence when giving instructions for collecting a 24-hour urine specimen?
2. A 26-year-old woman provides a random urine specimen that is reddish-colored, is turbid in appearance, and shows large blood on the reagent strip. What question(s) might you ask this patient that could provide significant information about these test results?
3. What types of casts may be seen in the microscopic examination of urine specimens, and what is their significance?

## Application Activities

1. Using a doll, demonstrate the correct method for applying a urine collection bag to a female infant.
2. Demonstrate the correct method for performing a reagent strip urinalysis.
3. Working with another student acting in the role of patient, explain the recommended procedure for collecting a 24-hour urine specimen. Ask appropriate questions to ensure that the "patient" understands the procedure. Then switch roles so that each student has the opportunity to play each role.

## Virtual Fieldtrip

*Visit the McGraw-Hill Higher Education Medical Assisting website at www.mhhe.com/medicalassisting3 to complete the following activity:*

Use the National Institutes of Health website, National Institute of Diabetes and Digestive and Kidney Diseases. Answer the following questions:

1. What type of information is available on this website?
2. How might the information be useful to you as a medical assistant?

Open the CD and complete this chapter's practice activities, play the games, listen to the key terms, and test yourself with the interactive review. Email, print, and/or save your results to document your proficiency.

# Collecting, Processing, and Testing Blood Specimens

## MEDICAL ASSISTING COMPETENCIES

**In preparation for the certification examination, you should know the following areas of competence:**

| COMPETENCY | CMA | RMA |
|---|---|---|
| **Clinical** | | |
| Apply principles of aseptic techniques and infection control, including hand washing | X | X |
| Dispose of biohazardous materials | X | X |
| Practice Standard Precautions | X | X |
| Perform venipuncture | X | X |
| Perform capillary puncture | X | X |
| Perform selected CLIA-waived tests (e.g., "kit tests") | X | X |
| Perform hematologic testing | X | X |
| Perform chemistry testing | X | X |
| Perform immunology testing | X | X |
| Screen and follow up on patient test results | X | X |
| **General/Legal/Professional** | | |
| Recognize and respond to verbal and nonverbal communications by being attentive and adapting communication to the recipient's level of understanding | X | X |
| Perform risk management procedures | | X |
| Instruct individuals according to their needs | X | X |
| Operate and maintain facilities, and perform routine maintenance of administrative and clinical equipment safely | X | X |
| Perform quality control procedures | X | X |
| Conduct work within scope of education, training, and ability | | X |
| Be impartial and show empathy when dealing with patients | | X |

## KEY TERMS

- agranular leukocyte
- B lymphocyte
- buffy coat
- capillary puncture
- erythrocyte sedimentation rate (ESR)
- formed elements
- granular leukocyte
- hematology
- hemolysis
- lancet
- micropipette
- morphology
- packed red blood cells
- phlebotomy
- plasma
- pyrogen
- serum
- T lymphocyte
- venipuncture
- whole blood

## CHAPTER OUTLINE

- The Role of the Medical Assistant
- The Functions and Composition of Blood
- Collecting Blood Specimens
- Responding to Patient Needs
- Performing Common Blood Tests

# LEARNING OUTCOMES

After completing Chapter 35, you will be able to:

**35.1** Discuss the composition and function of blood.

**35.2** Describe the process for collecting a blood specimen.

**35.3** Explain the importance of confirming patients' identities and correctly identifying blood samples.

**35.4** Describe how to perform venipuncture and capillary puncture procedures.

**35.5** Identify the equipment and supplies required for blood-drawing procedures.

**35.6** Discuss the correct procedures for disposing of waste generated during blood-drawing procedures.

**35.7** Discuss common fears and concerns of patients and how to ease these fears.

**35.8** Develop techniques for helping patients with special needs, including children, the elderly, patients at risk for uncontrolled bleeding, and difficult patients.

**35.9** Identify common blood tests and explain their purposes.

**35.10** Perform certain blood tests.

# Introduction

In many health-care settings, the medical assistant is responsible for collecting blood specimens from patients and even performs some waived testing. In order to properly collect the specimens, you will need to review the circulatory system and the function of blood. You will be introduced in this chapter to venipuncture and capillary collection procedures, and you will learn the appropriate supplies and equipment needed to perform these procedures. You will also learn techniques for dealing with different types of patients and how to efficiently and effectively obtain blood samples. Additionally, you will receive instruction on the performance and screening of common blood tests.

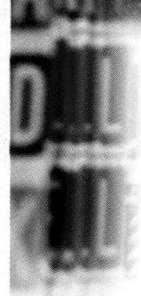

## CASE STUDY

A young man comes into the office to have a PT drawn. As you examine the antecubital fossa in his arm, you don't feel confident with the vein but you attempt the phlebotomy anyway, using an evacuated system. However, the vein collapses and you are unsuccessful in your attempt. As you turn away to gather your supplies to try the collection again, he informs you that he is bleeding rather heavily from the venipuncture site and requires your attention.

As you read this chapter, consider the following questions:

1. What and where is the antecubital fossa?
2. What is the principle of the evacuated collection system?
3. How should you attempt to collect the blood on the second try?
4. What type of a blood test is a PT?
5. What could have caused the extensive bleeding this patient experienced after the venipuncture?

# The Role of the Medical Assistant

The examination of blood can provide extensive information about a patient's condition. You may be asked to collect and process blood specimens for examination in your work as a medical assistant. A basic understanding of the anatomy and physiology of the circulatory system will help you properly perform these tasks. You will also need a working knowledge of the functions of blood and the kinds of cells that make up blood tissue.

You will use several techniques to obtain blood specimens. **Phlebotomy** is the insertion of a needle or cannula (small tube) into a vein for the purpose of withdrawing blood. Phlebotomists receive special training in phlebotomy; drawing blood is the main task in their work. Smaller blood samples may be obtained by using a small, disposable instrument to pierce surface capillaries. You must be able to perform such procedures accurately so that the sample is appropriate for the ordered tests. You must also be skilled in putting the patient at ease during this procedure. Your reassuring manner, ability to handle technical problems, and careful preparation for answering many kinds of questions will be important to your success in this area.

You must understand how to process blood specimens and conduct various blood tests, particularly if you work in a laboratory. Finally, to make sure the test results are handled efficiently and accurately, you must be able to complete the necessary paperwork. All these skills are essential, regardless of whether you collect blood specimens in a physician's office laboratory (POL), hospital, or laboratory drawing station.

# The Functions and Composition of Blood

The circulatory system transports blood throughout the body. The heart of the average adult pumps 8 to 12 pints of blood through more than 70,000 miles of veins, arteries, and capillaries each day. Blood is a complex and dynamic tissue that is essential to life and health.

**Hematology** is the study of blood, and hematologists study its functions and composition. Blood has many functions, all of which are important to the overall health of the body. Blood does all of the following:

- Distributes oxygen, nutrients, and hormones to body cells
- Eliminates waste products from body cells
- Attacks infecting organisms or pathogens
- Maintains acid-base balance
- Regulates body temperature

Blood is composed of four parts: **plasma** (the liquid in which other components are suspended), red blood cells, white blood cells, and platelets (thrombocytes). The plasma, or fluid part of blood, forms about 55% of blood volume.

The red blood cells, white blood cells, and platelets comprise the other 45% of blood volume, which is known as the **formed elements** (Figure 35-1). **Whole blood** is the total volume of plasma and formed elements.

## Red Blood Cells

Red blood cells (RBCs, or erythrocytes, play a vital role in internal respiration (the exchange of gases between blood and body cells). Blood transports oxygen to body cells in two forms. About 98% of the oxygen is bound to hemoglobin, the main component of erythrocytes. The other

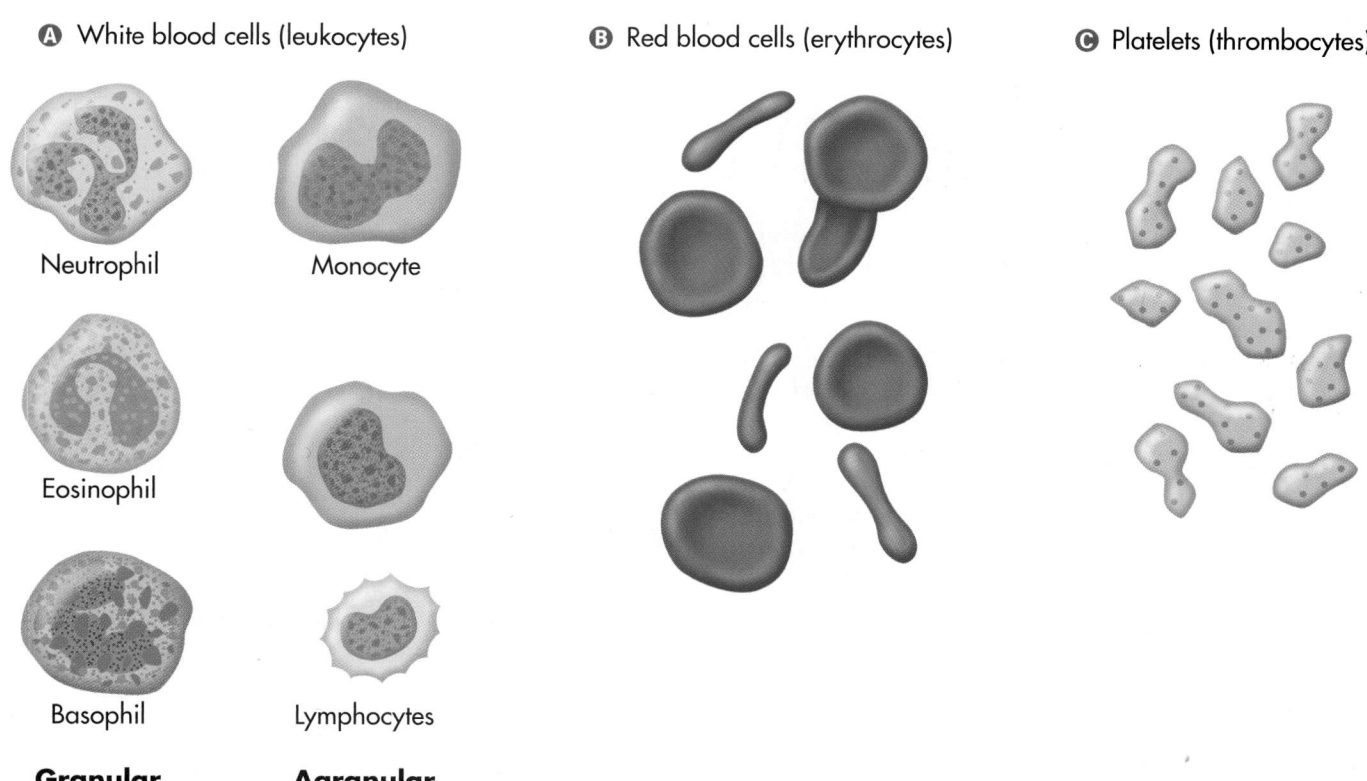

**(A)** White blood cells (leukocytes)

Neutrophil

Monocyte

Eosinophil

Basophil

Lymphocytes

**Granular**

**Agranular**

**(B)** Red blood cells (erythrocytes)

**(C)** Platelets (thrombocytes)

**Figure 35-1.** The formed elements of the blood are (A) white blood cells, (B) red blood cells, and (C) platelets.

2% to 3% of the oxygen is dissolved in plasma. In addition, erythrocytes transport carbon dioxide from body cells to the lungs, although most carbon dioxide is carried in plasma. Healthy RBCs are disk-shaped and have concave sides (biconcave). Hemoglobin, a protein that contains iron, gives RBCs their rusty red color. A mature erythrocyte contains no nucleus.

## White Blood Cells

White blood cells (WBCs), or leukocytes, protect the body against infection. (The function of WBCs as part of the body's defense against disease is discussed in Chapter 19.) Leukocytes are divided into two primary groups: **granular leukocytes** (also known as polymorphonuclear leukocytes) and **agranular leukocytes** (also known as mononuclear leukocytes). The division is based on the type of nucleus and cytoplasm in the cell. Each type of leukocyte performs a specific defense function, and the shape of each is suited to its role.

**Granular Leukocytes.** Granular, or polymorphonuclear, leukocytes have segmented nuclei and granulated cytoplasm. The three types of granular leukocytes are basophils, eosinophils, and neutrophils. Basophils produce the chemical histamine, which aids the body in controlling allergic reactions and other exaggerated immunologic responses. Eosinophils capture invading bacteria and antigen-antibody complexes through phagocytosis, or the engulfing of the invader. The number of eosinophils increases during allergic reactions and in response to parasitic infections. Neutrophils aid in phagocytosis by attacking bacterial invaders. They are also responsible for the release of **pyrogens,** which cause fever.

**Agranular Leukocytes.** Agranular leukocytes have solid nuclei and clear cytoplasm. The two types of agranular leukocytes are lymphocytes and monocytes. Lymphocytes are divided into two groups: B lymphocytes and T lymphocytes. **B lymphocytes** produce antibodies to combat specific pathogens. **T lymphocytes** regulate immunologic response. T lymphocytes are further classified as helper T cells and suppressor T cells. T cells are the cells attacked by human immunodeficiency virus (HIV), the virus that causes acquired immunodeficiency syndrome (AIDS). Monocytes are large WBCs with oval or horseshoe-shaped nuclei. They also defend the body by phagocytosis, recognizing and destroying foreign organisms and particles. Monocytes have a unique ability to pass through capillary walls into the body's tissues, where they perform phagocytosis.

## Platelets

Platelets, or thrombocytes, are fragments of cytoplasm (the part of the cell that surrounds the nucleus) of megakarocytes. Thrombocytes are smaller than either RBCs or WBCs. They are irregular in shape and have no nucleus. These cell fragments are crucial to clot formation.

## Plasma and Serum

Plasma is a clear, yellow liquid in which the formed elements of blood are suspended. Plasma is nearly 90% water; it also contains about 9% protein and 1% other substances in suspension (Figure 35-2). These other substances include carbohydrates, fats, gases, mineral salts, protective substances, and waste products.

**Serum** is the clear, yellow liquid that remains after a blood clot forms. It differs from plasma in that it does not contain fibrinogen, a protein involved in clotting. The fibrinogen converts into fibrin (a sticky protein) and traps formed elements of the blood in a clot. The process of clotting is called coagulation.

## Blood Types or Groups

An individual's RBCs may carry one or both of two major antigens on their surface. These antigens are known as A and B. The presence or absence of these antigens determines the blood type or group to which that person's blood belongs. Blood that contains neither A nor B antigen is designated O.

In addition to antigens, an individual's blood may contain certain antibodies. Blood that carries only the A antigen contains anti-B antibodies, and blood that carries only the B antigen contains anti-A antibodies. Blood that carries neither antigen contains both anti-A and anti-B antibodies, whereas blood that carries both antigens contains neither anti-A nor anti-B antibodies.

Blood is carefully matched before a blood transfusion. If a patient is given incompatible blood, the antibodies in the patient's blood will combine with the antigens in the transfused blood. This reaction leads to clumping of the RBCs and possible **hemolysis** (the rupturing of RBCs, which releases hemoglobin). The released hemoglobin can block the renal tubules and cause kidney failure and death.

# Collecting Blood Specimens

There is a standard process for drawing blood specimens. Following these steps will enable you to perform the procedure smoothly, accurately, and safely and ensure that documentation is completed properly.

## Reading and Interpreting the Test Order

The first steps in preparing to draw blood for testing are to review the written testing request and to assemble the equipment and supplies. The patient should arrive with a laboratory request form if you are working in a physician's office laboratory or a laboratory drawing station.

## Phlebotomist

*To gain medical assistant credentials, you must fulfill the requirements of either the American Association of Medical Assistants (for a Certified Medical Assistant) or the American Medical Technologists (for a Registered Medical Assistant). After obtaining your medical assistant certification or registration, you may wish to acquire additional skills in specialty areas through course work or on-the-job training. Although this course work or training may not lead to an additional certification or degree, it will enable you to expand your role in the medical office and advance your career as the demand for skilled health professionals increases.*

### Skills and Duties

Traditionally, a phlebotomist's job has been to draw blood from patients for analysis. Today, however, phlebotomists perform many additional duties. Many phlebotomists now perform simple tests on blood samples at the patient's hospital bedside or in close proximity to the patient. This "point of care" testing speeds physician diagnoses, often reducing the length of a patient's stay in the hospital.

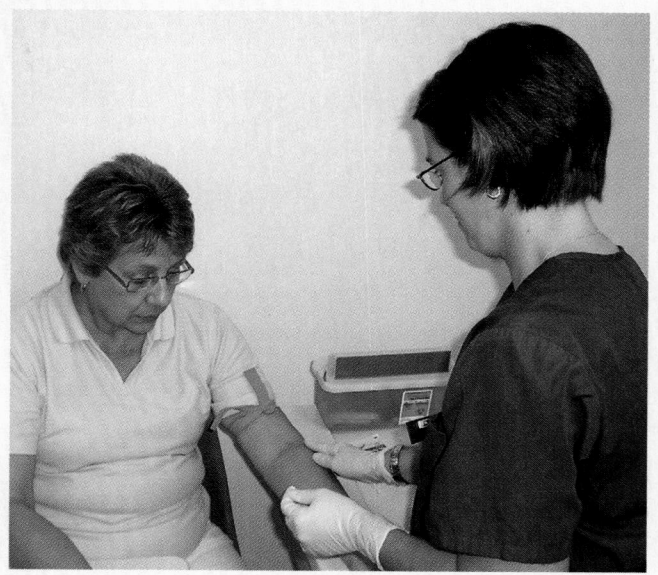

Other phlebotomists are trained to perform patient care functions, which differ from hospital to hospital. For example, they may run electrocardiogram equipment, change beds, deliver trays, or transport patients. Although phlebotomists in the past worked primarily in the hospital laboratory, today's phlebotomists work closely with the nursing department and have more direct contact with patients.

Blood collection remains the mainstay of a phlebotomist's job. As part of this process, a phlebotomist performs administrative duties such as documenting the collected blood samples and labeling specimens. A phlebotomist may also administer a health-related questionnaire to the patient if one is required by the physician or an insurance company.

### Workplace Settings

Most phlebotomists work in a hospital setting. Others are employed in laboratories, physicians' offices, and health departments. Some phlebotomists work with homebound individuals in nursing homes or private residences.

The job market for phlebotomists is good, provided that they are cross-trained in other specialties. Most institutions prefer phlebotomists who have additional training in areas such as performing blood tests.

### Education

Most states require phlebotomists to be certified. The American Society of Phlebotomy Technicians (ASPT) is one of the bodies that provides certification.

To take the ASPT's national phlebotomy examination, you must either have 6 months of full-time work experience (or 1 year of part-time work experience), or graduate from an accredited phlebotomy training program. A high school diploma or general equivalency diploma (GED) is needed to enroll in such a program. To receive full certification, candidates must have at least 100 successful, documented vein punctures and 25 successful, documented skin punctures.

### Where to Go for More Information

American Society for Clinical Pathologists
33 West Monroe, Suite 1600
Chicago, IL 60603
(800)267-2727

American Society of Phlebotomy Technicians
P.O. Box 1831
Hickory, NC 28603
(828)294-0078

National Phlebotomy Association
1901 Brightseat Road
Landover, MD 20785
(866)329-9108

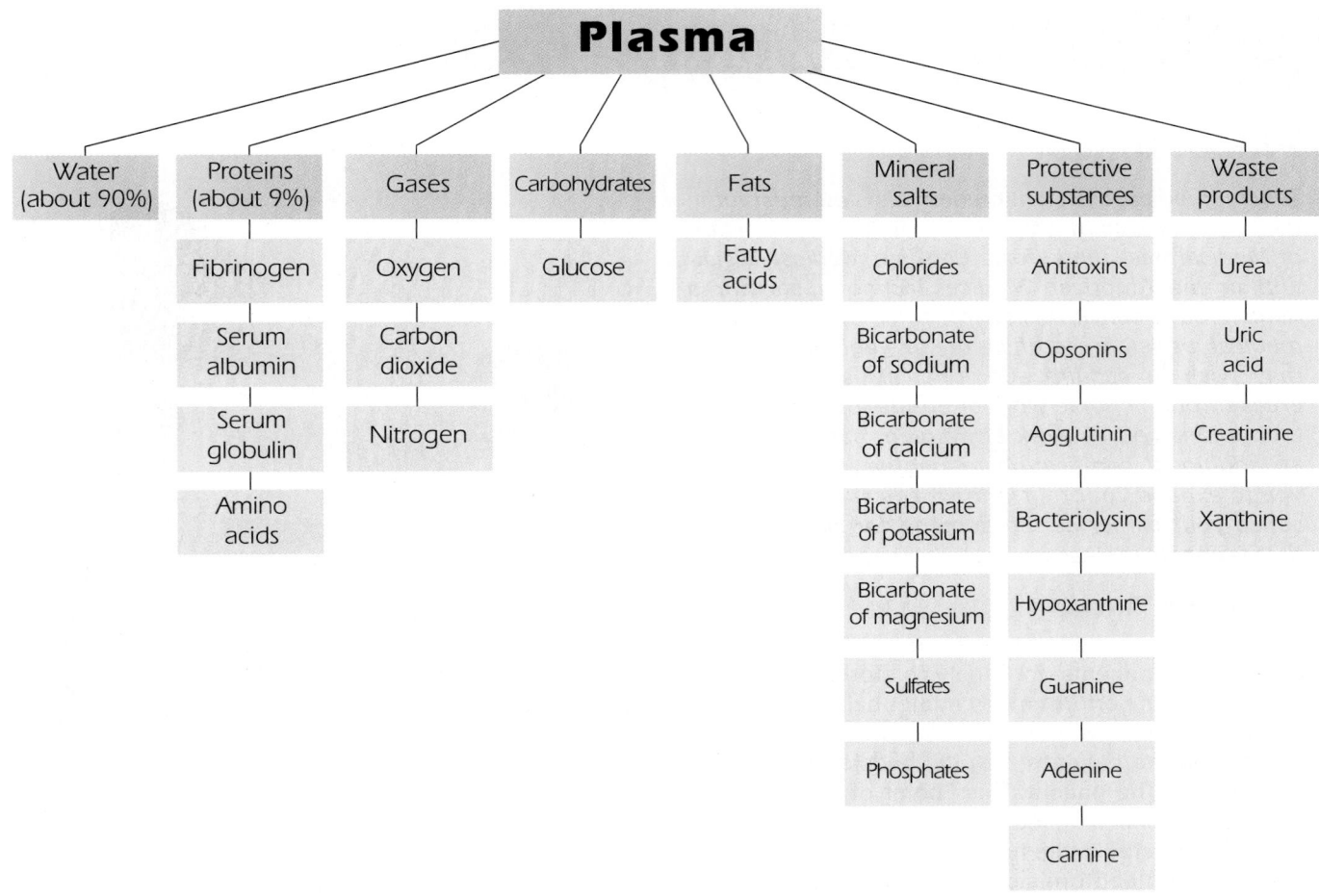

**Figure 35-2.** A wide variety of substances account for about 10% of plasma by volume. The remainder is water.

**Reviewing the Test Order.** It is essential to first review the patient's blood-collection order to determine what tests will be run. Many tests require expedited or special handling to ensure accurate results.

Your office will have specific collection procedures for each type of test. If you have any questions about these procedures, ask your supervisor. If you will be sending the blood specimen to a reference laboratory for testing, make sure you know its requirements. The cost of re-processing a test far surpasses the extra time needed to be sure of the process requirements.

When reviewing the test order, you will need to know the meaning of certain abbreviations. Many abbreviations used in laboratory work and their meanings are presented in Table 35-1. If you are ever in doubt or if the resources in your office or laboratory do not provide the answers you need, ask the doctor or your supervisor.

**Assembling the Equipment and Supplies.** Specific blood-drawing equipment and collection devices vary with the type of test. Make sure you have the appropriate equipment to collect all necessary samples if more than one test is ordered. All specimen-collection tubes, slides, and other containers should be labeled immediately after

collection with the patient's name, the date and time of collection, the initials of the person collecting the specimen, and other information as required by the test procedure or your office. Some offices use an identification code for each patient.

Alcohol and cotton balls or alcohol wipes, sterile gauze, and adhesive bandages are standard supplies for procedures during which blood is drawn from a vein or capillaries. Alcohol causes inaccurate results for certain tests, however, so for these tests, povidone iodine or benzalkonium chloride is used. You will need a tourniquet (a flat, broad length of vinyl or rubber or a piece of fabric with a Velcro closure) for **venipuncture,** the puncture of a vein—performed with a needle for the purpose of drawing blood.

## Preparing Patients

After you review the test order and assemble the necessary equipment and supplies, take a moment to relax, gather your thoughts, and consider your purpose. This may strike you as odd advice, but your calm and positive demeanor helps establish the best possible relationship

## TABLE 35-1    Common Abbreviations Routinely Used in Blood Tests

| | | | | |
|---|---|---|---|---|
| Ab | antibody | | CA | cancer antigen |
| ABO | classification system for four blood groups | | CBC | complete blood (cell) count |
| AcAc | acetoacetate | | CEA | carcinoembryonic antigen |
| ACE | angiotensin-converting enzyme | | CHE | cholinesterase |
| ACT | activated coagulation time | | CK | creatine kinase |
| ACTH | adrenocorticotropic hormone | | CMV | cytomegalovirus |
| ADH | antidiuretic hormone | | $CN^-$ | cyanide anion |
| AFB | acid-fast bacillus | | CO | carbon monoxide |
| AFP | alpha-fetoprotein | | $CO_2$ | carbon dioxide |
| Ag | antigen | | COHb | carboxyhemoglobin |
| AG | anion gap | | Cr | creatinine |
| A/G R | albumin-globulin ratio | | CrCl | creatinine clearance |
| AHF | antihemolytic factor | | CT | calcitonin |
| Alb | albumin | | DAF | decay accelerating factor |
| Alc | alcohol | | DHEA | dehydroepiandrosterone, unconjugated |
| ALG | antilymphocyte globulin | | Diff | differential (blood cell count) |
| ALP; alk phos | alkaline phosphatase | | EBNA | Epstein-Barr virus nuclear antigen |
| ALT | alanine aminotransferase | | EBV | Epstein-Barr virus |
| ANA | antinuclear antibody | | EDTA | ethylenediaminetetraacetic acid |
| APAP | acetaminophen | | Eos | eosinophil |
| APTT | activated partial thromboplastin time | | EP | electrophoresis |
| ASA | acetylsalicylic acid (aspirin) | | Eq | equivalent |
| AST | aspartate aminotransferase | | ERP | estrogen receptor protein |
| AT-III | antithrombin III | | ESR | erythrocyte sedimentation rate |
| B | blood (whole blood) | | FBS | fasting blood sugar |
| Baso | basophil | | FFA | free fatty acids |
| BCA | breast cancer antigen | | FSH | follicle-stimulating hormone (follitropin) |
| BJP | Bence Jones protein | | $FT_4$ | free thyroxine |
| BT | bleeding time | | $FT_4I$ | free thyroxine index |
| BUN | blood urea nitrogen | | GFR | glomerular filtration rate |
| Ca; $Ca^{++}$ | calcium | | GH | growth hormone |

continued →

| | | | | |
|------|------------------------------|---|-------|---------------------------------|
| GHRH | growth hormone–releasing hormone | | MetHb | methemoglobin |
| GnRH | gonadotropin-releasing hormone | | MLC | mixed lymphocyte culture |
| GTT | glucose tolerance test | | MONO | monocyte |
| HA | hemagglutination | | MPV | mean platelet volume |
| HAI | hemagglutination inhibition test | | MSAFP | maternal serum alpha-fetoprotein |
| HAV | hepatitis A virus | | NE | norepinephrine |
| Hb; Hgb | hemoglobin | | NPN | nonprotein nitrogen |
| HbCO | carboxyhemoglobin | | OGTT | oral glucose tolerance test |
| HBV | hepatitis B virus | | P | plasma |
| HCG; hCG | human chorionic gonadotropin | | PAP | prostatic acid phosphatase |
| Hct | hematocrit | | PB | protein binding |
| HCV | hepatitis C virus | | PBG | porphobilinogen |
| HDL | high-density lipoprotein | | PCT | prothrombin consumption time |
| HDV | hepatitis delta virus | | PCV | packed cell volume (hematocrit) |
| HGH; hGH | human growth hormone | | Pi | inorganic phosphate |
| HIV | human immunodeficiency virus | | PKU | phenylketonuria |
| HLA | human leukocyte antigen | | PLT | platelet |
| HPV | human papilloma virus | | PMN | polymorphonuclear (leukocyte; neutrophil) |
| HSV | herpes simplex virus | | PRL | prolactin |
| HTLV | human T-cell lymphotrophic virus | | PSA | prostate-specific antigen |
| Ig | immunoglobulin | | PT | prothrombin time |
| IgE | immunoglobulin E | | PTH | parathyroid hormone |
| INH | inhibitor | | PTT | partial thromboplastin time |
| IV | intravenous | | PV | plasma volume |
| L | liver | | PZP | pregnancy zone protein |
| LD; LDH | lactate dehydrogenase | | RAIU | thyroid uptake of radioactive iodine |
| LDL | low-density lipoprotein | | RBC | red blood cell; red blood (cell) count |
| LH | luteinizing hormone | | RBP | retinol-binding protein |
| LMWH | low-molecular-weight heparin | | RCM | red cell mass |
| Lytes | electrolytes | | RCV | red cell volume |
| MCV | mean cell volume | | RDW | red cell distribution of width |

*continued* ⟶

## TABLE 35-1 Common Abbreviations Routinely Used in Blood Tests *(concluded)*

| | | | | |
|---|---|---|---|---|
| Retic | reticulocyte | | TBG | thyroxine-binding globulin |
| RF | rheumatoid factor; relative fluorescence unit | | TBV | total blood volume |
| Rh | rhesus factor | | TG | triglyceride |
| RIA | radioimmunoassay | | TRH | thyrotropin-releasing hormone |
| $rT_3$ | reverse triiodothyronine | | TSH | thyroid-stimulating hormone |
| S | serum | | VDRL | Venereal Disease Research Laboratory (test for syphilis) |
| Segs | segmented polymorphonuclear leukocyte | | VLDL | very-low-density lipoprotein |
| SPE | serum protein electrophoresis | | WB | Western blot |
| $T_3$ | triiodothyronine | | WBC | white blood cell; white blood (cell) count |
| $T_4$ | thyroxine | | | |

Source: Adapted from Norbert W. Tietz, ed., *Clinical Guide to Laboratory Tests*, 3d ed. (Philadelphia: W. B. Saunders, 1995).

with a patient who may be uneasy about having blood drawn. The moment you use to relax and focus may save you time and save patients unnecessary discomfort by contributing to a quick, efficient procedure.

**Greeting and Identifying Patients.** Greet patients pleasantly, introduce yourself, and explain that you will be drawing some blood. It is essential to identify patients correctly before you begin the procedure. Ask patients to state their full name, and be sure you hear both the first and last names correctly. Verify that the name the patient gives is the name on the order. (In some facilities, the phlebotomist may ask for a patient ID or chart number to further identify the patient.)

**Confirming Pretest Preparation.** The presence and level of certain substances in blood are affected by food and fluid intake or by other activities in daily life. Some tests require that the patient follow certain pretest restrictions. The purpose behind these restrictions is either to minimize the influence of the restricted food on the blood or to stress the body to see how it responds, as indicated by the blood.

One test that requires patients to follow pretest instructions closely is the glucose tolerance test, which measures a patient's ability to metabolize carbohydrates. This test is used to detect hypoglycemia and diabetes mellitus. You instruct the patient to eat a diet high in carbohydrates for the 3 days before the test and to fast for the 8 to 12 hours before the appointment. After initial blood and urine samples are taken, the patient ingests a measured

dose of glucose solution. Blood and urine samples are then taken at prescribed intervals as ordered by the physician. The glucose levels in the samples are often graphed for the physician's review.

Before you draw blood for any test, determine whether the patient has complied with pretest instructions. If the patient has not followed pretest instructions, explain that the test cannot be performed. Make a note on the order, and report the information to the physician or your supervisor.

**Explaining the Procedure and Safety Precautions.** Explain to the patient the procedure you will use to obtain the blood specimen for testing. Be clear and brief when you describe what you will do; too much detail leaves some patients queasy. You must follow Standard Precautions during all phlebotomy procedures, as described in the Caution: Handle With Care section. These precautions may be second nature to you, but they may raise concerns in the patient. Explain the need for each of the preventive measures you are taking in language the patient can understand. Assure the patient that these measures protect against exposure to infection.

**Establishing a Chain of Custody.** You will need to follow specific guidelines to establish a chain of custody for blood samples drawn for drug and alcohol analysis. (Chapter 30 explains general chain of custody procedures.) Because donating a specimen for drug and alcohol testing is potentially self-incriminating, the patient must sign a consent form for the testing. (This form is discussed in Chapter 34.) Although the clerical procedures for blood tests for drug and alcohol analysis are similar to those for urine tests, blood tests differ because you can confirm by direct observation that a blood specimen has been taken from the patient in question.

**Handling an Exposure Incident.**   When you adhere to Standard Precautions, the risk of exposure to blood-borne pathogens is very small. Accidents can occur, however. If you suffer a needlestick or other injury that results in exposure to blood or blood products from another person, you must report the incident to the appropriate staff members immediately. Wash the injured area carefully and apply a sterile bandage. Record the time and date of the incident, the names of the people involved, and the nature of the exposure. Depending on the situation, you may receive medications. You and the other person involved will be asked to undergo blood testing and be involved in follow-up studies. The Occupational Safety and Health Administration (OSHA) requires every employer to have an established procedure for handling exposure incidents.

## Drawing Blood

Some, but not all, states permit medical assistants to obtain blood samples. Your office will clarify which duties, if any, you may perform related to phlebotomy procedures. If your duties include collecting blood samples, you will obtain them either through venipuncture or capillary puncture. You must understand when these techniques are used and know how to perform them. Procedure 35-1 details quality control procedures for collecting blood specimens.

**Venipuncture.**   Venipuncture requires puncturing a vein with a needle and collecting blood into either a tube or a syringe. The most common sites for venipuncture are the median cubital and cephalic veins

---

### CAUTION *Handle With Care*

## Phlebotomy and Personal Protective Equipment

The Centers for Disease Control and Prevention (CDC) has classified all phlebotomy procedures as a risk for exposure to contaminated blood or blood products. You must use appropriate protective equipment during all phlebotomy procedures. Remember, it is up to you to protect yourself and the patient.

### Gloves

Gloves are the first line of defense during a phlebotomy procedure. They protect against spills and splashing of contaminated blood. Wash your hands and put on clean exam gloves that fit snugly before you work with each patient. Remove the gloves, dispose of them in a biohazardous waste container, and wash your hands after working with each patient.

### Garments

Garments such as laboratory coats and aprons can protect your clothing from spills and splashes and provide a measure of protection from contaminated materials. Some garments are designed to resist penetration by blood or blood products. You may find it necessary to wear such garments when drawing blood or performing blood tests.

### Masks and Protective Eyewear

Mucous membranes are especially vulnerable to invasion by infectious agents. Use masks and protective eyewear to help safeguard mucous membranes in your mouth, nose, and eyes from infection.

Masks help protect your mouth and nose from splashes or sprays of blood or blood products. You cannot predict when exposure to blood may occur. Accidental puncture of an artery during a phlebotomy procedure could result in a spray of blood. Blood may also spray or splash accidentally during some testing protocols. Most medical assistants do not routinely wear masks for phlebotomy procedures, however, once they have achieved proficiency in performing them.

Goggles can protect your eyes from splashing and spraying during blood drawing or testing. Healthcare workers in dental offices often wear goggles because patient treatments can easily expose workers to contaminated blood or bloody saliva.

Clear plastic face shields combine the protection of masks and goggles. They are often used during major surgical procedures. You may use a face shield if you do extensive testing on blood specimens. Face shields are not usually worn when drawing blood.

Personal protective equipment works two ways: it protects you from a patient's contaminated blood, and it also protects the patient from infectious agents you may be carrying. By using PPE correctly, you will make your workplace a safer place for you and the patients.

---

# PROCEDURE 35.1

## Quality Control Procedures for Blood Specimen Collection

**Procedure Goal:** To follow proper quality control procedures when taking a blood specimen

**Materials:** Necessary sterile equipment, specimen-collection container, paperwork related to the type of blood test the specimen is being drawn for, requisition form, marker, proper packing materials for transport

**Method:**

1. Review the request form for the test ordered, verify the procedure, prepare the necessary equipment and paperwork, and prepare the work area.

2. Identify the patient and explain the procedure. Confirm the patient's identification. Ask the patient to spell her name. Make sure the patient understands the procedure that is to be performed, even if she has had it done before.

3. Confirm that the patient has followed any pretest preparation requirements such as fasting, taking any necessary medication, or stopping a medication. For example, if a fasting specimen is being taken, the patient should not have eaten anything after midnight of the day before. Some doctors' offices will let the patient drink water or black coffee, however. It often depends on the type of specimen being taken.

### Rationale
The test may be invalid if the patient did not follow the pretest instruction

4. Collect the specimen properly. Collect it at the right time intervals if that applies. Use sterile equipment and proper technique.

5. Use the correct specimen-collection containers and the right preservatives, if required. For example, blood collected into a test tube with additives should be mixed immediately.

### Rationale
To prevent clotting

6. Immediately label the specimens. The label should include the patient's name, the date and time of collection, the test's name, and the name of the person collecting the specimen. Do not label the containers before collecting the specimen.

### Rationale
To keep from wasting tubes if there is a problem drawing the blood

7. Follow correct procedures for disposing of hazardous specimen waste and decontaminating the work area. Used needles, for instance, should immediately be placed in a biohazard sharps container.

8. Thank the patient. Keep the patient in the office if any follow-up observation is necessary.

9. If the specimen is to be transported to an outside laboratory, prepare it for transport in the proper container for that type of specimen, according to OSHA regulations. Place the container in a clear plastic bag with a zip closure and dual pockets with the international biohazard label imprinted in red or orange. The requisition form should be placed in the outside pocket of the bag. This ensures protection from contamination if the specimen leaks. Have a courier pick up the specimen and place it in an appropriate carrier (such as an insulated cooler) with the biohazard label. Place specimens to be sent by mail in appropriate plastic containers, and then place the containers inside a heavy-duty plastic container with a screw-down, nonleaking lid. Then place this container in either a heavy-duty cardboard box or nylon bag. The words *Human Specimen* or *Body Fluids* should be imprinted on the box or bag. Seal with a strong tape strip.

### Rationale
To protect the courier or anyone who handles the package from exposure to blood-borne pathogens

---

of the forearm, although other sites may be used if the primary site is unacceptable. Figure 35-3 shows the veins in the antecubital fossa (the small depression inside the bend of the elbow) and the forearm that are used for venipuncture.

Various instruments are used to perform venipuncture. Practice using the devices so that your technique is smooth, steady, and competent.

***Evacuation Systems.*** Evacuation systems, the most common of which is the VACUTAINER system (manufactured

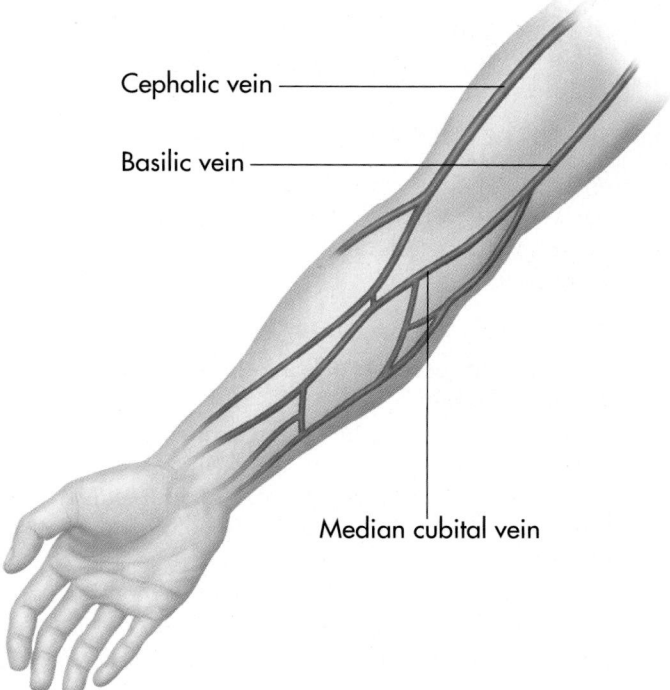

**Figure 35-3.** Veins commonly used for venipuncture include the cephalic vein, the basilica vein, and the median cubital vein.

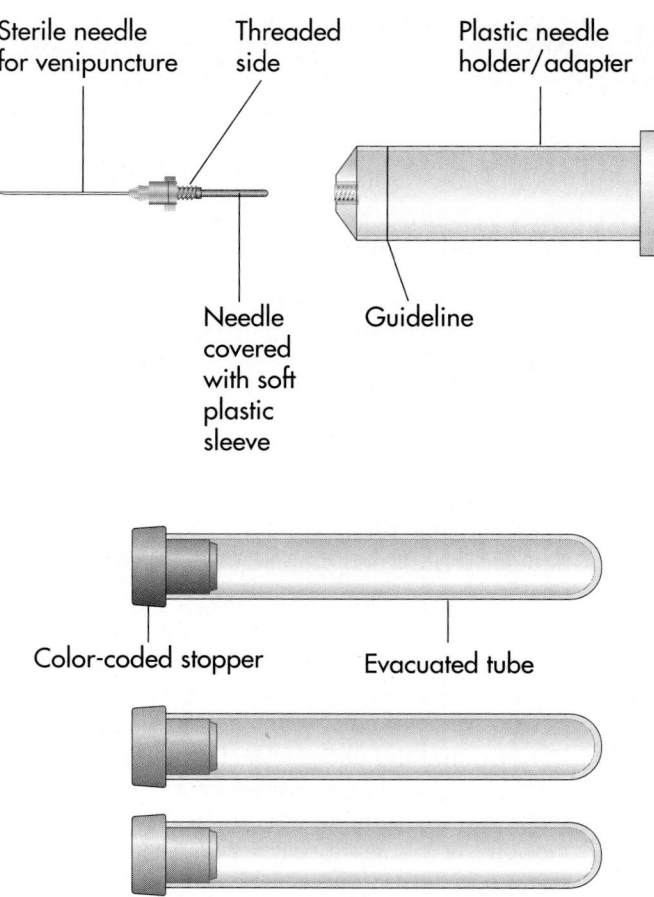

**Figure 35-4.** The VACUTAINER system uses interchangeable collection tubes that allow you to draw several blood specimens from the same venipuncture site.

by Becton Dickinson VACUTAINER Systems, Franklin Lakes, New Jersey), use a special double-pointed needle, a plastic needle holder/adapter, and collection tubes (Figure 35-4). The collection tubes are sealed to create a slight vacuum. You insert the covered inner point of the needle into one end of the holder/adapter and the first collection tube into the other end. Remove the plastic cap from the outer needle of the assembled system. Hold the needle at a 15-degree angle to the patient's arm, and puncture the patient's vein with the needle. Then press the collection tube fully onto the covered needle tip, piercing the stopper and allowing the vacuum to help draw blood into the collection tube. Procedure 35-2 explains how to use an evacuation system to draw a blood sample.

An evacuation system has several advantages over other methods of blood collection. It is easy to collect several samples from one venipuncture site using the interchangeable vacuum collection tubes. Tubes are calibrated by evacuation to collect the exact amount of blood required. Some collection tubes are prepared with additives needed to correctly process the blood sample for testing, such as anticoagulants. Finally, because there is no need to transfer blood from a collection syringe to a sample tube, the potential for exposure to contaminated blood is reduced.

**Needle and Syringe Systems.** An evacuation system is not the best choice for drawing blood in every case. For example, if the patient has small or fragile veins, the

vacuum created when the collection tube is pressed over the needle point can cause the veins to collapse. You may collect blood using a sterile needle and syringe assembly when an evacuation system is not suitable, such as when the patient is difficult to stick. You can use a smaller needle and control the vacuum in the syringe by pulling the plunger back slowly. The smaller needle should be no less than 23 gauge so that you do not hemolyze the blood. Other aspects of the procedure are essentially the same, except that the blood sample is collected in the syringe and must immediately be transferred to a collection tube.

**Butterfly Systems.** You may also use a butterfly system, or winged infusion set, when you work with patients who have small or fragile veins. Flexible wings attached to the needle simplify needle insertion. A length of flexible tubing (either 5 or 12 inches, approximately) connects the needle to the collection device. The inserted needle remains completely undisturbed while the collection device is manipulated. Because it is motionless, the needle causes less trauma to the vein and surrounding tissue than do other systems for venipuncture. A butterfly system generally uses a smaller needle (23 gauge) than other venipuncture techniques do. A butterfly system can be used with an evacuated collection tube or a syringe (Figure 35-5).

**Collection Tubes.** No matter which method is used to collect blood, the samples must immediately be mixed with the appropriate additives in the correct collection tubes before they are transported to the laboratory for testing. The stoppers of the tubes are different colors, each color identifying the type of additives (if any) they contain (Figure 35-11). These additives must be compatible with the laboratory process that the sample will undergo. Each laboratory may choose which tubes to use for a particular test.

Additives include anticoagulants and other materials that help preserve or process a sample for particular types of testing. When you collect a blood sample, double-check that you are using the appropriate collection tubes for the tests ordered. You must also fill the tubes in a specific order to preserve the integrity of the blood sample. Each laboratory requires a specific order of draw for collection tubes. The National Committee for Clinical Laboratory Standards also publishes its recommended order of draw. Table 35-2, identifies collection tube stopper colors, additives present in the tubes, and types of tests, in a typical order of draw.

**Engineered Safety Devices.** In response to the Needlestick Safety and Prevention Act, a number of engineered safety devices have been developed. These devices are intended to reduce the possibility of needlestick injuries (Figure 35-12). According to the National Institute for

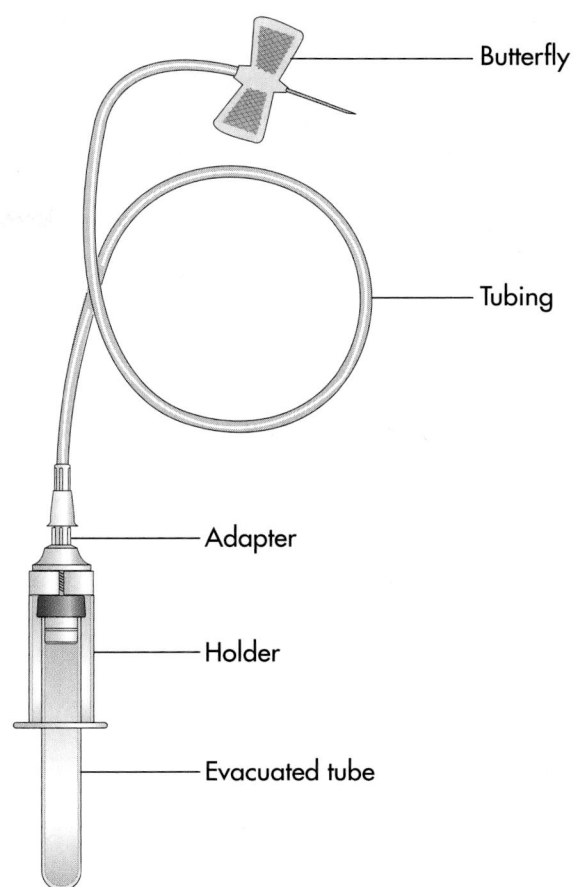

**Figure 35-5.** Once inserted, the needle of a butterfly system remains undisturbed during specimen collection.

# PROCEDURE 35.2

## Performing Venipuncture Using an Evacuation System

**Procedure Goal:** To collect a venous blood sample using an evacuation system

### OSHA Guidelines

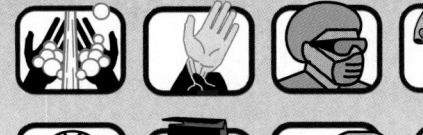

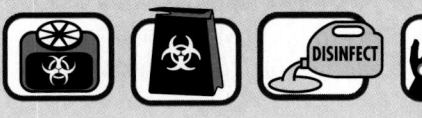

**Materials:** VACUTAINER components (safety needle, needle holder/adapter, collection tubes), antiseptic and cotton balls or antiseptic wipes, tourniquet, sterile gauze squares, sterile adhesive bandages

**Method:**

1. Review the laboratory request form, and make sure you have the necessary supplies.

2. Greet the patient, confirm the patient's identity, and introduce yourself.

3. Explain the purpose of the procedure, and confirm that the patient has followed the pretest instructions.

*Rationale*

To ensure the test will be valid

4. Make sure the patient is sitting in a venipuncture chair or is lying down.

5. Wash your hands. Put on exam gloves.

6. Prepare the safety needle holder/adapter assembly by inserting the threaded side of the

*continued* ⟶

**Collecting, Processing, and Testing Blood Specimens**    **845**

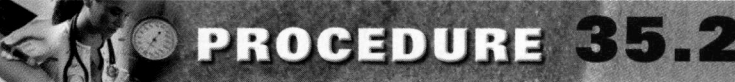
## Performing Venipuncture Using an Evacuation System *(continued)*

needle into the adapter and twisting the adapter in a clockwise direction. Push the first collection tube into the other end of the needle holder/adapter until the outer edge of the collection tube stopper meets the guideline.

### *Rationale*

So that the tube is stabilized but not completely punctured

7. Ask the patient whether one arm is better than the other for the venipuncture. The chosen arm should be positioned slightly downward (Figure 35-6).

8. Apply the tourniquet to the patient's upper arm midway between the elbow and the shoulder. Wrap the tourniquet around the patient's arm and cross the ends. Holding one end of the tourniquet against the patient's arm, stretch the other end to apply pressure against the patient's skin. Pull a loop of the stretched end under the end held tightly against the patient's skin, as shown in Figure 35-7. The tourniquet should be tight enough to cause the veins to stand out but should not stop the flow of blood. You should still be able to feel the patient's radial pulse. Ask the patient to make a fist and release it several times.

### *Rationale*

To make the veins in the forearm stand out more prominently

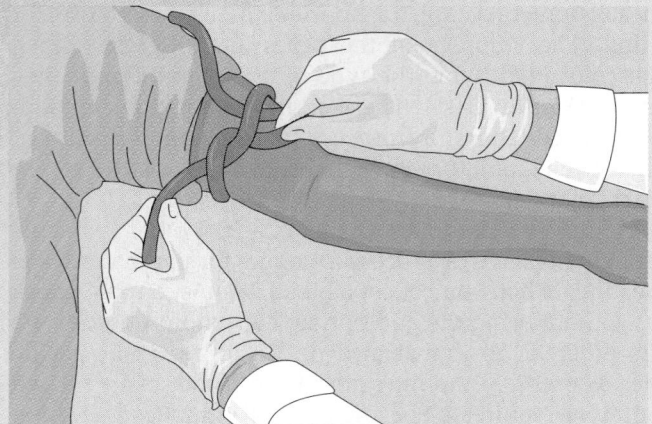

**Figure 35-7.** Applying a tourniquet makes it easier to find a patient's vein when you are drawing blood.

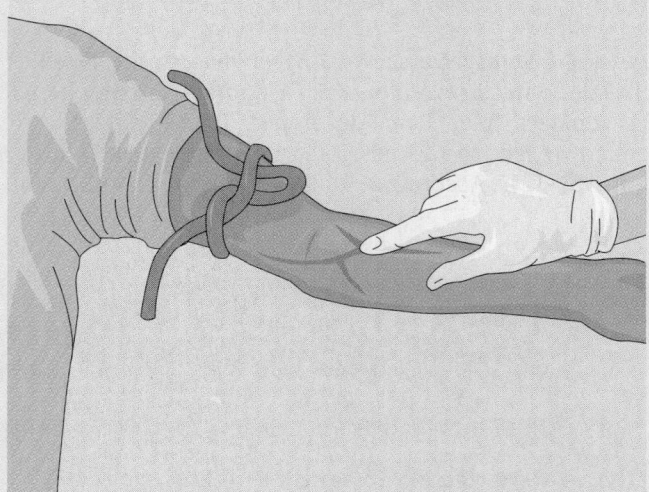

**Figure 35-8.** Use your index finger to locate the vein.

9. Palpate the proposed site, and use your index finger to locate the vein, as shown in Figure 35-8. The vein will feel like a small tube with some elasticity. If you feel a pulsing beat, you have located an artery. Do not draw blood from an artery. If you cannot locate the vein within 1 minute, release the tourniquet and allow blood to flow freely for 1 to 2 minutes. Then reapply the tourniquet and try again to locate the vein.

10. After locating the vein, clean the area with a cotton ball moistened with antiseptic or an antiseptic wipe. Use a circular motion to clean

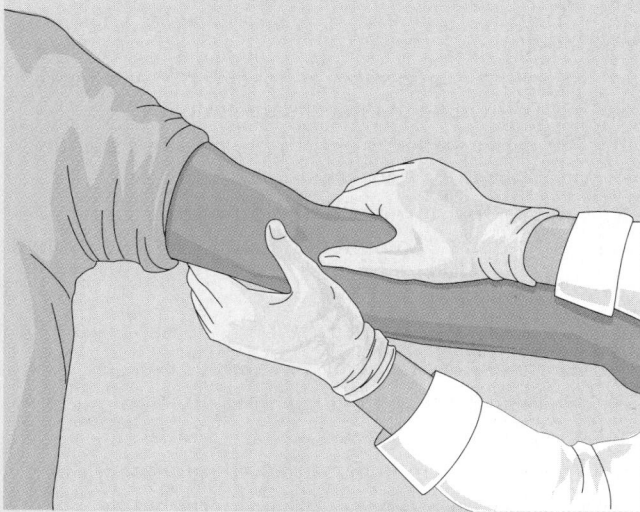

**Figure 35-6.** The patient's arm should be positioned slightly downward for a venipuncture.

*continued* ⟶

## Performing Venipuncture Using an Evacuation System *(continued)*

the area, starting at the center and working outward. Allow the site to air-dry.

### *Rationale*

The alcohol could interfere with some of the tests.

11. Remove the plastic cap from the outer point of the needle cover, and ask the patient to tighten the fist. Hold the patient's skin taut below the insertion site.

### *Rationale*

To anchor the vein so that it doesn't roll

12. With a steady and quick motion, insert the needle—held at a 15-degree angle, bevel side up, and aligned parallel to the vein—into the vein (Figure 35-9). You will feel a slight resistance as the needle tip penetrates the vein wall. Penetrate to a depth of ¼ to ½ inch. Grasp the holder/adapter between your index and great (middle) fingers. Using your thumb, seat the collection tube firmly into place over the needle point, puncturing the rubber stopper. Blood will begin to flow into the collection tube.

13. Fill each tube until the blood stops running to ensure the correct proportion of blood to additives. Switch tubes as needed by pulling one tube out of the adapter and inserting the next in a smooth and steady motion. (The soft plastic cover on the inner point of the needle retracts as each tube is inserted and recovers the needle point as each tube is removed.)

14. Once blood is flowing steadily, ask the patient to release the fist, and untie the tourniquet

by pulling the end of the tucked-in loop. The tourniquet should, in general, be left on no longer than 1 minute.

### *Rationale*

Longer periods may cause hemoconcentration, an increase in the blood-cell-to-plasma ratio, and invalidate test results.

You must remove the tourniquet before you withdraw the needle from the vein.

### *Rationale*

Removing the tourniquet releases pressure on the vein.

15. As you withdraw the needle in a smooth and steady motion, place a sterile gauze square over the insertion site (Figure 35-10). Immediately activate the safety device on the needle if it is not self-activating. Properly dispose of the needle immediately. Instruct the patient to hold the gauze pad in place with slight pressure. The patient should keep the arm straight and slightly elevated for several minutes.

### *Rationale*

To reduce the possibility of a hematoma

16. If the collection tubes contain additives, you will need to invert them slowly several times.

### *Rationale*

To mix the chemical agent and the blood sample

17. Label specimens and complete the paperwork.

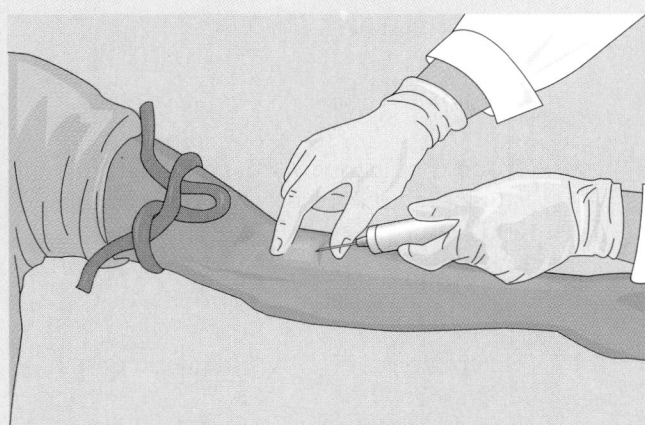

**Figure 35-9.** When performing venipuncture, hold the needle at a 15-degree angle.

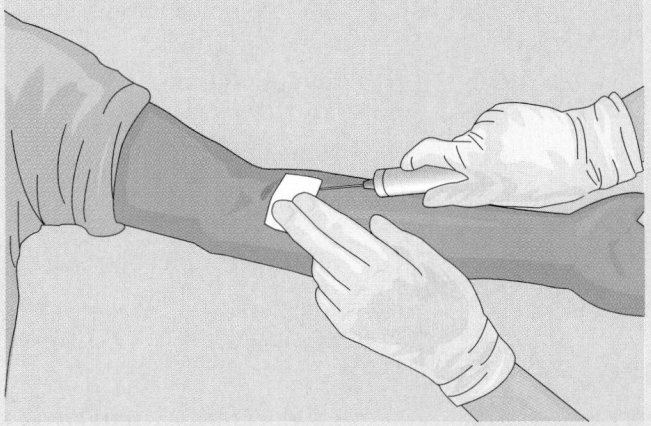

**Figure 35-10.** Place a sterile gauze square over the insertion site as you withdraw the needle.

*continued* ——➔

# Performing Venipuncture Using an Evacuation System *(concluded)*

18. Check the patient's condition and the puncture site for bleeding. Replace the sterile gauze square with a sterile adhesive bandage.

19. Properly dispose of used supplies and disposable instruments, and disinfect the work area.

20. Remove the gloves and wash your hands.

21. Instruct the patient about care of the puncture site.

22. Document the procedure in the patient's chart.

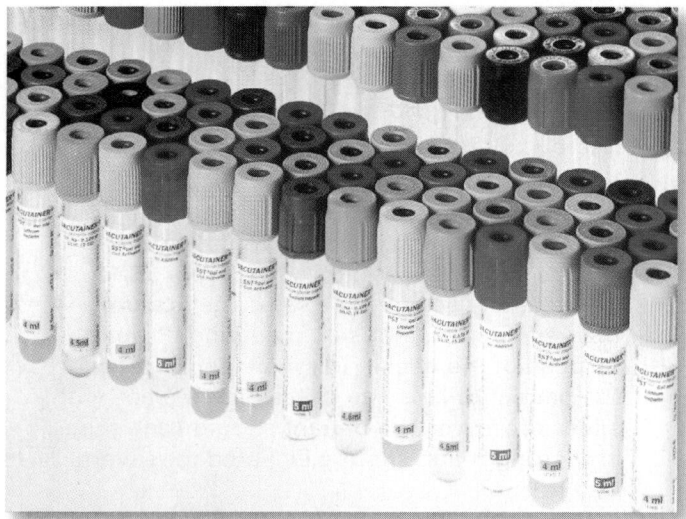

**Figure 35-11.** Special color-coded stoppers on collection tubes indicate which additives are present and, therefore, which types of laboratory tests may be performed on each blood specimen.

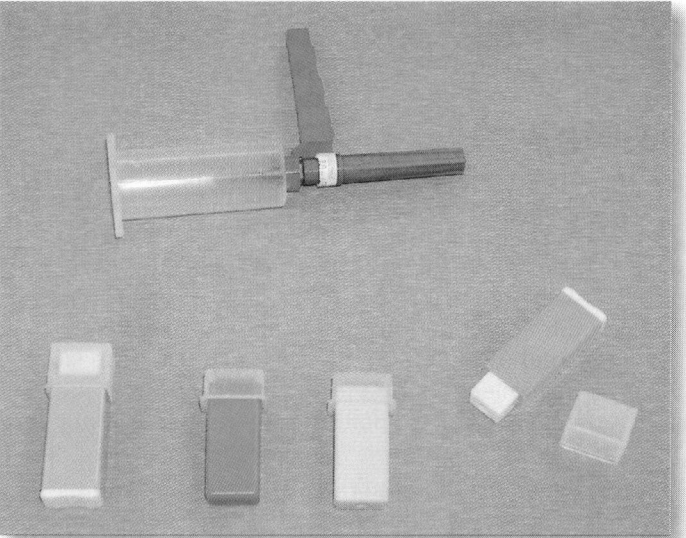

**Figure 35-12.** Various venipuncture and capillary puncture safety devices.

| TABLE 35-2 | Blood Collection Tubes | |
|---|---|---|
| **Stopper Color** | **Additive** | **Test Types** |
| Yellow | Sodium polyanetholsulfonate | Blood cultures |
| Light blue | Sodium Citrate | Coagulation studies |
| Red | None | Blood chemistries, AIDS antibody, viral studies, serologic tests, blood grouping and typing |
| Gold or Red/Black | Silicone serum separator | Tests requiring blood serum |
| Green | Heparin | Electrolyte studies, arterial blood gases |
| Lavender | Ethylenediaminetetraacetic acid (EDTA) (anticoagulant) | Hematology studies |
| Gray | Potassium oxalate or sodium fluoride (anticoagulant) | Blood glucose |

*Note:* Tubes are listed in the order they should be collected (Order of Draw).

Occupational Safety and Health (NIOSH), the desired characteristics of engineered safety devices include the following:

- The performance of the device is reliable
- The device is easy to use, safe, and effective
- The device should be needleless when possible
- The device should either not have to be activated by the user or may be activated using only one hand
- Once the safety feature is activated, it cannot be deactivated

Procedure 35-1 details quality control procedures for collecting blood specimens.

In certain circumstances, some of these characteristics are not feasible. Drawing blood from an artery or a vein is not possible without the use of a needle. Several types of safety devices for collecting blood specimens have been developed. These include:

- Retracting needles
- Hinged or sliding shields that cover phlebotomy and winged-steel (butterfly) needles
- Self-blunting phlebotomy and winged-steel needles
- Retractable lancets

Studies show that these devices, when used properly, have reduced needlestick injuries. NIOSH reports a 76% reduction of injuries with self-blunting needles, a 66% reduction with hinged needle shields, and a 23% reduction with sliding shields.

In addition to advocating the use of appropriate engineered safety devices, NIOSH also recommends that health-care workers follow these precautions:

- Use the safety devices provided to you by your employer.
- Only use needles if there is no effective alternative available.
- Participate in workplace programs that evaluate safety features.
- Recap needles only when absolutely necessary.
- Ensure the safe handling and disposal of sharps prior to beginning a procedure.
- Dispose of used sharps promptly using approved sharps containers.
- Report all needlestick injuries.
- Inform their employer of workplace hazards.
- Attend yearly blood-borne pathogen training.
- Follow recommended infection control practices.

**Capillary Puncture.** **Capillary puncture** requires a superficial puncture of the skin with a sharp point. Compared with venipuncture, capillary puncture releases a smaller amount of blood. The blood may be collected in small, calibrated glass tubes. It may also be collected on glass microscope slides or applied to reagent strips (or dipsticks), which are specially treated paper or plastic strips used in specific diagnostic tests.

Capillary puncture in adults and children is usually performed on the great (middle) finger or the ring finger. (Use the patient's nondominant hand for this procedure if possible.) The puncture should be made slightly off center on the pad of the fingertip. The center of the pad is usually more sensitive. Capillary puncture in infants is usually performed on one of the outer edges of the under-side of the heel (Figure 35-13). An alternate site for both children

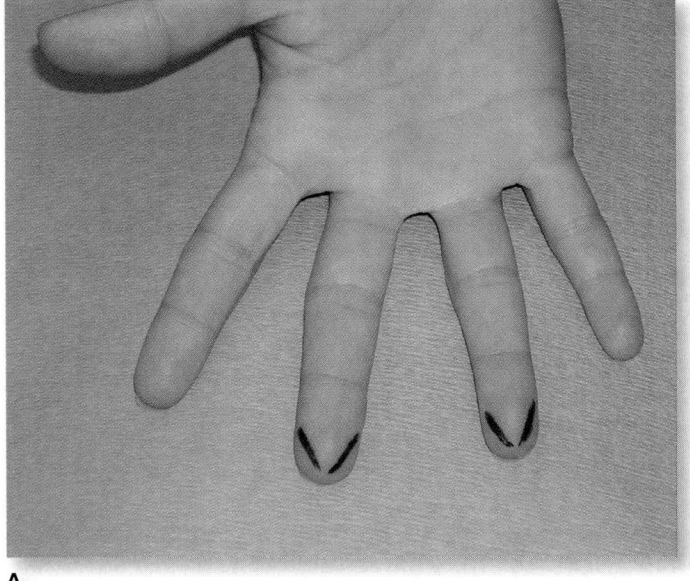
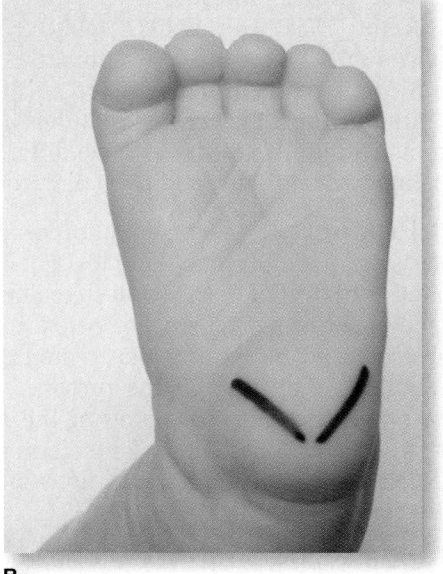

**Figure 35-13.** Capillary puncture sites for (A) an adult and (B) an infant.

and adults is the lower part of the earlobe, unless the patient's ear is pierced.

***Lancets.*** Lancets are used in the capillary puncture technique. This technique is employed when the amount of blood required for a specific procedure is not very large or when technical difficulties prevent use of the venipuncture technique. A **lancet** is a small, disposable instrument with a sharp point used to puncture the skin and make a shallow incision (between 2.0 and 3.0 mm deep for an adult and no deeper than 2.4 mm for an infant). The blood welling up from the incision is then collected.

***Automatic Puncturing Devices.*** Automatic puncturing devices are loaded with a lancet. Because the depth to which they puncture the skin is mechanically controlled, they are more accurate and comfortable than the traditional lancet method. These spring-loaded devices have disposable platforms that rest on the finger. Different platforms are used, depending on the desired depth of the puncture. Both the lancet and the platform should be discarded after use. There are also pen-like devices that hold a lancet inside. The device is held against the skin and activated by pushing a button. The advantages of these devices are that they are easy to use, the depth of the puncture can be easily adjusted, and there is an automatic ejection button for lancet disposal. Some companies also manufacture completely disposable devices, which come individually wrapped and are used only once.

***Micropipettes.*** A pipette is a calibrated glass tube for measuring fluids. A **micropipette** is a small pipette that holds a small, precise volume of fluid. You will use micropipettes to collect capillary blood for some tests. Capillary tubes, with a single calibration mark, are also used to collect capillary blood for certain tests. Procedure 35-3 explains how to perform a capillary puncture and collect a sample of capillary blood.

***MICROTAINER Tubes.*** MICROTAINER tubes (manufactured by Becton Dickinson VACUTAINER Systems) are small plastic tubes that have a widemouthed collector, similar to a funnel, which allows blood to flow quickly and freely into the tube. Like collection tubes in an evacuation system, MICROTAINER tubes have different colored tops indicating which, if any, additives they contain.

**Reagent Products.** Several common tests do not require processing of fluid blood samples. For these tests, you may apply droplets of freshly collected blood to chemically treated paper or plastic reagent strips (dipsticks) or add freshly collected blood droplets to small containers holding chemicals that react in the presence of specific substances or microorganisms. Some of the blood tests performed in this way are those for determining blood glucose levels, sickle cell anemia, infectious mononucleosis, and rheumatoid arthritis.

**Smear Slides.** You may need to apply a drop of freshly collected blood to a prepared microscope slide for some tests. More commonly, a smear slide is prepared in the laboratory from a blood sample containing an anticoagulant, for examination under a microscope.

# Responding to Patient Needs

Many patients are anxious when they have a blood test, and some patients have special needs or present special problems that make drawing blood challenging. Anxiety about blood tests may stem from a variety of concerns. Special needs may be related to a patient's age group or a medical condition. Some problems involve difficulty obtaining a blood sample or the patient's physiological or emotional response to a procedure. Being aware of possible sources of patient anxiety and understanding a wide range of special concerns can help you respond to patient needs with sensitivity and competence.

## Patient Fears and Concerns

Some patients express their fears or concerns directly. Other patients ask questions that highlight their fears. Providing more information or a complete understanding is reassuring to many patients. For others, the information serves only to confuse, overwhelm, or create more fear. You must decide how much information to give each patient and be prepared to answer questions.

Patients sometimes ask questions that are not appropriate for you to answer. A patient may ask you about his prognosis, medical condition, blood type, or other medical information. It is not appropriate for you to discuss these topics with the patient. Encourage the patient to discuss these issues with the physician. There are some commonly expressed fears and concerns to which you should respond, however.

**Pain.** The question that medical assistants performing phlebotomy probably hear most often is, Will this hurt? Never lie to a patient who asks this question. Inform the patient that he will feel a stick just as the lancet or point of the needle is inserted but that this pain goes away almost immediately. Tell a patient who seems particularly nervous to take a deep breath and let it out slowly. Also suggest that the patient focus on something else in the room or close his eyes and relax during the procedure.

A patient may express concern and report a previous unpleasant experience with blood testing. Listen to the patient's concerns. Describe what you will do to reduce discomfort and what the patient can do to be more at ease. Let the patient know that you will help him sit comfortably or lie down while the blood sample is being obtained. Tell the patient to let you know if he begins to feel light-headed. You might also ask the patient whether one arm is better to use than the other. Many patients have had blood drawn before and can tell you which sites were successful. Consulting the patient helps the patient feel more in control and provides you with important information.

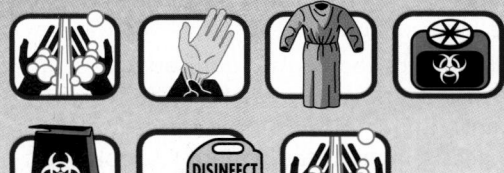

# PROCEDURE 35.3

## Performing Capillary Puncture

**Procedure Goal:** To collect a capillary blood sample using the finger puncture method

### OSHA Guidelines

**Materials:** Capillary puncture device (safety lancet or automatic puncture device such as Autolet or Glucolet), antiseptic and cotton balls or antiseptic wipes, sterile gauze squares, sterile adhesive bandages, reagent strips, micropipettes, smear slides

### Method:

1. Review the laboratory request form, and make sure you have the necessary supplies.
2. Greet the patient, confirm the patient's identity, and introduce yourself.
3. Explain the purpose of the procedure, and confirm that the patient has followed the pretest instructions, if indicated.

   *Rationale*

   The test may be invalid if the patient did not follow the pretest instructions.
4. Make sure the patient is sitting in the venipuncture chair or is lying down.
5. Wash your hands. Put on exam gloves.
6. Examine the patient's hands to determine which finger to use for the procedure. Avoid fingers that are swollen, bruised, scarred, or calloused. Generally, the ring and great (middle) fingers are the best choices. If you notice that the patient's hands are cold, you may want to warm them between your own, have the patient put them in a warm basin of water or under warm running water, or wrap them in a warm cloth.

   *Rationale*

   Warming the patient's hands improves circulation.
7. Prepare the patient's finger with a gentle "massaging" or rubbing motion toward the fingertip. Keep the patient's hand below heart level so that gravity helps the blood flow.

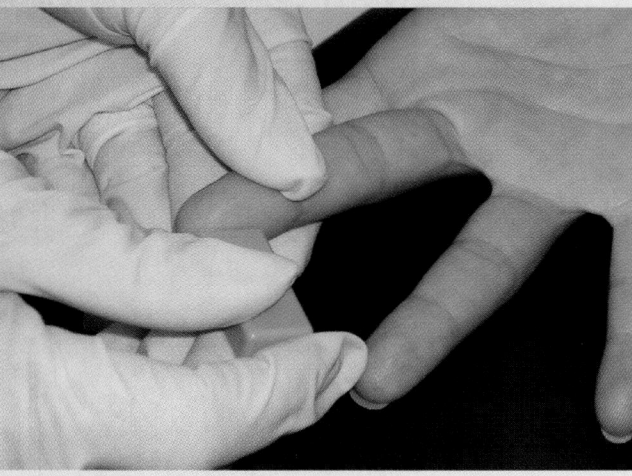

**Figure 35-14.** Hold the lancet or automatic puncture device at a right angle to the patient's fingerprint.

8. Clean the area with a cotton ball moistened with antiseptic or an antiseptic wipe. Allow the site to air-dry.

   *Rationale*

   The alcohol may interfere with some tests.
9. Hold the patient's finger between your thumb and forefinger. Hold the safety lancet or automatic puncture device at a right angle to the patient's fingerprint, as shown in Figure 35-14. Puncture the skin on the pad of the fingertip with a quick, sharp motion. The depth to which you puncture the skin is generally determined by the length of the lancet point. Most automatic puncturing devices are designed to penetrate to the correct depth.
10. Allow a drop of blood to form at the end of the patient's finger. If the blood droplet is slow in forming, apply steady pressure (Figure 35-15). Avoid milking the patient's finger.

    *Rationale*

    It dilutes the blood sample with tissue fluid and causes hemolysis.
11. Wipe away the first droplet of blood. (This droplet is usually contaminated with tissue fluids released when the skin is punctured.) Then fill the collection devices, as described.

*continued* ⟶

## Performing Capillary Puncture *(concluded)*

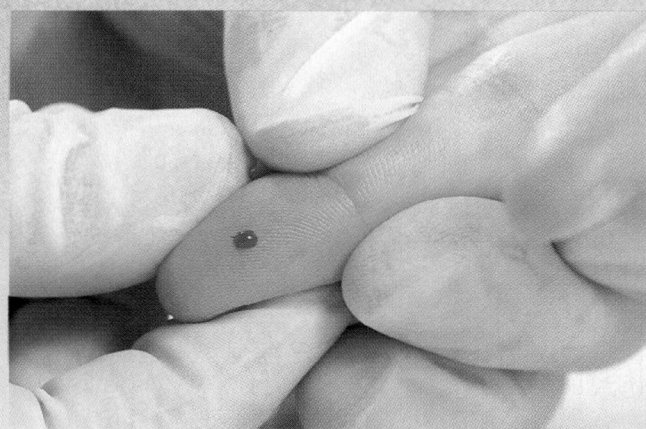

**Figure 35-15.** Apply steady pressure to the patient's finger, but do not milk it.

*Micropipettes:* Hold the tip of the tube just to the edge of the blood droplet. The tube will fill through capillary action (Figure 35-16). If you are preparing microhematocrit tubes, you need to seal one end of each tube with clay sealant. (See Procedure 35-5 for this process.)

*Reagent strips:* With some reagent strips (dipsticks), you must touch the strip to the blood drop but not smear it; with other strips, you must smear it. Follow the manufacturer's guidelines.

*Smear slides:* Gently touch the blood droplet to the smear slide and process the slide as described in Procedure 35-4.

12. After you have collected the required samples, dispose of the lancet immediately. Then wipe the patient's finger with a sterile gauze square (Figure 35-17). Instruct the patient to apply pressure to stop the bleeding.

13. Label specimens and complete the paperwork. Some tests, such as glucose monitoring, must be completed immediately.

14. Check the puncture site for bleeding. If necessary, replace the sterile gauze square with a sterile adhesive bandage.

15. Properly dispose of used supplies and disposable instruments, and disinfect the work area.

16. Remove the gloves and wash your hands.

17. Instruct the patient about care of the puncture site.

18. Document the procedure in the patient's chart. (If the test has been completed, include the results.)

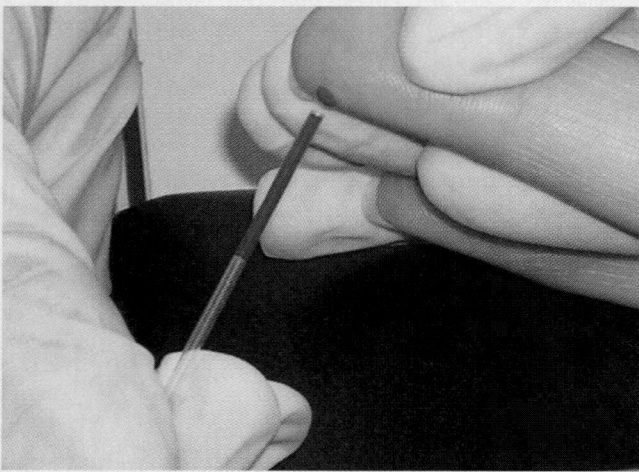

**Figure 35-16.** Touch the tube to the drop of blood to fill it.

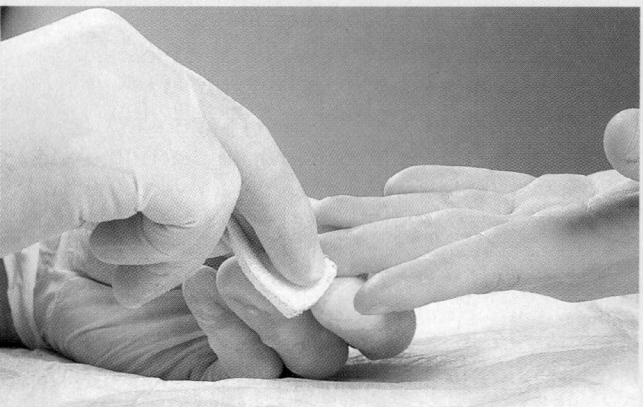

**Figure 35-17.** Use a sterile gauze square to wipe remaining blood from the patient's finger.

**Bruises or Scars.** Some patients may express fear of getting a bruise or scar from a blood test. Explain that some bruising is possible but that it will fade within a few days. Most bruising is caused by a hematoma, which occurs when blood leaks out of the vein and collects under the skin. Hematomas can be prevented by releasing the tourniquet before withdrawing the needle and applying proper pressure over the puncture site after the needle has been withdrawn. Bruising is common with fair-skinned patients. Scars, on the other hand, are unlikely.

**Serious Diagnosis.** Patient fears are not always rational. One fear that patients express is that the more tubes of blood you require, the more serious their condition must be. Patients may also fear that a blood test is being done to help the doctor diagnose an extremely serious disease.

You can help relieve a patient's fears by explaining that a blood test is one of the best ways to obtain an overall picture of health (emphasize health, not disease). Note that blood tests show what is normal about the blood as well as any abnormalities. You might also explain that several samples are being taken because the blood used in blood tests is processed in different ways; the blood collected for one test cannot be used in another.

Blood testing may also be done to determine how well and at what levels medications are acting in the blood. Explain that the doctor may want to see how much medication is in the blood to better manage the prescribed dosage. When a patient needs repeated tests for drug levels, explain that the tests show how the body is using the medication.

**Contracting a Disease From the Procedure.** Probably the greatest fear of patients undergoing blood tests is contracting HIV, AIDS, or hepatitis B virus (HBV). Although many people are now well informed about how AIDS and other serious diseases are contracted, it is understandable for a patient to worry about blood-borne pathogens. Do not dismiss the patient's concerns, and do not downplay the importance of following Standard Precautions.

Explain the precautions you will take to prevent the spread of infection. Allow the patient to see you wash your hands and put on new gloves before you begin to take the blood sample. Stress that the needle is sterile. Explain that you have not touched the needle and that it will be discarded when you finish. Let the patient see you put the needle in the sharps container.

Use this opportunity to educate the patient about the transmission of AIDS. Emphasize that AIDS, and other infections transmitted by blood, can be transmitted only when there is direct contact with contaminated blood or other body fluids. Explain that your gloves protect both you and the patient by providing a barrier to infection transmission from one person to another.

Explain that your other protective equipment, such as goggles or a mask, also helps prevent the spread of infection.

## Special Considerations

As you collect blood specimens, you will encounter a variety of patients, some of whom have special needs. You will find yourself in many different situations, some of them problematic. Some special needs and problematic situations are fairly common, and you must be prepared to deal with them.

**Children.** It is a challenge to explain blood-drawing procedures to children. Many children become visibly upset by the situation. If possible, it is best to talk with the parents or caregivers before working with the child. The adults can provide the best insight into how their child handles stressful situations.

Your primary concern when working with infants is to complete tests correctly. Because an infant's veins are often too small for adequate blood collection, the best site for drawing blood is usually the heel.

When working with children, address them directly. Speak clearly in a calm, soothing voice, and explain the procedure briefly in terms they can understand. If they ask whether the process will hurt, be honest. Very young children should be held by their parent or guardian or a coworker during a venipuncture or capillary puncture to prevent them from moving. If a child is extremely distressed, it may be best to go on to another patient while the child calms down.

After you have begun the procedure, give the child status reports such as, "We're almost finished!" and "You've been very brave." This information helps calm nervous parents or caregivers as well.

When the procedure is complete, offer a compliment on some aspect of the child's behavior. Gather your supplies and samples as quickly as possible to avoid alarming the child with the sight of blood-collection tubes. If parents or caregivers have questions, encourage them to discuss the tests with the child's physician.

**Elderly Patients.** The challenges presented by elderly patients may test your technical skills as well as your interpersonal skills. Physically, some older adults are frail and may not withstand blood-drawing procedures as easily as younger patients. Changes in skin condition often make elderly patients more prone to bruising and other injuries. Decreased circulation may make it difficult to collect enough blood for an adequate sampling. Elderly patients with impaired hearing may have trouble understanding instructions and answering questions. Patients with dementia may also be unable to understand what you are saying.

When you communicate with an elderly patient, speak in clear, low-pitched tones. High-pitched voices are more difficult for people with hearing impairments to understand. When asking questions, give the patient time to answer, and confirm the response to prevent misunderstandings. Avoid both overly simple yes or no questions that the patient might answer without thinking and overly complex questions that might confuse the patient. Take your time with the procedure, and explain it in language the patient can understand.

**Patients at Risk for Uncontrolled Bleeding.** Patients who have hemophilia or are taking blood-thinning medications are at risk for uncontrolled bleeding at the collection site. (Hemophilia is a disorder in which the blood does not coagulate at a wound or puncture site.) Be especially careful and alert as you follow the standard procedures for collecting a blood specimen. In addition, hold several gauze squares over the puncture site for at least 5 minutes to make sure bleeding has stopped completely. If uncontrolled bleeding does occur, call the physician immediately.

**Difficult Patients.** You may encounter a particular challenge in working with a patient either because of technical problems or because of personality issues. Being prepared for these situations is the best method for coping with them.

***The Difficult Venipuncture.*** There will be times when you simply cannot get a good blood sample. If your first attempt at drawing blood fails, try again at another site. Give the patient (and yourself) a short break, and make an attempt on the other arm, for instance. Sometimes the veins in one arm are easier to work with than the veins in the other arm. If you cannot get a good sample on the second try, stop. Ask for assistance from your supervisor or the doctor.

***Fainting Patients.*** It is impossible to predict which patients will have a reaction to a blood-drawing procedure. Generally, however, an ill patient is more likely to experience a reaction than a well patient. The best way to deal with this potential problem is to position every patient so that, if fainting does occur, no injury will result.

Have patients sit in a special venipuncture chair (Figure 35-18). These chairs are designed to help prevent patients from sliding to the floor in the event of fainting. If your office is not equipped with a venipuncture chair, have patients lie down on an examining table. A patient who has a history of fainting or feels ill should lie down with feet elevated or knees drawn up while you complete the procedure. Sometimes just talking with the patient, asking him or her simple questions, will help keep the patient from fainting.

If a patient does faint and the needle is still in the vein, release the tourniquet and withdraw the needle quickly and steadily. Apply pressure to the site. Most people revive promptly, and no other action is required. Do not leave the patient alone. Notify the doctor that the patient fainted, and ask the doctor whether you should continue with the procedure.

If there is a more severe reaction, notify the appropriate staff member and remain with the patient. If the

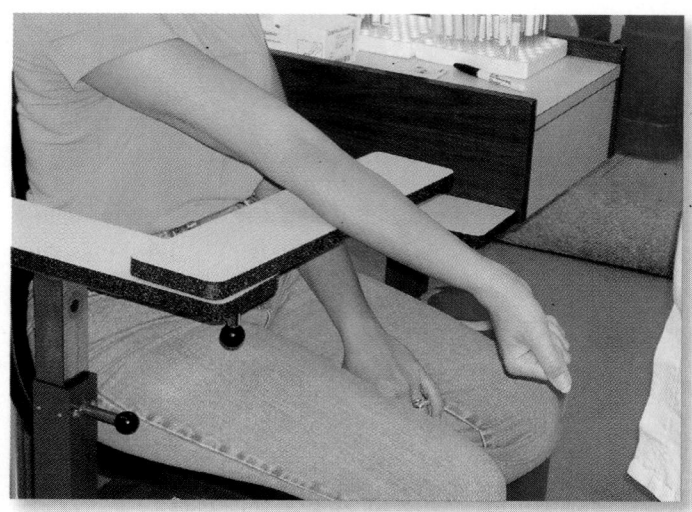

**Figure 35-18.** Venipuncture chairs are designed to make blood drawing easier and to prevent patients from falling if they should faint.

patient is in a chair and begins to slide out, raise the safety arm and gently lower the patient to the floor. Protect the patient's head at all times, and make sure the patient is breathing. The doctor should examine the patient before the patient is moved. Follow the doctor's instructions.

When the patient begins to recover, assist the person into a sitting position and then to a chair or couch. The patient should rest until feeling strong enough to walk—usually about 15 minutes. When the patient feels steady, take the patient to another area of the office, such as the patient reception area. At this point another staff member usually becomes responsible for the patient's care and determines when it is safe for the patient to leave. Additional information about venipuncture complications is found in the *Caution: Handle with Care* section.

***Angry or Violent Patients.*** Some patients are extremely resistant to having blood drawn. Although their objections may seem illogical, remember that people often do not think as clearly in moments of high emotion as they normally do.

Encourage a patient who is mildly upset and wants to argue about the need for the blood test to let you take the sample and then discuss the situation with the doctor. If you convince the patient to submit to the test, complete the procedure quickly and accurately. Avoid arguing with the patient.

Do not force the issue with a patient who becomes violent or refuses outright to submit to the procedure. A patient does have the right to refuse testing or treatment. Under no circumstances should you attempt to physically force a patient to give a blood sample. Never endanger yourself, other patients, or your colleagues by refusing to back down from an angry or violent patient. Report the problem to the appropriate staff, make a note on the order, and follow other established procedures.

## Venipuncture Complications

Venipuncture is, in general, a safe procedure. Most of the complications you encounter are mild and more of a nuisance than anything. There are some serious complications of venipuncture but they are rare. You must be aware of possible complications and ways to avoid them. You should also understand how to deal with these complications if they occur.

Some of the more serious complications you may encounter are:

- *Hematoma.* A collection of blood will sometimes form under the skin. This is especially a problem in patients who have bleeding disorders, are elderly, or are taking anticoagulants. To avoid hematomas, hold the needle as still as possible while filling and changing the tubes. You may need to use a butterfly collection device. Hold pressure on the venipuncture site as soon as you remove the needle. Have the patient elevate her arm but not bend the elbow. If a hematoma does form, apply extra gauze to the puncture site and wrap with stretch bandage. Watch the patient and alert the doctor if necessary.

- *Latex Allergy.* Some patients may have an allergy to latex. Make sure you ask the patient if he has any allergies before you begin the procedure. If the patient has a latex allergy, make sure you use nonlatex gloves, tourniquet, and bandages. If the patient has an unexpected allergic reaction to latex, alert the physician and follow her instructions.

- *Nerve Injury.* It is essential that you know the anatomy of the antecubital fossa so that you can accurately locate the proper veins for venipuncture. Inserting a needle into a nerve can cause nerve damage. Permanent sensory and/or motor damage to the arm and hand can occur if the venipuncture is done incorrectly. If you suspect you have stuck the patient's nerve, withdraw the needle immediately and alert the physician.

- *Infections.* Though quite rare, infections after venipuncture do occur and can be very serious. Use only approved single-use venipuncture equipment. Cleanse the venipuncture site well before the procedure. An infection at the venipuncture site may not be evident for several days after the procedure. If the patient calls complaining of redness, heat, or drainage at the site, have her return to the office to see the physician. A more serious blood infection (sepsis) may first seem like the patient has the flu. Fever and chills are the first symptoms of sepsis. A patient with a blood infection can go into shock if left untreated. If you suspect the patient has a blood infection, have her see the physician immediately.

# Performing Common Blood Tests

Many blood tests are routinely ordered as part of a complete general exam to determine a patient's overall health. The results of individual tests can provide information that aids in the diagnosis of specific conditions, diseases, and disorders, as noted in Table 35-3.

The number of blood tests routinely performed in POLs has declined since the implementation of Clinical Laboratory Improvement Amendments of 1988 (CLIA '88) regulations. Many POLs now perform only waived tests. Each POL is different, however, and regulations do change. Check with your employer about what tests your office performs regularly. You should be familiar with a wide range of tests and the steps involved with each even if you do not anticipate performing them.

You may encounter several chemical substances while performing your responsibilities in the laboratory. Chemicals you might encounter in laboratory work include the following:

- Anticoagulants, which cause the blood to remain in a liquid, uncoagulated state
- Serum separators, which form a gel-like barrier between serum and the clot in a coagulated blood sample
- Stains, which color particular cells, making microscopic studies easier to complete

Anticoagulants or serum separators are always present in blood-collection tubes and do not need to be added to the sample.

You must be absolutely clear about which chemicals are used for which tests and the precise amounts involved. It is also important to understand the purpose of blood tests so you can educate patients. You must, in addition, know the range of normal test values so you can be aware of potential problems and note them for the doctor's attention. Table 35-4 shows the normal ranges for a variety of blood tests.

## TABLE 35-3  Common Blood Tests and the Conditions They Help Identify

| Substance Identified or Quantified | Stopper Color and Additive | Part of Blood Tested | Indication, Disease, or Disorder |
|---|---|---|---|
| Alanine aminotransferase (ALT) | None / Silicone serum separator | Serum | Liver disorders |
| Alpha-fetoprotein (AFP) | None / Silicone serum separator | Fetal serum | Fetal liver and gastrointestinal tract status, hepatitis |
| Amylase | None / Silicone serum separator | Serum | Drug toxicity, parotid or pancreas disorders |
| Angiotensin-converting enzyme (ACE) | None / Silicone serum separator | Serum | Lung cancer, sarcoidosis, acute or chronic bronchitis |
| Antidiuretic hormone (ADH) | None / Silicone serum separator | Plasma | Syndrome of inappropriate ADH, Guillain-Barré syndrome, brain tumor |
| Aspartate aminotransferase (AST) | None / Silicone serum separator | Serum | Liver disease (including viral hepatitis), infectious mononucleosis, damaged heart or skeletal muscle |
| Bilirubin | None / Silicone serum separator | Serum | Liver disease, fructose intolerance, hypothyroidism |
| Blood urea nitrogen (BUN) | None / Silicone serum separator | Serum or plasma | Kidney disorders |
| Cancer antigens (numbers 125, 15-3, 549, 72-4), tumor-associated glycoprotein (TAG) | None / Silicone serum separator | Serum | Specific cancers identified, depending on antigen tested |
| Calcium, total (fasting) | None / Silicone serum separator | Serum | Hyperparathyroidism, malignant disease with bone involvement |
| Carbon dioxide, total | None / Silicone serum separator | Venous serum or plasma | Acidosis or alkalosis (acid-base balance) |

continued ⟶

## TABLE 35-3 Common Blood Tests and the Conditions They Help Identify (concluded)

| Substance Identified or Quantified | Stopper Color and Additive | Part of Blood Tested | Indication, Disease, or Disorder |
|---|---|---|---|
| Cholesterol, total | None / Silicone serum separator | Serum or plasma | Hyperlipoproteinemia, coronary artery disease, atherosclerosis |
| Creatine kinase (CK) | EDTA | Serum | Muscular dystrophies, Reye's syndrome, heart disease, shock, some neoplasms |
| Erythrocyte count (RBC) | EDTA | Whole blood | Anemia |
| Erythrocyte sedimentation rate (ESR) | EDTA | Whole blood | Infectious diseases, malignant neoplasms, sickle cell anemia |
| Glucose (fasting) | Potassium oxalate or sodium fluoride | Whole blood | Pancreatic function, ability of intravenous insulin to offset diet in diabetes mellitus |
| Glucose (fasting—tolerance test) | Potassium oxalate or sodium fluoride | Serum | Diabetes mellitus, hypoglycemia |
| Lactate dehydrogenase (LD) | None / Silicone serum separator | Serum | Anemia, viral hepatitis, shock, hypoxia, hyperthermia |
| Leukocyte count (WBC) | EDTA | Whole blood | Leukemia, infection, leukocytosis |
| Phenylalanine | Heparin or Newborn screening card | Plasma | Hyperphenylalaninemia, obesity, phenylketonuria |
| Potassium ($K^+$) and sodium ($Na^+$) | None / Silicone serum separator | Serum | Fluid-electrolyte balance |
| Prostate specific antigen (PSA) | None / Silicone serum separator | Serum | Prostatic cancer, BPH |
| Sickle cells | EDTA | Whole blood | Sickle cell anemia |
| Thyroid-stimulating hormone (TSH), triiodothyronine ($T_3$), thyroxine ($T_4$) | None / Silicone serum separator | Serum | Thyroid function |
| Uric acid | None / Silicone serum separator | Serum | Gout, leukemia |

*Note:* Various laboratories may have different testing protocols and require other tube tops than those represented in this table. Consult your laboratory procedures manual for additional information regarding required collection tubes.

## TABLE 35-4   Normal Ranges for Blood Tests

| Blood Test | Stopper Color and Additive | Blood Component Tested | Normal Range |
|---|---|---|---|
| ***Blood Counts*** | | | |
| Red blood cells (erythrocytes) | ⭕ EDTA | | |
|   Men | | Whole blood | $4.3–5.7 \times 10^6$ cells/μL |
|   Women | | Whole blood | $3.8–5.1 \times 10^6$ cells/μL |
| White blood cells (leukocytes) | ⭕ EDTA | Whole blood | $4.5–11.0 \times 10^3$ cells/μL |
| Platelets | | Whole blood | $150–400 \times 10^3$ cells/μL |
| Differential | | | |
|   Neutrophils | | Whole blood | 60%–70% |
|   Eosinophils | | Whole blood | 1%–4% |
|   Basophils | | Whole blood | 0%–0.5% |
|   Lymphocytes | | Whole blood | 20%–30% |
|   Monocytes | | Whole blood | 2%–6% |
| Hematocrit (Hct) | ⭕ EDTA | Whole blood | |
|   Men | | | 39%–49% |
|   Women | | | 35%–45% |
| Hemoglobin (Hb, Hgb) | ⭕ EDTA | Whole blood | |
|   Men | | | 13.2–17.3 g/dL |
|   Women | | | 11.7–16.0 g/dL |
| ***Erythrocyte Sedimentation Rate (ESR)*** | | | |
| Wintrobe | ⭕ EDTA | Whole blood | |
|   Men | | | 0–5 mm/hour |
|   Women | | | 0–15 mm/hour |
| Westergren | | Whole blood | |
|   Men | | | 0–15 mm/hour |
|   Women | | | 0–20 mm/hour |
| ***Coagulation Tests*** | | | |
| Prothrombin time (PT) | ⭕ Sodium citrate | Plasma | 11–15 seconds |
| Bleeding time | ⭕ Sodium citrate | Whole blood | 2–7 minutes |
| ***Electrolytes*** | | | |
| Bicarbonate ($HCO_3^-$) | ⚫ None | Arterial plasma | 21–28 mEq/L |
| | | Venous plasma | 27–29 mEq/L |
| Calcium ($Ca^{++}$) | | Serum | 8.6–10.0 mg/dL |
| Chloride ($Cl^-$) | | Serum, plasma | 98–108 mEq/L |
| Potassium ($K^+$) | ⚪⚫ Silicone serum separator | Serum | 3.5–5.1 mEq/L |
| Sodium ($Na^+$) | | Serum | 136–145 mEq/L |
| ***Chemical and Serologic Tests*** | | | |
| Alpha-fetoprotein (AFP) | ⚫ None | Serum | |
|   Fetal, first trimester | | | 20–400 mg/dL |
|   Adult | ⚪⚫ Silicone serum separator | | <15 ng/mL |

*continued* ⟶

**TABLE 35-4 Normal Ranges for Blood Tests** *(continued)*

| Blood Test | Stopper Color and Additive | Blood Component Tested | Normal Range |
|---|---|---|---|
| Alanine aminotransferase (ALT) | | Serum | |
| Men | | | 10–40 U/L |
| Women | Silicone serum separator | | 7–35 U/L |
| Aspartate aminotransferase (AST, formerly SGOT) | None | Serum | |
| Men | Silicone serum separator | | 11–26 U/L |
| Women | | | 10–20 U/L |
| Bilirubin, total direct | None | Serum | 0.3–1.2 mg/dL |
| | Silicone serum separator | | |
| Blood urea nitrogen (BUN) | None | Serum, plasma | 6–20 mg/dL |
| | Silicone serum separator | | |
| Carcinoembryonic antigen (CEA) | None | Serum | < 5.0 ng/mL |
| | Silicone serum separator | | |
| Cholesterol, total | None | Serum, plasma | |
| Men | | | 158–277 mg/dL |
| Women | | | 162–285 mg/dL |
| High-density lipoproteins (HDLs) | | Serum, plasma | |
| Men | | | 28–63 mg/dL |
| Women | | | 37–92 mg/dL |
| Low-density lipoproteins (LDLs) | Silicone serum separator | Serum, plasma | |
| Men | | | 89–197 mg/dL |
| Women | | | 88–201 mg/dL |
| Creatine kinase (CK) | EDTA | Serum, plasma | |
| Men | | | 38–174 U/L |
| Women | | | 26–140 U/L |
| Creatinine | None | Serum, plasma | |
| Men | | | 0.9–1.3 mg/dL |
| Women | Silicone serum separator | | 0.6–1.2 mg/dL |
| Cytomegalovirus (CMV) | None | Serum | None |
| | Silicone serum separator | | |
| Epstein-Barr virus (EBV) | None | Whole blood | None |
| | Silicone serum separator | | |

*continued* ⟶

## TABLE 35-4    Normal Ranges for Blood Tests *(concluded)*

| Blood Test | Stopper Color and Additive | Blood Component Tested | Normal Range |
|---|---|---|---|
| Glucose (fasting blood sugar, FBS) | Potassium oxalate or sodium fluoride | Serum | 74–120 mg/dL |
| Group A beta-hemolytic streptococci | None / Silicone serum separator | Serum | None |
| Human immunodeficiency virus (HIV) antibodies | None / Silicone serum separator | Serum, plasma | None |
| Insulin | None / Silicone serum separator | Serum | <17 µU/mL |
| Iron, total Men Women | None / Silicone serum separator | Serum | 65–175 µg/dL 50–170 µg/dL |
| Lactate dehydrogenase (LD) | None / Silicone serum separator | Serum, plasma | 140–280 U/L |
| pH | None / Silicone serum separator | Arterial blood Venous blood | 7.35–7.45 7.32–7.43 |
| Proteins Total Albumin | None / Silicone serum separator | Serum | 6.2–8.0 g/dL 3.4–4.8 g/dL |
| Fibrinogen | Sodium citrate | Plasma | 200–400 mg/dL |
| Uric acid Men Women | None / Silicone serum separator | Serum | 4.4–7.6 mg/dL 2.3–6.6 mg/dL |

*Note:* Various laboratories may have different testing protocols and require other tube tops than those represented in this table. Consult your laboratory procedures manual for additional information regarding required collection tubes.

## Hematologic Tests

Hematologic tests are commonly performed in routine blood testing. These tests can be performed on venous or capillary whole blood samples. Hematologic tests include blood cell counts, morphologic studies, coagulation tests, and the nonautomated erythrocyte sedimentation rate test.

**Blood Counts.** Whole blood, as described earlier, contains the formed elements (RBCs, WBCs, platelets) and the fluid portion (plasma). The total number of blood cells and the percentage of the whole sample that each type represents can tell the physician a great deal about a patient's condition. A physician can order an individual test or a complete blood (cell) count (CBC), which includes the following tests:

- Red blood (cell) count, which is the total number of RBCs in a sample
- White blood (cell) count, which is the total number of WBCs in a sample

- Differential WBC count, which is the percentage of each type of WBC (basophils, eosinophils, neutrophils, lymphocytes, and monocytes) in the first 100 leukocytes of a sample
- Platelet count (automated), which is the number of platelets in a sample, or a platelet estimate, which indicates whether the amount of platelets is adequate
- Hematocrit determination, which identifies how much of the volume of a sample is made up of RBCs after the sample has been spun in a centrifuge; expressed as a percentage
- Hemoglobin determination, which measures the amount of hemoglobin by weight per volume in the sample

Most POLs use automated equipment for performing blood counts, but you need to understand how to perform blood counts manually. Check your state regulations and office policy to find out if you are allowed to perform differential blood counts. This competency provides a backup for the automated instrumentation and puts you in a better position to recognize unusual findings among automated results. All manual counts are estimates. The types of blood cell counts differ in sample preparation and in the equipment and methods used.

***Differential Cell Counts.*** You will prepare a blood smear slide and stain the smear for a differential cell count. Procedure 35-4 details preparation of a blood smear slide. When you carry out this process correctly, there will be a region of the slide where blood cells are dense but lie in a single plane (not stacked or bunched together.) This is the region where the cells are counted.

A polychromatic (multicolored) stain such as Wright's stain simplifies a differential cell count. The blue and red-orange dyes (methylene blue and eosin, respectively) stain cell structures in ways that identify each of the five types of WBCs. When stained, neutrophils have a dark purple nucleus and pale pink cytoplasm containing fine pink or lavender granules. Basophils have a purple nucleus and light purple cytoplasm that contains large, blue-black granules. Eosinophils can be identified by the purple nucleus and the bright orange granules in pink cytoplasm. Lymphocytes appear as a large, dark purple nucleus surrounded by a small amount of blue cytoplasm. The fifth type of leukocytes, monocytes, are the largest and have gray-blue cytoplasm. There are several types of blood staining kits. Follow the manufacturer's instructions when performing this procedure.

Figure 35-19 shows the zigzag pattern for counting leukocytes visible in the field when using the microscope's oil-immersion objective. A total of 100 leukocytes are counted and recorded on a differential counter. Each cell type is expressed as a percentage of the 100 leukocytes counted. The platelet count is averaged in 10 to 15 fields.

***Hematocrit.*** You measure a patient's hematocrit percentage by collecting a small sample of the patient's blood in a microhematocrit tube, sealing the tube, and spinning it in a centrifuge. This process is described in Procedure 35-5.

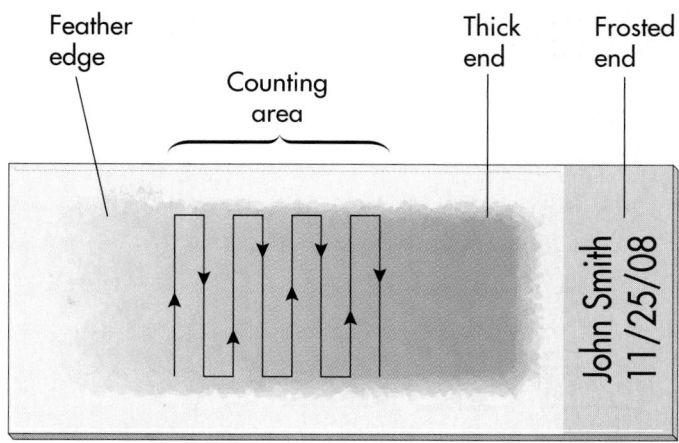

**Figure 35-19.** Follow this pattern when counting leukocytes visible in the field under the oil-immersion objective of the microscope.

During this process heavier RBCs move to one end of the tube, whereas lighter plasma moves to the other end. Between the RBCs, also called the **packed red blood cells,** and the plasma is the buffy coat (Figure 35-24). The **buffy coat** contains the WBCs and platelets.

Always run two samples of the patient's blood specimen. After removing each sample from the centrifuge, compare the column of packed RBCs with a standard hematocrit gauge. Read on the gauge the percentage of total blood volume represented by the RBCs. Average the readings of the two patient samples. (The samples should be within 2% of each other. If they are not, repeat the test.)

***Hemoglobin.*** Hemoglobin resides within the RBCs. You will determine the concentration of hemoglobin in the blood by lysing (rupturing) the RBCs (hemolysis) and evaluating the color of the sample. This procedure may be done with a hemoglobinometer—a handheld device that makes color evaluation less subjective than older methods of visual matching with color samples. Blood specimens mixed with a reagent, such as Drabkin's reagent, undergo a color reaction that can be quantified by reading color intensity in a photoelectric colorimeter.

Several automated hemoglobin analyzers are now included on the CLIA '88 waived list. These analyzers measure the amount of hemoglobin in a whole blood sample using a photometer (an instrument used to measure absorbed light). The blood sample can be obtained from a finger stick or from venous blood. Examples of the automated hemoglobin analyzers are HemoCue HB 301 Analyzer® (HemoCue AB) and the HemoPoint H2 Hemoglobin Measurement System® (Stanbio Laboratory). You should follow the manufacturer's instructions when performing these tests.

**Morphologic Studies.** **Morphology** is the study of the shape or form of objects. A morphologic study of a blood sample can provide important information about a patient's condition. During a morphologic study on blood,

# PROCEDURE 35.4

## Preparing a Blood Smear Slide

**Procedure Goal:** To prepare a blood specimen to be used in a morphologic or other study

### OSHA Guidelines

**Materials:** Blood specimen (either from a capillary puncture or a specimen tube containing anticoagulated blood), capillary tubes, sterile gauze squares, slide with frosted end, wooden applicator sticks

### Method:

1. Wash your hands and put on exam gloves.

2. If you will be using blood from a capillary puncture, follow the steps in Procedure 35-3 to express a drop of blood from the patient's finger. If you will be using a venous sample, check the specimen for proper labeling, carefully uncap the specimen tube, and use wooden applicator sticks to remove any coagulated blood from the inside rim of the tube. You may use a special safety transfer device if available.

### Rationale

Uncapping the specimen tube puts you at risk of exposure to blood-borne pathogens. The blood can spray or splatter or the tube could break. The safety device decreases the likelihood of exposure.

3. Touch the tip of the capillary tube to the blood specimen either from the patient's finger or the specimen tube. The tube will take up the correct amount through capillary action.

4. Pull the capillary tube away from the sample, holding it carefully to prevent spillage. Wipe the outside of the capillary tube with a sterile gauze square.

### Rationale

To remove excess blood

5. With the slide on the work surface, hold the capillary tube in one hand and the frosted end of the slide against the work surface with the other.

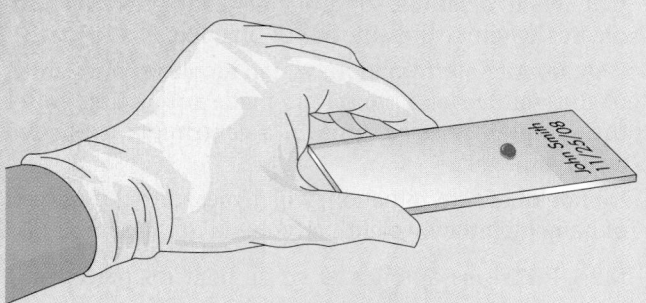

**Figure 35-20.** Apply a drop of blood to the slide about ¾ inch from the frosted end.

6. Apply a drop of blood to the slide, about ¾ inch from the frosted end, as shown in Figure 35-20. Place the capillary tube in the sharps container.

7. Pick up the spreader slide with your dominant hand. Hold the slide at approximately a 30- to 35-degree angle. Place the edge of the spreader slide on the smear slide close to the unfrosted end. Pull the spreader slide toward the frosted end until the spreader slide touches the blood drop (Figure 35-21). Capillary action will spread the droplet along the edge of the spreader slide.

### Rationale

So the sample can be thinly spread on the slide

8. As soon as the drop spreads out to cover most of the spreader slide edge, push the spreader slide back toward the unfrosted end of the smear slide, pulling the sample across the slide behind it, as shown in Figure 35-22. Maintain the 30- to 35-degree angle.

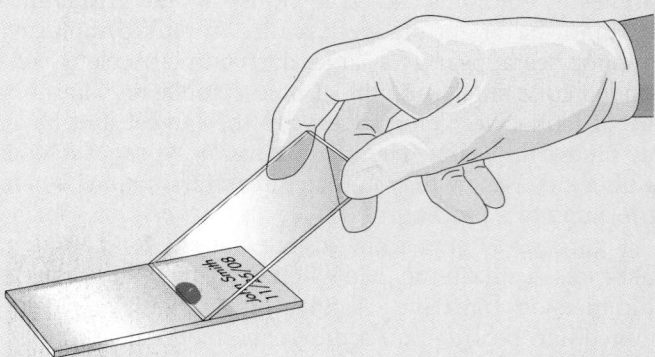

**Figure 35-21.** Hold the spreader slide at a 30-degree to 35-degree angle. Pull the spreader slide toward the frosted end until it touches the drop of blood.

*continued* ⟶

# PROCEDURE 35.4

## Preparing a Blood Smear Slide *(concluded)*

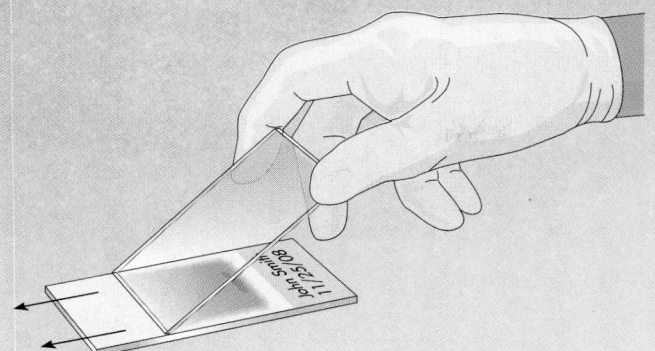

**Figure 35-22.** When the drop covers most of the spreader slide edge, push the spreader slide back toward the unfrosted end of the smear slide.

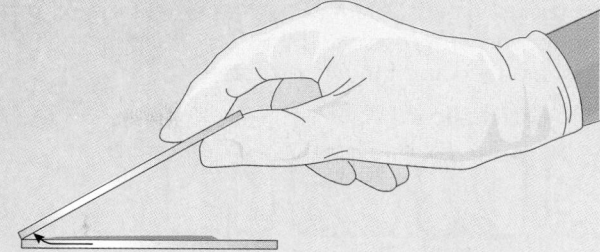

**Figure 35-23.** Push the spreader slide off the end of the smear slide, maintaining a 30-degree to 35-degree angle. The smear should be thicker on the frosted end of the slide.

9. Continue pushing the spreader until you come off the end, still maintaining the angle, as shown in Figure 35-23. The resulting smear should be approximately 1½ inches long, preferably with a margin of empty slide on all sides. The smear should be thicker on the frosted end of the slide.

10. Properly label the slide, allow it to dry, and follow the manufacturer's directions for staining it for the required tests.
11. Properly dispose of used supplies, and disinfect the work area.
12. Remove the gloves and wash your hands.

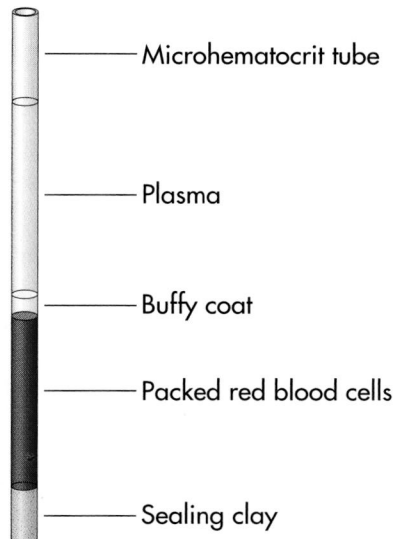

Microhematocrit tube

Plasma

Buffy coat

Packed red blood cells

Sealing clay

**Figure 35-24.** Blood in a centrifuged microhematocrit tube separates into packed red blood cells, the buffy coat, and plasma.

a blood smear is examined, and the appearance and shape of cells in the sample are recorded. Special note is made of abnormal cell size, shape, or content and abnormal organization of cells. A morphologic study is often performed just after the differential count and platelet estimate on the same blood smear slide. Morphologic studies require special training and are not routinely done by medical assistants.

**Coagulation Tests.** A physician may order coagulation tests to identify potential bleeding problems before surgical procedures. A regular schedule of coagulation tests may be ordered to monitor therapeutic drug levels when a patient is receiving medications such as heparin or warfarin (Coumadin). Coagulation studies include the prothrombin time (PT) and partial thromboplastin time (PTT) tests. These tests are usually performed using automated devices such as the Coaguchek Plus® (Boehringer Mannheim Diagnostics)or the Hemoshare INRatio System® (HemoSense, Inc.). These systems monitor the changing pattern of light transmission through the sample as coagulation occurs and calculate the INR (International Normalized Ratio). The INR measures the amount of time it takes for the test sample to clot and compares it to a reference average. This method was developed by the World Health Organization (WHO) so that samples from different labs can be compared. The INR is used to evaluate patients who are taking blood thinners such as warfarin. Medical assistants sometimes perform such coagulation studies.

# Measuring Hematocrit Percentage After Centrifuge

**Procedure Goal:** To identify the percentage of a blood specimen represented by RBCs after the sample has been spun in a centrifuge

## OSHA Guidelines

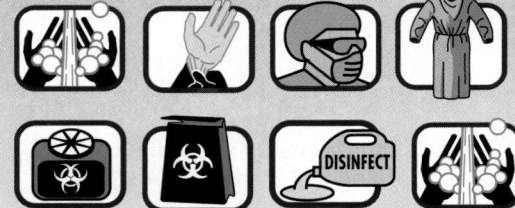

**Materials:** Blood specimen (either from a capillary puncture or a specimen tube containing anticoagulated blood), microhematocrit tube, sealant tray containing sealing clay, centrifuge, hematocrit gauge, wooden applicator sticks, gauze squares

## Method:

1. Wash your hands and put on exam gloves.

2. If you will be using blood from a capillary puncture, follow the steps in Procedure 35-3 to express a drop of blood from the patient's finger. If you will be using a venous blood sample, check the specimen for proper labeling, carefully uncap the specimen tube, and use wooden applicator sticks to remove any coagulated blood from the inside rim of the tube. Alternately, use a special safety transfer device if available.

*Rationale*
The safety device decreases the likelihood of exposure to blood-borne pathogens.

3. Touch the tip of one of the microhematocrit tubes to the blood sample, as shown in Figure 35-25. The tube will take up the correct amount through capillary action.

4. Pull the microhematocrit tube away from the sample, holding it carefully to prevent spillage. Wipe the outside of the microhematocrit tube with a gauze square.

*Rationale*
To remove excess blood

5. Hold the microhematocrit tube in one hand with a gloved finger over one end to prevent leakage, and press the other end of the tube gently into the clay in the sealant tray (Figure 35-26). The clay plug must completely seal the end of the tube.

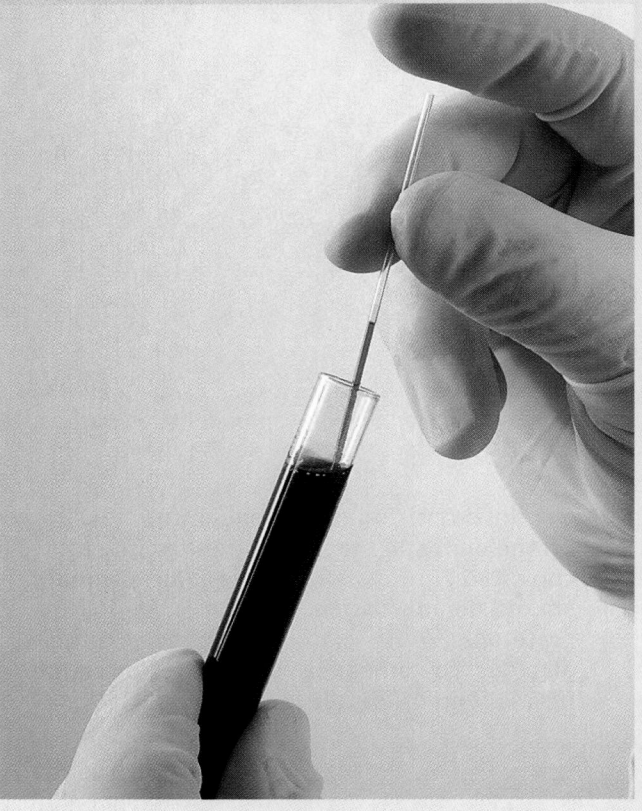

**Figure 35-25.** Touch the tip of one of the microhematocrit tubes to the blood specimen.

*Rationale*
The tube must be sealed to prevent the sample from being forced out of the tube during the spinning process.

6. Repeat the process to fill another microhematocrit tube. Tubes must be processed in pairs.

*Rationale*
To maintain a balance in the centrifuge

7. Place the tubes in the centrifuge, with the sealed ends pointing outward (Figure 35-27). If you are processing more than one sample, record the position identification number in the patient's chart to track the sample.

8. Seal the centrifuge chamber.

9. Run the centrifuge for the required time, usually between 3 and 5 minutes. Allow the centrifuge to come to a complete stop before unsealing it.

*continued* ⟶

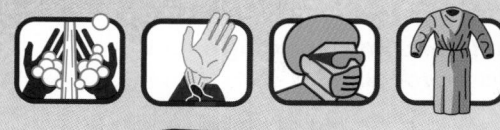

# PROCEDURE 35.6

## Measuring Blood Glucose Using a Handheld Glucometer

**Procedure Goal:** To measure the amount of glucose present in a blood sample.

### OSHA Guidelines

 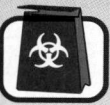 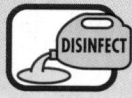 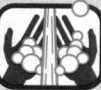

**Materials:** Safety engineered capillary puncture device (automatic puncture device or other safety lancet), antiseptic and cotton balls or antiseptic wipes, sterile gauze squares, sterile adhesive bandages, handheld glucometer, reagent strips appropriate for the device.

### Method:

1. Wash your hands and put on exam gloves.
2. Review the manufacturer's instructions for the specific device used.
3. Check the expiration date on the reagent strips.

### Rationale

To make sure they are not outdated

4. Code the meter to the reagent strips if required.

### Rationale

Some machines will need to be coded to account for small differences in the strips that occur during the manufacturing process.

5. Turn the device on according to the manufacturer's instructions.
6. Perform the required quality control procedures.

### Rationale

To ensure the machine is working as expected

7. Perform a capillary puncture following the steps outlined in Procedure 35-3.
8. Touch the drop of blood to the reagent strip, allowing it to be taken up by the strip.
9. Read the digital result after the required amount of time.
10. Record the time of the test and result on the laboratory slip.
11. Discard the reagent strip and used supplies according to OSHA standards.
12. Disinfect the equipment and area.
13. Remove the gloves and wash your hands.
14. Document the test results in the patient's chart. Record the quality control tests in the laboratory control log.

---

test in the office laboratory. These results are usually available in less than 10 minutes. Several home tests have recently become available. The patient can monitor his own HgBA1c levels, thus keeping a close watch on the efficiency of his diabetes treatment. FDA-approved home tests include:

- Bio-rad Micromat II Hemoglobin A1c Prescription Home Use Test
- Metrika InView A1c Multitest Monitor (for OTC Use)
- Provalis Diagnostics Glycosal II HBA1c
- Flex Site Diagnostics A1c at Home

Testing of HgBA1c should always be done in conjunction with routine blood glucose monitoring. Daily monitoring of blood glucose helps the patient with insulin therapy and diet maintenance. HgBA1c monitoring is important in assessing the patient's overall glucose levels. The advantages of this testing include:

- No pretesting preparation. The test may be done without regard to meals.

- Better overall assessment of long-term blood glucose control. Blood glucose testing gives information about glucose levels at one point in time. HgBA1c gives information over a period of 2 to 3 months.

Patients should have their HgBA1c levels checked two to four times per year. The target range for HgBA1c levels is less than 7%. Patients whose HgBA1c levels exceed 8% are at a greater risk for the complications associated with diabetes.

**Cholesterol Tests** Blood cholesterol tests are performed on a routine basis in the POL. There are several automated devices used for metabolic chemistry testing. Some of the analyzers test a variety of blood chemicals, including glucose, total cholesterol, HDL cholesterol, and triglycerides. Several of these devices may be used both in the POL and at home. The sample required is minimal and can be obtained with a capillary puncture.

FDA-approved waived tests include:

- Polymer Technology Systems CardioChek Analyzer® (Polymer Technology Systems, Inc.)

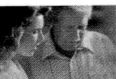
## Managing Diabetes

Diabetes affects an estimated 6 percent of the population, with more than 1 million newly diagnosed cases each year. In order to reduce the complications associated with diabetes, it is important for patients to maintain stable blood sugar. Proper patient education and medical care will help patients achieve this goal. As a medical assistant, you can assist patients and their families by providing them with information about diabetes that includes:

1. The risks and consequences associated with uncontrolled blood sugar. Patients whose blood sugar is unstable are at greater risk of developing the following conditions:
   - Loss of vision
   - Kidney failure
   - Heart disease
   - Nerve damage
   - Stroke

2. The patient's type of diabetes. Patients need to know the type of diabetes they have so that they can understand the type of treatment prescribed. The types of diabetes are:
   - Type I diabetes—An autoimmune disorder characterized by the body's inability to make enough insulin. Insulin is required for glucose utilization. Patients with Type I diabetes will need to take insulin daily.
   - Type II diabetes—The most common type of diabetes. Insulin is still being produced at normal levels but can no longer be utilized by the cells of the body. This causes a buildup of unused glucose in the blood. This type of diabetes is often controlled with careful diet management and increased exercise. There are also a number of oral medications used in the treatment of Type II diabetes.
   - Gestational diabetes—Develops only during pregnancy. This type of diabetes is generally managed through proper diet and exercise. Careful monitoring is important to reduce the risk of fetal complications. Women who have had gestational diabetes have an increased risk of developing Type II diabetes.

3. Maintaining proper diet and exercise. This should include:
   - Making proper food choices
   - Keeping a food diary
   - Reading food labels
   - Choosing proper food exchanges
   - Creating and implementing a routine exercise program

4. Routine self-monitoring of blood sugar and Hemoglobin A1c levels. Information should include:
   - The types of blood glucose monitors available. Figure 35-30 illustrates one type of blood glucose monitor, a glucometer.
   - Instructions on obtaining monitoring supplies
   - The number of times and the specific intervals at which blood sugar should be checked, based on individual needs and the physician's recommendations
   - Instructions on performing blood glucose testing
   - Guidelines on how to maintain a chart of blood glucose levels, including the time of

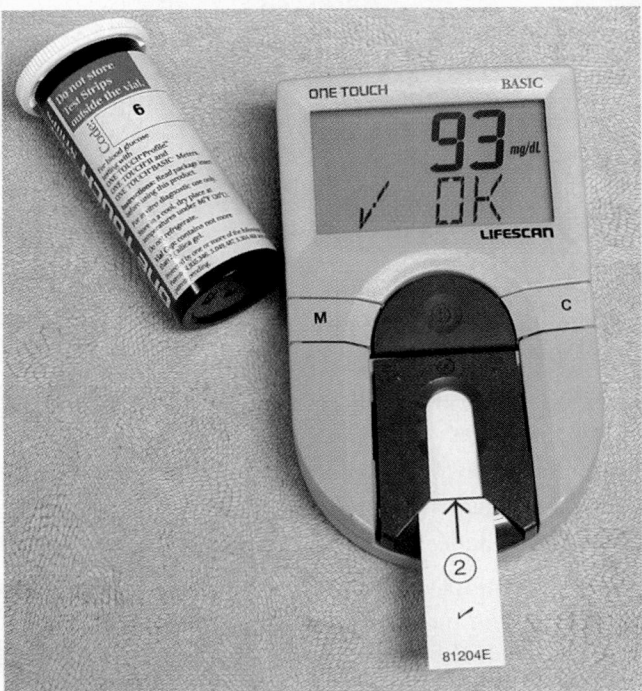

**Figure 35-30.** A handheld glucometer is an important tool in helping patients manage diabetes.

*continued* ⟶

## Managing Diabetes *(concluded)*

day, associated meals and activities, and actual blood sugar values

- Hemoglobin A1c monitoring. The patient should understand what Hemoglobin A1c is and why it is important to monitor these values.
- Normal (target) values for blood glucose and Hemoglobin A1c:
  - Blood glucose levels should remain between 90 and 130 mg/dL before meals and remain less than 180 mg/dL for 1 to 2 hours after a meal. Target ranges may be different for each patient. Consult with the physician about individual blood glucose levels.
  - Hemoglobin A1c is a test that shows the average amount of glucose in the blood over a three-month period. Ideally, this value should be less than 7%.

5. **Symptoms of uncontrolled blood sugar.** Patients need to be aware of the symptoms of both high and low blood sugar, both of which require immediate attention. Patients should test their blood sugar if any of the following occur:
   - Nausea, vomiting, or abdominal pain
   - Feeling tired all the time
   - Excessive thirst or dry mouth
   - Flushed skin
   - Confusion or difficulty thinking

6. **Self-screening for complications of diabetes.** Patients should be aware of the complications associated with diabetes and how to recognize them. Patients should be instructed to do the following:

- Perform a daily foot inspection for sores
- Recognize changes in vision
- Recognize the symptoms of kidney failure, which include nausea, vomiting, yellow skin, and swelling of the hands and feet
- Recognize early signs of nerve damage, which include numbness and tingling of the arms, hands, feet, or legs; dizziness; double vision; and drooping of the eyelid or lip

7. **Additional sources of information.** Patients should be encouraged to continue their education about diabetes. Providing patients with additional sources of information encourages them to take an active role in controlling their diabetes. Additional sources of information include:

   American Association of Diabetes Educators
   1-800-338-DMED

   American Diabetes Association
   1-800-DIABETES

   American Dietetic Association
   1-800-877-1600
   1-800-877-0877 (nutrition information hotline in English and Spanish)

   Centers for Disease Control and Prevention
   Diabetes Public Health Resource
   1-800-CDC-INFO (232-4636)

   Juvenile Diabetes Research Foundation
   International
   1-800-JDF-CURE

   National Institute of Diabetes and Digestive and Kidney Diseases
   National Diabetes Information Clearinghouse
   800-860-8747

---

- SpotChem HDL, Total Cholesterol, and Triglyceride® (Arkray, Inc.)
- Piccolo Total Cholesterol Test System® (Abaxis, Inc.)

## Serologic Tests

Serologic tests detect the presence of specific substances in a blood sample. The terms serologic test and immunoassay refer to the introduction of an antigen or antibody into the specimen and the detection of a specific reaction to the antigen or antibody. Serologic testing methods can be used to detect disease antibodies, drugs, hormones, and vitamins in the blood and to determine blood types. They are also used to test urine and other body fluids.

**Immunoassays.** Although medical assistants usually do not perform immunoassays, you should be familiar with several immunoassay methods that have common applications. These methods include:

- Western blot, in which antigens are blotted onto special filter paper for examination. Western blot tests are generally used to confirm HIV infection diagnosis.

- Radioimmunoassay (RIA), in which radioisotopes are used to "tag" antibodies. RIA tests are extremely sensitive and generally performed in a reference laboratory.
- Enzyme-linked immunosorbent assay (ELISA), in which enzyme-labeled antigens and substances that can absorb antigens generate reactions to specific antibodies. These reactions are identified through visual or photoelectric color detection. HIV infection is diagnosed using an ELISA test.
- Immunofluorescent antibody (IFA) test, in which dye, visible when the sample is examined under a fluorescent microscope, colors specific antibodies.

**Rapid Screening Tests.** Several serologic tests have been developed for quick processing. Some, such as early pregnancy tests performed on urine, are available for home use. There are also rapid screening tests for detecting antibodies to certain infections. Some of the rapid screening tests available for detection of antibodies are:

- Infectious Mononucleosis
  - LifeSign Status Mono (Princeton Boimeditech Corp.)
  - BioStar Acceava Mono II (Acon Laboratories, Inc.)
- HIV
  - Clearview HIV ½ Stat-Pak (Chembio Diagnostic Systems, Inc.)
  - Uni-gold Recombigen HIV Test (Trinity Biotech plc)

- *Helicobacter pylori*
  - Rapid Response *H. pylori* Rapid Test Device (Acon Laboratories, Inc.)
  - Beckman Coulter ICON HP Test (Princeton Biomedtech Corp.)

When you use tests of these types or explain their use to a patient, keep in mind that the manufacturer's guidelines must be carefully followed to ensure accurate results.

# Summary

Successful phlebotomy procedures require not only superior technical skills but also excellent interpersonal communication skills. When you are confident in your ability to perform venipuncture and capillary puncture techniques and in your understanding of common blood tests, you impart confidence to the patient. You should know what pretest instructions the patient should follow and what the patient can expect during the test.

As a medical assistant, you may be called on to complete certain testing procedures or to explain the purpose of tests to the patient. Therefore, it is important to understand the basics of blood composition and the common blood tests a patient might undergo. You can make the difference between a successfully drawn, accurately evaluated blood specimen and one that must be drawn again from a confused, unhappy patient.

# REVIEW

## CHAPTER 35

## CASE STUDY QUESTIONS

Now that you have completed this chapter, review the case study at the beginning of the chapter and answer the following questions:

1. What and where is the antecubital fossa?
2. What is the principle of the evacuated collection system?
3. How should you attempt to collect the blood on the second try?
4. What type of a blood test is a PT?
5. What could have caused the extensive bleeding this patient experienced after the venipuncture?

## Discussion Questions

1. Describe the medical assistant's role in the POL.
2. Identify the different methods of obtaining blood from a patient.
3. Describe the PPE you should use during phlebotomy procedures.
4. Identify the major components of whole blood.

## Critical Thinking Questions

1. How would you adequately prepare a patient for drawing a blood test?
2. Identify the different blood collection tubes by their stopper color, additive, and the testing usually performed with those tubes.
3. What complications may arise as a result of a venipuncture?

## Application Activities

1. With a partner, practice each step of the capillary puncture process on each other until you can smoothly execute each step. Critique each other's work.
2. Practice creating a smoothly drawn smear slide. Have a classmate critique your work.
3. Using a handheld glucometer, demonstrate the proper procedure for obtaining a blood glucose reading.

## Virtual Fieldtrip

*Visit the McGraw-Hill Higher Education Medical Assisting website at www.mhhe.com/medicalassisting3 to complete the following activity:*

Use the National Institute for Occupational Safety and Health, Bloodborne Infectious Diseases HIV/AIDS, Hepatitis B Virus, and Hepatitis C Virus website to research laws in your state that add additional safeguards for health-care workers at the state level.

Open the CD and complete this chapter's practice activities, play the games, listen to the key terms, and test yourself with the interactive review. Email, print, and/or save your results to document your proficiency.

# SECTION 5

# NUTRITION, PHARMACOLOGY, AND DIAGNOSTIC EQUIPMENT

# Nutrition and Special Diets

## MEDICAL ASSISTING COMPETENCIES

*In preparation for the certification examination, you should know the following areas of competence:*

| COMPETENCY | CMA | RMA |
|---|---|---|
| **General/Legal/Professional** | | |
| Determine the needs for documentation and reporting, and document accurately and appropriately | X | X |
| Instruct individuals according to their needs | X | X |
| Provide patients with methods of health promotion and disease prevention | X | X |
| Identify community resources and information for patients and employers | X | X |

## KEY TERMS

amino acid
anabolism
anorexia nervosa
antioxidant
behavior modification
bulimia
calorie
cholesterol
complete protein
complex carbohydrate
fiber
food exchange
incomplete protein
mineral
parenteral nutrition
saturated fat
skinfold test
unsaturated fat
vitamin

## CHAPTER OUTLINE

- The Role of Diet in Health
- Daily Energy Requirements
- Nutrients
- Dietary Guidelines
- Assessing Nutritional Levels
- Modifying Diets
- Eating Disorders
- Patient Education

## LEARNING OUTCOMES

After completing Chapter 36, you will be able to:

**36.1** Explain why a medical assistant needs to understand the role of diet in health.

**36.2** Describe how the body uses food.

**36.3** Explain the role of calories in the diet.

**36.4** Identify the seven basic food components and explain the major functions of each.

**36.5** List the Dietary Guidelines for Americans.

**36.6** Explain how the Food Guide Pyramid can be used to plan a nutritious, well-balanced diet.

**36.7** Describe the test used to assess body fat.

**36.8** Identify types of patients who require special diets and the modifications required for each group.

**36.9** Identify specific modified diets that may be ordered to treat or prevent certain conditions.

**36.10** Describe the warning signs, symptoms, and treatment for eating disorders.

**36.11** Describe techniques the medical assistant can use to effectively educate different types of patients about nutritional requirements.

**36.12** Explain the medical assistant's role in educating patients about nutrition and describe the proper documentation of patient education.

# Introduction

Nutrition is the process of how the body takes in and utilizes food and other sources of nutrients. It is a five-part process that includes intake, digestion, absorption, metabolism, and elimination. This chapter gives you an understanding of how a well-planned diet can lead to optimal health and well-being for your patients. You will also gain the knowledge needed to recognize the signs of illness related to diet.

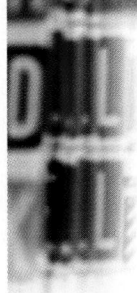

## CASE STUDY

A 17-year-old female cheerleader is brought to her family doctor by her parents. As the medical assistant, you take her history and physical, noting that she has no medical problems. The patient mentions that she has a lack of interest in food because she is being "careful not to eat too many calories" so she can keep her weight down and have a chance to be head cheerleader next year. She tells you she plans to try out for a cheerleading scholarship next fall and is preparing for the competition.

You note her vital signs:

Blood pressure: 100/60
Height: 5' 1"
Weight: 78 lbs.
Pulse rate: 40

She appears dehydrated and exhibits signs of muscle weakness.

As you read this chapter, consider the following questions:

1. What is the patient's probable diagnosis?
2. Do you think that the patient's attention to calorie intake is simply, as she says, preparation for the cheerleading competition?
3. Why is this patient experiencing muscle weakness?

# The Role of Diet in Health

You need to know what effect food has on health so that you can help patients meet their dietary requirements. Food is the body's source of nutrients, or substances the body needs to function properly. As you study nutrition, you learn how the body uses nutrients as well as how and why people eat. People need specific types of foods to stay healthy or to regain their health after illness or surgery. People with specific conditions may also need to follow special diets.

You will work closely with the rest of the medical team to ensure that patients understand the role of diet in health and that they adhere to any diet prescribed by their physician or dietitian. A registered dietitian (RD) is a professional who uses the science of nutrition to design ways for people to obtain their optimal nourishment. Dietetics plays an important role in the health field. Dietitians work with physicians and the rest of the medical team to plan diets that are both therapeutic and realistic for patients.

# Daily Energy Requirements

The human body requires the nutrients in food for three major purposes:

1. To provide energy
2. To build, repair, and maintain body tissues
3. To regulate body processes

A person's daily energy requirements depend on many factors. To understand the relationship of food to good health, you need to understand how the body uses food.

## Metabolism

Food must be broken down before the body can use it. This process is an integral part of metabolism. Metabolism is the sum of all the cellular processes that build, maintain, and supply energy to living tissue. During metabolism

## TABLE 36-1 Calories Burned per Hour in Selected Activities

| Activity | 120-lb Person | 190-lb Person |
|---|---|---|
| Bicycling | 360 | 570 |
| Football (touch) | 288 | 456 |
| Calisthenics | 324 | 516 |
| Handball | 456 | 720 |
| Hiking | 300 | 480 |
| Running (10 mph) | 720 | 1140 |
| Skiing<br>    (downhill)<br>    (cross-country) | <br>426<br>564 | <br>672<br>888 |
| Soccer | 456 | 720 |
| Swimming | 228 | 366 |
| Tennis | 330 | 522 |
| Volleyball | 258 | 408 |
| Walking (2 mph) | 156 | 252 |

Source: Adapted from Marvin R. Levy et al., *Life & Health: Targeting Wellness* (New York: McGraw-Hill, 1992).

body tissue is built up and broken down, and heat and energy are produced.

Metabolism takes place in two phases. In **anabolism,** substances such as nutrients are changed into more complex substances and used to build body tissues. In catabolism, complex substances, including nutrients and body tissues, are broken down into simpler substances and converted into energy. The body uses this energy to maintain and repair itself. Of the energy people get from the food they eat, about 25% is directly used for bodily functions, and the rest becomes heat.

Each person's body requires a minimal amount of nutrients to carry on a basic level of metabolism to live. Each person's daily nutritional requirements vary with age, weight, percentage of body fat, activity level, state of health, and other variables. The body's metabolic rate, or speed of metabolism, can also be affected by many factors, such as pregnancy, malnutrition, and disease.

## Calories

The amount of energy a food produces in the body is measured in kilocalories. A kilocalorie, commonly called a **calorie,** is the amount of energy needed to raise the temperature of 1 kilogram of water by 1°C. Foods differ in the number of calories they contain. The more calories in a food, the more available energy it has. Calories are also used to measure the energy the body uses during all activities and metabolic processes.

As mentioned, people's daily nutritional needs differ, depending on variables of age, weight, percentage of

body fat, activity level, and state of health. If people eat an excess of calories—more than the body can use—the excess is stored as fat in the body. Conversely, lowering caloric intake causes the body to burn off stored fat for energy.

Depending on the food's weight (in grams) or volume, each food has a value in calories. Therefore, you can count the number of calories a person consumes by monitoring food intake and adding up the calories in each food serving. You can use a food calorie counter, such as those often found in cookbooks and in nutrition books, to look up caloric values. A calorie counter tells you, for instance, that 1 cup of cooked carrots contains 50 calories or that 1 cup of cooked corn kernels contains 130 calories. Calories are also listed on the labels of food packages.

You can estimate the number of calories a person burns during certain activities by consulting a chart similar to Table 36-1. You can see how many more calories a 190-pound person burns than a 120-pound person does during the same activity.

## Nutrients

The body needs a variety of nutrients for energy, growth, repair, and basic processes. Seven basic food components provide these nutrients and work together to help keep the body healthy:

1. Proteins
2. Carbohydrates
3. Fiber

4. Lipids
5. Vitamins
6. Minerals
7. Water

As the body digests foods that contain these components, it breaks them down so that it can use them. Of the seven components, only proteins, carbohydrates, and fats contain calories and provide the body with energy. The rest perform a variety of other essential functions.

## Proteins

Protein is the most essential nutrient for building and repairing cells and tissue. Therefore, it is especially important for people to get enough protein during illness and healing. Other major functions of protein are to:

- Help maintain the body's water balance
- Assist with antibody production and disease resistance
- Help maintain body heat

The body makes protein out of **amino acids,** which are natural organic compounds found in plant and animal foods. Besides being used to build and maintain tissue, protein can be broken down to produce energy, especially if other energy sources are low. Each gram of protein contains 4 calories. Excess protein is broken down by the body and contributes to fat stores.

The optimal level of protein in a healthy person's diet is 10% to 20% of total caloric intake. More protein may be required during illnesses and recovery from injury. A deficiency in protein leads to weight loss and fatigue, malnutrition, extremely dry skin, lowered resistance to infection, and interference with normal growth processes.

**Complete Proteins.** There are 20 amino acids that are absolutely necessary to the body. The body can make 11 of them itself, but the remaining 9—called the essential amino acids—must be obtained through diet. Proteins that contain all 9 essential amino acids are called **complete proteins.** Complete proteins are found in animal food sources such as meat, fish, poultry, eggs (both the yolk and the white), and milk. (See Figure 36-1.)

Adults who eat meat products are advised to eat lean meats to avoid ingesting too much fat, which can be harmful. For instance, poultry, especially if it is eaten without the skin and prepared by a low-fat cooking method such as grilling, is a good lean-meat choice. Low-fat or skim milk can be substituted for whole milk (except for children younger than the age of 2, who need more fat in their diet than do older children and adults).

**Incomplete Proteins.** Individual plant sources of food do not provide complete proteins. They provide **incomplete proteins**—proteins that lack one or more of the essential amino acids. Various plant sources such as nuts, dry beans, grains, and vegetables can be

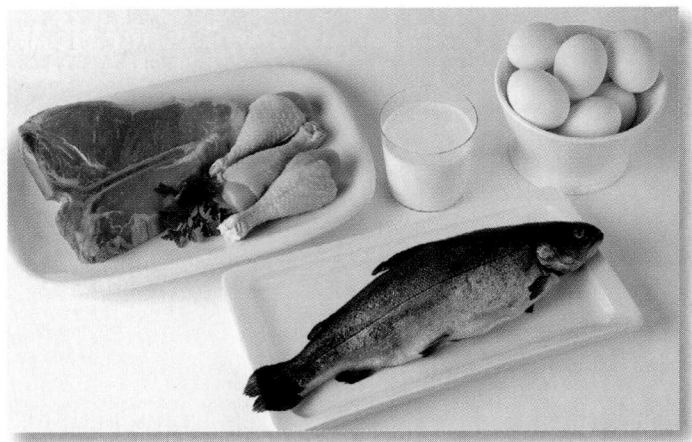

**Figure 36-1.** Foods such as meat, fish, poultry, eggs, and milk are complete proteins because they contain all the essential amino acids.

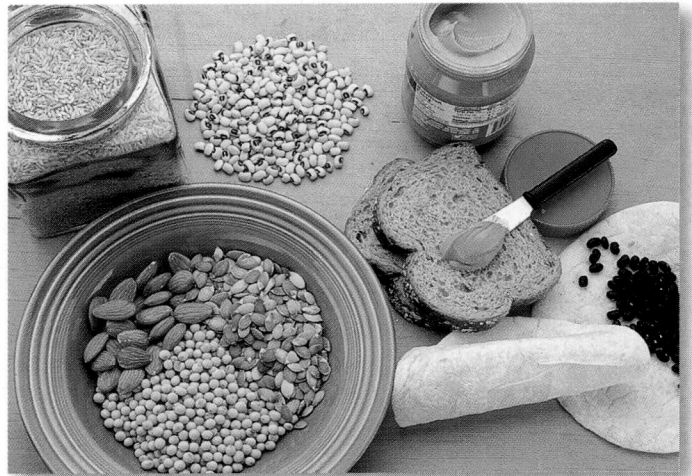

**Figure 36-2.** These foods, which contain incomplete protein, can be combined to make complete proteins.

combined, however, to provide all nine essential amino acids.

Planning for adequate protein intake and learning to combine protein foods to obtain all the essential amino acids are especially important for vegetarians (people who do not eat meat). Types of vegetarians include lacto-ovo-vegetarians, who eat no animal products except eggs and dairy products, and vegans, who eat no animal or dairy products at all. Although vegetarians may have to eat a larger quantity of foods than nonvegetarians to meet their daily nutritional needs, their diet offers advantages that include greater fiber intake and less fat. Figure 36-2 shows types of incomplete protein foods, such as rice and beans that can be used in combination to provide complete proteins.

# Carbohydrates

Carbohydrates in food provide about two-thirds of a person's daily energy needs. Carbohydrates also provide heat, help metabolize fat, and help reserve protein for uses other than supplying energy. Each gram of carbohydrate contains 4 calories. The daily requirement for carbohydrates is 50% to 60% of total caloric intake. Carbohydrate deficiency leads to weight loss, protein loss, and fatigue.

There are two basic types of carbohydrates:

1. Simple sugars, found in fruits, some vegetables, milk, and table sugar
2. Complex carbohydrates, found in grain foods, such as breads, pastas, cereals, and rice; in some fruits and vegetables, such as potatoes, corn, broccoli, apples, and pears; and in legumes, such as peas, peanuts, and beans

Simple sugars are small molecules that consist of 1 or 2 sugar (saccharide) units. **Complex carbohydrates,** or polysaccharides, are long chains of sugar units. Starch is a type of complex carbohydrate that is a major source of energy from foods of plant origin. Fiber, another type of complex carbohydrate, is discussed in the next section.

Carbohydrates used for immediate fuel are converted to glucose, a simple sugar that cells use for energy. An excess of carbohydrates is either stored in the liver and muscle cells as glycogen (long chains of glucose units—the animal equivalent of starch) or converted into and stored as fat. After the body's carbohydrate reserves are depleted, it starts burning fat. Healthful, nutritive sources of carbohydrates include fruits and vegetables, pasta, cereal, and potatoes (Figure 36-3). The American Dietetic Association suggests natural sources of carbohydrates with an emphasis on complex carbohydrates, such as vegetables, legumes, and whole grain breads and cereals. Sugary foods, such as sweet desserts, candy, and soft drinks, also contain carbohydrates, but they are high in calories and low in nutritional value.

# Fiber

**Fiber** is in a separate category, although it is a type of complex carbohydrate. Fiber does not supply energy or heat to the body. It is the tough, stringy part of vegetables and grains. Fiber is not absorbed by the body, but it serves these important digestive functions:

- Increasing and softening the bulk of the stool, thus promoting normal defecation
- Absorbing organic wastes and toxins in the body so that they can be expelled
- Decreasing the rate of carbohydrate breakdown and absorption

Therapeutically, fiber can help treat and prevent constipation, hemorrhoids, diverticular disease, and irritable bowel syndrome. It is linked to reduced blood cholesterol levels, reduction of gallstone formation, control of diabetes, and reduction in the risk of certain types of cancer and other diseases. Too little fiber can result in an increased risk of colon cancer, hypercholesterolemia (high blood cholesterol), and increased blood glucose levels after eating. Too much fiber can cause constipation, diarrhea, and other gastrointestinal disorders and can impair mineral absorption.

The recommended amount of fiber for adults is 20 to 35 grams a day. Because fiber works in conjunction with other substances and nutrients, it is advisable to get dietary fiber from a variety of food sources (Figure 36-4). Adequate water intake is especially important for fiber to work properly.

Fiber can be classified as soluble or insoluble. Soluble fiber, found in foods such as oats, dry beans, barley, and some fruits and vegetables, is the type that tends to absorb fluid and swell when eaten. It slows the absorption of food from the digestive tract, helps control the blood sugar level of diabetics, lowers blood cholesterol levels, and softens and increases the bulk of stools. Insoluble fiber, found in the bran in whole wheat bread and brown rice, for example, promotes regular bowel movements by contributing to stool bulk.

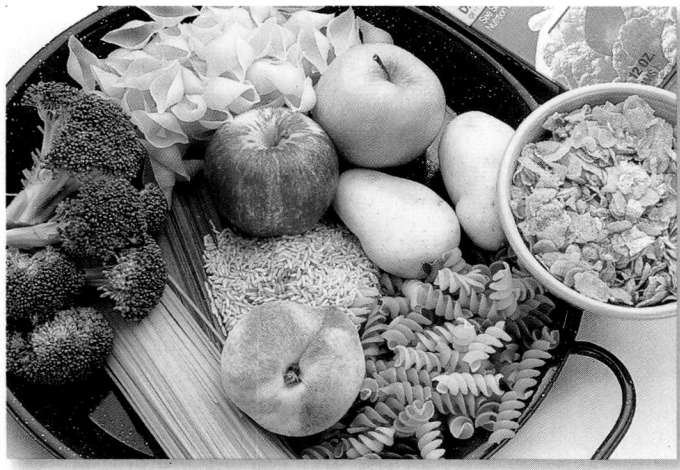

**Figure 36-3.** Healthful sources of carbohydrates are plentiful.

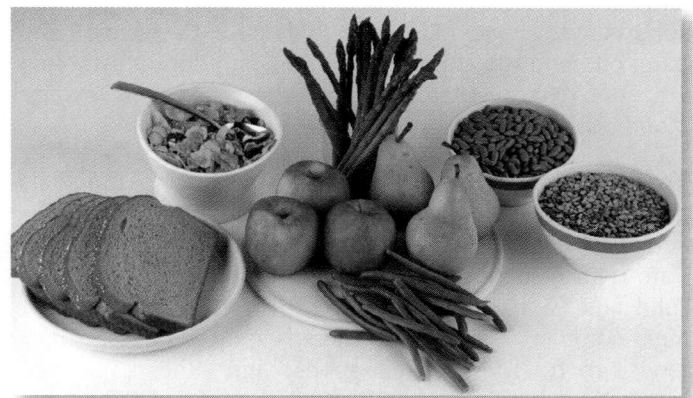

**Figure 36-4.** Dietary fiber serves many functions in the human body and is considered a basic food component.

# Lipids

Lipids in the diet include dietary fats and fat-related substances. Fats are a concentrated source of energy that the body can store in large amounts. Each gram of fat contains 9 calories (more than twice the calorie content of proteins and carbohydrates). About 95% of the lipids from plant and animal sources of food are fats. These simple lipids, or triglycerides, consist of glycerol (an alcohol) and three fatty acids. Chemical qualities of the fatty acids in a triglyceride determine the fat's characteristic flavor and texture. About 5% of dietary lipids are compound lipids such as cholesterol. Compound lipids are fat-related substances that are important components of cell membranes, nervous tissue, and some hormones. Compound lipids are vital to the transport of all fatlike substances within the body. Lipids assist with important body functions and are essential to growth and metabolism. Among this nutrient's jobs are the following:

- Providing a concentrated source of heat and energy
- Transporting fat-soluble vitamins
- Storing energy in the form of body fat, which insulates and protects the organs
- Providing a feeling of satiety, or fullness, because it is digested more slowly than other nutrients

A lipid deficiency can interfere with the body's absorption and utilization of vitamins and can cause fatigue and dry skin. An excess of lipids, particularly some dietary fats, however, can lead to increased levels of triglycerides and cholesterol in the blood and an increased risk of heart and artery disease and other diseases. It is recommended that adults obtain no more than 30% of their daily calories from fat sources. Cholesterol intake should be limited to 300 milligrams per day. People with heart disease and certain other diseases or risks may benefit from even lower levels of lipid intake.

**Saturated and Unsaturated Fats.** The fats in food can be classified as either saturated fats or unsaturated fats (Figure 36-5). **Saturated fats** are derived primarily from animal sources and are usually solid at room temperature. They are found in meats and animal products such as butter, egg yolks, and whole milk. Coconut oil and palm oil are also saturated fats. Consumption of saturated fats should be restricted because these fats tend to raise blood cholesterol levels.

**Trans Fats.** Also known as trans fatty acids, trans fats are a specific type of fat that is formed when hydrogen is added to vegetable oil through a process called hydrogenation. Hydrogenation is a process that turns liquid oils into solid fats. Trans fats can be found in vegetable shortenings, some margarines, crackers, candy, cookies, snack foods, fried foods, baked goods, and other processed foods. The U.S. Food and Drug Administration (FDA) recommends that individuals consume as close to zero grams as possible on a daily basis. The FDA currently requires that trans fat is displayed on all food labels.

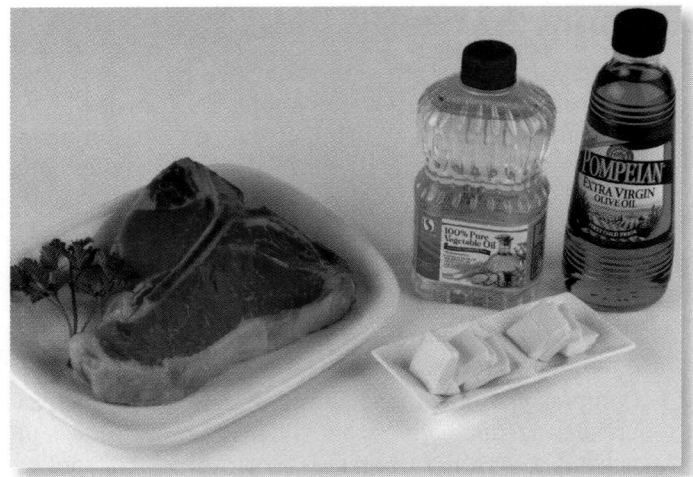

**Figure 36-5.** Foods that contain saturated fats include meat and butter. Most vegetable oils contain unsaturated fats.

**Unsaturated fats** are usually liquid at room temperature. They include most vegetable oils. Unsaturated fats can be divided into two classes:

1. Polyunsaturated fats, such as corn, soya, safflower, and sunflower oils
2. Monounsaturated fats, such as peanut, canola, and olive oils

Unsaturated fats can also be hydrogenated (have hydrogen added to their structures) so that they become solid at room temperature, as with margarine. Unsaturated fats tend to lower blood cholesterol.

The body needs essential fatty acids (primarily linoleic acid) for building and maintaining tissues. Because the body cannot produce these fatty acids, they must be supplied by food. Saturated fats in butter, egg yolks, and milk and unsaturated fats in corn, canola, sunflower, and safflower oils are good sources of essential fatty acids.

**Cholesterol.** **Cholesterol** is a fat-related substance produced by the liver that can also be obtained through dietary sources. Only animal-based foods contain cholesterol. It is essential to health because it:

- Serves as an integral part of cell membranes
- Provides the structural basis for all steroid hormones and vitamin D
- Serves as a constituent of bile, which aids in digestion

**Lipid Levels in the Blood.** Lipids, like other nutrients, are carried throughout the body in the bloodstream. When blood lipid levels become excessive, however, they pose certain risks. Doctors often order blood tests to determine the level of triglycerides and cholesterol in their patients' blood as a measure of overall health. High levels of cholesterol, especially if accompanied by high levels of triglycerides, may indicate an increased risk of heart disease, stroke, and peripheral vascular disease.

## TABLE 36-2  Saturated Fat and Cholesterol Contents of Various Foods

| Food | Saturated Fat (g) | Cholesterol (mg) |
|---|---|---|
| Cheddar cheese (1 oz) | 6.0 | 30 |
| Mozzarella, part skim (1 oz) | 3.1 | 15 |
| Whole milk (1 c) | 5.1 | 33 |
| Skim milk (1 c) | 0.3 | 4 |
| Butter (1 tbsp) | 7.1 | 31 |
| Mayonnaise (1 tbsp) | 1.7 | 8 |
| Tuna in oil (3 oz) | 1.4 | 55 |
| Tuna in water (3 oz) | 0.3 | 48 |
| Lean ground beef, broiled (3 oz) | 6.2 | 74 |
| Leg of lamb, roasted (3 oz) | 5.6 | 78 |
| Bacon (3 slices) | 3.3 | 16 |
| Chicken breast, roasted (3 oz) | 0.9 | 73 |

Source: U.S. Department of Agriculture.

Lipids are not soluble in water; fats (or oil) and water do not mix. Because the fluid portion of blood is 90% water, lipids are encased in large molecules that are fat-soluble on the inside and water-soluble on the outside. These large molecules, called lipoproteins, carry lipids such as cholesterol and triglycerides through the bloodstream. Low-density lipoproteins (LDLs) and high-density lipoproteins (HDLs) are the two main types of lipoproteins. Cholesterol in blood is identified as HDL or LDL, depending on which type of lipoprotein carries it. High levels of LDL cholesterol in blood are a primary risk factor for heart attacks. High levels of LDL cholesterol most commonly occur in people whose diets are high in saturated fats. HDL cholesterol, commonly referred to as good cholesterol, carries excess cholesterol away from arteries and back to the liver for breakdown and elimination. Patients can often reduce elevated cholesterol levels by increasing exercise and intake of soluble fiber and decreasing the dietary intake of saturated fats. These measures tend to elevate the level of HDL cholesterol in the bloodstream and reduce the level of LDL cholesterol. (Table 36-2 lists the saturated fat and cholesterol contents of various foods.)

## Vitamins

**Vitamins** are organic substances that are essential for normal body growth and maintenance and resistance to infection. Vitamins also help the body use other nutrients and assist in various body processes.

Most vitamins are absorbed directly through the digestive tract. They can be either water-soluble or fat-soluble. Water-soluble vitamins, such as vitamin C and the B vitamins, are not stored by the body and therefore must be replaced every day. Fat-soluble vitamins, such as vitamins A, D, E, and K, are stored for longer periods.

The amounts of vitamins the body needs are relatively small; however, a vitamin deficiency through lack of ingestion or absorption can lead to disease. Some vitamins can also cause health problems if taken in excess. Toxic levels of vitamin A, for example, can produce effects ranging from headache to liver damage. Because the level of vitamin intake is so essential to health, the Food and Nutrition Board of the National Research Council has established recommended dietary allowances (RDAs) for vitamins. For detailed information on specific vitamins, see Table 36-3.

Eating a well-balanced, nutritious diet minimizes the likelihood of vitamin deficiency. Many manufactured foods are also vitamin-fortified. Even so, some people choose to augment their diets with vitamin supplements (Figure 36-6). A physician or other member of the medical team may, in some instances, prescribe vitamin supplements for patients.

## Minerals

**Minerals** are natural, inorganic substances the body needs to help build and maintain body tissues and carry on life functions. Depending on the relative amounts the body requires, minerals fall into two categories:

1. Major minerals that the body needs in fairly large quantities, including calcium, magnesium, and phosphorus
2. Trace minerals that the body needs in tiny amounts, including iron, iodine, zinc, selenium, copper, fluoride, chromium, manganese, and molybdenum

## TABLE 36-3　Vitamins

| Vitamin | Functions | Adult RDA* | Food Sources | Deficiencies and/or Toxicities |
|---|---|---|---|---|
| Vitamin A (retinol, provitamin, carotene) | Aids in night vision; cell growth and maintenance; normal reproductive function; health of skin, mucous membranes, and internal tracts | Males: 900 µg retinol equivalents Females: 700 µg retinol equivalents | Milk fat; butter; egg yolks; meat; fish liver oil; liver; green, yellow, and orange leafy vegetables; yellow and orange fruits | Deficiency: night blindness; dry, rough skin; risk of internal infection Toxicity: headache, vomiting, joint pain, hair loss, jaundice, liver damage |
| Vitamin B$_1$ (thiamine) | Aids enzymes in breaking down and using carbohydrates; helps the nerves, muscles, and heart function efficiently | Males: 1.2 mg Females: 1.1 mg | Whole grains, brewer's yeast, organ meats, lean pork, beef, liver, legumes, seeds, nuts | Deficiency: beriberi with appetite loss, digestive problems, muscle weakness and deterioration, nervous disorders, heart failure |
| Vitamin B$_2$ (riboflavin) | Aids enzymes in metabolism of fats and proteins | Males: 1.3 mg Females: 1.1 mg | Dairy products, organ meats, green leafy vegetables, enriched and fortified grain products | Deficiency: cracks at lip corners, irritations at nasal angles, inflammation of the tongue, seborrheic dermatitis, anemia |
| Vitamin B$_3$ (niacin) | Aids enzymes in metabolism of carbohydrates and fats | Males: 16 mg Females: 14 mg | Meat, fish, poultry, enriched and fortified grain products | Deficiency: pellagra with dermatitis, diarrhea, inflammation of mucous membranes, dementia Toxicity: dilation of blood vessels; if sustained, abnormal liver function |
| Vitamin B$_6$ (pyridoxine) | Aids enzymes in synthesis of amino acids | Males: 1.7 mg Females: 1.3–1.5 mg | Chicken, fish, pork, liver, kidney, some vegetables, grains, nuts, legumes | Deficiency: convulsions, dermatitis, anemia Toxicity: loss of muscle coordination, severe sensory neuropathy |
| Folate (compounds) | Works with cobalamins in nucleic acid synthesis and metabolism of amino acids; maintains red blood cells | Males: 400 µg Females: 400 µg | Liver, yeast, legumes, green leafy vegetables, some fruits | Deficiency: glossitis, diarrhea, anemia, lethargy |
| Vitamin B$_{12}$ (cobalamins) | Works with folate in nucleic acid synthesis and metabolism of amino acids; coenzyme in metabolism of fatty acids | 2.4 µg | Seafood, meat, milk, eggs, cheese, brewer's yeast, blackstrap molasses | Deficiency: pernicious anemia, irreversible liver damage |

*continued* ⟶

TABLE 36-3 Vitamins *(concluded)*

| Vitamin | Functions | Adult RDA* | Food Sources | Deficiencies and/or Toxicities |
|---|---|---|---|---|
| Vitamin C (ascorbic acid) | Coenzyme involved in collagen production, capillary integrity, use of iron in hemoglobin, and synthesis of many hormones; improves absorption of iron; is an antioxidant | Males: 90 mg Females: 75 mg | Citrus fruits, mangoes, strawberries, green peppers, broccoli, potatoes, green leafy vegetables | Deficiency: scurvy with hemorrhages, loose teeth, poor wound healing Toxicity: stomachache, diarrhea |
| Vitamin D (calciferol) | Builds bones and teeth; helps maintain calcium-phosphorus balance in blood | 5–15 µg | Egg yolks; butter; liver; fortified milk, margarine, and prepared cereals | Deficiency: rickets in children, osteomalacia in adults Toxicity: excess blood calcium and phosphorus, calcium deposits in soft tissue, bone pain, irreversible kidney and cardiovascular damage |
| Vitamin E (group) | Is an intracellular antioxidant; maintains cell structure; aids in formation of red blood cells | 15 mg | Vegetable oils, margarine, shortening, wheat germ, nuts, green leafy vegetables | Deficiency: damage to cells, hemolytic anemia |
| Vitamin K (compounds) | Aids in blood clotting and bone growth | Males: 120 µg Females: 90 µg | Green leafy vegetables, milk, dairy products, meat, eggs, cereals, fruits, vegetables | Deficiency: slow blood clotting; hemorrhagic disease in newborns |

*RDAs may vary for different age groups.

Source: National Research Council, *Recommended Dietary Allowances*, 10th ed. (Washington, DC: National Academy Press, 1989).

Source for *Adult RDA:* National Academy of Sciences, 2002.

Minerals essential to good health include calcium, iron, iodine, zinc, copper, magnesium, phosphorus, fluoride, manganese, chromium, molybdenum, and selenium. Calcium, iron, and iodine are the minerals in which people are most often deficient. Most minerals are absorbed in the intestines, and any excess is eliminated.

**Minerals With Recommended Dietary Allowances.** There are several minerals for which RDAs have been established. These minerals are calcium, iron, iodine, zinc, magnesium, phosphorus, and selenium.

*Calcium.* Calcium builds healthy bones and teeth, aids in blood clotting, and helps nerves and muscles function properly. It is found in dairy products, green leafy vegetables, broccoli, legumes, and the soft bones of sardines and salmon (Figure 36-7).

Calcium deficiency can cause poor bone growth and tooth development in children, osteoporosis in adults, and poor blood clotting. The normal requirement is 800 to 1200 milligrams per day.

*Iron.* Iron, one of the most important nutrients, is essential for the production of red blood cells, which transport oxygen throughout the body. It is also a component of enzymes needed for energy production. Although iron is found in a wide variety of foods, it is the most frequently deficient nutrient in people's diets. Liver, meat, poultry, fish, egg yolks, fortified breads and cereals, dark green vegetables, and dried fruits are good dietary sources of iron (Figure 36-8), although less than 20% of it is usually absorbed.

Iron deficiency can cause anemia, a blood disorder that results in fatigue, weakness, and impaired mental abilities. At toxic levels iron may increase the risk of coronary heart disease (CHD). The daily requirement is 10 to 15 milligrams.

*Iodine.* Iodine plays a vital role in the activities of the thyroid hormones, which are involved in reproduction,

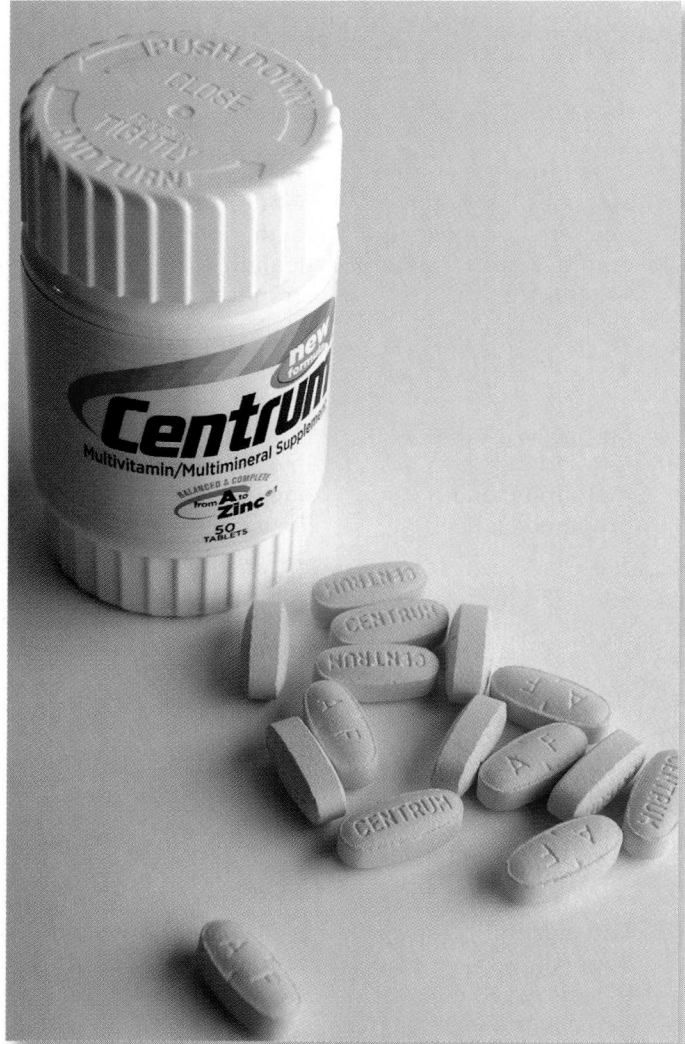

**Figure 36-6.** Some people use supplements to augment their dietary intake of vitamins.

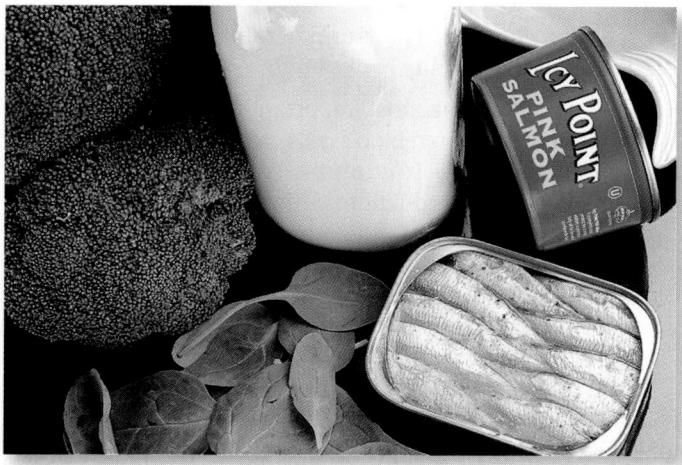

**Figure 36-7.** These foods are excellent sources of calcium, a mineral that is necessary for strong bones and teeth.

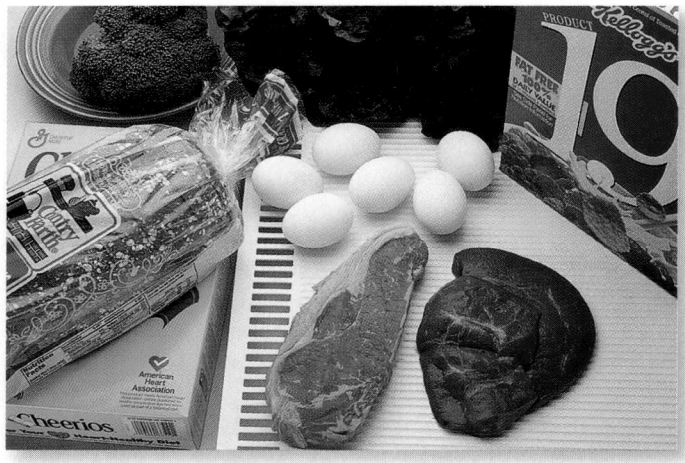

**Figure 36-8.** Iron, a mineral that is needed in small amounts, is found in a wide variety of foods.

growth, nerve and muscle function, and the production of new blood cells. Deficiency can cause an enlarged thyroid gland, known as goiter. Iodine can be obtained in seafood, iodized salt, and seaweed products. The daily requirement is 150 micrograms.

*Zinc.* Zinc promotes normal growth and wound healing and participates in many cell activities that involve proteins, enzymes, and hormones. It is found in liver, lamb, beef, eggs, oysters, and whole grain breads and cereals, although it is not always easily absorbed. Deficiency can result in growth retardation, impaired taste and smell, and reduced immune function. The daily requirement is 12 to 15 milligrams.

*Magnesium.* Magnesium activates cell enzymes, helps metabolize proteins and carbohydrates, maintains the structural integrity of the heart and other muscles, and aids in muscle contraction. Good sources include green leafy vegetables, nuts, legumes, bananas, and whole grain products. A deficiency may result from persistent vomiting or diarrhea, kidney disease, general malnutrition, alcoholism, and the use of certain medications. The daily requirement is 280 milligrams for women and 350 milligrams for men.

*Phosphorus.* Phosphorus is involved in bone and tooth formation, chemical reactions in the body, and energy production. It is found in dairy foods, animal foods, fish, cereals, nuts, and legumes. A deficiency of phosphorus can cause gastrointestinal, blood cell, and other disorders. Toxicity is harmful as well. The daily requirement is 800 milligrams for adults 25 and over.

*Selenium.* Selenium works with vitamin E to aid metabolism, growth, and fertility. It is found in seafood, kidney, liver, meats, grain products, and seeds. A daily dietary intake of 55 micrograms for women and 70 micrograms for men is recommended.

**Minerals With Estimated Safe and Adequate Dietary Intakes.** When data were sufficient to estimate a range of requirements—but insufficient for developing an RDA—the Food and Nutrition Board established a category of safe and adequate intakes for essential nutrients. The minerals in this category are copper, fluoride, chromium, manganese, and molybdenum.

***Copper.*** Copper interacts with iron to form hemoglobin and red blood cells. It can be obtained through a wide variety of foods, such as liver, seafood, nuts and seeds, and whole grain products. Copper deficiency can cause anemia and central nervous system problems. The safe and adequate range of dietary copper for adults is 1.5 to 3.0 milligrams per day.

***Fluoride.*** Fluoride is another contributor to bone and tooth formation, and it protects against tooth decay. Many municipal water supplies are fluoridated, and the mineral is also contained in saltwater fish, tea, and fluoridated toothpaste. Fluoride deficiency may predispose people to cavities and osteoporosis. Excess fluoride can cause discoloration and pitting of the teeth as well as other conditions. The range of safe and adequate intakes for adults is 1.5 to 4.0 milligrams per day.

***Chromium.*** Chromium is essential for the body to use glucose, the primary food of cells. Foods containing chromium include calf's liver, American cheese, and wheat germ. A range of intakes between 50 and 200 micrograms per day is considered safe and adequate for adults.

***Manganese.*** Manganese is part of several cell enzymes. It is also essential for bone formation and maintenance, insulin production, and nutrient metabolism. It is found in whole grain products, fruits, vegetables, and tea. A daily dietary intake of 2 to 5 milligrams for adults is recommended.

***Molybdenum.*** Molybdenum helps in the metabolism of the mineral sulfur and the production of uric acid. The best sources are legumes, whole grains, milk, and organ meats such as liver and kidneys. The recommended range for dietary intake is 75 to 250 micrograms per day for adults.

## Water

Water has no caloric value, but it contributes about 65% of body weight and is essential to the body's normal functioning. In general, water helps provide the body with other nutrients it needs and helps rid the body of what it does not need. Water has many functions, including these:

- Helping to maintain the balance of all the fluids in the body
- Lubricating the body's moving parts
- Dissolving chemicals and nutrients
- Aiding in digestion
- Helping to transport nutrients and secretions throughout the body
- Flushing out wastes
- Regulating body temperature through perspiration

The amount of water in the body directly affects the concentration and distribution of body fluids and all the functions related to them. The body maintains a careful balance between water consumed (in foods and beverages) and water lost (through urination, perspiration, and respiration). In a healthy fluid balance, water input equals water output. Measuring an ill person's level of water intake and output can help determine the best fluid replacement regimen to use.

People obtain most of their water from beverages such as tap water, milk, and fruit juices as well as coffee, tea, and soft drinks. On average, a person needs to drink six to eight glasses of water a day to maintain a healthy water balance. The daily need for water varies with size and age, the temperatures to which someone is exposed, the degree of physical exertion, and the water content of the foods one eats. Someone who is eating mostly foods with a high water content, such as fruits and vegetables, can drink a little less water than someone who is eating mostly foods with a low water content.

If people get too little water or lose too much water through vomiting, diarrhea, burns, or perspiration, they become dehydrated. Signs and symptoms of dehydration include dry lips and mucous membranes, weakness, lethargy, decreased urine output, and increased thirst. Severe dehydration can lead to hypovolemia, a reduction in the volume of blood in the body. Severe hypovolemia can result in inadequate blood pressure that affects the functioning of the heart, central nervous system, and various organs—a condition known as hypovolemic shock. If dehydration progresses so that water is lost from body cells, death usually occurs within a few days.

Procedure 36-1 explains how to educate patients to drink the right amount of water each day to prevent dehydration. Make sure patients know whether they are to drink extra fluids to replace fluids lost in an illness or to help rid the body of waste.

## Principal Electrolytes and Other Nutrients of Special Interest

The principal electrolytes are essential to normal body functioning. Other nutrients, such as antioxidants, also merit special mention.

**Principal Electrolytes.** Although the principal electrolytes in the body—sodium, potassium, and chloride—are often excluded from lists of nutrients, they are essential dietary components. Electrolytes play an important role in maintaining body functions, such as normal heart rhythm.

Sodium (Na) maintains fluid and acid-base balances, assists in the transport of glucose, and maintains normal conditions inside and outside cells. Salt is the main dietary source of sodium, and high salt intakes are normally associated with a diet high in processed foods. Too much sodium can be associated with high blood pressure in salt-sensitive individuals. Although many Americans consume far more, it is recommended that daily sodium intake be limited to 2.4 grams or less.

Potassium (K) is a crucial element in the maintenance of muscle contraction and fluid and electrolyte balance. It contributes to acid-base balance and the transmission of

# Educating Adult Patients About Daily Water Requirements

**Procedure Goal:** To teach patients how much water their bodies need to maintain health

**OSHA Guidelines:** This procedure does not involve exposure to blood, body fluids, or tissues.

**Materials:** Patient education literature, patient's chart, pen

**Method:**

1. Explain to patients the importance of water to the body. Point out the water content of the body and the many functions of water in the body: maintaining the body's fluid balance, lubricating the body's moving parts, transporting nutrients and secretions.

2. Add any comments applicable to an individual patient's health status—for example, issues related to medication use, physical activity, pregnancy, fluid limitation, or increased fluid needs.

### Rationale

Some elderly patients purposely limit their fluid intake because of incontinence or physical limitations that make getting to a bathroom difficult, so it is necessary to provide specific comments about their exact fluid needs.

3. Explain that people obtain water by drinking water and other fluids and by eating water-containing foods. On average, an adult should drink six to eight glasses of water a day to

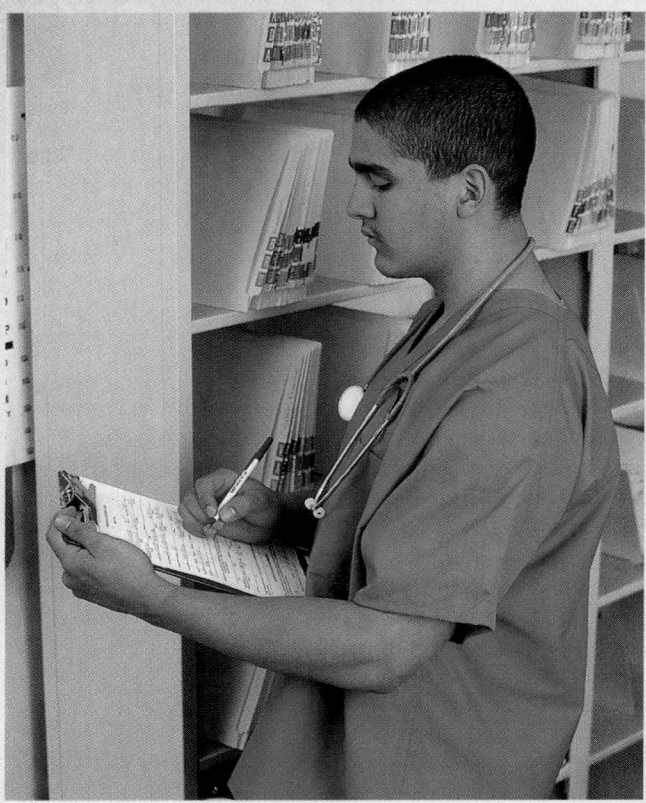

**Figure 36-10.** Always document patient education sessions in the patient's chart.

maintain a healthy water balance in which intake equals excretion. People's daily need for water varies with size and age, the temperatures to which they are exposed, degree of physical exertion, and the water content of foods eaten. Make sure you reinforce the physician's or dietitian's recommendations for a particular patient's water needs.

4. Caution patients that soft drinks, coffee, and tea are not good substitutes for water and that it would be wise to filter out any harmful chemicals contained in the local tap water or to drink bottled water, if possible.

5. Provide patients with tips about reminders to drink the requisite amount of water. Some patients may benefit from using a water bottle of a particular size, so they know they have to drink, say, three full bottles of water each day (Figure 36-9).

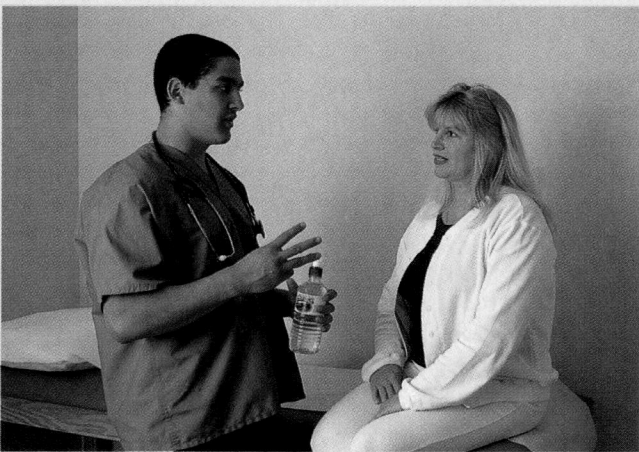

**Figure 36-9.** Using a personal water bottle that holds 16 ounces, the patient can make a point of drinking three to four full bottles daily.

*continued* ⟶

## Educating Adult Patients About Daily Water Requirements *(concluded)*

Another helpful tip is to make a habit of drinking a glass of water at certain points in the daily routine, such as first thing in the morning and before lunch.

6. Remind patients that you and the physician are available to discuss any problems or questions.

7. Document any formal patient education sessions or significant exchanges with a patient in the patient's chart, noting

whether the patient understood the information presented. Then initial the entry (Figure 36-10).

### Rationale

Many insurance companies require evidence of preventative health counseling and documentation is an important aspect of patient insurance coverage.

---

nerve impulses. Its role in fluid balance helps regulate blood pressure. Potassium occurs in unprocessed foods, particularly in fruits such as bananas, raisins, and oranges; many vegetables; and fresh meats (Figure 36-11). The minimum requirement is 1600 to 2000 milligrams per day. Chloride (Cl) is essential in maintaining fluid and electrolyte balance, and it is a necessary component of hydrochloric acid, secreted into the stomach during digestion of food. Because dietary chloride comes almost entirely from sodium chloride, sources are essentially the same as those of sodium.

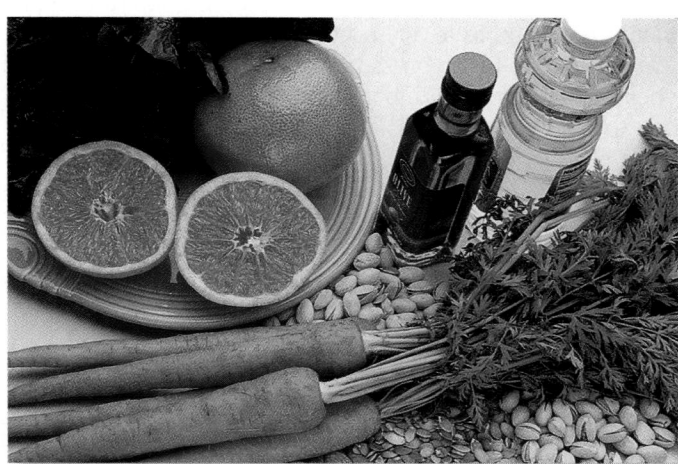

**Figure 36-12.** Antioxidants are substances in food that may offer protection against certain chronic diseases. Foods rich in beta-carotene, vitamin C, vitamin E, and selenium contain antioxidants.

**Antioxidants.** **Antioxidants** are chemical agents that fight certain cell-destroying chemical substances called free radicals. In fact, antioxidants may help ward off cancer and heart disease by neutralizing free radicals, by-products of normal metabolism that may also form as a result of exposure to various damaging factors such as cigarette smoke, alcohol, or x-rays. Antioxidants may be added to foods and cosmetics as preservatives. The nutrients beta-carotene, vitamin C, vitamin E, and selenium (Figure 36-12) are natural antioxidants.

## Dietary Guidelines

A variety of dietary guidelines exist to help people get proper nutrition, reduce the occurrence of disease, and control their weight. These recommendations, which are

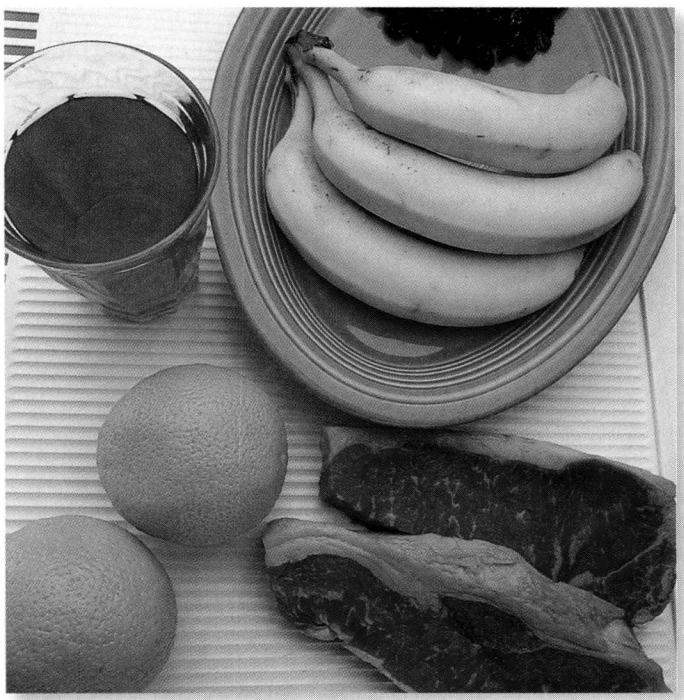

**Figure 36-11.** These foods are a good source of potassium.

issued by governmental agencies or private associations, are designed to encourage healthy eating habits.

Dietary guidelines suggest the types and quantities of food that people should eat each day. They may also contain recommendations about which types of foods to limit and which types of foods to increase.

## USDA Dietary Guidelines for Americans

The U.S. Department of Agriculture and the U.S. Department of Health and Human Services updated their Dietary Guidelines for Americans in 2005. These guidelines encourage people to eat a balanced diet, limit consumption of less nutritious foods, increase physical activity, and make good nutritional decisions consistently.

**Key Recommendations.** The 2005 USDA Dietary Guidelines recommend that you balance the food you eat with physical activity. They also recommend that you maintain or improve your weight to help reduce your chances of high blood pressure, heart disease, stroke, some types of cancer, and diabetes. Specific recommendations are the following:

*Maintain an adequate nutrient intake while monitoring caloric needs.*
- Consume a variety of nutritious foods from the basic good groups.
- Avoid foods that contain saturated fat, trans fat, sugar, and salt.
- Restrict alcoholic beverages.

*Weight Management*
- Maintain body weight in a healthy range.
- Balance calorie consumption with physical activity.
- Prevent gradual weight gain over time.

*Physical Activity*
- Engage in regular physical activity and reduce sedentary activities to promote health, psychological well-being, and a healthy body weight.

*Food Groups to Encourage*
- Consume a sufficient amount of fruits and vegetables while staying within energy needs.
- Choose a variety of fruits and vegetables each day.
- Consume three or more whole grains per day.
- Consume 3 cups of fat-free or low-fat milk or equivalent each day.

*Fats*
- Limit intake of fats and oils high in saturated and/or trans fatty acids. Choose foods that are low in such fats and oils.

*Carbohydrates*
- Choose fiber-rich fruits, vegetables, and whole grains often.

- Choose and prepare foods and beverages with little sugars.

*Sodium and Potassium*
- Consume less than 2300 mg (approximately 1 tsp of salt) of sodium per day.

*Alcoholic Beverages*
- Those who choose to drink alcoholic beverages should do so sensibly and in moderation.
- Alcoholic beverages should not be consumed by pregnant or lactating women, individuals who take medication that can interact, and children and adolescents.
- Avoid alcoholic beverages if engaging in activities that require skill and coordination.

*Food Safety*
- Take precautions while handling food, such as washing hands, disinfecting food surfaces, and washing fruit and vegetables.
- Separate raw, cooked, and ready to eat foods while shopping, preparing, and storing.
- Cook foods to a safe temperature.
- Refrigerate foods promptly and defrost foods properly.
- Avoid raw or partially raw foods such as eggs, meat, and unpasteurized milk or juices.

## USDA Food Guide Pyramid

In 2005, the U.S. Department of Agriculture introduced a new food pyramid. Continued research on obesity by the U.S. Department of Agriculture and the U.S. Department of Human Services led to the redesign of the food pyramid to include emphasis on eating more fruits, vegetables, whole grain foods, beans, and nuts, and to include less emphasis on carbohydrates. The new food pyramid is designed to help balance nutritional and physical activity needs (Figure 36-13). The new pyramid is color coded, with each color representing a food group:

- Orange represents grains
- Green represents vegetables
- Red represents fruits
- Yellow represents oils
- Blue represents milk products
- Purple represents meat and beans

In addition, the action figure represents physical activity.

To help patients plan a balanced diet, you will need to know how much of a food equals a serving. For example, one serving of fruit equals one medium apple or orange, ½ cup canned fruit, or ¾ cup (6 ounces) fruit juice. You should refer to a chart similar to Table 36-4, which lists serving sizes for foods in each of the basic food groups. Serving sizes for young children are smaller; for example, serving sizes for toddlers and preschoolers are about half the sizes listed in the table.

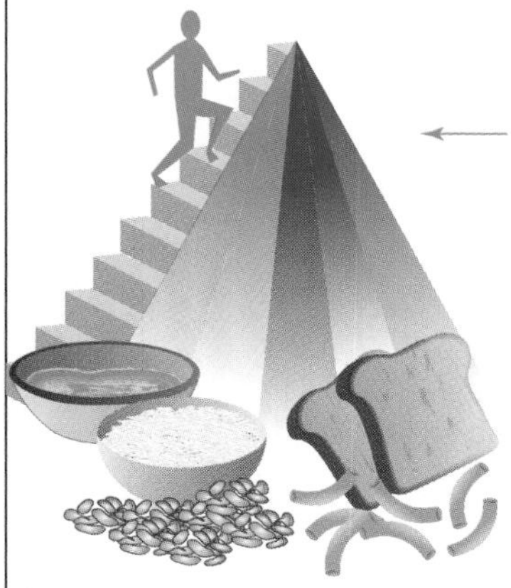

## Grains
**Make half your grains whole**

- Eat at least 3 ounces of whole grain bread, cereal, crackers, rice, or pasta every day

- Look for "whole" before the grain name on the list of ingredients

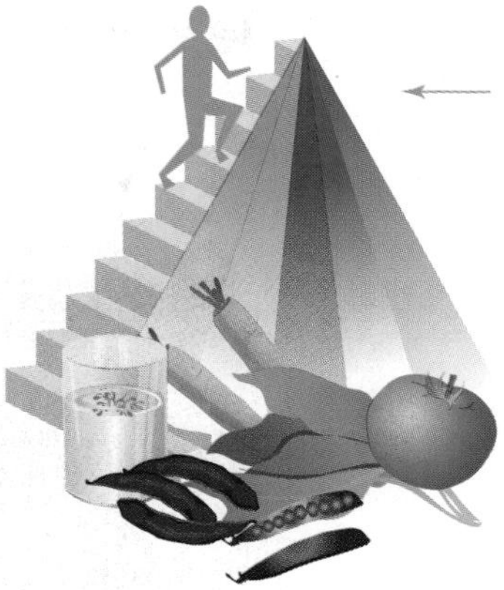

## Vegetables
**Vary your veggies**

- Eat more dark green veggies

- Eat more orange veggies

- Eat more dry beans and peas

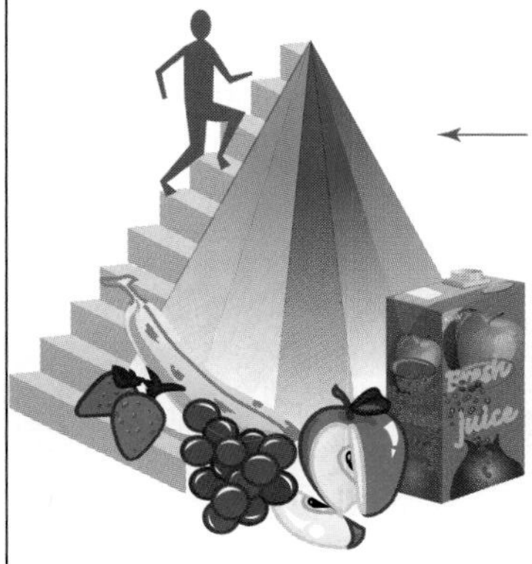

## Fruits
**Focus on fruits**

- Eat a variety of fruit

- Choose fresh, frozen, canned, or dried fruit

- Go easy on fruit juices

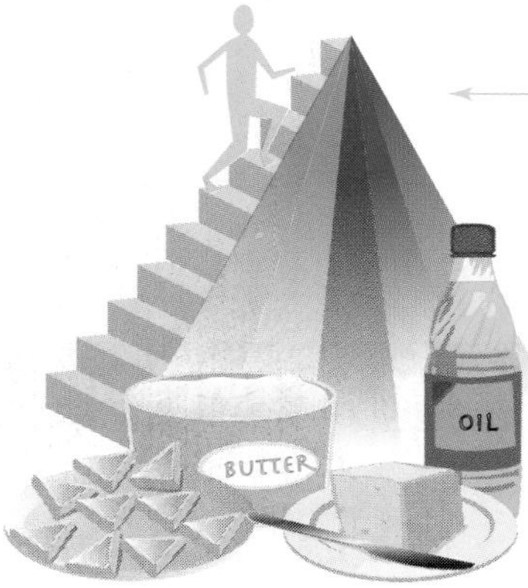

## Oils
**Know your fats**

- Make most of your fat sources from fish, nuts, and vegetable oils

- Limit soild fats like butter, stick margarine, shortening, and lard

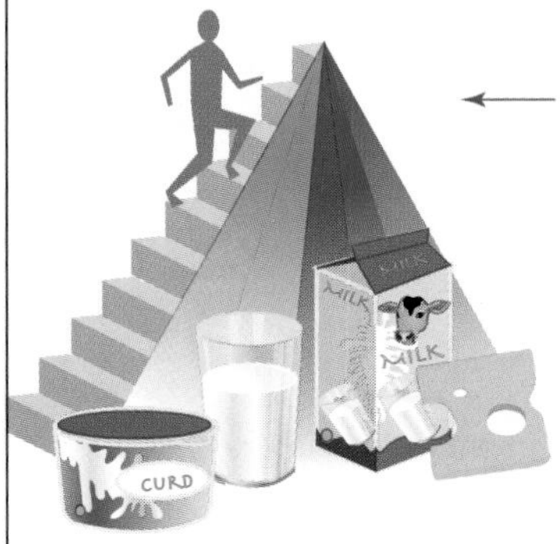

## Milk
**Get your calcium-rich foods**

- Go low-fat or fat-free

- If you don't or can't consume milk, choose lactose-free products or other calcium sources

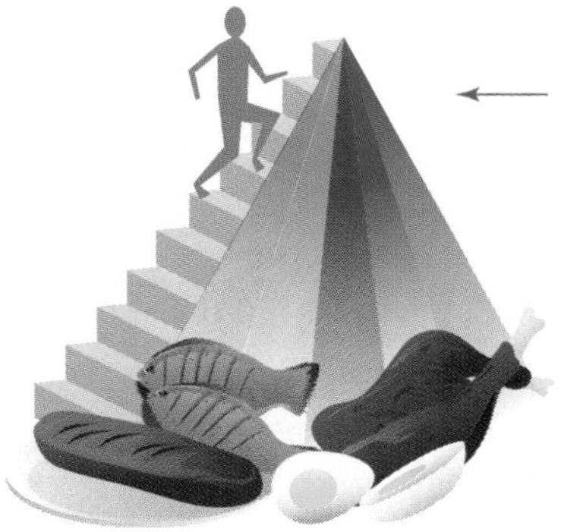

## Meat & Beans
**Go lean on protein**

- Choose low-fat or lean meats and poultry

- Bake it, broil it, or grill it

- Vary your choices—with more fish, beans, peas, nuts, and seeds

**Figure 36-13.** The U.S. Department of Agriculture's Food Guide Pyramid can be used to plan a nutritious, well-balanced diet.

## TABLE 36-4 What Counts as a Serving?

| Food Group | Food and Quantity |
|---|---|
| Bread, cereal, rice, and pasta | 1 slice bread<br>1 oz ready-to-eat cereal<br>½ c cooked cereal, rice, or pasta |
| Vegetable | 1 c raw leafy vegetables<br>½ c other vegetables, cooked or raw<br>¾ c vegetable juice |
| Fruit | 1 medium apple, banana, or orange<br>½ c chopped, cooked, or canned fruit<br>¾ c fruit juice |
| Milk, yogurt, and cheese | 1 c milk or yogurt<br>1½ oz natural cheese<br>2 oz processed cheese |
| Meat, poultry, fish, dry beans, eggs, and nuts | 2–3 oz cooked lean meat, poultry, or fish<br>½ c cooked dry beans or 1 egg counts as 1 oz lean meat<br>2 tbsp peanut butter or ⅓ c nuts counts as 1 oz meat |

Source: Nutrition and Your Health: *Dietary Guidelines for Americans*, 5th ed. (Washington, DC: U.S. Department of Agriculture and U.S. Department of Health and Human Services, 2000).

## TABLE 36-5 Number of Servings Required for Different Calorie Levels

| Calorie Level (Common Individuals in Group) | About 1600 (Many Women, Older Adults) | About 2200 (Children, Teen Girls, Most Men, Active Women) | About 2800 (Teen Boys, Active Men) |
|---|---|---|---|
| Grain products group servings | 5 | 7 | 10 |
| Vegetable group servings | 4 | 6 | 7 |
| Fruit group servings | 3 | 4 | 5 |
| Milk group servings | 3* | 3* | 3* |
| Meat and Beans group servings | 5 oz | 6 oz | 7 oz |
| Total Fat (g) | 20 g | 29 g | 36 g |

*Women who are pregnant or breast-feeding, teenagers, and young adults to age 24 need 3 servings.

Source: *Nutrition and Your Health: Dietary Guidelines for Americans*, 5th ed. (Washington, DC: U.S. Department of Agriculture and U.S. Department of Health and Human Services, 2005).

The Food Guide Pyramid is a general guideline. It does not provide exact information about what to eat. Nutritional needs vary from person to person, depending on age, gender, and activity level (see Table 36-5). That is why the pyramid lists ranges of servings.

Some patients may have special dietary preferences or choices. Vegetarians do not eat meat, poultry, and fish. In order to provide vegetarians with guidelines for healthful eating, the American Dietetic Association has developed a Food Guide Pyramid specifically for these individuals (Figure 36-14).

The U.S. government has developed a website that allows individuals to obtain a recommendation about their daily caloric and physical activity requirements by

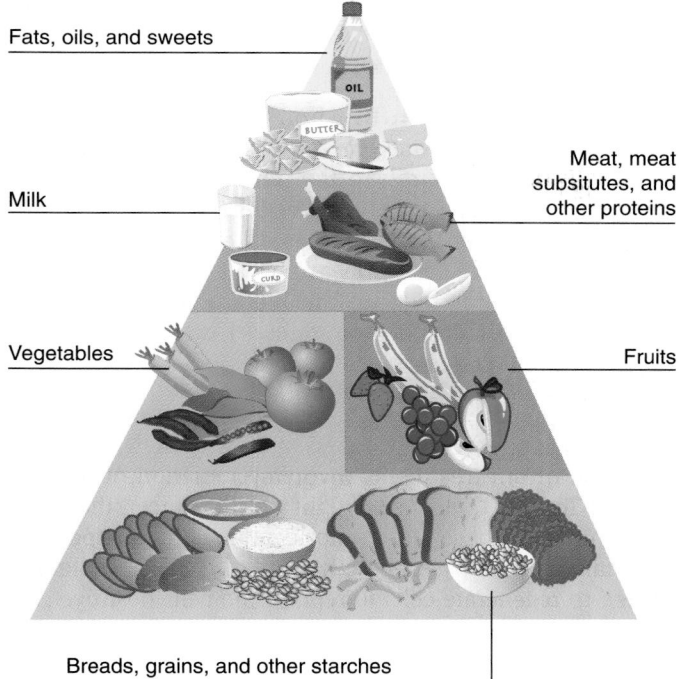

Fats, oils, and sweets

Milk

Vegetables

Meat, meat subsitutes, and other proteins

Fruits

Breads, grains, and other starches

**Figure 36-14.** The American Dietetic Association's Food Guide Pyramid for Vegetarian Meal Planning can provide vegetarians with suggestions for healthy, balanced nutrition.

entering information regarding their age, gender, and activity level.

## American Cancer Society Nutritional and Physical Activity Guidelines

The American Cancer Society updated their nutritional and physical activity guidelines in 2006 to aid in the prevention of cancer. Their suggestions include:

- Eating more high-fiber foods such as fruits, vegetables, and whole-grain cereals
- Eating five or more servings of a variety of vegetables and fruits each day
- Limiting the consumption of processed and red meats
- Adopting a physically active lifestyle
- Achieving and maintaining a healthy weight if overweight or obese
- Limiting the consumption of alcoholic beverages

The American Cancer Society advises that eating a healthy diet of fruits, vegetables, and whole grains each day, as well as limiting red meats and alcohol and engaging in at least 30 minutes of moderate to vigorous activity 5 or more days per week reduces a person's chances of getting cancer.

## Assessing Nutritional Levels

Doctors assess a patient's nutritional status by analyzing age, health status, height, weight, type of body frame, body circumference, percentage of body fat, nutritional and exercise patterns, and energy needs. They accomplish this assessment through direct measurement as well as through questionnaires and interviews. During the analysis, doctors take into account individual factors such as culture, beliefs, lifestyle, and education.

To measure fat as a percentage of body weight, doctors may perform a **skinfold test,** measuring the thickness of a fold of skin with a caliper (Figure 36-15). This measurement is often made on the triceps, midway between the shoulder and elbow. The test indicates the total percentage of fat, because about 50% of body fat is just below the skin and the volume of fat below the skin is related to the volume of inner fat. A trained individual must perform this test, which must be precise to be reliable.

The optimal percentage of body fat differs between men and women. For males younger than age 50, it is 10% to 14%; older than 50, 12% to 19%. In females younger than age 50, it is 14% to 23%; older than 50, 16% to 25%.

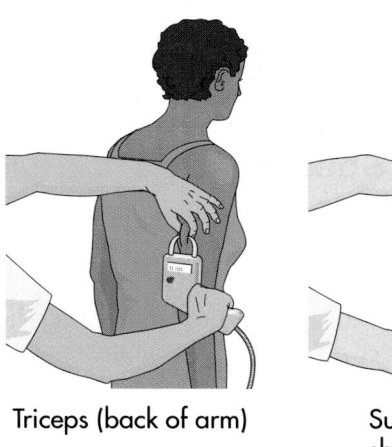

Triceps (back of arm)

Subscapular (below shoulder blade)

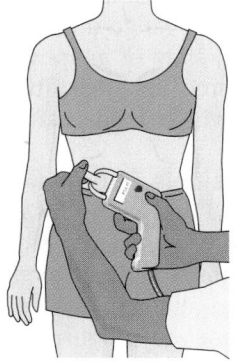

Suprailiac (above hipbone)

Thigh (front)

**Figure 36-15.** To estimate an individual's body fat percentage, a professional uses a tool called a caliper to measure the thickness of a fold of skin at one or more points on the body.

Aging usually changes the ratio a bit because some muscle tissue is replaced by fat, even if weight remains constant.

# Modifying Diets

A person's diet has a significant effect on health, appearance, and recovery from disease. After a physician or dietitian has established a patient's nutritional status, any necessary or beneficial dietary adjustments can be instituted. Dietary modification may be used alone or in combination with other therapies to prevent or treat illness. Factors affecting people's specific dietary needs may include pregnancy, injury, disease, vegetarianism, aging, genetic disorders, and substance abuse.

Adjustments in diet may involve any of the following:

- Restricting certain foods
- Emphasizing particular foods
- Changing daily caloric intake
- Changing the amount of a specific nutrient
- Changing textures of foods
- Altering the number of daily meals
- Changing variables such as bulk or spiciness

Physicians work with dietitians to determine the best diet therapy to initiate for individual patients. Diet therapy is based on many factors, including particular foods and nutrients associated with different diseases or body states.

## Patients With Specific Nutritional Needs

Patients may have a variety of conditions that require special diets. In situations such as those that follow, you may need to educate patients about their diets and answer their questions. You may need to provide encouragement and emotional support and teach patients' caregivers how to perform physical tasks, such as holding utensils for patients during meals.

**Patients With Allergies.** Some patients have food allergies. Allergic reactions to food can range from sneezing or a rash to the potentially fatal state of anaphylaxis, described in Chapter 30. The scratch test described in Chapter 27 is used to determine which foods cause an allergic reaction.

Usually specific foods must be eliminated from or restricted in an allergic patient's diet. Procedure 36-2 provides information on discussing with the patient potential dangers of common foods and reactions to those foods.

Some of the most common food allergens are wheat, milk, eggs, and chocolate. The doctor may confirm an allergy by eliminating and then reintroducing the patient's suspect foods one by one. The patient's allergy may decrease over time through systematic desensitization by means of allergy shots and other regimens.

If a food that is being eliminated or restricted was a primary source of nutrients for the patient, then the doctor must adjust the diet to include another source of those nutrients. For example, if a baby is allergic to milk, the doctor recommends a milk-substitute formula.

**Patients With Anemia.** Iron deficiency anemia, the most common type of anemia, is usually caused by chronic blood loss, a lack of iron in the diet, impaired intestinal absorption of iron, or an increased need for iron, as in pregnancy. A patient may need to take iron supplements and ingest more dietary iron as part of the treatment for this disorder. Foods high in iron include liver, egg yolks, dark green vegetables, beans, some dried fruits, and fortified breads and cereals.

**Patients With Cancer.** Most patients being treated for cancer undergo weight loss resulting both from the cancer and from treatments involving radiation or chemotherapy. To help their bodies fight off the cancer, these patients must increase their caloric intake. It is especially important that they get enough protein, because protein is needed to regenerate cells to replace the cells destroyed by the cancer and cancer treatments. These patients may also need to increase their intake of B vitamins and vitamins A, C, D, and E to support tissue growth and repair and promote efficient metabolism and use of all nutrients in the diet.

Encourage patients with cancer to follow the diet the physician sets for them. Patients may find this difficult, because cancer often produces loss of appetite. They may also experience nausea and vomiting. Educate patients about ways to make food more appealing and easier to digest. Consuming small meals at frequent intervals may help. Patients may also follow a liquid diet. Bringing food to room temperature or chilling it slightly may reduce food odors that can trigger nausea.

**Patients With Diabetes.** A special diet is one of the foundations of treatment for diabetes. Dietary guidelines for patients with diabetes must not only provide them with adequate nutrition but also keep their blood sugar level under control and interact appropriately with medication. Patient education is especially important, because patients with diabetes must comfortably maintain the dietary modifications over a lifetime.

The diet a physician or dietitian prescribes for someone with diabetes includes a specific number of calories, meals per day, amount of carbohydrates, and amounts of other nutrients. As a way to simplify the diet, a system of **food exchanges** is used. All food exchanges in a particular food category provide the same amounts of protein, fat, and carbohydrates. Food exchange lists can be obtained from a registered dietitian or the American Diabetes Association.

The list of exchanges is divided into seven categories—vegetables, fruits, starches, meats, fats, and milk—and indicates how large a portion of each food in a category is equal to one "exchange" of food in that category. This information tells patients what portions of specific foods are interchangeable and whether they are eating the correct amounts of those foods. The list includes a variety of foods from which patients make their selections. It is

# PROCEDURE 36.2

## Alerting Patients with Food Allergies to the Dangers of Common Foods

**Procedure Goal:** To explain how patients can eliminate allergy-causing foods from their diets

**OSHA Guidelines:** This procedure does not involve exposure to blood, body fluids, or tissues.

**Materials:** Results of the patient's allergy tests, patient's chart, pen, patient education materials

**Method:**

1. Identify the patient and introduce yourself.

2. Discuss the results of the patient's allergy tests (if available), reinforcing the physician's instructions. Provide the patient with a checklist of the foods that the patient has been found to be allergic to and review this list with the patient.

3. Discuss with the patient the possible allergic reactions those foods can cause.

   *Rationale*

   The patient should know what signs to look for in the event an allergic reaction to food occurs so that he or she can react quickly and appropriately.

4. Discuss with the patient the need to avoid or eliminate those foods from the diet. Point out that the patient needs to be alert to avoid the allergy-causing foods not only in their basic forms but also as ingredients in prepared dishes and packaged foods. (Patients allergic to peanuts, for example, should avoid products containing peanut oil as well as peanuts.)

5. Tell the patient to read labels carefully and to inquire at restaurants about the use of those ingredients in dishes listed on the menu.

6. With the physician's or dietitian's consent, talk with the patient about the possibility of finding adequate substitutes for the foods if they are among the patient's favorites. Also discuss, if necessary, how the patient can obtain the nutrients in those foods from other sources (for example, the need for extra calcium sources if the patient is allergic to dairy products). Provide these explanations to the patient in writing, if appropriate, along with supplementary materials such as recipe pamphlets, a list of resources for obtaining food substitutes, and so on.

7. Discuss with the patient the procedures to follow if the allergy-causing foods are accidentally ingested.

   *Rationale*

   Do not assume a patient will know what to do in the event of an allergic reaction.

8. Answer the patient's questions and remind the patient that you and the rest of the medical team are available if any questions or problems arise later on.

9. Document the patient education session or interchange in the patient's chart, indicate the patient's understanding, and initial the entry.

   *Rationale*

   Many insurance companies require evidence of preventative health counseling and documentation is an important aspect of patient insurance coverage.

---

important that patients with diabetes not skip a meal, because skipping meals disturbs the balance of blood sugar and metabolism. Table 36-6 provides the food exchanges recommended for diabetics.

Patients with diabetes who are dependent on insulin should eat regular meals at consistent times. Skipping or delaying meals can result in hypoglycemia or an insulin reaction. Patients should work with a registered dietitian and their physician to create a meal plan that keeps blood glucose levels as close to normal as possible. The medical team specifies the proportion of carbohydrates and calories in meals, depending on the type of insulin patients use and the timing of injections.

Fiber is also important for patients who have diabetes. Fiber can sometimes prevent a sharp rise in blood glucose after a meal and may reduce the amount of insulin needed. It is therefore recommended that people with diabetes gradually increase their fiber intake until it is at about 45 grams per day.

***Diabetes Food Pyramid.*** The diabetes pyramid is a little different than the USDA 2005 Food Guide because it groups foods into categories based on their carbohydrate and protein content instead of by their food classification. The diabetes pyramid allows for a range of servings. The lower end of the range represents a 1600-calorie diet and the higher end of the range represents a 2800-calorie diet.

## TABLE 36-6 Diabetic Food Exchange Table

| Food Exchange | U.S. Unit | Comments |
|---|---|---|
| **Starches (6 or more exchanges)** | | |
| 15g Carb, 3g Protein, 1g Fat | | • Most starches are a good source of B vitamins |
| • Bread | 1 slice | |
| • Breads, other | 1 oz | • Choose whole grain foods such as 100% whole wheat bread and flour, brown rice, tortillas, etc., for nutrients and fiber |
| • Tortilla | 1 (6") | |
| • Crackers | 4–6 (¾ oz) | |
| • Cooked cereals | ½ cup | |
| • Dry cereals | ¾ cup | |
| • Dry cereals, unsweetened | ½ cup | • Combine beans (starch and meat) with grains (starch) for their complimentary proteins and fiber |
| • Dry flour or grain | 3 Tbsp | |
| • Pasta | ½ cup | |
| • Rice | ½ cup | • Combine grains (starch) with milk (milk) or cheese (meat) to compliment proteins |
| • Corn | ½ cup | |
| • Popcorn | 3 cups | |
| • Potato (small) | 1 (3 oz) | • Add 1 fat exchange for starchy foods prepared with fat |
| • Potato, mashed | ½ cup | |
| • Sweet potato | ⅓ cup | |
| • Squash, winter | 1 cup | |
| • Cooked beans, peas, lentils (add 1 meat exchange) | ½ cup | |
| **Vegetables (3–5 exchanges)** | | |
| 5g Carb, 2g, Protein | | |
| • Raw vegetables | 1 cup | • Choose more dark green leafy and deep yellow vegetables such as spinach, broccoli, carrots, and peppers |
| • Cooked vegetables | ½ cup | |
| • Tomato or vegetable juice | ½ cup | |
| **Fruit (2–4 exchanges)** | | |
| 15g Carb | | |
| • Fresh fruit | 1 small | • Choose whole fruits for fiber |
| • Melon (cubes) | 12 oz (1 cup) | • Choose citrus fruits such as oranges, grapefruits, or tangerines |
| • Canned fruit | ½ cup | |
| • Dried fruit | ¼ cup | |
| • Fruit juice | ½ cup | |
| **Meat & Substitutes (5–7 exchanges)** | | |
| 7g Protein, 0–13g Fat | | |
| • Meat, poultry, fish | 1 oz | • Choose leaner meats such as chicken, fish, and lean cuts of meat; add fat exchange for higher-fat meats and substitutes |
| • Cheese | 1 oz | |
| • Cottage cheese | ¼ cup | |
| • Egg | 1 | |
| • Peanut butter | 1.5 Tbsp | • Remove skin from poultry |
| • Tofu | 4 oz (½ cup) | • Limit frying or adding fat |
| • Cooked beans, peas, lentils (add 1 starch) | ½ cup | • Have 2 servings of fish per week for Omega 3 fatty acid |
| **Milk (2–3 exchanges)** | | |
| 12g Carb, 8g Protein, 0–8g Fat | | |
| • Milk | 1 cup | • Choose lower-fat milks; add fat exchange for higher-fat milk |
| • Yogurt | 1 cup | |

*continued* ⟶

## TABLE 36-6 Diabetic Food Exchange Table (concluded)

| Food Exchange | U.S. Unit | Comments |
|---|---|---|
| **Fat (use sparingly)** | | |
| 5g Fat | | |
| • Oil | 1 tsp | • Eat less fat |
| • Mayonnaise | 1 tsp | • Eat less saturated fat such as animal |
| • Cream cheese | 1 Tbsp | fat found in fattier meat, cheese, and |
| • Salad dressing | 1 Tbsp | butter. Also eat less hydrogenated fat |
| • Peanuts | 10 | • Check Nutrition Facts on food labels; |
| • Avocado | ⅛ | 5g Fat = 1 Fat exchange |
| • Butter or margarine | 1 tsp | |
| • Higher fat exchange | 1 exchange | |
| **Sweets (use sparingly)** | | |
| 15g Carb, Protein & Fat varies | | |
| • Ice cream | ½ cup | • Choose sweets sparingly because |
| • Cookies | 2 small | they are high in fat or sugar |
| • Syrup | 1 Tbsp | • Can be substituted for 1 Starch, |
| • Jam or jelly | 1 Tbsp | Fruit, or Milk exchange |
| • Sugar | 2 Tbsp | • Add 1 or 2 Fat exchanges for sweets |
| • Pudding | ¼ cup | containing fat |
| • Muffin or cupcake | ½ small | |

Women tend to eat at the lower end of the range, whereas men tend to eat at the middle to upper end of the range, depending upon their activity level.

The diabetes pyramid divides food into six categories. The separate categories of the pyramid vary in size, with the largest category representing grains, beans, and starchy vegetables and the smallest category represents fats, oils, and sweets. Translated, this means that a diabetic should eat more servings of grains, and beans, instead of sweets and fats. Table 36-7 provides the food groups from the diabetes food pyramid and the daily recommendations of servings of each group.

**Patients Who Are Elderly.** Universal nutritional guidelines for aging patients have not been developed. It is known, however, that energy and metabolic requirements usually decline with age, which calls for some dietary modification. The Food and Nutrition Board of the National Academy of Science recommends a 10% decrease in caloric intake for people over age 50 compared with that of young adults. Men and women older than age 75 should decrease their intake another 10% to 15%. The exact adjustment, however, depends on the individual patient's condition and needs.

Because protein requirements do not change, elderly patients should select foods that provide ample protein in a smaller quantity of food. To achieve daily nutritional goals, patients may require supplements for iron, calcium, and other minerals, such as phosphorus and magnesium.

Because aging is often accompanied by decreased gastrointestinal muscle tone, elderly patients should increase their intake of high-fiber foods and drink plenty of water. Although all people need a certain amount of fat in their diet to help the body absorb vitamins, too much may lead to atherosclerosis. Elderly individuals should therefore keep fat intake to 20% of their total calories.

Certain factors can impair or impede eating in this age group and may even lead to malnutrition. If you recognize any of these factors, discuss them with the patient's doctor:

- Physical factors, such as chewing difficulty caused by tooth loss or poorly fitting dentures, swallowing difficulty, and lack of appetite caused by altered taste, smell, or sight
- Medications, which may adversely affect food intake or nutrient use
- Social factors, including apathy toward food caused by depression, grief, or loneliness
- Economic factors, including homelessness or lack of money for food or transportation

**Patients With Heart Disease.** Coronary heart disease is caused by atherosclerosis, which usually results from hyperlipidemia, or an excess of lipids in the bloodstream. Left untreated, this condition can lead to angina, heart attack, or stroke.

Patients can significantly lower their risk by reducing their blood cholesterol levels and losing weight if they are

## TABLE 36-7 Diabetes Food Pyramid

| Food Group | Serving Size | Daily Recommendation |
|---|---|---|
| Grains and Starches | 1 slice of bread<br>¼ of a bagel<br>½ English muffin or pita<br>1 six-inch tortilla<br>¾ cup dry cereal<br>½ cup cooked cereal<br>½ cup potato, yam, peas, corn, or cooked beans<br>1 cup winter squash<br>⅓ cup of rice or pasta | Choose 6–11 servings per day |
| Vegetables | 1 cup raw vegetables<br>½ cup cooked vegetables | Choose 3–5 servings per day |
| Fruit | ½ cup canned fruit<br>1 small fresh fruit<br>2 tbs dried fruit<br>1 cup of melon or raspberries<br>1¼ cup whole strawberries | Choose 2–4 servings per day |
| Milk | 1 cup of non-fat or low fat milk<br>1 cup of yogurt | Choose 2–3 servings per day |
| Meat and Meat Substitutes | 4–6 oz per day<br>beef, chicken, turkey, fish, eggs, tofu, dried beans, cheese, cottage cheese, peanut butter<br>Meat substitutes equal to 1 oz of meat:<br>¼ cup cottage cheese<br>1 egg<br>1 tbsp peanut butter<br>½ cup tofu | Choose 4–6 oz per day divided between meals |
| Fats, Sweets, and Alcohol | ½ cup ice cream<br>1 small cupcake or muffin<br>2 small cookies | Use sparingly as a special treat and keep serving sizes small |

overweight. Patients who have coronary heart disease usually must reduce their consumption of fats to a level that provides less than 30% of their total caloric intake. Saturated fats should provide less than 10% of caloric intake. Patients who have had a heart attack or are at increased risk for a heart attack are also encouraged to increase their consumption of soluble fiber.

As a medical assistant, your role with these patients is to encourage them to follow the nutritional regimen prescribed by the doctor. Do not recommend other dietary changes. Instead, educate patients about ways to reduce the amount of fat in their diets, such as by substituting skim milk for whole milk.

**Patients With Hypertension.** Hypertension (high blood pressure) is a condition that affects more than 20% of American adults. Nutritional therapy for patients with hypertension involves the following:

- Restricting sodium intake to 2 to 3 grams per day, especially in salt-sensitive individuals
- Increasing potassium intake through consumption of fresh fruits and vegetables
- Ensuring adequate calcium intake to meet an RDA of 800 milligrams
- Eliminating or reducing alcohol use
- Decreasing total fat intake and obtaining no more than 10% of calories from saturated fats

**Patients With Lactose Sensitivity.** Lactose is the sugar contained in human and animal milk. It must be broken down in the body by the enzyme lactase to enable the body to digest dairy products. In people from some parts of the world, lactase is present in the body until age 3 or 4, after which it all but disappears. As a result, after early childhood many people have trouble digesting foods that contain lactose and eliminate these foods from their diets. People who are especially sensitive to dietary lactose are often referred to as being lactose intolerant.

Chemical preparations can help a person digest lactose. Those preparations may be added to certain foods, such as ice cream, for lactose-sensitive people. If people with a lactose sensitivity choose to avoid dairy products, they need to be sure to obtain protein and calcium from other sources.

**Patients Who Are Overweight.** More than one-third of American adults are overweight. Overweight patients weigh 10% to 20% more than is recommended for their height and gender. Patients who are more than 20% overweight are considered obese. Obesity can lead to medical complications such as elevated blood cholesterol levels, hypertension, diabetes, joint problems, respiratory problems, and heart disease.

*Approaches to Weight Loss.* Weight reduction may be approached with dietary modification alone, but an exercise program is usually included. Behavior modification is also a common element of weight-loss programs. In a weight-loss program, foods should be proportioned in accordance with the Food Guide Pyramid, and the diet should be appealing and enjoyable. The goal is to have the patient decrease daily caloric intake and increase physical activity at an appropriate rate while remaining comfortable and healthy.

Weight loss will not occur unless patients expend more energy than they consume. A physician or dietitian can calculate each person's daily caloric needs and determine how many calories must be cut from the diet and how much activity must be increased to result in weight loss. Foods that are high in nutrients but low in calories are desirable.

The **behavior modification** facet of weight loss includes such methods as keeping a food diary to pinpoint overeating patterns, controlling the stimuli associated with overeating, and providing rewards for successful behavior.

You can help overweight patients in their weight-loss efforts by teaching them to:

- Eat slowly, because the message that the stomach is full takes 20 minutes to register with the brain
- Eat five or six small meals daily
- Be patient—reliable weight loss occurs over time, not immediately

*Motivation and Education.* Because patients who are trying to lose weight may have trouble with motivation, they need as much support as possible. You can provide encouragement and education. You may be able to introduce the patient to low-calorie or low-fat recipes, for instance, and positively reinforce the patient's efforts by complimenting small, gradual successes.

You will no doubt need to explain that fad diets and diet drugs are seldom successful. Fad weight-loss methods can lead to vitamin, mineral, and protein deficiency; serious medical disorders; and even death. Tell patients to use the following criteria to identify fad diets:

- They promise ease and comfort in weight loss
- They include only a few foods, such as grapefruit or low-protein foods
- They require the purchase of some secret ingredient or pill
- They are often published in a book or magazine

Truly effective weight-loss regimens usually possess the following qualities:

- They include a variety of foods that contain adequate nutrients
- They include an activity component
- They may be safely followed over a long period of time

An effective program should be one in which the patient is able to lose weight (including fat) gradually and constantly, with some plateaus, and then maintain the loss indefinitely afterward. You can help patients with the challenge of maintaining their weight loss by recommending a reputable weight-loss group or a support group that will help them make the necessary lifestyle changes and remain motivated.

**Pediatric Patients.** During the first year of life, an infant experiences the most rapid period of growth and development that occurs during the life span. Breast milk and commercially prepared formula contain the balance of nutrients that infants' bodies need during that period. Cow's milk does not meet these standards.

The pace of growth is steadier and slower during childhood, with growth spurts throughout. Nutritional needs change to reflect growth, maturation, and increasing activity levels. Vitamin D and calcium are critical to tooth and bone formation, and fluoride strengthens teeth. Hunger regulates food intake in young children, but forcing children to eat can promote eating habits that lead to obesity.

**Patients Who Are Pregnant or Lactating.** Nutrition is especially important during pregnancy, when it provides for normal growth and health of the baby as well as the health of the pregnant woman. Doctors recommend that pregnant women gain a certain amount of weight during each trimester of pregnancy, with a total weight gain of about 25 to 35 pounds. The rate of weight gain should be 2 to 5 pounds in the first trimester and about 1 pound per week after that. Gaining too little or too much weight during pregnancy can result in serious complications.

Here are some nutritional suggestions for pregnant women:

- An additional 10 to 15 grams of protein a day in the form of meat, poultry, fish, eggs, and dairy products
- 1200 milligrams of calcium a day, preferably in the form of low-fat dairy products such as skim milk

- 30 milligrams of iron a day through meat, liver, egg yolks, grains, leafy vegetables, nuts, dried fruits, legumes, and supplements (it is difficult to meet the daily need with food alone)
- Folic acid intake of 400 micrograms a day through leafy vegetables, yeast, and liver as well as supplements
- Adequate fiber intake to prevent the constipation that often accompanies pregnancy
- Recommendations consistent with the Food Guide Pyramid and normal sodium and water intake

Breast-feeding has specific nutritional and dietary requirements as well, because breast milk is nutrient-rich and the body requires considerable energy and nutrients to produce it. The infant depends on this milk for the extensive growth that takes place during the first months of life. Lactating women need to consume an additional 500 calories and an additional 12 to 19 grams of protein per day as well as 260 to 280 micrograms of folic acid and 1200 milligrams of calcium.

## Specific Modified Diets

Physicians may modify a patient's diet to treat or prevent certain conditions. Specific types of modified diets include changes in texture, nutrient level, frequency and timing of meals, and exclusions.

**Texture.** A patient may need changes in food consistency as a result of swallowing, chewing, or other gastrointestinal problems or to fulfill short-term needs that result from such events as laboratory tests or surgical procedures. The following special diets are based on texture.

- A clear-liquid diet consists solely of foods such as tea, broth, noncitrus juices, carbonated beverages, popsicles, and gelatin. A full-liquid diet is less restrictive and includes strained cooked cereals, plain ice cream, sherbet, pudding, and strained soups.
- A soft diet includes foods that are easy to chew, swallow, and digest. Foods that patients cannot tolerate and those high in fiber are eliminated from this diet.
- All foods in a pureed diet are put through a strainer so that they are in the form of a semisolid. Pureed foods are easy to chew and swallow.
- A high-fiber diet contains large amounts of fiber (greater than 40 grams) from sources such as fresh fruits, vegetables, and bran cereal. Physicians may prescribe this diet for patients with conditions such as diverticulosis and constipation. The diet increases the bulk of fecal matter and stimulates peristalsis (waves of alternating contraction and relaxation of the intestine that move contents through the intestine).

**Nutrient Level.** Doctors may make nutrient-level modifications in patients' diets before or after surgical or medical procedures or for patients who have specific conditions. The following special diets are based on nutrient levels.

- Doctors may prescribe low-sodium diets for patients who suffer from disease conditions affecting the cardiovascular system, liver, pancreas, and gallbladder, including edema and hypertension. The typical American diet contains 2 to 5 grams of sodium daily. For mild sodium restriction, daily intake is limited to 2 to 3 grams; the patient reduces salt in cooking, adds no salt at the table, and avoids processed foods. Moderate sodium restriction allows 1 gram per day; the patient adds no salt in cooking or at the table and limits high-sodium vegetables, meat, and milk. Severe restriction allows 500 milligrams per day and greatly limits high-sodium vegetables, meat, milk, and eggs.
- Doctors recommend low-cholesterol diets for patients with high blood cholesterol levels. Such diets involve replacing saturated fats with unsaturated fats, using low-fat or nonfat cooking methods, and restricting fatty foods.
- Doctors may prescribe reduced-calorie diets to promote weight loss in patients who are overweight.
- Doctors may recommend low-tyramine diets for patients who have migraine headaches and patients who are taking certain antidepressant drugs. The compound tyramine is found in aged cheeses, red wine, beer, cream, chocolate, and yeast.
- Doctors may order high-calorie, high-protein diets for patients who have infections, are recovering from burns or surgery, or have had weight loss caused by a severe illness. Food intake is increased to provide 3000 to 5000 calories per day. Protein usually accounts for the greatest caloric increase in these diets.
- Doctors may prescribe high-carbohydrate diets for patients with kidney diseases and some cardiac conditions.

You can help patients who need to make nutrient-level modifications by teaching them how to read food labels. All packaged foods carry a Nutrition Facts label that contains information on the ingredients, major nutrients, and recommended amounts of key nutrients in daily diets. Procedure 36-3 explains how to educate patients about reading food labels. You can also teach patients how to interpret the terms on food labels (Table 36-8). Understanding marketing terms simplifies the process of buying the right foods to meet special dietary needs.

**Frequency and Timing of Meals.** A patient's diet may also be modified by adjusting the standard three-meal pattern. The goal may be to eat six small meals rather than three large meals to minimize stress on organs affected by disease conditions—as in patients with an ulcer or hiatal hernia. In other cases meals may simply be timed to follow tests or therapeutic procedures.

## TABLE 36-8　Food Label Terms and Definitions

| Term | Definition |
|------|-----------|
| Low calorie | Less than or equal to 40 calories per serving |
| Reduced calorie | At least 25% fewer calories per serving than the food it replaces |
| Cholesterol free | Less than or equal to 2 mg cholesterol per serving |
| Low cholesterol | Less than or equal to 20 mg cholesterol per serving |
| Reduced cholesterol | At least 25% less cholesterol per serving than the food it replaces |
| Low fat | Less than or equal to 3 g fat per serving |
| Reduced fat | At least 25% less fat per serving than the food it replaces |
| Sodium free | Less than or equal to 5 mg sodium per serving |
| Very low sodium | Less than or equal to 35 mg sodium per serving |
| Low sodium | Less than or equal to 140 mg sodium per serving |
| Reduced sodium | At least 25% less sodium per serving than the food it replaces |

Source: U.S. Department of Health and Human Services, Food and Drug Administration.

lactose, the sugar in milk, is fairly common. Intolerance to the amino acid phenylalanine—a condition present at birth—is fairly rare but very serious. Infants born in hospitals in the United States are tested for this intolerance because if these infants were to receive a standard diet, they would develop severe mental retardation. People with this condition, known as phenylketonuria (PKU), must be vigilant about checking labels on prepared foods as well as knowledgeable about the phenylalanine content of fresh foods.

## Using Supplements and Parenteral Nutrition

When a patient has a loss or lack of appetite or cannot tolerate a normal meal, the doctor may prescribe a specially formulated food supplement that provides protein, carbohydrates, fat, vitamins, and minerals. A patient who is chronically ill, underweight, or anemic or who has just undergone surgery may take supplements orally or through a tube to the stomach or small intestine. If the supplement is being taken orally, encourage the patient to follow the prescribed directions.

When patients cannot tolerate receiving supplements enterally (by way of the digestive tract), they may be fed parenterally. **Parenteral nutrition** is provided to patients as specially prepared nutrients injected directly into their veins rather than given by mouth. Because a parenteral feeding bypasses the digestive system, the nutrients it contains must already be in a form the body can use as they enter the blood.

## Patients Undergoing Drug Therapy

Drugs may change a patient's nutritional status and needs. Long-term drug therapy and multiple prescriptions make close nutritional monitoring a high priority.

Drug therapy can cause a change in food intake, a change in the body's absorption of a nutrient, or both. Likewise, foods can interfere with the metabolism and action of a drug. For example, laxatives and certain other types of drugs may suppress the appetite. Antihistamines, alcohol, insulin, thyroid hormones, and some other drugs can stimulate appetite. Anesthetics can interfere with taste. Calcium in milk can diminish the absorption of some antibiotics. Be sure to discuss any possible interactions with the physician or dietitian before discussing diet and drug regimens with a patient.

## Eating Disorders

Eating disorders, characterized by extremely harmful eating behavior, can lead to health problems. These disorders can damage the body and even cause death. They are most common in adolescent girls and young women, although 10% to 15% of patients with eating disorders are male. Refer to the Points on Practice feature to identify the signs and symptoms of common eating disorders.

### Anorexia Nervosa

**Anorexia nervosa** is an eating disorder in which people starve themselves. They fear that if they lose control of eating, they will become grossly overweight. They lose an excessive amount of weight and become malnourished,

## Recognizing the Signs and Symptoms of Common Eating Disorders

As a medical assistant, one of your primary responsibilities is to interview patients about their medical histories. Chapter 23 explains patient interviewing in detail. It is important to know signs and symptoms of eating disorders in order to accurately form questions to gain complete medical information for the physician.

### Anorexia Nervosa

- Unexplained weight loss of at least 15%
- Self-starvation
- Excessive fear of gaining weight
- Malnourishment
- Cessation of menstruation in women
- Drastic reduction in food consumption
- Denial of feeling hungry
- Ritualistic eating habits
- Overexercising
- Unrealistic self-image as being obese
- Extremely controlled behavior

### Bulimia

- Eating large quantities of food in a short period, followed by purging
- Pretexts for going to the bathroom after meals
- Using laxatives or diuretics to control weight
- Buying and consuming large quantities of food
- Feeling out of control while eating
- Maintaining a constant weight while eating a large amount of fattening foods
- Mood swings
- Awareness of having a disorder, but fear of not being able to stop
- Depression, self-deprecation, and guilt following the episodes

### Binge Eating

- Bingeing on food, not followed by purging
- Weight gain

---

and women often stop menstruating. The typical patient with anorexia nervosa is a high-achieving, white female in her teens or early 20s. The numbers of children and middle-aged women who suffer from the disorder, however, have been increasing. The cause of anorexia remains unknown, but risk factors include the following:

- Coming from a family that has problems with alcoholism
- Suffering a childhood trauma, such as sexual abuse (20% to 50% of patients were sexually abused)
- Having a high stress level
- Suffering from depression
- Suffering from shame and low self-esteem
- Having an extreme need to be in control

It has also been noted that anorexia tends to run in families. The victim of anorexia often uses food as a way to deal with the psychological effects of trauma by numbing the emotions or as a means of getting some measure of control in life. Anorexia can be precipitated by any major life change.

This disorder can be fatal. The first stage of treatment is to restore normal nutrition. Patients may need to be hospitalized and fed intravenously or by nasogastric tube, which enters through the nose and delivers food into the stomach. Hospitalization may be necessary, because patients with excessive weight loss may develop cardiac

and other medical disorders. These patients may also be at risk for suicide. The hospital stay may eventually provide patients with the structure and support they need to establish healthy eating patterns.

Psychotherapy is a cornerstone of treatment protocol. Therapy usually involves a combination of one-on-one and group therapy. Therapy groups that are single-sex rather than coed are preferable because of the different gender and peer group issues men and women face. Doctors may prescribe medication for depression and anxiety. The later stages of treatment include teaching patients and their families about nutrition concepts.

## Bulimia

**Bulimia** is an eating disorder in which people eat a large quantity of food in a short time (bingeing) and then attempt to counter the effects of bingeing by self-induced vomiting, use of laxatives or diuretics, and/or excessive exercise. People with bulimia may use such behavior to try to gain control of their lives and weight.

Bulimia can be triggered when a slightly overweight person diets but fails to achieve the goal. Episodes are usually frequent, rapid, and uncontrollable. The behavior may occur only during periods of stress.

People with bulimia often diet when not bingeing. Psychologically, they believe their worth depends on being thin. Behind their cheerful exterior, they usually feel depressed, lonely, ashamed, and empty.

Most bulimics who seek help are in their early 20s and report that they have been bulimic for 4 to 6 years. Because they are more likely to want and seek help, they are slightly easier to treat than anorexics are.

Bulimia is usually not life-threatening, but it can cause the following serious health problems:

- Erosion of tooth enamel
- Enlarged salivary glands
- Lesions in the esophagus
- Stomach spasms
- Chemical and hormonal imbalances

As with anorexia, treatment for bulimia involves a combination of psychotherapy and medication. Dental work, medication for depression and anxiety, nutritional counseling, and support groups may be used. The goal is to establish a healthy weight and good eating patterns as well as to resolve the psychosocial triggers.

## Getting Help

Studies show an unsatisfactory rate of recovery from eating disorders; only about half of anorexic patients fully recover. The disorders can become chronic, with periods of remission and relapse. Chronic anorexia can be fatal, and many people who do recover from eating disorders remain preoccupied with food.

If you suspect that a patient has an eating disorder, be alert for the following eating or activity patterns that the patient might mention in conversation:

- Skipping two or more meals a day or limiting caloric intake to 500 or fewer calories a day
- Eating a very large amount of food in an uncontrollable manner over the course of 2 hours
- Eating large quantities of food without being hungry
- Using laxatives, excessive exercise, vomiting, diuretics, or other purges for weight control
- Avoiding social situations because they may interfere with a diet or exercise
- Feeling disgust, depression, and guilt after a binge
- Feeling that food controls life

## Patient Education

Whenever you teach patients about nutrition and diet, you help them take steps to improve their health. In most instances a physician or dietitian gives the patient instructions, which you then reinforce. Patients may feel more comfortable asking you questions about their diet than asking other members of the medical team. They may think their concerns are too trivial or simple for the physician or dietitian.

Because of your frequent contact with patients, you can play a major role in education. You can teach patients about the role of nutrition in helping to prevent specific medical conditions. You can also teach patients how to be wise consumers when they shop by reading food package labels. You will be better equipped to educate patients and answer their questions if you have a solid knowledge of diet and nutrition and if you stay current with recent research findings. See the Educating the Patient section for information on the relevance of such research. Before discussing a diet with any patient, be sure you understand the regimen the physician or dietitian is recommending as well as how to implement it.

If you are unsure of answers to any patient's questions, always ask the physician. Refer patients who have questions about meal patterns and food selections to the registered dietitian, if one is available.

## Your Role in Patient Education

When discussing dietary requirements with a patient, keep in mind that the patient is always the focus of nutritional care. Specific factors to take into account include the following:

- Any psychological or lifestyle factors that affect food choices and behaviors. Learn about the patient's dietary likes and dislikes, as well as religious or cultural restrictions, before you suggest the use of specific foods in meeting dietary requirements.
- The patient's age and family circumstances. For example, parents need to know the specifics about an infant's or a child's diet. An elderly person's diet needs to be physically and economically manageable as well as nutritious.
- Diseases and disorders. For example, if the patient has chewing or breathing problems or is nauseous, the doctor will have to prescribe treatments or medications to address those problems.
- The patient's psychological condition. You can learn a great deal about psychological status through discussion and nonverbal cues. For instance, you might look for signs that the patient is frustrated with the dietary changes or is in denial about a problem. The greater the rapport you develop with a patient, the more you will be able to help.

Remind patients that eating healthfully will help them feel and look better and help their bodies work better. When the doctor prescribes therapeutic diets, be sure patients are fully aware of the reasons they must follow the diets. Help patients set realistic goals, and praise them for even the smallest accomplishments. Offer positive reinforcement for current and new good food habits.

As with all patient education, teaching methods such as role playing, repetition of concepts, and the use of literature and other media reinforce your discussion. Use printed and audiovisual materials. Patient education sessions can be formal or informal and can take place at any appropriate time and place, such as in the office, over the telephone, or during a treatment or procedure. If possible, let patients decide which arrangements they prefer, or let them know the schedule in advance.

Patients need your support and empathy in working toward diet and nutrition goals, whether preventive or therapeutic. Follow these guidelines for best results when discussing diets with patients.

- Treat each patient as an individual with unique eating habits, knowledge of nutrition, and ability to learn
- Teach a small amount of material at a time; 15- to 30-minute sessions are better than hour-long ones
- Keep explanations at the level of the patient's understanding and vocabulary

- Emphasize the patient's good eating behavior to reinforce it
- Let the patient play an active role in the learning process—for example, by helping to plan the diet
- Give the patient a written diet plan to take home as well as any other helpful materials you have to offer
- Suggest that the patient contact local support groups for people who are trying to maintain the same kind of diet

Keep in mind that patient education has become increasingly important for patients receiving managed care. Managed care providers want to see documentation of preventive care in patients' charts. Failure to provide documentation can jeopardize a patient's insurance coverage.

## Educating the Patient

## Changes in Nutritional Recommendations

In the field of nutrition—as in other scientific fields—research continues to provide people with additional information. How that information is used and the speed with which it is communicated often depend on public service agencies and federal agencies responsible for nutritional guidance.

You can help answer patients' questions about the potential usefulness of new information by understanding the difference between initial research findings and those evaluated and endorsed by the government. In many cases information is not officially released or endorsed until the government has studied the facts and determined that they are accurate and concrete enough for public consideration. For example, initial findings have suggested the following information.

- Beta-carotene supplements may provide no benefit and may even be harmful.
- Certain fruit-derived flavenoids—pigmented antioxidants—may help halt the growth of cancer cells.
- Dark beer may reduce the risk of coronary artery disease (CAD).
- Vitamin D may reduce the risk of certain cancers.

Patients may read about research studies and ask whether they should make whatever dietary changes the findings suggest. You need to explain that such findings are preliminary and not formally approved by a government agency. Although the approval process is lengthy—requiring a significant amount of data and test results—it provides a system for protecting consumers from false nutritional claims.

Tell patients that once the government determines that a nutritional recommendation is warranted, it often acts on it. One example is the case of folate. Since the 1960s a number of studies have been conducted on the importance of folate in the diet. Over the years, those studies have yielded the following results.

- Folate offers protection from neural tube defects in unborn babies.
- Folate can reverse certain anemias.
- Folate may reduce the risk of cervical dysplasia.
- Folate appears to lower the likelihood of heart attacks.

As a result of these studies, the Department of Health and Human Services' Food and Drug Administration considered folate to be so important to all people that it approved the addition of folate to flour. Several nutrients have long been added to certain products to improve the products' nutritional value and to increase people's intake of important nutrients lacking in the general diet:

- Vitamin A and vitamin D, added to dairy products
- Iodine, added to salt
- Niacin, added to milled grain products
- Various vitamins and minerals, added to processed cereals

Explain to patients that nutritional recommendations change as scientists learn more about the ways various foods affect the human body and the exact amount of nutrients the body requires. Keep up to date on nutrition research so you can provide patients with the latest information and help them steer clear of unsubstantiated claims.

## TABLE 36-9 Sources of Information About Specific Diet and Nutrition Issues

| Organization | Address/Telephone Number |
|---|---|
| American Cancer Society | 777 Third Avenue<br>New York, NY 10017<br>(212) 586-8700 |
| American Diabetes Association | 1701 North Beauregard Street<br>Alexandria, VA 22311<br>(800) 342-2383 |
| American Dietetic Association | 120 S. Riverside Plaza<br>Suite 2000<br>Chicago, IL 60606-6995<br>(800) 877-1600<br>(800) 366-1655 |
| American Heart Association | 7320 Greenville Avenue<br>Dallas, TX 75231<br>(214) 373-6300 |
| Anorexia Nervosa and Related Eating Disorders | Box 7<br>Highland Park, IL 60035<br>(847) 831-3438 |
| National Association of Anorexia Nervosa and Associated Disorders | Box 7<br>Highland Park, IL 60035<br>(847) 831-3438 |
| National Eating Disorders Association | 603 Stewart Street<br>Suite 803<br>Seattle, WA 98101<br>(206) 382-3587 |
| Overeaters Anonymous (OA) | P.O. Box 44020<br>Rio Rancho, NM 87174<br>(505) 891-2664 |

## Cultural Considerations

Eating is a personal and social activity, and cultural issues play an especially important part in diet and nutrition. A person's cultural heritage, religious background, family traditions, socioeconomic status, and personal beliefs help determine eating habits and preferences. Culture and lifestyle also help shape food purchasing and serving habits, likes and dislikes, meal timing and frequency, attitude toward food supplements, and tendency to snack.

Dietitians and nutritionists who design diets and recipes for patients know that to design successful diets, they must take into account cultural and lifestyle factors. You can increase the effectiveness of your patient education if you become familiar with the food habits and beliefs common to your patients' cultural backgrounds. Learn to recognize the eating patterns belonging to different cultures, and make a special effort to familiarize yourself with the food preferences of the ethnic groups most commonly represented among the patients in the practice where you work.

## Outside Resources for Patient Education

Many community health agencies and organizations offer patient education materials and information about specific diet and nutrition issues. Some of them are listed in Table 36-9. Investigate your own community to find others, and keep the information on file.

## Summary

Nutrition is a complex, highly technical topic that touches people's daily lives. It is part of your job to make good nutrition understandable and achievable for patients. You will play a major role in educating patients about special diets and in helping them implement dietary changes as instructed by physicians and dietitians. Your knowledge of basic nutritional principles and current nutritional findings will help you perform these tasks with confidence and competence.

The more you learn about foods and their nutritional value, the better able you will be to educate patients about meeting their particular nutritional needs. Your knowledge about nutrition will help you teach patients a major means of supporting and improving their overall health. In some cases, your work in this area will help patients avoid or recover from life-threatening medical conditions.

Whenever you work with patients, be alert for body weights significantly above or below the ideal. It is also important to recognize indications of eating patterns that may lead to health problems such as obesity, anorexia nervosa, and bulimia.

## CASE STUDY *QUESTIONS*

Now that you have completed this chapter, review the case study at the beginning of the chapter and answer the following questions:

1. What is the patient's probable diagnosis?
2. Do you think that the patient's attention to calorie intake is simply, as she says, preparation for the cheerleading competition?
3. Why is this patient experiencing muscle weakness?

## Discussion Questions

1. Name a disease that can occur with either deficiencies of or toxicities from the vitamins listed below:
   a. Vitamin A
   b. Vitamin D
   c. Vitamin C
   d. Folate
2. An adult patient reads you his food journal for the previous week. His average daily intake of calcium is 540 milligrams. Is he getting enough calcium to supply his body's needs?
3. Using a normal clinical range of 90 to 171 for LDL cholesterol and a normal clinical range of 31 to 59 for HDL cholesterol, should you tell your patient that he is effectively controlling his cholesterol levels if he has readings of LDL 99 and HDL 56?

## Critical Thinking Questions

1. Should an insulin-dependent patient follow the recommended diabetic diet from the American Diabetes Association?
2. What are some suggestions you could make to a patient who has recently been diagnosed with borderline hypertension?
3. A patient informs you that she has discontinued all of her prescribed sleep and blood pressure medication and has started using herbal supplements as a replacement, such as St. Johns Wort and an herbal remedy for hypertension. What should you say to the patient?

## Application Activities

1. Plan a well-balanced, health-promoting diet for 1 day for a 45-year-old man recently diagnosed with cardiovascular disease; do the same for a diabetic patient using the exchange system.
2. Have each member of the class report on the typical diet of a particular culture—Mexican, Asian, Mediterranean, Saudi, and so on. How does the diet satisfy nutritional requirements? In what areas is it outstanding or inadequate? How does the diet differ from a typical American diet?
3. Choose a popular weight-loss supplement and research its benefits and contraindications. Share with the class your findings and lead a discussion.

## Virtual Fieldtrip

*Visit the McGraw-Hill Higher Education Medical Assisting website at www.mhhe.com/medicalassisting3 to complete the following activity:*

Using the U.S. Department of Agriculture website, access MyPyramid and enter the requested information about your dietary needs. Analyze the results and prepare a personal 3-day diet, using the suggestions within the 2005 Dietary Guidelines table.

Open the CD and complete this chapter's practice activities, play the games, listen to the key terms, and test yourself with the interactive review. Email, print, and/or save your results to document your proficiency.

## CHAPTER 37

# Principles of Pharmacology

## KEY TERMS

- absorption
- administer
- controlled substance
- dispense
- distribution
- dosage
- dose
- efficacy
- excretion
- generic name
- indication
- labeling
- narcotic
- opioid
- pharmaceutical
- pharmacodynamics
- pharmacognosy
- pharmacokinetics
- pharmacology
- pharmacotherapeutics
- prescribe
- prescription
- prescription drug
- toxicology
- trade name

## MEDICAL ASSISTING COMPETENCIES

*In preparation for the certification examination, you should know the following areas of competence:*

| COMPETENCY | CMA | RMA |
|---|:---:|:---:|
| **Clinical** | | |
| Screen and follow up on patient test results | X | X |
| Apply pharmacology principles to prepare and administer oral and parenteral (excluding IV) medications as directed by the physician | X | X |
| Maintain medication and immunization records | X | X |
| Initiate IV and administer IV medications with appropriate training and as permitted by state law | X | X |
| Recognize emergencies; perform first aid and CPR | | X |
| **General/Legal/Professional** | | |
| Be aware of and perform within legal and ethical boundaries | X | X |
| Determine the needs for documentation and reporting, and document accurately and appropriately | X | X |
| Demonstrate knowledge of and monitor current federal and state health-care legislation and regulations; maintain licenses and accreditation | X | X |
| Follow established policy in initiating or terminating medical treatment | | X |
| Perform risk management procedures | | X |
| Perform an inventory of supplies and equipment | X | X |
| Explain general office policies and procedures | X | X |
| Instruct individuals according to their needs | X | X |
| Exhibit initiative | | X |
| Conduct work within scope of education, training, and ability | | X |
| Dispose of controlled substances in compliance with government regulations | | X |
| Provide patients with methods of health promotion and disease prevention | X | X |

# CHAPTER OUTLINE

- The Medical Assistant's Role in Pharmacology
- Drugs and Pharmacology
- Sources of Drugs
- Pharmacodynamics
- Pharmacokinetics
- Pharmacotherapeutics

- Toxicology
- Sources of Drug Information
- The Food and Drug Administration (FDA) Regulatory Function
- Vaccines
- Patient Instructions about Medications

# LEARNING OUTCOMES

After completing Chapter 37, you will be able to:

**37.1** Describe the five categories of pharmacology.

**37.2** Differentiate between chemical, generic, and trade names for drugs.

**37.3** Describe the major drug categories.

**37.4** List the main sources of drug information.

**37.5** Contrast over-the-counter (OTC) and prescription drugs.

**37.6** Compare the five schedules of controlled substances.

**37.7** Describe how to register a physician with the Drug Enforcement Administration (DEA) for permission to administer, dispense, and prescribe controlled drugs.

**37.8** Describe how to telephone a medication refill.

**37.9** Describe how vaccines work in the immune system.

**37.10** Identify patient education topics related to the use of nonprescription and prescription drugs.

# Introduction

Pharmacology, which is the science of drugs, is a great responsibility to any allied health professional. Medication mistakes made can injure or even cause the death of a patient. It is important to begin with a good working knowledge of the foundations of pharmacology. This chapter provides an overview of the role of drugs in ambulatory medical facilities.

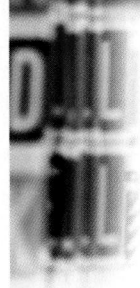

## CASE STUDY

You are a medical assistant working in a busy family practice office. You have been employed by this office for only 1 month. Your office manager tells you that because your performance to date has been excellent, you are being given the responsibility of maintaining the sample drug inventory and the office medications. The office has a space that is dedicated to the samples and office medications, but the area is very disorganized and your first task is to organize and implement an inventory system for the drugs.

As you read through this chapter, think about the steps you will take to design and implement an inventory system for your office's medications.

# The Medical Assistant's Role in Pharmacology

As a medical assistant, you will be expected to have a basic knowledge of medications. This includes knowledge of prescription drugs and over-the-counter (OTC) drugs. **Prescription drugs** require a physician's written order to authorize the dispensing (and, sometimes, administering) of drugs to a patient. OTC drugs, which are available in pharmacies and supermarkets, are purchased by people to treat themselves for ailments ranging from arthritis to colds to stomach ulcers. As a medical assistant you will need to:

- Be attentive to ensure that the physician is aware of all medications, both prescription and OTC, that a patient is taking.

- Ask each patient about use of alcohol and recreational drugs (both past and present) as well as herbal remedies.
- Educate the patient about the purpose of a drug and how to take the drug for maximum effectiveness and minimum adverse effects.

As your state permits, you may also be asked to give drugs to a patient. Safe and effective drug therapy requires advanced skills that you will want to attain. These are described in the Points on Practice section.

To handle these important functions, you must understand pharmacologic principles, be able to translate prescriptions, and be prepared to answer basic patient questions (Figure 37-1). You must also adhere to legal requirements and keep accurate records.

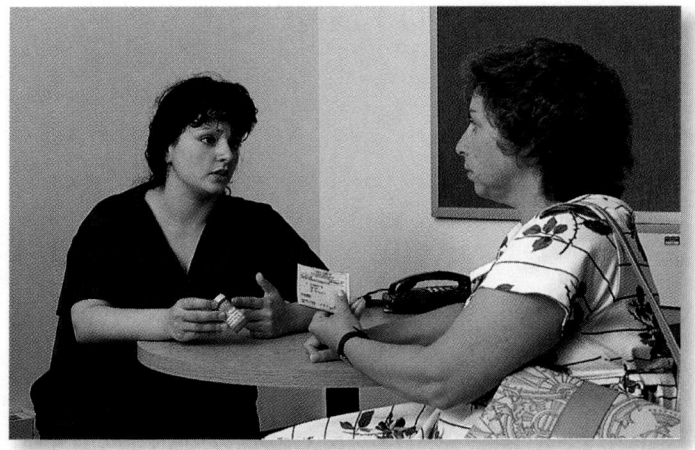

**Figure 37-1.** A medical assistant may need to be prepared to answer the patient's questions about a drug the doctor is prescribing.

# Drugs and Pharmacology

A drug is a chemical compound used to prevent, diagnose, or treat a disease or other abnormal condition. The study of drugs is called **pharmacology.** A specialist in pharmacology is called a pharmacologist. Included in pharmacology are **pharmacognosy** (the study of characteristics of natural drugs and their sources), **pharmacodynamics** (the study of what drugs do to the body), **pharmacokinetics** (the study of what the body does to drugs), **pharmacotherapeutics** (the study of how drugs are used to treat disease), and **toxicology** (the study of poisons or poisonous effects of drugs).

According to the Department of Justice's Drug Enforcement Administration (DEA) guidelines, a doctor **prescribes** a drug when he gives a patient a prescription to be filled by a pharmacy. To **administer** a drug is to give it directly by injection, by mouth, or by any other route that introduces the drug into a patient's body. A healthcare professional **dispenses** a drug by distributing it, in a properly labeled container, to a patient who is to use it.

# Sources of Drugs

Many drugs originate as natural products. Other drugs originate in the chemical laboratory, as chemists seek to improve existing drugs.

## Points on Practice

### Expanding Your Knowledge of Medications

Before you can administer medications safely, you must have a full knowledge of pharmacologic principles, be able to read and understand all medical terms and abbreviations that appear on a prescription, and maintain medication records.

Because controlled drugs are subject to many laws, you will be legally responsible for adhering to all related regulations. Laws require such activities as physician registration with the DEA, tight inventory control for drugs, and proper disposal of controlled drugs. These laws make it necessary for you to apply legal concepts to the practice on a daily basis.

Whenever a patient takes a nonprescription or prescription drug, your ability to provide helpful instructions will be vital. By educating the patient about how to use a drug properly, you will not only help the patient improve medically but also increase the probability of patient safety and compliance.

The most efficient way to prepare for all these responsibilities is to read the package inserts (Figure 37-2) and drug labels that accompany all medications, whether they are drugs from drug company representatives (the samples given to the practice to acquaint physicians with new drugs) or drugs ordered by the practice. Another excellent source of information is the *Physicians' Desk Reference,* or *PDR,* which most practices receive free of charge. To learn more about how drugs act in the body, you may want to read articles in professional journals or use the Internet.

*continued* ⟶

## Expanding Your Knowledge of Medications *(concluded)*

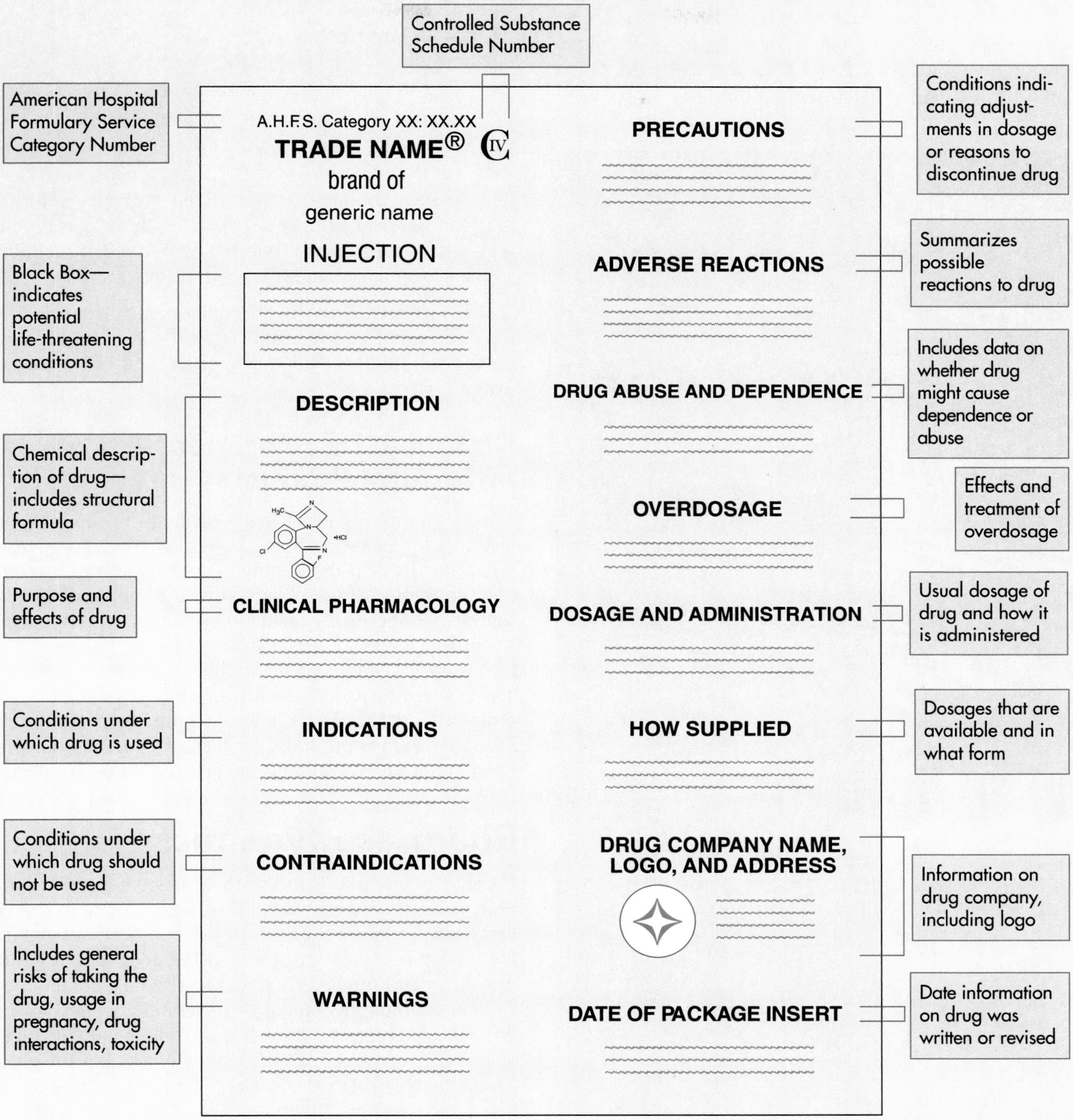

Controlled Substance
Schedule Number

American Hospital
Formulary Service
Category Number

A.H.F.S. Category XX: XX.XX

**TRADE NAME® ⒸIV**

brand of

generic name

**INJECTION**

Black Box—
indicates
potential
life-threatening
conditions

**DESCRIPTION**

Chemical descrip-
tion of drug—
includes structural
formula

Purpose and
effects of drug

**CLINICAL PHARMACOLOGY**

Conditions under
which drug is used

**INDICATIONS**

Conditions under
which drug should
not be used

**CONTRAINDICATIONS**

Includes general
risks of taking the
drug, usage in
pregnancy, drug
interactions, toxicity

**WARNINGS**

**PRECAUTIONS**

Conditions indi-
cating adjust-
ments in dosage
or reasons to
discontinue drug

**ADVERSE REACTIONS**

Summarizes
possible
reactions to drug

**DRUG ABUSE AND DEPENDENCE**

Includes data on
whether drug
might cause
dependence or
abuse

**OVERDOSAGE**

Effects and
treatment of
overdosage

**DOSAGE AND ADMINISTRATION**

Usual dosage of
drug and how it
is administered

**HOW SUPPLIED**

Dosages that are
available and in
what form

**DRUG COMPANY NAME,
LOGO, AND ADDRESS**

Information on
drug company,
including logo

**DATE OF PACKAGE INSERT**

Date information
on drug was
written or revised

**Figure 37-2.** Use the package insert to become familiar with a drug's indications, contraindications, dosage, and adverse effects. Here is a representation of a package insert for an injectable drug.

## Natural Products

Most often, drugs originate as substances from natural products, such as plants, animals, minerals, bacteria, or fungi. Figure 37-3 shows examples of natural sources of drugs.

**Plants.** Perhaps the oldest source of drugs is plants. For hundreds of years, drugs have been made from seeds, bulbs, roots, stems, buds, leaves, or other parts of plants. Two examples of plant-derived drugs are digitoxin, which comes from the foxglove plant, and quinine, which comes from cinchona tree bark. There are countless others, and new drugs are developed from plants almost daily.

**Animals.** Animals are also used as a source of drugs. Certain animal substances have been shown to be compatible with human physiology. Some examples of animal substances used as drugs are:

- Glandular substances, such as insulin and thyroid hormones
- Fats and oils, such as cod-liver oil
- Enzymes, such as pancreatin and pepsin
- Antiserums and antitoxins for vaccines

**Minerals.** Mineral sources yield various substances that can be used as they occur naturally or can be mixed with other substances. Two drugs derived from mineral sources are potassium chloride and mineral oil.

**Bacteria and Fungi.** Simple organisms, such as bacteria and fungi, produce substances that are used to make certain antibiotics. Cephalosporins and penicillins are examples.

## Chemical Development of Natural Products

After a pharmacognosist has identified the chemical properties of a natural product, a chemist conducts investigations that lead to the synthesis (chemical duplication) of one or more drugs, based on the pharmacognosist's findings. Some drugs are synthesized by strictly chemical methods. Others are duplicated by manipulating genetic information in a host organism. These types of manipulations can cause a host organism to produce a biologic product ordinarily produced only in another organism. For example, human insulin is produced by these means, also known as recombinant deoxyribonucleic acid (DNA) techniques.

# Pharmacodynamics

Pharmacodynamics is the study of what a drug does to the body, that is, the mechanism of action or how the drug works to produce a therapeutic effect. Pharmacodynamics includes the interaction between the drug and target cells or tissues and the body's response to that interaction.

For example, when a patient with diabetes takes insulin, the drug acts by allowing the movement of glucose across cell membranes. This movement makes the glucose available to cells to use as an energy source. The end effect is a decrease in the blood glucose level.

# Pharmacokinetics

Pharmacokinetics is what the body does to a drug—that is, how the body absorbs, distributes, metabolizes, and excretes the drug. It is important to understand these processes so that you will be able to explain to patients the

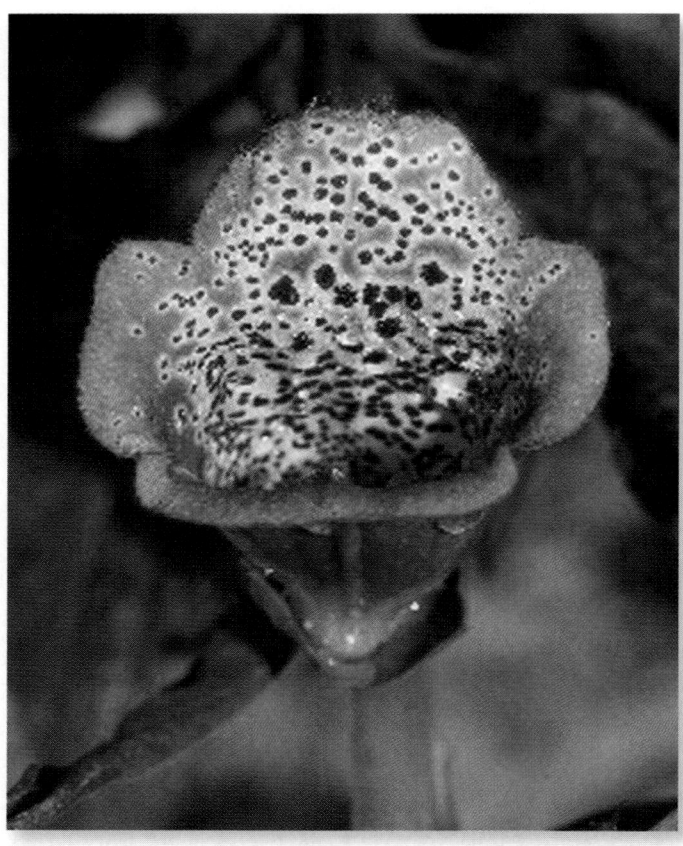

A

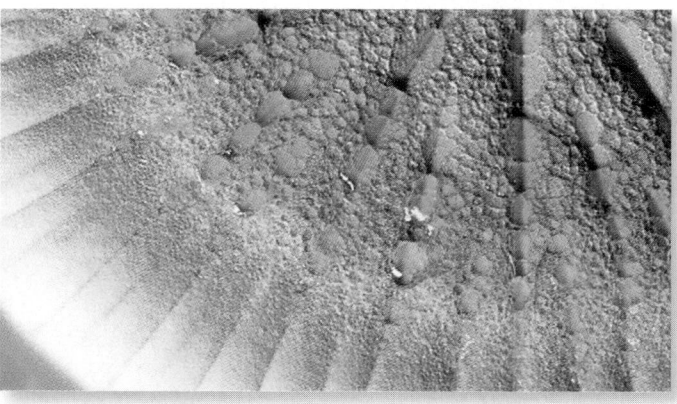

B

**Figure 37-3.** Many drugs originate as natural products. (A) The foxglove plant is the source of digitoxin. (B) Bacteria and yeasts are sources of many antibiotics.

reasons for taking a particular drug with food or for drinking plenty of water while taking a drug.

## Absorption

**Absorption** is the process of converting a drug from its dose form, such as a tablet or capsule, into a form the body can use. For example, tablets or capsules are absorbed through the stomach or intestines into the bloodstream. Water, food, or a particular food may either hinder or assist the absorption of a specific drug through the stomach or intestines. Some drugs may irritate the digestive organs if they are taken without food or water. Because of such possible reactions, patients must precisely follow instructions for taking a drug with plenty of water, with food, or without food.

Injected drugs are absorbed through the skin (intradermally), through the tissue just beneath the skin (subcutaneously), or through muscle (intramuscularly), depending on the type of injection. Absorption allows the drug to enter the bloodstream and pass into tissues. Drugs that are administered intravenously are directly available to target cells from the bloodstream. The extent and rate of drug absorption depend on several factors. One factor is the route of administration (see Chapter 38). When the drug is administered by mouth, for example, coatings on tablets or capsules and the amount and type of food consumed with the drug may affect absorption. Other factors involve the characteristics of the drug itself. For example, insulin products vary in rate of absorption, depending on their mode of preparation.

## Distribution

**Distribution** is the process of transporting a drug from its administration site, such as the muscle of an injection site, to its site of action. Distribution also pertains to the length of time a drug takes to achieve maximum or peak plasma levels, that is, the length of time between dosing and availability in the bloodstream.

## Metabolism

Drug metabolism is the process by which drug molecules are transformed into simpler products called metabolites. This transformation usually occurs in the liver, where enzymes break down the drug. Some drugs, however, are metabolized in the kidneys. Metabolism can be affected by disease, a patient's age or genetic makeup, characteristics of the drug, or other factors.

When drugs metabolized in the liver are prescribed for either children or the elderly, the dose is likely to be lower than that prescribed for young adults. Metabolism in children and the elderly is different from metabolism in other patients; the drugs may remain in the body longer and possibly reach harmful levels. The same concern holds true for any patient with impaired liver or kidney function if prescribed drugs are metabolized in the affected organ.

## Excretion

**Excretion** describes the manner in which a drug is eliminated from the body. Most drugs are eliminated in urine. Drugs may also be excreted in feces, perspiration, saliva, bile, exhaled air, and breast milk.

# Pharmacotherapeutics

Pharmacotherapeutics is the study of how drugs are used to treat disease. This area of pharmacology is sometimes called clinical pharmacology.

## Drug Names

One drug may have several different names, including the drug's official name (also known as the **generic name**), international nonproprietary name, chemical name, and **trade name** (brand or proprietary name). To demonstrate, the trade-name antibacterial drug prescribed by physicians as Keflex® or Biocef is also identified by the following names:

- Cephalexin (generic name)
- Cefalexin (international nonproprietary name)
- 7-(D-α-amino-α-phenylacentomido)-3-methyl-3-cephem-4-carboxylic acid, monohydrate (chemical name)

As a medical assistant, you will probably need to use only generic or trade names. In general, think of the generic name of a drug as a simple form of its chemical name. For each new drug marketed by a drug manufacturer, the United States Adopted Names (USAN) Council selects a generic name. This name is nonproprietary; that is, it does not belong to any one manufacturer. A generic name is also considered a drug's official name, which is listed in the *United States Pharmacopeia/National Formulary*. The 25 drugs most commonly dispensed in 2005 are listed in Table 37-1 by generic name, trade name, and category of pharmacologic activity. Notice that a drug may appear in the table more than once if the dispensing record was high for multiple trade names or for generic and trade names.

A drug's trade name is selected by its manufacturer. It is protected by copyright and is the property of the manufacturer. When a new drug enters the market, its manufacturer has a patent on that drug, which means that no other manufacturer can make or sell the drug for 17 years. When the patent runs out, any manufacturer can sell the drug under the generic name or a different trade name. The original manufacturer, however, is the only one allowed to use the drug's original trade name. For example, the antibiotic cephalexin has two trade names, Keflex® and Biocef. These names are owned by different manufacturers.

A physician may prescribe a drug by its generic or trade name. Because generic drugs are usually less expensive, most physicians try to prescribe them if possible. Many states allow pharmacists to substitute a generic

## TABLE 37-1 The 25 Drugs Most Commonly Dispensed in U.S. Community Pharmacies in 2005 Grouped by Drug Category

| Category of Pharmacologic Activity | Trade Name | Generic |
|---|---|---|
| Analgesic | Hydrocodone/Acetaminophen | Hydrocodone/Acetaminophen |
| | Propoxyphene-N/Acetaminophen | Propoxyphene-N/Acetaminophen |
| Antianxiety | Xanax® | Alprazolam |
| Antiasthmatic | Singulair® | Montelukast sodium |
| Antibiotic | Amoxil® | Amoxicillin |
| | Zithromax® | Azithromycin |
| | Keflex® | Cephalexin |
| Antidepressant | Zoloft® | Sertraline Hydrochloride |
| | Lexapro® | Escitalopram Oxalate |
| Antidiabetic | Glucophage® | Metformin Hydrochloride |
| Antihypertensive | Prinivil® | Lisinopril |
| | Tenormin® | Atenolol |
| | Toprol XL® | Metoprolol succinate |
| | Norvasc® | Amlodipine Besylate |
| Antiulcer | Nexium® | Esomeprazole Magnesium |
| Bronchodilator | Ventolin | Albuterol Aerosol |
| Diuretic | Hydrochlorothiazide (HCTZ) | Hydrochlorothiazide (HCTZ) |
| | Lasix® | Furosemide |
| Diuretic/Antihypertensive | Dyazide® | Triamterenew/Hctz |
| Hypnotic | Ambien® | Zolpidem |
| Nonsteroidal anti-inflammatory agent (NSAID) | Motrin® | Ibuprofen |
| Statin | Lipitor® | Atorvastatin Calcium |
| | Zocor® | Simvastatin |
| Steroid | Deltasone | Prednisone |
| Thyroid hormone | Synthroid® | Levothyroxine |

Source: Adapted from "The Top 300 Prescriptions for 2005 by Number of U.S. Prescriptions Dispensed," Rx List: The Internet Drug Index, www.rxlist.com.

drug for a trade-name drug unless the physician specifies otherwise. In fact, most health insurance prescription plans now require the substitution of generic drugs for trade-name drugs (unless otherwise specified by a physician). Frequently, they also require the pharmacy to charge a higher copay amount for trade-name drugs than for generic drugs. Some prescription plans now offer a mail-in pharmacy through which a patient can obtain generic drugs with a reduced copayment or without any copayment.

## Drug Categories

Drugs are categorized by their action on the body, general therapeutic effect, or the body system affected. Table 37-2 lists a variety of drug categories.

## Indications and Labeling

An **indication** is the purpose or reason for using a drug. The Food and Drug Administration (FDA) must approve

## TABLE 37-2  Selected Drug Categories

| Drug Category | Action of Drug | Examples* Generic Name (Trade Name) |
|---|---|---|
| Analgesic | Relieves mild to severe pain | Acetaminophen (Tylenol®)* <br> Acetylsalicylic acid, or aspirin <br> Morphine sulfate (MS Contin®)* <br> Oxycodone HCl (Percocet)* |
| Anesthetic | Prevents sensation of pain (generally, locally, or topically) | Lidocaine HCl (Xylocaine®, Lidoderm®)* <br> Tetracaine HCl (Pontocaine) |
| Antacid/Antiolcer | Neutralizes stomach acid | Calcium carbonate (Tums®) <br> Esomeprazole (Nexium®) <br> Lansoprazole (Prevacid®) |
| Anthelmintic | Kills, paralyzes, or inhibits the growth of parasitic worms | Mebendazole (Vermox®) <br> Pyrantel pamoate (Combantrin, Antiminth) |
| Antiarrhythmic | Normalizes heartbeat in cases of certain cardiac arrhythmias | Disopyramide phosphate (Norpace®) <br> Propafenone hydrochloride (Rythmol®) <br> Propranolol HCl (Inderal®)* |
| Antibiotics (Anti-infectives) | Kills microorganisms or inhibits or prevents their growth | Amoxicillin (Amoxil®)* <br> Azithromycin (Zithromax®)* <br> Cefprozil (Cefzil®)* <br> Ciprofloxacin (Cipro®)* <br> Clarithromycin (Biaxin® XL)* <br> Levofloxacin (Levaquin®)* |
| Anticholinergic | Blocks parasympathetic nerve impulses | Atropine sulfate (Isopto® Atropine) <br> Diclomine HCl (Bentyl®) |
| Anticoagulant | Prevents blood from clotting | Enoxaparin sodium (Lovenox®) <br> Heparin sodium (Hep-Lock) <br> Warfarin sodium (Coumadin®)* |
| Anticonvulsant | Relieves or controls seizures(convulsions) | Clonazepam (Klonopin®)* <br> Divalproex (Depakote®)* <br> Phenobarbital sodium* (Luminol® Sodium)* <br> Phenytoin (Dilantin®)* |
| Antidepressant (three types) <br>   Tricyclic | Relieves depression | Amitriptyline HCl (Elavil)* <br> Doxepin HCl (Sinequan)* |
|   Monoamine oxidase (MAO) inhibitors | | Phenelzine sulfate (Nardil®) <br> Tranylcypromine sulfate (Parnate®) |
|   Selective serotonin reuptake inhibitors (SSRIs) | | Escitalopram (Lexapro®)* <br> Fluoxetine HCl (Prozac®)* <br> Paroxetine (Paxil®)* <br> Sertraline HCl (Zoloft®)* |

*continued* ⟶

## TABLE 37-2 Selected Drug Categories *(continued)*

| Drug Category | Action of Drug | Examples* Generic Name (Trade Name) |
|---|---|---|
| Antidiabetic | Treats diabetes by reducing glucose | Metformin (Glucophage®)*<br>Glipizide (Glucotrol®)*<br>Glyburide (Micronase®)* |
| Antidiarrheal | Relieves diarrhea | Bismuth subsalicylate (Pepto-Bismol®)<br>Kaolin and pectin mixtures (Kaopectate®)<br>Loperamide HCl (Imodium®) |
| Antidote | Counteracts action of specific drug class | Acetylcysteine (Mucosil) for acetaminophen (Tylenol®)<br>Flumazenil (Romazicon) for benzodiazepines, such as diazepam (Valium®) or alprazolam (Xanax®)<br>Naloxone HCl (Narcan) for narcotics, such as morphine |
| Antiemetic | Prevents or relieves nausea and vomiting | Prochlorperazine (Compazine®)<br>Promethazine (Phenergan®)*<br>Trimethobenzamide HCl (Tigan) |
| Antifungal | Kills or inhibits growth of fungi | Amphotericin B (Fungizone®)<br>Fluconazole (Diflucan®)*<br>Nystatin (Mycostatin®)*<br>Terbinafine (Lamisil®)* |
| Antihistamine | Counteracts effects of histamine and relieves allergic symptoms | Cetirizine HCl (Zyrtec®)*<br>Diphenhydramine HCl (Benadryl®)<br>Fexofenadine (Allegra®)*<br>Desloratadine (Clarinex®)* |
| Antihypertensive | Reduces blood pressure | Amlodipine (Norvasc®)*<br>Diltiazem hydrochloride (Cartia XL®)<br>Quinapril (Prinivil®)* |
| Anti-inflammatory (two types)<br>  Nonsteroidal (NSAIDs)<br><br><br><br>  Steroids | Reduces inflammation | Naproxen (Aleve)<br>Colchicine*<br>Ibuprofen (Motrin®, Advil®)*<br><br>Dexamethasone (Decadron®)<br>Methylprednisolone (Medrol®)*<br>Prednisone (Deltasone)*<br>Triamcinoline (Kenalog®) |
| Antilipidemic | Lowers blood lipids such as triglyeride | Gemfibrozil<br>Atorvastatin (Lipitor®)*<br>Fenofibrate (TriCor®)* |
| Antineoplastic | Poisons cancerous cells | Bleomycin sulfate (Blenoxane®)<br>Dactinomycin (Cosmegen®)<br>Paclitaxel (Taxol®)<br>Tamoxifen citrate (Nolvadex®)* |

*continued* →

**TABLE 37-2** **Selected Drug Categories** *(continued)*

| Drug Category | Action of Drug | Examples* Generic Name (Trade Name) |
|---|---|---|
| Antipsychotic | Controls psychotic symptoms | Chlorpromazine HCl (Thorazine®)<br>Clozapine (Clozaril®)<br>Haloperidol (Haldol®)<br>Risperidone (Risperdal®)<br>Thioridazine HCl (Mellaril®) |
| Antipyretic | Reduces fever | Acetaminophen (Tylenol®)<br>Acetylsalicylic acid, or aspirin |
| Antiseptic | Inhibits growth of microorganisms | Isopropyl alcohol, 70%<br>Povidone-iodine (Betadine)<br>Chlorhexidine gluconate (PerioChip) |
| Antitussive | Inhibits cough reflex | Codeine<br>Dextromethorphan hydrobromide (component of Robitussin® DM) |
| Bronchodilator | Dilates bronchi (airways in the lungs) | Albuterol (Proventil®)*<br>Epinephrine (Epinephrine Mist)<br>Salmeterol (Severent) |
| Cathartic (laxative) | Induces defecation, alleviates constipation | Bisacodyl (Dulcolax®)<br>Casanthranol (Peri-Colace)<br>Magnesium hydroxide (Milk of Magnesia®) |
| Contraceptive | Reduces risk of pregnancy | Ethinyl estradiol and norgestimate (Ortho Tri-Cyclen®)*<br>Norethindrone and ethinyl estradiol (Ortho-Evra®)*<br>Norgestrel (Ovrette) |
| Decongestant | Relieves nasal swelling and congestion | Oxymetazoline HCl (Afrin)<br>Phenylephrine HCl (Neo-Synephrine®)<br>Pseudoephedrine HCl (Sudafed®) |
| Diuretic | Increases urine output, reduces blood pressure and cardiac output | Bumetanide (Bumex®)<br>Furosemide (Lasix®)*<br>Hydrochlorothiazide (Hydrodiuril®)*<br>Mannitol |
| Expectorant | Liquefies mucus in bronchi; allows expectoration of sputum, mucus, and phlegm | Guaifenesin (component of Robitussin®) |
| Hemostatic | Controls or stops bleeding by promoting coagulation | Aminocaprocic acid (Amicar)<br>Phytonadione or vitamin $K_1$ (Mephyton®)<br>Thrombin (Thrombogen) |
| Hormone replacement | Replaces or resolves hormone deficiency | Insulin (Humulin)* for pancreatic deficiency<br>Levothyroxine sodium (Synthroid®)* for thyroid deficiency |

*continued* ⟶

## TABLE 37-2 Selected Drug Categories *(concluded)*

| Drug Category | Action of Drug | Examples* Generic Name (Trade Name) |
|---|---|---|
| Hypnotic (sleep-inducing) or sedative | Induces sleep or relaxation (depending on drug potency and dosage) | Chloral hydrate (Noctec®)<br>Ethchlorvynol (Placidyl)<br>Secobarbital sodium (Seconal® Sodium)<br>201 pidem (Ambien®)* |
| Muscle relaxant | Relaxes skeletal muscles | Carisoprodol (Rela or Soma®)<br>Cyclobenzaprine HCl (Flexeril)* |
| Mydriatic | Constricts vessels of eye or nasal passage, raises blood pressure, dilates pupil of eye in ophthalmic preparations | Atropine sulfate (Allergan) for ophthalmic use<br>Phenylephrine HCl (Alcon Efrin) for ophthalmic use or (Neo-Synephrine® HCl) for nasal use |
| Stimulant (central nervous system) | Increases activity of brain and other organs, decreases appetite | Amphetamine sulfate (Benzadrine)<br>Caffeine (No-Doz); also component of many analgesic formulations and coffee |
| Vasoconstrictor | Constricts blood vessels, increases blood pressure | Dopamine HCl (Intropin)<br>Norepinephrine bitartrate (Levophed) |
| Vasodilator | Dilates blood vessels, decreases blood pressure | Enalopril (Vasotec®)<br>Lisinopril (Prinivil®)*<br>Nitroglycerin (Nitrostat®*, NitroQuick®) |

*Indicates one of the top 300 prescription medications for 2005 by number of U.S. prescriptions dispensed.

*Note:* Some drugs have a secondary category. When in doubt, check the *PDR* or other drug Reference.

Sources: *Physicians' Desk Reference; (PDR)* 2006.

indications before they can become part of a drug's **labeling.** The FDA is an agency of the Department of Health and Human Services. It regulates the manufacture and distribution of every drug used in the United States. Labeling also includes the form of the drug, such as tablet or liquid.

Regardless of category, some drugs may be used to treat several different conditions. Multiple uses are possible if the drug affects several body systems at once or if the drug's primary effect produces significant secondary effects in other body systems.

When a drug is used for multiple indications, one or more indications may not be in its labeling. Off-label prescribing is legal. Doctors who do it usually know from continuing education (seminars or journal articles) that such uses are generally accepted. For example, Benadryl (diphenhydramine) is an antihistamine used to treat allergic symptoms in both children and adults. Because it tends to make a patient sleepy but is safe for children, a pediatrician may use a low dose of Benadryl as a temporary sedative for a young child. Its use as a sedative, however, is not part of the labeling for Benadryl.

Another example of a drug with multiple uses is minoxidil. As a trade-name tablet, it is known as the antihypertensive Loniten; as a trade-name topical solution, it is known as the hair-growth stimulant Rogaine. In the case of minoxidil, both indications are approved, but the tablet labeling is for hypertension and the topical solution labeling is for hair growth.

It is important to be aware of these labeling considerations when dealing with questions from patients. Never assume that a drug is appropriate for only one use or that it is administered in only one form. Always consult the doctor or other sources of drug information before answering a patient's question.

## Safety

The safety of a drug is determined by how many and what kinds of adverse effects are associated with it. Some adverse effects are common, whereas others are rare. An adverse effect may require immediate attention. It is not uncommon for a patient to call the physician's office with complaints of new symptoms soon after beginning therapy with a drug. Be alert for such complaints, because they could be signs of an adverse reaction to the drug or an interaction with another medication. These calls should be brought to the physician's attention.

## Efficacy

A patient may complain that a newly prescribed drug is not doing what the doctor said it would. There are a variety of explanations for such a complaint, including the following:

- The drug is working adequately, but the patient does not understand how it works.
- The **dosage** (size, frequency, and number of doses) needs to be adjusted.
- The patient is not taking the medication according to the directions.
- The drug has not yet reached a therapeutic level in the bloodstream.
- The wrong drug was prescribed, or the wrong drug was dispensed by the pharmacy (this is rare, but possible).
- Some drugs work better in some patients than in others; not every drug is for everyone (this is particularly true of antihistamines).
- Some forms of a drug work better than others, such as tablets versus injection.
- The generic drug does not work, but the trade-name drug does.

## Kinds of Therapy

There are several descriptive terms for drug therapy. Depending on a patient's condition, the physician may use drugs for any of the following kinds of therapy:

- Acute: Drug is prescribed to improve a life-threatening or serious condition, such as epinephrine for severe allergic reaction
- Empiric: Drug is prescribed according to experience or observation until blood or other tests prove another therapy to be appropriate, such as penicillin for suspected strep throat
- Maintenance: Drug is prescribed to maintain a condition of health, especially in chronic disease, such as an anti-inflammatory medication for inflammatory bowel disease
- Palliative: Drug is prescribed to reduce the severity of a condition or its accompanying pain, such as morphine for cancer
- Prophylactic: Drug is prescribed to prevent a disease or condition, such as immunizations or birth control drugs
- Replacement: Drug is prescribed to provide chemicals otherwise missing in a patient, such as hormone replacement therapy for a woman in menopause
- Supportive: Drug is prescribed for a condition other than the primary disease until that disease resolves, such as a corticosteroid for severe allergic reactions.
- Supplemental: Drug or nutrients are prescribed to avoid deficiency, such as iron for a woman who is pregnant

## Toxicology

Toxicology is the study of the poisonous effects, or toxicity, of drugs, including adverse effects and drug interactions.

Because you are likely to see evidence of immediate toxic effects only when administering a drug, this topic will be discussed in more detail in Chapter 38. You must be aware, however, of some possible toxic effects that may not be apparent right away:

- An adverse effect on a fetus when the drug crosses the placenta
- An adverse effect on infants when the drug passes easily into breast milk
- Adverse reactions reported in clinical trials, such as headache, drowsiness, gastric upset, or other effects
- An adverse effect in immunocompromised patients who are unable to metabolize a drug normally
- An adverse effect in pediatric or elderly patients or in patients with hypertension, diabetes mellitus, or other serious chronic conditions
- An adverse drug interaction when the drug is taken with another drug that is incompatible
- A carcinogenic (cancer-causing) effect in some patients

Nearly always, an adverse effect has been encountered in the clinical trials of a drug, and there will be mention of the adverse effect under that heading in the package insert or in accepted drug reference works. In the reports of clinical trials, however, the drug company must report *all* adverse effects noted during testing. As a result, effects that, at least theoretically, could not be caused by the drug are included. In dealing with patients who are about to begin drug therapy, it is best to use discretion when mentioning specific adverse effects associated with drugs. The patient must be informed; however, you do not want to cause undue alarm or discourage patients from taking the needed medication. Always ask patients if they have any questions, and have the doctor answer patients' questions if they are drug-related. Because patients will receive lists of adverse effects from the pharmacist, encourage them to discuss concerns with the pharmacist or to call the doctor's office. Also encourage patients to inform the doctor of adverse effects they experience after beginning drug therapy.

## Sources of Drug Information

It is important to keep several up-to-date sources of drug information in the office for when you or the doctor need detailed information about a specific drug. In addition to books, many sources for drug information are available online or through personal digital assistant (PDA) devices. Books to refer to include the *Physicians' Desk Reference* (Figure 37-4), *Drug Evaluations, United States Pharmacopeia/National Formulary,* and *American Hospital Formulary Service.*

### *Physicians' Desk Reference (PDR)*

The *Physicians' Desk Reference,* or *PDR,* publishes annually, along with supplements twice a year. It sends the book

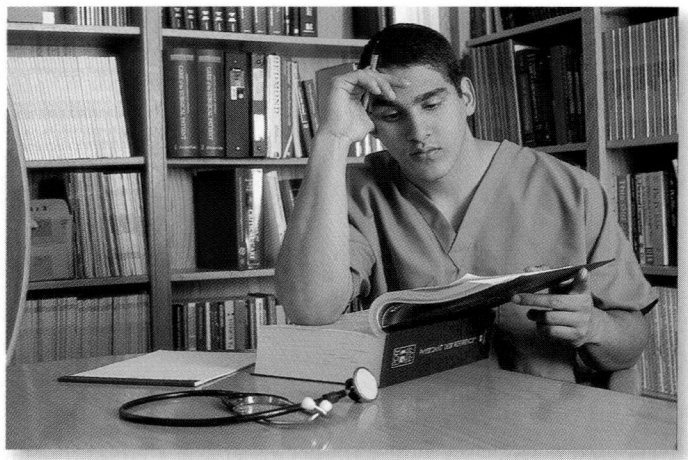

**Figure 37-4.** The *Physician's Desk Reference* is one of several publications in which you can find current information on specific drugs.

free to doctors' offices and sells it through bookstores. The company also publishes separate editions for generic, nonprescription, and ophthalmologic drugs as well as a guide to drug interactions, adverse effects, and indications. It is also available online.

The *PDR* presents information provided by pharmaceutical companies about more than 2500 prescription drugs. The *PDR* has the following sections:

- Section 1–Manufacturer's index (color-coded white), which includes the pharmaceutical company's name, address, emergency telephone number, and available products
- Section 2–Brand- and generic-name index (color-coded pink)
- Section 3–Product category index (color-coded blue)
- Section 4–Product identification guide with full-color photos of more than 2400 actual medications
- Section 5–Product information
- Section 6–Diagnostic product information

The product information section is divided according to manufacturer, and the drugs are then grouped alphabetically within each manufacturer's subsection. The information is provided for the PDR by the manufacturer and is either the drug package insert or closely resembles it. The package insert for each drug describes the drug, its purpose and effects (clinical pharmacology), indications, contraindications (conditions under which the drug should not be administered), warnings, precautions, adverse reactions, drug abuse and dependence, overdosage, dosage and administration, and how the drug is supplied (for example, tablets in different doses, or liquid). (Review the package insert illustration, Figure 37-2, included in the earlier Points on Practice section.)

After the large product information section, various smaller other sections are provided. These sections include diagnostic product information, state drug information centers, ratings for drug use in pregnancy, a state DEA directory, state-aided drug-assistance programs, patient assistance programs, drugs that should not be crushed, dosing instructions in Spanish, and the system for reporting adverse reactions to medications. All of these plus the PDR Internet site and PDR electronic library on the CD that comes with the PDR could be important resources for you.

## Epocrates

Epocrates is a software program that can be loaded on to a PDA. This electronic resource includes more that 3,300 brand and generic drugs, alternative medicines, a drug-drug interaction checker, an IV compatibility checker, health insurance Medicare Part D formularies, and an infectious disease treatment guide.

## United States Pharmacopeia/National Formulary

The *United States Pharmacopeia/National Formulary,* or *USP/NF,* is the official source of drug standards in the United States and is published about every 5 years. As the official public standards-setting authority for all prescription medications, OTC drugs, dietary supplements, and other health-care products, by law, every product sold under a name listed in the *USP/NF* must meet the strict standards of the *USP.*

The *USP/NF* describes each product approved by the federal government and lists its standards for purity, composition, and strength as well as its uses, dosages, and storage. The *NF* portion of the book provides the chemical formulas of the drugs.

## American Hospital Formulary Service (AHFS)

The American Society of Hospital Pharmacists in Bethesda, Maryland, publishes the *American Hospital Formulary Service,* or *AHFS.* It sells the two-volume set by subscription and provides four to six supplements each year. The *AHFS* lists generic names and is divided into sections based on drug actions.

## The Food and Drug Administration (FDA) Regulatory Function

The Food and Drug Administration (FDA) requires that drug manufacturers perform clinical tests on new drugs before the drugs are used by humans. These tests include toxicity tests in laboratory animals, followed by clinical studies (frequently called clinical trials) in controlled groups of volunteers, such as the one shown in Figure 37-5. Some volunteers are patients; others are healthy subjects.

Clinical tests are designed to consider the ratio of benefits to the risk of adverse side effects. If the clinical tests

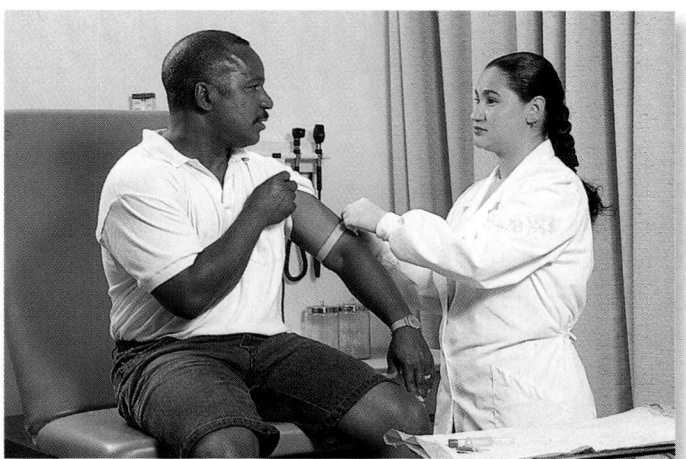

**Figure 37-5.** Tests such as blood tests provide baseline data on volunteers at the start of clinical trials.

prove that the drug is safe and effective, the FDA approves it for marketing. The manufacturer must continue to demonstrate the drug's safety and **efficacy** (therapeutic value) and must submit reports whenever it discovers unexpected adverse reactions. The FDA can withdraw a drug from the market at any time if evidence suggests that it is no longer safe or effective.

During the clinical trials the **pharmaceutical** (drug) company studies all aspects of the pharmacology of the new drug. When the company seeks approval from the FDA, it must document the pharmacodynamics, pharmacokinetics, safety (how many and what kind of adverse effects), and efficacy of the drug. In addition, it must present data regarding the **dose,** the amount of drug given at one time.

After the FDA approves a drug, it continues its regulatory function to protect patients and consumers. The FDA reviews new-indication proposals (applications from companies for new indications for a drug), OTC proposals (applications for OTC status of a prescription drug), and further clinical trial results. If an adverse effect appears many times, for example, the FDA may withdraw the causative drug from the market.

## Drug Manufacturing

The FDA also regulates drug manufacturing. It ensures that drugs shipped between states have the proper identity, strength, purity, and quality. Each manufacturer must consistently identify each drug by a particular color, form, shape, size, and label. It must produce every dose at the same tested strength, using the exact formula approved by the FDA. The manufacturer must also use high-quality, contaminant-free ingredients.

## Nonprescription, or Over-the-Counter, Drugs

A nonprescription, or OTC, drug is one that the FDA has approved for use without the supervision of a licensed health-

care practitioner. The consumer must follow the manufacturer's directions to use the drug safely. Some drugs, such as aspirin and vitamin supplements, have been OTC drugs for many years. The number of prescription drugs that have been granted OTC status is increasing. Although OTC drugs are safe when used as directed on the package, patient education contributes significantly to their safe use.

## Prescription Drugs

A prescription drug is one that can be used only by order of a physician and must be dispensed by a licensed healthcare professional, such as a pharmacist, physician, podiatrist, or licensed midwife. Some prescription drugs are dispensed as OTC medications at much lower strengths.

## Pregnancy Categories

Because clinical trials are not typically done on pregnant women, most of the data about the effect of medications on pregnant women is obtained after FDA approval. Some drugs can cause physical defects to the fetus if the mother takes them during pregnancy, especially during the first trimester. To assist physicians who are prescribing medications for pregnant women, the FDA has created the categories A, B, C, D, and X based upon the degree to which available information has ruled out risk to the fetus. See Table 37-3.

Most medications are typically Category C, although a medication can change categories after approval based upon adverse reactions. Also, some medications are placed into a different category based upon the trimester of the pregnancy.

## Controlled Substances

A **controlled substance** is a drug or drug product that is categorized as potentially dangerous and addictive. The greater the potential, the more severe the limitations on prescribing it. Use of these controlled drugs is strictly regulated by federal laws. States, municipalities, and institutions must adhere to these laws but may also impose their own regulations.

**Comprehensive Drug Abuse Prevention and Control Act.** The Comprehensive Drug Abuse Prevention and Control Act, also known as the Controlled Substances Act (CSA) of 1970, is the federal law that created the Drug Enforcement Administration (DEA) and strengthened drug enforcement authority. The CSA designates five schedules, according to degree of potential for a substance to be abused or used for a nontherapeutic effect. The five schedules and examples of substances in each are outlined in Table 37-4.

Sometimes the DEA reclassifies drugs. For example, a Schedule III drug may eventually be found to be less addictive than originally determined and therefore reclassified as a Schedule IV drug.

***Schedule I Drugs.*** Drugs that are Schedule I substances have a high abuse potential or pose unacceptable dangers. Heroin, LSD, and peyote fall into this category. These drugs have no accepted medical use in the United States.

## TABLE 37-3  Categories for Drug Use in Pregnancy

| Category | Description |
|---|---|
| A | *Controlled studies show no risk.* Adequate, well-controlled studies in pregnant women have not shown an increased risk of fetal abnormalities. |
| B | *No evidence of risk in humans.* Either animal findings show risk while human findings do not, or, if no adequate human studies have been done, animal findings are negative. |
| C | *Risk cannot be ruled out.* Human studies are lacking, and animal findings are either positive for fetal risk or lacking as well. Potential benefits may outweigh the risks. |
| D | *Positive evidence of risk.* Studies in pregnant women, either adequate and well-controlled or observational, have demonstrated a risk to the fetus. Potential benefits may outweigh the risks. |
| X | *Contraindicated in pregnancy.* Studies in animals or pregnant women, either adequate and well-controlled or observational, have demonstrated positive evidence of fetal abnormalities. |
| NR | *No rating is available* |

## TABLE 37-4  Schedule of Controlled Substances

| Schedule | Description | Prescription and Legal Considerations | Examples |
|---|---|---|---|
| I | High abuse (no accepted medical use) | No prescriptions written | GHB, Heroin, LSD, Mescaline |
| II | High abuse (accepted medical use; abuse may lead to dependence) | • Must be written by DEA licensed physician and include DEA number<br>• Multiple and/or special forms may be required<br>• Must be filled in 7 days and cannot be refilled<br>• Must be stored under lock and key<br>• Dispensing records are kept for two years | Opioids—morphine (MS-Contin), meperidine (Demerol), fentanyl, barbiturates—secobarbital, amphetamines—methylphenidate (Ritalin®) |
| III | Lower abuse than Schedule I and II drugs (accepted medical use; abuse may lead to moderate dependence) | • Five refills are allowed in 6 months<br>• Handwritten by physician<br>• Can only be telephoned by physician | Anabolic steroids, hydrocodone/codeine (Vicodin®, Tylenol 3®), barbiturate—talbutal, paregoric |
| IV | Lower abuse than Schedule III drugs (accepted medical use; abuse may lead to limited dependence) | • Five refills are allowed in 6 months<br>• Must be signed by physician<br>• Refills may be authorized over the phone | Benzodiazepines– alprazolam (Xanax®), chloridiazepoxide (Librium®), diazepam (Valium®), zolpidem (Ambien®), pentazocine (Talwin®) |
| V | Lower abuse than Schedule IV drugs (accepted medical use; very limited physical dependence) | • Inventory records must be kept on these drugs<br>• Five refills are allowed in 6 months<br>• Must be signed by physician<br>• Refills may be authorized over the phone | Antitussive and antidiarrheals that combine small amounts of opioids including (Lomotil®), (Kaolin), and (Robitussin A-C®) |

Source: U.S. Department of Justice Drug Enforcement Administration Office of Diversion Control, www.deadiversion.usdoj.gov.

**Schedule II Drugs.** Drugs that are Schedule II substances have a high potential for abuse and may cause physical or psychological dependence. They do have therapeutic uses for which they require written prescriptions. Prescriptions for these drugs may not be renewed. Examples of these drugs include dextroamphetamines (Dexedrine® ), secobarbital (Seconal), and opioids. **Opioids** are natural or synthetic drugs that produce opium-like effects, such as codeine, morphine, and meperidine (Demerol® ). Government agencies use the popular term **narcotics** for opioids.

**Schedule III Drugs.** Drugs that are Schedule III substances have a lower abuse potential than do drugs that are Schedule I or II substances and may cause moderate-to-low physical or psychological dependence. Prescriptions for these drugs may be given orally or in writing. Prescriptions may include refills, but refills are limited to five refills within 6 months of the original prescription. Schedule III drugs include certain stimulants, depressants, anabolic steroids, and narcotics in limited strengths. Benzphetamine (Didrex), butabarbital (Butisol), and methyltestosterone (Virilon) are specific examples of Schedule III drugs.

**Schedule IV Drugs.** Drugs that are Schedule IV substances have a lower abuse potential than do drugs that are Schedule III substances and have various therapeutic uses. Prescriptions may include refills, but refills are limited to five refills within 6 months of the original prescription. These drugs include pentazocine (Talwin), fenfluramine, and diazepam (Valium).

**Schedule V Drugs.** Drugs that are Schedule V substances have a lower abuse potential than do drugs that are Schedule IV substances and have varied therapeutic uses. Most Schedule V drugs are dispensed like other nonopioid prescription drugs, but some may be dispensed without a prescription, depending on state regulations. Most of these drugs are antidiarrheals or antitussives that contain small amounts of opioids, such as codeine, dihydrocodeine, or diphenoxylate.

**Controlled Substance Labeling.** The Controlled Substances Act also set up a labeling system to identify controlled substances. An example of this label is shown in Figure 37-6. The large C means that the drug is a controlled

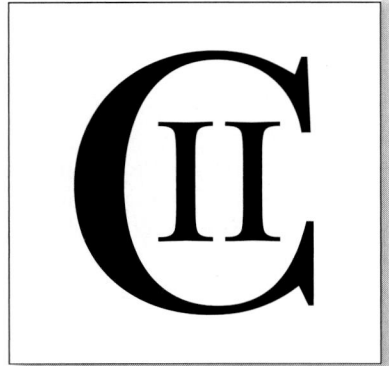

**Figure 37-6.** This symbol indicates that the drug is a Schedule II controlled substance.

substance, and the Roman numeral inside the C corresponds to the DEA schedule to which the drug belongs.

**Doctor Registration.** Under the CSA, doctors who administer, dispense, or prescribe any controlled substance must register with the DEA and must have a current state license to practice medicine and, if required, a state controlled substance license. They must also comply with all aspects of the CSA, as outlined in Procedure 37-1.

To register the doctor with the DEA, submit DEA Form 224 (Figure 37-7), called the Application for Registration Under Controlled Substances Act of 1970. This form is available online. Once complete, send the form and fee to the Drug Enforcement Administration at the address provided. This registration must be renewed every 3 years with DEA Form 224a. The renewal steps are outlined in Procedure 37-2. Renewal is done by mail or through the Internet through a log-in process.

Doctors who administer or dispense drugs at more than one office must register at each location. Each registration is assigned a unique number, which identifies to suppliers and pharmacies that the doctor is properly authorized.

**Ordering Drugs That Are Controlled Substances.** A doctor who needs Schedule II drugs for the practice must order them by using the U.S. Official Order Forms—Schedules I & II (DEA Form 222), which you can obtain from the DEA through the mail or by Internet (Figure 37-8). One copy of the form goes to the DEA for overall surveillance of drug distribution. In most states this form can be used to obtain Schedule II drugs from the normal drug supplier.

When Schedule II drugs are ordered from an out-of-state company, some states require the doctor to send a copy of the purchase agreement (not the DEA Form 222) to the state attorney general's office within 24 hours of placing the order.

Schedules III through V drugs require less complicated ordering. They require only the doctor's DEA registration number.

**Drug Security.** Always store drugs that are controlled substances in a locked cabinet or safe. If required by state law, use double locks for opioids. The doctor or other licensed practitioner should keep the key(s) at all times, except when asking you to add to or take from the stock (if this is a task medical assistants are permitted to perform in your state). If controlled drugs are stolen from the doctor's office, call the regional DEA office at once. Also notify the state bureau of narcotic enforcement and the local police. File all reports required by the DEA and other agencies as a follow-up.

**Record Keeping.** A doctor who administers or dispenses (as opposed to prescribing) controlled drugs to patients must maintain two types of records: dispensing records and inventory records. Note that these requirements don't apply to doctors who only prescribe drugs but who do not administer or dispense controlled drugs.

**Dispensing Records.** The dispensing record for Schedule II drugs must be kept separate from the patient's regular medical record. Each time a drug is administered or dispensed, the doctor must note the date, the patient's name and address, the drug, and the quantity dispensed.

The dispensing record for Schedules III through V drugs must include the same information. The record for these drugs may be kept in the patient's medical record unless the doctor charges for the drugs dispensed. All dispensing records must be kept for 2 years and are subject to inspection by the DEA.

**Inventory Records.** A doctor who regularly dispenses controlled drugs must also keep inventory records of all stock on hand. This regulation applies to all scheduled drugs. To take an inventory, count the amount of each drug on hand. Compare this amount with the amount of the drug ordered and the amount dispensed to patients.

The controlled drug inventory must be repeated every 2 years. You must include copies of invoices from drug suppliers in the inventory record. All inventories and records of Schedule II drugs must be kept separate from other records. Inventories and records of other controlled drugs must be separate or easily retrievable from ordinary business and professional records. All records on controlled drugs must be retained for 2 years and made available for inspection and copying by DEA officials if requested.

**Disposing of Drugs.** If the doctor asks you to dispose of any outdated, non-controlled drugs, you will most likely use the disposal company that takes your biohazardous waste. The DEA does not allow businesses to flush any medications and medications should not be placed in the trash. In some cases, you may work with a larger health-care facility or pharmacy to ensure proper disposal so that medications do not pollute the environment or end up in the trash where they can be taken by someone.

## PROCEDURE 37.1

## Helping the Physician Comply With the Controlled Substances Act of 1970

**Procedure Goal:** To comply with the Controlled Substances Act of 1970

**OSHA Guidelines:** This procedure does not involve exposure to blood, body fluids, or tissues.

**Materials:** DEA Form 224, DEA Form 222, DEA Form 41, pen

**Method:**

1. Use DEA Form 224 (shown in Figure 37-7) to register the physician with the Drug Enforcement Administration. Be sure to register each office location at which the physician administers or dispenses drugs covered under Schedules II through V. Renew all registrations every 3 years using DEA Form 224a. Form 224 can be printed from the U.S. Department of Justice website. Renewal application (Form 224a) can be completed through registration at this site.

2. Order Schedule II drugs using DEA Form 222, shown in Figure 37-8, as instructed by the physician. (Stocks of these drugs should be kept to a minimum.)

   *Rationale*
   Accurate instruction from the physician is necessary to ensure safety

3. Include the physician's DEA registration number on every prescription for a drug in Schedules II through V.

   *Rationale*
   The DEA number is required or prescriptions will not be accepted.

4. Complete an inventory of all drugs in Schedules II through V every 2 years (as permitted in your state; this task may be reserved to other health-care professionals).

5. Store all drugs in Schedules II through V in a secure, locked safe or cabinet (as permitted in your state).

   *Rationale*
   To prevent theft

6. Keep accurate dispensing and inventory records for at least 2 years.

7. Dispose of expired or unused drugs according to the DEA regulations. Always complete DEA Form 41 (shown in Figure 37-9) when disposing of controlled drugs.

*continued* ⟶

# Helping the Physician Comply With the Controlled Substances Act of 1970 *(continued)*

| Form-224 | APPLICATION FOR REGISTRATION<br>Under the Controlled Substances Act | APPROVED OMB NO 1117-0014<br>FORM DEA-224 (10-06)<br>Previous editions are obsolete |

**INSTRUCTIONS**  Save time—apply on-line at *www.deadiversion.usdoj.gov*

1. To apply by mail complete this application. Keep a copy for your records.
2. Print clearly, using black or blue ink, or use a typewriter.
3. Mail this form to the address provided in Section 7 or use enclosed envelope.
4. Include the correct payment amount. FEE IS NON-REFUNDABLE.
5. If you have any questions call 800-882-9539 prior to submitting your application.

IMPORTANT: DO NOT SEND THIS APPLICATION AND APPLY ON-LINE.

DEA OFFICIAL USE:

Do you have other DEA registration numbers?
☐ NO   ☐ YES

**MAIL-TO ADDRESS**   Please print mailing address changes to the right of the address in this box.

FEE FOR THREE (3) YEARS IS $551
**FEE IS NON-REFUNDABLE**

---

**SECTION 1**  APPLICANT IDENTIFICATION   ☐ Individual Registration   ☐ Business Registration

Name 1   (Last Name of individual -OR- Business or Facility Name)

Name 2   (First Name and Middle Name of individual -OR- Continuation of business name)

Street Address Line 1 (if applying for fee exemption, this must be address of the fee exempt institution)

Address Line 2

City   State   Zip Code

Business Phone Number   Point of Contact

Business Fax Number   Email Address

**DEBT COLLECTION INFORMATION**
Mandatory pursuant to Debt Collection Improvements Act

Social Security Number (*if registration is for individual*)

Provide **SSN** or **TIN.**
See additional information note #3 on page 4.

Tax Identification Number (*if registration is for business*)

FOR Practitioner or MLP ONLY:

Professional Degree: *select from list only*

Professional School:

Year of Graduation:

National Provider Identification:

Date of Birth (*MM-DD-YYYY*):

---

**SECTION 2**
**BUSINESS ACTIVITY**

Check one business activity box only

☐ Central Fill Pharmacy
☐ Retail Pharmacy
☐ Nursing Home
☐ Automated Dispensing System

☐ Practitioner<br>(DDS, DMD, DO, DPM, DVM, MD or PHD)
☐ Practitioner Military<br>(DDS, DMD, DO, DPM, DVM, MD or PHD)
☐ Mid-level Practitioner (MLP)<br>(DOM, HMD, MP, ND, NP, OD, PA, or RPH)
☐ Euthanasia Technician

☐ Ambulance Service
☐ Animal Shelter
☐ Hospital/Clinic
☐ Teaching Institution

FOR Automated Dispensing System (ADS) ONLY:

DEA Registration # of Retail Pharmacy for this ADS

An ADS is automatically fee-exempt.
Skip Section 6 and Section 7 on page 2.
You must attach a notarized affidavit.

---

**SECTION 3**
**DRUG SCHEDULES**

Check all that apply

☐ Schedule II Narcotic
☐ Schedule II Non-Narcotic

☐ Schedule III Narcotic
☐ Schedule III Non-Narcotic

☐ Schedule IV
☐ Schedule V

**Figure 37-7.**   DEA Form 224 must be completed to register the physician with the Drug Enforcement Administration. *(continued)*

*continued* ⟶

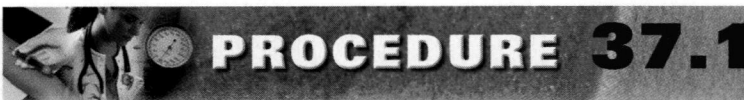

# Helping the Physician Comply With the Controlled Substances Act of 1970 *(continued)*

**SECTION 4**

**STATE LICENSE(S)**

Be sure to include both state license numbers if applicable

You MUST be currently authorized to prescribe, distribute, dispense, conduct research, or otherwise handle the controlled substances in the schedules for which you are applying under the laws of the **state** or jurisdiction in which you are operating or propose to operate.

State License Number (required)

What state was this license issued in? _____

Expiration Date (required) ___ / ___ / ___ MM - DD - YYYY

State Controlled Substance License Number (if required)

What state was this license issued in? _____

Expiration Date ___ / ___ / ___ MM - DD - YYYY

---

**SECTION 5**

**LIABILITY**

**IMPORTANT**

All questions in this section must be answered.

1. Has the applicant ever been **convicted of a crime** in connection with controlled substance(s) under state or federal law, or is any such action pending?    YES ☐   NO ☐

   Date(s) of incident MM-DD-YYYY: ☐☐ – ☐☐ – ☐☐☐☐

2. Has the applicant ever surrendered (for cause) or had a **federal** controlled substance registration revoked, suspended, restricted, or denied, or is any such action pending?    YES ☐   NO ☐

   Date(s) of incident MM-DD-YYYY: ☐☐ – ☐☐ – ☐☐☐☐

3. Has the applicant ever surrendered (for cause) or had a **state** professional license or controlled substance registration revoked, suspended, denied, restricted, or placed on probation, or is any such action pending?    YES ☐   NO ☐

   Date(s) of incident MM-DD-YYYY: ☐☐ – ☐☐ – ☐☐☐☐

4. If the applicant is a **corporation** (other than a corporation whose stock is owned and traded by the public), association, partnership, or pharmacy, has any officer, partner, stockholder, or proprietor been **convicted of a crime** in connection with controlled substance(s) under state or federal law, or ever surrendered, for cause, or had a **federal** controlled substance registration revoked, suspended, restricted, denied, or ever had a **state** professional license or controlled substance registration revoked, suspended, denied, restricted or placed on probation, or is any such action pending?    YES ☐   NO ☐

   Date(s) of incident MM-DD-YYYY: ☐☐ – ☐☐ – ☐☐☐☐    *Note: If question 4 does not apply to you, be sure to mark 'NO'. It will slow down processing of your application if you leave it blank.*

- - - - - - - - - - - - - - - - - - - - - - - - - - - - - - - - - - - - - - - - - - - - - - - - - - - - - - - - - - - -

**EXPLANATION OF "YES" ANSWERS**

Applicants who have answered "YES" to any of the four questions above **must provide a statement to explain each "YES" answer.**

Use this space or attach a separate sheet and return with application

Liability question # _____

Location(s) of incident: _____

Nature of incident:

Disposition of incident:

---

**SECTION 6**   **EXEMPTION FROM APPLICATION FEE**

☐ Check this box if the applicant is a federal, state, or local government official or institution. Does not apply to contractor-operated institutions.

Business or Facility Name of Fee Exempt Institution. **Be sure to enter the address of this exempt institution in Section 1.**

The undersigned hereby certifies that the applicant named hereon is a federal, state or local government official or institution, and is exempt from payment of the application fee.

**FEE EXEMPT CERTIFIER**

Provide the name and phone number of the certifying official

Signature of certifying official (other than applicant)     Date

Print or type name and title of certifying official     Telephone No. (required for verification)

---

**SECTION 7**

**METHOD OF PAYMENT**

Check one form of payment only

☐ Check   Make check payable to: **Drug Enforcement Administration**   See page 4 of instructions for important information.

☐ American Express   ☐ Discover   ☐ Master Card   ☐ Visa

Credit Card Number     Expiration Date ☐☐ – ☐☐

Sign if paying by credit card

Signature of Card Holder

Printed Name of Card Holder

*Mail this form with payment to:*

U.S. Department of Justice
Drug Enforcement Administration
P.O. Box 28083
Washington, DC 20038-8083

**FEE IS NON-REFUNDABLE**

---

**SECTION 8**

**APPLICANTS SIGNATURE**

Sign in ink

I certify that the foregoing information furnished on this application is true and correct.

**Signature of applicant (sign in ink)**     Date

Print or type name and title of applicant

**WARNING:** Section 843(a)(4)(A) of Title 21, United States Code states that any person who knowingly or intentionally furnishes false or fraudulent information in this application is subject to imprisonment for not more than four years, a fine of not more than $30,000,00 or both.

**Figure 37-7.** *(concluded)*

*continued* →

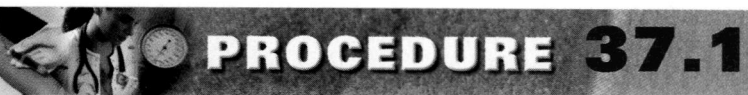

# PROCEDURE 37.1

## Helping the Physician Comply With the Controlled Substances Act of 1970 *(continued)*

**DEA Form-222**
**(Oct. 1992)**

### U.S. OFFICIAL ORDER FORMS - SCHEDULES I & II
Drug Enforcement Administration
**SUPPLIER'S Copy 1**

| See Reverse of PURCHASER'S Copy for Instructions | No order form may be issued for Schedule I and II substances unless a completed application form has been received. (21 CFR 1305.04). | OMB APPROVAL No. 1117-0010 |
|---|---|---|

To: (Name of Supplier)

Street Address

Address

City                                                    State

Date (MM-DD-YYYY)                                        Suppliers DEA Registration No.

**To Be Filled in By PURCHASER**

| Line No. | No. of Packages | Size of Package | Name of Item |
|---|---|---|---|
| 1 | | | |
| 2 | | | |
| 3 | | | |
| 4 | | | |
| 5 | | | |
| 6 | | | |
| 7 | | | |
| 8 | | | |
| 9 | | | |
| 10 | | | |

**To Be Filled in By SUPPLIER**

| National Drug Code | Packages Shipped | Date Shipped |
|---|---|---|
| | | |
| | | |
| | | |
| | | |
| | | |
| | | |
| | | |
| | | |
| | | |
| | | |

◀ **LAST LINE COMPLETED**     *(MUST BE 10 OR LESS)*

Signature of **PURCHASER** or Attorney or Agent

Date Issued                                             DEA Registration No.

Schedules                                               Name and Address of Registrant

Registered As a

No. of This Order Form

**Figure 37-8.** Use DEA Form 222 to order Schedule II drugs. The renewal can be completed online.

*continued* ⟶

# Helping the Physician Comply With the Controlled Substances Act of 1970 *(concluded)*

| OMB Approval No. 1117-0007 | U.S. Department of Justice/Drug Enforcement Administration **REGISTRANTS INVENTORY OF DRUGS SURRENDERED** | PACKAGE NO. |
|---|---|---|

The following schedule is an inventory of controlled substances which is hereby surrendered to you for proper disposition.

**FROM:** *(Include Name, Street, City, State and ZIP Code in space provided below.)*

Signature of applicant or authorized agent

Registrant's DEA Number

Registrant's Telephone Number

**NOTE:** CERTIFIED MAIL (Return Receipt Requested) IS REQUIRED FOR SHIPMENTS OF DRUGS VIA U.S. POSTAL SERVICE. See instructions on reverse (page 2) of form.

| NAME OF DRUG OR PREPARATION<br><br>Registrants will fill in Columns 1, 2, 3, and 4 ONLY. | Number of Con-tainers | CONTENTS *(Number of grams, tablets, ounces or other units per con-tainer)* | Con-trolled Sub-stance Con-tent, *(Each Unit)* | FOR DEA USE ONLY | | |
|---|---|---|---|---|---|---|
| | | | | DISPOSITION | QUANTITY | |
| | | | | | GMS. | MGS. |
| 1 | 2 | 3 | 4 | 5 | 6 | 7 |
| 1 | | | | | | |
| 2 | | | | | | |
| 3 | | | | | | |
| 4 | | | | | | |
| 5 | | | | | | |
| 6 | | | | | | |
| 23 | | | | | | |
| 24 | | | | | | |

The controlled substances surrendered in accordance with Title 21 of the Code of Federal Regulations, Section 1307.21, have been received in _____ packages purporting to contain the drugs listed on this inventory and have been: **(1) Forwarded tape-sealed without opening; (2) Destroyed as indicated and the remainder forwarded tape-sealed after verifying contents; (3) Forwarded tape-sealed after verifying contents.

DATE _____    DESTROYED BY: _____

**Strike out lines not applicable.    WITNESSED BY: _____

### INSTRUCTIONS

1. List the name of the drug in column 1, the number of containers in column 2, the size of each container in column 3, and in column 4 the controlled substance content of each unit described in column 3; e.g., morphine sulfate tabs., 3 pkgs., 100 tabs., 1/4 gr. (16 mg.) or morphine sulfate tabs., 1 pkg., 83 tabs., 1/2 gr. (32 mg.), etc.
2. All packages included on a single line should be identical in name, content and controlled substance strength.
3. Prepare this form in quadruplicate. Mail two (2) copies of this form to the Special Agent in Charge, under separate cover. Enclose one additional copy in the shipment with the drugs. Retain one copy for your records. One copy will be returned to you as a receipt. No further receipt will be furnished to you unless specifically requested. Any further inquiries concerning these drugs should be addressed to the DEA District Office which serves your area.
4. There is no provision for payment for drugs surrendered. This is merely a service rendered to registrants enabling them to clear their stocks and records of unwanted items.
5. Drugs should be shipped tape-sealed via prepaid express or certified mail (**return receipt requested**) to Special Agent in Charge, Drug Enforcement Administration, of the DEA District Office which serves your area.

### PRIVACY ACT INFORMATION

AUTHORITY: Section 307 of the Controlled Substances Act of 1970 (PL 91-513).
PURPOSE: To document the surrender of controlled substances which have been forwarded by registrants to DEA for disposal.
ROUTINE USES: This form is required by Federal Regulations for the surrender of unwanted Controlled Substances. Disclosures of information from this system are made to the following categories of users for the purposes stated.
   A. Other Federal law enforcement and regulatory agencies for law enforcement and regulatory purposes.
   B. State and local law enforcement and regulatory agencies for law enforcement and regulatory purposes.
EFFECT: Failure to document the surrender of unwanted Controlled Substances may result in prosecution for violation of the Controlled Substances Act.

Under the Paperwork Reduction Act, a person is not required to respond to a collection of information unless it displays a currently valid OMB control number. Public reporting burden for this collection of information is estimated to average 30 minutes per response, including the time for reviewing instructions, searching existing data sources, gathering and maintaining the data needed, and completing and reviewing the collection of information. Send comments regarding this burden estimate or any other aspect of this collection of information, including suggestions for reducing this burden, to the Drug Enforcement Administration, FOI and Records Management Section, Washington, D.C. 20537; and to the Office of Management and Budget, Paperwork Reduction Project no. 1117-0007, Washington, D.C. 20503.

**Figure 37-9.** Use DEA Form 41 to report disposal of controlled drugs.

# PROCEDURE 37.2

## Renewing the Physician's DEA Registration

**Procedure Goal:** To accurately complete DEA Form 224a to renew the physician's DEA registration on time

**OSHA Guidelines:** This procedure does not involve exposure to blood, body fluids, or tissues.

**Materials:** Calendar, tickler file (optional), pen, DEA Form 224a or Internet connected computer for electronic renewal.

**Method:**

1. Calculate a period of 3 years from the date of the original registration or the most recent renewal. Note that date as the expiration date of the physician's DEA registration.

2. Subtract 45 days from the expiration date, and mark this date on the calendar or create a reminder in your electronic calendar program. You might also put a reminder to submit renewal forms in the physician's tickler file for that date.

### Rationale

A reminder will help ensure renewal is done in the timely manner.

3. If you receive registration renewal paperwork (DEA Form 224a) from the DEA well before the submission date, put it in a safe place until you can complete it and have the physician sign it.

4. Before the expiration deadline, complete DEA Form 224a as instructed on the form, and have the physician sign it. Prepare or request a check for the fee.

5. Submit the original and one copy of the completed form with the appropriate fee to the DEA so that it will arrive before the deadline. Keep one copy for the office records.

6. Applicants are encouraged to use the online forms system for electronic renewal. Search the Internet for DEA Form 224A Note: The DEA form website is for renewals only and Internet renewals should not be done if you have already sent a paper application or renewal. Update and complete the areas of the form including Personal Information, Activity, State License(s), Background Information, Payment, and Confirmation. You will be able to print copies of the form once completed.

### Rationale

Using the Internet provides a quick, convenient, and secure method for renewal.

---

If the doctor needs to dispose of controlled drugs, such as expired samples, obtain DEA Form 41 (see Figure 37-9), called Registrants Inventory of Drugs Surrendered, which is available from the nearest DEA office or on the Internet. Complete the form in quadruplicate, have the doctor sign it, and call the DEA to obtain instructions for disposal of the drugs. If you must ship them, use registered mail. After the drugs have been destroyed, the DEA will issue the doctor a receipt, which you should keep in a safe place.

If doctors terminate their medical practice, they must return their DEA registration certificate and any unused copies of DEA Form 222 to the nearest DEA office. To prevent unauthorized use, write the word *VOID* across the front of these forms. Regional DEA offices will tell doctors how to dispose of any remaining controlled drugs.

## Writing Prescriptions

Any drug that is not available over the counter requires a **prescription.** According to the Controlled Substances Act, doctors may issue prescriptions for controlled drugs only in the schedules for which they are registered with the DEA.

You must be familiar with the terms and abbreviations used in prescriptions. See Table 37-5. You must become familiar with the doctor's style of writing or the electronic prescription process at your facility. With this knowledge, you will be able to administer the prescribed drugs accurately (if allowed in your state) and to discuss the prescription accurately with a patient or pharmacist.

Every prescription has four basic parts: the superscription, inscription, subscription, and signature. See Figure 37-10.

1. The superscription includes the date, the patient's full name and address, and the symbol ℞, which means "take thou" in Latin.

2. The inscription is the name of the drug (either generic or trade name) and the amount of drug per dose. It usually specifies each dose of capsules, tablets, or suppositories in milligrams, such as "Banthine 50 mg." The inscription for oral liquid drugs typically uses milligrams per milliliter, such as "codeine sulfate 15 mg/5 mL." The inscription usually gives the amount for creams, ointments, and topical liquids as a percentage, such as "Spectazole 1% cream."

# TABLE 37-5 Common Abbreviations Physicians Use When Writing Prescriptions

| Abbreviation | Meaning | Abbreviation | Meaning |
|---|---|---|---|
| ṫ | one | NS | normal saline |
| ṫṫ | two | O.D., OD | right eye |
| ṫṫṫ | three | oint | ointment |
| a | before | O.S., OS | left eye |
| A̅A̅, a̅a̅ | of each | O.U., OU | both eyes |
| a.c., ac | before meals | oz | ounce |
| ad lib | as desired | p̅ | after, past |
| amt | amount | p.c., pc | after meals |
| aq. | aqueous | per | by or with |
| b.i.d., BID, bid | twice a day | po, per os | by mouth |
| c̅ | with | PRN, p.r.n., prn | whenever necessary |
| cap, caps | capsules | pt | pint |
| d | day | Pt | patient |
| Dil, dil | dilute | pulv | powder |
| dr | dram | q. | every |
| Dr | doctor | q.a.m., qam | every morning |
| D/W | dextrose in water | q.h., qh | every hour |
| Dx, dx | diagnosis | q2h, q2 | every 2 hours |
| Fl, fl, fld | fluid | qhs | every night |
| gal | gallon | q.i.d., qid | four times a day |
| gm, Gm, g | gram | qns, QNS | quantity not sufficient |
| gr | grain | qs | quantity sufficient |
| gt, gtt | drop(s) | ℞ Rx | prescription, take |
| H, hr, h | hour | s̅ | without |
| HS, h.s., hs | hour of sleep or at bedtime | sub-Q, subq, SubQ | subcutaneous |
| IM | intramuscular | Sig | directions |
| IV | intravenous | sol | solution |
| kg | kilogram | ss | one-half |
| L, l | liter | stat, STAT | immediately |
| liq | liquid | subling, SL | sublingual |
| m, min | minim | S/W | saline in water |
| mcg | microgram | tab | tablet |
| mEq | milliequivalent | Tbsp, tbsp | tablespoon |
| mEq/L | milliequivalents per liter | t.i.d., tid | three times a day |
| mg | milligram | tinc, tr, tinct | tincture |
| mL | milliliter | top | topically |
| mm | millimeter | tsp | teaspoon |
| noc, noct | night | ung, ungt | ointment |
| npo, NPO | nothing by mouth | wt | weight |

3. The subscription contains the directions to the pharmacist. It includes the amount of each dose, if necessary (for example, 15 mL), the total number or amount of the drug to be dispensed for this prescription, and the form of the drug, such as tablets.

4. The signature, or transcription, refers to patient instructions. These are nearly always written using the abbreviations shown in Table 37-5. Instructions generally follow the abbreviation Sig, which means "mark" in Latin. The pharmacist includes the translated patient instructions on the prescription drug label.

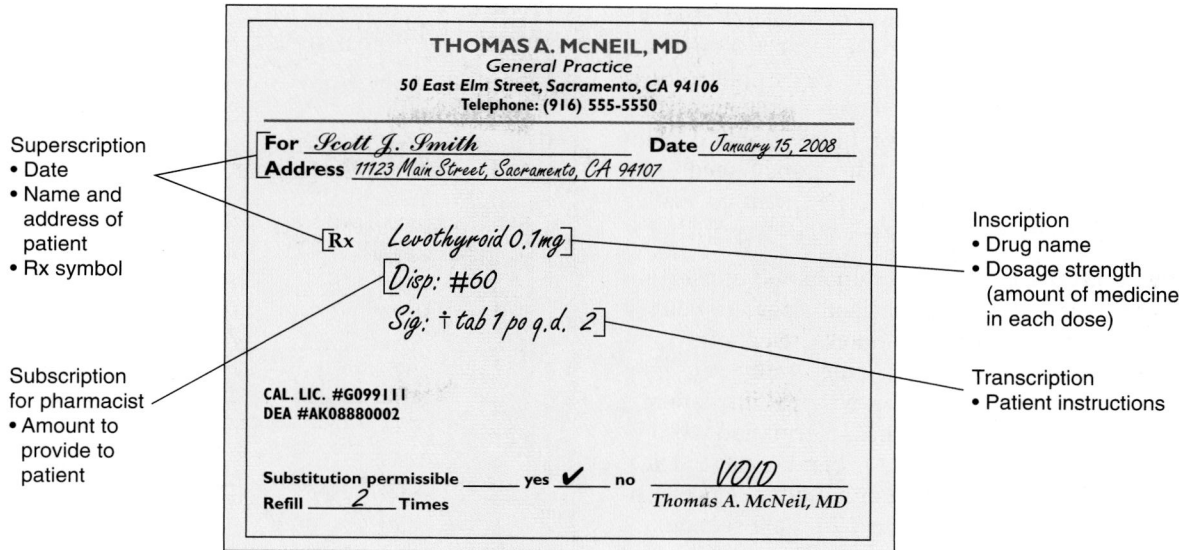

Superscription
- Date
- Name and address of patient
- Rx symbol

Subscription for pharmacist
- Amount to provide to patient

Inscription
- Drug name
- Dosage strength (amount of medicine in each dose)

Transcription
- Patient instructions

**Figure 37-10.** A complete prescription should include all the elements pictured here.

A prescription also includes these items:

- Doctor's name, office address and telephone number, and DEA registration number
- Doctor's signature
- Number of times the prescription can be refilled
- Indication of whether the pharmacist may substitute a generic version of a trade-name drug at the patient's request

Prescriptions may be typed or handwritten in ink or indelible pencil on a prescription blank. They may also be entered and received electronically. The physician can enter the prescription to be printed for the patient (Figure 37-11)

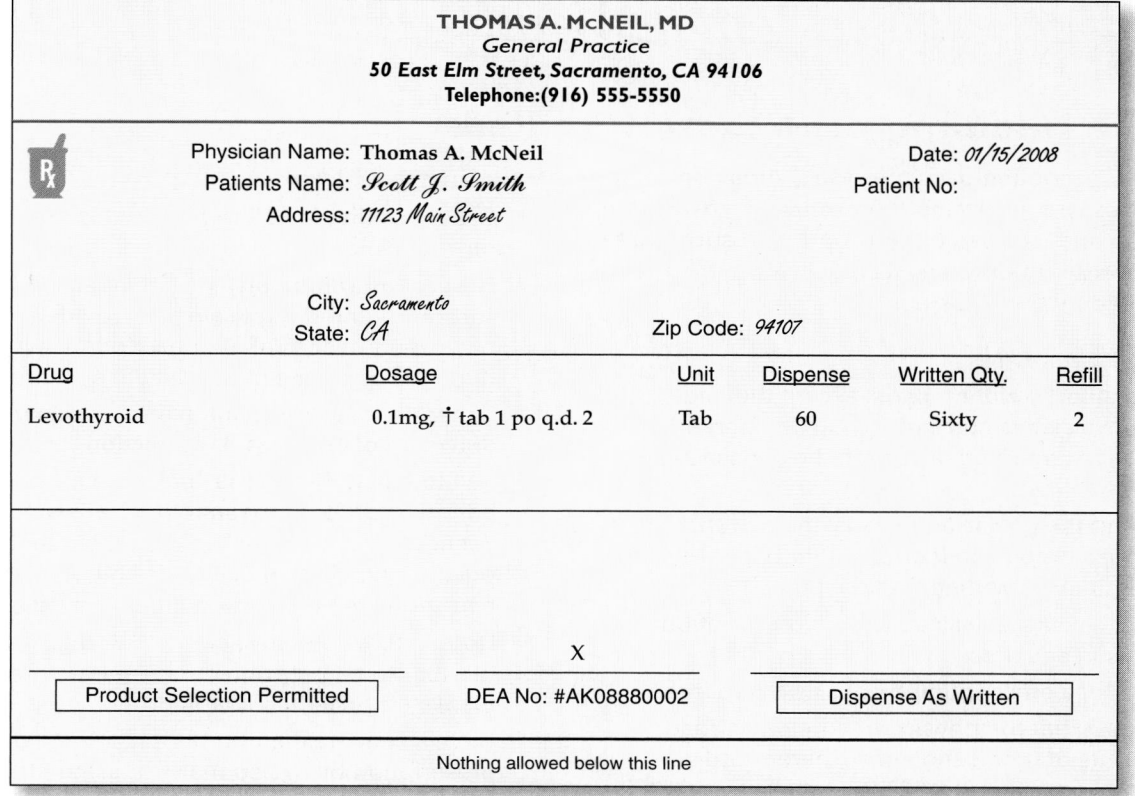

**Figure 37-11.** Electronic prescriptions, like this one, can be printed and given to the patient or sent electronically to the pharmacy to be filled.

or the information is received at the pharmacy and the actual prescription is never in the hands of the patient. Prescriptions for multiple medications may be completed on a different form than that used for a single medication (Figure 37-12). Schedule II medications require special consideration. Prescriptions for Schedule II drugs may need to be prepared in triplicate on an official Department of Justice prescription form or using an approved security printer.

**Prescription Blanks.** Prescription blanks make prescription writing convenient and efficient. They are usually preprinted with the doctor's name, address, telephone number, state license number, and DEA registration number. Most blanks also provide space for writing the patient's name and address, the date, and other information. To prevent unauthorized use of prescription blanks, never leave them unattended. For points on secures handling of prescription blanks, read the Caution: Handle With Care section.

If something about a prescription arouses suspicion, the pharmacist who receives it may call the doctor's office to verify it. You should be able to check the patient's records and tell the pharmacist whether the doctor wrote a prescription for that patient. If the prescription is a forgery, notify the doctor and, if she gives you authorization, notify the DEA.

The doctor should not use a prescription to obtain drugs for office stock. When the office needs drugs (other than Schedule II drugs), they should be obtained from a pharmacy with an order form. When the drugs are delivered, you should receive an invoice from the pharmacist.

THOMAS A. McNEIL, MD
General Practice
CAL. LIC. #G099111 50 East Elm Street, Sacramento, CA 94106
DEA #AK08880002 Telephone: (916) 555-5550

For Marjorie Smith Date January 7, 2008
Address 11123 Main Street, Sacramento, CA 94107

| SIG: | LABEL MEDICATION | MG/CC | QUANTITY | REFILLS |
|---|---|---|---|---|
| Rx 1. | Cyclobenzaprine | † tab 10mg po t.i.d. | 90 | ∅ |
| Rx 2. | Voltaren | † tab 50mg po b.i.d. | 100 | 2 |
| Rx 3. | Hydrocodone c̄ APAP | † tab 5/500mg po q4h prn pain | 30 | ∅ |
| Rx 4. | | | | |
| Rx 5. | | | | |

Substitution Permissible ______ yes ✔ no

McNeil
Thomas A. McNeil, MD

**Figure 37-12.** The physician may order multiple medications on one prescription blank like this one.

**Telephone Prescriptions.** If requested by the doctor, you may telephone a new or renewal prescription to

## CAUTION *Handle With Care*

### Secure Handling of Prescription Pads

Because prescription pads are small, substance abusers can easily steal a single prescription sheet or an entire pad and use it to obtain controlled substances. To keep prescription pads secure, handle them with caution and follow these tips.

#### Storage and Use

- Keep all prescription pads, except the pad the physician is currently using, in a locked cabinet or a locked drawer in the physician's desk.
- Remind the physician to carry the current pad at all times or to keep it out of sight but easily accessible for writing prescriptions.
- Never ask the physician to sign prescription blanks in advance.
- Never use prescription blanks as notepaper.
- Suggest that the physician write prescribed amounts of medication in numerals and words—for example, "25 (twenty-five) capsules."

#### Printing and Preparation

- Order printing in colored ink that is not reproducible.
- Order prescription blanks with attached no-carbon-required duplicates to provide a permanent record of all prescriptions written. Keep the duplicate in the patient's record.
- Order tinted prescription blanks to allow easy detection of erasures or correction fluid.
- See to it that the phrase "not valid for narcotics, barbiturates, or amphetamines" or "Not valid for Schedule II or III drugs" is preprinted in the center of each prescription blank. Use higher security and separate prescription blanks for these drugs.
- Do *not* allow the physician's DEA registration number to be preprinted on separate prescription blanks for Schedule II or III drugs.
- Have a sequencing number preprinted on all prescription blanks so that a missing blank will be noticed quickly.

the patient's pharmacy. You may not, however, telephone a prescription for a Schedule II drug. In an emergency situation, when a patient needs a drug immediately and no alternative is available, the doctor may telephone a prescription for a Schedule II drug. The amount must be limited to the period of emergency, and a written prescription must be sent to the pharmacist within 72 hours. The pharmacist must notify the DEA if a written prescription does not arrive within the specified time.

Telephone prescription renewals are called in on a daily basis from patients and pharmacies. See Procedure 37-3. The renewal requests may be called into the receptionist or left on a designated phone mail system. It is the medical assistant's responsibility to handle the prescription renewals in an appropriate manner.

# Vaccines

A vaccine is a special preparation made from microorganisms and administered to a person to produce reduced sensitivity to, or increased immunity to, an infectious disease. Vaccines are stored with the office supply of drugs and require similar handling. If you work in a pediatrician's office, you will handle the vaccines for childhood diseases. In an adult practice you can expect to see influenza vaccines and vaccines for diseases to which patients might be exposed in foreign travel.

It is important to know how vaccines work in the immune system. Immunity is discussed in detail in Chapter 19. Immunizations, particularly those for children, are discussed in Chapter 20. Adverse reactions to medications and vaccines are discussed in Chapter 38.

## PROCEDURE 37.3

### Renewing a Prescription by Telephone

**Procedure Goal:** To ensure a complete and accurate prescription is received by the patient.

**OSHA Guidelines:** This procedure does not involve exposure to blood, body fluids, or tissues.

**Materials:** Telephone, appropriate phone numbers, message pad or prescription refill request form, pen and patient chart with prescription order

**Method:**

1. Take the message from the call or the message system. For the prescription to be complete, you must obtain the patient's name, date of birth, phone number, pharmacy name and/or phone number, medication, and dosage.

2. Follow your facility policy regarding prescription renewals. Typically, the prescription is usually called into the pharmacy the day they are requested. An example policy may be posted at the facility and may state "Non-emergency prescriptions refill requests must be made during regular business hours. Please allow 24 hours for processing."

3. Communicate the policy to the patient. You should know the policy and the time when the refills will be reviewed. For example, you might state, "Dr. Alexander will review the prescription between patients and it will be telephoned within one hour to the pharmacy. I will call you back if there is a problem."

4. Obtain the patient's chart or reference the electronic chart to verify you have the correct patient and that the patient is currently taking the medication. Check the patient's list of medications, which are usually part of the chart.

5. Give the prescription refill request and the chart to the physician or prescriber. Do not give a prescription refill request to the physician without the chart or chart access information. Wait for an authorization from the physician before you proceed.

*Rationale*

All prescription refills must be authorized by the physician.

6. Once the physician authorizes the prescription, call the pharmacy with the renewal information. You cannot call in Schedule II or III medications. However, renewals can be called in for Schedule IV and V medications. Be certain to have the physician order, the patient's chart, and the refill request in front of you when you make the call.

7. Document the prescription renewal in the chart after the medication has been called into the pharmacy. Include the date, the time, the name of pharmacy, and the person taking your call. Also include the medication, dose, amount, directions, and number of refills. Sign your first initial, last name, and title.

An example of charting is as follows:

*5/03/08 Rx telephoned to Beth Stone at Noname Pharmacy: Zyrtec 10 mg, one tablet daily at bedtime, #30, 6 refills _____ K. Buckwalter, RMA*

Through the action of the immune system, a patient can be protected from—or made not susceptible to—a disease. This immunity results from the formation of antibodies that destroy or alter disease-causing agents.

## Antibody Formation

The human body creates antibodies in response to an invasion by an antigen (foreign substance). When an antigen enters the body, specialized white blood cells (lymphocytes) produce antibodies, which in turn combine with the antigens to neutralize them. This action arrests or prevents the reaction or disease that the antigen otherwise would cause. Specific antibodies always fight specific antigens.

Antigens can be bacteria, viruses, or other organisms that enter the body in spite of its natural defenses. Toxins, pollens, and drugs can also be antigens if the body reacts to them by forming antibodies. (Allergens are antigens that induce an allergic reaction.)

Vaccines contain organisms that have been killed or attenuated (weakened) in a laboratory. Because the organisms have been weakened, they stimulate antibody formation but do not overpower the body and cause disease. They may, however, still be strong enough to cause slight inflammation at the injection site and a fever. Some vaccines, such as those for the influenza viruses, may even produce some of the lesser effects of the disease against which they provide protection.

Immunizations made from organisms are called vaccines. Those made from the toxins of organisms are called toxoids. Some immunizations, such as polio vaccine, last a lifetime. Others, such as tetanus toxoid, do not. In the latter case, booster immunizations must be used to stimulate the lymphocytes to produce antibodies again.

## Immunizations

The Advisory Committee on Immunization Practices, the American Academy of Pediatrics, and the American Academy of Family Physicians jointly publish a schedule for immunizations as discussed in Chapter 20 and included in Figure 20-17, Recommended Childhood and Adolescent Immunization Schedule on page 432. This schedule covers children from infancy through 16 years of age. Just as children receive immunizations before exposure to disease, adults may receive immunizations for influenza or other diseases, including those to which an adult could be exposed during travel.

Patients are sometimes immunized after exposure. For example, if patients have been exposed to a serious disease and there is too little time for them to produce antibodies, they may receive an antiserum that contains antibodies to the disease-carrying organism. These immunizations are made from human or animal serum. If bacterial toxins (rather than bacteria) cause the disease, the patient may receive an antitoxin.

Antiserums and antitoxins must be used cautiously. They are usually reserved for life-threatening infectious diseases. Because patients can be allergic to substances in animal antiserums and antitoxins, human serums are usually preferred.

An example of a postexposure immunization is one given to a patient who has been exposed to hepatitis B virus (HBV). This patient should be given the antiserum hepatitis B immune globulin (HBV-Ig) within 7 days after exposure and again 28 to 30 days later. Because HBV-Ig is made from human serum, it causes relatively few adverse reactions. Another example involves a patient who may have been exposed to tetanus (lockjaw) organisms as the result of an injury such as a puncture wound. This patient may receive tetanus immune globulin (T-Ig, a human product) or tetanus antitoxin. Because tetanus antitoxin is made from horse serum, it may cause serious reactions in patients who are allergic to horses or horsehair.

For every vaccine in your medical office, you must be familiar with the indications, contraindications, dosages, administration routes, potential adverse effects, and methods of storage and handling. You must carefully read the package insert provided with each vaccine and, when necessary, consult drug reference books for further information. Specific information about administering vaccines is included in Chapter 38.

# Patient Instruction about Medications

As a medical assistant, you have an important role in patient instruction about medications. This role may vary depending upon your state, training, or place of employment but should not be underestimated with regard to drug education. In addition to providing specific instructions about different categories of drugs, you need to give your attention to all the drugs a patient is taking, whether prescription or OTC.

## Over-the-Counter Drugs

Even though patients can obtain OTC drugs without a prescription, they need to know several important facts to use them safely. Patients should not treat themselves with OTC drugs as a way to avoid medical care. For example, OTC drugs are available to treat recurrent yeast infections. Nonetheless, a patient should consult a doctor the first time she develops an infection.

Patients should also know that OTC drugs may not produce enough therapeutic benefit in some cases or be dangerous when used in combination with other substances. For example, a combination of the OTC medication acetaminophen (Tylenol®) and alcohol can cause liver damage. In addition, some OTC drugs may even mask symptoms or aggravate a problem.

Many OTC drugs contain more than one active ingredient. These extra ingredients, such as aspirin or caffeine, can cause allergic or other undesirable effects.

It is important to advise patients that interactions can occur when a person takes more than one OTC drug at a time or takes an OTC and a prescription drug or other substance, such as an herbal or supplement together. These interactions can lead to adverse reactions. For example, a patient who takes the prescription blood modifier (anticoagulant) warfarin (Coumadin®) to prevent blood clots must avoid taking aspirin for pain relief. Taking these drugs together increases the risk of uncontrolled bleeding.

## Prescription Drugs

Before patients begin drug therapy, they should be informed of certain considerations (such as when to take the drug) and drug safety precautions. As part of your patient education, provide instructions orally and, if possible, in writing. For commonly prescribed drugs, you may use pre-printed information sheets published by the American Medical Association. Some pharmacies now routinely provide an information sheet with each dispensed drug. Figure 37-13 shows a sample of a drug information sheet.

**Encouraging the Complete Medication List.** Patients must inform the doctor of all substances they use regularly or periodically. This includes prescription and OTC drugs, plus herbals and supplements. It also includes past and present use of alcohol and recreational drugs. When patients have more than one doctor, tell them to inform each doctor about all medications they are taking. Encourage them to keep up-to-date medication lists with dosages (some patients keep this information on their home computers). This information can help patients and health-care professionals prevent and monitor for drug interactions. The list should be kept on the patient chart and updated with every visit to the physician's office.

**Encouraging the Complete Adverse Reaction List.** Tell patients to inform each of their doctors of any adverse reactions (including allergic reactions) they have had to drugs. Previous adverse reactions may prompt a doctor to adjust a dosage or select a different drug. A history of drug allergies may contraindicate the use of a particular drug.

**Patient Compliance.** To help ensure that patients comply with instructions, confirm that they completely understand the name, dosage, and purpose of each drug prescribed for them. If patients must take more than one drug at a time, be sure they know the correct and relevant information for each one. Also teach patients to inform other health-care providers whenever there is a change in their medication regimen. In addition, cover each of the following points when educating patients about drugs.

- Explain how and when to take each drug to ensure its safety and effectiveness. Some drugs should be taken

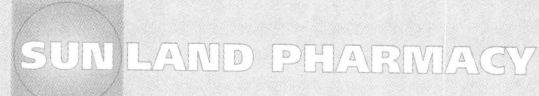

**Patient Name:** Jean Cranston
**RX#:** 711428172
**Drug:** Albuterol Inhalation Aerosol

*COMMON USES:*
To treat asthma, bronchitis, and other lung diseases.

*HOW SHOULD I USE IT?*
Follow your doctor's and/or the package instructions. Shake well before each use. Rinse mouth after each inhalation to avoid dryness. If breathing has not improved in 20 minutes, call doctor.

*ARE THERE ANY SIDE EFFECTS?*
Very unlikely, but report: Flushing, trembling, headache, nausea, vomiting, rapid heartbeat, chest pain, weakness, dizziness.

*HOW DO I STORE THIS?*
Store at room temperature away from moisture and sunlight. Do not puncture. Do not store in the bathroom. Rinse and clean inhaler regularly as described in package instructions.

**Figure 37-13.** Many pharmacies provide consumers with drug information sheets that accompany their prescriptions.

with food to minimize gastrointestinal irritation. Others should be taken on an empty stomach for proper absorption and metabolism. Some drugs must be taken once a day in the morning; others should be taken three or four times a day. If patients' medication schedules are complex, suggest that they create a chart, calendar, or diary to remind them of what drug to take and when, or create a schedule for them.

- Tell patients how long to take each drug. In the case of antibiotics, advise them to take the entire drug as scheduled, even if they feel better before finishing it. In the case of medicines prescribed for chronic disease, advise patients that they will need to continue taking the medication unless the doctor tells them to stop. Be aware that some drugs, such as prednisone, must be tapered off slowly to prevent adverse reactions.

## Preventing Medication Errors

Medication errors are the most common medical mistake. Sometimes this mistake is due to poor communication with the patient during education. A November 2006 study in the Annals of Internal Medicine indicated that many patients, especially those with low literacy, do not understand the directions on prescription containers (the Sig line on the prescription). When a prescription is given to the patient, you must ensure he or she understands it. You should review verbally and in writing how and when the medication should be taken. Use language the patient will understand. If necessary, demonstrate the process of preparing the medication. Also be certain to review any warnings about the medication, since this study also indicates that patients tend to ignore these.

- Explain how to identify possible adverse effects of each drug and safety measures related to adverse effects. For example, instruct patients to avoid certain activities, such as driving or operating machinery, while taking a drug that causes drowsiness. Also tell them to call the doctor if they experience adverse effects or any unusual reactions. If appropriate, inform patients that misuse of the drug may lead to dependence, and mention the dangers of drug dependence.

- Tell patients not to save medications that are over one year old or share them with anyone else. Old medications and those taken by people other than the patient for whom they were prescribed can cause severe, unexpected adverse effects. Advise patients to check the expiration date on all drugs and to discard them by wrapping in a tightly sealed or childproof container and placing in the trash. Flushing is not recommended due to possible water contamination.

- Suggest that patients avoid alcohol when taking a drug unless the doctor or pharmacist indicates otherwise. Alcohol interacts with some drugs, causing adverse effects such as lethargy, confusion, or coma.

- Tell patients to ask their pharmacists where to store each medication. Some drugs must be refrigerated. Others should be kept in a dry, cool area. Drugs should not usually be kept in a hot, damp place, such as a bathroom. They must always be kept out of the reach of children.

- Tell patients to take their drugs in a well-lit area so they can read each drug label carefully before taking each dose. They should never assume that they are taking the right medication without reading the label on the container. If patients have poor vision, print the name of the drug and the dosage schedule clearly on a separate piece of paper or card to attach to the medication container.

- Instruct patients to call the doctor if they have any questions about their drug therapy.

## Summary

Pharmacology is the study of drugs, or pharmaceuticals. The pharmacologist studies pharmacognosy, pharmacokinetics, pharmacodynamics, pharmacotherapeutics, and toxicology. Pharmacognosy is the study of the characteristics of natural drugs and their sources. Pharmacokinetics pertains to how the body absorbs, metabolizes, distributes, and excretes a drug. Pharmacodynamics relates to a drug's mechanism of action, or how it affects the body. Pharmacotherapeutics addresses the use of drugs to prevent or treat disease. Toxicology is the study of poisons and the toxic effects of drugs, including adverse effects or drug interactions.

Every drug has several names, including chemical, generic, and trade names. Based on its action, a drug can belong to one of many classifications. These data can be found in the *Physicians' Desk Reference* and other sources of drug information.

Patients can obtain nonprescription (OTC) drugs without a physician's order. For prescription drugs, patients must have a physician's written (or oral) order. For drugs that have been classified as controlled substances because they are potentially dangerous and addictive, extensive regulations apply. The physician must be registered with the Drug Enforcement Administration and follow the legal requirements of the Controlled Substances Act of 1970 to administer, dispense, and prescribe these drugs.

Immunizations usually contain killed or weakened organisms. They are used to provide immunity against specific diseases. Childhood immunizations should follow a recommended schedule. Other immunizations should be given as the need arises.

No matter what type of drug a patient must take, your role is an important one. Patients should be given instruction about specific drugs and required safety precautions. When you instruct a patient carefully and thoroughly about a drug, you enhance the likelihood of patient compliance and safety.

## CASE STUDY *QUESTIONS*

Now that you have completed this chapter, review the case study at the beginning of the chapter and detail the steps you will take to design and implement an inventory system for your office's medications.

## Discussion Questions

1. How would you teach a patient about medication use?
2. What is the best method to expand your knowledge of medications?
3. Distinguish between the chemical, generic, and trade names of a drug.
4. What is the protocol for prescription renewal for controlled substances?
5. What are the prescribing requirements for controlled drugs in your state?

## Critical Thinking Questions

1. What do you think is most important aspect of pharmacology in direct patient care?
2. Why should children be immunized against diseases such as diphtheria and hepatitis B?
3. Why is patient education especially important for a patient who is receiving drug therapy?

## Application Activities

1. Using the abbreviations in Table 37-5, translate the following prescriptions:
   - triamterene 100 mg po b.i.d. p.c.
   - Benadryl® 25–50 mg po hs prn insomnia
   - Rocephin® 250 mg IM STAT
   - Levothyroxine® 100 mcg po daily in am
2. Using the *Physicians' Desk Reference,* find the information on indications, contraindications, warnings, drug abuse and dependence, and overdosage for each of the following drugs: Clinoril®, fenfluramine hydrochloride, mirtazapine, Lipitor®, Zocor®, Lorazepam®, Darvocet®, and Serevent®.
3. Examine and complete samples of the forms required for controlled substances in your state and/or the facility where you will be working.

## Virtual Fieldtrip

*Visit the McGraw-Hill Higher Education Medical Assisting website at www.mhhe.com/medicalassisting3 to complete the following activities:*

Take a virtual field trip to the U.S. Department of Justice Drug Enforcement Administration Office of Diversion Control website and create a table of at least five medications from each of the controlled substances schedules. Include the DEA number, trade name, and classification with each identified controlled substance.

Open the CD and complete this chapter's practice activities, play the games, listen to the key terms, and test yourself with the interactive review. Email, print, and/or save your results to document your proficiency.

## CHAPTER 38

# Drug Administration

## KEY TERMS

- buccal
- diluent
- douche
- infusion
- intradermal (ID)
- intramuscular (IM)
- intravenous (IV)
- ointment
- route
- solution
- sublingual
- transdermal
- volume
- Z-track method

## MEDICAL ASSISTING COMPETENCIES

*In preparation for the certification examination, you should know the following areas of competence:*

| COMPETENCY | CMA | RMA |
|---|---|---|
| **Clinical** | | |
| Apply principles of aseptic techniques and infection control, including hand washing | X | X |
| Practice Standard Precautions | X | X |
| Apply pharmacology principles to prepare and administer oral and parenteral (excluding IV) medications as directed by the physician | X | X |
| Maintain medication and immunization records | X | X |
| Screen and follow up on patient test results | X | X |
| **General/Legal/Professional** | | |
| Respond to and initiate written communications by using correct grammar, spelling, and formatting techniques | X | X |
| Recognize and respond to verbal and nonverbal communications by being attentive and adapting communication to the recipient's level of understanding | X | X |
| Identify and respond to issues of confidentiality by maintaining confidentiality at all times and following appropriate guidelines when releasing records or information | X | X |
| Be aware of and perform within legal and ethical boundaries | X | X |
| Determine the needs for documentation and reporting, and document accurately and appropriately | X | X |
| Follow established policy in initiating or terminating medical treatment | | X |
| Dispose of controlled substances in compliance with government regulations | | X |
| Instruct individuals according to their needs | X | X |
| Provide patients with methods of health promotion and disease prevention | X | X |
| Exercise efficient time management | | X |
| Project a positive attitude | | X |
| Exhibit initiative | | X |
| Adapt to change | | X |
| Evidence a responsible attitude | | X |
| Be courteous and diplomatic | | X |
| Conduct work within scope of education, training, and ability | | X |
| Be impartial and show empathy when dealing with patients | | X |

# CHAPTER OUTLINE

- Drug Administration and Scope of Practice
- Dosage Calculations
- Preparing to Administer a Drug
- Techniques of Administering Drugs

- Educating the Patient About Drug Administration
- Special Considerations
- Charting Medications
- Nonpharmacologic Pain Management

# LEARNING OUTCOMES

After completing Chapter 38, you will be able to:

**38.1** Discuss your responsibilities regarding drug administration.

**38.2** Perform dosage calculations accurately.

**38.3** Describe how to assess the patient before administering any drug.

**38.4** Identify the seven rights of drug administration.

**38.5** Describe the various techniques of drug administration.

**38.6** Compare different types of needles and syringes.

**38.7** Explain how to administer an intradermal, subcutaneous, or intramuscular injection.

**38.8** Explain what information you need to teach the patient about drug use, interactions, and adverse effects.

**38.9** Describe special considerations related to drug administration.

**38.10** Describe nonpharmacologic ways to manage pain.

# Introduction

Drug administration is one of the most important and most dangerous duties for a medical assistant. By following the procedures for proper drug administration, you can help restore patients to health. If you calculate dosages inaccurately, measure drugs incorrectly, or administer drugs improperly, patients' medications may have no therapeutic effect, may worsen their disease or abnormal condition, or may cause them to die.

To administer drugs safely and effectively to all patient groups, including pediatric, pregnant, and elderly patients, you must know and understand the principles of pharmacology as presented in Chapter 37. Chapter 38 prepares you to understand the fundamentals of drug administration, including the following:

- Routes of medication administration
- Dosage calculations

- Techniques involved with various types of parenteral injections
- Seven rights of drug administration
- Patient education

Because drug administration is a vital and common aspect of your job, you must familiarize yourself with the uses, contraindications, interactions, and adverse effects of common drugs. You should be familiar with the medications frequently prescribed in your practice. Furthermore, to be able to assume a role in patient education, you must be comfortable with all aspects of drug administration so that you can instruct patients about the drugs prescribed to them.

Your responsibility in drug administration is great. Your critical thinking skills are important when performing this function. Self-directed lifelong learning is a key concept in direct patient care and drug administration.

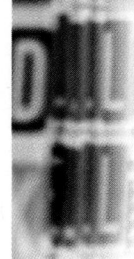

## CASE STUDY

Jennifer has been a medical assistant for a year. She works with one physician in a busy multi-specialty medical facility. She is very competent in her job and has a good working relationship with her physician based on mutual respect.

On one busy Monday morning, the physician orders injections and various procedures in three different exam rooms. Injections were ordered for two of the three patients. Jennifer is uncomfortable because she is unsure of what injections were ordered for each patient.

As you read through this chapter, think about what the medical assistant should do next and why.

# Drug Administration and Scope of Practice

Many states have medical practice acts that define medical assistants' exact duties in drug administration. For example, an act may specify which drugs you are allowed to administer and by which routes. Because state laws vary, you need to research the scope of practice for medical assistants in the state where you will work.

# Dosage Calculations

Before you can administer a drug, you may need to calculate the dose prescribed by the physician. To do so, you must understand various systems of measurement and ways to convert from one system to another.

## Measurement Systems

In the United States three systems of measurement are used in pharmacology and drug administration.

1. Metric
2. Apothecaries'
3. Household

Most drug manufacturers and doctors use the metric system. Some doctors still use the older apothecaries system. You must also be familiar with the household system, because most patients use household measures when taking medicines at home.

To understand drug measurement, focus primarily on remembering the basic unit of volume and weight for each system, as shown in Table 38-1. **Volume** refers to the amount of space a drug occupies. Weight refers to its heaviness.

**Metric System.** The basic units of volume and weight in the decimal-based metric system are liters (L) to measure volume and grams (g) to measure weight. Prefixes are added to these basic units of measurement to indicate multiples—such as dekaliter or kilogram—or fractions—such as milliliter or microgram. Common metric equivalents are presented in Table 38-2. Note that a cubic centimeter (cc) is the amount of space occupied by 1 mL. Although these two measurements are equal, the accepted medical abbreviation is mL. The abbreviation "cc" should not be used, even if you may sometimes see it in practice.

**Apothecaries' System.** The apothecaries' system uses units such as a fluidounces, fluidrams, pints, and quarts for volume, and drams, ounces, and pounds for weight. Apothecaries' equivalents you may come across in

---

| TABLE 38-1 | Comparing Selected Metric and Apothecaries' Measures (Approximate Values) | |
|---|---|
| **Measures of Volume** | **Measures of Weight** |
| Metric vs. Apothecaries' | Metric vs. Apothecaries' |
| 1 milliliter (mL) = 15–16 minims (min, ℳ) | 0.06 gram (g) or 60 milligrams (mg) = 1 grain (gr) |
| 4 mL = 1 fluidram (fl dr, f℥) | 0.5 g or 500 mg = 7¾ gr |
| 30 mL = 1 fluidounce (fl oz, f℥) | 1 g or 1000 mg = 15 gr |
| 500 mL = 1 pint (pt) | 4 g = 1 dram (dr, ℥) |
| 1000 mL or 1 liter (L) = 1 quart (qt) | 30 g = 1 ounce (oz, ℥) |

---

| TABLE 38-2 | Common Metric Equivalents | |
|---|---|
| **Measures of Volume** | **Measures of Weight** |
| 0.001 liter (L) = 1 milliliter (mL) or 1 cubic centimeter | 0.001 gram (g) or 1000 micrograms (µg) = 1 milligram (mg) |
| 0.01 L = 1 centiliter (cL) | 0.01 g = 1 centigram (cg) |
| 0.1 L = 1 deciliter (dL) | 0.1 g = 1 decigram (dg) |
| 1 L = 1000 mL | 1 g = 1000 mg or 0.001 kilogram (kg) |
| 10 L = 1 dekaliter (daL) | 10 g = 1 dekagram (dag) |
| 100 L = 1 hectoliter (hL) | 100 g = 1 hectogram (hg) |
| 1000 L = 1 kiloliter (kL) | 1000 g = 1 kg |

## TABLE 38-3 Common Apothecaries' Equivalents

| Measures of Volume | Measures of Weight |
|---|---|
| 8 fl dr = 1 fluidounce (fl oz, f℥) | 60 gr = 1 dram (dr, ℨ) |
| 16 fl oz = 1 pint (pt) | 8 dr = 1 ounce (oz, ℥) |
| 2 pt = 1 quart (qt) | 16 oz = 1 pound (lb) |
| 4 qt = 1 gallon (gal) | |

## TABLE 38-4 Common Household Measurements

| Measures of Volume |
|---|
| 60 drops (gtt) = 1 teaspoon (tsp) |
| 3 tsp = 1 tablespoon (tbsp) |
| 6 tsp = 1 ounce (oz) or 2 tbsp |
| 8 oz = 1 cup (c) |
| 2 c = 1 pint (pt) |
| 4 c = 1 quart (qt) or 2 pt |

practice are outlined in Table 38-3. The apothecaries' system also uses Roman numerals to indicate the amount of the drug. For example, ASA gr X means "10 grains of acetylsalicylic acid (aspirin)." Note that in the metric system, the amount precedes the unit, whereas in the apothecaries' system, the amount follows the unit.

**Household System.** The only household units of measurement that are used to measure drugs are units of volume. These include drops, teaspoons, tablespoons, ounces, cups, pints, quarts, and gallons. Common household equivalents are shown in Table 38-4.

## Conversions Between Measurement Systems

At times you may need to convert from one measurement system to another. Because of the difference in basic units of measure, you must remember that conversions between systems are only approximate equivalents. If you use a conversion chart, read it carefully before administering a drug. Check it several times, and place a ruler under the line you are reading to be absolutely sure you are reading the chart properly. When you must calculate conversions instead of using a conversion chart, use either the ratio or the fraction method.

**Basic Calculations.** In some instances, you can use a basic formula to calculate drugs that have the same labels—such as milligrams and milligrams—and therefore do not require a conversion. The basic calculation that you would use looks like this:

$$\frac{\text{desired dose}}{\text{dose on hand}} \times \text{quantity of dose on hand}$$

Suppose that the physician orders acetaminophen, 650 milligrams (mg). However, all that the office has on hand are 325-mg Tylenol tablets (tabs). Follow these steps to perform the basic calculation:

1. Verify that no conversion is necessary. In this example, because both measures are in milligrams, you do not need to convert the measurement.
2. Use the following formula and label all the parts:

$$\frac{\text{desired dose}}{\text{dose on hand}} \times \text{quantity of dose on hand}$$

$$\frac{650 \text{ mg}}{325 \text{ mg}} \times 1 \text{ tablet (tab)}$$

3. Cancel units and solve:

$$\frac{650 \text{ mg}}{325 \text{ mg}} \times 1 \text{ tablet (tab)} = \frac{650}{325} \times 1 \text{ tab} = 2 \text{ tablets}$$

Now let's say the physician asks you to administer and inject 10 mg of Compazine. The Compazine label notes 5 mg/mL, which means there are 5 milligrams (mg) in every 1 milliliter (mL). Follow the same steps to perform the basic calculation:

1. Verify that no conversion is necessary. In this example, because both measures are in milligrams, you do not need to convert the measurement.
2. Use the following formula and label all the parts:

$$\frac{\text{desired dose}}{\text{dose on hand}} \times \text{quantity of dose on hand}$$

$$\frac{10 \text{ mg}}{5 \text{ mg}} \times 1 \text{ mL}$$

3. Cancel units and solve:

$$\frac{10 \text{ mg}}{5 \text{ mg}} \times 1 \text{ mL} = \frac{10}{5} \times 1 \text{ mL} = 2 \text{ mL}$$

**Ratio Method.** Suppose the doctor orders ASA gr X. Although this translates to 10 grains of aspirin in the apothecaries' system, the available tablets come in milligrams, a metric measurement. To convert from apothecaries' to metric measure, you must set up a ratio to solve for $x$, the unknown dose in milligrams. Follow these steps to convert the measurement.

1. Set up the first ratio:

$$x : \text{gr } 10$$

2. Next set up the second ratio with the standard equivalent between the available and ordered measurements:

$$60 \text{ mg} : \text{gr } 1$$

3. Then use both ratios in a proportional equation that reads, $x$ is to gr 10 as 60 mg is to gr 1. Mathematically, this is written:

$$x : \text{gr } 10 :: 60 \text{ mg} : \text{gr } 1$$

4. Multiply the outer and then the inner parts of the proportion:

$$x \times \text{gr } 1 = \text{gr } 10 \times 60 \text{ mg}$$

5. To solve for $x$, divide both sides of the equation by gr 1, then do the arithmetic, canceling out like terms in each numerator (top of the fraction) and denominator (bottom of the fraction):

$$\frac{x \times \cancel{\text{gr } 1}}{\cancel{\text{gr } 1}} = \frac{\cancel{\text{gr }} 10 \times 60 \text{ mg}}{\cancel{\text{gr } 1}}$$

$$x = \frac{10 \times 60}{1}$$

$$x = \frac{600 \text{ mg}}{1}$$

$$x = 600 \text{ mg}$$

**Fraction Method** Suppose the physician orders 5 milliliters of Benadryl elixir in the metric system. However, there is only a teaspoon (tsp) available to measure the dose. To make this conversion, follow these steps.

1. Set up a fraction with the ordered dose on the top and the unknown amount on the bottom:

$$\frac{5 \text{ mL}}{x}$$

2. Next set up a fraction with the standard equivalent. Make sure that for this fraction you use units of measure on the top and the bottom that match the units of measure on the top and the bottom of the first fraction:

$$\frac{5 \text{ mL}}{1 \text{ tsp}}$$

3. Then set up a proportion with both fractions:

$$\frac{5 \text{ mL}}{x} = \frac{5 \text{ mL}}{1 \text{ tsp}}$$

4. Now cross multiply. Multiply the bottom left number by the top right number, and multiply the top left number by the bottom right number:

$$x \times 5 \text{ mL} = 5 \text{ mL} \times 1 \text{ tsp}$$

5. To solve for $x$, divide both sides of the equation by 5, then do the arithmetic, canceling out like terms in the top and bottom of each fraction:

$$\frac{x \times \cancel{5 \text{ mL}}}{\cancel{5 \text{ mL}}} = \frac{\cancel{5 \text{ mL}} \times 1 \text{ tsp}}{\cancel{5 \text{ mL}}}$$

$$x = 1 \text{ tsp}$$

## Calculations and Drug Doses

You may need to do some calculations to provide a prescribed drug dose. The ratio or fraction method can be used. No matter what method you use, you must be aware that the patient's health or life can depend on your calculations. Always take the time to check and recheck your arithmetic. If you have a question or you are not sure about your calculations, check the problem again and then have a coworker check. If you need extra practice in calculations, consider buying and using a dosage calculation workbook or searching the Internet to perform extra practice.

**Ratio Method.** Suppose the doctor orders 500 mg of ampicillin, but each tablet contains only 250 mg. To calculate how to provide this dose, follow these steps.

1. Set up a ratio with the unknown number of tablets and the amount of the drug ordered:

$$x : 500 \text{ mg}$$

2. Next set up a ratio with a single tablet and the amount of drug in a single tablet:

$$1 \text{ tab} : 250 \text{ mg}$$

3. Now put both of these ratios in a proportion:

$$x : 500 \text{ mg} :: 1 \text{ tab} : 250 \text{ mg}$$

4. Multiply the outer and then the inner parts of the proportion:

$$x \times 250 \text{ mg} = 500 \text{ mg} \times 1 \text{ tab}$$

5. To solve for $x$, divide both sides of the equation by 250 mg, then do the arithmetic, canceling out like terms in the top and bottom of each fraction:

$$\frac{x \times \cancel{250 \text{ mg}}}{\cancel{250 \text{ mg}}} = \frac{500 \cancel{\text{ mg}} \times 1 \text{ tab}}{250 \cancel{\text{ mg}}}$$

$$x = \frac{500 \text{ tabs}}{250}$$

$$x = 2 \text{ tabs}$$

As another example, the doctor orders 30 mg of Adalat, but each capsule (cap) contains only 10 mg. To calculate the prescribed drug dose using the ratio method, you would set up these equations:

$$x : 30 \text{ mg}$$

$$1 \text{ cap} : 10 \text{ mg}$$

$$x : 30 \text{ mg} :: 1 \text{ cap} : 10 \text{ mg}$$

$$x \times 10 \text{ mg} = 30 \text{ mg} \times 1 \text{ cap}$$

$$\frac{x \times \cancel{10 \text{ mg}}}{\cancel{10 \text{ mg}}} = \frac{30 \cancel{\text{ mg}} \times 1 \text{ cap}}{10 \cancel{\text{ mg}}}$$

$$x = \frac{30 \text{ caps}}{10}$$

$$x = 3 \text{ caps}$$

**Fraction Method.** For the same problem, you could use the fraction method to calculate how to provide the prescribed dose. Follow these steps for the fraction method.

1. Set up the first fraction with the dose ordered and the unknown number of capsules:

$$\frac{30 \text{ mg}}{x}$$

2. Set up the second fraction with the amount of drug in a capsule and a single capsule:

$$\frac{10 \text{ mg}}{1 \text{ cap}}$$

3. Then use both fractions in a proportion:

$$\frac{30 \text{ mg}}{x} = \frac{10 \text{ mg}}{1 \text{ cap}}$$

4. Cross multiply. Remember to multiply the bottom left number by the top right number and multiply the top left number by the bottom right number:

$$x \times 10 \text{ mg} = 30 \text{ mg} \times 1 \text{ cap}$$

5. To solve for $x$, divide both sides of the equation by 10 mg, then do the arithmetic, canceling out like terms in the top and bottom of each fraction:

$$\frac{x \times \cancel{10 \text{ mg}}}{\cancel{10 \text{ mg}}} = \frac{30 \cancel{\text{ mg}} \times 1 \text{ cap}}{10 \cancel{\text{ mg}}}$$

$$x = \frac{30 \text{ caps}}{10}$$

$$x = 3 \text{ caps}$$

As another example, the doctor orders 120 mg of Armour thyroid but each tablet contains only 30 mg. To calculate the prescribed drug dose using the fraction method, you would set up these equations:

$$\frac{120 \text{ mg}}{x}$$

$$\frac{30 \text{ mg}}{1 \text{ tab}}$$

$$\frac{120 \text{ mg}}{x} = \frac{30 \text{ mg}}{1 \text{ tab}}$$

$$x \times 30 \text{ mg} = 120 \text{ mg} \times 1 \text{ tab}$$

$$\frac{x \times \cancel{30 \text{ mg}}}{\cancel{30 \text{ mg}}} = \frac{120 \cancel{\text{ mg}} \times 1 \text{ tab}}{30 \cancel{\text{ mg}}}$$

$$x = \frac{120 \text{ tabs}}{30}$$

$$x = 4 \text{ tabs}$$

## Pediatric and Geriatric Dosage Calculations

The risk of harm from medication is far greater in pediatric and geriatric patients because of the way they break down and absorb medications. The calculations must be precise. Most pediatric and geriatric dosage calculations are based on body surface area (BSA) or weight. Calculations based upon BSA require a complex formula or the use of a *nomogram* (Figure 38-1). These calculations are typically done by the physician or other licensed health-care personnel. However you may be asked to perform calculations based upon a patient's weight or BSA, depending upon your area of practice.

An order based upon weight will often state the amount of medication per weight of the patient per unit of

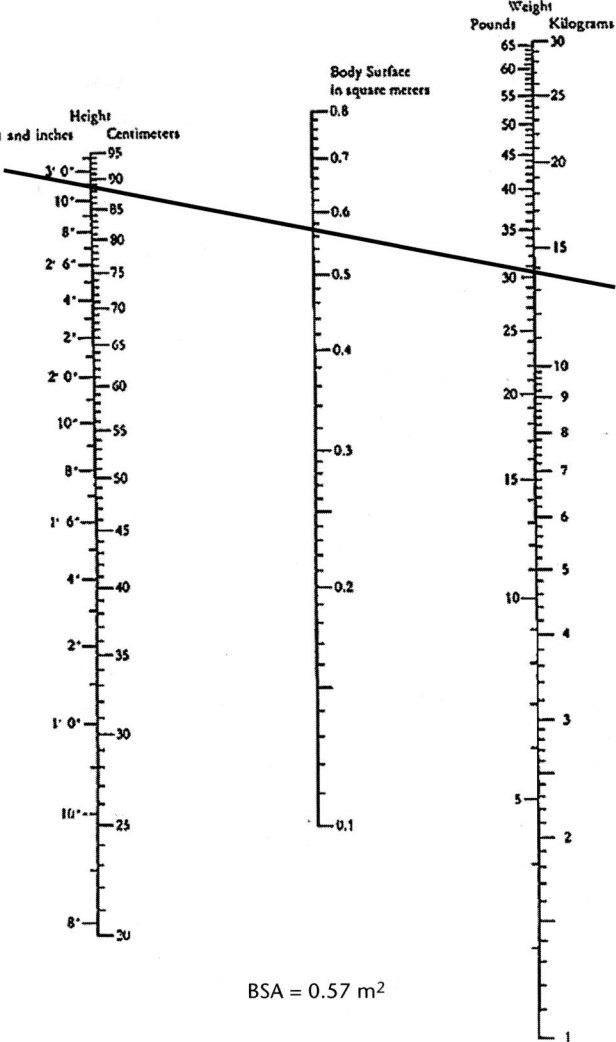

**Figure 38-1.** A nomogram is used to determine the BSA in order to calculate a medication dose. In this metrix nomogram, the child weighs 13.9 kg and is 85 cm tall.

time. For example "8 mg/kg/day PO q6h" means over 24 hours the patient should receive 8 mg of medication for every kilogram (kg) he or she weighs and it is to be given every six (6) hours or four (4) times during a 24-hour period. If the patient weighs 34 pounds (lbs), perform the calculation as follows:

1. Convert the patient's weight to kilogram using either the fraction or ratio method. For accuracy when converting, round to the nearest hundredths (two decimal places).

   **Fraction Method:**
   a. Set up the equation. (Recall 1 lb = 2.2 kg)

   $$\frac{34 \text{ lbs}}{x} = \frac{1 \text{ lb}}{2.2 \text{ kg}}$$

   b. Cross multiply. Remember to multiply the bottom left number by the top right number and multiply the top left number by the bottom right number:

   $$x \times 1 \text{ lb} = 34 \text{ lbs} \times 2.2 \text{ kg}$$

**c.** Solve for $x$

$$x = 74.8 \text{ kg}$$

2. Calculate the desired dose (D) for 24 hours by multiplying the dose ordered by the weight in kilograms.

$$8 \text{ mg} \times 74.8 \text{ kg} = \text{desired dose (D)}$$

$$598.4 \text{ mg} = D$$

3. Calculate the desired dose (D) for one dose by dividing the amount to be received by the number of times the medication will be received in 24 hours.

In this case the medication is to be given four times in 24 hours.

$$598.4 \text{ mg divided by } 4 = 149.6 \text{ mg}$$

# Preparing to Administer a Drug

Drugs may be administered for either local or systemic effects. Generally, drugs that have local effects are applied directly to the skin, tissues, or mucous membranes. Drugs that produce systemic effects are administered by **routes** that allow the drug to be absorbed and distributed in the bloodstream throughout the body. The importance of extreme care with drug dose and route is described in the Caution: Handle With Care section. The different routes of administration are described in Table 38-5 and discussed later in this chapter.

## TABLE 38-5  Routes and Methods of Drug Administration

| Route and Drug Forms | Method |
|---|---|
| Buccal route<br>  Tablets | Place drug between patient's gum and cheek. To ensure absorption, tell patient to leave tablet there until it dissolves and not to chew or swallow it. Tell the patient not to eat, drink, or smoke until tablet is completely dissolved. |
| Intradermal route<br>  Solutions<br>  Powders for reconstitution | Administer drug by injection between the upper layers of patient's skin. |
| Intramuscular route<br>  Solutions<br>  Powders for reconstitution | Administer drug by injection into muscle. |
| Intravenous route<br>  Solutions (often in bags of 250, 500, or 1000 mL)<br>  Powders for reconstitution<br>  Blood and blood products | Administer drug by injection or infusion into vein. |
| Inhalation therapy (nasal or oral)<br>  Aerosols<br>  Sprays<br>  Mists or steam | Administer drug by inhalation to reach respiratory tract. |
| Oral route<br>  Tablets<br>  Capsules<br>  Liquids<br>  Lozenges | Give drug to patient to swallow. |
| Ophthalmic (eye) or otic (ear) route<br>  Solutions<br>  Ointments | Apply drug, usually as drops, in patient's eye or ear. |
| Rectal route<br>  Suppositories<br>  Solutions | Insert suppository into rectum. Administer solution as enema, using tube and nozzle. |
| Subcutaneous route<br>  Solutions<br>  Powders for reconstitution | Administer drug by injection into subcutaneous layer of skin. |

*continued ⟶*

## TABLE 38-5 Routes and Methods of Drug Administration (concluded)

| Route and Drug Forms | Method |
|---|---|
| Sublingual route<br>  Tablets<br>  Sprays | Place drug under patient's tongue. To ensure absorption, tell patient to leave tablet there until it dissolves and not to chew or swallow it. Tell the patient not to eat, drink, or smoke until tablet is completely dissolved. |
| Topical route<br>  Ointments<br>  Lotions<br>  Creams<br>  Tinctures<br>  Powders<br>  Sprays<br>  Solutions | Apply drug to patient's skin or rub into skin. |
| Transdermal route<br>  Patches | Apply drug to clean, dry, nonhairy area of skin. |
| Urethral route<br>  Solutions | Administer drug by instilling in bladder, using catheter. |
| Vaginal route<br>  Solutions<br>  Suppositories<br>  Ointments<br>  Foams<br>  Creams | Administer solution as douche, using tube and nozzle. Administer other forms by inserting into vagina with applicator. |

## Assessment

Although the doctor gives the order to administer a drug, much of the responsibility is yours. Because you will often interview the patient, you must be alert to—and inform the doctor of—any change in the patient's condition that could affect drug therapy.

**Injection Site.** Part of your assessment is to locate and inspect the injection site. Find the injection site by using anatomical landmarks. Inspect the skin by checking for the following conditions:

- Moles
- Birthmarks
- Traumatic injury
- Redness
- Rash
- Edema
- Cyanosis
- Burns
- Tattoos
- Side of a mastectomy
- Paralyzed areas
- Warts

If you are unsure about any of these conditions, inform the physician.

**Drug Allergies.** During the assessment, it is important to ask the patient about any drug allergies. Even though you may see a patient on a regular basis, be in the habit of asking about drug allergies at every patient visit. Patients often see other physicians or specialists, who may have prescribed different medications. A patient could have had a drug reaction to a medication that has been prescribed by another physician. If applicable, document in the patient chart "NKDA" or "no known drug allergies."

**Patient Condition.** Before administering a drug, assess the patient's overall condition. For example, does the patient have a viral infection? Vaccines are not recommended if the patient has a viral infection such as a common cold. In addition, review the patient's drug list to ensure that any medications already being taken will not interfere with the ordered drug or route of administration. Also verify again that the ordered dose is appropriate for the patient's age and weight.

**Patient Consent Form.** Many physicians require that a patient sign a consent form before receiving an injection. This form provides general information regarding the medication or vaccine and lists the possible side effects or adverse reactions. If your physician requires a consent form, make sure that the patient signs the form and that you have answered any questions prior to giving the injection.

## Preventing Errors During Drug Administration

Medication errors are a serious problem in health care. As a medical assistant, you can do your part to help prevent errors by giving close attention to the dose and route of administration. You must also check and recheck the ordered form of the drug (for example, tablet or extended release capsule). In the following examples, this crucial relationship is illustrated.

1. Prochlorperazine (Compazine) is an antiemetic drug for acute nausea and vomiting. It is given to both children and adults. When the vomiting is so severe that a tablet or capsule cannot be swallowed, the drug is administered in injectable or suppository form. This drug is available in the following forms:

   - 10 mL multidose vials with 5 mg of drug per mL, written as 5 mg/mL
   - 2 mL single-dose vials 5 mg/mL
   - 4 fl oz bottles of syrup 5 mg/5 mL (5 mg/1 tsp)
   - 5 mg tablets
   - 10 mg tablets
   - 2 mL prefilled disposable syringes 5 mg/mL
   - 2½ mg suppositories
   - 5 mg suppositories
   - 25 mg suppositories
   - 10 mg extended release capsules
   - 15 mg extended release capsules

   Because so many forms of this drug are available, there is a high risk of error in choosing the correct form. In addition, the route of administration can determine how much drug is delivered in one dose. For example, note that suppositories are available in 2½-mg, 5-mg, and 25-mg forms. If the 2½-mg dose were written as 2.5 mg, there might be confusion with the 25-mg dose suppository. Thus the 2½-mg suppository is

   always written this way, even in the PDR. This clarification helps prevent a child's receiving the adult dose of 25 mg, which could result in serious complications to the central nervous system. This possible confusion is a one example of how much difference a decimal point can make.

   Note also that in the syrup there is a 5-mg dose of drug per 5 mL (1 tsp), whereas in the other liquid forms (vials and prefilled syringes), there is a 5-mg dose of drug per 1 mL. The injectable form is five times more concentrated than the syrup. Therefore, if you were to administer the same amount of injectable liquid as syrup to a patient, you would give the patient five times more drug than in the syrup. Just as a child could be endangered with the 25-mg suppository, an adult could be endangered with the wrong form of liquid. Because elderly patients often receive syrup forms of medication, this instruction could be particularly confusing.

2. Allergy shots must be administered subcutaneously rather than intramuscularly to allow slower absorption of the serum. Within 30 minutes, a wheal and redness will appear if the patient has an allergic reaction. In such a case the patient requires further close monitoring. If the serum were injected intramuscularly, this reaction would not only be hidden (because of the deeper administration), it would also occur more rapidly (because of the faster rate of absorption). In fact, the patient could go into anaphylaxis, or anaphylactic shock, without any warning. Check and recheck every order and drug label to prevent confusion and incorrect administration. This procedure is always worth the time it takes and could prevent you from making a serious medication error.

## Rules for Drug Administration

No matter what drug or administration route is ordered, follow these general rules when administering drugs.

- Give only the drugs the physician has ordered. Written orders are preferable, but oral orders are appropriate for emergencies. If you are unfamiliar with any aspect of a drug the physician orders, consult a drug reference work.

- Wash your hands before handling the drug. Prepare the drug in a well-lit area, away from distractions. Focus only on the task at hand.

- Calculate the dose if necessary. If you are unsure of your computation, ask another medical assistant, a nurse, or the physician to check it.

- Avoid leaving a prepared drug unattended, and never administer a drug that someone else has prepared.

## Using an Epinephrine Autoinjector

If you are working in a medical office that treats people with allergies, you must be familiar with epinephrine so that you can teach patients how to self-administer the drug. Epinephrine is a drug used to treat allergies so severe that exposure to the allergen may be life-threatening. The following reactions indicate the possibility of anaphylaxis, or anaphylactic shock, a severe allergic reaction:

- Flushing
- Sharp drop in blood pressure
- Hives
- Difficulty breathing
- Difficulty swallowing
- Convulsions
- Vomiting
- Diarrhea and abdominal cramps

If a patient with a severe allergy experiences any or all of these symptoms, the reaction can be fatal unless emergency treatment is given immediately. Therefore, patients who cannot always control their exposure to an allergen—for example, bee or wasp venom—must have access to an epinephrine autoinjector for emergency intramuscular use.

These injectors, which are prepackaged (Figure 38-2), deliver either 0.3 mg of epinephrine—a single dose for an adult—or 0.15 mg of epinephrine— a single dose for a child. A patient who is exposed to the allergen should use the injector if the allergy is confirmed or if the allergy is suspected and signs of anaphylaxis appear.

Teach the patient to follow these steps when using an autoinjector.

1. Remove the autoinjector from the packaging (box and/or plastic tube).
2. Pull back the gray cap.
3. Place the black tip of the injector on the outside of the upper thigh. (The injector can go through clothing.)

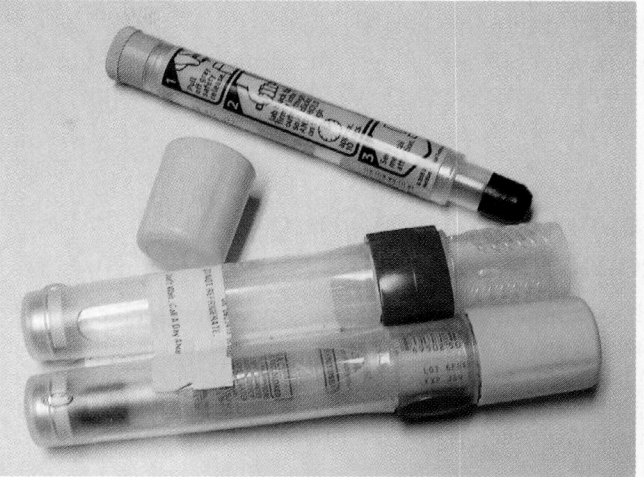

**Figure 38-2.** Epinephrine autoinjectors come prepackaged, containing the correct amount of the drug for an adult or a child.

4. Press firmly into the thigh and hold for 10 seconds.
5. Remove the autoinjector and massage the injection site for a few minutes.
6. Call your physician or go to the emergency room of a nearby hospital. An autoinjector is designed as emergency supportive therapy only. It is not a replacement or substitute for immediate medical or hospital care.

Make sure the patient is thoroughly familiar with the parts of the autoinjector, how to activate it, how to use it, and what to do next. Ask the patient to explain the use of the autoinjector to you, as if you had never seen one. This approach not only reinforces the patient's understanding of the process but also improves the patient's self-confidence and points out any possible misconceptions. If the patient is very young or otherwise unable to use the autoinjector reliably, teach a family member or companion how to perform the process.

- Ask the patient to state his name and date of birth to ensure correct identification. Also ask the patient to tell you about any possible drug allergies. Do not rely on documentation in his chart; he may have developed a new allergy that has not yet been added to the record. Then verify any drug allergies in the chart.
- Be sure the physician is in the office when you administer a drug or vaccine. If the patient develops an anaphylactic reaction (sudden, severe allergic reaction) to the drug or vaccine, the physician must administer epinephrine. Some patients need to know how to administer this drug themselves. For information about epinephrine, see the Educating the Patient section.
- After administering the drug, ask the patient to remain in the facility for 10 to 20 minutes so that you can observe the patient for any unexpected effects. Give the patient specific instructions about the effects of the drug as well as general information about drug use.

- If the patient refuses to take the drug, discard it according to your facility policy. Do not flush it down the toilet or return it to the original container. Be sure to document the refusal in the patient's record and tell the physician.
- If you make an error in drug administration, tell the physician immediately.
- Document immediately the drug and dose administered; never document administration before giving medicine.

## Seven Rights of Drug Administration

When administering any drug, whether medication or vaccine, observe the seven "rights" of drug administration. *Never* deviate from these seven steps. Adhering to these rights helps ensure that you administer the drug correctly. The seven rights refer to the:

1. Right patient
2. Right drug
3. Right dose
4. Right time
5. Right route
6. Right technique
7. Right documentation

**Right Patient.** Always check the name and date of birth on the order for a drug or vaccine in the patient's chart; then ask the patient to state his or her name and date of birth. Do not call the patient by name, because a forgetful or confused patient might answer to any name. Always have the patient state his or her name and date of birth, or have an attending caregiver or family member state the name and date of birth if the patient is unable.

**Right Drug.** Carefully compare the name of the prescribed drug or vaccine in the patient's chart with the label on the drug container. As you check the drug name on the label, look at the expiration date. Never use a drug that has passed this date (Figure 38-3).

If you are unfamiliar with the drug, look it up in the *PDR* or other drug reference. Also, never prepare a drug from a container with a damaged or handwritten label. To ensure accuracy, read the label three times, performing a "triple check" every time you prepare a medication. This triple check is done by checking:

1. When you obtain the drug container from the cabinet
2. When you pour or prepare the drug from the container
3. When you put the container back in the cabinet (before leaving the medication room)

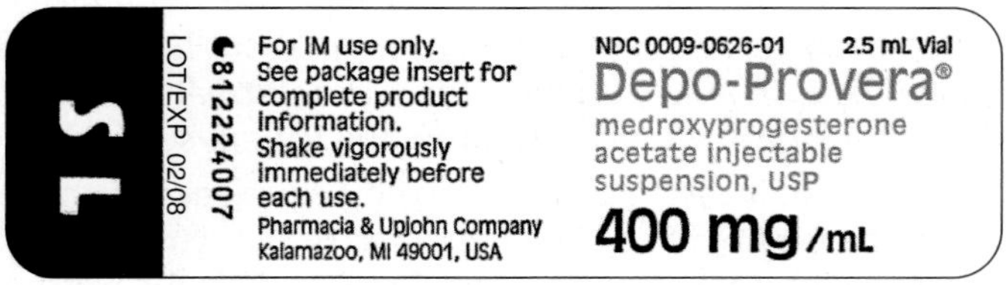

**Right Dose.** Compare the dose on the order in the patient's chart with the dose you prepare. To obtain the right dose, read the label closely. Do not confuse the dose contained in one tablet with the number of tablets in the container.

**Right Time.** Be sure to give the drug at the right time. If it must be given after meals, make sure the patient has eaten recently. For certain drugs, you must ensure that it is the correct time of day and the correct time in a series of doses. Timing is crucial with allergy shots because of possible reactions.

**Right Route.** Double-check to make sure the administration route you are preparing to use matches the route the doctor ordered. Also check that the medication you are using can be administered by that route ordered. For example do not confuse ear (otic) drops, with eye (optic) drops. Check that the patient can receive the drug by this route and that the route seems appropriate. For example, if the patient has an injury at the specified injection site, consult the doctor for a possible alternative site or a different route.

**Right Technique.** Always use the proper administration technique. If you have not given a drug or vaccine by the ordered route recently, review the technique before administering the drug.

**Right Documentation.** Document the procedure immediately after administering the drug or vaccine to the patient. Do not wait until later, and do not document before administration. Be sure to include the date, time, drug or vaccine name, dose, administration route, patient reaction, patient education about the drug, and your first initial and last name. If the drug is a controlled substance, also document it on the controlled substance inventory record. Remember that correct documentation demands neat handwriting that others who care for the patient can read easily. If using computer documentation, check your entry carefully before submitting it.

**For IM use only.** See package insert for complete product information. Shake vigorously immediately before each use. Pharmacia & Upjohn Company Kalamazoo, MI 49001, USA

LOT/EXP 02/08 812224007

NDC 0009-0626-01 2.5 mL Vial
**Depo-Provera®**
medroxyprogesterone acetate injectable suspension, USP
**400 mg/mL**

**Figure 38-3.** Check the label for the expiration date before administering a drug.

## Techniques of Administering Drugs

The doctor may ask you to administer drugs by one of the routes outlined in Table 38-5. Most patients take a prescription to a pharmacy to be filled and then take oral drugs at home, so you will rarely need to administer these

# Reflecting On . . . Legal and Ethical Issues

## Handling Medication Errors

Medication errors are a serious yet inevitable problem. Great care should always be taken to prevent them, including following the "Seven Rights or Drug Administration," performing the "triple check," and ensuring accurate calculations. However, if an error does occur, no matter the cause, it must be reported. Not reporting an error is unethical and in some cases could be illegal, especially if a serious consequence occurs.

Most facilities require that an incident report be completed. This form documents the error. It is completed and then signed by everyone involved, as well as your supervisor. Errors are also reported online through an online program developed by the U.S. Pharmacopeia and the Institute for Safe Medical Practices. Reporting errors at these sites provide information to assist in the prevention of errors.

drugs in the office. However, you are likely to be asked to do the following.

- Place drugs in the patient's mouth between the cheek and gum or under the tongue
- Administer a drug by any means other than by mouth (if permitted in your state)
- Demonstrate how to use an inhaler
- Apply topical drugs (those applied to the skin)
- Administer or assist in administering drugs into the urethra, vagina, or rectum
- Administer medications to the eye or ear

These duties require you to master a variety of techniques to give drugs safely by any route.

## Oral Administration

Drugs for oral administration include tablets, capsules, lozenges, and liquids. These drugs are absorbed relatively slowly as they travel along the gastrointestinal (GI) tract.

Oral administration is contraindicated in patients who have severe nausea, are comatose, or cannot swallow. Certain drugs are ineffective when administered orally, because the digestive process changes them chemically to an ineffective form or does not deliver them to the bloodstream quickly enough.

Many drugs, however, are most effective when given orally. These include antibiotics, vitamins, throat lozenges, and cough syrups. Although these drugs are familiar to most people, as a medical assistant, you must follow certain steps to ensure that the patient understands the drug and that the drug is administered safely and effectively. The steps for oral administration are outlined in Procedure 38-1.

## Buccal and Sublingual Administration

Although **buccal** and **sublingual** drugs are placed in the mouth, they do not continue along the GI tract. Instead, they dissolve and are absorbed in the buccal area (between the cheek and gum) or the sublingual area (under the tongue), where they are placed. The medication is absorbed through tissue that is rich in capillaries, and the drug enters the bloodstream directly. Because the drug does not pass into the stomach or intestines before absorption, it produces a therapeutic effect more quickly than do oral drugs.

Specially formulated tablets may be given by the buccal or sublingual routes. When you administer buccal or sublingual medications, your role usually includes teaching the patient how to administer these medications at home. See Procedure 38-2, Administering Buccal or Sublingual Drugs.

## Parenteral Administration

Parenteral administration is the administration of a substance such as a drug by muscle, vein, or any means other than through the GI tract. Although the parenteral route offers the advantage of rapid drug action, it has several potential drawbacks.

Parenteral administration poses more safety risks for the patient because after the drug has been injected, it cannot be retrieved. To reduce the risks, you must administer the drug expertly and observe the seven rights meticulously.

Parenteral administration increases your risk of potential exposure to blood-borne pathogens when performing injections and disposing of used needles. To minimize risks, follow Universal Precautions during injections. Also adhere to Occupational Safety and Health Administration (OSHA) and Environmental Protection Agency (EPA) regulations for disposing of contaminated needles and sharp items, as discussed in Chapter 20. Most offices provide a rigid, puncture-proof container for collecting disposable sharp instruments. This container should be self-sealing and have a lock-tight cap and a safety neck.

After using a needle, lancet, or syringe, engage the safety mechanism, then immediately place it in the sharps container. To avoid puncturing yourself, always ensure the safety mechanism is engaged and do not force the needle,

# Administering Oral Drugs

**Procedure Goal:** To safely administer an oral drug to a patient

**OSHA Guidelines:** This procedure does not involve exposure to blood, body fluids, or tissues.

**Materials:** Drug order (in patient chart), container of oral drug, small paper cup (for tablets, capsules, or caplets) or plastic calibrated medicine cup (for liquids), glass of water or juice, straw (optional), package insert or drug information sheet

**Method:**

1. Identify the patient and wash your hands.
2. Select the ordered drug (tablet, capsule, or liquid).
3. Check the seven rights, comparing information against the drug order.

   *Rationale*

   To ensure necessary accuracy

4. If you are unfamiliar with the drug, check the PDR or other drug reference, read the package insert, or speak with the physician. Determine whether the drug may be taken with or followed by water or juice.

5. Ask the patient about any drug or food allergies. If the patient is not allergic to the ordered drug or other ingredients used to prepare it, proceed.

   *Rationale*

   To prevent a reaction to the medication

6. Perform any calculations needed to provide the prescribed dose. If you are unsure of your calculations, check them with a coworker or the physician.

## If You Are Giving Tablets or Capsules

7. Open the container and tap the correct number into the cap (Figure 38-4). Do not touch the inside of the cap because it is sterile. If you pour out too many tablets or capsules and you have not touched them, tap the excess back into the container.

8. Tap the tablets or capsules from the cap into the paper cup.

9. Recap the container immediately.

   *Rationale*

   Recapping immediately protects the medication from exposure to air that can break down the medication.

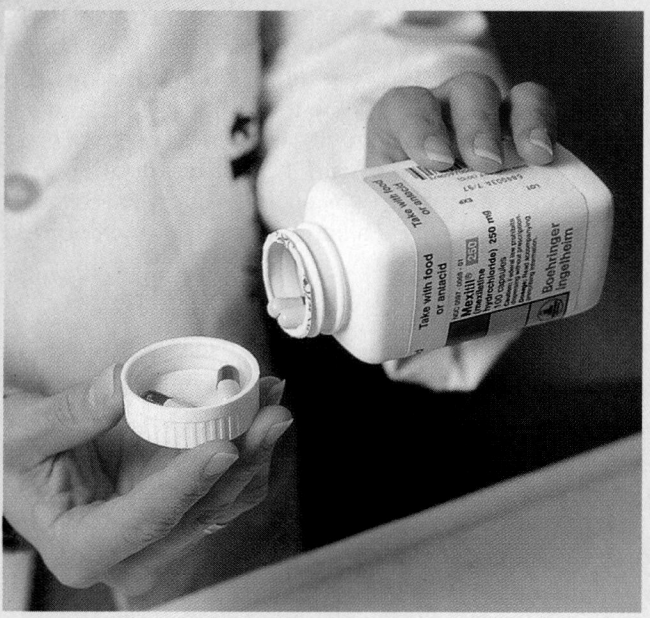

**Figure 38-4.** Tap tablets gently into the cap.

10. Give the patient the cup along with a glass of water or juice. If the patient finds it easier to drink with a straw, unwrap the straw and place it in the fluid. If patients have difficulty swallowing pills, have them drink some water or juice before putting the pills in the mouth.

    *Rationale*

    Additional fluid makes the pills float in the mouth and allows patients to swallow quickly.

## If You Are Giving a Liquid Drug

7. If the liquid is a suspension, shake it well.

8. Locate the mark on the medicine cup for the prescribed dose. Keeping your thumbnail on the mark, hold the cup at eye level and pour the correct amount of the drug. Keep the label side of the bottle on top as you pour (Figure 38-5), or put your palm over it.

   *Rationale*

   To prevent liquid drips from obscuring the label

9. After pouring the drug, place the cup on a flat surface, and check the drug level again. At eye

*continued* ⟶

## Administering Oral Drugs *(concluded)*

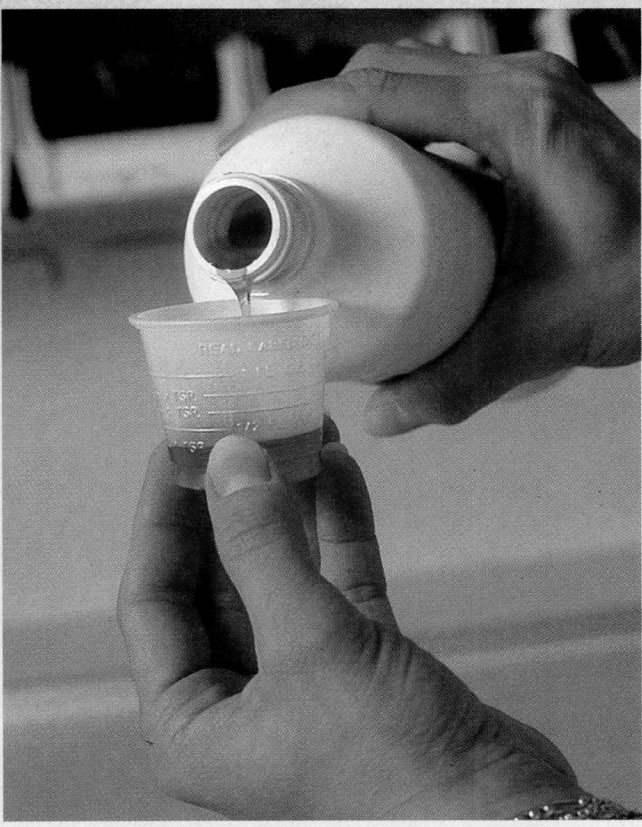

**Figure 38-5.** Pour a liquid drug into a calibrated medication cup.

level the base of the meniscus (the crescent-shaped form at the top of the liquid) should align with the mark that indicates the prescribed dose (Figure 38-6). If you poured out too much, discard it.

### Rationale

Do not return it to the container because medicine cups are not sterile.

10. Give the medicine cup to the patient with instructions to drink the liquid. If appropriate, offer a glass of water or juice to wash down the drug.

### *After You Have Given an Oral Drug*

11. Wash your hands.

12. Give the patient an information sheet about the drug. Discuss the information with the patient and answer any questions she may have. If the patient has questions you cannot answer, refer her to the physician.

13. Document the drug administration with the date, time, drug name, dosage, expiration date, lot number, manufacturer, route, site, significant patient reactions, and any patient education in the patient's chart.

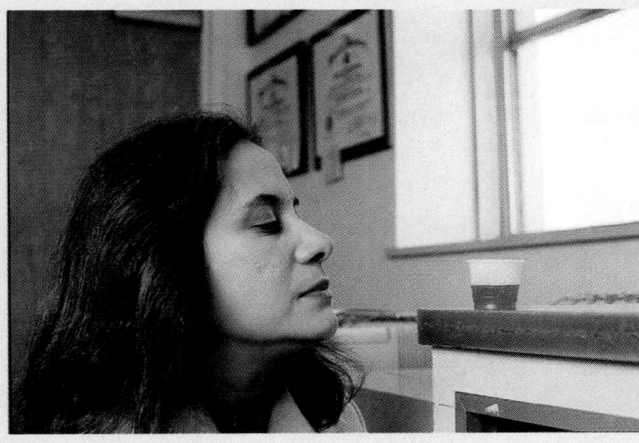

A

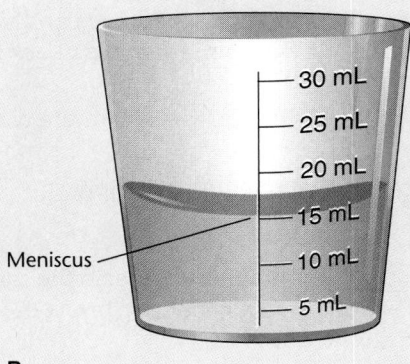

30 mL
25 mL
20 mL
Meniscus
15 mL
10 mL
5 mL

B

**Figure 38-6.** Read the measurement at eye level. You are looking for the meniscus or the crescent-shaped form at the top of the liquid for the correct measure.

# PROCEDURE 38.2

## Administering Buccal or Sublingual Drugs

**Procedure Goal:** To safely administer a buccal or sublingual drug to a patient

**OSHA Guidelines:** This procedure does not involve exposure to blood, body fluids, or tissues.

**Materials:** Drug order (in patient chart), container of buccal or sublingual drug, small paper cup, package insert or drug information sheet

**Method:**

1. Identify the patient and wash your hands.
2. Select the ordered drug.
3. Check the seven rights, comparing information against the drug order.

   *Rationale*

   To ensure necessary accuracy

4. If you are unfamiliar with the drug, check the PDR or other drug reference, read the package insert, or speak with the physician.
5. Ask the patient about any drug or food allergies. If the patient is not allergic to the ordered drug or other ingredients used to prepare it, proceed.

   *Rationale*

   To prevent a reaction to the medication

6. Perform any calculations needed to provide the prescribed dose. If you are unsure of your calculations, check them with a coworker or the physician.
7. Open the container and tap the correct number into the cap (see Figure 38-4). Do not touch the inside of the cap because it is sterile. If you pour out too many tablets or capsules and you have not touched them, tap the excess back into the container.
8. Tap the tablets or capsules from the cap into the paper cup.
9. Recap the container immediately.

   *Rationale*

   Recapping immediately protects the medication from exposure to air that can break down the medication.

### If You Are Giving Buccal Medication

10. Provide patient instruction, including:
    - Tell the patient not to chew or swallow the tablet.
    - Place the medication between the cheek and gum until it dissolves (Figure 38-7).

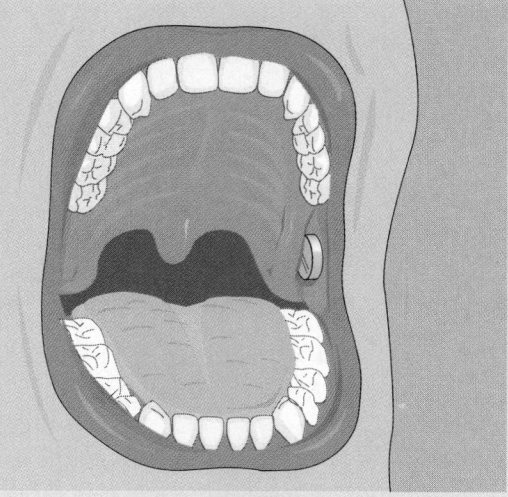

**Figure 38-7.** Place a buccal drug between the cheek and gum.

*Rationale*

This area is rich in blood supply to promote rapid absorption of the drug.

- Instruct the patient not to eat, drink, or smoke until the tablet is completely dissolved.

*Rationale*

Food and fluids wash the drug into the gastrointestinal (GI) tract, slowing absorption or allowing gastric juices to destroy it. Smoking increases salivation, causing impaired absorption of the drug.

### If You Are Giving a Sublingual Drug

10. Provide patient instruction including:
    - Tell the patient not to chew or swallow the tablet.
    - Place the medication under the tongue until it dissolves (Figure 38-8).

*Rationale*

The capillaries in this area promote rapid absorption of the drug.

- Instruct the patient not to eat, drink, or smoke until the tablet is completely dissolved.

*Rationale*

Food and fluids wash the drug into the GI tract, slowing absorption or allowing gastric juices

*continued* ⟶

## Administering Buccal or Sublingual Drugs *(concluded)*

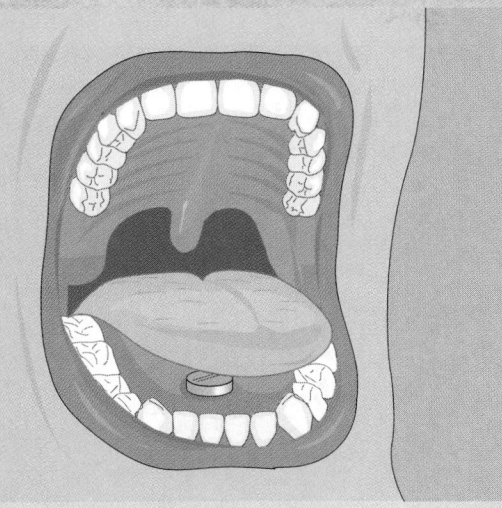

**Figure 38-8.** Place a sublingual drug under the tongue.

to destroy it. Smoking increases salivation, causing impaired absorption of the drug.

### *After You Have Given a Buccal or Sublingual Medication*

11. Remain with patients until their tablet dissolves to monitor for possible adverse reaction and to ensure that patients have allowed the tablet to dissolve in the mouth instead of chewing or swallowing it.

12. Wash your hands.

13. Give the patient an information sheet about the drug. Discuss the information with the patient and answer any questions she may have. If the patient has questions you cannot answer, refer her to the physician.

14. Document the drug administration with the date, time, drug name, dosage, expiration date, lot number, manufacturer, route, site, significant patient reactions, and any patient education in the patient's chart.

**A.** Intradermal (ID)

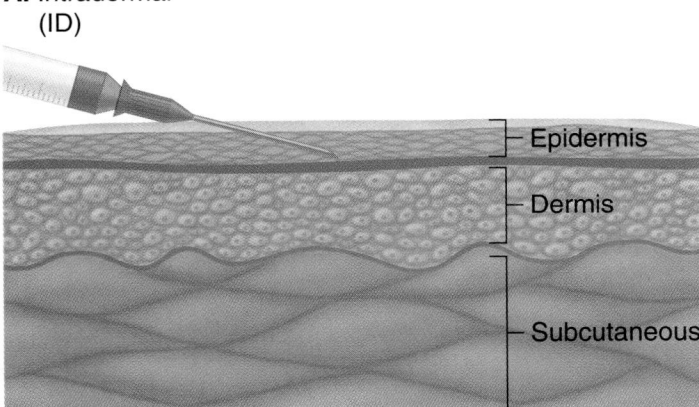

**B.** Subcutaneous (sub-Q)  **C.** Intravenous (IV)  **D.** Intramuscular (IM)

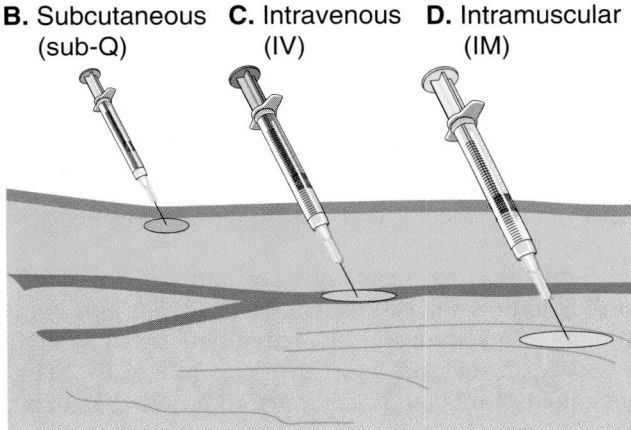

**Figure 38-9.** Injection needles are placed into separate areas under the skin. (A) intradermal (ID), (B) subcutaneous (sub-Q), (C) intravenous (IV), and (D) intramuscular (IM).

lancet, or syringe into the container. If you do accidentally stick yourself, notify the physician at once so you can be treated. OSHA requires medical follow-up for all workers who have been accidentally punctured.

Never let a sharps container become full. When the container is two-thirds full, seal it and follow your office procedure for container disposal.

**Needles.** When you administer a parenteral drug, you must select the appropriate needle, syringe, and drug form

to use on the basis of the type of injection. The following are methods of injection:

- Intradermal (ID), or within the upper layers of the skin
- Subcutaneous (sub-Q), or beneath the skin
- Intramuscular (IM), or within a muscle
- Intravenous (IV), or directly into a vein (Figure 38-9)

Needles consist of a hub, hilt, shaft, lumen, point, and bevel (Figure 38-10). The hub of the needle fits onto the

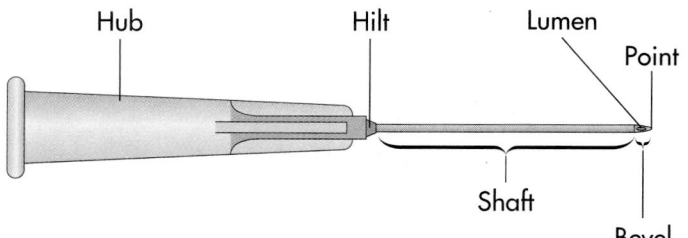

Figure 38-10. Understanding the parts of a needle will help you use it correctly.

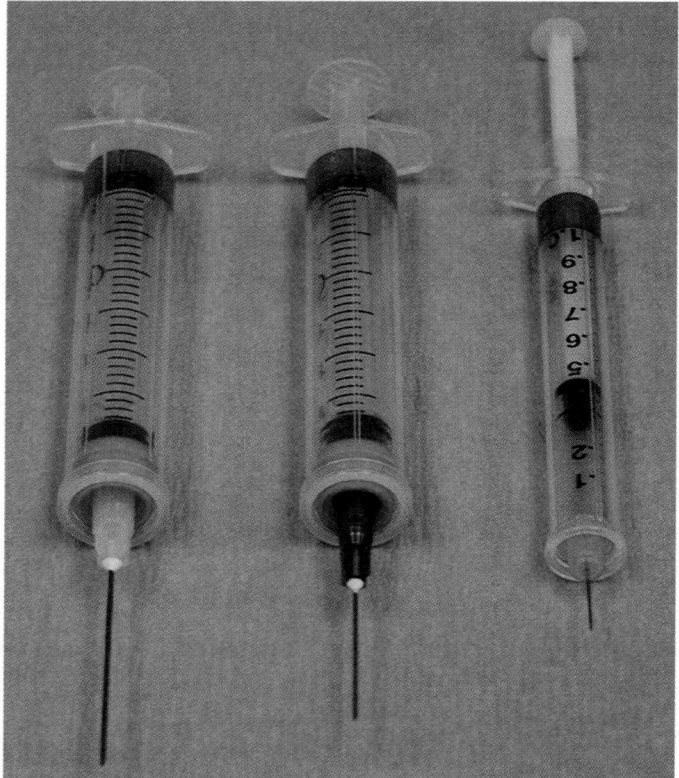

**B**

Figure 38-11. (A) The gauge of the needle relates to the diameter. Notice the larger the number the smaller the needle diameter. (B) Always choose a needle with a length and gauge appropriate to the type of injection, the drug being injected, and the patient receiving the injection.

syringe. The needle tip is beveled (sloped at the opening). The bevel helps the needle cut through the skin with minimum trauma.

Needles are available in various gauges (inside diameters) and lengths (Figure 38-11). A needle's gauge is expressed with numbers. The smaller the number, the larger the gauge. For example, a 25-gauge needle is smaller than an 18-gauge needle. Use the right gauge for the type of injection and the viscosity (thickness) of the drug to be administered. For example, use a large-gauge needle for a highly viscous drug.

When selecting a needle, also consider its length. It must be long enough to penetrate the appropriate layers of tissue but not so long as to go too deep. Choose the correct needle length on the basis of the type of injection as well as the patient's size, amount of fatty tissue, and injection site. Table 38-6 lists the approximate ranges of needle gauge and length typically used for intradermal, subcutaneous, and intramuscular injections.

**Syringes.** Syringes have two basic parts: a barrel and a plunger. The barrel is the calibrated cylinder that holds the drug. The plunger forces the drug through the barrel and out the needle, as shown in Figure 38-12. The syringe may be packaged with the needle attached and a guard cap over the needle, or the syringe and needle may be packaged separately.

Syringes come in many sizes and are calibrated according to how the syringe will be used. For example, the common 3-mL syringe is divided into tenths of a milliliter. It is used to measure most drugs. A tuberculin (TB) syringe holds 1 mL and is calibrated in hundredths of a milliliter (Figure 38-13A). Insulin syringes are calibrated in units (U), commonly either 50 U or 100 U (Figure 38-13B). Unlike other syringes, insulin syringes have permanently attached needles and no dead space (fluid remaining in

the needle or syringe after the plunger is depressed fully). These differences help the patient self-administer the correct amount of insulin.

**Forms of Packaging for Parenteral Drugs.** Parenteral drugs are supplied in the forms shown in Figure 38-14. They are ampules, cartridges, and vials.

| TABLE 38-6 Suggested Needle Gauges and Lengths | | |
|---|---|---|
| **Type of Injection** | **Gauge of Needle** | **Length of Needle** |
| Intradermal | 25–26 gauge | 3/8–1/2 inch |
| Subcutaneous | 23–27 gauge | 1/2–3/4 inch |
| Intramuscular | 18–23 gauge | 1–3 inches |

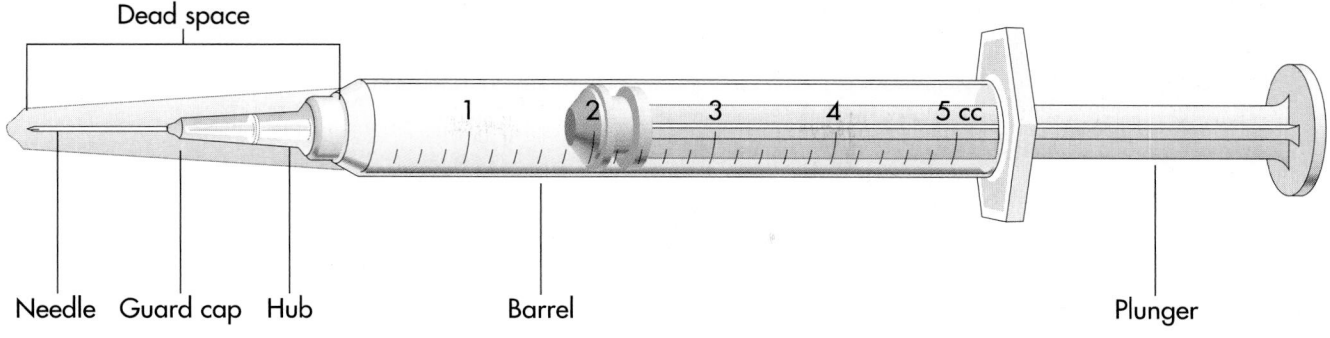

**Figure 38-12.** Know the parts of a standard syringe.

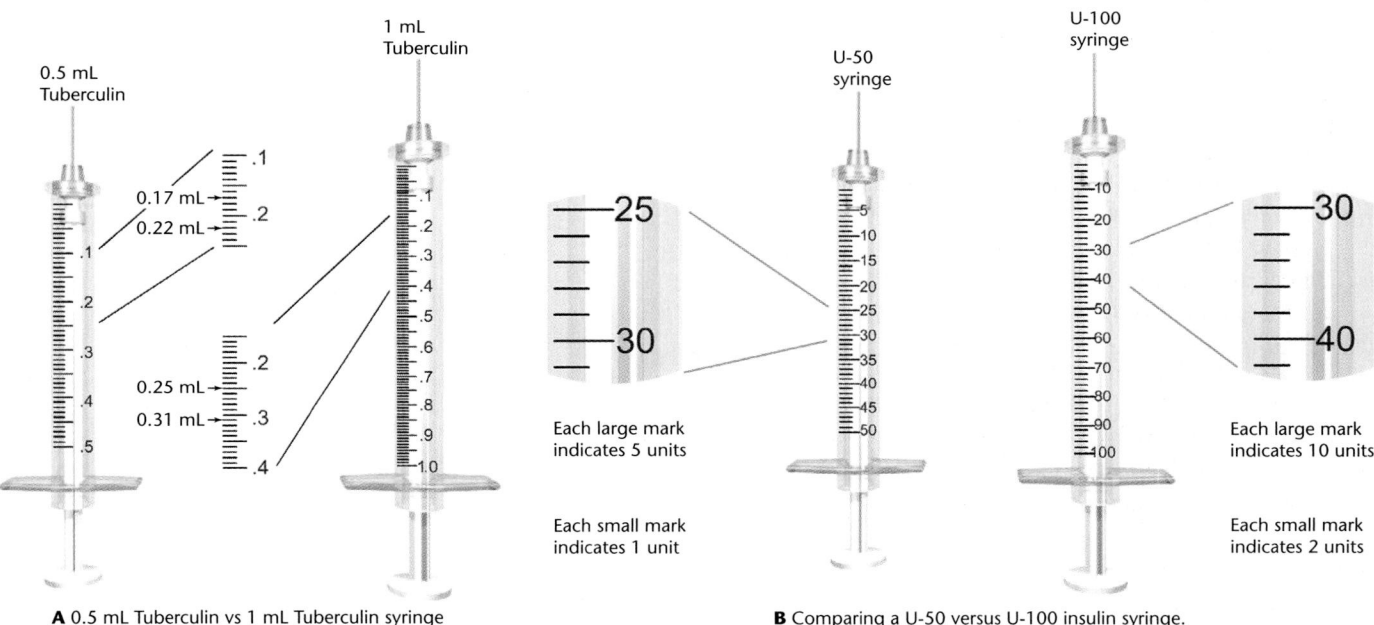

**A** 0.5 mL Tuberculin vs 1 mL Tuberculin syringe

**B** Comparing a U-50 versus U-100 insulin syringe.

**Figure 38-13.** (A) You may use the tuberculin syringe to deliver small doses (up to 1.0 mL) of drugs. (B) This insulin syringe delivers precisely 100 U of insulin when filled with insulin of the proper concentration (100 U per mL).

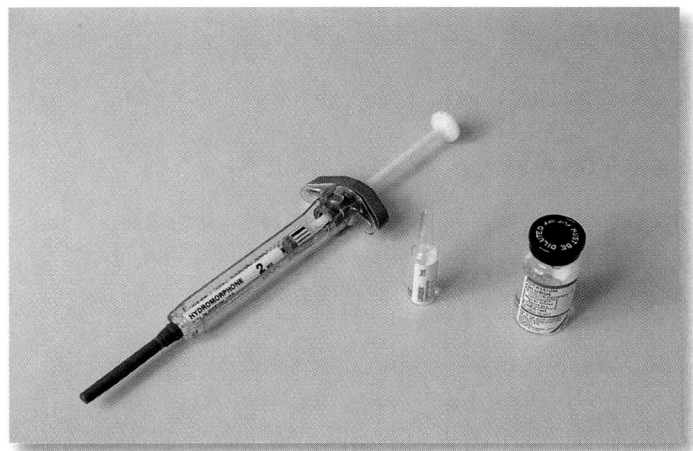

**Figure 38-14.** Injectable drugs may come in a cartridge (left), an ampule (center), or a vial (right).

- An ampule is a small glass or plastic container that is sealed to keep its contents sterile. It must be opened and used with care, as described in Procedure 38-3.

- A cartridge is a small barrel prefilled with a sterile drug. It slips into a special, reusable syringe assembly.

- A vial is a small bottle with a rubber diaphragm that can be punctured by needle. A vial contains a liquid or powder, which must first be reconstituted with a **diluent** (liquid used to dissolve and dilute a drug), as described in Procedure 38-4. It may contain a single or multiple doses. This procedure requires two needles and syringe sets—one for inserting the diluent into the vial and another to draw and administer the reconstituted drug—to avoid using a contaminated needle. The first needle is considered contaminated when you set it down to mix the diluent and the drug.

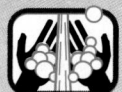 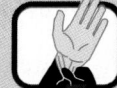 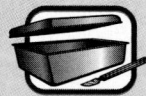

# Drawing a Drug from an Ampule

**Procedure Goal:** To safely open an ampule and draw a drug, using sterile technique

## OSHA Guidelines

**Materials:** Ampule of drug, alcohol swab, 2-by-2-inch gauze square, small file (provided by the drug manufacturer), sterile filtered needle, sterile needle, and a syringe of the appropriate size

## Method:

1. Wash your hands and put on exam gloves.
2. Gently tap the top of the ampule with your forefinger to settle the liquid to the bottom of the ampule.
3. Wipe the ampule's neck with an alcohol swab.
4. Wrap the 2-by-2-inch gauze square around the ampule's neck. Then snap the neck away from you (Figure 38-15). If it does not snap easily, score the neck with the small file and snap it again.
5. Insert the filtered needle into the ampule without touching the side of the ampule.

### Rationale

A filtered needle will prevent contamination of the medication.

6. Pull back on the plunger to aspirate (remove by vacuum or suction) the liquid completely into the syringe.

7. Replace with the regular needle and push the plunger on the syringe until the medication just reaches the tip of the needle. The drug is now ready for injection.

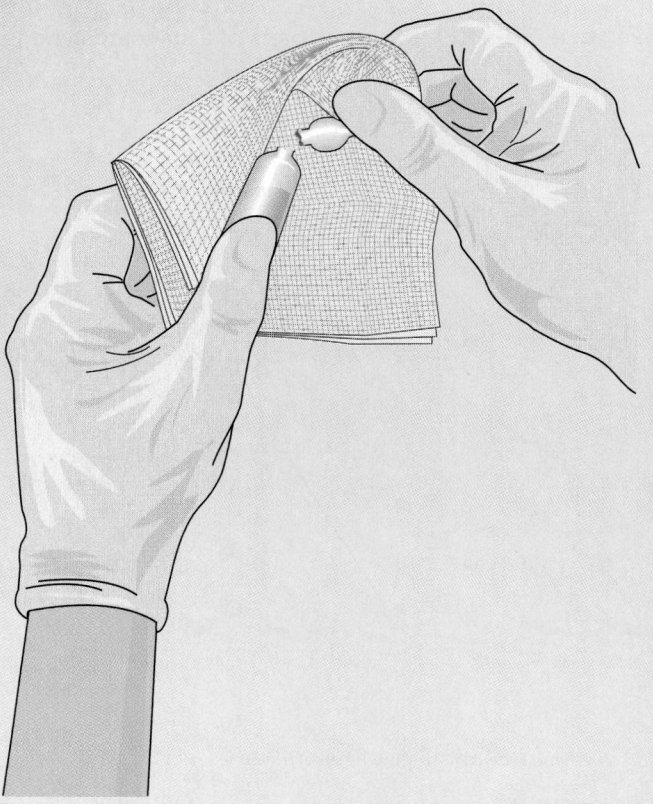

**Figure 38-15.** You must snap the neck of the ampule before inserting the needle.

# Reconstituting and Drawing a Drug for Injection

**Procedure Goal:** To reconstitute and draw a drug for injection, using sterile technique

## OSHA Guidelines

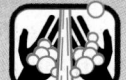 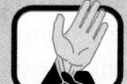 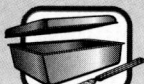

**Materials:** Vial of drug, vial of diluent, alcohol swabs, two disposable sterile needle and syringe sets of appropriate size, sharps container

## Method:

1. Wash your hands and put on exam gloves.
2. Place the drug vial and diluent vial on the countertop. Wipe the rubber diaphragm of each with an alcohol swab.

*continued* ⟶

# PROCEDURE 38.4

## Reconstituting and Drawing a Drug for Injection *(concluded)*

3. Remove the cap from the needle and the guard from the syringe. Pull the plunger back to the mark that equals the amount of diluent needed to reconstitute the drug ordered.

### Rationale

This action aspirates air into the syringe.

4. Puncture the diaphragm of the vial of diluent with the needle, and inject the air into the diluent (Figure 38-16).

### Rationale

This action creates positive pressure that lets you draw the diluent easily. If you do not add air, a vacuum forms, making it difficult to draw the diluent.

5. Invert the vial and aspirate the diluent.
6. Remove the needle from the diluent vial, inject the diluent into the drug vial, and withdraw

the needle. Properly dispose of this needle and syringe.

7. Roll the vial between your hands to mix the drug and diluent thoroughly. Do not shake the vial unless so directed on the drug label. When completely mixed, the solution in the vial should have no flakes. The solution will be clear or cloudy when completely mixed (depending on the drug).

8. Remove the cap and guard from the second needle and syringe.

9. Pull back the plunger to the mark that reflects the amount of drug ordered. Inject the air into the drug vial.

10. Invert the vial and aspirate the proper amount of the drug into the syringe (Figure 38-17). The drug is now ready for injection.

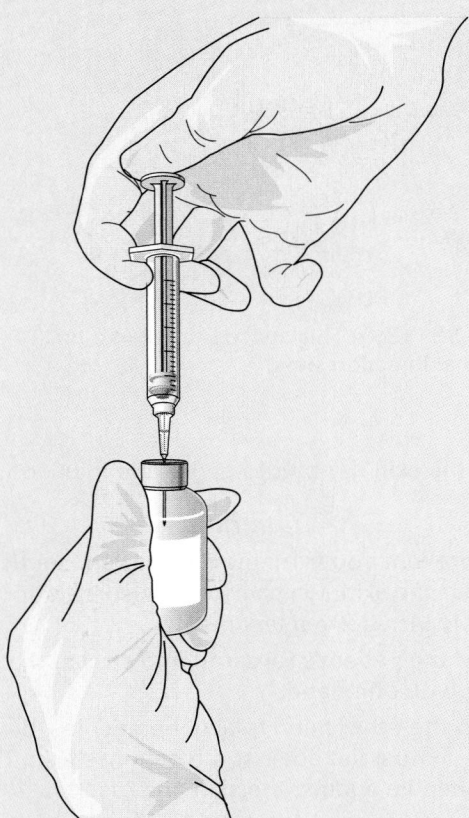

**Figure 38-16.** Injecting air into the diluent makes it easier to draw.

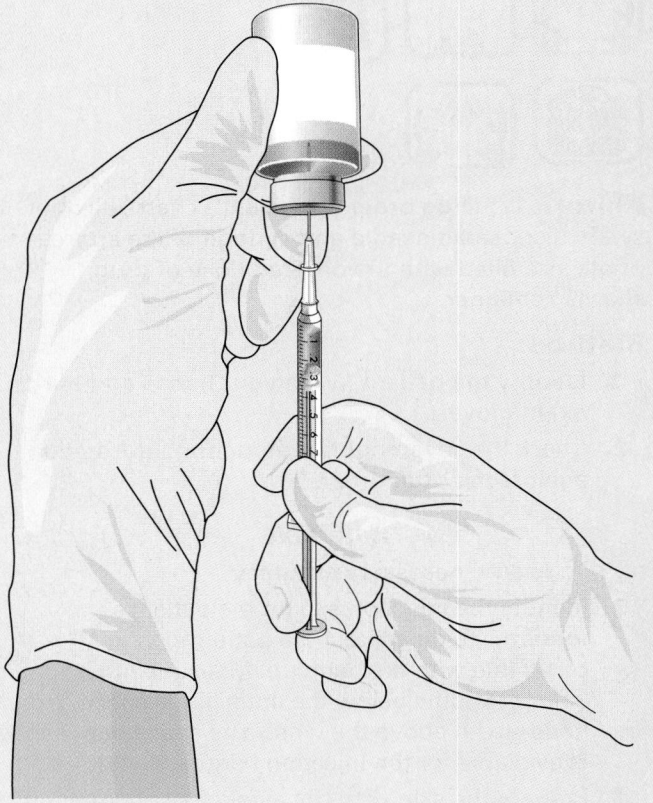

**Figure 38-17.** Invert the vial and draw the reconstituted drug.

**Methods of Injection.** Injections are the most common method of drug administration in a medical office. You need to be knowledgeable about all injection methods: intradermal, subcutaneous, intramuscular, and intravenous. You may also need to be skilled in these procedures as permitted by your state.

*Intradermal.* An **intradermal (ID)** injection is administered into the upper layer of skin at an angle almost parallel to the skin, as described in Procedure 38-5. Common sites for intradermal injections are the forearm and back. Intradermal injections are usually used to administer a skin test, such as an allergy test or a TB test. When choosing an injection site on patients, avoid scarred, blemished, or hairy areas, because those features interfere with your ability to interpret test results on the skin.

The drug is injected under the top skin layer, and a little bubble or wheal is raised. If the body reacts to the drug, erythema (redness) and induration (hardening) occur. This reaction generally takes place 15 to 20 minutes after an allergy test and from 48 to 72 hours after a TB test.

*Subcutaneous.* Frequently called sub-Q by health-care professionals, a subcutaneous injection provides a slow, sustained release of a drug and a relatively long duration of action. Generally, 1 mL or less of a drug can be delivered by a sub-Q injection (Procedure 38-6). Various drugs, such as insulin and heparin, are commonly administered by a sub-Q injection.

Common subcutaneous injection sites include an area on the back between the shoulder blades, the outer sides of the upper arms and thighs, and the abdomen (except for a 2-inch area around the umbilicus). To prepare for a

## PROCEDURE 38.5

## Giving an Intradermal Injection

**Procedure Goal:** To administer an intradermal injection safely and effectively, using sterile technique

### OSHA Guidelines

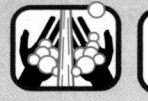 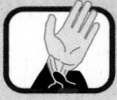 
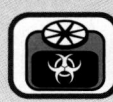 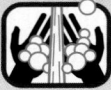

**Materials:** Drug order (in patient's chart), alcohol swab, disposable needle and syringe of the appropriate size filled with the ordered dose of drug, sharps container

### Method:

1. Identify the patient. Wash your hands and put on exam gloves.

2. Check the seven rights, comparing information against the drug order.

   *Rationale*
   To ensure necessary accuracy

3. Identify the injection site on the patient's forearm. To do so, rest the patient's arm on a table with the palm up. Measure 2 to 3 finger-widths below the antecubital space and a hand-width above the wrist. The space between is available for the injection (Figure 38-18).

4. Prepare the skin with the alcohol swab, moving in a circle from the center out.

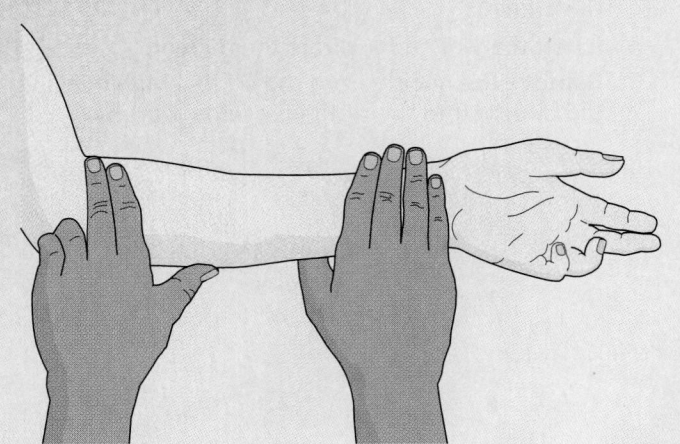

**Figure 38-18.** This space is available for intradermal injection sites.

5. Let the skin dry before giving the injection.

   *Rationale*
   To prevent you from introducing antiseptic under the skin, which could cause irritation and falsify intradermal test results

6. Hold the patient's forearm, and stretch the skin taut with one hand.

7. With the other hand, place the needle—bevel up—almost flat against the patient's skin. Press the needle against the skin and insert it.

8. Inject the drug slowly and gently. You should see the needle through the skin and feel

*continued* ⟶

## PROCEDURE 38.5

### Giving an Intradermal Injection *(concluded)*

resistance. As the drug enters the upper layer of skin, a wheal (raised area of the skin) will form (Figure 38-19).

9. After the full dose of the drug has been injected, withdraw the needle. Properly dispose of used materials and the needle and syringe immediately.

10. Remove the gloves and wash your hands.

11. Stay with the patient to monitor for unexpected reactions.

12. Document the injection with the date, time, drug name, dosage, expiration date, lot number, manufacturer, route, site, significant patient reactions, and any patient education in the patient's chart.

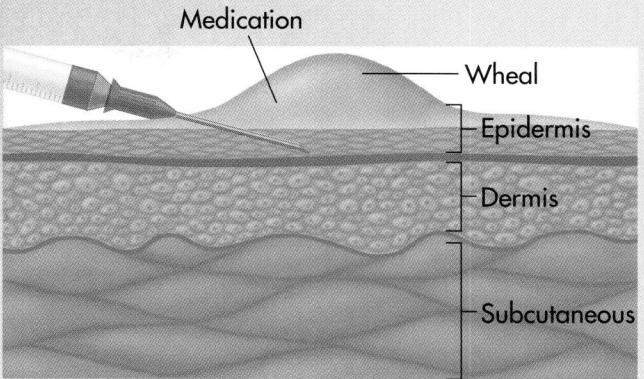

**Figure 38-19.** Medication collects under the skin, forming a wheal during an intradermal injection.

## PROCEDURE 38.6

### Giving a Subcutaneous (Sub-Q) Injection

**Procedure Goal:** To administer a subcutaneous injection safely and effectively, using sterile technique

**OSHA Guidelines**

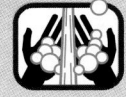 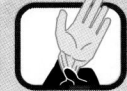 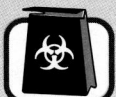
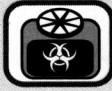 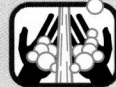

**Materials:** Drug order (in patient's chart), alcohol swabs, sterile 2 × 2 gauze or cotton ball, container of the ordered drug, disposable needle and syringe of the appropriate size, sharps container

**Method:**

1. Identify the patient. Wash your hands and put on exam gloves.

2. Check the seven rights, comparing information against the drug order.

   *Rationale*
   To ensure necessary accuracy

3. Prepare the drug and draw it up to the mark on the syringe that matches the ordered dose.

4. Choose a site (Figure 38-20) and clean it with an alcohol swab, moving in a circle from the center out. Let the area dry.

5. Pinch the skin firmly to lift the subcutaneous tissue.

6. Position the needle—bevel up—at a 45-degree angle to the skin.

   *Rationale*
   The angle of the needle helps ensure the medication is administered into the correct location.

7. Insert the needle in one quick motion. Then release the skin and inject the drug slowly (Figure 38-21).

8. After the full dose of the drug has been injected, place a 2 × 2 gauze over the site, and withdraw the needle at the same angle you inserted it.

9. Apply pressure at the puncture site with the gauze or cotton ball.

10. Massage the site gently to help distribute the drug, if indicated. Do not massage insulin, heparin, or other anticoagulant medications.

*continued* ⟶

## Giving a Subcutaneous (Sub-Q) Injection *(concluded)*

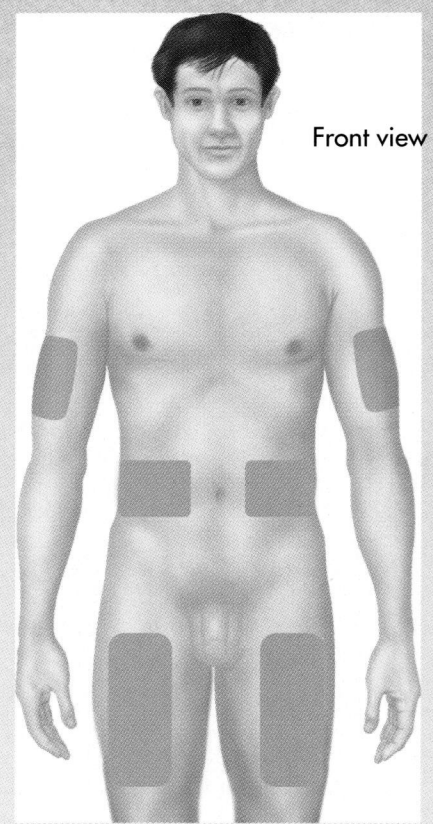

Front view

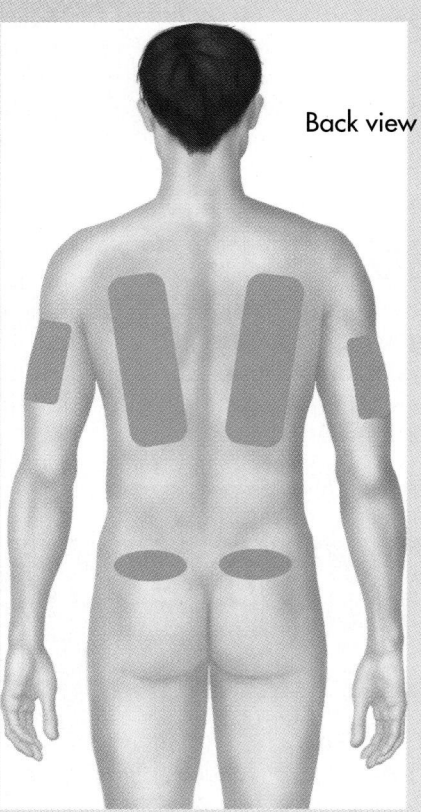

Back view

**Figure 38-20.** Many sites are available for subcutaneous injection.

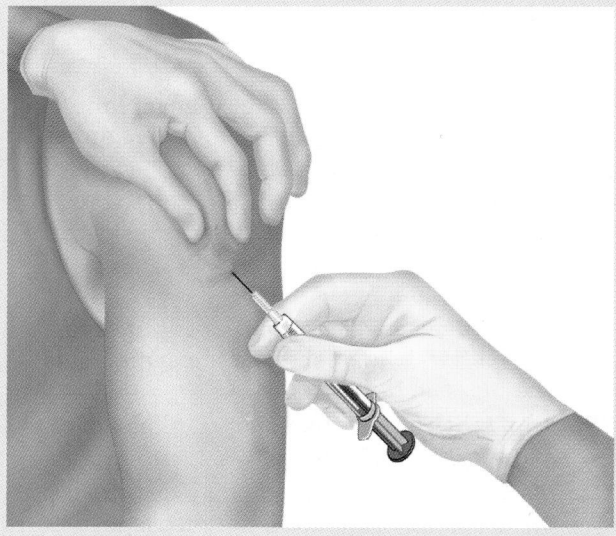

**Figure 38-21.** The bevel of the needle should be up and at a 45-degree angle when performing a subcutaneous injection.

*Rationale*

Massaging a site for heparin can cause bruising.

11. Properly dispose of the used materials and the needle and syringe.

12. Remove the gloves and wash your hands.

13. Stay with the patient to monitor for unexpected reactions.

14. Document the injection with the date, time, drug name, dosage, expiration date, lot number, manufacturer, route, site, significant patient reactions, and any patient education in the patient's chart.

sub-Q injection, select a site away from bones and blood vessels. Do not use an area that is edematous (swollen), scarred, or hardened or one that has a large amount of fat, because these areas may not have the capillary network needed for absorption. When patients need regular sub-Q injections, remember to rotate injection sites systematically. Begin the rotation pattern by giving injections in rows in the same area of the body (such as the abdomen). After all those sites have been used once, proceed to the next area on the body (such as the right leg), and follow a similar pattern there. Rotating sites promotes drug absorption and prevents hard subcutaneous lumps from forming.

At the injection site, ensure that you can pinch at least a 1-inch skin fold for the injection. If a patient is frail, dehydrated, or thin, you may need to use a site other than the back or abdomen to provide the necessary fold of skin.

***Intramuscular.*** When a patient requires rapid drug absorption, you may be asked to administer an **intramuscular (IM)** injection, as described in Procedure 38-7. An IM injection usually irritates a patient's tissues less than a sub-Q injection and allows administration of a larger amount of drug, usually 3 to 5 mL in an adult.

Common IM injection sites include the dorsogluteal, ventrogluteal, vastus lateralis, and deltoid muscles, illustrated

## PROCEDURE 38.7

# Giving an Intramuscular Injection

**Procedure Goal:** To administer an intramuscular injection safely and effectively, using sterile technique

## OSHA Guidelines

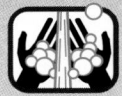 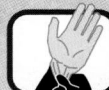 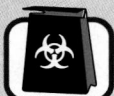
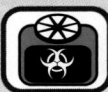 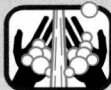

**Materials:** Drug order (in patient's chart), alcohol swabs, sterile 2 × 2 gauze or cotton ball, container of the ordered drug, disposable needle and syringe of the appropriate size, sharps container

## Method:

1. Identify the patient. Wash your hands and put on exam gloves.
2. Check the seven rights, comparing information against the drug order.

### Rationale

To ensure necessary accuracy

3. Prepare the drug and draw it up to the mark on the syringe that matches the ordered dose.
4. Choose a site (Figure 38-22) and gently tap it. Tapping stimulates the nerve endings and reduces pain caused by the needle insertion.
5. Clean the site with an alcohol swab, moving in a circle from the center out. Let the site dry.
6. Stretch the skin taut over the injection site.

7. Hold the needle and syringe at a 90-degree angle to the skin. Then insert the needle with a quick, dart-like thrust.

### Rationale

The angle of the needle helps ensure the medication is administered into the correct location.

8. Release the skin and aspirate by pulling back slightly on the plunger to check the needle placement. If pulling back on the plunger produces blood, placement is incorrect and you must begin again with a fresh needle and syringe. If pulling back on the plunger produces no blood, placement is correct. Inject the drug slowly.

### Rationale

Injecting an intramuscular drug into the bloodstream can cause severe side effects for the patient.

9. After the full dose of the drug has been injected, place a 2 × 2 gauze over the site. Then quickly remove the needle at a 90-degree angle.
10. Use the 2 × 2 gauze to apply pressure to the site and massage it, if indicated.
11. Properly dispose of used materials and the needle and syringe.
12. Remove the gloves and wash your hands.
13. Stay with the patient to monitor for unexpected reactions.
14. Document the injection with the date, time, drug name, dosage, expiration date, lot number, manufacturer, route, site, significant patient reactions, and any patient education in the patient's chart.

*continued* ⟶

# Giving an Intramuscular Injection *(concluded)*

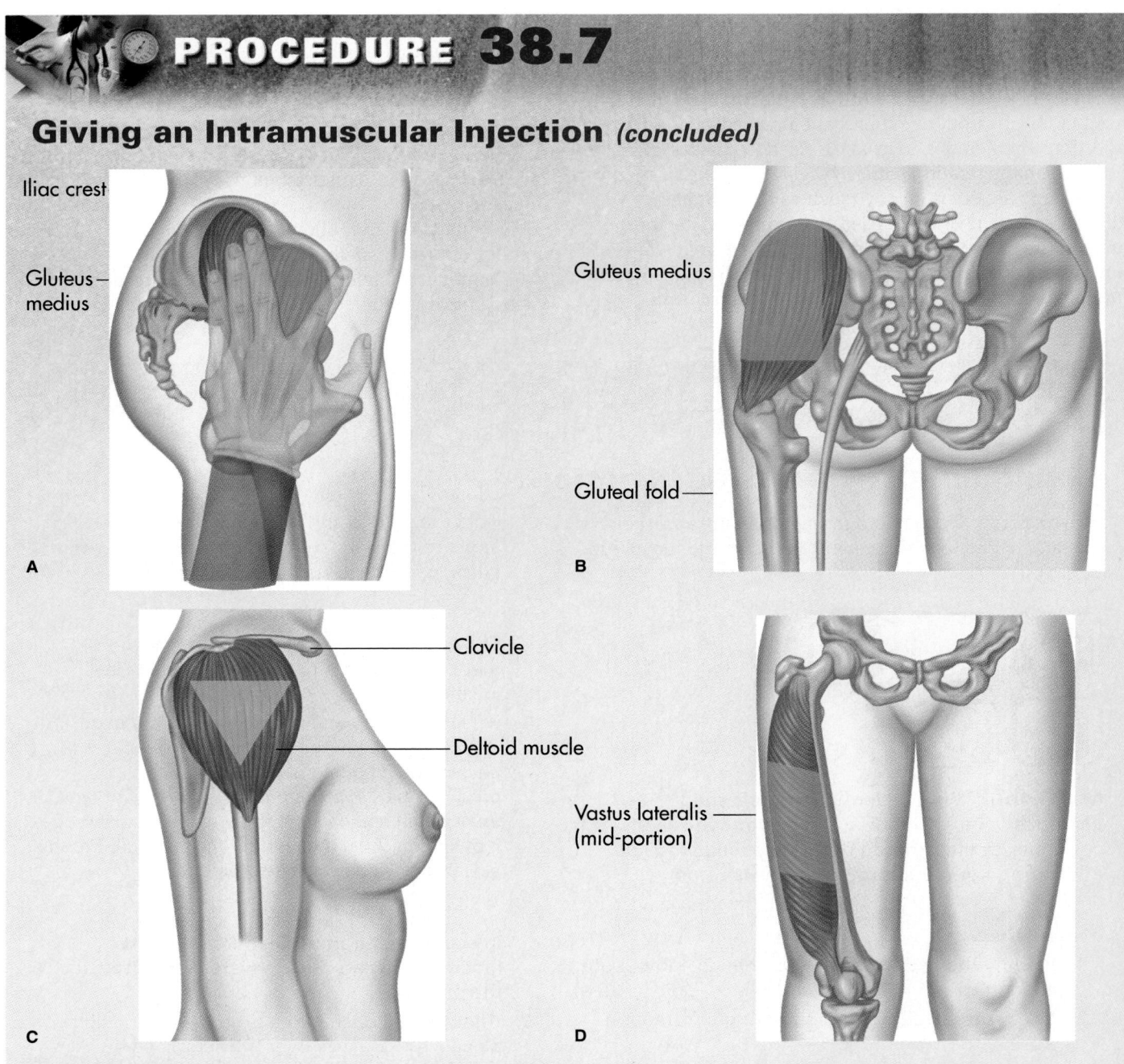

**Figure 38-22.** For intramuscular injection in an adult, use (A) the ventrogluteal site, (B) the dorsogluteal site, (C) the deltoid site, or (D) the vastus lateralis site.

in Figure 38-22. Before giving an IM injection, identify the site carefully to prevent injury to blood vessels and nerves in the area. As with sub-Q injections, rotate sites if the patient must receive regular or multiple IM injections.

Take into consideration the patient's layer of fat when choosing an IM injection site. You want the injection to penetrate beyond the fat layer to muscle. If, for example, a patient is heavy in the buttocks and thighs, the deltoid may be the best site for administering an IM injection.

When giving an IM injection to a pediatric patient, use the smallest gauge needle, usually 22 to 25 gauge. Also

use the shortest length needle that will allow you to reach muscle, usually 1 inch.

Injection sites vary with age. For an infant or toddler, use the vastus lateralis muscle. For a child who has been walking for about a year, use the ventrogluteal or dorsogluteal site. For an older, well-developed child, use any adult site.

When injecting an IM drug that can irritate subcutaneous tissues, such as iron dextran (Imferon), use the **Z-track method,** illustrated in Figure 38-23. To do this, pull the skin and subcutaneous tissue to the side before inserting the needle at the site. After the drug is injected,

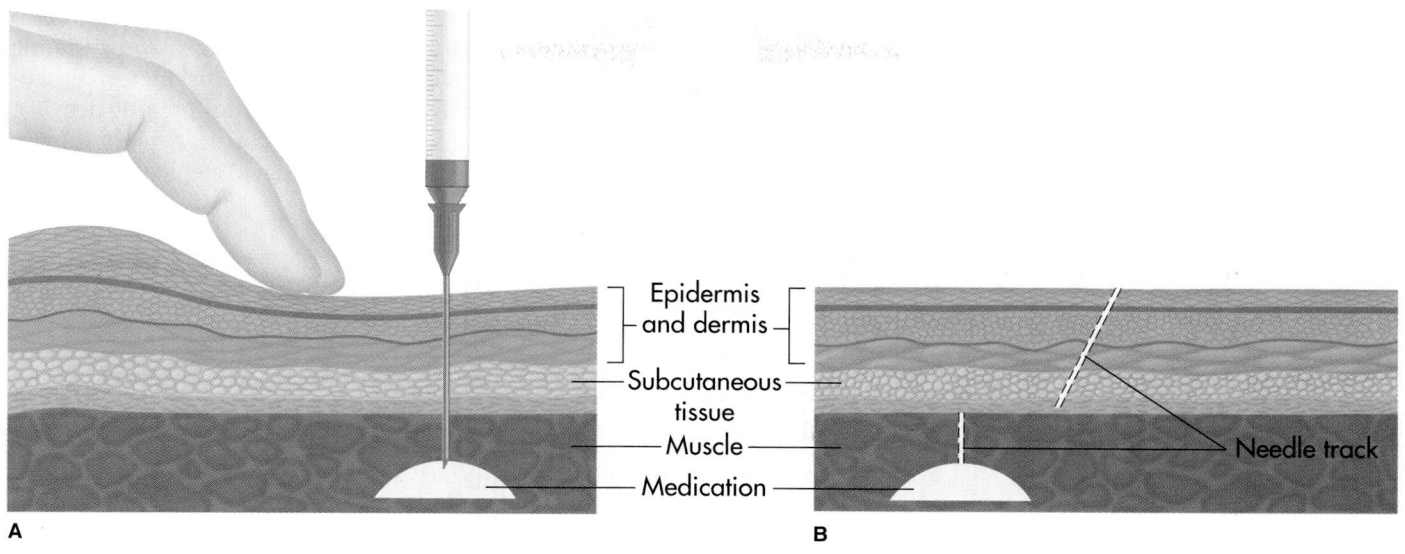

**Figure 38-23.** Use the Z-track method for IM injection of irritating solutions. (A) Pull the skin to one side before inserting the needle. (B) After injecting the drug, release the skin to seal off the needle track.

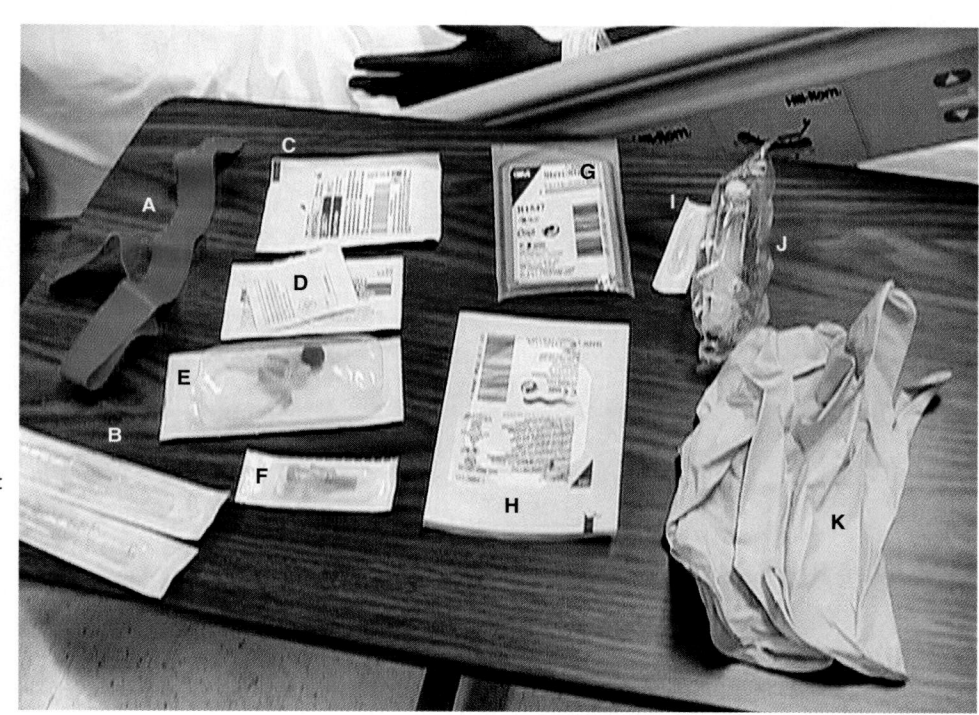

A. Tourniquet
B. Two venous access devices
C. 2 X 2 gauze
D. Alcohol prep pad
E. Extension tubing
F. PRN cap
G. Tape strips
H. Semitransparent dressing
I. Needleless access tip for saline syringe
J. Saline flush
K. Gloves

**Figure 38-24.** You may be required to gather the equipment for an intravenous medication to be infused.

release the tissue. This technique creates a zigzag path in the tissue layers, which prevents the drug from leaking into the subcutaneous tissue and causing irritation.

***Intravenous.*** Although **intravenous (IV)** injections are not commonly performed in a medical office or by medical assistants, certain drugs may be administered this way. Drugs may also be mixed and dissolved into a **solution** (a homogeneous mixture of a solid, liquid, or gaseous substance in a liquid) and given by IV **infusion** (slow drip) into a vein. Examples of IV drugs include powerful antibiotics, chemotherapeutic drugs, emergency drugs, and electrolytes. Because these drugs are introduced directly into the bloodstream, they produce an almost immediate effect. They also can cause sudden adverse reactions.

Although in most cases a doctor or nurse must administer an IV drug, you may assist by laying out supplies and equipment. When assisting with any intravenous medications, gather the ordered drug and a tourniquet, bedsaver pad, gloves, iodine and alcohol swabs, venipuncture device, tape, and gauze pad, as ordered. Obtain other supplies and equipment, depending on the specific type of infusion or injection being administered (Figure 38-24).

## Inhalation Therapy

Inhalation therapy can be administered through the mouth or nose. There are a number of disorders for which the physician may order an inhaler or aerosol form of medication. For example, an oral inhaler is frequently used by patients with asthma, whereas a nasal inhaler is frequently used for local treatment of nasal congestion. Nasal inhalers are also used to administer medicines for systemic effect, such as a vasopressin derivative for nocturnal bedwetting. Package inserts for inhaled drugs provide detailed descriptions of the exact procedure for the type of inhalation. Procedure 38-8 provides the basic steps of the procedure plus patient education.

# PROCEDURE 38.8

## Administering Inhalation Therapy

**Procedure Goal:** To administer inhalation therapy safely and effectively

**OSHA Guidelines:** This procedure does not involve exposure to blood, body fluids, or tissues.

**Materials:** Drug order (in patient's chart), container of the ordered drug, tissues, package insert or patient education sheet about medication

**Method:**

1. Identify the patient. Wash your hands.
2. Check the seven rights, comparing information against the drug order. Make sure you have the correct type of inhaler based upon the order (oral or nasal).

### Rationale
To ensure necessary accuracy.

3. Prepare the container of medication as directed. Use the package insert and show the directions to the patient.
4. Shake the container as directed and stress this step to the patient.

### Rationale
The drug must be evenly distributed in the inhaler to ensure its effectiveness.

### For a Nasal Inhaler

5. Instruct the patient to complete the following steps:
   - Have the patient blow the nose to clear the nostrils.
   - Tilt the head back, and with one hand, place the inhaler tip about ½ inch into the nostril.
   - Point the tip straight up toward the inner corner of the eye.

   ### Rationale
   Angling the inhaler downward makes the drug run down the back of the throat, causing a burning sensation.
   - Use the opposite hand to block the other nostril.
   - Inhale gently while quickly and firmly squeezing the inhaler.
   - Remove the inhaler tip and exhale through the mouth.
   - Shake the inhaler and repeat the process in the other nostril.
   - If indicated in the package insert, instruct patients to keep the head tilted back and not to blow their nose for several minutes.

### For an Oral Inhaler

5. Instruct the patient to complete the following steps:
   - Warm the canister by rolling it between the palms of your hands.
   - Uncap the mouthpiece and assemble the inhaler as directed on the package insert.
   - Hold the mouth open and place the canister in the mouth or about 1 inch from the mouth.
   - Check the package insert for the proper placement.
   - Exhale normally and inhale through the canister as he or she depresses it. The medication must be inhaled.
   - Breathe in until the lungs are full and hold the breath for 10 seconds
   - Breathe out normally.

### After You Have Given an Inhalation Medication

6. Remain with the patient to monitor for changes and possible adverse reaction.
7. Recap and secure the medication container. Instruct the patient in this procedure.
8. Wash your hands.
9. Give the patient an information sheet about the drug. Discuss the information with the patient and answer any questions she may have. If the patient has questions you cannot answer, refer her to the physician.
10. Document the drug administration with the date, time, drug name, dosage, expiration date, lot number, manufacturer, route, site, significant patient reactions, and any patient education in the patient's chart.

## Topical Application

Topical application is the direct application of a drug on the skin. Topical drugs can take the form of creams, lotions, **ointments** (salves), tinctures, powders, sprays, and solutions, which are used for their local effects. They include antibacterial and antifungal drugs as well as corticosteroids.

To apply a cream, lotion, or ointment, use long, even strokes with a cotton-tipped applicator and/or a gloved finger when rubbing it into the skin. Follow the direction of the hair growth to avoid irritating the hair follicles and skin. To apply a powder, shake it on but do not rub it in.

A specialized type of topical administration that produces a systemic effect is the **transdermal** system (or patch). A drug administered through the transdermal patch is absorbed through the skin directly into the bloodstream. The patch slowly and evenly releases a systemic drug, such as scopolamine, nitroglycerin, estrogen, or fentanyl, through the skin. The patient receives a timed-release dose, usually over a day or several days. See Procedure 38-9.

## PROCEDURE 38.9

## Administering and Removing a Transdermal Patch and Providing Patient Instruction

**Procedure Goal:** To safely administer and remove a transdermal patch drug to a patient

**OSHA Guidelines:** This procedure does not involve exposure to blood, body fluids, or tissues.

**Materials:** Drug order (in patient chart), transdermal patch medication, gloves, package insert or drug information sheet, patient chart

**Method:**

1. Identify the patient, wash your hands, and put on gloves.

   *Rationale*

   Gloves prevent the medication from being absorbed through your skin.

2. Select the ordered transdermal patch and check the seven rights, comparing information against the drug order.

   *Rationale*

   To ensure necessary accuracy.

3. Ask the patient about any drug or food allergies. If the patient is not allergic to the ordered drug or other ingredients used to prepare it, proceed.

   *Rationale*

   To prevent a reaction to the medication

4. If you are unfamiliar with the drug, check the PDR or other drug reference, read the package insert, or speak with the physician. The package insert is extremely detailed for transdermal medications and should be used when applying the medication and/or doing patient teaching.

5. Perform any calculations needed to provide the prescribed dose. If you are unsure of your calculations, check them with a coworker or the physician.

### Applying the Transdermal Medication

6. Remove the patch from its pouch. The plastic backing is easily peeled off once the patch is removed from the pouch. For patches without a protective pouch, bend the sides of the transdermal unit back and forth until the clear plastic backing snaps down the middle.

7. For either type of patch, demonstrate how to peel off the clear plastic backing to expose the sticky side of the patch.

8. Apply the patch to a reasonably hair-free site, such as the abdomen. Figure 38-25 shows how to apply both types of patches. Note that Estrogen patches are usually placed on the hip.

9. Instruct the patient how to apply the patch. Advise the patient to avoid using the extremities below the knee or elbow, skin folds, scar tissue, or burned or irritated areas.

   *Rationale*

   These areas do not absorb the medication as well because of the reduced blood supply.

### Removing the Transdermal Patch

6. Gently lift and slowly peel the patch back from the skin. Wash the area with soap and dry it with a towel. Instruct the patient on this technique.

7. Explain to the patient that the skin may appear red and warm, which is normal. Reassure the patient that the redness will disappear. In some

*continued* ⟶

# Administering and Removing a Transdermal Patch and Providing Patient Instruction (concluded)

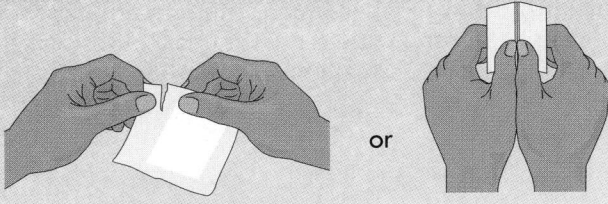

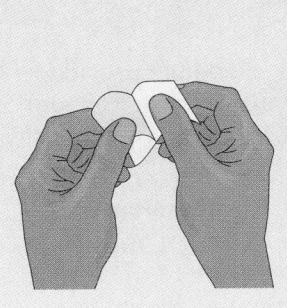

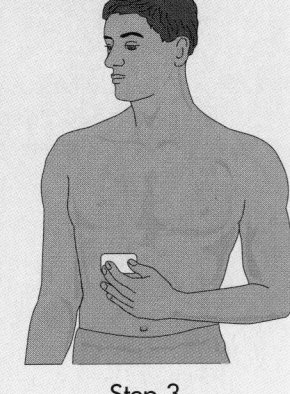

Step 1

Step 2

Step 3

**Figure 38-25.** To apply a transdermal patch, first (1) either remove it from the pouch, or bend the sides back and forth until the backing snaps; then (2) peel the backing off the patch; and (3) apply the patch, sticky side down, to a clean, relatively hairless site.

cases, lotion may be applied to the skin if it feels dry.

8. Instruct the patient to notify the doctor if the redness does not disappear in several days or if a rash develops.

9. *Never* apply a new patch to the site just used. It is best to allow each site to rest between applications. Some transdermal systems call for waiting 7 days before using a site again. Be sure to check the package directions regarding site rotation.

### After You Have Applied and/or Removed the Transdermal Patch

10. Wash your hands and instruct the patient they should do the same after applying or removing a transdermal system at home.

11. Give the patient an information sheet about the drug. Discuss the information with the patient and answer any questions she may have. If the patient has questions you cannot answer, refer her to the physician.

12. Document the drug administration with the date, time, drug name, dosage, expiration date, lot number, manufacturer, route, site, significant patient reactions, and any patient education in the patient's chart.

## Urethral Administration

The urethral route is used when antibiotic and antifungal drugs are needed locally—that is, at the site of infection—for some urinary tract infections. Depending on the nature of the infection and the duration of drug action, the physician or a nurse may instill liquid drugs only one time or several times a day for a week. Urethral administration is used in both men and women.

Urethral drug administration requires passing a small-diameter urinary catheter into the bladder, instilling a drug through it, and clamping the catheter to let the drug bathe the urinary bladder walls. See Procedure 38-10.

## Vaginal Administration

Physicians usually prescribe vaginal drugs to treat local fungal infections. The drugs may also be used for local bacterial infections. They are usually packaged as suppositories (the most common form), solutions, creams, ointments, and foams. The liquid form of vaginal medication is administered by performing a **douche** (vaginal irrigation). This process is similar to giving a urethral drug, but it requires a special irrigating nozzle. Patients frequently ask about administering vaginal medications, and they usually administer such medications at home. Therefore, you must be prepared to provide detailed patient education for this route of administration. The physician may ask you to administer the first dose as a means of teaching a patient the method to use at home, or you may be asked to administer a one-time-only dose. See Procedure 38-11.

## Rectal Administration

Certain medications, such as drugs used to treat constipation, nausea, and vomiting, may be administered by the rectal route. These medications may be given in the form of suppositories or enemas and may produce local or systemic effects. See Procedure 38-12.

# PROCEDURE 38.10

## Assisting with Administration of an Urethral Drug

**Procedure Goal:** To assist with an urethral administration

**OSHA Guidelines**

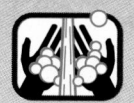 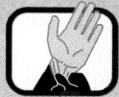 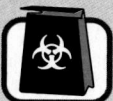
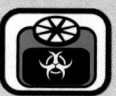 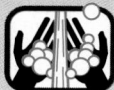

**Materials:** Urinary catheter kit, either a syringe without a needle or tubing and a bag (depending on the amount of drug to be administered), sterile gloves, the prescribed drug, a drape, and a bedsaver pad

**Method:**

1. Wash your hands and use sterile technique to assemble the equipment.
2. Check the seven rights, comparing information against the drug order, and explain the procedure and the drug order to the patient.

### Rationale

To ensure necessary accuracy.

3. Assist the patient into the lithotomy position (shown in Chapter 25, Figure 25-1D), and drape her to preserve her modesty while exposing the vulva.
4. Place a bedsaver pad under the buttocks.
5. Open the catheter kit.

6. Put on sterile gloves.
7. Cleanse the vulva as you would to perform catheterization, using the materials in the kit. As you sweep down with the antiseptic swab, watch for the urethral opening to "wink."

### Rationale

The wink helps you accurately locate the urethral opening.

8. The physician or nurse will insert the lubricated catheter. Tell the patient that she should feel pressure, not pain, and that the physician or nurse is going to attach the syringe to the catheter and insert the drug (or attach the tubing and bag to the catheter and let the drug run in by gravity).
9. After instilling the drug, the physician or nurse will clamp the catheter and leave the drug in place for the ordered amount of time.
10. Stay with the patient not only to ensure that she remains still but also to reassure her that the full feeling in the bladder is normal. She may also say she feels the need to urinate. Advise her that this feeling, too, is normal and is caused by the catheter.
11. When the time is up, unclamp the catheter, gently remove it, and allow the patient to urinate. Assist the patient as needed.
12. While the patient is dressing, immediately document the drug instillation with date, time, drug, dose, route, and any significant patient reactions.

# PROCEDURE 38.11

## Administering a Vaginal Medication

**Procedure Goal:** To safely administer a vaginal medication with patient instruction

**OSHA Guidelines**

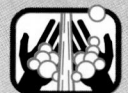 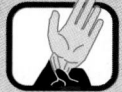 
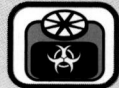 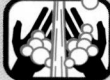

**Materials:** Prescription or drug order in the patient's chart, a cloth or paper drape, a bedsaver pad, gloves, cotton balls, water-soluble lubricant, and the prescribed drug

**Method:**

1. Wash your hands.
2. Check the seven rights, comparing information against the drug order, and explain the procedure and the drug order to the patient.

*continued* ⟶

## PROCEDURE 38.11

## Administering a Vaginal Medication *(concluded)*

### Rationale

To ensure necessary accuracy.

3. Give the patient the opportunity to empty her bladder before beginning.

4. Assist the patient into the lithotomy position (shown in Chapter 25, Figure 25-1D), and drape her.

### Rationale

To preserve her modesty while exposing the vulva

5. Place a bedsaver pad under the buttocks.

6. Put on gloves.

7. Cleanse the perineum with soap and water, using one cotton ball per stroke, and cleanse the center last, while spreading the labia.

### Rationale

This technique prevents contamination to areas cleaned.

8. Lubricate the vaginal suppository applicator in lubricant spread on a paper towel. For vaginal drugs in the forms of creams, ointments, gels, and tablets, use the appropriate applicator, preparing it according to the package insert.

9. While spreading the labia with one hand, insert the applicator with the other (the applicator should be about 2 inches into the vagina and angled toward the sacrum).

10. Release the labia and push the applicator's plunger to release the suppository into the vagina.

11. Remove the applicator, and wipe any excess lubricant off the patient.

12. Help her to a sitting position, and assist with dressing if needed.

13. Document the administration with date, time, drug, dose, route, and any significant patient reactions.

## PROCEDURE 38.12

## Administering a Rectal Medication

**Procedure Goal:** To safely administer a rectal medication

### OSHA Guidelines

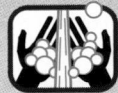 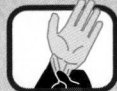 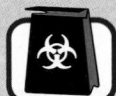

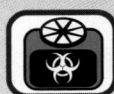 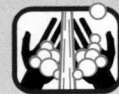

**Materials:** Prescription or drug order in the patient's chart, a cloth or paper drape, a bedsaver pad, gloves, water-soluble lubricant, and the prescribed drug

### Method:

1. Check the seven rights, comparing information against the drug order.

### Rationale

To ensure necessary accuracy.

2. Explain the procedure and the drug order to the patient.

3. Give the patient the opportunity to empty the bladder before beginning.

4. Help the patient into Sims' position (shown in Chapter 25, Figure 25-1H). Place a bedsaver pad under the patient.

5. Lift the patient's gown to expose the anus.

6. Wash your hands, put on gloves, and prepare the medication.

### *When Administering a Suppository*

7. Lubricate the tapered end of the suppository with about 1 tsp of lubricant.

8. While spreading the patient's buttocks with one hand, insert the suppository—tapered end first—into the anus with the other hand.

9. Gently advance the suppository past the sphincter with your index finger. Before it passes the sphincter, the suppository may feel as if it is being pushed back out the anus. When it passes the sphincter, it seems to disappear.

10. Use tissues to remove excess lubricant from the area.

*continued* ⟶

## Administering a Rectal Medication *(concluded)*

11. Remove your gloves and ask the patient to lie quietly and retain the suppository for at least 20 minutes. When the treatment is completed, help the patient to a sitting, then standing, position.

### Rationale
To ensure the maximum effectiveness of the medication.

### When Administering a Retention Enema

7. Place the tip of a syringe into a rectal tube. Let a little rectal solution flow through the syringe and tube. While holding the tip up, clamp the tubing.

8. Lubricate the end of the tube and spread the patient's buttocks, and slide the tube into the rectum about 4 inches.

9. Slowly pour the rectal solution into the syringe, release the clamp, and let gravity move the solution into the patient. When you have administered the ordered amount of solution, clamp the tube and then remove it.

10. Using tissues, apply pressure over the anus for 20 seconds to stifle the patient's urge to defecate, and then wipe any excess lubricant or solution from the area. Encourage the patient to retain the enema for the time ordered.

### Rationale
To ensure the maximum effectiveness of the medication.

11. When the time has passed, help the patient use a bedpan or direct the patient to a toilet to expel the solution.

### After the Administration Is Complete

12. Remove your gloves and wash your hands.

13. Immediately document the drug administration with date, time, drug, dose, route, and any significant patient reactions.

---

## Administering Medications to the Eye or Ear

Doctors commonly administer eye medications or perform eye irrigations to assist patients in eye tests, reduce pressure in the eyes, relieve eye pain, and treat eye infections and inflammation. Refer to Procedures 38-13 and 38-14 for instructions. Although most eye medications are administered for local effect, some contain drugs that are absorbed systemically. To prevent systemic absorption, the doctor may request that you apply pressure with one finger just below the inner corner of each eye after instilling medications. Continue applying pressure for 2 to 3 minutes, as directed.

Doctors often administer eardrops or perform ear irrigations to treat patients' ear infections or inflammation, relieve ear pain, or loosen earwax. Like eye medications, eardrops are ordered primarily for their local effects. They are not usually absorbed systemically, nor do they cause systemic effects. Procedures 38-15 and 38-16 provide instructions for these two procedures.

---

## Administering Eye Medications

**Procedure Goal:** To instill medication into the eye for treatment of certain eye disorders

### OSHA Guidelines

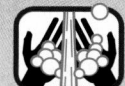 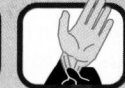  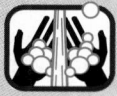

**Materials:** Medication (drops, cream, or ointment), tissues, eye patch (if applicable)

**Method:**

1. Identify the patient, introduce yourself, and explain the procedure.

2. Review the doctor's medication order. This should include the patient's name, drug name, concentration, number of drops (if a liquid), into which eye(s) the medication is to be administered, and the frequency of administration.

*continued* ⟶

# Administering Eye Medications *(continued)*

*Rationale*

The physician's order must be followed exactly.

3. Compare the drug with the medication order three times, checking the seven rights of medication administration.

*Rationale*

To ensure necessary accuracy.

4. Ask whether the patient has any known allergies to substances contained in the medication.

5. Wash your hands and put on gloves.

6. Assemble the supplies.

7. Ask the patient to lie down or to sit back in a chair with the head tilted back.

8. Give the patient a tissue to blot excess medication as needed.

9. Remove an eye patch, if present.

10. Ask the patient to look at the ceiling. Instruct the patient to keep both eyes open during the procedure.

11. With a tissue, gently pull the lower eyelid down by pressing downward on the patient's cheekbone just below the eyelid with your nondominant hand. This pressure will open a pocket of space between the eyelid and the eye (Figure 38-26).

## Eyedrops

12. Resting your dominant hand on the patient's forehead, hold the filled eyedropper or bottle approximately ½ inch from the conjunctiva (Figure 38-27).

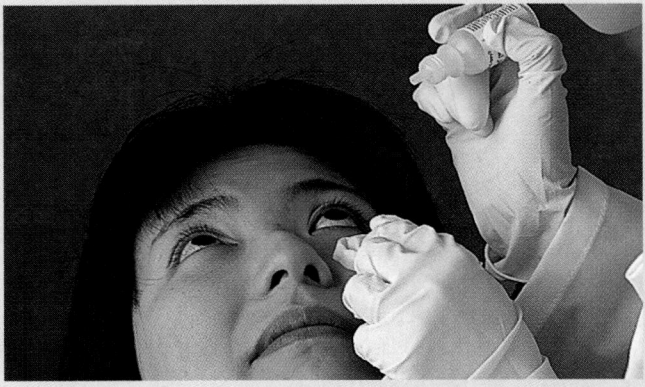

**Figure 38-26.** Use a tissue to press down on the patient's cheekbone just below the eyelid, opening up a pocket of space between the eyelid and the eye.

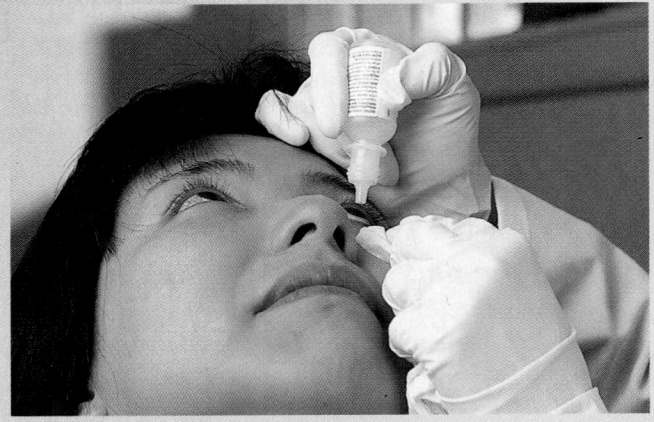

**Figure 38-27.** The medication container should be approximately ½ inch from the conjunctiva as you prepare to instill drops in the patient's eye.

*Rationale*

Touching patient's skin with dropper or bottle tip will cause contamination.

13. Drop the prescribed number of drops into the pocket. If any drops land outside the eye, repeat instilling the drops that missed the eye.

## Creams or Ointments

12. Rest your dominant hand on the patient's forehead, and hold the tube or applicator above the conjunctiva.

13. Without touching the eyelid or conjunctiva with the applicator, evenly apply a thin ribbon of cream or ointment along the inside edge of the lower eyelid on the conjunctiva, working from the medial (inner) to the lateral (outer) side (Figure 38-28).

*Rationale*

Touching the patient's skin with the applicator will cause contamination.

## All Medications

14. Release the lower lid and instruct the patient to gently close the eyes.

15. Repeat the procedure for the other eye as necessary.

16. Remove any excess medication by wiping each eyelid gently with a fresh tissue from the medial to the lateral side (Figure 38-29).

17. Apply a clean eye patch to cover the entire eye as necessary.

*continued* ⟶

# PROCEDURE 38.13

## Administering Eye Medications (concluded)

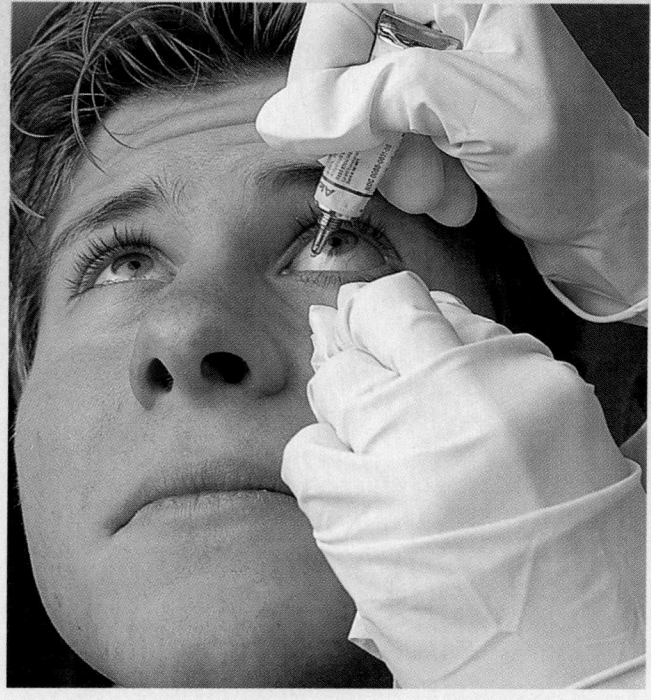

**Figure 38-28.** Apply a thin ribbon of cream or ointment along the inside of the lower eyelid on the conjunctiva.

18. Ask whether the patient felt any discomfort and observe for any adverse reactions. Notify the doctor as necessary.

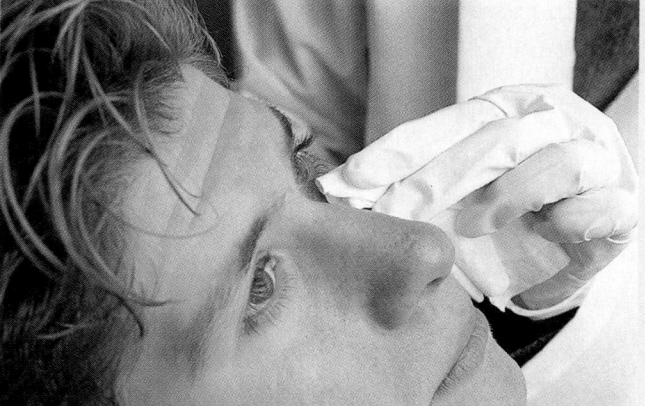

**Figure 38-29.** Use a tissue to remove excess medication from the eyelid.

19. Instruct the patient on self-administration of medication and patch application as necessary.
20. Ask the patient to repeat the instructions.
21. Provide written instructions.
22. Properly dispose of used disposable materials.
23. Remove gloves and wash your hands.
24. Document administration in the patient's chart. Include the drug, concentration, the number of drops, the time of administration, and the eye(s) that received the medication.

# PROCEDURE 38.14

## Performing Eye Irrigation

**Procedure Goal:** To flush the eye to remove foreign particles or relieve eye irritation

**OSHA Guidelines**

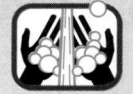 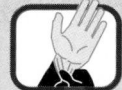 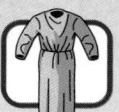 

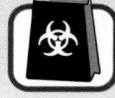 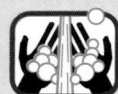 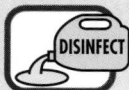

**Materials:** Sterile irrigating solution, sterile basin, sterile irrigating syringe and kidney-shaped basin, tissues

**Method:**
1. Identify the patient, introduce yourself, and explain the procedure.
2. Review the physician's order. This should include the patient's name, the irrigating solution, the volume of solution, and for which eye(s) the irrigation is to be performed.

*continued* ⟶

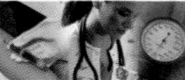

# PROCEDURE 38.14

## Performing Eye Irrigation *(concluded)*

3. Compare the solution with the instructions three times, checking the seven rights of medication administration.

   *Rationale*
   To ensure necessary accuracy.

4. Wash your hands and put on gloves, a gown, and a face shield.

   *Rationale*
   Splashing is possible when a syringe is used.

5. Assemble supplies.

6. Ask the patient to lie down or to sit with the head tilted back and to the side that is being irrigated. The solution should not spill over into the other eye.

   *Rationale*
   Cross-contamination between the eyes must be avoided.

7. Place a towel over the patient's shoulder (or under the head and shoulder, if the patient is lying down). Have the patient hold the kidney-shaped basin at the side of the head next to the eye to be irrigated.

8. Pour the solution into the sterile basin.

9. Fill the irrigating syringe with solution (approximately 50 mL).

10. Hold a tissue on the patient's cheekbone below the lower eyelid with your nondominant hand, and press downward to expose the eye socket.

11. Holding the tip of the syringe ½ inch away from the eye, direct the solution onto the lower conjunctiva from the inner to the outer aspect of the eye. (Avoid directing the solution against the cornea because it is sensitive; do not use excessive force.)

    *Rationale*
    To avoid contamination, do not let the tip touch the eye or skin.

12. Refill the syringe and continue irrigation until the prescribed volume of solution is used or until the solution is used up.

13. Dry the area around the eye with tissues.

14. Properly dispose of used disposable materials.

15. Remove your gloves, gown, and face shield, and wash your hands.

16. Record in the patient's chart the procedure, the amount of solution used, the time of administration, and the eye(s) irrigated.

17. Put on gloves and clean the equipment and room according to OSHA guidelines.

# PROCEDURE 38.15

## Administering Eardrops

**Procedure Goal:** To instill medication into the ear to treat certain ear disorders

**OSHA Guidelines**

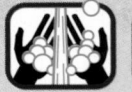 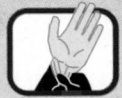 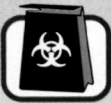 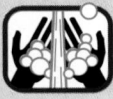

**Materials:** Liquid medication, cotton balls

**Method:**

1. Identify the patient, introduce yourself, and explain the procedure.

2. Check the physician's medication order. It should include the patient's name, drug name, concentration, the number of drops, into which ear(s) the medication is to be administered, and the frequency of administration.

3. Compare the drug with the instructions three times, checking the seven rights of medication administration.

   *Rationale*
   To ensure necessary accuracy.

*continued* ⟶

## Administering Eardrops *(continued)*

4. Ask whether the patient has any allergies to ear medications.
5. Wash your hands and put on gloves.
6. Assemble supplies.
7. If the medication is cold, warm it to room temperature with your hands or by placing the bottle in a pan of warm water.

### Rationale

Internal ear structures are very sensitive to extreme heat or cold. Administering cold medications can result in vertigo (dizziness) or nausea.

8. Have the patient lie on the side with the ear to be treated facing up.
9. Straighten the ear canal by pulling the auricle upward and outward for adults (Figure 38-30), down and back for infants and children (Figure 38-31).

### Rationale

Straightening the ear canal assures the medication reaches its destination.

10. Hold the dropper ½ inch above the ear canal.

### Rationale

The dropper must not be contaminated by touching patient's skin or any other surface.

11. Gently squeeze the bottle or dropper bulb to administer the correct number of drops (Figure 38-32).
12. Have the patient remain in this position for 10 minutes.
13. If ordered, loosely place a small wad of cotton in the outermost part of the ear canal.
14. Note any adverse reaction, notifying the physician as necessary.
15. Repeat the procedure for the other ear if ordered.
16. Instruct the patient on how to administer the drops at home.
17. Ask the patient to repeat the instructions.

### Rationale

For maximum effectiveness, it is important that the patient understands how to correctly continue treatment at home.

18. Provide written instructions.
19. Remove the cotton after 15 minutes.
20. Properly dispose of used disposable materials.

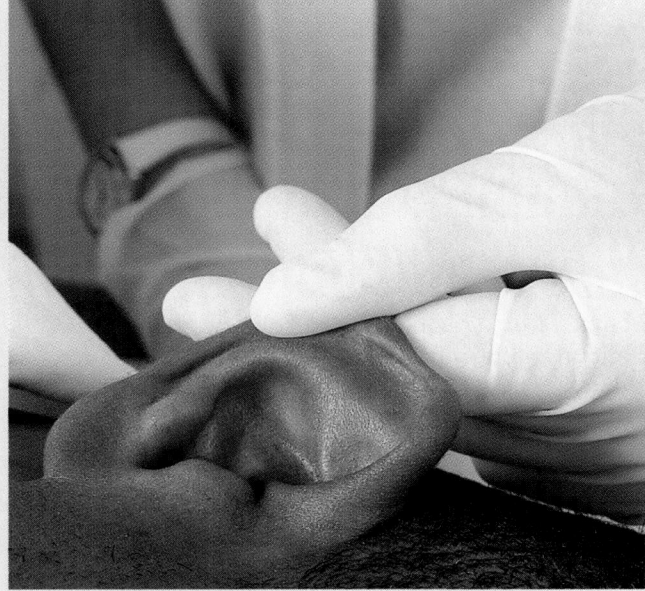

**Figure 38-30.** Straighten an adult's ear canal by pulling the auricle upward and outward.

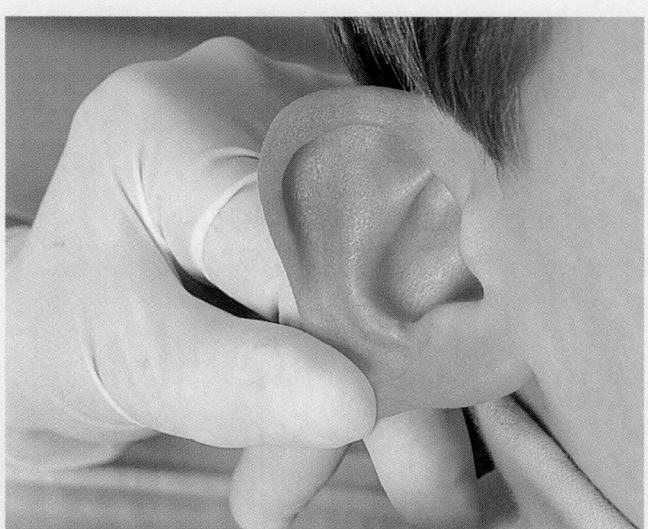

**Figure 38-31.** Straighten an infant's or child's ear canal by pulling the auricle downward and back.

*continued* ⟶

## Administering Eardrops *(concluded)*

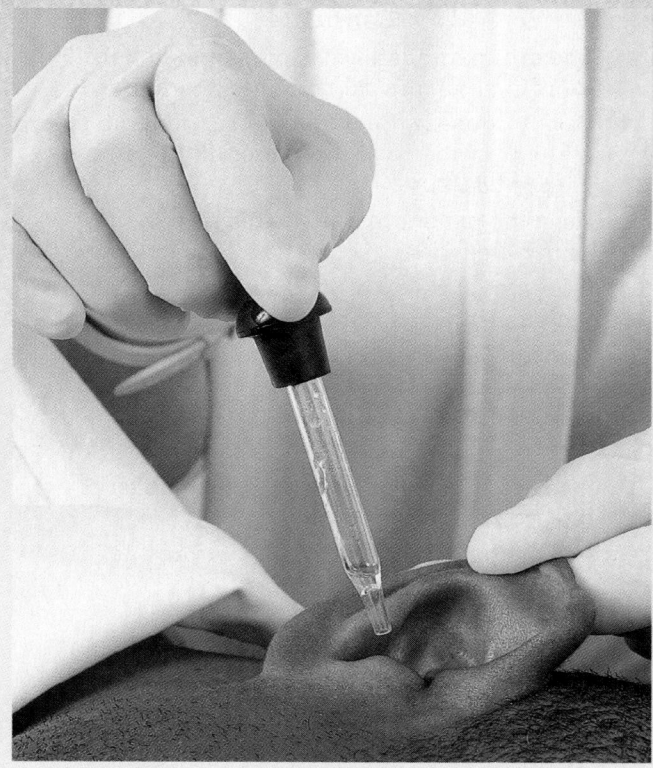

**Figure 38-32.** Apply slow gentle pressure to the dropper bulb so you can count the drops and administer the prescribed number.

21. Remove gloves and wash your hands.
22. Record in the patient's chart the medication, concentration, the number of drops, the time of administration, and which ear(s) received the medication.

## Performing Ear Irrigation

**Procedure Goal:** To wash out the ear canal to remove impacted cerumen, relieve inflammation, or remove a foreign body

**OSHA Guidelines**

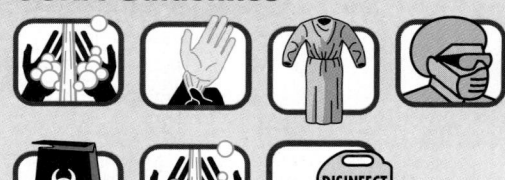

**Materials:** Fresh irrigating solution, clean basin, clean irrigating syringe, towel or absorbent pad, kidney-shaped basin, cotton balls

**Method:**

1. Identify the patient, introduce yourself, and explain the procedure.
2. Check the doctor's order. It should include the patient's name, the irrigating solution, the volume of solution, and for which ear(s) the irrigation is to be performed. If the doctor has not specified the volume of solution, use the amount needed to remove the wax.

*continued* ⟶

## Performing Ear Irrigation *(concluded)*

3. Compare the solution with the instructions three times, checking the seven rights of medication administration.

   *Rationale*

   To ensure necessary accuracy.

4. Wash your hands and put on gloves, a gown, and a face shield.

   *Rationale*

   Splashing is possible when a syringe is used.

5. Look into the patient's ear to identify if cerumen or a foreign body needs to be removed. You will know when you have completed the irrigation when the cerumen or foreign body is removed.

6. Assemble the supplies.

7. If the solution is cold, warm it to room temperature by placing the bottle in a pan of warm water.

   *Rationale*

   Internal ear structures are very sensitive to extreme heat or cold. Administering cold liquids can result in vertigo or nausea.

8. Have the patient sit or lie on her back with the ear to be treated facing you.

9. Place a towel over the patient's shoulder (or under the head and shoulder if she is lying down), and have her hold the kidney-shaped basin under her ear.

10. Pour the solution into the other basin.

11. If necessary, gently clean the external ear with cotton moistened with the solution.

12. Fill the irrigating syringe with solution (approximately 50 mL).

13. Straighten the ear canal by pulling the auricle upward and outward for adults, down and back for infants and children.

    *Rationale*

    Straightening the ear canal allows solution to reach its destination.

14. Holding the tip of the syringe ½ inch above the opening of the ear, slowly instill the solution into the ear. Allow the fluid to drain out during the process.

    *Rationale*

    Do not contaminate the syringe by allowing it to touch the patient or by allowing the draining fluid to touch it.

15. Refill the syringe and continue irrigation until the canal is cleaned or the solution is used up.

16. Dry the external ear with a cotton ball, and leave a clean cotton ball loosely in place for 5–10 minutes.

17. If the patient becomes dizzy or nauseated, allow her time to regain balance before standing up. Assist her as needed.

18. Properly dispose of used disposable materials.

19. Remove your gloves, gown, and face shield, and wash your hands.

20. Record in the patient's chart the procedure and result, the amount of solution used, the time of administration, and the ear(s) irrigated.

21. Put on gloves and clean the equipment and room according to OSHA guidelines.

# Educating the Patient About Drug Administration

Educating patients about what drugs do to the body and what the body does to drugs is discussed in detail in Chapter 37. You need to provide additional patient education, however, with regard to routes of administration. This education is extremely important; a patient who does not administer a drug correctly or safely may put health or life at risk.

# Reading the Drug Package Label

You must check the *PDR* or package insert for information about any drug with which you are not familiar. Likewise, before you teach a patient how to administer a drug, you must review the specific administration instructions for the drug in the *PDR* or on the package insert. An important aspect of this kind of information is teaching the patient how to read a prescription drug label. Instruct the patient to be particularly alert for special instructions and warning labels, such as those shown in Figure 38-33.

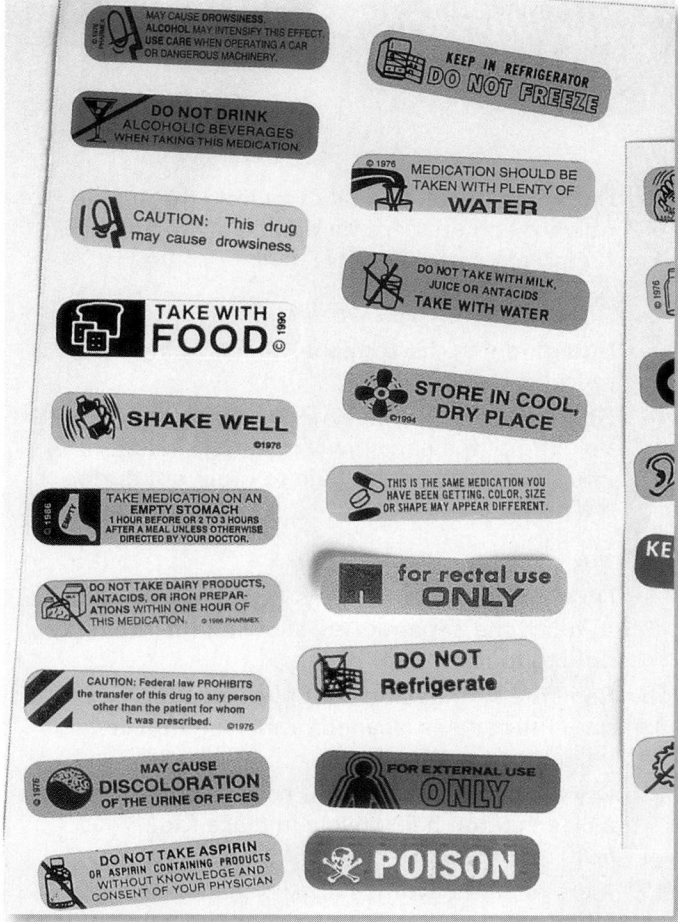

**Figure 38-33.** Teach the patient to heed warning labels and instructions on drug bottles.

## Interactions

Drug interactions should not be confused with adverse effects of drugs, discussed in Chapter 37. Patient education with regard to interactions is important. Interactions may occur between two prescription or nonprescription drugs or between a drug and food and may cause serious effects. Explain that the greater the number of drugs the patient takes, including over-the-counter medications or supplements, the greater the chance of a drug interaction.

**Drug-Drug Interactions.** When two drugs are taken at the same time, there are several possible interactions.

The effects of both drugs are increased, causing either a toxic or beneficial effect. For example, when alcohol is combined with diazepam (Valium), there is the potential toxic effect of severe central nervous system depression, because one drug intensifies the effect of the other. An example of a beneficial effect is the combination of acetaminophen and codeine, which increases the activity of both drugs, allowing the physician to prescribe a lower dose of each. In fact, this combination of drugs is available in one tablet (Tylenol® with codeine).

The effects of both drugs are decreased, or one drug cancels out the effect of the other. For example, combining propranolol (Inderal®) with albuterol (Proventil®) causes each drug to lose its effectiveness.

The effect of one of the drugs is increased by the other. For example, the effect of digoxin (Lanoxin®) is increased by the presence of furosemide (Lasix®), but the furosemide still works at the same degree of effectiveness as when administered alone.

To help prevent unintentional drug interactions, thoroughly assess the patient's medication use. Be sure to ask about medications prescribed by specialists as well as over-the-counter (OTC) drugs and supplements. Question the patient about past and present use of alcohol and recreational drugs as well as herbal remedies. Update the chart as needed. If you detect a potential for drug interactions, notify the physician. Drug interaction checkers are available online.

Also teach patients about possible drug interactions and how to avoid or minimize them. For example, patients may need to take certain drugs at least 2 hours apart. Instruct patients to call the office if they think their drugs are interacting adversely.

**Drug-Food Interactions.** Interactions between a drug and food can alter a drug's therapeutic effect. For example, taking tetracycline with milk can reduce the drug's effectiveness because of decreased absorption from the GI tract. The drug-food interaction between a monoamine oxidase (MAO) inhibitor (such as Parnate®, an antidepressant drug) and aged cheese or meat or other foods containing high levels of tyramine can produce a toxic effect. This interaction can cause a dangerous hypertensive crisis in which the patient's blood pressure rises quickly to dangerous levels, possibly leading to stroke and death.

A food that may interact with drugs is grapefruit and grapefruit juice. Interactions with some heart or blood pressure medications, such as Nifedipine, might cause irregularities in heartbeat, called arrhythmia.

Some drug-food interactions can affect the body's use of nutrients. For example, the cholesterol-lowering drugs cholestyramine resin and colestipol HCl may reduce the body's absorption of fat-soluble vitamins (A, D, E, and K) from food.

When teaching a patient about drug-food interactions, specify exactly which foods to avoid and when. For example, a patient may drink milk or eat food several hours before or after taking tetracycline, whereas a patient taking an MAO inhibitor must avoid foods that contain high levels of tyramine at all times. Explain what to expect if an interaction occurs, and describe how to deal with it. Make sure to check the package insert, PDR, or reliable Internet resource for specific guidelines for each medication.

## Adverse Effects

Adverse effects or reactions associated with a drug and reported in the PDR are discussed briefly in the section on toxicology in Chapter 37. These responses are somewhat predictable and range from mild adverse reactions, such as stomach upset, to severe or life-threatening allergic responses. For example, certain cholesterol-lowering medications, called statins (e.g., Lipitor®), can increase the likelihood of painful muscle disorders. Unpredictable adverse effects can also occur; they are unique to each patient. Always advise the patient to report any change in overall health, because that change could be drug-related.

Elderly patients and patients with liver or kidney disease are more susceptible than others to adverse effects because these conditions affect drug metabolism and excretion. When drugs are not metabolized properly or excreted from the body quickly enough, drugs can reach toxic levels, even with normal doses.

To help prevent adverse effects, teach the patient to take the drug at the right time, in the right amount, and under the right circumstances. For example, the patient may need to take a cephalosporin with food to avoid nausea and diarrhea. Also teach the patient to recognize significant adverse effects and to call the office if any of them occur.

# Special Considerations

Pediatric, pregnant, breast-feeding, or elderly patients or patients from different cultures require special considerations. When giving a drug to these patients, you must adjust patient care as needed.

## Pediatric Patients

Children pose special challenges in drug administration and use. Their physiology and immature body systems may make drug effects less predictable because drugs are absorbed, distributed, metabolized, and excreted differently in children than in adults. Therefore, plan to observe a pediatric patient closely for adverse effects and interactions.

A child's small size may also increase the risk of overdose and toxicity. These factors require dosage adjustments and careful measurement of small doses. To help administer drugs safely to pediatric patients, always check your calculations for providing a prescribed dose, and then ask a nurse or the doctor to double-check them.

Remember that administration sites and techniques for a child may differ from those for an adult. For example, fewer IM injection sites can be used for a young child. Also, the technique for eardrop administration varies slightly.

When dealing with an infant or young child, teach the parents—not the patient—about the drug. With an older child, include parents and patient in the teaching session. Be sure to use age-appropriate language when speaking to children.

Pediatric patients are not like adults—they often have difficulty adjusting to medical procedures or illnesses. Children who do not understand what is happening to them can become problematic; some may see a physician visit as a punishment. It is important for you to be sensitive to the needs and reactions of pediatric patients. The first memorable exposure to an office visit will often determine how the child will react to physician visits for years to come.

Patience is important when working with pediatric patients. Infants and children can sense when you are irritated or annoyed. Pay close attention to your nonverbal communication as well as your verbal communication. New mothers are often apprehensive about invasive procedures when it concerns their children. Empathy and compassion are needed to ensure that the office visit is a pleasant one.

Administering medications to a pediatric patient may become a challenge if the child is not cooperative. It is important to ensure that the child receives the full dose as ordered.

**Oral Medications.** When administering oral medications to children, follow these guidelines:

- Use a calibrated dropper or spoon device to measure the ordered dose.
- Administer the medication to the side of the tongue; this method prevents the child from spitting out the medication.
- Hold the child until you are sure the medication is swallowed.
- If a small amount dribbles from the mouth, do not attempt to give more medication to the child.
- If the child vomits within 5 minutes and you can see the medication in the vomitus, you should readminister the medication after the child is calm. If you are unsure of readministering medication, consult with the physician.
- If the medication only comes in tablet form and the child is unable to swallow a tablet or capsule, verify in a drug reference to see if the medication can be crushed and given with food, such as applesauce.

**Injections.** Stress and anxiety will differ from child to child. When giving injections to pediatric patients, the following steps will help to ensure a smooth procedure:

- Distract the patient. Talk to the child while giving the injection. Often the injection is performed and over before the child realizes it.
- Praise the child. Say things that promote maturity and self-esteem.
- Use an anesthetic topical agent prior to the injection. This can be applied in the office or at home before the patient arrives in the office.
- Be swift. Do not allow a lot of time to pass before giving the injection. The faster the better.
- Try not to allow the child to see the syringe before giving the injection.

*Pediatric Injection Sites.* Pediatric patients have less muscle development than adults do, which limits the sites for intramuscular injections. The deltoid muscle is not developed enough for an injection and can be painful for the child. The sciatic nerve is larger in children; dorsogluteal injections are therefore not recommended because of the danger of hitting the sciatic nerve.

The vastus lateralis and ventrogluteal sites are recommended for infants and children. The vastus lateralis site is good because it is a large and thick muscle that is developed before the child begins to walk. It is also the most desirable site for infants and children because it is not near major nerves and blood vessels. The vastus lateralis site is an easier site if you need to incorporate restraining methods.

The most common injections given to pediatric patients are vaccines. Most vaccines are given intramuscularly with a 25-gauge, ⅝-inch needle. The gauge and length varies based upon the size of the patient. Use your critical thinking and best judgment when selecting a needle and always check the package insert to ensure the correct amount and route is used.

In many cases, pediatric patients will require more than one vaccine injection in a single limb (vastus lateralis). When this is the case, the injections should be at least one inch apart on the site and the specific location of each vaccine should be documented.

***Restraining Methods.*** Sometimes a pediatric patient will need to be restrained in order for you to administer an injection. Two medical assistants may be needed to safely restrain a child while giving an injection. Common restraining methods include the following:

- Have the child "hug the mother." The mother holds the child in front of her, with the child's thighs extended on either side of her torso. As the mother is talking to her child, make the injection in the vastus lateralis.
- Weight-bearing restraining is better than muscular control. Have the child sit on the edge of the examining table and use your weight to immobilize the child's legs against the table.

## Pregnant Patients

When dealing with pregnant patients, remember that you are caring for two patients at once: the mother and her fetus. When you give the mother a drug, you may also be giving it to the fetus.

It is extremely important to double-check the drug in the *PDR* for toxicology or pregnancy warnings and to assess the patient carefully for therapeutic and adverse effects of the drug.

Some drugs can cause physical defects in the fetus if the mother takes them during pregnancy (especially in the first trimester). For this reason, you must be aware of the pregnancy drug risk categories, which were discussed in Chapter 37. If the physician orders a drug for a pregnant patient, double-check the order against the pregnancy drug risk categories. If it is a high-risk drug, check with the physician before administering the drug.

## Patients Who Are Breast-Feeding

Some drugs are excreted in breast milk and can thus be ingested by a breast-feeding infant. This ingestion can be dangerous because infants have immature body systems and cannot metabolize and excrete drugs that are safe for the mother. Some drugs, such as sedatives, diuretics, and hormones, can reduce the mother's flow of breast milk.

Whenever a drug is ordered for a patient who is breast-feeding, check a drug reference to see whether the drug is contraindicated during lactation. If so, consult the doctor. If not, teach the mother to recognize signs of adverse drug effects in her infant. If a mother must take a drug that affects lactation, advise her to supplement breast-feedings with infant formula.

## Elderly Patients

Age-related changes in the body can affect drug absorption, metabolism, distribution, and excretion. These normal changes can be exaggerated by various diseases or disorders. Therefore, as people age, they have an increased risk of drug toxicity, adverse effects, or lack of therapeutic effects. Because of this risk, be especially alert when assessing an elderly patient who is on drug therapy.

Many elderly patients have complex, chronic diseases with unusual symptoms. This situation can make it difficult to tell whether a problem is caused by a drug. Listen closely to elderly patients and their family members; they are more likely to notice subtle changes than you are.

Patient and family education is important with elderly patients, particularly if they engage in polypharmacy (take several medications concurrently). Polypharmacy is common in elderly patients, and possible drug-drug interactions can be severe. See the Caution: Handle With Care section.

If an elderly patient is forgetful or confused, talk to the doctor about simplifying the medication schedule to reduce the risk of drug administration errors or omissions. Suggest the use of pill-organizing devices to help prevent forgotten doses or overdoses (Figure 38-34). If the patient has vision problems, provide drug instruction sheets in large type. To do this, either type instructions on a word processor in a large type size, enlarge the instructions on a photocopier, or clearly handwrite the instructions in large block letters. You might also contact a local association for the blind or visually impaired for devices and tips.

## Patients From Different Cultures

Although cultural background is not likely to affect a drug's action in the body, it can affect a patient's understanding of drug therapy and compliance with it. For example, a patient who speaks little or no English cannot benefit from instructions given in English. To remedy this problem, obtain drug information sheets in the languages that are commonly spoken by patients of the practice. Use simple gestures and drawings to clarify difficult words or

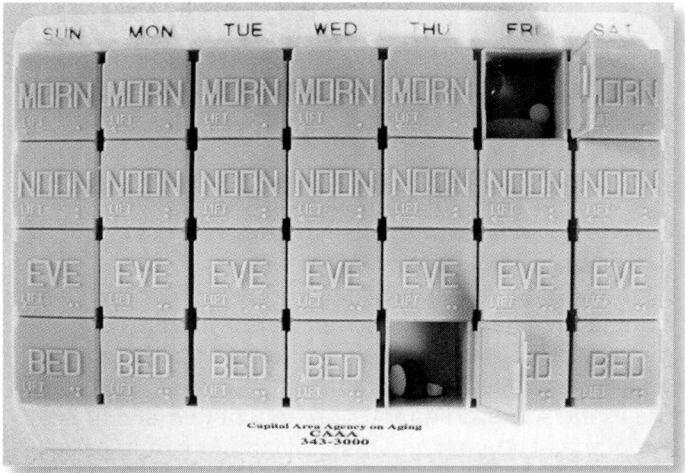

**Figure 38-34.** A pill organizer like this one would be very useful for a patient taking multiple daily medications.

concepts. Also try to find a caregiver or family member who speaks English.

To improve compliance, ask about and discuss the patient's feelings regarding medications and home remedies. Depending on cultural background, the patient may be more likely to use teas, poultices, and other home remedies than prescription or nonprescription drugs. Home remedies may or may not affect the prescribed medication, so the physician should be aware of any practices. These practices should also be included in the patient's chart or medication record. If the remedies do not affect the prescribed medication, tell the patient that it is all right to continue using the home remedies. You may suggest adding the drug to the patient's usual routine to help it work better. Your cultural sensitivity may greatly increase the patient's compliance.

## Charting Medications

Whenever a patient receives some form of treatment, such as medication, a record is kept of that treatment. Special problems or circumstances are also recorded, such as new symptoms, the patient's own statements, and how the patient tolerated the medications or treatment.

Most charting in the physician's office is documented on a progress note. As you learned in Chapter 9, a progress note is a document that is organized in a chronological sequence by date, usually with the most recent date on top. The progress note is important because it serves as a communication tool that is utilized by all allied health-care members who are connected to that patient. The medical record is considered a legal document and is taken as proof that care was administered to the patient. All chart entries must be factual, accurate, complete, current, organized, and confidential. Avoid using words or statements that can be interpreted as your opinion. For example, if a patient gags and spits up cough syrup that you just administered, you would not write that the patient did not like the taste of the medication; you would simply state, "patient experienced difficulty in swallowing medication and expelled medication." Avoid terms like "appear" or "seems," which can lead you to draw assumptions without objective data to support them. Use abbreviations when appropriate because they allow you to say a great deal in a small space. Learn and use the proper medical terms for symptoms and body functions.

Charting is not difficult, but it requires some practice. Review your office's charts to keep consistent with the charting methods used in them. Your own charting will be appropriate if you follow a few simple rules:

- Before you begin, make sure you have the right chart.
- Chart medications directly from the physician order.
- Be specific. Do not write "Gave Demerol for pain in the evening." Instead, write "(Date), Demerol 100 mg given IM in right upper outer quadrant of gluteus maximus for c/o sharp pain, rated 7 on a scale of 10, in left arm, lot number, expiration date, initials."
- Do not leave gaps or skip lines. If an entry does not fill a complete line, draw a straight line to fill the gap. Put your signature or first initial and last name and title at the right side directly after the note.
- If you make an error, do not erase it. Draw a line through the mistake. It should still be visible, so do not black it out. Initial it and then rechart the information correctly.
- Never use ditto marks.
- Write only in blue ink, never in pencil or another color ink.
- Write neatly in longhand or carefully enter into the electronic chart and check your note before submitting it.
- Spelling must be accurate.
- Use abbreviations and correct symbols. Most facilities will have an approved abbreviation list to use as a reference.
- When you are unsure about charting, ask the physician. Here is an example of a charted medication on a progress note:

| Date | Patient Name: Jane Doe | DOB 12/12/63 | Progress Note |
|------|------------------------|--------------|---------------|
| 11/29/08 | PPD, 0.1cc given ID, Rt. Forearm, Lot # 222-01, Exp. Date 12/05, ABC Pharmaceutical Co. Pt to return to office in 48–72 hours for screening results<br>Patient tolerated well-------------------------------------------------------------------------------------------------------------------ST/RMA | | |
| | | | |
| | | | |

## CAUTION *Handle With Care*

### Avoiding Unsafe Polypharmacy

Before administering any drug by any route, you must know every drug, both prescription and nonprescription, that the patient is taking. Many patients, especially elderly ones, visit several doctors. It is entirely possible that each doctor may prescribe one or more drugs without being aware of other drugs the patient is taking. This practice can result in polypharmacy, which means taking several drugs at once. Polypharmacy can be safe, but if the doctor is unaware of the total drug profile, serious drug interactions can result.

When asking patients to identify *all* other drugs they are taking, including OTC drugs, keep in mind that patients may forget to mention all their medicines, OTC drugs, supplements, or herbal remedies to the doctor. Drugs that patients often forget to mention include antacids (such as Tums or Rolaids), birth control pills (some women do not think of these as medication), medicines that are used only as needed, such as medicine for migraine headaches, vitamins, and herbal remedies such as glucosamine and chondroitin.

To help prompt patients about drugs they may have forgotten, ask patients who have seen an orthopedist or cardiologist whether pain medication has been prescribed. Ask women who have seen a gynecologist if they are using a patch or other form of hormone replacement therapy. Ask women of an appropriate age whether there is any chance they are pregnant. Ask a pregnant woman whether she is taking prenatal vitamin and mineral supplements. Ask all patients if they take any other dietary supplement, OTC medication, and/or herbal remedy. If a patient has been referred to any other doctor for any reason, ask whether that doctor prescribed medication.

After determining the total drug profile, you should:

- Update the patient's record. (This should be done with every visit to your facility.)
- Consider possible drug interactions, consulting the *PDR* or other drug reference if needed.
- Inform the doctor of your findings.

## Nonpharmacologic Pain Management

Because of drug interactions, adverse effects, or the risk of dependence, many patients may either prefer not to or should not take drugs to relieve chronic pain. The overuse and abuse of pain medications can be a problem for patients. To meet their needs, some practices now offer nonpharmacologic methods for managing pain, such as biofeedback, guided imagery, and relaxation exercises, in addition to traditional drug therapy. (For other alternative treatments, see Chapter 31.)

Biofeedback can help a patient learn to evoke relaxation, which helps block pain perception. Guided imagery helps patients relax by teaching them to envision themselves in a calm, nurturing, wonderful place. Some cancer patients are taught to envision the cancer cells being eaten by healthy cells. Audiotapes and videotapes are available to help lead patients through these mental exercises. Relaxation exercises involve learning special breathing techniques. Patients also learn how to relax different muscle groups.

## Summary

As a medical assistant, you must be prepared to administer drugs safely and effectively. Before you can do so, however, you must be familiar with the metric, apothecaries', and household systems of measurement. You must also be able to convert measures from one system to another and perform calculations to provide a prescribed dose. For these skills, you can use the ratio or fraction method or a formula.

When preparing to administer a drug, assess the patient for contraindications, and observe the general rules and seven rights of drug administration. Depending on the prescription, the drug may be administered by the oral, buccal, sublingual, intradermal, subcutaneous, intramuscular, nasal, topical, transdermal, vaginal, or rectal routes or as eyedrops or eardrops. If directed, assist the physician or nurse with urethral administration and IV drug injection or infusion.

Patient education is an important responsibility related to drug administration. You may need to instruct patients in the proper use of a prescribed drug. In addition, you may have to teach them to prevent or to recognize and report drug interactions and adverse effects.

Some patients require special consideration when receiving drugs. These include pediatric, pregnant, breastfeeding, and elderly patients as well as patients from different cultures.

Nonpharmacologic methods for managing chronic pain are gaining acceptance. Patients who are interested in learning about such methods should ask the physician for further information.

## CASE STUDY QUESTIONS

Now that you have completed this chapter, review the case study at the beginning of the chapter. Detail what you think the medical assistant should do next and why.

## Discussion Questions

1. What effects may drug interactions produce?
2. Why should you observe the seven rights every time you prepare and administer a drug?
3. Compare subcutaneous and intramuscular drug administration in terms of technique and possible dosage levels.
4. Why is proper needle selection important when administering an injection?

## Critical Thinking Questions

1. A foreign patient is in the office, and the physician has ordered a PPD. You ask the patient if he has had a reaction to a TB screen before, and the patient responds by telling you he has had the BCG vaccination as a child. What is BCG? What should you do? What can happen if you administer the PPD?
2. A patient in her first trimester of pregnancy calls the office saying she has acid indigestion. She says that before her pregnancy, she used to take Tagamet for acid indigestion and wants to know if it is safe to take it now. How can you find this information, and what should you do once you find it?
3. Mr. Lance, age 29, visits the office for his regular IM injection. As you are making a routine assessment, he tells you that the last time the drug was administered, he had a bad reaction to it. What should you do?

## Application Activities

1. Perform the necessary calculations for the following conversions. Use a table of equivalents, if needed.
   a. 350 mL _____ L
   b. 0.17 g _____ mg
   c. 3 tbsp _____ tsp
   d. ½ tsp _____ gtt
   e. 2 fl dr _____ mL
   f. 45 mL _____ ounces
   g. 1 tsp _____ mL
2. Using the ratio or fraction method, calculate the following to provide a prescribed drug dose.
   a. The doctor orders 60 mg of acetaminophen with codeine, but each tablet contains only 15 mg. How many tablets should the patient take?
   b. The doctor orders 300 mg of theophylline anhydrous, but each tablet contains only 100 mg. How many tablets should the patient take?
   c. The doctor orders 5 mg of glyburide, but each tablet contains only 1.25 mg. How many tablets should the patient take?
   d. A 5-year-old child weighs 44 lbs. The physician orders him to receive Zinacef 50 mg/kg/day IM q6h. How many milligrams of medication should the child receive in one dose?
3. Using the basic formula of dose desired/dose on hand × quantity = dose, calculate the following to provide a prescribed drug dose.
   a. The doctor orders 250 mg of a drug. You have 100-mg scored tablets on hand. How many tablets will you give the patient?
   b. An injectable antibiotic is packaged as 100,000 units per mL. The doctor orders 400,000 units. How many packages will you administer parenterally to the patient?
   c. The physician orders Ceclor 0.375 g PO bid. You have on hand Ceclor Oral suspension 187 mg per 5 mL.

**d.** The physician wants you to give the patient an IM injection of 100 mcg of Cyanocobalamin. You have on hand the medication pictured below. How many mL of medication would you inject?

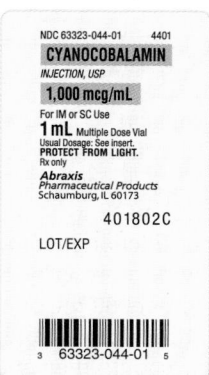

**e.** You need to give Engerix-B 10 mcg IM now. You have on hand the medication pictured below. How much medication would you administer?

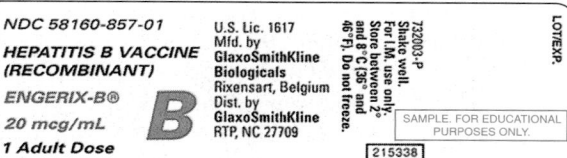

### Virtual Fieldtrip

*Visit the McGraw-Hill Higher Education Medical Assisting website at www.mhhe.com/medicalassisting3 to complete the following activities:*

1. Drug-drug and food-drug interactions can be a serious concern for some patients and are many times overlooked or misunderstood. Take a trip to the Food and Drug Administration Internet site and search for drug-drug interactions or drug-food interactions. Identify at least five interactions of concern. Create a table or chart of your findings to use while practicing as a clinical medical assistant.

2. Travel the U.S. Pharmacopeia and the Institute of Safe Medication Practice websites and research some common medication errors. Go to the USP Medication Errors Reporting Program and download the error reporting form. Using what you have learned about medication errors, complete the form you downloaded using information about a possible medication error that could occur. Be prepared to discuss your medication error report.

Open the CD and complete this chapter's practice activities, play the games, listen to the key terms, and test yourself with the interactive review. Email, print, and/or save your results to document your proficiency.

# Electrocardiography and Pulmonary Function Testing

## MEDICAL ASSISTING COMPETENCIES

*In preparation for the certification examination, you should know the following areas of competence:*

| COMPETENCY | CMA | RMA |
|---|---|---|
| **Clinical** | | |
| Apply principles of aseptic techniques and infection control, including hand washing | X | X |
| Dispose of biohazardous materials | X | X |
| Practice Standard Precautions | X | X |
| Perform electrocardiography | X | X |
| Perform respiratory testing | X | X |
| **General/Legal/Professional** | | |
| Recognize and respond to verbal and nonverbal communications by being attentive and adapting communication to the recipient's level of understanding | X | X |
| Be aware of and perform within legal and ethical boundaries | X | X |
| Determine the needs for documentation and reporting, and document accurately and appropriately | X | X |

## KEY TERMS

calibration syringe
cardiac cycle
deflection
depolarization
electrocardiogram (ECG)
electrocardiograph
electrocardiography
electrode
forced vital capacity (FVC)
Holter monitor
lead
polarity
pulmonary function test
sleep apnea
spirometer
spirometry
stylus

## CHAPTER OUTLINE

- The Medical Assistant's Role in Electrocardiography and Pulmonary Function Testing
- Anatomy and Physiology of the Heart
- The Conduction System of the Heart
- The Electrocardiograph
- Preparing to Administer an ECG
- Applying the Electrodes and the Connecting Wires
- Operating the Electrocardiograph
- Troubleshooting: Artifacts and Other Problems
- Completing the Procedure
- Interpreting the ECG
- Exercise Electrocardiography (Stress Testing)
- Ambulatory Electrocardiography (Holter Monitoring)
- Anatomy and Physiology of the Respiratory System
- Pulmonary Function Testing
- Spirometry
- Performing Spirometry
- Peak Expiratory Flow Rate (PEFR)
- Pulse Oximetry

## LEARNING OUTCOMES

After completing Chapter 39, you will be able to:

**39.1** Describe the anatomy and physiology of the heart.

**39.2** Explain the conduction system of the heart.

**39.3** Describe the basic patterns of an electrocardiogram (ECG).

**39.4** Identify the components of an electrocardiograph and what each does.

**39.5** Explain how to position the limb and precordial electrodes correctly.

**39.6** Describe in detail how to obtain an ECG.

**39.7** Identify the various types of artifacts and potential equipment problems and how to correct them.

**39.8** Discuss how the ECG is interpreted

**39.9** Identify common arrhythmias.

**39.10** Define exercise electrocardiography.

**39.11** Explain the procedure of Holter monitoring.

**39.12** Describe forced vital capacity.

**39.13** Describe the procedure of performing spirometry.

**39.14** Describe the procedure for obtaining peak expiratory flow rate.

**39.15** Describe the procedure for performing pulse oximetry testing.

## Introduction

It is not uncommon for patients to have cardiovascular or respiratory problems when they consult physicians. As a medical assistant, you may be responsible for performing screening and/or diagnostic testing in the physician's office. To correctly perform testing on the cardiac or respiratory system, you need to review the anatomy and physiology of the heart and the respiratory system. This chapter introduces you to the electrocardiograph instrument and how to administer an electrocardiogram. You will also learn how to apply electrocardiograph electrodes and wires, operate the instrument, and troubleshoot problems that can occur while recording the heart's electrical activity. Because many physicians perform more complex cardiac diagnostic testing, you will also learn about Holter monitors and stress testing. Pulmonary function testing is a procedure performed in physician's offices, and this chapter introduces you to the basics of performing respiratory procedures, such as spirometry, peak flow, and pulse oximetry.

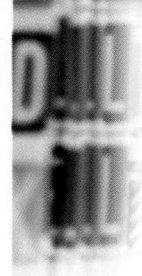

## CASE STUDY

A 57-year-old woman has been having chest pain, discomfort in the chest, and a slight shortness of breath since the previous morning. She chose to come to the office where you are employed rather than the emergency room because she didn't think her symptoms were too severe. The physician orders an ECG and spirometry after reviewing the patient's history. The ECG reveals nonspecific wave changes, and the spirometry shows that the FVC is slightly decreased. The physician then orders a Holter monitor to be placed on the patient and requests that she be scheduled for an exercise electrocardiography.

As you read this chapter, consider the following questions:

1. What does the abbreviation ECG stand for? What is the diagnostic value of the ECG?
2. What is another name for a spirometry? What does FVC designate?
3. Why were the Holter monitor and stress tests ordered for this patient?

## The Medical Assistant's Role in Electrocardiography and Pulmonary Function Testing

Electrocardiography and pulmonary function testing are two procedures you may be required to perform in a medical office. **Electrocardiography** is the process by which a graphic pattern is created from the electrical impulses generated within the heart as it pumps. It is often performed to evaluate symptoms of heart disease, to detect abnormal heart rhythms, to evaluate a patient's progress after a heart attack, or to check the effectiveness or side effects of certain medications. Electrocardiography is sometimes performed as part of a general examination.

**Pulmonary function tests** (PFTs) measure and evaluate a patient's lung capacity and volume. Such tests are commonly performed when a person suffers from shortness of breath, but they may also be performed as part of a general examination. Pulmonary function tests can help detect and diagnose pulmonary problems. They are also used to monitor certain respiratory disorders and to evaluate the effectiveness of treatment.

# Anatomy and Physiology of the Heart

A description of the anatomy and physiology of the heart will help you better understand electrocardiography. It will also help you make sense of the electrical activity that electrocardiography records.

## Anatomy of the Heart

The heart is a muscular pump that circulates blood throughout the body, carrying oxygen and nutrients to the tissues and removing waste products. The pumping action begins in the muscle tissue of the heart, called the myocardium.

The heart is actually a double pump. The right side of the heart receives blood from the body by way of the superior vena cava and the inferior vena cava. From there, the pulmonary arteries deliver blood to the lungs, where the blood exchanges carbon dioxide for oxygen. Oxygenated blood flows into the left side of the heart through the pulmonary veins. Once in the heart, blood is pumped into the aorta, which pumps oxygenated blood to all parts of the body.

The heart has four sections, or chambers: two upper receiving chambers, the atria (singular, atrium), and two lower pumping chambers, the ventricles (Figure 39-1). Valves between each atrium and ventricle prevent blood from regurgitating (backing up) into the atrium while the ventricle contracts. Similar valves between the ventricles and the arteries into which they pump (the aorta and the pulmonary arteries) prevent blood from regurgitating into the ventricles when they relax. A partition, the septum, divides the heart into right and left sides.

## Physiology of the Heart

The heart is divided into separate chambers that work as a single unit. Contraction of the atria, followed by contraction of the ventricles, moves the blood. This contraction phase is called systole. Systole is followed by a relaxation phase, called diastole. When you take someone's blood pressure, you are measuring the pressure during the contraction (systolic) and relaxation (diastolic) phases. This sequence of contraction and relaxation makes up a complete heartbeat,

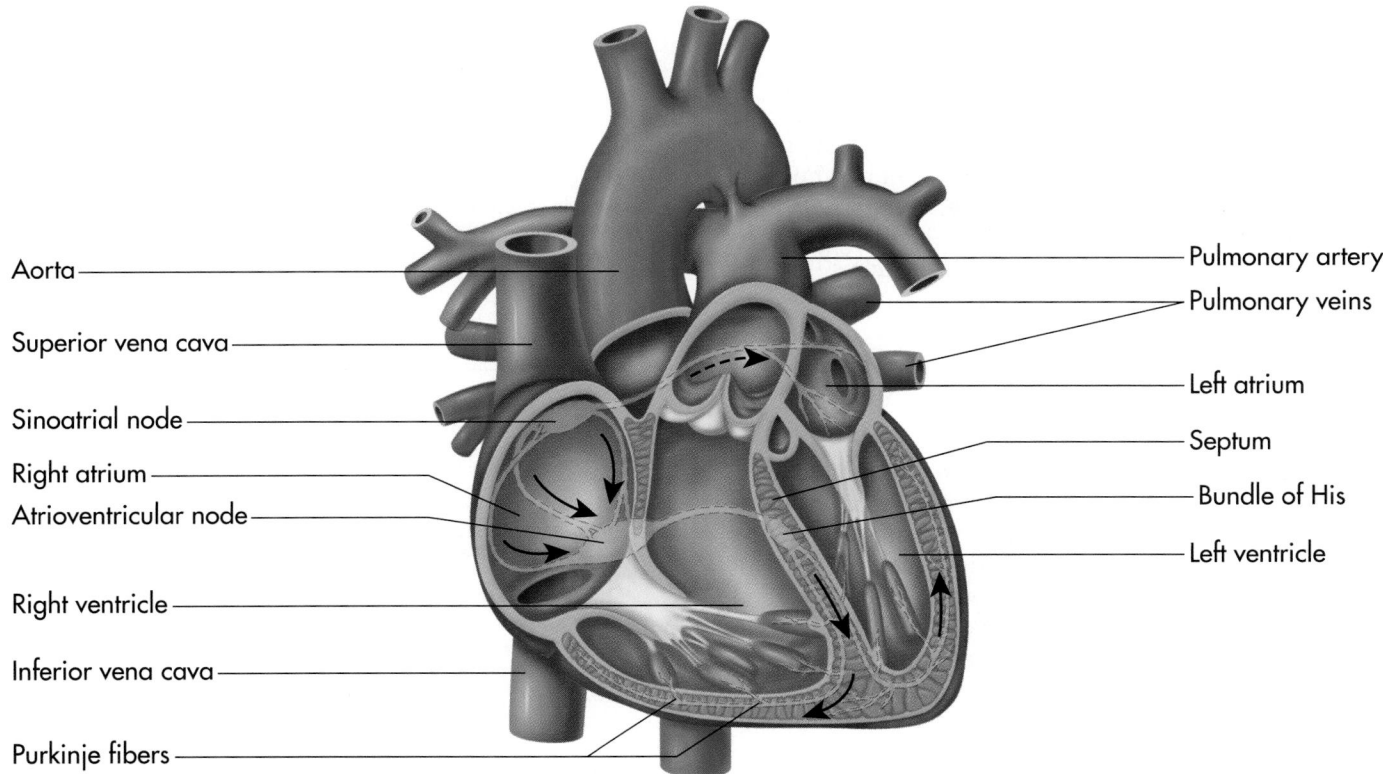

**Figure 39-1.** Electrical impulses control the cardiac conduction system. Each impulse begins in the sinoatrial node, progresses to the atrioventricular node, and then travels through the bundle of His, the right and left bundle branches, and the Purkinje fibers.

known as the **cardiac cycle.** Each cycle lasts an average of 0.8 second.

All the fibers in the cardiac muscle are interconnected and act as one muscle. Consequently, when one fiber is stimulated to contract, the entire group of fibers contracts. This property plays an important role in the conduction system of the heart.

# The Conduction System of the Heart

The cardiac cycle is regulated by specialized tissues in the heart wall, shown in Figure 39-1, that transmit electrical impulses. These electrical impulses cause the heart muscle to contract and relax.

Transmission of electrical impulses in the heart begins in the sinoatrial (SA) node, also called the sinus node or the pacemaker of the heart. The SA node is a small bundle of heart muscle tissue in the superior wall of the right atrium that specializes in producing electrical impulses. The SA node sets the rhythm of the heart's contractions.

When the electrical impulse for muscle contraction is generated, it travels throughout the muscle of each atrium, causing atrial contraction. The impulse then travels to the atrioventricular (AV) node, another mass of specialized conducting cells, similar to those of the SA node. The AV node is located at the bottom of the right atrium, near the junction of the ventricles (the septum), where transmission of the impulse is slightly delayed. This delay gives the atria time to completely contract and fill the ventricles with blood.

The atrioventricular node then passes the impulse to the bundle of His, located in the septum between the ventricles. The bundle of His acts as a relay station, sending the impulse through a series of bundle branches to a network of cardiac conducting muscle fibers. These specialized muscle fibers, called Purkinje fibers, are located in the ventricle walls. When the impulse reaches the Purkinje fibers, the ventricles contract.

## Conduction and Electrocardiography

Electrocardiography records the transmission, magnitude, and duration of the various electrical impulses of the heart. Before you can understand how electrocardiography works, you must understand **polarity,** the condition of having two separate poles, one of which is positive and the other negative. A resting cardiac cell is polarized; that is, there is a negative charge inside and a positive charge outside. When the cardiac cell loses its polarity (a natural occurrence), depolarization occurs. **Depolarization** is the electrical impulse that initiates a chain reaction resulting in contraction. This wave of depolarization flows from the SA node to the ventricles and can be detected by **electrodes,** or electrical impulse sensors, that are placed on specific areas on the surface of the body. During electro-cardiography, electrodes detect and record the electrical activity of the heart, including disturbances or disruptions in its rhythm.

Depolarization is always followed by a period of electrical recovery called repolarization, when polarity is restored. Following repolarization, the heart returns to a resting, polarized state. The electrical cycle is then repeated, leading to another cardiac cycle.

# The Basic Pattern of the Electrocardiogram

The waves of electrical impulses responsible for the cardiac cycle produce a series of waves and lines on an **electrocardiogram** (abbreviated **ECG** or EKG), which is the tracing made by an **electrocardiograph,** an instrument that measures and displays these impulses (Figure 39-2). These peaks and valleys, called waves or **deflections,** are labeled with the letters P, Q, R, S, T, and U. Each letter represents a specific part of the pattern, as explained in Table 39-1. The recognition of abnormalities in the size of the waves or the various time intervals can aid in the diagnosis of certain types of heart problems.

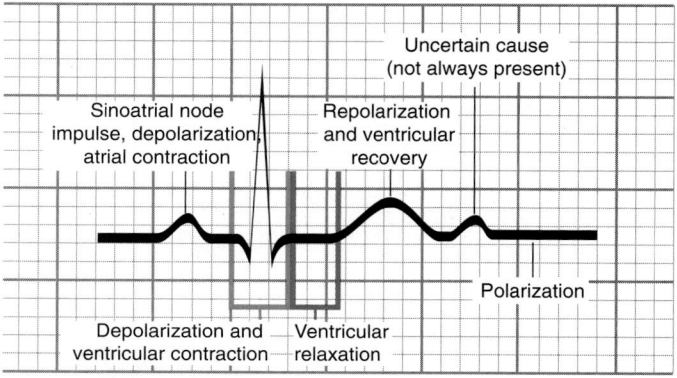

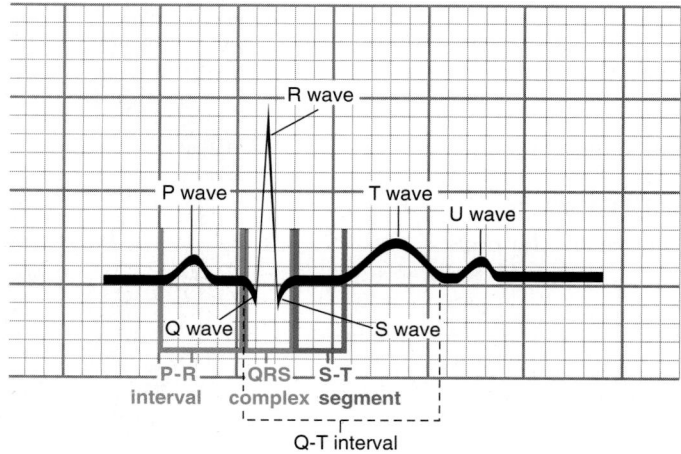

**Figure 39-2.** This ECG tracing shows the pattern of one cardiac cycle in a normal heart. These specific electrical impulses (top) represent the cycle of cardiac contraction and relaxation. The waves and lines (bottom) represent specific parts of the pattern.

## TABLE 39-1    Parts of the ECG

| Name | Appearance | Represents |
|------|-----------|-----------|
| P wave | Small upward curve | Sinoatrial node impulse, wave of depolarization through atria, and resultant contraction |
| QRS complex | Includes Q, R, and S waves | Contraction (following depolarization) of ventricles; QRS complex is larger than P wave because ventricles are larger than atria |
| Q wave | Downward deflection | Impulse traveling down septum toward Purkinje fibers |
| R wave | Large upward spike | Impulse going through left ventricle |
| S wave | Downward deflection | Impulse going through both ventricles |
| T wave | Upward curve | Recovery (repolarization) of ventricles; repolarization of atria is not obvious because it occurs while ventricles are contracting and producing QRS complex |
| U wave | Small upward curve sometimes found after T wave | May be seen in normal individuals, in patients who experience slow recovery of Purkinje fibers, or in patients who have low potassium levels or other metabolic disturbances |
| P–R interval | Includes P wave and straight line connecting it to QRS complex | Time it takes for electrical impulse to travel from SA node to AV node |
| Q–T interval | Includes QRS complex, S–T segment, and T wave | Time it takes for ventricles to contract and recover, or repolarize |
| S–T segment | Connects end of QRS complex with beginning of T wave | Time between contraction of ventricles and recovery |

# The Electrocardiograph

Each type of electrocardiograph works in the same way. The electrical impulses produced by the heart can be detected through the skin; these impulses are measured, amplified, and recorded on the ECG. Detection begins with electrodes that conduct and transmit the electrical impulses to the electrocardiograph through insulated wires. An amplifier increases the signal, making the heartbeat visible. The **stylus,** a pen-like instrument, records this movement on the ECG paper. The impulses received through various combinations of electrodes constitute different **leads,** or views of the electrical activity of the heart, that are recorded on the ECG.

## Types of Electrocardiographs

Several different types of electrocardiographs are in use today. Two types are shown in Figure 39-3. The standard machine is a 12-lead electrocardiograph, which records the electrical activity of the heart simultaneously from 12 different views. A single-channel electrocardiograph records the electrical activity of one lead, and consequently, one view of the heart's electrical activity at a time. The record is printed on a long, thin strip of ECG paper. The most common single-channel units allow you to attach all electrodes at the same time and obtain a manual or automatic printout of individual leads. This is sometimes referred to as a rhythm strip The multichannel units record more than one lead at a time. These machines use wider paper and more than one stylus to record the leads. Some models of multichannel ECGs provide a diagnosis or an interpretation of the electrocardiogram. The interpretive option can be turned on or off. Even though the interpretive electrocardiograph can provide a diagnosis, the physician will review the tracing and confirm the diagnosis before treatment is ordered. Larger medical facilities may use an electronic health records (EHR) software program so that electrocardiograms can be inserted into the patient medical record and transmitted to specialists to interpret. Electrocardiograms can be transmitted by fax or telephone, depending on the software and model of the electrocardiograph.

## Electrodes and Electrolyte Products

Electrodes are attached to the patient's skin during electrocardiography. Disposable electrodes (Figure 39-4) are the most widely used.

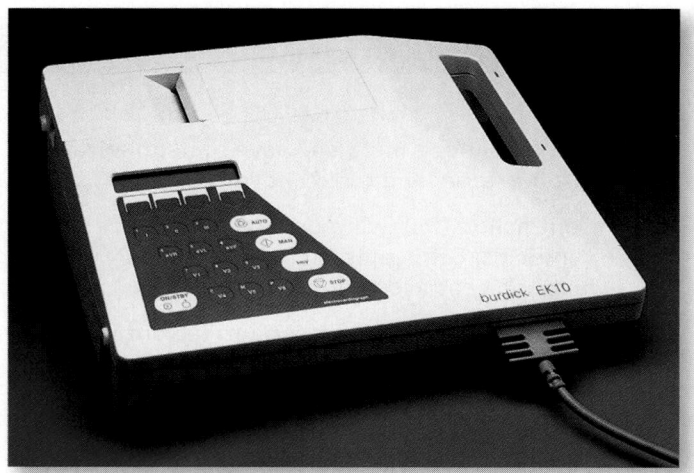
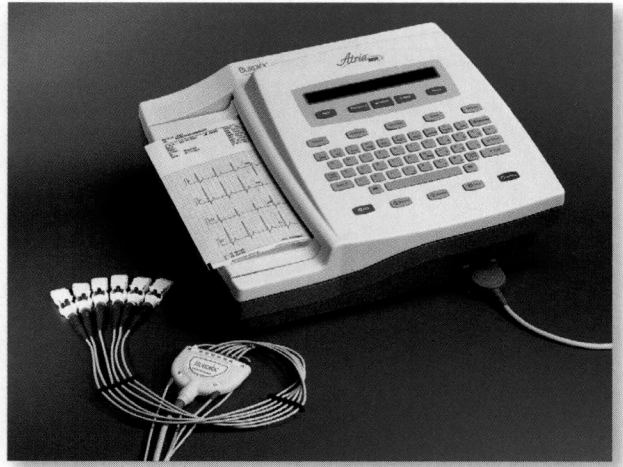

**Figure 39-3.** Single-channel (left) and multichannel (right) electrocardiographs are used to obtain an ECG.

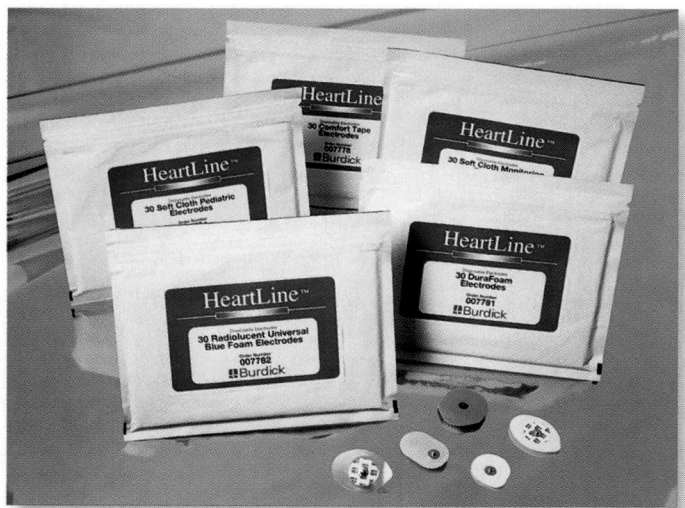

**Figure 39-4.** Disposable electrodes are available in several varieties.

The skin does not conduct electricity well. Consequently, an electrolyte (a substance that enhances transmission of electric current) is needed with each electrode. Disposable electrodes come with an electrolyte preparation in place.

When performing routine electrocardiography, you place electrodes on ten areas of the body: one each on the right arm (RA), left arm (LA), right leg (RL), and left leg (LL) and six on specific locations on the chest wall. The right leg is designated as the ground. Evaluating different leads, that is, the electrical activity measured through various combinations of electrodes, enables the physician to pinpoint the origin of certain problems.

## Leads

Each lead provides an image of the electrical activity of the heart from a different angle. Together, the images give the doctor a full picture of electrical activity moving up and down, left and right, and forward and backward through

the heart. Monitoring the electrodes on the arms and legs in two different ways produces six leads that record electrical impulses that move up and down and left and right. The electrodes that are placed on the chest provide six more leads, showing electrical activity moving forward and backward (from the front of the body toward the back and vice versa).

Each lead is given a specific designation and code. The 12 leads are usually marked automatically on the ECG.

**Limb Leads.** Of the six leads that directly monitor electrodes on the arms and legs, three are standard leads and three are augmented leads. The standard leads each monitor two limb electrodes, recording electrical activity between them. These leads are also called bipolar leads, because they monitor two electrodes. The augmented leads monitor one limb electrode and a point midway between two other limb electrodes, recording electrical activity between the monitored electrode and the midway point. Because they directly monitor only one electrode, augmented leads are also called unipolar leads. The electrical activity recorded by these leads is very slight, requiring the machine to augment (amplify) the tracings to produce readable waves and lines on the ECG paper. The standard limb leads appear on the ECG as I, II, III and the augmented limb leads appear as AVF (augmented voltage-foot), AVR (augmented voltage-right), and AVL (augmented voltage-left).

**Precordial Leads.** The six precordial, or chest, leads are unipolar leads. The electrodes are placed across the chest in a precise specific pattern (Figure 39-5). Each precordial lead monitors one electrode and a point within the heart. The precordial leads are each designated by a letter and a number: $V_1$ through $V_6$. The designations for the 12 leads of a routine ECG are shown in Table 39-2. The table also indicates which electrodes and points are monitored by each lead. A common system of marking codes completes the information in the table. Other coding systems are in use; be sure to follow office policy or the doctor's preference when you code an ECG.

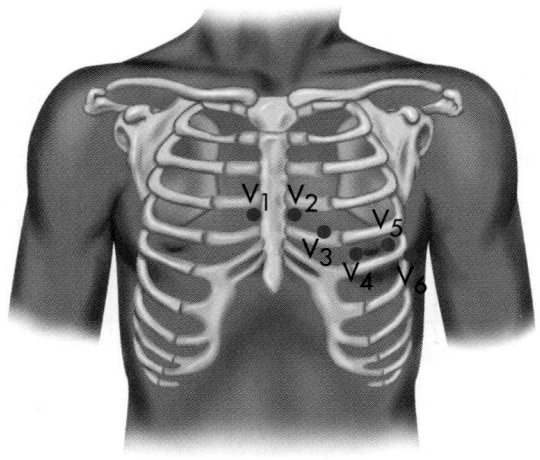

V$_1$ Fourth intercostal space (between the ribs), to the right of the sternum (breastbone)

V$_2$ Fourth intercostal space, to the left of the sternum

V$_4$ Fifth intercostal space, on the left midclavicular line

V$_3$ Fifth intercostal space, midway between V$_2$ and V$_4$

V$_6$ Fifth intercostal space, on the left midaxillary line

V$_5$ Fifth intercostal space, midway between V$_4$ and V$_6$

**Figure 39-5.** Six precordial electrodes are arranged in specific positions on the chest. Notice that electrode V$_4$ must be positioned before V$_3$ and V$_6$ before V$_5$.

## ECG Paper

ECG paper is provided in a long, continuous roll or pad. If the paper is designed for use with a single-channel electrocardiograph, it is just wide enough for a single trace.

Other ECG papers can accommodate several traces at once; these papers are used with multichannel electrocardiography. ECG paper consists of two layers and is both heat- and pressure-sensitive. The heated stylus on the electrocardiograph serves as a "pen" that records the ECG pattern on the paper. Handle the paper carefully to reduce the likelihood of making errant marks that might affect the tracing.

ECG paper (Figure 39-6) is marked with light and dark lines or with dots and lines. The pattern is standardized to permit uniform interpretation by any physician. Each small square, or square area delineated by dots, measures 1 mm by 1 mm. Each large square measures 5 mm by 5 mm.

The vertical, or short, axis of the paper records the voltage, or strength of the impulse; the horizontal axis measures time. Normally the paper moves through the machine at a speed of 25 mm per second. This means that the distance across 1 small square represents 0.04 second. The distance across 1 large square represents 0.2 second. The distance across 5 large squares represents 1.0 second. In 1 minute (60 seconds), the paper advances 300 large squares, or 1500 mm (150 cm).

Each electrocardiograph is standardized before use so that one small square represents 0.1 millivolt (mV). One large square represents 0.5 mV, and two large squares represent 1.0 mV.

## Electrocardiograph Controls

The location of certain knobs and buttons on an electrocardiograph may vary from model to model. Certain features, however, are common to most machines. These include the standardization control, speed selector, sensitivity

| TABLE 39-2 ECG Lead Designations and Marking Codes | | |
|---|---|---|
| **Lead** | **Electrodes and Points Monitored** | **Marking Codes** |
| **Standard limb** | | |
| I | RA and LA | • |
| II | RA and LL | •• |
| III | LA and LL | ••• |
| **Augmented limb** | | |
| aVR | RA and (LA-LL) | - |
| aVL | LA and (RA-LL) | -- |
| aVF | LL and (RA-LA) | --- |
| **Precordial** | | |
| V$_1$ | V$_1$ and (LA-RA-LL)* | -• |
| V$_2$ | V$_2$ and (LA-RA-LL)* | -•• |
| V$_3$ | V$_3$ and (LA-RA-LL)* | -••• |
| V$_4$ | V$_4$ and (LA-RA-LL)* | -•••• |
| V$_5$ | V$_5$ and (LA-RA-LL)* | -••••• |
| V$_6$ | V$_6$ and (LA-RA-LL)* | -•••••• |

*The point within the heart is identified by averaging the readings from the electrodes.

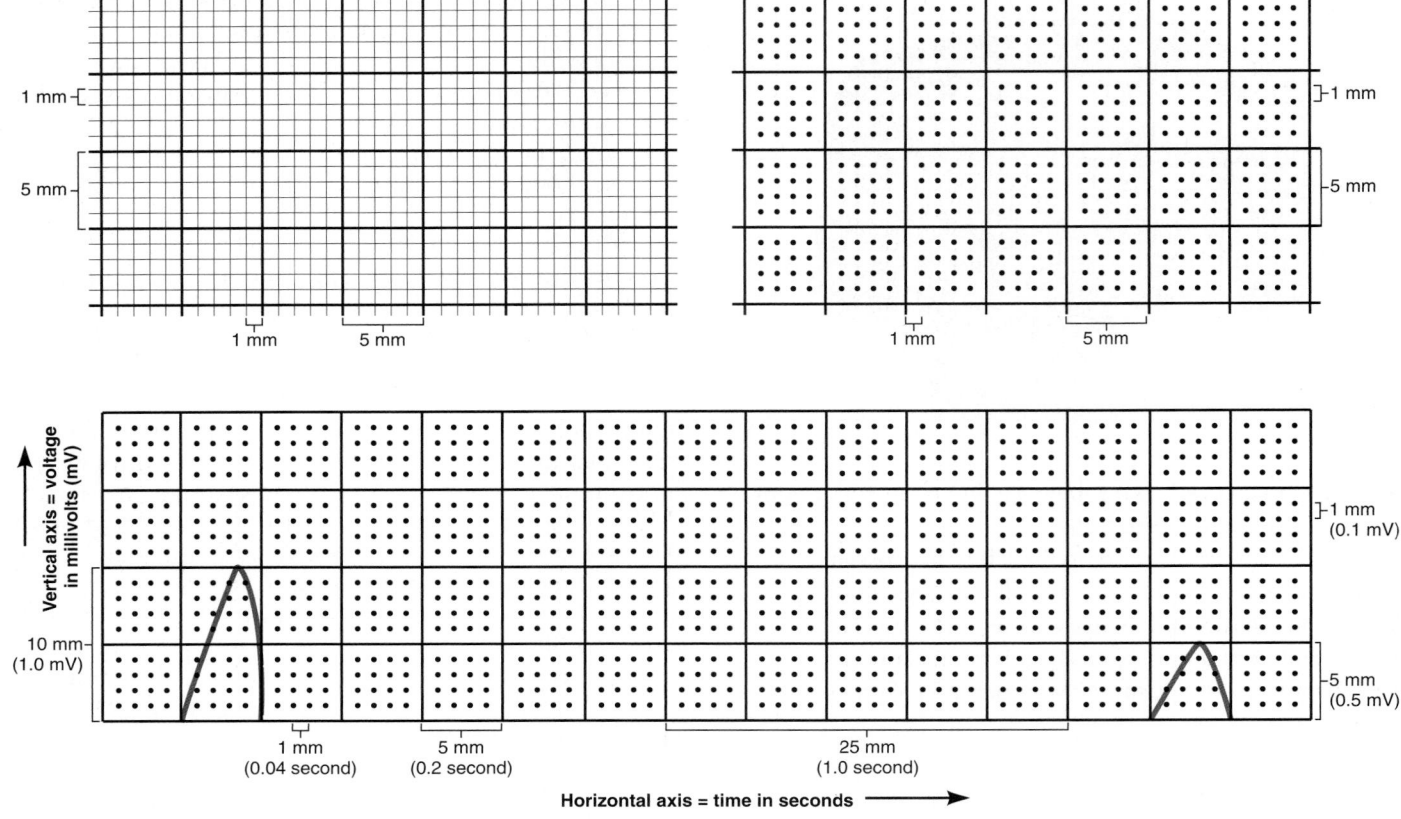

**Figure 39-6.** The pattern and spacing of lines or lines and dots on ECG paper are standardized and represent specific units of voltage and time.

control, lead selector, centering control, stylus temperature control, marker control, and on/off switch.

**Standardization Control.** Before you obtain an ECG, you must correctly standardize the machine. The standardization control uses a 1-mV impulse to produce a standardization mark on the ECG paper. When you press the standardization control, the stylus should move up ten small squares, or 10 mm (1 cm) and remain there for 0.08 second (two small squares, or 2 mm). If it does not, the instrument must be adjusted before you use it.

**Speed Selector.** The paper is normally set to run at 25 mm per second for adults. When you run an ECG on infants and children or on adults with a rapid heartbeat, the deflections may appear too close together. In these cases you may need to adjust the speed to 50 mm per second to separate the peaks and create a tracing that is easier to read. If you must set the speed at 50 mm per second, note it on the strip. Otherwise, a speed of 25 mm per second is assumed. In any case do not change the speed selection unless the doctor directs you to do so.

**Sensitivity Control.** The sensitivity control adjusts the height of the standardization mark and the tracing. It is normally set on 1. When the height of an ECG tracing is too high to fit completely on the paper, however, adjust this control to ½ to reduce the size of

both the standardization mark and the tracing by one-half. For tracings that have very low peaks, set this control on 2 to double the standardization mark and the height of the tracing. Note this change on the ECG.

**Lead Selector.** Most electrocardiographs have a setting that enables a standard 12-lead tracing to run automatically. All machines, however, have a lead selector that allows you to run each lead individually, in case you need to repeat a strip containing artifacts (erroneous marks or defects).

**Centering Control.** The centering control allows you to adjust the position of the stylus, which must be centered on the paper. (Centering the stylus simplifies the process of measuring wave heights for the person who interprets the ECG.)

**Stylus Temperature Control.** Another control allows you to adjust the temperature of the stylus. A higher temperature results in a heavier line, whereas a lower temperature results in a lighter, thinner line. The line should be clear without being so dark that it bleeds or smears on the ECG paper.

**Marker Control.** Most older machines have a marker control that allows you to place marking codes (Table 39-2) on the ECG paper to identify the lead during each run. Current machines do this automatically.

**On/Off Switch.** The on/off switch turns the machine on and off. Most machines have an indicator light that signals when the power is on.

# Preparing to Administer an ECG

You must obtain a good-quality tracing when performing electrocardiography. To do so, you must be able to recognize an artifact or a generally defective ECG tracing when you see one. Proper technique is also essential to help you obtain the best-quality tracing. The following sections guide you through the process. The steps in obtaining a standard 12-lead ECG using a single-channel electrocardiograph are listed in Procedure 39-1.

# Preparing the Room and Equipment

Be sure the room and equipment are properly set up before you begin to administer an electrocardiogram. The accuracy of an ECG can sometimes be affected by electric currents emitted from nearby machines. Although some electrocardiographs have filters to minimize outside electrical interference, it is always a good idea to perform electrocardiography in a room where all other electrical equipment is turned off. This equipment includes air conditioners, refrigerators, and fans as well as laboratory and diagnostic equipment.

## PROCEDURE 39.1

## Obtaining an ECG

**Procedure Goal:** To obtain a graphic representation of the electrical activity of a patient's heart

**OSHA Guidelines**

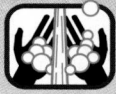 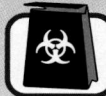 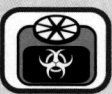 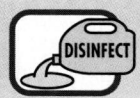 

**Materials:** Electrocardiograph, ECG paper, electrodes, electrolyte preparation, wires, patient gown, drape, blanket, pillows, gauze pads, alcohol, moist towel, scissors for trimming hair (if needed)

**Method:**

1. Turn on the electrocardiograph and, if necessary, allow the stylus to heat up.
2. Identify the patient, introduce yourself, and explain the procedure.
3. Wash your hands.
4. Ask the patient to disrobe from the waist up and remove jewelry, socks or stockings, bra and shoes. If the electrodes will be placed on the patient's legs, have the patient roll up his or her pant legs. Sometimes the electrodes are placed on the sides of the lower abdomen—check the manufacturer's instructions. Provide a gown if the patient is female, and instruct her to wear the gown with the opening in front.

*Rationale*

Making sure the patient knows exactly what clothing to remove and the correct way to put on the gown will make the process more efficient.

5. Assist the patient onto the table and into a supine position. Cover the patient with a drape (and a blanket if the room is cool). If the patient experiences difficulty breathing or cannot tolerate lying flat, use a Fowler's or semi-Fowler's position, adjusting with pillows under the head and knees for comfort if needed.
6. Tell the patient to rest quietly and breathe normally. Explain the importance of lying still to prevent false readings.
7. Wash the patient's skin, using gauze pads moistened with alcohol. Then rub it vigorously with dry gauze pads to promote better contact of the electrodes.

*Rationale*

If a patient has applied lotion in the areas where electrodes are placed, it may cause conduction problems.

8. If the patient's leg or chest hair is dense, use a small pair of scissors to closely trim the hair where you will attach the electrode.
9. Apply electrodes to fleshy portions of the limbs, making sure that the electrodes on one arm and leg are placed similarly to those on the other arm and leg (Figure 39-7). Attach electrodes to areas that are not bony or muscular. The arm lead tabs on the electrode point downward and the electrode tabs for the leg leads point upward. Peel off the backings of the disposable electrodes and press them into place.

*continued* ⟶

## Obtaining an ECG *(concluded)*

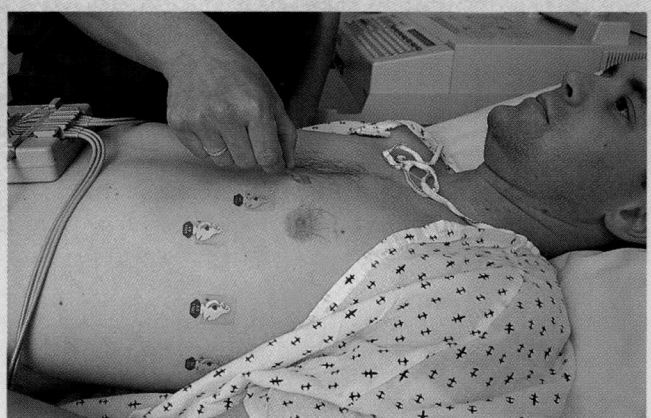

**Figure 39-7.** Place electrodes at the specified locations on the chest, arms, and legs.

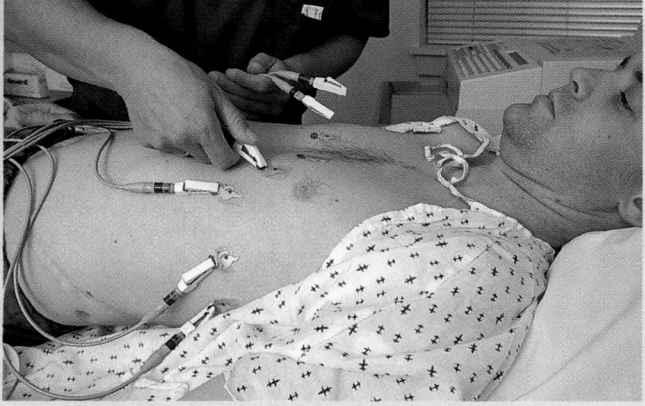

**Figure 39-8.** Attach wires and cables, draping wires over the patient to avoid tension that canresult in artifacts.

### Rationale

Using the correct tab position will reduce tension on the limb wires. Artifacts can occur when electrodes are placed on bones and muscles.

10. Apply the precordial electrodes at specified locations on the chest. Precordial electrode tabs point downward.

11. Attach wires and cables, making sure all wire tips follow the patient's body contours.

12. Check all electrodes and wires for proper placement and connection; drape wires over the patient to avoid creating tension on the electrodes that could result in artifacts (Figure 39-8).

13. Enter the patient data into the electrocardiograph. Press the on, run, or record button. Standardize the machine, if necessary, by following these steps:

    a. Set the paper speed to 25 mm per second or as instructed.

    b. Set the sensitivity setting to 1 or as instructed.

    c. Turn the lead selector to standardization mode.

    d. Adjust the stylus so the baseline is centered.

    e. Press the standardization button. The stylus should move upward above the baseline 10 mm (two large squares).

14. Run the ECG.

    a. If the machine has an automatic feature, set the lead selector to automatic.

    b. For manual tracings, turn the lead selector to standby mode. Select the first lead (I), and record the tracing. Switch the machine to standby, and then repeat the procedure for all 12 leads.

15. Check tracings for artifacts.

16. Correct problems and repeat any tracings that are not clear.

17. Disconnect the patient from the machine.

18. Remove the tracing from the machine, and label it with the patient's name, the date, and your initials.

19. Disconnect the wires from the electrodes, and remove the electrodes from the patient.

20. Clean the patient's skin with a moist towel.

21. Assist the patient into a sitting position.

22. Allow a moment for rest, and then assist the patient from the table.

### Rationale

Some patients may experience postural hypotension after lying and may feel dizzy.

23. Assist the patient in dressing if necessary, or allow the patient privacy to dress.

24. Wash your hands.

25. Record the procedure in the patient's chart.

26. Properly dispose of used materials and disposable electrodes.

27. Clean and disinfect the equipment and the room according to OSHA guidelines.

## CAUTION *Handle With Care*

### Allaying Patient Anxiety About Having Electrocardiography

The most common reason for a patient's anxiety is not knowing what to expect from electrocardiography. The patient may be fearful of being hooked up to an electrical device and worried about receiving an electric shock.

Calmly and simply explain the procedure in detail, both before you begin and while you prepare the patient for the test. Assure her that it is a safe procedure that will last about 10 to 15 minutes. Explain that the machine measures the electrical activity of the heart and that no outside electricity will pass through the body. It is also helpful to explain why the doctor has ordered the procedure, without giving any diagnosis or prognosis.

Above all, talk to and listen to the patient. Encourage her to express her concerns and ask questions. Respond to the patient's concerns and questions calmly, fully, and respectfully.

#### Ensuring Patient Comfort

Ensuring that the patient is comfortable will help her feel more at ease. It will also result in less body movement and a more accurate ECG.

Each patient is an individual. You will need to find out from the patient what is and is not comfortable for her. First make sure the room temperature is right for the patient. If she says the room feels too cool, provide an extra blanket to prevent chills. Being chilly can make a patient shiver and increase her anxiety. Shivering can cause muscle tremor artifacts. Next ensure that the patient is comfortable on the examining table. Placing a small pillow under the head can help. Make sure, however, that the pillow does not touch the shoulders or raise them off the table. For most patients, placing a pillow under the knees helps relax the abdomen and lower extremities and prevents lower-back pain. Try this arrangement and let the patient decide whether it contributes to or detracts from her comfort. If the patient has trouble breathing, shift her into a Fowler's or semi-Fowler's position. Ask the patient which position is more comfortable, and use the position she chooses. If the patient chooses a position other than supine, be sure to note the position in her chart.

---

The room should be in a quiet, private location, protected from interruptions. Because the patient must partially disrobe, adjust the room temperature to a comfortable level.

The examining table should be sturdy and comfortable. Make sure the table paper is fresh and the table is disinfected after each patient's use.

Before using the electrocardiograph, check the date of its last inspection. Each machine should be periodically inspected and certified safe to use for a specific period of time. Using a machine only within this time period helps ensure your safety and that of the patient. Be sure to turn the machine on ahead of time to allow the stylus to warm up. It is good practice to check the ECG paper and ECG electrodes, restocking them if necessary. Verifying that you have adequate supplies prior to preparing the patient will save time for you and the physician.

### Preparing the Patient

Introduce yourself to the patient, explain the procedure, and answer any questions the patient has. Follow the steps described in Procedure 39-1 as you prepare the patient for electrocardiography. Keep in mind that some patients are apprehensive about undergoing electrocardiography. Anxiety often stems from the fear of receiving an electric shock from the machine. See the Caution: Handle

With Care section for ways to allay a patient's anxiety about having an ECG.

## Applying the Electrodes and the Connecting Wires

You must prepare the patient's skin before applying the electrodes. Proper contact between an electrode and the skin allows for proper conduction of the impulses. Follow the steps described in Procedure 39-1 as you prepare the patient's skin. Depending on your office policy, you may be required to trim chest or leg hair if it is dense to ensure proper contact.

### Electrodes

Disposable electrodes are the most commonly used type of electrode. Disposable electrodes come with the electrolyte product already applied. Simply remove the adhesive backing and press the electrode firmly into place on the skin. This type of electrode has largely replaced the metal plate and suction bulb electrodes from previous models. Because the electrolyte gel is prepackaged and measured, artifacts occurring from the placement of unequal amounts of electrolyte have been minimized.

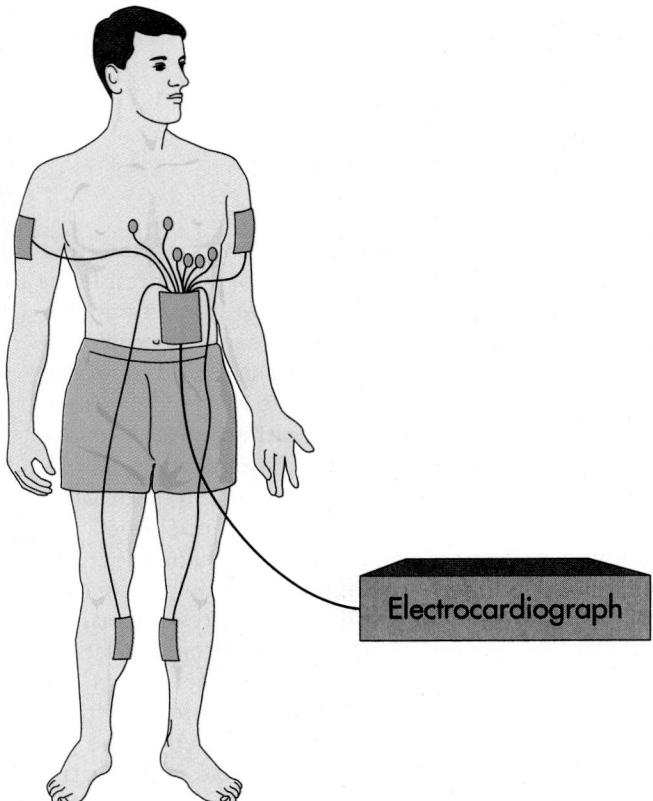

**Figure 39-9.** There are ten electrode positions for electrocardiography.

## Positioning the Electrodes

You must position electrodes at ten locations on the body (Figure 39-9). If the electrocardiograph has only five electrodes, you will need to move the fifth electrode to six different positions on the patient's chest to obtain the necessary tracings.

**Limb Electrodes.** Limb electrodes are most commonly placed on the inside of the fleshy part of the calf muscle and on the outside of the upper arm, but they are sometimes placed on the thigh, abdomen, and above the wrist. Follow office policy on limb placement, but remember that a consistent technique will ensure that all ECGs will be standardized, even with different equipment models. It is generally better to place arm electrodes on the upper arm because this reduces the amount of artifact caused by arm movement. Attach the electrodes to a smooth and fleshy part of each limb to ensure optimal conduction of impulses. Limb electrodes must always be placed at the same level on both arms and on both legs. If a patient has had a leg amputated, both leg electrodes should be placed on the thighs or abdomen.

**Precordial Electrodes.** Unlike the limb electrodes, the precordial electrodes must be placed at precise specific locations on the chest to obtain accurate readings. These locations specify intercostal spaces, the spaces between the ribs. Intercostal spaces are numbered from top to bottom. Refer to Figure 39-5 for the exact description of each location.

Determine the position for the first precordial electrode ($V_1$) by counting to the fourth intercostal space to the right of the sternum (breastbone). The $V_1$ electrode should be placed over this space, directly adjacent to the sternum. After you have this electrode in place, use it as a guide to position the other electrodes.

Place the $V_2$ electrode in the fourth intercostal space to the left of the sternum in the same manner. Note that the $V_1$ and $V_2$ positions may not line up exactly; one may be higher than the other. Perfect symmetry is rare in the human body.

Next place the $V_4$ electrode in the fifth intercostal space, where it intersects an imaginary line drawn straight down from the middle of the clavicle (midclavicular line). When the $V_4$ electrode is in place, place the $V_3$ electrode midway between $V_2$ and $V_4$ in the fifth intercostal space.

Place the $V_6$ electrode in the fifth intercostal space, directly below the middle of the armpit (midaxillary line). Place the last electrode ($V_5$) in the fifth intercostal space, midway between $V_4$ and $V_6$.

## Attaching the Wires

After placing the electrodes, attach the wires that connect the electrodes to the electrocardiograph. Numbers and letters on the wires correspond to numbers and letters for the electrodes. For example, RA stands for right arm, LL stands for left leg, and so on. The precordial electrode wires are labeled $V_1$ through $V_6$. Connect the limb wires first, then the precordial wires, in the sequence already described. Some wires are also color-coded.

Depending on the type of electrodes you use, connect the wires to the electrodes by snapping, clipping, or screwing the wire tips tightly in place. Wires should follow the patient's body contours and lie flat against the body. Drape the wires over the patient to avoid putting tension on the electrodes, which could cause interference. You may also bundle the wires together to form a single cable.

# Operating the Electrocardiograph

Before running the ECG, remind the patient to remain as still as possible and not to talk. Be sure the patient is comfortable. A comfortable patient is less likely to move around and cause artifacts on the ECG tracing.

## Standardizing the Electrocardiograph

Follow the steps described in Procedure 39-1 if you need to standardize the electrocardiograph. Some machines have automatic standardization. The stylus should move upward above the baseline 10 mm (two large squares) when you

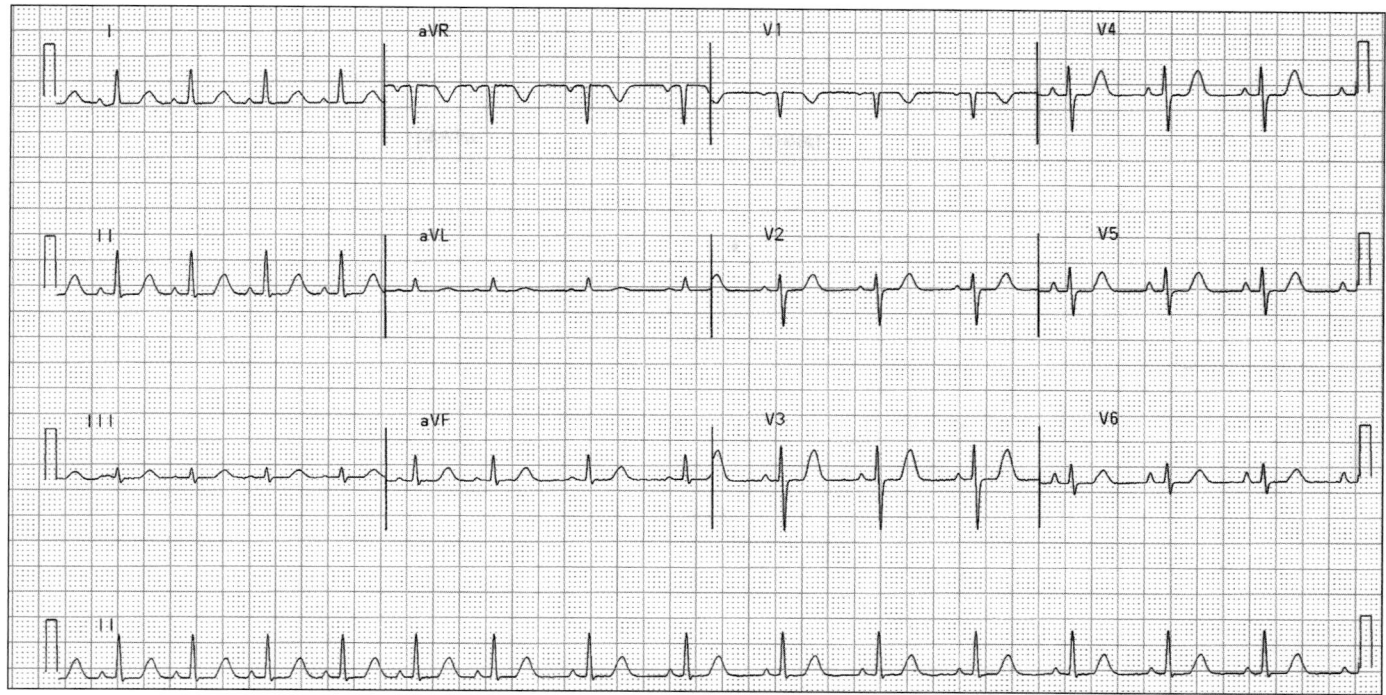

**Figure 39-10.** The tracing from each lead will differ. The long tracing of a single lead along the bottom is the rhythm strip.

Source: Courtesy of Cardiac Science Corporation, Milton, Wisconsin.

press the standardization button. If it does not, you must see to it that the instrument is adjusted before continuing.

## Running the ECG

You can now run the ECG. On most machines, turning the lead selector to the automatic mode produces a standard 12-lead strip. Because each lead provides a specific view of the heart's electrical activity, each of the 12 leads has a characteristic tracing (Figure 39-10).

**Manual ECGs.** If your office has a machine without an automatic setting, you must manually run the ECG for each of the 12 leads. You may also be required to repeat certain leads manually if artifacts are detected. Most of the ECG machines are able to run single channel or multi-channel ECGs.

To run a manual ECG, standardize the machine as already outlined. Then turn the lead selector to standby mode. Some older machines may require you to stop the paper before selecting the first lead (I) using the lead selector. Push the marking button on the machine to indicate the lead if the machine does not do this automatically. Allow the strip to run for four to five cardiac cycles, taking about 3 to 5 seconds. Turn the machine back to the standby mode; stop the paper if necessary, and repeat the procedure for leads II and III, the augmented leads, and the precordial leads. Remember to standardize the machine for consistency before running each lead.

Many physicians request another strip on lead II to assess for rhythm. Some physicians choose a different lead

for the rhythm strip. Run the rhythm strip on the requested lead to produce a strip that is at least 2 feet long so rhythmic abnormalities can be easily recognized.

**Multiple-Channel Electrocardiographs.** Some electrocardiographs have multiple channels that can record three, four, or six leads simultaneously (Figure 39-11). Electrode placement is the same for these types of electrocardiographs.

## Checking the ECG Tracing

After running the 12 leads and before disconnecting the patient from the machine, check all tracings to make sure they are clear and free of artifacts. If any of the leads do not appear on a tracing, it may mean that a wire has come loose. In this case reconnect the wire, and repeat the tracing. Repeat any tracings that are not clear.

Also check that all tracings are contained within the boundaries of the paper and that no waves peak above the edges of the paper. If this happens, recenter the stylus if it is positioned too high, or set the sensitivity selector to ½ before repeating the tracing. In the reverse situation—where very low peaks appear—set the sensitivity selector to 2 to increase the height of the peaks.

If the peaks in a tracing are too close together, increase the paper speed to 50 mm per second. Increasing the speed separates the peaks and makes the tracing easier to read.

Make a note on the ECG tracing whenever it is necessary to adjust sensitivity or speed settings. This information is vital to the interpretation of the test.

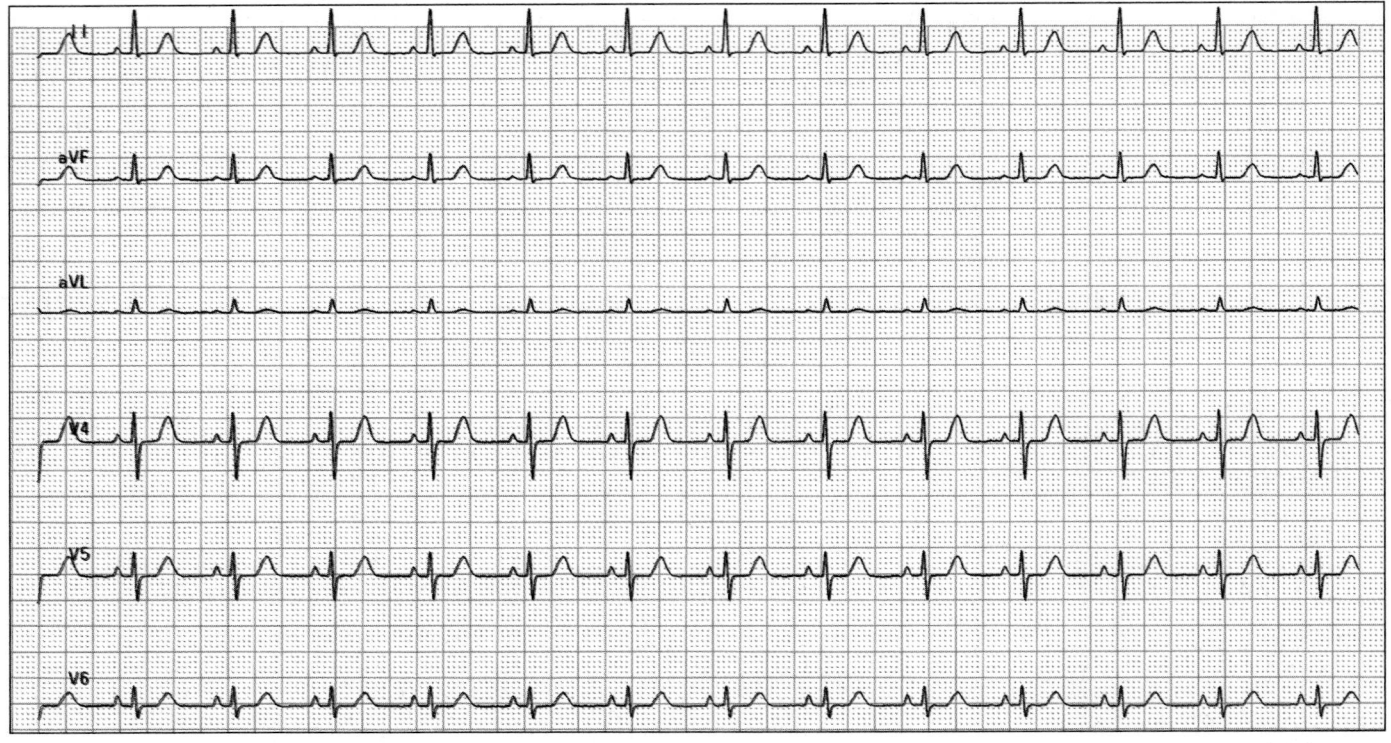

**Figure 39-11.** Some electrocardiographs allow you to run six leads at the same time.

Source: Courtesy of Cardiac Science Corporation, Milton, Wisconsin.

# Troubleshooting: Artifacts and Other Problems

To ensure high-quality tracings, it is essential to recognize artifacts and identify sources of interference. You must also know how to correct them.

## Artifacts

Artifacts are caused by improper technique, poor conduction, outside interference, or improper handling of a tracing. If artifacts are present on an ECG tracing, the doctor may not be able to make an accurate diagnosis of the patient's condition. Recognizing the presence of an artifact in the baseline during setup allows you to correct the problem before the tracing is recorded.

There are several types of artifacts. Among the common ones you may see are a wandering baseline or a flat line. You may also see marks that are not characteristic of a tracing; large, erratic spikes; or uniform, small spikes. Table 39-3 outlines these artifacts and summarizes possible causes and solutions.

**Wandering Baseline.** A wandering baseline, shown in Figure 39-12, is identified by a shift in the baseline from the center position for that lead. Causes include somatic interference and a variety of mechanical problems. Mechanical problems may be an inadequately warmed stylus, improper application of electrodes (too loose or incorrectly placed), tension on electrodes caused by a dangling wire, inadequate electrolyte, inadequate skin preparation, or the presence of creams or lotions on the skin.

Having the patient lie still can reduce somatic interference. Proper skin preparation and electrode placement are also essential. When the appointment for electrocardiography is made, instruct the patient to use no creams or lotions, deodorant, perfume, or powder. Be sure to include specific instructions in patient education materials, and ask the patient whether any of these substances were used before the procedure. If so, clean each area of electrode placement thoroughly with alcohol to avoid conduction disturbances.

**Flat Line.** A flat line on the tracing of one of the leads (Figure 39-13) is typically caused by a loose or disconnected wire. If flat lines occur on more than one lead, two of the wires may have been switched. If flat lines occur on all leads, the patient cable may be loose or disconnected, or there may be a break (short) somewhere in the unit. On the other hand, a flat line on all leads can be an indication of cardiac arrest. Always assess the patient's pulse and respiration first when flat lines occur on all leads.

**Extraneous Marks.** Because ECG graph paper is sensitive to heat and pressure, it can easily be damaged. Any marks on the paper that are not part of the tracing are referred to as extraneous marks. These marks can be caused by careless handling, such as using paper clips to hold the tracing together or handling the tracing with wet hands.

## TABLE 39-3 Correcting ECG Artifacts

| Problem | Possible Causes | Solutions |
|---|---|---|
| Wandering baseline | Inadequately warmed stylus | Allow electrocardiograph to warm up |
| | Poor skin preparation | Repeat skin preparation and electrode placement |
| | Loose electrode | Reapply electrode |
| | Improper electrode placement | Reapply electrode |
| | Dirty or corroded electrode | Clean and reapply electrode/replace electrode |
| | Somatic interference | Help patient relax and be comfortable |
| | Pickup of breathing movement | Reposition electrode |
| | Tension on electrode | Drape wires over patient |
| Flat line | Detached/loose wire or cable | Reattach wires/cable |
| | Wrong selector switch setting | Check/change selector switch setting |
| | Crossed wires | Check/switch wires |
| | Short circuit in wires | Check/replace broken equipment |
| | Cardiac arrest | Check pulse/respiration; begin CPR |
| Marks not part of tracing | Careless handling | Handle carefully |
| | Use of paper clips | Use a rubber band |
| | Wet hands | Ensure hands are dry |
| | Improper mounting | Mount properly |
| Uniform, small spikes | AC interference | Turn off/unplug other electrical equipment; remove patient's watch |
| | Improper electrode placement | Reapply electrode |
| | Inadequate grounding | Check grounding |
| | Dirty electrode | Clean and reapply electrode |
| Large, erratic spikes | Somatic interference | Help patient relax and be comfortable |
| | Loose/dry electrode | Reapply electrode |
| | Electrode placed over bone | Reposition electrode |

## Causes of Artifacts

You can use the line of the tracing to identify the cause of artifacts. Then you can take steps to eliminate the particular type of interference involved.

**Alternating Current (AC) Interference.** AC interference occurs when the electrocardiograph picks up a small amount of electric current given off by another piece of electrical equipment. The line of the tracing will be jagged, consisting of a series of uniform, small spikes (Figure 39-14). Many of the newer electrocardiographs have filters to reduce or eliminate most of this interference. AC interference can often be eliminated by turning off or unplugging other appliances in the room. It is also helpful to keep the examining table away from the wall, because wiring in the wall can contribute to AC interference. If the wires are crossed and the lead wires are not following the patient's body contour, this can cause AC interference. Make sure that the ECG cable is not underneath the examination table. If these remedies do not work, check to see whether the electrodes are dirty or attached improperly or whether the machine is incorrectly grounded.

**Somatic Interference.** Somatic interference is caused by muscle movement. Tensing of voluntary muscles, shifting of body position, tremors, or even talking requires muscular contractions that generate electrical impulses. A sensitive electrocardiograph detects these impulses. The result is erratic movement of the stylus during the tracing, leading to large, erratic spikes and a shifting baseline (Figure 39-15).

Eliminate this type of interference by reminding the patient to remain still and to refrain from talking. To reduce the chance of shivering, be sure the room temperature is comfortable. Make the patient comfortable to reduce shifting and moving.

Placing the limb electrodes closer to the trunk of the body—on the upper arms, close to the shoulder, and on the upper thighs—can reduce interference. Reducing patient anxiety by explaining the procedure can also help reduce somatic interference.

Certain nervous system disorders, such as Parkinson's disease, cause patients to experience involuntary movements that can cause interference. Placing the limb electrodes closer to the trunk of the body is often helpful;

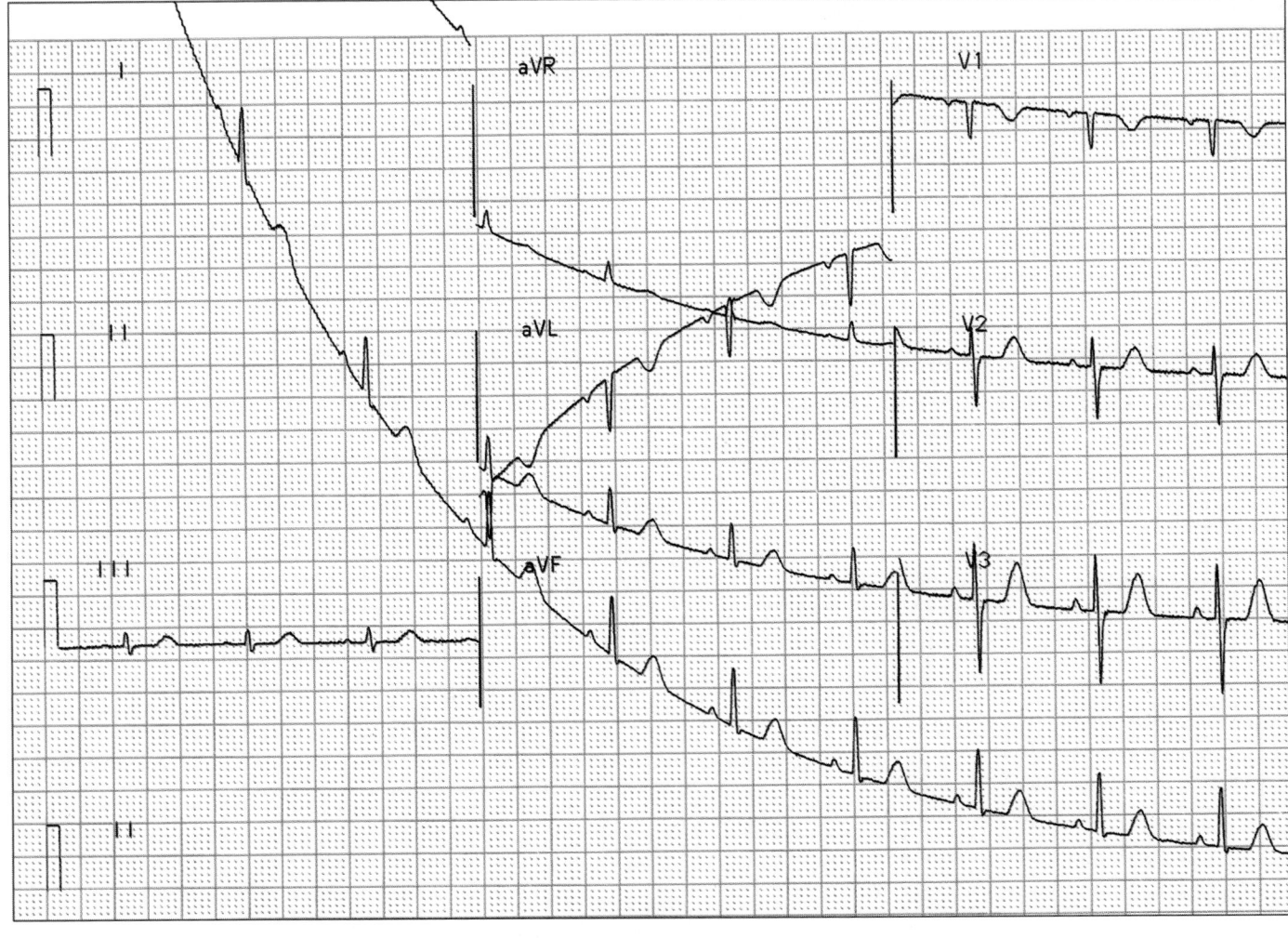

**Figure 39-12.** A wandering baseline may be caused by somatic interference or a mechanical problem.
Source: Courtesy of Cardiac Science Corporation, Milton, Wisconsin.

however, it may be necessary to interrupt the tracing until the tremors subside.

## Identifying the Source of Interference

The source of interference on an ECG can often be identified by checking the tracings obtained on leads I, II, and III. If there is a problem with a particular limb electrode, the interference will be prominent in two leads. For prominent interference in the following pairs of leads, check the limb electrode indicated:

- Leads I and II, right arm electrode
- Leads I and III, left arm electrode
- Leads II and III, left leg electrode

If the cause of the artifact or the source of interference cannot be determined, stop the machine and notify your supervisor or the physician of the problem. Do not disconnect the patient from the electrocardiograph.

## Completing the Procedure

When you are sure the quality of all ECG tracings is acceptable, disconnect the patient from the machine. First remove the tracing from the machine, and label it with the patient's name, the date, and your initials. If using a single channel ECG, loosely roll long tapes from single-channel machines with the printed side facing in, and secure them with a rubber band. Do not use paper clips because they can cause extraneous marks on the tracing.

Next, disconnect the wires from the electrodes, and remove the electrodes from the patient. Wipe excess electrolyte from the patient's skin with a moist towel. Assist the patient to a sitting position, allowing a moment's rest before assisting the patient from the table. Help the patient dress if necessary, or allow the patient privacy to dress. Remove disposable paper covers from the table and pillows, clean surfaces according to OSHA guidelines, and discard all disposable materials in a biohazardous waste container.

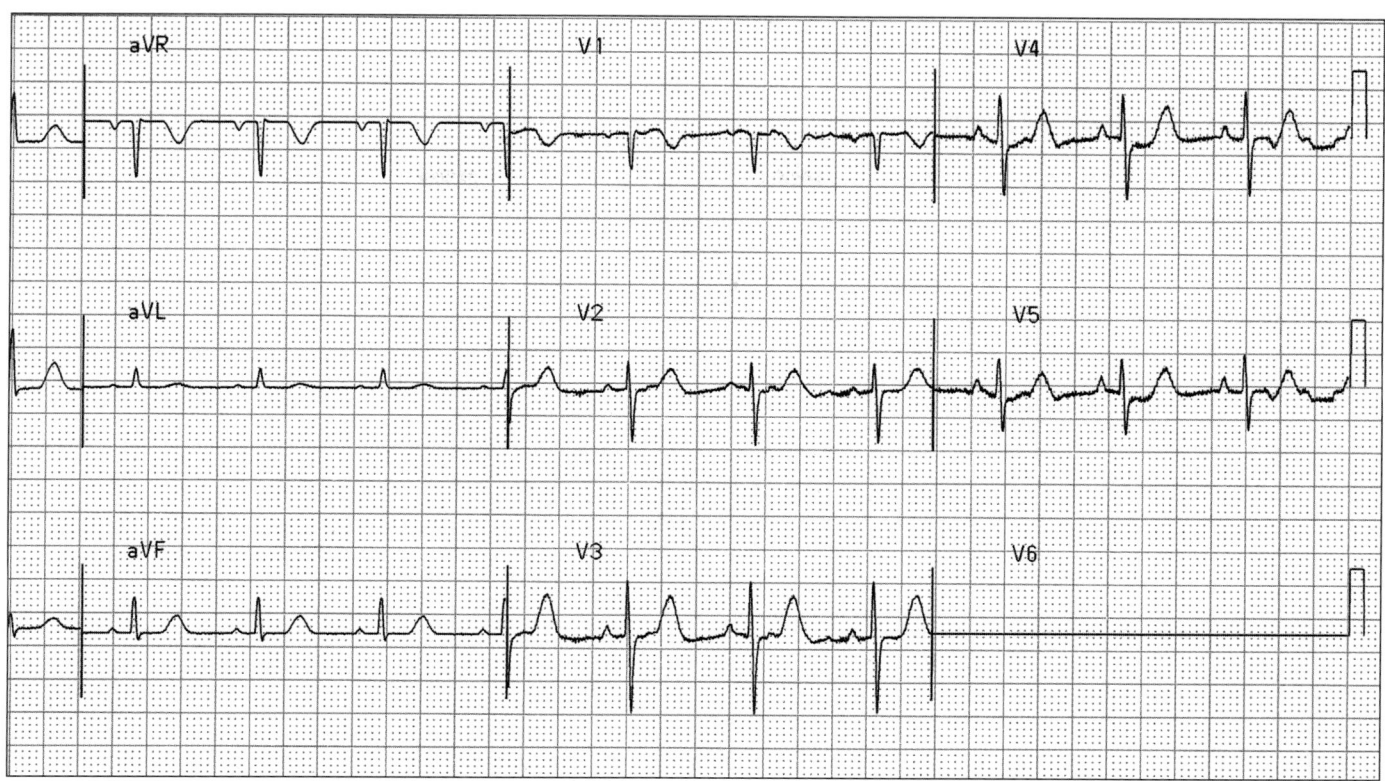

**Figure 39-13.** A flat line on one of the leads is caused by a loose or disconnected wire.
Source: Courtesy of Cardiac Science Corporation, Milton, Wisconsin. (ECG tracing represents earlier model from Burdick, Inc.)

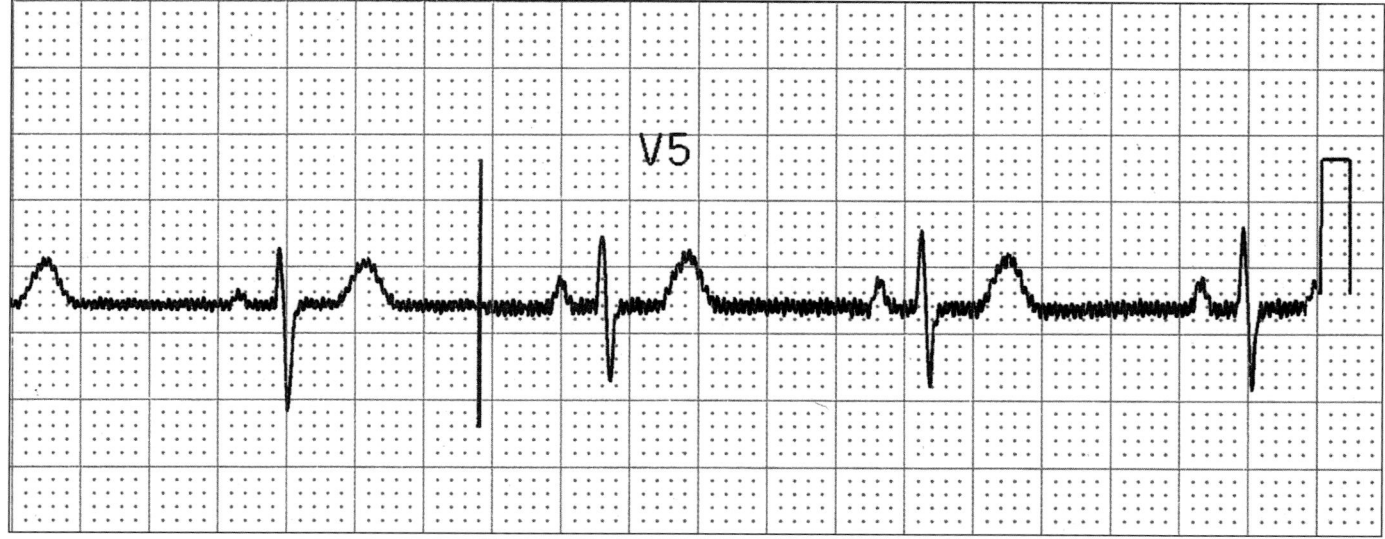

**Figure 39-14.** This type of artifact is caused by AC interference.
Source: Courtesy of Cardiac Science Corporation, Milton, Wisconsin.

## Mounting the Tracing

There are many types of ECG mounts or holders for single-channel ECG tracings. These mounts form a permanent record of the ECG and allow the doctor to read tracings from all 12 leads at once. Mounts are not typically necessary for multiple-channel ECG tracings because these are compact records of several leads. Several types of mounts are available, including slotted folders and folders with self-adhesive surfaces.

## Interpreting the ECG

As a medical assistant, you are not responsible for interpreting an ECG. Knowing something about how ECGs are interpreted, however, may allow you to recognize a problem

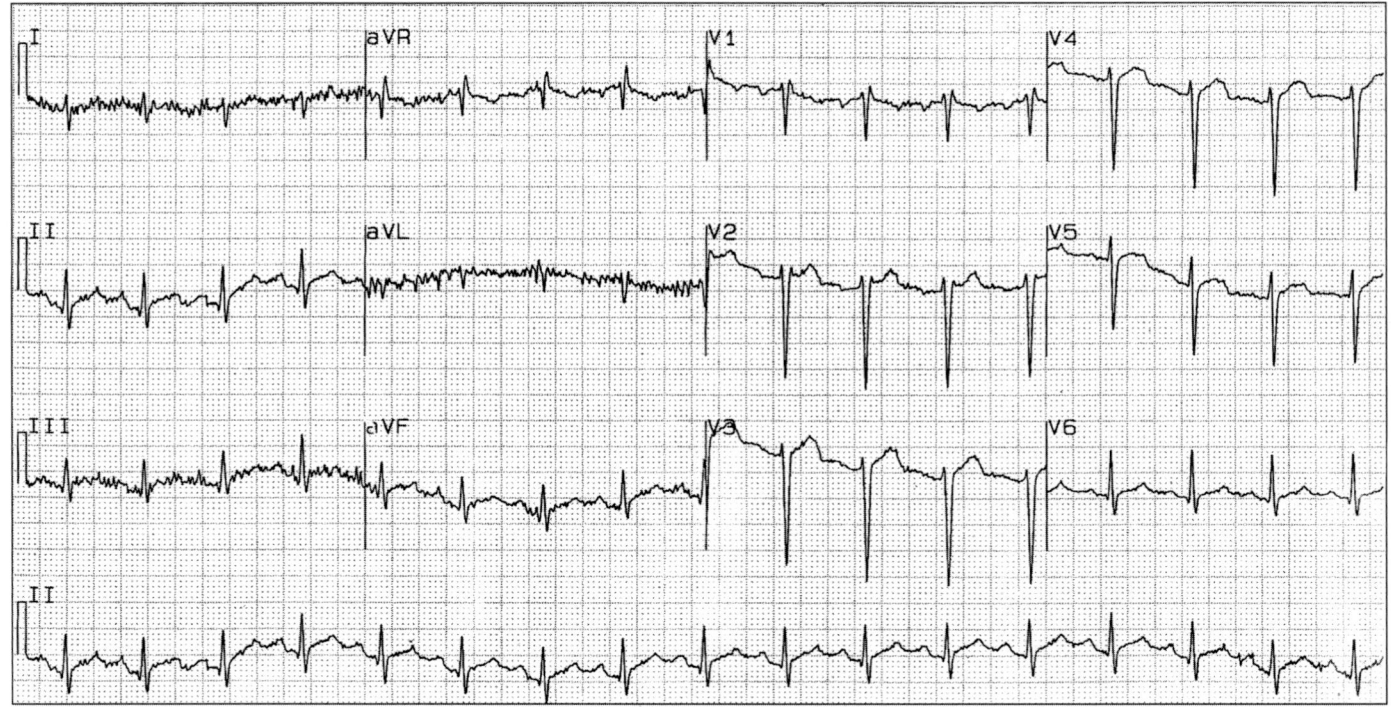

**Figure 39-15.** The somatic interference in this ECG was caused by patient tremors.
Source: Courtesy of Cardiac Science Corporation, Milton, Wisconsin.

that requires immediate attention. Some of the features that are assessed by means of an ECG include heart rhythm, heart rate, the length and position of intervals and segments, and wave changes. A series of ECGs are often taken before a physician makes a diagnosis. The tracings are compared for changes in a patient's condition, progress, or response to a specific medication.

## Heart Rhythm

The ECG is the best way to assess heart rhythm—the regularity of the heartbeat. A normal heart rhythm is indicated on the ECG by regularly spaced complexes. In a regularly spaced complex, the distance between one P wave and the next P wave—or one R wave and the next R wave—is consistent. The physician assesses the patient's rhythm by viewing the rhythm strip you obtain from lead II.

## Heart Rate

The heart rate can easily be determined by counting the number of QRS complexes in a 6-second strip of the tracing (30 large squares at 25 mm per second) and multiplying by 10. Irregularities in heart rate may result from conduction abnormalities or reactions to certain drugs.

## Intervals and Segments

Variations in the length and position of the intervals and segments can indicate many heart conditions, including conduction disturbances and myocardial infarction, or

heart attack. For example, following a heart attack, the ST segment will be elevated in the tracing for a period of time. Thus, the ECG can be used to determine not only the occurrence of a heart attack but also the approximate time it occurred. Electrolyte disturbances in the blood and drug reactions can also affect intervals and segments.

## Wave Changes

The direction of certain waves may vary, depending on which lead is being viewed. Normally each wave should have a similar appearance in each of the leads. Changes in the height, width, or direction of a wave may indicate a problem. During the early stages of a heart attack, for example, the T wave forms a large peak. Not long afterward the T wave inverts and appears below the baseline.

## Cardiac Arrhythmias

Irregularities in heart rhythm are called arrhythmias. Some arrhythmias do not cause problems, but many of them can be dangerous. It is important, therefore, to detect these irregularities with an ECG.

**Ventricular Fibrillation (V-Fib).** Ventricular fibrillation, commonly referred to as v-fib, is a life-threatening heart condition in which the ventricles of the heart appear to "quiver" and there is no cardiac output. The patient will quickly lose consciousness and cardioversion (defibrillation) must be used to stop the arrhythmia. Ventricular fibrillation is seen in patients experiencing a myocardial infarction. The tracing is often described as a "saw tooth" image (Figure 39-16).

## Premature Ventricular Contractions (PVC).

Premature ventricular contractions (PVCs) are premature heartbeats that originate from the ventricles of the heart. A PVC is identified as a beat that occurs early in the cycle and is followed by a pause before the next cycle (Figure 39-17). PVCs are premature because they occur before the regular heartbeat. PVCs are the result of an irritability of the heart muscle in the ventricles. PVCs can be caused by myocardial infarctions, electrolyte imbalances, lack of oxygen, or certain medications. A PVC appears on the ECG as having no P wave, a wide QRS complex, and T waves that deflect in an opposite direction than the R wave.

## Atrial Fibrillation.

Atrial arrhythmias occur because of electrical disturbances in the atria and/or the AV node, which leads to fast heart beats (tachycardia). Atrial fibrillation is a common atrial arrhythmia that causes rapid, multiple electrical signals that fire rapidly from different areas in the atria rather than from the SA node. The causes of atrial fibrillation can include myocardial infarction; hypertension; heart failure; mitral valve diseases, such as MVP; overactive thyroid; pulmonary embolisms (blood clots); excessive alcohol consumption; emphysema; and pericarditis. Atrial fibrillation is seen on the ECG as small, irregular, uncoordinated complexes that are difficult to interpret because the P waves can't be identified (Figure 39-18).

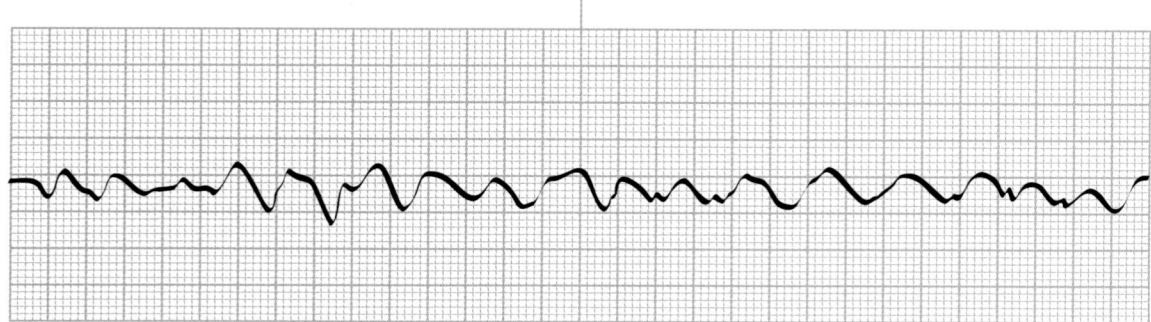

**Figure 39-16.** Ventricular fibrillation resembles and is sometimes referred to as a "saw tooth" pattern.

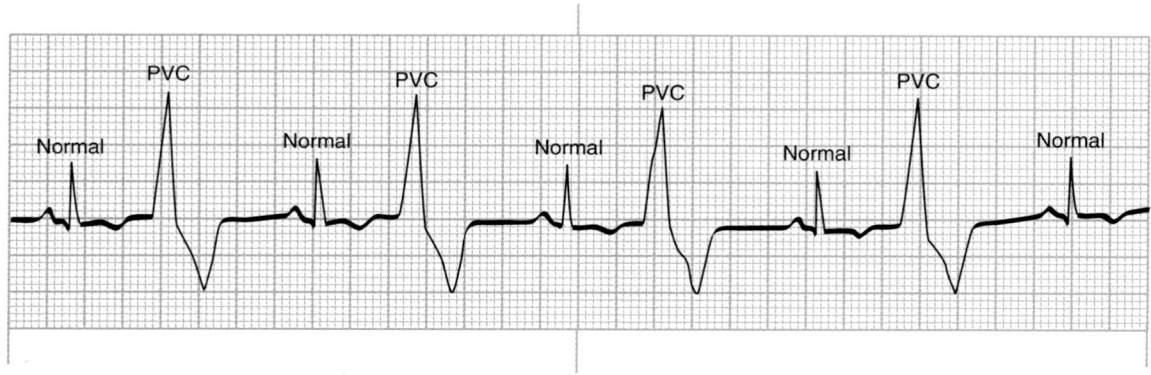

**Figure 39-17.** This rhythm strip compares a normal deflection to a premature ventricular contraction (PVC).

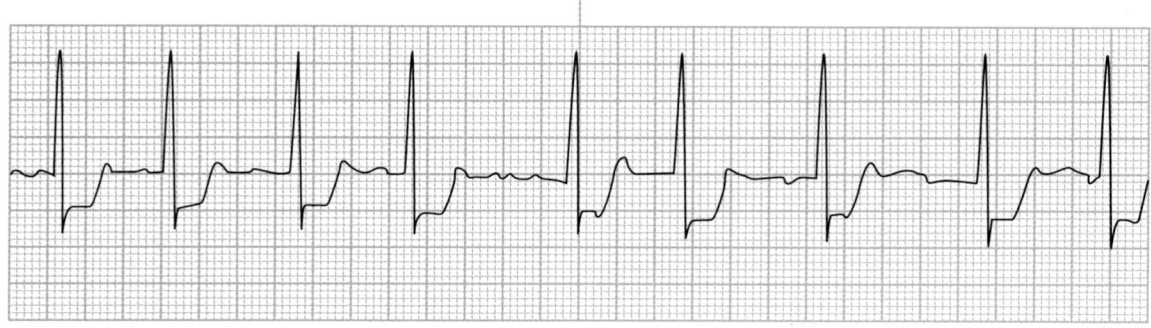

**Figure 39-18.** Atrial fibrillation.

# Exercise Electrocardiography (Stress Testing)

The resting ECG doesn't always provide a doctor with enough information to diagnose a problem. Exercise electrocardiography, more commonly known as a stress test, assesses the heart's conduction system during exercise, when the demand for oxygen increases. This test measures a patient's response to a constant or increasing workload.

A stress test may be performed on a patient who has had surgery or a heart attack to determine how the heart is functioning. It is sometimes used to screen a patient for heart disease and to determine a patient's ability to undertake an exercise program.

During the procedure the patient is required to walk on a treadmill, pedal a stationary bicycle, or walk on a stair-stepping ergonometer while ECG readings are taken (Figure 39-19). An ergonometer measures work performed. You are responsible for preparing the patient for electrocardiography and monitoring blood pressure throughout the procedure. The test continues until the patient reaches a target heart rate, experiences chest pain or fatigue, or develops complications, such as tachycardia or dysrhythmia.

A patient who undergoes stress testing is often suspected of having a heart problem or is recovering from a heart attack or surgery. Consequently, there may be a risk of cardiac distress, heart attack, or cardiac arrest during testing. Because of the risks, the patient must be monitored by a physician throughout the test. Emergency medication and equipment, such as a defibrillator, must always be present in the room. The patient must sign an informed consent form before the procedure.

Because of the potential risk, patients may be apprehensive about the test. As a medical assistant, you can be instrumental in helping them feel comfortable about undergoing the procedure and in making the procedure as safe as possible for them. See the Caution: Handle With Care section for ways to help a patient safely undergo stress testing.

# Ambulatory Electrocardiography (Holter Monitoring)

Patients who experience intermittent chest pain or discomfort may have a normal resting ECG and a normal stress test. When this is the case, the electrical activity of the patient's heart can be monitored over a 24-hour period of normal activity to help diagnose the problem. A special monitor, the Holter monitor, is used for this purpose.

## Function of the Holter Monitor

The **Holter monitor** is an electrocardiography device that includes a small cassette or microchip recorder worn around a patient's waist or on a shoulder strap to record the heart's electrical activity. The monitor is connected to electrodes on the patient's chest (Figure 39-20). During

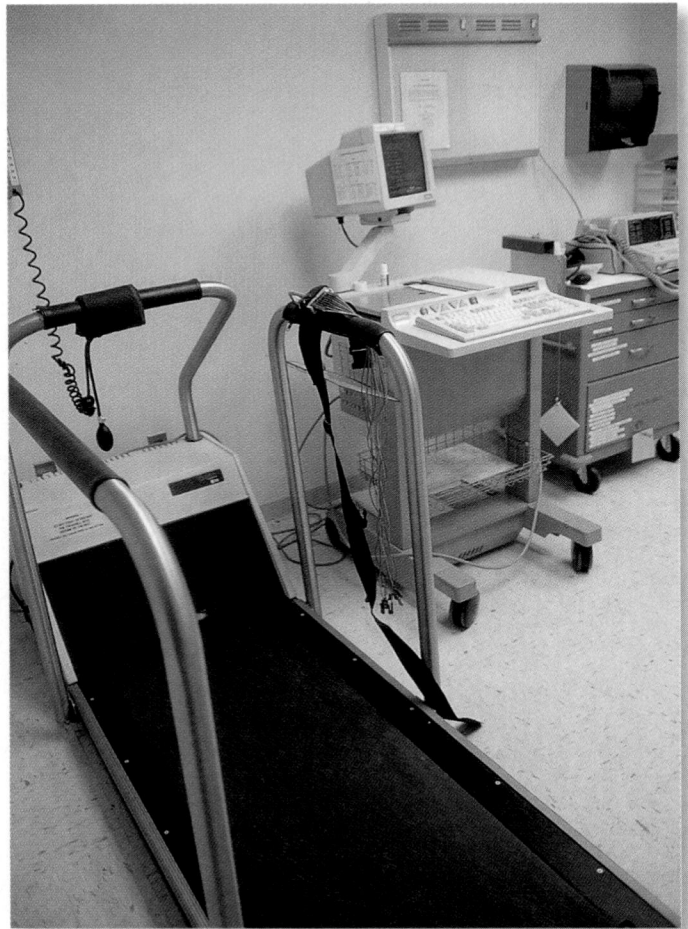

**Figure 39-19.** During a stress test, the patient exercises on special equipment to see how well the heart handles increased physical demands.

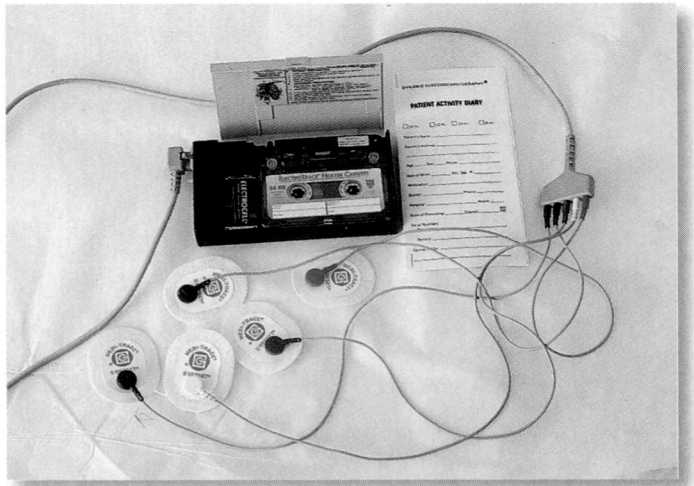

**Figure 39-20.** The Holter monitor is used to determine electrical activity of a patient's heart over a 24-hour period.

## CAUTION *Handle With Care*

### Ensuring Patient Safety During Stress Testing

Some risk is involved in exercise electrocardiography, because patients who most commonly undergo the test may either already have cardiac problems or be suspected of having them. The risk of having a heart attack during a stress test, however, is less than 1 in 500, and the risk of death is less than 1 in 10,000. Still, some patients may be apprehensive about the procedure because of the risks.

You can help educate and prepare patients for stress tests and assist them during the procedure. One way to help is to ask patients to wear comfortable shoes and clothes. In addition, there are several ways to help these patients be less fearful of the procedure while helping to ensure their safety.

A patient who has recently suffered a heart attack may be particularly afraid to undergo stress testing. A stress test may, however, be the only way the physician can accurately determine the functional ability of the patient's heart and assess his physical limitations. This information is vital to preventing future heart attacks.

By informing the patient of what symptoms he may expect during the test—including fatigue, slight breathlessness, an increased heart rate, and increased perspiration—the patient will be better able to cope with the test. Make it clear that an advance warning of adjustments in the procedure, such as an increased workload, will be given.

Assure the patient that there are few risks associated with the test and that the test may be stopped if he experiences chest pain or extreme fatigue. Patients will relax and follow instructions better when they know that the procedure can be controlled. Tell the patient that both you and the physician will be monitoring his vital signs during and after the procedure and that all safety precautions will be taken. Explain the presence of the safety equipment—for example, the crash cart with medication, equipment, and supplies.

During the test, remember to talk to and listen to the patient. Even symptoms not related to cardiac symptoms should be reported, and the patient should be encouraged to report any symptoms. Observe the patient for signs of distress and inform the physician immediately if such symptoms appear.

---

the testing period, the patient is asked to perform usual daily activities and to keep a written log of activities undertaken and of stress or symptoms experienced. To aid in the diagnosis, some monitors allow patients to press an event button to mark the area on the recording whenever symptoms appear.

The patient returns to the office at the end of the 24-hour test period to have the monitor and electrodes removed. The tape is analyzed by a microcomputer in the office or at a reference laboratory, and a printout of the results is prepared. When the tracing has been evaluated, the doctor can correlate cardiac irregularities, such as arrhythmias or ST segment changes, with the activities and symptoms listed in the patient's diary.

In addition to its role as a diagnostic tool, Holter monitoring can be used to evaluate the status of a patient who is recovering from a heart attack. It can indicate progress or the need to change therapy or modify the rehabilitation plan.

## Patient Education

It is absolutely essential that the patient continue normal activities during Holter monitoring. Give the patient the following additional instructions.

- Record all activities, emotional upsets, physical symptoms, and medications taken.

- Wear loose-fitting clothing that opens in the front while wearing the monitor.

- Avoid going near magnets, metal detectors, and high-voltage areas, and avoid using electric blankets during the monitoring period. These devices and areas can interfere with the recording.

- Avoid getting the monitor wet. Do not take a bath or shower. A sponge bath is permissible.

- Show the patient how to check the monitor to make sure it is working properly. This step is particularly important if any of the electrodes seem loose. Instruct the patient to inform the office if there are any problems.

## Connecting the Patient

Holter monitors have either three or five electrodes, depending on the unit. As with a resting ECG, correct placement of the electrodes is necessary for accurate readings.

Because the electrodes must stay in place for 24 hours, you may need to shave the areas where the electrodes are attached to permit optimum adherence. The wires may be connected to the electrodes before they are attached to minimize patient discomfort.

After the electrodes and wires are attached and the monitor is in place, tape the wires to the patient's chest to eliminate tension on the wires or electrodes (Figure 39-21). Be sure that the unit has a fresh battery, that a cassette

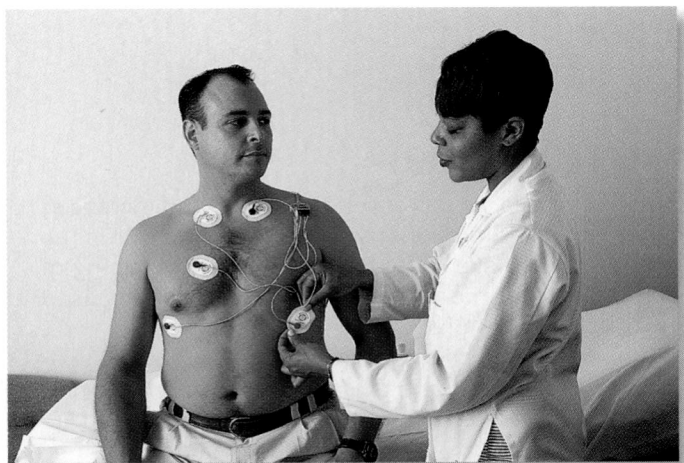

**Figure 39-21.** Taping the wires to the patient's chest reduces the chance that tension on a wire or electrode will produce artifacts on the ECG.

tape has been inserted, and that the unit is turned on. The steps in performing Holter monitoring are outlined in Procedure 39-2.

# Anatomy and Physiology of the Respiratory System

Pulmonary function tests are used to evaluate a patient's lung volume and capacity. A description of the anatomy and physiology of the respiratory system will help clarify pulmonary function testing and the problems it is used to diagnose.

## Anatomy of the Respiratory System

The respiratory system is composed of the nose, pharynx, larynx, trachea, two bronchi, and the lungs. The bronchi branch into bronchioles and eventually into alveoli. In the

## PROCEDURE 39.2

### Holter Monitoring

**Procedure Goal:** To monitor the electrical activity of a patient's heart over a 24-hour period to detect cardiac abnormalities that may go undetected during routine electrocardiography or stress testing

**OSHA Guidelines**

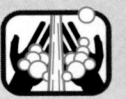 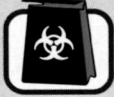 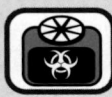 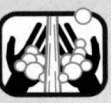

**Materials:** Holter monitor, battery, cassette tape, patient diary or log, alcohol, gauze pads, disposable shaving supplies, disposable electrodes, hypoallergenic tape, drape, electrocardiograph

**Method:**

1. Identify the patient, introduce yourself, and explain the procedure.
2. Ask the patient to remove clothing from the waist up; provide a drape if necessary.
3. Wash your hands and assemble the equipment.
4. Assist the patient into a comfortable position (sitting or supine).
5. If the patient's body hair is particularly dense, put on examination gloves and trim the areas where the electrodes will be attached.

*Rationale*
Trimming the area will ensure that the electrodes will stay secure during the 24-hour period.

6. Clean the electrode sites with alcohol and gauze.
7. Rub each electrode site vigorously with a dry gauze square.

*Rationale*
To help electrodes adhere to the skin

8. Attach wires to the electrodes, and peel off the paper backing on the electrodes. Apply as indicated (Figure 39-22), pressing firmly to ensure that each electrode is securely attached and is making good contact with the skin.

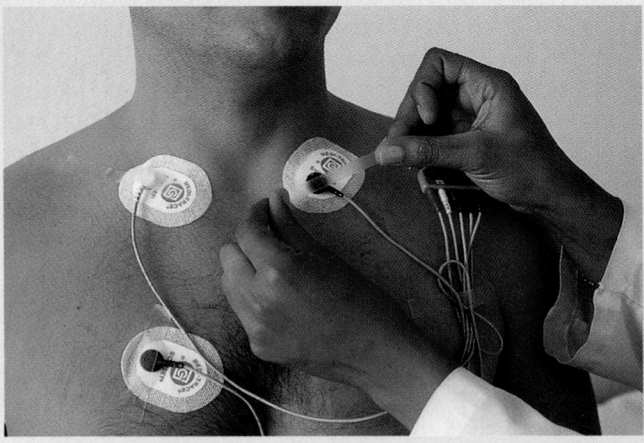

**Figure 39-22.** Correctly connecting the patient to the Holter monitor is essential.

*continued* ⟶

# Holter Monitoring *(concluded)*

### Rationale

Good skin contact is essential to obtaining an accurate reading.

9. Attach the patient cable.

10. Insert a fresh battery, and position the unit (Figure 39-23).

11. Tape wires, cable, and electrodes as necessary to avoid tension on the wires as the patient moves.

12. Insert the cassette tape, and turn on the unit.

13. Confirm that the cassette tape is actually running (Figure 39-24). Indicate the start time in the patient's chart.

### Rationale

If the cassette tape is not running, results will not be recorded and the test will have to be repeated.

14. Instruct the patient on proper use of the monitor and how to enter information in the diary. Caution the patient not to alter any diary entries; it is crucial to know what the patient is doing at all times.

15. Schedule the patient's return visit for the same time on the following day.

16. On the following day remove the electrodes, discard them, and clean the electrode sites.

17. Wash your hands.

18. Remove the cassette and obtain a printout of the tracing according to office procedure.

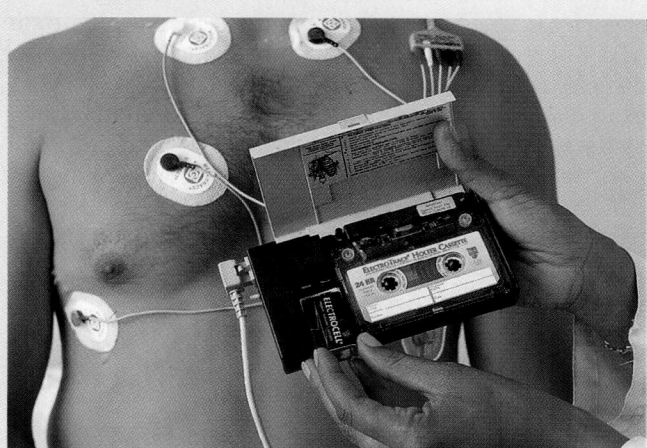

**Figure 39-23.** Make sure the monitor has a fresh battery and cassette tape.

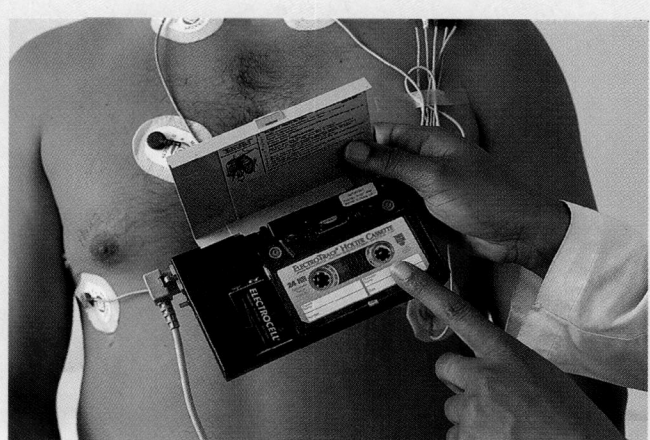

**Figure 39-24.** Observe the cassette to make sure the tape is moving through the recording unit.

alveoli, external respiration—the exchange of gases between the air and the blood—occurs. Figure 39-25 shows the lungs, bronchi, and alveoli in detail.

## Physiology of the Respiratory System

There are two levels of respiration: external and internal. External respiration involves two processes: ventilation and diffusion. Ventilation is the movement of air in and out of the lungs. It results from the contraction and relaxation of the respiratory muscles. The major respiratory muscle is the diaphragm. Other respiratory muscles, including the intercostal muscles (between the ribs), are found in the walls of the chest and back.

Inspiration, or breathing in, results when the respiratory muscles contract. The diaphragm pushes down toward the abdomen when it contracts, while the other respiratory muscles help expand the chest outward and upward. Both actions serve to decrease the pressure within the alveoli so that it is less than the atmospheric pressure. The result is the flow of air into the lungs.

Expiration, or breathing out, results from relaxation of the respiratory muscles and a consequent increase in

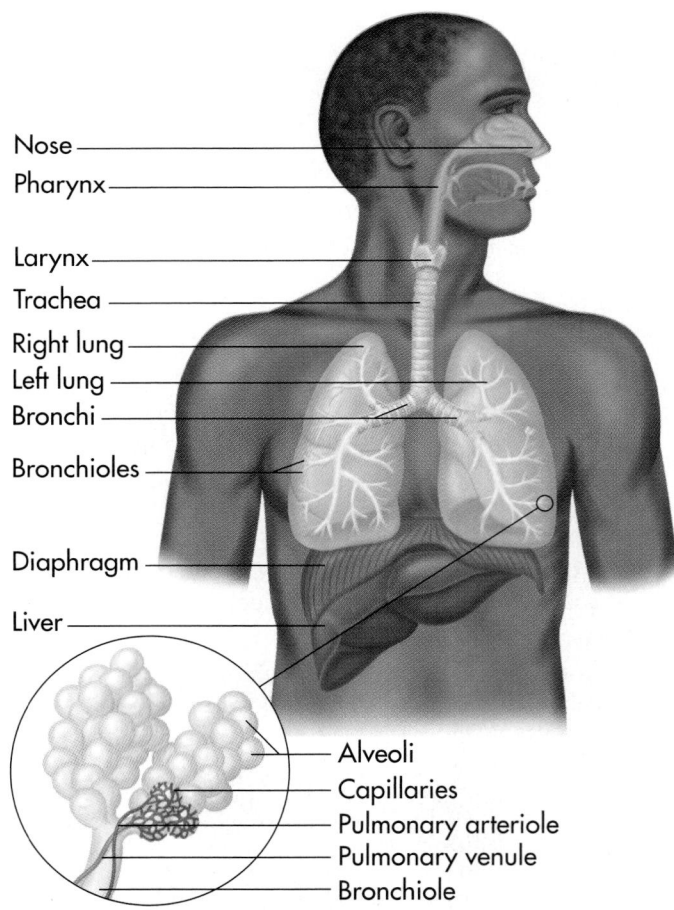

Nose
Pharynx
Larynx
Trachea
Right lung
Left lung
Bronchi
Bronchioles
Diaphragm
Liver

Alveoli
Capillaries
Pulmonary arteriole
Pulmonary venule
Bronchiole

**Figure 39-25.** Knowing how the respiratory system works will help you understand the application of spirometry.

pressure within the alveoli. As a result, air flows out of the lungs. Expiration is normally a passive process. During fast, hard breathing, however, the abdominal muscles push the diaphragm upward, and certain chest and back muscles pull the ribs downward and inward to decrease the size of the chest cavity and help force the air out.

Diffusion is a passive process wherein oxygen and carbon dioxide cross the capillary and alveolar membranes to enter the capillaries or alveoli. Oxygen diffuses from the alveolar air into the blood, because there is a higher concentration in the alveoli than in the blood. Carbon dioxide, at a higher concentration in the blood, diffuses across the membranes into the alveoli. Perfusion, or internal respiration, is the exchange of oxygen in the blood for carbon dioxide in the cells of body tissues and organs. Perfusion, diffusion, and ventilation occur simultaneously, as the circulatory system moves the blood from the lungs to the body cells and back.

## Pulmonary Function Testing

Pulmonary function tests (PFTs) evaluate lung volume and capacity. These tests are commonly used to evaluate shortness of breath and can help detect and classify pulmonary disorders. They may also be performed as part of a general examination. PFTs are used to monitor conditions such as asthma, certain allergies, cystic fibrosis, and chronic obstructive pulmonary disease (COPD), a chronic lung disorder. The tests are also used to evaluate the effectiveness of particular treatments on a patient's lung function.

## Career Opportunities

### Respiratory Therapist

*To gain medical assistant credentials, you must fulfill the requirements of either the American Association of Medical Assistants (for a Certified Medical Assistant) or the American Medical Technologists (for a Registered Medical Assistant). After obtaining your medical assistant certification or registration, you may wish to acquire additional skills in specialty areas through course work or on-the-job training. Although this course work or training may not lead to an additional certification or degree, it will enable you to expand your role in the medical office and advance your career as the demand for skilled health professionals increases.*

### Skills and Duties

A respiratory therapist diagnoses, treats, and cares for people who have difficulty breathing. Some of his

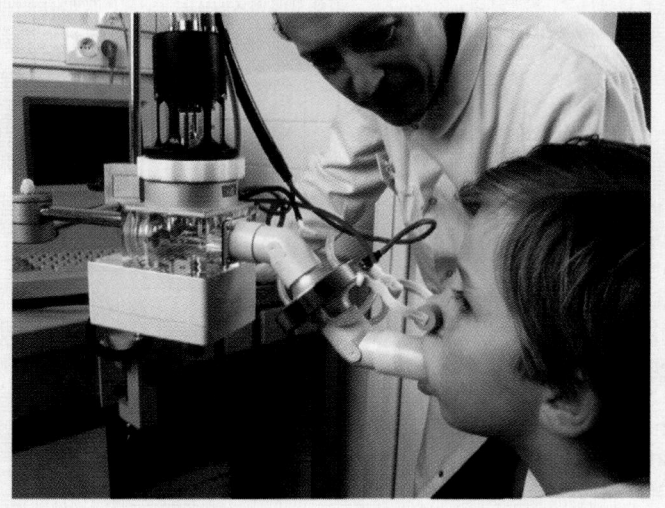

*continued ⟶*

# Career Opportunities

## Respiratory Therapist *(concluded)*

patients are people with chronic lung problems, such as asthma, bronchitis, emphysema, and chronic obstructive pulmonary disease (COPD). Others may have difficulty breathing as the result of complications caused by a heart attack, an accident, cystic fibrosis, lung cancer, or acquired immunodeficiency syndrome (AIDS). Some infants who are born prematurely have difficulty breathing and may need respiratory therapy, which may include the use of apnea monitors and oxygen tents.

A respiratory therapist works under the supervision of a physician. Duties include both diagnostic and therapeutic tasks. For example, to diagnose a breathing problem, the therapist analyzes samples of a patient's breath or blood for levels of oxygen, carbon dioxide, and other gases. He also measures the capacity of a patient's lungs to determine whether they are working properly and performs stress tests and other studies of the cardiopulmonary system.

Once a problem is diagnosed, the respiratory therapist may use a variety of treatment options. He may use equipment such as oxygen respirators and oxygen tents to administer oxygen to help the patient breathe. He may administer medication in aerosol form to treat breathing disorders. The respiratory therapist may also set up and maintain mechanical ventilation, such as artificial airways, for patients who cannot breathe on their own.

In addition to diagnosis and treatment of breathing disorders, the respiratory therapist may be responsible for patient education to promote healthy breathing. Education duties may include:

- Teaching smoking cessation programs to help prevent breathing problems associated with smoking.
- Conducting rehabilitation activities, such as low-impact aerobics, to help patients increase their lung capacity.

The respiratory therapist is also often responsible for testing equipment to make sure it is operating effectively. He may make minor repairs to faulty respiratory equipment or arrange for major repair work.

### Workplace Settings

Most respiratory therapists work in hospitals. Sometimes, in emergency situations, they also work in ambulances. Increasing numbers of respiratory therapists, however, work in locations outside the hospital. These locations include nursing homes, physicians' offices, home health-care agencies, rehabilitation centers, clinics, medical equipment supply companies, and patients' homes.

### Education

Approximately 400 colleges and universities in the United States offer respiratory care programs. To qualify for a program, you must be a high school graduate with a background in math and science.

The National Board for Respiratory Therapists has established two levels of respiratory care practitioners. A Certified Respiratory Therapy Technician (CRTT) has graduated from an approved program (usually 12 to 18 months), has 1 year of work experience, and has passed a voluntary written examination. A Registered Respiratory Therapist (RRT) has completed either a 2-year or 4-year approved program, has 1 year of work experience, and has passed a written and practical examination.

### Where to Go for More Information

American Association for Respiratory Care
9425 McArthur Blvd., Suite 100
Irving, TX 75063
(972) 243-2272

American Lung Association
61 Broadway, 6th Floor
New York, NY 10006
(212) 315-8700 or 1-800-LUNGUSA

## Spirometry

**Spirometry** is a test used to measure breathing capacity. An instrument called a **spirometer** measures the air taken in by and expelled from the lungs. Several different measurements related to lung volume and capacity can be made with a spirometer (Table 39-4). Some of these measurements are made directly by the spirometer; others are calculated.

## Forced Vital Capacity

Many measurements can be obtained during one particular maneuver—obtaining the **forced vital capacity (FVC),** the greatest volume of air that can be expelled when a person performs rapid, forced expiration. To obtain the FVC, ask the patient to take as deep a breath as possible and to exhale into the spirometer as quickly and completely as possible. You can determine the lung's ability to

## TABLE 39-4    Pulmonary Function Tests

| Lung Capacity Tests | Definition |
| --- | --- |
| Vital capacity (VC) | Total volume of air that can be exhaled after maximum inspiration |
| Inspiratory capacity (IC) | Amount of air that can be inhaled after normal expiration |
| Functional residual capacity (FRC) | Amount of air remaining in lungs after normal expiration |
| Total lung capacity (TLC) | Total volume of lungs when maximally inflated |
| Forced vital capacity (FVC) | Greatest volume of air that can be expelled when person performs rapid, forced expiratory maneuver |
| Forced expiratory volume (FEV) | Volume of air expelled in first, second, or third second of FVC maneuver |
| Peak expiratory flow rate (PEFR) | Greatest rate of flow during forced expiration |
| Forced expiratory flow (FEF) | Average rate of flow during middle half of FVC |
| Maximal voluntary ventilation (MVV) | Greatest volume of air breathed per unit of time |
| Tidal volume ($T_V$) | Amount of air inhaled or exhaled during normal breathing |
| Minute volume (MV) | Total amount of air expired per minute |
| Inspiratory reserve volume (IRV) | Amount of air inspired over above-normal inspiration |
| Expiratory reserve volume (ERV) | Amount of air exhaled after normal expiration |
| Residual volume (RV) | Amount of air remaining in lungs after forced expiration |

Source: Adapted from *Illustrated Guide to Diagnostic Tests* (Springhouse, PA: Springhouse, 1998).

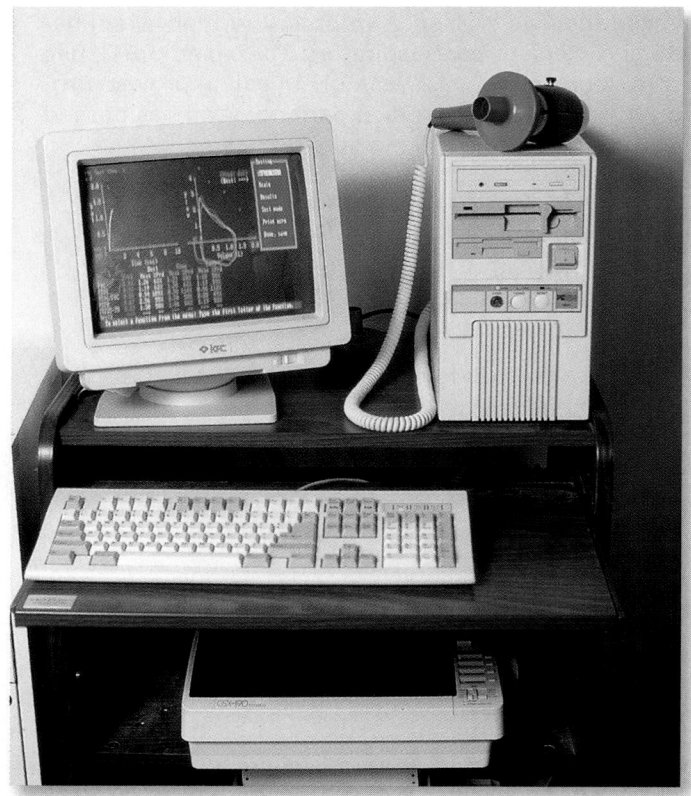

**Figure 39-26.** This computerized spirometer measures air volume and airflow.

function by taking into account the volume of air expelled and the time it takes to perform this maneuver.

## Types of Spirometers

Many models of computerized spirometers are used in physicians' offices. Each consists of a mouthpiece or a mouthpiece and a tube to carry air to the machine, a mechanism to measure the volume or flow of air, and a means of calculating and printing the results.

Computerized spirometers measure air volume and airflow, perform various calculations, and print a graphic representation of the information. Figure 39-26 shows a computerized spirometer.

Although seldom used, mechanical spirometers directly measure either the air volume displaced or airflow. Spirometers that directly measure airflow calculate air volume using flow rate and time values. The flow-sensing spirometer illustrated in Figure 39-27 calculates airflow by counting the rotations of a turbine.

## Performing Spirometry

The technique for performing pulmonary function testing is similar for all types of spirometers. Successful spirometry depends on proper patient preparation and consistent technique in performing the procedure and analyzing the

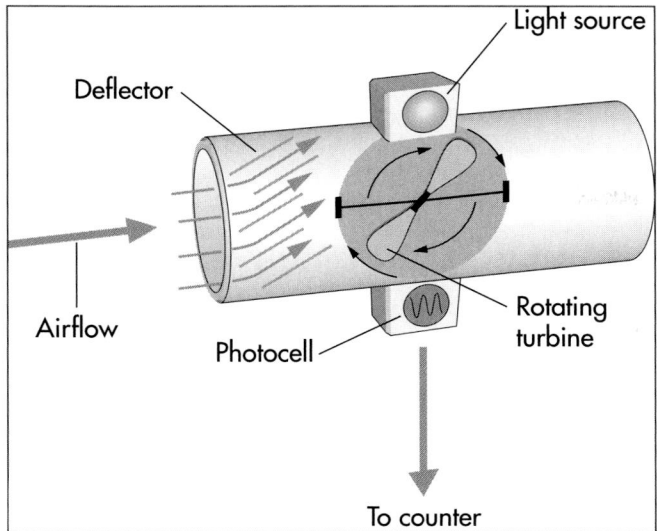

Figure 39-27. One type of flow-sensing spirometer uses a turbine to measure airflow directly from the lungs.

Light source

Deflector

Airflow

Photocell

Rotating turbine

To counter

results. The steps involved in measuring forced vital capacity using a spirometer are described in detail here and outlined in Procedure 39-3.

## Patient Preparation

When patients are scheduled for pulmonary function tests, inform them that the following conditions and activities may affect the test's accuracy:

- Viral infection or acute illness within the previous 2 to 3 weeks
- Serious medical condition, such as a recent heart attack
- Recent use of a prescribed medication if test order calls for spirometry before and after prescribed medication
- Use of a sedative or opioid substance before the test
- Smoking or eating a heavy meal within 1 hour of taking the test

# PROCEDURE 39.3

## Measuring Forced Vital Capacity Using Spirometry

**Procedure Goal:** To determine a patient's forced vital capacity using a volume-displacing spirometer

### OSHA Guidelines

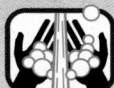 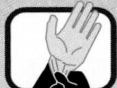  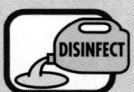 

**Materials:** Adult scale with height bar, spirometer, patient tubing (tubing that runs from the mouthpiece to the machine), mouthpiece, nose clip, disinfectant

### Method:

1. Prepare the equipment. Ensure that the paper supply in the machine is adequate.
2. Calibrate the machine as necessary.
3. Identify the patient and introduce yourself.
4. Check the patient's chart to see whether there are special instructions to follow.
5. Ask whether the patient has followed instructions.
6. Wash your hands and put on examination gloves.
7. Measure and record the patient's height and weight.
8. Explain the proper positioning.
9. Explain the procedure.
10. Demonstrate the procedure.

### Rationale

Explanations and demonstrations are effective patient teaching methods.

11. Turn on the spirometer, and enter applicable patient data and the number of tests to be performed.
12. Ensure that the patient has loosened any tight clothing, is comfortable, and is in the proper position. Apply the nose clip.
13. Have the patient perform the first maneuver, coaching when necessary.
14. Determine whether the maneuver is acceptable.
15. Offer feedback to the patient and recommendations for improvement if necessary.
16. Have the patient perform additional maneuvers until three acceptable maneuvers are obtained.
17. Record the procedure in the patient's chart, and place the chart and the test results on the physician's desk for interpretation.
18. Ask the patient to remain until the physician reviews the results.

### Rationale

The physician may want to speak with the patient regarding results or may want to order additional testing.

19. Properly dispose of used materials and disposable instruments.
20. Sanitize and disinfect patient tubing and reusable mouthpiece and nose clip.
21. Clean and disinfect the equipment and room according to OSHA guidelines.

Review the conditions and activities with patients again on the day of the test to ensure that none apply. If there are no contraindications, weigh and measure patients. Use simple terms to explain the procedure and its purpose. Have them loosen tight clothing so they will be comfortable and their breathing will not be restricted in any way. The procedure is performed with patients sitting down. Make sure their legs are not crossed and that both feet are flat on the floor.

Explain that they need to wear a nose clip or hold the nose tightly closed to be sure that they will inhale and exhale through the mouth. The mouthpiece of the unit may be a disposable cardboard tube or a reusable rubber one that can be disinfected after use. If disposable mouthpieces are used, instruct patients to avoid biting down on them, because that will obstruct the flow of air. Be sure patients form a tight seal around the mouthpiece with their lips. Dentures normally help maintain a tight seal; however, they should be removed if they hinder the process.

**Proper Positioning.** Instruct patients to keep their chin and neck in the correct position during the procedure. The chin should be slightly elevated and the neck slightly extended. Bending the chin to the chest tends to restrict the flow of air and should be avoided (Figure 39-28). Some bending at the waist is acceptable.

**Explaining and Demonstrating the Procedure.** Tell patients to take the deepest breath possible, insert the mouthpiece into the mouth, form a tight seal, and then blow into the mouthpiece as hard and as fast as possible to completely exhale. Tell them to exhale as long as they can to force air from the lungs. Remind them that the initial force of their exhalation must be strong to get a valid reading. Demonstrate the procedure to show how the test is done correctly.

## Performing the Maneuver

You can improve patients' performance during the maneuver by actively and forcefully coaching them. Urge patients to blow hard and to continue blowing. After a maneuver, give them feedback on their performance, and indicate corrective actions they can take to improve the next maneuver.

Some spirometers indicate whether a particular maneuver was of adequate force and duration to be measured. Adequate force does not, however, indicate that the maneuver was acceptable. An acceptable maneuver must have the following five features:

1. No coughing, particularly during the first second
2. A quick and forceful start
3. An adequate length of time (a minimum of 6 seconds)
4. A consistent and fast flow with no variability
5. Consistency with other maneuvers

Spirometry tracings plot volume and time. You will need to obtain three acceptable maneuvers, which may require more than three attempts. Observe the patient for

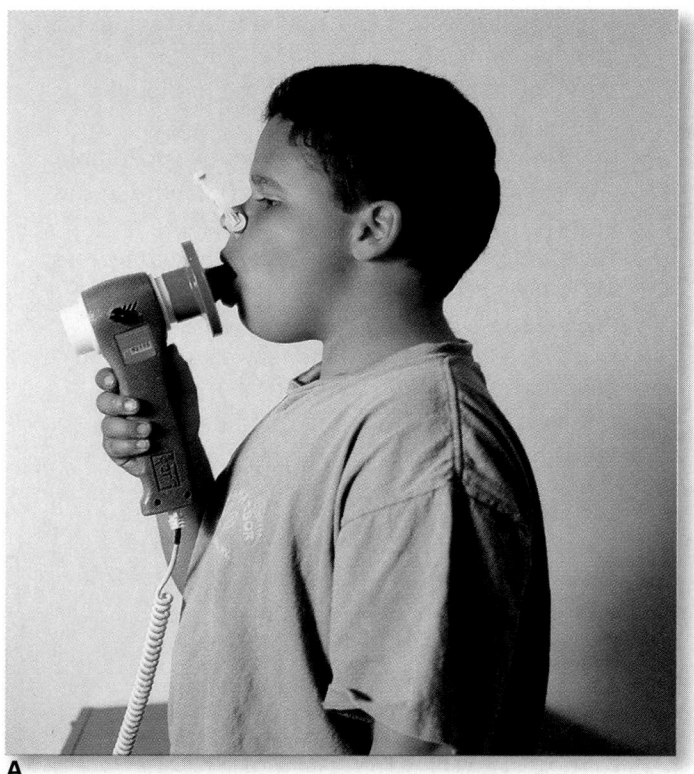

A

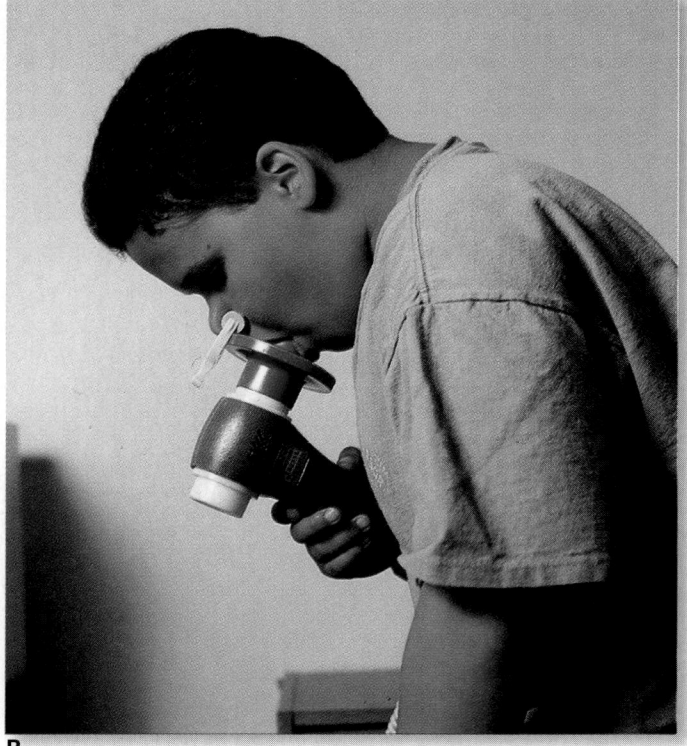

B

**Figure 39-28.** The patient must maintain the proper position during a pulmonary function test: (A) The chin should be slightly elevated and the neck slightly extended. (B) The chin should not approach the chest.

signs of breathing difficulty, dizziness, light-headedness, or changes in pulse and blood pressure. If necessary, allow the patient to rest briefly before continuing. Notify the physician immediately if symptoms are severe.

**Determining the Effectiveness of Medication.** Spirometry is often used to determine the effectiveness of certain medications that a patient is taking. You will perform two sets of maneuvers if this determination is required. Instruct the patient to refrain from taking the prescribed medication on the day of the test. Before performing the test, confirm that the patient has followed this instruction. Conduct the first set of maneuvers, ensuring that they are acceptable. After obtaining the results, instruct the patient to take the prescribed medication. Allow the medication to take effect, and then perform a second set of maneuvers. Comparing the two sets of readings shows whether the medication has effectively improved the patient's lung function. Some computerized spirometers can graph both sets of readings together to simplify the comparison (Figure 39-29).

**Special Considerations.** On occasion you may have to deal with an uncooperative patient, one who cannot understand or follow directions, or one who cannot perform the procedure. In these situations patience and skill are essential to obtaining an acceptable spirometry tracing.

The doctor may be able to convince an uncooperative patient to perform the maneuver. You can help by taking a no-nonsense approach, perhaps stating that the doctor needs these test results to help the patient. Patients who cannot understand or follow directions—the very young, the very old, those who have limited proficiency in English, or those with a hearing impairment—may need extra attention and patience to obtain acceptable results. Explain the procedure in simple terms, and repeat instructions as necessary. If, after eight attempts, the patient is unable to perform the procedure, stop and report the situation to the doctor.

## The Importance of Calibration

Spirometers should be calibrated each day they are used to ensure accurate readings. You may be required to perform this procedure. Calibration of a spirometer requires the use of a standardized measuring instrument called a **calibration syringe** (Figure 39-30). When the plunger is pulled back, this syringe contains a fixed volume of air. Connect the syringe to the patient tubing (the tubing that runs from the mouthpiece to the machine), and depress the plunger to inject the entire volume of air. The reading on the spirometer should be within 3 % of the stated volume. It is important to keep a calibration logbook for each spirometer.

While calibrating the spirometer, you can detect leaks by checking the volume/time graph. The volume should remain at a steady reading. If the volume declines with time, there is a leak somewhere in the system.

## Infection Control

After a patient completes the pulmonary function test, you must clean the spirometer and other pulmonary function devices thoroughly to prevent transmission of microorganisms. If disposable mouthpieces and nose clips are used, discard them in a biohazardous waste container. If reusable mouthpieces and nose clips are used, clean and disinfect them between patients. Also change patient tubing between patients. Thoroughly clean and disinfect patient tubing before reusing it. Most important, wash your hands thoroughly before and after performing a pulmonary function test.

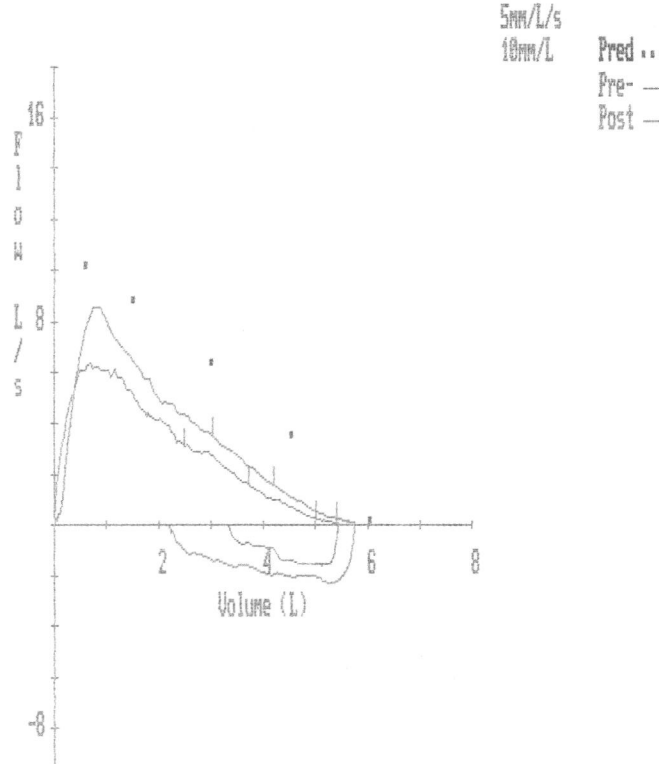

**Figure 39-29.** These spirometry tracings show air volume per second before and after use of a medication.

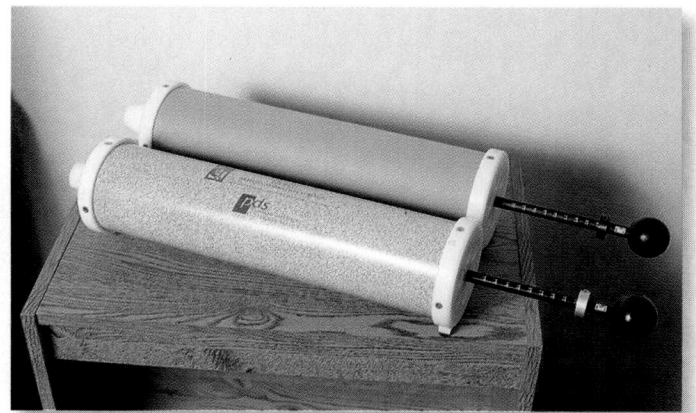

**Figure 39-30.** A calibration syringe delivers a fixed volume of air.

## What the Results Reveal

Pulmonary function tests help the doctor evaluate ventilatory function of the lungs and chest wall. They are good screening tools for pulmonary disorders, such as pulmonary edema, chronic obstructive pulmonary disease, and asthma. These tests also help the doctor determine the nature of a patient's disorder, such as narrowing or obstruction of the airways. Pulmonary function tests can determine the severity of a patient's problem and response to therapy or medication.

## Peak Expiratory Flow Rate (PEFR)

A peak expiratory flow rate (PEFR) is a measurement taken to determine the amount of air that can be quickly forced from the lungs. A peak flow meter is often used to obtain a PEFR. A peak flow meter is a small handheld device that can be used in the medical office or the patient's home (Figure 39-31). Patients who suffer from asthma are commonly asked to monitor their asthma by using a peak flow meter and recording their results. During an asthma flare-up, the large airways of the lungs begin to narrow. This narrowing slows the speed of air leaving the lungs. A peak flow meter, when used properly, can reveal narrowing of the airways in advanced of an asthma attack. Peak flow meters can help determine:

- When to seek emergency medical care
- The effectiveness of an asthma management treatment plan

- When to stop or add medication as directed by a physician
- Asthma triggers, such as stress or exercise

Procedure 39-4 explains the procedure of obtaining a peak expiratory rate using a peak flow meter.

## Peak Flow Zones

After obtaining a peak expiratory flow rate, the type of patient care given will be determined based on the individual's results. The physician will instruct the patient about the peak flow zones and how to respond to each zone. Peak flow zones are different for each patient and will be determined by the physician. The three peak flow zones are green, yellow, and red (Figure 39-32).

**Green Zone.** The green zone indicates good control of asthma, with peak flow rates of 80% to 100% of the highest peak flow rate. Measurements in this zone indicate that air moves well through the large airways and that the patient's usual activities can be continued.

**Yellow Zone.** Peak flow rates in the yellow zone range from 50% to 80% of the highest peak flow rate. Measurements in the yellow zone indicate that the large airways are beginning to narrow and medication is needed. Patient symptoms include tiredness and tightening of the chest.

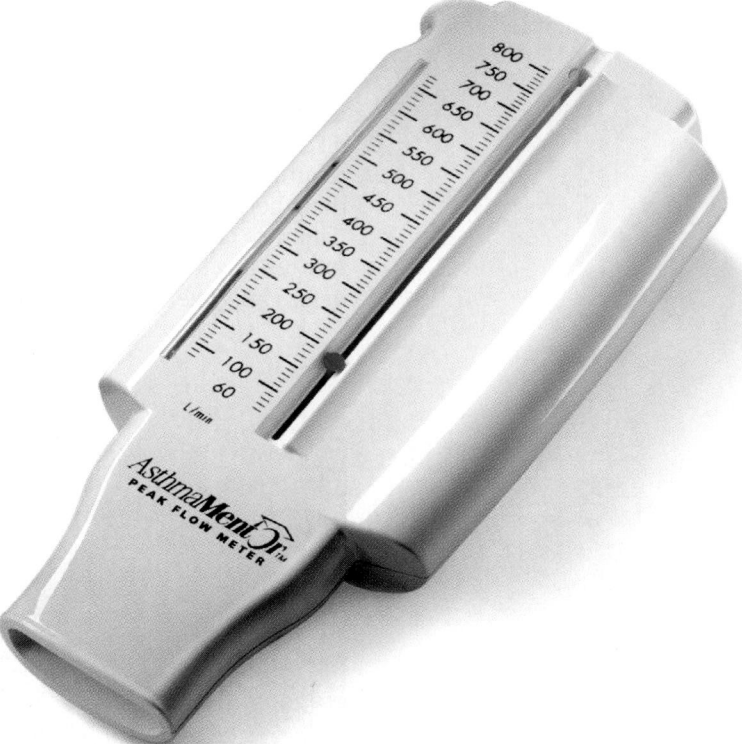

**Figure 39-31.** Peak expiratory flow meter markings will determine the patient's treatment based on accurate readings.

# PROCEDURE 39.4

## Obtaining a Peak Expiratory Flow Rate

**Procedure Goal:** To determine a patient's peak expiratory flow rate

### OSHA Guidelines

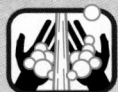 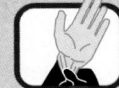  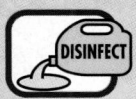 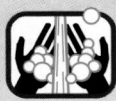

**Materials:** Peak flow meter, disposable mouthpiece

### Method:

1. Assemble all necessary equipment and supplies for the test.
2. Wash your hands and identify the patient.
3. Explain and demonstrate the procedure to the patient.

### Rationale

Patient education and understanding is crucial for getting accurate test results.

4. Position the patient in a sitting or standing position with good posture. Make sure that any chewing gum or food is removed from the patient's mouth.
5. Set the indicator to zero.

### Rationale

Helps to ensure accurate results.

6. Ensure that the disposable mouthpiece is securely placed onto the peak flow meter.
7. Hold the peak flow meter with the gauge uppermost and ensure that your fingers are away from the gauge.

8. Instruct patient to take as deep a breath as possible.
9. Instruct the patient to place the mouthpiece into her mouth and close her lips tightly around the mouthpiece, sealing her lips around the mouthpiece.
10. Instruct the patient to blow out as fast and as hard as possible.

### Rationale

A fast blast is better than a slow blow.

11. Observe the reading where the arrowhead is on the indicator.
12. Reset the indicator to zero and repeat the procedure two times, for a total of three readings. You will know the technique is correct if the reading results are close. If coughing occurs during the procedures, repeat the step.
13. Document the readings into the patient's chart. The highest reading will be peak flow rate.

### Rationale

The highest reading represents the personal best reading for the patient, and future measurements are based upon this result. Do not average the results.

14. Dispose of mouthpiece in a biohazardous waste container.
15. Disinfect or dispose of the peak flow meter per office policy.
16. Wash your hands.

---

**Red Zone.** Peak flow rates in the red zone are less than 50% of the highest or best personal reading recorded. Narrowing of the largest airways has occurred and is considered a medical emergency and medical treatment should be sought right away. Patients are usually directed to take a bronchodilator or other medication that will open the airway and call their physician. Patient symptoms include wheezing, shortness of breath, and trouble walking and talking.

## Pulse Oximetry

Pulse oximetry is a non-invasive test that measures the saturation of oxygen in a patient's arterial blood. A sensor is placed on a patient's finger, earlobe, toe, or bridge of the nose (Figure 39-33). A red infrared light is shone through one side of the appendage to the other. The amount of light absorbed by the hemoglobin is detected using a pulse oximeter. Any reading less than 95% indicates hypoxemia (low blood oxygen). Pulse oximetry is performed on patients with pulmonary or cardiac conditions, and during post-operative patient observation. It is also used to help diagnose **sleep apnea,** a condition characterized by pauses in breathing during sleep. The pauses are often long enough to cause a drop in blood oxygen levels. Some medications after surgery can slow down breathing rates and it is important that their blood oxygen levels be carefully monitored. Procedure 39-5 explains the procedure of obtaining a pulse oximetry reading.

## The Peak Flow Zone System

**% Personal Best**

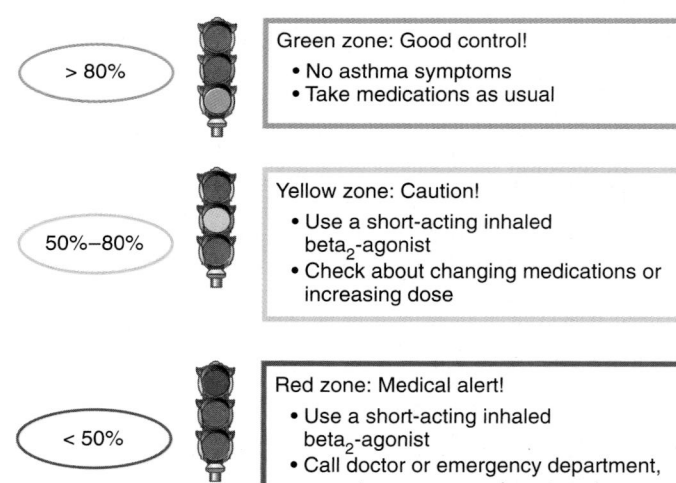

> 80%

**Green zone: Good control!**
- No asthma symptoms
- Take medications as usual

50%–80%

**Yellow zone: Caution!**
- Use a short-acting inhaled beta₂-agonist
- Check about changing medications or increasing dose

< 50%

**Red zone: Medical alert!**
- Use a short-acting inhaled beta₂-agonist
- Call doctor or emergency department, or go to emergency department

**Figure 39-32.** The peak flow zone system alerts patients about when to seek medical treatment.

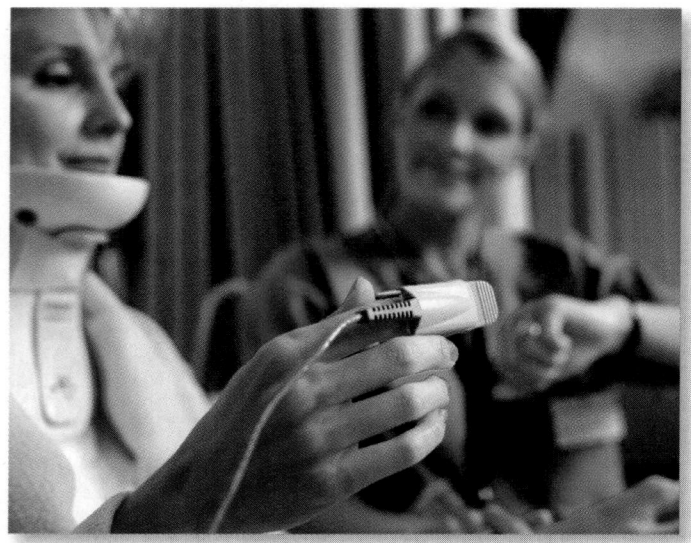

**Figure 39-33.** A pulse oximeter is a portable, handheld device used by many medical facilities.

# PROCEDURE 39.5

## Obtaining a Pulse Oximetry Reading

**Procedure Goal:** To obtain a pulse oximetry reading

### OSHA Guidelines

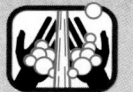 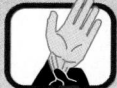  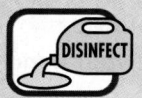 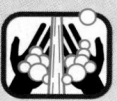

**Materials:** Pulse oximeter

### Method:

1. Assemble all the necessary equipment and supplies.
2. Wash your hands and correctly identify the patient.
3. Select the appropriate site to apply the sensor to by assessing capillary refill in the patient's toe or finger.

   *Rationale*

   If the patient has poor circulation in his fingers or toes, use the bridge of his nose or an earlobe.

4. Prepare the selected site, removing nail polish or earrings if necessary. Wipe the selected site with alcohol and allow it to air dry.

   *Rationale*

   Nail polish can alter the test results.

5. Attach the sensor to the site (if a finger is used, placed in the clip).
6. Instruct the patient to breathe normally.
7. Attach the sensor cable to the oximeter. Turn on the oximeter and listen to the tone.
8. Set the alarm limits for high and low oxygen saturations and high and low pulse rates as directed by the physician's order and turn on the oximeter.
9. Read the saturation level and document it in the patient's chart. Report to the physician readings that are less than 95%. Manually check the patient's pulse and compare it to the pulse oximeter. Document all the readings and the application site in the patient's medical chart.
10. Wash your hands.
11. Rotate the patient's finger sites every four hours if using a pulse oximeter long-term.

# Summary

Electrocardiography and pulmonary function testing play a vital role in the diagnosis and treatment of cardiac and pulmonary disease. As a medical assistant, you may be required to perform these procedures in the medical office.

To understand electrocardiography, you need to know the basics of the conduction system of the heart and the components of an electrocardiograph. To obtain accurate electrocardiogram readings, you must properly place the electrodes and be able to recognize artifacts and correct them.

Likewise, to provide accurate assessments of pulmonary function, you must use proper technique and recognize the acceptability of a spirometric maneuver, peak expiratory flow, and pulse oximetry. Because patient compliance is crucial for accurate results, effective patient education is vital to the process.

# REVIEW

## CHAPTER 39

## CASE STUDY QUESTIONS

Now that you have completed this chapter, review the case study at the beginning of the chapter and answer the following questions:

1. What does the abbreviation ECG stand for? What is the diagnostic value of the ECG?
2. What is another name for a spirometry? What does FVC designate?
3. Why were the Holter monitor and stress tests ordered for this patient?

## Discussion Questions

1. Describe the zone systems related to peak expiratory flow and why it is important for the patient to understand each zone.
2. For what reasons might a physician order an electrocardiogram?
3. Describe where to place the six precordial chest leads.
4. List the placement sites for pulse oximetry testing.

## Critical Thinking Questions

1. For what reasons could a wandering ECG baseline occur? What are the solutions for these problems?
2. Stress testing is often ordered for patients suspected of having cardiac problems. Are there special precautions to consider for these patients, and if so, what are they?
3. What conditions or activities could affect the accuracy of a pulmonary function test?
4. What is meant by forced vital capacity?
5. Why is patient education important when using a peak expiratory flow meter?

## Application Activities

1. Practice obtaining ECGs on volunteers from the class. Practice confidentiality and maintain patient modesty during practice ECGs.
2. Explain to another student how to use and care for a Holter monitor.
3. Practice explaining and demonstrating the procedure of obtaining a forced vital capacity to someone who is not familiar with the procedure.
4. Practice obtaining and documenting a pulse oximetry test.
5. Practice obtaining and documenting a peak expiratory flow rate.

## Virtual Fieldtrip

*Visit the McGraw-Hill Higher Education Medical Assisting website at www.mhhe.com/medicalassisting3 to complete the following activity:*

Access the American Heart Association website and research the warning signs of heart attack, stroke, or cardiac arrest. Create an information poster that can be used at a health fair. The information should include the warning signs of and appropriate actions taken during heart attack, stroke, or cardiac arrest.

Open the CD and complete this chapter's practice activities, play the games, listen to the key terms, and test yourself with the interactive review. Email, print, and/or save your results to document your proficiency.

## CHAPTER 40

# X-Rays and Diagnostic Radiology

## MEDICAL ASSISTING COMPETENCIES

*In preparation for the certification examination, you should know the following areas of competence:*

| COMPETENCY | CMA | RMA |
|---|---|---|
| **Administrative** | | |
| Schedule and oversee appointments | X | X |
| Schedule inpatient and outpatient admissions and procedures | X | X |
| Prepare, organize, and maintain medical records | X | X |
| File medical records | X | X |
| **Clinical** | | |
| Apply principles of aseptic techniques and infection control, including hand washing | X | X |
| Perform telephone and in-person screening | X | X |
| Interview the patient to obtain and record the patient's history | X | X |
| Prepare the patient for and assist the physician with routine and specialty exams, treatments, and minor office surgeries | X | X |
| Screen and follow up on patient test results | X | X |
| **General/Legal/Professional** | | |
| Identify and respond to issues of confidentiality by maintaining confidentiality at all times and following appropriate guidelines when releasing records or information | X | X |
| Be aware of and perform within legal and ethical boundaries | X | X |
| Determine the needs for documentation and reporting, and document accurately and appropriately | X | X |
| Instruct individuals according to their needs | X | X |
| Conduct work within scope of education, training, and ability | | X |
| Be impartial and show empathy when dealing with patients | | X |
| Serve as a liaison between the physician and others | | X |
| Interview effectively | | X |
| Use appropriate medical terminology | | X |
| Receive, organize, prioritize, and transmit information appropriately | | X |

## KEY TERMS

arthrography
barium enema
barium swallow
brachytherapy
cholangiography
contrast medium
diagnostic radiology
intravenous pyelography (IVP)
invasive
KUB radiography
mammography
MUGA scan
myelography
noninvasive
nuclear medicine
PET
radiation therapy
retrograde pyelography
SPECT
stereoscopy
teletherapy
thermography
ultrasound
xeroradiography

# CHAPTER OUTLINE

# LEARNING OUTCOMES

# Introduction

Diagnostic radiology has evolved immensely since the discovery of the simple x-ray beam. It has become a valuable screening and clinical diagnosis tool for physicians. In this chapter, you will learn the basics of noninvasive and invasive radiology as well as your role as a medical assistant in this testing. Safety issues for the administration of radiologic testing are discussed, as is the proper handling and storage of the actual films. In addition, you learn about preparing and instructing patients for the more common radiology procedures.

## CASE STUDY

A 42-year-old woman has arrived at the office for her annual physical, part of which involves scheduling her to have a mammogram performed. The patient completes the procedure, which comes back revealing a small, abnormal density. The physician asks you to schedule the patient for a CT scan of the breast, which also reveals an abnormal mass. The patient decides that she wants to be more aggressive in determining if the small mass is cancerous, so you now schedule a mammotest, which is used to determine that the mass is benign with no evidence of cancer.

As you read this chapter, consider the following questions:

1. What special instructions should be given to the patient before her mammogram?
2. How is a CT scan performed?
3. When preparing a patient for a CT scan, what allergies should be disclosed during the patient interview?
4. Why was a mammotest requested by the physician?
5. What education requirements must you fulfill in order to work as a radiographer/sonographer?

# Brief History of the X-Ray

In 1895 Wilhelm Konrad Roentgen (1845–1923) discovered the x-ray, or roentgen ray, a type of electromagnetic wave. It has a high energy level, traveling at the speed of light (186,000 miles per second), and an extremely short wavelength (one-billionth of an inch) that can penetrate solid objects. X-rays react with photographic film to produce a permanent record (x-ray, or radiograph). The x-ray image is lightest where the film is struck by the most x-ray energy. Differences in tissue densities produce the x-ray image, with the least dense being lightest and the most dense being darkest on the film.

Today there are both diagnostic and therapeutic uses for x-rays and radioactive substances. Radiologic technologists are trained medical personnel who are certified to perform certain radiologic procedures upon completion of a radiology curriculum lasting 2 to 4 years. Some radiologic technologists receive further training in radiology subspecialties, such as ultrasound, mammography, magnetic resonance imaging, and nuclear medicine. Radiographers, sonographers, radiation therapists, and nuclear medicine technologists are all radiologic technologists. Invasive radiologic procedures or procedures requiring a high degree of expertise are nearly always performed by a radiologist, a physician who specializes in radiology. A radiologist is also the physician who interprets the films for other physicians. Other specialists who perform radiologic procedures, either alone or with the assistance of a radiologist, include cardiologists, orthopedists, obstetricians, and oncologists.

## Diagnostic Radiology

**Diagnostic radiology** is the use of x-ray technology for diagnostic purposes. Radiologic tests sometimes use contrast media as well as special techniques or instruments for viewing internal body structures and functions. A **contrast medium** is a substance that makes internal organs denser and blocks the passage of x-rays to the photographic film. Introducing contrast media into certain structures or areas of the body can provide a clearer image of organs and tissues and indications of how well they are functioning. Contrast media include gases (air, oxygen, or carbon dioxide), heavy metal salts (barium sulfate or bismuth carbonate), and iodine compounds. They can be administered orally, parenterally (for example, intravenously), or by routes that introduce them into an organ or body cavity (for example, by insertion). Types of diagnostic imaging include x-rays, computed tomography (CT), nuclear medicine, magnetic resonance imaging (MRI), and ultrasound.

### Invasive Procedures

Diagnostic tests can be invasive or noninvasive. An **invasive** procedure (such as angiography) requires a radiologist to insert a catheter, wire, or other testing device into a patient's blood vessel or organ through the skin or a body orifice. All invasive tests require surgical aseptic technique. Some procedures, including angiography, are performed in a hospital or same-day surgical facility. The patient may need general anesthesia for some procedures. The anesthetist must closely monitor the patient who is under anesthesia during and after the test for life-threatening complications, such as anaphylaxis.

### Noninvasive Procedures

**Noninvasive** procedures, such as standard x-rays or ultrasonography, use other technologies to view internal structures. They do not require inserting devices, breaking the

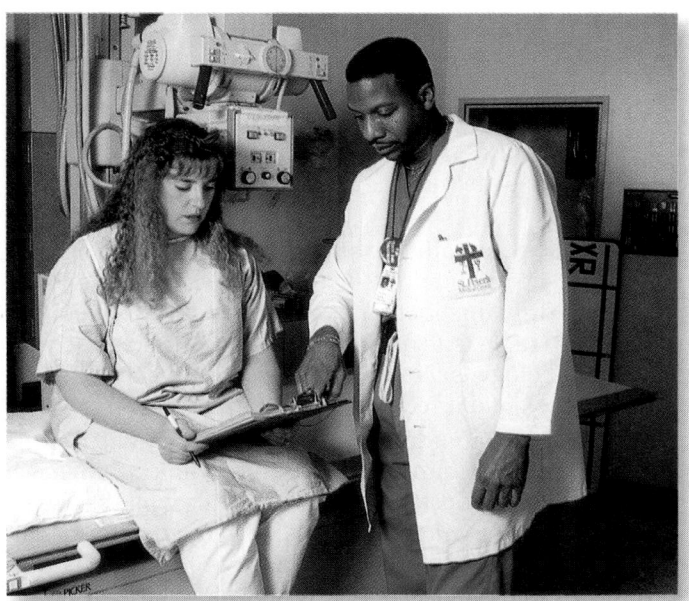

**Figure 40-1.** A standard x-ray is one of the most frequently performed radiologic tests.

skin, or the degree of monitoring needed with invasive procedures.

The most familiar equipment used for diagnostic imaging is the conventional x-ray machine, as shown in Figure 40-1. This machine consists of a table, an x-ray tube, a control panel, and a high-voltage generator. Other equipment used for diagnostic radiology includes instruments specifically designed for the test. Examples are a mammography unit, a scanner for CT, and a transducer for ultrasound.

## The Medical Assistant's Role in Diagnostic Radiology

You may work with diagnostic radiology in a radiology facility or in a medical office. Your duties in a radiology facility will include assisting a radiologic technologist or a radiologist in performing diagnostic radiologic procedures. Depending on the scope of practice in your state, you may be allowed to learn how to operate certain x-ray equipment. Even if you are not allowed to assist with an x-ray procedure or to operate x-ray equipment, you will probably provide preprocedure and postprocedure care of the patient. Your duties in a medical facility, such as an orthopedic office, may include assisting a radiologic technologist in performing x-ray procedures. In an obstetric practice, you might assist a physician in performing an ultrasound examination of a pregnant woman. Even if you work in a medical office that does not perform radiologic testing, you must still provide a certain amount of preprocedure care and education. In order to properly explain a test to a patient and to assist a radiologic technologist or radiologist in performing a test, you must have a basic understanding of x-ray technology. You may also need in-service training to ensure accuracy and patient safety for some procedures.

## Preprocedure Care

Preprocedure care varies somewhat, depending on the test. In general, however, you may do the following:

- Schedule the patient's appointment, if necessary. Inform the patient of the location, date, and time of the procedure.
- Provide preparation instructions. Advise the patient about diet restrictions or requirements (such as fasting or drinking liquids) as well as medication requirements (such as taking a laxative). Always check with the radiology facility for specific requirements, and be sure the patient receives this information.
- Explain the procedure to the patient briefly and clearly. Use proper terminology and non-technical language. Reinforce the doctor's reason for requesting the procedure, and provide any available written information about the test. Inform the patient about the length of the examination, about possible side effects or safety precautions and warnings, and about injections or uncomfortable steps. Check for clarity and understanding by using the mirroring communication technique when communicating with the patient. You must ensure the patient understands the preprocedure directions.
- Ask pertinent questions. Obtain a medication history from the patient (current medications could interfere with some procedures). If the patient is a woman of childbearing age, ask whether she is pregnant or whether there is any chance she could be pregnant. Report the answers to the physician in a medical office or to the radiologic technologist in a radiology facility.

## Care During and After the Procedure

If you work in a radiology facility, your responsibilities include preparing and guiding the patient through the procedure. You may also assist the radiologic technologist or the radiologist in performing the procedure by placing, removing, and developing film in the x-ray machine. Procedure 40-1 describes the general process of assisting with a radiologic procedure.

You may care for a patient and assist the radiologic technologist or radiologist during a wide variety of x-ray and other diagnostic imaging tests. Although requirements vary depending on the procedure, you will probably be asked to perform many of the duties described in Procedure 40-1. Although you are unlikely to position the patient, you should know that the position relative to the x-ray source determines the path of the x-rays and the sorts of images that result. Figure 40-2 illustrates common x-ray pathways and the images produced.

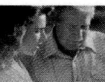

## Educating the Patient

### Providing Patient Instruction for Radiologic Procedures

It is crucial for patients to thoroughly understand the pre- and postprocedural instructions because accurate and focused diagnoses depend on correct radiology images. Provide patient instructions orally, observing for understanding and soliciting feedback from the patient. Follow the oral instructions with written instructions. Review the written instructions and encourage questions to clarify patient understanding. A collection of instructions for common radiological tests ordered by your facility can be obtained from the radiology facility that is most frequently used by the facility. Keep a library of patient instructions for a variety of diagnostic procedures.

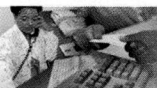

## Points on Practice

### Verifying Insurance for Radiologic Procedures

Managed care health insurance plans are the most common type of insurance you will encounter in the office. Managed care plans often have facilities in which they are contracted. Patients with HMOs are often required to use the services of certain radiology facilities. Ensure that the patient is sent to a radiology facility that is contracted with their health insurance. If needed, verify and complete the necessary referrals for all radiology testing. Make insurance verification a regular step in preprocedure care.

# PROCEDURE 40.1

## Assisting With an X-Ray Examination

**Procedure Goal:** To assist with a radiologic procedure under the supervision of a radiologic technologist

**OSHA Guidelines:** This procedure does not involve exposure to blood, body fluids, or tissue. You must wear a radiation exposure badge (dosimeter), however, and will be required to wear a garment containing a lead shield if you remain in the room during the operation of x-ray equipment

**Materials:** X-ray examination order, x-ray machine, x-ray film and holder, x-ray film developer, drape, patient shield

**Method:**

1. Check the x-ray examination order and equipment needed.
2. Identify the patient and introduce yourself.
3. Determine whether the patient has complied with the preprocedure instructions. Do not depend on the patient to inform you, but ask the patient if and how they prepped for the procedure.

### Rationale

If a patient has not been compliant with preprocedural directions, then the test ordered may not be as effective as it should and will need to be rescheduled.

4. Explain the procedure and the purpose of the examination to the patient.
5. Instruct the patient to remove clothing and all metals (including jewelry) as needed, according to body area to be examined, and to put on a gown. Explain that metals may interfere with the image. Ask whether the patient has any surgical metal or a pacemaker, and report this information to the radiologic technologist. Leave the room to ensure patient privacy.

*Note:* Steps 6 through 11 are nearly always performed by a radiologic technologist.

6. Position the patient according to the x-ray view ordered.
7. Drape the patient and place the patient shield appropriately.
8. Instruct the patient about the need to remain still and to hold the breath when requested.
9. Leave the room or stand behind a lead shield during the exposure.
10. Ask the patient to assume a comfortable position while the films are developed. Explain that x-rays sometimes must be repeated.
11. Develop the films.
12. Determine if the x-ray films are satisfactory by allowing the radiologist to review the films.

### Rationale

The radiologist may want another film or view.

13. Instruct the patient to dress and tell the patient when to contact the physician's office for the results.
14. Label the dry, finished x-ray films, place them in a properly labeled envelope, and file them according to the policies of your office.
15. Record the x-ray examination, along with the final written findings, in the patient's chart.

# Common Diagnostic Radiologic Tests

A variety of radiologic imaging tests are available. Table 40-1 identifies some of the most frequently ordered tests and the disorders they are used to diagnose.

## Contrast Media in Diagnostic Tests

Various procedures involve the use of contrast media to visualize body structures and observe their function. These procedures include angiography, arthrography, barium enema, barium swallow, cholangiography, cholecystography, cystography, fluoroscopy, intravenous pyelography, magnetic resonance imaging (sometimes), myelography, nuclear medicine studies, and retrograde pyelography.

As mentioned, contrast media can be administered by mouth, by needle or catheter into a blood vessel, or by a route that introduces the medium into an organ or body cavity (for example, into the colon). A contrast medium can cause adverse effects in some patients. Common adverse effects with oral agents include mild and transient abdominal cramping, constipation, nausea, vomiting, diarrhea, skin rashes, itching, heartburn, dizziness, and headache. Intravenous agents cause some of the same adverse effects as well as localized injection-site reactions and more serious reactions such as anaphylaxis. Because many contrast media contain iodine, a common allergen, patients should be questioned about known allergies to

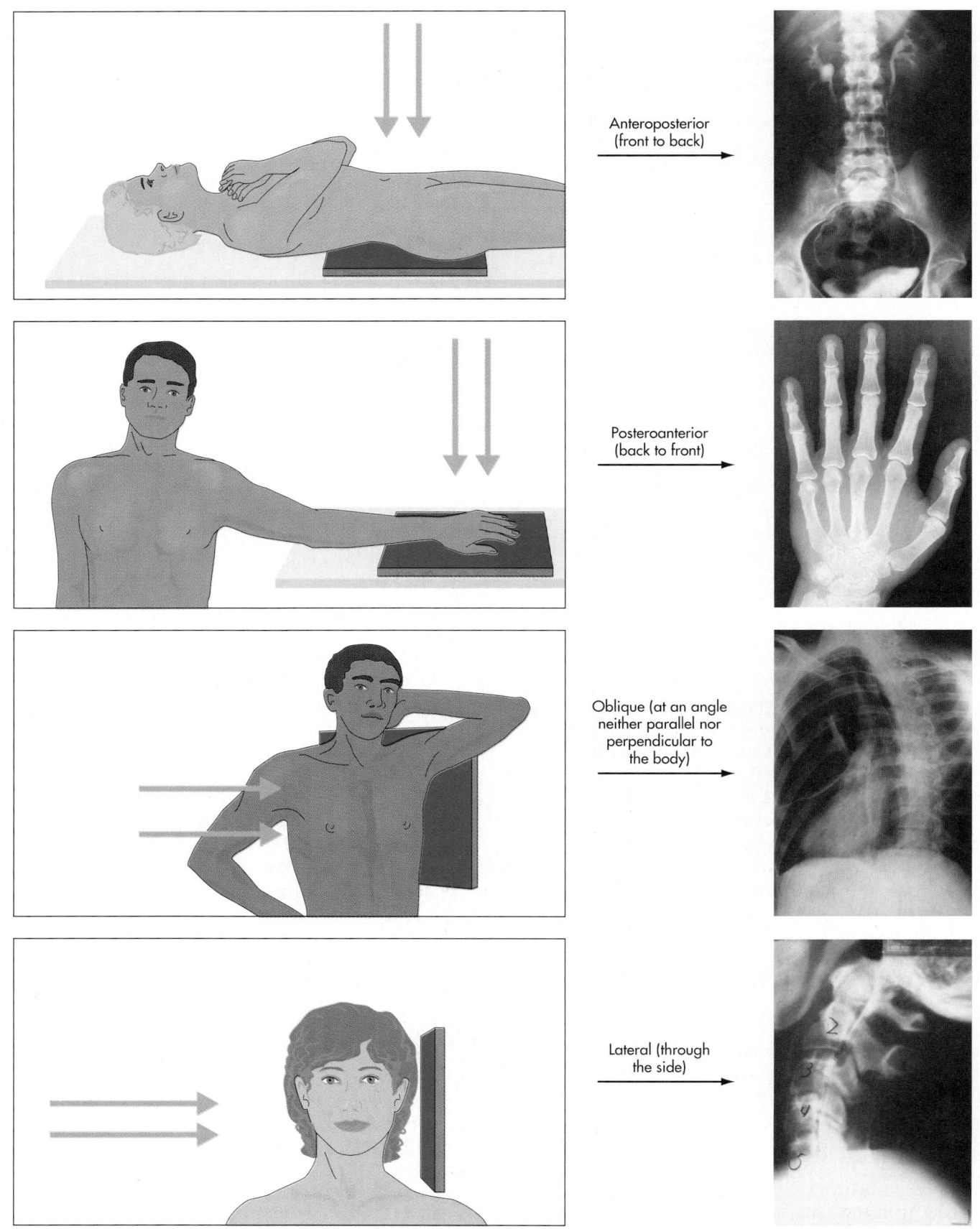

**Figure 40-2.** These are the x-ray pathways and resulting projections for the most common types of x-rays.

## TABLE 40-1  Common Radiologic Tests and Disorders Diagnosed

| Test | Disorders Diagnosed/Treated |
|---|---|
| Angiography | |
|   Cardiovascular | Status of blood flow, collateral circulation, malformed vessels, aneurysm, narrowing or blockages of vessels, presence of hemorrhage |
|   Cerebral | Aneurysm, hemorrhage, evidence of cerebrovascular accident, arteriosclerosis |
|   Gastrointestinal (GI) | Upper gastrointestinal bleeding |
|   Pulmonary | Pulmonary emboli (especially when lung scan is inconclusive), evaluation of pulmonary circulation in some heart conditions before surgery |
|   Renal | Abnormalities of blood vessels in urinary system |
| Arthrography | Joint conditions |
| Barium enema (lower GI series) | Obstructions, ulcers, polyps, diverticulosis, tumor, and motility problems of colon or rectum |
| Barium swallow (upper GI series) | Obstructions, ulcers, polyps, diverticulosis, tumor, and motility problems of esophagus, stomach, duodenum, and small intestine |
| Cholangiography, cholecystography | Gallstones, gallbladder or common bile duct stones or obstructions; ability of gallbladder to concentrate and store dye |
| Computed tomography (CT) | Aortic and heart aneurysms, disorders of liver and biliary systems, renal and pulmonary tumors, brain abnormalities (tumors, blood clots, evidence of cerebrovascular accident, outlines of brain ventricles), GI tract lesions, GI disorders (acute pseudocyst of pancreas, abdominal abscesses, biliary obstruction), breast diseases and disorders, spinal disorders; to guide biopsy procedures |
| Fluoroscopy | Structure, process, and function of organs in motion to detect abnormalities |
| Intravenous pyelography (IVP) (excretory urography) | Urinary system abnormalities, including renal pelvis, ureters, and bladder (for example, kidney stones); abnormal size, shape, or structure of kidneys, ureters, or bladder; space-occupying lesions; pyelonephrosis; hydronephrosis; trauma to the urinary system |
| KUB (kidneys, ureters, bladder) radiography | Size, shape, and position of urinary organs; urinary system diseases or disorders; kidney stones |
| Magnetic resonance imaging (MRI) | Cancerous tissue, atherosclerotic tissue, blood clots, tumors, and deformities, particularly of the heart valves, brain, spine, and joints |
| Mammography | Breast tumors and lesions |
| Myelography | Irregularities or compression of spinal cord |
| Nuclear medicine (radionuclide imaging) | Abnormal function (defects), lesions, or disorders of bone, brain, lungs, kidneys, liver, pancreas, thyroid, and spleen |
| Radiation therapy | Treatment of cancer |
| Retrograde pyelogram | Obstruction of ureters, bladder, or urethra (including tumors, stones, strictures, or blood clots); perinephritic abscess |
| Stereoscopy | Fractures, dense areas that indicate a tumor or increased pressure within the skull |
| Thermography | Breast tumors, breast abscesses, fibrocystic breast disease |
| Ultrasound | Abnormalities of gallbladder, liver, spleen, heart, kidneys, gonads, blood vessels, and lymph system; fetal conditions (including number of fetuses; age and sex of fetus; fetal development, position, and deformities) |
| Xeroradiography | Breast cancer, abscesses, lesions, calcifications |

iodine or shellfish, which contain iodine, before procedures involving the use of contrast media. All patients should be observed during such procedures for signs of allergic reaction.

## Fluoroscopy

X-rays can cause certain chemicals to fluoresce, or emit visible light. When x-rays penetrate a body structure and are directed onto a fluorescent screen, they produce an image the radiologist can view either directly or through special glasses. Usually, fluoroscopic procedures are performed by a radiologist rather than by a radiology technician or a medical assistant.

Many diagnostic procedures involve fluoroscopy, which allows viewing of internal organ movement or the movement of a contrast medium, such as barium sulfate, while the contrast medium travels through the alimentary canal. Fluoroscopy also guides the radiologist in locating a precise internal area that needs to be recorded on film or digitally.

Fluoroscopic images are sometimes photographed for further study. Photofluorography is a series of these photographs that records the body's internal movements over time. Cinefluorography is a motion picture of the images.

## Hysterosalpingography

Hysterosalpingography, also called uterosalpingography, is a radiologic examination of a women's uterus and fallopian tubes using fluoroscopy. Hysterosalpingography is used to examine women who have difficulty becoming pregnant. A hysterosalpingogram assists the radiologist to evaluate the shape and structure of the uterus, the openness (patency) of the fallopian tubes, and any scarring within the fallopian tubes and peritoneal cavity. Hysterosalpingography is sometimes ordered when the woman has a history of miscarriages that result from congenital abnormalities of the uterus or as part of a fertility exam. It is also used to determine the presence and severity of tumor masses or adhesions, uterine fibroids, and fallopian tube adhesions or obstructions. Hysterosalpingography is usually performed on an outpatient basis (Figure 40-3).

## Angiography

Angiography requires a physician (usually a radiologist) to insert a catheter into the patient's vein (venography) or artery (arteriography). The test may be performed jointly by a radiologist and a vascular surgeon or other specialist. The test is used to evaluate the vessels of the heart, (coronary angiography), the brain (cerebral angiography), and the femoral, brachial, or carotid artery. The physician guides the catheter tip to the vessel being examined. Then the physician injects a contrast medium through the catheter and takes a series of x-rays to assess the vessel's blood flow and condition (Figure 40-4).

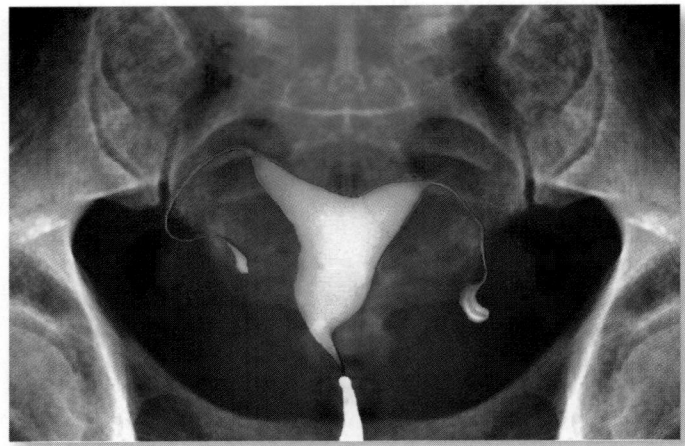

**Figure 40-3.** A hysterosalpingogram of the uterus and fallopian tubes.

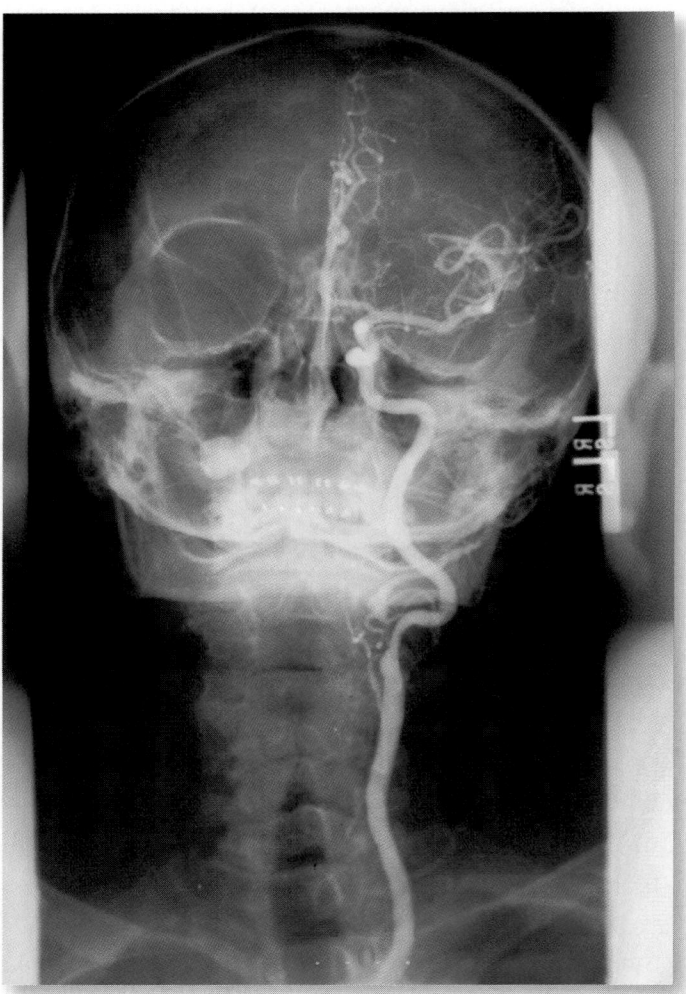

**Figure 40-4.** Carotid angiogram. In intra-arterial catheter is inserted and a contrast media is injected to create an image of the arteries.

Because this procedure requires insertion of a catheter into a blood vessel and the use of local anesthesia, the patient is admitted to a hospital or same-day surgical facility.

The physician who performs the examination provides the patient with instructions immediately before the procedure. You will, however, schedule the procedure, and you can encourage the patient to ask questions. Radiology facilities usually have information sheets for each procedure. If the patient has questions you cannot answer or if you have any doubt about preprocedure instructions, check with your supervisor.

## Arthrography

**Arthrography** is performed by a radiologist, who uses a contrast medium and fluoroscopy to help diagnose abnormalities or injuries in the cartilage, tendons, or ligaments of the joints—usually the knee or shoulder. When preparing patients for arthrography or assisting with the procedure, follow these guidelines:

- Describe the procedure to patients, and inform them that the examination will take about 1 hour. Ask patients about possible allergies to contrast media, iodine, or shellfish. If they have any of these allergies, inform the radiologist immediately.

- Explain to patients that no special preprocedure preparations are necessary.

- Tell patients the doctor will first inject a local anesthetic to numb the area being examined. Then the doctor will inject the contrast medium (dye, air, or both) into the joint and will use a fluoroscope to evaluate the joint's function. Inform patients who are having a knee examined that the doctor may ask them to walk a few steps to spread the contrast medium.

- After the test is completed, advise patients that for 1 or 2 days they may experience some pain or swelling, particularly if the joint is exercised. Tell them to rest and avoid putting strain on the joint.

## Barium Enema (Lower GI Series)

A **barium enema** is performed by a radiologist, who instills barium sulfate through the anus into the rectum and then into the colon, to help diagnose and evaluate obstructions, ulcers, polyps, diverticulosis, tumors, or motility problems of the colon or rectum. This procedure is called a lower GI (gastrointestinal) series, a series of x-rays of the colon and rectum. The two types of barium enema techniques are single-contrast, in which only barium is instilled into the colon, and double-contrast, in which air is forced into the colon to distend the tissue. The air may be added while the barium is present, after it has been expelled, or both. The double-contrast technique makes structures more visible by fluoroscopy and allows identification of small lesions. The digestive tract must be totally empty, requiring the patient to thoroughly cleanse the tract with a series of preparatory steps and to have nothing by mouth for 8 hours before the test, except for one cup of clear liquid on the morning of the test. In most facilities a radiologic technologist assists with a barium enema, but you may assist the patient before and after the procedure. If you do assist with a barium enema, you will have various responsibilities before, during, and after the procedure.

**Before the Procedure.** Include the following steps when you instruct a patient about the preparation for a barium enema:

- Schedule the patient's appointment in the morning so he can sleep through most of the period during which his digestive tract must be empty and thus avoid experiencing hunger unnecessarily.

- Describe the procedure to the patient, and tell him the examination will take 1 to 2 hours. Ask about possible allergies to contrast media, iodine, or shellfish, and report such allergies to the radiologist.

- Explain to the patient the importance of following the preparation instructions so the colon and rectum are free of residual material. (Residual material in the colon or rectum could cause blockages or shadows, resulting in an inaccurate test.) Preprocedure preparation on the day before the examination includes following an clear liquid diet beginning in the morning (coffee, tea, carbonated beverages, clear gelatin, strained fruit juice, bouillon, or clear broths; milk is not permitted) and taking prescribed amounts of electrolyte solution or other laxative preparations and fluids on a specified schedule. Tell the patient he may have one cup of coffee, tea, or water on the morning of the examination.

**During the Procedure.** Follow these steps when assisting during a barium enema:

- Have the patient undress and put on a gown.

- Tell the patient to expect some discomfort during the examination, as well as frequent side-to-side turning.

- Have the patient lie on his side. The radiologist inserts the enema tip, which is designed to help the patient hold the liquid, into the rectum and instills the barium sulfate into the colon. If the patient experiences cramping or the urge to defecate during instillation of the barium, instruct him to relax the abdominal muscles by breathing slowly and deeply through the mouth.

- Instruct the patient to remain still and hold his breath when x-rays are taken. Using a fluoroscope, the doctor observes the barium as it flows through the lower bowel and periodically takes x-rays while the patient is placed in various positions. You may be asked to assist with placing the patient in these positions.

- Tell the patient if a double-contrast study is being performed. Explain that air will be introduced into the colon to expand the colon tissue. Also tell the patient that the combination of air and barium provides a clearer view of structures than only one contrast medium would provide and allows possible identification of small lesions if they are present.

- Tell the patient that when the doctor has completed the barium portion of the examination, including x-rays with both barium and air, the patient should use the toilet and expel as much barium as possible. Explain that if enough barium is expelled, the doctor may take a final x-ray of the empty colon.
- Have the patient wait to dress until the doctor tells you that no additional x-rays are needed.

**After the Procedure.** After the radiologist has completed the barium enema, instruct the patient in postprocedure care. Tell the patient the following:

- He may now have a regular meal.
- The residual barium may make his stools appear whitish or lighter than usual, but this is normal.
- The barium may cause constipation, so he should drink extra water to help relieve constipation and to eliminate remaining barium sulfate. The physician may order a laxative to be taken if constipation is not relieved within 1 or 2 days.

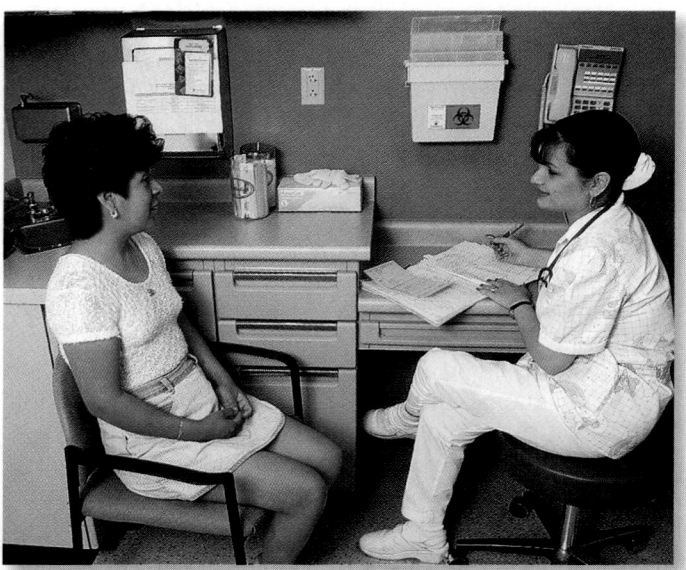

**Figure 40-5.** Preprocedure instruction is essential to a successful barium swallow procedure.

## Barium Swallow (Upper GI Series)

A **barium swallow** involves oral administration of a barium sulfate drink to help diagnose and evaluate obstructions, ulcers, polyps, diverticulosis, tumors, or motility problems of the esophagus, stomach, duodenum, and small intestine. This test is called an upper GI series. In preparation for this test, the patient can have nothing by mouth for at least 8 hours before the test. You will have various responsibilities before, during, and after the procedure.

**Before the Procedure.** When instructing a patient about the preparation for an upper GI series (Figure 40-5), include the following steps:

- Schedule the patient's appointment in the morning so she can sleep through most of the period during which her digestive tract is empty and thus avoid experiencing hunger unnecessarily.
- Describe the procedure to the patient, and tell her the examination will take about 1 hour. If x-rays of the small bowel are needed, the test may take several hours. Ask about possible allergies to contrast media, iodine, or shellfish, and report such allergies to the radiologist.
- Explain to the patient the importance of following the preparation instructions so that the stomach is empty. Preprocedure requirements include having nothing by mouth (food or liquids) after midnight the night before the examination and no breakfast the morning of the examination. If the patient's small bowel is to be evaluated, also tell her to take the prescribed laxative preparation between 2:00 and 4:00 P.M. the day before the examination.
- Instruct the patient not to swallow water when brushing her teeth or rinsing her mouth and, if applicable, to stop smoking, because nicotine stimulates gastric secretions and can affect the test results.

**During the Procedure.** When assisting during an upper GI series, take the following steps:

Have the patient undress and put on a gown.

- Explain to the patient that she will be drinking a barium sulfate drink that tastes chalky and resembles a milk shake.
- Have the patient stand and drink part of the barium.
- The radiologist will use a fluoroscope to observe the flow of the barium and to assess the functioning of the esophagus, stomach, duodenum, and small intestine as the barium passes through the structures. (The doctor will then direct the patient to drink additional barium and continue to observe the function of the various structures.)
- Place the patient on the x-ray table, and move her to different positions (if medical assistants are permitted to do so in your state) as instructed by the doctor, to allow x-rays to be taken of the upper digestive tract. Instruct the patient to remain still and hold her breath when x-rays are taken.

**After the Procedure.** After the physician completes the upper GI series, instruct the patient in postprocedure care. Give the patient the following information:

- She may now have a regular meal.
- Her stools may appear whitish or lighter than usual as the barium is eliminated, but this is normal.
- Sometimes another examination may be required after 24 hours to determine whether the barium has

## Radiographer/Sonographer

*To gain medical assistant credentials, you must fulfill the requirements of either the American Association of Medical Assistants (for a Certified Medical Assistant) or the American Medical Technologists (for a Registered Medical Assistant). After obtaining your medical assistant certification or registration, you may wish to acquire additional skills in specialty areas through course work or on-the-job training. Although this course work or training may not lead to an additional certification or degree, it will enable you to expand your role in the medical office and advance your career as the demand for skilled health professionals increases.*

### Skills and Duties

Radiographers and sonographers obtain images of internal organs, tissues, bones, and blood vessels. Physicians use these images to diagnose disease or to monitor health status.

A radiographer uses x-rays to produce the images. The radiographer positions the patient for imaging, covering parts of the body that are not to be x-rayed with a lead drape to protect them from the radiation. She then positions the x-ray machine, sets the controls, and makes the requested number of exposures.

The resulting black-and-white images can reveal whether a patient has a broken bone, tumor, ulcer, or other condition. Sometimes the radiographer or a physician administers a special material before the imaging process to make organs and blood vessels more visible on the x-ray film. The physician, usually a radiologist, examines the film and makes a diagnosis.

Sonographers use ultrasound machines that rely on sound waves rather than electromagnetic radiation to produce the images. The images are displayed on a television screen and can be videotaped or printed on film for further review by the physician.

The sonographer prepares the patient by applying a sound-enhancing gel. She then strokes the machine's handheld pad across the gel to create the image. She must be well-versed in anatomy to determine which parts of the image are important as she records measurements and data from the examination. Again, the physician uses the image to make a diagnosis and prescribe treatment if needed.

Sonographers can specialize in a variety of fields. Because sound waves are considered safe, sonography is frequently used in obstetrics and gynecology to

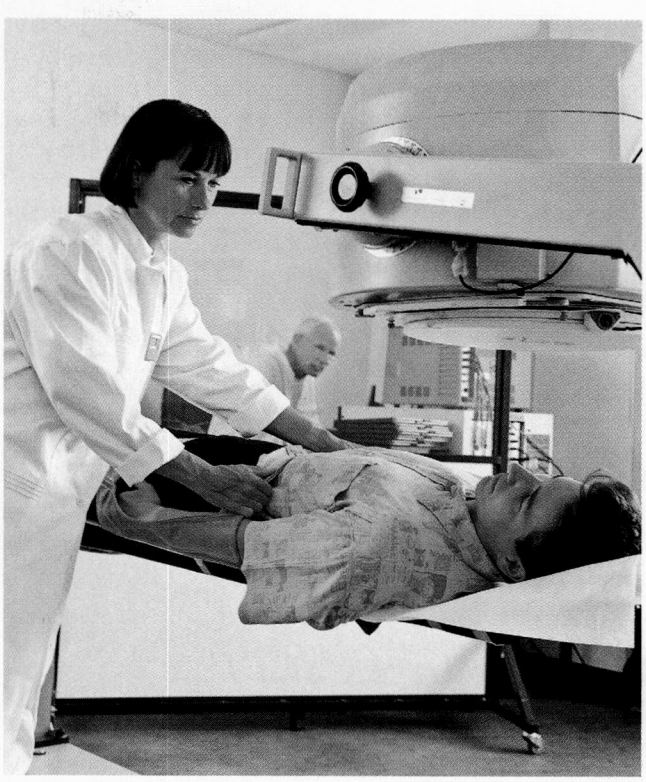

take pictures of a fetus in the womb. Sonographers may also specialize in echocardiography, where they focus on heart problems.

### Workplace Settings

Radiographers and sonographers most often work in hospitals. Some are employed in clinics, physicians' offices, and imaging centers. Radiographers may also work in dentists' offices, in mobile units, or in private industry. People in this field generally work 40-hour weeks, including some nights, weekends, and holidays.

### Education

To become a radiographer or sonographer, you must complete an accredited 2- to 4-year program in radiography/sonography from an accredited vocational school, college, or university. (For those who are already employed in health care, a 1-year certificate program may be available.) Typically, such a program provides instruction in physics, biology, anatomy, medical terminology, radiation safety, and imaging techniques. The program may also include brief

*continued* ⟶

## Radiographer/Sonographer *(concluded)*

courses in nuclear medicine, computed tomography, magnetic resonance imaging, and radiation therapy—each of which can be further studied as a specialty.

After completing the program, you may take a national registry exam from the American Registry of Radiologic Technologists. The disciplines of sonography, nuclear medicine, and radiation therapy require a national registration exam for entry-level work. Radiographers must also have a license from the state to practice.

**Where to Go for More Information**

American Society of Radiologic Technologists
15000 Central Avenue SE
Albuquerque, NM 87123
(505) 298-5063 or (800) 444-2778

Society of Diagnostic Medical Sonography
2745 Dallas Pkwy
Suite 350
(214) 473-8057 or (800) 229-9506

---

moved into the large intestine. If this test is indicated, tell the patient to follow a clear liquid diet (coffee, tea, carbonated beverages, clear gelatin, strained fruit juices, bouillon, or clear broths; milk is not permitted) and to return in 24 hours.

## Cholecystography and Cholangiography

Two similar tests performed by a radiologist are cholecystography and cholangiography. Both tests involve use of a contrast medium to view parts of the gallbladder.

**Cholecystography.** A radiologist uses cholecystography to detect gallstones and other abnormalities of the gallbladder. The doctor x-rays the patient's gallbladder after the patient has ingested an oral contrast medium. Cholecystography is usually used when ultrasound does not provide enough information for a diagnosis. You will be responsible for preparing the patient for the procedure and assisting during the procedure.

**Before the Procedure.** When instructing a patient about preparing for a cholecystography, follow these guidelines:

- Schedule the patient's appointment in the morning so he can sleep through most of the period during which his digestive tract is empty and thus avoid experiencing hunger unnecessarily.

- Describe the procedure to the patient, and explain that the examination will take about 1 to 2 hours. Ask the patient about possible allergies to contrast media, iodine, or shellfish, and report them to the radiologist.

- Explain to the patient the diet restrictions necessary to prepare for the test. Tell the patient to have a fat-free dinner (dry toast, tea, fruit, gelatin dessert) the evening before the examination. He should not smoke or

have any food or liquids after midnight, and he should have no breakfast the morning of the examination.

- Instruct the patient to take the oral contrast medium (usually in tablet form) beginning about 2 hours after dinner or as prescribed by the doctor. The tablets should be taken one at a time, 5 minutes apart, with a small amount of water, until six tablets have been taken. Explain to the patient that the contrast agent may cause nausea or diarrhea but that nothing should be taken for these conditions. In the case of severe nausea, the doctor may prescribe an antiemetic; diarrhea is an expected result of the contrast medium used for this test.

- Some doctors also order a laxative for the patient to take the day before the examination.

**During and After the Procedure.** When assisting during a cholecystography, take the following steps:

- Have the patient undress and put on a gown.

- Have the patient lie on the x-ray table in the supine position (face up).

- Explain that the radiologist will take x-rays of the gallbladder, which will be filled with the contrast medium the patient took the night before. Then the radiologist will use a fluoroscope to study the gallbladder's function. A functioning gallbladder absorbs the contrast agent properly.

- Next give the patient a specially prepared fatty meal, which should stimulate the gallbladder to empty bile into the duodenum. After about 1 hour, the doctor takes more x-rays to study the gallbladder's function. A functioning gallbladder empties the contrast medium properly. A nonfunctioning gallbladder may indicate, for example, the presence of gallstones or obstruction of the bile ducts.

- After the examination advise the patient to return to a normal diet and to drink plenty of fluids to replace those lost with diarrhea.

**Cholangiography.** Cholangiography is similar to cholecystography and is performed by a radiologist to evaluate the function of the bile ducts. It involves injection of the contrast medium directly into the common bile duct (during gallbladder surgery) or through a T tube (after gallbladder surgery or during radiologic testing). X-rays are taken immediately after injection. Use the guidelines for cholecystography. In addition, follow these steps:

- Describe the procedure to the patient, and tell him the examination will take about 2 to 3 hours. Ask the patient about possible allergies to contrast media, iodine, or shellfish, and report them to the radiologist.
- Explain the preparation instructions to the patient. Tell the patient to eat a light evening meal the night before the examination, to take a laxative (as prescribed by the doctor), and to have no food or liquids after midnight. He should also have no solid food the morning of the examination.

## Conventional Tomography and Computed Tomography

Conventional tomography produces tomograms, and computed tomography produces CT scans. These two techniques are frequently confused. Computers are involved in producing both kinds of images, but the computers are different and have different functions.

Conventional tomography uses a computerized x-ray camera that moves back and forth in an arc over the patient to produce a series of views of a body part. The computer sets the angle and layer for each arc; the camera produces one view per arc.

In CT scans produced by computed tomography, the x-ray camera rotates completely around the patient, and the computer compiles one cross-sectional view from each rotation of the camera. The patient is lying on a special table that gradually moves through the doughnut-shaped machine containing the rotating camera.

The preparation is essentially the same for the two procedures. Reassure the patient that he will not be inserted into an enclosed space, as is the case in magnetic resonance imaging. The patient will be able to see around the room during the test.

Tomograms and CT scans are used to diagnose abnormalities in almost all body structures, including the head, kidneys, heart, chest, liver, biliary tract, pancreas, GI tract, spine, pelvis, bones, and breast. When preparing the patient for a tomogram or a CT scan, use the following guidelines:

- Ask the patient about possible allergies to contrast media, iodine, or shellfish, and report them to the radiologist.
- Tell the patient that he will be placed on a table that moves through the scanner for CT scans or on an x-ray table for tomograms.

- Inform the patient that the procedure will last about 45 to 90 minutes and that he must lie still while the scans are taken. The patient may breathe normally while the CT scans are taken but must hold his breath for each of the tomograms.
- If a contrast medium will be used, advise the patient that it will be injected into a vein in the arm or on the back of the hand (except with a CT scan of the spine) to enhance detail of the structure being evaluated.
- If the patient is having a CT scan of the head or chest, instruct him not to eat anything for 4 hours or drink any liquids for 2 hours before the examination. Explain that he may experience mild nausea after injection of the contrast medium if the stomach is too full.
- If the patient is having tomograms or a CT scan of the abdomen or pelvis, tell him to obtain a preparation kit from the office or hospital the day before the examination. This kit includes a special drink the patient must take the night before the examination that helps outline the intestines. Inform the patient that the drink should not produce a laxative effect or any discomfort.
- Tell the patient to remove metallic objects that could interfere with the path of the x-rays. Also, ask if the patient has skin staples or metallic prostheses that could interfere.
- Inform the patient that a written report of the results should be available within 24 hours of the test and that a report will be sent to his primary care physician (or the referring physician).

## Heart X-Ray

An x-ray of the heart, using a contrast medium, may be necessary to show the configuration of the heart and to reveal cardiac enlargement and aortic dilation. Angiography of the heart is called angiocardiography, in which a contrast medium is injected into a major blood vessel. X-rays are taken while the medium flows through the heart, lungs, and major vessels. Coronary arteriography uses a dye inserted through a catheter that has been passed through an artery to the heart. Both procedures require hospital admission, usually in a day surgery or ambulatory surgery unit.

## Intravenous Pyelography

Also known as excretory urography, **intravenous pyelography (IVP)** is performed by a radiologist who injects a contrast medium into a vein. The doctor then takes a series of x-rays as the contrast medium travels through the kidneys, ureters, and bladder. IVP is used to evaluate urinary system abnormalities or trauma to the urinary system. In most facilities a nurse assists with IVP, but you may assist the patient before the procedure. If you assist with IVP, you will have several responsibilities both before and during the procedure.

**Before the Procedure.** When instructing a patient about the preparation for an IVP, include the following steps:

- Schedule the patient's appointment in the morning so she can sleep through most of the period during which her digestive tract is empty and thus avoid experiencing hunger unnecessarily.

- Describe the procedure to the patient, and tell her that the examination will take about 1½ hours. Ask about possible allergies to contrast media, iodine, or shellfish, and report such allergies to the radiologist.

- Explain the importance of adhering to the preparation instructions, so that the bowel is free of any material that could obstruct the view of the urinary organs. Tell the patient to follow a liquid diet (coffee, tea, carbonated beverages, clear gelatin, strained fruit juice, bouillon, or clear broths, but no milk) the day before the examination. The patient should take the prescribed amount of electrolyte solution or other laxative preparation as specified the night before the examination and have no food or liquids after midnight and no breakfast the morning of the examination. Some physicians also order an enema to be taken about 2 hours before the examination.

**During and After the Procedure.** When assisting during an IVP, you will generally proceed in this manner:

- Have the patient undress and put on a gown.

- Explain that a contrast medium will be injected into her vein (usually in the arm). Instruct her to inform the physician if she notices shortness of breath or itching after injection of the dye. This type of symptom can indicate an allergic reaction.

- Have the patient lie on the x-ray table, and move her to different positions as instructed by the physician, to allow x-rays to be taken of the urinary tract as the contrast medium is excreted. Instruct the patient to remain still and hold her breath when x-rays are taken.

- Note that some physicians place a compression device on the abdomen, which helps hold the contrast medium in the kidneys and ureters by exerting moderate pressure.

- After the physician takes the series of x-rays to evaluate urinary system function, ask the patient to urinate, and explain that a final x-ray will be taken.

- Inform the patient that she may resume a normal diet after the test and that the contrast medium will be eliminated in the urine.

## Retrograde Pyelography

**Retrograde pyelography** is similar to the IVP, except that the doctor injects the contrast medium through a urethral catheter. This procedure, which evaluates function of the ureters, bladder, and urethra, is often used for patients with poor kidney function. Follow the same preparation and assistance instructions as for the IVP.

## KUB (Kidneys, Ureters, and Bladder) Radiography

Also called a flat plate of the abdomen, **KUB radiography** is an x-ray of the abdomen used to assess the size, shape, and position of the urinary organs; to evaluate urinary system diseases or disorders; and to determine the presence of kidney stones. It can also be helpful in determining the position of an intrauterine device (IUD) or in locating foreign bodies in the digestive tract. No patient preparation is required. A KUB x-ray is taken by a radiologic technologist; thus, you follow the guidelines you would use for a patient having any type of standard, noninvasive x-ray.

## Magnetic Resonance Imaging (MRI)

Nonionizing radiation (radio frequency signals) and a strong magnetic field are combined in magnetic resonance imaging to allow the physician to examine internal structures and soft tissues of any area of the body. The combination of nonionizing radiation and magnetic field, which allows the MRI scanner to produce images based primarily on the water content of tissues, appears to have no harmful effects on the patient. The test may be performed with or without contrast. You will be responsible for preparing the patient for an MRI and assisting with the procedure.

High-speed MRI scanners scan four times faster than other MRIs, which makes the procedure more tolerable by the patient and produces clear, high-resolution images that assist physicians to improve diagnoses for conditions like common knee and shoulder conditions and abdominal and brain disorders.

**Before the Procedure.** When instructing a patient about preparing for an MRI, include the following steps:

- If a contrast medium is going to be used, ask the patient and inform the radiologist about possible allergies to contrast media, iodine, or shellfish.

- Screen the patient to determine whether any internal metallic materials are present. (This is especially important because a strong magnetic field is involved in creating the image.) Ask about a pacemaker, brain or aneurysm clips, brain or heart surgery, shunts and heart valves, other surgeries, and shrapnel or metal fragments (particularly in an eye).

- Ask the patient whether he is or has been a metalworker. If so, he may carry metal slivers, chips, or filings under his nails or skin.

- Describe the procedure to the patient, and explain that the examination will take between 45 minutes and 2 hours.

- Tell the patient he does not need to fast before the examination or follow any preprocedure diet, unless he is having an MRI of the pelvis. In that case instruct him to have no solid food for 6 hours and no liquids for 4 hours before the examination. Inform the patient that he may take prescription medications.

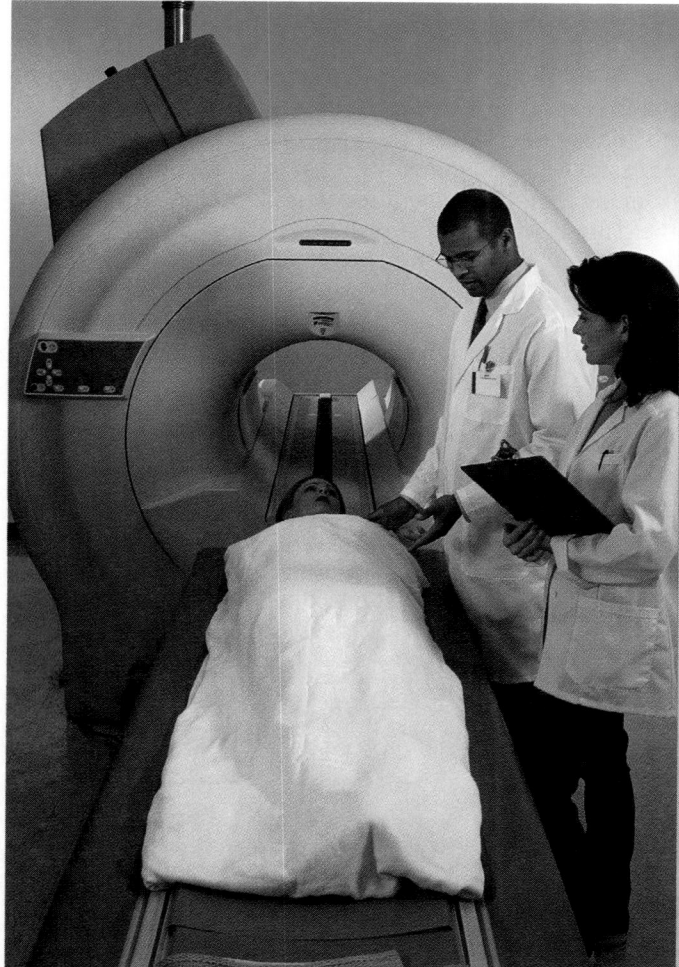

**Figure 40-6.** A patient who is claustrophobic or unable to lie still may require sedation during an MRI.

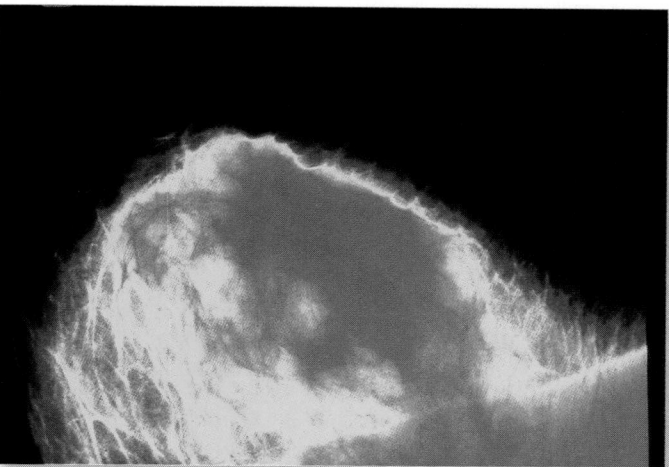

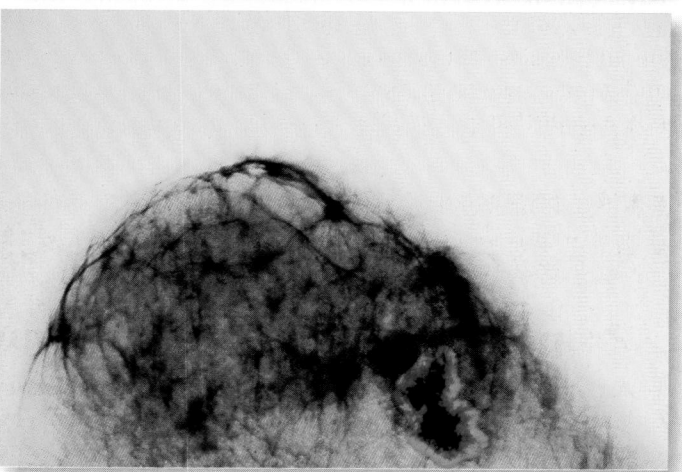

**Figure 40-7.** Mammograms can reveal the presence of tumors that are not detected by other means. The upper mammogram indicates normal breast tissue, whereas the lower suggests a malignancy.

- Explain that he will not be required to drink an oral contrast preparation but that he should avoid caffeine for 4 hours before the examination. (Instruct women not to wear eye makeup the day of the examination, because eye makeup often contains metallic ingredients.)
- Tell the patient that he will probably have no side effects from the examination but that some nausea may occur as a result of the contrast medium.

**During and After the Procedure.** When assisting during an MRI, you will need to follow these specific steps:

- Inform the patient that he may wear street clothing, unless it has metallic thread, metal stays or grippers, or thick elastic. Tell the patient that he will probably be asked to undress, however, and put on a gown.
- Have the patient lie on the padded table.
- Explain that the table will be placed inside a long, narrow tube about 22 inches in diameter and that he will hear a loud knocking noise as the machine scans. Offer the patient hearing protection devices (ear plugs or headphones) during the test. Warn the patient to re-

main still to avoid blurring the image and the consequent need for a retake. Note that physicians commonly order sedation for patients who are claustrophobic or cannot lie still for a long period (Figure 40-6).

- Advise the patient that although the technician will not be in the scanning room during the examination, she will maintain contact with a camera and a microphone. The patient may speak to the technician at any time in case of a problem, but he is encouraged to be still for each series.
- Inform the patient that his primary care physician or referring doctor should have a preliminary report of test results within about 24 hours.

## Mammography

**Mammography,** the x-ray exam of the internal breast tissues, helps in diagnosing breast abnormalities (Figure 40-7). A specially trained radiologic technologist takes mammograms. Types of mammography include film-screen, thermography, and ultrasonography (ultrasound).

You will have several responsibilities during both setup and patient care before and after mammography. A medical assistant does not assist during mammography in most states. Instead, you will prepare the patient for the procedure and ease her fears. The Educating the Patient section provides information on this topic.

## Mammotest Biopsy Procedure

When a mammogram reveals an abnormality in the breast tissue, it is often treated in one of two ways—either the abnormality is followed for a period of time to see if there are any significant changes or a surgical excision biopsy is performed. Because so many abnormalities revealed by mammography are benign and present no health risk, physicians now perform stereotactic breast biopsies, which are less painful and less invasive than conventional excisional biopsies. The procedure is performed by a physician and a radiologic technologist and is similar to mammography except that the patient is lying face down rather than standing. The breast is compressed with a compression paddle to confirm that the area of the breast with the lesion is correctly centered in the paddle window. A computer is used to help determine the exact positioning of the biopsy needle, and the physician takes a small sample of tissue to be examined by a pathologist for the presence of malignant cells. The attending physician later contacts the patient with the test results.

## Myelography

**Myelography** is a kind of fluoroscopy of the spinal cord. The physician performs a lumbar puncture, removes some cerebrospinal fluid (CSF), and instills a contrast medium to evaluate spinal abnormalities, such as compression of the spinal cord. Sometimes the physician performs pneumoencephalography, which involves instilling air after removal of the CSF to allow visualization of the cerebral cavities.

The physician who performs myelography or pneumoencephalography must be skilled in performing lumbar

## Educating the Patient

### Preprocedure Care for Mammography

A patient who is scheduled for mammography must know the guidelines to follow before the exam. You can help educate the patient by instructing her in the following preprocedure care:

- The mammography should be scheduled for the first week after the patient's menstrual cycle. This timing helps minimize discomfort from compression of the breasts and ensures that the breasts are in their most normal state.

- No special preprocedure diet or medication requirements are necessary, but the patient should consider avoiding caffeine for 7 to 10 days before the exam (in some patients caffeine may cause swelling and soreness that would heighten discomfort during the procedure). Have the patient decrease caffeine intake gradually, however, to avoid getting headaches.

- The patient should shower or bathe as close as possible to the time of the mammography and wear loose clothing that is easy to remove. A blouse and pants or skirt work best to allow undressing only to the waist.

- The patient should not use deodorants, powders, or perfumes on the breasts or underarm areas before the examination, because these products could produce a false result on the x-ray.

- Inform the patient that the radiologist will want films from a prior mammogram if the mammogram was obtained from a different facility. Some radiologists may not read the films for an impression if a comparison study is not possible.

- In addition to providing these instructions, you may need to reassure a patient who is fearful about mammography. Explain that although mammography is uncomfortable, it is usually not painful. Describing how the procedure is performed may alleviate the patient's fears. Provide the patient with the following information:

- The procedure usually takes 15 to 20 minutes. A lead apron will be placed on the patient's abdominal area to protect her from unnecessary radiation exposure.

- The patient will be positioned in front of the machine. The technician will compress the left breast between the machine plates and take two x-rays—one horizontal view and one vertical view—of the left breast.

- The technician will then position and compress the right breast between the machine plates. Two x-rays will be taken of the right breast.

- If needed, the physician may order a mild pain reliever after the procedure to alleviate discomfort or aching.

puncture—most likely a radiologist, neurologist, neurosurgeon, or anesthetist. A radiologic technologist is typically the only other person present for the test. Although myelography is not used as frequently as it was before the invention of CT and MRI, it is still performed when these newer techniques do not provide enough information about the spinal canal. Myelography may be reserved for cases in which the clinical findings are unusual or the scanning results uncertain.

## Nuclear Medicine

Also known as radionuclide imaging, **nuclear medicine** involves use of radionuclides, or radioisotopes (radioactive elements or their compounds). The radionuclides are administered orally, intravenously, or through routes that introduce them into organs or body cavities. The purpose is to evaluate the bone, brain, lungs, kidneys, liver, pancreas, thyroid, or spleen. Sometimes the entire body is scanned for "hot spots," or places where the radioisotope is concentrated.

For common nuclear medicine scans, the technician uses a scanner called a gamma camera. This scanner detects radiation from the radioisotope and converts it into an image (called a scintiscan or scintigram) to be photographed or displayed on a screen (see Figure 40-8). Some images are produced immediately, whereas others may take up to several days. Radionuclide imaging exposes patients to lower doses of radiation than some radiologic

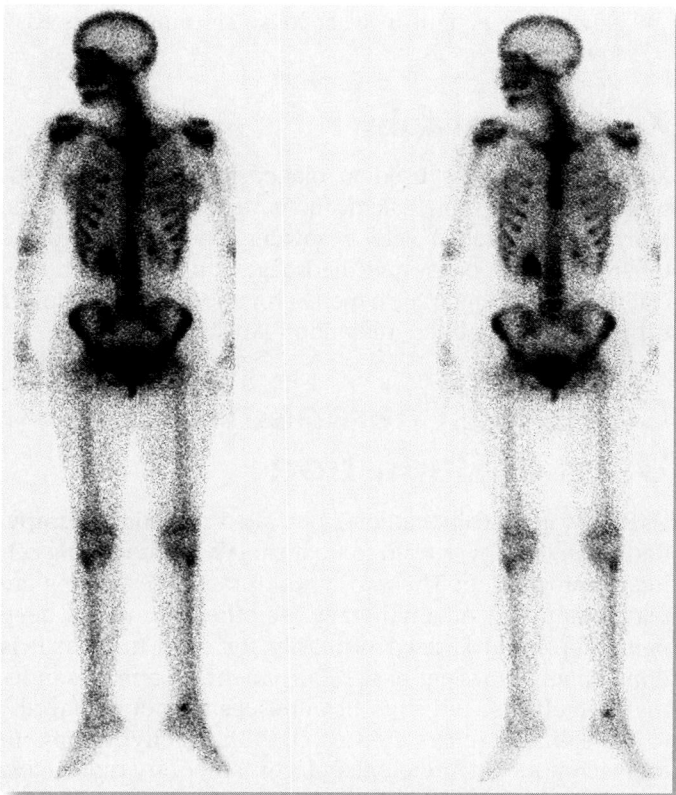

**Figure 40-8.** This bone scan shows the uptake of the radioactive contrast medium.

techniques, because the amount of ionizing radiation in the isotope is less than that emitted from x-ray cameras.

Other nuclear medicine procedures include single photon emission computed tomography (SPECT), positron emission tomography (PET), and MUGA (multiple gated acquisition) scan.

- **SPECT** is often used to locate and determine the extent of brain damage from a stroke. The gamma camera detects signals induced by gamma radiation, and a computer converts these signals into either two- or three-dimensional images that are displayed on a screen.

- **PET** entails injecting isotopes combined with other substances involved in metabolic activity, such as glucose. These special isotopes emit positrons, which a computer processes and displays on a screen. PET is especially useful for diagnosing brain-related conditions, such as epilepsy, mental illnesses, and Parkinson's disease.

- The **MUGA scan** evaluates the condition of the heart's myocardium. It can be done while the patient is at rest or in stress (exercise) and involves the injection of radioisotopes that concentrate in the myocardium. The gamma camera allows the physician to measure ventricular contractions to evaluate the patient's heart wall.

When preparing a patient for a nuclear medicine procedure, describe the procedure and tell her how long the examination will take. Explain any preparation requirements and other special instructions, and tell the patient she will need to wait the required length of time for the uptake of the radioisotope. Length of examination and requirements for common scans are as follows:

- A bone scan lasts about 1 hour; it is done 2 to 3 hours after a 15-minute injection; the patient drinks 1 quart of liquid between the injection and the scan; a normal diet is permitted

- A liver/spleen or lung scan lasts approximately 1 hour; there are no diet restrictions

- A kidney scan lasts about 2 hours; there are no diet restrictions

- A thyroid uptake and scan test usually requires 2 days; the patient takes a capsule of contrast medium in the morning and has the scan on the first day; the patient returns 24 hours later for the second scan; there are no diet restrictions, except that the patient must have no fish because of its natural iodine content

## Stereoscopy

Used primarily to study the skull, **stereoscopy** is an x-ray procedure that uses a specially designed microscope (stereoscopic, or Greenough, microscope) with double eyepieces and objectives to take films at different angles. Stereoscopy identifies fractures and dense areas to produce three-dimensional images. The images, which have depth as well as height and width, can indicate a tumor or increased pressure within the skull. No special preparation is required. Follow the guidelines you would use with any other noninvasive x-ray.

## Thermography

**Thermography** is performed to diagnose breast tumors, breast abscesses, and fibrocystic breast disease. The procedure uses an infrared camera to take photographs that record variations in skin temperature as dark (cool areas), light (warm areas), or shades of gray (areas with temperatures between cool and warm). Tumors or inflammations produce more heat than healthy tissues and therefore show up lighter on these photographs; areas with lack of circulation are cooler than tissues with adequate circulation and show up as dark. Because no preparation requirements are necessary for this test, you need only to schedule the procedure and to assist as needed with reassurance during the examination.

## Ultrasound

**Ultrasound** directs high-frequency sound waves through the skin over the area of the body being examined and produces an image based on the echoes. A radiologist or an ultrasound sonographer coats the body area with a special gel and passes a transducer (instrument similar to a microphone) over the area. As the transducer passes back and forth over the area, it picks up echoes from the sound waves, which a computer converts into an image on a screen. The image produced is sometimes called a sonogram. Ultrasound is used to detect abnormalities in the gallbladder, liver, spleen, heart, and kidneys. It is also safe to use in obstetrics to evaluate the developing fetus or to detect multiple fetuses, because it does not expose the patient (or the fetus) to radiation (Figure 40-9). In this case the obstetrician may perform the test in the office.

One form of ultrasound, called Doppler echocardiography, involves sound waves that echo against the flow of blood through vessels. Doppler echocardiography is usu-

ally performed by a cardiologist to determine whether blood flow is laminar (normal) or turbulent (disturbed).

Echocardiography, a type of ultrasound test, is used to study the structure and function of the heart. The test is usually performed while the patient is resting and again after exercising on a treadmill or bicycle. Images of the heart before and after exercise help the physician diagnose abnormalities of the structure and function of the heart and heart valves.

When preparing the patient for an ultrasound or assisting with the examination, follow these guidelines:

- Describe the procedure to the patient and inform her that the examination will take about ½ to 2 hours, depending on the type of ultrasound. For example, a cardiac ultrasound takes about 1½ hours; pelvic, 1 to 2 hours; and abdominal, ½ to 1 hour.

- Explain the preparation requirements, which vary according to the type of ultrasound. Tell a patient who is having a gallbladder or liver ultrasound not to eat for several hours before the test. Tell a pregnant patient to drink the prescribed amount of water 1 hour before the examination and not to void. Advise a patient having a pelvic ultrasound to take the prescribed laxative (if indicated), drink three to four glasses of water within 1 hour, and not to void within 1 hour of the test. If the patient is having an abdominal ultrasound, instruct her to take a laxative the night before the examination and not to have any food or fluids for 8 hours before the test.

- Advise the patient to wear loose clothing that is easy to remove.

## Xeroradiography

**Xeroradiography** is used to diagnose breast cancer, abscesses, lesions, and calcifications. The xeroradiographic x-rays are developed with a powder toner, similar to the toner in photocopiers, and the image is processed on specially treated xerographic paper. Xeroradiography uses lower exposure times and less radiation than standard x-rays.

# Common Therapeutic Uses of Radiation

Used therapeutically, radiology is called **radiation therapy.** Radiation therapy is used to treat cancer by preventing cellular reproduction. The two types of radiation therapy are teletherapy and brachytherapy. **Teletherapy** allows deep penetration and is used primarily for deep tumors; it is done on an outpatient basis. The patient experiences minimal side effects, and superficial tissues are not damaged.

Localized cancers are treated with **brachytherapy.** In this technique the radiologist places temporary radioactive implants close to or directly into cancerous tissue. Both the staff and patient are subject to radiation exposure. Therefore, radiation safety precautions must be closely

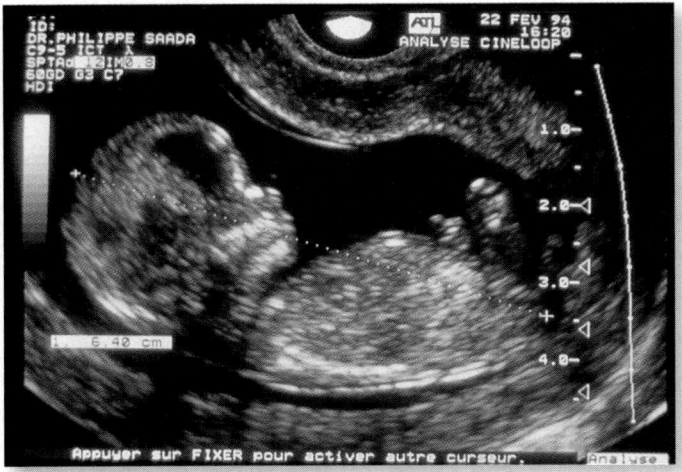

**Figure 40-9.** Ultrasound is commonly used to evaluate the health of a developing fetus.

followed. When preparing the patient for radiation therapy, follow these guidelines:

- Describe the procedure to the patient, and explain how long the procedure will take, as determined by the radiologist and oncologist according to the diagnosis and the condition of the patient.
- Inform the patient that the radiologist or oncologist will explain the possible side effects of the treatment. Common side effects include nausea, vomiting, hair loss, ulceration of mucous membranes, weakness, and malaise. Other possible effects include localized burns on tissue and damage to organs in the path of treatment. Encourage the patient to discuss with the doctor (or the oncology nurse specialist) measures to relieve or minimize stress and discomfort.
- Advise the patient to immediately report any other symptoms to the doctor.

# Radiation Safety and Dose

For many years after the discovery of the x-ray, the seriousness of radiation hazards was not addressed. In the 1920s the government of Great Britain took the first steps to limit x-ray exposure. Since World War II, studies have been performed, mostly on the effects of high-dose radiation.

Other studies on the effects of background radiation and nonradiologic versus radiologic (x-ray–related) risks have enabled scientists to assess the risks of diagnostic x-rays. Results from these studies show the risk of excess radiation from routine x-rays to be minimal.

## Reducing Patient Exposure

Advances in diagnostic imaging technology, as well as limits to radiation exposure, have helped reduce the dose of radiation to which a patient is exposed during a diagnostic procedure. Another way to reduce the risk of excessive radiation exposure lies with the physician, who must assess the benefit-to-risk ratio when recommending a diagnostic radiology procedure. Because radiation has a cumulative effect, the physician must have valid medical reasons for ordering the test, particularly if the patient has recently had other x-rays. Some types of x-rays, such as mammograms, should be repeated regularly, however, because of their potential to prevent or promote treatment of life-threatening disorders.

According to a 1993 report by the National Council on Radiation Protection and Measurements (NCRP) titled *Limitation of Exposure to Ionizing Radiation,* one of the earliest pieces of legislation in the United States to limit occupational radiation exposure was enacted in the 1930s. The first legislation to limit public exposure, however, was not enacted until the 1950s. The NCRP report of 1993 set guidelines for protection from radiation in and out of the workplace. The two primary objectives outlined in the report are to prevent serious general tissue damage from radiation by limiting radiation dose to levels below known

thresholds for such damage and to reduce the risk of cancer and genetic effects to a level that is balanced by potential benefits to the individual and society.

Because exposure to radiation always poses some degree of risk, the NCRP recommends that any activity involving radiation exposure be justified, or balanced against the expected benefits to society. Furthermore, the NCRP recommends that the cost, or detriment, to society from such activities be kept *as low as reasonably achievable* (ALARA) and that individual dose limits be applied to ensure that justification and ALARA principles do not result in unacceptable levels of risk for individuals or groups.

The NCRP has developed detailed lists on radiation doses to achieve the primary objectives stated in the report. There are separate specific limits for occupational exposure and public exposure.

## Safety Precautions

Understanding and following standard safety precautions are crucial for protection from radiation exposure. These precautions are essential to the health and safety of both medical personnel and patients.

**Personnel Safety.** If you work in a medical facility that performs radiologic tests, you are at risk for excessive radiation exposure. To protect yourself from radiation exposure, you must adhere to the following specific guidelines:

- You (and other members of the medical staff) must always wear a radiation exposure badge, or dosimeter, which is a sensitized piece of film in a holder (Figure 40-10). You must have the badge checked regularly by specially qualified personnel, who measure the

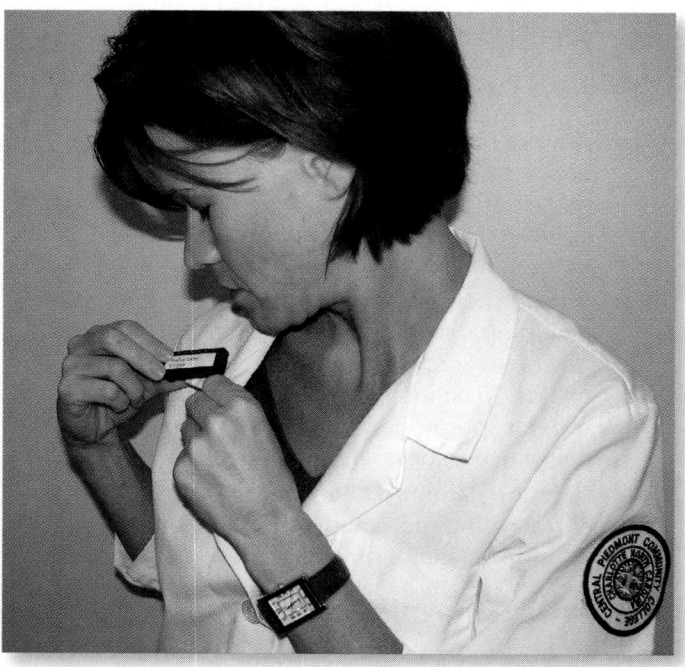

**Figure 40-10.** A radiation exposure badge contains a film that registers the levels of radiation to which a medical staff member is exposed at work.

# Educating the Patient

## Safety With X-Rays

You are responsible for teaching the patient about x-ray safety. You will need to obtain pertinent patient history data, answer questions, and provide basic information on x-rays, possible side effects, and other important guidelines. Consider the following points when teaching the patient about x-ray safety.

### Patient History

- Ask the patient about x-rays received in the past, including how many and what type, and about the possibility of exposure to radiation in the home, school, or workplace. Explain that the effects of radiation exposure are cumulative; that is, the effects are related to total exposure over the lifetime as well as to exposure from each procedure.

- Ask a female patient about the possibility of pregnancy. Use the 10-day rule—take an x-ray only within 10 days of the last menstrual period to avoid taking an x-ray of a patient who is unknowingly pregnant. If the patient knows that she is pregnant, do not schedule an x-ray unless approved by the radiologist.

- Inform the patient about possible side effects of radiation exposure. These effects include fetal abnormality or genetic mutation in a fetus (when a patient is pregnant) and the depression of bone marrow activity, which decreases the production of red blood cells and white blood cells.

### Patient Questions

- Always answer questions in simple, easy-to-understand language; make explanations brief and clear. Do not use complex medical terms; however, do include proper terminology. Offer written information about the test, if available.

- Answer fully any questions about examinations, including descriptions of procedures; the doctor's reason for ordering them; their length, side effects, injections, or other uncomfortable aspects; preprocedure requirements; cost and insurance issues; and availability of test results.

- Help the patient reduce fear or anxiety surrounding the scheduled test and feel comfortable and informed about the procedure.

### General X-Ray Information

- Be aware of the most current guidelines established by the American College of Radiology. Always keep up with new studies on the risks of radiation exposure.

- Encourage the patient to ask questions about the need for x-rays ordered by the doctor and risks associated with those x-rays.

- If the patient's employer requires annual x-rays or a potential employer asks for pre-employment x-rays, advise the patient to question the necessity of these tests. Suggest that the patient find out whether the doctor has x-rays on file that could be submitted.

- Advise the patient to discuss testing options with the doctor. For instance, if the doctor orders fluoroscopy, the patient might ask whether standard x-rays can be taken instead, because fluoroscopy often represents a higher risk for exposure to radiation than do standard x-rays. (Mobile x-ray exams often pose a higher exposure risk as well.)

- Advise the patient to ask questions about x-ray safety standards in the office or hospital in which the tests are to take place.

- Tell the patient to avoid dental x-rays that are performed with wide-beamed plastic cones; narrow-beamed cones are more exact and less dangerous. In addition, educate the patient about the opinions of the American Dental Association and the National Conference of Dental Radiology, both of which believe that x-rays should not be performed solely for insurance claim purposes. Advise the patient to always ask for a lead apron over organs not being studied. Tell the patient to avoid retakes of x-rays because of blurriness or shadows (which are caused by movements or breathing) by remaining still when instructed to do so during x-ray exams.

- Explain to the patient the importance of x-rays in proper diagnosis of disorders. Inform the patient about the constant improvements in equipment and x-ray procedures and the much lower doses of radiation now used in these procedures.

- Advise the patient to keep a family record of x-ray exams.

- Educate a female patient without breast disease on the correct schedule for mammography exams. The patient should have a baseline mammogram between ages 35 and 40; a mammogram every 1 to 2 years between ages 40 and 49; and an annual mammogram after age 50.

- Also tell the patient to see a doctor immediately if she notices a breast mass, lump, or nipple discharge.

degree of radiation uptake on the film to determine the amount of radiation to which you have been exposed.

- Make sure that all equipment is in good working order and is checked routinely for radiation leakage and any other problems.
- Be aware that the technician and any other staff members present when equipment is operating should always wear a garment that contains a lead shield.

**Patient Safety.** You must follow all rules governing patient safety from radiation exposure. The Educating the Patient section explains safety measures and information that help protect a patient from exposure to unnecessary radiation.

# Storing and Filing X-Rays

You will be responsible for storing x-ray films if you work in a radiology facility. Follow these guidelines for proper storage of x-rays:

- Keep fresh film on hand at all times.

- Maintain new and exposed films in as good a condition as possible by keeping them at a temperature between 50°F and 70°F (between 10°C and 20°C) and a relative humidity between 30% and 50%. Radiology facilities usually have one or more special rooms for films.
- Prevent pressure marks and keep expiration dates visible by storing packages on end; do not stack them on top of each other.
- Use a first-in, first-out method for using film (that is, use the oldest film first).
- Open film packages or boxes only in the darkroom.
- Do not store film near acid or ammonia vapors.

You will also be responsible for providing accurate record keeping of x-rays. See Procedure 40-2 for guidelines on documentation and filing techniques.

Remember that x-ray films are the property of the radiology facility or the doctor's office where they are taken. Although the films may be sent (or taken by the patient) to a hospital or another doctor for consultation, they

# PROCEDURE 40.2

## Documentation and Filing Techniques for X-Rays

**Procedure Goal:** To document x-ray information and file x-ray films properly

**OSHA Guidelines:** This procedure does not involve exposure to blood, body fluids, or tissues.

**Materials:** X-ray film(s), patient x-ray record card or book, label, film-filing envelopes, film-filing cabinet, inserts, marking pen

**Method:**

1. Document the patient's x-ray information on the patient record card or in the record book (Figure 40-11). Include the patient's name, the date, the type of x-ray, and the number of x-rays taken.
2. Verify that the film is properly labeled with the referring doctor's name, the date, and the

### X-RAY EXAMINATIONS RECORD

| Patient | Date | Type X-Ray | No. Taken | Referring Doctor | Comments |
|---------|------|-----------|-----------|------------------|----------|
| | | | | | |
| | | | | | |
| Jill Cabot | 2/16 | Chest | 4 | Wapnir | |
| M. C. Gaines | 2/16 | Right knee | 8 | Wright | |
| J. Hale | 2/19 | Right wrist | 6 | McCarthy | |
| L. Becker | 2/23 | Left hip | 4 | Wright | |
| R. Bell | 2/24 | Chest | 4 | Wapnir | |
| Donna Lin | 2/24 | Sinuses | 6 | Harris | |
| Jon Carey | 2/26 | Right hand | 2 | Cohen | |

**Figure 40-11.** Keeping accurate records of patient x-ray information is an important duty of the medical assistant.

*continued* ⟶

# Documentation and Filing Techniques for X-Rays *(concluded)*

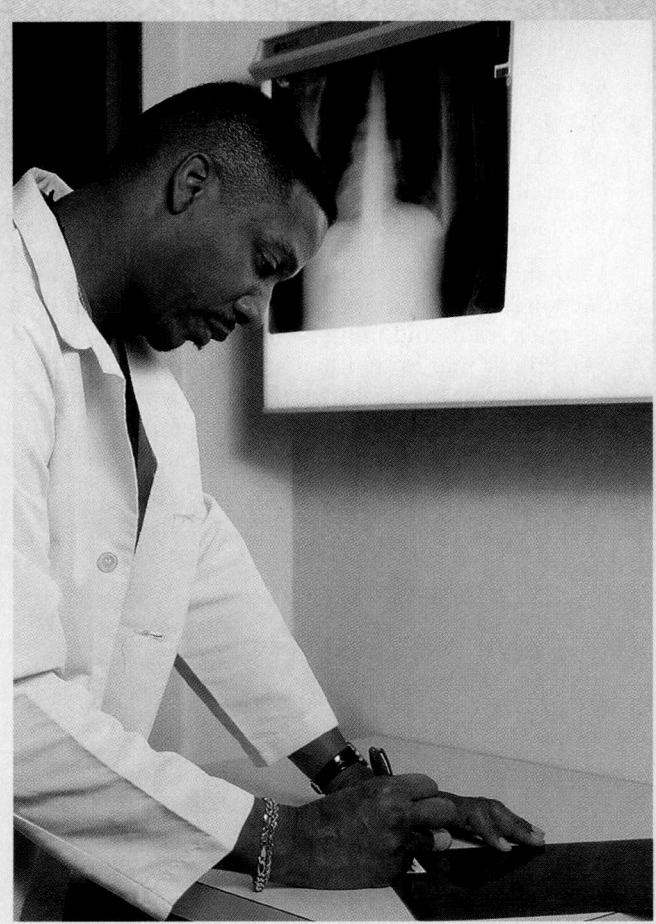

**Figure 40-12.** You may need to provide labeling information on an x-ray film before you file it.

patient's name. To note corrections or unusual positions or to identify a film that does not include labeling, attach the appropriate label and complete the necessary information (Figure 40-12). Some facilities also record the name of the radiologist who interpreted the x-ray.

*Rationale*

To reduce the likelihood of misidentifying a patient's x-ray.

3. Place the processed film in a film-filing envelope. File the envelope alphabetically or chronologically (or according to your office's protocol) in the filing cabinet.

4. If you remove an envelope for any reason, put an insert or an "out card" in its place until it is returned to the cabinet.

*Rationale*

Proper filing techniques save time and prevent litigation.

should be returned to the original facility (for example, the radiologist's office). In some facilities, the images are stored on a specialized computer disk, and the patient receives a copy of films to take to another doctor or medical facility. The information, however, is the property of the patient. Thus, the patient need not return reports.

# Electronic Medicine

Recent major advances in telemedicine technology, including rapid video and computer-based communications of medical information, enable physicians to "examine" a patient in another city or country, view highly detailed medical images, consult with specialists in other cities, and supervise complex medical procedures. In addition, health-care personnel, including medical assistants, can

participate in interactive teaching conferences by means of closed-circuit television.

In some cities emergency medical technicians (EMTs) are able to transmit an electrocardiogram (ECG) electronically to an emergency room physician to obtain lifesaving directives from the physician. These directives may involve administration of drugs or other measures the EMTs otherwise would not be permitted to perform without a physician's order. Similarly, some patients are monitored by cardiologists by the transmission of daily ECGs through telephone lines to the cardiologist's office.

Another new technology is stereotaxis, a magnetic neurosurgery procedure that allows surgeons to treat or remove brain tissue safely while being guided by a computer screen. Traditionally, neurosurgeons risked causing severe damage while gaining access to an affected area of a patient's brain. With stereotaxis, however, the computer screen shows a view of the brain containing a surgically implanted magnetic pellet in a safe area of the brain. The neurosurgeon then uses magnetic resonance imaging to guide the pellet, which is the size of a grain of rice, toward a critical area. Using this technique, the surgeon can avoid critical neurons and deliver treatment to the high-risk area. The pellet can be used to move a catheter, probe, or other implement into place to remove tissue or deliver a drug. Researchers hope to expand this technology to other parts of the body, such as the liver or blood vessels.

## Digital Imaging

With the emergence of electronic health records (EHR), technology in health care is expanding rapidly. However, no department is affected more than radiology because it is the only specialty that is completely technology driven. Digital radiology (DR) devices are integrated with the EHR system to provide quality images, rapid access, and to eliminate the time and equipment that is associated with film processing and development. A large benefit of digital radiology is that the amount of radiation is decreased, therefore reducing risks to the patient and technician (Figure 40-13).

**Digital Imaging and Communications in Medicine (DICOM).** Digital Imaging and Communications is a communications protocol or standard for handling, storing, printing and transmitting information in medical imaging. DICOM was designed as part of the Integrating the Healthcare Enterprise (IHE) initiative that makes it easier for medical systems to share information. A Picture

Archive and Communication System (PAC) is the digital storage area where digital images are sent and stored for diagnostic viewing and electronic image storage and distribution (Figure 40-14).

## Advances in Radiology

As radiology continues to experience technological changes, more advances are occurring to enhance the quality of digital imaging. Some major advances include 3D/4D ultrasound.

This type of ultrasound provides "live-action" images that allow physicians to observe fetal movement, study body organs, and guide needle biopsies (Figure 40-15).

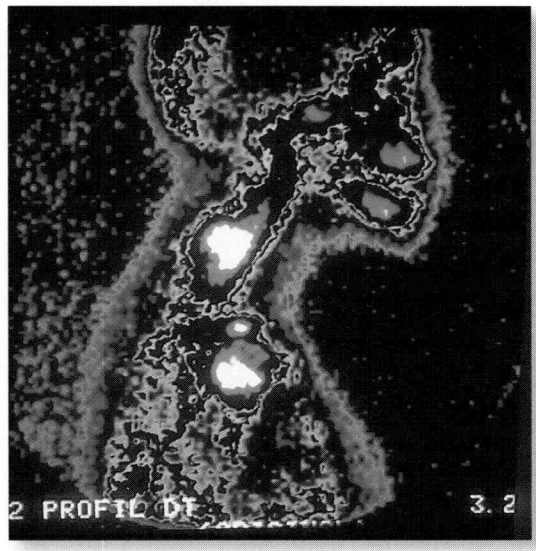

**Figure 40-14.** A digital bone scan of the neck and skull showing malignant tumors.

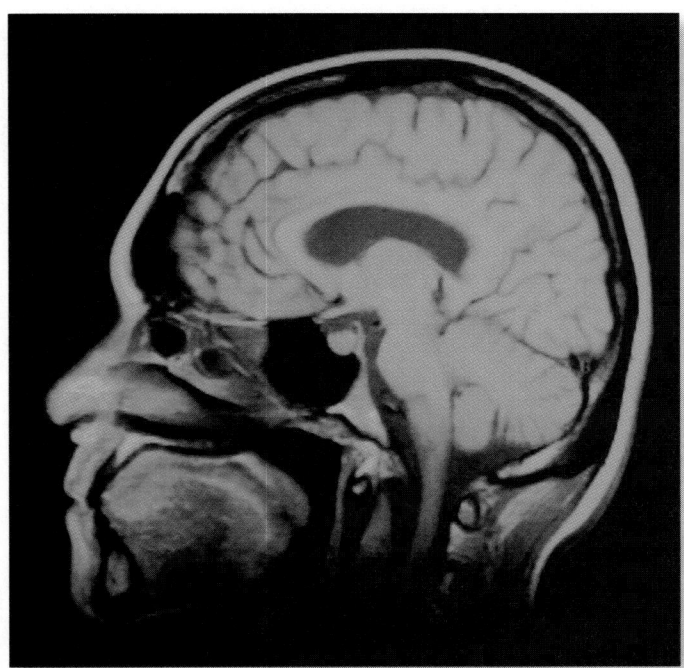

**Figure 40-13.** A digital lateral MRI image of the brain.

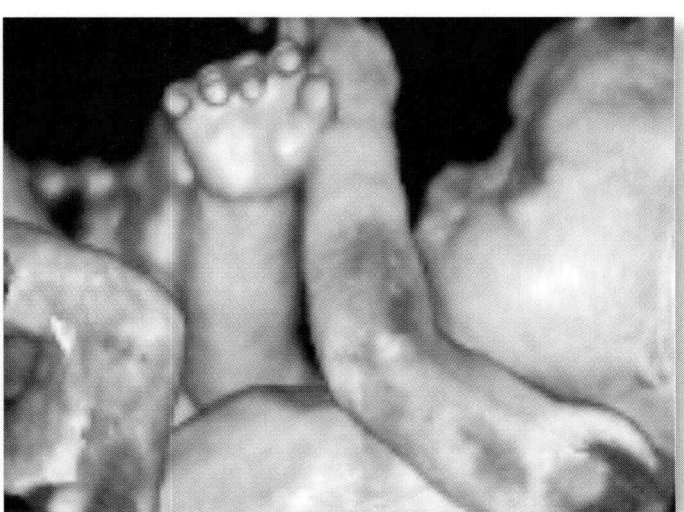

**Figure 40-15.** A 3-D ultrasound shows the fetus in great detail

# Summary

Diagnostic tests are an important part of medical care because they help doctors diagnose a variety of diseases and disorders. As a medical assistant, you will be asked to assist with patient care before, and sometimes during and after, diagnostic radiology procedures. Your responsibilities include providing instructions and explanations to patients, preparing patients for various tests, and assisting the doctor or technician with the procedures. Your duties may also include storing and filing x-rays.

Safety is a vital concern with radiologic tests. Understanding and following safety precautions will help you ensure your patients' health and well-being as well as your own.

## CASE STUDY *QUESTIONS*

Now that you have completed this chapter, review the case study at the beginning of the chapter and answer the following questions:

1. What special instructions should be given to the patient before her mammogram?
2. How is a CT scan performed?
3. When preparing a patient for a CT scan, what allergies should be disclosed during the patient interview?
4. Why was a mammotest requested by the physician?
5. What education requirements must you fulfill in order to work as a radiographer/sonographer?

## Discussion Questions

1. What types of problems might a hysterosalpingogram diagnose?
2. What special preprocedure instructions should be provided to a patient scheduled for a mammogram?
3. What guidelines must be followed for the proper storage of x-rays?
4. What are the advantages of digital imaging technology?

## Critical Thinking Questions

1. What are the differences between invasive and noninvasive diagnostic radiology tests?
2. In general, what preprocedure care should be given to patients for whom radiology procedures have been ordered?
3. When scheduling a patient for an MRI, you must note whether the patient has any internal metallic elements (such as a pacemaker, clips, pins, shrapnel, etc.). Explain why this information is important.
4. The office manager asks you to retrieve a mammogram film from the PAC. What does PAC mean and what device is used to retrieve the mammogram?

## Application Activities

1. Write a list of instructions to give to a patient who is going to have an upper GI series. Exchange lists with a classmate, and evaluate each other's work.
2. With another student, role-play a situation in which a medical assistant is preparing a patient for an MRI of the pelvis. Then switch roles and critique each other's technique.
3. With another student, role-play a situation in which a medical assistant is training a new coworker in how to document and file x-rays. Have your classmate evaluate the thoroughness of your instructions.

## Virtual Fieldtrip

*Visit the McGraw-Hill Higher Education Medical Assisting website at www.mhhe.com/medicalassisting3 to complete the following activity:*

Use the National Library of Medicine's reference website. Search for information about mammography. Research information regarding digital mammography and write a 500-word summary of your findings.

Open the CD and complete this chapter's practice activities, play the games, listen to the key terms, and test yourself with the interactive review. Email, print, and/or save your results to document your proficiency.

# SECTION 6

# EXTERNSHIP

# Medical Assisting Externships and Preparing to Find a Position

## AREAS OF COMPETENCE

*In preparation of the certification examination, you should know the following areas of competence:*

| COMPETENCY | CMA | RMA |
|---|---|---|
| **General/Legal/Professional** | | |
| Respond to and initiate written communications by using correct grammar, spelling, and formatting techniques | X | X |
| Recognize and respond to verbal and nonverbal communications by being attentive and adapting communication to the recipient's level of understanding | X | X |
| Demonstrate proper telephone techniques | X | X |
| Identify and respond to issues of confidentiality by maintaining confidentiality at all times and following appropriate guidelines when releasing records or information | X | X |
| Be aware of and perform within legal and ethical boundaries | X | X |
| Utilize computer software and electronic technology to maintain office systems | X | X |
| Project a positive attitude | | X |
| Be a "team player" | | X |
| Exhibit initiative | | X |
| Adapt to change | | X |
| Evidence a responsible attitude | | X |
| Be courteous and diplomatic | | X |
| Conduct work within scope of education, training, and ability | | X |
| Be impartial and show empathy when dealing with patients | | X |
| Serve as a liaison between the physician and others | | X |
| Interview effectively | | X |

## KEY TERMS

affiliation agreement
chronological résumé
clinical coordinator
constructive criticism
functional résumé
networking
portfolio
reference
targeted résumé

## CHAPTER OUTLINE

- Externships
- Preparing to Find a Position
- Interviewing
- On the Job

## LEARNING OUTCOMES

After completing Chapter 41, you will be able to:

**41.1** Perform as a professional in all externship scenarios.

**41.2** Discuss employment services and methods of obtaining a position.

**41.3** Create a résumé.

**41.4** Create a cover letter.

**41.5** Create a follow-up letter.

**41.6** Explain key factors for a successful interview

# Introduction

After completing a medical assisting program, you may be excited and apprehensive about beginning your new career. In this chapter, you learn how to maximize your externship experience and gain the hands-on experience you need for securing a position in medical assisting. Your externship is an opportunity for you to explore the different responsibilities that are required of a medical assistant.

After completing this chapter, you will begin to search for a position; you will be able to complete a résumé, a cover letter, and a thank-you letter. You will form a strategic plan on how to secure a position in medical assisting, and you will gain interviewing techniques needed to compete in today's health-care world.

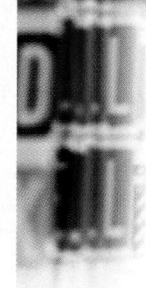

## CASE STUDY

Sarah has completed the didactic portion of her comprehensive medical assisting program. She has been assigned to a family practice office that was highly recommended to her by her clinical advisor. She is excited but apprehensive about her performance in this facility. She fears she will forget everything she has learned.

The first week of her externship, she observes the flow of the office and some medical procedures ordered by the physician. She is blending in with the office staff and manager. The second week of her externship, she begins to perform basic clinical procedures such as vital signs and measurements. She completes these procedures with minimal direction. The third week of her externship, she is introduced to the laboratory and is observed performing venipuncture. After ten successful draws, she is able to perform a venipuncture without supervision.

By the fourth week of her externship, she is performing basic laboratory testing, venipuncture, ECGs, and other clinical patient care duties, and she is feeling comfortable and excited that she has gained the skills needed to work as a medical assistant. During the fourth week, the physician asks her to perform an ear irrigation and leaves to examine the next patient. She is unsure of this skill and does not remember the procedure.

As you read this chapter, consider the following questions:

1. What should Sarah do about the ear irrigation?
2. How has she remembered all the previous procedures and not this one?
3. Will the clinical preceptor be disappointed or angry with her?

# Externships

An externship is the opportunity to work within a medical facility to gain the on-the-job experience that is essential for beginning your new career. It is an opportunity to apply in an actual medical environment the knowledge and skills that you have learned.

Most externships are measured by hours attended. The minimum amount of hours for a medical assisting externship is 160 hours. Externships are a mandatory requirement of fulfilling a medical assisting program in educational institutions that are accredited by the Accrediting Bureau of Health Education Schools (ABHES) and the Commission on Accreditation of Allied Health Education Programs (CAAHEP). Some externships are completed after the didactic portion of the curriculum (for example, during the last module or semester), and some are completed during the last semester. Medical assisting externships may be performed at physician offices, laboratories, hospitals, administrative billing offices, and clinics.

# The Externship Process

The educational institution partners with local medical facilities throughout the area surrounding the school. Most schools have a **clinical coordinator** who is familiar with medical assisting and the medical community. The clinical coordinator procures externship sites and qualifies them to ensure that they provide a thorough educational experience. A checklist is often designed to ensure that medical assisting extern students are given a well-rounded, safe experience (Figure 41-1). All student externships are unpaid, and the student should be positive about the experience and appreciate the opportunity to train with the facility.

**Externship Requirements.** Externship sites are required to review and sign an **affiliation agreement.** The affiliation agreement states the expectations of the facility and the expectations of the student. Some examples of the expectations of the externship site are as follows:

- Retaining complete responsibility for the patient care that is totally under its control and supervision
- Providing reasonable opportunities for clinical instruction by qualified facility personnel for students participating in the program
- Supervising students in a manner that will provide safe practice and meaningful clinical education

In addition, the expectations of the educational institution may include the following:

- Reinforcing patient confidentiality by having the student sign a statement of confidentiality

---

## CLINICAL SITE ASSESSMENT

NAME OF SITE _____

ADDRESS _____

SPECIALITY _____ SUPERVISOR _____

TELEPHONE # _____ FAX # _____

NUMBER OF STAFF _____

ADMINISTRATIVE/CLINICAL EXPERIENCE AVAILABLE TO STUDENTS
(*CHECK ALL THAT APPLY*)

____ FRONT OFFICE SKILLS

____ WORD PROCESSING SKILLS

____ MEASURE/RECORD VITAL SIGNS

____ BLOOD DRAWING (VENIPUNCTURE, FINGERSTICKS)

____ INJECTIONS

____ ELECTROCARDIOGRAMS

____ SPECIMEN COLLECTION/DIAGNOSTIC PROCEDURES
(urinalysis, blood sugar, cholesterol, etc.)

____ ASSISTING WITH MINOR SURGICAL PROCEDURES

I HAVE DETERMINED THAT THIS SITE MEETS THE NEED OF THE STUDENTS IN THE MEDICAL ASSISTING PROGRAM.

PRINT NAME OF UDS EVALUATOR _____

SIGNATURE OF EVALUATOR _____

DATE _____

**Figure 41-1.** A form such as this clinical site assessment is often used by the clinical coordinator to help determine if a clinical site will be appropriate for medical assisting externships.

- Providing professional liability insurance for the student, the educational institution, and the faculty
- Ensuring that the student is medically able to perform the assigned duties of the extern facility by providing proof of immunizations and health physicals

The clinical coordinator is the liaison between the externship site and the educational institution.

**Screening.** Students are placed in externship clinical sites by the clinical coordinator. It is not uncommon for the clinical site to screen students prior to their externship. This screening can include the following:

- Interviewing students prior to their externship.
- Asking students to provide a urine or hair sample for drug screening prior to the externship.
- Asking students to consent to a criminal background check prior to beginning their externship. Some medical facilities check only for felony convictions, whereas others check for misdemeanors and felonies. Honesty is the best policy for criminal background checks. Some institutions will waive some convictions as long as the student is honest and truthful about the conviction early in the process.
- Accepting students only if employment at the facility is the end result. The student may be asked to fill out an application and participate in a new employee orientation prior to beginning the externship.

**Time Sheets.** Students are given time sheets to be completed on a daily basis and faxed to the educational facility at the end of every week. The clinical preceptor and the student both sign the time sheet (Figure 41-2). The student is monitored by the clinical coordinator and the program director for the duration of the externship. Weekly telephone calls and site visits are performed by the educational institution for each student. Some schools require weekly progress reports from each student. Figure 41-3 provides an example of this report. When students finish their externships, the preceptors will complete a final evaluation and the students will be graded on their externship performance (Figure 41-4).

# Expectations of Externship Candidates

While in an externship, you are expected to be and look professional, report to the externship site as scheduled, and display initiative and a willingness to learn.

**Professionalism.** You are expected to conduct yourself in a professional manner at all times while attending your externship. You may feel that you are often criticized by the site preceptor. This normal part of learning is called **constructive criticism.** Constructive criticism is aimed at giving you feedback about your performance in order to improve that performance. You are not expected to know everything on your externship, but you are expected to be open to suggestions and ideas. It is not considered professional to question clinical preceptors during the learning experience. You may be exposed to some procedures that are not performed exactly as you were taught. Do not argue with preceptors about their skills. There is usually more than one way to get the desired result in patient care.

Your behavior is expected to be as professional as if you were an employee there. Foul language and inappropriate conversation is not tolerated in any workplace. You are expected to be professional with the patients under all circumstances. Medical facilities expect you to demonstrate empathy and compassion to every patient. Proper verbal skills and grammar are expected at all times. Do not use slang when communicating with office staff and patients. Personal phone calls should not be made during working hours; do not use the facility phone. Cell phones and pagers should be turned off during working hours. Do not park your car in areas that are convenient for patients. Many patients are older and have difficulties walking long distances. It is a professional courtesy and good customer practice to allow the patients the parking spots closest to the entrances.

**Attendance.** You are expected to report to your externship *every day* that you are assigned to a schedule. It is your responsibility to have several alternates to babysitting and transportation. Employers are seeking dependable and punctual medical staff and would not tolerate attendance problems with their own staff. In the event of an emergency, you are expected to report a call-off to the medical facility and the school 2 hours before the beginning of your shift, as would any other employee. Many medical facilities will not tolerate absenteeism or tardiness from an externship student, and they may ask the school to remove the student from the site.

Adhere to the facility's policy regarding breaks. Take breaks only when it is appropriate to do so. If you smoke, refrain from smoking during working hours and do not smoke in patient entrances. Lunch breaks are permitted under facility policies.

**Professional Appearance.** Medical facilities expect you to appear as a medical professional. Most require a uniform that consists of a scrub top and bottom and a lab jacket. Your scrubs should be clean, pressed, and well fitting. Shoes should be clean, white, and in good repair. Your name tag or badge should always be worn and visible to patients. Nails should be trimmed and polished in good taste in pale and neutral colors. Many medical facilities will not accept students with artificial nails, such as acrylics. Facial and tongue piercings are not acceptable when working with patients, and visible tattoos must be covered. Your hair should be a natural color and pulled back from your face and off your collar. Makeup should be conservative and in good taste. Perfumes and colognes should be avoided because patients with respiratory conditions or allergies may not be able to tolerate them.

# Clinical Externship Timesheet
## Medical Assistant Program

**Instructions:**

Students are expected to attend their clinical site for a minimum of 32 hours per week, and will not receive credit for more than ten hours per day. **For shifts greater than four hours, you must include a thirty-minute meal break.**

- Complete the log daily and fax the log each week to the school no later than 5 p.m. Friday.
- For each day attended, please include a brief description of the duties performed.
- The Timesheet must be signed and dated by both the student and the Clinical Site Supervisor.

**Student Information**

Name: _____

Program: _____

Home Phone: _____

Alt. Phone: _____

**Clinical Site Information**

Name: _____

Phone: _____

Rotation: _____

Assignment Dates: _____

Site Supervisor's Name: _____

| | Date | Time In | Time Out | Total Hours | General Duties Performed * |
|---|---|---|---|---|---|
| Monday | | | | | |
| Tuesday | | | | | |
| Wednesday | | | | | |
| Thursday | | | | | |
| Friday | | | | | |
| Saturday | | | | | |
| TOTAL HOURS | | | | | |

* Examples of General Duties include: Billing, Vital Signs, Lab Work, Filing, Charting, etc.

Student Signature: _____     Supervisor: _____

Date: _____     Supervisor Signature: _____

Date: _____

**Figure 41-2.** Students participating in an externship complete a weekly timesheet.

## STUDENT WEEKLY PROGRESS REPORT

This form needs to be completed and signed each week. It must be faxed with the timesheet on Friday afternoon. It is designed to help you maximize your clinical externship experience. Having recognizable goals is the surest way to succeed!

Name: _____     Date: _____

Class Code: _____

Clinical Site: _____

Supervisor Signature: _____

Student Signature: _____

I.   Goals for next week:
  1. _____
  2. _____
  3. _____

II.  Personal assessment of progress this week:
  _____
  _____
  _____

III. Supervisor's assessment of progress this week:
  _____
  _____
  _____

IV.  Identify one task/item/event you are most proud of that occurred this week:
  _____
  _____

V.   Did you meet your goals for this week? Why or why not?
  _____
  _____

**Figure 41-3.**   A weekly progress report is a helpful way for students to track their externship goals and achievements.

Remember that you as a medical assisting student on an externship represent several things:

- The school you attend. It is important to maintain a good reputation in the medical community. You will depend on the reputation of the school to obtain a job.
- The profession of medical assisting. Participating in a medical assisting externship gives you an opportunity to represent the profession of medical assisting to patients and the community.
- Yourself. First impressions are lasting impressions. Make your first impression to the medical community an outstanding one.

**Initiative and Willingness to Learn.** During your externship, accept all assignments with enthusiasm and grace, no matter how mundane. These tasks are often a test on how well you accept orders and work within a medical team. Ask for additional work if you are idle, and look for tasks that need to be done. Keep a notebook and record the office policies and procedures. Be prepared to observe and participate in office procedures.

## Preparing to Find a Position

The next phase of beginning your new career is seeking a position as a medical assistant. Most accredited schools have a career services department. Its primary focus is job placement after graduation. The department's counselors will assist you in writing your résumé, improving your interviewing skills, and learning about positions in your

# MEDICAL ASSISTANT PROGRAM

## EXTERNSHIP TRAINING PLAN

| NAME: | INTERNSHIP PERIOD:<br>/ / TO / / |
|---|---|
| SITE NAME: | ADDRESS: |
| ON-SITE EMPLOYER REPRESENTATIVE: | PHONE #: |

DIRECTIONS: THIS TRAINING PLAN WILL SERVICE TO SPECIFY THE APPLICATIONS AND EXPERIENCES THAT ARE TO BE SECURED DURING THEIR TRAINING. UPON COMPLETION OF THEIR TRAINING, PLEASE INDICATE YOUR APPRAISAL OF THE STUDENTS' PERFORMANCE BY DRAWING A CIRCLE AROUND THE NUMBER CORRESPONDING WITH THE ACHIEVEMENT LEVEL AS FOLLOWS:

1 = UNSATISFACTORY, 2 = FAIR, 3 = VERY GOOD, 4 = OUTSTANDING.

CIRCLE THE UA IF THE STUDENT WILL BE UNAVAILABLE TO DO THIS PROCEDURE, AND THE NA IF THIS IS NOT APPLICABLE TO THE STUDENTS' STUDIES.

## EXTERNSHIP GOALS & OBJECTIVES/PERFORMANCE RATING SCALE

### DURING THE EXTERNSHIP PERIOD, THE STUDENT WILL:

| | | | | | | | |
|---|---|---|---|---|---|---|---|
| A. | DEVELOP EFFECTIVE "FRONT OFFICE" SKILLS INCLUSIVE OF SUCH ACTIVITIES AS; PATIENT COMMUNICATION, MEDICAL RECORDS, BILLING & COLLECTIONS, INSURANCE PROCESSING, AND COMPUTERIZED BUSINESS FUNCTIONS | 1 | 2 | 3 | 4 | UA | NA |
| B. | ACCURATELY MEASURE AND RECORD VITAL SIGNS, UTILIZING PROPER TECHNIQUE | 1 | 2 | 3 | 4 | UA | NA |
| C. | PERFORM STANDARD EKG RECORDING/ MOUNTING PER SITE PROTOCOL | 1 | 2 | 3 | 4 | UA | NA |
| D. | DEVELOP PROFICIENCY IN PARENTERAL MEDICATION ADMINISTRATION (INTRADERMAL, SUBQ, INTRAMUSCULAR) | 1 | 2 | 3 | 4 | UA | NA |
| E. | DEVELOP PROFICIENCY AND TECHNIQUE IN PERFORMING VENIPUNCTURE USING THE EVACUATED TUBE SYSTEM | 1 | 2 | 3 | 4 | UA | NA |
| F. | DEMONSTRATE EFFECTIVE SPECIMEN COLLECTION TECHNIQUE AND DIAGNOSTIC PROCEDURES (i.e., URINALYSIS, BLOOD SUGAR, CHOLESTEROL, ETC.) | 1 | 2 | 3 | 4 | UA | NA |

SIDE 1 OF 2

*(continues)*

**Figure 41-4.** A form such as this one may be used by the clinical preceptor to evaluate a student's externship performance.

```
PROFESSIONAL ATTRIBUTES                                    PERFORMANCE RATING SCALE

A.    ORAL COMMUNICATIONS                          1      2      3      4      UA     NA

B.    ORGANIZATION & SAFETY                        1      2      3      4      UA     NA

C.    DEPENDABILITY & SELF-DIRECTION               1      2      3      4      UA     NA

D.    COOPERATIVENESS                              1      2      3      4      UA     NA

E.    RECORDKEEPING                                1      2      3      4      UA     NA

F.    COLLABORATIVENESS/TEAMWORK                   1      2      3      4      UA     NA

G.    PATIENT RAPPORT/CONSIDERATION                1      2      3      4      UA     NA

H.    ATTENDANCE/PUNCTUALITY                       1      2      3      4      UA     NA


WHAT IS YOUR OVERALL OPINION OF THIS STUDENT'S PERFORMANCE?

( ) UNSATISFACTORY  ( ) POOR  ( ) FAIR  ( ) GOOD  ( ) VERY GOOD  ( ) OUTSTANDING


THIS WILL CERTIFY THAT THE INTERN HAS COMPLETED ( ) HOURS AT THE SITE.


COMMENTS:

ON-SITE EVALUATOR'S SIGNATURE: _____

  DATE: _____

                              SIDE 2 OF 2
```

```
              THIS PAGE IS STRICTLY FOR THE USE OF EDUCATION

TOTAL GOALS AND OBJECTIVE POINTS                    _____/_____
# OBJECTIVES EVALUATED              =               _____ AVG POINTS


TOTAL ATTRIBUTE POINTS                              _____/_____
# ATTRIBUTES EVALUATED              =               _____ AVG POINTS

AVERAGE OF TOTAL POINTS                   =         _____

GRADE POINT SCALE

A = 3.5–4.0

B = 2.5–3.4

C = 2.0–2.4

F = 1.9 OR LESS              FINAL GRADE = _____

PROGRAM DIRECTOR SIGNATURE: _____

DATE: _____
```

**Figure 41-4.** *(concluded)*

field. Many employers will contact a school's career services department to recruit medical personnel. It is important to work closely with the career services department in the beginning of your career to assist you in obtaining your first position.

# Seeking Employment

In addition to working with a career services department, you can take advantage of a number of other resources in seeking employment within the field of medical assisting. These

## Make a Good Impression

Often a shy and passive medical assisting extern will appear to the preceptor and facility as unmotivated or lacking initiative. It is important to be assertive and confident when working in health care. Remember: Every day on your externship is "show time"! You may have to "step out of your comfort zone" to make a good impression.

resources include classified ads, Internet sites, employment services, and networking with classmates and others.

**Classified Ads and Internet Sites.** Many prospective employers use classified advertisements in area newspapers to alert potential applicants to a career opportunity within their organization. The advertisement usually describes the duties and responsibilities of the position as well as the type of education and experience preferred.

When you are first beginning to seek a medical assisting position, don't become discouraged if you see advertisements asking for a specified amount of experience, such as 2 years. You must realize that employers place ads seeking an experienced candidate, but many will consider a new graduate because experienced candidates are not always available. Becoming credentialed will help you bridge the gap of experience. A local newspaper's classified advertisements are often a good place to start your search. There is usually a separate section listing health-related jobs.

It is important to explore all the possibilities when seeking employment opportunities. A medical assistant is qualified for a number of positions. New graduates can apply for the following positions:

- Unit secretary in hospitals
- Phlebotomist in labs
- Patient care associate or patient care technician in hospitals
- Entry-level medical coding and billing
- Customer service representative in medical-related companies
- Clinical or administrative position in physician offices

The Internet is another useful tool when seeking employment. Websites often allow job seekers to post résumés online and to respond to advertisements that are posted by employers locally or statewide. Many hospitals will not accept paper or faxed résumés and require that all applicants fill out an electronic application and post résumés on the facility website. Newly graduated medical assistants should post their résumé and cover letter on all local hospitals websites during their externships to start circulating their résumés.

**Employment Services.** Employment and temporary agencies provide assistance in locating a specific job. Both types of agencies have a variety of job openings on file. Agencies also place classified ads. You should call to make an appointment with an employment counselor. Agencies usually require you to fill out an application, take a basic health-care knowledge test, and provide a résumé. If the agency has positions that match your skills, it contacts the employer. If the service has no appropriate listings, it will place your résumé on file.

Employment services are an excellent way to gain experience and select a position. You are given an opportunity to try out the office or facility at little commitment on your part. Many permanent opportunities can result from a temporary job assignment.

**Networking.** **Networking** involves making contacts with relatives, friends, and acquaintances that may have information about how to find a job in your field. People in your network may be able to give you job leads or tell you about openings. Word-of-mouth referrals—finding job information by talking with other people—can be very helpful. Other people may be able to introduce you to others who work in, or know people who work in, your field. Networking is a valuable tool. It can advance your career even while you are employed.

Joining a medical assisting organization and attending conferences are the easiest ways to network. Attend an organization's local chapter meetings, such as the AAMA county or state chapters, and talk with as many people as possible. Remember to bring a pen and a notebook. Be prepared to exchange information with other attendees. Remember, networking is an exchange of information—it is not one-sided. What you learn through networking may enable you to provide others with information to help their job search or further their career.

Your classmates are often a good source of networking. It is important to build lasting friendships with your classmates and keep in touch after graduation. Oftentimes they will know of positions as they gain employment. Networking begins in the classroom.

## Creating a Résumé

Your résumé is a vital part of the employment process. It provides potential employers with information about your educational and work history and other aspects of your background.

**Components of a Résumé.** In order to create a well-rounded, informative résumé, you need to include a wide variety of information about your background.

***Personal Information.*** Include your name, address, telephone number, cell phone number, and e-mail address. Do not include your marital status or the number of children you have. You should not include your height, weight, interests, or hobbies unless you think they are relevant to the position.

***Professional Objective.*** A professional objective is a brief, general statement that demonstrates a career goal. An example of an effective, professional objective is the following: "To work as a medical assistant, applying skills in patient relations and laboratory work while gaining increasing responsibility." If you want to list a specific career objective, such as applying your medical assisting skills in a pediatric medical facility, it would be best to mention it in the cover letter and not on your résumé.

***Employment Experience.*** List the title of your most recent or last job first, the dates you were employed there, and a brief description of your duties. Choose jobs that have been the most beneficial to your working career. Do not clutter your résumé with needless details or irrelevant jobs. You can elaborate on specific duties in your cover letter and in the interview. Only include jobs you have held for a longer period of time, such as 6 months to a year.

***Educational Background.*** In providing your educational history, list your highest degree first, the school attended, the dates, and the major field of study. Include educational experience that may be relevant to the job, such as certification, licensing, advanced training, and intensive seminars. Do not list individual classes on your résumé. If you have taken special classes that relate directly to the job you are seeking, list them in your cover letter.

***Awards and Honors.*** List the awards and honors that are related to your career or that indicate excellence. Perfect attendance, academic honors, and student of the month are excellent traits that employers are seeking. Highlight this information prominently rather than writing it as an afterthought. You can make the most impact by displaying your best qualities at the beginning of this section.

***Campus and Community Activities.*** List activities that show leadership abilities and a willingness to contribute. Include any volunteer work that you may have performed.

***Professional Memberships and Activities.*** List any professional memberships that are related to your career. Student memberships are available through the American Medical Technologists (AMT) and the American Association of Medical Assistants (AAMA). You can contact the AMT and request a copy of the student by-laws and directions on how to form a student membership in your school. The AAMA provides continuing education through their local chapters. They sponsor local meetings periodically throughout the year. Employers like medical professionals who are involved in their disciplines. It demonstrates a commitment and dedication to their chosen field.

***Summary of Skills.*** As you learn clinical and administrative skills, you will want to list them on your résumé. Under headings such as "Clinical Skills" or "Administrative Skills," list the skills you have acquired in school and on your externship. Some examples of clinical skills are the following:

- ECG
- Venipuncture
- Urinalysis
- Parenteral injections
- Aseptic technique and blood-borne pathogens
- First aid and bandaging
- CPR
- Triage and vital statistics
- Spirometry

Some examples of administrative work include the following:

- Diagnostic and procedural insurance coding
- Insurance claim form processing and reimbursement
- Practice management software (for example, Medisoft)
- Medical office accounting practices
- Typing speed
- Microsoft Office software

**Choosing a Résumé Style.** Three different résumé styles have been developed, each of which has specific advantages and disadvantages. You will want to choose a style or combination of styles that best describes your strengths and skills.

***Functional Résumé.*** A **functional résumé** highlights specialty areas of your accomplishments and strengths. You can organize these in an order that supports your objective. Functional résumés are useful when you change careers, reenter the job market after an absence, or have had a variety of different, unconnected work experiences. Functional résumés are often not appropriate in highly traditional fields such as teaching, law, or health care, where the specific employers are the main interest. A sample of a functional résumé is shown in Figure 41-5.

***Chronological Résumé.*** A **chronological résumé** is used by individuals who have job experience. List your most recent job first, and end with your first job. Chronological résumés are best when you stay in the same field as your prior jobs and when your employment history shows growth and development. Do not use a chronological résumé if you have gaps in your work history, if you have changed careers, if you have been in the same job for many years, or if you are looking for your first job. Figure 41-6 illustrates a chronological résumé.

***Targeted Résumé.*** A **targeted résumé** is best if you are focused on a specific job target. The résumé should contain a clear, concise objective about what you are looking for. This résumé should list your skills, academic achievements, student honors, and other pertinent information that correlates with your objective. This type of information adds substance to your résumé when you

**Donna Turner-Smith**
**18 Kingsley Road**
**Olmsted Falls, OH 44138**
**(440) 555-4279**

**PUBLIC HEALTH EDUCATION:**
> Instructed community groups on HIV awareness.
> Instructed volunteers on how to set up community programs on domestic violence
> Facilitated workshops for parents of teenagers
> Provided in-services for public school teachers on signs and symptoms of substance abuse

**COUNSELING:**
> Consulted with social workers on individual cases for suspected child abuse
> Worked with parents from abused homes
> Counseled individual abused children

**ORGANIZATIONAL:**
> Grant writing for federal funds for HIV awareness programs
> Served as a liaison for transitional shelters for victims of domestic violence
> Served as a liaison between community health agencies and public schools

**PROFESSIONAL WORK HISTORY:**
> 1995–2001    Project SAFE, Plymouth, Michigan
> HIV Public Health Instructor
>
> 2001–2005    Department of Child Health and Safety, Cleveland, Ohio
> Public Health Educator

**EDUCATION:**
> 1994 B.S. Sociology, Eastern Michigan University, Ypsilanti, Michigan

**References available upon request**

**Figure 41-5.** A functional résumé is often used by people who are reentering the job market.

have just graduated and do not have relevant job experience. Because the targeted résumé is an academic-type résumé, your skills, achievements, and community and volunteer work—your most significant assets—should be listed first. A sample of a targeted résumé is shown in Figure 41-7.

## Writing the Résumé

One of the most daunting tasks of completing the résumé process is writing the résumé. The language that you use in your résumé will affect its success, so it is important to be careful and conscientious when choosing your words. Translate the facts of your academic and employment history into an active and precise résumé that will keep the reader's interest and highlight your major accomplishments in a concise, effective manner.

Résumé writing is different from any other form of writing. You should use a direct, functional writing style that focuses on the use of verbs and other words that imply action on your part. Writing with action words and strong verbs portrays you as an energetic, active person who is able to achieve results in his or her work. Choose words that display your strengths and demonstrate your initiative. Table 41-1 provides a list of commonly used verbs that help create a strong, active résumé.

Below are two writing samples that differ only in their writing style. The first example is ineffective because it does not use action words to accent the applicant's work experiences.

Anthony Dalton
1234 West 25<sup>th</sup> Street
Park Ridge, NJ 07656
(201) 555-8311

**WORK EXPERIENCE:**

September, 2005–Present   NORTH BERGEN CLINIC FOUNDATION

Lead Medical Assistant for Cardiology practice
Patient preparation
EKG and Holter Monitor
Assist with Stress Testing
Patient follow-up

June, 2002–September, 2005   ST. JOSEPH HOSPITAL

Phlebotomist–inpatient and outpatient

March, 2002–June, 2002   ST. JOSEPH HOSPITAL

Medical Assisting Externship
Administrative and clinical responsibilities utilizing all
medical assisting skills in the Emergency department.

- Patient Triage
- Foley catheters
- EKG
- Specimen collection
- Patient intake
- Insurance verification

**EDUCATION AND CERTIFICATIONS:**

Associate of Applied Science Degree, June 2002, Bergen Community College,
Paramus, New Jersey, 07645

Certified Medical Assistant, August, 2002

**References available upon request**

**Figure 41-6.** A chronological résumé lists a person's job history in chronological order.

*Example #1*

**WORK EXPERIENCE**

**Medical Assistant**
Manager of eight medical assistants from three offices. Office Manager of three offices located east and west side. In charge of the daily operations of the medical office. Trainer of all new medical assistants.

**Special Projects:** Coordinator and Secretary for Cuyahoga County Chapter of the American Association of Medical Assistants.

**Accomplishments:** Daily patient census went up 25% by implementing the "Patient First" customer service program. Patient-facility relations improved.

In the second example, below, the first paragraph has been rewritten. Notice how the tone has changed. The paragraph now sounds stronger and more active. This person accomplished goals and really did things.

**Kelly Adamson**
**220 Terrace Avenue**
**Mooresburg, TN 37811**
**(423) 555-2657**

**CAREER OBJECTIVE:**

To obtain a challenging position as a medical assistant in a growth oriented ambulatory care facility

**ACHIEVEMENTS:**

Registered Medical Assistant
Certified Phlebotomy Technician
Registered Medical Office Specialist
Graduate of an Accredited Medical Assistant Program
OSHA Compliance Officer
American Heart BLS Instructor

**SKILLS AND CAPABILITIES:**

Front office and Clinical Medical Assistant Patient Triage
Specimen Collection Venipuncture
EKG and Holter Monitor Parenteral Injections
ICD-9 and CPT Coding Medical Billing

**PROFESSIONAL EXPERIENCE:**

September, 2005–Present   Affiliated Physician Network, Mooresburg, Tennessee
    Medical Assistant/Office Coordinator
June, 2001–September, 2005,   Partners in Internal Medicine, Mooresburg, Tennessee
    Medical Assistant

**EDUCATION:**

Sanford Brown Institute, Diploma, Medical Assisting 2001

**AFFILIATIONS:**

American Medical Technologists

**References available upon request**

**Figure 41-7.**   A targeted résumé is often used by a person who is focusing on a specific job target.

*Example #2*

**WORK EXPERIENCE**

**Medical Assistant**
Managed eight medical assistants from 3 different offices. Oversaw three offices in the Greater Cleveland area. Directed the daily operations of the medical offices. Coordinated events and served as Secretary for the Cuyahoga County Chapter of the American Association of Medical Assistants. Increased daily patient census by 25% due to the success of a customer service model, "Patient First," which improved patient-facility relations during my tenure.

## Résumé Writing Tips

Pay close attention to detail as you create your résumé. Here are some suggestions to help you:

- Organize your information by using a worksheet (Figure 41-8). List all the addresses, dates, phone numbers,

**TABLE 41-1    Effective Résumé Terms**

| | |
|---|---|
| administered | inspected |
| advised | introduced |
| analyzed | maintained |
| billed | managed |
| carried out | motivated |
| compiled | negotiated |
| completed | operated |
| conducted | ordered |
| contacted | organized |
| coordinated | oversaw |
| counseled | performed |
| designed | planned |
| developed | prepared |
| directed | presented |
| distributed | produced |
| established | reviewed |
| functioned as | supervised |
| implemented | taught |
| improved | trained |

and supervisors of previous positions that you have held. Write down brief descriptions of all the responsibilities and duties of your positions.

- List your educational institutions and their addresses, your dates of attendance, and the type of diploma or degree, including your major.

- Choose a résumé format that best describes your experience, education, and achievements.

- Use a computer and save your résumé on a disk or flash drive.

- Proofread all spelling and grammar. Your completed résumé should be perfect. Do not rely on the spell-checking feature of your computer. Proofread your résumé line by line, and request that someone else also proofread your résumé.

- Select a high-quality résumé paper that is the standard size of 8½ by 11, with a weight between 16 and 25 pounds. Use an ivory or white paper with matching envelopes.

- Use clear and concise statements and sentences. Your writing should reflect a positive and confident tone. For example, if you are describing your duties as a server, use sentences that focus on customer service, cash management, and the training and development of new servers. Avoid using the word "I" because the reader already knows that the résumé is referring to you.

- Be truthful and honest about your strengths and abilities. Do not mislead or exaggerate any skills, talents, or experience.

Procedure 41-1 provides information on how to write a résumé.

## Writing a Cover Letter

A cover letter is an introduction to your résumé. It is a tool that markets your résumé as well as your skills and abilities. Cover letters are just as important as your résumé in your job search. An effective cover letter motivates the employer to review the résumé and interview the candidate.

Your cover letter should be direct and to the point. It should be no longer than one page and is typed on paper that matches your résumé. If possible, your cover letter should be addressed to a specific person in the organization. You can call the hospital or facility and ask to whom you should address the letter. If a name is not available, it is acceptable to address the letter to "Human Resource Manager" or "Recruitment Manager." Research the facility or hospital prior to writing the letter. This information can help you tailor your letter to show how your qualifications and interests directly relate to the needs of the company or medical facility. Make sure the description of your qualifications and interests reflects the words used by the company in the advertisement. Always be truthful about the information in the cover letter; employers often verify all facts presented in your résumé and cover letter. Check each cover letter for errors in spelling, grammar, and punctuation. An example of a cover letter is shown in Figure 41-9.

## Sending a Résumé

When sending a résumé, make sure you have the correct name, address, and zip code of the facility. This information should be typed on a matching envelope. Many software programs have an envelope template feature that allows you to print an envelope using the address in your cover letter. Do not hand-write envelopes; professionally appearing mail is often opened first. Make sure that you attach sufficient postage.

When you fax a résumé, verify the fax number and person or department you are faxing to. Make sure your name is on all the faxed pages. If your fax machine provides a fax completion printout, save it to verify that the fax was delivered.

Some classified ads request that you send your résumé via e-mail. In order to send your résumé in electronic form, you must first have an account with an Internet service provider (ISP). You will be asked by the ISP to select a log-in, or screen, name. Do not use a casual name for your log-in; prospective employers will see your log-in name in their in-box. Instead, choose a name that is conservative and professional. Most e-mail programs have an attachment feature that will allow you to send a Microsoft Word document via e-mail. Verify that your e-mail was sent by checking your sent items.

Post your résumé and cover letter on the Internet by using a career job search Internet site. Most Internet job

# EMPLOYMENT WORKSHEET

Job Title _____

Dates _____

Employer _____

City, State _____

Major Duties _____

_____

_____

_____

_____

_____

_____

_____

_____

Special Projects _____

_____

_____

_____

Accomplishments _____

_____

_____

_____

_____

_____

_____

**Figure 41-8.** An employment worksheet can be a useful tool in drafting a résumé.

sites have local employers posting positions daily. A job search Internet site will provide clear directions on how to post your résumé and cover letter. Some school career services departments host online job fairs and will assist you in posting your résumé.

## Obtaining a Reference

Prior to the end of your externship, meet with your preceptor and ask for a **reference.** A reference is a recommendation for employment from the facility and the preceptor.

## Résumé Writing

**Objective:** To develop a résumé that defines your career objective and highlights your skills

**OSHA Guidelines:** This procedure does not involve exposure to blood, body fluids, or tissues.

**Materials:** Paper; pen; dictionary; thesaurus; computer

**Method:**

1. Type your full name, address (temporary and permanent, if you have both), and telephone number (include the area code).

2. List your general career objective. You may also choose to summarize your skills. If you want to phrase your objective to fit a specific position, you should include that information in a cover letter to accompany the résumé.

3. List the highest level of education or the most recently obtained degree first. Include the school name, degree earned, and date of graduation. Be sure to list any special projects, courses, or participation in overseas study programs.

4. Summarize your work experience. List your most recent or most relevant employment first. Describe your responsibilities, and list job titles, company names, and dates of employment. Summer employment, volunteer work, and student externships may also be included. Use short sentences with strong action words such as *directed, designed, developed,* and *organized.* For example, condense a responsibility into

"Handled insurance and billing" or "Drafted correspondence as requested."

*Rationale*

Action verbs give the impression that you are an energetic and results-oriented employee.

5. List any memberships and affiliations with professional organizations. List them alphabetically or by order of importance.

6. Do not list references on your résumé.

*Rationale*

It is easier to update your reference list if you maintain it in a separate file.

7. Do not list the salary you wish to receive in a medical assisting position. Salary requirements should not be discussed until a job offer is received. If the ad you are answering requests that you include a required salary, it is best to state a range (no broader than $5,000 from lowest to highest point in the range for an annual salary).

8. Print your résumé on an 8½- by 11-inch sheet of high-quality white, off-white, or gray bond paper. Carefully check your résumé for spelling, punctuation, and grammatical errors. Have someone else double-check your résumé whenever possible.

*Rationale*

Your résumé is a printed reflection of you, so ensuring its accuracy and completeness is essential.

A reference can be in the form of a letter from the facility, preceptor, or physician, or it can be a request to include these people on your reference list. It is professional to always ask before you list someone as a reference. References are important to career building because employers often like to inquire about a person prior to offering them employment. Your first references in medical assisting are your instructors and then the externship facility.

You will want three to five references, including employment, academic, and character references. Ask instructors for a general letter before you finish your program. Fellow members of professional associations or your classmates can provide character references, and your externship can provide an employment reference. Make certain that you ask your references for permission to use their names and phone numbers. Do not print your references on the bottom of your

résumé. List them on a separate sheet of paper so that you can update the list as needed.

## Preparing a Portfolio

Prior to the interviewing phase, you should organize all your employment documentation into a portfolio. A **portfolio** is a collection of documents such as your résumé, cover letter, reference list or reference letters, awards for volunteer service in a health-related field, and student recognition certificates for student of the year or month, perfect attendance, or academic honors. Include a copy of your transcript, diploma or degree, and medical assisting credentials such as your CMA or RMA. You can also include any other certifications you hold, such as a CPR card or phlebotomy certification. Some employers request proof

**Your Street Address**
**City, State, Zip Code**

**Date**

**Name of person to whom you are writing**
**Title**
**Company or Organization**
**Street Address**
**City, State, Zip Code**

Dear Dr., Mr., Mrs., Miss, or Ms. _____:

<u>1st Paragraph:</u>  Tell why you are writing. Name the position or general area of work that interests you. Mention how you learned about the job opening. State why you are interested in the job.

<u>2d Paragraph:</u>  Refer to the enclosed résumé and give some background information. Indicate why you should be considered as a candidate, focusing on how your skills can fulfill the needs of the company. Relate your experiences to their needs and mention results/achievements. Do not restate what is said on your résumé—you want to pull together all the information and tell how your background fits the position.

<u>3d Paragraph:</u>  Close by making a specific request for an interview. Say that you will follow up with a phone call to arrange a mutually convenient interview time. Offer to provide any additional information that may be needed. Thank the employer for his/her time and consideration.

Sincerely,

(your handwritten signature)

Type your name

Enclosure

**Figure 41-9.**   The object of a cover letter is to convince the recipient to read your résumé.

of immunizations, so include that in your portfolio. Give your portfolio a professional presentation by printing your documents on a high-quality printer and organizing them in a nice binder. A professional portfolio can help you obtain employment. If needed, look for a service that specializes in creating professional portfolios.

# Interviewing

Preparation for your interview begins long before the interview itself. After you send your cover letters and résumés, you must make sure that prospective employers can reach you by telephone. You must practice how you are going to handle your interview, and you must plan what to wear and how to present yourself in the most professional way.

Before starting your job search, invest in an answering machine or voice mail to receive calls when you are not available. Be sure the outgoing message is clear, concise, and professional. Avoid cute messages or background music. An appropriate message would be "I'm unable to take your call at the moment, but your call is important to me. Please leave your name, number, the time you called, and a brief message after the tone, and I will call you back as soon as I can. Thank you." Also, make sure all household members who answer the phone (especially children) know proper phone etiquette and how to take a written message. When a prospective employer calls with an interview invitation, write down the interviewer's name, company or practice name, day, time, and location of the interview.

## Interview Planning and Strategies

Just as the résumé is important for opening the door to opportunity, the job interview itself is critical for allowing you to present yourself professionally and to clearly articulate why you are the best person for the job. As you learned in Chapter 4, being successful in a medical assisting career is centered on communication—both verbal and nonverbal. These communication skills will be assets during your job interviews. The following list provides some strategies that will help you improve your interviewing skills:

- Practice interviewing. Rehearse possible questions and be prepared to answer them directly. Have a friend or family member interview you as you sit in front of a mirror and observe your body language.
- Anticipate question types. Expect open-ended questions such as, What are your strengths? What are your weaknesses? Tell me about your best work experience. Can you give me an example how you have worked with others to solve a problem? Decide in advance what information and skills are pertinent to the position and reveal your strengths. For example, you could say, "While I was at school, I learned to get along with a diverse group of people."
- Learn about the company. Be prepared; research the company or medical facility. What is the type of specialty? How many physicians are there?

- Dress appropriately. Because much communication is nonverbal, dressing appropriately for the interview is important. In most situations, you will be safe if you wear clean, pressed, conservative business clothes in neutral colors. Do not wear current fashions or fad clothing to an interview. Pay special attention to grooming. Keep makeup light, and wear little jewelry. Make sure that your hair and nails are clean and styled conservatively. Do not carry a large purse, backpack, books, coat, or hat. Leave extra clothing in an outside office, and simply carry a pen, your portfolio with extra copies of your résumé, and a small pad for taking notes.
- Be punctual. A good first impression is important and can be lasting. If you arrive late for the interview, a prospective employer may conclude that you will be late in arriving to work. Make certain you know the location and the time of the interview. Allow time for traffic, parking, and other preliminaries.
- Be professional. Being too familiar in your manner can be a barrier to a professional interview. Never call anyone by his or her first name unless you are asked to.
- Know the interviewer's title and the pronunciation of his or her name. Do not sit down until the interviewer does.
- Exhibit appropriate interview behavior. Always greet the interviewer with a smile. The interview is an opportunity to sell yourself to the employer. Offer your hand for a firm, confident handshake, and be alert to the interviewer's body language. The flow of conversation during an interview should be natural. Maintain eye contact, pay attention to the interviewer, and show interest. Ask intelligent questions that you have prepared before the interview. Remember, the interview is an opportunity for both the prospective employer and the prospective employee to gather information and make a good impression. In addition to reviewing the experience listed on your résumé, the interviewer will evaluate your personality and behavior. At the same time, you will be observing the office and learning more about the position. Try to be aware of the office's atmosphere, its equipment and supplies, and the attitudes of the staff. Does it seem like a pleasant, professional place to work? Request a tour of the facility, and ask yourself if you would be happy in that work environment.
- Be poised and relaxed. Avoid nervous habits such as tapping your pencil, playing with your hair, or covering your mouth with your hand. Watch language such as "you know," "ah," "stuff like that." Use proper grammar and pronunciation as you talk with the interviewer—do not use slang. Do not smoke, chew gum, fidget, or bite your nails.
- Maintain comfortable eye contact. Look the interviewer in the eye and speak with confidence. Your eyes reveal much about you; use them to show interest, confidence, poise, and sincerity. Use other nonverbal techniques such as a firm handshake to reinforce your confidence.

- Relate your experience to the job. Use every question as an opportunity to show how your skills relate to the job. Use examples taken from school, previous jobs, your externship, volunteer work, leadership in student organizations, and personal experience to indicate that you have the personal qualities, aptitude, and skills needed for this job.

- Be honest. While it is important to be confident and stress your strengths, it is equally important to your sense of integrity to be honest. Dishonesty always catches up to you sooner or later. Someone will verify your background, so do not exaggerate your accomplishments, grade point average, or experience.

- Focus on how you can benefit the company. Don't ask about benefits, salary, or vacations until you are offered the job. During a first interview, try to show how you can contribute to the organization. Do not appear to be too eager to move up through the company or suggest that you are more interested in gaining experience than in contributing to the company.

- Close the interview on a positive note. Thank the interviewer for his or her time, shake hands, and say that you are looking forward to hearing from him or her. On the way out of the office, thank the staff members involved in the interview. Ask for a business card from anyone whom you think you might want to send a thank-you note. After leaving the interview, write down any additional information you want to remember. Every interview provides you with information about the medical assisting profession. Even if an interview does not result in a job, you will have met new people, developed a larger network of professional contacts, and gained valuable interviewing experience.

- Follow up with a letter. After an interview, it is professional to send a thank-you letter to the person or persons from the company who conducted your interview. You should send this letter within two days of the interview. It may be brief, but it should express your appreciation for the opportunity to have met with the interviewer, reaffirm your interest in the organization, and state your desire to remain a part of the selection process. By sending a thank-you letter, you display common business courtesy, which can make a difference in the employer's hiring decision. Even if you are not interested in continuing the interview and selection process, you should thank the employer for holding the interview. Procedure 41-2 explains how to write and send a thank-you letter.

- Complete an application. Some employers ask you to complete an employment application at an interview even when you provide a résumé. You can use your résumé to help you complete the application. Fill out the application neatly. Spell all words correctly, and read and follow the instructions on the form carefully. Your application represents you; it must make a good first impression. Fill in all sections of the application—do not write "see résumé." An example of an application is shown in Figure 41-10.

- Comply with other aspects of the application process. As part of the application process, employers are required by federal law to request documents that prove your identity and eligibility to work in the United States. To maintain the safety and confidentiality of the medical office, hospital, or laboratory, employers may also check your police record, credit rating, and history of chemical or alcohol abuse. A drug screen may be requested. You may be asked to provide the needed documents or to give the employer authorization too obtain them.

- Do not excessively contact the interviewer by telephone or e-mail after the interview. Prior to leaving the interview, it is acceptable to ask the interviewer when a decision will be made, and if the interviewer will call whether or not an offer of employment will be made. It is acceptable to ask permission to contact the interviewer to follow up on the position.

## Interview Questions

In order to prepare for your interview, you can anticipate that you may be asked any of the following questions:

- I see from your résumé that you graduated from ABC School. What did that school have to offer you that others did not?
- What is your five-year goal?
- Tell me about yourself.
- What do you consider to be your greatest strengths and weaknesses?
- How would your instructors describe you?
- What qualifications do you have that make you a good candidate for this position?
- How could you make a contribution to this facility?
- How well do you work with others?
- What is your concept of a team environment?
- How well do you work under pressure?
- Will you be able to work overtime?
- Do you have the flexibility to work various shifts?
- What has been your major accomplishment to date?
- Why did you choose medical assisting as your career?
- Do you have any questions that you would like to ask?

It is helpful to be prepared with any questions that you may have for the interviewer about the position or the facility. Questions about salary and benefits are not appropriate in a first interview.

An interviewer may ask you questions that you are not obligated to answer. These questions refer to age, race, sexual orientation, marital status, or number of children. Even if the questions sound harmless or the interviewer seems nonjudgmental, these questions have nothing to do with your skills or abilities. If the interviewer asks even

# PROCEDURE 41.2

## Writing Thank-You Notes

**Objective:** To develop an appropriate, professional thank-you note after an interview or externship

**OSHA Guidelines:** This procedure does not involve exposure to blood, body fluids, or tissues.

**Materials:** Paper; pen; dictionary; thesaurus; computer; #10 business envelope

**Method:**

1. Complete the letter within 2 days of the interview or completion of the externship. Begin by typing the date at the top of the letter.

### Rationale

It is considered professional behavior to follow up in a prompt manner and will assist the interviewer to remember you during employment selection.

2. Type the name of the person who interviewed you (or who was your mentor in the externship). Include credentials and title, such as Dr. or Director of Client Services. Include the complete address of the office or organization.

3. Start the letter with "Dear Dr., Mr., Mrs., Miss, or Ms. _____ :"

4. In the first paragraph, thank the interviewer for his time and for granting the interview. Discuss some specific impressions, for example, "I found the interview and tour of the facilities an enjoyable experience. I would welcome the

opportunity to work in such a state-of-the-art medical setting." If you are writing to thank your mentor for her time during your externship and for allowing you to perform your externship at her office, practice, or clinic, discuss the knowledge and experience you gained during the externship.

5. In the second paragraph, mention the aspects of the job or externship that you found most interesting or challenging. For a job interview thank-you note, state how your skills and qualifications will make you an asset to the staff. When preparing an externship thank-you letter, mention interest in any future positions.

6. In the last paragraph, thank the interviewer for considering you for the position. Ask to be contacted at his earliest convenience regarding his employment decision.

7. Close the letter with "Sincerely," and type your name. Leave enough space above your typewritten name to sign your name.

8. Type your return address in the upper left corner of the #10 business envelope. Then type the interviewer's name and address in the envelope's center, apply the proper postage, and mail the letter. You can also e-mail your thank-you letter. Proper letter format and professional tone and appearance still apply. Send the thank-you letter as an attachment.

---

one of these questions, you should reconsider whether you want to work for the organization.

If you are asked an inappropriate question during an interview, be polite and remain professional in declining to answer. You may simply state that you do not believe the requested information is necessary for the employer to evaluate your qualifications for the job. Try to move the discussion onto a more relevant topic.

## Reasons for Not Being Hired

Employers in business were asked to list reasons for not hiring a job candidate. The 15 biggest complaints are the following:

1. Poor appearance, not being dressed properly, and being poorly groomed
2. Acting like a know-it-all
3. Not communicating clearly as well as poor voice, diction, and grammar
4. Lack of planning for the interview, with no purpose or goals communicated
5. Lack of confidence or poise
6. No interest in or enthusiasm for the job
7. Not being active in extracurricular school programs
8. Being interested only in the best salary offer
9. Poor school record, either in academics, attendance, or both
10. Unwillingness to begin in an entry-level position
11. Making excuses about an unfavorable record
12. No tact
13. No maturity
14. No curiosity about the job
15. Being critical of past employers

| Date Called | Type of Work Applied For | Appointment Date | Appointment Time | Reschedule Date | Reschedule Time | Availability | No Phone | GR | PC | Credentials | Pay Rate | Surplus Skill |
|---|---|---|---|---|---|---|---|---|---|---|---|---|
| | | | | | | | | | | | | |

| Last Name | First | M.I. | Applicant Profile | Service Code | Pay Rate | Last Hiring Process Step |
|---|---|---|---|---|---|---|
| | | | | | | |

Address

City | State | Zip Code

Telephone No. | Social Security No. | Today's Date

*Please print. Do not complete shaded areas.*

**EMPLOYMENT APPLICATION**

*EQUAL OPPORTUNITY EMPLOYER*

KELLY Assisted Living

**FOR SUPERVISOR USE ONLY**

Are you at least 18? ☐YES ☐NO

Are you familiar with the way a temporary help service works? *(Explain to applicant)* ☐YES ☐NO

Have you ever worked for a temporary help service? ☐YES ☐NO

Did you work for Kelly Assisted Living Services? ☐YES ☐NO

Where? ______

How long ago? ______

When could you start working for us? ______

How long do you plan to work on a temporary basis?

Can you work Monday through Friday? ☐YES ☐NO

Can you work Saturday? ☐YES ☐NO

Can you work Sunday? ☐YES ☐NO

Are you available ☐DAYS ☐EVENINGS ☐NIGHTS

Are you available as a Live-in? ☐YES ☐NO

What hours are you available? From______ To______

What form of transportation would you usually use to get to work? *(Car, Public transportation, Other)*

Did you bring your professional credentials with you today? ☐YES ☐NO ☐NONE REQUIRED

***Check ☑ T if Trained; ☑ E if Experienced; ☑ T and E if Trained and Experienced.***

T E

☐ ☐ Home Health Aide

☐ ☐ Homemaker

☐ ☐ Nurse Aide

☐ ☐ Registered Nurse

☐ ☐ Licensed Practical Nurse or Licensed Vocational Nurse

T E

☐ ☐ Other health-related positions

*Specify:* ______

Do you have experience as a Live-in? ☐YES ☐NO

***Check ☑ where work experience was obtained.***

☐ Hospital ☐ Home ☐ Industry

☐ Nursing Home ☐ Clinic/Office ☐ Other ______

☐ Community Health

©1990 Kelly Assisted Living Services, Inc. 816 R9/90

**Figure 41-10.** Job applicants are often asked to fill out an application form like the one shown here.

Source: Reprinted with permission from Kelly Assisted Living Services, Inc.

## Salary Negotiations

Medical assisting salaries are varied and differ by geographic area. When you are a new graduate, you will begin your career as an entry-level medical assistant. As you gain experience, your compensation will reflect that. Salary ranges are determined by geographic location, medical specialty, and years of experience, credentialing, and the job description.

The first step in determining your compensation needs is to know how much income is required to meet your living expenses. You will need to prepare a budget. Keep track of your overall expenditures and living expenses. Itemizing your basic living expenses can help you to prepare a budget. These living expenses can include:

- Rent
- Car payments or anticipated car payments
- Car insurance
- Food
- Utilities
- Student loans
- Credit cards
- Clothing
- Child care
- Other

Establishing a budget will give you an idea of the amount of income you may need. Once your budget is established, you have a negotiating benchmark. Employers will often ask you what you are looking for with regard to salary. If you answer directly, you may risk either quoting yourself out of a job or leaving money on the table. The best response to this question is to ask the employer the range of the position. Most positions have a low-to-high range. For example, the range for a specific position could be between $23,000 and $32,000 annually. Once you know the range, quote a little higher than what your budgetary amount is, which will give the employer room to negotiate down if necessary. Allow the employer to bring up salary first.

## On the Job

Once you have a job, you must learn how to be an effective employee. There are many ways that your initiative enables the medical team in the office, hospital, clinic, or laboratory to function effectively. You must identify the important skills in your daily duties, stay competitive and marketable through continuing education, and integrate constructive criticism from your employee evaluations into your daily work and annual goals.

## Job Description

During the initial paperwork process when you begin as a new employee, you will be asked to read and sign a job description for the position for which you have been hired. The job description will list and describe the expectations of the position and the duties to be performed. A job description includes detailed information, such as:

- Essential duties and responsibilities
- Qualifications
- Education and experience
- Certificates, licenses, and registrations
- Physical demands
- Description of the work environment

The purpose of a job description is to provide the standard benchmarks of your position. It communicates to you what will be expected of your in your position.

## Employee Evaluations

Employee evaluations are usually held annually. An initial employment review generally occurs after a probationary period of 90 days. Evaluations describe an employee's performance. A completed evaluation is placed in an official record of employment. In most situations, the employee and the employer meet to discuss the employee's performance. The purpose of an annual evaluation should be to check the goals and values of both the employer and the employee to make sure they support each other.

An employee evaluation form typically outlines the most important qualities and abilities needed for the job. It evaluates the employee's strengths and weaknesses. This form may help determine whether an employee is worthy of a merit raise, which is a raise based on performance (as opposed to a cost-of-living raise). The quantity and quality of work are assessed on this form, as are initiative, judgment, and cooperation.

## Continuing Education

After completing a medical assisting program, you should continue your education, setting specific educational advancement goals on a yearly basis. For example, you may decide to obtain further education to learn more about the medical specialty in which you work.

As medical research expands its discoveries and as new technologies emerge, the necessity for self-education increases. You must read to stay abreast of updates in medicine. The need for more highly specialized training presents you with an opportunity for growth in your education and career. Medical publications are the best source for the latest medical information (Figure 41-11). Local and state medical assisting meetings also provide

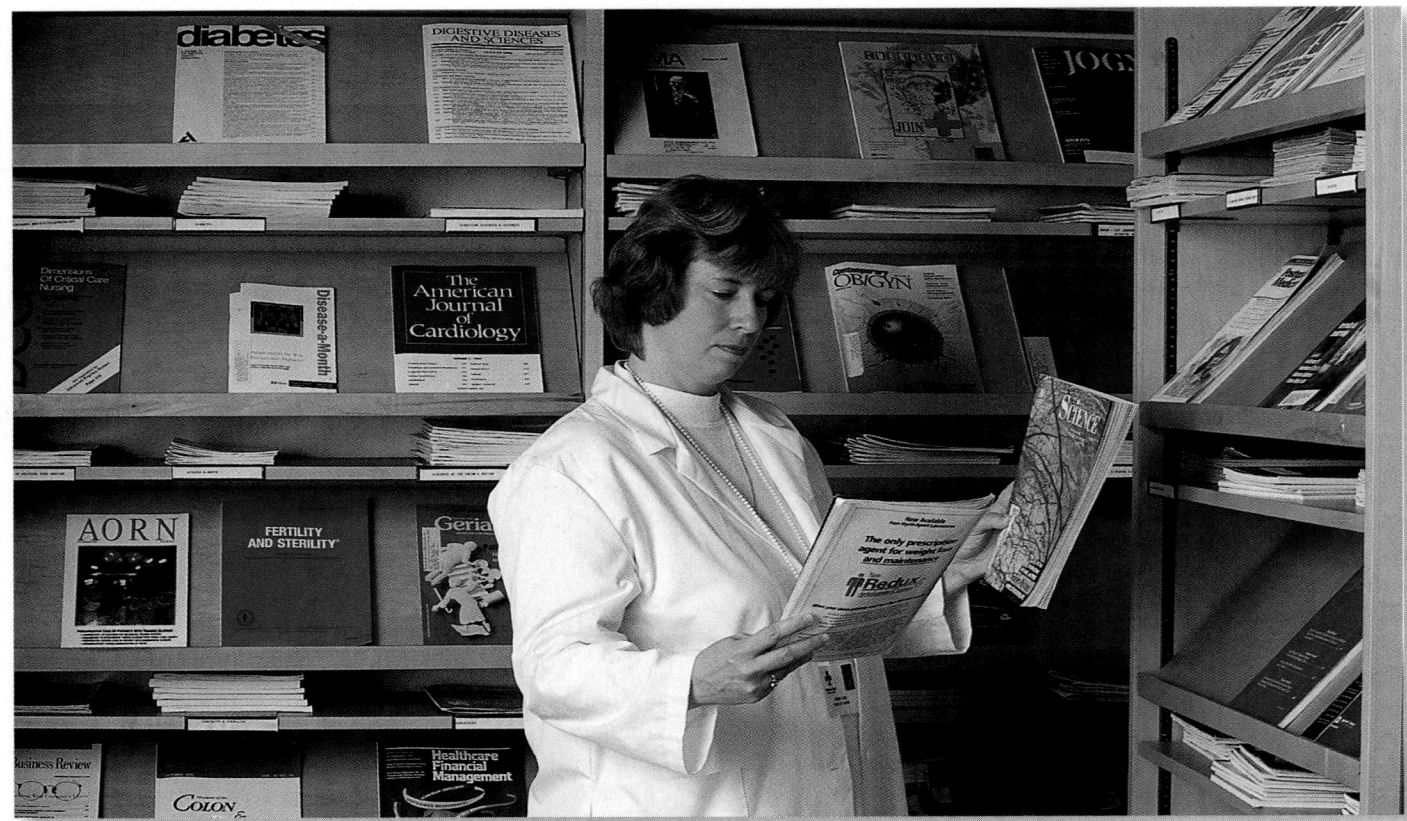

**Figure 41-11.** Part of self-education involves reading articles in professional and lay magazines about topics that relate to the medical practice in which you work.

information about advances in the field. The Internet is a valuable source for staying current about today's technological advances. Self-education is an important skill for the medical assistant. Stay up-to-date in topics about medicine, health care, wellness, insurance products, and pharmaceuticals. Patients may ask questions about information they have read or about the effectiveness of certain new treatments.

## Summary

Medical assisting is an exciting field with many opportunities available to you. It is important to realize that the career phase begins with the externship and will continue for the duration of your career. Your résumé will be a lifelong document that summarizes your career endeavors. Your professionalism will become your reputation, and employment offers may cross your path even if you are not actively seeking them. Continuing education and credentialing will enhance your career, so you should make education and credentialing your short-term goal after completing your medical assisting program.

The profession of medical assisting allows you many directions to take your career and will enable you to make many career changes within this profession. For example, you may choose academics and teaching future medical assistants or you may choose to pursue customer service or management positions in different areas within health care. Because medical assisting is one of the fastest-growing occupations, if you manage your career with professionalism and diligence and continue to learn, you will have many options for satisfying and successful employment.

# REVIEW

## CHAPTER 41

### CASE STUDY QUESTIONS

Now that you have completed this chapter, review the case study at the beginning of the chapter and answer the following questions:

1. What should Sarah do about the ear irrigation?
2. How has she remembered all the previous procedures and not this one?
3. Will the clinical preceptor be disappointed or angry with her?

### Discussion Questions

1. What specialty of medicine would provide an overall, well-rounded externship experience? Refer to Chapter 2 if needed.
2. What accreditation does your school have, and how long is the externship requirement?
3. Describe constructive criticism.
4. List some ways in which you can become more confident in interviewing.
5. What might be some factors that could prevent you from being hired for an externship?

### Critical Thinking Questions

1. Describe an effective medical assistant, and explain two ways that a new medical assistant can learn to be an efficient and effective employee.
2. What are among the most important skills prospective employers seeks?
3. What is the best résumé type for a new graduate of a medical assisting program?

### Application Activities

1. Bring in current classified advertisements from your local newspaper. Highlight all the positions that a medical assistant is qualified for. Discuss the different positions and describe how your qualifications would benefit the organization.
2. Stage mock interviews in your class in which the instructor interviews each student and the classmates critique the interview. Have students look for poise, confidence, and the ability to answer open-ended questions.
3. Invite a local recruiter to talk about interviewing skills. Stage an interview between the instructor and the recruiter. The instructor should behave in ways that are inappropriate for an interview. Write a paper describing what was wrong with the interview.
4. Practice answering interview questions in front of a mirror. Take a personal inventory of what you see. Write a one-page paper describing areas that need improvement as well as your best answers to interview questions.

### Virtual Fieldtrip

*Visit the McGraw-Hill Higher Education Medical Assisting website at www.mhhe.com/medicalassisting3 to complete the following activity:*

Once you have completed your résumé and cover letter, post both documents to job search engines and apply for at least one position.

Open the CD and complete this chapter's practice activities, play the games, listen to the key terms, and test yourself with the interactive review. Email, print, and/or save your results to document your proficiency.

# APPENDIX I

## AAMA/CAAHEP Competencies for the Medical Assistant

The Entry-Level Competencies for the medical assistant include, but are not limited to:

### a. Administrative Competencies:

1. **Perform Clerical Functions**
   a. Schedule and manage appointments
   b. Schedule inpatient and outpatient admissions and procedures
   c. Organize a patient's medical record
   d. File medical records
2. **Perform Bookkeeping Procedures**
   a. Prepare a bank deposit
   b. Post entries on a daysheet
   c. Perform accounts receivable procedures
   d. Perform billing and collection procedures
   e. Post adjustments
   f. Process credit balance
   g. Process refunds
   h. Post NSF checks
   i. Post collection agency payments
3. **Process Insurance Claims**
   a. Apply managed care policies and procedures
   b. Apply third party guidelines
   c. Perform procedural coding
   d. Perform diagnostic coding
   e. Complete insurance claim forms

### b. Clinical Competencies:

1. **Fundamental Procedures**
   a. Perform hand washing
   b. Wrap items for autoclaving
   c. Perform sterilization techniques
   d. Dispose of biohazardous materials
   e. Practice Standard Precautions
2. **Specimen Collection**
   a. Perform venipuncture
   b. Perform capillary puncture
   c. Obtain specimens for microbiological testing
   d. Instruct patients in the collection of a clean-catch midstream urine specimen
   e. Instruct patients in the collection of fecal specimens
3. **Diagnostic Testing**
   a. Perform electrocardiography
   b. Perform respiratory testing
   c. CLIA Waived Tests:
      (i) Perform urinalysis
      (ii) Perform hematology testing
      (iii) Perform chemistry testing
      (iv) Perform immunology testing
      (v) Perform microbiology testing

4. **Patient Care**
   a. Perform telephone and in-person screening
   b. Obtain vital signs
   c. Obtain and record patient history
   d. Prepare and maintain exam and treatment areas
   e. Prepare patient for and assist with routine and specialty exams
   f. Prepare patient for and assist with procedures, treatments, and minor office surgeries
   g. Apply pharmacology principles to prepare and administer oral and parenteral (excluding IV) medications
   h. Maintain medication and immunization records
   i. Screen and follow-up test results

### c. General Competencies

1. **Professional Communications**
   a. Respond to and initiate written communications
   b. Recognize and respond to verbal communications
   c. Recognize and respond to nonverbal communications
   d. Demonstrate telephone techniques
2. **Legal Concepts**
   a. Identify and respond to issues of confidentiality
   b. Perform within legal and ethical boundaries
   c. Establish and maintain the medical record
   d. Document appropriately
   e. Demonstrate knowledge of federal and state health-care legislation and regulations
3. **Patient Instruction**
   a. Explain general office policies
   b. Instruct individuals according to their needs
   c. Provide instruction for health maintenance and disease prevention
   d. Identify community resources
4. **Operational Functions**
   a. Perform an inventory of supplies and equipment
   b. Perform routine maintenance of administrative and clinical equipment
   c. Utilize computer software to maintain office systems
   d. Use methods of quality control

*General Competencies may be addressed in clinical, administrative, or both areas.*

# APPENDIX II

## AMT Registered Medical Assistant (RMA) Certified Examination Topics Correlation Chart

### Examination Topics

I. **GENERAL MEDICAL ASSISTING KNOWLEDGE**
   A. *Orientation*
      1. Introduction and review of program
      2. Employment outlook
      3. General responsibilities
   B. *Anatomy and Physiology*
      1. Anatomy and Physiology
      2. Diet and nutrition
      3. Study of diseases and etiology
      4. All body systems
      5. Diagnostic/treatment modalities
   C. *Medical Terminology*
      1. Basic structure of medical words (roots, prefixes, suffixes, spelling, and definitions)
      2. Combining word elements to form medical words
      3. Medical specialties and short forms
      4. Medical abbreviations
   D. *Medical Law and Ethics*
      1. Ethical decisions, medical jurisprudence, and confidentiality
      2. Legal terminology pertaining to office practice
      3. Medical/ethical issues in today's society
      4. Risk management
   E. *Psychology of Human Relations*
      1. Dealing with difficult patients with normal/abnormal behavior
      2. Caring for patients with special and specific needs
      3. Caring for cancer and terminally ill patients
      4. Emotional crisis/patients and/or family
      5. Various treatment protocols
      6. Basic principles
      7. Developmental stages of the life cycle
      8. Hereditary, cultural, and environmental influences on behavior standards
   F. *Career Development*
      1. Instruction regarding internship rules, regulations
      2. Job search, professional development, and success
      3. Goal setting, time management, and employment opportunities
      4. Resume writing, interviewing techniques, and follow-up
      5. Dress for success
      6. Professionalism

II. **ADMINISTRATIVE MEDICAL ASSISTING**
   A. *Medical Office Business Procedures/Management*
      1. Manual and computerized records management
         (1) Patient case histories (confidentiality)
         (2) Filing
         (3) Appointments and scheduling
         (4) Inventory/Control

   2. Financial Management
      (1) Basic bookkeeping
      (2) Billing and collections
      (3) Purchasing
      (4) Banking and payroll
   3. Insurance (including HMOs, PPOs, co-pays, CPT coding, etc.)
   4. Equipment and Supplies (including ordering/maintaining/storage/inventory)
   5. Reception, public, and interpersonal relations
      (1) Telephone techniques
      (2) Professional conduct and appearance
      (3) Professional office environment and safety
   6. Office safety and security
   B. *Basic Keyboarding*
      1. Office machines, transcriptions, computerized systems/medical data processing
      2. Transcribing medical correspondence and medical reports
      3. Medical terminology review

III. **CLINICAL MEDICAL ASSISTING**
   A. *Medical Office Clinical Procedures*
      1. Basic clinical skills (e.g., vital signs)
      2. Basic skills and procedures used in medical emergencies
      3. Patient exam
         (1) Patient histories
         (2) Patient preparation
         (3) Physical exam
         (4) Instruments
         (5) Assisting the physician
         (6) Housekeeping
      4. Medical Equipment
         (1) Electrocardiogram, centrifuge, etc.
         (2) Physical therapy
         (3) Radiology
            (a) Safety
            (b) Patient preparation
            (c) Radiography of chest and extremities
         (4) Medical asepsis/sterilization and minor office surgery
         (5) Specialties
         (6) First Aid, CPR
         (7) Injections (dosage calculations)
            (a) IM
            (b) Subq
            (c) ID
         (8) Universal precautions in the medical office
   B. *Medical Laboratory Procedures*
      1. Orientation
         (1) Laboratory equipment and maintenance
         (2) Safety

        (3) Storage of chemicals and supplies
        (4) Fire safety
        (5) Care of microscope (introduction)
    2. Urinalysis
        (1) Specimen collection
        (2) Physical exam
        (3) Chemical analysis
        (4) Microscopic exam
    3. Hematology
        (1) Personal protection equipment
        (2) Specimen collection
            (a) Venipuncture
            (b) Finger puncture
        (3) Hemoglobin
        (4) Hematocrit
        (5) WBC
        (6) RBC

        (7) Slide preps
        (8) Serology
            (a) Blood typing
            (b) Blood morphology
        (9) Quality control
    4. Basic blood chemistries
    5. HIV/AIDS and blood-borne pathogens
    6. OSHA compliance rules and regulations
C. *Pharmacology*
    1. Occupational math and metric conversions (drug calculations)
    2. Use of PDRs and medication books
    3. Common abbreviations used in prescription writing
    4. Legal aspects of writing prescriptions
    5. FDC and state laws
    6. Medications prescribed for the treatment of illness and disease based on a systems method

# APPENDIX III

## National Healthcareer Association (NHA)

## Medical Assisting Duty/Task List

**Duties:**

A. DISPLAY PROFESSIONALISM

B. APPLY COMMUNICATION SKILLS

C. DEMONSTRATE KEYBOARDING SKILLS AND COMPUTER AWARENESS

D. PERFORM BUSINESS SOFTWARE APPLICATIONS

E. WORK WITHIN COMPUTER OPERATING ENVIRONMENTS

F. PERFORM ADMINISTRATIVE DUTIES

G. PERFORM CLINICAL DUTIES

H. APPLY LEGAL, ETHICAL, AND CONFIDENTIALITY CONCEPTS TO PRACTICE

I. MANAGE THE OFFICE

J. PROVIDE PATIENT INSTRUCTION

K. MANAGE PRACTICE FINANCES

### Duty A: Display Professionalism

A. 01 Project a Positive Attitude

A. 02 Demonstrate Ethical Behavior

A. 03 Practice Within the Scope of Education, Training and Personal Capabilities

A. 04 Maintain Confidentiality

A. 05 Work as a Team Member

A. 06 Conduct Oneself in a Courteous and Diplomatic Manner

A. 07 Adapt to Change

A. 08 Show Initiative and Responsibility

A. 09 Promote the Profession

A. 10 Apply Critical Thinking Skills to Workplace Situations

A. 11 Manage stress

### Duty B: Apply Communication Skills

B. 01 Listen and Observe

B. 02 Treat all Patients with Empathy and Impartiality

B. 03 Adapt Communication to Individual's Abilities to Understand

B. 04 Recognize and Respond to Verbal and Nonverbal Communication

B. 05 Serve as Liaison Between Physician and Others

B. 06 Evaluate Understanding of Communication

B. 07 Receive, Organize, Prioritize and Transmit Information

B. 08 Use Proper Telephone Technique

B. 09 Interview Effectively

B. 10 Use Medical Terminology Appropriately

B. 11 Compose Written Communication Using Correct Grammar, Spelling and Format

### Duty C: Demonstrate Keyboarding Skill and Computer Awareness

C. 01 Perform Keyboarding by Touch on a Microcomputer

C. 01 Use Basic Terminology Common in the Computer Industry

C. 02 Demonstrate Care and Routine Maintenance of Computer Systems

C. 03 Identify the Types and Functions of Hardware and Peripheral Components

C. 04 Identify the Types of Operating Systems

C. 05 Define Differences in the Application of Microcomputer Software

### Duty D: Perform Business Software Applications

D. 01 Explain the Characteristics and Components of Word Processing

D. 02 Start Up Word Processing Software

D. 03 Produce and Format Common Business Documents Such as Letters, Memos, and Reports

D. 04 Edit a Document

D. 05 Print a Document

D. 06 Retrieve a Document

D. 07 Enhance a Document

D. 08 Utilize Software Reference/Documentation

D. 09 Explain the Uses of Database Management Concepts and Applications

D. 10 Perform Basic Database Operations

D. 12 Index and/or Sort Databases

D. 13 Link Databases

D. 14 Design Reports

D. 15 Integrate Software Applications

D. 16 Utilize Software Reference/Documentation

### Duty E: Work Within Computer Operating Environments

E. 01 Use Operating System Commands

E. 02 Work with Directories and Subdirectories

E. 03 Demonstrate File Naming Conventions

E. 04 Understand the Basic Function of Batch Files

E. 07 Explain the Characteristics and Components of Graphical User Interface Software

E. 08 Start Up Graphical User Interface Software

E. 09 Utilize the Programs in the Standard Graphical User Interface Software Groups

E. 10 Build and Use Icons

E. 11 Perform Basic File Commands on Network Drive

E. 12 Print Using a Network Printer

**Duty F: Perform Administrative Duties**

F. 01 Perform Records Management

F. 02 Use and Maintain Office Equipment

F. 03 Handle Incoming Mail

F. 04 Schedule and Monitor Appointments

F. 05 Prepare and Maintain Medical Records

F. 06 Implement a Health Care Software System

F. 07 Operate a Health Care Software System

F. 08 Information for Patients and Employers

F. 11 Manage Calendar/Itineraries

F. 12 Organize Meetings and Presentations

**Duty G: Perform Clinical Duties**

G. 01 Apply Principles of Aseptic Technique

G. 02 Apply Principles of Infection Control

G. 03 Vital Signs

G. 04 Recognize Emergencies

G. 05 Perform First-Aid and CPR

G. 06 Prepare and Maintain Examination and Treatment Area

G. 07 Interview and Take Patient History

G. 08 Prepare Patients for Procedures

G. 09 Assist Physician with Examinations and Treatments

G. 10 Use Quality Control

G. 11 Collect and Process Specimens

G. 12 Perform Selected Tests That Assist With Diagnosis and Treatment

G. 13 Perform Immunological Tests and Record Results

G. 14 Perform Microbiological Tests and Record Results

G. 15 Perform Tuberculosis Screen and Record Results

G. 16 Run an Electrocardiogram and Record Results

G. 17 Perform Vision Testing and Record Results

G. 18 Screen and Follow Up Patient Test Results

G. 19 Prepare and Administer Medications as Directed by Physician

G. 20 Maintain Medication Records

G. 21 Utilize Proper Body Mechanics

G. 22 Apply Basic Math to Medically Related Problems.

G. 25 Use Formulas and Equations to Solve Health-Related Math Problems

G. 26 Transfer and Transport Patients With or Without Assistive Devices Using Proper Body Mechanics

**Duty H: Apply Legal, Ethical, and Confidentiality Concepts**

H. 01 Document Accurately

H. 02 Determine Needs for Documentation and Reporting

H. 03 Use Appropriate Guidelines When Releasing Records or Information

H. 04 Follow Established Policy in Initiating, Withdrawing, Withholding, or Terminating Medical Treatment

H. 05 Dispose of Controlled Substances in Compliance With Government Regulations

H. 06 Maintain Licenses and Certification

H. 07 Monitor Legislation Related to Current Health Care and Practice

H. 08 Perform Within Ethical Boundaries

**Duty I: Manage the Office**

I. 01 Maintain the Physical Plant

I. 02 Operate and Maintain Facilities and Equipment Safely

I. 03 Maintain and Operate Medical Equipment

I. 04 Observe Safety Precautions in the Office

I. 05 Inventory Equipment and Supplies

I. 06 Identify Supply Resources

I. 07 Evaluate and Recommend Equipment and Supplies

I. 08 Maintain Liability Coverage

I. 09 Maintain Documentation of Continuing Education

I. 10 Exercise Efficient Time Management

**Duty J: Provide Patient Instruction**

J. 01 Orient Patients to Office Policies and Procedures

J. 02 Instruct Patients With Special Needs

J. 03 Teach Patients Methods of Health Promotion and Disease Prevention

J. 04 Provide Verbal and Written Information

J. 05 Orient and Train Personnel

**Duty K: Manage Practice Finances**

K. 01 Use Bookkeeping Systems

K. 02 Implement Current Diagnostic/Procedural Coding Systems (CPT and ICD-9-CM coding)

K. 03 Analyze and Use Current Third-Party Guidelines for Reimbursement

K. 04 Manage Accounts Receivable

K. 05 Manage Accounts Payable

K. 06 Maintain Records for Accounting and Banking Purposes

# APPENDIX IV
## Prefixes and Suffixes Commonly Used in Medical Terms

**a-, an-** without, not
**ab-** from, away
**ad-, -ad** to, toward
**adeno-** gland, glandular
**aero-** air
**-aesthesia** sensation
**-al** characterized by
**-algia** pain
**ambi-, amph-, amphi-** both, on both sides, around
**andr-, andro-** man, male
**angio-** blood vessel
**ano-** anus
**ante-** before
**antero-** in front of
**anti-** against, opposing
**arterio-** artery
**arthro-** joint
**-ase** enzyme
**-asthenia** weakness
**auto-** self
**bi-** twice, double
**bili-** bile
**bio-** life
**blasto-, -blast** developing stage, bud
**brachy-** short
**brady-** slow
**broncho-** bronchial (windpipe)
**cardio-** heart
**cata-** down, lower, under
**-cele** swelling, tumor
**-centesis** puncture, tapping
**centi-** hundred
**cephal-, cephalo-** head
**cerebr-, cerebro-** brain
**chol-, chole-, cholo-** gall
**chondro-** cartilage
**chromo-** color
**-cidal** killing
**-cide** causing death
**circum-** around
**-cise** cut
**co-, com-, con-** together, with
**-coele** cavity
**colo-** colon
**colp-, colpo-** vagina
**contra-** against
**cost-, costo-** rib

**crani-, cranio-** skull
**cryo-** cold
**cysto-, -cyst** bladder, bag
**-cyte, cyto-** cell, cellular
**dacry-, dacryo-** tears, lacrimal apparatus
**dactyl-, dactylo-** finger, toe
**de-** down, from
**deca-** ten
**deci-** tenth
**demi-** half
**dent-, denti-, dento-** teeth
**derma-, dermat-, dermato-, -derm** skin
**dextro-** to the right
**di-** double, twice
**dia-** through, apart, between
**dipla-, diplo-** double, twin
**dis-** apart, away from
**dorsi-, dorso-** back
**dynia-** pain
**dys-** difficult, painful, bad, abnormal
**e-, ec-, ecto-** away, from, without, outside
**-ectomy** cutting out, surgical removal
**em-, en-** in, into, inside
**-emesis** vomiting
**-emia** blood
**encephalo-** brain
**endo-** within, inside
**entero-** intestine
**ento-** within, inner
**epi-** on, above
**erythro-** red
**esthesio-, -esthesia** sensation
**eu-** good, true, normal
**ex-, exo-** outside of, beyond, without
**extra-** outside of, beyond, in addition
**fibro-** connective tissue
**fore-** before, in front of
**-form** shape
**-fuge** driving away
**galact-, galacto-** milk
**gastr-, gastro-** stomach
**-gene, -genic, -genetic, -genous** arising from, origin, formation
**glosso-** tongue
**gluco-, glyco-** sugar, sweet
**-gram** recorded information
**-graph** instrument for recording

**-graphy** the process of recording
**-gravida** pregnant female
**gyn-, gyno-, gyne-, gyneco-** woman, female
**haemo-, hemato-, hem-, hemo-** blood
**hemi-** half
**hepa-, hepar-, hepato-** liver
**herni-** rupture
**hetero-** other, unlike
**histo-** tissue
**homeo, homo-** same, like
**hydra-, hydro-** water
**hyper-** above, over, increased, excessive
**hypo-** below, under, decreased
**hyster-, hystero-** uterus
**-ia** condition
**-iasis** condition of
**-ic, -ical** pertaining to
**ictero-** jaundice
**idio-** personal, self-produced
**ileo-** ileum
**im-, in-, ir-** not
**in-** in, into
**infra-** beneath
**inter-** between, among
**intra-, intro-** into, within, during
**-ism** condition, process, theory
**-itis** inflammation of
**-ium** membrane
**-ize** to cause to be, to become, to treat by special method
**juxta-** near, nearby
**karyo-** nucleus, nut
**kata-, kath-** down, lower, under
**kera-, kerato-** horn, hardness, cornea
**kineto-, -kinesis, -kinetic** motion
**lact-** milk
**laparo-** abdomen
**latero-** side
**-lepsis, -lepsy** seizure, convulsion
**leuco-, leuko-** white
**levo-** to the left
**lipo-** fat
**lith-, -lith** stone
**-logy** science of, study of
**-lysis** setting free, disintegration, decomposition

**macro-** large, long
**mal-** bad
**-malacia** abnormal softening
**-mania** insanity, abnormal desire
**mast-, masto-** breast
**med-, medi-** middle
**mega-, megalo-** large, great
**meio-** contraction
**melan-, melano-** black
**meno-** month
**mes-, meso-** middle
**meta-** beyond
**-meter** measure
**metro-, metra-** uterus
**-metry** process of measuring
**micro-** small
**mio-** smaller, less
**mono-** single, one
**multi-** many
**my-, myo-** muscle
**myel-, myelo-** marrow
**narco-** sleep
**nas-, naso-** nose
**necro-** dead
**neo-** new
**nephr-, nephro-** kidney
**neu-, neuro-** nerve
**niter-, nitro-** nitrogen
**non-, not-** no
**nucleo-** nucleus
**-nuli** none
**ob-** against
**oculo-** eye
**odont-** tooth
**-odynia** pain
**-oid** resembling
**-ole** small, little
**olig-, oligo-** few, less than normal
**-oma** tumor
**onco-** tumor
**oo-** ovum, egg
**oophor-** ovary
**ophthalmo-** eye
**-opia** vision
**-opsy** to view
**orchid-** testicle
**ortho-** straight
**os-** mouth, bone
**-osis** disease, condition of
**oste-, osteo-** bone
**-ostomy** to make a mouth, opening
**oto-** ear

**-otomy** incision, surgical cutting
**-ous** having
**oxy-** sharp, acid
**pachy-** thick
**paedo, pedo-** child
**pan-** all, every
**par; para-** alongside of, with; woman who has given birth
**path-, patho-, -pathy** disease, suffering
**ped-, pedi-, pedo-** foot
**-penia** too few, lack, decreased
**per-** through, excessive
**peri-** around
**pes-** foot
**-pexy** surgical fixation
**phag-, phagia, phago-, -phage** eating, consuming, swallowing
**pharyng-** throat, pharynx
**phlebo-** vein
**-phobia** fear, abnormal fear
**-phylaxis** protection
**-plasia** formation or development
**-plastic** molded
**-plasty** operation to reconstruct, surgical repair
**-plegia** paralysis
**pleuro-** side, rib
**pluri-** more, several
**pneo-, -pnea** breathing
**pneumo-** air, lungs
**-pod** foot
**poly-** many, much
**post-** after, behind
**pre-, pro-** before, in front of
**presby-, presbyo-** old age
**primi-** first
**procto-** rectum
**proto-** first
**pseudo-** false
**psych-** the mind
**pulmon-, pulmono-** lung
**pyelo-** pelvis (renal)
**pyo-** pus
**pyro-** fever, heat
**quadri-** four
**re-** back, again
**reni-, reno-** kidney
**retro-** backward, behind
**rhino-** nose
**-rrhage, -rrhagia** abnormal or excessive discharge, hemorrhage, flow
**-rrhaphy** suture of

**-rrhea** flow, discharge
**sacchar-** sugar
**sacro-** sacrum
**salpingo-** tube, fallopian tube
**sarco-** flesh
**sclero-** hard, sclera
**-sclerosis** hardening
**-scopy** examining
**semi-** half
**septi-, septic-, septico-** poison, infection
**-spasm** cramp or twitching
**-stasis** stoppage
**steno-** contracted, narrow
**stereo-** firm, solid, three-dimensional
**stomato-** mouth
**-stomy** opening
**sub-** under
**super-, supra-** above, upon, excess
**sym-, syn-** with, together
**tachy-** fast
**tele-** distant, far
**teno-, tenoto-** tendon
**tetra-** four
**-therapy** treatment
**thermo-, -thermy** heat
**thio-** sulfur
**thoraco-** chest
**thrombo-** blood clot
**thyro-** thyroid gland
**-tome** cutting instrument
**tomo-, -tomy** incision, section
**trans-** across
**tri-** three
**-tripsy** surgical crushing
**tropho-, -trophy** nutrition, growth
**-tropy** turning, tendency
**ultra-** beyond, excess
**uni-** one
**-uria** urine
**urino-, uro-** urine, urinary organs
**utero-** uterus, uterine
**vaso-** vessel
**ventri-, ventro-** abdomen
**xanth-** yellow

# APPENDIX V
## Latin and Greek Equivalents Commonly Used in Medical Terms

**abdomen**  venter
**adhesion**  adhaesio
**and**  et
**arm**  brachium; brachion (Gr)
**artery**  arteria
**back**  dorsum
**backbone**  spina
**backward**  retro; opistho (Gr)
**bend**  flexus
**bile**  bilis; chole (Gr)
**bladder**  vesica, cystus
**blister**  vesicula
**blood**  sanguis; haima (Gr)
**body**  corpus; soma (Gr)
**bone**  os, ossis; osteon (Gr)
**brain**  encephalon
**break**  ruptura
**breast**  mamma; mastos (Gr)
**buttock**  gloutos (Gr)
**cartilage**  cartilago; chondros (Gr)
**cavity**  cavum
**chest**  pectoris, pectus; thorax (Gr)
**child**  puer, puerilis
**choke**  strangulo
**corn**  clavus
**cornea**  kerat (Gr)
**cough**  tussis
**deadly**  lethalis
**death**  mors
**dental**  dentalis
**digestive**  pepticos
**disease**  morbus
**dislocation**  luxatio
**doctor**  medicus
**dose**  dosis (Gr)
**ear**  auris; ous (Gr)
**egg**  ovum
**erotic**  erotikos (Gr)
**exhalation**  exhalatio, expiro
**external**  externus
**extract**  extractum
**eye**  oculus; ophthalmos (Gr)
**eyelid**  palpebra
**face**  facies
**fat**  adeps; lipos (Gr)
**female**  femella

**fever**  febris
**finger (or toe)**  digitus
**flesh**  carnis, caro
**foot**  pes
**forehead**  frons
**gum**  gingiva
**hair**  capillus, pilus; thrix (Gr)
**hand**  manus; cheir (Gr)
**harelip**  labrum fissum; cheiloschisis (Gr)
**head**  caput; kephale (Gr)
**health**  sanitas
**hear**  audire
**heart**  cor; kardia (Gr)
**heat**  calor; therme (Gr)
**heel**  calx, talus
**hysterics**  hysteria
**infant**  infans
**infectious**  contagiosus
**injection**  injectio
**intellect**  intellectus
**internal**  internus
**intestine**  intestinum; enteron (Gr)
**itching**  pruritis
**jawbone**  maxilla
**joint**  vertebra; arthron (Gr)
**kidney**  ren, renis; nephros (Gr)
**knee**  genu
**kneecap**  patella
**lacerate**  lacerare
**larynx**  guttur
**lateral**  lateralis
**limb**  membrum
**lip**  labium, labrum; cheilos (Gr)
**listen**  auscultare
**liver**  jecur; hepar (Gr)
**loin**  lapara
**looseness**  laxativus
**lung**  pulmo; pneumon (Gr)
**male**  masculinus
**malignant**  malignons
**milk**  lac
**moisture**  humiditas
**month**  mensis
**monthly**  menstruus
**mouth**  oris, os; stoma, stomato (Gr)

**nail**  unguis; onyx (Gr)
**navel**  umbilicus; omphalos (Gr)
**neck**  cervix; trachelos (Gr)
**nerve**  nervus; neuron (Gr)
**nipple**  papilla; thele (Gr)
**no, none**  nullus
**nose**  nasus; rhis (Gr)
**nostril**  naris
**nourishment**  alimentum
**ointment**  unguentum
**pain**  dolor; algia
**patient**  patiens
**pectoral**  pectoralis
**pimple**  pustula
**poison**  venenum
**powder**  pulvis
**pregnant**  praegnans, gravida
**pubic bone**  os pubis
**pupil**  pupilla
**rash**  exanthema (Gr)
**recover**  convalescere
**redness**  rubor
**rib**  costa
**ringing**  tinnitus
**scaly**  squamosus
**sciatica**  sciaticus; ischiadikos (Gr)
**seed**  semen
**senile**  senilis
**sheath**  vagina; theke (Gr)
**short**  brevis; brachys (Gr)
**shoulder**  omos (Gr)
**shoulder blade**  scapula
**side**  latus
**skin**  cutis; derma (Gr)
**skull**  cranium; kranion (Gr)
**sleep**  somnus
**solution**  solutio
**spinal**  spinalis
**stomach**  stomachus; gaster (Gr)
**stone**  calculus
**sugar**  saccharum
**swallow**  glutio
**tail**  cauda
**taste**  gustatio
**tear**  lacrima
**testicle**  testis; orchis (Gr)

*Parenthetical "Gr" means the preceding term is Greek. Other terms in the column are Latin.

**thigh**   femur
**throat**   fauces; pharynx (Gr)
**tongue**   lingua; glossa (Gr)
**tooth**   dens; odontos (Gr)
**touch**   tactus
**tremor**   tremere
**twin**   gemellus

**ulcer**   ulcus
**urine**   urina; ouran (Gr)
**uterus**   hystera (Gr)
**vagina**   vagina; kolpos (Gr)
**vein**   vena; phlebos, phleps (Gr)
**vertebra**   spondylos (Gr)
**vessel**   vas

**wash**   diluere
**water**   aqua
**wax**   cera
**weak**   debilis
**windpipe**   arteria aspera
**wrist**   carpus; karpos (Gr)

# APPENDIX VI

## Abbreviations Commonly Used in Medical Notations

**a**  before
**a.c.**  before meals
**ADD**  attention deficit disorder
**ADL**  activities of daily living
**ad lib**  as desired
**ADT**  admission, discharge, transfer
**AIDS**  acquired immunodeficiency syndrome
**a.m.a.**  against medical advice
**AMA**  American Medical Association
**amp.**  ampule
**amt**  amount
**aq., AQ**  water; aqueous
**ausc.**  auscultation
**ax**  axis
**Bib, bib**  drink
**b.i.d., bid, BID**  twice a day
**BM**  bowel movement
**BP, B/P**  blood pressure
**BPC**  blood pressure check
**BPH**  benign prostatic hypertrophy
**BSA**  body surface area
**c̄., c̄**  with
**Ca**  calcium; cancer
**cap, caps**  capsules
**CBC**  complete blood (cell) count
**C.C., CC**  chief complaint
**CDC**  Centers for Disease Control and Prevention
**CHF**  congestive heart failure
**chr**  chronic
**CNS**  central nervous system
**Comp, comp**  compound
**COPD**  chronic obstructive pulmonary disease
**CP**  chest pain
**CPE**  complete physical examination
**CPR**  cardiopulmonary resuscitation
**CSF**  cerebrospinal fluid
**CT**  computed tomography
**CV**  cardiovascular
**d**  day
**D&C**  dilation and curettage
**DEA**  Drug Enforcement Administration
**Dil, dil**  dilute
**DM**  diabetes mellitus
**DOB**  date of birth
**DTP**  diptheria-tetanus-pertussis vaccine

**Dr.**  doctor
**DTs**  delirium tremens
**D/W**  dextrose in water
**Dx, dx**  diagnosis
**ECG, EKG**  electrocardiogram
**ED**  emergency department
**EEG**  electroencephalogram
**EENT**  eyes, ears, nose, and throat
**EP**  established patient
**ER**  emergency room
**ESR**  erythrocyte sedimentation rate
**FBS**  fasting blood sugar
**FDA**  Food and Drug Administration
**FH**  family history
**Fl, fl, fld**  fluid
**F/u**  follow-up
**Fx**  fracture
**GBS**  gallbladder series
**GI**  gastrointestinal
**Gm**  gram
**gr**  grain
**gt, gtt**  drops
**GTT**  glucose tolerance test
**GU**  genitourinary
**GYN**  gynecology
**HB, Hgb**  hemoglobin
**HEENT**  head, ears, eyes, nose, throat
**HIV**  human immunodeficiency virus
**HO**  history of
**h.s., hs, HS**  hour of sleep/at bedtime
**Hx**  history
**ICU**  intensive care unit
**I&D**  incision and drainage
**I&O**  intake and output
**IM**  intramuscular
**inf.**  infusion; inferior
**inj**  injection
**IT**  inhalation therapy
**IUD**  intrauterine device
**IV**  intravenous
**KUB**  kidneys, ureters, bladder
**L1, L2, etc.**  lumbar vertebrae
**lab**  laboratory
**liq**  liquid
**LLL**  left lower lobe
**LLQ**  left lower quadrant
**LMP**  last menstrual period
**LUQ**  left upper quadrant

**MI**  myocardial infarction
**mL**  millileter
**MM**  mucous membrane
**MRI**  magnetic resonance imaging
**MS**  multiple sclerosis
**NB**  newborn
**NED**  no evidence of disease
**no.**  number
**noc, noct**  night
**npo, NPO**  nothing by mouth
**NPT**  new patient
**NS**  normal saline
**NSAID**  nonsteroidal anti-inflammatory drug
**NTP**  normal temperature and pressure
**N&V**  nausea and vomiting
**NYD**  not yet diagnosed
**OB**  obstetrics
**OC**  oral contraceptive
**OD**  overdose
**O.D., OD**  right eye
**oint**  ointment
**OOB**  out of bed
**OPD**  outpatient department
**OPS**  outpatient services
**OR**  operating room
**O.S., OS**  left eye
**OTC**  over-the-counter
**O.U., OU**  both eyes
**P&P**  Pap smear (Papanicolaou smear) and pelvic examination
**PA**  posteroanterior
**Pap**  Pap smear
**Path**  pathology
**p.c., pc**  after meals
**PE**  physical examination
**per**  by, with
**PH**  past history
**PID**  pelvic inflammatory disease
**p/o**  postoperative
**POMR**  problem-oriented medical record
**PMFSH**  past medical, family, social history
**PMS**  premenstrual syndrome
**p.r.n., prn, PRN**  whenever necessary
**Pt**  patient
**PT**  physical therapy
**PTA**  prior to admission

**PVC** premature ventricular contraction
**pulv** powder
**q.** every
**q2, q2h** every 2 hours
**q.a.m., qam** every morning
**q.h., qh** every hour
**qhs** every night, at bedtime
**q.i.d., QID** four times a day
**qns, QNS** quantity not sufficient
**qs, QS** quantity sufficient
**RA** rheumatoid arthritis; right atrium
**RBC** red blood cells; red blood (cell) count
**RDA** recommended dietary allowance, recommended daily allowance
**REM** rapid eye movement
**RF** rheumatoid factor
**RLL** right lower lobe
**RLQ** right lower quadrant
**R/O** rule out
**ROM** range of motion
**ROS/SR** review of systems/systems review
**RUQ** right upper quadrant
**RV** right ventricle
**Rx** prescription, take

**SAD** seasonal affective disorder
**SIDS** sudden infant death syndrome
**Sig** directions
**sig** sigmoidoscopy
**SOAP** subjective, objective, assessment, plan
**SOB** shortness of breath
**sol** solution
**S/R** suture removal
$\overline{ss}$, $\overline{ss}$ one-half
**Staph** staphylococcus
**stat, STAT** immediately
**STD** sexually transmitted disease
**Strep** streptococcus
**subling, SL** sublingual
**subq, SubQ** subcutaneously
**surg** surgery
**S/W** saline in water
**SX** symptoms
**T1, T2, etc.** thoracic vertebrae
**T & A** tonsillectomy and adenoidectomy
**tab** tablet
**TB** tuberculosis
**TBS, tbs.** tablespoon
**TIA** transient ischemic attack

**t.i.d., tid, TID** three times a day
**tinc, tinct, tr** tincture
**TMJ** temporomandibular joint
**top** topically
**TPR** temperature, pulse, and respiration
**TSH** thyroid stimulating hormone
**tsp** teaspoon
**Tx** treatment
**UA** urinalysis
**UCHD** usual childhood diseases
**UGI** upper gastrointestinal
**ung, ungt** ointment
**URI** upper respiratory infection
**US** ultrasound
**UTI** urinary tract infection
**VA** visual acuity
**VD** venereal disease
**Vf** visual field
**VS** vital signs
**WBC** white blood cells; white blood (cell) count
**WNL** within normal limits
**wt** weight
**y/o** year old

# APPENDIX VII

## Symbols Commonly Used in Medical Notations

### Apothecaries' Weights and Measures

ʒ   dram
℥   ounce
fʒ   fluidounce
O   pint
lb   pound

### Other Weights and Measures

\#   pounds
°   degrees
′   foot; minute
″   inch; second
μm   micrometer
μ   micron (former term for micrometer)
mμ   millimicron; nanometer
mEq   milliequivalent
mL   milliliter
dL   deciliter
mg%   milligrams percent; milligrams per 100 mL

### Abbreviations

$\overline{aa}$, $\overline{AA}$   of each
$\overline{c}$   with
M   mix (Latin *misce*)
*m*-   meta-
*o*-   ortho-
*p*-   para-
$\overline{p}$   after
$\overline{s}$   without
ss, $\overline{ss}$   one-half (Latin *semis*)

### Mathematical Functions and Terms

\#   number
+   plus; positive; acid reaction
−   minus; negative; alkaline reaction
±   plus or minus; either positive or negative; indefinite
×   multiply; magnification; crossed with, hybrid
÷ , /   divided by
=   equal to
≈   approximately equal to
>   greater than; from which is derived
<   less than; derived from
≮   not less than
≯   not greater than
≤   equal to or less than
≥   equal to or greater than
≠   not equal to
√   square root
³√   cube root
∞   infinity
:   ratio; "is to"
∴   therefore

%   percent
π   pi (3.14159)—the ratio of circumference of a circle to its diameter

### Chemical Notations

Δ   change; heat
⇌   reversible reaction
↑   increase
↓   decrease

### Warnings

Ⓒ   Schedule I controlled substance
Ⓒ   Schedule II controlled substance
Ⓒ   Schedule III controlled substance
Ⓒ   Schedule IV controlled substance
Ⓒ   Schedule V controlled substance
☠   poison
☢   radiation
☣   biohazard

### Others

℞   prescription; take
□, ♂   male
○, ♀   female
†   one
††   two
†††   three

# APPENDIX VIII

## Professional Organizations and Agencies

**American Academy of Dental Practice Administrators**
1063 Whippoorwill Lane
Palatine, IL 60067
(847) 934-4404

**American Academy of Medical Administrators**
30555 Southfield Road, Suite 150
Southfield, MI 48076
(313) 540-4310

**American Academy of Ophthalmology**
655 Beach Street
San Francisco, CA 94109
(415) 561-8500

**American Academy of Pediatrics**
141 Northwest Point Blvd.
Elk Grove, IL 60007-1098
(847) 434-4000

**American Academy of Professional Coders (AAPC)**
2480 South 3850 West, Suite B
Salt Lake City, UT. 84120
(800) 626-CODE (2633)

**American Association for Medical Transcription**
PO Box 576187
Modesto, CA 95355
(209) 527-9620

**American Association for Respiratory Care**
9425 McArthur Blvd, Suite 100
Irving, TX 75063
(972) 243-2272

**American Association of Medical Assistants**
20 N. Wacker Drive
Suite 1575
Chicago, IL 60606
(312) 899-1500

**American Cancer Society**
777 Third Avenue
New York, NY 10017
(212) 586-8700

**American Collectors Association International**
ACA International
P.O. Box 390106
Minneapolis, MN 55439
(952) 926–6547

**American College of Cardiology**
9111 Old Georgetown Road
Bethesda, MD 20814
(301) 897-5400

**American College of Physicians**
2011 Pennsylvania Avenue NW
Washington, DC 20006
(202) 261-4500

**American Diabetes Association**
1701 North Beauregard Street
Alexandria, VA 22311
(800) 342-2383

**American Dietetic Association**
120 South Riverside Plaza, Suite 2000
Chicago, Illinois 60606-6995
(800) 877-1600

**American Health Information Management Association (formerly the American Medical Record Association)**
233 N. Michigan Avenue, 21st Floor
Chicago, IL 60601-5800
(312) 233-1100

**American Heart Association**
National Center
7272 Greenville Avenue
Dallas, TX 75231-4596
(800) 242-8721, or call your local center

**American Hospital Association**
One North Franklin
Suite 2706
Chicago, IL 60606-3421
(312) 422-3000

**American Lung Association**
61 Broadway, 6th Floor
New York, NY 10006
(212) 315-8700 or 1-800-LUNGUSA

**American Medical Association Division of Allied Health Education and Accreditation**
515 North State Street
Chicago, IL 60610
(800) 621-8335

**American Medical Technologists**
10700 West Higgins Road
Suite 150
Rosemont, IL 60018
(847) 823-5169

**American Occupational Therapy Association**
4720 Montgomery Lane
PO Box 31220
Bethesda, MD 20824-1220
(301) 652-2682
TDD: (800) 377-8555

**American Pharmacists Association**
2215 Constitution Avenue NW
Washington, DC 20037-2985
(202) 628-4410

**American Physical Therapy Association/Foundation for Physical Therapy**
1111 North Fairfax Street
Alexandria, VA 22314
(703) 684-2782

**American Red Cross**
2025 E Street, NW
Washington, DC 20006
(202) 303-4498, or call your local chapter

**American Red Cross**
HIV/AIDS Education, Health and Safety Services
8111 Gatehouse Road
6th Floor
Falls Church, VA 22042
(703) 206-7180

**American Society for Cardiovascular Professionals**
120 Falcon Drive, Unit 3
Fredericksburg, VA 22408
(540) 891-0079

**American Society for Clinical Laboratory Science**
7910 Woodmont Avenue
Suite 1301
Bethesda, MD 20814
(301) 657-2768

**American Society of Clinical Pathologists**
33 West Monroe, Suite 1600
Chicago, IL 60603
(312) 541-4999

**American Society of Hand Therapists**
401 North Michigan Avenue
Chicago, IL 60611-4267
(312) 321-6866

**American Society of Phlebotomy Technicians**
PO Box 1831
Hickory, NC 28603
(704) 322-1334

**American Society of Radiologic Technologists**
15000 Central Avenue SE
Albuquerque, NM 87123
(505) 298-4500

**Anorexia Nervosa and Related Eating Disorders**
Box 7
Highland Park, IL 60035
(847) 831-3438

**The Arthritis Foundation**
1314 Spring Street, NW
Atlanta, GA 30309
(404) 872-7100

**Association of Surgical Technologists**
6 West Dry Creek Circle
Littleton, CO 80120
(303) 694-9130

**Association of Technical Personnel in Ophthalmology**
50 Lee Road
Chestnut Hill, MA 02167
(617) 232-4433

**Asthma and Allergy Foundation of America**
1717 Massachusetts Avenue
Suite 305
Washington, DC 20036
(202) 265-0265

**International Society for Clinical Laboratory Technology**
818 Olive Street
Suite 918
St. Louis, MO 63101
(314) 241-1445

**Joint Commission on Allied Health Personnel in Ophthalmology**
2025 Woodlane Drive
St. Paul, MN 55125-2995
(800) 284-3937

**Medical Collection Agency**
517 S. Livingston Ave.
Livingston, NJ 07039
Toll Free: 1-877-77-Collect
Phone: 1-973-740-0044

**Medical Group Management Association**
104 Inverness Terrace East
Englewood Cliffs, CA 80112
(313) 799-1111

**National Accrediting Agency for Clinical Laboratory Services**
8410 West Bryn Mawr Avenue
Suite 670
Chicago, IL 60631
(773) 714-8880

**National AIDS Hotline**
215 Park Avenue South, Suite 714
New York, NY 10003
(800) 342-AIDS
(800) 344-SIDA (Spanish)

**National Association of Anorexia Nervosa and Associated Disorders**
Box 7
Highland Park, IL 60035
(847) 831-3438

**National Association of Medical Staff Services**
PO Box 23590
Knoxville, TN 37933-1590
(615) 531-3571

**National Cancer Institute**
9000 Rockville Pike Building 31
Room 10A18
Bethesda, MD 20205
(800) 4-CANCER

**National Clearinghouse for Alcohol and Drug Information**
PO Box 2345
Rockville, MD 20852
(301) 468-2600

**National Eating Disorders Association**
603 Stewart Street
Suite 803
Seattle, WA 98101
(206) 382-3587

**National Healthcare Association**
134 Evergreen Place, 9th Floor
East Orange, NJ 07018
(800) 499-9092

**National Health Council**
1730 Street NW
Suite 500
Washington, DC 20036
(202) 785-3910

**National Health Information Center**
PO Box 1133
Washington, DC 20013-1133
(800) 336-4797

**National Institute of Mental Health Office of Communications**
6001 Executive Boulevard
Room 8184, MSC 9663
Bethesda, MD 20892-9663
(301) 443-4513

**National Institute on Aging**
Building 31, Room 5C27
31 Center Drive, MSC 2292
Bethesda, MD 20892
(301) 496-1752

**National Kidney Foundation**
30 East 33rd Street
New York, NY 10016
(212) 889-2210

**National Mental Health Association**
2001 N. Beauregard Street, 12th Floor
Alexandria, VA 22311
(703) 684-7722

**National Organization for Rare Disorders**
100 Route 37
PO Box 8923
New Fairfield, CT 06812
(800) 999-NORD

**National Phlebotomy Association**
1901 Brightseat Road
Landover, MD 20785
(866) 329-9108

**National Rehabilitation Association**
633 South Washington Street
Alexandria, VA 22314
(703) 836-0850

**National Society for Histotechnology**
4201 Northview Drive
Suite 502
Bowie, MD 20716-1073
(301) 262-6221

**Overeaters Anonymous (OA)**
P. O. Box 44020
Rio Rancho, NM 87174
(505) 891-2664

**President's Council on Physical Fitness and Sports**
Department of Health and Human
    Services
Washington, DC 20001
(202) 272-3421

**Society of Diagnostic Medical Sonographers**
2745 Dallas Pkwy, Suite 350
Plano, TX 75093-8730
(214) 473-8057 or (800) 229-9506

# GLOSSARY

*Note:* (†) Pronunciation from *Stedman's Medical Dictionary*, 26th edition; all others from *American Heritage*, 4th edition, in case you need to consult.

**10× lens (těn)** A magnifying lens in the ocular of a microscope that magnifies an image ten times.

**24-hour urine specimen (twĕn'tē fôr our yŏŏr' in spĕs' ə-mən)** A urine specimen collected over a 24-hour period and used to complete a quantitative and qualitative analysis of one or more substances, such as sodium, chloride, and calcium.

**abandonment (ə-băn'dən-mənt)** A situation in which a health-care professional stops caring for a patient without arranging for care by an equally qualified substitute.

**ABA number (nŭm'ber)** A fraction appearing in the upper right corner of all printed checks that identifies the geographic area and specific bank on which the check is drawn.

**abduction (ab-dŭk'shuň)(†)** Movement away from the body.

**abscess (ăb'sĕs')** A collection of pus (white blood cells, bacteria, and dead skin cells) that forms as a result of infection.

**absorption (əb-sôrp'shən)** The process by which one substance is absorbed, or taken in and incorporated, into another, as when the body converts food or drugs into a form it can use.

**abuse (ə-byŏŏz')** A practice or behavior that is not indicative of or in line with sound medical or fiscal activity.

**access (ăk'sĕs)** The way patients enter and exit a medical office.

**accessibility (ăk-sĕs'ə-bĭl'ĭ-tē)** The ease with which people can move into and out of a space.

**accommodation (ă-kom'ə-dā-shən)** The ability of the lens to change shape, allowing the eye to focus images of objects that are near or far away.

**accounts payable (ə-kounts' pā'-ə-bəl)** Money owed by a business; the practice's expenses.

**accounts receivable (ə-kounts' rĭ-sē'və-bəl)** Income or money owed to a business.

**accreditation (ə-krĕd'ĭ-tā'shən)** The documentation of official authorization or approval of a program.

**acetabulum (as'ətab'yələm)** The hip socket.

**acetylcholine (as-e-til-kō'lēn)(†)** A neurotransmitter released by the parasympathetic nerves onto organs and glands for resting and digesting.

**acetylcholinesterase (as'e-til-kō-lin-es'ter-ās)** An enzyme within the nervous system that hydrolyzes acetylcholine to acetate and choline.

**acid-fast stain (ăs'ĭd făst stān)** A staining procedure for identifying bacteria that have a waxy cell wall.

**acids (ăs'ĭds)** Electrolytes that release hydrogen ions in water.

**acinar cells (as'i-nar sĕlz)(†)** Cells in the pancreas that produce pancreatic juice.

**acquired immunodeficiency syndrome (AIDS) (ə-kwīrd im'yū-nō-dē-fish'en-sē sĭn'drōm')(†)** The most advanced stage of HIV infection; it severely weakens the body's immune system.

**acromegaly (ak-rō-meg'ă-lē)(†)** A disorder in which too much growth hormone is produced in adults.

**acrosome (ak'rō-sōm)(†)** An enzyme-filled sac covering the head of a sperm that aids in the penetration of the egg during fertilization.

**action potential (ăk'shən pə-těn'shəl)** The flow of electrical current along the axon membrane.

**active file (ăk'tĭv fĭl)** A file used on a consistent basis.

**active listening (ăk'tĭv lĭs'ənĭng)** Part of two-way communication, such as offering feedback or asking questions; contrast with **passive listening.**

**active transport (ak'-tĭv trans-pórt)** The movement of a substance across a cell membrane from an area of low concentration to an area of high concentration.

**acupressure (ak-you-presh-er)** Pressure applied by hands to various areas of the body to restore balance in the body's energy flow.

**acupuncture (ak-you-punk-chūr)** The practice of inserting needles into various areas of the body to restore balance in the body's energy flow.

**acupuncturist (ăk'yŏŏ-pŭngk'chər-ĭst)** A practitioner of acupuncture. The acupuncturist uses hollow needles inserted into the patient's skin to treat pain, discomfort, or systemic imbalances.

**acute (ə-kyŏŏt')** Having a rapid onset and progress, as acute appendicitis.

**addiction** (ă-dĭk´shun)(†)   A physical or psychological dependence on a substance, usually involving a pattern of behavior that includes obsessive or compulsive preoccupation with the substance and the security of its supply, as well as a high rate of relapse after withdrawal.

**Addison's disease** (ă-dĭsuns dĭzēz)   A condition in which the adrenal glands fail to produce enough corticosteroids.

**add-on code** (ăd´on´ kōd)   A code indicating procedures that are usually carried out in addition to another procedure. Add-on codes are used together with the primary code.

**adduction** (ă-dŭk´shŭn)(†)   Movement toward the body.

**adenoids** (ăd´n-oidz´)   See **pharyngeal tonsils.**

**adjustment** (ə-jŭst´-ment)   Manual treatments given by a chiropractor that move the joints of the spine and other joints into proper alignment.

**administer** (ăd-mĭn´ĭ-stər)   To give a drug directly by injection, by mouth, or by any other route that introduces the drug into the body.

**adrenocorticotropic hormone (ACTH)** (ă-drē´nō-kōr´ti-kō-trō´pik hor´mōn)   Hormone that stimulates the adrenal cortex to release its hormones.

**advance scheduling** (ăd-văns skēj´ōōl-ĭng)   Booking an appointment several weeks or even months in advance.

**aerobes** (âr´ōbs´)   Bacteria that grow best in the presence of oxygen.

**aerobic respiration** (â-rō´bĭk rĕs´pə-rā´shən)   A process that requires large amounts of oxygen and uses glucose to make ATP.

**afebrile** (ā-feb´ril)(†)   Having a body temperature within one's normal range.

**afferent arterioles** (ăf´ər-ənt ar-tēr´ē-ōlz)(†)   Structures that deliver blood to the glomeruli of the kidneys.

**afferent nerves** (ăf´ər-ənt nûrvs)   A type of sensory nerves are responsible for detecting sensory information from the environment or even from inside the body and bringing it to the CNS for interpretation.

**affiliation agreement** (ə-fĭl´ē-ā´shən ə-grē´mənt)   An agreement that externship participants must sign that states the expectations of the facility and the expectations of the student.

**agar** (ā´gär´)   A gelatin-like substance derived from seaweed that gives a culture medium its semisolid consistency.

**age analysis** (āj ə-năl´ĭ-sĭs)   The process of clarifying and reviewing past due accounts by age from the first date of billing.

**agenda** (ə-jĕn´də)   The list of topics discussed or presented at a meeting, in order of presentation.

**agent** (ā´-jənt)   (legal) A person who acts on a physician's behalf while performing professional tasks; (clinical) an active principal or entity that produces a certain effect, for example, an infectious agent.

**agglutination** (ă-glū-ti-nā´shŭn)(†)   The clumping of red blood cells following a blood transfusion.

**aggressive** (ə-grĕs´ĭv)   Imposing one's position on others or trying to manipulate them.

**agonist** (ăg´ənist)   See **antagonist.**

**agranular leukocyte** (ă-gran´-yulər lū´kō-sīt)(†)   A type of leukocyte (white blood cell) with a solid nucleus and clear cytoplasm; includes lymphocytes and monocytes.

**agranulocyte** (ă-gran´yū-lō-sīt)(†)   See **agranular leukocyte.**

**albumins** (ăl-byōō´mĭns)   The smallest of the plasma proteins. Albumins are important for pulling water into the bloodstream to help maintain blood pressure.

**aldosterone** (al-dos´ter-ōn)(†)   A hormone produced in the adrenal glands that acts on the kidney. It causes the body to retain sodium and excrete potassium. Its role is to maintain blood volume and pressure.

**alimentary canal** (ăl´ə-mĕn´tə-rē kə-năl´)   The organs of the digestive system that extend from the mouth to the anus.

**allele** (ə-lēl´)   Any one of a pair or series of **genes** that occupy a specific position on a specific **chromosome.**

**allergen** (ăl´ər-jən)   An antigen that induces an allergic reaction.

**allergic rhinitis** (al´ərjik rīni´tis)   A hypersensitivity reaction to various airborne allergens.

**allergist** (ăl´ər-jĭst)   A specialist who diagnoses and treats physical reactions to substances including mold, dust, fur, pollen, foods, drugs, and chemicals.

**allopathy** (ə-lō-păth-ē)   The usual medical practice of physicians and other health professionals; also known as conventional medicine.

**allowed charge** (ə-loud´ chärj)   The amount that is the most the payer will pay any provider for each procedure or service.

**alopecia** (ăl´ə-pē´shə)   The clinical term for baldness.

**alphabetic filing system** (ăl´fə-bĕt´ĭk fī´lĭng sis´təm)   A filing system in which the files are arranged in alphabetic order, with the patient's last name first, followed by the first name and middle initial.

**Alphabetic Index** (ăl´fə-bĕt´ĭk ĭn´dĕks´)   One of two ways diagnoses are listed in the ICD-9-CM. They appear in alphabetic order with their corresponding diagnosis codes.

**alternative medicine** (ôl-tûr´-nə-tĭv mĕd´-ĭ-sĭn)   The type of medicine used in place of conventional medicine to promote health and treat disease.

**alveolar glands (al-vē´ō-lăr glăndz)(†)** Glands that make milk under the influence of the hormone **prolactin.**

**alveoli (ăl-vē´ə-lī´)** Clusters of air sacs in which the exchange of gases between air and blood takes place; located in the lungs.

**American Association of Medical Assistants (AAMA) (ə-měr´ĭkən ə-sō´sē-ā´shən měd´ĭ-kəl ə-sĭs´tənts)** The professional organization that certifies medical assistants and works to maintain professional standards in the medical assisting profession.

**Americans With Disabilities Act (ADA) (ə-měr´ĭ-kəns dĭs´ə-bĭl´ĭ-tēs ăkt)** A U.S. civil rights act forbidding discrimination against people because of a physical or mental handicap.

**amblyopia (am-blē-ō´pē-ă)(†)** Poor vision in one eye without a detectable cause.

**amino acids (ə-mē´nō ăs´ĭds)** Natural organic compounds found in plant and animal foods and used by the body to create protein.

**amnion (ăm´nē-ən)** The innermost membrane enveloping the embryo and containing amniotic fluid.

**anabolism (ənab´əlĭz´əm)** The stage of metabolism in which substances such as nutrients are changed into more complex substances and used to build body tissues.

**anaerobe (ăn´ə-rōb´)** A bacterium that grows best in the absence of oxygen.

**anal canal (ā´nəl kə-năl´)** The last few centimeters of the rectum.

**anaphase (an´əfāz)** The period of mitosis when the centromeres divide and pull the chromosomes (formerly chromatids) toward the centrioles at opposite sides of the cell.

**anaphylaxis (an´ă-fī-lak´sis)** A severe allergic reaction with symptoms that include respiratory distress, difficulty in swallowing, pallor, and a drastic drop in blood pressure that can lead to circulatory collapse.

**anatomical position (ăn´ə-tŏm´ĭ-kəl pə-zĭsh´ən)** When the body is standing upright and facing forward with the arms at the side and the palms of the hands facing forward.

**anatomy (ə-năt´ə-mē)** The scientific term for the study of body structure.

**anemia (ə-nē´mē-ə)** A condition characterized by low red blood cell count. This condition decreases the ability to transport oxygen throughout the body.

**anergic reaction (an-er´jik rē-ăk´shən)** A lack of response to skin testing that indicates the body's inability to mount a normal response to invasion by a pathogen.

**anesthesia (ăn´ĭs-thē´zhə)** A loss of sensation, particularly the feeling of pain.

**anesthetic (ăn´ĭs-thět´ik)** A medication that causes anesthesia.

**anesthetist (ă-nes´thĕ-tist)(†)** A specialist who uses medications to cause patients to lose sensation or feeling during surgery.

**aneurysm (ăn´yə-rĭz´əm)** A serious and potentially life-threatening bulge in the wall of a blood vessel.

**angiography (an-jē-og´ră-fē)(†)** An x-ray examination of a blood vessel, performed after the injection of a contrast medium, that evaluates the function and structure of one or more arteries or veins.

**annotate (ăn´ō-tāt´)** To underline or highlight key points of a document or to write reminders, make comments, and suggest actions in the margins.

**anorexia nervosa (ăn´ə-rěk´sē-ə nûr-vō´sə)** An eating disorder in which people starve themselves because they fear that if they lose control of eating they will become grossly overweight.

**antagonist (ăn-tăg´ə-nĭst)** A muscle that produces the opposite movement of the **prime mover.**

**antecubital space (an-te-kyū´bi-tăl spās)** The inner side or bend of the elbow; the site at which the brachial artery is felt or heard when a pulse or blood pressure is taken.

**anterior (ăn-tîr´ē-ər)** Anatomical term meaning toward the front of the body; also called ventral.

**anthracosis (an´thrə kō´sis)** Chronic lung disease caused by the inhalation of coal deposits; also known as Black Lung Disease.

**antibodies (ăn´tĭ-bod´ēs)** Highly specific proteins that attach themselves to foreign substances in an initial step in destroying such substances, as part of the body's defenses.

**antidiuretic hormone (ADH) (an´tē-dī-yū-ret´ik hôr´mōn´)(†)** A hormone that increases water reabsorption, which decreases urine production and helps to maintain blood pressure.

**antigen (an´tĭ-jən)** A foreign substance that stimulates white blood cells to create antibodies when it enters the body.

**antihistamines (ăn´tē-hĭs´tə-mēnz)** Medications used to treat allergies.

**antimicrobial (an´tē-mī-krō´bē-ăl)(†)** An agent that kills microorganisms or suppresses their growth.

**antioxidants (ăn´tē-ŏk´sĭ-dənt)** Chemical agents that fight cell-destroying chemical substances called free radicals.

**antiseptic (ăn´tĭ-sěp´tĭk)** A cleaning product used on human tissue as an anti-infection agent.

**anuria (an-yū´rē-ă)(†)** The absence of urine production.

**aortic semilunar valve (ā ôr´tĭk sem´ē loonər valv)** Heart valve that is a semilunar valve and that is situated between the left ventricle and the aorta.

**apex (ā´pĕks)** The left lower corner of the heart, where the strongest heart sounds can be heard.

**apical (ap´i-kăl)(†)** Located at the **apex** of the heart.

**apnea (an´nēə)** The absence of respiration.

**apocrine gland (ap´ō-krin glănd)(†)** A type of sweat gland. It produces a thicker type of sweat than other sweat glands and contains more proteins.

**aponeurosis (ap´ō-nū-rō´sis)(†)** A tough, sheet-like structure that is made of fibrous connective tissue. It typically attaches muscles to other muscles.

**appendicitis (ə-pĕn´dĭ-sī´tĭs)** Inflammation of the appendix.

**appendicular (ap´en-dik´yū-lăr)** The division of the skeletal system that consists of the bones of the arms, legs, pectoral girdle, and pelvic girdle.

**approximate (a-prŏk´s i māt)** To bring the edges of a wound together so the tissue surfaces are close in order to protect the area from further contamination and to minimize scar and scab formation.

**aqueous humor (a´kwē-əs hyo͞o´mər)** A liquid produced by the eye's ciliary body that fills the space between the cornea and the lens.

**arbitration (är´bĭ-trā´shən)** A process in which opposing sides choose a person or persons outside the court system, often someone with special knowledge in the field, to hear and decide a dispute.

**areflexia (ā-rē-flek´sē-ă)(†)** The absence of reflexes.

**areola (ă-rē´ō-lă)(†)** The pigmented area that surrounds the nipple.

**aromatherapy (a-rō´-mə-thēr´-ə-pē)** The use of essential oil extracts or essences from flowers, herbs, and trees to promote health and well-being.

**arrector pili (ă-rek´tōr pī´lī)(†)** Muscles attached to most hair follicles and found in the dermis.

**arrhythmia (ə-rĭth´mē-ə)** Irregularity in heart rhythm.

**arterial blood gases (är-tîr´ē-əl blŭd găs´ses)** A test that measures the amount of gases, such as oxygen and carbon dioxide, dissolved in arterial blood.

**arthritis (arth rīt´is)** A general term meaning joint inflammation.

**arthrography (ar-throg´ră-fē)(†)** A radiologic procedure performed by a radiologist, who uses a contrast medium and fluoroscopy to help diagnose abnormalities or injuries in the cartilage, tendons, or ligaments of the joints—usually the knee or shoulder.

**arthroscopy (är-thŏs´kə-pē)** A procedure in which an orthopedist examines a joint, usually the knee or shoulder, with a tubular instrument called an arthroscope; also used to guide surgical procedures.

**articular cartilage (ar-tik´yu-lăr kär´tl-ĭj) (†)** The cartilage that covers the **epiphysis** of long bones.

**articulations (ärtik´yəla´shəns)** The area where bones are joined together; joints.

**artifact (är´tə-făkt´)** Any irrelevant object or mark observed when examining specimens or graphic records that is not related to the object being examined; for example, a foreign object visible through a microscope or an erroneous mark on an ECG strip.

**asbestosis (asbestō´sis)** Chronic lung disease caused by the inhalation of asbestos fibers.

**ascending colon (ə-sĕnd´ĭng ko´lən)** The segment of the large intestine that runs up the right side of the abdominal cavity.

**ascending tracts (ə-sĕnd´ĭng trăkts)** The tracts of the spinal cord that carry sensory information to the brain.

**asepsis (ă-sep´sis)(†)** The condition in which pathogens are absent or controlled.

**assault (ə-sôlt´)** The open threat of bodily harm to another.

**assertive (ə-sûrt´tĭv)** Being firm and standing up for oneself while showing respect for others.

**asset (ăs´ĕt´)** An item owned by the practice that has a dollar value, such as the medical practice building, office equipment, or accounts receivable.

**assignment of benefits (ə-sīn´mənt bĕn´ə-fĭts)** An authorization for an insurance carrier to pay a physician or practice directly.

**asthma (az´mə)** A condition in which the tubes of the bronchial tree become obstructed due to inflammation.

**astigmatism (ə-stĭg´mə-tĭz´əm)** A condition in which the cornea has an abnormal shape, which causes blurred images during near or distant vision.

**astrocytes (ăs´-tro-sīts)** Star-shaped cells within the nervous system that anchor blood vessels to the nerve cells.

**atelectasis (at´ilek´təsis)** The collapse of a lung because of fluid, air, pus, or blood.

**atherosclerosis (ăth´-ə-rō-sklə-rō´sĭs)** The accumulation of fatty deposits along the inner walls of arteries.

**atlas (ăt´ləs)** The first cervical vertebra.

**atoms (ăt´əmz)** The simplest units of all matter.

**atria (ā´trē-ă)(†)** [*Singular:* **atrium**] Chambers of the heart that receive blood from the veins and circulate it to the ventricles.

**atrial natriuretic peptide (ā´trē-ăl nā´trēyū-ret´ik pep´tīd)(†)** A hormone secreted by the heart that regulates blood pressure.

**atrioventricular bundle (ā´trē-ō-ventrik´yū-lar bŭn´dl)(†)** A structure that is located between the ventricles of the heart and that sends the electrical impulse to the Purkinje fibers.

**atrioventricular node (ā´trē-ō-ventrik´yū-lar nōd)** A node that is located between the atria of the heart. After the electrical impulse reaches the atrioventricular node, the atria contract and the impulse is sent to the ventricles.

**atrioventricular septum (a´treo-ventrik´yu-lar səp´təm)** The wall separating the upper atrial chambers from the lower ventricular chambers of the heart.

**audiologist (aw-dē-ol´ōjist)(†)** A health-care specialist who focuses on evaluating and correcting hearing problems.

**audiometer (aw-dē-om´ĕ-ter)** An electronic device that measures hearing acuity by producing sounds in specific frequencies and intensities.

**auricle (ôr´ĭ-kəl)** The outside part of the ear, made of cartilage and covered with skin.

**auscultated blood pressure (ô´skəl-tāt-ĕd blŭd prĕsh´ər)** Blood pressure as measured by listening with a stethoscope.

**auscultation (ô´skəl-tā´shən)** The process of listening to body sounds.

**authorization (ô´thər-ĭ-zā´shən)** A form that explains in detail the standards for the use and disclosure of patient information for purposes other than treatment, payment, or health-care operations.

**autoclave (aw´tō-klāv)(†)** A device that uses pressurized steam to sterilize instruments and equipment.

**autoimmune disease (aw´tō-ĭmyoŏn di-zēz´)** Any condition in which the body attacks its own antigens, causing illness to the patient.

**automated external defibrillator (AED) (ô´tə-mā´tĭd ĭk-stûr´nəl dē-fib´ri-lā-ter)** A computerized defibrillator programmed to recognize lethal heart rhythms and deliver an electrical shock to restore a normal rhythm.

**autonomic (ô´tə-nŏm´ĭk)** A division of the peripheral nervous system that connects the central nervous system to viscera such as the heart, stomach, intestines, glands, blood vessels, and bladder.

**autonomic nervous system (ANS) (ô´tə-nŏm´ĭk nūr´vəs sĭs´təm)** A system that is in charge of the body's automatic functions, such as the respiratory and gastrointestinal systems.

**autopsy (ô-top´-sē)** The examination of a cadaver to determine or confirm the cause of death.

**autosome (ô´tə-sōm´)** A chromosome that is not a sex chromosome.

**axial (ăk´sē-əl)** The division of the skeletal system that consists of the skull, vertebral column, and rib cage.

**axilla (ăk-sĭl´ə)** Armpit; one of the four locations for temperature readings.

**axis (ak´-səs)** The second vertebra of the neck on which the head turns.

**axon (ăk´sŏn´)** A type of nerve fiber that is typically long and branches far from the cell body. Its function is to send information away from the cell body.

**Ayurveda (eye-yer-vay-duh)** A form of medicine, originated in India, that uses herbal preparations, dietary changes, exercises, and meditation to restore health and promote well-being.

**bacillus (ba-sil´ŭs)(†)** A rod-shaped bacterium.

**bacterial spore (băk-tîr´ēăl spôr)** A primitive, thick-walled reproductive body capable of developing into a new individual; resistant to killing through disinfection.

**balance billing (băl´əns bĭl´ĭng)** Billing a patient for the difference between a higher usual fee and a lower allowed charge.

**balloon angioplasty (buh-loon an´je-o-plas´te-)** A procedure using a slender, hollow tube passed through a coronary artery

to compress a blockage in the artery.

**bandwidth (bānd´wĭdth´)** A measurement, calculated in bits or bytes, of how much information can be sent or processed with one single instruction.

**barium enema (bâr´ē-əm ĕn´ə-mə)** A radiologic procedure performed by a radiologist who administers barium sulfate through the anus, into the rectum, and then into the colon to help diagnose and evaluate obstructions, ulcers, polyps, diverticulosis, tumors, or motility problems of the colon or rectum; also called a lower GI (gastrointestinal) series.

**barium swallow (bâr´ē-əm swŏl´ō)** A radiologic procedure that involves oral administration of a barium sulfate drink to help diagnose and evaluate obstructions, ulcers, polyps, diverticulosis, tumors, or motility problems of the esophagus, stomach, duodenum, and small intestine; also called an upper GI (gastrointestinal) series.

**baroreceptors (bar´ō-rē-sep´ters)(†)** Structures, located in the aorta and carotid arteries, that help regulate blood pressure.

**Bartholin's glands (bär´ tə linz glăndz)** Glands lateral to the vagina that produce mucus for lubrication of the vagina.

**bases (bā´sēz´)** Electrolytes that release hydroxyl ions in water.

**basophil (bā-sō-fil)(†)** A type of granular leukocyte that produces the chemical histamine, which aids the body in controlling allergic reactions and other exaggerated immunologic responses.

**battery (băt´ə-rē)** An action that causes bodily harm to another.

**behavior modification (bĭ-hāv´yər mŏd´-ə-fī-kā-shən)** The altering of personal habits to promote a healthier lifestyle.

**benefits (bĕn´ə-fĭts)** Payments for medical services.

**benign (bē-nīn´)** A noncancerous or nonmalignant growth or condition.

**benign prostatic hypertrophy (bē nīn´ pros-tat´ik hī pur´trə fē)** A noncancerous enlargement of the prostate gland.

**bicarbonate ions (bī-kar´bon-āt ī´onz)** Elements formed when carbon dioxide gets into the bloodstream and reacts with water. In the alimentary canal, these ions neutralize acidic chyme arriving from the stomach.

**bicuspids (bī-kŭs´pĭds)** Teeth with two cusps. There are two in front of each set of molars.

**bicuspid valve (bī-kŭs´pĭd vălv)** Heart valve that has two cusps and that is located between the left atrium and the left ventricle. Also known as the mitral valve.

**bile (bīl)** A substance created in the liver and stored in the gallbladder. Bile is a bitter yellow-green fluid that is used in the digestion of fats.

**bilirubin (bili-rū´bin)(†)** A bile pigment formed by the breakdown of hemoglobin in the liver.

**bilirubinuria (bil´i-rū-bi-nū´rē-ă)(†)** The presence of bilirubin in the urine; one of the first signs of liver disease or conditions that involve the liver.

**biliverdin (bil-i-ver´din)(†)** A pigment released when a red blood cell is destroyed.

**biochemistry (bĭ´ō-kĕm´ĭ-strē)** The study of matter and chemical reactions in the body.

**bioelectromagnetic-based therapies (bĭ´ō-ī-lĕk´trĭk basĕd thĕr´-ə-pēs)** The use of measurable energy fields in such things as magnetic therapy, millimeter wave therapy, sound energy therapy, and light therapy.

**bioethics (bī-ō-ĕth´ĭks)** Principles of right and wrong in issues that arise from medical advances.

**biofeedback (bī-ō-fēd´-bāk)** A type of therapy in which an individual learns how to control involuntary body responses in order to promote health and treat disease.

**biofield therapies (bī-ō-field thĕr´-ə-pēs)** Treatments that affect the energy fields that surround and penetrate the human body in order to promote health and well-being.

**biohazard symbol (bī-ō-hăz´ərd sĭm´bəl)** A symbol that must appear on all containers used to store waste products, blood, blood products, or other specimens that may be infectious.

**biohazardous materials (bī-ō-hăz´ərd-əs mə-tîr´ə-əls)** Biological agents that can spread disease to living things.

**biohazardous waste container (bī-ō-hăz´ərd-əs wāst kən-tā´nər)** A leakproof, puncture-resistant container, color-coded red or labeled with a special biohazard symbol, that is used to store and dispose of contaminated supplies and equipment.

**biopsy (bī-op´-sē)** The removal and examination of a sample of tissue from a living body for diagnostic purposes.

**biopsy specimen (bī´ŏp´sē spĕs´ə-mən)** A small amount of tissue removed from the body for examination under a microscope to diagnose an illness.

**bioterrorism (bī-ō´tĕr´ə-rĭz´əm)** The intentional release of a biologic agent with the intent to harm individuals.

**birthday rule (bûrth´dā´rŏŏl)** A rule that states that the insurance policy of a policyholder whose birthday comes first in the year is the primary payer for all dependents.

**blastocyst (blas´tō-sist)** A morula that travels down the uterine tube to the uterus and is invaded with fluid. It then implants into the wall of the uterus.

**blood-borne pathogen (blŭd-bôrn păth´ə-jən)** A disease-causing microorganism carried in a host's blood and transmitted through contact with infected blood, tissue, or body fluids.

**blood-brain barrier (blŭd brān băr´ē-ər)** A structure that is formed from tight capillaries to protect the tissues of the central nervous system from certain substances.

**B lymphocyte (bē lĭm´fə-sīt´)** A type of nongranular leukocyte that produces antibodies to combat specific pathogens.

**body (bod-ee)** Single-spaced lines of text that are the content of a business letter.

**body language (bŏd´ē lăng´gwĭj)** Nonverbal communication, including facial expressions, eye contact, posture, touch, and attention to personal space.

**bolus (bō´ləs)** The mass created when food is combined with saliva and mucus.

**bone conduction (bōnkən-dŭk´shən)** The process by which sound waves pass through the bones of the skull directly to the inner ear, bypassing the outer and middle ears.

**bookkeeping (bŏŏk´kē´pĭng)** The systematic recording of business transactions.

**botulism (bŏch´ə-lĭz´əm)** A life-threatening type of food poisoning that results from eating improperly canned or preserved foods that have been contaminated with the bacterium *Clostridium botulinum*.

**Bowman's capsule (bō´mənz kap´səl)** A capsule that surrounds the **glomerulus** of the kidney.

**brachial artery (brāk´ē-ăl är´tə-rē)** An artery that provides a palpable pulse and audible vascular sounds in the antecubital space (the bend of the elbow).

**brachytherapy (brak-ē-thăr´ă-pe´)(†)** A radiation therapy technique in which a radiologist places temporary radioactive implants close to or directly into cancerous tissue; used for treating localized cancers.

**bradycardia (braid uh card e uh)** A slow heart rate; usually less than 60 beats per minute.

**brain stem (brān stēm)** A structure that connects the cerebrum to the spinal cord.

**breach of contract (brēch kŏn´trăkt´)** The violation of or failure to live up to a contract's terms.

**bronchi (brŏn-kī)** The two branches of the trachea that enter the lungs.

**bronchial tree (brŏng´kē-al trē)** A series of tubes that begins where the distal end of the trachea branches.

**bronchioles (brŏng´kē-ōlz)** A part of the respiratory tract that branches from the tertiary bronchi.

**buccal (bŭk´ăl)(†)** Between the cheek and gum.

**buffy coat (buf´ē kōt)** The layer between the packed red blood cells and plasma in a centrifuged blood sample; this layer contains the white blood cells and platelets.

**bulbourethral glands (bŭl´bō-yū-rē´thrăl glăndz)(†)** Glands that lie beneath the prostate and empty their fluid into the urethra. Their fluid aids in sperm movement.

**bulimia (boo-lē´mē-ə)** An eating disorder in which people eat a large quantity of food in a short period of time (bingeing) and then attempt to counter the effects of bingeing by self-induced vomiting, use of laxatives or diuretics, and/or excessive exercise.

**bundle of His (bēn´ dl ov hiss)** Also known as the AV bundle, this is the node located between the ventricles of the heart that carries the electrical impulse from the AV node to the bundle branches.

**burnout (´bər-naút)** The end result of prolonged periods of stress without relief. Burnout is an energy-depleting condition that can affect one's health and career. It can be common for those who work in health care.

**bursitis (bər-sī´tĭs)** Inflammation of a bursa.

**calcaneus (kal-kā´nē-ŭs)(†)** The largest tarsal bone; also called the heel bone.

**calcitonin (kal-si-tō´nin)** A hormone produced by the thyroid gland that lowers blood calcium levels by activating osteoblasts.

**calibrate (kīal´-brat)** To determine the caliber of; to standardize a measuring instrument.

**calibration syringe (kăl´ə-brā´shənsə-rĭnj)** A standardized measuring instrument used to check and adjust the volume indicator on a spirometer.

**calorie (kăl´ə-rē)** A unit used to measure the amount of energy food produces; the amount of energy needed to raise the temperature of 1 kg of water by 1°C.

**calyces (kă´lĭ-sēz´)** Small cavities of the renal pelvis of the kidney.

**CAM (kăm)** The acronym for complementary and alternative medicine. Complementary medicine is used with conventional medicine. Alternative medicine is used in place of conventional medicine.

**canaliculi (kan-ă-lik´yū-lī)** Tiny canals that connect lacunae to each other.

**cancellous (kan´siləs)** Bone also known as spongy bone. It contains spaces within it containing the red bone marrow.

**capillary (kăp´ə-lĕr´ē)** Branches of arterioles and the smallest type of blood vessel.

**capillary puncture (kăp´ə-lĕr´ē pŭngk´chər)** A blood-drawing technique that requires a superficial puncture of the skin with a sharp point.

**capitation (kăp´ĭ-tā´shən)** A payment structure in which a health maintenance organization prepays an annual set fee per patient to a physician.

**carboxyhemoglobin (kärbok´sēhē´məglō´bin)** The term used when the hemoglobin of red blood cells is carrying carbon dioxide.

**carboxypeptidase (kar-bok-sē-pep´ti-dās) (†)** A pancreatic enzyme that digests proteins.

**carcinogen (kär-sĭn´ə-jən)** A factor that is known to cause the formation of cancer.

**cardiac catheterization (kär´dē-ăk´ kath´ē-ter-ī-zā´shun) (†)** A diagnostic method in which a catheter is inserted into a vein or artery in the arm or leg and passed through blood vessels into the heart.

**cardiac cycle (kär´dē-ăk´ sī´kəl)** The sequence of contraction and relaxation that makes up a complete heartbeat.

**cardiac sphincter (kär´dē-ăk sfingk´tər)** The valve-like structure composed of a circular band of muscle at juncture of the esophagus and stomach. Also known as the esophageal sphincter.

**cardiologist (kär´dē-ŏl´ə-jĭst)** A specialist who diagnoses and treats diseases of the heart and blood vessels (cardiovascular diseases).

**carditis (kar-dī´tis)(†)** Inflammation of the heart.

**carpal (kär´pəl)** Bones of the wrist.

**carpal tunnel syndrome (kär´pəl tŭn´əl sĭn´drōm´)** A painful disorder caused by compression of the median nerve in the carpal tunnel of the wrist.

**carrier (kăr´ē-ər)** A reservoir host who is unaware of the presence of a pathogen and so spreads the disease while exhibiting no symptoms of infection.

**cast (kăst)** A rigid, external dressing, usually made of plaster or fiberglass, that is molded to the contours of the body part to which it is applied; used to immobilize a fractured or dislocated bone.

Cylinder-shaped elements with flat or rounded ends, differing in composition and size, that form when protein from the breakdown of cells accumulates and precipitates in the kidney tubules and is washed into the urine.

**catabolism (kə tab′əliz′am)** The stage of metabolism in which complex substances, including nutrients and body tissues, are broken down into simpler substances and converted into energy.

**cataracts (kăt′ə-răkts′)** Cloudy areas that form in the lens of the eye that prevent light from reaching visual receptors.

**cash flow statement (kăsh flō stā′mənt)** A statement that shows the cash on hand at the beginning of a period, the income and disbursements made during the period, and the new amount of cash on hand at the end of the period.

**cashier's check (kă-shîrz′ che′k)** A bank check issued by a bank on bank paper and signed by a bank representative; usually purchased by individuals who do not have checking accounts.

**catheterization (kath′ĕ-ter-ī-ză′shun)(†)** The procedure during which a catheter is inserted into a vessel, an organ, or a body cavity.

**caudal (kôd′l)** See **inferior.**

**CD-ROM (sē′dē′rŏm′)** A compact disc that contains software programs; an abbreviation for "compact disc—read-only memory."

**cecum (sē′kəm)** The first section of the large intestine.

**cell body (sĕl bŏd′ē)** The portion of the neuron that contains the nucleus and organelles.

**cell membrane (sĕl mĕm′brăn′)** The outer limit of a cell that is thin and selectively permeable. It controls the movement of substances into and out of the cell.

**cells (sĕlz)** The smallest living units of structure and function.

**cellulitis (sel-yū-lī′tis)** Inflammation of cellular or connective tissue.

**cellulose (sĕl′yə-lōs′)** A type of carbohydrate that is found in vegetables and cannot be digested by humans; commonly called fiber.

**Celsius (centigrade) (sĕl′sē-əs)** One of two common scales for measuring temperature; measured in degrees Celsius, or °C.

**Centers for Medicare and Medicaid Services (CMS) (sĕn′tərs mĕd′ĭ-kâr′ mĕd′ĭ-kād′ sûr′vĭs-əz)** A congressional agency designed to handle Medicare and Medicaid insurance claims. It was formerly known as the Health Care Financing Administration.

**central nervous system (CNS) (sĕn′trəl nûr′vəs sĭs′təm)** A system that consists of the brain and the spinal cord.

**central processing unit (CPU) (sĕn′trəl prŏs′es′ĭng yōō′nĭt)** A microprocessor, the primary computer chip responsible for interpreting and executing programs.

**centrifuge (sĕn′trə-fyōōj′)** A device used to spin a specimen at high speed until it separates into its component parts.

**centrioles (sen′trē ōz)** Two cylinder-shaped organs near the cell nucleus that are essential for cell division, by equally dividing chromosomes to the daughter cells.

**cerebellum (sĕr′ə-bĕl′əm)** An area of the brain inferior to the cerebrum that coordinates complex skeletal muscle coordination.

**cerebrospinal fluid (CSF) (ser′ĕ-brō-spĭ′-năl flōō′ĭd)** The fluid in the subarachnoid space of the meninges and the central canal of the spinal cord.

**cerebrovascular accident (ser′əbrovas′kyələr ak′sidənt)** A stroke. Caused by a hemorrhage in the brain or more often by a clot lodged in a cerebral artery.

**cerebrum (sĕr′ə-brəm)** The largest part of the brain; it mainly includes the cerebral hemispheres.

**Certificate of Waiver tests (sər-tĭf′ĭ-kĭt wā′vər tĕsts)** Laboratory tests that pose an insignificant risk to the patient if they are performed or interpreted incorrectly, are simple and accurate to such a degree that the risk of obtaining incorrect results is minimal, and have been approved by the Food and Drug Administration for use by patients at home; laboratories performing only Certificate of Waiver tests must meet less stringent standards than laboratories that perform tests in other categories.

**certified check (sûr′tə-fīd′ chĕk)** A payer's check written and signed by the payer, which is stamped "certified" by the bank. The bank has already drawn money from the payer's account to guarantee that the check will be paid.

**Certified Medical Assistant (CMA) (sûr′tə-fīd′ mĕd′ĭ-kəl ə-sĭs′tənt)** A medical assistant whose knowledge about the skills of medical assistants, as summarized by the 2003 AAMA Role Delineation Study areas of competence, has been certified by the Certifying Board of the American Association of Medical Assistants (AAMA).

**cerumen (sə-rōō′mən)** A wax-like substance produced by glands in the ear canal; also called earwax.

**cervical enlargement (sûr′vĭ-kəl in-lär′j-mənt)** The thickening of the spinal cord in the neck region.

**cervical orifice (sûr′vĭ-kəl ôr′ə-fĭs)** The opening of the uterus through the cervix into the vagina.

**cervicitis (ser-vi-sī′tis)** Inflammation of the cervix.

**cervix (sûr′vĭks)** The lowest portion of the uterus that extends into the vagina.

**cesarean section (si zer´ē ən sak´ shən)** A surgical incision of the abdomen and uterus to deliver a baby transabdominally.

**chain of custody (chān kŭs´tə-dē)** A procedure for ensuring that a specimen is obtained from a specified individual, is correctly identified, is under the uninterrupted control of authorized personnel, and has not been altered or replaced.

**CHAMPVA (Civilian Health and Medical Program of the Veterans Administration)(sĭ-vĭl´yən hĕlth mĕd´ĭ-kəl prō´ğram vĕtər-enz ăd-mĭn´ĭ-strā´shən)** A type of health insurance that covers the expenses of families (dependent spouses and children) of veterans with total, permanent, and service-connected disabilities. It also covers the surviving families of veterans who die in the line of duty or as a result of service-connected disabilities.

**chancre (shang´ker)(†)** A painless ulcer that may appear on the tongue, the lips, the genitalia, the rectum, or elsewhere.

**charge slip (chärj slĭp)** The original record of services performed for a patient and the charges for those services.

**check (chĕk)** A bank draft or order written by a payer that directs the bank to pay a sum of money on demand to the payee.

**chemistry (kĕm´ĭ-strē)** The study of the composition of matter and how matter changes.

**chemoreceptor (kē´mo-rī-sĕp´tôr)** Any cell that is activated by a change in chemical concentration and results in a nerve impulse. The olfactory or smell receptors in the nose are an example of a chemoreceptor.

**Cheyne-Stokes respirations (chain stokes RES per ra shuns)** A pattern of breathing that gradually alternates between deep and shallow breaths with a period of apnea or no breathing that can last from 5 to 40 seconds.

**chief cells (chēf sĕlz)** Cells in the lining of the stomach that secrete **pepsinogen.**

**chief complaint (chēf kəm-plān´t)** The patient's main issue of pain or ailment.

**chiropractor (kī´rə-prăk´tôr)** A physician who uses a system of therapy, including manipulation of the spine, to treat illness or pain. This treatment is done without drugs or surgery.

**chlamydia (klə mid´ē ah)** A common bacterial STD caused by bacterium *Chlamydia trachomatis* that can lead to PID in women.

**cholangiography (kō-lan-jē-og´rǎ-fĕ)(†)** A test that evaluates the function of the bile ducts by injection of a contrast medium directly into the common bile duct (during gallbladder surgery) or through a T-tube (after gallbladder surgery or during radiologic testing) and taking an x-ray.

**cholecystography (kō-lē-sis-tog´rǎ-fĕ)(†)** A gallbladder function test performed by x-ray after the patient ingests an oral contrast agent; used to detect gallstones and bile duct obstruction.

**cholesterol (kə-lĕs´tə-rôl)** A fat-related substance that the body produces in the liver and obtains from dietary sources; needed in small amounts to carry out several vital functions. High levels of cholesterol in the blood increase the risk of heart and artery disease.

**chordae tendineae (kōr´dĕ ten-din´ā)(†)** Cord-like structures that attach the cusps of the heart valves to the papillary muscles in the ventricles.

**choroid (kôr´oid´)** The middle layer of the eye, which contains the iris, the ciliary body, and most of the eye's blood vessels.

**chromosome (krō´mə-sōm´)** Thread-like structures composed of DNA.

**chronic (krŏn´ĭk)** Lasting a long time or recurring frequently, as in chronic osteoarthritis.

**chronic obstructive pulmonary disease (COPD) (krŏn´ĭk ob-strŭk´tiv pŏolmə-nĕr´ē dĭ-zēz´)** A disease characterized by the presence of airflow obstruction as a result of chronic bronchitis or emphysema. It is typically progressive. Cigarette smoking is the leading cause.

**chronological résumé (krŏn´ə-lŏj´ĭ-kəl rĕzŏo-mā´)** The type of résumé used by individuals who have job experience. Jobs are listed according to date, with the most recent being listed first.

**chylomicron (kī-lō-mi´kron)** The least dense of the lipoproteins; it functions in lipid transportation.

**chyme (kīm)(†)** The mixture of food and gastric juice.

**chymotrypsin (kī-mō-trip´sin)(†)** A pancreatic enzyme that digests proteins.

**cilia (sil´ēa)** Hair-like projections from the outside of the cell membrane on some cell types.

**ciliary body (sĭl´ē-ēr´ē bŏd´ē)** A wedge-shaped thickening in the middle layer of the eyeball that contains the muscles that control the shape of the lens.

**circumduction (ser-kŭm-dŭk´shŭn)** Moving a body part in a circle; for example, tracing a circle with your arm.

**cirrhosis (sĭ-rō´sĭs)** A long-lasting liver disease in which normal liver tissue is replaced with nonfunctioning scar tissue.

**civil law (sĭv´əl lô)** Involves crimes against persons. A person can sue another person, business, or the government. Judgments often require a payment of money.

**clarity (klār´i-tē)** Clearness in writing or stating a message.

**class action lawsuit (klăs-ăk´shən lô´sōōt)** A lawsuit in which one or more people sue a company or other legal entity that allegedly wronged all of them in the same way.

**clavicle (klăv′ĭ-kəl)** A slender, curved long bone that connects the sternum and the scapula; also called the collar bone.

**clean-catch midstream urine specimen (klēn-kăch mĭd′strēm yŏŏr′ĭn spĕs′əmən)** A type of urine specimen that requires special cleansing of the external genitalia to avoid contamination by organisms residing near the external opening of the urethra and is used to identify the number and types of pathogens present in urine; sometimes referred to as midvoid.

**clearinghouse (klîr′ĭng-hous′)** A group that takes nonstandard medical billing software formats and translates them into the standard EDI formats.

**cleavage (klē′vĭj)** The rapid rate of mitosis of a zygote immediately following fertilization.

**clinical coordinator (klĭn′ĭ-kəlkō-ôr′dn-ā′tor)** The person associated with the medical assisting school that procures externship sites and qualifies them to ensure that they provide a thorough educational experience.

**clinical diagnosis (klĭn′ĭ-kəl dī′əg-nō′sĭs)** A diagnosis based on the signs and symptoms of a disease or condition.

**clinical drug trial (klĭn′ĭ-kəl drŭg trī′əl)** An internationally recognized research protocol designed to evaluate the efficacy or safety of drugs and to produce scientifically valid results.

**Clinical Laboratory Improvement Amendments of 1988 (CLIA '88) (klē′ə)** A law enacted by Congress in 1988 that placed all laboratory facilities that conduct tests for diagnosing, preventing, or treating human disease or for assessing human health under federal regulations administered by the Health Care Financing Administration (HCFA) and the Centers for Disease Control and Prevention (CDC).

**clitoris (klĭt′ər-ĭs)** Located anterior to the urethral opening in females. It contains erectile tissue and is rich in sensory nerves.

**clock speed (klŏk spēd)** A measurement of how many instructions per second that a CPU can process. Clock speed is measured in megahertz (MHz) or gigahertz (GHz).

**closed file (klōzd fīl)** A file for a patient who has died, moved away, or for some other reason no longer consults the office for medical expertise.

**closed posture (klōzd pŏs′chər)** A position that conveys the feeling of not being totally receptive to what is being said; arms are often rigid or folded across the chest.

**cluster scheduling (klŭs′tər skĕj′ōol-ĭng)** The scheduling of similar appointments together at a certain time of the day or week.

**coagulation (kō-ăg′yə-lā′shən)** The process by which a clot forms in blood.

**coccus (kŏk′əs)** A spherical, round, or ovoid bacterium.

**coccyx (kŏk′sĭks)** A small, triangular-shaped bone consisting of three to five fused vertebrae.

**cochlea (kŏk′lē-ă)** A spiral-shaped canal in the inner ear that contains the hearing receptors.

**code linkage (kōd lĭng′kĭj)** Analysis of the connection between diagnostic and procedural information in order to evaluate the medical necessity of the reported charges. This analysis is performed by insurance company representatives.

**coinsurance (kō-ĭn-shŏŏr′əns)** A fixed percentage of covered charges paid by the insured person after a deductible has been met.

**colitis (kə-lī′tĭs)** Inflammation of the colon.

**colonoscopy (kō-lon-os′ kŏ-pē)(†)** A procedure used to determine the cause of diarrhea, constipation, bleeding, or lower abdominal pain by inserting a scope through the anus to provide direct visualization of the large intestine.

**colony (kōl′ə-nē)** A distinct group of microorganisms, visible with the naked eye, on the surface of a culture medium.

**color family (kūl′ər făm′ə-lē)** A group of colors that share certain characteristics, such as warmth or coolness, allowing them to blend well together.

**colposcopy (kol-pos′ kŏ-pē)(†)** The examination of the vagina and cervix with an instrument called a colposcope to identify abnormal tissue, such as cancerous or precancerous cells.

**common bile duct (kŏm′ən bīl dŭkt)** Duct that carries bile to the duodenum. It is formed from the merger of the cystic and hepatic ducts.

**compactible file (kəm-păkt′-əbəl fīl)** Files kept on rolling shelves that slide along permanent tracks in the floor and are stored close together or stacked when not in use.

**complement (kŏm′plə-mənt)** A protein present in serum that is involved in specific defenses.

**complementary medicine (kŏm′-plə-mĕn-tə-rē mĕd′-ĭ-sĭn)** A type of medicine that is used with conventional medicine.

**complete proteins (kəm-plēt′ prō′ten′)** Proteins that contain all nine essential amino acids.

**complex carbohydrates (kəm-plĕks′ kär′bō-hī′drāt′s)** Long chains of sugar units; also known as polysaccharides.

**complex inheritance (kəm-plĕks′ ĭn-hĕr′ĭ-təns)** The inheritance of traits determined by multiple genes.

**compliance plan (kəm-plī′əns plăn)** A process for finding, correcting, and preventing illegal medical office practices.

**complimentary closing (kom-pluh-men-tuh-ree kloh-zing)** The closing remark of a business letter found two spaces below the last line of the body of the letter.

**compound (kŏm′pound′)** A substance that is formed when

two or more atoms of more than one element are chemically combined.

**compound microscope (kŏm′pound′ mī′krə-skōp′)** A microscope that uses two lenses to magnify the image created by condensed light focused through the object being examined.

**computed tomography (kəm-pyo͞ot′ ĕd tō-mogra-fē)(†)** A radiographic examination that produces a three-dimensional, cross-sectional view of an area of the body; may be performed with or without a contrast medium.

**concise (k n-sīs′)** Brevity; the use of no unnecessary words.

**concussion (kən-kŭsh′ən)** A jarring injury to the brain; the most common type of head injury.

**conductive hearing loss (kon-dŭk-tiv′hēr′ing lôs)(†)** A type of hearing loss that occurs when sound waves cannot be conducted through the ear. Most types are temporary.

**condyle (kon′dīl)(†)** Rounded articular surface on a bone.

**cones (kōnz)** Light-sensing nerve cells in the eye, at the posterior of the retina, that are sensitive to color, provide sharp images, and function only in bright light.

**conflict (kŏn′flīkt′)** An opposition of opinions or ideas.

**conjunctiva (kŏn′jŭngk-tī′və)** The protective membrane that lines the eyelid and covers the anterior of the sclera, or the white of the eye.

**conjunctivitis (kən-jŭngk′tə-vī′tĭs)** A contagious infection of the conjunctiva caused by bacteria, viruses, and allergies. The symptoms may include discharge, red eyes, itching, and swollen eyelids; also commonly called pinkeye.

**connective tissue (kə-nĕk′tĭv)** A tissue type that is the framework of the body.

**consent (kən-′sēnt)** A voluntary agreement that a patient gives to allow a medically trained person the permission to touch, examine, and perform a treatment.

**constructive criticism (kən-stre′k-tiv kr′i-tə-si-zəm)** A type of critique that is aimed at giving an individual feedback about his or her performance in order to improve that performance.

**consumable (kən-so͞o′mə-bəl)** Able to be emptied or used up, as with supplies.

**consumer education (kən-so͞o′mər ĕj′ə-ka′shən)** The process by which the average person learns to make informed decisions about goods and services, including health care.

**contagious (kən-tā′jəs)** Having a disease that can easily be transmitted to others.

**contaminated (kən-tăm′ə-nāt′ĕd)** Soiled or stained, particularly through contact with potentially infectious substances; no longer clean or sterile.

**contract (kŏn′trăct′)** A voluntary agreement between two parties in which specific promises are made.

**contraindication (kŏn′trə-ĭn′dĭ-kā′-shən)** A symptom that renders use of a remedy or procedure inadvisable, usually because of risk.

**contrast medium (kŏn′trast′ mē′dē-əm)** A substance that makes internal organs denser and blocks the passage of x-rays to photographic film. Introducing a contrast medium into certain structures or areas of the body can provide a clear image of organs and tissues and highlight indications of how well they are functioning.

**controlled substance (kən-trōld′ sūb′stəns)** A drug or drug product that is categorized as potentially dangerous and addictive and is strictly regulated by federal laws.

**control sample (kən-trol′ săm′pəl)** A specimen that has a known value; used as a comparison for test results on a patient sample.

**contusion (kon-tŭ′shŭn) (†)** A closed wound, or bruise.

**conventional medicine (kən-vĕn′-shən-əl mĕd′-ĭ-sĭn)** The usual practice of physicians and other allied health professionals, such as physical therapists, psychologists, medical assistants, and registered nurses. Also known as allopathy.

**conventions (kən-vĕn′shənz)** A list of abbreviations, punctuation, symbols, typefaces, and instructional notes appearing in the beginning of the ICD-9. The items provide guidelines for using the code set.

**convolutions (kŏn′və-lo͞o′shənz)** The ridges of brain matter between the sulci; also called gyri.

**coordination of benefits (kō-ôr′dn-ā′shən bĕn′ə-fĭts)** A legal principle that limits payment by insurance companies to 100% of the cost of covered expenses.

**co-payment (kō-pā′mənt)** A small fee paid by the insured at the time of a medical service rather than by the insurance company.

**cornea (kôr′nē-ə)** A transparent area on the front of the outer layer of the eye that acts as a window to let light into the eye.

**coronary artery bypass graft (CABG) (kor′-uh-ner-ee, ahr′-tuh-ree, bahy′-pas, grahft)** A surgery performed to bypass a blockage within a coronary artery with a vessel taken from another area.

**coronary sinus (kôr′ə-nĕr′ē sī′nəs)** The large vein that receives oxygen-poor blood from the cardiac veins and empties it into the right atrium of the heart.

**corporation (kôr-pə-′rā-shən)** A type of business group, such as a medical practice, that is established by law and managed by a board of directors.

**corpus callosum (kôr′pəs ka-l′ō-səm)** A thick bundle of nerve fibers that connects the cerebral hemispheres.

**corpus luteum (kôr´pŭs lū-tē´ŭm)(†)** A ruptured follicle cell in the ovary following ovulation.

**cortex (kôr´təks´)** The outermost layer of the cerebrum.

**cortisol (kōr´ti-sol) (†)** A steroid hormone that is released when a person is stressed. It decreases protein synthesis.

**coryza (côrī´zə)** Another name for an upper respiratory tract infection. The common cold.

**costal (kos´tăl)(†)** Cartilage that attaches true ribs to the sternum.

**counter check (koun´tər chĕk)** A special bank check that allows a depositor to draw funds from his own account only, as when he has forgotten his checkbook.

**courtesy title (kûr´tĭ-sē tīt´l)** A title used before a person's name, such as Dr., Mr., or Ms.

**cover sheet (kŭr´ər shēt)** A form sent with a fax that provides details about the transmission.

**covered entity (kūv´ərd en-tə-tē)** Any organization that transmits health information in an electronic form that is related in any way with a HIPAA-covered business.

**Cowper's glands (kou´ pərz glāndz)** Bulbourethral glands.

**coxal (koks-al´)(†)** Pertaining to the bones of the pelvic girdle. The coxa is composed of the ilium, ischium, and pubis.

**CPT** See *Current Procedural Terminology.*

**cranial (krā´-nē-ăl)(†)** See **superior.**

**cranial nerves (krā´nē-ăl nûrvs)(†)** Peripheral nerves that originate from the brain.

**crash cart (krăsh kärt)** A rolling cart of emergency supplies and equipment.

**creatine phosphate (krē´ă-tēn fos´fāt)(†)** A protein that stores extra phosphate groups.

**credit (krĕd´ĭt)** An extension of time to pay for services, which are provided on trust.

**credit bureau (krē´-dit byür´-o)** A company that provides information about the credit worthiness of a person seeking credit.

**cricoid cartilage (krī´koyd kär´tl-ĭj)(†)** A cartilage of the larynx that forms most of the posterior wall and a small part of the anterior wall.

**crime (krīm)** An offense against the state committed or omitted in violation of public law.

**criminal law (krĭm´ə-nəl lô)** Involves crimes against the state. When a state or federal law is violated, the government brings criminal charges against the alleged offender.

**cross-reference (krôs´rĕf´ər-əns)** The notation within the ICD-9 of the word *see* after a main term in the index. The *see* reference means that the main term first checked is not correct. Another category must then be used.

**cross-referenced (krôs´rĕf´ər-ənsd)** Filed in two or more places, with each place noted in each file; the exact contents of the file may be duplicated, or a cross-reference form can be created, listing all the places to find the file.

**cross-training (krós-trā´-ning)** The acquisition of training in a variety of tasks and skills.

**cryosurgery (krī´ō-sûr´jə-rē)** The use of extreme cold to destroy unwanted tissue, such as skin lesions.

**cryotherapy (krī´ō-thĕr´ə-pē)** The application of cold to a patient's body for therapeutic reasons.

**cryptorchidism (kriptôr´kidiz´əm)** Congenital failure of the testes to descend into the scrotal sac.

**crystals (krĭs´təls)** Naturally produced solids of definite form; commonly seen in urine specimens, especially those permitted to cool.

**culture (kŭl´chər)** In the sociologic sense, a pattern of assumptions, beliefs, and practices that shape the way people think and act.

To place a sample of a specimen in or on a substance that allows microorganisms to grow in order to identify the microorganisms present.

**culture and sensitivity (C and S) (kŭl´chər sĕn´sī-tĭv´ə-tē)** A procedure that involves culturing a specimen and then testing the isolated bacteria's susceptibility (sensitivity) to certain antibiotics to determine which antibiotics would be most effective in treating an infection.

**culture medium (kŭlchər mē´de-əm)** A substance containing all the nutrients a particular type of microorganism needs to grow.

*Current Procedural Terminology* **(CPT) (kûr´ənt prə-sē´jər-əl tûr´mə-nŏl´ə-jē)** A book with the most commonly used system of procedure codes. It is the HIPAA-required code set for physicians' procedures.

**cursor (kûr´sər)** A blinking line or cube on a computer screen that shows where the next character that is keyed will appear.

**Cushing's disease (kush´ingz dĭ-zēz´)** A condition in which a person produces too much **cortisol** or has used too many steroid hormones. Some of the signs and symptoms include buffalo hump obesity, a moon face, and abdominal stretch marks; also called hypercortisolism.

**cuspids (kūs´pĭdz)** The sharpest teeth; they act to tear food.

**cyanosis (sī´ə-no´sīs)** A bluish color of skin that results when the supply of oxygen is low in the blood.

**cycle billing (sī´kəl bĭl´ing)** A system that sends invoices to groups of patients every few days, spreading the work of billing all patients over the month while billing each patient only once.

**cystic duct (sĭs´tĭk dŭkt)** The duct from the gallbladder that merges with the hepatic duct to form the common bile duct.

**cystitis (sis-tī′tis)(†)** Inflammation of the urinary bladder caused by infection.

**cytokines (sī′tō-kīnz)** A chemical secreted by T lymphocytes in response to an antigen. Cytokines increase T- and B-cell production, kill cells that have antigens, and stimulate red bone marrow to produce more white blood cells.

**cytokinesis (sī′tō-ki-nē′sis)(†)** Splitting of the cytoplasm during cell division.

**cytoplasm (sī′tə-plăz′əm)** The watery intracellular substance that consists mostly of water, proteins, ions, and nutrients.

**damages (dăm′ĭjz)** Money paid as compensation for violating legal rights.

**database (dā′tə-bās)** A collection of records created and stored on a computer.

**dateline (dāt′līn′)** The line at the top of a letter that contains the month, day, and year.

**debridement (dā-brēd-mont′)(†)** The removal of debris or dead tissue from a wound to expose healthy tissue.

**decibel (děs′ə-bəl)** A unit for measuring the relative intensity of sounds on a scale from 0 to 130.

**deductible (dĭ-dŭk′tə-bəl)** A fixed dollar amount that must be paid by the insured before additional expenses are covered by an insurer.

**deep (dēp)** Anatomical term meaning closer to the inside of the body.

**defamation (děf′ə-mā′shən)** Damaging a person's reputation by making public statements that are both false and malicious.

**defecation reflex (def-ē-kā′shŭn rē′flěks′)** The relaxation of the anal sphincters so that feces can move through the anus in the process of elimination.

**deflection (dĭ-flěk′shən)** A peak or valley on an electrocardiogram.

**dehydration (dē-hī′drā′shən)** The condition that results from a lack of adequate water in the body.

**dementia (dĭ-měn′shə)** The deterioration of mental faculties from organic disease of the brain.

**dendrite (děn′drīt′)** A type of nerve fiber that is short and branches near the cell body. Its function is to receive information from the neuron.

**deoxyhemoblobin (dē-oks-ē-hē-mō-glō′bin)(†)** A type of hemoglobin that is not carrying oxygen. It is darker red in color than hemoglobin.

**dependent (dĭ-pěn′dənt)** A person who depends on another person for financial support.

**depolarization (dē-pō′lăr-i-za-shŭn)(†)** The loss of polarity, or opposite charges inside and outside; the electrical impulse that initiates a chain reaction resulting in contraction.

**depolarized (dē-pō′lăr-īzd)(†)** A state in which sodium ions flow to the inside of the cell membrane, making the outside less positive. Depolarization occurs when a neuron responds to stimuli such as heat, pressure, or chemicals.

**depression (di′-pre-shan)** The lowering of a body part.

**dermatitis (dûr′mə-tī′tĭs)** Inflammation of the skin.

**dermatologist (der-mă-tol′ō-jist)(†)** A specialist who diagnoses and treats diseases of the skin, hair, and nails.

**dermatome (dur′mə tōm)** An area of skin innervated by a spinal nerve.

**dermis (dûr′mĭs)** The middle layer of the skin, which contains connective tissue, nerve endings, hair follicles, sweat glands, and oil glands.

**descending colon (dĭ-sěnd′ĭng kō′lən)** The segment of the large intestine after the transverse colon that descends the left side of the abdominal cavity.

**descending tracts (dĭ-sěnd′ĭng trăkts)** Tracts of the spinal cord that carry motor information from the brain to muscles and glands.

**detrusor muscle (dē-trŭs′or mŭs′əl)** A smooth muscle that contracts to push urine from the bladder into the urethra.

**diabetes insipidus (dī′ə bētĭs ĭn′sĭp′ĭdəs)** The condition of excessive thirst and excessive urination related to hyposecretion of ADH so that water is not retained by the kidney.

**diabetes mellitus (dī′ə-bē′tĭs mə-lī′təs)** Any of several related endocrine disorders characterized by an elevated level of glucose in the blood, caused by a deficiency of insulin or insulin resistance at the cellular level.

**diagnosis (Dx) (dī′əg-nō′sĭs)** The primary condition for which a patient is receiving care.

**diagnosis code (dī′əg-nō′sĭs kōd)** The way a diagnosis is communicated to the third-party payer on the health-care claim.

**diagnostic radiology (dī′əg-nos′tik rā′dē-ōl′ə-jē)** The use of x-ray technology to determine the cause of a patient's symptoms.

**diapedesis (dī′ă-pě-dē′sis)(†)** The squeezing of a cell through a blood vessel wall.

**diaphoresis (dī′əfarē′sis)** Excessive sweating as a result of illness or injury.

**diaphragm (dī′ə-frăm′)** A muscle that separates the thoracic and abdominopelvic cavities.

**diaphysis (dī′-af′i-sis)** The shaft of a long bone.

**diastolic pressure (dī′ə-stŏl′ĭk prěsh′ər)** The blood pressure measured when the heart relaxes.

**diathermy (dī′ə-thŭr′mē)** A type of heat therapy in which a machine produces high-frequency waves that achieve deep heat penetration in muscle tissue.

**diencephalon (dī-en-sef´ă-lon)(†)** A structure that includes the thalamus and the hypothalamus. It is located between the cerebral hemispheres and is superior to the brain stem.

**dietary supplement (dī´-ĭ-tĕr-ē sŭp´-lə-mənt)** Vitamins, minerals, herbals, and other substances taken by mouth without a prescription to promote health and well-being.

**differential diagnosis (dĭf´ə-rĕn´shəl dī´ag-nō´sĭs)** The process of determining the correct diagnosis when two or more diagnoses are possible.

**differently abled (dĭf´ər-ənt-lē ā´bəld)** Having a condition that limits or changes a person's abilities and may require special accommodations.

**diffusion (di-fyū´zhŭn)(†)** The movement of a substance from an area of high concentration to an area of low concentration.

**digital examination (dĭj´ĭ-tl ĭg-zam´ə-nā´shən)** Part of a physical examination in which the physician inserts one or two fingers of one hand into the opening of a body canal such as the vagina or the rectum; used to palpate canal and related structures.

**diluent (dĭl´yōō-ənt)** A liquid used to dissolve and dilute another substance, such as a drug.

**disability insurance (dĭs´ə-bĭlĭ-tē ĭn-shōōr´əns)** Insurance that provides a monthly, prearranged payment to an individual who cannot work as the result of an injury or disability.

**disaccharide (dī-sak´ă-rīd) (†)** A type of carbohydrate that is a simple sugar.

**disbursement (dĭs-bûrs´mənt)** Any payment of funds made by the physician's office for goods and services.

**disclaimer (dĭs-klā´mər)** A statement of denial of legal liability or that refutes the authenticity of a claim.

**disclosure (dĭ-sklō´zhər)** The release of, the transfer of, the provision of access to, or the divulgence in any manner of patient information.

**disclosure statement (dĭ-sklō´zhər stāt´mənt)** A written description of agreed terms of payment; also called a federal Truth in Lending statement.

**discrimination (dĭs-´skrĭm-ə-´nā-shən)** Unequal and unfair treatment.

**disinfectant (dĭs´ĭn-fĕk´tănt)** A cleaning product applied to instruments and equipment to reduce or eliminate infectious organisms; not used on human tissue.

**dislocation (dĭs´lō-kā´shən)** The displacement of a bone end from a joint.

**dispense (dĭ-spĕns´)** To distribute a drug, in a properly labeled container, to a patient who is to use it.

**distal (dĭs´tal)** Anatomic term meaning farther away from a point of attachment or farther away from the trunk of the body.

**distal convoluted tubule (dĭs´tal kon´vō-lū-ted tū´byūl)** The last twisted section of the renal tubule; it is located after the loop of Henle. Several of these tubules merge together to form collecting ducts.

**distribution (dĭs´trĭ-byōō´shən)** The biochemical process of transporting a drug from its administration site in the body to its site of action.

**diverticulitis (dī´ver-tik-yū-li´tis)(†)** Inflammation of the diverticuli, which are abnormal dilations in the intestine.

**diverticulosis (dī´ver-tik-yū-lō-sis)** Abnormal outpouchings or dilations of the intestine.

**DNA (dē´ĕn-ā´)** A nucleic acid that contains the genetic information of cells.

**doctor of osteopathy (dok´tər ŏs´tē-ŏp´ə-thē)** A doctor who focuses special attention on the musculoskeletal system and uses hands and eyes to identify and adjust structural problems, supporting the body's natural tendency toward health and self-healing.

**doctrine of informed consent (dōk-´trĭn of ĭn-fôrmd´ kən-´sēnt)** The legal basis for informed consent, usually outlined in a state's medical practice act.

**doctrine of professional discretion (dōk-´trĭn of prə-fĕsh´ə-nəl dĭ-skĕsh´ən)** A principle under which a physician can exercise judgment as to whether to show patients who are being treated for mental or emotional conditions their records.

**documentation (dōk´yə-mən-tā´shən)** The recording of information in a patient's medical record; includes detailed notes about each contact with the patient and about the treatment plan, patient progress, and treatment outcomes.

**dorsal (dôr´səl)** See **posterior**.

**dorsal root (dôr´səl rōōt)** A portion of a spinal nerve that contains axons of sensory neurons only.

**dorsiflexion (dôr-si-flek´shŭn)(†)** Pointing the toes upward.

**dosage (dōs´āj)** The size, frequency, and number of doses.

**dose (dōs)** The amount of a drug given or taken at one time.

**dot matrix printer (dŏt mā´trĭks prĭn´tər)** An impact printer that creates characters by placing a series of tiny dots next to one another.

**double-booking system (dŭb´əl bōōk´ing sĭs´təm)** A system of scheduling in which two or more patients are booked for the same appointment slot, with the assumption that both patients will be seen by the doctor within the scheduled period.

**douche (dōōsh)** Vaginal irrigation, which can be used to administer vaginal medication in liquid form.

**drainage catheter (drā´nĭj kăth´ĭ-tər)** A type of catheter used to withdraw fluids.

**dressing (drĕs´ĭng)** A sterile material used to cover a surgical or other wound.

**DSL (digital subscriber line) (dĭj´ĭ-tl səb-skrīb´ līn)** A type of modem that operates over telephone lines but uses a different frequency than a telephone, allowing a computer to access the Internet at the same time that a telephone is being used.

**ductus arteriosus (dŭk´tŭs ar-tēr´ ē-ō´sus)(†)** The connection in the fetus between the pulmonary trunk and the aorta.

**ductus venosus (duk´tŭs ven-ō´sus)(†)** A blood vessel that allows most of the blood to bypass the liver in the fetus.

**duodenum (dōō´ə-dē´nəm)** The first section of the small intestine.

**durable item (dōōr´ə-bəl ī´təm)** A piece of equipment that is used repeatedly, such as a telephone, computer, or examination table; contrast with **expendable item.**

**durable power of attorney (dōōr´ə-bəl poúər ə-tûr´nē)(†)** A document naming the person who will make decisions regarding medical care on behalf of another person if that person becomes unable to do so.

**dwarfism (dwôrf´ĭzm)** A condition in which too little growth hormone is produced, resulting in an abnormally small stature.

**dysmenorrhea (dis-men-ōr-ē´ä)(†)** Severe menstrual cramps that limit daily activity.

**dyspnea (disp-nē´ä)(†)** Difficult or painful breathing.

**ear ossicles (îr os´ĭ-kl)(†)** Three tiny bones called the malleus, the incus, and the stapes located in the middle ear cavity. They are the smallest bones of the body.

**eccrine gland (ek´rin glănd)(†)** The most numerous type of sweat gland. Eccrine sweat glands produce a watery type of sweat

and are activated primarily by heat.

**echocardiography (ek´ō-kar-dē-og´rǎ-fē)(†)** A procedure that tests the structure and function of the heart through the use of reflected sound waves, or echoes.

**E code (ē kŏd)** A type of code in the ICD-9. E-codes identify the external causes of injuries and poisoning.

**ectoderm (ek´tō-derm)(†)** The primary germ layer that gives rise to nervous tissue and some epithelial tissue.

**ectropian (ek-trō´pē-ŭn)** Eversion of the lower eyelid.

**eczema (ĕk´sə-mə)** Inflammatory condition of the skin.

**edema (ĭ-dē´mə)** An excessive buildup of fluid in body tissue.

**editing (ĕd´ĭt-ĭng)** The process of ensuring that a document is accurate, clear, and complete; free of grammatical errors; organized logically; and written in the appropriate style.

**effacement (i fās´mənt)** Thinning of the cervix in preparation for childbirth.

**effectors (ĭ-fĕk´tərs)** Muscles and glands that are stimulated by motor neurons in the peripheral nervous system.

**efferent arterioles (ĕf´ər-ənt ar-tēr´ē-ōlz)(†)** Structures that deliver blood to peritubular capillaries that are wrapped around the renal tubules of the nephron in the kidneys.

**efferent nerves (ĕf´ər-ənt nûrvs)** Motor nerves that bring information or impulses from the Central nervous System to the Peripheral nervous System to allow for the movement or action of a muscle or gland.

**efficacy (ĕf´ĭ-kə-sē)** The therapeutic value of a procedure or therapy, such as a drug.

**efficiency (ĭ-fĭsh´ən-sē)** The ability to produce a desired result with the least effort, expense, and waste.

**elective procedure (ĭ-lĕk´tĭv prə-sē´jər)** A medical procedure that is not required to sustain life but is requested for payment to the third-party payer by the patient or physician. Some elective procedures are paid for by third-party payers, whereas others are not.

**electrocardiogram (ECG or EKG) (ĭ-lĕk´trō-kär´dē-ə-grăm´)** The tracing made by an **electrocardiograph.**

**electrocardiograph (ĭ-lĕk´trō-kär´dē-ə-grăf´)** An instrument that measures and displays the waves of electrical impulses responsible for the cardiac cycle.

**electrocardiography (ĭ-lĕk´trō-kär´dē-ŏg´rə-fē)** The process by which a graphic pattern is created to reflect the electrical impulses generated by the heart as it pumps.

**electrocauterization (ĭ-lĕk´trō-kô´tər-ĭ-zā´shən)** The use of a needle, probe, or loop heated by electric current to remove growths such as warts, to stop bleeding, and to control nosebleeds that either will not subside or continually recur.

**electrodes (ĭ-lĕk´trōds´)** Sensors that detect electrical activity.

**electroencephalography (ĭ-lĕk´trō-ĕn-sĕf´ə-lŏg´rə-fē)** A procedure that records the electrical activity of the brain as a tracing called an electroencephalogram, or EEG, on a strip of graph paper.

**electrolytes (ĭ-lĕk´trə-līts)** Substances that carry electrical current through the movement of ions.

**electromyography (ĭ-lĕk´trō-mī-ŏg´rə-fē)** A procedure in which needle electrodes are inserted into some of the skeletal muscles and a monitor records the nerve impulses and measures conduction time; used to detect neuromuscular disorders or nerve damage.

**electronic data interchange (EDI) (ĭ-lĕk-trŏnʹĭk dāʹtə ĭnʹtər-chānjʹ)** Transmitting electronic medical insurance claims from providers to payers using the necessary information systems.

**electronic mail (ĭ-lĕkʹtrŏnʹĭks)** A method of sending and receiving messages through a computer network; commonly known as e-mail.

**electronic media (i-lek-tron-ik meeʹ-dee-uh)** Any transmissions that are physically moved from one location to another through the use of magnetic tape, disk, compact disk media, or any other form of digital or electronic technology.

**electronic transaction record (ĭ-lĕkʹtrŏnʹĭk trăn-săkʹshən rĭ-kôrd)** The standardized codes and formats used for the exchange of medical data.

**elevation (e-lə-vʹā-shən)** The raising of a body part.

**embolism (ĕmʹbə-lĭzʹəm)** An obstruction in a blood vessel.

**embolus (ĕmʹbə-ləs)** A portion of a thrombus that breaks off and moves through the bloodstream.

**embryonic period (em-brē-onʹik pîrʹē-əd)(†)** The second through eighth weeks of pregnancy.

**E/M code (ēʹ/ĕm kōd)** Evaluation and management codes that are often considered the most important of all CPT codes. The E/M section guidelines explain how to code different levels of services.

**empathy (ĕmʹpə-thē)** Identification with or sensitivity to another person's feelings and problems.

**emphysema (emʹfəsēmə)** A chronic lung condition consisting of damage to the alveoli of the lungs. It is heavily associated with smoking, which causes stretching of the spaces between the alveoli and paralyzes the cilia of the respiratory system.

**employment contract (ĕm-ploiʹmənt kŏnʹtrăktʹ)** A written agreement of employment terms between employer and employee that describes the employee's duties and the considerations (money, benefits, and so on) to be given by the employer in exchange.

**empyema (emʹpīēʹmə)** A collection of pus in the pleural cavity.

**enclosure (ĕn-klōʹzhərz)** Materials that are included in the same envelope as the primary letter.

**encounter form (en-ʹkaun-tər form)** A form that combines the charges for services rendered, an invoice for payment or insurance copayment, and all the information for submitting an insurance claim; also known as a superbill.

**endocardium (en-dō-karʹdē-ŭm)(†)** The innermost layer of the heart.

**endochondral (en-dō-konʹdrăl)(†)** A type of ossification in which bones start out as cartilage models.

**endocrine gland (ĕnʹdə-kra-n glănd)** A gland that secretes its products directly into tissue, fluid, or blood.

**endocrinologist (ĕnʹdə-kra-nŏlʹə-jĭst)** A specialist who diagnoses and treats disorders of the endocrine system, which regulates many body functions by circulating hormones that are secreted by glands throughout the body.

**endoderm (ĕnʹdō-derm)(†)** The primary germ layer that gives rise to epithelial tissues only.

**endogenous infection (ĕnʹ-dŏjʹə-nəs ĭn-fĕkʹshən)** An infection in which an abnormality or malfunction in routine body processes causes normally beneficial or harmless microorganisms to become pathogenic.

**endolymph (ĕnʹdō-limf)(†)** A fluid in the inner ear. When this fluid moves, it activates hearing and equilibrium receptors.

**endometriosis (enʹdō-mē-trē-ōʹsis)(†)** A condition in which tissues that make up the lining of the uterus grow outside the uterus.

**endometrium (enʹdō-mēʹtrē-ŭm)(†)** The innermost layer of the uterus. It undergoes significant changes during the menstrual cycle.

**endomysium (enʹdō-mizʹē-ŭm)(†)** A connective tissue covering that surrounds individual muscle cells.

**endoplasmic reticulum (enʹdoplazʹmik ritikʹyəlum)** The organelles of the endoplasmic reticulum is composed of both smooth and rough types. The rough type contains ribosomes on its surface. The smooth type has no ribosomes. Both types create a network of passageways throughout the cytoplasm.

**endorse (ĕn-dôrsʹ)** To sign or stamp the back of a check with the proper identification of the person or organization to whom the check is made out, to prevent the check from being cashed if it is stolen or lost.

**endoscopy (ĕn-dôsʹkə-pē)** Any procedure in which a scope is used to visually inspect a canal or cavity within the body.

**endosteum (en-dosʹtē-ŭm)(†)** A membrane that lines the medullary cavity and the holes of spongy bone.

**entropion (en-trōʹpē-ūn)** Inversion of the lower eyelid.

**enunciation (ĭ-nŭnʹsē-āʹshən)** Clear and distinct speaking.

**enzyme immunoassay (EIA) (ĕnʹzīm imʹyū-nō-asʹā)(†)** The detection of substances by immunologic methods. This method involves an antigen, an antibody specific for the antigen, and a second antibody conjugated to an enzyme.

**enzyme-linked immunosorbent assay (ELISA) test (ĕnʹzīm-lĭngkt imʹyū-nō-sôrʹbent ăsʹā tĕst)(†)** A blood test that confirms the presence of antibodies developed by the body's immune system in response to an initial HIV infection.

**eosinophil (ē-ō-sinʹō-fil)(†)** A type of granular leukocyte that captures invading bacteria and antigen-antibody complexes through phagocytosis.

**epicardium (ep-i-kar´dē-ŭm)(†)** The outermost layer of the wall of the heart. Also known as the **visceral pericardium.**

**epidermis (ĕp´ĭ-dûr´mĭs)** The most superficial layer of the skin.

**epididymis (ep-i-did´i-mis) (†)** An elongated structure attached to the back of the testes and in which sperm cells mature.

**epididymitis (ep-i-did-i-mī´tis)(†)** Inflammation of an **epididymis.** Most cases result from infection.

**epiglottic cartilage (ep-i-glot´ik kär´tl-ĭj)(†)** A cartilage of the larynx that forms the framework of the epiglottis.

**epiglottis (ep-i-glot-ī´tis)(†)** The flap-like structure that closes off the larynx during swallowing.

**epilepsy (ĕp´ə-lĕp´sē)** A condition that occurs when parts of the brain receive a burst of electrical signals that disrupt normal brain function; also called **seizures.**

**epimysium (ep-i-mis´-ē-ŭm)(†)** A thin covering that is just deep to the fascia of a muscle. It surrounds the entire muscle.

**epinephrine (ĕp´ə-nĕf´rĭn)** An injectable medication used to treat anaphylaxis by causing vasoconstriction to increase blood pressure.
A hormone secreted from the adrenal glands. It increases heart rate, breathing rate, and blood pressure.

**epiphyseal disk (ep-i-fiz´ē-ăl dĭsk)(†)** A plate of cartilage between the **epiphysis** and the **diaphysis.**

**epiphysis (e-pif´i-sis)(†)** The expanded end of a long bone.

**episiotomy (epē´zēot´əmē)** A surgical incision of the female perineum to enlarge the vaginal opening for delivery.

**epistaxis (ĕp´i-stak´sis)** Nosebleed.

**epithelial tissue (ep-i-thē´lē-ĕl tĭsh´oo)(†)** A tissue type that lines the tubes, hollow organs, and cavities of the body.

**erectile tissue (ĭ-rĕk´təl tĭsh´oo)** A highly specialized tissue located in the shaft of the penis. It fills with blood to achieve an erection.

**erythema (er-i-thē´mă)** Redness of the skin.

**erythroblastosis fetalis (ĕ-rith´rō-blas-tō´sis fe´tăl-is)(†)** A serious anemia that develops in a fetus with Rh-positive blood as a result of antibodies in an Rh-negative mother's body.

**erythrocytes (ĭ-rĭth´rə-sīt´s)** Red blood cells.

**erythrocyte sedimentation rate (ESR) (ĭ-rĭth´rə-sīt´ sĕd´ə-mən-tā´shən rāt)** The rate at which red blood cells, the heaviest blood component, settle to the bottom of a blood sample.

**erythropoietin (ĕ-rith-rō-poy´ē-tin)(†)** A hormone secreted by the kidney and is responsible for regulating the production of red blood cells.

**esophageal hiatus (ĭ-sŏf´ə-jē´əl)** Hole in the diaphragm through which the esophagus passes.

**established patient (ĭ-stăb´lĭsht pā´shənt)** A patient who has seen the physician within the past 3 years. This determination is important when using E/M codes.

**estrogen (ĕs´trə-jən)** A female sex hormone; when produced during ovulation, estrogen causes a buildup of the lining of the uterus (womb) to prepare it for a possible pregnancy.

**ethics (ĕth´ĭks)** General principles of right and wrong, as opposed to requirements of law.

**ethmoid (ĕth´moyd)(†)** Bones located between the sphenoid and nasal bone that form part of the floor of the cranium.

**etiologic agent (ē´tē-ə-lŏj´ĭkā´jənt)** A living microorganism or its

toxin that may cause human disease.

**etiquette (ĕt´ĭ-ket´)** Good manners.

**eustachian tube (yoo-stā´shən toob)** An opening in the middle ear, leading to the back of the throat, that helps equalize air pressure on both sides of the eardrum.

**eversion (ē-ver´zhŭn)(†)** Turning the sole of the foot laterally.

**exclusion (ĭk-skloozh´ən)** An expense that is not covered by a particular insurance policy, such as an eye examination or dental care.

**excretion (ĭk-skrē´shən)** The elimination of waste by a discharge; in drug metabolism, the manner in which a drug is eliminated from the body.

**exocrine gland (ĕk´sə-krĭn glănd)** A gland that secretes its product into a duct.

**exogenous infection (ĕk-sŏj´ə-nəs ĭn-fĕk´shən)** An infection that is caused by the introduction of a pathogen from outside the body.

**exophthalmos (k´s f´th lm s)** Bulging of the eyeballs, often related to hyperthyroidism.

**expendable item (ĭk-spĕn´dəbəl ī´təm)** An item that is used and must then be restocked; also known collectively as supplies. Contrast with **durable item.**

**expiration (ĕk´spə-rā´shən)** The process of breathing out; also called exhalation.

**explanation of benefits (EOB) (ĕk´splə-nā´shən ŭv bĕn´ə-fits)** Information that explains the medical claim in detail; also called **remittance advice (RA).**

**expressed contract (ĭk-sprĕst´ kŏn´trăct)** A contract clearly stated in written or spoken words.

**extension (ĭk-stĕn´shən)** An unbending or straightening movement of the two elements of a jointed body part.

**external auditory canal (ĭk-stûr′nəl ô′dĭ-tôr′ē kə-năl′)** Canal that carries sound waves to the tympanic membrane; commonly called the ear canal.

**externship (ĭk-stûrn′shĭp)** A period of practical work experience performed by a medical assisting student in a physician's office, hospital, or other health-care facility.

**extrinsic eye muscles (ĭk-strĭn′ sĭk ĭ-mūs′əlz)** The skeletal muscles that move the eyeball.

**facsimile machine (făk-sĭm′ə-lē mə-shēn′)** A piece of office equipment used to send a facsimile, or fax, over telephone lines from one modem to another; more commonly called a fax machine.

**facultative (fak-ŭl-tā′tiv)(†)** Able to adapt to different conditions; in microbiology, able to grow in environments either with or without oxygen.

**Fahrenheit (făr′ən-hīt)** One of two common scales used for measuring temperature; measured in degrees Fahrenheit, or °F.

**fallopian tubes (fə-lō′-pē-ən tūbz)** Tubes that extend from the uterus on each side and that open near an ovary.

**family practitioner (făm′ə-lē prăk-tĭsh′ə-nər)(†)** A physician who does not specialize in a branch of medicine but treats all types and ages of patients; also called a general practitioner.

**fascia (fash′e-ă)(†)** A structure that covers entire skeletal muscles and separates them from each other.

**fascicle (făs′ĭ-kəl)** Sections of a muscle divided by connective tissue called perimysium.

**febrile (fĕb′rəl)** Having a body temperature above one's normal range.

**feces (fē′sēz)** Material found in the large intestine and made from leftover chyme. Faces are eventually eliminated through the anus.

**Federal Unemployment Tax Act (FUTA)** This act requires employers to pay a percentage of each employee's income up to a certain dollar amount.

**feedback (fēd′băk′)** Verbal and nonverbal evidence that a message was received and understood.

**feedback loop (fēd′băk lōōp)** A mechanism to control hormone levels. The two types are positive and negative feedback loops.

**fee-for-service (fēfôr sûr′vĭs)** A major type of health plan. It repays policyholders for the costs of health care that are due to illness and accidents.

**fee schedule (fē skĕj′ōōl)** A list of the costs of common services and procedures performed by a physician.

**felony (fĕl′ə-nē)** A serious crime, such as murder or rape, that is punishable by imprisonment. In certain crimes, a felony is punishable by death.

**femoral (fem′ŏ-răl)(†)** Relating to the femur or thigh.

**femur (fē′mər)** The bone in the upper leg; commonly called the thigh bone.

**fenestrated drape (fĕn′ĭ-strāt′ĕd drāp)** A drape that has a round or slit-like opening that provides access to the surgical site.

**fertilization (fer′til-i-zā′shŭn)** The process in which an egg unites with a sperm.

**fetal period (fĕt′l pîr′ē-əd)** A period that begins at week nine of pregnancy and continues through delivery of the offspring.

**fiber (fī′bər)** The tough, stringy part of vegetables and grains, which is not absorbed by the body but aids in a variety of bodily functions.

**fibrinogen (fī-brin′ō-jen)(†)** A protein found in plasma that is important for blood clotting.

**fibroid (fī′broid)** A benign tumor in the uterus composed of fibrous tissue.

**fibromyalgia (fī-brō-mī-al′jē-ă)(†)** A condition that exhibits chronic pain primarily in joints, muscles, and tendons.

**fibula (fĭb′yə-lə)** The lateral bone of the lower leg.

**file guide (fīlgīd)** A heavy cardboard or plastic insert used to identify a group of file folders in a file drawer.

**filtration (fĭl-trā′shən)** A process that separates substances into solutions by forcing them across a membrane.

**fimbriae (fĭm-brē-ə)** Fringe-like structures that border the entrances of the **fallopian tubes.**

**first morning urine specimen (fûrst môr′nĭng yōōr′in spĕs′ə-mən)** A urine specimen that is collected after a night's sleep; contains greater concentrations of substances that collect over time than specimens taken during the day.

**fixative (fĭk′sə-tĭv)** A solution sprayed on a slide immediately after the specimen is applied. It is used to preserve and hold the cells in place until a microscopic examination is performed.

**flaccid (flak′sid)** Weak, soft; not erect.

**flagellum (flajel′əm)** The "tail-like" structure on some cell membranes that provides cell movement.

**flexion (flek′shŭn)(†)** A bending movement of the two elements of a jointed body part.

**floater (flō′tər)** A nonsterile assistant who is free to move about the room during surgery and attend to unsterile needs.

**fluidotherapy (flōō′id-ōthĕr′ə-pē)** A technique for stimulating healing, particularly in the hands and feet, by placing the affected body part in a container of glass beads that are heated and agitated with hot air.

**follicle (fŏl′ĭ-kəl)** An accessory organ of the skin that is found in the dermis and the sites at which hairs emerge.

**follicle-stimulating hormone (FSH) (fŏl´ĭ-kəl stĭm´yū-lā-tĭng hôr´mōn)** A hormone that in females stimulates the production of estrogen by the ovaries; in males, it stimulates sperm production.

**follicular cells (fə-lĭ´-kyə-lər selz)** Small cells contained in the primordial follicle along with a large cell called a primary **oocyte.**

**folliculitis (fŏ-lĭk-yū-lī´tĭs)(†)** Inflammation of the hair follicle.

**fomite (fō´mīt)(†)** An inanimate object, such as clothing, body fluids, water, or food, that may be contaminated with infectious organisms and thus serve to transmit disease.

**fontanel (fän-tə-n´el)** The soft spot in an infant's skull that consists of tough membranes that connect to incompletely developed bone.

**food exchange (fōōd ĭks-chānj´)** A unit of food in a particular food category that provides the same amounts of protein, fat, and carbohydrates as all other units of food in that category.

**foramen magnum (fə-rā´-mən mag-nəm)** The large hole in the occipital bone that allows the brain to connect to the spinal cord.

**foramen ovale (fō-rā´men ō-va´lē)(†)** A hole in the fetal heart between the right atrium and the left atrium.

**forced vital capacity (FVC) (fôrst vīt´l kə-păs´ĭ-tē)** The greatest volume of air that a person is able to expel when performing rapid, forced expiration.

**formalin (fōr-mă-lin)(†)** A dilute solution of formaldehyde used to preserve biological specimens.

**formed elements (fôrmd ĕl´ə-mənts)** Red blood cells, white blood cells, and platelets; compose 45% of blood volume.

**formulary (fōr´myū-lā-rē)(†)** An insurance plan's list of approved prescription medications.

**fracture (frăk´chər)** Any break in a bone.

**fraud (frôd)** An act of deception that is used to take advantage of another person or entity.

**frequency (frē´kwən-sē)** The number of complete fluctuations of energy per second in the form of waves.

**frontal (frŭn´tl)** Anatomic term that refers to the plane that divides the body into anterior and posterior portions. Also called coronal.

**fulgurated (ful´gy ə rā təd)** The ise of heat or laser to burn or destroy tissue.

**full-block letter style (fōōl blŏk lĕt´ə̄r stīl)** A letter format in which all lines begin flush left; also called block style.

**functional résumé (fŭngk´shə-nəl rĕz´ōō-mā´)** A résumé that highlights specialty areas of a person's accomplishments and strengths.

**fundus (fun´dus)** The upper domed portion of an organ.

**fungus (fŭng´gəs)** A eukaryotic organism that has a rigid cell wall at some stage in the life cycle.

**gait (gāt)** The way a person walks, consisting of two phases: stance and swing.

**ganglia (găng´glē-ə)** Collections of neuron cell bodies outside the central nervous system.

**gastic juice (găs´trĭk jüs)** Secretions from the stomach lining that begin the process of digesting protein.

**gastritis (gă-strī´tĭs)** Inflammation of the stomach lining.

**gastroenterologist (găs´trō-ĕn-ter-ol´ō-jist)(†)** A specialist who diagnoses and treats disorders of the entire gastrointestinal tract, including the stomach, intestines, and associated digestive organs.

**gastroesophageal reflux disease (GERD) (gas´trō-ē-sof´ă-jē´ăl rē´flĕks dĭ-zēz´)** A condition that occurs when stomach acids are pushed into the esophagus and cause heartburn.

**gene (jēn)** A segment of DNA that determines a body trait.

**general physical examination (jĕn´ər-əl fĭz´ĭ-kəl ĭg-zăm´ə-nā´shən)** An examination performed by a physician to confirm a patient's health or to diagnose a medical problem.

**generic name (jə-nĕr´ĭk nām)** A drug's official name.

**gerontologist (jĕr´ən-tŏl´ə-jĭst)** A specialist who studies the aging process.

**giantism (jī´an-tizm)(†)** A condition in which too much growth hormone is produced in childhood, resulting in an abnormally increased stature.

**glans penis (glanz pē´nĭs)** A cone-shaped structure at the end of the penis.

**glaucoma (glou-kō´mə)** A condition in which too much pressure is created in the eye by excessive aqueous humor. This excess pressure can lead to permanent damage of the optic nerves, resulting in blindness.

**global period (glō´bəl pîr´ē-əd)** The period of time that is covered for follow-up care of a procedure or surgical service.

**globulins (glob´yū-lin)(†)** Plasma proteins that transport lipids and some vitamins.

**glomerular filtrate (glō-mār´yū-lăr fĭl´trāt´)(†)** The fluid remaining in the **glomerular capsule** after **glomerular filtration.**

**glomerular filtration (glō-mār´yū-lăr fĭl-trā´shən)(†)** The process by which urine forms in the kidneys as blood moves through a tight ball of capillaries called the glomerulus.

**glomerulonephritis (glō-mār´yū-lō-nef-rī´tis)(†)** An inflammation of the glomeruli of the kidney.

**glomerulus** (glō-mār´yū-lŭs)(†)　A group of capillaries in the renal corpuscle.

**glottis** (glot´is)(†)　The opening between the vocal cords.

**glucagon** (glōō´kə-gŏn´)　A hormone that increases glucose concentrations in the bloodstream and slows down protein synthesis.

**glycogen** (glī´kə-jən)　An excess of glucose that is stored in the liver and in skeletal muscle.

**glycosuria** (glī-kō-sū´rē-ă)(†)　The presence of significant levels of glucose in the urine.

**goiter** (goi´tər)　Enlargement of the thyroid gland, which causes swelling of the neck, often related to iodine insufficiency in the diet.

**Golgi apparatus** (gôl´jē ap´ərat´es)　The cell's Golgi apparatus synthesizes carbohydrates and also appears to prepare and store secretions for discharge from the cell.

**gonadotropin-releasing hormone (GnRH)** (gō´na-dō-trō´pinr ĭ-lēs´ĭng hôr´mōn´)　Hormone that stimulates the anterior pituitary gland to release **follicle-stimulating hormone (FSH).**

**gonads** (gō´nădz)　The reproductive organs; namely, in women, the ovaries, and in men, the testes.

**goniometer** (gō-nē-ă´-me-tər)　A protractor device that measures range of motion.

**gout** (gowt)(†)　A medical condition characterized by an elevated uric acid level and recurrent acute arthritis.

**G-protein** (jē-prō´tēn)(†)　A substance that causes enzymes in the cell to activate following the activation of the hormone-receptor complex in the cell membrane.

**gram-negative** (grăm´nĕg´ə-tĭv)　Referring to bacteria that lose their purple color when a decolorizer has been added during a Gram's stain.

**gram-positive** (grăm´pŏz´ ĭ-tĭv)　Referring to bacteria that retain their purple color after a decolorizer has been added during a Gram's stain.

**Gram's stain** (grămz stăn)　A method of staining that differentiates bacteria according to the chemical composition of their cell walls.

**granular leukocyte** (grăn´yə-lər lōō´kəsīt´)　A type of leukocyte (white blood cell) with a segmented nucleus and granulated cytoplasm; also known as a polymorphonuclear leukocyte.

**granulocyte** (gran´yū-lō-sīt)(†)　See **granular leukocyte.**

**Grave's disease** (grāvz dĭ-zēz´)　A disorder in which a person develops antibodies that attack the thyroid gland.

**gray matter** (grā măt´ər)　The inner tissue of the brain and the spinal cord that is darker in color than **white matter.** It contains all the bodies and dendrites of nerve cells.

**gross earnings** (grōs ûr´nĭngz)　The total amount an employee earns before deductions.

**group practice** (grōōp prăk´ tĭs)　A medical management system in which a group of three of more licensed physicians share their collective income, expenses, facilities, equipment, records, and personnel. (3)

**growth hormone (GH)** (grōth hôr´mōn´)　A hormone that stimulates an increase in the size of the muscles and bones of the body.

**gustatory receptors** (gə´s-tə-tör-ē ri-se´p-tər)　Taste receptors that are found on taste buds.

**gynecologist** (gĭ´n ĭ-kŏi´ə-jĭst)　A specialist who performs routine physical care and examinations of the female reproductive system.

**gyri** (jī´rī)(†)　The ridges of brain matter between the sulci; also called **convolutions.**

**hairy leukoplakia** (hâr´ē lū-kō-plā´ kē-ă)(†)　A white lesion on the tongue associated with AIDS.

**hapten** (hap´tĕn)(†)　Foreign substances in the body too small to start an immune response by themselves.

**hard copy** (härd´ kŏp´ē)　A readable paper copy or printout of information.

**hardware** (härd´wâr´)　The physical components of a computer system, including the monitor, keyboard, and printer.

**hazard label** (hăz´ərd lā´bəl)　A shortened version of the Material Safety Data Sheet; permanently affixed to a hazardous substance container.

**HCPCS Level II codes** (āch sē pē sē ĕs lĕv´əl tōō kōdz)　Codes that cover many supplies such as sterile trays, drugs, and durable medical equipment; also referred to as national codes. They also cover services and procedures not included in the CPT.

**Health Care Common Procedure Coding System (HCPCS)** (hĕlth kâr kŏm´ən prə-sē´jər kōd´ĭng sĭs´təm)　A coding system developed by the Centers for Medicare and Medicaid Services that is used in coding services for Medicare patients.

**health fraud** (hĕlth frôd)　A deception or trickery related to health prevention or care for profit.

**health maintenance organization (HMO)** (hĕlth măn´tə-nəns ôr´ gə-nĭ-zā´shən)　A health-care organization that provides specific services to individuals and their dependents who are enrolled in the plan. Doctors who enroll in an HMO agree to provide certain services in exchange for a prepaid fee.

**helper T-cells** (hĕl´pər tē´ sĕlz)　White blood cells that are a key component of the body's immune system and that work in coordination with other white blood cells to combat infection.

**hematemesis** (hē´-mă-tem´ĕ-sis)　The vomiting of blood.

**hematocrit (hē′mă-tō-krit)(†)** The percentage of the volume of a sample made up of red blood cells after the sample has been spun in a centrifuge.

**hematology (hē′mə-tŏl′ə-jē)** The study of blood.

**hematoma (hē′mə-tō′me)** A swelling caused by blood under the skin.

**hematopoiesis (hēmətōpōē′sis)** The process of new blood cell formation in the red bone marrow of cancellous bone.

**hematuria (hē-mă-tu′rē-ă)(†)** The presence of blood in the urine.

**hemocytoblast (hē′mă-sī′tō-blast)(†)** Cells of the red bone marrow that produce most red blood cells.

**hemoglobin (hē′mə-glō′bĭn)** A protein that contains iron and bonds with and carries oxygen to cells; the main component of erythrocytes.

**hemoglobinuria ((hē′mō-glō-bi-nū′rē-ă) (†)** The presence of free **hemoglobin** in the urine; a rare condition caused by transfusion reactions, malaria, drug reactions, snake bites, or severe burns.

**hemolysis (hē-mol′ĭ-sis)(†)** The rupturing of red blood cells, which releases hemoglobin.

**hemolytic anemias (hē mō lit′ ik ənē′mēə)** Types of anemia that cause red blood cells to be destroyed faster than they can be made.

**hemoptysis (hi mop′ ti sis)** The spitting up of blood from the respiratory tract.

**hemorrhoids (hĕm′ə-roidz′)** Varicose veins of the rectum or anus.

**hemostasis (hē′mō-stā-sis)(†)** The stoppage of bleeding.

**hemothorax (hē′ mō thôr′ aks)** Blood collection in the pleural cavity causing collapse of the lung.

**hepatic duct (hĭ-păt′ĭk dŭkt)** A duct that leaves the liver carrying bile and merges with the cystic duct to form the common bile duct.

**hepatic lobule (he-păt′ĭk lob′yūl)(†)** Smaller divisions within the lobes of the liver.

**hepatic portal system (he-pat′ik pôr′tl sĭs′təm)(†)** The collection of veins carrying blood to the liver.

**hepatic portal vein (hĭ-păt′ĭk pôr′tl vān)** A blood vessel that carries blood from the other digestive organs to the **hepatic lobules.**

**hepatitis (hĕp′ə-tī′tĭss)** Inflammation of the liver usually caused by viruses or toxins.

**hepatocytes (hep′ă-tō-sītz)(†)** The cells within the lobules of the liver. Hepatocytes process nutrients in the blood and make bile.

**hernia (hûr′nē-ə)** The protrusion of an organ through the wall that usually contains it, such as a hiatal or inguinal hernia.

**herpes simplex (her′pēz sĭm′plĕks)(†)** A medical condition characterized by an eruption of one or more groups of vesicles on the lips or genitalia.

**herpes zoster (her′pēz zos′ter)(†)** A medical condition characterized by an eruption of a group of vesicles on one side of the body following a nerve root.

**hierarchy (hī′ə-rär′kē)** A term that pertains to Abraham Maslow's hierarchy of needs. This hierarchy states that human beings are motivated by unsatisfied needs and that certain lower needs must be satisfied before higher needs can be met.

**hilum (hī′lŭm)(†)** The indented side of a lymph node. The entrance of the renal sinus that contains the renal artery, renal vein, and ureter.

**HIPAA (Health Insurance Portability and Accountability Act) (hĭp′ə)** A set of regulations whose goals include the following: (1) improving the portability and continuity of health-care coverage in group and individual markets; (2) combating waste, fraud, and abuse in health-care insurance and health-care delivery; (3) promoting the use of a medical savings account; (4) improving access to long-term care services and coverage; and (5) simplifying the administration of health insurance.

**Holter monitor (hol′tər mŏn′ĭ-tər)** An electrocardiography device that includes a small portable cassette recorder worn around a patient's waist or on a shoulder strap to record the heart's electrical activity.

**homeopathic medicine (hō-mē-ō-păth′-ĭk mĕd′-ĭ-sĭn)** A system of medicine that uses remedies in an attempt to stimulate the body to recover itself.

**homeostasis (hō′mē-ō-stā′sĭs)** A balanced, stable state within the body.

**homologous chromosome (hō-mŏl′ō-gŭs krō′mə-sōm′)(†)** Members in each pair of chromosomes.

**hormone (hôr′mōn′)** A chemical secreted by a cell that affects the functions of other cells.

**hospice (hŏs′pĭs)** Volunteers who work with terminally ill patients and their families.

**human chorionic gonadotropin (HCG) (hyo͞o′mən kō-rē-on′ik gō′nad-ōtrō′pin)** A hormone secreted by cells of the embryo after implantation. It maintains the corpus luteum in the ovary so it will continue to secrete estrogen and progesterone.

**human immunodeficiency virus (HIV) (hyo͞o′mən im′yū-nō-dē-fish′en-sē vī′rəs)** A retrovirus that gradually destroys the body's immune system and causes AIDS.

**humerus (hyü′-mə-rəs)** The bone of the upper arm.

**humors (hyo͞o′mərz)** Fluids of the body.

**hydrotherapy (hī′drə-thĕr′ə-pē)** The therapeutic use of water to treat physical problems.

**hydrothorax** (hī' drō thôr' aks) Fluid collection in the pleural cavity causing collapse of the lung.

**hyoid** (hī'-òid) The bone that anchors the tongue.

**hyperextension** (hī'per-eks-ten'shŭn)(†) Extension of a body part past the normal anatomic position.

**hyperglycemia** (hī'pər-glī-sē'mē-ə) High blood sugar.

**hyperopia** (hī-per-ō'pē-ă) A condition that occurs when light entering the eye is focused behind the retina; commonly called farsightedness.

**hyperpnea** (hī-per-nē'ă)(†) Abnormally deep, rapid breathing.

**hyperpyrexia** (hy per py rex' e a) An exceptionally high fever.

**hyperreflexia** (hī'per-rē-flek'sē-ă) Reflexes that are stronger than normal reflexes.

**hypertension** (hī'pər-těn'shən) High blood pressure.

**hyperventilation** (hī'pər-věn'tl-ā'shən) The condition of breathing rapidly and deeply. Hyperventilating decreases the amount of carbon dioxide in the blood.

**hypnosis** (hīp-nō'-sĭs) A trance-like state usually induced by another person to access the subconscious mind and promote healing.

**hypodermis** (hī'pə-dûr'mĭs) The subcutaneous layer of the skin that is largely made of adipose tissue.

**hypoglycemia** (hī'pō-glī-sē'mē-ə) Low blood sugar.

**hyporeflexia** (hī'pō-rē-flek'sē-ă)(†) A condition of decreased reflexes.

**hypotension** (hī'pō-těn'shən) Low blood pressure.

**hypothalamus** (hī'pō-thăl'ə-məs) A region of the **diencephalon**. It maintains homeostasis by regulating many vital activities such as heart rate, blood pressure, and breathing rate.

**hypovolemic shock** (hī'per-vō-lē'mē-ă shŏk)(†) A state of shock resulting from insufficient blood volume in the circulatory system.

**hypoxia** (hī pôk' sē ə) Inadequate oxygenation of the cells of the body.

**hysterectomy** (hĭs'tə-rĕk'tə-mē) Surgical removal of the uterus.

**ICD-9** See *International Classification of Diseases, Ninth Revision, Clinical Modification.*

**icon** (ī'kŏn') A pictorial image; on a computer screen, a graphic symbol that identifies a menu choice.

**identification line** (ī-děn'tə-fĭ-kā'shən līn) A line at the bottom of a letter containing the letter writer's initials and the typist's initials.

**idiopathic** (ĭd-ē-ō-path'ik) A disease or condition of unknown cause.

**ileocecal sphincter** (ĭl'ē ō sē'kəl sfĭngk'ter) A structure that controls the movement of **chime** from the ileum to the **cecum.**

**ileum** (ĭl'ē-əm) The last portion of the small intestine. It is directly attached to the large intestine.

**ilium** (ĭ'-lē-əm) The most superior part of the hip bone. It is broad and flaring.

**immunity** (ĭ-myoōn'ĭ-tē) The condition of being resistant or not susceptible to pathogens and the diseases they cause.

**immunization** (ĭm'yū-nī-zā-shən) The administration of a vaccine or toxoid to protect susceptible individuals from communicable diseases.

**immunocompromised** (ĭm'yū-nōkom'pro-mīzd)(†) Having an impaired or weakened immune system.

**immunofluorescent antibody (IFFA) test** (ĭm'yū-nō-flūr-es'ent ăn'tĭ-bŏd-ē těst)(†) A blood test used to confirm enzyme-linked immunosorbent assay (ELISA) test results for HIV infection.

**immunoglobulins** (ĭm'yū-nō-glob'yū-linz)(†) A class of structurally related proteins that include IgG, IgA, IgM, and IgE; also called **antibodies.**

**impetigo** (ĭm'pĭ-tī'gō) A contagious skin infection usually caused by germs commonly called staph and strep.

**implied contract** (ĭm-plīd kŏn'trăct') A contract that is created by the acceptance or conduct of the parties rather than the written word.

**impotence** (ĭm'pŏ-tens)(†) A disorder in which a male cannot maintain an erect penis to complete sexual intercourse; also called erectile dysfunction.

**inactive file** (ĭn-ăk'tĭv fīl) A file used infrequently.

**incision** (ĭn-sĭzh'ən) A surgical wound made by cutting into body tissue.

**incisors** (ĭn-sī'zərz) The most medial teeth. They act as chisels to bite off food.

**incomplete proteins** (ĭn'kəm-plēt' prō'tēnz') Proteins that lack one or more of the essential amino acids.

**incontinence** (in-kon'ti-nens)(†) The involuntary leakage of urine.

**incus** (ĭng'kəs) A small bone in the middle ear, located between the malleus and the stapes; also called the anvil.

**indexing** (n'dēks' ing) The naming of a file.

**indexing rules** (n'dĕks' ing rōōls) Rules used as guidelines for the sequencing of files based on current business practice.

**indication** (ĭn'dĭ-kā'shən) The purpose or reason for using a drug, as approved by the FDA.

**individual identifiable health information (IIHI)** (in-duh-vij-oo-uh ahy-den-tuh-fahy-able hĕlth ĭn'fər-mā'shən) Any part of an individual's health information, including demographic information, collected from an individual that is received by a covered entity (e.g., a health-care provider).

**induration (in-də-´rā-shən)** The process of hardening or of becomming hard.

**infection (ĭn-fĕk´shən)** The presence of a pathogen in or on the body.

**infectious waste (ĭn-fĕk´shəs wāst)** Waste that can be dangerous to those who handle it or to the environment; includes human waste, human tissue, and body fluids as well as potentially hazardous waste, such as used needles, scalpels, and dressings, and cultures of human cells.

**inferior (ĭn-fîr´ē-ər)** Anatomic term meaning below or closer to the feet; also called caudal.

**inflammation (ĭn´flə-mā´shən)** The body's reaction when tissue becomes injured or infected. The four cardinal signs are redness, heat, pain, and swelling.

**inflammatory phase (in-flam'-a-tor-ee fāz)** The initial phase of wound healing in which bleeding is reduced as blood vessels in the affected area constrict.

**informed consent (ĭn-fôrmd´ kən-sĕnt)** The patient's right to receive all information relative to his or her condition and then make a decision regarding treatment based upon that knowledge.

**informed consent form (ĭn-fôrmd´ kən-sĕnt fôrm)** A form that verifies that a patient understands the offered treatment and its possible outcomes or side effects.

**infundibulum (in-fŭn-dib´yū-lŭm)(†)** The funnel-like end of the uterine tube near an ovary. It catches the secondary oocyte as it leaves the ovary.

**infusion (in-fyū´zhŭn)(†)** A slow drip, as of an intravenous solution into a vein.

**ink-jet printer (ĭngk´jĕt´ prĭn´tər)** A nonimpact printer that forms characters by using a series of dots created by tiny drops of ink.

**innate immunity (ĭn āt ĭmyoōn'ītē)** The body's mechanisms to protect itself against pathogens in general; also called nonspecific defenses.

**inner cell mass (ĭn´ər sĕl măs)** A group of cells in a blastocyte that gives rise to an embryo.

**inorganic (ĭn´ôr-găn´ĭk)** Matter that generally does not contain carbon and hydrogen.

**insertion (ĭn-sûr´shən)** An attachment site of a skeletal muscle that moves when a muscle contracts.

**inside address (ĭn-sĭd' ə-drĕs')** The name and address of the person to whom the letter is being sent. It appears on a business letter two to four spaces down from the date. It should be two, three, or four lines in length.

**inspection (ĭn-spĕk´shən)** The visual examination of the patient's entire body and overall appearance.

**inspiration (in-spə-rā´-shən)(†)** The act of breathing in; also called inhalation.

**instruction set (ĭn-strŭk'shən set)** Includes the groups of instructions from installed programming that a CPU can implement.

**insulin (ĭn´sə-lĭn)** A hormone that regulates the amount of sugar in the blood by facilitating its entry into the cells.

**integrative medicine (ĭn´-tĭ-grāt´-tĭv mĕd´-ĭ-sĭn)** The combination of components of conventional medicine with complementary and alternative medicine modalities.

**interactive pager (ĭn´tər-ăk´tĭv pāj´ər)** A pager designed for two-way communication. The pager screen displays a printed message and allows the physician to respond by way of a mini keyboard.

**interatrial septum (in´tər ā´trē əl səp´təm)** The wall separating the right and left atria from each other.

**intercalated disc (in-ter´kă-lā-ted disk)(†)** A disk that connects groups of cardiac muscles. This disc allows the fibers in that group to contract and relax together.

**interferon (in-ter-fēr´on)(†)** A protein that blocks viruses from infecting cells.

**interim room (ĭn´tər-ĭm roōm)** A room off the patient reception area and away from the examination rooms for occasions when patients require privacy.

***International Classification of Diseases, Ninth Revision, Clinical Modification* (ICD-9) (ĭn´tər-năsh´ə-nəl klăs´ə-fīkā´ shən dĭ-zēz´əz nīnth rĭ-vĭzh´ən klĭn´ĭ-kəl mŏd´ə-fī-kā´shən)** Code set that is based on a system maintained by the World Health Organization of the United Nations. The use of the ICD-9 codes in the health-care industry is mandated by **HIPAA** for reporting patients' diseases, conditions, and signs and symptoms.

**Internet (ĭn´tər-nĕt´)** A global network of computers.

**interneuron (in´ter-nū´ron)(†)** A structure found only in the central nervous system that functions to link sensory and motor neurons together.

**internist (ĭn-tûr´nĭst)** A doctor who specializes in diagnosing and treating problems related to the internal organs.

**interpersonal skills (ĭn´tər-pûr´sə-nəl skĭlz)** Attitudes, qualities, and abilities that influence the level of success and satisfaction achieved in interacting with other people.

**interphalangeal (intərfəlan´jeal)** Pertaining to the joints between the phalangeal bones.

**interphase (in´ter-fāz)(†)** The state of a cell carrying out its normal daily functions and not dividing.

**interstitial cell (in-ter-stish´ăl sĕl)** A cell located between the seminiferous tubules that is responsible for making testosterone.

**interstitial fluid (in-ter-stish´ăl flōō ĭd)** Fluid found between tissue cells that is absorbed by lymph capillaries to become lymph.

**interventricular septum (in´tər ventrik´yələr səp´təm)** The wall separating the right and left ventricles from each other.

**intestinal lipase (ĭn-tĕs´tĭ-n lip´ās)** An enzyme that digests fat.

**intradermal (ID) (in´tră-der´măl)** Within the upper layers of the skin.

**intradermal test (in´tră-der´măl tĕst)** An allergy test in which dilute solutions of allergens are introduced into the skin of the inner forearm or upper back with a fine-gauge needle.

**intramembranous (in-tra-me´m-brə-nəs)** A type of ossification in which bones begin as tough fibrous membranes.

**intramuscular (IM) (in´tră-mŭs´kyū-lăr)** Within muscle; an IM injection allows administration of a larger amount of a drug than a subcutaneous injection allows.

**intraoperative (in´tră-ŏp´ər-ə-tĭv)** Taking place during surgery.

**intravenous IV (in´trə-vē´nəs)** Injected directly into a vein.

**intravenous pyelography (IVP) (in´trə-vē´nəs pī´ĕ-log´ră-fē)(†)** A radiologic procedure in which the doctor injects a contrast medium into a vein and takes a series of x-rays of the kidneys, ureters, and bladder to evaluate urinary system abnormalities or trauma to the urinary system; also known as excretory urography.

**intrinsic factor (ĭn-trĭn´zĭk făk´tər)** A substance secreted by **parietal cells** in the lining of the stomach. It is necessary for vitamin B₁₂ absorption.

**invasive (ĭn-vā´sĭv)** Referring to a procedure in which a catheter, wire, or other foreign object is introduced into a blood vessel or organ through the skin or a body orifice. Surgical asepsis is required during all invasive tests.

**inventory (ĭn´vən-tôrē)** A list of supplies used regularly and the quantities in stock.

**inversion (ĭn-vûr´zhən)** Turning the sole of the foot medially.

**invoice (ĭn´vois´)** A bill for materials or services received by or services performed by the practice.

**ions (ī´ənz)** Positively or negatively charged particles.

**iris (ī´rĭs)** The colored part of the eye, made of muscular tissue that contracts and relaxes, altering the size of the pupil.

**ischium (is´-kē-əm)** A structure that forms the lower part of the hip bone.

**islets of Langerhans (ī´lĭt lan´ger-hans)** Structures in the pancreas that secrete insulin and glucagon into the bloodstream.

**itinerary (ī-tĭn´ə-rĕr´ē)** A detailed travel plan listing dates and times for specific transportation arrangements and events, the location of meetings and lodgings, and phone numbers.

**jaundice (jôn´dĭs)** A condition characterized by yellowness of the skin, eyes, mucous membranes, and excretions; occurs during the second stage of hepatitis infection.

**jejunum (jə-jōō´nəm)** The midportion and the majority of the small intestine.

**journalizing (jûr´nə-līz´ĭng)** The process of logging charges and receipts in a chronological list each day; used in the single-entry system of bookkeeping.

**juxtaglomerular apparatus (jŭks´tă-glŏmer´yū-lăr ăp´ə-răt´əs)(†)** A structure contained in the nephron and made up of the macula densa and **juxtaglomerular cells.**

**juxtaglomerular cells (jŭks´tă-glŏmer´yū-lăr sĕlz)** Enlarged smooth muscle cells in the walls of either the afferent or efferent arterioles.

**Kaposi's sarcoma (kap´ō-sēz sar-kō´mă)** Abnormal tissue occurring in the skin, and sometimes in the lymph nodes and organs, manifested by reddish-purple to dark blue patches or spots on the skin.

**keratin (kĕr´ə-tĭn)** A tough, hard protein contained in skin, hair, and nails.

**keratinocyte (kĕ-rat´i-nō-sīt)(†)** The most common cell type in the epidermis of the skin.

**key (kē)** The act of inputting or entering information into a computer.

**KOH mount (kā´ō-ăch mount)** A type of mount used when a physician suspects a patient has a fungal infection of the skin, nails, or hair and to which potassium hydroxide is added to dissolve the keratin in cell walls.

**Krebs cycle (krēbz sī´kəl)** Also called the citric acid cycle. This cycle generates ATP for muscle cells.

**KUB radiography (kā´yōō-bē rā´dēog´ră-fē)(†)** The process of x-raying the abdomen to help assess the size, shape, and position of the urinary organs; evaluate urinary system diseases or disorders; or determine the presence of kidney stones. It can also be helpful in determining the position of an intrauterine device (IUD) or in locating foreign bodies in the digestive tract; also called a flat plate of the abdomen.

**kyphosis (kī-fō´sis)** A deformity of the spine characterized by a bent-over position; more commonly called humpback.

**labeling (lā´bəl-ĭng)** Information provided with a drug, including FDA-approved indications and the form of the drug.

**labia majora (lā´bē-ă mă´jôr-ă)** The rounded folds of adipose tissue and skin that serve to protect the other female reproductive organs.

**labia minora (lā´bē-ă mĭ´nôr-ă)** The folds of skin between the labia majora.

**labyrinth (lăb´ə-rĭnth´)** The inner ear.

**laceration (lăs´ə-rā´shən)** A jagged, open wound in the skin that can extend down into the underlying tissue.

**lacrimal apparatus (lăk´rə-məl ăp´ə-răt´əs)** A structure that consists of the lacrimal glands and nasolacrimal ducts.

**lacrimal gland (lăk´rə-məl glănd)** A gland in the eye that produces tears.

**lactase (lăk´tās)(†)** An enzyme that digests sugars.

**lactic acid (lăk´tĭk ăs´ĭd)** A waste product that must be released from the cell. It is produced when a cell is low on oxygen and converts pyruvic acid.

**lactiferous (lak-tif´ə rus)** Pertaining to producing milk.

**lactogen (lak´tō-jen)** Substance secreted by the placenta that stimulates the enlargement of the mammary glands.

**lacunae (1-kü-na)** Holes in the matrix of bone that hold osteocytes.

**lamella (lə-me´-lə)** Layers of bone surrounding the canals of osteons.

**LAN (lăn)** Abbreviation for Local Area Network.

**lancet (lăn´sĭt)** A small, disposable instrument with a sharp point used to puncture the skin and make a shallow incision; used for capillary puncture.

**laryngopharynx (lă-ring´gō-far-ingks) (†)** The portion of the pharynx behind the **larynx.**

**larynx (lăr´ĭngks)** The part of the respiratory tract between the pharynx and the trachea that is responsible for voice production; also called the voice box.

**laser printer (lā´zər prĭn´tər)** A high-resolution printer that uses a technology similar to that of a photocopier. It is the fastest type of computer printer and produces the highest-quality output.

**lateral (lăt´ər-əl)** A directional term that means farther away from the midline of the body.

**lateral file (lăt´ər-əl fīl)** A horizontal filing cabinet that features doors that flip up and a pull-ut drawer, where files are arranged with sides facing out.

**law (lô)** A rule of conduct established and enforced by an authority or governing body, such as the federal government.

**law of agency (lô ā´jən-sē)** A law stating that an employee is considered to be acting on the physician's behalf while performing professional duties.

**lead (lēd)** A view of a specific area of the heart on an electrocardiogram.

**lease (lēs))** To rent an item or piece of equipment.

**legal custody (lēgəl kŭs´tə-dē)** The court-decreed right to have control over a child's upbringing and to take responsibility for the child's care, including health care.

**lens (lēnz)** A clear, circular disc located in the eye, just posterior to the iris, that can change shape to help the eye focus images of objects that are near or far away.

**letterhead (lĕt´ər-hĕd´)** Formal business stationery, with the doctor's (or office's) name and address printed at the top, used for correspondence with patients, colleagues, and vendors.

**leukemia (lōō-kē´mē-ə)** A medical condition in which bone marrow produces a large number of white blood cells that are not normal.

**leukocyte (lōō-kə-sīt)** White blood cells.

**leukocytosis (lū´kō-sī-tō´sis)(†)** A white blood cell count that is above normal.

**leukopenia (lū´kō-pē´nē-ă)(†)** A white blood cell count that is below normal.

**liability insurance (lī´ə-bĭl´ĭ-tē ĭn-shōōr´əns)** A type of insurance that covers injuries caused by the insured or injuries that occurred on the insured's property.

**liable (lī´ə-bəl)** Legally responsible.

**libel (lī´bəl)** A false publication, as in writing, print, signs, or pictures, that damages a person's reputation.

**lifetime maximum benefit (līf´tīm´ măk´sə-məm bĕn´ə-fĭt)** The total sum that a health plan will pay out over the patient's life.

**ligament (lĭg´ə-mənt)** A tough, fibrous band of tissue that connects bone to bone.

**ligature (lĭg´ə-chōōr´)** Suture material.

**limbus (lĭm bŭs)** The corneal-scleral junction, which is the area where the sclera (the white of the eye) gives way to the clear covering of the iris (cornea).

**limited check (lĭm´ĭ-tĭd chĕk)** A check that is void after a certain time limit; commonly used for payroll.

**lingual frenulum (ling´gwăl fren´yūlŭm)(†)** A flap of mucosa that holds the body of the tongue to the floor of the oral cavity.

**lingual tonsils (ling´gwăl ton´silz)(†)** Two lumps of lymphatic tissue on the back of the tongue that act to destroy bacteria and viruses.

**linoleic acid (lin-ō-lē´ik as´id)(†)** An essential fatty acid found in corn and sunflower oils.

**lipoproteins (lip-ō-prō´tēnz)** Large molecules that are fat-soluble on the inside and water-soluble on the outside and carry lipids such as cholesterol and triglycerides through the bloodstream.

**living will (lĭv´ĭng wĭl)** A legal document addressed to a patient's family and health-care providers stating what type of treatment the patient wishes or does not wish to receive if he becomes terminally ill, unconscious, or permanently comatose; sometimes called an advance directive.

**lobe (lōb)**   The frontal, parietal, temporal, or occipital regions of the cerebral hemisphere.

**locum tenens (lō´kum těn´ens)(†)**   A substitute physician hired to see patients while the regular physician is away from the office.

**loop of Henle (lōōp hen´lē)**   The portion of the renal tubule that curves back toward the renal corpuscle and twists again to become the distal convoluted tubule.

**lubricant (loo-bri-*kuh* nt)**   A water-soluble gel used during examination of the rectum or vaginal cavity.

**lumbar enlargement (lŭm´bər ěnlärj´mənt)**   The thickening of the spinal cord in the low back region.

**lunula (lū´nū-lă)**   The white half-moon–shaped area at the base of a nail.

**luteinizing hormone (LH) (lū´tē-in-izing hôr´mōn´)(†)**   Hormone that in females stimulates ovulation and the production of estrogen; in males, it stimulates the production of testosterone.

**lymphedema (limf´e-dē´mă)**   The blockage of lymphatic vessels that results in the swelling of tissue from the accumulation of lymphatic fluid.

**lymphocyte (lĭm´fō-sīt)(†)**   An agranular leukocyte formed in lymphatic tissue. Lymphocytes are generally small. See **T lymphocyte** and **B lymphocyte**.

**lymphokines (lĭmf´ō kĭnz)**   A type of cytokine secreted by T cells that increases T-cell production and directly kill cells with antigens.

**lysosomes (lī´səsōmz)**   Structures that are known to perform the digestive function of the cells.

**lysozyme (lī´sō-zīm)(†)**   An enzyme in tears that destroys pathogens on the surface of the eye.

**macrophage (măk´rə-făj´)**   A type of phagocytic cell found in the liver, spleen, lungs, bone marrow, and connective tissue. Macrophages play several roles in humoral and cell-mediated immunity, including presenting the antigens to the lymphocytes involved in these defenses; also known as monocytes while in the bloodstream.

**macula densa (mak´yū-lă den´sa)(†)**   An area of the distal convoluted tubule that touches afferent and efferent arterioles.

**macular degeneration (mak´yū-lăr dējen-er-ā´shŭn)(†)**   A progressive disease that usually affects people older-than the age of 50. It occurs when the retina no longer receives an adequate blood supply.

**magnetic resonance imaging (MRI) (măgnět´ĭk rěz´ə-nəns ĭ-măj´ing)**   A viewing technique that uses a powerful magnetic field to produce an image of internal body structures.

**magnetic therapy (măg-nět´-ĭk thěr´-ə-pē)**   A type of therapy in which magnets are placed on the body to penetrate and correct the body's energy fields.

**maintenance contract (mān´tə-nəns kŏn´trăkt´)**   A contract that specifies when a piece of equipment will be cleaned, checked for worn parts, and repaired.

**major histocompatibility complex (MHC) (mā´jər his´tō-kom-pat-ĭ-bil´i-tē kəm-plěks)**   A large protein complex that plays a role in T-cell activation.

**malignant (mə-lĭg´nənt)**   A type of tumor or neoplasm that is invasive and destructive and that tends to metastasize; it is commonly known as cancerous.

**malleus (măl´ē-əs)**   A small bone in the middle ear that is attached to the eardrum; also called the hammer.

**malpractice claim (măl-prăk´tĭs klām)**   A lawsuit brought by a patient against a physician for errors in diagnosis or treatment.

**maltase (mawl-tās)**   An enzyme that digests sugars.

**mammary glands (mam´ă-rē glăndz)**   Accessory organs of the female reproductive system that secrete milk after pregnancy.

**mammography (mă-mŏg´rə-fē)**   X-ray examination of the breasts.

**managed care organization (MCO) (măn´ĭjd kâr ôr´gə-nĭ-zā´shən)**   A health-care business that, through mergers and buyouts, can deliver health care more cost-effectively.

**mandible (man´-də-bəl)**   A bone that forms the lower portion of the jaw.

**manipulation (mə-nĭp´yə-la´shən)**   The systematic movement of a patient's body parts.

**margin (mahr-jin)**   The space or measurement around the edges of a form or letter that is left blank.

**marrow (mer´-ō)**   A substance that is contained in the medullary cavity. In adults, it consists primarily of fat.

**massage (mə-sāzh)**   The use of pressure, kneading, stroking, and the human touch to alleviate pain and promote healing through relaxation.

**massage therapist (mə-säzh´thěr´ə-pĭst)**   An individual who is trained to use pressure, kneading, and stroking to promote muscle and full-body relaxation.

**mastoid process (mas´-to´id pr´ä-ses)**   A large bump on each temporal bone just behind each ear. It resembles a nipple, hence the name mastoid.

**Material Safety Data Sheet (MSDS) (mə-tîr´e-əl sāf´tē dā´tə shēt)**   A form that is required for all hazardous chemicals or other substances used in the laboratory and that contains information about the product's name, ingredients, chemical characteristics, physical and health hazards, guidelines for safe handling, and procedures to be followed in the event of exposure.

**matrix (mā′trĭks)** The basic format of an appointment book, established by blocking off times on the schedule during which the doctor is able to see patients. The material between the cells of connective tissue.

**matter (măt′er)** Anything that takes up space and has weight. Liquids, solids, and gases are matter.

**maturation phase (măch′ə-rā′shən fāz)** The third phase of wound healing, in which scar tissue forms.

**maxillae (mak-si′-lə)** A bone that forms the upper portion of the jaw.

**Mayo stand (mā′ō stănd)** A movable stainless steel instrument tray on a stand.

**medial (mē′dē-əl)** A directional term that describes areas closer to the midline of the body.

**Medicaid (mĕd′ĭ-kād′)** A federally funded health cost assistance program for low-income, blind, and disabled patients; families receiving aid to dependent children; foster children; and children with birth defects.

**medical asepsis (mĕd′ĭ-kəl ə-sĕp′sĭs)** Measures taken to reduce the number of microorganisms, such as hand washing and wearing examination gloves, that do not necessarily eliminate microorganisms; also called clean technique.

**medical practice act (mĕd′ĭ-kəl prăk′tĭs ăkt)** A law that defines the exact duties that physicians and other health-care personnel may perform.

**Medicare (mĕd′ĭ-kâr′)** A national health insurance program for Americans aged 65 and older.

**Medicare + Choice Plan (mĕd′ĭ-kâr′ chois plăn)** Medicare benefit in which beneficiaries can choose to enroll in one of three major types of plans instead of the **Original Medicare Plan.**

**Medigap (mĕd′ĭ-găp′)** Private insurance that Medicare recipients can purchase to reduce the gap in coverage—the amount they would have to pay from their own pockets after receiving Medicare benefits.

**meditation (mĕd′-ĭ-tā-shən)** A state in which the body is consciously relaxed and the mind becomes calm and focused.

**medullary cavity (me′-de-ler-ē ka′-və-tē)** The canal that runs through the center of the **diaphysis.**

**megakaryocytes (meg-ă-kar′ē-ō-sīts)(†)** Cells within red blood marrow that give rise to platelets.

**meiosis (mī-ō′sis)(†)** A type of cell division in which each new cell contains only one member of each chromosome pair.

**melanin (mĕl′ə-nĭn)** A pigment that is deposited throughout the layers of the epidermis.

**melanocyte (mĕl′ă-nō-sīt)(†)** A cell type within the epidermis that makes the pigment **melanin.**

**melanocyte-stimulating hormone (MSH) (məl′ən ō sīt stim′ yū lāting hôr mōn′)** A hormone released from the anterior pituitary to stimulate melanin production in the skin's epidermal cells.

**melatonin (mĕl′ə-tō′nĭn)** A hormone that helps to regulate circadian rhythms.

**membrane potential (mĕm′brān′ pə-tĕn′shəl)** The potential inside a cell relative to the fluid outside the cell.

**menarche (me-nar′ke)** The first menstrual period.

**Meniere's disease (Mən′erz dĭzēz)** An inner ear disease characterized by attacks of vertigo, tinnitus, and nausea. Permanent hearing loss may result.

**meninges (mĕ-nin′jēz)(†)** Membranes that protect the brain and spinal cord.

**meningitis (mĕn′ĭn-jī′tĭs)** An inflammation of the **meninges.**

**meniscus (mə-nĭs′kəs)** The curve in the air-to-liquid surface of a liquid specimen in a container.

**menopause (mĕn′ə-pôz′)** The termination of the menstrual cycle due to the normal aging of the ovaries.

**menses (mĕn′sēz)** The clinical term for menstrual flow.

**menstrual cycle (mĕn′strōō-əl sī′kəl)** The female reproductive cycle. It consists of regular changes in the uterine lining that lead to monthly bleeding.

**mensuration (mĕn′sə-rā′-shən)** The process of measuring.

**meridian (mə-rĭd′-ē-ən)** Pathways of energetic flow that are distributed symmetrically throughout the body. These pathways are used in acupuncture, traditional Chinese medicine, and Ayurveda.

**mesentery (me′sen′tərē)** The fan-like tissue that attaches the jejunum and ileum to the posterior abdominal wall.

**mesoderm (mez′ō-derm)(†)** The primary germ layer that gives rise to connective tissue and some epithelial tissue.

**metabolism (mĭ-tăb′ə-lĭz′əm)** The overall chemical functioning of the body, including all body processes that build small molecules into large ones (anabolism) and break down large molecules into small ones (catabolism).

**metacarpals (me-tə-k′är-pəl)** The bones that form the palms of the hand.

**metacarpophalangeal (met′əkar′ pōfəlan′jēəl)** Pertaining to the joints that join the phalanges to the metacarpals.

**metaphase (met´əfāz)** Period of mitosis when the chromosomes line up on the spindle fibers created by the centrioles during prophase.

**metastasis (mə-tăs´tə-sĭs)** The transfer of abnormal cells to body sites far removed from the original tumor; the spread of tumor cells.

**metatarsals (mĕt´ə-tär´salz)** The bones that form the front of the foot.

**metatarsophalangeal (met´ətar´sōfəlan´jēəl)** Pertaining to the joints that join the phalanges to the metatarsals.

**microbiology (mī´krō-bī-ŏl´ə-jē)** The study of microorganisms.

**microfiche (mī´krō-fēsh´)** Microfilm in rectangular sheets.

**microfilm (mī´krə-fĭlm´)** A roll of film stored on a reel and imprinted with information on a reduced scale to minimize storage space requirements.

**microglia (mī-krŏg´lēa)** Small cells within the nervous system that act as phagocytes, watching for and engulfing invaders.

**microorganism (mī´krō-ôr´gə-nĭz´əm)** A simple form of life, commonly made up of a single cell and so small that it can be seen only with a microscope.

**micropipette (mī´krō-pĭ-pet´)** A small pipette that holds a small, precise volume of fluid; used to collect capillary blood.

**microvilli (mī´krō-vil´-ī)(†)** Structures found in the lining of the small intestine. They greatly increase the surface area of the small intestine so it can absorb many nutrients.

**micturition (mik-chū-rish´ŭn)(†)** The process of urination.

**middle digit (´mi-dəl ´di-jət)** A small group of two to three numbers in the middle of a patient

number that is used as an identifying unit in a filing system.

**midsagittal (mid´saj´i-tǎl)(†)** Anatomical term that refers to the plane that runs lengthwise down the midline of the body, dividing it into equal left and right halves.

**minerals (mĭn´ər-əlz)** Natural, inorganic substances the body needs to help build and maintain body tissues and carry on life functions.

**minors (mī-nərs)** Anyone under the age of majority—18 in most states, 21 in some jurisdictions.

**minutes (mi-nətz´)** A report of what happened and what was discussed and decided at a meeting.

**mirroring (mĭr´ər-ĭng)** Restating in your own words what a person is saying.

**misdemeanor (mĭs´dĭ-mē´nər)** A less serious crime such as theft under a certain dollar amount or disturbing the peace. A misdemeanor is punishable by fines or imprisonment.

**mitochondria (mīto´kon´drēə)** Structures that provide energy for cells and are the respiratory centers for the cell.

**mitosis (mī-tō´sĭs)** A type of cell division that produces ordinary body, or somatic, cells; each new cell receives a complete set of paired chromosomes.

**mitral valve (mī´trəl vălv)(†)** See **bicuspid valve.**

**mobility aid (mō´bəl-ə-tē ād)** Device that improve one's ability to move from one place to another; also called mobility assistive device.

**modeling (mŏd´l-ĭng)** The process of teaching the patient a new skill by having the patient observe and imitate it.

**modem (mō´dəm)** A device used to transfer information from one computer to another through telephone lines.

**modified-block letter style (mŏd´ə-fīd blŏk lĕt´ər stīl)** A letter

format similar to full-block style, except that the dateline, complimentary closing, signature block, and notations are aligned and begin at the center of the page or slightly to the right of center.

**modified-wave schedule (mŏd´ə-fīd wāv skĕj´ool)** A scheduling system similar to the wave system, with patients arriving at planned intervals during the hour, allowing time to catch up before the next hour begins.

**modifier (mŏd´ə-fī´ər)** One or more two-digit codes assigned to the five-digit main code to show that some special circumstance applied to the service or procedure that the physician performed.

**molars (mō´lərz)** Back teeth that are flat and are designed to grind food.

**mold (mōld)** Fungi that grow into large, fuzzy, multicelled organisms that produce spores.

**molecule (mŏl´ĭ-kyool´)** The smallest unit into which an element can be divided and still retain its properties; it is formed when atoms bond together.

**money order (mŭn´ē ôr´dər)** A certificate of guaranteed payment, which may be purchased from a bank, a post office, or some convenience stores.

**monocyte (mon´-o-s-īt)(†)** A type of phagocyte that is formed in bone marrow and circulates throughout the blood for a very short period of time. It then migrates to specific tissues and is called a macrophage.

**monokines (mon´ō kīnz)** A type of cytokine secreted by lymphocytes and macrophages that assists in regulating the immune response by increasing B-cell production and stimulating red bone marrow to produce more white blood cells.

**mononucleosis (mon´ō noo klē ō´sis)** A highly contagious viral infection caused by the Epstein-Barr virus (EBV).

**monosaccharide (mon-ō-sakʹă-rīd)(†)** A type of carbohydrate that is a simple sugar.

**mons pubis (mʹänz pyʹü-bəs)** A fatty area that overlies the public bone.

**moral values (môrʹəl vălʹyōoz)** Values or types of behavior that serve as a basis for ethical conduct and are formed through the influence of the family, culture, or society.

**mordant (môrʹdnt)** A substance, such as iodine, that can intensify or deepen the response a specimen has to a stain.

**morphology (môr-fŏlʹə-jē)** The study of the shape or form of objects.

**morula (mōrʹū-lă)(†)** A zygote that has undergone cleavage and results in a ball of cells.

**motherboard (mŭthʹər-bôrdʹ)** The main circuit board of a computer that controls the other components in the system.

**motility (mōʹti li tē)** To be capable of movement.

**motor (mōʹtər)** Efferent neurons that carry information from the central nervous system to the effectors.

**mouse (mous)** A pointing device that can be added to a computer that directs activity on the computer screen by positioning a pointer or cursor on the screen. It can be directly attached to the computer or can be wireless.

**moxibustion (mŏk-ĭ-bŭsʹ-chən)** The application of heat at the points where the needles are inserted during acupuncture.

**mucocutaneous exposure (myü-kō-kyüʹ-tā-nē-əs ik-spōʹ-zhər)** Exposure to a pathogen through mucous membranes.

**mucosa (myōo-kōʹsə)** The innermost layer of the wall of the alimentary canal.

**mucous cells (myōoʹ-kəs sĕlz)** Cells that are found in the salivary glands and the lining of the stomach and that secrete mucous.

**MUGA scan (mŭgʹə skăn)** A radiologic procedure that evaluates the condition of the heart's myocardium; it involves injection of radioisotopes that concentrate in the myocardium, followed by the use of a gamma camera to measure ventricular contractions to evaluate the patient's heart wall.

**multimedia (mŭlʹtē-mēʹdē-ə)** More than one medium, such as in graphics, sound, and text used to convey information.

**multitasking (mŭlʹtē-tăsʹkĭng)** Running two or more computer software programs simultaneously.

**multi-unit smooth muscle (mŭlʹtə-yōoʹnĭt smōoth mŭsʹəl)** A type of smooth muscle that is found in the iris of the eye and in the walls of blood vessels.

**murmur (mûrʹmər)** An abnormal heart sound heard when the ventricles contract and blood leaks back into the atria.

**muscle fatigue (mŭsʹəl fa-tēgʹ)** A condition caused by a buildup of lactic acid.

**muscle fiber (mŭsʹəl fīʹbər)** Muscle cells that are called fibers because of their long lengths.

**muscle tissue (mŭsʹəl tĭshʹōo)** A tissue type that is specialized to shorten and elongate.

**muscular dystrophy (mŭsʹkyə-lər disʹtrō-fē)(†)** A group of inherited disorders characterized by a loss of muscle tissue and by muscle weakness.

**mutation (myōo-taʹshən)** An error that sometimes occurs when DNA is duplicated. When it occurs, it is passed to descendent cells and may or may not affect them in harmful ways.

**myasthenia gravis (mī-as-thēʹnē-ă gravʹis)** An autoimmune disorder that is characterized by muscle weakness.

**myelin (mīʹə-lĭn)** A fatty substance that insulates the axon and allows it to send nerve impulses quickly.

**myelography (mīʹě-logʹră-fē)** An x-ray visualization of the spinal cord after the injection of a radioactive contrast medium or air into the spinal subarachnoid space (between the second and innermost of three membranes that cover the spinal cord). This test can reveal tumors, cysts, spinal stenosis, or herniated disks.

**myocardial infarction (mīʹō-kärʹ dē-ăl ĭn-farkʹshən)** A heart attack that occurs when the blood flow to the heart is reduced as a result of blockage in the coronary arteries or their branches.

**myocardium (mīʹō-kärʹdē-əm)** The middle and thickest layer of the heart. It is made primarily of cardiac muscle.

**myocytes (mīō sīts)** Muscle cells; also called muscle fibers.

**myofibrils (mī-ō-fīʹbrils)(†)** Long structures that fill the sarcoplasm of a muscle fiber.

**myoglobin (mī-ō-glōʹbin)(†)** A pigment contained in muscle cells that stores extra oxygen.

**myoglobinuria (mīʹō-glō-bi-nūrē-ă)** The presence of myoglobin in the urine; can be caused by injured or damaged muscle tissue.

**myometrium (mīʹō-mēʹtrē-ŭm)(†)** The middle, thick muscular layer of the uterus.

**myopia (mī-ōʹpē-ə)** A condition that occurs when light entering the eye is focused in front of the retina; commonly called nearsightedness.

**myxedema (mik-se-dēʹmă)(†)** A severe type of hypothyroidism that is most common in women older than the age of 50.

**nail bed (nāl bĕd)** The layer beneath each nail.

**narcotic (när-kŏtʹĭk)** A popular term for an opioid and term of choice in government agencies; see **opioid**.

**nares (nerʹēz)** The openings of the nose or nostrils.

**nasal** (nāʹzəl) Relating to the nose. The nasal bones fuse to form the bridge of the nose.

**nasal conchae** (nāʹzəl konʹkē)(†) Structures that extend from the lateral walls of the nasal cavity.

**nasal mucosa** (nāʹzəl myoo-kōʹsə) The lining of the nose.

**nasal septum** (nāʹzəl sĕpʹtəm) A structure that divides the nasal cavity into a left and right portion.

**nasolacrimal duct** (nā-zō-lăkʹrə-məl dŭkt) A structure located on the medial aspect of each eyeball. These ducts drain tears into the nose.

**nasopharynx** (nāʹzō-farʹingks)(†) The portion of the pharynx behind the nasal cavity.

**National Center for Complementary and Alternative Medicine (NCCAM)** (năshʹə-nəl sĕnʹtər for kŏmʹ -plə-mĕn-tə-rē and ôl-tûrʹ-nə-tĭv mĕdʹ-ĭ-sĭn) National organization that conducts and supports CAM research and provides CAM information to healthcare providers and the public.

**natural killer (NK) cells** (năchʹər-el kĭlʹər selz) Non-B and non-T lymphocytes. NK cells kill cancer cells and virus-infected cells without previous exposure to the antigen.

**naturopathic medicine** (nă-chə-rŏpʹ-ə-ĭk mĕdʹ-ĭ-sĭn) A system of medicine that relies on the healing power of the body and supports that power through various healthcare practices, such as nutritional counseling, lifestyle counseling, and exercise.

**needle biopsy** (nēdʹl bīʹŏpʹsē) A procedure in which a needle and syringe are used to aspirate (withdraw by suction) fluid or tissue cells.

**negligence** (nĕgʹlĭ-jəns) A medical professional's failure to perform an essential action or performance of an improper action that directly results in the harm of a patient.

**negotiable** (nĭ-gōʹshē-ə-bəl) Legally transferable from one person to another.

**neonatal period** (nē-ō-nāʹtăl pîrʹē-əd)(†) The first 4 weeks of the postnatal period of an offspring.

**neonate** (nēʹə-nātʹ) An infant during the first 4 weeks of life.

**nephrologist** (ne-frolʹō-jĭst)(†) A specialist who studies, diagnoses, and manages diseases of the kidney.

**nephrons** (nefʹronz)(†) Microscopic structures in the kidneys that filter blood and form urine.

**nerve fiber** (nûrv fīʹbər) A structure that extends from the cell body. It consists of two types: axons and dendrites.

**nerve impulse** (nûrv ĭmʹpŭlsʹ) Electrochemical messages transmitted from neurons to other neurons and effectors.

**nervous tissue** (nûrʹvəs tĭshʹoo) A tissue type located in the brain, spinal cord, and peripheral nerves.

**net earnings** (nĕt ûrʹnĭngz) Take-home pay, calculated by subtracting total deductions from gross earnings.

**network** (nĕtʹwûrkʹ) A system that links several computers together.

**networking** (nĕtʹwûrkʹĭng) Making contacts with relatives, friends, and acquaintances that may have information about how to find a job in your field.

**neuralgia** (noo-rălʹjə) A medical condition characterized by severe pain along the distribution of a nerve.

**neuroglia** (nûr-ŏgʹlēə) Structures that function as support cells for other neurons, including astrocytes, microglia, and oligodendrocytes. See also **neuroglial cells.**

**neuroglial cell** (nū-rogʹlē-ăl sĕl)(†) Non-neuronal type of nervous tissue that is smaller and more abundant than neurons. Neuroglial cells support neurons.

**neurologist** (noo-rəlʹə-jēst) A specialist who diagnoses and treats disorders and diseases of the nervous system, including the brain, spinal cord, and nerves.

**neuron** (noorʹŏnʹ) A nerve cell; it carries nerve impulses between the brain or spinal cord and other parts of the body.

**neurotransmitter** (noorʹō-trănsʹmĭt-ər) A chemical within the vesicles of the synaptic knob that is released into the postsynaptic structures when a nerve impulse reaches the synaptic knob.

**neutrophil** (nūʹtrō-fil)(†) A type of granular leukocyte that aids in phagocytosis by attacking bacterial invaders; also responsible for the release of pyrogens.

**new patient** (noo pāʹshənt) Patient that, for CPT reporting purposes, has not received professional services from the physician within the past 3 years.

**nocturia** (nok-tūʹrē-ă)(†) Excessive nighttime urination.

**noncompliant** (nŏnʹkəm-plīʹent) The term used to describe a patient who does not follow the medical advice given.

**noninvasive** (non-in-vāʹsiv)(†) Referring to procedures that do not require inserting devices, breaking the skin, or monitoring to the degree needed with invasive procedures.

**nonsteroidal hormone** (non-stērʹoyd-al hôrʹmōnʹ)(†) A type of hormone made of amino acids and proteins.

**norepinephrine** (nōrʹep-i-nefʹrin)(†) A neurotransmitter released by sympathetic neurons onto organs and glands for fight-or-flight (stressful) situations.

**no-show** (nō shō) A patient who does not call to cancel and does not come to an appointment.

**nosocomial infection** (nos-ō-kōʹmē-ăl in-fĕk-shən) An infection contracted in a hospital.

**notations** (nō-tā′shən)   Information found at the end of a business letter indicating enclosures included with the letter and the names of other people who will be receiving copies of the letter.

**Notice of Privacy Practices (NPP)** (nō′tĭs prī′və-sē prăk′tis-əs)   A document that informs patients of their rights as outlined under **HIPAA**.

**nuclear medicine** (nōō′klē-ər mĕd′ĭ-sĭn)   The use of radionuclides, or radioisotopes (radioactive elements or their compounds), to evaluate the bone, brain, lungs, kidneys, liver, pancreas, thyroid, and spleen; also known as radionuclide imaging.

**nucleases** (nū′klē-ās-ez)   Pancreatic enzymes that digest nucleic acids.

**nucleus** (nōō′klē-əs)(†)   The control center of a cell; contains the chromosomes that direct cellular processes.

**numeric filing system** (nōō-mĕr′ĭk fĭl′ĭng sĭs′təm)   A filing system that organizes files by numbers instead of names. Each patient is assigned a number in the order in which she joins the practice.

**nystagmus** (nis-tag′mŭs)   Rapid involuntary eye movements that may be the result of drug or alcohol use, brain injury or lesion, or cerebrovascular accident (CVA).

**O&P specimen** (ō ənd pē spĕs′ə-mən)   An ova and parasites specimen, or a stool sample, that is examined for the presence of certain forms of protozoans or parasites, including their eggs (ova).

**objective** (əb-jĕk′tĭv)   Pertaining to data that is readily apparent and measurable, such as vital signs, test results, or physical examination findings.

**objectives** (ob-jek′tĭvs)   The set of magnifying lenses contained in the nosepiece of a compound microscope.

**occipital** (ŏk-sĭp′ĭ-tl)   Relating to the back of the head. The occipital bone forms the back of the skull.

**occult blood** (ə-kŭlt blŭd)   Blood contained in some other substance, not visible to the naked eye.

**ocular** (ŏk′yə-lər)   An eyepiece of a microscope.

**oil-immersion objective** (oil ĭ-mûr′zhənəb-jĕk′tĭv)   A microscope objective that is designed to be lowered into a drop of immersion oil placed directly above the prepared specimen under examination, eliminating the air space between the microscope slide and the objective and producing a much sharper, brighter image.

**ointment** (oint′mənt)   A form of topical drug; also known as a salve.

**Older Americans Act of 1965** (ōl′dər ə-mĕr′ĭ-kəns ăkt)   A U.S. law that guarantees certain benefits to elderly citizens, including health care, retirement income, and protection against abuse.

**olfactory** (ŏl-făk′tə-rē)   Relating to the sense of smell.

**oligodendrocytes** (ōl′igōden′drəsit)   Specialized neuroglial cells that assist in the production of the myelin sheath.

**oliguria** (ol′i-gu′re-ah)   Insufficient production (or volume) of urine.

**oncologist** (ŏn-kŏl′ə-jĭst)   A specialist who identifies tumors and treats patients who have cancer.

**onychectomy** (ŏn-i-kek′tō-mē)   The removal of a fingernail or toenail.

**oocyte** (ō′ō-sīt)(†)   The immature egg.

**oogenesis** (ō-ō-jen′ĕ-sis)(†)   The process of egg cell formation.

**open-book account** (ō′pən bŏōk ə-kount′)   An account that is open to charges made occasionally as needed.

**open-hours scheduling** (ō′pən ourz skĕj′ōōl-ĭng)   A system of scheduling in which patients arrive at the doctor's office at their convenience and are seen on a first-come, first-served basis.

**open posture** (ōpən pŏs′chər)   A position that conveys a feeling of receptiveness and friendliness; facing another person with arms comfortably at the sides or in the lap.

**ophthalmologist** (ŏf-thəl-mŏl′ə-jĭst)   A medical doctor who is an eye specialist.

**ophthalmoscope** (of-thal′mōskōp)(†)   A hand-held instrument with a light; used to view inner eye structures.

**opioid** (ō′-pē-oid)   A natural or synthetic drug that produces opium-like effects.

**opportunistic infection** (ŏp′ər-tōōn ĭs′tĭk ĭn-fĕk-shən)   Infection by microorganisms that can cause disease only when a host's resistance is low.

**optical character reader (OCR)** (ŏp′tĭ-kəl kār′ək-tər-rek-tər rēdər)   An electronic scanner that can "read" typed letters.

**optical character recognition (OCR)** (ōp′tĭ-kəl kār′ək-tər rek-uh g-nish-uh n)   The process or technology of reading data in printed form by a device that scans and identifies characters.

**optical microscope** (op′ti-kăl mī′krə-skōp′)   A microscope that uses light, concentrated through a condenser and focused through the object being examined, to project an image.

**optic chiasm** (ŏp′tĭk kī′azm)(†)   A structure located at the base of the brain where parts of the optic nerves cross. It carries visual information to the brain.

**optician** (ōp-tĭ′shən)   An eye professional who fills prescriptions for eyeglasses and contact lenses.

**optometrist** (ŏp-tŏm´ĭ-trĭst)   A trained and licensed vision specialist who is not a physician.

**orbicularis oculi** (ōr-bik´yū-lā´ris ok´yū-lī)   The muscle in the eyelid responsible for blinking.

**orbit** (ôr´bĭt)   The eye socket, which forms a protective shell around the eye.

**organ** (ôr´gan)   Structure formed by the organization of two or more different tissue types that carries out specific functions.

**organ of Corti** (ôr´gən əv kôr´tē)   The organ of hearing, located within the cochlea of the inner ear.

**organelle** (ôr´gə-nəl´)   A structure within a cell that performs a specific function.

**organic** (ôr-găn´ĭk)   Pertaining to matter that contains carbon and hydrogen.

**organism** (ôr´gə-nĭz´əm)   A whole living being that is formed from organ systems.

**organ system** (ôr´gən sĭs´təm)   A system that consists of organs that join together to carry out vital functions.

**orifice** (ôr´i fis)   An opening.

**origin** (ôr´ə-jĭn)   An attachment site of a skeletal muscle that does not move when a muscle contracts.

**Original Medicare Plan** (ə-rĭj´ə-nəl mĕd´ĭ-kâr´ plăn)   The Medicare fee-for-service plan that allows the beneficiary to choose any licensed physician certified by Medicare.

**oropharynx** (ōr´ō-far´ingks)(†)   The portion of the pharynx behind the oral cavity.

**orthopedist** (ôr´thə-pēd´ĭst)   A specialist who diagnoses and treats diseases and disorders of the muscles and bones.

**orthopnea** (ôr thop´nē a)   Condition of difficulty breathing except while in an upright position.

**orthostatic hypotension** (ôr´-thə-stăt´-ĭk hi´po-tĕn´shən)   A situation in which blood pressure

becomes low and the pulse increases when a patient is moved from a lying to standing position; also known as postural hypotension.

**OSHA (Occupational Safety and Health Act)** (ō´shə)   A set of regulations designed to save lives, prevent injuries, and protect the health of workers in the United States.

**osmosis** (ŏz-mō´sĭs)   The diffusion of water across a semipermeable membrane such as a cell membrane.

**ossification** (ä-sə-fə-kā´-shən)   The process of bone growth.

**osteoblast** (os´tē-ō-blast)(†)   Bone-forming cells that turn membrane into bone. They use excess blood calcium to build new bone.

**osteoclast** (os´tē-ō-klast)(†)   Bone-dissolving cells. When bone is dissolved, calcium is released into the bloodstream.

**osteocyte** (äs´-tē-ə-sīt)   A cell of osseous tissue; also called a bone cell.

**osteon** (äs´-tē-ən)   Elongated cylinders that run up and down the long axis of bone.

**osteopathic manipulative medicine (OMM)** (ŏs´tē-ō-păth´ĭk mə-nĭp´ū-lă´tĭv mĕd´ĭ-sĭn)   A system of hands-on techniques that help relieve pain, restore motion, support the body's natural functions, and influence the body's structure. Osteopathic physicians study OMM in addition to medical courses.

**osteoporosis** (ôs´tē-ō-pə-rō´sĭs)   An endocrine and metabolic disorder of the musculoskeletal system, more common in women than in men, characterized by hunched-over posture.

**osteosarcoma** (os´tē-ō-sar-kō´mă)   A type of bone cancer that originates from osteoblasts, the cells that make bony tissue.

**otologist** (ō-tol´ō-jist)(†)   A medical doctor who specializes in the health of the ear.

**otorhinolaryngologist** (ō-tō-rī´nōlar-ing-gol´ŏ-jist)   A specialist who diagnoses and treats diseases of the ear, nose, and throat.

**otosclerosis** (ō-tō-sklŭ rōsis)   Hardening or immobilization of the stapes within the inner ear.

**out guide** (out gīd)   A marker made of stiff material and used as a placeholder when a file is taken out of a filing system.

**ova** (ō va)   Eggs.

**oval window** (ō´vəl wĭn´dō)   The beginning of the inner ear.

**overbooking** (ō´vər-bŏŏk´ĭng)   Scheduling appointments for more patients than can reasonably be seen in the time allowed.

**oviduct** (ō´və´duct)   A Fallopian tube.

**ovulation** (ō´vyə-lā´shən)   The process by which the ovaries release one ovum (egg) approximately every 28 days.

**ovum** (ō vəm)   One egg. The female "egg" that unites with the male sperm to begin reproduction.

**oxygenated** (ok´səjənātəd)   Oxygenated blood refers to blood that has been to the lungs and is carrying oxygen in the hemoglobin.

**oxygen debt** (ok´sĭ-jən)   A condition that develops when skeletal muscles are used strenuously for a minute or two.

**oxyhemoglobin** (oks-ē-hē-mō-glō´bin)(†)   Hemoglobin that is bound to oxygen. It is bright red in color.

**oxytocin OT** (ok-sē-tō´sin)(†)   A hormone that causes contraction of the uterus during childbirth and the ejection of milk from mammary glands during breast-feeding.

**packed red blood cells** (păkt rĕd blud sĕlz)   Red blood cells that collect at the bottom of a centrifuged blood sample.

**palate** (pal´ăt)(†)   The roof of the mouth.

**palatine** (pa´-lə-tīn) Bones that form the anterior potion of the roof of the mouth and the **palate.**

**palatine tonsils** (pal´ă-tīn tŏn´sils)(†) Two masses of lymphatic tissue located at the back of the throat.

**palpation** (păl-pā´shən) A type of touch used by health-care providers to determine characteristics such as texture, temperature, shape, and the presence of movement.

**palpatory method** (pal-pa´tôr´ē mĕth´əd) Systolic blood pressure measured by using the sense of touch. This measurement provides a necessary preliminary approximation of the systolic blood pressure to ensure an adequate level of inflation when the actual auscultatory measurement is made.

**palpitations** (păl´pĭ-tā´shənz) Unusually rapid, strong, or irregular pulsations of the heart.

**pancreatic amylase** (pan-krē-at´ik am´il-ās)(†) An enzyme that digests carbohydrates.

**pancreatic lipase** (pan-krē-at´ik lip´ās) (†) An enzyme that digests lipids.

**panel** (păn´əl) Tests frequently ordered together that are organ or disease oriented.

**papillae** (pə-pĭl´ē) The "bumps" of the tongue in which the taste buds are found.

**paranasal sinuses** (par-ă-nā´zəl sī´nŭs-ĕz) Air-filled spaces within skull bones that open into the nasal cavity.

**parasite** (păr´ə-sīt´) An organism that lives on or in another organism and relies on it for nourishment or some other advantage to the detriment of the host organism.

**parasympathetic** (păr´ə-sĭm´pə-thĕt´ĭk) (†) A division of the autonomic nervous system that prepares the body for rest and digestion.

**parathyroid glands** (para-ă-thī royd glăndz) Four small glands embedded in the posterior thyroid gland that secrete parathyroid hormone (PTH); also known as parathormone.

**parathyroid hormone PH** (par-ă-thī´royd hôr´mōn´)(†) A hormone that helps regulate calcium levels in the bloodstream. It increases blood calcium by decreasing bone calcium.

**parenteral nutrition** (pă-ren´ter-ăl nōō-trĭsh´ən) Nutrition obtained when specially prepared nutrients are injected directly into patients' veins rather than taken by mouth.

**paresthesias** (par-es-thē´zē-ăs)(†) Abnormal sensations ranging from burning to tingling.

**parietal** (pă-rī´ē-tăl) Bones that form most of the top and sides of the skull.

**parietal cells** (pă-rī´ē-tăl sĕlz) Stomach cells that secrete hydrochloric acid, which is necessary to convert **pepsinogen** to **pepsin.** Parietal cells also secrete **intrinsic factor,** which is necessary for vitamin $B_{12}$ absorption.

**parietal pericardium** (pă-rī´ē-tăl per-i-kar´dē-ŭm)(†) The layer on top of the visceral pericardium.

**parietal peritoneum** (pă-rī´ē-tăl per-ə-tōnē´əm) The lining of the abdominal cavity.

**parotid glands** (pă-rot´id glăndz)(†) The largest of the salivary glands. The parotid glands are located beneath the skin just in front of the ears.

**participating physicians** (pär-tĭs´ə-pāt´ĭng fĭ-zĭsh´ənz) Physicians who enroll in managed care plans. They have contracts with MCOs that stipulate their fees.

**partnership** (pärt´n r shĭp) A form of medical practice management in which two or more parties practice together under a written agreement, specifying the rights, obligations, and responsibilities of each partner.

**parturition** (pär´ tur ish´ ən) The act of giving birth.

**passive listening** (păs´ĭv lĭs´ən-ĭng) Hearing what a person has to say without responding in any way; contrast with **active listening.**

**patch test** (păch tĕst) An allergy test in which a gauze patch soaked with a suspected allergen is taped onto the skin with nonallergenic tape; used to discover the cause of contact dermatitis.

**patella** (pə-té-lə) The bone commonly referred to as the kneecap.

**pathogen** (păth´ə-jən) A microorganism capable of causing disease.

**pathologist** (pă-thŏl´ə-jĭst) A medical doctor who studies the changes a disease produces in the cells, fluids, and processes of the entire body.

**patient compliance** (pā´shənt kəm-plī´əns) Obedience in terms of following a physician's orders.

**patient ledger card** (pā´shənt lĕj´ər kärd) A card containing information needed for insurance purposes, including the patient's name, address, telephone number, Social Security number, insurance information, employer's name, and any special billing instructions. It also includes the name of the person who is responsible for charges if this is anyone other than the patient.

**patient record/chart** (pā´shənt rĕk´ərd/chärt) A compilation of important information about a patient's medical history and present condition.

**pay schedule** (pā skĭej´ool) A list showing how often an employee is paid, such as weekly, biweekly, or monthly.

**payee** (pā-ē´) A person who receives a payment.

**payer** (pā´ər) A person who pays a bill or writes a check.

**pectoral girdle (pěk´tər əl)** The structure that attaches the arms to the axial skeleton.

**pediatrician (pē´dē-ə-trĭshən)** A specialist who diagnoses and treats childhood diseases and teaches parents skills for keeping their children healthy.

**pediculosis (pədik´yoolō´sis)** The medical term for lice.

**pegboard system (pěg´bôrd sĭs´təm)** A bookkeeping system that uses a lightweight board with pegs on which forms can be stacked, allowing each transaction to be entered and recorded on four different bookkeeping forms at once; also called the one-write system.

**pelvic girdle (pĕl´vik)** The structure that attaches the legs to the axial skeleton.

**pepsin (pep´sin)(†)** An enzyme that allows the body to digest proteins.

**pepsinogen (pep-sin´ō-jen)(†)** Substance that is secreted by the chief cells in the lining of the stomach and becomes **pepsin** in the presence of acid.

**peptidases (pep´ti-dās-ez)(†)** Enzymes that digest proteins.

**percussion (pər-kŭsh´ən)** Tapping or striking the body to hear sounds or feel vibration.

**percutaneous exposure (per-kyūtā´ nē-ŭs ĭk-spō´zhər)(†)** Exposure to a pathogen through a puncture wound or needlestick.

**pericardium (per-i-kar´dē-ŭm)(†)** A membrane that covers the heart and large blood vessels attached to it.

**perilymph (per´i-limf)(†)** A fluid in the inner ear. When this fluid moves, it activates hearing and equilibrium receptors.

**perimetrium (peri-mē´trēŭm)** The thin layer that covers the myometrium of the uterus.

**perimysium (per-i-mis´ē-ŭm)(†)** The connective tissue that divides a muscle into sections called fascicles.

**perineum (per i nē´üm)** In the male, the area between the scrotum and anus; in the female, the area between the vagina and rectum.

**periosteum (pĕr´ē ŏs´tē əm)** The membrane that surrounds the **diaphysis** of a bone.

**peripheral nervous system (PNS) (pə-rĭf´ər-əl nûr´vəs sĭs´təm)** A system that consists of nerves that branch off the central nervous system.

**peristalsis (pĕr´ĭ-stôl´sĭs)** The rhythmic muscular contractions that move a substance through a tract, such as food through the digestive tract and the ovum through the fallopian tube.

**personal protective equipment (PPE) (pur-suh-nl pruh-tek-tiv i-kwip-muh nt)** Any type of protective gear worn to guard against physical hazards.

**personal space (pûr´sə-nəl spās)** A certain area that surrounds an individual and within which another person's physical presence is felt as an intrusion.

**petty cash fund (pět´ē kăsh fŭnd)** Cash kept on hand in the office for small purchases.

**phagocyte (făg´ə-sīt´)** A specialized white blood cell that engulfs and digests pathogens.

**phagocytosis (fag´ō-sī-tō´sis)(†)** The process by which white blood cells defend the body against infection by engulfing invading pathogens.

**phalanges** The bones of the fingers.

**pharmaceutical (färˈmə-soo´tĭ-kəl)** Pertaining to medicinal drugs.

**pharmacodynamics (far´mă-kō-dīnam´iks)(†)** The study of what drugs do to the body: the mechanism of action, or how they work to produce a therapeutic effect.

**pharmacognosy (far-mă-kog´nō-sē)(†)** The study of characteristics of natural drugs and their sources.

**pharmacokinetics (far´mă-kō-kinet´iks) (†)** The study of what the body does to drugs: how the body absorbs, metabolizes, distributes, and excretes the drugs.

**pharmacology (fär´ma-kŏl´ə-jē)(†)** The study of drugs.

**pharmacotherapeutics (far´mă-kō-thĕr´ə-pyoo´tĭks)** The study of how drugs are used to treat disease; also called clinical **pharmacology.**

**pharyngeal tonsils (fă-rin´jē-ăl tŏn´səls) (†)** Two masses of lymphatic tissue located above the palatine tonsils; also called adenoids.

**pharynx (făr´ĭngks)** Structure below the mouth and nasal cavities that is an organ of the respiratory system as well as the digestive system.

**phenylketonuria (PKU) (fen´il-kē´tō-nū´rē-ă)(†)** A genetically inherited disorder in which the body cannot properly metabolize the nutrient phenylalanine, resulting in the buildup of phenylketones in the blood and their presence in the urine. The accumulation of phenylketones results in mental retardation.

**philosophy (fĭ-lŏs´ə-fē)** The system of values and principles an office has adopted in its everyday practice.

**phlebotomy (flĭ-bŏt´ə-mē)** The insertion of a needle or cannula (small tube) into a vein for the purpose of withdrawing blood.

**photometer (fō-tŏm´ĭ-tər)** An instrument that measures light intensity.

**physiatrist (fiz-ī´ă-trist)(†)** A physical medicine specialist, who diagnoses and treats diseases and disorders with physical therapy.

**physical therapy (fĭz´ĭ-kəl thĕr´ə-pē)** A medical specialty that uses cold, heat, water, exercise, massage, traction, and other physical means to treat musculoskeletal, nervous, and cardiopulmonary disorders.

**physician assistant (PA) (fĭ-zĭsh´ən ə-sĭs´tənt)** A health-care provider who practices medicine under the supervision of a physician.

**physician's office laboratory (POL) (fĭ-zĭsh´ənz ô´fĭs lăb´rə-tôr´ē)** A laboratory contained in a physician's office; processing tests in the POL produces quick turnaround and eliminates the need for patients to travel to other test locations.

**physiology (fĭz´ē-ŏl´ə-jē)** The science of the study of the body's functions.

**pineal body (pĭn´ē-ăl bŏd´ē)** A small gland located between the cerebral hemispheres that secretes melatonin.

**pitch (pĭch)** The high or low quality in the sound of a person's speaking voice.

**placebo effect (plə´-sē-bō ĭ-fĕkt´)** The belief that a medication or treatment works even though it is not scientifically substantiated. In research, a placebo is an inactive substance or preparation used as a control to determine the effectiveness of a medicinal drug.

**placenta (plə-sĕn´tə)** An organ located between the mother and the fetus. It permits the absorption of nutrients and oxygen. In some cases, harmful substances such as viruses are absorbed through the placenta.

**plantar flexion (plan´tăr flek´shŭn)(†)** Pointing the toes downward.

**plasma (plăz´mə)** The fluid component of blood, in which formed elements are suspended; makes up 55% of blood volume.

**plastic surgeon (plăs´tĭk sûr´jən)** A specialist who reconstructs, corrects, or improves body structures.

**platelets (plāt´lĭts)** Fragments of cytoplasm in the blood that are crucial to clot formation; also called thrombocytes.

**pleura (plŭr´ă)(†)** The membranes that surround the lungs.

**pleural effusion (plŏŏr´əl if yōō´ zhən)** A buildup of fluid within the pleural cavity.

**pleurisy (plŏŏr´əsē)** Also known as pleuritis; this is an inflammation of the parietal pleura of the lungs.

**pleuritis** A condition in which the **pleura** become inflamed, which causes them to stick together. It can also cause an excess amount of fluid to form between the membranes.

**plexus (plĕk´səs)** A structure that is formed when spinal nerves fuse together. It includes the cervical, brachial, and lumbosacral nerves.

**pneumoconiosis (nŏŏ mŏ kō´nē ō´sis)** This is the name given to lung diseases that result from years of exposure to different environmental or occupational types of dust.

**pneumothorax (nū-mō-thōr´aks)(†)** The presence of air or gas in the pleural cavity. The lung typically collapses with pneumothorax.

**polar body (pō´lər bŏd´ē)** A nonfunctional cell that is one of two small cells formed during the division of an oocyte.

**polarity (pō-lăr´ĭ-tē)** The condition of having two separate poles, one of which is positive and the other, negative.

**polarized (pō´lə-rīzd´)** The state in which the outside of a cell membrane is positively charged and the inside is negatively charged. Polarization occurs when a neuron is at rest.

**polysaccharide (pol-ē-sak´ă-rīd)(†)** A type of carbohydrate that is a starch.

**POMR (pē´ō-ĕm-är)** The problem-oriented medical record system for keeping patients' charts. Information in a POMR includes the database of information about the patient and the patient's condition, the problem list, the diagnostic and treatment plan, and progress notes.

**portfolio (pôrt-fō´lē-ō´)** A collection of an applicant's résumé, reference letters, and other documents of interest to a potential employer.

**positive tilt test (pŏz´-ĭ-tĭv tĭlt tĕst)** When the pulse rate increases more than 10 beats per minute (bpm) and the blood pressure drops more than 20 points while taking vital signs in the lying, sitting, and standing positions.

**positron emission tomography (PET) (pah´-zih-tron ee-mih´-shun toh-mah´-gruh-fee)** A radiologic procedure that entails injecting isotopes combined with other substances involved in metabolic activity, such as glucose. These special isotopes emit positrons, which a computer processes and displays on a screen.

**posterior (pŏ-stîr´ē-ar)** Anatomic term meaning toward the back of the body. Also called dorsal.

**postnatal period (pōst-nā´tăl pîr´ē-əd)(†)** The period following childbirth.

**postoperative (pōst-ŏp´ər-ə-tĭv)** Taking place after a surgical procedure.

**postural hypotension (pŏs-chĕr-ăl hī-pō-tĕn-shŭn)** A situation in which blood pressure becomes low and the pulse increases increases when a patient is moved from a lying to standing position; also known as orthostatic hypotension.

**posture (pŏs´chər)** Body position and alignment.

**power of attorney (pou´ər ə-tûr´nē)** The legal right to act as the attorney or agent of another person, including handling that person's financial matters.

**practitioner (prăk-tĭsh´ə-nər)** One who practices a profession.

**pre-authorization (prē ô´thər-ĭ-zā´shən)** Authorization or approval for payment from a third-party payer requested in advance of a specific procedure.

**pre-certification (prē sûr´tə-fĭ-kā´shən)** A determination of the amount of money that will be paid by a third-party payer for a specific procedure before the procedure is conducted.

**preferred provider organization (PPO) (prĭ-fûrd′ prə-vīd′ər or′ gə-nĭ-zā′shən)**　A managed care plan that establishes a network of providers to perform services for plan members.

**premenstrual syndrome (PMS) (prē-mĕn′-strə-wal sin′-drōm)(†)**　A syndrome that is a collection of symptoms that occur just before the menstrual period.

**premium (prē′mē-əm)**　The basic annual cost of health-care insurance.

**prenatal period (prē-nā′tăl pîr′ē-əd)(†)**　The period that includes the embryonic and fetal periods until the delivery of the offspring.

**preoperative (prē-ŏp′ər-ə-tĭv)**　Taking place prior to surgery.

**prepuce (prē′pūs)(†)**　A piece of skin in the uncircumcized male that covers the glans penis.

**presbyopia (prez-bē-ō′pē-ă)**　A common eye disorder that results in the loss of lens elasticity. Presbyopia develops with age and causes a person to have difficulty seeing objects close up.

**prescribe (prĭ-skrīb′)**　To give a patient a prescription to be filled by a pharmacy.

**prescription (prĭ-skrĭp′shən)**　A physician's written order for medication.

**prescription drug (prĭ-skrĭp′shən drŭg)**　A drug that can be legally used only by order of a physician and must be administered or dispensed by a licensed health-care professional.

**primary care physician (prī′mĕr′ē kâr fĭ-zĭsh′ən)**　A physician who provides routine medical care and referrals to specialists.

**primary germ layer (prī′mĕr′ē jûrm lā′ər)**　An inner cell mass that organizes into layers: the ectoderm, mesoderm, and endoderm.

**prime mover (prīm moo′vər)**　The muscle responsible for most of the movement when a body movement is produced by a group of muscles.

**primordial follicle (prī-mōr′dĕl-ăl fŏl′ĭ-kəl)(†)**　A structure that develops in the ovarian cortex of a female infant before she is born.

**Privacy Rule (prī′və-sē rool)**　Common name for the **HIPAA** Standard for Privacy of Individually Identifiable Health Information, which provides the first comprehensive federal protection for the privacy of health information. The Privacy Rule creates national standards to protect individuals' medical records and other personal health information.

**procedure code (prə-sē′jər kōd)**　Codes that represent medical procedures, such as surgery and diagnostic tests, and medical services, such as an examination to evaluate a patient's condition.

**proctoscopy (prok-tos′kō-pē)**　An examination of the lower rectum and anal canal with a 3-inch instrument called a proctoscope to detect hemorrhoids, polyps, fissures, fistulas, and abscesses.

**proficiency testing program (prə-fĭ′shən-cē tĕst′ĭng prō′grăm′)**　A required set of tests for clinical laboratories; the tests measure the accuracy of the laboratory's test results and adherence to standard operating procedures.

**progesterone (prō-jĕs′tə-rōn′)**　A female steroid hormone primarily produced by the ovary.

**prognosis (prŏg-nō′sĭs)**　A prediction of the probable course of a disease in an individual and the chances of recovery.

**prolactin (PRL) (prō-lak′tin)(†)**　A hormone that stimulates milk production in the mammary glands.

**proliferation phase (prə-lĭf′ər-ā′shən fāz)**　The second phase of wound healing, in which new tissue forms, closing off the wound.

**pronation (prō-nā′shŭn)(†)**　Turning the palms of the hand downward.

**pronunciation (prə-nun′cē-ā′shən)**　The sounding out of words.

**proofreading (proof′rēd′ing)**　Checking a document for formatting, data, and mechanical errors.

**prophase (prō′faz)**　Movement of the replicated centrioles to the opposite ends of the cell, creating spindle-like fibers during mitosis.

**prostaglandin (pros-tă-glan′din)(†)**　A local hormone derived from lipid molecules. Prostaglandins typically do not travel in the bloodstream to find their target cells because their targets are close by. This hormone has numerous effects, including uterine stimulation during childbirth.

**prostate gland (prŏs′tāt′ glănd)**　A chestnut-shaped gland that surrounds the beginning of the urethra in the male.

**prostatitis (pros-tă-tī′tis)**　Inflammation of the prostate gland, which can be acute or chronic.

**protected health information (PHI) (prə-tĕkt-əd hĕlth ĭn′fər-mă′shən)**　Individually identifiable health information that is transmitted or maintained by electronic or other media, such as computer storage devices. The core of the **HIPAA Privacy Rule** is the protection, use, and disclosure of protected health information.

**proteinuria (prō-tē-nū′rē-ă)**　An excess of protein in the urine.

**protozoan (prō′-tə-zō′ən)**　A single-celled eukaryotic organism much larger than a bacterium; some protozoans can cause disease in humans.

**protraction (prō-trăk′shən)**　Moving a body part anteriorly.

**proximal (prok′si-măl)(†)**　Anatomic term meaning closer to a point of attachment or closer to the trunk of the body.

**proximal convoluted tubule (prok´simăl kon´vō-lū-ted tū´byūl)(†)** The portion of the renal tubule that is directly attached to the glomerular capsule and becomes the loop of Henle.

**psoriasis (sə-rī´ə-sĭs)** A common skin condition characterized by reddish-silver scaly lesions most often found on the elbows, knees, scalp, and trunk.

**puberty (pyōō´bər-tē)** The period of adolescence when a person begins to develop secondary sexual traits and reproductive functions.

**pulmonary circuit (pōōl´mə-nĕr´ē sûr´kĭt)** The route that blood takes from the heart to the lungs and back to the heart again.

**pulmonary semilunar valve (p ŭl´ mənerē sem´ē loonər valv)** A heart valve that is a semilunar valve. It is situated between the right ventricle and the pulmonary trunk.

**pulmonary trunk (pōōl´mə-nĕr´ētrŭngk)** A large artery that branches into the pulmonary arteries and carries blood to the lungs.

**pubis (pyü´-bəs)** The area that forms the front of a hip bone.

**pulmonary function test (pōōl´mə-nĕr´ēfŭngk´shən tĕst)** A test that evaluates a patient's lung volume and capacity; used to detect and diagnose pulmonary problems or to monitor certain respiratory disorders and evaluate the effectiveness of treatment.

**puncture wound (pŭngk´chər wound)** A deep wound caused by a sharp, pointed object.

**punitive damages (pyōō´nĭ-tĭv dăm´ĭjz)** Money paid as punishment for intentionally breaking the law.

**pupil (pyōō´pəl)** The opening at the center of the iris, which grows smaller or larger as the iris contracts or relaxes, respectively;

it regulates the amount of light that enters the eye.

**purchase order (pûr´chĭs ôr´dər)** A form that authorizes a purchase for the practice.

**purchasing groups (pur´chĭs-ĭng grōōps)** Groups of medical offices associated with a nearby hospital that order supplies through the hospital to obtain a quantity discount.

**Purkinje Fibers (per´kin-jē fī´bərz)** Cardiac fibers that are located in the lateral walls of the ventricles.

**pyelonephritis (pī´ĕ-lō-ne-frī-tis)(†)** A urinary tract infection that involves one or both of the kidneys.

**pyloric sphincter (pī-lôrīk sfingk´ tər)** The valve-like structure composed of a circular band of muscle at the juncture of the stomach and small intestine.

**pyothorax (pī ōt hôr´ aks)** Pus or infected fluid in the pleural cavity causing collapse of the lung.

**pyrogens (pī´ō-jenz)(†)** Fever-producing substances released by neutrophils.

**qi (chē)** According to traditional Chinese medicine, a vital energy that flows throughout the body.

**quadrants (kwŏd´rəntz)** Four equal sections, such as those into which the abdomen is figuratively divided during an examination.

**qualitative analysis (kwŏl´ĭ-tā´tĭv-ənăl´ĭ-sĭs)** In microbiology, identification of bacteria present in a specimen by the appearance of colonies grown on a culture plate.

**qualitative test response (kwŏl´ĭ-tā´tĭvtĕst rĭ-spŏns´)** A test result that indicates the substance tested for is either present or absent.

**quality assurance program (kwŏl´ĭ-tēə-shōōr´əns prō´gram´)** A required program for clinical laboratories designed to monitor the quality of patient care, including quality control, instrument and equipment

maintenance, proficiency testing, training and continuing education, and standard operating procedures documentation.

**quality control (QC) (kwōl´ĭ-tē kən-trōl´)** An ongoing system, required in every physican's office, to evaluate the quality of medical care provided.

**quality control program (kwōl´ĭ-tē kəntrōl´ prō´gram´)** A component of a quality assurance program that focuses on ensuring accuracy in laboratory test results through careful monitoring of test procedures.

**quantitative analysis (kwŏn´tĭ-tā´tĭvə-năl´ĭ-sĭs)** In microbiology, a determination of the number of bacteria present in a specimen by direct count of colonies grown on a culture plate.

**quantitative test results (kwŏn´tĭ-tā´tĭvtĕst rĭ-zŭlt´)** The concentration of a test substance in a specimen.

**quarterly return (kwŏr´tar-lē rĭ-tûrn´)** The Employer's Quarterly Federal Tax Return, a form submitted to the IRS every 3 months that summarizes the federal income and employment taxes withheld from employees' paychecks.

*qui tam* **(k -´t m)** Latin, meaning "to bring action for the king and for one's self."

**radial artery (rā´dē-əl är´tə-rē)** An artery located in the groove on the thumb side of the inner wrist, where the pulse is taken on adults.

**radiation therapy (rā´dē-ā´shən thĕr´ə-pē)** The use of x-rays and radioactive substances to treat cancer.

**radiologist (rā´dē-ŏl´ ə-jĭst)** A physician who specializes in taking and reading x-rays.

**radius (rā-dā-əs)** The lateral bone of the forearm.

**rales (ralz)** Noisy respirations usually due to blockage of the bronchial tubes.

**random access memory (RAM) (răn′dəmăk′sĕs mĕm′ə-rē)** The temporary, or programmable, memory in a computer.

**random urine specimen (răn′dəm yoor′ĭn spĕs′ə-mən)** A single urine specimen taken at any time of the day; the most common type of sample collected.

**range of motion (ROM) (rānj mō′sh ən)** The degree to which a joint is able to move.

**rapport (ră-pôr′)** A harmonious, positive relationship.

**read only memory (ROM) (rēd ōn′lēmĕm′ə-rē)** A computer's permanent memory, which can be read by the computer but not changed. It provides the computer with the basic operating instructions it needs to function.

**reagent (rē-ā′jənt)** A chemical or chemically treated substance used in test procedures and formulated to react in specific ways when exposed under specific conditions.

**reconciliation (rĕk′ən-sĭl′ē-ā′shən)** A comparison of the office's financial records with bank records to ensure that they are consistent and accurate; usually done when the monthly checking account statement is received from the bank.

**records management system (rĭ-kôrdz măn′ĭj-mənt sĭs′təm)** How patient records are created, filed, and maintained.

**recovery position (rĭ-kŭv′ər-ē pə-zĭsh′ən)** The position a person is placed in after receiving first aid for choking or cardiopulmonary resuscitation.

**rectum (rĕk′təm)** The last section of the sigmoid colon that straightens out and becomes the anal canal.

**reference (rĕf′ər-əns)** A recommendation for employment from a facility or a preceptor.

**reference laboratory (rĕf′ər-əns lăb′rə-tôr′ē)** A laboratory owned and operated by an organization outside the physician's practice.

**referral (rĭ-fûr′əl)** An authorization from a medical practice for a patient to have specialized services performed by another practice; often required for insurance purposes.

**reflex (rē′flĕks′)** A predictable automatic response to stimuli.

**reflexology (rē -flĕk-sōl′-ə-jē)** Manual therapy to the foot and/or hand in which pressure is applied to "reflex" points mapped out on the feet or hands.

**refraction (rī-frāk′shən)** The bending of light by the cornea, lens, and eye fluids to focus light onto the retina.

**refraction examination (rĭ-frāk′shən ĭg-zăm′ə-nā′shən)** An eye examination in which the patient looks through a succession of different lenses to find out which ones create the clearest image.

**refractometer (rē-frak-tom′ē-ter)(†)** An optical instrument that measures the refraction, or bending, of light as it passes through a liquid.

**Registered Medical Assistant (RMA) (rĕj′ĭ-stərd mĕd′ĭ-kəl ə-sĭs′tənt)** A medical assistant who has met the educational requirements and taken and passed the certification examination for medical assisting given by the American Medical Technologists (AMT).

**Reiki (ray-key)** The use of visualization and touch to balance energy flow and bring healthy energy to affected body parts.

**relaxin (rē-lak′sin)(†)** A hormone that comes from the corpus luteum. It inhibits uterine contractions and relaxes the ligaments of the pelvis in preparation for childbirth.

**remedy (rĕm′-ī-dē)** A treatment prescribed by a homeopath in small amounts that in large doses would produce the same symptoms seen in the patient.

**remittance advice (RA) (rĭ-mĭt′ns˘ ad-vīz′)** A form that the patient and the practice receive for each encounter that outlines the amount billed by the practice, the amount allowed, the amount of subscriber liability, the amount paid, and notations of any service not covered, including an explanation of why that service is not covered; also called an explanation of benefits.

**renal calculi (rē′nəl kăl′kyə-lī′)** Kidney stones.

**renal column (rē′nəl kŏl′əm)** The portion of the **renal cortex** between the **renal pyramids.**

**renal corpuscle (rē′nəl kôr′pə-səl)** Corpuscle that is composed of the glomerulus and the glomerular capsule. The filtration of blood occurs here.

**renal cortex (rē′nəl kôr′tĕks′)** The outermost layer of the kidney.

**renal medulla (rē′nəl mĭ-dŭl′ə)** The middle portion of the kidney.

**renal pelvis (rē′nəl pĕl′vĭs)** The internal structure of the kidney. Urine flows from the renal pelvis down the ureter.

**renal pyramids (rē′nəl pĭr′ə-mĭdz)** Triangular-shaped areas in the medulla of the kidney.

**renal sinus (rē′nəl sī′nəs)** The medial depression of a kidney.

**renal tubule (rē′nəl tū′byūl)** Structure that extends from the glomerular capsule of a nephron and is composed of the proximal convoluted tubule, the loop of Henle, and the distal convoluted tubule.

**renin (ren′in)(†)** A hormone secreted by the kidney that helps to regulate blood pressure.

**repolarization (rē′pō-lăr-i-zā′shŭn)(†)** The process of returning to the original polar (resting) state.

**reputable (rĕpyə-tə-bəl)** Having a good reputation.

**requisition (rĕk′wĭ-zĭsh′ən)** A formal request from a staff member or doctor for the purchase of equipment or supplies.

**res ipsa loquitur (reez ip-suh loh-kwi-ter)** Latin, meaning "the thing speaks for itself," which is also known as the doctrine of common knowledge.

**reservoir host (rĕz´ər-vwär´ hōst)** An animal, insect, or human whose body is susceptible to growth of a pathogen.

**resident normal flora (´re-zə-dənt, ´nōr-məl, ´flōr-ə)** Bacteria, fungi, and protozoa that have taken up residence either in or on the human body. Some of these organisms neither help nor harm the host and some are beneficial, creating a barrier against pathogens.

**resource-based relative value scale (RBRVS) (rē´sôrs´ bāst rĕl´ə-tĭvvăl´yōō skāl)** The payment system used by Medicare. It establishes the relative value units for services, replacing the providers' consensus on usual fees.

**respiratory distress syndrome (res´pərətôr´ə distres sin´drəm)** Condition found usually in premature babies, who lack the substance surfactant in their lungs, causing the lungs to collapse on expiration.

**respiratory volume (rĕs´pər-ə-tôr´ē vŏl´yōōm)** The different volumes of air that move in and out of the lungs during different intensities of breathing. These volumes can be measured to assess the healthiness of the respiratory system.

**respondeat superior (rehs-pond-dee-at soo-peer-e-or)** Latin, meaning "let the master answer," a doctrine under which an employer is legally liable for the acts of his or her employees, if such acts were performed within the scope of the employee's duties.

**résumé (rĕz´ōo-mā´)** A typewritten document summarizing one's employment and educational history.

**retention schedule (rĭ-tĕn´shən skĕj´ōol)** A schedule that details how long to keep different types of patient records in the office after they have become inactive or closed and how long the records should be stored.

**retina (rĕt´n-ə)** The inner layer of the eye; contains light-sensing nerve cells.

**retraction (rĭ-trăk´shən)** Moving a body part posteriorly.

**retrograde pyelography (rĕt´rə-grād´pī´ĕ-log´ră-fē)(†)** A radiologic procedure in which the doctor injects a contrast medium through a urethral catheter and takes a series of x-rays to evaluate function of the ureters, bladder, and urethra.

**retroperitoneal (re-trō-per-ə-ə-nē´-əl)** An anatomic term that means behind the peritoneal cavity. It is where the kidneys lie.

**return demonstation (rĭ-tûrn´ dĕm´ən-strā´shən)** Participatory teaching method in which the technique is first described to the patient and then demonstrated to the patient; the patient is then asked to repeat the demonstration.

**rhabdomyolysis (rab´dō-mī-ol´i-sis)(†)** A condition in which the kidneys have been damaged due to toxins released from muscle cells.

**Rh antigen (är´ach an´tĭ-jən)** A protein first discovered on the red blood cells of rhesus monkeys, hence the name Rh.

**RhoGAM (rō´găm)** A medication that prevents an Rh-negative mother from making antibodies against the Rh antigen.

**ribosomes ((rībəsomz)** The organelle within the cytoplasm responsible for protein synthesis.

**RNA (är´ĕn-ā´)** A nucleic acid used to make protein.

**rods (rŏdz)** Light-sensing nerve cells in the eye, at the posterior of the retina, that function in dim light but do not provide sharp images or detect color.

**rosacea (rō-zā´shē-ă)(†)** A condition characterized by chronic redness and acne over the nose and cheeks.

**rotation (rō-tā´shən)** Twisting a body part.

**route (rōōt)** The way a drug is introduced into the body.

**rugae (rōō´gā)** The expandable folds of an organ. The folds of the stomach lining.

**sacrum (sa´-krəm)** A triangular-shaped bone that consists of five fused vertebra.

**sagittal (saj´i-tăl)(†)** An anatomic term that refers to the plane that divides the body into left and right portions.

**salutation (săl´yə-tā´shən)** A written greeting, such as "Dear," used at the beginning of a letter.

**sanitization (săn´ĭ-tĭ-zā´shən)(†)** A reduction of the number of microorganisms on an object or a surface to a fairly safe level.

**sarcolemma (sar´kō-lem´ă)** The cell membrane of a muscle fiber.

**sarcoplasm** The cytoplasm of a muscle fiber.

**sarcoplasmic reticulum (sar-kō-plaz´mik re-tik´yū-lŭm)** The endoplasmic reticulum of a muscle fiber.

**SARS (severe acute respiratory syndrome) (särz; sivēr əkyōot res´pərətôr´ē sin´drəm)** A severe and acute respiratory illness characterized by fever and a nonproductive cough that progresses to the point at which insufficient oxygen is present in the blood.

**saturated fat (săch´ə-rā´tĭd făt)** Fats, derived primarily from animal sources, that are usually solid at room temperature and that tend to raise blood cholesterol levels.

**scabies (skā´bēz)** Skin lesions that are very itchy and caused by a burrowing mite. Scabies is most commonly found between the fingers and on the genitalia.

**scanner (skăn´ər)** An optical device that converts printed matter into a format that can be read by the computer and inputs the converted information.

**scapula (sk´a-pyə-la)** Thin, triangular-shaped, flat bones located on the dorsal surface of the rib cage; also called shoulder blades.

**Schwann cell (shwahn sĕl)(†)** A neuroglial cell whose cell membrane coats the axons.

**sciatica (sī-ăt´ĭ-kə)** Pain in the low back and hip radiating down the back of the leg along the sciatic nerve.

**sclera (sklîr´ə)** The tough, outermost layer, or "white," of the eye, through which light cannot pass; covers all except the front of the eye.

**scoliosis (skō´lē-ō´sĭs)** A lateral curvature of the spine, which is normally straight when viewed from behind.

**scratch test (skrăch tĕst)** An allergy test in which extracts of suspected allergens are applied to the patient's skin and the skin is then scratched to allow the extracts to penetrate.

**screening (skrēn´ĭng)** Performing a diagnostic test on a person who is typically free of symptoms.

**screen saver (skrēn sāv´ər)** A program that automatically changes the monitor display at short intervals or constantly shows moving images to prevent burn-in of images on the computer screen.

**scrotum (skrō´təm)** In a male, the sac of skin below the pelvic cavity that contains the testes.

**sebaceous (sĭ-bā´shəs)** A type of oil gland found in the dermis.

**sebum (sē´bŭm)(†)** An oily substance produced by sebaceous glands.

**Security Rule (sĭ-kyŏŏr´ĭ-tē rŏŏl)** The technical safeguards that protect the confidentiality, integrity, and availability of health information covered by **HIPAA.** The Security Rule specifies how patient information is protected on computer networks, the Internet, disks, and other storage media.

**seizure (sē´zhər)** A series of violent and involuntary contractions of the muscles; also called a convulsion.

**sella turcica (sel´ă tŭr´sē-kă)(†)** A deep depression in the sphenoid bone where the pituitary gland sits.

**semen (sē´mən)** Sperm and the various substances that nourish and transport them.

**semicircular canals (sĕm´ē-sûr´kyə-lər kə-nălz´)** Structures in the inner ear that help a person maintain balance; each of the three canals is positioned at right angles to the other two.

**seminal vesicles (sem´-năl ves´i-klz)(†)** A pair of convoluted tubes that lie behind the bladder. These tubes secrete a fluid that provides nutrition for the sperm.

**seminiferous tubules (sem´i-nif´er-ŭs tū´byūlz)(†)** These tubes contain spermatogenic cells and are located in the lobules of the testes.

**sensorineural hearing loss (sen´sōr-i-nūr´ăl hîr´ĭng lôs)** This type of hearing loss occurs when neural structures associated with the ear are damaged. Neural structures include hearing receptors and the auditory nerve.

**sensory (sĕn´sə-rē)** Afferent neurons that carry sensory information from the periphery to the central nervous system.

**sensory adaptation (sĕn´sə-rē ăd´ăp-tā´shən)** A process in which the same chemical can stimulate receptors only for a limited amount of time until the receptors eventually no longer respond to the chemical.

**septic shock (sĕp´tĭk shŏk)** A state of shock resulting from massive, widespread infection that affects the blood vessels' ability to circulate blood.

**sequential order (sĭ´kwĕn´shəl ôr´dər)** One after another in a predictable pattern or sequence.

**serosa (se-rō´să)(†)** The outermost layer of the alimentary canal; also known as the visceral peritoneum.

**serous cells (sēr´ŭs sĕlz)(†)** One of two types of cells that make up the salivary glands. These cells secrete a watery fluid that contains amylase.

**serum (sēr´ŭm)(†)** The liquid portion of blood (plasma) when all of the clotting factors have been removed.

**service contract (sûr´vĭs kŏn´trăkt´)** A contract that covers services for equipment that are not included in a standard maintenance contract.

**sex chromosome (sĕks krō´mə-sōm´)** Chromosome of the 23rd pair.

**sex-linked trait (sĕks lĭngk trāt)** Traits that are carried on the sex chromosomes, or X and Y chromosomes.

**sigmoid colon (sig-mŏid ko-lən)** An S-shaped tube that lies between the **descending colon** and the **rectum.**

**sigmoidoscopy (sig´moy-dos´kŏ-pē)** A procedure in which the interior of the sigmoid area of the large intestine, between the descending colon and the rectum, is examined with a sigmoidoscope, a lighted instrument with a magnifying lens.

**sign (sīn)** An objective or external factor, such as blood pressure, rash, or swelling, that can be seen or felt by the physician or measured by an instrument.

**signature block (sig´-nuh-cher blok´)** The writer's name and business title found four lines

**below** the complimentary closing in a business letter.

**silicosis (sĭl´ i kō´ sis)** Chronic lung disease caused by the inhalation of silica dust.

**simplified letter style (sĭm´plə-fīd´ lĕt´ər stīl)** A modification of the full-block style in which the salutation and complimentary closing are omitted and a subject line typed in all capital letters is placed between the address and the body of the letter.

**single-entry account (sĭng´gəl-ĕn´trē-ə-kount´)** An account that has only one charge, usually for a small amount, for a patient who does not come in regularly.

**sinoatrial node (sī´nō-ā´trē-ăl nōd)(†)** A small bundle of heart muscle tissue in the superior wall of the right atrium that sets the rhythm (or pattern) of the heart's contractions; also called sinus node or pacemaker.

**sinusitis (sī´nə-sī´tĭs)** Inflammation of the lining of a sinus.

**skinfold test (skĭn´ fōld tĕst)** A method of measuring fat as a percentage of body weight by measuring the thickness of a fold of skin with a caliper.

**slander (slăn´ dər)** The speaking of defamatory words intended to prejudice others against an individual in a manner that jeopardizes his or her reputation or means of livelihood.

**sleep apnea (slēp ap-ne´ah)** A condition characterized by pauses in breathing during sleep.

**slit lamp (slĭt lămp)** An instrument composed of a magnifying lens combined with a light source; used to provide a minute examination of the eye's anatomy.

**smear (smîr)** A specimen spread thinly and unevenly across a slide.

**SOAP (sōp)** An approach to medical records documentation that documents information in the following order: S (**subjective** data), O (**objective** data),

A (assessment), P (plan of action).

**software (sôft´wâr´)** A program, or set of instructions, that tells a computer what to do.

**sole proprietorship (sōl prə -prī´-tər shĭp)** A form of medical practice management in which a physician practices alone, assuming all benefits, and liabilities for the business.

**solution (sə-lōō´shən)** A homogeneous mixture of a solid, liquid, or gaseous substance in a liquid, such as a dissolved drug in liquid form.

**somatic (sō-măt´ĭk)** A division of the peripheral nervous system that connects the central nervous system to skin and skeletal muscle.

**somatic nervous system (SNS) (sō-măt´ĭk nûr´vəs sĭs´təm)** A system that governs the body's skeletal or voluntary muscles.

**SPECT (spĕkt)** Single photon emission computed tomography; a radiologic procedure in which a gamma camera detects signals induced by gamma radiation and a computer converts these signals into two- or three-dimensional images that are displayed on a screen.

**speculum (spĕk´yə-ləm)** An instrument that expands the vaginal opening to permit viewing of the vagina and cervix.

**spermatids (sper´mă-tidz)(†)** Immature sperm before they develop their flagella (tails).

**spermatocytes (sper´mă-tō-sīts)(†)** The cells that result when spermatogonia undergo mitosis.

**spermatogenesis (sper´mă-tō-jen´ĕ-sis)(†)** The process of sperm cell formation.

**spermatogenic cells (sper´mă-tō-jen´ik sĕlz)(†)** The cells that give rise to sperm cells.

**spermatogonia (sper´mă-tō-gō´nē-ă)(†)** The earliest cell in the process of **spermatogenesis.**

**sphenoid** A bone that forms part of the floor of the cranium.

**sphincter (sfĭngk´tər)** A valve-like structure formed from circular bands of muscle. Sphincters are located around various body openings and passages.

**sphygmomanometer (sfig´mō-mănom´ĕter)(†)** An instrument for measuring blood pressure; consists of an inflatable cuff, a pressure bulb used to inflate the cuff, and a device to read the pressure.

**spinal nerves (spī´năl nûrvs)(†)** Peripheral nerves that originate from the spinal cord.

**spirillum (spī-ril´ŭm)(†)** A spiral-shaped bacterium.

**spirometer (spī-rom´ĕ-ter)(†)** An instrument that measures the air taken in and expelled from the lungs.

**spirometry (spī-rom´ĕ-trē)(†)** A test used to measure breathing capacity.

**splenectomy (splən ek´ tō me)** Surgical removal of the spleen.

**splint (splĭnt)** A device used to immobilize and protect a body part.

**splinting catheter (splĭnt´ĭng kăth´ĭ-tər)** A type of catheter inserted after plastic repair of the ureter; it must remain in place for at least a week after surgery.

**sprain (sprān)** An injury characterized by partial tearing of a ligament that supports a joint, such as the ankle. A sprain may also involve injuries to tendons, muscles, and local blood vessels and contusions of the surrounding soft tissue.

**stain (stān)** In microbiology, a solution of a dye or group of dyes that impart a color to microorganisms.

**standard (stăn´dərd)** A specimen for which test values are already known; used to calibrate test equipment.

**standardization (stăn-dər-dĭ-zā´-shən)** The consistency of the active ingredient(s) in a supplement from batch to batch and from manufacturer to manufacturer.

**Standard Precautions (stăn´dərd prĭ-kô´shənz)** A combination of Universal Precautions and Body Substance Isolation guidelines; used in hospitals for the care of all patients.

**stapes (stā´pēz)** A small bone in the middle ear that is attached to the inner ear; also called the stirrup.

**statement (stāt´mənt)** A form similar to an invoice; contains a courteous reminder to the patient that payment is due.

**State Unemployment Tax Act (SUTA)** Some states are also governed by this act; these taxes are filed along with FUTA taxes.

**statute of limitations (stăch´ōot lĭm´ĭ-tā´shənz)** A state law that sets a time limit on when a collection suit on a past-due account can legally be filed.

**stent (stěnt-)** A metal mesh tube used to hold a vessel open.

**stereoscopy (ster-ē-os´kŏ-pē) (†)** An x-ray procedure that uses a specially designed microscope (stereoscopic, or Greenough, microscope) with double eyepieces and objectives to take films at different angles and produce three-dimensional images; used primarily to study the skull.

**sterile field (stěr´əl fēld)** An area free of microorganisms used as a work area during a surgical procedure.

**sterile scrub assistant (stěr´əl skrŭb ə-sĭs´tənt)** An assistant who handles sterile equipment during a surgical procedure.

**sterilization (stěr´ə-lĭ-zā´shən)** The destruction of all microorganisms, including bacterial spores, by specific means.

**sterilization indicator (stěr´ə-lĭ-zā´shən ĭn´dĭ-kā´shən)** A tag, insert, tape, tube, or strip that confirms that the items in an autoclave have been exposed to

the correct volume of steam at the correct temperature for the correct amount of time.

**sternum (st´ər-nəm)** A bone that forms the front and middle portion of the rib cage; also called the breastbone or breast plate.

**steroid al hormone (stîr´oid´ə hôr´mōn´)** A hormone derived from steroids that are soluble in lipids and can cross cell membranes very easily.

**stethoscope (stěth´ə-skōp´)** An instrument that amplifies body sounds.

**strabismus (strə-bĭz´məs)** A condition that results in a lack of parallel visual axes of the eyes; commonly called crossed eyes.

**strain (strān)** A muscle injury that results from overexertion or overstretching.

**stratum basale (strat´ŭm bā-sā´le)(†)** The deepest layer of the epidermis of the skin.

**stratum corneum (strat´ŭm kōr´nē ŭm) (†)** The most superficial layer of the epidermis of the skin.

**stratum germinativum (strat´ŭm jur´minə tē´vūm)** The deepest layer of the epidermis; also known as staratum basale.

**stressor (stres´or)(†)** Any stimulus that produces stress.

**stress test (strĕs tĕst)** A procedure that involves recording an electrocardiogram while the patient is exercising on a stationary bicycle, treadmill, or stair-stepping ergometer, which measures work performed.

**striations (strī-ā´shŭns)(†)** Bands produced from the arrangement of filaments in myofibrils in skeletal and cardiac muscle cells.

**stroke (strōk)** A condition that occurs when the blood supply to the brain is impaired. It may cause temporary or permanent damage.

**stylus (stī´ləs)** A pen-like instrument that records electrical impulses on ECG paper.

**subarachnoid space (sŭb-ă-rak´noydspās)(†)** An area between the arachnoid mater and the pia mater.

**subclinical case (sŭb-klin´i-kăl kās) (†)** An infection in which the host experiences only some of the symptoms of the infection or milder symptoms than in a full case.

**subcutaneous (SC) (sŭb´kyoo-tā´nē -əs)** Under the skin.

**subject line (sŭb´jĭkt līn)** Optional line of two to three words that appear three lines below the inside address of a business letter.

**subjective (səb-jĕk´tĭv)** Pertaining to data that is obtained from conversation with a person or patient.

**sublingual (sŭb-ling´gwăl) (†)** Under the tongue.

**sublingual gland (sŭb-ling´gwăl glănd)(†)** The smallest of the salivary glands.

**submandibular gland (sŭb-man-dib´yu-lăr glănd)(†)** The gland that is located in the floor of the mouth.

**submucosa (sŭb-mū-kō´s ă)(†)** The layer of the alimentary canal located between the mucosa and the muscular layer.

**subpoena (sə-pē´nə)** A written court order that is addressed to a specific person and requires that person's presence in court on a specific date at a specific time.

*subpoena duces tecum* **(suh-pee-nuh doo-seez tee-kuh)** Latin; a legal document that requires the recipient to bring certain written records to court to be used as evidence in a lawsuit.

**substance abuse (sŭb´stəns ə-byooz´)** The use of a substance in a way that is not medically approved, such as using diet pills to stay awake or consuming large quantities of cough syrup that contains codeine. Substance abusers are not necessarily addicts.

**sucrase (sū′krās)(†)** An enzyme that digests sugars.

**sudoriferous (soo′dərif′ərəs)** The sweat glands.

**sulci (sŭl′si)(†)** The grooves on the surface of the cerebrum.

**superbill (soo′pər-bĭl′)** A form that combines the charges for services rendered, an invoice for payment or insurance copayment, and all the information for submitting an insurance claim; also known as an encounter form.

**superficial (soo′pər-fĭsh′əl)** Anatomic term meaning closer to the surface of the body.

**superior (soo′-pîr′-ē-ər)** Anatomic term meaning above or closer to the head; also called cranial.

**supernatant (sū-per-nā′tănt)(†)** The liquid portion of a substance from which solids have settled to the bottom, as with a urine specimen after centrifugation.

**supination (sū′pi-nā′shŭn)(†)** Turning the palm of the hand upward.

**surfactant (sər fak′ tənt)** Fatty substance secreted by some alveolar cells that helps maintain the inflation of the alveoli so that they do not collapse in on themselves between inspirations.

**surgeon (sûr′jən)** A physician who uses hands and medical instruments to diagnose and correct deformities and treat external and internal injuries or disease.

**surgical asepsis (sûr′jə-kəl ă-sep′sis)(†)** The elimination of all microorganisms from objects or working areas; also called sterile technique.

**susceptible host (sə-sĕp′təbal hōst)** An individual who has little or no immunity to infection by a particular organism.

**suture (soo′chər)** Fibrous joints in the skull. (25) A surgical stitch made to close a wound.

**symmetry (sĭm′ĭ-trē)** The degree to which one side of the body is the same as the other.

**sympathetic (sĭm′pə-thĕt′ĭk)** A division of the autonomic nervous system that prepares organs for fight-or-flight (stressful) situations.

**symptom (sĭm′təm)** A subjective, or internal, condition felt by a patient, such as pain, headache, or nausea, or another indication that generally cannot be seen or felt by the doctor or measured by instruments.

**synaptic knob (si-nap′tik nŏb)(†)** The end of the axon branch.

**synergist (sĭn′ər-jist′)** Muscles that help the **prime mover** by stabilizing joints.

**synovial (sin-ō-vā-əl)** A type of joint, such as the elbow or knee, that is freely moveable.

**systemic circuit (sĭ-stĕm′ĭk sûr′kĭt)** The route that blood takes from the heart through the body and back to the heart.

**systemic lupus erythematosus (SLE) (si-stĕm′ĭk loo′p s er the′to′s s)** An autoimmune disorder in which a person produces antibodies that target the person's own cells and tissues.

**systolic pressure (sĭ-stŏl′ĭk prĕsh′ər)** The blood pressure measured when the left ventricle of the heart contracts.

**tab (tăb)** A tapered rectangular or rounded extension at the top of a file folder.

**Tabular List (tăb′yə-lər lĭst)** One of two ways that diagnoses are listed in the **ICD-9.** In the Tabular List, the diagnosis codes are listed in numerical order with additional instructions.

**tachycardia (tak′i-kar′dē-ă)(†)** Rapid heart rate, generally in excess of 100 beats per minute.

**tachypnea** Abnormally rapid breathing.

**targeted résumé (tär′gĭt-əd rĕz′oo-mā′)** A résumé that is focused on a specific job target.

**tarsals (tär′-səlz)** Bones of the ankle.

**taste bud (tāst bŭd)** A structure that is made of taste cells (a type of chemoreceptor) and supporting cells.

**tax liability (tăk lī′ə-bĭl′ĭ-tē)** Money withheld from employees' paychecks and held in a separate account that must be used to pay taxes to appropriate government agencies.

**telephone triage (tĕl′ə-fōn′ trē-äzh′)** A process of determining the level of urgency of each incoming telephone call and how it should be handled.

**teletherapy (tel-ĕ-thăr′ăpē)(†)** A radiation therapy technique that allows deeper penetration than brachytherapy; used primarily for deep tumors.

**teletype (TTY) device (tĕl′ə-tīp)** A specially designed telephone that looks very much like a laptop computer with a cradle for the receiver of a traditional telephone. It is used by the hearing impaired to type communications onto a keyboard.

**telophase (tel′əfāz)** The final stage of mitosis; chromosomes reach the centrioles and the division creating two cells, each with a complete set of chromosomes is completed.

**template (tĕm′plĭt)** A guide that ensures consistency and accuracy.

**temporal (tem′-p(a)-rəl)** Bones that form the lower sides of the skull.

**temporal scanner (temp′-or-al skăn-ĕr)** An instrument used to measure the body temperature by scanning the temporal artery in the forehead.

**tendon (tĕn′dən)** A cord-like fibrous tissue that connects muscle to bone.

**tendonitis (ten dŭn ĭ tis)** Inflammation of a tendon.

**terminal (tûr′mə-nəl)** Fatal.

**terminal digit (tûrmə-nəl dĭjĭt)** A small group of two to three numbers at the end of a patient number that is used as an identifying unit in a filing system.

**testes (těs´tēz)** The primary organs of the male reproductive system. Testes produce the hormone **testosterone.**

**testosterone (těs-tŏs´tə-rōn´)** A hormone produced by the testes that maintains the male reproductive structures and male characteristics such as deep voice, body hair, and muscle mass.

**tetanus (tět´n-əs)** A disease caused by *clostridium tetani* living in the soil and water; more commonly called lockjaw.

**thalamus (thăl´ə-məs)** Structure that acts as a relay station for sensory information heading to the cerebral cortex for interpretation; a subdivision of the **diencephalon.**

**thalassemia (thal´əē´mēaə)** An inherited form of anemia with a defective hemoglobin chain causing micocytic (small), hypochromic (pale), and short-lived red blood cells.

**therapeutic team (thĕr´ə-pyo͞o´tĭk tēm)** A group of physicians, nurses, medical assistants, and other specialists who work with patients dealing with chronic illness or recovery from major injuries.

**therapeutic touch (thĕr´ -ə-pyo͞o-tĭk tŭch)** The use of touch to detect and correct an person's energy fields, thus promoting healing and health.

**thermography (ther-mog´ră-fē)(†)** A radiologic procedure in which an infrared camera is used to take photographs that record variations in skin temperature as dark (cool areas), light (warm areas), or shades of gray (areas with temperatures between cool and warm); used to diagnose breast tumors, breast abscesses, and fibrocystic breast disease.

**thermometer (ther-mom´ə-ter)** An instrument, either electronic or disposable, that is used to measure body temperature.

**thermotherapy (ther´mō-thär´ă-pē) (†)** The application of heat to the body to treat a disorder or injury.

**third-party check (thûrd pär´tē chĕk)** A check made out to one recipient and given in payment to another, as with one made out to a patient rather than the medical practice.

**third-party payer (thûrd pär´tē pā´ər)** A health plan that agrees to carry the risk of paying for patient services.

**thoracocentesis (thôr´ə kō´sen tē´ sis)** Medical procedure where a sterile needle is introduced into the chest to remove fluid and pus.

**thoracostomy (thor´ə kos´ tə mē)** The surgical insertion of a chest tube to provide continuous drainage of the thoracic (chest) cavity.

**thorax (thôr´aks)** The chest cavity.

**thrombocytes (throm´bō-sīts)** See **platelets.**

**thrombophlebitis (thrŏm´bō-flĕ-bī´tis) (†)** A medical condition that most commonly occurs in leg veins when a blood clot and inflammation develop.

**thrombus (thrŏm´bəs)** A blood clot that forms on the inside of an injured blood vessel wall.

**thymosin (thī´mō-sin)(†)** A hormone that promotes the production of certain lymphocytes.

**thymus gland (thī´məs glănd)** A gland that lies between the lungs. It secretes a hormone called **thymosin.**

**thyroid cartilage (thī´roid´ kär´tl-ĭj)** The largest cartilage in the larynx. It forms the anterior wall of the larynx.

**thyroid hormone (thī´roid´ hôr´mōn´)** A hormone produced by the thyroid gland that increases energy production, stimulates protein synthesis, and speeds up the repair of damaged tissue.

**thyroid-stimulating hormone (TSH) (thī´roid´stim´yū-lā-ting hôr´mōn´)** A hormone that stimulates the thyroid gland to release its hormone.

**tibia (ti-bē-ə)** The medial bone of the lower leg; commonly called the shin bone.

**tickler file (tĭk´lər fīl)** A reminder file for keeping track of time-sensitive obligations.

**timed urine specimen (tīmd yo͞or´ĭn spĕs´ə-mən)** A specimen of a patient's urine collected over a specific time period.

**time-specified scheduling (tīm spĕs´ə-fīd skĕj´o͞ol-ing)** A system of scheduling where patients arrive at regular, specified intervals, assuring the practice a steady stream of patients throughout the day.

**tinea (tin ē´ă)** A fungal infection.

**tinnitus (ti-nī´tus)(†)** An abnormal ringing in the ear.

**tissue (tĭsh´o͞o)** A structure that is formed when cells of the same type organize together.

**T lymphocyte (tē lĭm´fə-sīt)** A type of nongranular leukocyte that regulates immunologic response; includes helper T cells and suppressor T cells.

**topical (tŏp´ĭ-kəl)** Applied to the skin.

**tort (tôrt)** In civil law, a breach of some obligation that causes harm or injury to someone.

**torticollis (tôr´tikol´is)** A muscular disease causing a cervical deformity in which the head bends toward the affected side while the chin rotates to the opposite side.

**touchpad (tŭch păd)** A type of pointing device common to laptop and notebook computers that directs activity on the computer screen by positioning a pointer or cursor on the screen. It is a small, flat device or surface that is highly sensitive to touch.

**touch screen (tūch skrēn)** A type of computer monitor that acts as an intake device, receiving information thought the touch of a pen, wand, or hand directly to the screen.

**tower case (tou´ər kās)** A vertical housing for the system unit of a personal computer.

**toxicology (tŏk´sĭ-kŏl´ə-jē)** The study of poisons or poisonous effects of drugs.

**trachea (trā´kē-ə)** The part of the respiratory tract between the larynx and the bronchial tree that is tubular and made of rings of cartilage and smooth muscle; also called the windpipe.

**trackball (trăk bôl)** A pointing device with a ball that is rolled to position a pointer or cursor on a computer screen. It can be directly attached to the computer or can be wireless.

**tracking (trăk´ĭng)** (financial) Watching for changes in spending so as to help control expenses.

**traction (trăk´shən)** The pulling or stretching of the musculoskeletal system to treat dislocated joints, joints afflicted by arthritis or other diseases, and fractured bones.

**trade name (trād nām)** A drug's brand or proprietary name.

**traditional Chinese medicine (TCM) (trə-dĭsh´-ə-nəl chĭ-nĕz mĕd´-ĭ-sĭn)** An ancient system of medicine originating in China that involves herbal and animal source preparations to treat illness. TCM includes various treatments such as acupuncture and acupressure.

**transcription (trăn-skrĭp´shən)** The transforming of spoken notes into accurate written form.

**transcutaneous absorption (trans-kyū-tā´nē-ŭs əb-sorp´shən)(†)** Entry (as of a pathogen) through a cut or crack in the skin.

**transdermal (trans-der´mel)** A type of topical drug administration that slowly and evenly releases a systemic drug through the skin directly into the bloodstream; a transdermal unit is also called a patch.

**transfer (trăns-fûr´)** To give something, such as information, to another party outside the doctor's office.

**transurethral resection of prostate (trans´yŏŏ rĕ thrəl rĕ-sək´ shən)** Removal of the prostate through the urethra.

**transverse (trăns-vûrs´)** Anatomic term that refers to the plane that divides the body into superior and inferior portions.

**transverse colon (trăns-vûrs´ kō´lən)** The segment of the large intestine that crosses the upper abdominal cavity between the ascending and descending colon.

**traveler's check (trăv´əlz chĕk)** A check purchased and signed at a bank and later signed over to a payee.

**treatment, payments and operations (TPO) (trēt´mənt pā´mənts ŏp´ə-rā´shəns)** The portion of **HIPAA** that allows the provider to use and share patient health-care information for treatment, payment, and operations (such as quality improvement).

**triage (trē-äzh´)** To assess the urgency and types of conditions patients present as well as their immediate medical needs.

**TRICARE (trī´kâr)** A program that provides health-care benefits for families of military personnel and military retirees.

**trichinosis (trik-i-nō´sis)(†)** A disease caused by a worm that is usually ingested from under-cooked meat.

**tricuspid valve (trī-kŭs´pid vălv)(†)** A heart valve that has three cusps and is situated between the right atrium and the right ventricle.

**triglycerides (trī-glĭs´ə-rīd´z)** Simple lipids consisting of glycerol (an alcohol) and three fatty acids.

**trigone (trī´gōn)(†)** The triangle formed by the openings of the two ureters and the urethra in the internal floor of the bladder.

**troubleshooting (trŭb´əl-shoo´tĭng)** Trying to determine and correct a problem without having to call a service supplier.

**trypsin (trip´sin)(†)** A pancreatic enzyme that digests proteins.

**tubular reabsorption (tū´byū-lăr)(†)** The second process of urine formation in which the glomerular filtrate flows into the proximal convoluted tubule.

**tubular secretion (tū´byū-lăr sĭ-krē´shən)(†)** The third process of urine formation in which substances move out of the blood in the peritubular capillaries into renal tubules.

**tutorial (too-tôr´ē-əl)** A small program included in a software package designed to give users an overall picture of the product and its functions.

**tympanic membrane (tĭm-păn´ĭk mĕm´brăn´)** A fibrous partition located at the inner end of the ear canal and separating the outer ear from the middle ear; also called the eardrum.

**tympanic thermometer (tim-pan´ik ther-mom´ē-ter)** A type of electronic thermometer that measures infrared energy emitted from the tympanic membrane.

**ulna (əl´-nə)** The medial bone of the lower arm.

**ultrasonic cleaning (ŭl´trə-sŏn´ĭk klēn´ĭng)** A method of sanitization that involves placing instruments in a cleaning solution in a special receptacle that generates sound waves through the cleaning solution, loosening contaminants. Ultrasonic cleaning is safe for even very fragile instruments.

**ultrasound** The noninvasive theraputic or diagnostic use of ultrasound for examination of internal body structures.

**umami (oo-mom´ē)** Savory taste produced by glutamic acid

(monosodium glutamate), recognized as the fifth taste sensation.

**umbilical cord** (ŭm-bĭl´ĭ-kəl kôrd) The rope-like connection between the fetus and the placenta. It contains the umbilical blood vessels.

**underbooking** (ŭn´dər-bŏŏkĭng) Leaving large, unused gaps in the doctor's schedule; this approach does not make the best use of the doctor's time.

**uniform donor card** (yōō´nə-fôrm´ dō´nər kärd) A legal document that states a person's wish to make a gift upon death of one or more organs for medical research, organ transplants, or placement in a tissue bank.

**unit** (yōō´nĭt) A part of an individual's name or title, described in indexing rules.

**unit price** (yōō´nĭt prīs) The total price of a package divided by the number of items that comprise the package.

**Universal Precautions** (yōō´nə-vur´səl prĭ-kô´shənz) Specific precautions required by the Department of Health and Human Services' Centers for Disease Control and Prevention (CDC) to prevent health-care workers from exposing themselves and others to infection by blood-borne pathogens.

**unsaturated fats** (ŭn-săch´ə-rā´tĭd făts) Fats, including most vegetable oils, that are usually liquid at room temperature and tend to lower blood cholesterol.

**upper respiratory (tract) infection** (upper res´pərətôr´ē tract infek´ shən) The common cold.

**urea** (yŏŏ-rē´ə) Waste product formed by the breakdown of proteins and nucleic acids.

**ureters** (yŏŏ-rē´tərz) Long, slender, muscular tubes that carry urine from the kidneys to the urinary bladder.

**urethra** (yŏŏ-rē´thrə) The tube that conveys urine from the bladder during urination.

**uric acid** (yŏŏr´ĭk as´id) Waste product formed by the breakdown of proteins and nucleic acids.

**urinalysis** (yŏŏr´ə-năl´ĭ-sĭs) The physical, chemical, and microscopic evaluation of urine to obtain information about body health and disease.

**urinary catheter** (yŏŏr´ə-nĕr´ē kăth´ĭ-tər) A sterile plastic tube inserted to provide urinary drainage.

**urinary pH** (yŏŏr´ə-nĕr´ē pē´äch) A measure of the degree of acidity or alkalinity of urine.

**urine specific gravity** (yŏŏr´ĭn spĭ-sĭf´ĭk grăv´ĭ-tē) A measure of the concentration or amount (total weight) of substances dissolved in urine.

**urobilinogen** (yūr-ō-bī-lin´ō-jen)(†) A colorless compound formed by the breakdown of hemoglobin in the intestines. Elevated levels in urine may indicate increased red blood cell destruction or liver disease, whereas lack of urobilinogen in the urine may suggest total bile duct obstruction.

**urologist** (yŏŏ-rŏl´ə-jĭst) A specialist who diagnoses and treats diseases of the kidney, bladder, and urinary system.

**use** (yōōz) The sharing, employing, applying, utilizing, examining, or analyzing of individually identifiable health information by employees or other members of an organization's workforce.

**uterus** (yōō´tər-əs) A hollow, muscular organ that functions to receive an embryo and sustain its development; also called the womb.

**uvula** (yōō´vyə-lə) The part of the soft palate that hangs down in the back of the throat.

**uvulotomy** (yoo´vyəlot´əmē) Surgical procedure removing all or part of the uvula of the soft palate.

**vaccine** (văk-sēn´) A special preparation made from microorganisms and administered to a person to produce reduced

sensitivity to, or increased immunity to, an infectious disease.

**vagina** (və-jī´nə) A tubular organ that extends from the uterus to the labia.

**vaginal introitus** (vaj´i-nəl in trō´ təs) The vaginal os or orifice. The opening of the vagina to the outside of the body.

**vaginitis** (vaj-i-nī´tis)(†) Inflammation of the vagina characterized by an abnormal vaginal discharge.

**varicose veins** (văr´i-kōs vānz)(†) Distended veins that result when vein valves are destroyed and blood pools in the veins, causing these veins to dilate.

**vas deferens** (văs´ dĕf´ər-ənz) A tube that connects the epididymis with the urethra and that carries sperm.

**vasectomy** (və-sĕk´tə-mē) A male sterilization procedure in which a section of each vas deferens is removed.

**vasoconstriction** (vā´sō-kon-strik´shŭn)(†) The constriction of the muscular wall of an artery to increase blood pressure.

**vasodilation** (vā-sō-dī-lā´shŭn)(†) The widening of the muscular wall of an artery to decrease blood pressure.

**V code** (vē kōd) A code used to identify encounters for reasons other than illness or injury, such as annual checkups, immunizations, and normal childbirth.

**vector** (vĕk´tər) A living organism, such as an insect, that carries microorganisms from an infected person to another person.

**venipuncture** (ven´i-pŭnk-chŭr)(†) The puncture of a vein, usually with a needle, for the purpose of drawing blood.

**ventilation** (vĕn´tə-lā´shən) Moving air in and out of the lungs; also called breathing.

**ventral** (vĕn´trəl) See **anterior**.

**ventral root** (vĕn´trəl rōōt) A portion of the spinal nerve that contains axons of motor neurons only.

**ventricle (věn´trĭ-kəl)** Interconnected cavities in the brain filled with cerebrospinal fluid.

**ventricular fibrillation (VF) (ven-trik´yū-lăr fī-bri-lā´shŭn)** An abnormal heart rhythm that is the most common cause of cardiac arrest.

**verbalizing (vûr´bə-līz´-ĭng)** Stating what you believe the patient is suggesting or implying.

**vermiform appendix (ver´mi-fŏrm ə-pĕn´dĭks)(†)** A structure made mostly of lymphoid tissue and projecting off the cecum. It is commonly referred to as simply the appendix.

**vertical file (vûr´tĭ-kəl fīl)** A filing cabinet featuring pull-out drawers that usually contain a metal frame or bar equipped to handle letter- or legal-sized documents in hanging file folders.

**vertigo (vûr´tĭ g ō)** Dizziness.

**vesicles (věs´ĭ-kəlz)** Small sacs within the synaptic knobs that contain chemicals called neurotransmitters.

**vestibule (ves ti b´yule)** The space enclosed by the labia minora.

**vestibule (věs´tə-byōōl´)** The area in the inner ear between the semicircular canals and the cochlea.

**vial (vī´əl)** A small glass bottle with a self-sealing rubber stopper.

**vibrio (vib´rē-ō) (†)** A comma-shaped bacterium.

**Virtual Private Network (VPN) (vur - choo-ul prahy-vit net-wurk)** These are used to connect two or more computer systems.

**virulence (vîr´yə-ləns)** A microorganism's disease-producing power.

**virus (vī´rəs)** One of the smallest known infectious agents, consisting only of nucleic acid surrounded by a protein coat; can live

and grow only within the living cells of other organisms.

**visceral pericardium (vis´er-ăl per-i-kar´dē-ŭm)(†)** The innermost layer of the pericardium that lies directly on top of the heart; also known as the epicardium.

**visceral peritoneum (vīs´er-ăl per-ə-tōne´əl)** Also known as the serosa, the outermost layer of the abdominal organs that secretes serous fluid to keep the organs from sticking to each other.

**visceral smooth muscle (vĭs´ər-əl smōōth mŭs´əl)** A type of smooth muscle containing sheets of muscle that closely contact each other. It is found in the walls of hollow organs such as the stomach, intestines, bladder, and uterus.

**vitamins (vī´tə-mĭnz)** Organic substances that are essential for normal body growth and maintenance and resistance to infection.

**vitreous humor (vĭt´rē-əs hyōō´mər)** A jelly-like substance that fills the part of the eye behind the lens and helps the eye keep its shape.

**voice mail (vois māl)** An advanced form of answering machine that allows a caller to leave a message when the phone line is busy.

**void (void)** (legal) A term used to describe something that is not legally enforceable.

**volume (vŏl´yōōm)** The amount of space an object, such as a drug, occupies.

**vomer (vō´-mər)** A thin bone that divides the nasal cavity.

**voucher check (vou´chər chĕk)** A business check with an attached stub, which is kept as a receipt.

**vulva (vul´ vah)** External female genitalia.

**vulvovaginitis (vul vō vaj´i-nī´tis)** Inflammation of the external female genitalia and vagina.

**walk-in (wôk´ĭn)** A patient who arrives without an appointment.

**WAN (wŏn)** Abbreviation for Wide Area Network.

**warranty (wôr´ən-tē)** A contract that specifies free service and replacement of parts for a piece of equipment during a certain period, usually a year.

**warts (wôrts)** Flesh-colored skin lesions with distinct round borders that are raised and often have small finger-like projections; also called verruca.

**wave scheduling (wāv skĕj´ōōl-ĭng)** A system of scheduling in which the number of patients seen each hour is determined by dividing the hour by the length of the average visit and then giving that number of patients appointments with the doctor at the beginning of each hour.

**Western blot test (wĕs´tərn blŏt tĕst)** A blood test used to confirm enzyme-linked immunosorbent assay (ELISA) test results for HIV infection.

**wet mount (wĕt mount)** A preparation of a specimen in a liquid that allows the organisms to remain alive and mobile while they are being identified.

**white matter (hwīt măt´ər)** The outer tissue of the spinal cord that is lighter in color than **gray matter**. It contains myelinated axons.

**whole blood (hōl blŭd)** The total volume of plasma and formed elements, or blood in which the elements have not been separated by coagulation or centrifugation.

**whole-body skin examination (hōl bŏd´ē skĭn ĭg-zăm´ə-nā´shən)** An examination of the visible top layer of the entire surface of the skin, including the scalp, genital area, and areas between the toes, to look for lesions, especially suspicious moles or precancerous growths.

**Wood's light examination (wŏŏdz līt ĭg-zăm´ə-nā´shən)** A type of dermatologic examination in which a physician inspects the patient's skin under an ultraviolet lamp in a darkened room.

**written-contract account (rĭt´n kŏn´trăkt´ ə-kount´)** An agreement between the physician and patient stating that the patient will pay a bill in more than four installments.

**X12 837 Health Care Claim (hĕlth kâr klām)** An electronic claim transaction that is the **HIPAA** Health Care Claim or Equivalent Encounter Information ("HIPAA claim").

**xeroradiography (zē´rō-rā´dē-og´ră-fē)(†)** A radiologic procedure in which x-rays are developed with a powder toner, similar to the toner in photocopiers, and the x-ray image is processed on specially treated xerographic paper; used to diagnose breast cancer, abscesses, lesions, or calcifications.

**xiphoid process (zif´oyd prŏs´ĕs)(†)** The lower extension of the breastbone; the cartilaginous tip of the sternum.

**yeast (yēst)** A fungus that grows mainly as a single-celled organism and reproduces by budding.

**yoga (yō´-gə)** A series of poses and breathing exercises that provide awareness of the unity of the whole being. The practice of yoga also increases flexibility and strength.

**yolk sac (yōk săk)** The sac that holds the materials for the nutrition of the embryo.

**zip drive (zĭp drīv)** A Zip drive is a high-capacity floppy disk drive developed by Iomega®. Zip drives are slightly larger and about twice as thick as a conventional floppy disk. Zip drives can hold 100 to 750 MB of data. They are durable and relatively inexpensive. They may be used for backing up hard disks and transporting large files.

**zona pellucida (zō´nă pe-lū´sid-ă)(†)** A layer that surrounds the cell membrane of an egg.

**Z-track method (zē´trăk mĕth´əd)** A technique used when injecting an intramuscular (IM) drug that can irritate subcutaneous tissue; involves pulling the skin and subcutaneous tissue to the side before inserting the needle at the site, creating a zigzag path in the tissue layers that prevents the drug from leaking into the subcutaneous tissue and causing irritation.

**zygomatic (zī-gə-m´a-tik)** The bones that form the prominence of the cheeks.

**zygote (zī´gōt)** The cell that is formed from the union of the egg and sperm.

# PHOTO CREDITS

**CHAPTER 1**
Fig. 1.1: Courtesy of Total Care Programming, Inc.; Fig. 1.2, Page 13, Fig. 1.3: © David Kelly Crow.

**CHAPTER 2**
Fig. 2.1: © Kathy Sloane; Fig. 2.2: © David Kelly Crow; Fig. 2.3: © Ron Neubauer/PhotoEdit Inc.; Page 28: © John Cole/Photo Researchers, Inc.; Fig. 2.4, Fig. 2.5: © David Kelly Crow; Fig. 2.6: © K. Glaser & Associates/Custom Medical Stock Photo; Fig. 2.7: © Will and Deni McIntrye.

**CHAPTER 3**
Fig. 3.2: © Volker Steger/Peter Arnold; Fig. 3.3, Fig. 3.4: © Cliff Moore.

**CHAPTER 4**
Fig. 4.2, Fig. 4.3, Fig. 4.4, Fig. 4.5: © Cliff Moore.

**CHAPTER 5**
Fig. 5.1: © Terry Wild Studio; Fig. 5.3: © Comstock Images/Alamy; Fig. 5.5: © Terry Wild Studio; Fig. 5.6: © David Kelly Crow; Fig. 5.7: Courtesy of Total Care Programming, Inc.; Fig. 5.8, Fig. 5.9: © Terry Wild Studio.

**CHAPTER 6**
Fig. 6.2, Fig. 6.4, Fig. 6.7, Fig. 6.8: Courtesy of Total Care Programming, Inc.; Fig. 6.10: © Terry Wild Studio; Fig. 6.11: Courtesy of Total Care Programming, Inc.; Fig. 6.12: © Terry Wild Studio.

**CHAPTER 7**
Fig. 7.1: Courtesy of Total Care Programming, Inc.; Fig. 7.8, Fig. 7.9: © Cliff Moore.

**CHAPTER 8**
Fig. 8.1, Fig. 8.5: © David Kelly Crow.

**CHAPTER 9**
Fig. 9.1: © Hank Morgan/Photo Researchers, Inc.; Fig. 9.5: © David Kelly Crow; Fig. 9.6: Courtesy of Total Care Programming, Inc.; Fig. 9.8: © David Kelly Crow; Page 193: © Kathy Sloane; Fig. 9.9: © David Kelly Crow.

**CHAPTER 10**
Fig. 10.1: © Terry Wild Studio, Fig. 10.2, Fig. 10.4: Courtesy Bibbero Systems, Inc. Petaluma, CA (800) 242.2376, www.bibbero.com; Fig. 10.5: © Terry Wild Studio; Fig. 10.7: © David Kelly Crow; Page 218: © Terry Wild Studio.

**CHAPTER 11**
Fig. 11.2: Courtesy of Total Care Programming, Inc.; Fig. 11.3: © Terry Wild Studio.

**CHAPTER 12**
Fig. 12.6, Fig. 12.7: © Terry Wild Studio.

**CHAPTER 13**
Fig. 13.1, Page 259: Courtesy of Total Care Programming, Inc.; Fig. 13.2, Fig. 13.3: © Terry Wild Studio; Fig. 13.4: © Cliff Moore; Fig. 13.6: © Terry Wild Studio; Fig. 13.7: © Shirley Zeiberg; Fig. 13.8: © Terry Wild Studio.

**CHAPTER 14**
Fig. 14.1: © Terry Wild Studio; Fig. 14.2: © Kathy Sloane; Fig. 14.5: © Terry Wild Studio; Page 287: © Ken Lax.

**CHAPTER 15**
Fig. 15.2: © David Kelly Crow; Fig. 15.7: © Terry Wild Studio.

**CHAPTER 17**
Fig. 17.4: © Terry Wild Studio.

**CHAPTER 18**
Fig. 18.8: Courtesy of Total Care Programming, Inc.; Fig. 18.10: © Terry Wild Studio.

**CHAPTER 19**
Fig. 19.2: © Biology Media/Photo Researchers, Inc.; Fig. 19.4: © Tony Freeman/PhotoEdit, Inc.; Fig. 19.5: © Stephen Dalton/Photo Researchers, Inc.

**CHAPTER 20**
Fig. 20.1: © David Kelly Crow; Fig. 20.2, Fig. 20.3: © The McGraw-Hill Companies, Inc./Jill Braaten, photographer; Fig. 20.4: © Cliff Moore; Fig. 20.5: Leesa Whicker; Fig. 20.6: © Vol. 43 PhotoDisc/Getty; Fig. 20.7: Courtesy of Total Care Programming, Inc.; Fig. 20.8, Fig. 20.10: © Cliff Moore; Fig. 20.11: Courtesy of Total Care Programming, Inc.; Fig. 20.12: Courtesy Tyco Healthcare/Kendall; Fig. 20.13: © Cliff Moore; Fig. 20.15, Fig. 20.16: © David Kelly Crow.

**CHAPTER 21**
Page 442: © EP063 Eyewire/Getty; Fig. 21.2: © Gary Watson/SPL/Photo Researchers, Inc.; Fig. 21.4: © SIU/Photo Researchers, Inc.; Fig. 21.10: © RF Getty.

**CHAPTER 22**
Fig. 22.1: © David Kelly Crow; Fig. 22.2, Fig. 22.3, Fig. 22.4: © Cliff Moore; Fig. 22.6, Fig. 22.7, Fig. 22.8, Fig. 22.9: © David Kelly Crow.

**CHAPTER 23**
Fig. 23.1, Fig. 23.2, Fig. 23.3: © David Kelly Crow.

**CHAPTER 24**
Fig. 24.1: Courtesy ALARIS Medical Systems, Inc.; Fig. 24.2: Courtesy of Total Care Programming, Inc.; Fig. 24.3: Courtesy of Exergen, www.exergen.com; Fig. 24.4: NexTemp® is a registered trademark of Medical Indicators, Inc.; Fig. 24.6: © 2007, Keith Eng, Photographer; Fig. 24.7: Courtesy of Exergen, www.exergen.com; Fig. 24.10, Fig. 24.11, Fig. 24.13, Fig. 24.15: Courtesy of Total Care Programming, Inc.; Fig. 24.17: © Mark Richards/PhotoEdit, Inc.; Fig. 24.18: © Shirley Zeiberg.

**CHAPTER 25**
Fig. 25.2, Fig. 25.3, Fig. 25.4, Fig. 25.5, Fig. 25.6, Fig. 25.7: © Terry Wild Studio; Fig. 25.8: Courtesy of Total Care Programming, Inc.; Fig. 25.11: © The McGraw-Hill Companies, Inc./Rick Brady, photographer; Fig. 25.12: Courtesy Richmond Products, Inc.; Fig. 25.13: © Ken Lax; Fig. 25.14, Fig. 25.15, Fig. 25.16: Courtesy Richmond Products, Inc.; Fig. 25.17: Welch Allyn, Inc.

**CHAPTER 26**
Fig. 26.2: © Vol. 58 PhotoDisc/Getty; Fig. 26.3: © CDC/Peter Arnold, Inc.; Fig. 26.4: © David Kelly Crow; Fig. 26.5: © Ken Lax; Fig. 26.6: Aaron Haupt, Photo Researchers, Inc.; Fig. 26.7: © Ken Lax; Fig. 26.10: © Vol. 113 PhotoDisc/Getty.

**CHAPTER 27**
Fig. 27.1: © Cliff Moore; Fig. 27.3: © John Radcliffe/SPL/Photo Researchers, Inc.; Fig. 27.5: © Shirley Zeiberg; Fig. 27.6: © BrandX 122/Getty; Fig. 27.7: © Martin M. Rotker; Fig. 27.8: © BioPhoto/Photo Researchers, Inc.; Fig. 27.9: © Tom Meyers/Photo Researchers, Inc.; Fig. 27.10: © Ken Lax; Fig. 27.12: © CNRI/SPL/Photo Researchers, Inc.; Fig. 27.13: © The McGraw-Hill Companies, Inc./Bob Coyle, photographer; Fig. 27.14: © Grant Pix/Photo Researchers, Inc.; Fig. 27.15, Fig. 27.16, Fig. 27.17: © Ken Lax; Fig. 27.18: © BioPhoto/Photo Researchers, Inc.; Fig. 27.20: © Herb Snitzer.

**CHAPTER 28**
Page 626: © Stockbyte/Punchstock; Fig. 28.1: © Barry Slaven/PMODE Photography; Fig. 28.6, Fig. 28.7, Fig. 28.8: © David Kelly Crow; Figure 28.13, Fig. 28.14, Fig. 28.15: © Cliff Moore; Fig. 28.16: Courtesy of Total Care Programming; Fig. 28.17, Fig. 28.18, Fig. 28.19, Fig. 28.21, Fig. 28.22, Fig. 28.23, Fig. 28.24: © Cliff Moore.

**CHAPTER 29**
Fig. 29.3: Courtesy of Total Care Programming, Inc.; Page 665: © Vol. 59 PhotoDisc/Getty; Fig. 29.4: © David Kelly Crow; Fig. 29.6: © SS36 PhotoDisc/ Getty; Fig. 29.7: © RF Corbis; Fig. 29.8: Courtesy of Total Care Programming, Inc.

**CHAPTER 30**
Fig. 30.9: © National Safety Council/Rick Brady photographer; Fig. 30.10: © Cliff Moore; Fig. 30.15: Courtesy of Total Care Programming, Inc.

**CHAPTER 31**
Fig. 31.4: © The McGraw-Hill Companies, Inc./ Shaana Pritchard, photographer; Fig. 31.5, Fig. 31.6: © The McGraw-Hill Companies, Inc./Jan L. Saeger, photographer.

**CHAPTER 32**
Fig. 32.1: © David Kelly Crow; Page 745: © Ken Lax; Fig. 32.3, Fig. 32.4, Fig. 32.5, Fig. 32.6, Fig. 32.7, Fig. 32.8: Leesa Whicker; Fig. 32.12: © Cliff Moore; Fig. 32.13: Leesa Whicker; Fig. 32.15: Courtesy Safetec of America, Buffalo, NY 14215.

**CHAPTER 33**
Fig. 33.1a: © NIBSC/Photo Researchers, Inc.; Fig. 33.1b: © SPL/Photo Researchers, Inc.; Fig. 33.1c: © R.J. Erwin/Photo Researchers, Inc.; Fig. 33.2a-b: © Oliver Meckes/Photo Researchers, Inc.; Fig. 33.2c: © Volker Stegner/Peter Arnold, Inc.; 33.2d: © Morendum Animal Health, Ltd./Photo Researchers Inc.; Fig. 33.3: © Morendum Animal Health, Ltd./Photo Researchers Inc.; Fig. 33.4: © David Scharf/Peter Arnold, Inc.; Fig. 33.5a: © J. H. Robinson/Photo Researchers, Inc.; Fig. 33.5b: © Dickson Despommier/Photo Researchers, Inc.; Fig. 33.5c: © Dr. Tony Brian/SPL/Photo Researchers, Inc.; Fig. 33.5d: © Scott Camazine/Photo Researchers, Inc.; Fig. 33.5e: © SIU/Peter Arnold; Fig. 33.6a-e: © Cliff Moore; Fig. 33.6f: © RF CD338/Corbis; Fig. 33.7, Fig. 33.8, Fig. 33.9: © Cliff Moore; Fig. 33.13: © Cliff Moore; Fig. 33.14: © Martin M. Rotker; Fig. 33.16: Courtesy Orion Diagnostica, OY, Finland/Life Sign, LLC; Fig. 33.18: © John Durham/ SPL/Photo Researchers, Inc.; Fig. 33.20: © Dr. E. Bottone/Peter Arnold, Inc.; Fig. 33.21: Courtesy Becton Dickinson Diagnostic Systems; Fig. 33.22: © Cliff Moore.

**CHAPTER 34**
Fig. 34.5, Fig. 34.7, Fig. 34.8: Leesa Whicker.

**CHAPTER 35**
Page 837: Courtesy Total Care Programming, Inc.; Fig. 35.11: © Courtesy Becton Dickinson; Fig. 35.12, Fig. 35.13, Fig. 35.14: Leesa Whicker; Fig. 35.15: © Terry Wild Studio; Fig. 35.16: Leesa Whicker; Fig. 35.17: © Terry Wild Studio; Fig. 35.18: Leesa Whicker; Fig. 35.25, Fig. 35.26, Fig. 35.27, Fig. 35.28: © Terry Wild Studio; Fig. 35.29: Leesa Whicker; Fig. 35.30: Courtesy of Total Care Programming, Inc.

**CHAPTER 36**
Fig. 36.1: © The McGraw-Hill Companies, Inc./Jill Braaten, photographer; Fig. 36.2, Fig. 36.3: © Ken Lax; Fig. 36.4, Fig. 36.5, Fig. 36.6: © The McGraw-Hill Companies, Inc./Jill Braaten, photographer; Fig. 36.7, Fig. 36.8: © Ken Lax; Fig. 36.9, Fig. 36.10: © David Kelly Crow; Fig. 36.11, Fig. 36.12: © Ken Lax; Fig. 36.16, Fig. 36.17: © The McGraw-Hill Companies, Inc./Jill Braaten, photographer.

**CHAPTER 37**
Fig. 37.1: © David Kelly Crow; Fig. 37.3a: © R.J. Erwin/Photo Researchers, Inc.; Fig. 37.3b: © Andrew McClenaghan/SPL/Photo Researchers, Inc.; Fig. 37.4: © David Kelly Crow; Fig. 37.5: © Terry Wild Studio.

**CHAPTER 38**
Fig. 38.2: Leesa Whicker; Fig. 38.4, Fig. 38.5, Fig. 38.6a: © Cliff Moore; Fig. 38.11b: Courtesy of Total Care Programming, Inc.; Fig. 38.14:

© Cliff Moore; Fig. 38.24: Courtesy of Total Care Programming, Inc.; Fig. 38.26, Fig. 38.27, Fig. 38.28, Fig. 38.29: © Ken Lax; Fig. 38.30, Fig. 38.31, Fig. 38.32: © Terry Wild Studio; Fig. 38.33: © Cliff Moore; Fig. 38.34: Courtesy Total Care Programming, Inc.

**CHAPTER 39**

Fig. 39.3, Fig. 39.4: Courtesy Burdick/Quinton Cardiology, Inc.; Fig. 39.7, Fig. 39.8: © David Kelly Crow; Fig. 39.19: © Cliff Moore; Fig. 39.20: Fig. 39.21, Fig. 39.22, Fig. 39.23, Fig. 39.24: © David

Kelly Crow; Page 1004: © Edwige/BSIP/Phototake; Fig. 39.26, Fig. 39.28, Fig. 39.30: © Cliff Moore; Fig. 39.31: Image Courtesy of Respironics, Inc. Murrysville, PA; Fig. 39.33: © Dynamic Graphics/Jupiter Images.

**CHAPTER 40**

Fig. 40.1: © David Kelly Crow; Fig. 40.2: © Martin M. Rotker; Fig. 40.3: © Sovereign/ISM/Phototake; Fig. 40.4: © Corbis R-F; Fig. 40.5: © Cliff Moore; Page 1025: © Comstock Images/Picture Quest; Fig. 40.6: © Corbis R-F; Fig. 40.7a: © Stephen Gerard/

Science Source/Photo Researchers, Inc.; Fig. 40.7b: © Scott Camazine/Photo Researchers, Inc.; Fig. 40.8: © Vol. 59 PhotoDisc/Getty; Fig. 40.9: © Cliff Moore; Fig. 40.10: Courtesy of Total Care Programming, Inc.; Fig. 40.12: © Cliff Moore; Fig. 40.13: © Vol. 41/Corbis; Fig. 40.14, Fig. 40.15: © SPL/Photo Researchers, Inc.

**CHAPTER 41**

Fig. 41.11: © David Kelly Crow.

# TEXT AND LINE ART CREDITS

**CHAPTER 4**

Table 4-2: Adapted from Alberti, Robert E., and Emmons, Michael, *Your Perfect Right: A Guide to Assertive Behavior*, San Luis Obispo, California: Impact Publishing, 1970.

**CHAPTER 5**

Fig. 5-4: Reprinted with permission of Heavenly Office. www.heavenlyoffice.com.

**CHAPTER 6**

Fig. 6-9: Manage Bytes Software; support@managebytes.com.

**CHAPTER 7**

Fig. 7-5: Reprinted with permission from English Plus. Copyright © English Plus. All rights reserved.

**CHAPTER 8**

Fig. 8-6: Reprinted with permission from Bibbero Systems, Inc., Petaloma, CA (800)242-2376, www.bibbero.com.

**CHAPTER 23**

Fig. 23-6: Reprinted with permission from Bibbero Systems, Inc., Petaloma, CA (800)242-2376, www.bibbero.com.

**CHAPTER 24**

Fig. 24-12: From Booth, *Health Care Science Technology: Career Technology*, 1st edition. Peoria, IL: Glencoe/McGraw-Hill, 2004.

**CHAPTER 25**

Fig. 25-12: Reprinted with permission of Richmond Products, Inc.; Fig. 25-14: Reprinted with permission

of Richmond Products, Inc.; Fig. 25-15: Reprinted with permission of Richmond Products, Inc.; Fig. 25-16: Reprinted with permission of Richmond Products, Inc.

**CHAPTER 29**

Fig. 29-5: From Booth, *Health Care Science Technology: Career Technology*, 1st edition. Peoria, IL: Glencoe/McGraw-Hill, 2004; Fig. 29-9: From Booth, *Health Care Science Technology: Career Technology*, 1st edition. Peoria, IL: Glencoe/McGraw-Hill, 2004.

**CHAPTER 30**

Fig. 30-19: From Booth, *Health Care Science Technology: Career Technology*, 1st edition. Peoria, IL: Glencoe/McGraw-Hill, 2004; Fig. 30-20: From Booth, *Glencoe Health Care Science Technology*, p. 101, Fig 4.8. Copyright © 2004 the McGraw-Hill Companies.

**CHAPTER 31**

Fig. 31-1: From Booth, *Health Care Science Technology: Career Technology*, 1st edition. Peoria, IL: Glencoe/McGraw-Hill, 2004; Fig. 31-3: Adapted from/reprinted with permission of Christopher Shirley, Pacific Institute of Reflexology, www.pacificreflexology.com; Fig. 31-7: From Booth, *Health Care Science Technology: Career Technology*, 1st edition. Peoria, IL: Glencoe/McGraw-Hill, 2004.

**CHAPTER 38**

Fig. 38-1: From Booth & Whaley, *Math and Dosage Calculations for Medical Careers*, 2nd edition, pp. 402, Fig. 11.10; Fig. 38-3: Phizer Corporation;

Fig. 38-6b: From Booth & Whaley, *Math and Dosage Calculations for Medical Careers*, 2nd edition, pp. 105, Fig. 4.2; Text Art 51-7: Reprinted with permission of Abraxis BioScience, Inc.; Fig. 38-8: Reprinted with permission of GlaxoSmithKline; Fig. 38-13: From Booth/Whaley, *Math and Dosage Calculations for Medical Careers*, 2nd edition, pp. 114-115, Fig. 4-14 & 4-17.

**CHAPTER 39**

Fig. 39-10: Courtesy of Cardiac Science Corporation, Milton, Wisconsin; Fig. 39-11: Courtesy of Cardiac Science Corporation, Milton, Wisconsin; Fig. 39-12: Courtesy of Cardiac Science Corporation, Milton, Wisconsin; Fig. 39-13: Courtesy of Cardiac Science Corporation, Milton, Wisconsin (ECG tracing represents earlier model from Burdick, Inc.); Fig. 39-14: Courtesy of Cardiac Science Corporation, Milton, Wisconsin; Fig. 39-15: Courtesy of Cardiac Science Corporation, Milton, Wisconsin; Fig. 39-16: From Shade, B., Wesley, K. Fast and Easy, *ECGs: A Self-Paced Learning Program*, pp. 344, Fig. 11.17. Copyright © 2007 by The McGraw-Hill Companies; Fig. 39-17: From Shade, B., Wesley, K. Fast and Easy, *ECGs: A Self-Paced Learning Program*, pp. 333, Fig. 11.6a. Copyright © 2007 by The McGraw-Hill Companies; Fig. 39-18: From Shade, B., Wesley, K. Fast and Easy, *ECGs: A Self-Paced Learning Program*, pp. 226, Fig. 7.12. Copyright © 2007 by The McGraw-Hill Companies; Fig. 39-32: PCCA.

# INDEX

Page numbers in **boldface** indicate figures. Page numbers followed by (b) indicate box features, (p) procedures, and (t) tables, respectively.

Herpes zoster, 529(t), 600, 608(t)
 AIDS/HIV infection, 451
HEV. *See* Hepatitis E virus
Hiatal hernia, 605(t)
Hibiclens, 642
HID. *See* Herniated intervertebral disk (HID)
Hierarchy of needs, 68–69
High-complexity tests, 51
High-density lipoproteins (HDL), 859(t), 879
Highly active anti-retroviral therapy (HAART), 452
High-risk procedures, 429
HIPAA. *See* Health Insurance Portability and Accountability Act (HIPAA)
HIPAA claim, 307, 313(b)
Hippocrates, 724
Hippocratic oath, 60
Hispanic HIV/AIDS Program, 442(b)
Hispanic patients
 AIDS/HIV infection and, 448
 communicating with, 77
HIV. *See* AIDS/HIV infection
*HIV/AIDS Surveillance Report*, 448
HIV antibodies, testing blood, 52(t)
Hold, putting telephone call on, 232
Holmes, Oliver Wendell, 394(t)
Holter monitor, 593, **593**, 1000–1002, 1002(p)–1003(p)
Home, preventing injury at, 276(t)
Homeopathic medicine, 721–722, 722(t)
Homeopathy, 720(t)
Homeostasis, 68
Homosexual population, AIDS/HIV infection and, 448
Honesty, of medical assistant, 17
Honeymoon Phase, 85
Horizontal files, 202
Hormone replacement, 915(t)
Horticultural therapy, 655(b)
Hospice, 79, 295
Hospital discharge summary form, 180
Hospitals
 isolation guidelines for, 431, 431(t)
 recycling procedure, 15(b)
 Standard Precautions, 424, 427
Hot compress, 664
Hot pack, 664
Hot soak, 664
Hot-water bottle, 662(p)–663(p), 663
Houseflies, transmission of infection, 406
Household system, 939, 939(t)
Housekeeping
 examination room, 467, 470
 in laboratory, 759
 for reception area, 261–262
 storing office supplies, 163
Human bites, 683, 685
Human chorionic gonadotropin (HCG), 576
Human immunodeficiency virus. *See* AIDS/HIV infection
Human papilloma virus (HPV), 566
Human T-cell lymphotrophic virus (HTLV-1), 453
Humpback, 542
Hyaline casts, 828, **828**
Hydrocele, 620
Hydrochloric acid, as defense mechanism, 401
Hydrocodone, 920(t)
Hydrotherapy, 664
Hypercalcemia, urine test for, 817(t)
Hyperglycemia, 600, 703
Hypericum, 722(t)
Hyperlipidemia, 564, **564**
Hyperopia, **614**, 614–615
Hyperpnea, 514
Hypertension, 515, 567(t), 596(t)
 dietary guidelines for, 894
 urine test for, 817(t)
Hyperthyroidism, 601
Hyperventilation, 701
Hypnosis, 720(t), 724–725

Hypnotic, 912(t), 915(t)
Hypoglycemia, 703
Hypotension, 515
 postural, 519
Hypothermia, 696–697
Hypothetical questions, 486(t)
Hypothyroidism, 601
Hypovolemic shock, 710
Hysterectomy, 578, 580
Hysterosalpingography, 577

# I

IBM-compatible computers, 122
ICD-9-CM, 57, 317–322, 352(b)
 Alphabetic Index, **318**, 318–319
 code structure, 319–320
 conventions of, 321–322
 E codes, 320–321
 locating code, 322(p)
 new revision of, 322–323
 Tabular List, 318, **318**, 319–321, 320(t)
 V codes, 320–321
Ice pack, 660
Icons, 122, **122**
Identification line, of business letter, **138**, 139
Ignatia, 722(t)
Illnesses. *See also* Diseases and disorders
 common for emergency medical intervention, 700–701
 cultural differences in view of, 77(b)
 less common for emergency medical intervention, 701–711
 stages of, 401
Imaging procedures, 606–607
IM injections, 959–961, 959(p)–960(p)
Immune system
 active immunity, 404, **404**
 cell-mediated defenses, 403, 404
 humoral defenses, 403–404
 microbial diseases of, 783(t)–784(t)
 nonspecific defenses of, 403
 passive immunity, 404, **404**
 phagocytosis, 403, **403**
 wound healing and, 628(b)
Immunity, defined, 401
Immunization. *See also* Vaccinations
 administering, 434
 antibody formation, 932
 contraindications, 434
 defined, 431
 elderly patients, 434–435
 immunocompromised patients, 435–436
 as infection-control technique, 431–436
 informed consent, 434
 pediatric, 434, 569–570
 pregnant patients, 434
 procedure codes, 326
 recommendations, 432, **432–433**, 434
 record of, 434
 timing of, 932
Immunoassay, 869–870
Immunocompromised patients, 269–270, 451
 immunizations and, 435–436
Immunofluorescent antibody (IFA) test, 446
Impetigo, 571(t), 600
Implied contract, 41
Impotence, 620
Inactive files, 214
Incidental supplies, 161
Incident report, 757, **758**, 759
Incision, 625, 697, **698**
Income, statement of, 375
Income tax
 as payroll deduction, 378
 submitting federal, 382

Incoming calls
 managing, 224–225, 226(b)
 types of, 227–231
Incomplete fracture, 691, **692**
Incomplete proteins, 876
Incontinence, 812
 elderly patients, 553
Incubation of culture plate, 798–799
Incubation period, 401
Incubation phase of HIV infection, 446
Inderal, 974
Indexing, in filing process, 211
Indexing rules, 205–207, 206(t)
Indications, drugs, 912, 916
Indirect transmission, 405
Individual identifiable health information (IIHI), 184(b)
Induration, 168, 400
Industry vs. inferiority stage, 69(t)
Indwelling catheter, 810, **811**
Infants. *See also* Children; Pediatrics
 breast-feeding, 583
 choking, 688, 689(p)–690(p)
 developmental stage, 69(t)
 dosage calculations for, 941–942
 intramuscular injections, 960
 newborn function test, 583
 rule of nines for, **687**
 urine specimen collection, 812, 813(p)
 weight, height, head circumference, 519, 521, 523(p)–524(p)
Infection
 antibiotic-resistant, 400
 breaking cycle of infection, 407
 cycle of, **405**, 405–407
 diagnosis of, 779–780, 784
 endogenous, 405
 environmental factors in transmission, 407
 exogenous, 405
 nosocomial, 429
 opportunistic, 403, 448–451
 toxic shock syndrome, 710–711
 venipuncture complication, 855(b)
 wound healing and, 628(b)
Infection-control techniques, 409–436
 autoclave, 416–423
 Bloodborne Pathogens Standard, 424, 425(t), 429
 disinfection, 414–416
 in examination room, 466–467, 468(p)
 exposure incident, 429
 guidelines for isolation precautions in hospitals, 431, 431(t)
 history of infectious disease prevention, 394–395
 immunization, 431–436
 infectious laundry waste disposal, 424, 425(b)–426(b)
 medical assistant's role in, 411
 patient education about disease prevention, 435(b), 436
 sanitization, 412, 414, **414**
 in spirometer, 1009
 Standard Precautions, 424, 427–428
 sterilization, 416–423
 transmission from health-care worker to patient, 429–430
 Universal Precautions, 424, 427
Infectious conjunctivitis, 571(t)
Infectious diseases, 395–400. *See also* Blood-borne pathogens
 AIDS/HIV infection as, 445–448
 body's defense against, 401–404
 CDC reporting guidelines for, 430, 430(t)
 chickenpox, 395–396
 common cold, 396
 croup, 396
 diphtheria, 396
 disease process of, 400–401
 environmental factors in transmission, 407

# DISEASES AND DISORDERS INDEX

Page numbers in **boldface** indicate figures. Page numbers followed by (b) indicate box features, (p) procedures, and (t) tables, respectively.